TEXTBOOK OF PEDIATRIC
EMERGENCY PROCEDURES

TEXTBOOK OF PEDIATRIC EMERGENCY PROCEDURES

Second Edition

EDITORS ▶

CHRISTOPHER KING, MD, FACEP

Associate Professor
Departments of Emergency Medicine
  and Pediatrics
University of Pittsburg School of Medicine
Attending Physician
UPMC-Presbyterian Hospital
Children's Hospital of Pittsburgh
Pittsburgh, Pennsylvania

FRED M. HENRETIG, MD, FAAP

Professor
Departments of Pediatrics and Emergency Medicine
University of Pennsylvania School of Medicine
Director, Section of Clinical Toxicology
Division of Emergency Medicine
The Children's Hospital of Philadelphia
Philadelphia, Pennsylvania

ASSOCIATE EDITORS ▶

BRENT R. KING, MD
JOHN M. LOISELLE, MD
RICHARD M. RUDDY, MD
JAMES F. WILEY, II, MD

ILLUSTRATOR ▶

CHRISTINE D. YOUNG, AMI

Wolters Kluwer | Lippincott Williams & Wilkins
Health

Philadelphia • Baltimore • New York • London
Buenos Aires • Hong Kong • Sydney • Tokyo

Acquisitions Editor: Frances DeStefano
Managing Editor: Nicole Dernoski
Project Manager: Nicole Walz
Manufacturing Coordinator: Kathleen Brown
Marketing Manager: Angela Panetta
Creative Director: Doug Smock
Cover Designer: Larry Didona
Production Services: Aptara, Inc.

2nd Edition
© 2008 by LIPPINCOTT WILLIAMS & WILKINS, a Wolters Kluwer business
© 1997 by Williams & Wilkins

Printed in the United States

Library of Congress Cataloging-in-Publication Data

Textbook of pediatric emergency procedures/editors, Christopher King, Fred M. Henretig; associate editors, Brent R. King . . . [et al.]; illustrator, Christine D. Young.—2nd ed.
        p. ; cm.
Includes bibliographical references and index.
ISBN-13: 978-0-7817-5386-9
ISBN-10: 0-7817-5386-4
    I. Pediatric emergencies.   2. Pediatric intensive care.   I. King, Christopher, 1959-   II. Henretig, Fred M.
    [DNLM: I. Emergencies.   2. Child.   3. Emergency Medicine—methods.   4. Infant.
WS 205 P371 2008]
    RJ370.P456 2008
    618.92'0025—dc22
                                                                        2007022934

Care has been taken to confirm the accuracy of the information presented and to describe generally accepted practices. However, the authors, editors, and publisher are not responsible for errors or omissions or for any consequences from application of the information in this book and make no warranty, expressed or implied, with respect to the currency, completeness, or accuracy of the contents of the publication. Application of this information in a particular situation remains the professional responsibility of the practitioner; the clinical treatments described and recommended may not be considered absolute and universal recommendations.

The authors, editors, and publisher have exerted every effort to ensure that drug selection and dosage set forth in this text are in accordance with current recommendations and practice at the time of publication. However, in view of ongoing research, changes in government regulations, and the constant flow of information relating to drug therapy and drug reactions, the reader is urged to check the package insert for each drug for any change in indications and dosage and for added warnings and precautions. This is particularly important when the recommended agent is a new or infrequently employed drug.

Some drugs and medical devices presented in this publication have Food and Drug Administration (FDA) clearance for limited use in restricted research settings. It is the responsibility of health care providers to ascertain the FDA status of each drug or device planned for use in their clinical practice.

The publishers have made every effort to trace copyright holders for borrowed material. If they have inadvertently overlooked any, they will be pleased to make the necessary arrangements at the first opportunity.

To purchase additional copies of this book, call our customer service department at (800) 638-3030 or fax orders to 1-301-223-2400. Lippincott Williams & Wilkins customer service representatives are available from 8:30 am to 6:00 pm, EST, Monday through Friday, for telephone access. Visit Lippincott Williams & Wilkins on the Internet: http://www.lww.com.

20 19 18 17

Since the publication of the first edition of the *Textbook of Pediatric Emergency Procedures*, we have had the pleasure of hearing from many clinicians working in clinics, offices, and emergency departments in widely diverse geographies about times that they used the book and found just what they needed to positively impact the care of an ill or injured child. At the same time, we have also received numerous suggestions about possible improvements we could make, such as procedures that should be added or dropped, illustrations that should be "tweaked" to make them better, tables that could be improved, etc. Both types of comments have been deeply appreciated, although perhaps in different ways, and have motivated us to present this revised and hopefully improved resource for our colleagues. We are grateful that our publisher, Lippincott Williams & Wilkins has given us this opportunity.

Just as the practice of medicine has changed necessitating a second edition of this text, so have there been many changes in our chosen subspecialty. Still a comparatively young field, pediatric emergency medicine is now among the most popular choices of graduating pediatric residents seeking subspecialty training. The number of candidates receiving subspecialty certification from the American Board of Pediatrics and the American Board of Emergency Medicine has continued to grow, but the demand for these physicians has grown even faster. This reflects a rapid change occurring in the delivery of emergency care to children in general, as confidence in the quality of care provided in the emergency department has steadily increased. Far more patients are referred to hospital emergency departments for acute care problems that in years past would likely have been handled by office-based practitioners, and an ever larger segment of the public sees the emergency department as a preferred setting to seek medical care, rather than (as in the past) a place to be avoided. This has resulted in busier and busier emergency departments—which has been both curse and sincere compliment—and an even greater need for clinically useful reference materials.

The years since the publication of the first edition of this text have also seen changes in our professional career tracks. In particular, one of us (FMH), has reached that stage of life and practice when it seems prudent to him to "slow down" a bit, and allow the younger generation to step into the driver's seat at trauma resuscitations, and textbook editing. At the same time, the other (CK) is still going full speed and capable of taking on ever increasing challenges. These differing career trajectories are reflected by the switch in order of editorship for this edition.

This second edition maintains and builds on those strengths the first sought to achieve. It is still intended primarily for use by all who provide medical care to acutely ill and injured children in hospital emergency departments. We hope it will also remain a useful adjunct to office-based pediatricians and family practitioners. In the first edition, we strived to maintain a balance between authoritative reference work and user-friendly bedside procedural guide. To that end, we have kept and updated the basic chapter structure, detailing each procedure's scientific background, indications, equipment needs, procedural technique, potential complications, and strategies to minimize those complications. The sources of both background information and procedural approach are thoroughly referenced. Chapter illustrations and "Summary" and "Clinical Tips" boxes allow a quick overview for the more experienced clinician. A number of new illustrations are included in this edition, and many from the first have been improved by our superb illustrator, Christine Young, to allow a better "view" of the correct technique. The textbook's original structure of organization by sections, beginning with general topics, followed by organ system-based procedures and then concluding with an overview of the rapidly expanding field of emergency ultrasonography, has been retained. A few chapters have been deleted where current practice has rendered them obsolete (e.g., use of military antishock trousers), and others have been added if the procedure has taken on a more prominent role in everyday emergency care (e.g., use of tissue adhesives).

We hope this second edition of the *Textbook of Pediatric Emergency Procedures* will prove a worthy successor to the first edition. As before, our greatest hope remains that it will serve as a useful aid to front-line clinicians in pursuing their mission of providing quality emergency care to their pediatric patients.

FMH
CK
July 2007

In a small conference room on the second floor of the Children's Hospital of Philadelphia, Fred Henretig introduced us to the vivid writing of William Carlos Williams. It was a routine emergency medicine morning conference in 1982. Somehow, of all of the conferences given on all the mornings, this one is remembered. Fred's topic was "How to Perform Procedures on Pediatric Patients." He began by reading from Williams' essay entitled "The Use of Force." The words were magic. They described young Dr. Williams encountering a flushed and febrile little girl who he suspected of having diphtheria at a time when diphtheria was killing children in his practice. It was imperative that he perform the procedure of examining the child's throat in order to make the diagnosis and provide the correct therapy. The treatment room was the family's kitchen, for this was in the time of the $3.00 house call.

"Well I said, suppose we take a look at the throat first. I smiled in my best professional manner and asking for the child's first name I said, come on, Mathilda, open your mouth and let's take a look at your throat.

Nothing doing."

We had all been in that very same situation. Anyone who has worked with children has faced the same awful dilemma. Those of us who had dedicated our careers to pediatric emergency medicine had faced a similar predicament on a daily basis. The conference room was filled with staff, residents, and students, who listened on.

"Aw, come on, I coaxed, just open your mouth wide and let me take a look. Look, I said opening both hands wide. I haven't anything in my hands. Just open up and let me see."

Fred read on, and we smiled as we listened to the common scenario. But soon the coaxing turned more serious. As Dr. Williams became more aggressive the child parried with even more determined resistance. The parents tried to coax her as well, but the child's mouth remained tightly clenched and resolute.

"As I moved my chair a little nearer, suddenly with one cat like movement both her hands clawed instinctively for my eyes and she almost reached them too. In fact she knocked my glasses flying and they fell, though unbroken, several feet away from me on the kitchen floor."

The conference room fell silent. Now this was getting serious. I think we all began to reflect on similar moments of confrontation in our past. I need to get the job done and the child will not let me. Do I push on? Do I try another technique? And through it all, perhaps a bit of anger is starting to infiltrate my professional demeanor. It is an uncomfortable feeling. I am there to help my young patients, not to be angry with them—they are only kids. Yes, but sometimes they are provoking. Yes, but always they seem to be so fragile, so dependent. Around the room, some smiles were gone, some heads were downed. As the story continued Dr. Williams saw that the child was breathing fast and appearing more ill. He decided to do what we had often done, appeal to the parents.

"I had to have a throat culture for her own protection. But first I told the parents that it was entirely up to them. I explained the danger but said that I would not insist on a throat examination so long as they would take responsibility."

This too was an all too familiar vignette. Shift the responsibility to the parents. Force them into action. Make them sign out against medical advice when we have failed. But it often works and the parents may put on the pressure, as they did in the case of Mathilda.

"If you don't do what the doctor says you'll have to go to the hospital the mother admonished her severely."

And then finally, it had to be done, the way no one prefers to perform a procedure, by the use of force. The father was asked to hold the child. The child started shrieking.

"Stop it! You're killing me!"

Williams grew furious. He tried first with a wooden tongue blade, but she splintered it. Determined to go through with the procedure, he asked the mother for a spoon. The child's tongue was cut and bleeding. She shrieked. Our conference room was spellbound by Fred and his choice of reading and by our own remembering.

"The damned little brat must be protected against her own idiocy, one says to oneself at such times. Others must be protected against her. It is a social necessity. And all these things are true. But a blind fury, a feeling of adult shame, bred of a longing for muscular release are the operatives. One goes to the end.

In the final unreasoning assault I overpowered the child's neck and jaws. I forced the heavy silver spoon back of her teeth and down her throat until she gagged. And there it was—both tonsils covered with membranes. She had fought valiantly to keep me from knowing her secret. She had been hiding the sore throat for three days at least and lying to her parents in order to escape such an outcome as this."

Dr. Henretig now confronted an audience as involved as an audience could be about the difficult role we have in performing procedures on children. As a master teacher, he had recognized the components needed to perform any procedure:

the knowledge, the equipment, and, most importantly, the attitude. He had given us a profound lesson in the latter. The emotion in the room was heavy. People began to speak of their experiences—their victories and their defeats. Most of all they began to talk about their feelings and how difficult it was to have to hurt in order to heal.

We were then ready to learn about the specifics that Fred had to teach us. It was one of those teaching/learning experiences that you never forget. William Carlos Williams, a University of Pennsylvania medical student who graduated in 1906, and Fred Henretig, a University of Pennsylvania faculty member in 1982, had teamed up to teach us something about pediatric procedures and how to perform them.

In later years, Chris King joined us from the Medical College of Pennsylvania. He also focused us on procedures and brought the world of general emergency medicine to our pediatric hospital setting. Chris also proved to be an excellent teacher and highly skilled clinician.

Both Dr. Henretig and Dr. King taught us that performing procedures takes more than the correct psychological mindset and caution in working with children. It takes information about the indications and contraindications for performing the task. It takes the proper equipment. It takes a step-by-step approach. These elements are all important, whether the procedure is the removal of a wayward fishhook or the placement of a central venous catheter. In these times, correct procedural technique also includes gaining the appropriate, informed parental consent and protecting oneself and staff colleagues from possible hazardous exposures.

Dr. Williams wrote more than 40 volumes of poems, fiction, essays, and plays. Dr. Henretig and Dr. King, along with our other colleagues, have prepared this excellent volume on pediatric procedures. It embodies all the strong teaching principles and dedication to the needs of our young patients, characterized by that single emergency medicine conference previously described. The authors have not been theorists working in their laboratories; they have all been front-line combatants in the battle to improve the lives of ill and injured children. Each has spent countless hours tending to his or her patients whenever the need was felt. Each has also been a master educator in training students, residents, fellows, and colleagues in the science and in the art of medical practice. This book reflects their knowledge and their spirit. It is comprehensive in scope, meticulous in detail, and presented with the beautiful illustrations of Christine Young, as well as with many photographs. We are proud that Henretig & King's *Textbook of Pediatric Emergency Procedures* follows the *Textbook of Pediatric Emergency Medicine* as part of a series of books published by Williams & Wilkins. We salute the editors, illustrator, and authors, and thank them for their magnificent accomplishment.

Stephen Ludwig, M.D.
Gary Fleisher, M.D.

This book is intended for physicians who care for children with acute illness or injury. Virtually all of these patients will require some type of procedural intervention, whether it is as simple as an otoscopic examination or as complex as endotracheal intubation. We have attempted to codify both the experience of clinicians and the medical literature relating to the various hands-on techniques used in treating pediatric patients. In deciding what constitutes an "emergency" procedure, we have used procedures that are performed routinely in a hospital emergency department (ED) as a general criterion. This obviously includes the more invasive techniques involved in the emergency management of life-threatening processes. Yet since a great deal of primary care takes place in every ED, this definition also encompasses most procedures performed in other acute care settings, as well as office-based practice. We hope this book will be an equally useful resource for the emergency physician, pediatrician, and family practitioner.

Why produce an entire textbook devoted to pediatric emergency procedures? Why now? The answer reflects in part the evolution of our respective background disciplines (pediatrics for FH, emergency medicine for CK) and, more specifically, the recent growth and development of our chosen hybrid subspecialty of pediatric emergency medicine (PEM). The past 15 years have witnessed the publication of several authoritative texts on PEM and emergency medicine. In 1983, the appearance of Fleisher & Ludwig's *Textbook of Pediatric Emergency Medicine* served as a milestone in the recognition of PEM as a legitimate subspecialty. The Fleisher & Ludwig book is now in its third edition. Over this same period, a proliferation of titles in emergency medicine kept pace with the rapid development and subspecialization of that field, including procedural titles covering the encyclopedic approach to a previously underrepresented aspect of emergency medicine. We consider these pioneering texts as landmarks in the evolution of their respective disciplines, and believe that the *Textbook of Pediatric Emergency Procedures* owes a debt of ancestry to these foundational works.

In 1992, the American Board of Pediatrics and the American Board of Emergency Medicine jointly offered the first examination for certification in the newly recognized subspecialty of PEM. We believe that this recognition will cause a further expansion in the PEM body of literature, serving as

the infrastructure in building this new discipline. The scope of PEM is broad, spanning the entire pediatric age range and the gamut of medical and surgical conditions of every organ system. It provides the opportunity for critical life support interventions, as well as a full range of diagnostic and therapeutic ambulatory care challenges. Furthermore, the procedural nature of PEM is an innate part of its appeal. Achieving technical proficiency is an essential component of its practice, and striving for mastery in this realm is an ongoing quest for all its practitioners. A textbook focused on this aspect of the discipline therefore seems appropriate at this time, and we hope that the publication of this effort will be a timely contribution toward expanding the academic foundation of the field.

One of our primary aims for this book was to achieve a balance between the dual roles of a comprehensive reference and a "user-friendly," clinically useful procedural guide. On the one hand, we have endeavored to produce an authoritative, well-referenced text, with sufficient detail for the reader to fully appreciate relevant basic science, indications, equipment requirements, comparative approaches, and potential complications for each procedure described. We believe the novice practitioner will find all the depth needed to provide a complete resource for learning about a given procedure de novo, while the more experienced clinician will find enough information to enhance one's knowledge or skill. At the same time, each chapter affords the senior physician a quick and easy review of the key points of a procedure just prior to performing it (for those who want a brief reminder about a technique not done in some time, or who wish to cast a few "pearls" while teaching a resident, etc.). A lengthy reading of the text should not be necessary in this situation. The format of this book was designed to meet this need through the liberal use of step-by-step illustrations combined with highlighted tables containing a distillation of the important information in the chapter. A quickly directed review of the figures and tables for each procedure should allow the practitioner to "just do it."

We feel especially fortunate in having had the privilege of working from the inception of this endeavor with a talented and experienced medical illustrator. Christine Young has illustrated all three editions of Fleisher & Ludwig's book, as well as several titles in pediatric surgery. We believe her ability to "see" how procedures are done and to convey this in her artwork is masterful and will be immediately obvious to the reader perusing the illustrations in each chapter.

The contents of this book are organized into chapters covering one or more techniques and procedures relevant to specific clinical situations. The chapters are grouped into sections, which have overlapping areas of focus. Each chapter is structured similarly in order to provide a familiar format for the reader, allowing information to be retrieved quickly and efficiently. The background anatomy, physiology, and other relevant science is briefly reviewed. Issues regarding the likely setting for the procedure are addressed, as are specific indications and contraindications. Available equipment options are listed and compared. The procedure is then detailed in a step-by-step fashion, linked closely with illustrations to provide an "at-the-bedside" view of the methods involved. Where appropriate, various approaches for performing the procedure are presented and contrasted, with the authors indicating their prioritization of choices. Potential complications are described, along with suggestions for minimizing their likelihood of occurrence. Summary tables and tables providing "clinical tips" (i.e., focused suggestions for optimizing technique) are included to facilitate a rapid review of the key points. Finally, each chapter is fully referenced, so that the interested reader can critically pursue the scientific basis of the procedural recommendations.

The first section includes chapters related to the general care of the pediatric patient in the emergency and acute care settings. Sections 2 and 3 provide in-depth discussions of medical and trauma life support procedures. Section 4 focuses on methods of sedation and anesthesia. Section 5 describes procedures relevant to managing neonatal emergencies that may require intervention in the ED. Sections 6–14 detail procedures classified by disorders of the various major organ systems. The last several sections are devoted to more generic emergency procedures, including those related to minor outpatient procedures, bedside laboratory investigations, toxicologic and environmental exposures, the use of ultrasonography in the ED, and pediatric transport procedures.

This textbook is respectfully offered to our fellow practitioners with the hope that it will enhance the capabilities—and, ideally, the resultant professional satisfaction experienced—of those who care for pediatric patients. Ultimately, it will be the sick and injured children who stand to benefit the most from skillfully and compassionately performed procedures. If this book were to make even a small contribution to this end, we would consider that the most gratifying accomplishment.

Fred M. Henretig, M.D.
Christopher King, M.D.

▶ ACKNOWLEDGMENTS

We wish to thank all those who in various ways have helped to bring this second edition of the *Textbook of Pediatric Emergency Procedures* into being. We express our gratitude to our clinical colleagues at both the Children's Hospital of Pittsburgh and the Children's Hospital of Philadelphia for the support they have offered on many levels. We also thank our mentors and students who challenge us and give us fresh perspectives on the art and science of medicine. We wish to acknowledge the talent and hard work of those involved with the actual creation of this edition, including Anne Sydor, Sarah Granlund, and Nicole Dernoski of Lippincott Williams & Wilkins, and Wendy Druck of Aptara Inc. Finally, we thank our families, whose forbearance, love, and support make all of our creative endeavors both possible and worthwhile.

Evaline A. Alessandrini, MD, MSCE
Associate Professor
Department of Pediatrics and Emergency Medicine
University of Pennsylvania School of Medicine
Attending Physician
Division of Emergency Medicine
The Children's Hospital of Philadelphia
Philadelphia, Pennsylvania

Michael Altieri, MD, FAAP (Deceased)
Associate Clinical Professor
Department of Pediatrics and Emergency Medicine
George Washington University School of Medicine
Georgetown University School of Medicine
Washington, DC
Chief of Pediatric Emergency Medicine
Fairfax Hospital
Falls Church, Virginia

Angela C. Anderson, MD, FAAP
Associate Professor
Departments of Emergency Medicine and Pediatrics
Brown Medical School
Attending Physician
Departments of Emergency Medicine
    and Pediatrics
Hasbro Children's Hospitals
Providence, Rhode Island

Peter M. Antevy, MD
Fellow
Department of Pediatric Emergency Medicine
Children's Hospital of Pittsburgh
Pittsburgh, Pennsylvania

Magdy W. Attia, MD
Associate Professor
Department of Pediatrics
Jefferson Medical College
Philadelphia, Pennsylvania
Emergency Medicine Fellowship Program
    Director
Department of Pediatrics
AI duPont Hospital for Children
Wilmington, Delaware

David T. Bachman, MD
Associate Professor
Department of Surgery
University of Vermont School of Medicine
Burlington, Vermont
Attending Physician
Department of Emergency Medicine
Central Maine Medical Center
Lewiston, Maine

M. Douglas Baker, MD
Professor of Pediatrics
Department of Pediatrics
Yale University
Chief
Department of Pediatric Emergency Services
Yale-New Haven Children's Hospital
New Haven, Connecticut

Steven Baldwin, MD
Associate Professor
Department of Pediatrics
University of Alabama at Birmingham
Pediatric Emergency Medicine
Children's Hospital of Alabama
Birmingham, Alabama

Jill M. Baren, MD, MBE, FACEP, FAAP
Associate Professor
Departments of Emergency Medicine and Pediatrics
University of Pennsylvania School of Medicine
Attending Physician
Department of Emergency Medicine and the Division
    of Pediatric Emergency Medicine
Hospital of the University of Pennsylvania and The
    Children's Hospital of Philadelphia
Philadelphia, Pennsylvania

Louis M. Bell, MD
Professor
Department of Pediatrics
University of Pennsylvania
Division Chief
Division of General Pediatrics
The Children's Hospital of Philadelphia
Philadelphia, Pennsylvania

Jonathan E. Bennett, MD
Assistant Professor
Department of Pediatrics
Jefferson Medical College
Philadelphia, Pennsylvania
Attending Physician
Division of Emergency Medicine
AI duPont Hospital for Children
Wilmington, Delaware

Suzanne Beno, MD
Fellow
Pediatric Emergency Medicine
Division of Emergency Medicine
The Children's Hospital of Philadelphia
Philadelphia, Pennsylvania

Mananda S. Bhende, MD, FAAP, FACEP
Professor
Department of Pediatrics
University of Pittsburgh School of Medicine
Attending Physician
Emergency Department
Children's Hospital of Pittsburgh
Pittsburgh, Pennsylvania

A. Felipe Blanco, MD
Professor and Instructor
Department of Pediatrics and Emergency
    Medicine
University of Costa Rica
Attending
Emergency Department
Hospital Nacional de Niños
San José, Costa Rica

G. Randall Bond, MD
Professor
Departments of Pediatrics and Emergency
    Medicine
University of Cincinnati
Medical Director
Cincinnati Drug and Poison Information Center
Cincinnati Children's Hospital Medical Center
Cincinnati, Ohio

John A. Brennan, MD
Core Faculty
Emergency Department
Newark Beth Israel
Senior Vice President for Clinical and Emergency
    Services
Emergency Department
Newark Beth Israel Medical Center
Newark, New Jersey

Kathleen Brown, MD
Assistant Professor
Department of Pediatrics and Emergency
    Medicine
George Washington University School of
    Medicine
Medical Director
Emergency Department
Children's National Medical Center
Washington, DC

John H. Burton, MD
Professor of Emergency Medicine
Residency Program Director
Department of Emergency Medicine
Albany Medical Center
Albany, New York

Diane P. Calello, MD
Instructor in Pediatrics
The Department of Pediatrics
University of Pennsylvania School of Medicine
Fellow, Division of Emergency Medicine
Department of Medicine, Section of Medical
    Toxicology
The Children's Hospital of Philadelphia
Philadelphia, Pennsylvania

James M. Callahan, MD
Associate Professor
Department of Pediatrics
University of Pennsylvania School of Medicine
Director, Medical Education
Division of Emergency Medicine
The Children's Hospital of Philadelphia
Philadelphia, Pennsylvania

Carolyn M. Carey, MD, MBA, FACS, FAAP
Affiliate Assistant Professor
Department of Pediatric Neurological Surgery
University of South Florida
Tampa, Florida

Meta Carroll, MD
Pediatric Emergency Medicine
Northwest Acute Care Specialist, PC
Legacy Emanuel Children's Hospital
Legacy Salmon Creek Hospital
Vancouver, Washington

Patricia Chambers, MD
Research Fellow
Division of Emergency Medicine
Cincinnati Children's Hospital Medical Center
Cincinnati, Ohio

Vidya T. Chande, MD
Adjunct Associate Professor
Department of Pediatrics
University of Iowa, Carver College of
   Medicine
Iowa City, Iowa
Medical Director
Department of Pediatric Emergency
Blank Children's Hospital
Des Moines, Iowa

Christine S. Cho, MD, MPH
Assistant Clinical Professor
Department of Pediatrics
University of California San Francisco
San Francisco, California
Attending
Division of Emergency Medicine
Children's Hospital and Research Center
   Oakland
Oakland, California

Cindy W. Christian, MD
Associate Professor
Department of Pediatrics
University of Pennsylvania School of
   Medicine
Chair, Child Abuse and Neglect
   Prevention
Department of Pediatrics
The Children's Hospital of Philadelphia
Philadelphia, Pennsylvania

Andrew T. Costarino, Jr., MD
Professor
Department of Anesthesiology and Pediatrics
Jefferson Medical College
Philadelphia, Pennsylvania
Chairman
Department of Anesthesiology and Critical
   Care Medicine
Nemours/AI duPont Hospital for
   Children
Wilmington, Delaware

Kathleen M. Cronan, MD
Associate Professor
Department of Pediatrics
Jefferson Medical College
Philadelphia, Pennsylvania
Chief, Division of Emergency
   Medicine
Department of Pediatrics
AI du Pont Hospital for Children
Wilmington, Delaware

Sandra J. Cunningham, MD
Associate Professor
Department of Pediatrics and Emergency
   Medicine
Albert Einstein College of Medicine
Associate Director
Division of Pediatric Emergency Medicine
Department of Pediatrics
Jacobi Medical Center
Bronx, New York

James D'Agostino, MD
Clinical Assistant Professor
Department of Emergency Medicine
Upstate Medical University
Syracuse, New York

Lauren Daly, MD
Clinical Instructor
Department of Pediatrics
Thomas Jefferson University
Philadelphia, Pennsylvania
Attending Physician
Department of Emergency Medicine
AI duPont Hospital for Children
Wilmington, Delaware

Reza J. Daugherty, MD
Assistant Professor of Pediatrics
Department of Pediatrics
Thomas Jefferson University
Philadelphia, Pennsylvania
Attending Physician
Pediatric Emergency Medicine
AI duPont Hospital for Children
Wilmington, Delaware

Holly W. Davis, MD
Associate Professor
Department of Pediatrics
University of Pittsburgh School
   of Medicine
Senior Attending Physician
Department of Pediatrics
Children's Hospital of Pittsburgh
Pittsbugh, Pennsylvania

Allan de Caen, MD, FRCP(c)
Clinical Associate Professor
Department of Pediatrics
University of Alberta
Pediatric Intensivist
Department of Pediatric Critical Care Medicine
Stollery Children's Hospital
Edmonton, Canada

Michael DeAngelis, MD
Assistant Professor
Department of Emergency Medicine
Temple University School of Medicine
Academic Faculty
Department of Emergency Medicine
Temple University Hospital
Philadelphia, Pennsylvania

Joanne M. Decker, MD (Deceased)
Assistant Professor
Department of Pediatrics
University of Pennsylvania School of Medicine
Attending Physician
Division of Emergency Medicine
The Children's Hospital of Philadelphia
Philadelphia, Pennsylvania

Andrew D. DePiero, MD
Assistant Professor
Department of Pediatrics
Jefferson Medical College
Philadelphia, Pennsylvania
Attending Physician
Division of Emergency Medicine
AI duPont Hospital for Children
Wilmington, Delaware

Maria Carmen G. Diaz, MD, FAAP
Assistant Professor of Pediatrics
Department of Pediatrics
Thomas Jefferson University/Jefferson Medical
    College
Philadelphia, Pennsylvania
Attending Physician
Division of Emergency Medicine
AI duPont Hospital for Children
Wilmington, Delaware

Douglas S. Diekema, MD, MPH
Professor
Department of Pediatrics
University of Washington
Attending Physician
Department of Emergency Medicine
Children's Hospital and Regional Medical
    Center
Seattle, Washington

Gregg A DiGiulio, MD
Attending Physician
Cincinnati Children's Hospital Medical Center
Division of Emergency Medicine
Cincinnati, Ohio

Nanette C. Dudley, MD
Associate Professor
Department of Pediatrics
University of Utah School of Medicine
Attending Physician
Emergency Department
Primary Children's Medical Center
Salt Lake City, Utah

Susan Duffy, MD MPH
Assistant Professor
Department of Emergency Medicine and Pediatrics
Brown University
Attending Physician
Department of Pediatric Emergency Medicine
Hasbro Children's Hospital/Rhode Island Hospital
Providence, Rhode Island

Ann-Christine Duhaime, MD
Professor
Department of Surgery (Neurosurgery)
Dartmouth Medical School
Director
Department of Pediatric Neurosurgery
Children's Hospital at Dartmouth
Dartmouth Hitchcock Medical Center
Lebanon, New Hampshire

Yamani Durani, MD
Fellow
Department of Pediatric Emergency Medicine
Thomas Jefferson University
Philadelphia, Pennsylvania
Fellow
Department of Pediatric Emergency Medicine
AI duPont Children's Hospital
Wilmington, Delaware

Mirna M. Farah, MD
Assistant Professor
Department of Clincal Pediatrics
University of Pennsylvania School of Medicine
Attending Physician
Department of Pediatrics
Division of Emergency Medicine
The Children's Hospital of Philadelphia
Philadelphia, Pennsylvania

Joel A. Fein, MD
Associate Professor
Department of Pediatrics
University of Pennsylvania School of Medicine
Attending Physician
Emergency Department
The Children's Hospital of Philadelphia
Philadelphia, Pennsylvania

Deborah M. Fernon, DO
Assistant Professor
Department of Emergency Medicine
University of Texas - Health Science Center at
    Houston
Attending Physician
Department of Emergency Medicine
Memorial Hermann Hospital
Houston, Texas

Scott H. Freedman, MD, FAAP
Clinical Educator
Department of Emergency Medicine and Pediatrics
Georgetown University
Washington, DC
Medical Director
Department of Pediatric Emergency Medicine
Shady Grove Adventist Hospital
Rockville, Maryland

Janet H. Friday, MD
Assistant Clinical Professor
Department of Pediatrics
University of California School of Medicine, San Diego
La Jolla, California
Attending Physician
Division of Emergency Medicine
Rady Children's Hospital,
San Diego, California

Eron Y. Friedlaender, MD
Assistant Professor
Department of Pediatrics
University of Pennsylvania School of Medicine
Attending Physician
Department of Pediatrics
The Children's Hospital of Philadelphia
Philadelphia, Pennsylvania

Howard Friedland, DO, FACEP, FACOEP
Osteopathic Program Director
Department of Emergency Medicine
Newark Beth Israel Medical Center
Newark, New Jersey
Clinical Assistant Professor
New York College of Osteopathic Medicine
Old Westbury, New York

Marla J. Friedman, MD
Attending Physician
Division of Pediatric Emergency Medicine
Miami Children's Hospital
Miami, Florida

Susan M. Fuchs, MD
Professor
Department of Pediatrics
Feinberg School of Medicine, Northwestern
    University
Associate Director
Division of Pediatric Emergency Medicine
Children's Memorial Hospital
Chicago, Illinois

Ronnie S. Fuerst, MD
Clinical Associate Professor
Department of Pediatrics and Medicine
University of South Carolina School of
    Medicine
Medical Director, Children's Emergency Center
Department of Emergency Medicine
Palmetto Health Richland
Columbia, South Carolina

Alan Fujii, MD
Associate Professor
Department of Pediatrics
Boston University
Medical Director, NICU
Department of Pediatrics
Boston Medical Center
Boston, Massachusetts

Aris C. Garro, MD
Teaching Fellow
Department of Pediatric Emergency Medicine
Brown University Medical School
Fellow
Department of Pediatric Emergency Medicine
Rhode Island Hospital
Providence, Rhode Island

Gary Geis, MD
Assistant Professor
Department of Pediatrics
University of Cincinnati, College of Medicine
Assistant Professor of Clinical Pediatrics
Division of Emergency Medicine
Cincinnati Children's Hospital Medical Center
Cincinnati, Ohio

Angelo P. Giardino, MD, PhD
Clinical Associate Professor
Department of Pediatrics–Administration
Baylor College of Medicine
Medical Director
Texas Children's Health Plan
Texas Children's Hospital
Houston, Texas

Mark A. Ginsburg, DO
Resident Physician
Department of Otolaryngology Facial Plastic Surgery
Philadelphia College of Osteopathic Medicine
Philadelphia, Pennsylvania

Timothy G. Givens, MD
Associate Professor
Department of Emergency Medicine and
    Pediatrics
Vanderbilt University Medical Center
Associate Medical Director
Pediatric Emergency Department
Monroe Carell, Jr. Children's Hospital at
    Vanderbilt
Nashville, Tennessee

Javier A. Gonzalez del Rey, MD
Professor
Department of Pediatrics
University of Cincinnati College of Medicine
Director, Pediatric Residency Programs
Associate Director
Division of Emergency Medicine
Cinicinnati Children's Hospital Medical Center
Cincinnati, Ohio

Marc H. Gorelick, MD, MSCE
Professor and Chief
Department of Pediatrics Emergency Medicine
Medical College of Wisconsin
Jon E. Vice Chair and Medical Director
Emergency Department
Children's Hospital of Wisconsin
Milwaukee, Wisconsin

John W. Graneto, DO, FACEP, FAAP
Assistant Professor
Education Director
Department of Emergency Medicine
Midwestern University Chicago College of
    Osteopathic Medicine
Emergency Physician
Department of Emergency Medicine
Swedish Covenant Hospital
Chicago, Illinois

Daniel A. Green, MD
Assistant Professor
Department of Pediatrics
Baylor College of Medicine
Attending Physician
Pediatric Emergency Center
Texas Children's Hospital
Houston, Texas

Hazel Guinto-Ocampo, MD
Assistant Professor
Department of Pediatrics
Jefferson Medical College
Philadelphia, Pennsylvania
Attending Physician
Division of Emergency Medicine
AI duPont Hospital for Children, Nemours Children's Clinic
Wilmington, Delaware

Waseem Hafeez, MD
Associate Professor
Department of Pediatrics
Albert Einstein College of Medicine
Attending Physician
Division of Pediatric Emergency Medicine
Children's Hospital at Montefiore
Bronx, New York

Carin A. Hagberg, MD
Professor
Department of Anesthesiology
University of Texas Medical School at Houston
Director, Neuroaneshtesia and Advanced
    Airway Management
Department of Anesthesiology
Memorial Hermann Hospital
Houston, Texas

Elliott M. Harris, MD
Associate Professor
Department of Emergency Medicine
UMDNJ-Robert Wood Johnson School of Medicine
Piscataway, New Jersey
Attending Physician
Division of Pediatric Emergency Medicine
Cooper University Hospital
Camden, New Jersey

Mary Hegenbarth, MD, FAAP, FACEP
Associate Professor
Department of Pediatrics
University of Missouri–Kansas City School of Medicine
Pediatrician
Division of Emergency Medicine
Children's Mercy Hospitals and Clinics
Kansas City, Missouri

Fred M. Henretig, MD
Professor
Departments of Pediatrics and Emergency
    Medicine
University of Pennsylvania School of
    Medicine
Director, Section of Clinical Toxicology
Division of Emergency Medicine
The Children's Hospital of Philadelphia
Philadelphia, Pennsylvania

Robert Hickey, MD
Associate Professor
Department of Pediatrics
University of Pittsburgh
Attending Physician
Division of Pediatric Emergency Medicine
Children's Hospital of Pittsburgh
Pittsburgh, Pennsylvania

Dee Hodge, III, MD
Associate Professor
Department of Pediatrics
Washington University School of Medicine
Associate Director, Clinical Affairs Emergency
    Services
Department of Emergency Services
St. Louis Children's Hospital
St. Louis, Missouri

Judd E. Hollander, MD
Professor
Department of Emergency Medicine
University of Pennsylvania
Professor
Department of Emergency Medicine
Hospital of the University of Pennsylvania
Philadelphia, Pennsylvania

Frank A. Illuzzi, MD
Vice Chair
Department of Emergency Medicine
St. Vincent's Medical Center,
Bridgeport, Connecticut

Sonia O. Imaizumi, MD
Associate Professor
Department of Pediatrics
Robert Wood Johnson Medical School
University of Medicine and Dentistry of
    New Jersey
Assistant Division Head
Division of Neonatology
Cooper University Hospital
Camden, New Jersey

Srikant B. Iyer, MD
Assistant Professor
Department of Pediatrics
University of Cincinnati College of
    Medicine
Department of Emergency Medicine
Cincinnati Children's Hospital Medical
    Center
Cincinnati, Ohio

Deitrich Jehle, MD
Associate Professor and Vice Chair
Department of Emergency Medicine
State University of New York at Buffalo
Director of Emergency Services
Department of Emergency Medicine
Erie County Medical Center
Buffalo, New York

Frederick C. Johnson, DO
Attending Physician
Department of Emergency Medicine
Medical City Children's Hospital
Dallas, Texas

Jean Marie Kallis, MD
Associate Professor
Department of Pediatrics
University of Louisville
Kosair Children's Hospital
Louisville, Kentucky

Zach Kassutto, MD, FAAP
Assistant Professor
Department of Emergency Medicine
Drexel University College of Medicine
Philadelphia, Pennsylvania
Director
Department of Pediatric Emergency
    Medicine
Capital Health System
Trenton, New Jersey

Kathleen P. Kelly, MD
Attending Physician
Department of Emergency Medicine
Inova Alexandria Hospital
Alexandria, Virginia

Valerie McDougall Kestner, MD
Fellow
Department of Pediatric Emergency
    Medicine
Children's Hospital of Pittsburgh
Pittsburgh, Pennsylvania

Jason Y. Kim, MD
Attending Physician
Division of Infectious Diseases
The Children's Hospital of Philadelphia
Philadelphia, Pennsylvania

Christopher King, MD, FACEP
Associate Professor
Department of Emergency Medicine and Pediatrics
University of Pittsburg School of Medicine
Attending Physician
Department of Emergency Medicine
UPMC-Presbyterian Hospital
Children's Hospital of Pittsburgh
Pittsburgh, Pennsylvania

Brent R. King, MD FACEP, FAAP, FAAEM
Professor and Chairman
Department of Emergency Medicine
The University of Texas Houston Medical
    School
Chief of Emergency Medicine
Department of Emergency Medicine
Memorial Hermann Hospital
Houston, Texas

**Niranjan Kissoon, MD, FRCPC(c), FAAP,
    FCCM, FACPE**
Professor and Associate Head
Department of Pediatrics
University of British Columbia
Senior Medical Director
Acute and Critical Care Program
British Columbia's Children's Hospital
Vancouver, British Columbia

Bruce L. Klein, MD
Associate Professor
Department of Pediatrics and Emergency
    Medicine
The George Washington University School of
    Medicine and Health Sciences
Chief
Division of Transport Medicine
Children's National Medical Center
Washington, DC

Jean E. Klig, MD
Assistant Professor
Department of Pediatrics
Boston University School of Medicine
Attending in Pediatric Emergency
    Medicine
Department of Pediatrics
Boston Medical Center
Boston, Massachusetts

Christine E. Koerner, MD
Associate Professor
Department of Emergency Medicine
University of Texas Health Science Center at
    Houston
Chief, Division of Pediatric Emergency
    Medicine
Department of Emergency Medicine
University of Texas Health Science Center Emergency
    Medicine
Lyndon B. Johnson General Hospital
Houston, Texas

Tadeusz Korzun, MD
Resident
Department of Emergency Medicine
North Shore University Hospital at Manhassett
Manhassett, New York

Susanne I. Kost, MD
Associate Professor
Department of Pediatrics
Jefferson Medical College
Philadelphia, Pennsylvania
Attending Physician
Division of Emergency Medicine
AI duPont Hospital for Children
Wilmington, Delaware

Mary E. Lacher, MD
Associate Professor
Division of Pediatric Emergency Medicine
University of Louisville
Kosiar Hospital
Louisville, Kentucky

Natalie E. Lane, MD
Assistant Professor
Department of Emergency Medicine
Medical College of Georgia
Attending Faculty
Children's Medical Center
Medical College of Georgia Hospitals and
    Clinics
Augusta, Georgia

Bernard J. Larson, DDS
Affiliate Dental Practitioner
Department of Pediatric Dentistry
University of Washington
Seattle, Washington
Medical Staff
Department of Surgery
Skagit Valley Hospital
Mount Vernon, Washington

Jane M. Lavelle, MD
Associate Professor
Department of Pediatrics
University of Pennsylvania School of Medicine
Associate Director
Department of Pediatric Emergency Medicine
The Children's Hospital of Philadelphia
Philadelphia, Pennsylvania

David C. Lee, MD
Assistant Professor
Department of Emergency Medicine
New York University School of Medicine
New York, New York
Director of Research
Department of Emergency Medicine
North Shore University Hospital
Manhasset, New York

**Alex V. Levin, MD, MHSc, FAAP,
   FAAO, FRCSC**
Professor
Pediatrics and Opthalmology and Vision Sciences
University of Ontario
Staff Ophthalmologist
Departments of Pediatrics, Genetics and
   Ophthalmology and Vision Science
Hospital for Sick Children
Toronto, Ontario

William Lewander, MD
Professor
Department of Emergency Medicine and
   Pediatrics
Brown Medical School
Director
Department of Pediatric Emergency Medicine
Hasbro Children's Hospital of Rhode Island
Providence, Rhode Island

Rhett Lieberman, MD, MPH
Assistant Professor
Department of Pediatric Emergency Medicine
Children's Hospital of Pittsburgh
Pittsburgh, Pennsylvania

Kathleen A. Lillis, MD
Clinical Associate Professor
Department of Pediatrics
University of Buffalo School of Medicine
   and Biomedical Sciences
Emergency Department Attending
Department of Pediatrics
Women and Children's Hospital of
   Buffalo
Buffalo, New York

James G. Linakis, MD
Associate Professor
Department of Emergency Medicine and Pediatrics
Brown Medical School
Associate Director
Department of Pediatric Emergency Medicine
Hasbro Children's Hospital/Rhode Island
   Hospital
Providence, Rhode Island

Jordan D. Lipton, MD, FACEP
Physician and COO
Signature Healthcare, PLLC
Charlotte, North Carolina

John M. Loiselle, MD
Associate Professor
Department of Pediatrics
Thomas Jefferson University
Philadelphia, Pennsylvania
Assistant Director
Department of Emergency Medicine
AI duPont Hospital for Children
Wilmington, Delaware

Joseph W. Luria, MD
Associate Professor
Department of Pediatrics
University of Cincinnati
Division of Emergency Medicine
Cincinnati Children's Hospital Medical
   Center
Cincinnati, Ohio

Robert Luten, MD
Professor
Department of Pediatrics and Emergency
   Medicine
University of Florida
Faculty
Department of Emergency Medicine
Shands Hospital
Jacksonville, Florida

Charles G. Macias, MD, MPH
Associate Professor
Department of Pediatrics
Baylor College of Medicine
Attending Physician
Emergency Department
Texas Children's Hospital
Houston, Texas

Mioara D. Manole, MD
NIH Research Scholar
Department of Pediatrics
University of Pittsburgh
Attending Physician
Department of Pediatrics
Division of Pediatric Emergency Medicine
Children's Hospital of Pittsburgh
Pittsburgh, Pennsylvania

Nestor J. Martinez, MD
Fellow
Department of Emergency Medicine
Miami Children's Hospital
Miami, Florida

James R. Mateer, MD, FACEP
Associate Professor
Department of Emergency Medicine
Director
Department of Emergency Medicine Ultrasonography
    Fellowship
Medical College of Wisconsin
Milwaukee, Wisconsin

Constance M. McAneney, MD
Associate Professor of Clinical Pediatrics
Department of Pediatrics
University of Cincinnati College of Medicine
Associate Director
Division of Emergency Medicine
Director
Pediatric Emergency Medicine Fellowship
Cincinnati Children's Hospital Medical
    Center
Cincinnati, Ohio

Audra McCreight, MD, FAAP
Fellow in Training
Department of Pediatrics
University of Texas Southwestern Medical Center of
    Dallas
Fellow in Training
Division of Pediatric Emergency Medicine
Children's Medical Center of Dallas
Dallas, Texas

Michele McKee, MD
Attending Physician
Pediatric Emergency Medicine
Boston Medical Center
Boston, Massachussetts

Robert McNamara, MD, FAAEM
Professor and Chairperson
Department of Emergency Medicine
Temple University School of Medicine
Temple University Hospital
Philadelphia, Pennsylvania

Manoj K. Mittal, MD, MRCP, FAAP
Instructor
Department of Pediatrics
University of Pennsylvania School of Medicine
Fellow
Pediatric Emergency Medicine
The Children's Hospital of Philadelphia
Philadelphia, Pennsylvania

Colette C. Mull, MD
Assistant Professor
Director in Pediatric Emergency Medicine Fellowship
    Program
Department of Emergency Medicine and Pediatrics
Drexel University College of Medicine
Department of Pediatric Emergency Medicine
St. Christopher's Hospital for Children
Philadelphia, Pennsylvania

Fran Nadel, MD, MSCE
Assistant Professor
Department of Pediatrics
University of Pennsylvania School of Medicine
Attending Physician
Division of Emergency Medicine
The Children's Hospital of Philadelphia
Philadelphia, Pennsylvania

Leo G. Niederman, MD, MPH
Associate Professor
Department of Pediatrics
University of Illinois at Chicago
Medical Director
Children and Adolescent Center
University of Illinois Medical Center at
    Chicago
Chicago, Illinois

Karen J. O'Connell, MD
Assitant Professor
Department of Pediatrics
The George Washinton School of Medicine
Attending Physician
Emergency Medicine and Trauma Center
Children's National Medical Center
Washington, DC

Pamela J. Okada, MD
Assistant Professor
Department of Pediatric Emergency
    Medicine
The University of Texas Southwestern Medical Center at
    Dallas
Attending Physician
Department of Emergency Services
Children's Medical Center of Dallas
Dallas, Texas

Kevin C. Osterhoudt, MD, MSCE, FAAP, FACMT
Associate Professor
Department of Pediatrics
University of Pennsylvania School of
    Medicine
Medical Director
The Poison Control Center
The Children's Hospital of
    Philadelphia
Philadelphia, Pennsylvania

Floyd S. Ota, MD, FAAP
Attending Physician
Department of Pediatric Emergency
    Medicine
Cook Children's Medical Center
Fort Worth, Texas

James F. Parker, MD
Assistant Professor
Department of Pediatrics and Emergency
    Medicine/Traumatology
University of Connecticut School of Medicine
Farmington, Connecticut
Attending Physician
Department of Pediatric Emergency
Connecticut Children's Medical Center
Hartford, Connecticut

Kala Parker, MD
Fellow
Pediatric Emergency Medicine
Children's Hospital Pittsburgh
Pittsburgh, Pennsylvania

Parul B. Patel, MD
Clinical Instructor
Department of Pediatrics
Thomas Jefferson University
Attending Physician
Department of Pediatric
    Emergency
AI duPont Hospital for Children
Wilmington, Delaware

Ronald I. Paul, MD
Professor
Department of Pediatrics
University of Louisville
Chief
Pediatric Emergency Medicine
Kosair Children's Hospital
Louisville, Kentucky

Barbara M. G. Peña, MD, MPH
Research Director
Division of Emergency Medicine
Miami Children's Hospital
Miami, Florida

Erin D. Phrampus, MD
Assistant Professor
Department of Pediatrics
Children's Hospital of Pittsburgh
Pittsburgh, Pennsylvania

Raymond D. Pitetti, MD, MPH
Assistant Professor
Department of Pediatrics
University of Pittsburgh School of Medicine
Assistant Clinical Director
Department of Pediatric Emergency Medicine
Children's Hospital of Pittsburgh
Pittsburgh, Pennsylvania

Melanie Pitone, MD
Clinical Instructor
Department of Pediatrics
Jefferson Medical College
Philadelphia, Pennsylvania
Attending
Department of Pediatric Emergency Medicine
AI duPont Hospital for Children
Wilmington, Delaware

Shari L. Platt, MD, FAAP
Assistant Professor
Department of Pediatrics
Weill Medical College of Cornell University
Director
Division of Pediatric Emergency Medicine
Departments of Pediatrics and Emergency Medicine
New York Presbyterian Hospital
New York, New York

Michael P. Poirier, MD, FAAP
Associate Professor
Department of Pediatrics
Eastern Virginia Medical School
Attending Physician
Division of Emergency Medicine
Children's Hospital of The King's Daughters
Norfolk, Virginia

Wendy J. Pomerantz, MD, MS
Assistant Professor of Clinical Pediatrics
Department of Pediatrics
University of Cincinnati
Attending Physician
Division of Emergency Medicine
Cincinnati Children's Hospital Medical Center
Cincinnati, Ohio

Amanda Pratt, MD
Assistant Professor
Department of Pediatrics
Robert Wood Johnson Medical School
Assistant Professor/Attending Physician
Department of Pediatric Emergency Medicine
University of Medicine & Dentistry of
   New Jersey
New Brunswick, New Jersey

Juliette Quintero-Solivan, MD
Assistant Professor
Department of Pediatrics
UMDNJ – Robert Wood Johnson Medical School
Assistant Professor
Department of Pediatrics
UMDNJ – Robert Wood Johnson University
   Hospital
New Brunswick, New Jersey

Lara Davidovic Rappaport, MD, MPH
Assistant Professor
Department of Emergency Medicine
University of Colorado School of Medicine
Denver, Colorado
Children's Hospital of Pittsburgh
Pittsburgh, Pennsylvania

Jennifer L. Reed, MD
Assistant Professor
Department of Pediatrics
University of Cincinnati
Cincinnati, Ohio
Attending Physician
Division of Emergency Medicine
Cincinnati Children's Hospital Medical Center
Cincinnati, Ohio

Scott D. Reeves, MD
Assistant Professor
Department of Pediatrics
University of Cincinnati
Staff Physician
Division of Emergency Medicine
Cincinnati Children's Hospital Medical Center
Cincinnati, Ohio

Stacy L. Reynolds, MD
Fellow
Department of Pediatric Emergency Medicine
Children's Hospital of Pittsburgh
Pittsburgh, Pennsylvania

Richard M. Ruddy, MD
Professor
Department of Pediatrics
University of Cincinnati College of Medicine
Director
Division of Emergency Medicine
Department of Pediatrics
Cincinnati Children's Hospital Medical Center
Cincinnati, Ohio

Gail S. Rudnitsky, MD
Associate Professor
Department of Emergency Medicine
Drexel University College of Medicine
Philadelphia, Pennsylvania

Maia S. Rutman, MD
Teaching Fellow
Department of Pediatrics
Brown Medical School
Fellow
Department of Pediatric Emergency Medicine
Hasbro Children's Hospital
Providence, Rhode Island

Seema Sachdeva, MD, FAAP
Vice Chair
Division of Pediatrics
Pikeville College School of Osteopathic Medicine
Director
Physicians for Children and Adolescents
Pikeville, Kentucky

Richard A. Saladino, MD
Associate Professor
Department of Pediatrics
University of Pittsburgh School of Medicine
Chief
Division of Pediatric Emergency Medicine
Children's Hospital of Pittsburgh
Pittsburgh, Pennsylvania

Morton E. Salomon, MD
Professor and Associate Professor
Department of Clinical Emergency Medicine and Pediatrics
Albert Einstein College of Medicine
Bronx, New York
Chairman
Department of Emergency Medicine
St. Vincent's Medical Center
Bridgeport, Connecticut

Esther M. Sampayo, MD
Clinical Instructor
Department of Pediatrics
University of Pennsylvania School of Medicine
Fellow
Department of Pediatric Emergency Medicine
The Children's Hospital of Philadelphia
Philadelphia, Pennsylvania

Richard J. Scarfone, MD
Associate Professor
Department of Pediatrics
University of Pennsylvania School of Medicine
Medical Director of Disaster Preparedness
The Children's Hospital of Philadelphia
Philadelphia, Pennsylvania

Charles J. Schubert, MD
Associate Professor
Department of Pediatrics
University of Cincinnati
Attending
Division of Emergency Medicine
Cincinnati Children's Hospital Medical Center
Cincinnati, Ohio

Jeff E. Schunk, MD
Professor
Department of Pediatrics
University of Utah
Division Chief
Division of Pediatric Emergency Medicine
Primary Children's Medical Center
Salt Lake City, Utah

Sandra Schwab, MD
Fellow
Department of Pediatric Emergency Medicine
The Children's Hospital of Philadelphia
Philadelphia, Pennsylvania

Gary Schwartz, MD
Assistant Professor
Department of Emergency Medicine
Vanderbilt University
Nashville, Tennessee

Philip V. Scribano, DO, MSCE
Associate Professor
Department of Pediatrics
The Ohio State University College of Medicine
Medical Director
Center for Child and Family Advocacy
Columbus Children's Hospital
Columbus, Ohio

Michael Shannon, MD, MPH, FAAP, FACEP
Professor
Department of Pediatrics
Harvard Medical School
Chief and CHB Chair
Division of Emergency Medicine
Children's Hospital Boston
Boston, Massachusetts

Robert A. Shapiro, MD
Clinical Professor
Department of Pediatrics
University of Cincinnati
Medical Director
Mayerson Center for Safe & Healthy
   Children
Cincinnati Children's Hospital Medical Center
Cincinnati, Ohio

Kathy N. Shaw, MD, MSCE
Professor
Department of Pediatrics
University of Pennsylvania School
   of Medicine
Chief
Division of Emergency Medicine
The Children's Hospital of Philadelphia
Philadelphia, Pennsylvania

Harold K. Simon, MD, MBA
Associate Professor
Department of Pediatrics and Emergency
   Medicine
Emory University School of Medicine
Associate Division Director
Division of Pediatric Emergency Medicine
Children's Healthcare of Atlanta
Atlanta, Georgia

Sharon R. Smith, MD
Associate Professor
Department of Pediatrics and Division of Emergency
   Medicine
University of Connecticut School of Medicine
Associate Professor
Department of Pediatrics and Division of Emergency
   Medicine
Connecticut Children's Medical Center
Hartford, Connecticut

Philip R. Spandorfer, MD, MSCE
Attending Physician
Department of Emergency Medicine
Children's Healthcare of Atlanta at Scottish Rite
Atlanta, Georgia

Dale Steele, MD
Associate Professor
Department of Emergency Medicine and Pediatrics
Brown Medical School
Attending Physician and Fellowship
    Director
Department of Pediatric Emergency Medicine
Hasbro Children's Hospital
Providence, Rhode Island

Maria Stephan, MD
Associate Professor
Department of Pediatrics Emergency
    Medicine
University of Texas Southwestern School of
    Medicine
Attending Physican
Division of Emergency
    Medicine
Children's Medical Center of Dallas
Dallas, Texas

Gary R. Strange, MD
Professor and Head
Department of Emergency Medicine
University of Illinois
Chicago, Illinois

Milton Tenenbein, MD
Professor
Department of Pediatrics and Pharmacology
University of Manitoba
Director of Emergency Services
Department of Pediatrics
Children's Hospital
Winnipeg, Manitoba

Thomas E. Terndrup, MD, FACEP, FAAEM
Professor
Department of Emergency Medicine
Associate Dean for Clinical Research
Milton S. Hershey Medical Center
    Chair
Department of Emergency Medicine
Penn State University College of
    Medicine
Hershey, Pennsylvania

Eric Tham, MD
Fellow
Department of Pediatrics
Division of Pediatric Emergency
    Medicine
Children's Hospital of Pittsburgh
Pittsburgh, Pennsylvania

Susan B. Torrey, MD
Assistant Clinical Professor
Department of Pediatrics
Harvard Medical School
Staff Physician
Department of Emergency Medicine
Children's Hospital Boston
Boston, Massachusetts

William Tsai, MD
Assistant Professor
Department of Pediatrics
George Washington University
Attending Physician
Department of Critical Care and Emergency
    Medicine
Children's National Medical Center
Washington, DC

Nicholas Tsarouhas, MD
Associate Professor
Department of Pediatrics
University of Pennsylvania School of Medicine
Medical Director of Emergency Transport Services
Attending Physician
Division of Emergency Medicine
The Children's Hospital of Philadelphia
Philadelphia, Pennsylvania

Brian D. Upham, MD
Instructor
Department of Pediatrics
University of Pennsylvania School of Medicine
Fellow Physician
Division of Pediatric Emergency Medicine
The Children's Hospital of Philadelphia
Philadelphia, Pennsylvania

Verena T. Valley, MD, RDMS
Associate Professor
Department of Emergency Medicine
University of Mississippi
Ultrasound Director
Department of Emergency Medicine
University of Mississippi
Jackson, Mississippi

Robert J. Vinci, MD
Professor
Department of Pediatrics
Boston University School of Medicine
Vice Chairman
Department of Pediatrics
Boston Medical Center
Boston, Massachusetts

Eva Vogeley, MD, JD (Deceased)
Assistant Professor
Department of Pediatrics
University of Pittsburgh
Division of Pediatric Emergency Medicine
Children's Hospital of Pittsburgh
Pittsburgh, Pennsylvania

Gary S. Wasserman, DO, FAAP, FACMT, FAACT, ABMT
Professor
Department of Pediatrics
University of Missouri–Kansas City, School of Medicine
Chief-Section of Medical Toxicology
Department of Pediatrics
Children's Mercy Hospitals and Clinics
Kansas City, Missouri

Winnie T. Whitaker, MD
Research Fellow
Division of Emergency Medicine
Cincinnati Children's Hospital Medical Center
Cincinnati, Ohio

James F. Wiley, II, MD, MPH
Professor
Departments of Pediatrics and Emergency Medicine/Traumatology
University of Connecticut School of Medicine
Farmington, Connecticut
Attending Physician
Department of Emergency Medicine
Connecticut Children's Medical Center
Hartford, Connecticut

George A. Woodward, MD, MBA
Professor
Department of Pediatrics
University of Washington School of Medicine
Chief
Division of Emergency Services
Children's Hospital & Regional Medical Center
Seattle, Washington

Robert F. Yellon, MD
Associate Professor
Department of Otolaryngology
University of Pittsburgh School of Medicine
Co-Director
Department of Pediatric Otolaryngology
Children's Hospital Pittsburgh
Pittsburgh, Pennsylvania

Kenneth Yen, MD, MS, FAAP
Assistant Professor
Department of Pediatrics
Medical College of Wisconsin
Milwaukee, Wisconsin
Attending Physician
Department of Pediatrics
Children's Hospital of Wisconsin
Wauwatosa, Wisconsin

Stephen A. Zderic, MD
Professor of Urology
Department of Surgery
University of Pennsylvania School of Medicine
Attending Urologist
Division of Urology
The Children's Hospital of Philadelphia
Philadelphia, Pennsylvania

Noel Zuckerbraun, MD, MPH
Assistant Professor
Department of Pediatrics
University of Pittsburgh
Attending
Division of Pediatric Emergency Medicine
Children's Hospital of Pittsburgh
Pittsburgh, Pennsylvania

▶ CONTENTS

◀ SECTION 1
GENERAL CONCEPTS
EDITOR
FRED M. HENRETIG

◀ SECTION 2
CARDIOPULMONARY
LIFE SUPPORT
PROCEDURES
EDITOR
CHRISTOPHER KING

SECTION 3 ▶ TRAUMA LIFE SUPPORT PROCEDURES
EDITOR
BRENT R. KING

SECTION 4 ▶ ANESTHESIA AND SEDATION PROCEDURES
EDITOR
BRENT R. KING

SECTION 9 ▶ DENTAL PROCEDURES

EDITOR

JOHN M. LOISELLE

SECTION 10 ▶ CARDIOVASCULAR PROCEDURES

EDITOR

RICHARD M. RUDDY

◀ SECTION 11
PULMONARY
PROCEDURES
EDITOR
RICHARD M. RUDDY

◀ SECTION 12
GASTROINTESTINAL
PROCEDURES
EDITOR
JAMES F. WILEY, II

◀ SECTION 13
GENITOURINARY
PROCEDURES
EDITOR
JAMES F. WILEY, II

SECTION 14 ▶
ORTHOPAEDIC
PROCEDURES
EDITOR
BRENT R. KING

SECTION 15 ▶
MINOR EMERGENCY
PROCEDURES
EDITOR
JOHN M. LOISELLE

SECTION 1 ▶ GENERAL CONCEPTS
SECTION EDITOR: FRED M. HENRETIG

1

MIRNA M. FARAH, FRED M. HENRETIG, AND
KAREN O'CONNELL

Patient and Family Issues

▶ INTRODUCTION

A child is rushed to the emergency department (ED) by anxious parents. This scenario unfolds tens of millions of times a year in the United States but remains a uniquely compelling event for all the persons involved: the patient, family, and medical staff. In the most dramatic of cases, the child's life depends on the skill of the ED staff in rapidly diagnosing the injury or illness, instituting life support, and initiating definitive treatment as a prelude to hospitalization. Unfortunately, some of these visits end tragically with the death of a child in the ED, despite a technically optimal resuscitation effort. In the vast majority of visits, the family returns home within a few hours, the child sporting some new sutures, or a new cast, or an antibiotic prescription for that unbearable middle-of-the-night ear infection. In every case, the child or family bears a lasting impression of the experience, even if the pathophysiologic aberration is readily corrected. Their pain and fear of the ED visit, and how these were addressed by the ED staff, may be remembered long after the physical wounds heal. Conversely, even an otherwise forgettable pediatric walk-in visit, perhaps one of dozens experienced during a busy shift, can be a residual source of frustration to the ED physician, who may have to battle to examine a screaming child or try five times to "get the i.v." The general approach to these psychosocial stresses on child, parent, and medical staff is the focus of this chapter.

All patients are potentially traumatized by an ED experience, but some factors pertain uniquely to the pediatric visit (1,2). Children vary enormously in age and developmental status, but as a group they have an innate fear of needles and procedures. The younger child in particular fears strangers (and especially physicians, who are often perceived as sources of pain). Parents are the natural protectors and sources of comfort for their children during a physical or emotional crisis. When their child is sick, parents feel an obligation to serve in a helping role. They may also feel some share of responsibility for having "allowed" the illness or injury to occur. Thus, parents are functioning in dual roles when their child visits the ED. On the one hand, they wish to be composed and to function as members of the helping team. On the other hand, they are stressed and anxious and may feel some guilt over their child's illness. In essence, they too are patients. Medical staff often diminish both of these parental roles in their zeal to get things done efficiently. This is generally a mistake. Parents, in most situations, are able to function as considerable sources of comfort and support for their children in the ED setting and belong at the bedside during the vast majority of interventions. This chapter explores background issues related to parental involvement in pediatric ED procedures. It offers an approach that allows the medical staff to take maximal advantage of the parents as allies in the effort to accomplish such procedures successfully from the child, the family, and the staff perspectives.

1

▶ BENEFITS OF FAMILY PRESENCE

Benefits to Patients

Psychologists consider the first year of life to be a period when children experience their world as an extension of their parents. Although toddlers aged 1 to 3 years begin to understand themselves as individuals, there is still a very close bond to parents that requires a nearly constant sense of parental presence within the immediate environment for maximal sense of security. Infants beyond 6 to 9 months of age have intense stranger anxiety, often lasting to the age of 3 years. Maintaining close contact with parents is crucial to optimizing psychological support during a stressful event in this age group (Table 1.1).

Although older preschool and school-aged children are obviously able to tolerate brief separations from their parents, they still derive a strong sense of comfort from ready access to them. Dentists have reported that children aged 41 to 49 months are less fearful and more cooperative when their parents stay with them (3). Pediatricians looked at the effects of family presence during i.v. placement in children 1 to 18 years of age and found that both the patients and their parents in the family presence group were significantly less distressed than those in the family absence group (4,5). Further surveys of health care providers and parents witnessing more invasive procedures done on their child showed family presence to be significantly helpful to the patient (6,7). When surveyed, more than 90% of children 9 to 12 years old reported that the "thing that helped most" during a painful procedure was to have their parents present (8). Other researchers observed that behavioral manifestations of discomfort may actually increase if the parents are present (9); this may reflect the child's perception that parental presence gives permission to verbalize his or her discomfort. However, the goal of pain management during procedures is obviously not to produce a cooperative child who bravely suffers in silence.

Not only is it essential to include the parents in the care plan, but it is equally important to involve the children and allow them to make choices when applicable (10). Examples of such choices range from a favorite cast color to a preferred i.v. site and to whether they want their parents to be present or absent during the procedure. Medical information should be explained using age-appropriate language, and any strong disagreement should not be ignored. Increasing the patients' knowledge about their care improves both their compliance with the treatment plan and their level of satisfaction and can thus improve the outcome (11).

Benefits to Parents

Parents play an integral role in the health and well-being of their child. Therefore, supporting and integrating the family into the emergency care process is crucial for meeting the full spectrum of the patient's needs. Family presence during resuscitation and procedures meets the family's emotional need to be informed, feel accepted, and be able to provide comfort to the patient.

Using theoretical scenarios, parents were surveyed on their preferences regarding being present during a variety of procedures done on their children. In one study, 400 parents completed anonymous surveys in the ED waiting area (12). The majority of parents (98%) wanted to be present during venipuncture, 87% during lumbar puncture, 81% during endotracheal intubation, and 83% during cardiopulmonary resuscitation (CPR) if the child was likely to die. Nearly all parents (94%) wanted to participate in the decision regarding their presence. In another study, from a Boston pediatric ED (13), 78% of parents surveyed indicated they would want to be present when their child had blood drawn or an i.v. was started. Of this group, 80% said it would make them personally feel better, 91% thought it would make their child feel better, and 73% felt it would help the physician. A follow-up study by the same authors (14) reported on actual observations of 50 venipunctures or intravenous cannulations. Parents remained with their children during 62% of the procedures. Many of the parents who did not stay indicated they would have preferred to but were either directly asked to leave or given nonverbal cues strongly suggesting that they should. Overall, only 10% of this group of parents stated they had not wanted to be with their child during the procedure.

Multiple other studies have shown that the majority of parents who witnessed procedures done on their child felt that their presence helped them and helped their child (4–7,15). Family presence reduced both the parents' and the patient's anxiety and sense of helplessness and eliminated the parents' agony of being left outside the treatment room without seeing what's really happening to their child. Even when the patient is likely to die, family presence remains extremely beneficial. Family presence allows parents to be beside their loved one until the last minute. Parents can touch their child, express their love, and say good-bye while there is still a chance that the patient can hear (16). Family presence also brings a sense of reality regarding the treatment efforts and clinical status of the patient, helping the family avoid a prolonged period of denial (17). Parents can see for themselves the tremendous effort put into the resuscitation attempt, and this has far more meaning then being told, "Everything possible was done" (18). In addition, family presence facilitates the grieving process and

TABLE 1.1	BENEFITS OF FAMILY PRESENCE

FP reduces the patient and the parents' anxiety level and sense of helplessness
FP allows parents to comfort and support their child
FP facilitates the grieving process when the patient dies
FP allows families to be by their loved one until the last minute and be able to say good bye
FP brings a sense of reality to the treatment efforts and clinical status of the patient
FP promotes collaboration and fosters trust between medical providers, patients and family members
FP may decrease litigation by improving communication and increasing openness

FP, family prsence.

may be one of the most powerful interventions that can be offered to a grieving family (18–21). The majority of family members who witness CPR feel that their presence helped them adjust more easily to the death and benefited the dying patient (18,19,21). Therefore, the manner in which we as health care providers care and respect the wishes of both the dying patients and their parents is crucial in helping the family accept the death and deal with the crisis.

Benefits to Health Care Providers

Including the family in the care plan promotes collaboration among medical providers, patients, and family members. When present, family members take on unique "patient helper" roles, providing support and security to the patient and medical information and translation to the staff (17). With loved ones present, patients become less anxious and more compliant; thus, the procedure has potential to go more smoothly (7). Regardless of the patient's condition, parents seem to focus on their child-comforting role rather than the standards of medical care (17,22). One father said, "The doctors and nurses were there for the procedures, but I was there for my daughter" (17). Emergency physicians and pediatricians should foster the parents' role as allies and partners in their child's treatment.

Family presence may also decrease litigation risks to health care providers (23–25). Many disputes and complaints are avoided by improving communication, increasing openness, and decreasing doubt about the adequacy of care (11,26,27). Too often, family members who are kept out of the room during a procedure or code cannot help but get suspicious (24). They may ask themselves, "Why don't they want us to see what they are doing?" If they do ask themselves this, they are more likely to seek legal advice, especially if they feel that the staff failed to show compassion and concern for their situation. When family members see with their own eyes that the team was working feverishly to save their loved one's life, they are far more inclined to view the team members as partners rather than adversaries (24). Even if the

parents decide not to be at their child's bedside, knowing that they have that option serves to foster trust and positive communication.

When family members are present, codes take on a more "personal" aspect, and team members develop an increased awareness of each other's feelings (19). This tends to strengthen the bond of camaraderie and support among health care providers (19). The patient is viewed as part of a loving family and not as a clinical challenge, thus reminding staff to consider the patient's dignity, privacy and need for pain management (9,17,28). Family presence encourages a more passionate and professional atmosphere and less nonessential talk and black humor (17).

▶ PERCEIVED BARRIERS TO FAMILY PRESENCE

Breaking the Tradition

Family presence challenges basic assumptions and longstanding practices (Table 1.2). There were times when parents were not allowed to visit their child during certain hours of the day or even stay overnight, let alone view procedures and resuscitations. The concept of family presence during resuscitation emerged in the mid-1980s, when the ED staff at Foote Hospital in Michigan questioned a hospital policy that excluded families from the resuscitation room (18). This was the first time family members were encouraged to attend resuscitation attempts on a systematic basis. Initially, opinions about family presence were mixed. However, the trend has moved toward the acceptance of this process as a result of new research. Now that the documented benefits have exceeded the perceived risks, several organizations promote family presence, including the American Academy of Pediatrics, the Emergency Nurses Association, the Emergency Medical Services for Children, and the American Heart Association (29–32). In general, the more informed health care providers are about the process of family presence, the higher the acceptance of family presence (33). Nurses were surveyed before and

TABLE 1.2	PERCEIVED BARRIERS TO FAMILY PRESENCE AND PROPOSED SOLUTIONS
Breaking a tradition	The more informed HCP are, the higher the acceptance of FP
Increasing staff anxiety or hindering performance	Confidence in procedural and CPR skills, and experience with FP quickly decrease anxiety level
Distracting or obstructing medical care	Screen and prepare families adequately
Harder to end a code	Address the family prior to ending the code and give them a moment to express themselves.
	FM can see for themselves that everything possible was done.
Too traumatic for the staff to witness grieving	Opportunity for support
Too traumatic for the family	Keep it a choice
Difficult to teach junior staff	New learning opportunity on how to comfort families
Trauma resuscitation	Family support person essential
Limited resources: adequate space, family support person, adequate staffing, staff education, follow-up services	Determine appropriateness of FP depending on the different circumstances

FSP, family support person; HCP, health care providers; FP, family presence; FM, family members.

after attending a class on family presence, and their approval ratings for family presence increased from 11% to 80% at the completion of the educational session (34). Several other studies showed that health care providers' acceptance of family presence was higher among nurses and experienced physicians than among residents (17,35–37).

Increasing Staff Anxiety or Hindering Performance

There is no doubt that it is harder for health care providers to work with an audience and that patient care should remain our priority. However, confidence in one's procedural and CPR skills and experience with family presence and dealing with distressed families quickly decreases that anxiety level (17,38). The majority of health care providers who offer family presence do not report a change in their performance or a change in the outcome of the procedure or CPR (4,6,7,15,17,38,39). In one survey (18), 30% of health care providers felt anxious about performing CPR in view of others; however, the hospital ACLS committee that reviews all CPR videotapes did not find a difference between family- and non-family-witnessed resuscitations.

Distraction from or Obstruction of Medical Care

Many health care providers fear that the family's uncontrollable emotions will disrupt the smooth functioning of the medical team or that family members may become physically involved in the procedure or the resuscitation attempt. Undoubtedly, the most stressful procedure is CPR. Foote hospital reported no instances of such interference during an entire 9-year period (28). Most family members seemed awed by the activity in the resuscitation room and frequently had to be led to the bedside and encouraged to touch and speak with their loved ones (28). Another hospital reported a similar experience during a 2-year observation period (19). Regardless of their background, family members understood the need for appropriate behavior at the bedside so that their presence would not impede the care of the person they are trying to help (17). However, proper assessment and preparation of the family prior to the performance of the procedure or their entry into the resuscitation room is fundamental (17,19,28).

Harder to End a Code

It may be harder for staff to end an unsuccessful code when they hear the family sobbing. However, turning toward the parents and stressing to them that every possible intervention has been done and giving them a moment to say what they need to say before ending the code may help them accept the reality of the situation. Witnessing CPR efforts helps family members understand how grave the patient's condition is and feel confident that everything was done to save the patient (17,18,28).

Traumatic for the Staff to Witness the Family Grieving

Identifying with family members is going to bring emotions closer to the surface, making it harder to forget and move on. However, taking time after a code to talk and vent these feelings can make the circumstances easier to deal with (19,28). Health care providers at Foote Hospital noted over the years that it was indeed difficult to remain distant and unemotional, and this had both positive and negative effects (28). Although more emotions were evoked, the staff continued to function professionally, and clinical tasks remained a priority. Health care providers developed informal support networking among themselves to help ease these feelings.

Traumatic for the Family

No matter how often people see blood and needles and watch anxious health care providers providing CPR on television, witnessing these procedures performed on a loved one is not the same. It is common for the parents' desire to stay along the bedside to decrease as the procedures become more invasive (12,40). However, the majority of family members want to participate in the decision regarding their presence, and when given the choice, they prefer to be present (12–14,22,40). Even those who witnessed CPR said that they would participate again (17,19,21,41). One mother said, "I want my daughter to know that I will be there for her no matter what." Nevertheless, this feeling is certainly not universal. Being present during invasive procedures or resuscitation is not something all families want. Patients who choose not to have family members present, or family members who desire not to participate, must be supported in their decision without judgment. Therefore, family presence should be offered as an "option" so parents can play a part in the decision about their presence. Parents should also be told that they can leave the room any time they wish to in order to prevent any undo stress. The majority of parents believe that for them and their child to be given an explanation of the procedure provides them with the most helpful means of coping (40).

A common example of a procedure that parents are typically averse to watching is the reduction of a displaced fracture. The combination of visual and auditory sensations, as well as the nearly unavoidable though very transient pain to the child, makes this an exceedingly difficult moment for most parents. The family could easily remain with their child during the initial evaluation, the intravenous line placement, and the initiation of conscious sedation. One method is to gently suggest to the parents that the reduction itself will be very brief and that the appropriately sedated and narcotized child would be unlikely to miss their short absence. The family might briefly leave or at least stand away from the bedside and then return immediately at the completion of the reduction, during the casting and subsequent re-evaluation. Some parents may still choose to stay, and such a decision should be supported with appropriate forewarnings of what they will see and hear.

Difficulty Teaching Junior Staff

Residents and students are not as comfortable with their procedural skills as seasoned professionals and have less experience with family presence. They also fear that attending physicians may not allow them to attempt a procedure if the parents are watching. However, assuring them and the parents that proper supervision and guidance will take place throughout the procedure may alleviate any fears. Family presence should also be viewed by junior staff as an opportunity for them to learn early on from experienced faculty how to approach and involve parents.

Family Presence during Trauma Resuscitations

Family member presence during pediatric trauma evaluation and resuscitation is an area of considerable controversy. We must remember that trauma is the leading cause of childhood mortality and has a profound and sustained impact on the lives of children and their families. Family members are frequently with their children at the time of injury and have been witness to the traumatic event from the beginning; however, when medical personnel arrive, family members are routinely separated from their children. Intuitively, it may strike many clinicians that the more traumatic the circumstances, the less appropriate it would be for parents to remain with their child during emergency procedures, such as those associated with significant anatomical disfigurement or potential death. In both adult and pediatric studies, trauma providers have expressed concerns about the potential adverse effects of allowing family members to be present during trauma resuscitation. Hesitation about involving family members stems from thoughts that witnessing trauma resuscitation may be psychologically damaging for family members, that family members may directly interfere with patient care, and that family presence may increase staff stress and decrease the quality of their performance (42).

Although few studies have assessed the impact of family presence on pediatric trauma resuscitation, data from medical resuscitation and adult trauma resuscitation have documented substantial potential benefits without medical interference. Some case reports have indicated that parents express gratitude and appreciation for having been allowed to be with their child and speak to him or her during an unsuccessful trauma resuscitation (16). Provider fears surrounding family presence during trauma resuscitation have not been substantiated in the literature. At our institution (a large tertiary care children's hospital with an abundance of medical and ancillary staff), we have a structured family presence program that involves screening family members for appropriateness and having a designated family support person whose sole responsibility is to the family members while in the resuscitation area. In a recent study of 171 trauma resuscitation evaluations with family presence over a 12-month period, there were no cases of interference with medical care noted. Only three family members were asked to leave the resuscitation area: one parent became emotionally overwhelmed, one provider preferred that family members not be present for an intubation, and one parent was asked to leave so that the team could better communicate their concerns regarding child abuse. Participating pediatric emergency medicine attendings and trauma surgeons rarely reported that family presence made it more difficult to make medical decisions (3%), institute medical care (3%), or communicate with other providers (7%) (43).

Special Resource Considerations

Adequate space. Certain procedures require extra personnel, which may restrict the space available for family members. When space is critically limited, it may be necessary to limit the number of family members to one at a time or ask the family to step out temporarily.

A family room. During resuscitation, having a family room adjacent to the resuscitation room allows family members easier contact with health care providers and with the patient.

A family support person (FSP). During certain invasive procedures (especially resuscitation), a predesignated family support person is essential to ensure that family members are continually assessed and supported and do not suffer adverse reactions. The FSP should have a good understanding of grief reactions and should be competent at supporting distressed families. The FSP should also be trained in the explanation of medical care and in the assessment and preparation of family members. The designated FSP can be a social worker, nurse, or chaplain. The FSP has no direct patient care responsibility and is assigned exclusively to assist the family.

Adequate staffing. The participating ED should be aware of the potential for a family member to sustain a stress-related event (e.g., syncope), although these events are uncommon. Therefore, the ED should establish a plan for such an occurrence, ideally designating a staff member who is not directly involved in the care of the patient and is instead assigned to assist the family. Also, security personnel need to be available in the building in the rare event a family member threatens staff or obstructs care.

Departmental specific guidelines. It is very important to establish a unified departmental philosophy regarding family presence during procedures. The guidelines help delineate staff roles and responsibilities during a family presence event. They also should specify health care provider involvement in both resuscitation situations and invasive procedures that vary in complexity and need for personnel. Support procedures must be addressed for all hours of the day.

Staff education. The purpose of this education is (a) to provide the multidisciplinary staff with the skills necessary to support distressed families and become familiar with grief reactions and (b) to introduce the guidelines and the roles of the staff in the process. Support personnel need to have a strong psychosocial background and some understanding of common invasive procedures and CPR. Other health care providers need to be comfortable assessing family needs and at least initiating appropriate interventions and consultation. A variety of formats may be used, including lectures, workshops, role-playing exercises, videotaped presentations, self-study modules, and case reviews.

Means to monitor progress, provide feedback, and customize the guidelines. Evaluation is essential for validating the efficacy of the strategies implemented. Ideally, input should be sought from health care providers, support staff, and families. Such input helps identify further educational needs, problems encountered, and required guideline revisions. The mechanisms for evaluation may include surveys, postevent questionnaires, interviews, and open forum discussions.

▶ APPROACH TO INVOLVING THE PARENTS

The first step in engaging parents is to offer them the opportunity to be with and to help their child during the procedure. It should be made clear that they are not being asked to take on a medical or nursing role; rather, they are being asked to remain as comforters of and empathizers with their child. Many parents who might faint during their own venipuncture can nurture their child through a complex and bloody laceration repair if they (a) know what to expect, (b) trust the physician's competence and sense of caring for their child, and (c) understand that everything medically possible will be done to relieve their child's pain. If, despite these conditions being met, parents continue to appear hesitant or express discomfort with remaining present, they should certainly not be made to feel inadequate. Such parents may remain with the child during the preparations for the procedure, be separated as short a time as possible, and be immediately ushered in as comforters at the procedure's completion.

Both parents and child need some preparation, including information about the technical and sensory aspects of the procedure (Fig. 1.1A). They need to know what the steps of the procedure will be and approximately how long it will take, to be given an honest estimation of the degree of discomfort the child may encounter, and to understand how that discomfort will be mitigated by the physician. Information on the sensory aspects includes describing the sights, sounds, smells, and physical sensations the child will experience during the procedure, and when appropriate, the child should be allowed to see and feel the equipment.

For those parents who have chosen to stay, their role should be made more explicit. They will be asked to position themselves so that their child may see them, if possible. Their job will be to talk soothingly to and touch their child as much as possible (Fig. 1.1B). Suggestions may be offered regard-

ing the content of the parents' comforting words, such as the narrating of a favorite adventure story, particularly one that might engage the child in a fantasy. Parents should not tell their child that the procedure will not hurt but rather should reaffirm the physician's assurances that significant pain will be avoided and/or treated pharmacologically as necessary. They will not be expected to participate in the medical or surgical aspects of the procedure or help with restraint (other than in the briefest, pain-free situations, such as an otoscopic examination). Parents are expected not to observe the procedure itself critically but rather to be fully engaged with comforting their child (Fig. 1-1C).

As the procedure begins, parents may need continued guidance and reinforcement of these points. The ED staff should help to position the parents at the head of the bed or as appropriate for the particular procedure. The parents need to be continuously updated and reassured about the procedure's steps toward completion and the child's condition. If the parents become anxious and falter, a second or two of directed interaction with them may suffice to help them back into their role. There may be some cases where it will be obvious that everyone would be better off if the parents left the room momentarily. Again, they should be supported in this decision and returned to the child as soon as feasible to resume their comforter role.

Parental anxiety about the procedure may influence the child's experience (44). For this reason, preparing the parents for the procedure may be as important as preparing the child. It is likely that the parental role of providing comfort to their child during the procedure can be enhanced by physician-directed preparation and guidance. Bauchner et al. studied the impact of a brief effort to educate parents with children who were less than 3 years old and required procedures in the ED (45,46). The educational intervention included instructions for the parents to situate themselves near the head of the bed and talk with and touch their child soothingly. They were not expected to help in restraint. They were also warned that their child might cry, and they were asked not to tell the child that the procedure would not hurt. Parents were randomized into three groups—those who stayed with their child and received the educational intervention (group 1), those who stayed for the procedure but did not receive the intervention (group 2), and those who did not stay (group 3). Of the 101 parents in the intervention group, 89% were effective in following the instructions, and 93% stated the instructions were helpful. Only 46% of the 101 parents who stayed but did not receive the specific guidelines (group 2) used similar strategies in comforting their child. Of the parents in group 1, 95% were satisfied with their child's care, compared with 81% in group 2. Among the parents who stayed, the vast majority reported they would be likely to stay with their child for a future procedure (93% of group 1, 95% of group 2), compared with only 53% of those who did not stay (group 3).

During resuscitation and certain more invasive procedures, a predesignated FSP whose job is to continually assess and

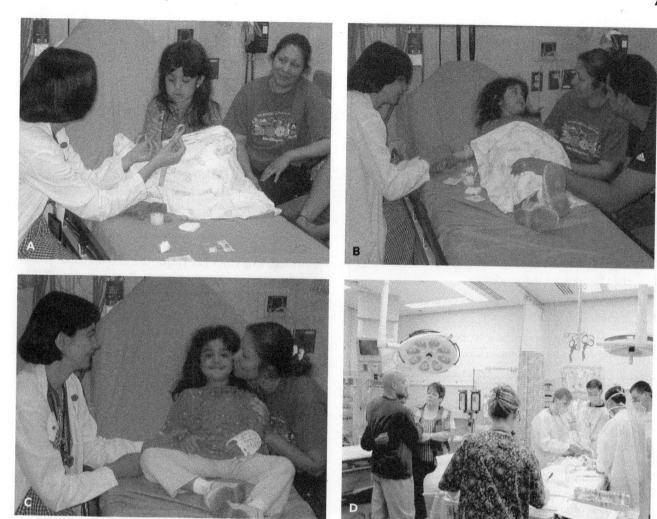

Figure 1.1
A. Health care provider explaining the procedure to the patient as the parents listen and watch.
B. Parents providing distraction, comfort and support to the patient during IV placement.
C. Patient, parents and HCP taking pride in their "accomplishments" despite requiring 2 attempts to achieve IV placement.
D. Parents present during resuscitation, helped by a family support person.

support family members to prevent adverse reactions is essential (Fig. 1.1D). The FSP screens and prepares the family prior to entering the treatment area. Acceptable family member behaviors in the treatment area include being quiet; being distressed or crying but consolable; being distracted but able to focus and answer questions; and being anxious or angry but cooperative and able to follow instructions. Worrisome behaviors include being uncooperative, physically aggressive, combative, threatening and argumentative, extremely unstable emotionally, hysterical, and loud; also of concern are parents who are unable to be redirected or calmed and parents who are intoxicated or have an altered mental status. Parents exhibiting such disruptive behaviors are not suitable for entry into the treatment room.

A family member's ability to participate can progress or regress throughout his or her presence in the room. Continuous assessment and intervention are critical to prevent

adverse reactions. Therefore, the FSP should be present with the family at all times while in the resuscitation room. Prior to entering the treatment room, the family should be told how many family members may enter the room at one time, where they will stand or sit initially, and when they will be able to move to the bedside. They should know that they may leave the room if they feel the need to step out and that they are welcome to re-enter. Also, they may be asked to step out of the room (a) at the request of the health care providers, (b) if they obstruct medical care, or (c) if they need medical assistance (if they faint, develop chest pain, etc.). If they do need medical assistance, a health care provider not involved in the care of their child should aid them (as noted above, this requires adequate health care provider availability for such a scenario). In the treatment room, the family must be clearly informed of the status of their loved one and be prepared for the interventions that are in progress. The FSP should explain

SUMMARY

1 Explain the procedure to the child and the parents using age-appropriate language.

2 Offer parents the option of staying with their child.

3 Explain to the parents that their presence, if calm and supportive, will help the child.

4 Prepare the parents for role as providers of emotional support, not technical assistants.

5 Position the parents, if possible, within the child's sight.

6 Ask the parents to speak soothingly and touch their child throughout the procedure.

7 Update and reassure the parents on procedural steps and child's condition.

8 Indicate to the parents how supportive their presence has been to their child.

the patient's role during the procedure (holding still, etc.) and the family members' role in providing comfort and reassurance. The FSP can describe the procedures performed and interpret medical jargon, but the physicians should explain indications and outcomes.

The issue of exactly which procedures are appropriate for parental presence is a complex one, and no arbitrary rules are offered here. Conditions vary for any given procedure. Physician experience, parental experience with previous emergency interventions, adequate staffing and resources, and the medical circumstances of the particular context in which the procedure is necessary all affect the determination of appropriateness. The reader is urged to seriously consider the value of parental presence in virtually any pediatric emergency procedure.

▶ SUMMARY

Parents should be encouraged and guided in remaining with their child through pediatric emergency procedures. Their presence will not only be comforting to the child but will also play a therapeutic role for the parents themselves and will often facilitate the successful completion of the procedure. ED staff should offer parents the option of remaining, prepare them for their comforter role, and provide continuing guidance to them during the procedure. During the more invasive procedures and in particular resuscitations, a predesignated FSP to continually assess and support family members to prevent adverse reactions is essential. When planned properly, family presence helps meet both the family's and patient's needs without disrupting medical care. The more experience health

care providers have with family presence, the greater their acceptance of family presence will be. As health care providers and patient advocates, we should strive for the widespread establishment of family presence.

▶ REFERENCES

1. Zeltzer LK, Jay SM, Fisher DM. The management of pain associated with pediatric procedures. *Pediatr Clin North Am.* 1989;36:941–964.
2. Selbst SM, Henretig FM. The treatment of pain in the emergency department. *Pediatr Clin North Am.* 1989;36:965–978.
3. Frankl S, Shiere F, Fogels H. Should the parent remain with the child in the dental operatory? *J Dent Child.* 1962;29:152–163.
4. Wolfram RW, Turner ED, Philput C. Effects of parental presence during young children's venipuncture. *Pediatr Emerg Care.* 1997;13: 325–328.
5. Wolfram RW, Turner ED. Effects of parental presence during children's venipuncture. *Acad Emerg Med.* 1996;3:58–64.
6. Powers KS, Rubenstein JS. Family presence during invasive procedures in the pediatric intensive care unit. *Arch Pediatr Adolesc Med.* 1999;153:955–958.
7. Sacchetti A, Lichenstein R, Carraccio CA, et al. Family member presence during pediatric emergency department procedures. *Pediatr Emerg Care.* 1996;12:268–271.
8. Ross DM, Ross SA. The importance of type of question, psychological climate and subject set in interviewing children about pain. *Pain.* 1984;19:71–79.
9. Shaw EG, Routh DK. Effect of mother presence on children's reduction of aversive procedures. *J Pediatr Psychol.* 1982;7:33–44.
10. American Academy of Pediatrics Committee on Bioethics. Informed consent, parental permission, and assent in pediatric practice. *Pediatrics.* 1995;95:314–317.
11. Rydman RJ, Roberts RR, Albrecht GL, et al. Patient satisfaction with an emergency department asthma observation unit. *Acad Emerg Med.* 1999;6:178–183.
12. Boie ET, Moore GP, Brummett C, et al. Do parents want to be present during invasive procedures performed on their children in the emergency department? A survey of 400 parents. *Ann Emerg Med.* 1999;34:70–74.
13. Bauchner H, Vinci R, Waring C. Pediatric procedures: do parents want to watch? *Pediatrics.* 1989;84:907–909.
14. Bauchner H, Waring C, Vinci R. Parental presence during procedures in an emergency room: results from 50 observations. *Pediatrics.* 1991;87:544–548.
15. Bauchner H, Vinci R, Bak S, et al. Parents and procedures: a randomized controlled trial. *Pediatrics.* 1996;98:861–867.
16. Eichhorn DJ, Meyers TA, Guzzetta CE. Family presence during resuscitation: it is time to open the door. *Capsules Comments Crit Care Nurs.* 1995;3:8–13.
17. Meyers TA, Eichhorn DJ, Guzzetta CE, et al. Family presence during invasive procedures and resuscitation. *Am J Nurs.* 2000;100:32–43.
18. Doyle CJ, Post H, Burney RE, et al. Family participation during resuscitation: an option. *Ann Emerg Med.* 1987;16:673–675.
19. Belanger MA, Reed S. A rural community hospital's experience with family-witnessed resuscitation. *J Emerg Nurs.* 1997;23:238–239.
20. Eichhorn DJ, Meyers TA, Mitchell TG, et al. Opening the doors: family presence during resuscitation. *J Cardiovasc Nurs.* 1996;10:59–70.
21. Robinson SM, Mackenzie-Ross S, Campbell Hewson GL, et al. Psychological effect of witnessed resuscitation on bereaved relatives. *Lancet.* 1998;352:614–617.

22. Barratt F, Wallis DN. Relatives in the resuscitation room: their point of view. *J Accid Emerg Med.* 1998;15:109–111.

23. Offord RJ. Should relatives of patients with cardiac arrest be invited to be present during cardiopulmonary resuscitation? *Intensive Crit Care Nurs.* 1998;14:288–293.

24. Brown JR. Letting the family in during a code: legally it makes good sense. *Nursing.* 1989;19:46.

25. Forster H, Schwartz J, Derenzo E. Reducing legal risk by practicing patient-centered medicine. *Arch Intern Med.* 2002;162:1217–1219.

26. Tsai E. Should family members be present during cardiopulmonary resuscitation? *N Engl J Med.* 2002;13:1019–1021.

27. Trout A, Magnusson R, Hedges JR. Patient satisfaction investigations and the emergency department: what does the literature say? *Acad Emerg Med.* 2000;7:695–709.

28. Hanson C, Strawser D. Family presence during cardiopulmonary resuscitation: Foote Hospital emergency department's nine-year perspective. *J Emerg Nurs.* 1992;18:104–106.

29. American Academy of Pediatrics. http://www.aap.org.

30. Emergency Nurses Association. Family presence at the bedside during invasive procedures and/or resuscitations. Available at: http//:www.ena.org.

31. Emergency Medical Services for Children. http//:www.emsc.org.

32. Guidelines 2000 for cardiopulmonary resuscitation and emergency cardiovascular care. *Circulation.* 2000;102 suppl I (8):1–370. Available at: http//:www.circulationaha.org.

33. Sacchetti A, Carraccio C, Leva E, et al. Acceptance of family member presence during pediatric resuscitations in the emergency department: effects of personal experience. *Pediatr Emerg Care.* 2000;16:85–87.

34. Bassler PC. The impact of education on nurse's beliefs regarding family presence in a resuscitation room. *J Nurs Staff Dev.* 1999;15:126–131.

35. Mitchell MH, Lynch MB: Should relatives be allowed in the resuscitation room? *J Accid Emerg Med.* 1997;14:366–369.

36. Fein JA, Ganesh J, Alpern ER. Medical staff attitudes toward family presence during pediatric procedures. *Pediatr Emerg Care.* 2004;20:224–227.

37. Waseem M, Ryan M. Parental presence during invasive procedures in children: what is the physician's perspective? *South Med J.* 2003;96:884–887.

38. O'Brien MM, Creamer KM, Hill EE, et al. Tolerance of family presence during pediatric cardiopulmonary resuscitation: a snapshot of military and civilian pediatricians, nurses, and residents. *Pediatr Emerg Care.* 2002;18:409–413.

39. Haimi-Cohen Y, Amir J, Harel L, et al. Parental presence during lumbar puncture: anxiety and attitude toward the procedure. *Clin Pediatr.* 1996;35:2–4.

40. Merrit KA, Sargent JR, Osborn LM. Attitudes regarding parental presence during medical procedures. *Am J Dis Child.* 1990;144:270–271.

41. Meyers TA, Eichhorn DJ, Guzzetta CE. Do families want to be present during CPR? A retrospective survey. *J Emerg Nurs.* 1998;24:400–405.

42. Helmer SD, Smith SR, Dort JM, et al. Family presence during trauma resuscitation: a survey of AAST and ENA members. *J Trauma.* 2000;48:1015–1024.

43. O'Connell K, Farah M, Spandorfer P, et al. Family presence during pediatric trauma resuscitation: an evaluation of a structured program. Washington, DC: Meeting of the Pediatric Academic Societies; May 2005.

44. Jay SM, Ozolins M, Elliot CH, et al. Assessment of children's distress during painful medical procedures. *Health Psychol.* 1983;2:133–147.

45. Bauchner H, Vinci R, Pearson C. Parental presence during procedures: satisfaction with care. *Am J Dis Child.* 1993;147:426–427.

46. Bauchner H, Vinci R, May A. Teaching parents how to comfort their children during common medical procedures. *Arch Dis Child.* 1994;70:548–550.

2

JANET H. FRIDAY AND FRED M. HENRETIG

Techniques for Examining the Fearful Child

▶ INTRODUCTION

In caring for children in the outpatient setting, most of us have been humbled at some time by the difficulty of examining an uncooperative child. Although no single fail-proof technique exists to avoid this problem, a calm and relaxed approach that incorporates knowledge of developmental stages can smooth the interaction (1–5). This method should not significantly increase the time spent on the examination. Instead, it will help to establish a relationship with the family, provide a basis for future interventions, and allow an optimal diagnostic evaluation in a timely manner. A related subject, minimizing fear and anxiety during procedures, is discussed in Chapter 33.

▶ PHYSIOLOGY: NORMAL DEVELOPMENTAL STAGES

Recognition of childhood developmental stages and their accompanying issues will help the examining physician to interact with the child in a way that optimizes patient comfort and acceptance of the examination (Table 2.1).

Infants (Birth to 1 Year)

Until the appearance of stranger anxiety around 8 to 9 months of age, the infant examination is not constrained by fear; however, infants are quite sensitive to their immediate environment. After stranger anxiety appears, the infant may be threatened by the physician's presence and will remain most cooperative in a parent's arms.

Toddlers (1 to 3 Years)

Although the young toddler may appear relatively nonverbal, the child's receptive language skills develop sooner than the expressive ones. Therefore, the physician must be careful of what is said in the child's presence. The toddler is most cognizant of his or her developing individuality and independence. The negativism of the "terrible twos" is prevalent. The child fears separation from the parents and will be best examined in a parent's lap.

Preschool-Age Children (3 to 5 Years)

The preschooler has developed expressive skills and a strong concept of self. Magical thinking and fantasy play become important during preschool years and can be incorporated into the examination.

School-Age Children (5 to 10 Years)

Development of logic and reason and a good grasp of language allow the older child to cooperate with the examination. An understanding of body function and structure can be incorporated during these years. Even before the development of sexual maturation, modesty will emerge and should be anticipated.

Adolescents (10 to 19 Years)

In general, cooperation with the physical examination is not an issue with the adolescent. However, appreciation for the importance of the adolescent's particular issues with autonomy, peer group importance, self-determination, and control will certainly ease the interaction.

TABLE 2.1	DEVELOPMENTAL APPROACH TO PEDIATRIC EMERGENCY CARE PATIENTS		
Age (yrs)	**Important development issues**	**Fears**	**Useful techniques**
Infancy (0–1)	Minimal language Feel an extension of parents Sensitive to physical environment	Stranger anxiety	Keep parents in sight and touch. Avoid hunger. Use warm hands. Keep room warm.
Toddler (1–3)	Receptive language more advanced than expressive See themselves as individuals Assertive will	Brief separation Pain	Maintain verbal communication. Examine in parent's lap. Allow some choices when possible.
Preschool (3–5)	Excellent expressive skills for thoughts and feelings Rich fantasy life Magical thinking Strong concept of self	Long separation Pain Disfigurement	Allow expression. Encourage fantasy and play. Encourage participation in care.
School-age (5–10)	Fully developed language Understanding of body structure and function Able to reason and compromise Experience with self-control Incomplete understanding of death	Disfigurement Loss of function Death	Explain procedures. Explain pathophysiology and treatment. Project positive outcome. Stress child's ability to master situation. Respect physical modesty.
Adolescence (10–19)	Self-determination Decision making Peer group important Realistic view of death	Loss of autonomy Loss of peer acceptance Death	Allow choices and control. Stress acceptance by peers. Respect autonomy. Stress confidentiality.

From Fleisher G, Ludwig S (eds). Textbook of Pediatric Emergency Medicine. 3rd ed. Baltimore: Williams & Wilkins, 1993, with permission.

▶ INDICATIONS

Every encounter with the child who is not critically ill will be enhanced by a few efforts to gain trust and cooperation. The ability to detect subtle but important physical findings (e.g., a heart murmur or friction rub, the presence of pulmonary rales or asymmetric air entry, or abdominal tenderness or mass) will certainly be optimized by examining a child who is cooperative (or at least not screaming and resisting).

In certain circumstances, the examiner may anticipate that a difficult situation will arise even before entering the examination room. This will allow him or her to take special care not to rush the interaction and to carefully apply the appropriate techniques. Such situations include children with chronic diseases, irritable toddlers, and any child who already has had difficult interactions with other members of the health care team. The obvious contraindication to using the following approaches would be a seriously ill or injured child where attention to immediate resuscitation or stabilization takes precedence over all else.

▶ EQUIPMENT

Every experienced pediatric specialist has a few tricks of the trade which he or she uses to put a child at ease. For infants,

one trick is to offer a pacifier or bottle during the examination. At around 3 months of age, babies will become enamored with simple noises such as lip smacking or jingling keys. In toddlers, any toy may work wonders in engaging the child (Fig. 2.1). Many examination tools can be incorporated into a game that will transition nicely into the actual examination. Part of the ascertainment of a child's well-being will be seeing him or her doing normal activities, so giving out crayons and paper during a waiting period is helpful in this regard.

For actual examination equipment, many pediatricians prefer long stethoscope tubing so the examination may be accomplished at some distance from the anxious child (Fig. 2.1). It has become dogma that children are afraid of the "white coat," which may be somewhat true. However, children are not easily fooled, and if afraid of doctors, they will notice the scrub suits, beepers, and stethoscopes that characterize them. In general, an unfamiliar examiner will be challenged to gain a child's trust no matter how he or she is attired.

▶ PROCEDURE

Infants

Ensuring a warm, quiet environment and offering a bottle when appropriate will typically provide a good milieu for the

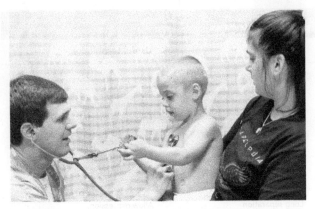

Figure 2.1 A simple toy may engage the toddler.

physical examination of an infant. Speaking to the parent in a soft, friendly voice and establishing a rapport with him or her before approaching the child will make the examination more accepted. Much of the examination can be accomplished while the parent is holding the infant in his or her lap (Fig. 2.2). Washing with hot water, in addition to its antimicrobial benefit, will warm the examiner's hands and thus avoid startling the infant. Instruments, especially the stethoscope, can be "rubbed up" to warm them as well. The examination should be ordered so that auscultation of the heart, lungs, and abdomen occur first, followed by palpation of the abdomen. Any disruptive or painful procedure (e.g., removal of the diaper or examination of the ears and mouth) should be done last.

Toddlers

In most cases, it is preferable to discuss the history with the parents first, keeping in mind that the child understands much of the conversation. For the fearful toddler, this discussion should occur prior to any threatening approach. When it comes time for the examination, most toddlers will be comforted by being held by the parents and will prefer not to sit on the table. In order to gain a toddler's trust, the examiner should begin with examining the feet or hands. The subsequent order should be the same as for infants (see previous section). Playing some simple games, such as auscultating the extremities while working up to the chest, may be helpful. The examiner should not offer choices when none exist and similarly should not ask any question unless prepared to hear the response "no" (e.g., not "Would you like to roll on your tummy now?" when it is preferable to say, "Roll over now, please"). When undergoing an ear and mouth examination, the toddler should be given a chance to cooperate, but noncompliance should be anticipated. Games such as blowing out the otoscope light or pretending to examine the doctor's ears can be attempted with older toddlers (Fig. 2.3A,B). However, they will usually require some restraint (Fig. 2.3C; see also Chapter 4). Overall, the examiner must seek assistance when necessary and move fast!

Preschool-Age Children

At the preschool age, the examination begins to become less difficult. A more direct interaction with the child is appropriate and accepted. For example, greeting the child and complementing the child's attire will no longer be a threat ("Hi! How are you today? I like those Mickey Mouse sneakers!"). Allowing the child to express fears or desires and participate will often lead to a better examination. Some of the magical thinking and fantasy can be incorporated into the examination (e.g., listening for french fries in the tummy or looking for monkeys in the ears). Again, it is preferable to leave any intrusive procedure until last.

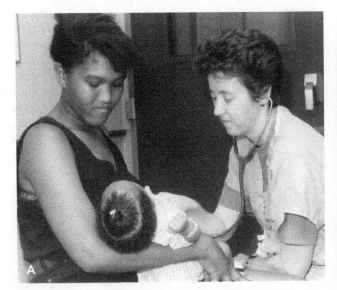
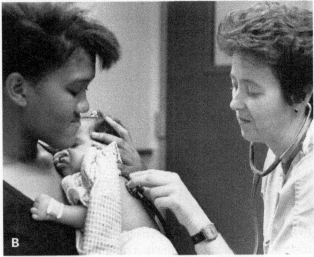

Figure 2.2 The infant examination is often begun on mother's lap or against her chest.

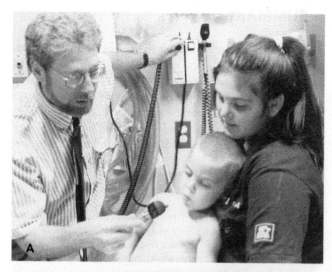
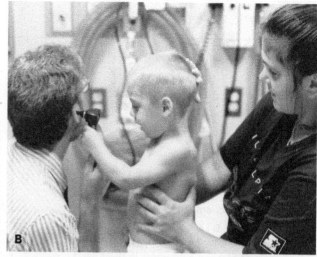
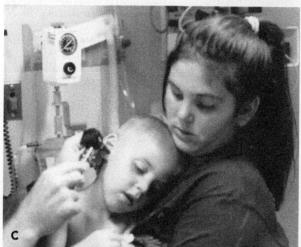
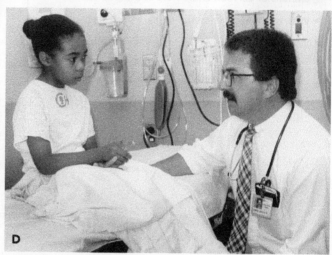

Figure 2.3
A. The toddler "blows out" the light prior to the otoscopic examination.
B. The toddler "examines" the physician's ears.
C. The toddler now allows an ear examination with minimal restraint from the mother.
D. Respect for modesty is crucial in school-age children.

School-Age Children

For the most part, the examination of a school-age child does not need to differ greatly in content from the examination of an adult. At this age, children become extraordinarily inquisitive and are interested in what the examiner is really doing and why. Explaining the examination as one proceeds may be helpful. Appreciation for modesty at this age is an absolute necessity (Fig. 2.3D).

Adolescents

Again, the examination of an adolescent is usually not different from that of an adult. Appreciation of autonomy and confidentiality and respect for modesty and decision making should be exhibited. Allowing for choices and control, when appropriate, may be helpful.

 SUMMARY

1 Use an age-related approach.

2 Techniques are applicable to all encounters except where the patient is critically ill.

3 Wash (and warm) hands.

4 With infants and toddlers, utilize the parents as much as possible.

5 With preschool-age children, encourage fantasy, play, and participation in the examination.

6 With school-age children, explain actions and respect modesty.

7 With adolescents, stress confidentiality and respect modesty and autonomy.

CLINICAL TIPS

▶ Perform the examination with an "unhurried" manner.

▶ Handwashing reassures parents and patients and warms hands.

▶ With infants, use props (e.g., pacifier, bottle, and jingling keys).

▶ With toddlers, play games (e.g., blow out the otoscope light and auscultate their shoes).

▶ With preschool-age children, utilize magical thinking and fantasy (e.g., auscultate or palpate favorite foods during the abdominal examination and look for animals or cartoon characters in their ears).

▶ With school-age children, explain each step.

▶ With adolescents, allow choices and control as possible.

▶ SUMMARY

In conclusion, it can be difficult to ease the fears of an unco-operative young child. The approach and techniques detailed here are no substitute for years of experience (and mistakes). However, used judiciously and with adaptation to unique situations, they will maximize the information that can only be obtained by a thorough examination. The trust established with the child and family will serve as a foundation for further care.

▶ REFERENCES

1. Algranati PS. Effect of developmental status on the approach to physical examination. *Pediatr Clin North Am.* 1998;45:1–23.
2. Fleisher GR, Ludwig S. *Textbook of Pediatric Emergency Medicine.* Baltimore: Williams & Wilkins; 1993:xxxvii–xi.
3. Hoekelman RA. The physical examination of infants and children. In: Bates B, ed. *A Guide to Physical Examination and History Taking.* 7th ed. Philadelphia: JB Lippincott; 1999:621–703.
4. Hughes WT, Buescher ES. Preparation of the patient. In: *Pediatric Procedures.* 2nd ed. Philadelphia: WB Saunders, 1980:1–25.
5. Selbst SM, Henretig FM. The treatment of pain in the emergency department. *Pediatr Clin North Am.* 1989;36:965–978.

JOEL A. FEIN AND REZA J. DAUGHERTY

3

Restraint Techniques and Issues

▶ INTRODUCTION

In the course of managing patients in an acute care setting, we sometimes find it necessary to restrain the violent or uncooperative patient. Approximately 50% of human service providers are victims of violence (1). Twenty-five percent of adult emergency departments restrain at least one patient per day (2). There are limited available data on use of restraints in children in the emergency department, leaving the practitioner only generalizations from the adult literature. In the absence of psychiatric illness, intoxication, or organic brain syndromes, the most common indication is the uncooperative child requiring an emergency procedure. It is therefore important that both the equipment and the overall approach used be safe, effective, and developmentally appropriate. Since restraint procedures are also used in the prehospital, inpatient, and intensive care settings, emergency medical technicians, nurses, physicians, and security personnel should be familiar with the risks, benefits, and proper use of these techniques. The various forms of restraint should be thought of as having a temporizing purpose, and frequent reassessment of the need and method of restraint is imperative. Although the actual application of physical restraints or sedation is straightforward, the ethical and legal issues surrounding these procedures are complex.

▶ ANATOMY AND PHYSIOLOGY

One must be familiar with and sensitive to the developmental level of the child in need of a potentially painful or anxiety-provoking procedure (see Table 2.1). Whereas 5- and 6-year-old children might be adept at the art of negotiation, they are not as adept at keeping their end of the bargain during a painful procedure. Most developmentally appropriate

10- and 11-year-old children have the ability to understand the necessity for a procedure in the abstract but will often require some help immobilizing during the procedure itself.

In contrast, the older patient who is uncooperative with emergency medical care or is combative may have some physiologic disturbance that can alter judgment, self-control, or the ability to assess pain. These patients may suffer from a variety of conditions, including organic brain syndrome, intoxication, functional psychosis, and personality disorder. In these cases, one must recognize that the patient may not stop struggling even if that struggle causes personal harm. A striking example of this is seen in adolescent patients with exposure to phencyclidine (PCP), which is discussed in the following section.

▶ INDICATIONS

Two situations exist in which health care professionals must consider the use of physical restraints or the rapid tranquilization (often referred to as "chemical restraint") of a patient. In the first, the patient will not or cannot cooperate with the performance of a medically necessary emergent procedure. As noted, this may be developmentally appropriate for a child or may represent an alteration of mental status in an older individual. A psychiatric consultant is helpful in the diagnosis and treatment of patients with psychosis or personality disorders and should always be involved if physical restraint or rapid tranquilization is required for these patients.

In the second situation, the patient's actions may be assessed as being either personally harmful or harmful to others. If the hospital personnel cannot verbally de-escalate the situation, physical restraint or rapid tranquilization reduces the risk of injury to the person and those around him or her.

15

There are few absolute contraindications to restraining patients in need of acute care. Restraints should only be used when deemed to be in the best interest of the patient or the safety of the staff. They should never be used punitively or for staff convenience. Furthermore, alternative methods should be considered if the use of chemical or physical restraints would exacerbate a medical condition and render the patient medically unstable or would inhibit the continuous monitoring required by a critically ill patient. In addition, one should not attempt to restrain a patient if there are not enough personnel or inadequate equipment to perform the technique safely and efficiently.

A special circumstance in which physical restraint may be harmful to the patient is after recreational drug use, such as with cocaine, amphetamine, or PCP, and/or overdose with a variety of sympathomimetic, anticholinergic, or other stimulative agents. Such patients can be unpredictable and are not aware of their behavior. Some authors have recommended that patients who are agitated after PCP use, in particular, do better with an environmental sensory deprivation approach and should be allowed to remain in a quiet, dark room with as little stimulation as possible (3). However, this approach has never been validated in controlled studies. Physical restraint should be applied if such intoxicated persons become a danger to themselves or others, as with any other severely agitated patient. Because patients are not aware of the tissue damage occurring as a result of fighting against the restraints, severe physical injury can occur if adequate pharmacologic sedation is not provided as well.

▶ EQUIPMENT

The equipment necessary for restraining patients appropriately is listed in Table 3.1. Equipment used for restraint should be easy to apply, size appropriate, padded, and contoured to minimize damage to the patient. Equipment specifically designed for restraining patients should be used, and "makeshift" methods (such as tying a patient down with sheets or towels) should be avoided, as they are difficult to implement and often require excessive force to maintain. A papoose board should have a portion for head immobilization that is part of the unit. In order to minimize the risk of the patient

TABLE 3.1	LIST OF EQUIPMENT NECESSARY FOR PATIENT RESTRAINT

▶ Papoose boards of various sizes (Fig. 3.1)
    Canvas flaps and Velcro fasteners
    (Olympic Medical, Seattle, WA)
▶ Leather four-point restraint bracelets with leather straps
    (Stuarts Drug and Surgical Supply, Greensburg, PA)
▶ Philadelphia collar
▶ Monitoring equipment
    CR monitor
    Pulse oximeter

getting free during a procedure, it is better to overestimate than to underestimate the board size. Leather restraints should be padded internally and have adjustable ring clips.

Appropriate monitoring equipment is mandatory to supplement the continuous observation required of the restrained patient. This includes continuous assessment of vital signs in potentially unstable patients and frequent assessment in all others. The exact requirements for monitoring are discussed later in this chapter. Further details regarding monitoring devices are reviewed in Chapter 5.

▶ RESTRAINT PROCEDURES

As mentioned, patients may require restraint for a variety of reasons. The approach to the uncooperative pediatric patient depends on the size and strength of the child. In addition, the overtly violent patient is more likely to require a systematic approach directed toward the protection of hospital or office personnel.

Consent Issues

Obtaining consent in order to restrain a patient may seem a contradiction in terms. However, in the absence of a medical emergency or risk of harm, one needs the consent of the patient or the parents before any treatment can be initiated. Simply informing the patient of how and when he or she is going to be restrained is a helpful and necessary part of the restraint procedure. Adolescent or adult patients with organic brain syndromes or psychiatric illness might not be considered competent to make a choice regarding their treatment. A more detailed discussion of consent and competence issues is contained in Chapter 9.

Techniques

The Violent Patient

During an interaction with a violent or potentially violent patient, the goal is to prevent injury to the patient and health care team while the appropriate medical treatments are provided. In order to prevent personal injury, the best positioning would allow both the patient and the interviewer to have access to the door; however, if this is not possible, then it is best to position the interviewer between the patient and the door. Speak calmly but definitively and first request the patient's cooperation in a nonthreatening manner. Explain that violence is unacceptable, and in a noncondescending tone make clear the consequences of the patient's actions. As these negotiations proceed, it may be helpful to provide a nonthreatening "show of force," using the restraint team, security personnel, and the local police if available. This often provides the patient with an excuse that he or she was outnumbered or that physical resistance was futile. Once the decision to physically restrain a patient is made, there is no further negotiation. At this point, the restraint

TABLE 3.2	APPROACH TO THE VIOLENT PATIENT

▶ Universal access to door
▶ Speak calmly but definitively request cooperation and explain consequences
▶ Show of force
▶ Five-point restraint technique
▶ Weapons search

team should use the five-point restraint technique described below. A thorough weapons search should be conducted as soon as the patient is immobilized (Table 3.2).

Papoose

For the uncooperative but otherwise nonviolent patient, monitoring systems should be placed before the restraint procedure. Infants or small children may only require immobilization of the body part on which the procedure is being performed. This is usually the case during intravenous catheter placement, when the person performing the procedure might provide his or her own immobilization or might only need the help of a colleague. For longer or more complex procedures, immobilization of the whole body can be accomplished using a papoose board, as shown in Figures 3.1 and 3.2. For this procedure, the board is placed on the stretcher or bed, and a sheet is folded and placed on top of the padded backing

inside the canvas straps. The child is then placed supine on top of the sheet, which prevents abrasions from developing after the canvas straps envelop the patient and connect. The child is initially restrained across the midabdomen, followed by trunk and arms and then by the legs, as necessary. Papoose boards come in a variety of sizes. If the board is appropriately sized, then holes in the fabric allow one or both arms to extrude from the papoose if necessary. Some brands of papoose boards contain additional straps for head immobilization. If a papoose board is not available, a folded sheet may be used to immobilize the child's arms and body, as shown in Figure 3.3. First, the child stands on the stretcher. Next, the sheet is folded on itself along its length to a width that covers the child's trunk and legs. It is then initially placed behind the back, with the short end tucked under the right axilla and folded around the right arm, ending behind the back (Fig. 3.3A). The long end is tucked under the left axilla, wrapped around the left arm, then behind the back and around the chest to behind the back again (Fig. 3.3B). Now the child can be placed prone or supine, as desired, and secured with several strips of wide adhesive tape to the sides of the stretcher (Fig. 3.3C). As previously mentioned, care should be taken when using equipment not expressly designed for the intent of restraint, as it may increase the risk of injury.

Five-Point Restraint

Older children or adolescents will often comply with painful procedures if the rationale and methods are described to them beforehand. If the patient requires immobilization for an emergency procedure or is a danger to him- or herself or others, a five-point restraint system should be used (Table 3.3). As with other medical emergencies, the most successful approach to this procedure involves a predesignated restraint team with well-defined roles and directed by one person. Using a minimum of five people, one team member is assigned to immobilize each extremity, and the fifth member controls the head and airway. The placement of a Philadelphia collar or soft neck collar helps to prevent injury to the patient or team members caused by the patient's thrashing or biting. A mask can be applied loosely to prevent the patient from biting or spitting. Extremities are best immobilized by holding down the large joints such as the shoulders, elbows, and knees. Leather restraints are first secured around the distal portion of each extremity and then secured to the stretcher. These restraints should be tight enough to hold down the extremity without causing neurovascular compromise (Fig. 3.4).

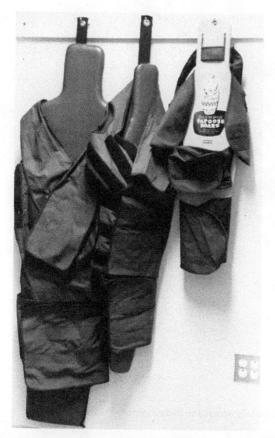

Figure 3.1 Papoose boards should be available in several sizes.

TABLE 3.3	FIVE-POINT RESTRAINT SYSTEM

▶ Four persons for extremities, one for head
▶ Immobilize major joints
▶ Philadelphia collar or soft collar
▶ Secure restraints around extremity first, then tie down
▶ Tight enough to hold extremity without causing NV compromise

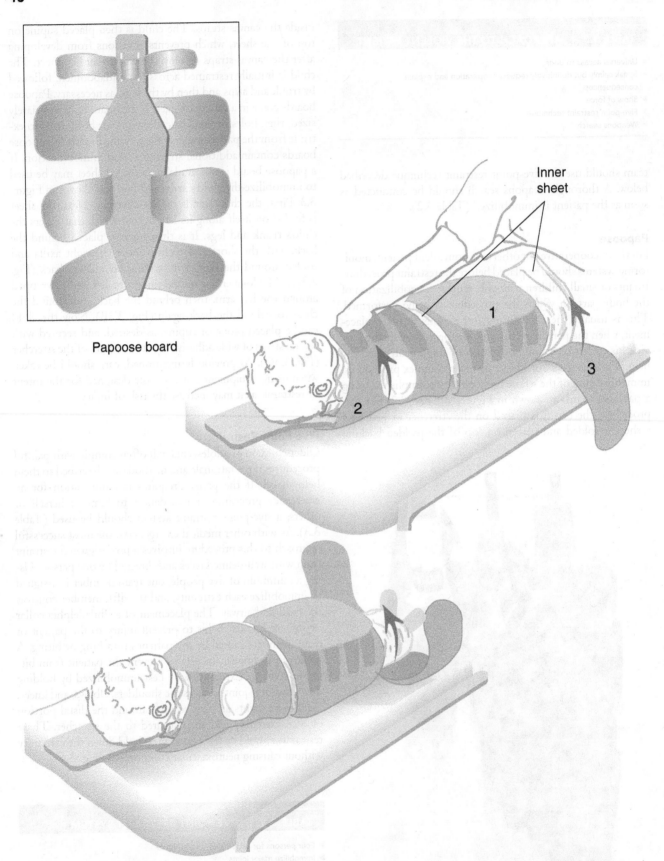

Papoose board

Figure 3.2 The child is restrained in a papoose board, initially across the midabdomen, followed by the trunk and arms and then the legs.

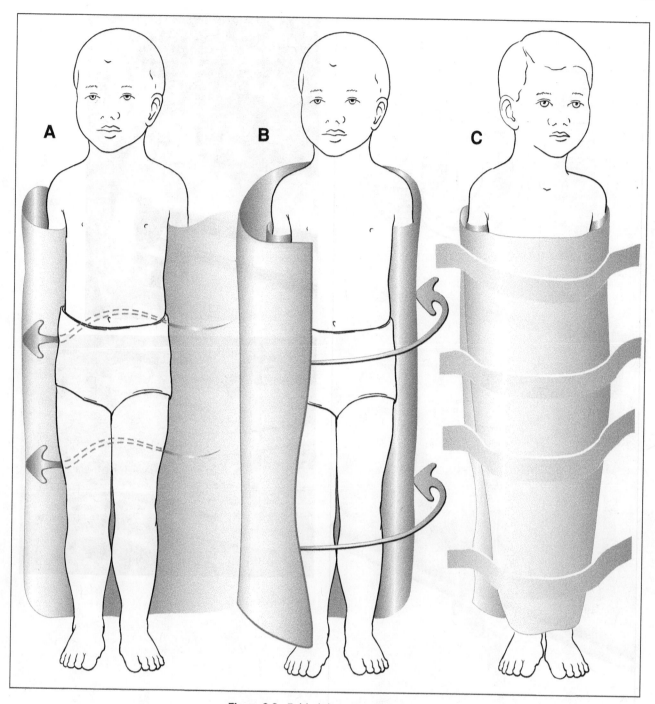

Figure 3.3 Folded sheet immobilization.

Rapid Tranquilization

"Chemical restraint," "drug used as a restraint," and "rapid tranquilization" are terms used in the literature to describe use of psychoactive medications to "restrict a person's freedom of movement, physical activity, or normal access to his or her body" (4). A list of the medications used to accomplish or supplement patient restraint, along with their dosage, indications, and most common side effects, is provided in Table 3.4. Prior to using these agents, health care providers should familiarize themselves with the most common complications, medication interactions, and contraindications to use. Anxiolytic medications, when used in conjunction with physical restraint procedures, can lessen the force necessary to restrain patients and thereby reduce the risk of injury. They are commonly used before anxiety-provoking procedures in children. Various forms can be given intravenously, intramuscularly, rectally, or intranasally (see also Chapter 33). Neuroleptic medications may obviate the need for prolonged

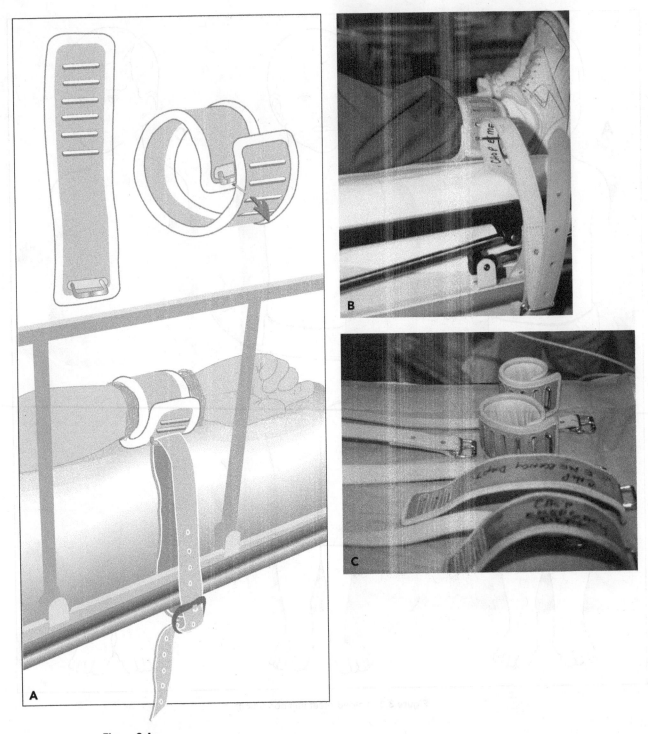

Figure 3.4
A. Leather restraints are first fastened to distal extremity, then tied down.
B. Restraints should be snug enough to hold down extremity without causing neurovascular compromise.
C. A set of leather restraints.

TABLE 3.4	MEDICATIONS FOR EMERGENT PEDIATRIC RESTRAINT		
Medication	**Dose range**	**Max dose**	**Side effects**
Benzodiazepines			
Lorazepam	P.O./I.M./I.V. 0.05–0.1 mg/kg	P.O./I.M./I.V. 2–4 mg	Sedation Respiratory depression Mild Hypotension
Midazolam	P.O. 0.25–1 mg/kg I.M. 0.1–0.5 mg/kg I.N. 0.2–0.4 mg/kg I.V. 0.05–0.1 mg/kg	P.O. 20 mg I.M. 10 mg I.N. 15 mg I.V. 10 mg	Sedation Respiratory depression Mild hypotension
Diazepam	P.O. 0.2–0.3 mg/kg I.M./I.V. 0.04–0.3 mg/kg	P.O./I.M./I.V. 10 mg	Sedation Respiratory depression Mild hypotension
Butyrophenones			
Haloperidol	P.O. 0.05–0.15 mg/kg I.V. 0.03–0.15 mg/kg	P.O. 10 mg I.M./I.V. 5 mg	Prolonged QT NMS EPS
Droperidol	I.M./I.V. 0.05–0.1 mg/kg	I.M./I.V. 2.5 mg	Prolonged QT NMS EPS

EPS, extrapyramidal symptoms; I.M., intramuscular; I.N., intranasal; NMS, neuroleptic malignant syndrome.

physical restraint. Barbiturates or antihistamines have poor side-effect profiles and have limited roles in emergency sedation.

Maintenance and Removal of Restraints

While physical restraints are in place, serial monitoring of vital signs and physical examination should occur in accordance with hospital and government regulations, as noted above. If signs of neurovascular compromise appear, restraints should be removed immediately from the affected extremity. Patients who require pharmacologic interventions such as anxiolytics or neuroleptics need to be monitored more closely. The sedative and anticholinergic effects of these medications can alone, or in conjunction with drugs of abuse and comorbid conditions, cause respiratory depression, neurologic depression, and extrapyramidal reactions.

Once the patient is deemed to be ready for removal of restraints, it should be made clear to him or her what behavior will be required for the restraints to remain off. The restraints may be removed sequentially, with a period of observation between to ensure the patient is ready and cooperative.

Documentation

There has been a recent scrutiny of restraint use as a result of disturbing media reports of deaths associated with this procedure. Government and regulatory organizations, namely, the Joint Commission on Accreditation of Healthcare Organizations (JCAHO) and the Health Care Financing Administration (HCFA), have developed strict regulations on the use of medical restraints. It is essential that any physician ordering or participating in the use of restraints be familiar with the requirements for their appropriate use, ordering, observation and monitoring, removal, and documentation (4,5).

Restraining a patient is similar to any other procedure, in that it requires meticulous documentation of the medical decision process, of the consent process (or the inappropriateness of consent if the patient is deemed incompetent), and of all efforts made to preserve the dignity of the individual. Also, the type of restraint used, the application times, the removal times, the patient's reaction to restraint, and the patient's eventual disposition must be documented (see also Chapter 11). Preprinted forms can facilitate this kind of documentation. Restraint performed against a patient's wishes has potential legal implications, and therefore the documentation should clarify the intent of and medical need for the procedure. This documentation need not be as comprehensive when implied or expressed consent is obtained from the patient's guardian, as is the case during a laceration repair in a young child. However, as the restraint mechanisms become more invasive, the consent and documentation requirements increase.

Complications

The complications that may occur secondary to restraint procedures range from mild psychological effects to life-threatening physiologic reactions. It is admittedly difficult for the patient, parents, and medical staff to avoid an emotional response to the restraint of a patient against his or her will. It is therefore important for the medical staff to understand the risks and benefits of performing the procedure and to communicate these to the patient, parents, and each other. In addition, all alternative methods of achieving the medical goals should be explored before restraining the patient.

In one prospective study of patients restrained in a general emergency department, 6.7% sustained "complications," including getting out of restraints, vomiting, injuring others, spitting, and self-injury. None required further care as a consequence (2). One of the most serious physical injuries that can occur involves respiratory compromise from improper airway positioning. Assigning one member of the restraint team to manage and monitor the airway can minimize this complication. In addition, noninvasive monitoring by cardiorespiratory monitor or pulse oximeter can supplement the information achieved through physical examination.

Cardiopulmonary compromise occurs more often in intoxicated patients, small children, and patients with underlying medical illness. Other potential complications include skin breakdown, rhabdomyolysis, aspiration pneumonia, cardiac stress, dehydration, extreme hyperthermia, and sudden death. Neurovascular injury can occur if the restraint materials are placed too tightly around an extremity or if the patient is struggling violently against the restraints. Frequent monitoring of the general appearance, pulses, capillary refill, and the range of motion of restrained extremities can prevent permanent injury. In addition, one should use only the force necessary to immobilize a patient quickly.

These tenets, along with the judicious use of medications, can prevent or allow early detection of these complications. Legal complications resulting from restraint procedures may be avoided or lessened by following the consent methods delineated in this chapter and documenting the thought processes and techniques used from beginning to end.

▶ SUMMARY

The restraint of patients for procedures or protection is at times a necessary part of providing the best care for our patients and families. However, it is important to determine beforehand the indications, equipment, techniques, and

---

 SUMMARY

1 Assess the potential for danger to the patient or the emergency department staff.

2 Use a verbal intervention first.

3 Use a papoose board for younger children, five-point restraint for others.

4 Form a standard restraint team with specific roles.

5 Use chemical restraint when indicated and safe.

6 Frequently monitor the patient's cardiopulmonary, neurovascular, and mental status.

7 Remove the restraints as soon as patient proves to be in control.

8 Document decisions, times, and monitoring.

---

personnel that will be used for restraint procedures in any given setting. A stepwise approach toward the violent or uncooperative patient is useful, beginning with verbal intervention and progressing to physical restraint and pharmacologic adjuncts if necessary. Careful monitoring and documentation is paramount in these situations and can be facilitated by preprinted forms. The proper technique for patient restraint involves a multidisciplinary approach that may make use of medical, security, and law enforcement personnel. In order to provide safe and effective care, all individuals involved should be aware of the psychological, physiologic, and legal issues surrounding restraint procedures.

▶ ACKNOWLEDGMENT

The authors would like to acknowledge the valuable contributions of M. Douglas Baker to the version of this chapter that appeared in the previous edition.

▶ REFERENCES

1. Rice MM, Moore GP. Management of the violent patient: therapeutic and legal considerations. *Emerg Med Clin North Am.* 1991;9:13–30.
2. Zun LS. A prospective study of the complication rate of use of patient restraint in the emergency department. *J Emerg Med.* 2003;24:119–124.
3. Neinstein LS, Heischober BS. Hallucinogens. In: Neinstein LS, ed. *Adolescent Health Care: A Practical Guide.* 4th ed. Baltimore: Williams & Wilkins, 2002.
4. Joint Commission on Accreditation of Healthcare Organizations. *2000 Hospital Accreditation Standards.* Oakbrok Terrace, IL: Joint Commission on Accreditation of Healthcare Organizations; 1996. TX-47.
5. Health Care Financing Administration. Hospital condition of participation in Medicare and Medicaid. 64 *Fed. Reg.* 36089 (1999).

 CLINICAL TIPS

▶ Have a plan of action before attempting restraint.

▶ Remove stethoscopes, loose jewelry, or anything that might be used as a weapon before performing a restraint procedure.

▶ Once the decision to restrain has been made, do not "bargain."

▶ Use the least amount of restraint necessary for patient and staff safety.

▶ Protect yourself and other health care team members.

▶ If a patient is able to pull his or her hands out of leather restraints, then roll a washcloth into a ball in each hand.

▶ Never leave a restrained patient alone.

ERON Y. FRIEDLAENDER AND FRED M. HENRETIG

Evaluation of Vital Signs

4

▶ INTRODUCTION

Accurate vital sign measurement is essential for appropriate triage, initial evaluation, and ongoing assessment and management of all patients presenting for care in an emergency department (ED). The systematic evaluation of respiratory and heart rates, blood pressure, body temperature, and peripheral capillary refill enables the rapid determination of specific organ dysfunction and allows for the estimation of severity of illness. Trends in vital sign measurements also help to reflect responses to medical intervention. Certain clinical situations may require continuous monitoring of vital signs rather than intermittent recordings; the use of electronic devices for this purpose is discussed in Chapter 5, which also contains a detailed discussion of the physiology and procedural aspects of blood pressure and tympanic thermometry monitoring. Importantly, under any circumstance, the measurement and interpretation of vital signs in children requires skills, equipment, and techniques suited to the size and age-specific needs of this population, just as the practice of pediatric emergency medicine involves specialized care tailored to the physiologic and developmental needs of young patients.

▶ ANATOMY AND PATHOPHYSIOLOGY

The consideration of several patient factors is important for the accurate measurement and interpretation of pediatric vital signs. More often with children than adults the patient's emotional state (anxiety, anger, pain), age, and weight and the methods used in obtaining measurements may influence the findings. In addition, significant variations exist in the normal ranges for blood pressure and respiratory and heart rates; failure to account for patient age in the interpretation of

vital signs may cause undue alarm or false reassurance of stability.

▶ INDICATION

Vital sign determination offers a fast, objective evaluation of patient disease and physiologic status. Vital sign measurements help the physician estimate the seriousness of current illness and assist in determining the need for various forms of medical intervention. In the apparently well patient, they may also serve as a screening tool, occasionally identifying patients with unsuspected pathologic conditions.

The extensive range of mechanisms and etiologies of emergency medical and traumatic conditions in children requires that providers approach the care of a sick child using a systematic schema for evaluating physical findings and vital signs. One system, currently advocated in the American Heart Association's Pediatric Advanced Life Support course (I), utilizes the "ABC" mnemonic approach. This system emphasizes the early recognition of problems related to the airway (**A**), the determination of the adequacy of breathing (**B**), and the determination of the status of patient circulation (**C**). This chapter will use a similar approach to the determination and interpretation of pediatric vital signs.

The most serious problem encountered in any medical setting is a patient with cardiac arrest. Unlike in adult patients, cardiac arrest in children is rarely the result of sudden cardiac dysrhythmia or infarction. Rather, cardiac arrest in pediatric patients is more likely the result of a compromised airway or failure of pulmonary ventilation. In addition, children in septic, distributive, or hypovolemic shock states display signs of reduced peripheral perfusion (delayed capillary refill) and persistent tachycardia before they manifest hypotension.

It follows, then, that recognition of the early signs of cardiorespiratory compromise allows for therapeutic intervention and possible prevention of further clinical deterioration.

▶ COMPLICATIONS

Although vital signs are an important component of the initial ED evaluation, medical staff should not permit the precise measurement of vital signs to delay the establishment of an unobstructed airway or support respirations or circulation for a patient in extremis. The temptation to measure patient vital signs at the expense of necessary emergency interventions can have disastrous consequences. A rapid survey of the ABCs and interventions necessary to correct any problems should always take precedence over detailed measurement of routine vital signs.

▶ PROCEDURES

Vital Impression

Evaluation of a patient begins with a general assessment. This rapid survey or "vital impression" includes an assessment of airway patency, the adequacy of respirations, the quality of cry, and skin color and a general visual assessment of the degree of patient illness. Level of consciousness, eye contact and visual tracking (especially in the young infant), and age-appropriate interaction with caregivers all contribute to this global assessment. This vital impression is helpful as a quick first screen in determining the need for emergency interventions.

Respiration

After establishing the patency of the airway, ensuring the adequacy of ventilation and oxygenation must take priority over all other medical interventions. The evaluation of respirations should include the rate, effectiveness, and pattern of breathing and the work of breathing. A patient's respiratory rate is the number of breaths taken in 1 minute. The effectiveness of respiration is clinically estimated by determining the adequacy of air movement, the presence or absence of cyanosis, and any changes in mental status.

Equipment and Procedure

The respiratory rate is routinely measured and recorded during the course of most ED evaluations. The respiratory rate should be taken while the patient is relaxed (asleep, if possible, in infants) and breathing at a rate unaffected by the process of evaluation. Attempts to calm or distract anxious or uncooperative patients prior to assessment will result in more accurate measurements. The respiratory rate may be measured directly by auscultation of breath sounds during a given length of time. In the young or uncooperative patient, the respiratory rate may sometimes be determined more accurately by simply counting chest or abdominal movements over a determined period. The accuracy of a counted respiratory rate improves when the period of time for determination is lengthened (1 minute is optimal).

The respiratory rate may also be determined by respiratory inductive plethysmography. By measuring changes in thoracic impedance between two cardiac chest leads, the number of chest wall movements over a set time can be determined. However, one must not rely on electronic measurement of respirations as the sole method in determining the respiratory rate of patients. Electronic measurement of chest wall movements may not accurately correlate with the number of effective respirations. Electronic measurement of respiratory rates may also be erroneously influenced by voluntary or involuntary patient movements, precordial cardiac activity, improper application or standardization of equipment, or equipment failure. In addition, chest wall movement does not ensure the presence of an unobstructed airway or the adequacy of air exchange. ED personnel should not rely solely on electronic monitors for the ongoing observation of severely ill children (see also Chapter 5). Failing to detect the presence of a respiratory emergency because of electronic monitor malfunction may have serious medical and legal ramifications.

Interpretation

The interpretation of respiratory rates among children requires consideration of patient age and emotional status at the time of measurement (Table 4.1). Normal resting respiratory rates vary between pediatric age groups (2). The respiratory rates of patients who are emotionally upset, in pain, or feel threatened by the interventions of medical personnel should be interpreted in the context of these stresses. As well, fever and crying will elevate respiratory rates transiently. Therefore, the ED record should reflect the presence of factors that may affect the measurement of respiratory rates.

An aberrant respiratory rate or pattern may be the result of abnormalities in the patient's airway, pulmonary ventilation, oxygen exchange, acid-base status, central nervous system (due to metabolic or toxicologic derangement), or emotional status; brain or spinal cord lesions; seizures; or lack of patient cooperation.

TABLE 4.1*	AGE-ADJUSTED RESPIRATORY RATES
Term infant	30–50
1 to 6 months	20–40
6 months to 2 years	20–30
2 to 12 years	16–24
Adolescent	12–20

*Adapted from Silverman BK. Practical information. In: Fleisher GR, Ludwig S, eds. *Textbook of Pediatric Emergency Medicine.* 3rd ed. Baltimore: Williams & Wilkins; 1993.

Heart Rate

As with respiratory rates, the measurement and interpretation of the heart rate in pediatric patients requires that clinicians consider patient age, clinical condition, and emotional state. Clinical evaluation of the heart rate may also provide the first indication of cardiac rhythm disturbances.

Equipment and Procedure

The heart rate and regularity of rhythm may be determined by several different methods: palpation of pulses, auscultation of heart sounds, observation or palpation of apical chest wall movement, and electronic ECG monitors. The latter technique is detailed in Chapter 5. Palpation of pulses provides additional information concerning pulse volume and has a time-honored mystique that may confer some significant advantages when dealing with older children, adolescents, and adults (3). If possible, the patient's heart rate should be determined while the patient is relaxed and unaffected by the process of evaluation, although this is typically difficult in the ED setting. Counting the number of heart beats over a defined period determines the beats per minute; counting the beats for a full 60 seconds helps to ensure accurate results. Measuring the rate for shorter periods of time may increase the chances of erroneous results and misguided clinical interventions.

Interpretation

The interpretation of heart rate and rhythm, like that of respiratory rate, depends on numerous physiologic and pathologic variables. Age-appropriate heart rates are listed in Table 4.2. Assuming an accurate measurement in a resting state, a heart rate significantly elevated for age may reflect numerous conditions, including fever, endocrine dysfunction, hypovolemia, hypoxia, hypoglycemia, acidosis, anemia, decreased cardiac function, tachyarrhythmia, vasodilatation, and increased sympathomimetic activity via any of a variety of exogenous or endogenous causes. Alternatively, bradycardia may reflect increased intracranial pressure, hypothermia, endocrine dysfunction, bradyarrhythmia, excess vagal tone, hypoxia, and poisoning, most commonly with digoxin, beta-blockers, or calcium channel blockers.

Pulse volume may be increased under the following conditions: patent ductus arteriosus, aortic insufficiency, hyperthyroidism, fever, and anemia. Decreased pulse volume may signify shock or aortic stenosis.

The approach to the diagnosis of an irregular pulse is beyond the scope of this chapter and has been summarized elsewhere (4). However, a common cause of benign heart rate irregularity in children is sinus arrhythmia. In this physiologic rhythm, the pulse rate increases with inspiration and decreases during expiration. If the relation to respiration is not easily apparent during the physical exam, an electrocardiographic rhythm strip will confirm the diagnosis.

Capillary Refill

The measurement of capillary refill time as an indicator of the adequacy of peripheral perfusion, although not a classic vital sign, is a useful complement to temperature, blood pressure, and heart and respiratory rates in the assessment of an ill child. Changes in capillary refill time may reflect decreased vascular volume or alteration in systemic vascular resistance. The capillary refill time is arguably the earliest measurable clinical indicator of inadequate peripheral circulation (5,6).

Procedure

The determination of capillary refill time is simple, reliable, and quick. The time required for the blanched nailbed to return to the normal color represents capillary refill (Fig. 4.1). It is most accurate in a fingernail depressed with gentle pressure for at least 3 seconds and under warm ambient conditions. When using capillary refill time as a reflection of response to medical therapy, serial determinations measured at the same anatomic location prove most reliable.

Interpretation

Normal capillary refill time for the pediatric patient is usually considered to be less than 2.0 seconds. The upper limit of normal for capillary refill time is slightly higher in adults. Schriger and Baraff reported an upper limit of normal of 2.0 seconds for adult men and 2.9 seconds for adult women (5). Skin temperature also plays a role in determining capillary refill time; capillary refill time may be significantly delayed with cool environmental conditions, including air-conditioning (7).

A delay in capillary refill of greater than 2.0 to 3.0 seconds may reflect inadequacy of peripheral perfusion. Saavedra et al. reported a correlation between the degree of dehydration in pediatric patients and prolongation of capillary refill time (6). In patients admitted to the hospital for diarrhea, a refill time of 1.5 to 3.0 seconds suggested a fluid deficit of greater than 100 mL/kg.

Other conditions that may result in a prolongation of capillary refill time include heart failure, hypothermia, electrolyte abnormalities, hypotension, and conditions resulting in alterations of circulatory regulation.

TABLE 4.2*	AGE-ADJUSTED HEART RATES
Age	Heart rate (per minute)
Neonate	80–180
1 week to 1 month	80–160
3 months to 2 years	80–150
2 to 10 years	75–110
10 years to adult	50–100

*Adapted from Silverman BK. Practical information. In: Fleisher GR, Ludwig S, eds. *Textbook of Pediatric Emergency Medicine*. 3rd ed. Baltimore: Williams & Wilkins; 1993.

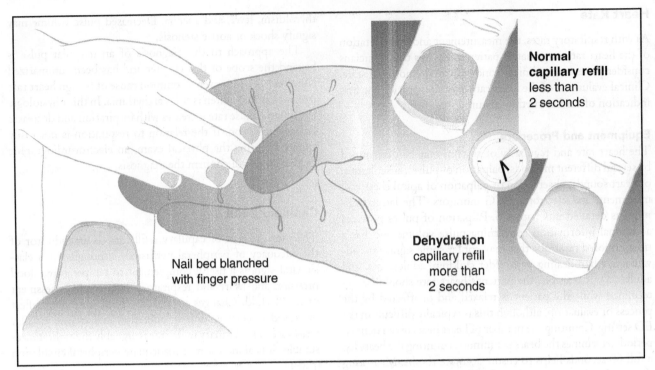

Normal capillary refill less than 2 seconds

Dehydration capillary refill more than 2 seconds

Nail bed blanched with finger pressure

Figure 4.1 The assessment of capillary refill time at the fingernail bed.

Blood Pressure

Routine measurement of blood pressure is occasionally omitted in pediatric patients due to inexperience, impatience, and, in many cases, lack of appropriate equipment. However, blood pressure alterations or instability may cause, complicate, or herald serious medical conditions in children as well as in adults. Although significant hypotension is usually accompanied by changes in sensorium, heart rate, pulse volume, skin color, and capillary refill, hypertension may be less clinically obvious in the young patient.

Several types of instruments to measure blood pressure are available, including mercury or aneroid sphygmomanometers using stethoscope- or ultrasound-based (Doppler) determinations of blood flow and oscillometric-based instruments such as the Dinamap. The mercury manometer remains the gold standard for blood pressure measurement; oscillometric devices are best suited for monitoring trends (8). Chapter 5 offers an overview of the physiologic basis of blood pressure measurement in general and proper Dinamap technique in particular. The main point emphasized here is that cuff size is of crucial importance in all forms of blood pressure determination. Whereas most authors focus on cuff width in relation to arm length (e.g., the former should be at least two-thirds of the latter), it is probably more accurate, especially in obese patients, to relate cuff width to arm *diameter* (9). Park et al. have shown that a cuff width 20% greater than arm diameter, which allows proper transmission of cuff bladder pressure to the level of the brachial artery in most patients, will obtain a blood pressure measurement that correlates closely with the measurement achieved using an intra-arterial catheter (Fig. 4.2). Cuff widths significantly narrower (e.g., less than 10% wider than arm diameter) will falsely elevate measured pressure by 10 to 15 mm Hg, and cuffs too large (e.g., 30% to 45% wider than arm diameter) will falsely lower pressure 3 to 6 mm Hg. The cuff length is also a consideration, and most authors favor a cuff length that completely encircles the arm. The ED should have cuffs in widths of 3, 5, 8, 12, and 18 cm to accommodate all sizes of pediatric patients (Fig. 4.3). If the proper size cuff is not available, folding down a larger cuff will suffice. When the choice is very limited, a cuff larger than optimal is probably preferable, because the discrepancy with overly wide cuffs is less than with those that are too narrow.

Procedure

The patient should be relatively calm and in a supine position or with the arm held at level of the heart (Fig. 4.4) during the measurement of blood pressure. The proper size cuff is wrapped snugly around the patient's arm (or leg) and then inflated. Consider first estimating systolic pressure by palpating the distal pulse. The cuff is reinflated to 10 to 20 mm Hg above the point of pulse disappearance and then deflated slowly, at a rate of no more than 2 to 4 mm Hg per second. Auscultation of the first Korotkoff sound indicates systolic pressure; muffling of sounds indicates diastolic pressure, although in some children distinct onset of muffling is difficult to appreciate, and disappearance of sounds is noted as the diastolic pressure. In busy and noisy EDs, the Dinamap approach is favored for accuracy of measurement and because, when left in place, the anxious child is more likely to become relaxed without the nurse's or physician's close proximity.

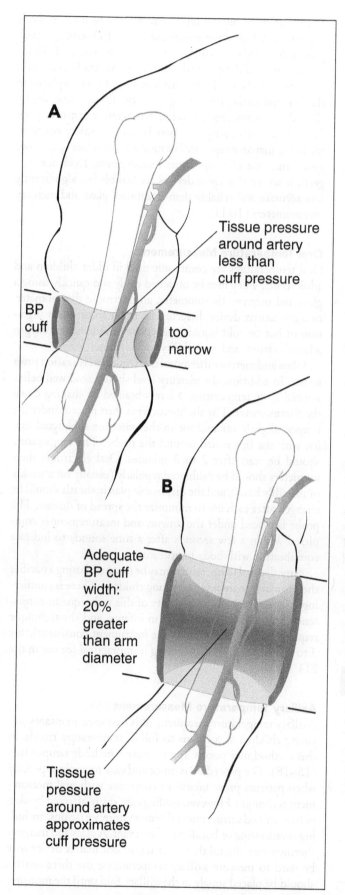

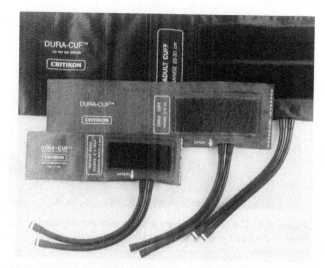

Figure 4.3 The pediatric ED should stock several different cuff sizes.

Interpretation

Numerous pathophysiologic states alter blood pressure. Hypotension is classically associated with hypovolemia, cardiac (pump) failure, or profound vasodilation from a variety of potential causes. Hypovolemia in children is most commonly secondary to dehydration from gastroenteritis or, less frequently, traumatic blood loss, a plasma deficit from large burns, or osmotic shift as might occur in adrenal insufficiency or diabetic ketoacidosis. Distributive shock (vasodilatation) is most frequently caused by sepsis in the pediatric population; other causes include anaphylaxis, drug overdoses, and spinal injury. Cardiogenic shock in children may be due to congenital cardiac defects, particularly those that are dependent on a patent ductus for systemic circulation, such as hypoplastic left heart syndrome. Other causes of cardiogenic shock in children include viral myocarditis, certain drug overdoses, and dysrhythmias.

Hypertension is being increasingly recognized as a pediatric problem. Generally, a blood pressure above the 95th percentile for age identifies hypertension, and a pressure greater than the 99th percentile represents severe hypertension. The most common etiologies for hypertension in the pediatric population include renal parenchymal and renovascular disease. Infants and young children should also be evaluated for aortic coarctation. Age-appropriate blood pressures are summarized in Table 4.3. A good rule of thumb for approximating

Figure 4.2

A. Cuff pressure is transmitted through the arm in a diminishing band.

B. An appropriate cuff width in relation to arm diameter is necessary for adequate transmission of cuff pressure to tissue pressure surrounding the brachial artery and thus is necessary for accurate blood pressure measurement. (Adapted from Park MK, Kawabori I, Guntheroth WG. Need for an improved standard for blood pressure cuff size. *Clin Pediatr.* 1976;15:784–787; Kirkendall WM, Burton AC, Epstein FH, et al. Recommendations for human blood pressure determination by sphygmomanometers. *Circulation.* 1967;36:980–988.)

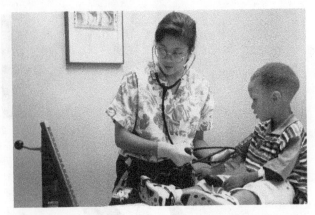

Figure 4.4 The blood pressure is taken with the arm held at the level of the heart and with the child (hopefully) relaxed and cooperative.

50th percentile systolic pressures by age (in mm Hg) is as follows: neonate = 70; infant to 1 year = 80; child older than 2 years = $90 + (2 \times$ age in years) (1).

Temperature

Body temperature measurement is a cornerstone of vital sign assessment. Alterations of body temperature, including hyperthermia and hypothermia, may result from infection, intoxication, malignancy, collagen vascular disease, thyroid disorders, nutritional insufficiency, or exposure to environmental temperature extremes.

Accurate body temperature measurement in the pediatric population is particularly important, as the presence of fever in a very young or immune-compromised individual dictates an algorithm for evaluation and management that is at times invasive and carries risk. Therefore, inaccurate estimations of body temperature may result in serious errors in diagnosis and treatment.

The ideal thermometer should be easy to use, accurately and reliably reflect core body temperature, minimize the spread of contagious diseases, provide rapid results, and cause minimal patient discomfort and embarrassment. At present,

a range of thermometer types may be used to measure body temperature. Those commonly used in the ED setting include probes designed for use in the oral cavity, the axillary fold, the rectal vault, and the external auditory canal. Traditional thermometers of glass and mercury have been largely replaced in the hospital setting by a new generation of electronic, digital clinical thermometers (including temperature-sensitive pacifiers and forehead strips) in part because of safety concerns related to mercury exposure but mostly in an effort to improve speed and ease of temperature measurement. Evidence suggests, however, that these devices are feasible but significantly less accurate and reliable than traditional glass and mercury thermometers (10,11).

Oral Temperature Measurements

Oral temperatures are commonly used in older children and adolescents. They may be obtained easily and quickly using a glass and mercury thermometer, an electronic thermometer, or a dot matrix device. Inaccuracies result from recent ingestion of hot or cold liquids, tachypnea, supplemental oxygen administration, and an inability to cooperate.

Glass and mercury thermometers require sterilization prior to use. In addition, the mercury level should read well below normal body temperature, a level obtained by shaking down the thermometer. The thermometer is then placed under the tongue, slightly off midline in the posterior sublingual cavity, with the lips sealed around the probe. The temperature should be read after 2 to 3 minutes. Oral electronic thermometers should be calibrated regularly (usually on a weekly or monthly basis), and the disposable plastic sheath should be changed after each use to minimize the spread of disease. The probe is placed under the tongue, and measurement is completed within a few seconds after a tone sounds to indicate equilibration with body temperature.

Supralingual temperatures may be measured using a pacifier thermometer in infants and young children. There is conflicting evidence regarding the ability of this technique to consistently and reliably detect fever in infants, and the technique requires the child to suck on the instrument consistently for 3 to 4 minutes (12–14), making it impractical for use in the ED.

Axillary Temperature Measurement

Axillary temperature measurement is best used in infants and young children as a means to follow temperature trends, as this method may poorly approximate core body temperature (15–18). The procedure is quick and easy to apply, especially when patients prove unable to cooperate with oral measurement technique. However, readings are easily affected by skin perfusion and environmental temperature variations, including overdressing or bundling of an infant. A glass and mercury thermometer, digital thermometer, or dot matrix device may be used to measure axillary temperatures; the thermometer should be placed snugly in the axillary fold until the measurement is completed.

TABLE 4.3*	AGE-ADJUSTED BLOOD PRESSURE	
Age	**Pressure (systolic/diastolic in mm Hg)**	
Neonate	Range 40–80/20–55	
	Percentile	
	50th	**95th**
2 years	96/60	112/78
6 years	98/64	116/80
9 years	106/68	126/84
12 years	114/74	136/88

*Adapted from Silverman BK. Practical information. In: Fleisher GR, Ludwig S, eds. *Textbook of Pediatric Emergency Medicine.* 3rd ed. Baltimore: Williams & Wilkins; 1993.

Rectal Temperature Measurement

Rectal temperature measurement has long been considered the gold standard for approximation of core body temperatures (13,19). However, recent evidence suggests that rectal temperature measurement may poorly reflect rapid changes in core body temperature (20–23). While it has generally been the method of choice in studies involving correlations between bacteremia and temperature in infants and young children (24), it has been determined that rectal temperature measurements lag behind core body temperature changes largely because of local vascular insulation (25). Although the measurement is easily obtained, the procedure is uncomfortable, may cause patient embarrassment in older children, carries the potential for transmission of stool-borne pathogens (26, 27), and poses a risk of traumatic injury to the rectum, especially in newborns (28,29). Despite these limitations, rectal thermometry remains the most accurate and reliable of the available noninvasive means by which to measure body temperature in the ambulatory care setting (13,19,30–32). Of note, rectal temperatures are contraindicated in patients with recent rectal surgery, neutropenia, or severe thrombocytopenia.

Rectal temperatures can be obtained via glass and mercury or digital thermometers. With the patient in a supine, prone, or lateral decubitus position with the hips flexed, the thermometer should be placed 2 to 3 cm into the rectal vault, with the nurse or parent securing the infant (Fig. 4.5). The temperature may be read in 2 to 3 minutes if a glass and mercury thermometer are used. With a digital thermometer, the rectal probe should be similarly inserted into the rectum and temperature equilibration will be reached within a few seconds. In either case, care should be taken to ensure the thermometer is not placed directly into a mass of fecal matter, which may falsely lower the temperature reading.

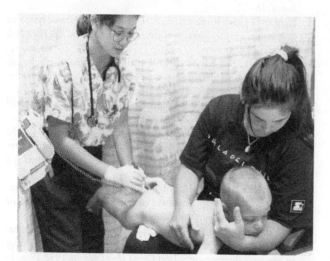

Figure 4.5 The rectal temperature is taken with the infant secured on mother's lap in the prone position and with hips flexed.

Tympanic Temperature Measurement

Tympanic membrane thermometers use an infrared probe to sense the temperature of the tympanic membrane (25,33). Theoretically, tympanic membrane temperatures most closely approximate true core body temperatures, as the hypothalamus and the tympanic membrane both receive their blood supply from the internal carotid artery (34). Proper technique for tympanic membrane temperature measurement parallels that for traditional otoscopy. The aural probe should be positioned within the external auditory canal and directed toward the tympanic membrane. Insertion is facilitated by gently pulling the pinna down and back in young children and up and back in the older child and young adult. These maneuvers serve to straighten the auditory canal and ease placement of the measuring device. However, tympanic membrane temperatures are less accurate in children under 3 months of age given their small and torturous auditory canals. As electronic devices used to monitor temperature, tympanic membrane thermometers are discussed further in Chapter 5.

Interpretation

Fever is an elevation of body temperature in response to a pathologic stimulus. It is difficult to ascertain the least elevation of temperature that is abnormal for all children under all circumstances. Temperature varies with environment, clothing, activity, digestion, and diurnal rhythms (35). Most children have a peak temperature in the early evening, between 5:00 and 7:00 PM. For a child at rest who has been appropriately dressed for the ambient temperature, we define fever as a rectal or tympanic temperature of 38°C (100.4°F). Oral temperatures are usually 0.6°C (1.0°F) lower than rectal temperatures, and axillary temperatures are usually 1.1°C (2.0°F) lower. The evaluation of febrile children in regard to the diagnosis of infectious diseases is a complex topic and will not be detailed here. Briefly, several factors play an important role in the evaluation of fever, including the patient's age, overall clinical appearance, and host defense status; evidence of focal infection on clinical evaluation; and degree of temperature elevation beyond normal (35). Infants under 8 to 12 weeks of age may have serious infections with normal or low-grade temperatures. In children 3 to 36 months of age, the likelihood of severe illness and bacteremia increases with the degree of temperature elevation.

Fever can also be a prominent symptom in many important noninfectious processes, such as malignancies, collagen vascular disease, endocrinologic abnormalities, drug intoxications, and environmental exposures.

Hypothermia, defined as a temperature of less than 35°C, is also an important sign of disease. In infants less than 8 weeks old and in immunocompromised patients, hypothermia can be the result of overwhelming sepsis and warrants aggressive investigation. Other causes of hypothermia include endocrinologic failure, nutritional insufficiency, erythrodermas, and environmental exposure. Hypothermia is also frequently seen in major resuscitations, especially in trauma victims. Patients suffering severe trauma often have prolonged cold exposure

SUMMARY

1 The careful evaluation of vital signs is crucial to every ED encounter.

2 The evaluation of pediatric vital signs includes a rapid global assessment and the determination of capillary refill time as well as the measurement of heart rate, respiratory rate, blood pressure, and temperature.

3 Heart rate, respiratory rate, and blood pressure vary considerably by age and by the child's anxiety level, so the most accurate assessment of physiologic status is gained in the calm, resting child.

4 Capillary refill is an excellent pediatric technique for estimating intravascular volume status.

5 Appropriate blood pressure cuff size is critical to an accurate determination of blood pressure.

6 Rectal temperature remains the gold standard for determining the presence of fever in the ambulatory setting, particularly in infants up to 3 months of age.

7 Tympanic temperature measurement is quick, accurate, and relatively noninvasive for the child over 3 months of age (see Chapter 5).

and aggressive fluid and blood replacement, which can lead to hypothermia if fluids and blood are not warmed. Hypothermia in trauma victims may lead to profound coagulopathy and poor outcome. Hypothermia is particularly compelling in small infants undergoing resuscitation from any cause and must be carefully avoided. The appropriately equipped ED should have access to delivery room–type overhead warmers, heated bedding, and/or blankets to be used as necessary for pediatric resuscitations.

▶ ACKNOWLEDGMENTS

The authors would like to acknowledge the valuable contributions of Jefrey Biehler and Brent Barnes to the version of this chapter that appeared in the previous edition.

▶ REFERENCES

1. American Heart Association. *Textbook of Pediatric Advanced Life Support.* Dallas, TX: American Heart Association; 1988.
2. Silverman BK. Practical information. In: Fleisher GR, Ludwig S, eds. *Textbook of Pediatric Emergency Medicine.* 3rd ed. Baltimore: Williams & Wilkins; 1993.
3. Athreya B, Silverman BK. *Pediatric Physical Diagnosis.* East Norwalk, CT: Appleton-Century-Crofts; 1985.
4. Gewitz MH, Vetter VL. Cardiac emergencies. In: Fleisher GR, Ludwig S, eds. *Textbook of Pediatric Emergency Medicine.* 3rd ed. Baltimore: Williams & Wilkins; 1993.
5. Schriger DL, Baraff LJ. Defining normal capillary refill: variation with age, sex, and temperature. *Ann Emerg Med.* 1988;17:932–935.
6. Saavedra JM, Harris GD, Li S, et al. Capillary filling (skin turgor) in the assessment of dehydration. *Am J Dis Child.* 1991;145:296–298.
7. Gorelick MH, Shaw KN, Baker MD. Effect of ambient temperature on capillary refill in healthy children. *Pediatrics.* 1993;62:699–702.
8. Jones DW, Appel LJ, Sheps SG, et al. Measuring blood pressure accurately. *JAMA.* 2003;289:1027–1030.
9. Park MK, Kawabori I, Guntheroth WG. Need for an improved standard for blood pressure cuff size. *Clin Pediatr.* 1976;15:784–787.
10. Latman NS. Clinical thermometry: possible causes and potential solutions to electronic, digital thermometer inaccuracies. *Biomed Instrum Technol.* 2003;37:190–196.
11. Jensen BN, Jensen FS, Madsen SN, et al. Accuracy of digital tympanic, oral, axillary, and rectal thermometers compared with standard rectal mercury thermometers. *Eur J Surg.* 2000;166:848–851.
12. Press S, Quinn BJ. The pacifier thermometer: comparison of supralingual with rectal temperatures in infants and young children. *Arch Pediatr Adolesc Med.* 1997;151:551–554.
13. Callanan D. Detecting fever in young infants: reliability of perceived, pacifier, and temporal artery temperatures in infants younger than 3 months of age. *Pediatr Emerg Care.* 2003;19:240–243.
14. Banco L, Jayashekaramurthy S, Graffam J. *Am J Dis Child.* 1988; 142:171–172.
15. Anagnostakis D, Matsaniotis N, Grarfakos S, et al. Rectal-axillary temperature difference in febrile and afebrile infants and children. *Clin Pediatr.* 1993;32:268–272.
16. Erickson RS, Woo TM. Accuracy of infrared ear thermometry and traditional temperature methods in young children. *Heart Lung.* 1994; 23:181–195.
17. Morley CJ, Hewson PH, Thornton AJ, et al. Axillary and rectal temperature measurements in infants. *Arch Dis Child.* 1992;67:122–125.
18. Muma BK, Treloar DJ, Wurmlinger K, et al. Comparison of rectal, axillary, and tympanic membrane temperatures in infants and young children. *Ann Emerg Med.* 1991;20:41–44.
19. Greenes DS, Fleisher GR. Accuracy of a noninvasive temporal artery thermometer for use in infants. *Arch Pediatr Adolesc Med.* 2001;155:376–381.
20. Terndrup T, Milewski A. The performance of two tympanic thermometers in a pediatric emergency department. *Clin Pediatr.* 1991:30[4 Suppl]:18–22.
21. Brennan D, Falk J, Rothrock SG, et al. Reliability of infrared tympanic thermometry in the detection of rectal fever in children. *Ann Emerg Med.* 1995;25:21–29.
22. Robinson JL, Seal RF, Spady DW, et al. Comparison of esophageal, rectal, axillary, bladder, tympanic, and pulmonary artery temperatures in children. *J Pediatr.* 1998;133:553–556.
23. Greenes DS, Fleisher GR. When body temperature changes, does rectal temperature lag? *J Pediatr.* 2004;144:824–826.
24. Baraff LJ, Bass JW, Fleisher GR, et al. Practice guidelines for the management of infants and children 0 to 36 months of age with fever without source. Agency for Health Care Policy and Research. *Ann Emerg Med.* 1993;22:1198–1210.
25. Chamberlain J, Grandner J, Rubinoff JL, et al. Comparison of a tympanic thermometer to rectal and oral thermometers in a pediatric emergency department. *Clin Pediatr.* 1991;30[4 Suppl]:24–29.
26. Brooks S, Khan A, Stoica D, et al. Reduction in vancomycin-resistant *Enterococcus* and *Clostridium difficile* infections following change to tympanic thermometers. *Infect Control Hosp Epidemiol.* 1998;19:333–336.

27. Samore MH. Epidemiology of nosocomial *Clostridium difficile* diarrhea. *J Hosp Infect*. 1999;43(suppl):S183–190.

28. Frank JD, Brown S. Thermometers and rectal perforations in the neonate. *Arch Dis Child*. 1978;53:824–825.

29. Horwitz MA, Bennett JV. Nursery outbreak of peritonitis with pneumoperitoneum probably caused by thermometer-induced rectal perforation. *Am J Epidemiol*. 1976;104:632–644.

30. Falzon A, Grech V, Caruana B, et al. How reliable is axillary temperature measurement? *Acta Paediatr*. 2003;92:309–313.

31. Jean-Mary MB, Dicanzio J, Shaw J, et al. Limited accuracy and reliability of infrared axillary and aural thermometers in a pediatric outpatient population. *J Pediatr*. 2002;141:671–676.

32. Craig J, Lancaster GA, Taylor S, et al. Infrared ear thermometry compared with rectal thermometry in children: a systematic review. *Lancet*. 2002;360:603–609.

33. Milewski A, Ferguson KL, Terndrup TE. Comparison of pulmonary artery, rectal, and tympanic membrane temperatures in adult intensive care unit patients. *Clin Pediatr*. 1991;30:13–16.

34. Childs C, Harrison R, Hodkinson C. Tympanic membrane temperature as a measure of core temperature. *Arch Dis Child*. 1999;80:262–266.

35. Alpern ER, Henretig FM. Fever. In: Fleisher GR, Ludwig S, eds. *Textbook of Pediatric Emergency Medicine*. 5th ed. Philadelphia: Lippincott Williams & Wilkins; 2006.

5

KENNETH YEN AND MARC H. GORELICK

Use of Monitoring Devices

▶ INTRODUCTION

Monitoring is the process of observing the clinical condition of a patient, typically by repeated measurement of vital signs. Although such monitoring may be done by human observers, the task is frequently performed by automated devices. In this section, methods and equipment for several of the most commonly monitored parameters in pediatric emergency medicine—heart rate and rhythm, blood pressure, and temperature—are discussed. Capnography is a commonly used type of monitoring but will not be covered here because it is the subject of Chapter 76. Pulse oximetry, which is also the subject of another chapter (Chapter 75), is briefly discussed below.

▶ PULSE OXIMETRY

The use of pulse oximetry, a noninvasive transcutaneous method of measuring the oxygen saturation of blood, has expanded rapidly since its introduction into clinical practice in the early 1980s.

Physiology

Noninvasive arterial oxygen saturation measurement is obtained by directing red and infrared light through a pulsating vascular bed. The pulsating arterioles in the path of the light beam cause a change in the amount of light detected by a photodiode. Different hemoglobin species (oxygenation) have different light absorption spectra (1). The oximeter measures within the pulse wave form the ratio of transmitted red to infrared light and uses it to determine the oxygen saturation of the blood. The nonpulsatile signal is removed electronically for the purpose of calculation, and therefore skin, bone, and other nonpulsating substances do not interfere with the calculation of arterial saturation.

Procedure

The pulse oximeter consists usually of a small and portable monitor and a sensing unit that clips or tapes onto the patient's finger. Toes and ear lobes are also often used. Along with the arterial oxygen saturation (SaO_2), the meter also typically provides a tracing of the pulse rate. The strength of the identified pulse rate can also help determine if the oximeter reading is accurate.

Indications for pulse oximetry include screening for the presence or development of hypoxemia, as well as continuous monitoring to measure response to therapy. It is commonly used in the assessment of children with acute respiratory illness such as pneumonia, asthma, and upper airway obstruction. It is also recommended for monitoring patients undergoing conscious sedation (2). The anatomy, physiology, and technology underlying pulse oximetry are detailed in Chapter 75, which also contains a discussion of proper technique and interpretation of findings.

Several things have to be kept in mind. Measurements in hypothermic patients and in patients with poor perfusion (e.g., decompensated shock) are often inaccurate. The reading can be falsely high in patients with carbon monoxide poisoning or in a chronic smoker who has elevated blood carbon monoxide levels. Other things that may affect pulse oximetry readings include extremely bright lights, dense fingernail polish, and patient movement.

▶ ELECTROCARDIOGRAPHIC MONITORING

Physiology

Electrocardiograph (ECG) monitors measure and display heart rate and rhythm by detecting the electrical activity of cardiac muscle. The device consists of a sensing component, the electrode, which when placed on the skin surface can detect changes in electrical potential (i.e., depolarization and repolarization) originating in the heart. Two electrodes comprised in a lead are required to detect cardiac activity by measuring the difference in electrical potential between two sites. Standard limb leads are placed on the left arm, right arm, and left leg. A right leg electrode serves as ground. Each lead detects a different view of the heart, and all the leads together give a complete picture of cardiac activity. A 12-lead ECG involves both limb and chest leads placed in a standard configuration and allows a look at the activity of a specific lead. Routine monitoring in the emergency department (ED) usually involves only three electrodes, one placed at the base of the heart, one at the apex, and a reference electrode on the upper left chest wall to reduce electrical interference (3).

Electrical potentials detected by leads require amplification to detect the low-voltage signal. The amplifier also has a filtration system to reduce electrical "noise." Cardiac activity can be displayed continuously on an oscilloscope and/or recorded on ECG graph paper as a plot of voltage versus time. Most monitors also have the capacity to freeze and record a tracing in the last few seconds before an abnormality activates the monitor alarm (4). Monitor alarms, both auditory and visual, indicate equipment problems, including loose or defective electrodes, heart rate parameters that have exceeded the programmed limits, and abnormal cardiac rhythms.

Procedure

Intended electrode sites are cleansed with alcohol. Conductive gel is used at each area of contact between the electrode surface and skin to stabilize the electrode. Most disposable electrodes are pre-gelled. The electrode and lead wire should be firmly applied to dry skin. As previously noted, for routine continuous monitoring, three thoracic sites (at the base and apex of the heart and on the upper left chest) are usually chosen (Fig. 5.1).

Potential sources of difficulty can be patient- or equipment-related. Any voluntary movement, involuntary shivering, seizure activity, or interference by nearby electronic devices can produce artifacts. Good contact must occur between the skin and the electrode to reduce artifacts and produce an accurate tracing. The machine must be standardized so that a given voltage activity produces a consistent deflection, and both patient and machine should be properly grounded.

As with all monitoring devices, the ECG must not replace frequent clinical assessment of the patient. The results of ECG monitoring can be normal in a patient with organic

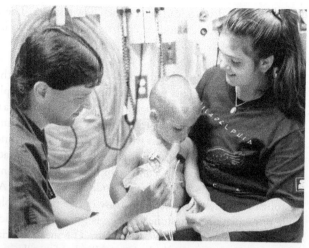

Figure 5.1 Electrocardiograph monitoring leads are placed at the three usual sites: the base and apex of the heart and the upper left chest.

heart disease or abnormal in a healthy individual. As with any laboratory test, ECG findings must be interpreted in conjunction with the clinical status of the patient.

▶ BLOOD PRESSURE

Monitoring of blood pressure in the ED is used as a screen to (a) assess the level of cardiovascular stability for patient triage, (b) follow clinical response or adverse reaction to therapy, and (c) follow clinical course in a potentially unstable condition. In the majority of cases, this can be done noninvasively with a blood pressure cuff and stethoscope or with an automated oscillometric device such as the Dinamap. Invasive blood pressure monitoring is reserved for those critically ill patients requiring intensive care unit admission, multiple repeated measurements of arterial blood gases, and continuous monitoring.

Physiology

Noninvasive blood pressure monitoring involves the use of a compression cuff applied to the limb and inflated with air to a pressure above systolic blood pressure, thereby terminating distal flow. Blood pressure is determined by detecting the pressure at which blood flow resumes as the cuff is deflated. Auscultatory methods include using a stethoscope to detect Korotkoff sounds, which are the result of turbulent blood flow as cuff pressure falls below arterial systolic pressure (see also Chapter 4). The first sound auscultated approximates systolic blood pressure. Diastolic blood pressure is the pressure at which muffling of sounds occurs. If auscultation is difficult because of noise level or a low-flow state, the arterial pulse can be palpated as the cuff is deflated or an ultrasonic flow detector can detect when flow resumes. These two latter methods cannot be used to determine diastolic pressure.

An alternative method of blood pressure detection is the oscillometric method utilized in equipment such as the Dinamap machines. This method is based on the principle that pulsatile blood flow through a blood vessel produces arterial wall oscillations that are transmitted to a blood pressure cuff (5). The machine operates with a pressure transducer and a microcomputer, both of which sense cuff pressure, initiate cuff inflation and deflation, control for motion artifacts, and record points of the changing amplitude of oscillations. At systolic blood pressure, a rapid increase occurs in the amplitude of oscillations. Diastolic pressure is the point at which a sudden decrease occurs in oscillations. The mean arterial pressure is the point at which the amplitude of oscillations reaches a maximum. These three independently measured values are typically displayed on the monitor at the completion of each inflation-deflation cycle.

Procedure

Errors in blood pressure measurement can be cuff- or patient-related (6). The most common error is incorrect cuff size—in particular, a cuff that is too small—which falsely elevates the blood pressure (see Figs. 4.2 and 4.3). The cuff should cover two thirds of the upper arm length, fully encircling the arm with a snug fit. In obese children, a cuff width 20% greater than arm diameter will provide a more accurate reading. Rapid deflation rate is another source of measurement error, creating falsely low blood pressure measurements. Cuff deflation rate should be no more than 2 to 3 mm Hg per second. Before cuff application and between determinations, ensure that all residual air is eliminated.

Patient-related sources of error include having a crying or anxious child and placing the extremity above or below heart level during measurement.

Use of Dinamap machine and other similar oscillometric blood pressure–monitoring equipment begins with placing the proper size cuff on the selected limb, which in most cases is the upper arm. Other sites, including the forearm and ankle, are more comfortable for prolonged periods of monitoring in the conscious patient but are less helpful when dealing with the patient with shock or peripheral vasoconstriction. Before the cuff is applied, all residual air must be squeezed out; the cuff is then put on snugly but not so tightly as to cause venous congestion. If residual air remains in the cuff or the cuff is not snug, blood pressure readings will be falsely elevated. The cuff and the patient's heart must be at the same level to avoid the effect of hydrostatic pressure on the reading, which is falsely high when the cuff is below the heart and falsely low when the cuff is above the heart. The conscious, cooperative patient must be told to remain quiet and avoid movement (Fig. 5.2; see also Fig. 4.4).

Problems with noninvasive blood pressure monitoring occur with shock and peripheral vasoconstriction. Palpation and

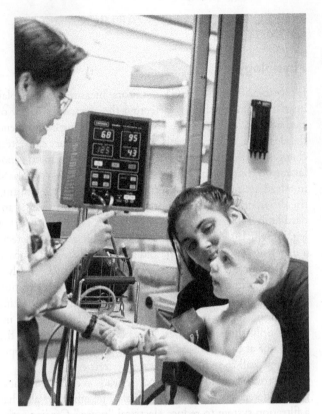

Figure 5.2 The child is relaxed and comfortable, with arm at heart level, for blood pressure monitoring.

auscultatory methods are insensitive in low-flow states. The Dinamap is more useful during shock because it measures pressure oscillations instead of sounds. In severe cases, only mean arterial pressure may be measurable, if even that, and invasive blood pressure monitoring may be warranted. Accurate noninvasive monitoring is also compromised in patients with frequent irregular heart rhythms; patients with significant tachycardia; and patients who are moving excessively (shivering) or on rapid cycling mechanical ventilators, when large variability in systolic blood pressures exists.

Recent studies that compare the newest Dinamap models (Dinamap model 8100, Critikon, Tampa, FL) with the auscultatory blood pressure method in children have found that the Dinamap systolic pressure readings are 10 mm Hg (95% CI, −4 to 24 mm Hg) higher than the auscultatory systolic pressure readings. The Dinamap diastolic readings were 5 mm Hg (95% CI, −14 to 23 mm Hg) higher. The authors recommend care when using automated devices to diagnose hypertension in children (7).

Despite the fact that the readings from these two methods cannot be used interchangeably, the automated oscillometric monitors have been adopted as the method of choice in the pediatric ED. The reasons are that the automated oscillometric method allows easier repeated measurements, is more useful in noisy environments like the ED, has less interobserver variability, and is often better able to measure blood pressure in low-flow states. It is recommended that values outside of normal range be confirmed by the auscultatory method and that all values be correlated with the rest of the clinical examination of the patient.

▶ TYMPANIC THERMOMETRY

Measurement of body temperature is essential in the evaluation of acutely ill children. The traditional method of temperature measurement uses a glass mercury or electronic thermometer at one of several sites: rectal, oral, or axillary. Oral thermometry is difficult to perform on infants and young children. Increased respiratory rate may alter the accuracy of this method. Axillary thermometry has been considered unsatisfactory in detecting fever in young children (8–10). Rectal thermometry has generally been considered the standard for measurement of temperature in infants. Rectal thermometry has several disadvantages, including discomfort for the patient and parent (11–13), risk of traumatic injury to the rectum (14–17), risk of transmission of stool-borne pathogens (18,19), relative contraindication in immunosuppressed children, and the need for time-consuming and increased effort (undressing) by the health care practitioner. Because of these disadvantages, devices have been developed that measure body temperature in less invasive manners. One such method uses infrared emission detection of the tympanic membrane. Tympanic thermometers, although popular with patients and parents and fairly reliable in adults (12), have uncertain reliability in infants and young children (9,10,20–23). This issue is discussed further below.

Physiology

Tympanic thermometers measure infrared emissions from the tympanic membrane, and these emissions are correlated with core body temperature (hypothalamic or pulmonic artery temperature) (24–26). Because core temperature is lower than rectal temperature, with which clinicians are most familiar, most ear thermometers use a microprocessor to add an "offset" to the tympanic temperature, yielding a rectal or oral equivalent. The algorithm for this offset is specific to each of the different ear thermometers currently marketed in the United States.

Procedure

To use the tympanic thermometer, a disposable cover is placed over the otoscope-like probe. This probe is then inserted in the auditory canal (Fig. 5.3). Care should be taken to aim the probe at the tympanic membrane for the most accurate results. An ear tug is recommended to straighten the canal as much as possible—posteriorly for infants and posteriorly and superiorly for older children (27). A reading is available in 1 to 3 seconds. Neither cerumen nor concomitant otitis media has a significant effect on the accuracy of tympanic temperature measurement (28–30). Extremes of ambient temperature will distort the results, particularly in infants with shallow ear canals (31).

A large number of studies of tympanic thermometry have been performed in adults and children, with varying results (10,25,30,32–35). Much of the discrepancy is the result of differences in technique, choice of different gold standards for comparison, and differences in offsets between devices.

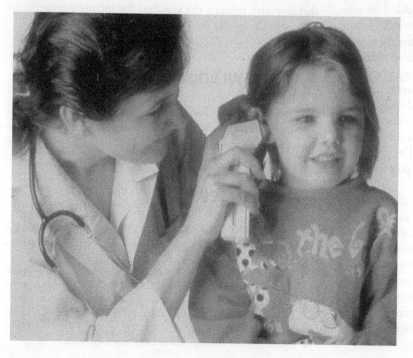

Figure 5.3 Using the tympanic thermometer. (Photograph courtesy of Thermoscan, Inc., San Diego, CA.)

Based on current literature, tympanic temperature is not recommended in infants less than 3 months of age. In older children, careful attention to technique as described previously is essential. In addition, because of the use of varying correction offsets, the interpretation of tympanic temperature can be problematic when treatment decisions are based on equivalent rectal temperature. Thus, familiarity with the particular device being used is also helpful.

▶ TEMPORAL ARTERY THERMOMETRY

Since tympanic thermometry has been shown to have questionable reliability in infants and young children, a need still exists for a form of thermometry that is well tolerated but gives results that are more closely in agreement with rectal temperature. The newer temporal artery (TA) thermometer has emerged as a possible candidate. This thermometer uses the arterial heat balance method for measurement.

Physiology

Temporal artery thermometers, like tympanic thermometers, use scanning infrared transmission and the arterial heat balance method. The arterial heat balance method concurrently and repeatedly measures the temperature of the skin surface over the temporal artery and the ambient temperature and then synthesizes these data by way of a patented algorithm to estimate the pulmonary artery temperature (36).

Procedure

The temporal artery thermometer sensor is placed over the center of the forehead, midway between the eyebrow and the hairline. The scan button is depressed and held. The sensor is then slid laterally across the forehead, with the sensor kept flat and in contact with the skin, until the hairline at the temple is reached. A beep will sound and/or an indicator light will blink to indicate a measurement is taking place. The scan button is then released and the thermometer removed from the head. The temperature is read on a display. These instructions apply to the temporal artery thermometers produced by Exergen, the makers of the most commonly used temporal artery thermometer (37) (Fig. 5.4). The procedure may differ with other brands; the instructions provided with other devices should be reviewed.

A number of factors have been found to affect the accuracy of the reading. Excessive perspiration can cause the thermometer reading to be lower. It is recommended that if there is sweating, the procedure should be performed as described above, but the button should be held depressed when reaching the temple. The probe is then lifted from the forehead and touched to the area on the neck behind the ear lobe. The button is then released and the temperature read. The thermometer also has to be acclimatized to the temperature of the room in which it is to be used.

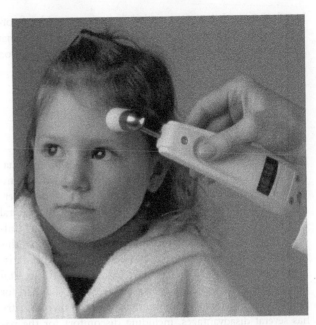

Figure 5.4 Using the temporal artery thermometer. (Photograph courtesy of Exergen Corporation, Watertown, MA.)

One study has found that temporal artery thermometry is more accurate than tympanic thermometry in infants and is better tolerated by infants than rectal thermometry (38). Temporal artery thermometry may also be able to measure defervescence faster that rectal thermometry (39). However, the sensitivity of temporal artery thermometers for detecting slight elevations of rectal temperature in young infants is questionable (38,40). It has been suggested, though, that a temporal artery temperature of less than 37.7°C can be safely used as a screen to exclude rectal temperature of greater than 38.3°C in infants 3 to 24 months of age (40,41). Rectal thermometry remains the standard for infants younger than 3 months of age (42).

▶ ACKNOWLEDGMENT

The authors would like to acknowledge the valuable contributions of Jacalyn S. Maller to the version of this chapter that appeared in the previous edition.

▶ REFERENCES

1. Alexander CM, Teller LE, Gross JB. Principles of pulse oximetry: theoretical and practical considerations. *Anest Analg.* 1989;68:368–376.
2. Sacchetti A, Schafermeyer R, Geradi M, et al. Pediatric analgesia and sedation. *Ann Emerg Med.* 1994;23:237–250.
3. Morriss FC, Mast CP. Electrocardiographic and respiratory monitors. In: Levin DL, ed. *A Practical Guide to Pediatric Intensive Care*. St. Louis: Mosby; 1984:474–478.
4. Nobel JJ. ECG monitors. *Pediatr Emerg Care.* 1993;9:52.

5. Park MK, Menard SM. Accuracy of blood pressure measurement by the Dinamap monitor in infants and children. *Pediatrics.* 1987;79:907–914.

6. Ramsey M. Knowing your monitoring equipment: blood pressure monitoring: automated oscillometric devices. *J Clin Monit.* 1991;7:56–67.

7. Park MK, Menard SW, Yuan C. Comparison of auscultatory and oscillometric blood pressures. *Arch Pediatr Adolesc Med.* 2001;155:50–53.

8. Kresch MJ. Axillary temperature as a screening test for fever in children. *J Pediatr.* 1984;104:596–599.

9. Morley CJ, Hewson PH, Thornton AJ, et al. Axillary and rectal temperature measurements in infants. *Arch Dis Child.* 1992;67:122–125.

10. Muma BK, Treloar DJ, Wurmlinger K, et al. Comparison of rectal, axillary, and tympanic membrane temperatures in infants and young children. *Ann Emerg Med.* 1991;20:41–44.

11. McCaffery M. Children's responses to rectal temperatures: an exploratory study. *Nurs Res.* 1971;20:32–45.

12. Barber N, Kilmon CA. Reactions to tympanic temperature measurement in an ambulatory setting. *Pediatr Nurs.* 1989;15:477–481.

13. McDonald R. Objection to taking rectal temperatures. *Clin Pediatr.* 1968;7:707.

14. Smiddy FG, Benson EA. Rectal perforation by thermometer. *Lancet.* 1969;2(7624):805–806.

15. Shaw EB. Rectal perforation by thermometer. *Lancet.* 1970;1(7643):416.

16. Merenstein GB. Rectal perforation by thermometer. *Lancet.* 1970;1(7654):1007.

17. Frank JD, Brown S. Thermometers and rectal perforations in the neonate. *Arch Dis Child.* 1978;53:824–825.

18. Im SW, Chow K, Chau PY. Rectal thermometer mediated cross-infection with *Salmonella wandsworth* in a paediatric ward. *J Hosp Infect.* 1981;2:171–174.

19. Brooks S, Khan A, Stoica D, et al. Reduction in vancomycin-resistant *Enterococcus* and *Clostridium difficile* infections following change to tympanic thermometers. *Infect Control Hosp Epidemiol.* 1998;19:333–336.

20. Brennan DF, Falk JL, Rothrock SG, et al. Reliability of infrared tympanic thermometry in the detection of rectal fever in children [see comment]. *Ann Emerg Med.* 1995;25:21–30.

21. Petersen-Smith A, Barber N, Coody DK, et al. Comparison of aural infrared with traditional rectal temperatures in children from birth to age three years. *J Pediatr.* 1994;125:83–85.

22. Freed GL, Fraley JK. Lack of agreement of tympanic membrane temperature assessments with conventional methods in a private practice setting [see comment]. *Pediatrics.* 1992;89:384–386.

23. Hooker EA. Use of tympanic thermometers to screen for fever in patients in a pediatric emergency department. *South Med J.* 1993;86:855–858.

24. Milewski A, Ferguson KL, Terndrup TE. Comparison of pulmonary artery, rectal, and tympanic membrane temperatures in adult intensive care unit patients. *Clin Pediatr.* 1991;30[4 Suppl]:13–16; discussion 34–35.

25. Terndrup TE. An appraisal of temperature assessment by infrared emission detection tympanic thermometry. *Ann Emerg Med.* 1992;21:1483–1492.

26. Nobel JJ. Infrared ear thermometry. *Pediatr Emerg Care.* 1992;8:54–58.

27. Pransky SM. The impact of technique and conditions of the tympanic membrane upon infrared tympanic thermometry. *Clin Pediatr.* 1991;30[4 Suppl]:50–52; discussion 60.

28. Terndrup TE, Wong A. Influence of otitis media on the correlation between rectal and auditory canal temperatures. *Am J Dis Child.* 1991;145:75–78.

29. Kelly B, Alexander D. Effect of otitis media on infrared tympanic thermometry. *Clin Pediatr.* 1991;30[4 Suppl]:46–48; discussion 49.

30. Chamberlain JM, Grandner J, Rubinoff JL, et al. Comparison of a tympanic thermometer to rectal and oral thermometers in a pediatric emergency department. *Clin Pediatr.* 1991;30[4 Suppl]:24–29; discussion 34–35.

31. Zehner WJ, Terndrup TE. The impact of moderate ambient temperature variance on the relationship between oral, rectal, and tympanic membrane temperatures. *Clin Pediatr.* 1991;30[4 Suppl]:61–64; discussion 71–72.

32. Kenney RD, Fortenberry JD, Surratt SS, et al. Evaluation of an infrared tympanic membrane thermometer in pediatric patients. *Pediatrics.* 1990;85:854–858.

33. Rhoads FA, Grandner J. Assessment of an aural infrared sensor for body temperature measurement in children. *Clin Pediatr.* 1990;29:112–115.

34. Talo H, Macknin ML, Medendorp SV. Tympanic membrane temperatures compared to rectal and oral temperatures. *Clin Pediatr.* 1991;30[4 Suppl]:30–33; discussion 34–35.

35. Terndrup TE, Milewski A. The performance of two tympanic thermometers in a pediatric emergency department. *Clin Pediatr.* 1991;30[4 Suppl]:18–23; discussion 34–35.

36. Pompei F, Pompei M. Arterial thermometry via heat balance at the ear. *Med Electron.* 1996;27:86–91.

37. *Exergen Temporal Artery Thermometer: Instructions for Use.* Watertown, MA, Exergen Corporation; 2002.

38. Greenes DS, Fleisher GR. Accuracy of a noninvasive temporal artery thermometer for use in infants. *Arch Pediatr Adolesc Med.* 2001;155:376–381.

39. Greenes DS, Fleisher G. When body temperature changes, does rectal temperature lag? *J Pediatr.* 2004;144:824–826.

40. Siberry GK, Diener-West M, Schappell E, et al. Comparison of temple temperatures with rectal temperatures in children under two years of age. *Clin Pediatr.* 2002;41:405–414.

41. Schuh S, Komar L, Stephens D, et al. Comparison of the temporal artery and rectal thermometry in children in the emergency department. *Pediatr Emerg Care.* 2004;20:736–741.

42. Callanan D. Detecting fever in young infants: reliability of perceived, pacifier, and temporal artery temperatures in infants younger than 3 months of age. *Pediatr Emerg Care.* 2003;19:240–243.

6

ROBERT C. LUTEN

Emergent Drug Dosing and Equipment Selection

▶ INTRODUCTION

Most procedures performed in the emergency department (ED) do not require rapid selection of drugs and equipment. Although the majority of ED procedures are of an urgent or nonelective nature, the clinician usually has adequate time for the measurement of a patient's weight, the selection of equipment, and the calculation of drug dosages required before performing a procedure. Examples include the suturing of lacerations, the reduction of fractures, and suprapubic aspirations.

Some procedures, however, do not afford the clinician the luxury of a preparation period. These procedures must be done immediately. Failure to act expeditiously can cause loss of life or limb. There is no time to obtain an accurate weight on a patient. Efforts spent in equipment selection and drug dosage calculation only exacerbate the lack of time. Anxiety produced when faced with this dilemma, as well as error from inaccurate drug dosage calculation and equipment selection, compounds the problem. An example is endotracheal intubation, which requires proper-sized laryngoscopes, endotracheal tubes, and suction catheters as well as medications for rapid sequence induction of anesthesia.

The advent of organized, educational, resuscitative efforts for adults (advanced cardiac life support [ACLS]) and children (pediatric advanced life support [PALS]) brought about attempts to solve drug dosage and equipment selection problems, as it became clear that this area of resuscitation was fraught with error and delays (I). The need to spend time addressing drug dosing and equipment selection in pediatric emergency situations is an added logistical difficulty not present in adult resuscitation, as drugs are usually packaged in prefilled syringes containing the standard resuscitation dose,

and equipment sizes vary little. The sum total of the difficulties encountered increases the provider's mental burden, referred to as the "cognitive load" of pediatric resuscitation (2). These logistical activities can detract from the provider's "critical thinking time" and hence his or her ability to evaluate, synthesize, and prioritize information and make decisions, which are necessary for successful resuscitation management. To the extent that resuscitation aids can reduce the logistics of pediatric resuscitation by eliminating calculations for drug dosing, equipment selection, and other size-related therapy issues, such as ventilator settings and fluid therapy, care can be facilitated and efforts optimized. Table 6.1 compares various types of resuscitation aids and their relative merits.

Following is a description the Broselow tape and its application in emergent therapy. The Broselow tape is a length-measuring tape that estimates patient weight (Fig. 6.1A). Emergent drug dosages and drug volumes, as well as equipment, can be read directly from the tape. Studies have validated the accuracy of the tape in weight estimation for drug dosing (3) and for equipment selection (4). A more recent enhancement to the tape, referred to as the "Broselow-Luten system," incorporates multiple additional medications and therapeutic information in various formats. In simulation studies, use of the system in common emergent situations has been demonstrated to reduce time and errors (5).

▶ PROCEDURE

The child is measured in the recumbent position, the likely posture during critical care interventions (Fig. 6.1B). The tape is stretched from the crown of the head to the heel. It is not crucial to measure to the nearest millimeter, nor to

TABLE 6.1	EVALUATION OF METHODS FOR SELECTION OF PEDIATRIC EQUIPMENT AND DRUG DOSAGES					
Weight-based methods			**Length-based methods**		
Memory	**Drug equipment cards**	**Precalculated equipment cards and computer printouts**	**Length-based chart (Table 6.2)**	**First 5 minutes**	**Broselow-Luten system**
3 steps	2 steps	1 step	2 steps	2+ steps	1 step
1. Recollection of dose 2. Weight estimation 3. Calculation 4. Associated with anxiety and error	Associated with anxiety and error Require calculation in crisis situation Associated with error, 1/10 or 10X common	Associated with anxiety and error	Measure and access chart Minimal anxiety and error	Measurement, determination of habitus, then reference to a book Minimal anxiety and error	Measure and read directly from tape or reference materials Minimal anxiety and error

Legend: Progressing from left to right increases accuracy and decreases anxiety, error, and time lost. All weight-based methods are only as accurate as the clinicians weight estimation. The same is true for formulas used to predict equipment size, which are based on age or weight.

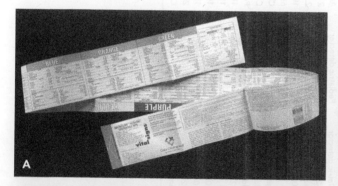

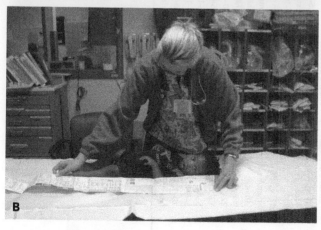

Figure 6.1
A. The Broselow tape.
B. The child is measured in the recumbent position, from crown to heel.
C. A page from the companion *Resuscitation Medication Manual* (the purple, or 10- to 11-kg, page), which provides respective drug volumes from available product concentrations and pertinent preparation and administration information.

TABLE 6.2   LENGTH-BASED EQUIPMENT SELECTION GUIDE

Item	Length (cm)							
	60-66	66-75	75-85	85-97	97-109	109-120	120-133	133-147
ET tube size (mm)	3.5	3.5	4.0	4.5	5.0	5.5	6.0	6.5
Lip-tip length (cm)	10-10.5	10.5-11	11-12	12.5-13.5	14-15	15.5-16.5	17-18	18.5-19.5
ETCO$_2$	Pediatric detector	Pediatric detector	Pediatric detector	Pediatric detector	Adult detector	Adult detector	Adult detector	Adult detector
LMA	1.5	1.5	1.5-2	2	2	2-2.5	2.5	3
Laryngoscope	1 straight	1 straight	1 straight	2 straight	2 straight or curved	2 straight or curved	2-3 straight or curved	3 straight or curved
Suction catheter	8F	8F	8-10F	10F	10F	10F	10F	12F
Stylet	6F	6F	6F	6F	6F	14F	14F	14F
Oral airway	Infant/small child	Infant/small child	Small child	Child	Child	Child/small adult	Child/small adult	Medium adult
Bag-valve-mask	Infant	Infant	Child	Child	Child	Child	Child/adult	Adult
O$_2$ mask	Newborn	Newborn	Child	Child	Pediatric	Adult	Adult	Adult
Vascular access	22-24/23-25	22-24/23-25	20-22/23-25	18-22/21-23	18-22/21-23	18-20/21-23	18-20/21-22	16-20/18-21
Intraosseus	18/15#	18/15#	15#	15#	15#	15#	15#	15#
Nasogastric tube	5-8F	5-8F	8-10F	10F	10-12F	12-14F	14-18F	18F
Urinary catheter	5-8F	5-8F	8-10F	10F	10-12F	10-12F	12F	12F
Chest tube	10-12F	10-12F	16-20F	20-24F	20-24F	24-32F	28-32F	32-40F
Blood pressure cuff	Newborn, infant	Newborn, infant	Infant, child	Child	Child	Child	Child/adult	Adult

DRUGS	**EQUIPMENT**	**FLUIDS**
Paralytic Agents	BVMs	Volume Expansion
Succinylcholine	ET Tubes	Maintenance Fluids
Pancuronium	Stylets	
Vecuronium	Suction Catheters	**OTHER**
Defasciculating	Oral Airway	**INFORMATION**
Agents	O2 Masks	Ventilator Settings
Pancuronium	NG Tubes	Pediatric Trauma
Vecuronium	Urinary Catheters	Score
Infusions	Chest Tubes	Abnormal Vital
Isoproterenol	Vascular Access	Signs
Epinephrine	Modalities	
Norepinephrine	Seizure	
Dopamine	Diazepam (IV & PR)	
Dobutamine	Phenobarbital	
Lidocaine	Phenytoin	
PGE	Lorazepam	
Nitroprusside	Resuscitation	
Nitroglycerine	Epinephrine	
Amrinone	Atropine	
ICP Agents	Sodium Bicarbonate	
Mannitol	Calcium Choride	
Furosemide	Lidocaine	
Overdose	Defibrillation Doses	
D25W	Cardioversion Doses	
Naloxone		

Figure 6.2 Drugs, equipment, and other emergency modalities contained on the Broselow tape.

TABLE 6.3 | EQUIPMENT SELECTION: CLINICAL GUIDELINES

The following suggested guidelines are specific to each piece of equipment to ensure that the appropriate size is used. Never use force to achieve fit.

Bag-valve-mask. The mask of the BVM apparatus should cover the nose and mouth of the patient (from the bridge of the nose to the cleft of the chin) and form a tight seal, not allowing air leaks. Regardless of the size of the bag or patient, one should always start with the smallest tidal volumes, increasing in increments quickly until chest rise is obtained.

Endotracheal tubes. Select one size larger (0.5 mm larger) and one size smaller for a backup. Do not force the tubes through the vocal cords.

Stylets/suction catheters. Tape and store the appropriate size suction catheters to the ET tube for quick access. The stylet should not extend beyond the end of the ET tube.

Oral airways. Size can be estimated by placing the proximal end of the airway at the teeth. The correct size will have the distal end at the level of the lower border of the angle of the mandible.

Blood pressure cuffs. In general, the width of the cuff should cover a minimum of two-thirds of the child's upper arm.

Nasogastric tubes. Tube length can be estimated by placing the tube in line externally from the tip of the nose to the ear and then from the ear to just below the rib cage. Position should be confirmed by injecting a volume of air while listening over the stomach.

Urinary catheters. The catheter should easily pass through the external meatus.

Chest tubes. In general, small-diameter tubes are used to evacuate air, and larger-diameter tubes are used to evacuate blood. The largest tube that fits comfortably between the ribs may be used if needed.

Vascular access. For shock, the largest possible catheter should be used, and ideally two lines should be inserted. For drug administration in cardiac arrest, catheter size is less of a concern. There are no established guidelines for the size of the intraosseus needle. Many clinicians prefer the smaller 18# needle for smaller children (pink, red, and purple zones) and the 15# needle for older children (white, blue, orange, and green zones). There are currently no age restrictions on the use of intraosseus needles.

Laryngeal mask apparatus (LMA). These guidelines are derived from the manufacturer's weight-based guidelines. Clinical judgment should be used with patients who are outliers (i.e., morbidly obese or emaciated).

End-tidal CO_2 colorimetric detectors. Use the pediatric end-tidal CO_2 detector for children up to approximately 14 kg (pink, red, purple, and yellow zones) and the adult detector for children who are 15 kg and above (white, blue, orange, and green zones). The pediatric detector can be used in the larger children but should be removed immediately after CO_2 detection, as the small caliber of the unit impedes air flow. The adult unit will not function reliably in smaller children, as relative gas flow is minimal.

SUMMARY

1 Access the Broselow tape, if available, and use it as described.

2 In lieu of the Broselow tape, measure the patient and access the length-based chart (Table 6.2) for the selection of appropriate resuscitation equipment.

3 Clinical guidelines can be used if no measurement system is available and are also helpful to confirm the fit of selected equipment.

obsess over perfect straightening of the child. There are 11 "weight spaces," including 3-, 4-, 5-kg zones and eight larger zones, ranging from a 6- to 7-kg zone to a zone spanning 30 to 36 kg. Each weight zone is assigned a color to distinguish it from the others. Drugs and other modalities incorporated into the Broselow tape are shown in Figure 6.2.

▶ SUMMARY

Table 6.2 may be used as an adjunct for equipment selection. Using a single length measurement in centimeters, the clinician can access pediatric equipment using this chart.

The Broselow tape permits immediate access to precalculated drug doses as well as the direct selection of equipment from the tape by means of a single length measurement. Table 6.3 gives clinical guidelines for equipment selection that can be used in the event that no measuring tape or Broselow tape is available, and these are also valuable as a way to confirm the measurement guidelines.

▶ REFERENCES

1. Oakley PA. Inaccuracy and delay in decision-making in pediatric resuscitation and a proposed reference chart to reduce error. *Br Med J.* 1988;297:817–819.

2. Luten R, Wears R, Broselow J, et al. Managing the unique size related issues of pediatric resuscitation: reducing cognitive load with resuscitation aids. *Acad Emerg Med.* 2002;9:840–847.

3. Lubitz DS, Seidel JA, Chameides L, et al. A rapid method for estimating weight and resuscitation drug dosages for length in the pediatric age group. *Ann Emerg Med.* 1988;17:576–581.

4. Luten RC, Wears RL, Broselow J, et al. Length-based endotracheal tube sizing for pediatric resuscitation. *Ann Emerg Med.* 1992;21: 900–904.

5. Shah AN, Frush KS. Reduction in error severity associated with use of a pediatric medication dosing system: a crossover trial involving simulated resuscitation events. *Arch Pediatr Adolesc Med.* 2003;157:229–236.

CHRISTINE S. CHO AND EVALINE A. ALESSANDRINI

7

Aseptic Technique

▶ INTRODUCTION

Aseptic technique is used to prevent the access of micro-organisms to a sterile field where a procedure or operation is being performed. The word "antisepsis" derives from the Greek and means "against putrefaction." The concept of antisepsis was recognized in the mid-19th century by Oliver Wendell Holmes when he observed that a physician performing an autopsy was infected and subsequently killed by the same disease as the patient being autopsied. This knowledge resulted in improved handwashing and changing of clothing during some procedures. In 1867, Lister published his first description of "antiseptic principles," coincident with the discovery of bacteria and their role in wound infection.

Aseptic technique employs several methods: the use of sterile instruments and antiseptic hand scrubs; the wearing of sterile gowns, gloves, caps, and masks by personnel; and the cleansing of the patient's skin with antiseptics. Other modalities are included in aseptic technique. *Sterilization* is the ultimate in disinfection, for it is defined as the process of killing all micro-organisms by either physical or chemical agents. Steam under pressure is the most commonly used method of sterilizing instruments for pediatric procedures. An *antiseptic* is a chemical agent applied to the body that kills or inhibits the growth of pathogenic organisms. A *disinfectant* is a chemical substance used on inanimate objects, such as floors and countertops, to eliminate bacteria.

Aseptic technique is an important prelude to many of the other procedures described in this text. Proper aseptic technique should be used by physicians, nurses, and other health professionals performing pediatric procedures to eliminate potentially serious infectious complications.

▶ ANATOMY AND PHYSIOLOGY

The anatomy of the skin and its microbial inhabitants must be understood in order to properly perform aseptic technique. Two types of micro-organisms are causative in both skin and wound infections and have been termed "resident flora" and "transient flora." Resident flora are those bacteria that live and grow in the skin and can be repetitively cultured from it. These micro-organisms live in the cracks and dead cells of the horny layer of the skin. Most organisms are of low virulence and include *Staphylococcus epidermidis*, micrococci, and diphtheroids such as *Propionibacterium acnes*. Transient skin flora coexist with the resident flora in the horny skin layer and are barred from deeper skin invasion by the cells of the tightly packed stratum corneum. The transient organisms are acquired by contact with colonized or infected materials, often in the hospital environment. Subsequently these organisms are more likely to be resistant to many antibiotics and responsible for nosocomial infections. *Staphylococcus aureus* and Gram-negative enterobacteria are frequently identified as transient flora. The goal of cleansing and preparing the skin with antiseptics is to remove the transient bacteria and reduce the levels of resident flora to a low level.

These potentially infectious micro-organisms must be removed from both the patient and the health care provider. It is important to understand the bacterial load of various areas of the body, for it has been determined that when organism counts exceed 10^5 per square centimeter, infection is more likely (1). Organisms are actually sparse on the palms and dorsa of the hands. However, most hand flora are harbored under the nails and around the lateral nail folds, achieving counts of 10^4 to 10^6 per square centimeter. Most of the body surface, including the trunk, arms, and legs, are colonized with only a few thousand organisms per square centimeter. Other moist places, such as the perineum, axilla, and intertriginous areas, harbor millions of bacteria per square centimeter. These bacterial counts must be considered in the preparation of a field during aseptic technique.

The physiology of the body and its relation to aseptic technique has been reviewed. The physical characteristics of barriers used in aseptic technique are also important. Various barrier methods are used in aseptic technique to eliminate the passage of micro-organisms onto the sterile field, including caps, masks, gloves, and gowns worn by the health care providers as well as sterile drapes to define and preserve the boundaries of the sterile field. Masks should be worn, especially by those with upper respiratory tract infections, to decrease the transmission of respiratory flora to the sterile field. Speaking while wearing a mask promotes leaking of respiratory flora from the sides of the mask and so should be kept at a minimum during procedures. Gowns and gloves are worn to provide a barrier to the transfer of the physicians' bacterial flora to patients. Gowns impermeable to moisture prevent the wicklike effect of transferring bacteria from one side of a gown to the other. Latex gloves, and to a lesser extent vinyl gloves, serve as protective barriers to the transmission of bacteria from health care workers' hands. However, bacteria multiply under moist gloves, and hand contamination can occur even when gloves are worn, so handwashing is recommended routinely after gloves are removed (2).

▶ INDICATIONS

Aseptic technique is indicated to minimize the risk of infectious complications from various invasive procedures. Such procedures in the pediatric emergency setting typically include lumbar puncture, urethral catheterization, suprapubic bladder aspiration, central venous and arterial access procedures, thoracentesis, chest tube placement, paracentesis, joint aspiration, tapping of a cerebrospinal fluid (CSF) shunt, and wound repair. The need for aseptic technique in laceration repair has never been proven, and one randomized trial found similar wound infection rates whether sterile or nonsterile gloves were used (3).

Good judgment, as well as specific institutional guidelines, should be used in determining the level of aseptic technique necessary for a given procedure. The following list details what level of aseptic technique is recommended for various procedures:

Full aseptic technique (cap, mask, gown, gloves, drapes, and skin preparation)
　　Central venous and arterial access procedures
　　Thoracentesis
　　Paracentesis
　　Chest tube placement

Aseptic technique, including skin preparation, draping, and sterile gloves
　　Lumbar puncture
　　Wound repair
　　Tapping a cerebrospinal fluid shunt
Partial aseptic technique (skin preparation and sterile gloves)
　　Suprapubic bladder aspiration
　　Urethral catheterization
　　Joint aspiration

There are no true contraindications to aseptic technique. Latex sensitivity must be considered in patients at risk, especially those with spina bifida. Although allergies to the various antiseptic solutions are rare, a history of sensitivity to povidone-iodine or other antiseptics must be elicited.

▶ EQUIPMENT

Cap
Disposable mask
Sterile gown
Sterile gloves
Antiseptic solution
Disposable sponges or gauze pads with hemostats
Sterile drapes

Sterile gowns and drapes may be purchased in disposable, single-use types, which are often made of waterproof material that is nonwoven and therefore not likely to be penetrated by bacteria. More traditional woven cloth can also be used. Woven gowns and drapes may be reused after laundering but should be washed no more than 75 times to maintain their barrier integrity (4).

If disposable sponges are not available, fine-pore (90 pores per inch) $4'' \times 4''$ gauze pads may be soaked in a disinfectant and used to cleanse the field.

Any type of sterile glove may be used, although studies have shown that latex gloves are more protective and resistant to organism penetration than vinyl gloves (2). The use of double gloving has been shown to improve barrier protection in the operating room and reduce occupational exposure to patients' bloodborne pathogens (5). Although it has not been studied in the emergency department, double gloving should be considered for full aseptic procedures and when trying to maximize protection against potential exposures.

Several types of antiseptic solutions are available for preparation of the sterile field and handwashing. The most commonly used antiseptics are summarized in Table 7.1. Povidone-iodine solution is often used for skin preparation because of its highly bactericidal effects against both Gram-positive and Gram-negative organisms (6,7). Chlorhexidine may also be used for skin preparation in the event that a hypersensitivity to povidone-iodine exists. Chlorhexidine is the

TABLE 7.1	TABLE OF SKIN ANTISEPTICS			
Antiseptic	**Uses**	**Antibacterial spectrum**	**Benefits**	**Drawbacks**
Povidone-iodine scrub "Betadine scrub"	Handwashing	Highly bactericidal against Gram-positive and Gram-negative organisms	Nontoxic	Minimally toxic to wound tissue
Povidone-iodine solution "Betadine solution"	Skin preparation	As above	Can be used for large body surface areas	Iodism rare Stains skin temporarily
Chlorhexidine "Hibiclens"	Handwashing	Highly bactericidal against Gram-positive organisms, less bactericidal against Gram-negative organisms	Persistent protective residue after single handwashing Rarely causes dermatitis	Ototoxicity or corneal damage if instilled in middle ear or eye
Chlorhexidine "ChloraPrep"	Skin preparation	As above	Superior to povidone-iodine for central line placement	As above Activity is formulation dependent
Hexachlorophene "pHisoHex"	Handwashing	Good activity against Gram-positive organisms, poor against Gram-negative organisms	Persistent protective residue after handwashing	Teratogenic CNS toxicity with repeated usage
Benzalkonium chloride "Zephiran"	Handwashing	Effective against Gram-positive and Gram-negative organisms	None; use not often recommended	Storage prone to contamination Inactivated by soaps and detergents
Alcohols	Skin preparation	Effective against Gram-positive and Gram-negative organisms	Organic solvent; removes oil and debris	Requires 2 minutes of moist application to achieve good antisepsis Drying effect on skin Volatile and flammable when stored
Para-chloro-meta-xylenol	Handwashing	Good activity against Gram-positive organisms, less active against Gram-negative organisms	Persistent protective residue after handwashing	May be less effective than chlorhexidine and povidone-iodine
Triclosan	Handwashing	Effective against Gram-positive and Gram-negative organisms	Persistent protective residue after handwashing	Activity is formulation dependent

antiseptic of choice for handwashing because it leaves a protective bactericidal residue on the skin after cleansing. It is also the antiseptic of choice for insertion of central venous or arterial access. Two percent chlorhexidine is superior to iodine in preventing line colonization and infection (8–10). Chlorhexidine does not stain or cause dermatitis, reactions which are often encountered when povidone-iodine scrub is used for handwashing (6,7). Hexachlorophene, benzalkonium chloride, para-chloro-meta-xylenol, triclosan, and alcohols are infrequently used, for reasons listed in Table 7.1 (11).

▶ PROCEDURE

Operator Preparation

An orderly approach to aseptic technique will ensure the best results. First, a cap is worn and a mask is placed snugly over the mouth and nose and tied securely behind the head. Use of an appropriate method of handwashing comes next. Friction with soap and water is adequate to remove transient flora for procedures such as urethral catheterizations and lumbar punctures. However, a scrub of several minutes with an antiseptic such as chlorhexidine has broad antibacterial activity, sustains suppressant action on the skin flora, and is beneficial in more invasive procedures such as chest tube placement (1). Special attention to the lateral nail folds and nail tips is necessary to

eliminate the majority of organisms. At this point, a sterile gown is donned.

Two methods of gloving are used for aseptic procedures. The first is the *closed method*, which is used in the operating room and will not be described further. The *open method* (12) is more commonly used in the ED and will be described here (Fig. 7.1). Before scrubbing or washing the hands, the outer wrapper of the gloves is opened. If the procedure requires gowning, it is done before glove placement, with the cuffs of the gown pulled over the hands from inside the sleeve by an assistant.

Placement of the Right Glove

First the inner glove cover is opened. By convention, the right glove is placed first. The right glove is grasped by the left fingers at the folded cuff end and lifted up. The right hand is then placed inside the right glove while the left hand continues to pull out the glove cuff until it hits the cuff of the gown. Avoid contamination of the gown with the nonsterile left hand.

Placement of the Left Glove

The left glove is picked up with the right fingers by the folded cuff. The right gloved fingers are then placed under the left glove cuff and the glove is pulled onto the left hand until it hits the gown cuff. The cuff of the left glove is unfolded by the right hand, which is still slid under the left glove cuff. Finally, the right glove cuff is turned by sliding the left gloved

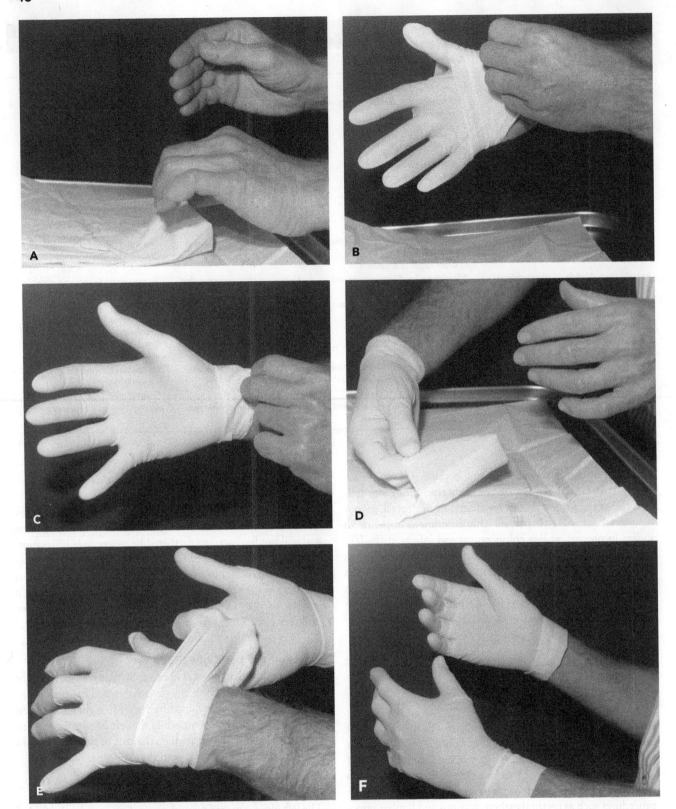

Figure 7.1
A. The operator picks up the cuffed end of the right glove.
B. The right glove is pulled over the right hand
C. and left cuffed.
D. The gloved right hand is placed under the left glove cuff.
E. The left glove is pulled over the left hand, and then the left glove is uncuffed with an unfolding motion by the right hand.
F. The left hand is now ready to uncuff the right glove by (*continued*)

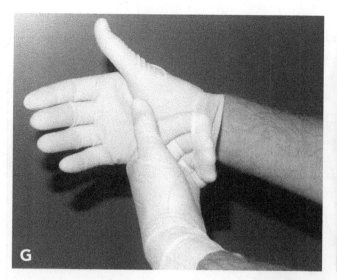

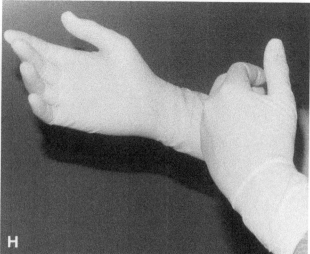

Figure 7.1 (*Continued*).
G. sliding into the right cuff
H. and unfolding it.

fingers under the right glove cuff and unfolding it over the right gown cuff.

Field Preparation

It is important to change gloves if they break or touch any non-sterile objects. Gloves should be kept at waist level or above and should always be easily visible to prevent any inadvertent contamination. Skin preparation is performed next (Fig. 7.2). It begins at the incision or procedure site with a concentric motion that starts centrally and moves peripherally. The antiseptic is placed on a sterile sponge and rubbed on firmly. A new sponge is used when returning to the central site, and the procedure is repeated four times. Preparation of a dirty or infected area, as in the incision and drainage of an abscess, is performed differently. It begins at the outer boundaries and continues toward the incision site (peripheral to central) so that bacteria are not spread from a dirty site to a clean surface. Each subsequent preparation begins approximately 0.5 cm inside the outer boundaries of the first wash (12). Draping is done immediately after the antiseptic preparation is completed.

Sterile drapes are used to establish a sterile field around the area in which a procedure is performed. They provide a barrier to minimize the passage of micro-organisms from nonsterile to sterile sites. Drapes should be held higher than the level of the physician's waist and the bed on which the procedure is performed. Draping is done from the operative or "clean" site to the periphery, using either two or three drapes, as illustrated in Figure 7.3.A,B. The draping material is cuffed back over the gloved hands to preserve the sterility of the gloves. Once a drape is in place, it should not be moved. Excessive handling, which may generate air currents and spread droplets or other particles, must be avoided. The physician should always face the sterile area. If the physician must face the nonsterile

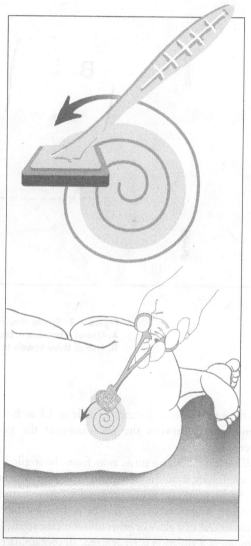

Figure 7.2 Skin preparation for a "clean" procedure such as a lumbar puncture.

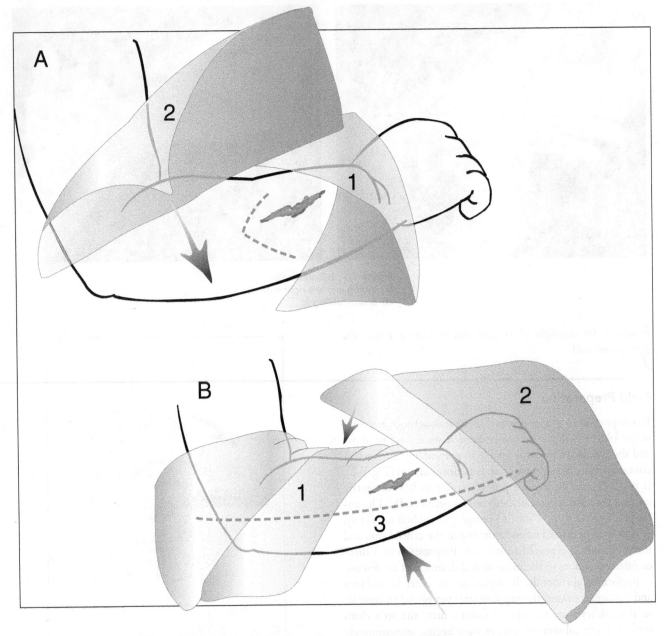

Figure 7.3 Sterile draping to prepare the procedural field.
A. Use of a two-towel technique to create a "diamond-shaped" field.
B. Use of three towels to create a "triangle-shaped" field.

area for any reason, a distance of at least 12 inches should be maintained between the physician and the nonsterile objects (12).

When the physician turns away from the sterile field, the physician's back should again remain 12 inches from the sterile area. At this point, the field is prepared for the initiation of the procedure. Aseptic technique may be violated by the contamination or tear of a glove or other object on the sterile field. At the moment a violation is recognized, all contaminated items must be replaced.

▶ COMPLICATIONS

Performing aseptic technique may potentially be complicated by allergic reactions to either latex gloves or an antiseptic solution. The complication may be minimized by taking a good history before initiation of aseptic technique.

The most unfavorable outcome of improperly performed aseptic technique is an infection at the site of the procedure. This may range from a urinary tract infection as the result of an improperly performed urethral catheterization to

SUMMARY

1 Elicit a history of relevant allergies, such as allergies to latex, antiseptics, etc.

2 Gauge the level of aseptic technique to the invasiveness of the procedure.

3 Perform handwashing with an emphasis on nail tips and lateral nail folds.

4 The proper order is as follows: cap, mask, handwashing, gown, gloves, skin preparation, and draping.

5 Prepare the skin from the procedure site to the periphery for "clean" procedures and from the periphery to the procedure site for "dirty" procedures.

a bacteremic illness as the result of an infection from central line placement. Clinicians may avoid complications by strict adherence to aseptic technique and rapid correction of any recognized violations.

▶ ACKNOWLEDGMENT

The authors would like to acknowledge the valuable contributions of Jacalyn S. Maller to the version of this chapter that appeared in the previous edition.

▶ REFERENCES

1. Steere AC, Mallison GF. Handwashing practices for the prevention of nosocomial infections. *Ann Intern Med.* 1975;83:683–690.
2. Olsen RJ, Lynch P, Coyle MB, et al. Examination gloves as barriers to hand contamination in clinical practice. *JAMA.* 1993;270:350–353.
3. Perelman VS, Francis GJ, Rutledge T, et al. Sterile versus nonsterile gloves for repair of uncomplicated lacerations in the emergency department: a randomized controlled trial. *Ann Emerg Med.* 2004;43:362–370.
4. Beck WC. Aseptic barriers in surgery: their present status. *Arch Surg.* 1981;116:240–244.
5. Graves PB, Twomey CL. The changing face of hand protection. *AORN J.* 2002;76:246–264.
6. Kaul AF, Jewett JF. Agents and techniques for disinfection of the skin. *Surg Gynecol Obstetr.* 1981;152:677–685.
7. Sebben JE. Surgical antiseptics. *J Am Acad Derm.* 1983;9:759–765.
8. Maki DG, Ringer M, Alvarado CJ. Prospective randomized trial of povidone-iodine, alcohol, and chlorhexidine for prevention of infection associated with central venous and arterial catheters. *Lancet.* 1991;338:339–343.
9. Mimoz O, Pieroni L, Lawrence C, et al. Prospective, randomized trial of two antiseptic solutions for prevention of central venous or arterial catheter colonization and infection in intensive care unit patients. *Crit Care Med.* 1996;24:1818–1823.
10. O'Grady NP, Alexander M, Dellinger P, et al. Guidelines for the prevention of intravascular catheter-related infections. *Pediatrics.* 2002;110(5):e51.
11. Larson EL. APIC Guideline for handwashing and hand antisepsis in health care settings. *Am J Infect Control.* 1995;23:251–269.
12. Brooks SM. *Fundamentals of Operating Room Nursing.* St. Louis: Mosby; 1975:65–69, 96–99, 100–102.

8

JASON Y. KIM AND LOUIS M. BELL

Protecting the Health Professional Against Hazardous Exposures

▶ INTRODUCTION

Health care workers (HCWs) practice medicine in a potentially dangerous environment. Occupational health hazards include infectious, chemical, and radioactive exposures. The high volume, high acuity, and unscheduled nature of emergency medicine practice make emergency health professionals unique in their potential for such exposures. This is particularly important in the practice of pediatric emergency medicine, where infectious disease and accidental poisoning are commonly encountered. HCWs need to be aware of and continually educated about their risks from hazardous exposures. This chapter provides an overview of the risks associated with occupational exposure to infectious, chemical, and radioactive agents. Guidelines for exposure prevention and control are discussed.

▶ INFECTIOUS DISEASE EXPOSURES

Microbiologic Considerations

HCWs are at risk of acquiring many different infectious diseases, which can be transmitted via blood, respiratory secretions, and other body fluids. Routes of exposure to infectious agents include percutaneous inoculation of and contact with nonintact skin or mucous membranes by contaminated blood or body fluids. More than 20 different infectious diseases can be transmitted via blood-contaminated or body fluid–contaminated needles. Of particular importance among these agents are human immunodeficiency virus (HIV), hepatitis C virus (HCV), and hepatitis B virus (HBV). Expo-

sure by aerosol droplets from the respiratory tract of infected patients and direct contact with infected secretions can place the HCW at risk of acquiring many serious infections. These include tuberculosis, measles, varicella, pertussis, cytomegalovirus, meningococcus, pneumococcus, and adenovirus infections.

Indications

The care of pediatric emergency department patients is highly procedure oriented. Medical and trauma resuscitations are particularly high-risk situations that place the HCW in close contact with blood and other body fluid secretions. Close patient contact makes occupational exposure to infectious diseases common for emergency medicine HCWs in their everyday practice. This is particularly true for pediatric emergency medicine HCWs because children do not routinely have good hygienic practices and, in comparison to adults, have an increased incidence of infections. Precautions to limit HCW exposure and prevent occupational acquisition of infectious diseases are indicated in virtually every emergency department (ED) encounter and rest on two fundamental principles: most infectious diseases are contagious before the patient and HCW are aware of the diagnosis, and following infection control guidelines will help prevent transmission.

Procedures

Guidelines for Infection Control
Hospital employee health services should provide annual or biannual screening for each HCW, including Mantoux skin

testing for tuberculosis, annual influenza vaccination, and, for those regularly exposed to blood, vaccination against HBV if the HCW is without HBV immunity. In addition, the HCW's immunity to varicella, rubella, measles, mumps, pertussis, and polio, either by history of disease or by immunization, should be documented. If protective immunity is lacking, the appropriate vaccine should be administered. For infections that are not preventable by vaccination, such as adenovirus conjunctivitis, the HCW should be counseled about the risks of exposure. Some infections pose increased risk for pregnant HCWs, and these are discussed later in this chapter.

Needlestick Injuries

There are approximately 384,000 needlestick injuries per year among all HCWs, and about 60% are associated with hollow-bore needles. (1). Despite a 6% to 30% risk of infection with HBV to a hepatitis B surface antibody-negative HCW following a needlestick exposure from a hepatitis B surface antigen-positive patient, HCWs paid little attention to needlestick injuries in the ED before the HIV-AIDS epidemic. In the current era, acquisition of HIV by needlestick injury is associated with significant morbidity, from either HIV infection itself or from antiretroviral therapy. Percutaneous exposure to the blood of an HIV-infected patient places the HCW at an approximate 0.3% risk of acquiring HIV infection (2,3). Nonparenteral (mucous membrane and nonintact skin) exposure to the blood of an HIV-infected patient is associated with a decreased rate of acquisition. The risk of acquisition following percutaneous exposure to certain other body fluids of an HIV-infected patient is unknown. The likelihood of a HCW becoming infected at work with HIV or other bloodborne pathogens depends on the rate of parenteral or nonparenteral exposure to the blood of an infected patient and the local prevalence of the infection. As of 2001, 57 HCWs have been reported to the Centers for Disease Control and Prevention (CDCP) with HIV seroconversion following an occupational exposure, and 88% of the cases were the result of percutaneous needlestick injury (4). Mucous membrane and skin exposure to blood is a commonplace event in the practice of pediatric emergency medicine (5). Virtually all hospital-related blood contacts involve the hand (5,6). Needlestick injury is less common but does occur. As the prevalence of HIV infection continues to rise, so does the rate at which recognized and unrecognized HIV-infected patients present for emergency care. Several reports from inner-city and non-inner-city EDs have focused attention on the high prevalence rates of HIV infection in adult patients (7–13). Published data on the prevalence rate of HIV among children presenting to the ED are limited (14). With continued adolescent participation in high-risk behaviors and increased survival of vertically infected infants, HIV-infected patients presenting to pediatric EDs are likely to increase in number and not be restricted to inner-city EDs.

Universal Precautions

Recognizing the risks of occupational exposure to HIV and other bloodborne pathogens in health care settings, in 1985 the CDCP published recommendations for preventing HIV transmission in the workplace (15). The CDCP referred to this approach as "universal blood and body fluid precautions" or "universal precautions." The CDCP has subsequently consolidated and updated its recommendations (16–19).

Universal precautions are essentially barrier precautions based on infection control principles designed to prevent parenteral, nonintact skin, and mucous membrane exposures to bloodborne pathogens (20). The tenets include routine use of gloves, masks, protective eyewear, and impervious gowns and ways of preventing injuries when handling needles and sharp instruments. Table 8.1 reviews infection control requirements for exposure to body fluids and procedures performed in the ED.

Universal precautions are currently our best strategy for preventing occupational exposure to blood and body fluids. While postexposure prophylaxis regimens have demonstrated efficacy in reducing the risk of transmission of HIV, their efficacy is not absolute.

Gloves should be worn during all vascular access procedures (e.g., phlebotomy, arterial blood sampling, and intravenous line placement), during examinations of nonintact skin and mucous membranes, and when touching blood and body fluids. Wearing gloves may provide some protection against needlestick injuries (21). Gloves should be changed and hands washed thoroughly after contact with each patient. Handwashing and, when appropriate, glove and gown use are very important procedures in preventing nosocomial infections (22).

Masks and protective eyewear (a face shield will work as both) should be worn to protect the mucous membranes of the face when procedures are performed that could generate a spray of blood or blood-containing body fluids (e.g., wound irrigation, endotracheal intubation, and naso/orogastric tube placement). Impervious gowns should be worn when there is profuse bleeding or procedures are performed that could create splashes of blood or blood-containing body fluids (e.g., arterial line placement, central line placement, cutdown, and thoracostomy tube placement) (Fig. 8.1). Mouth-to-mouth resuscitation should be avoided, and alternative ventilation devices should be used (e.g., bag-valve-mask ventilation).

Needles should never be recapped, bent, or broken by hand. All sharp objects should be handled with exceptional care. Puncture-resistant containers should be used for needle and sharp instrument disposal. These containers should be readily accessible and, if possible, within arm's reach of the working area (Figs. 8.2A,B).

Universal precautions will be useful in preventing the occupational transmission of bloodborne and other pathogens only if HCWs adhere to them. Studies from EDs and other health care settings have demonstrated that use of gloves and other barrier precautions by HCWs is far from universal (23–27). Educational interventions have been somewhat successful

TABLE 8.1	INFECTION CONTROL REQUIREMENTS FOR EXPOSURE TO BODY FLUIDS AND PROCEDURES PERFORMED IN THE EMERGENCY DEPARTMENT			
	Gloves	Mask and protective eyewear	Gown	No precautions required
Body Fluids				
Stool	Yes	No	No	
Urine	Yes	No	No	
Vomitus	Yes	No	No	
Blood	Yes	Optional	Optional	
Oral secretions	Yes	No	No	
Tears				Yes
Procedures				
Venipuncture	Yes	No	No	
Intravenous line	Yes	No	No	
Control of minor bleeding	Yes	No	No	
Control of profuse bleeding	Yes	Yes	Yes	
Endotracheal intubation	Yes	Yes	No	
Naso/orogastric tube placement	Yes	Yes	No	
Tracheostomy care	Yes	Yes	No	
Oral examination	Yes	No	No	
Wound irrigation	Yes	Yes	Optional	
Diaper changing	Yes	No	No	

in improving HCW compliance with universal precautions (28–30). The Occupational Safety and Health Administration (OSHA) issued regulations that mandate HCWs to wear gloves for all phlebotomy procedures in hospitals and that also mandate hospital personnel to train their employees annually regarding the reasons for wearing gloves during all phlebotomy procedures (31). HCWs can be fined for infractions.

The reasons for poor compliance with universal precautions by HCWs are numerous. They include lack of time to put on protective materials, uncomfortable protective materials, failure to remember, judging the patient not high risk, and interference with proficient performance of procedures. In particular, HCWs often complain that they cannot perform vascular access procedures when wearing gloves. However, investigators from Philadelphia reported no difference in the success rate on the first attempt at vascular access with

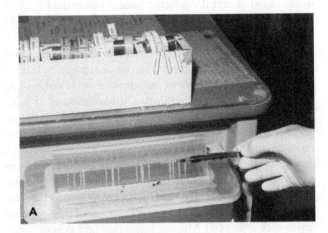

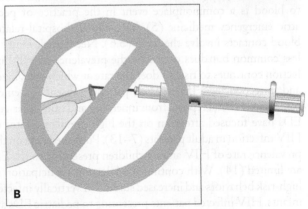

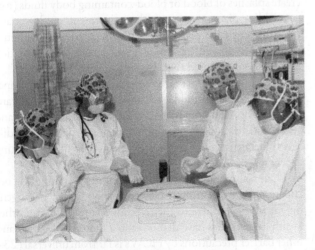

Figure 8.1 The pediatric trauma team prepares for patient arrival with gown, mask, goggles, and gloves.

Figure 8.2
A. The proper disposal of contaminated needles.
B. Needles should never be recapped before disposal.

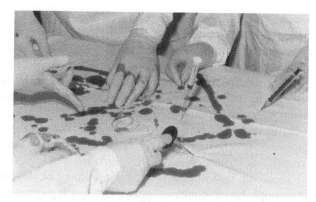

Figure 8.3 Improper, careless scattering of used needles and sharps, including their insertion into a mattress, creates a hazardous environment for health care workers.

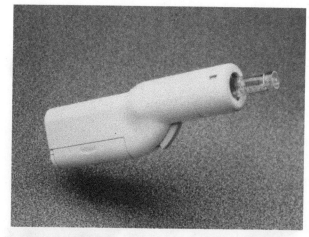

Figure 8.4 The Biojector 2000, an advanced needle-free system for intramuscular and subcutaneous injections, was engineered by Bioject Inc. of Portland, Oregon.

and without wearing gloves by nurses and residents in a pediatric ED (28). HCWs should be advised that retraining can be easily accomplished through practice and patience.

Universal precautions are very effective at protecting against cutaneous and mucous membrane exposures to blood and body fluids. However, percutaneous exposure from needlestick and sharp instrument injuries accounts for the vast majority of occupational HIV and HBV transmissions. In a study of 1,201 HCWs exposed to blood or body fluids of HIV-infected patients, needlestick injuries accounted for 80% of the exposures, and sharp instruments for 8% (32). Exposure causes included manipulating needles (36%), recapping needles (17%), and improper disposal of sharp objects (14%). Two exposures that led to HIV seroconversion resulted from needlestick injuries inflicted by coworkers during resuscitation procedures (Fig. 8.3).

Training and educating HCWs to take extraordinary precautions while handling sharp items is not sufficient. In ad-

dition to implementing universal precautions, hospitals must continue to create a safer working environment for HCWs, government bureaus must continue to enact safety regulation guidelines, and industry must create safer devices (33).

In 2000, the Needlestick Safety and Prevention Act became law, and in response OSHA revised Bloodborne Pathogens Standard 1910.1030. The standard requires employers to provide safer needle devices that have been developed and marketed (20,34,35) with input from HCWs. At least 340 patents for sharp safety devices had been issued, and the U.S. Food and Drug Administration (FDA) had approved for marketing at least 88 needlestick prevention devices (36). Examples of devices to perform procedures with fewer sharp instruments include compressed-air injection systems (Fig. 8.4), needleless i.v. and vial access systems (Fig. 8.5), and needles

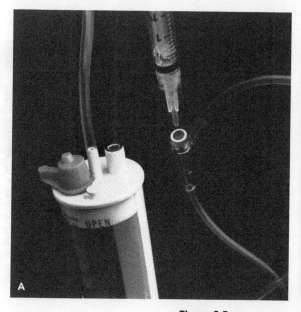
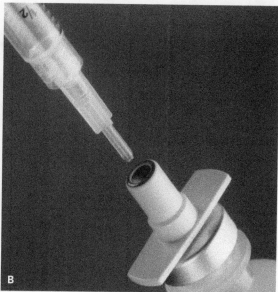

Figure 8.5
A. Representative needleless i.v. tubing system and
B. Needleless vial access system.

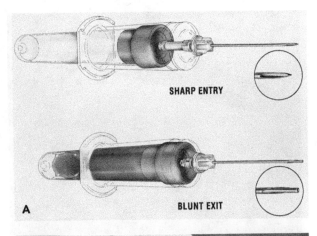

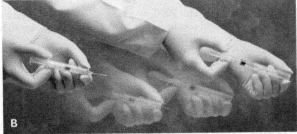

Figure 8.6
A. A "blunt" needle system.
B. A safety syringe with a protective shield.

that can be used and disposed with no risk of injury (Fig. 8.6A,B).

The vast majority of blood contacts by HCWs are cutaneous. Latex gloves provide reliable protection against cutaneous exposure to blood and body fluids; however, they do not preclude needlestick or sharp instrument injuries. Wearing two pair of gloves can decrease the risk of inner-glove perfo-

ration (21). Cut-resistant glove liners designed to be worn under latex gloves are available. Recently, manufacturers have redesigned the suture needle in an attempt to reduce inadvertent needlestick injuries. One product, the Ethiguard Blunt Point needle (Ethicon Products), claims to have reconfigured the tapered end of the needle to reduce needlesticks while maintaining tissue penetration during suturing.

In many EDs, a simple needleless device is used to irrigate wounds, which prevents splash of blood-contaminated irrigation fluid (Fig. 8.7A,B). This product is a clear plastic, parabolic cup that attaches to the tip of a Luer-Lok or slip-tip syringe. Its self-contained nozzle creates a high-pressure stream for irrigation, while the shield protects against contaminated splashback.

Disposable gloves, masks, protective eyewear, impervious gowns, sharp containers, and the newly developed safe needles and other safety devices are expensive, (37); however, they are currently our best protection against occupational acquisition of bloodborne and other pathogens. The benefit of possibly preventing cases of occupationally acquired HIV, HBV, or other infections far outweighs the costs of barrier protective materials and the new safer devices.

Selected Infections That Occur following Exposure to Blood or Secretions

Although the use of universal precautions is the recommended approach in caring for all patients, it is prudent to review some of the more common infections that could affect HCWs. Despite careful adherence to infection control procedures and policies during the management of acutely ill or injured patients, exposures will occur. In evaluating the risk of exposure and infection after exposure, the HCW should consider the infectious agent, the mode of transmission, his or her individual susceptibility, the type of contact exposure, and whether

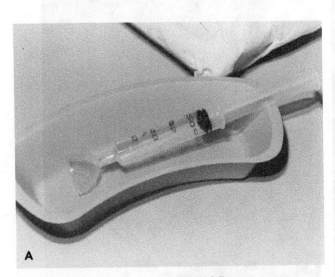

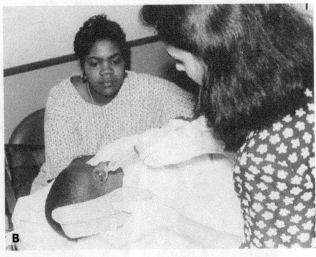

Figure 8.7
A. A clear plastic splash guard attached to an irrigation syringe.
B. Irrigation of a laceration using the syringe–splash guard technique.

TABLE 8.2	SUMMARY OF POTENTIAL INFECTIOUS DISEASES FOLLOWING EXPOSURE TO BLOOD AND SECRETIONS

Infectious agent	Source	Transmission and incubation	Risk of infection after exposure to contaminated blood (needlestick)
Human immunodeficiency virus (HIV)	Blood, bloody secretions, genital secretions of infected person	Intravenous inoculations Splash accidents	0.3% 0.09%[a]
Hepatitis B virus (HBV)	Blood, bloody secretions of infected person or carrier	Intravenous inoculations	26%
Hepatitis C virus (HCV)	Blood, bloody secretions of infected person	Intravenous inoculation	1.8%

[a]Ippolito et al. (ref. 40).

the patient or situation is high risk. Table 8.2 outlines the more common infectious diseases in terms of source of exposure, transmission and incubation, and risk of infection following exposure.

HIV

HCWs exposed to HIV-infected blood or secretions are rarely infected. As of December 2001, 57 HCWs had been reported to the CDC with HIV infection associated with an occupational exposure and no other risk factors. The risk of infection after a needlestick exposure to HIV-infected blood is approximately 0.3% (1,2,38). A case control study revealed that significant risk factors for HIV seroconversion following needlestick injury are deep injury, visible contamination with source patient's blood, procedure associated with needle placement into the patient's vein or artery, and exposure to a patient who died of AIDS within 2 months following the incident. HIV infection following mucous membrane exposure is approximately 0.09% (39,40). Proper handling and disposal of needles will prevent a majority of these exposures (41). In November 2002, the FDA approved OraQuick for point-of-care testing for HIV-1. Many studies have validated that the sensitivity and negative predictive value are equal to the traditional EIA for anti–HIV-1 IgG (42). If exposed, HCWs should contact the employee health department in their institution for counseling and testing. Table 8.3 outlines the steps to take after accidental exposure. All institutions should have a protocol in place to deal with needlestick injuries.

The use of zidovudine for postexposure prophylaxis has been associated with an 81% decrease in the risk of seroconversion following percutaneous needle injury (39). In animal models, both single-drug postexposure prophylaxis (PEP) and multidrug combination PEP have demonstrated efficacy in reducing transmission of HIV. Thus, the U.S. Public Health Service (PHS) recommends either a two- or three-drug regimen, and the selection of regimen depends on the risk of

HIV infection (see Tables 8.4 and 8.5). For percutaneous exposure to blood from a known HIV-infected patient who is asymptomatic or has a viral load less than 1,500 copies/mL or exposure to a small volume of blood from a known HIV-infected patient who is in acute seroconversion, is symptomatic for HIV infection, has AIDS, or has a viral load known to be greater than 1,500 copies/mL, the PHS recommends a regimen consisting of two nucleoside reverse transcriptase inhibitors (NRTI): zidovudine, lamivudine (3TC), or stavudine (d4T). The PHS recommends the addition of either a protease inhibitor or a non-nucleoside reverse transcriptase inhibitor (NNRTI) if the HCW has a large-volume exposure to a known HIV-infected patient who is in acute seroconversion, is symptomatic for HIV infection, has AIDS, or has a viral load greater than 1,500 copies/mL (43). PEP should be given for 4 weeks. PEP should be initiated only in consultation with an expert. There have been case reports of occupational acquisition of multidrug-resistant HIV-1 despite multidrug PEP. PEP is not recommended more than 48 hours after the exposure if the exposure was superficial (not bleeding) or was a mucous membrane exposure (44,45). Female HCWs of childbearing age should have a negative pregnancy test prior to initiation of PEP.

TABLE 8.3	MANAGEMENT OF EXPOSED HCW TO BLOOD OR BLOODY SECRETIONS FROM AN HIV POSITIVE PATIENT

▶ Confirm that the source patient is HIV positive.
▶ Determine HIV "class" of source patient:
 ▶ Class I: Asymptomatic HIV infection or known low viral load (<1,500 copies/mL)
 ▶ Class II: Symptomatic HIV infection, AIDS, acute seroconversion, or known high viral load
▶ If HCW is seronegative, consider PEP and initiate according to Table 8.4.
▶ Counsel about risk of infection and adverse events from PEP.
▶ Retest at 6 weeks, 3 months, and 6 months.[a]

Adapted from ref. 43.
[a] Retest at 12 months if the HCW is at risk for coinfection with HCV.

TABLE 8.4	RECOMMENDED HIV POSTEXPOSURE PROPHYLAXIS AGAINST HIV FOR PERCUTANEOUS INJURIES

Exposure type	Infection status of the source				
	HIV positive class I*	HIV positive class II*	Unknown HIV status†	Unknown source‡	HIV negative
Less severe§	Recommend 2 NRTI¶	Recommend 3 drug regimen#	None, but consider 2 NRTI** for source with known HIV risk factors††	None, but consider 2 NRTI** in setting where exposure to HIV-infected persons is likely	None
More severe‡‡	Recommend 3 drug regimen#	Recommend 3 drug regimen#	Same as above	Same as above	None

Adapted from ref. 43.
*Please see Table 8.3 for definitions.
†Source without known HIV status (e.g., deceased person with no samples for HIV testing).
‡For example, a needle from a sharps container.
§Less severe injury as represented by a solid needle and superficial injury.
¶May give a combination consisting of two of the following: AZT, 3TC, d4T.
#May add NNRTI (efavirenz, nevirapine) or PI (nelfinavir, indinavir, lopinavir/ritonavir).
**"Consider PEP" indicates that PEP is optional and should be individualized to the situation, HCW, and treating clinician.
††If PEP is taken and the source patient is HIV negative, then PEP should be discontinued.
‡‡More severe injury as represented by a large hollow-bore needle, deep puncture wound, visible blood on needle, or needle previously used in patient's artery or vein.

Hepatitis B

Hepatitis B virus infection is a major cause of acute and chronic hepatitis, cirrhosis, and primary hepatocellular carcinoma. The reported incidence of acute hepatitis B in the United States increased by 37% from 1979 to 1989, with an estimated 200,000 to 300,000 new infections occurring from 1980 to 1991 (46). Fortunately, with the advent of HBV vaccination programs and the implementation of universal precautions, there was a 95% decrease in infection with HBV from occupational exposures from 1983 to 1995 (47).

All HCWs who work in EDs should be immunized with hepatitis B vaccine. The chance of infection following percu-taneous exposure from blood contaminated with hepatitis B is approximately 85 times greater than the chance of infection from the same type of exposure but with HIV-contaminated blood (46). Table 8.6 outlines the recommendations for postexposure prophylaxis.

Protective antibody levels of 10 or more milli-international units develop in 85% to 96% of those receiving vaccine. The vaccine should be given in the deltoid muscle in adults—this site has the highest response rate. Vaccination with either Recombivax HB (Merck & Co.) or Energix B (Glaxo Smith Kline) is recommended. Adults over 20 years of age should be given 10 mg (1.0 mL) of hepatitis B surface antigen protein

TABLE 8.5	RECOMMENDED HIV POSTEXPOSURE PROPHYLAXIS FOR MUCOUS MEMBRANE EXPOSURES AND NONINTACT SKIN EXPOSURES

Exposure type	Infection status of the source				
	HIV positive class I*	HIV positive class II*	Unknown HIV status†	Unknown source‡	HIV negative
Small volume§	Consider 2 NRTI¶	Recommend 2 NRTI¶	None, but consider 2 NRTI# for source with known HIV risk factors**	None, but consider 2 NRTI# in setting where exposure to HIV-infected persons is likely	None
Large volume††	Recommend 2 NRTI¶	Recommend 3 drug regimen‡‡			None

Adapted from ref. 43.
Note: For skin exposures, follow-up is indicated when there is compromised skin integrity (e.g., abrasion, open wound).
*See Table 8.3 for definitions.
†Source without known HIV status (e.g., deceased person with no samples for HIV testing).
‡For example, a needle from a sharps container.
§A few drops.
¶May give a combination consisting of two of the following: AZT, 3TC, d4T.
#"Consider PEP" indicates that PEP is optional and should be individualized to the situation, HCW, and treating clinician.
**If PEP is taken and the source patient is HIV negative, then PEP should be discontinued.
††Major splash with a large volume.
‡‡May add NNRTI (efavirenz, nevirapine) or PI (nelfinavir, indinavir, lopinavir/ritonavir).

| TABLE 8.6 | RECOMMENDATIONS FOR HEPATITIS B PROPHYLAXIS AFTER PERCUTANEOUS EXPOSURE TO BLOOD THAT CONTAINS (OR MIGHT CONTAIN) HBsAg* |

	Treatment when source is found to be		
Exposed person	**HBsAg positive**	**HBsAg negative**	**Unknown or not tested**
Unvaccinated	Administer HBIG × 1[†] and initiate hepatitis B vaccine[‡]	Initiate hepatitis B vaccine[‡]	Initiate hepatitis B vaccine
Previously vaccinated Known responder	Test exposed person for anti HBs[§] 1. If adequate, no treatment 2. If inadequate, hepatitis B vaccine booster dose[‡]	No treatment	No treatment
Known nonresponder	HBIG × 2 or HBIG × 1 plus 1 dose of hepatitis B vaccine[‡]	No treatment	If known high-risk source, may treat as if source were HBsAg positive
Person for whom response is unknown	Test exposed person for anti-HBs[§] 1. If inadequate, HBIG × 1 plus hepatitis B vaccine booster dose[‡] 2. If adequate, no treatment	No treatment	Test exposed person for anti-HBs[§] 1. If inadequate, hepatitis B vaccine booster dose[‡] 2. If adequate, no treatment

*Reproduced from Centers for Disease Control and Prevention. *MMWR Morb Mortal Wkly Rep.* 1991;40(RR-13):22.
[†]Hepatitis B immune globulin (HBIG) dose 0.06 mL/kg intramuscularly.
[‡]See Recommendations American Academy of Pediatrics. In: Peter G, ed. *1994 Red Book: report of the Committee on Infectious Diseases.* 23rd ed. Elk Grove Village, IL: American Academy of Pediatrics; 1994:229, Table 3.12.
[§]Adequate anti-HBs is ≥10 milli-international units.

of the Recombivax HB or 20 mg (1.0 mL) of the Energix B intramuscularly at 0, 1, and 6 months (46).

After the series of immunizations, postvaccination testing should also be considered for persons at risk for exposure, such as ED HCWs. Such testing should be performed 1 to 6 months after completion of the series. For persons who do not respond, two to three additional doses will produce adequate antibody levels in up to 50% of adults (46).

Hepatitis C

The transmission of hepatitis C virus (HCV) occurs by exposure to parenteral blood or blood products that contain the virus. Although most cases of transfusion-related non-A, non-B hepatitis are due to HCV, infection by transfusion accounts for only 5% to 10% of the total number of clinical infections (38). The risk of infection is estimated to be 1.8% following percutaneous exposure to a person with known HCV infection (48). Infection during intravenous drug use and sexual transmission are thought to play major roles in the spread of HCV.

HCV RNA may be detected in the serum as early as 10 days after exposure (49–51). However, false-positive results do occur with the RNA polymerase chain reaction test, thus demonstrating the need for serial HCV RNA polymerase chain reaction tests as well as serologic studies (52). Seroconversion with anti-HCV IgG is detectable 50 to 70 days after exposure (53). However, the PHS recommends normal ALT and negative EIA for anti-HCV IgG at 4 to 6 months after exposure to definitively exclude HCV infection after exposure.

Approximately 15% to 20% of patients with acute HCV will clear viremia spontaneously. Multiple studies have

suggested that interferon therapy in the acute phase of HCV infection may prevent chronic HCV infection, but there are no data to suggest that therapy needs to begin in the first 6 months of HCV infection (54,55). In addition, there are no data concerning either the optimal antiviral regimen or duration of therapy for acute HCV infection. Thus, postexposure prophylaxis against HCV is not currently recommended acutely after occupational exposure.

Tuberculosis

Unlike HIV and hepatitis B and C, tuberculosis (TB) in HCWs occurs following exposure to the aerosolized secretions of infected patients or coworkers. Control of tuberculosis within a hospital setting depends on early identification and treatment of persons with TB, on the proper functioning and use of isolation rooms, and on an aggressive surveillance program to identify transmission of TB to HCWs (56).

TB surveillance is especially important for the HCWs in the ED. Because emergency medicine functions as the front line or interface with the community, exposure to TB may be frequent. Screening using the Mantoux technique (the intradermal injection of 5 tuberculin units of purified protein derivative) should be done at least yearly and perhaps every 6 months, depending on the prevalence of TB in the population served.

Control of TB in the ED also depends on engineering factors, including ventilation factors (e.g., the number of air exchanges within a defined space) and the direction of air flow (negative or low flow into the isolation room). The best movement and housing of the patient and family within the ED should be determined with these factors in mind (56).

▶ CHEMICAL EXPOSURES

Certain chemical materials may pose a hazard to patients via continuing contamination and to HCWs via cross-contamination. Cross-contamination may occur if hazardous chemicals gather on a HCWs' clothes or skin or ED equipment during the process of caring for patients involved in chemical incidents (e.g., chemical spills, explosions, gas leaks, fires, accidental poisonings, suicide attempts, and terrorist attacks). Preferably, a receiving ED will be notified by prehospital care providers before the arrival of any patients involved in chemical incidents. The ED team's preparation will be improved with prior knowledge about the chemical involved and the details of the incident. On notification, the ED team should contact both the hospital's safety officer and the regional poison control center. The poison control center can help determine the extent of acute or chronic medical problems that may arise from the chemical involved and if decontamination is necessary. This information also will assist the safety officer in readying possible special decontamination materials. Effective decontamination begins in the field and continues in the hospital (see also Chapter 128).

Toxicologic Considerations

Occupational exposure to hazardous chemicals may occur via three main routes: inhalation, ingestion, and skin absorption. Inhalation exposure occurs through the introduction of toxic compounds into the respiratory system. Examples include gases and vapors of volatile liquids, although solids and liquids can be inhaled as dusts and aerosols. Inhalation exposure usually results in a rapid systemic dosage because of the lung's large surface area and high vascularity. Ingestion is an uncommon source of exposure. One route is the incidental transfer of chemical materials when a HCW wipes his or her mouth with a hand or sleeve. Skin contamination is a common route of occupational exposure. It is estimated that one in four industrial chemicals carry hazards from skin absorption (57). Skin exposure can cause local as well as systemic effects. The systemic effects are usually not as rapid as those that result from inhalation exposure, although some chemicals are rapidly absorbed. In addition, some chemicals that come in contact with the eye can also be absorbed, in addition to causing ocular injury. Ocular decontamination is detailed in Chapter 48.

Procedures

Guidelines for Chemical Control

Decontamination is the removal or neutralization of hazardous chemicals collected on the clothes or skin of patients or HCWs or on ED equipment during the process of caring for patients involved in chemical incidents (58–60). Decontamination is important to HCW safety, and we recommend that ED HCWs regularly refamiliarize themselves with the decontamination process. Along with decontamination, the patients' medical needs also must be assessed, and appropriate resuscitative measures and antidotes initiated.

Decontamination procedures as they pertain to patient management, including the decontamination of HCWs who are inadvertently exposed, are detailed in Chapter 128. From the perspective of HCW protection, the primary goal is to avoid contact with the hazardous chemical as much as possible via the use of personal protective equipment (PPE). The choice of appropriate personal protective equipment for ED staff is an important consideration. It is thought that the chemical agent contaminating patients who arrive alive at the ED after most hazardous chemical exposures (including those related to an intentional terrorist attack) essentially consists of the agent on their skin and clothing and thus is of far lower concentration than rescue workers face at the scene of exposure. Most experts believe adequate protection in this context would be afforded to ED staff garbed in level C personal protective equipment, which consists of a nonencapsulated, chemically resistant body suit, gloves, and boots, with a full-face air purifier mask containing a cartridge with both an organic-vapor filter for chemical gases and vapors and a HEPA filter to trap aerosols of biological and chemical agents. Such personal protective equipment is considerably less cumbersome to work in than level A or B outfits (which use a self-contained breathing apparatus) and is much less expensive (60).

Choices regarding specific materials used in level C personal protective equipment are difficult because few such barrier materials have been tested against a wide variety of highly toxic agents. At least one such material, DuPont's Tyvek F, has been found effective against even military-grade organophosphate nerve agents.

▶ RADIOACTIVE EXPOSURES

Radiation exposure in the ED is another potential health hazard facing HCWs. Exposure is almost exclusively related to diagnostic radiographs or roentgenograms taken during resuscitation efforts. Although rare, radiation accidents do occur and may contaminate HCWs if proper procedures are not followed. From 1944 to October 1990, 331 radiation accidents occurred worldwide (61). Most of these were in the United States. Recent concerns about potential terrorism mandate ED capacity to manage radiologic casualties effectively and safely.

Radiation Biology

Radiation is energy released from a source and comes in two forms, nonionizing (light, microwaves, radio waves, ultraviolet radiation, etc.) and ionizing. Ionizing radiation is the most damaging to tissue and can be either nonparticulate (x-rays,

TABLE 8.7	HOSPITAL PLAN FOR EMERGENCY TREATMENT OF PATIENT CONTAMINATED WITH RADIOACTIVE MATERIALS

Goal

Hospital is prepared to provide care of patients contaminated with radioactive material in a manner that will minimize risk to staff and other patients.

Components

Notification:
- ▶ Related injuries, type of exposure, number of patients?
- ▶ Instruct ambulance crews to wait in ambulance on arrival
- ▶ Notify hospital radiation safety officer.
- ▶ Notify other HCWs.

Emergency department area preparation:
- ▶ Assign a buffer zone nurse.
- ▶ Ensure that the ED decontamination room is prepared.
- ▶ Secure the area.

HCW Preparation:
- ▶ Protective clothing and dosimeters are dispensed.
- ▶ Caps, surgical masks, water repellent gown, shoe covers, and gloves are put on.

Patient arrival:
- ▶ Meet patient at ambulance if condition permits. Remove and treat clothing as contaminated. Wrap clothing in sheet and transport with patient to decontamination room.
- ▶ Radiation officer measures radiation of patient and ambulance.
- ▶ Transport patient immediately to decontamination room by shortest route possible.
- ▶ Hold ambulance until determined free of radioactive contamination.

Patient treatment (see also Table 128.2):
- ▶ Proceed with medical needs
- ▶ Internal and external decontamination.

HCW decontamination:
- ▶ All HCWs should be carefully checked for contamination before leaving area and decontaminated if necessary.

TABLE 8.8	RULES TO PROTECT THE HEALTH CARE WORKER FROM RADIATION EXPOSURE IN THE EMERGENCY DEPARTMENT

The radiology technician should:
- ▶ set proper collination of the x-ray beam
- ▶ minimize retakes

The other health care workers should:
- ▶ use mechanical means of immobilization or adequate shielding
- ▶ maintain distance during procedure
- ▶ not order radiographs unless indicated

Procedures

Guidelines to Control the Exposure to Radiation

All hospitals are required to have an ED plan for handling radiation accidents. Main components of a plan are outlined in Table 8.7. Of course, each hospital will individualize its plan based on staffing and the physical plant. Care of life-threatening conditions must always take priority over containment of contamination. Because radiation accidents are rare, drills should be conducted periodically in order to evaluate and familiarize HCWs with the protocol.

Furthermore, adherence to a few simple rules will reduce risk of radiation exposure when diagnostic radiographs are required (Table 8.8). The amount of exposure to x-rays is governed by time, distance, and shielding. Time is not often a factor in the ED. Having distance between the clinician and the radiation source (i.e., the radiographic machine) is frequently the best course. X-rays are governed by the "inverse square law," which means that doubling the distance from a source of radiation reduces the amount of exposure to 25% of the amount at the original distance. Tripling the distance reduces the exposure to 1% (61).

However, following this "distance" rule requires having mechanical methods to immobilize the child during the radiographic procedure rather than relying on parents or HCWs as "holders." If the HCW or parent is required to restrain the patient, proper shielding is important. Finally, quality improvement programs to reduce the number of repeat or unnecessary radiographs will reduce exposures in the ED.

▶ SUMMARY

This chapter has provided an overview on how to protect HCWs from occupational exposures. Procedural details are summarized in Tables 8.1 to 8.8 and Figures 8.1 to 8.7.

▶ ACKNOWLEDGMENTS

The authors would like to acknowledge the valuable contributions of Leonard R. Friedland to the version of this chapter that appeared in the previous edition.

gamma rays) or particulate. Particulate ionizing radiation is further subdivided into uncharged radiation (neutrons) and charged radiation (alpha and beta rays).

Because of tissue penetration, radiation exposures can result in somatic and hereditary effects. Tissues most at risk following exposure are bone marrow and breast, thyroid, and gonadal tissues. The dose equivalent of radiation is a rem. One rad is approximately equal to 1 rem. For example, the maximum permissible occupational dose equivalent for the whole body is 5 rem per year. However, pregnant women are allowed only 0.5 rem during the gestational period. The hands can be exposed to 75 rem per year but no more than 25 rem in each quarter (62).

In a United Kingdom study from 1992, 143 patients required emergency radiographs during resuscitation (63). A total of 790 radiographs were taken, and 4% were repeated. Seven physicians and one nurse were monitored for the cumulative exposure to their hands. Although none received radiation exceeding the acceptable limits, shield gloves were used infrequently. In only 5 of 85 occasions were lead gloves worn by the physician during cross-table, lateral cervical radiographs.

▶ REFERENCES

1. *Occupational Safety: Selected Cost and Benefit Implications of Needlestick Prevention Devices for Hospitals.* Washington, DC: General Accounting Office; November 17, 2000. GAO-01-60R.

2. Tokars JI, Marcus R, Culver DH, et al. Surveillance of HIV and zidovudine use among health care workers after occupational exposure to HIV-infected blood. *Ann Intern Med.* 1993;118:913–919.

3. Henderson DK, Fahey BJ, Willy M. Risk of occupational transmission of human immunodeficiency virus type I (HIV-I) associated with clinical exposures. *Ann Intern Med.* 1990;113:740–746.

4. Do AN, Ciesielski CA, Metler RP, et al. Occupationally acquired human immunodeficiency virus (HIV) infection: national case surveillance data during 20 years of the HIV epidemic in the United States. *Infect Control Hosp Epidemiol.* 2003;24:86–96.

5. Marcus R, Bell D, Srivastava P, et al. Contact with HIV-infected blood among emergency care providers. Paper presented at: the Third International Conference on Nosocomial Infections; July 31–August 3, 1990; Atlanta, GA.

6. Wong ES, Stotka JL, Chinchilli VM, et al. Are universal precautions effective in reducing the number of occupational exposures among health care workers? A prospective study of physicians on a medical service. *JAMA.* 1991;265:1123–1128.

7. Baker JL, Kelen GD, Sivertson KT, et al. Unsuspected human immunodeficiency virus in critically ill emergency patients. *JAMA.* 1987;257:2609–2611.

8. Kelen GD, Fritz S, Qaquish B, et al. Unrecognized human immunodeficiency virus infection in emergency department patients. *N Engl J Med.* 1988;318:1645–1650.

9. Kelen GD, Fritz S, Qaquish B, et al. Substantial increase in human immunodeficiency virus (HIV-I) infection in critically ill emergency patients: 1986 and 1987 compared. *Ann Emerg Med.* 1989;18:378–382.

10. Lewandowski C, Ognjan A, Rivers E, et al. Health care worker exposure to HIV-I and HTLV I-II in critically ill, resuscitated emergency department patients. *Ann Emerg Med.* 1992;21:1353–1359.

11. Baraff LJ, Talan DA, Torres M. Prevalence of HIV antibody in a non-inner-city university hospital emergency department. *Ann Emerg Med.* 1991;20:782–786.

12. Rhee KJ, Albertson TE, Kizer KW, et al. The HIV-I seroprevalence rate of injured patients admitted through California emergency departments. *Ann Emerg Med.* 1991;20:969–972.

13. Sturm JT. HIV prevalence in a Midwestern emergency department. *Ann Emerg Med.* 1991;20:276–278.

14. Schweich PJ, Fosarelli PD, Duggan AK, et al. Prevalence of human immunodeficiency virus seropositivity in pediatric emergency room patients undergoing phlebotomy. *Pediatrics.* 1990;86:660–665.

15. Centers for Disease Control and Prevention. Recommendations for preventing transmission of infection with human T-lymphotropic virus type III/lymphadenopathy-associated virus in the workplace. *MMWR Morb Mortal Wkly Rep.* 1985;34:681–686, 691–695.

16. Centers for Disease Control and Prevention. Recommendations for the prevention of HIV transmission in health care settings. *MMWR Morb Mortal Wkly Rep.* 1987;36[Suppl 2S]:1–18.

17. Centers for Disease Control and Prevention. Update: universal precautions for prevention of transmission of human immunodeficiency virus, hepatitis B virus, and other bloodborne pathogens in health care settings. *MMWR Morb Mortal Wkly Rep.* 1988;37:377–382, 387–388.

18. Centers for Disease Control and Prevention. Guidelines for prevention of transmission of human immunodeficiency virus and hepatitis B virus to health care and public safety workers. *MMWR Morb Mortal Wkly Rep.* 1989;38[Suppl 6S]:1–37.

19. Centers for Disease Control and Prevention. Recommendations for preventing transmission of human immunodeficiency virus and hepatitis B virus to patients during exposure-prone invasive procedures. *MMWR Morb Mortal Wkly Rep.* 1991;40(RR-8):1–9.

20. Friedland LR. Universal precautions and safety devices which reduce the risk of occupational exposure to bloodborne pathogens: a review for emergency health care workers. *Pediatr Emerg Care.* 1991;7:356–362.

21. Mast ST, Gerberding JL. Factors predicting infectivity following needlestick exposure to HIV: an in vitro model. *Clin Res.* 1991;39:58A.

22. Leclair JM, Freeman J, Sullivan BF, et al. Prevention of nosocomial respiratory syncytial virus infections through compliance with glove and gown isolation precautions. *N Engl J Med.* 1987;317:329–334.

23. Kelen GD, DiGiovanna TA, Celentano DD, et al. Adherence to universal (barrier) precautions during interventions on critically ill and injured emergency department patients. *J Acquir Immune Defic Syndr.* 1990;3:987–994.

24. Baraff LJ, Talan DA. Compliance with universal precautions in a university hospital emergency department. *Ann Emerg Med.* 1989;18:654–657.

25. Hammond JS, Eckes JM, Gomez GA, et al. HIV, trauma, and infection control: universal precautions are universally ignored. *J Trauma.* 1990;30:555–558.

26. Courington KR, Patterson SL, Howard RJ. Universal precautions are not universally followed. *Arch Surg.* 1991;126:93–96.

27. Henry K, Campbell S, Maki M. A comparison of observed and self-reported compliance with universal precautions among emergency department personnel at a Minnesota public teaching hospital: implications for assessing infection control programs. *Ann Emerg Med.* 1991;21:940–946.

28. Friedland LR, Joffe M, Wiley JF, et al. Effect of educational program on compliance with glove use in a pediatric emergency department. *Am J Dis Child.* 1992;146:1355–1358.

29. Kelen GD, Green GB, Hexter DA, et al. Substantial improvement in compliance with universal precautions in an emergency department following institution of policy. *Arch Intern Med.* 1991;151:2051–2056.

30. Talan DA, Baraff LJ. Effect of education on the use of universal precautions in a university hospital emergency department. *Ann Emerg Med.* 1990;19:1322–1326.

31. Occupational Safety and Health Administration. Occupational exposure to bloodborne pathogens: final rule. *Fed. Reg.* 1991;56:64175–64182.

32. Marcus R, and the CDC Cooperative Needlestick Surveillance Group. Surveillance of health care workers exposed to blood from patients infected with the human immunodeficiency virus. *N Engl J Med.* 1988;319:1118–1123.

33. Jagger J, Hunt EH, Brand-Elnaggar J, et al. Rates of needlestick injury caused by various devices in a university hospital. *N Engl J Med.* 1988;319:284–288.

34. Emergency Care Research Institute. Needlestick prevention devices. *Health Dev.* 1991;20:154–180.

35. Schuman AJ. Preventing needlesticks and their consequences. *Contemp Pediatr.* 1992;9:76–106.

36. Owens-Schwab E, Fraser VJ. Needleless and needle protection devices: a second look at efficacy and selection. *Infect Control Hosp Epidemiol.* 1993;14:657–660.

37. Doebbeling BN, Wenzel RP. The direct costs of universal precautions in a teaching hospital. *JAMA.* 1990;264:2083–2087.

38. American Academy of Pediatrics. In: Pickering L, ed. *2003 Red Book: Report of the Committee on Infectious Diseases.* 26th ed. Elk Grove Village, IL: American Academy of Pediatrics; 2003. CD-ROM.

39. Cardo DM, Culver DH, Cielsielski CA, et al., and the Centers for Disease Control and Prevention Needlestick Surveillance Group. A case control study of HIV seroconversion in health care workers after percutaneous exposure. *N Engl J Med.* 1997;337:1485–1490.

40. Ippolito G, Puro V, De Carli G, and Italian Study Group on Occupational Risk of HIV Infection. The risk of occupational human immunodeficiency virus in health care workers. *Arch Int Med.* 1993;153:1451–1458.

41. Klontz KC, Gunn RA, Caldwell JS. Needlestick injuries and hepatitis B immunization in Florida paramedics: a statewide survey. *Ann Emerg Med.* 1991;20:1310–1313.

42. Salgado CD, Flanagan HL, Haverstick DM, et al. Low rate of false positive results with use of a rapid HIV test. *Infect Control Hosp Epidemiol.* 2002;23:335–337.

43. Centers for Disease Control and Prevention. Updated U.S. Public Health Service guidelines for the management of occupational exposures to HBV, HCV, and HIV and recommendations for postexposure prophylaxis. *MMWR Morb Mortal Wkly Rep.* 2001;50(RR-11):1–42.

44. Go GW, Baraff LJ, Schriger DL. Management guidelines for health care workers exposed to blood and body fluids. *Ann Emerg Med.* 1991;20:1341–1350.

45. Callaham ML. Prophylaxis with zidovudine (AZT) after exposure to human immunodeficiency virus: a brief discussion of the issues for emergency physicians. *Ann Emerg Med.* 1991;20:1351–1354.

46. Centers for Disease Control and Prevention. Hepatitis B virus: a comprehensive strategy for eliminating transmission in the U.S. through universal childhood vaccinations, recommendations of the ACIP. *MMWR Morb Mortal Wkly Rep.* 1991;40(RR-13):1.

47. Mahoney FJ, Stewart K, Hu H, et al. Progress toward the elimination of hepatitis B virus transmission among health care workers in the United States. *Arch Int Med.* 1997;157:2601–2603.

48. Lanphear BP. Trends and patterns in the transmission of bloodborne pathogens to health care workers. *Epidemiol Rev.* 1994;16:437–450.

49. Farci P, Alter HJ, Wong D, et al. A long-term study of hepatitis C virus replication in non-A, non-B hepatitis. *N Engl J Med.* 1991;325:98–104.

50. Shimizu YK, Weiner AJ, Rosenblatt J, et al. Early events in hepatitis C virus infection of chimpanzees. *Proc Natl Acad Sci U S A.* 1990;87:6441–6444.

51. Prince AM, Brotman B, Inchauspe G, et al. Patterns and prevalence of hepatitis C virus infection in post-transfusion non-A, non-B hepatitis. *J Infect Dis.* 1993;167:1296–1301.

52. Zaaijer HL, Cuypers HTM, Reesink HW, et al. Reliability of polymerase chain reaction for detection of hepatitis C virus. *Lancet.* 1993;341:722–724.

53. Courouce AM, LeMarrec N, Girault A, et al. Anti-hepatitis C virus (anti-HCV) seroconversion in patients undergoing hemodialysis. *Transfusion.* 1994;34:790–795.

54. Hwang SJ, Lee SD, Chan CY, et al. A randomized controlled trial of recombinant interferon alpha-2b in the treatment of Chinese patients with acute post-transfusion hepatitis C. *J Hepatol.* 1994;21:831–836.

55. Gursoy M, Gur G, Arslan H, et al. Interferon therapy in haemodialysis patients with acute hepatitis C virus infection and factors that predict response to treatment. *J Viral Hepat.* 2001;8:70–77.

56. Guidelines for preventing the transmission of tuberculosis in health care settings, with special focus on HIV-related issues. *MMWR Morb Mortal Wkly Rep.* 1990;39(RR-17):1–29.

57. Kay MM, Henschel AF, Butler J, et al, eds. *Occupational Diseases: A Guide to Their Recognition.* Washington, DC: U.S. Department of Health, Education, and Welfare; 1977:16.

58. Agency for Toxic Substances and Disease Registry. *Hospital Emergency Departments: A Planning Guide for the Management of Contaminated Patients.* Atlanta, GA: Agency for Toxic Substances and Disease Registry; 1992. *Managing Hazardous Materials Incidents*; vol. 2.

59. Walter FG, Flomenbaum NE. Hazmat incident response with pre- and interhospital care of the poisoned patient. In: Goldfrank LR, Flomenbaum NE, Lewin NA, et al., eds. *Toxicologic Emergencies.* Norwalk, CT: Appleton & Lange; 2002:1421–1437.

60. Henretig FM, Cieslak TJ, Madsen JM, et al. Emergency department awareness and response to incidents of biological and chemical terrorism. In: Fleisher GL, Ludwig S, Henretig FM, eds. *Textbook of Pediatric Emergency Medicine.* 5th ed. Philadelphia: Lippincott Williams & Wilkins, 2006:135–162.

61. Mettler FA, Royal HD, Drum DE. Radiation accidents. In: Fleisher GL, Ludwig S, Henretig FM, eds. *Textbook of Pediatric Emergency Medicine.* 5th ed. Philadelphia: Lippincott Williams & Wilkins; 2006:1033–1044.

62. National Institutes of Health. *Report of the National Institutes of Health Ad Hoc Working Group to Develop Radioepidemiological Tables.* Washington DC: U.S. Department of Health and Human Services; 1985. NIH Publication 85-2748.

63. Evans RJ, Cusack S, Parkek T. Exposure of the hands to ionizing radiation in the resuscitation room of an accident and emergency department. *Arch Emerg Med.* 1992;9:220–224.

9

JENNIFER L. REED AND RICHARD M. RUDDY

Informed Consent

▶ INTRODUCTION

Every person has the right to be informed regarding their medical care and then consent to or dissent from the proposed treatments. A person's age and mental capacity may impact on the degree of self-determination exercised in receiving medical care. In this chapter, the concept of informed consent is developed in relation to the pediatric emergency physician, the patient, and the parent or guardian. This chapter discusses the legal principles of informed consent and provides definitions of the concept of informed consent, minor consent, dissent, and leaving against medical advice. Specific informed consent issues relating to adolescents are discussed. The chapter concludes with some illustrative examples of common problems of informed consent in the pediatric emergency department (ED) and options for solution. References are provided for the reader seeking further in-depth discussion of informed consent.

▶ LEGAL PRINCIPLES

Consent for medical treatment is a fairly recent notion. As late as 1847, the American Medical Association Code of Ethics stated, "The obedience of a patient to the prescriptions of his physician should be prompt and implicit. He should never permit his own crude opinions as to their fitness to influence his attention to them" (1). In 1914, Justice Cardozo (*Schloendorff v. New York Hospital*) made a statement that began the ideal of consent: "Every human being of adult years and sound mind has a right to determine what shall be done with his own body." Later came an interest not just in consent but also in its quality (1,2). In 1957, the case of *Salvo v. Leland Stanford Jr. University Board of Trustees* resulted in a legal decision that is believed to be the birth of informed consent. The court

stated that it is the physician's duty to disclose "any facts which are necessary to form the basis of intelligent consent by the patient to the proposed treatment" (1). This simply means that for consent to be valid, the patient must be given sufficient information to understand the nature of the treatment. This decision marked the beginning of the shift of medicolegal cases based on assault, battery, and tort law to ones based on negligence or malpractice (Table 9.1).

In the early 1970s, another shift occurred, characterized by an emphasis on the requirement that disclosure of information regarding medical therapy fit the patient's needs. The 1972 *Canterbury v. Spence* decision stated that "the scope of the physician's communication to the patient . . . must be measured by the patient's need, and that need is the information material to the decision" (3). The American Medical Association endorsed this theory at that time, asserting that "the patient's right of self-decision can be effectively exercised only if the patient possesses enough information to enable an intelligent choice" (3).

The concept of informed consent is somewhat more complex, and often imprecise, when applied to consent for minors. Two centuries ago, English common law held that the father's right of custody of his children took precedence over the mother's and all other's (4). In colonial times, children had no constitutional rights, so parents had absolute control over them. This is known as "parental sovereignty" and is still widely applied by the courts today. In 1912, in the case of *Luka v. Lowrie*, the court decided that in an emergency any child may be treated without parental consent, which was a break from the traditional ideal of parental sovereignty (4). However, in 1933, in the case of *Zuman v. Schultz*, it was decided that non-emergency treatment of a child without the consent of a parent can give rise to assault and battery charges against the physician rendering care (4). This decision reinforced the ideal of parental control. In 1967, the Supreme Court ruled that a

TABLE 9.1	LEGAL TERMINOLOGY

Assault—unlawful placing of an individual in fear of immediate bodily harm
Battery—intentional touching of another person's body without authorization
Tort—intentional wrong
Negligence—omission of reasonable care or action

TABLE 9.2	COMPONENTS OF INFORMED CONSENT

1 Diagnosis and condition of the patient
2 "Reasonable patient standard":
  ▶ Nature and purpose of the proposed treatment
  ▶ Risks and consequences of the proposed treatment
  ▶ Probability of success
  ▶ Feasible alternatives, with benefits, risks, and success rates

child may be treated differently from an adult by a government entity (referring to a government-funded hospital) only if the difference accrues to the child's benefit (4). This means that lack of consent should not keep a minor from receiving medical care equivalent to the care that would be given to an adult. This has been interpreted to include treatment at all medical facilities, not just at ones that are federally funded. In 1971, the voting age dropped from 21 to 18 years of age, and subsequently the age of majority in each state dropped to 18.

▶ DEFINITIONS OF INFORMED CONSENT

According to Holder, *informed consent* is "the duty (of the physician) to warn a patient of the hazards, possible complications and expected and unexpected results of a proposed treatment" (4). Informed consent should contain the following five basic elements (5–7):

1 The patient and/or parent should be told the diagnosis and prognosis in lay terms.
2 The nature and purpose of the proposed treatment should be explained in detail.
3 The significant risks and consequences of the proposed treatment should be discussed. *Significant risk* is best interpreted to mean any consequent event of treatment with a high probability of occurring or with a devastating enough result that a person would want to know about it.
4 The probability and degree of success of the proposed treatment should be communicated.
5 All feasible alternative treatments and their benefits, risks, and success rates should be discussed.

The last four elements are referred to as the "reasonable patient standard" (6), which is the information that any reasonable patient and/or parent would need in order to make an informed decision about the treatment (Table 9.2).

The content of the communicated information can vary depending on the geographic location and the individual situation. Such variation results the existence of "local practice standards." Recently the court system has shifted away from local to more national standards for informed consent (4). Given the "information highway" that exists, as well as the greater access to information that most people now have, this shift toward national standards is not surprising. The specifics

of the information rendered should be adapted to the ability of the patient or parent to understand.

After discussing consent, the physician needs to ensure that these elements of informed consent are present: capacity, disclosure, comprehension, voluntariness, and consent or refusal (8). Each is important to document in the medical record, especially when consent is refused. Capacity is the patient's or parent's (or guardian's) ability to understand the information and make a decision. The physician must assess whether the patient or parent understands the options for treatment, the consequences of the options, and the personal costs and benefits of the treatment (1,7). The physician must also ensure that there is sufficient disclosure of the information required to make an informed decision, including the purpose, risks, and benefits of the proposed treatment and alternatives to the treatment. The physician should consider the apparent level of intelligence of the patient or parent and his or her ability to express choice. Evidence of patient and parent comprehension should be communicated back to the physician by the patient or the parent. Lastly, the physician must be assured that the patient or parent is voluntarily making the decision without external coercion. The physician should also seek to understand the reasonableness of the choice that is made when obtaining consent. Strictly speaking, if the patient lacks the capacity to give consent, the physician must obtain consent from a third party. The physician should not allow the lack of consent to unduly affect the patient's health.

In an emergency setting, other types of consent are important to understand for anyone providing care to children. Whenever a patient enters a hospital ED to be treated, he or she is asked to sign a *general consent* form (3). This usually involves signing the ED record and agreeing to evaluation and treatment. The giving of consent usually takes place at registration, and little or no information on medical care is exchanged before the form is signed. The general consent form should be thought of as a statement of willingness to be examined and have minor treatment done. It is not informed consent, and all significant interventions, unless immediately life saving, will require further consent by the patient or parent. In *expressed consent*, the patient or parent is aware of the proposed care, agrees to such, and in some manner demonstrates a willingness to proceed (3). This is common when the physician wants to obtain a blood sample and the parent approves of the test being done. An additional subtype is *implied consent* (2,5), which is consent implied by the actions of the patient but without specific agreement. An example is when a patient rolls up a sleeve to receive an injection. A subtype of implied consent is *implied parental consent*. For example, parents send their child to the ED for care of a laceration, and phone approval is obtained. It is reasonable to infer that the parents would want the care to be definitive at that visit. Physicians may treat any minor seeking emergency care if they believe that any reasonable parent would agree to treatment. The legal term for this implied parental consent is "in loco parentis." *Deferred consent* is consent after the fact. An example is treatment with epinephrine for severe bronchospasm given to an obtunded patient and getting consent after the patient has improved (3). There is legitimate debate as to whether this is informed consent or deferred assent to what already was done.

An important subtype of consent for an ED physician is *emergency consent* (3,5). The definition of an emergency is not uniform, but the term broadly applies to situations in which "immediate treatment is deemed necessary to prevent loss of life or permanent disability and the patient lacks the capacity to make independent decisions." The physician is allowed and expected to act in the patient's best interests. Most states have broadened this to include those conditions that require prompt treatment, such as alleviating pain, suturing, and fracture reduction (5). The physician does not have to be certain that harm will eventually result but only has to recognize that it is a reasonable possibility. The laws pertaining to emergency consent are deliberately broad to encourage treatment without fear of liability. States such as South Carolina, North Carolina, and Oklahoma require a second opinion if surgery is contemplated (5). Although a second opinion is not required by law elsewhere, if a short delay will not be critical, many institutions choose to obtain a second opinion.

In 1985, Congress passed the Emergency Medical Treatment and Active Labor Act (EMTALA). Passage of this act was in direct response to the patient "dumping" issue (9). Many private hospitals were refusing uninsured patients and sending them to public hospitals for economic reasons only. EMTALA applies to any hospital that receives federal funding. Since EMTALA is a federal law, it supersedes any state laws, including laws applying to minors. Under EMTALA, a medical screening exam (MSE) must be conducted on any patient (including a minor) regardless of the acuity of the complaint if that patient, or any person acting on the patient's behalf (including another minor), requests that an MSE be done. Attempts should be made to contact the parent or guardian, but an MSE exam should not be delayed if the physician is unable to obtain consent. If the physician deems no emergency medical condition exists after an MSE exam is performed, then he or she should delay further treatment until consent is obtained from the parent or guardian. It is key to use the commonsense principle that an acute though not serious condition can be treated (based on the principle of implied consent). If an emergency condition exists, a physician must render treatment under the stabilization requirement of EMTALA or state law. EMTALA empowers a physician to examine, treat, stabilize (including by means of surgical intervention if emergently necessary), and transfer to an appropriate higher-level hospital without the consent of the parent or guardian (9).

▶ ISSUES AND DEFINITIONS IN CONSENT FOR MINORS

A *minor* is defined by law to be a person who has not yet reached the age of 18 years. Minors are legally incapable of giving consent (6). Therefore, a parent or guardian must consent for them. However, there are no reported legal decisions that hold a physician liable for treating a minor for his or her own benefit in a nonelective situation without consent. Also, in most states, *minor treatment statutes* allow for older minors to consent to "ordinary medical treatment" (4). "Ordinary medical treatment" in this context refers to treatment with only minimal risk.

Additional confusion exists as to when minors are able to consent for themselves. Some exceptions are based on the minors themselves and on specific medical problems. Exceptions based on minors fall into two categories, the category of *emancipated minor* and the category of *mature minor*. The precise definition of each varies from state to state, but the following holds for most states. A minor is considered emancipated and able to give consent if he or she is living alone and/or financially independent, a high school graduate, serving in the military, married, pregnant, or a parent (Table 9.3) (3–6,10).

A minor can be considered mature and therefore able to give consent if he or she is 15 years old and understands the nature and risks of the treatment and if the physician believes the following are true: the minor can make an informed decision, the treatment is in the minor's best interest, and the treatment does not involve serious risks (Table 9.3) (3–6,10).

Exceptions to minor consent based on medical problems are in place in many states. These exceptions are based on the belief that the need to be treated outweighs the parents' right to consent in some medical situations in which treatment is in the minor's or society's best interest. An example is a sexually transmitted infection. The minor and society both benefit from treatment. The laws pertaining to these cases are known as *minor treatment statutes*. In order to encourage minors to seek medical care for these problems, the statutes allow for immediate and confidential treatment of the minor. Some states go so far as to forbid informing the parents unless not informing them puts the minor at undue risk. Common medical problems covered under the majority of state statutes are mental illness; substance abuse; pregnancy; contraception;

TABLE 9.3	MINOR ISSUES DEFINITIONS

Minor—any person under the age of 18 years
Emancipated minor—living alone and/or financially independent such as:
  ▶ high school graduate
  ▶ serving in the military
  ▶ married, pregnant, or parent
Mature minor—15 years old *and* understands nature and risks of the treatment and
physician believes all of the following:
  ▶ the patient can make an informed decision
  ▶ treatment is in the minor's best interest
  ▶ treatment does not involve serious risks

communicable and sexually transmitted infections, including HIV; emergencies; suspected child abuse; and medical problems resulting from a crime (4–6,8,10).

When a physician treats a minor as an emancipated or mature minor or under the minor treatment statues, the minor assumes responsibility for his or her own medical care as well as financial responsibility, except in the case of emergency or necessary medical care (11). One needs to communicate only with the minor when discussing his or her medical care and laboratory results to avoid breaching patient confidentiality. Additionally, a system needs to be in place to prevent financial breach of confidentiality, such as sending a medical bill to the minor's parents (12). Emergency departments need to have guidelines in place that address the consent of minors, financial responsibility, patient confidentiality, and the notification of parents.

In some circumstances, consent for treatment for minors can seem confusing and troublesome, especially when deciding which adult parent can give consent for the minor. A physician may treat a minor with consent of only one parent as long as there is no reason to believe the other parent would object (4,5). No cases are found of a physician being successfully sued under these circumstances. In divorce, the custodial parent retains the duty to provide care and give consent. However, the parent with actual physical control at the time the health need arises may give consent (4,5,10). In foster care, the foster parents or the institution or agency may give consent for routine health care. However, for elective or major treatment, which person or persons are empowered to give consent depends on whether the placement was voluntary or involuntary. If the placement was voluntary, the parents must give consent, and if involuntary, then the social agency gives consent and the foster parents may not (5,10). In detention facilities, the parents maintain custody and therefore the right to consent (5,10). When a child is away from the care of his or her parents, such as at school or camp, there is often a blanket consent form that the parents sign giving consent for treatment. This type of consent does not cover nonemergency care. Because support for true emergency care is implied by the law, these forms do not add additional support for nonemergency treatment without consent (4,5,10). When runaways are involved, the parents maintain custody and right of consent unless the child can be considered mature or emancipated (4,8). Lastly, if the parent is a minor, then the courts tend to view this parent like any other parent. The minor parent may then give his or her consent for treatment of his or her child if he or she has the capacity to understand (4–6).

▶ DISSENT

Dissent or refusal of treatment can be very troubling to ED staff. However, the reality is that if a patient has a right to consent, that patient has a right to dissent. The decision to dissent must be accepted just as readily as the decision to consent. Numerous reasons exist why people dis-

sent from treatment. Among the most common are religious beliefs. Patients and/or parents may refuse medical treatment on religious grounds as long as there is no threat to the health of others (6). An example when dissent is disallowed would be treatment for tuberculosis. Additionally, parents do not have the right to deny emergency medical care to their child (*State v. Perricone*, 1962) (10). However, at the same time, states will provide immunity from prosecution for medical neglect to parents who withhold consent for religious reasons (5).

Another difficult situation arises when consent is given by the parents but refused by the minor. Even if the parents consent, there are some circumstances where the minor's dissent takes priority. A minor's dissent must be accepted if he or she can be considered a mature or an emancipated minor or if the situation falls under specific treatment statutes (4).

Arguably the most difficult situation occurs when the parents refuse consent. Courts generally support parental control over the child's health care. Still, a child's health cannot be seriously jeopardized because of the parents' limitations or convictions (6,10). Additionally, parents do not have the authority to deny their child life-saving treatment. In cases where parents attempt to do this, the physician and the state depend on child abuse statutes for help in obtaining custody and rendering treatment (10).

The physician's role in a situation where a treatment has been refused varies according to the type of patient and the degree to which the treatment is needed and beneficial. The more serious the illness and the more beneficial the treatment, the greater the physician's involvement and efforts should be. With a *mature or emancipated minor*, the physician must first decide on the capacity of the patient. If the patient appears competent, then the physician should try to discover the reason(s) for the dissent. Often the dissent is related to anger and/or anxiety. The anger can come from the perception of a long wait and the attendant sense of frustration, rudeness by a staff member, the feeling of being used in an experiment, or a misunderstanding of the disease and its treatment. Anxiety can come from a lack of understanding of the disease or treatment, the observation of other occurrences in the ED, or a sense of loss of control.

Once the reason for dissent is known, addressing that reason may be all that is necessary to obtain consent. If discussion with the patient does not work, then involving an individual who the patient trusts, such as the primary caregiver, a friend, a family member, or a religious leader, may assist in obtaining consent.

If the physician fails to obtain consent, the refusal of treatment should be thoroughly documented as follows. A careful history and physical examination should be noted, assuming the patient allowed such a clinical evaluation. The reasons for considering the patient to be competent should be clearly stated. The patient must be competent for the refusal to be accepted. The risks and benefits of the proposed treatment and any alternative treatments, including no treatment, should be included. A brief explanation of why the physician feels the proposed treatment was refused should be given. The patient

TABLE 9.4	DOCUMENTATION OF DISSENT

▶ History and physical examination if obtained
▶ Reasons for considering the patient and/or guardian competent
▶ Risks and benefits of the proposed treatment
▶ Risks and benefits of alternative treatment, including no treatment
▶ Why the proposed treatment was refused
▶ That an offer was made to provide treatment at any future time if the patient and/or parent changes their mind
▶ Witness of refusal

should understand that if he or she has a change of mind at any time, treatment will be available, and the offer is documented. Lastly, the refusal and the documentation of the refusal should be witnessed. It is worthwhile to have the patient and a third party read and sign the documented refusal, if possible (Table 9.4).

The physician's role in a refusal of treatment involving an *immature or unemancipated minor* differs from his or her role in a refusal by an adult. Again the physician must decide on competency, but in this case the competency of the minor and the competency of the parents are both relevant. The physician should try to define exactly why the treatment is being refused and address the pertinent issues. If the refusal is maintained, then the physician should involve an individual trusted by the patient or parents. If, despite good efforts, the refusal persists, the physician must decide on the degree to which intervention is required. If the condition is life-threatening, the physician has four options. The best option depends on the urgency of the situation. The physician can (a) take temporary protective custody based on the child neglect statutes, (b) report to the hospital administrator and attorney, (c) contact the local child protective agency, or (d) obtain a court order to render care (5).

Taking custody is the quickest option, but the physician is usually treading on unfamiliar ground. If possible, it is best to engage someone who is more familiar with the legal system. Relying on the hospital attorney and/or administrator to settle the issue can take time. Regardless of the option chosen, hospital staff should be informed of the situation in a timely manner. The best option, if there is little time, is to involve the hospital social worker and the local child protective agency. They know the system and can work in a very efficient manner if need be. The last option, obtaining a court order, can be very time consuming. The reality is that in a difficult case all of these people, the child protective agency, and the courts may eventually become involved.

Most courts tend to prefer that a child protective agency seek the court order for treatment. If there is no time to involve the local child protective agency, the physician should seek the court order him- or herself. Historically, the courts have supported the parents' right to refuse care in the case of nonserious or non-life-threatening conditions. When the courts do get involved, they use a case-by-case analysis. Factors that are taken into account include whether the treatment will restore the patient to a normal life, whether the refusal has suicidal or homicidal motives, the competence of the patient and parent, the age of the patient (i.e., could the decision wait until the child can be considered mature, emancipated, or an adult), and whether the patient has dependent children. Conflicting medical opinions on the proposed treatment or alternative treatments can be an important factor in a court's denying or maintaining the parents' or a guardian's right to decide on medical care. Figure 9.1 illustrates one possible approach to parents who refuse consent for lumbar puncture on their infant even though he or she likely has meningitis.

▶ LEAVING AGAINST MEDICAL ADVICE

Another difficult situation for the emergency physician is when the patient wants to leave against medical advice or the parents want the patient to do this. An expressed desire to leave against medical advice can and should be handled in much the same manner as dissent. The physician needs to decide on the competence of the patient and/or the parents. If they are felt to be competent, then the reason behind the desire to leave needs to be discovered and specifically addressed. The approach to the parents and the patient needs to be one of compassion, sensitivity, and diplomacy. Involvement of a trusted family member can be very helpful. If the physician fails to persuade the patient to stay, then the physician must determine how imperative it is that the patient stay to be evaluated and treated. A parent may not leave with a child if a life-threatening condition exists, if there is suspected child abuse, or if the parent is incompetent (6,7,10). The same actions and documentation should occur as for the patient or parent who refuses treatment.

▶ OBTAINING AND DOCUMENTING INFORMED CONSENT

Ideally, the physician providing the treatment should obtain the consent, but there may be designees assigned to obtain consent from patients. It would be wise to first have the performing physicians obtain consent from patients while the designees observe the interaction. Then, when comfortable and knowledgeable about the procedure, the designees should be allowed to obtain consent while the performing physicians observe the process. This sequence allows education of the designees about the purpose and significant risks of the procedure, allows them to be mentored, and allows the performing physicians to become assured that the informed consent procedure will be performed completely and accurately even in their absence. When discussing a proposed treatment and obtaining informed consent from the parent or patient, the physician should address the five elements discussed in Table 9.2. The consent process should also be witnessed by a third party and documented in writing when appropriate.

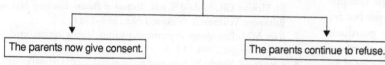

Figure 9.1 Parents who refuse consent for their child's lumbar puncture.

A 5-month-old infant presents to the ED with fever, irritability, and vomiting. After evaluation, the ED physician recommends lumbar puncture to exclude the diagnosis of meningitis. The parents initially refuse consent.

- The physician notes the child's ill appearance and abnormal examination findings and emphasizes that these are suggestive of meningitis.
- The physician explains the potential serious consequences of delayed diagnosis and treatment of meningitis.
- The relatively low risk and frequent experience in performing lumbar puncture are detailed.

The parents listen attentively and are assessed as competent to give informed consent but continue to refuse.

- The parents are asked to discuss their reluctance. It is revealed that in the father's family a relative had been ill, underwent lumbar puncture, and subsequently suffered paralysis. This event had occurred more than 50 years ago, and the story had been passed down through several generations.
- The physician attempts to put this family history into context, pointing out that the illness occurred during the poliomyelitis era and at a time when treatment for bacterial meningitis was not available. The likely relationship between the disease itself and the paralysis is noted. The rarity of neurologic complications from lumbar puncture in febrile infants is re-emphasized.

The parents now give consent.

The parents continue to refuse.

- Under these circumstances, it would be advisable to document the discussion in the medical record and obtain written consent.

- Options to the ED physician include:
  — Consider empiric antibiotic therapy without preceding lumbar puncture. This course may be more acceptable to this family without unduly delaying treatment. However, definitive diagnosis is delayed or lost, and hospitalization may be prolonged or have been unnecessary. Detailed documentation is necessary.
  — Initiate emergency assumption of protective custody, with hospital security assistance as necessary. Simultaneously, notify hospital attorney, social worker, child protective agency, or courts, as per community protocols. Perform lumbar puncture and start antibiotic treatment as indicated. Detailed documentation is necessary.

Documentation should ideally record exactly what was discussed. The more risky the treatment, the more detailed the documentation should be. Common and low-risk treatments, as many routine ED procedures are, need minimal informed consent and little or no written consent. This does not mean that consent should be overlooked in this situation, only that the process can be abbreviated. Additionally, physicians need to decide for themselves how comfortable they are with the amount of written documentation they obtain (see also Chapter 11).

In the case of uncommon, controversial, and high-risk treatments, more comprehensive written documentation should be obtained. The patient or the parent should read and sign a consent form that includes all risks and benefits. Remember that written consent does not substitute for the informed consent discussion between the physician and the patient or parent. The oral provision of appropriate informa-

tion to the patient or parent will do more to avert a future legal case than a signed consent form.

▶ WHEN INFORMED CONSENT IS NOT NECESSARY

There are five different situations in which full informed consent is not necessary. The first is when the patient or parents state they do not want to know the risks and will proceed with the treatment (1,5). It is still best for physicians to attempt to get informed consent in this situation, but they are not obligated to obtain it. A second situation in which informed consent can be waived is where the physician believes that disclosure of the risks would substantially or adversely affect the patient's health. This type of "therapeutic privilege" does not apply to minors, since the parents are the ones who must consent, and disclosure of the risks only to the parents may avoid harming the patient through discussion of the issues (1,4,5). The third situation is when the risks of the treatment are considered common knowledge (5). Examples include an injection or placement of an intravenous line. In such instances, the patient and parents should be informed as part of the procedure, but the amount of detail provided may be less than that indicated for more complex problems. The fourth situation is where informed consent is precluded because of an emergent problem, such as cardiac arrest (1). Last is the situation in which a physician assesses the patient and/or parents and determines that they lack the capacity to understand the problem and/or the proposed treatment (1). In this instance, the physician needs to fully document the assessment in the record.

▶ SUMMARY

Informed consent is a key element in the proper delivery of quality health care in the ED. As outlined, the components of good consent generally follow common sense but are predicated on the principle that patients or their guardians have the right to understand and concur with the therapies the patients are to receive. In true emergencies, the need to provide timely care can and should preclude a detailed explanation of the treatment in order to maximize the likelihood of a good outcome. Although documentation is important, providing thorough and easy-to-understand explanations to patients and parents is the most important component of informed consent. One should document thoroughly the discussions regarding consent and attempt to obtain consent from the parent or legal guardian and assent from the patient when necessary. However, both the American Academy of Pediatrics and the American College of Emergency Physicians support the principle that treatment of a minor for an urgent or emergent condition, including a medical screening examination, should not be delayed solely due to difficulties in obtaining consent (12,13).

▶ ACKNOWLEDGMENT

The authors would like to acknowledge the valuable contributions of Richard T. Strait to the version of this chapter that appeared in the previous edition.

▶ REFERENCES

1. Botkin JR. Informed consent for lumbar puncture. *Am J Dis Child.* 1989;143:899–904.
2. Iserson KV. Bioethics. In: Rosen P, Barkin RM, Braen GR, et al., eds. *Emergency Medicine: Concepts and Clinical Practice.* St. Louis: Mosby; 1992:37–48.
3. Seigel DM. Consent and refusal of treatment. *Emerg Med Clin North Am.* 1993;11:833–840.
4. Holder AR. *Legal Issues in Pediatrics and Adolescent Medicine.* New Haven, CT: Yale University Press; 1985.
5. Morrissey JM, Hofmann AD, Thorpe JC. *Consent and Confidentiality in the Health Care of Children and Adolescents: A Legal Guide.* New York: The Free Press; 1986.
6. Korin JB, Selbst SM. Legal aspects of emergency department pediatrics. In: Fleisher GR, Ludwig S, eds. *Textbook of Pediatric Emergency Medicine.* Baltimore: Williams & Wilkins; 1993:1559–1564.
7. Rice MM. Emergency department patients leaving against medical advice. *Foresight.* 1994;29:1–8.
8. Kassutto Z, Vaught W. Informed decision making and refusal of treatment. *Clin Pediatr Emerg Med.* 2003;4:285–291.
9. Bitterman RA. *Providing Emergency Care under Federal Law: EMTALA.* Dallas, TX: American College of Emergency Physicians; 2000:25, 35–36.
10. Sullivan DJ. Minors and emergency medicine. *Emerg Med Clin North Am.* 1993;11:841–851.
11. Tsai AK, Schafermeyer RW, Kalifon D, et al. Evaluation and treatment of minors: reference on consent. *Ann Emerg Med.* 1993;22:1211–1217.
12. American Academy of Pediatrics, Committee on Pediatric Emergency Medicine. Policy statement: consent for emergency medical services for children and adolescents. *Pediatrics.* 2003;111:703–706.
13. American College of Emergency Physicians. *Evaluation and Treatment of Minors.* Irving, TX: American College of Emergency Physicians; February 2001. ACEP Policy Statement 400129. Available at: http://www.acep.org/1,558,0.html. Accessed March 29, 2005.

FRAN NADEL AND GARY GEIS

10

Teaching Procedures in the Emergency Department

▶ INTRODUCTION

Teaching procedures in the emergency department (ED) offers many unique advantages and challenges. There are many opportunities to perform procedures, as initial patient assessment, evaluation, and management often occur in the ED. The diverse patient population that presents to the ED may require many different types of procedures, and the bedside presence of an attending and a resident creates many hands-on teaching moments.

However, barriers to teaching in the ED exist as well. Patient education should never interfere with patient safety. Clinical and administrative demands may also decrease the time available for teaching. The unpredictable workload requires flexibility and readiness to teach. The abilities and training of residents vary greatly as well, and the limited exposure to any one individual may make it harder to develop a sense of the learner's needs.

Teaching is a skill in itself, and as with any skill, it requires practice and refinement. The purpose of this chapter is to present a structured, systematic approach to teaching procedures that is based on principles of adult learning and psychomotor skill learning as well as to review the literature on different teaching methods.

▶ ADULT LEARNING PRINCIPLES

In the 1970s, Malcolm Knowles described characteristics of adult learners that seem especially applicable to skills teaching (I). It is important to incorporate an adult learner's own experiences and self-assessed needs into a teaching session (I). For example, a few simple questions about a resident's level

and kind of training and the number of times he or she has performed a specific procedure can give the teacher a sense of the resident's abilities and needs. In addition, adult learners want to learn practical, immediately relevant information through hands-on application, which makes the emergency department an excellent environment for teaching (I). Adult learners favor teaching that focuses on the process rather than rote memorization (I). For instance, describing a method for suture selection is more helpful than just giving the student the correct suture. The bedside presence of teacher and learner offers an excellent opportunity to give feedback, a crucial part of adult learning (2). In a survey of "successful" emergency medicine teachers, respondents identified teaching strategies that echo Knowles' adult learning principles (3). Additionally, they described good teachers as approachable, eager, prepared to teach, and respectful of the learner (3).

▶ PSYCHOMOTOR SKILLS

"See one, do one, teach one." Though the numbers may be grossly underestimated, this often-repeated method of teaching medical procedures contains some of the important concepts in psychomotor skill education, namely, observation, practice, and supervision. Three phases of psychomotor learning have been described (4). During the *cognitive phase*, the student intellectually analyzes the skill and develops a mental image (4). This is followed by the *fixation phase*, during which motor patterns are practiced until correct behaviors are well established (4). Finally, during the *autonomous phase*, the student becomes more expert and develops increasing speed and precision (4). The student moves from initially performing the procedure awkwardly under total conscious control to performing the procedure smoothly under total or near-total automatic control.

Three important conditions exist that influence the acquisition of new skills (4). *Contiguity* is the proper sequence and appropriate timing of motor responses. *Practice*, which comes second, involves rehearsal and fixation of the skill (4). The amount of practice required will vary depending on the ability of the student and the complexity of the task. *Feedback* is the third and possibly most important condition that influences the learning of psychomotor skills (4). Feedback reinforces accurate performance and corrects errors. Experience without feedback increases confidence but does not improve skill performance (5).

The process of teaching a skill can be similarly divided into three broad phases corresponding to the phases of psychomotor learning already discussed (4). The introductory (cognitive) phase allows the student to develop a mental plan for the procedure (4). During the practice (fixation) phase, the student is supervised while rehearsing the skill and is given feedback to reduce errors and strengthen correct responses (4). The perfecting (autonomous) phase is generally a more extended period during which the student performs the skill under realistic clinical conditions and improves speed and precision (4). A fourth phase that many would add is the teaching phase, which provides the student the opportunity to demonstrate mastery of the skill by successfully teaching it to a new student (6,7). Table 10.1 lists the first three phases divided into the component steps that might occur, for example, in the setting of a procedure workshop (4).

The steps listed in Table 10.1 may need to be slightly modified when at the bedside and depending on the time available. The instructor initiates a brief, focused discussion of the procedure that concentrates on the critical elements, such as surface anatomy; helpful hints; or common errors. Ideally, this discussion should not occur in front of the patient or family, but the family should know about the student-instructor relationship. This will make it easier to coach the student during the actual procedure. In addition, the instructor can surreptitiously guide the student through the procedure while explaining the procedure step by step to the patient or family. Although many families initially balk at having a resident perform a procedure on their child, many change their minds if a supervisor agrees to be there during the critical steps. It is also important to tell each family that even the best can "miss" a procedure. However, if a family refuses to allow the resident to perform the procedure, the supervisor must perform it.

When observing a procedure, the student should be placed as much as possible in the position from which he or she will perform the procedure. This often requires the resident to stand behind the instructor and view the procedure over the instructor's shoulder (Fig. 10.1). This method facilitates a better understanding of spatial orientation and handedness (8).

Besides the family's wishes, many other factors must be considered in allowing a trainee to perform a procedure on an actual patient. The patient's status, the urgency of the situation, the ratio of risks and benefits to the patient, the skill

TABLE 10.1	PHASES OF TEACHING A PROCEDURE

Introductory (Cognitive) Phase

1 Explicitly describe the objectve of the session and the expected performance outcome.
2 Describe the relevant anatomy and physiology, indications, contraindications, and potential complications.
3 Familiarize the student with the required equipment.
4 Demonstrate and simultaneously articulate how each sequential step of the procedure is currently performed.

Practice (Fixation) Phase

1 Both verbally and physically guide the first attempt of each student to perform the procedure.
2 Provide immediate feedback and/or allow peers to provide immediate feedback.
3 Allow time for independent practice.
4 Document that the student is able to correctly perform the procedure in the practice setting.

Perfecting (Autonomous) Phase

1 Provide the opportunity for students to practice and receive feedback under realistic clinical conditions.

SUMMARY

1 The three phases of psychomotor learning are cognitive, fixation, and autonomous.
2 The three critical conditions that influence procedural learning are contiguity, practice, and feedback.
3 Divide the procedure into small discrete steps.
4 Teach the procedure in three phases that correspond to the three phases of psychomotor learning: introductory (cognitive), practice (fixation), and perfecting (autonomous).
5 If possible, allow the student to observe the procedure from the position in which the student will actually perform the procedure (e.g., from over the instructor's shoulder). This facilitates a better understanding of spatial orientation and handedness (Fig. 10.1).
6 Teaching of a procedure in the ED requires a preprocedure discussion and demonstration, if possible. Explaining each step to the patient and/or family may further serve as additional guidance to the student.

levels of the teacher and trainee, and other clinical demands in the ED will all influence this decision. Although instructors should strive to facilitate every opportunity for students to practice procedures, many situations will require the student to observe or assist only. It is difficult to give universal guidelines, but the overarching principles are that patients should never be exposed to undue risk or discomfort and that residents should graduate with proficiency in the core procedural skills of their specialty.

▶ COMPETENCY

How to instill and measure skill competency is an important but unresolved issue. Trainees seem to follow a predictable "learning curve" when obtaining a new skill set (9). Initially, the curve rises rapidly as success with a skill improves with practice (9). The trainee subsequently may experience a decrease in success as he or she attempts more difficult cases before reaching a stable plateau of successful skill performance (9). Although the number of procedures performed

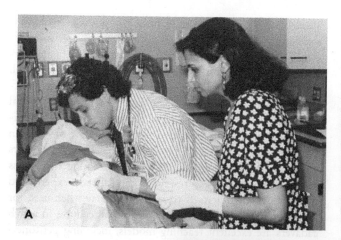
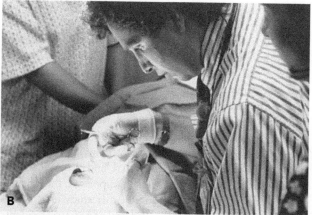
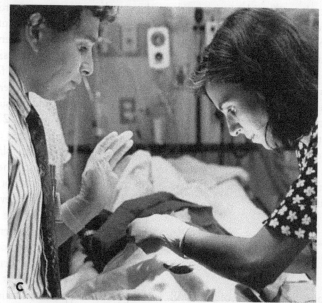

Figure 10.1
A, B. The student gains correct spatial orientation and an appreciation of each hand's movements during the procedure by observing over the instructor's shoulder.
C. The student has the opportunity to practice the procedure with direct observation and feedback from the instructor.

is often taken as a proxy for competency, a relationship between number of performances and competency has never been demonstrated in the literature. Some authors have suggested that a trainee needs to perform a skill 30 to 60 times before being considered proficient (10). The actual number needed to achieve competency will depend on the learner, the complexity of the procedure, and the frequency of procedure performance. The patient's condition and the immediacy of the situation may also influence procedure performance.

A related issue is the maintenance of procedural skills in practice. This may be particularly problematic for academic physicians, who have less clinical time and must allow trainees to perform procedures, although teaching may help prevent the deterioration of psychomotor skills. Proposed methods of skills maintenance and advancement include computer-based review and assessment, simulation workshops, and "mini-rotations" in specific clinical areas, such as anesthesia. Learn-

ing how to learn may be the most important skill of all to teach and live by.

Multiple studies have demonstrated that pediatric residents lack experience and skills in life-saving procedures. In 25% of pediatric programs, residents did not have the opportunity to place chest tubes, place central lines, perform rapid sequence intubation, or participate in trauma resuscitations (11). In a study of third-year pediatric residents, only 18% properly performed ancillary airway maneuvers, and 78% demonstrated errors in endotracheal intubation technique that may have precluded correct placement (12). Appropriate intraosseous access and Seldinger vascular technique were demonstrated by only one third of these residents, and 44% reported never having led resuscitations in residency. Several additional studies confirm the relative lack of formal procedural curricula, experience, and proficiency among pediatric residents (13,14).

With these deficiencies in mind, recent studies have looked at methods for teaching procedural skills in addition to one-on-one precepting and large-class didactics. Investigators showed an increased fund of knowledge, increased retention of skills, and increased procedural proficiency using an animal laboratory to teach tube thoracostomy (15). Another study of pediatric residents compared training that incorporated an added teaching videotape and use of a checklist with standard training in ankle and knee examination (16). The investigators showed an improvement in written test scores and examination techniques at both 1 and 9 months compared with baseline scores. Although important, the strength of the evidence is limited because neither study used a control group. A prospective controlled trial of pediatric residents compared routine training (control group) with routine training plus a brief resuscitation course and a minimum of three mock resuscitations (intervention group) (17). The intervention group performed significantly better in regard to fund of knowledge, success in technical skills, and assessment of critically ill patients. Another prospective controlled trial was performed in the prehospital setting. The authors examined field intubation success rates in two groups of paramedics, one trained on manikins only, the other trained on manikins plus cadavers (18). The overall success rates were 86% and 85%, respectively. The small numbers in each group precluded comparison of the groups, but the study highlighted the usefulness of manikins in procedural training.

▶ EDUCATIONAL SETTINGS AND EQUIPMENT

Although there are multiple opportunities for procedural skill teaching in the ED, there are many reasons that other resources can and should be used. To ensure patient safety as well as adequate practice in important skills for the trainee, various alternatives to live patients can be used, including manikins, models, animals, human cadavers, newly deceased human patients, and human volunteers.

Manikins and other models can be very useful tools in teaching procedures. Residents are introduced to this equipment right from the start, as manikins are used in basic and pediatric advanced life support classes, where large groups of learners assemble at one time. Manikins allow repetitive use for procedures such as intubation, bag-valve-mask ventilation, chest compressions, nasogastric tube placement, and urinary catheter placement. Additionally, there is no requirement for patient or family consent. However, they can have a large upfront cost, may require frequent maintenance, and do not offer complete realism. In addition, procedures that require frequent use of needles or incisions often damage the models and cannot be repeated multiple times. These would include central line placement, tube thoracostomy, suturing, and even peripheral line placement. The Vancouver model for simulating femoral line placement has been studied using emergency medicine physicians, pediatricians, and pediatric

residents (19). Although no control group was present, non-emergency physicians reported a significant change in confidence after practical experience using the model, and emergency physicians stressed the educational value of this model.

Using live and deceased animals for medical training offers a greater amount of realism but is highly controversial and strongly opposed by animal rights groups (20). Additionally, animals can be expensive and differ from human patients anatomically and physiologically. Human cadavers are routinely used in graduate medical training in a gross anatomy laboratory. As residents have already experienced this setting, it lends itself to less controversy when used for procedural training. There are multiple procedures in which cadavers are excellent teaching models, including peritoneal lavage, thoracotomy, pericardiocentesis, and cricothyrotomy (21). These procedures are infrequently encountered by emergency medicine residents even less frequently by pediatric residents (22). Drawbacks of using human cadavers include their limited availability, the need for appropriate preservation, and their expense. In addition, certain procedures, such as peripheral line placement and incision and drainage of abscesses, are impractical in this setting (21).

Newly deceased patients offer the most realistic anatomy, but their use brings into play ethical questions and the issue of informed consent. The practice of teaching procedures on the newly deceased is not uncommon in EDs and critical care settings (23,24). However, very few centers have written polices regarding use of the newly deceased or methods for family notification or consent. Interestingly, the majority of families indicate that they would be willing to consent to invasive procedures being performed on a newly deceased relative (25,26). The establishment of policies regarding appropriate procedures, potential trainees, and the obtaining of family consent could serve to improve the use of this important teaching tool (24).

Human volunteers obviate the need for consent; however, some ethical issues are raised when volunteers receive payment for the experience and when painful procedures are involved. Procedures like pelvic examinations, peripheral line placement, and extremity splinting or casting are commonly done with human volunteers.

Computer-based technologies have numerous applications in the teaching of emergency procedures. Multimedia technologies can deliver text information augmented with photographs, audio files, and video clips. Such technologies allow a more realistic presentation of the information. Included in the eight steps of procedural skill learning listed by Chapman is "developing a mental image of performing the procedure," which can be greatly aided by videodiscs and CD-ROM technology (27). Additionally, the use of web-based programs will allow individual learning away from the bedside, which is important given recent decreases in direct patient care opportunities resulting from work hour restrictions. The Educational Technology Section of the 2004 Academic Emergency Medicine Consensus Conference recommended that every emergency department have access to educational

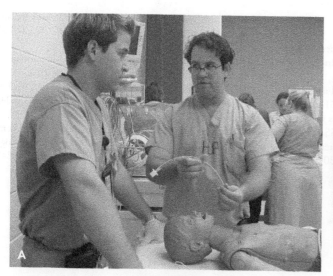
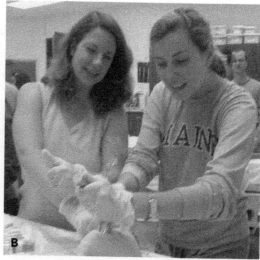

Figure 10.2
A. An intubation workshop utilizing manikin-based simulators.
B. Practicing endotracheal intubation on a manikin-based simulator.

materials via the Internet and that real-time automated tools be integrated for contemporaneous education (28).

The need for active learning and frequent practice, combined with the explosion of computer-based technology, has led to the recent development of high-fidelity manikin-based simulators (Fig. 10.2) The newer manikins generate more realistic physical exam findings, and the computer interface allows for the accurate programming of physiologic responses to interventions. The models are expensive and require a considerable time commitment in order to master the designing of effective scenarios. However, computer-controlled simulation for high-risk, low-frequency events appears promising (29).

▶ ACKNOWLEDGMENTS

The authors would like to acknowledge the valuable contributions of Roy M. Kulick to the version of this chapter that appeared in the previous edition.

▶ REFERENCES

1. Knowles MS. *The Modern Practice of Adult Education: Andragogy versus Pedagogy.* New York: Association Press; 1970.
2. Ende J. Feedback in clinical medical education. *JAMA.* 1983;250:777–781.
3. Bandiera G, Lee S, Tiberius R. Creating effective learning in today's emergency departments: how accomplished teachers get it done. *Ann Emerg Med.* 2005;45:253–261.
4. Whitman N, Lawrence P. Teaching procedures. In: *Surgical Teaching: Practice Makes Perfect.* Salt Lake City: University of Utah School of Medicine; 1991:65–80.
5. Marteau TM, Wynne G, Kaye W, et al. Resuscitation experience without feedback increases confidence but not skills. *BMJ.* 1990;300:849.
6. Thomas H Jr. Teaching procedural skills: beyond "see one-do one." *Acad Emerg Med.* 1994;1:398–401.
7. Weiss V, Needlman R. To teach is to learn twice: resident teachers learn more. *Arch Pediatr Adolesc Med.* 1998;152:190–192.
8. Hedges JR. Pearls for the teaching of procedural skills at the bedside. *Acad Emerg Med.* 1994;1:401–404.
9. Shysh AJ. Adult learning principles: you can teach an old dog new tricks. *Can J Anaesth.* 2000;47:837–842.
10. Shysh AJ, Carter K, Eagle CJ. The Canadian and U.S. perspective in setting the competency level for residents: minimum numbers of cases and procedures [abstract]. *Can J Anaesth.* 1998;45:A55-B.
11. Trainor JL, Krug SE. The training of pediatric residents in the care of acutely ill and injured children. *Arch Pediatr Adolesc Med.* 2000;154:1154–1159.
12. Nadel FM, LaVelle JM, Fein JA, et al. Assessing pediatric senior residents' training in resuscitation: fund of knowledge, technical skills, and perception of confidence. *Pediatr Emerg Care.* 2000;16:73–76.
13. Falck AJ, Escobedo MB, Baillargeon JG, et al. Proficiency of pediatric residents in performing neonatal endotracheal intubation. *Pediatrics.* 2003;112:1242–1247.
14. Fein JA, LaVelle J, Giardino AP. Teaching emergency medicine to pediatric residents: a national survey and proposed model. *Pediatr Emerg Care.* 1995;11:208–211.
15. Homan CS, Viccellio P, Thode HC, et al. Evaluation of an emergency-procedure teaching laboratory for the development of proficiency in tube thoracostomy. *Acad Emerg Med.* 1994;1:382–387.
16. Hergenroeder AC, Chorley JN, Laufman L, et al. Pediatric residents' performance of ankle and knee examinations after an educational intervention. *Pediatrics.* 2001;107(4):1–5.
17. Nadel FM, LaVelle JM, Fein JA, et al. Teaching resuscitation to pediatric residents: the effects of an intervention. *Arch Pediatr Adolesc Med.* 2000;154:1049–1054.
18. Stratton SJ, Kane G, Gunter CS, et al. Prospective study of manikin-only versus manikin and human subject endotracheal intubation training of paramedics. *Ann Emerg Med.* 1991;20:1314–1318.
19. Macnab AJ, Macnab M. Teaching pediatric procedures: the Vancouver model for instructing Seldinger's technique of central venous access via the femoral vein. *Pediatrics.* 1999;103(1):1–4.
20. Kaplan J. The use of animals in research. *Science.* 1998;242:839–840.

21. Nelson MS. Models for teaching emergency medicine skills. *Ann Emerg Med.* 1990;19:333–335.

22. Deveau JP, Lorenz JE, Hughes MJ. Emergency medicine resident work productivity and procedural accomplishment. *J Am Osteopath Assoc.* 2003;103:291–296.

23. Morhaim DK, Heller MB. The practice of teaching endotracheal intubation on recently deceased patients. *J Emerg Med.* 1991;9:515–518.

24. Burns JP, Reardon FE, Truog RT. Using newly deceased patients to teach resuscitation procedures. *N Engl J Med.* 1994;331:1652–1655.

25. Brattebo G, Wisborg T, Solheim K, et al. Public opinion on different approaches to teaching intubation techniques. *Br Med J.* 1993;307:1256–1257.

26. McNamara RM, Monti S, Kelly JJ. Requesting consent for an invasive procedure in newly deceased adults. *JAMA.* 1995;273:310–312.

27. Chapman DM. Use of computer-based technologies in teaching emergency procedural skills. *Acad Emerg Med.* 1994;1:404–407.

28. Vozenilek J, Huff JS, Reznek M, et al. See one, do one, teach one: advanced technology in medical education. *Acad Emerg Med.* 2004;11:1149–1154.

29. Mayo PH, Hackney JE, Mueck JT, et al. Achieving house staff competence in emergency airway management: results of a teaching program using a computerized patient simulator. *Crit Care Med.* 2004;32:2422–2427.

PHILIP V. SCRIBANO

Documentation

11

▶ INTRODUCTION

When encountering a pediatric patient in the emergency department (ED) who requires a diagnostic or therapeutic procedure, the medical provider must be able to accurately document the procedure. Clinical documentation has at least four purposes: recording of medical care and subsequent communication among providers, payment for services rendered, medicolegal concerns, and surveillance for public health or research purposes (1–5). The Joint Commission on Accreditation of Healthcare Organizations (JCAHO) requirement for the ED record at a minimum prescribes that a report of any procedure, including tests sent and results received, be documented appropriately on the ED chart.

In our high-technology era, medical informatics, including the use of electronic documentation of emergency department care, has become an active issue for many departments. It offers tremendous potential for improved patient care by enhancing patient care continuity, patient safety, and health care system efficiency; advancing research efforts; and supporting surveillance efforts. However, implementing a system of electronic documentation given the realities of limited standards and evolving technology is a major challenge (5,6). To provide additional information to assist with emergency department documentation guidelines, the Centers for Disease Control and Prevention developed Data Elements for Emergency Department Systems (DEEDS) (7). Lastly, an important medicolegal component of medical care is informed consent and the documentation of this process. Issues regarding informed consent are discussed in Chapter 9. Discussion of this topic here will focus on the recording of medical care and medicolegal issues. The topic will be elaborated by reviewing the appropriate documentation of surgical procedures, such as laceration repair (Fig. 11.1); of medical procedures, such as lumbar puncture (Fig. 11.2) and thoracentesis; and of the use

of restraints for specific behavioral health issues (Fig. 11.3). Specific information regarding restraint techniques is included in Chapter 3.

Briefly, informed consent in the pediatric patient raises some issues that do not apply to the competent adult patient. The law views the pediatric patient as incompetent to consent to treatment or procedures and is clear in providing that legal right to natural parents or legal guardians on behalf of the child. Although the competent adult patient has the legal and moral right to refuse consent to a procedure or treatment, parents are not given the absolute right to refuse treatment or to have a procedure performed on behalf of their child under the conditions of an emergency (8).

An *emergency* has been defined as "any condition that requires prompt medical intervention" but is not restricted to conditions that may cause death or disability. If the life or health of the child would be adversely affected by a delay caused by the parents' refusal, the situation is deemed an emergency (8). Limitations on parental authority have been supported by the Committee on Bioethics of the American Academy of Pediatrics and the President's Commission for the Study of Ethical Problems in Medicine and Biomedical and Behavioral Research. More detailed discussion of informed consent and refusal may be found in Chapter 9.

▶ THE DOCUMENTATION PROCESS

The purposes of documentation of procedures in the ED are many. First, any encounter with a patient should generate a record of that encounter and events surrounding it, especially when an action has the potential to adversely affect the patient's well-being. This record serves to protect both the patient and the physician. Second, documenting a procedure

Consent issues regarding repair and conscious sedation discussed with parent/guardian; risks and benefits of repair and sedation were explained and informed consent was obtained. Midazolam, 3 mg PO was given and continuous pulse oximetry and cardiac monitoring was used. In the supine position, under sterile conditions, a 2.5 linear laceration along the lateral aspect of the right thigh was irrigated with 200 ml NSS, followed by preparation of the site with povidine; topical anesthetic 3 ml (lidocaine 4%, epinephrine 0.05%, tetracaine 0.5%) was applied to the wound over 20 minutes. Three- 4.0 chromic, interrupted sutures were placed subcuticular to approximate the wound margins; Six- 4.0 interrupted nylon sutures were placed with good approximation of wound margins. Antibiotic ointment was applied with a sterile dressing. The patient tolerated the procedure well. No evidence of lasting sedative effects noted and the patient was stable for discharge from the E.D.

Figure 11.1 Sample laceration repair procedure note.

and its results maximizes communication with other health care professionals who may be caring for the patient, especially if verbal communication is not possible. Third, from an academic standpoint, the well-documented procedure note serves to educate other health care professionals regarding the approach to that particular procedure and the associated issues,

Consent issues discussed with parent/guardian; risks (e.g., infection, bleeding) and benefits (e.g., possible diagnosis of meningitis) of lumbar puncture explained and informed consent was obtained. In the lateral recumbent position and under sterile conditions, the child was prepped with povidine and 1 mL of 1% lidocaine without epinephrine was injected at the L3-4 interspace followed by a 2$\frac{1}{2}$ inch spinal needle in the usual fashion. Six mL of clear CSF fluid was obtained without difficulty. A sterile dressing was applied to the puncture site and the patient tolerated the procedure well.

Figure 11.2 Sample lumbar puncture procedure note.

2130: Patient exhibiting danger to others. Verbal de-escalation and seclusion attempted without success. Patient placed in supine position, and wrist and ankle (bilateral) restraints applied without difficulty after explanation to child and parent of need for procedure. Parents verbally communicate understanding of procedure. Will re-evaluate in 1 hour to determine continued application vs. restraint removal. Frequent nursing monitoring, per protocol.

Figure 11.3 Sample restraint procedure note.

such as use of sedation and/or analgesia, the use of specific equipment, and the positioning of the patient. It also affords researchers the opportunity to critically review certain aspects of a given technique and to suggest ways of improving the procedure in the future.

The documentation of the procedure itself should focus on several key features. First, the practitioner should describe in detail the area of interest. For instance, in the case of a laceration requiring repair, the practitioner should describe its length, the depth of the wound (e.g., through the dermis, through the fascia), the shape (e.g., curvilinear, jagged), the body area of involvement, the presence of active bleeding, and the overall integrity of the soft tissues (e.g., avulsed, intact).

Second, the practitioner should document the preparation of the wound area, including irrigation of the area with saline and/or povidone-iodine solution and débridement of devitalized skin or underlying soft tissue.

Third, the practitioner should note the use and type of anesthesia. The practitioner should record particular features, including the concentration and volume of the anesthetic (e.g., 3 mL of 1% lidocaine without epinephrine) and the route of administration (e.g., topical using preparations such as LET [lidocaine, epinephrine, tetracaine] or simple infiltration with lidocaine by needle). If sedation is required, it is recommended that the practitioner document the type of sedative used, the amount given, and its route of administration (e.g., oral, rectal, intranasal, intravenous), as well as the use of appropriate monitoring such as pulse oximetry and cardiac monitoring. Given the recent JCAHO focus on sedation and analgesia procedures, a more detailed documentation process is recommended (9), with a separate documentation form to adequately comply with the JCAHO guidelines. This topic is discussed further in Chapter 33.

Fourth, the practitioner should record the repair itself, including the materials used and the type and number of sutures (e.g., four #5.0 nylon interrupted sutures; two #4.0 nylon vertical mattress sutures; or three #4.0 chromic, subcuticular, interrupted sutures). The practitioner also should comment on the overall approximation of the repair (e.g., good approximation of the wound margins is observed). Lastly, the practitioner should document the wound dressing in the chart, including the use of antibiotic ointment, the type of sterile dressing applied, and the use and type of splints.

Documentation of a medical procedure such as a lumbar puncture, thoracentesis, or arthrocentesis requires some additional details that are less crucial than in most minor surgical procedures. More emphasis on the position of the patient, as well as a description of the approach to the procedure and the actual findings related to the procedure, is warranted. For example, when performing a lumbar puncture, the practitioner should document whether the patient was placed in a lateral recumbent position or seated upright for the procedure. This is especially important if opening and closing pressures will be assessed. As previously mentioned for surgical procedures, preparation of the needle entry site and the use and type of anesthesia should be documented. Again, special mention should be made if conscious sedation is being used, with a comment on the monitoring employed. The cerebrospinal fluid specimen as it is being obtained also should be described (e.g., CSF was noted to be clear or bloody). If multiple attempts have been made, this too should be documented. The description of the approach should include details such as the gauge of the needle used and the site of penetration (e.g., L3-L4 interspace). A comment on the patient's condition after the lumbar puncture has been performed should be included (e.g., the child tolerated the procedure well). Any adverse events related to or occurring at the time of the procedure should be recorded. After the appropriate studies have been sent, recording the laboratory findings on the chart is required.

Similarly, if an arthrocentesis is being performed, a description of the position of the patient (e.g., supine, prone) and the extremity (e.g., extension, flexion) is important. The description of the approach should include details such as the gauge of the needle used and the site of penetration (e.g., inferolateral to the patella). The synovial fluid specimen (e.g., straw-colored, turbid, sanguineous) should be described. As previously mentioned for surgical procedures, preparation of the site and the use and type of anesthesia should be documented. Again, special mention should be made if sedation and analgesia are being used, with a comment on the monitoring employed.

Documentation of a procedure such as thoracentesis requires slightly more vigilance than documentation of the procedures previously described, for several reasons. First, because of the upright positioning required, immobilization of the anxious pediatric patient may be less than optimal and may therefore lessen the overall success of the procedure. Second, some patients may have immediate life-threatening disease, putting them at higher risk, especially if a complication occurs. Third, the complications of a thoracentesis have a higher morbidity than the complications of the procedures previously discussed and may not be immediately apparent (e.g., pulmonary contusion, pneumothorax, hepatic or splenic trauma). The child's position (e.g., in the sitting position with the arms and head supported on a pillow) should be documented. The

SUMMARY

Key Features of a Well-Documented Medical or Surgical Procedure

1 Position of the patient

2 Preparation of the body area

3 Use of anesthetic/sedation

4 General technique

5 Specimen/gross findings

6 General condition of patient

7 Results of laboratory tests on specimens obtained

8 Potential complications

approach, including the preparation of the area, the use of anesthetics and sedation, the location of needle insertion (e.g., at the 7th intercostal space along the posterior axillary line), and the gauge of the needle, should be briefly described. Mention of the thoracentesis specimen findings, such as the volume of pleural fluid obtained and its color (e.g., serous, serosanguinous, sanguinous), should be made. A comment on the patient's condition after the procedure is recommended. Lastly, after successful completion of the procedure, the results of laboratory tests should be recorded and an upright chest radiograph taken to document the presence of any iatrogenic complications.

Another important JCAHO focus has been on patient restraint procedures (see Chapter 3). Documentation of patient restraint must include a description of the behavior requiring restraint or seclusion (e.g., danger to self or others); identification of the type of restraints (e.g., wrist restraints, ankle restraints); any explanation or information provided to the patient and/or guardian regarding the use of restraints and the criteria for their discontinuation; and documentation of the need for continued restraint versus restraint removal, along with hourly reassessments and recording of such. It is also very important for nursing staff to document the patient's condition (as often as every 15 to 30 minutes), including vital signs and the status of the areas (e.g., wrist, ankles) being restrained throughout the procedure (9,10).

▶ SUMMARY

Good documentation of emergency department procedures will provide the information necessary to maintain optimal communication to those caring for the patient after the procedure has been performed and can be helpful and instructional to those reviewing the medical record in the future. The basic elements of this documentation should support the purposes of clinical documentation and provide the reader with a clear understanding of the patient at the time of the procedure, the actual procedure performed, the results of the procedure, and any untoward events resulting from or temporally related to the procedure. These elements are summarized in the summary box.

▶ REFERENCES

1. Botkin J. Informed consent for lumbar puncture. *Am J Dis Child.* 1989;143:899–903.
2. Bukata WR. Emergency department medical record. In: Henry GL, ed. *Emergency Medicine Risk Management.* Dallas, TX: American College of Emergency Physicians; 1991:235–247.
3. Selbst S. Medicolegal considerations. In: Diekmann RA, Craven L, Eckhart C, et al., eds. *Pediatric Emergency Care Systems.* Baltimore: Williams and Wilkins; 1992:421–432.
4. Cordovan MB. Legal issues. In: Barkin R, Caputo G, Jaffe D, ed. *Pediatric Emergency Medicine: Concepts and Clinical Practice.* St. Louis, Mosby; 1997:81–94.
5. Davidson SJ, Zwemer FL, Nathanson LA, et al. Where's the beef? The promise and the reality of clinical documentation. *Acad Emerg Med.* 2004;11:1127–1134.
6. Coonan KM. Medical informatics standards applicable to emergency department information systems: making sense of the jumble. *Acad Emerg Med.* 2004;11:1198–1205.
7. Centers for Disease Control and Prevention. *Data Elements for Emergency Department Systems.* Available at: http://www.cdc.gov/ncipc/pubres/pdf/deeds.pdf. Accessed February 5, 2007.
8. Weintraub MI. Documentation and informed consent. *Neurol Clin.* 1999;17:371–381.
9. Joint Commission on Accreditation of Healthcare Organizations. *Comprehensive Accreditation Manual for Hospitals: The Official Handbook.* Oakbrook Terrace, IL: Joint Commission on Accreditation of Healthcare Organizations; 2005:PC25–43.
10. Dorfman DH. The use of physical and chemical restraints in the pediatric emergency department. *Pediatr Emerg Care.* 2000;16:355–360.

SECTION 2 ▶ CARDIOPULMONARY LIFE SUPPORT PROCEDURES

SECTION EDITOR: CHRISTOPHER KING

12

CONSTANCE M. McANENEY

Basic Life Support

▶ INTRODUCTION

Basic life support (BLS) encompasses early recognition and intervention for respiratory and cardiopulmonary arrest. The goal of BLS is to artificially supply oxygen to the body, most importantly to the brain and heart, through the use of rescue breathing and chest compressions. BLS can represent either a definitive intervention (since spontaneous respirations and normal cardiac activity will sometimes resume) or a temporizing measure until advanced life support (ALS) can be administered (the usual case). BLS is a crucial component of the overall emergency medical system for children, which includes bystander cardiopulmonary resuscitation (CPR), rapid response by appropriately trained prehospital personnel, and transport to a hospital emergency department (ED). Prompt initiation of BLS is critical for a good outcome. Consequently, all individuals responsible for the care of children—including parents and other caregivers, emergency medical personnel, nurses, and physicians—should have training in this procedure.

Cardiopulmonary arrest in the pediatric population is an uncommon event. In fact, only 10% to 15% of all arrest victims are younger than 19 years of age (1). The age range most commonly affected is children under 1 year, representing approximately half of all pediatric arrests. Among the remaining patients, children between the ages of 1 and 4 years account for 15% to 30% of pediatric arrests, school-age children

(5 to 12 years) 15% to 20%, and teenagers 10% to 15% (1–5). With children younger than 4 years of age, the causative event is most likely to occur in or around the home, including apparent life-threatening events (formerly called "near-miss sudden infant death syndrome"), household injuries, respiratory illnesses, drownings, and neurologic disorders. For school-age children, the streets and recreational areas are more common sites, with injuries and drownings representing the most common causes (2,6–8).

Asystole is by far the most common arrest rhythm seen among pediatric patients, accounting for 75% to 90% of documented cases (1,5,7,9,10). However, ventricular fibrillation (VF) also occurs. Two studies suggest that from 6% to 11% of children and young adults who experience a pulseless arrest have VF (11,12). Pediatric patients presenting with VF are likely to have a specific insult to the heart, such as accidental ingestion of a cardiotonic medication, metabolic abnormalities, or underlying cardiac disease (2,7,9,10). Unlike in the case of adults, coronary artery insufficiency is a rare cause of pediatric arrest. As a result, whereas adult patients usually suffer a sudden primary cardiac arrest, cardiopulmonary arrest in children generally represents a "final common pathway" after progressively worsening compromise as a result of other illnesses. Indeed, respiratory etiologies of arrest are far more likely among pediatric patients than are cardiac etiologies.

Most studies of out-of-hospital normothermic cardiac arrest in children report survival averages of 10%, although most of these victims suffer permanent neurologic impairment (4,5,8,13,14). Not surprisingly, the highest rate of intact survival is achieved with witnessed arrests when there has been prompt institution of BLS and ALS procedures (2,3,6,9). In a study of out-of-hospital arrest in children, Hickey et al. found an overall 27% survival rate; all but one of the survivors had return of spontaneous circulation prior to arrival in the ED (15). Conversely, the intact survival rate for respiratory arrest alone may exceed 50% with rapid intervention (4,10,13). This relatively high rate of survival underscores the importance of early recognition and resuscitation for pediatric patients who suffer a primary respiratory arrest.

This chapter focuses exclusively on the CPR component of BLS for children. Although traditionally included with BLS procedures, the initial management of upper airway foreign bodies (back blows, Heimlich maneuver, etc.) is not discussed in this chapter. A complete description of both the basic and advanced techniques for managing upper airway foreign bodies is found in Chapter 51.

▶ ANATOMY AND PHYSIOLOGY

Airway/Breathing

Various techniques for attempted resuscitation of the dead or near-dead have been described since ancient times (16). Proposed methods for reviving victims have included rolling on a barrel, bouncing on a galloping horse, and using a bellows to blow air into the lungs. Manual methods of ventilation using either back pressure arm-lift or chest pressure arm-lift date back almost 150 years (17,18). The Schafer "prone pressure method" was taught by the American Red Cross until the late 1950s, when mouth-to-mouth resuscitation was recognized as being more effective.

References to mouth-to-mouth ventilation date as far back as biblical times. In 1771, Tossach described inflating a person's lungs using the rescuer's expired air (19). Yet it was the pivotal studies by Safar and Gordon published in the 1950s that demonstrated that mouth-to-mouth ventilation was superior to other methods for all age groups in providing rescue breathing (20–22). These reports, along with the landmark publication by Kouwenhoven et al. describing closed chest compression (23), began the modern era of CPR.

A number of important differences exist between pediatric patients and adults that are relevant to airway control and rescue breathing (24,25) (Fig. 12.1). For one, the occiput of an infant is more prominent, which may cause a flexed airway when the infant is lying in the supine position. In addition, when compared with adults, infants and younger children have a larger tongue relative to the size of the hypopharynx and greater laxity of the pharyngeal soft tissues. These characteristics contribute to the fact that pediatric patients are prone to develop airway obstruction simply from lying supine. More-

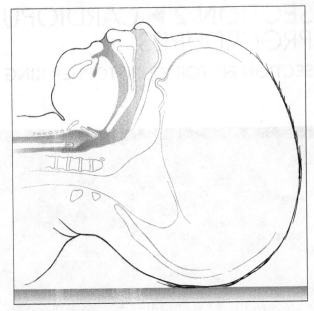

Figure 12.1 Anatomy of the infant airway. The infant has a more prominent occiput than an adult, resulting in neck flexion and potential airway obstruction when the patient is lying supine on a flat surface. The tongue of an infant is also large in relation to the size of the oropharynx, as well as being more superiorly positioned. Both characteristics increase the likelihood of airway obstruction by the tongue.

over, the neck is short and chubby, making appropriate positioning more difficult. The tracheal cartilage is soft and easily compressible; as a result, hyperextension of the infant's head and neck can produce airway obstruction. There is also greater airway resistance caused by the narrower luminal diameter of the pediatric airway. According to Poiseuille's law, resistance to gas flow is inversely proportional to the fourth power of the radius (25). A pediatric airway one-half the diameter of an adult airway will therefore have a 16-fold greater resistance to flow. For this reason, even small changes in airway diameter (e.g., due to inflammation, edema, or improper positioning) may cause severe respiratory compromise in a younger patient. Further discussion of this concept and other aspects of pediatric airway anatomy can be found in Chapters 14 and 16.

Many aspects of the mechanics of breathing are also unique to infants and children. Because the pediatric rib cage is very pliable and more horizontally oriented, it does not provide the same degree of support as with an adult, and therefore the residual capacity of the lungs is decreased. If there is diminished air entry resulting from intrinsic lung disease or upper airway obstruction, the negative pressure created during inspiration causes paradoxical movement of the chest. In addition, infants and younger children are more dependent on diaphragmatic excursion for ventilation. Any conditions that hamper movement of the diaphragm (abdominal distension, masses, etc.) can therefore significantly impair gas exchange. Children also develop hypoxemia in response to respiratory insults more rapidly than adults due in part to differences in the work of breathing and alveolar surface area. Efficient respiratory effort takes place when a minimum of energy is expended to provide an adequate respiratory rate and tidal volume. Increased airway resistance and greater chest wall compliance cause children to achieve efficient breathing at higher relative rates than adults, disproportionately increasing the metabolic demands of respiration (25). Furthermore, the smaller alveolar surface area of a pediatric patient results in a diminished reserve for gas exchange. As a result, processes that cause mismatching of ventilation and perfusion in the lungs are more likely to produce hypoxemia in children.

As mentioned previously, respiratory failure is the primary cause of cardiopulmonary arrest among pediatric patients. Respiratory failure results from inadequate oxygenation of blood and/or inadequate ventilation. Inadequate oxygenation, which is usually caused by either intrinsic lung disease or upper airway obstruction, leads to a succession of adverse effects, including tissue hypoxia, lactic acid production, and metabolic acidosis. Initially the patient attempts to compensate by increasing the respiratory effort and rate; when this can no longer be sustained, the patient develops progressively worsening hypoxemia and acidosis, resulting eventually in full cardiopulmonary failure. By contrast, ventilatory dysfunction impairs excretion of CO_2 (hypercarbia), producing a respiratory acidosis. This is generally a more gradual process and results from conditions that inhibit the normal functioning of the "respiratory pump" (i.e., those systems of the body responsible for producing effective ventilation) (see also Chapter 16). With progressively increasing levels of CO_2 in the blood, fatigue and mental status depression cause respiratory effort to wane and finally cease altogether. The patient develops worsening hypoxemia as well as hypercarbia, profound acidosis, and ultimately cardiac arrest.

Circulation

Although adults typically have abrupt cardiovascular collapse caused by arrhythmia as a prelude to arrest, pediatric patients often experience a more gradual worsening of circulatory compromise and shock. Simply stated, the shock state is characterized by delivery of oxygen and substrate to tissues that is insufficient to meet metabolic demands. This outcome depends on the circulating blood volume, cardiac output, and vasomotor tone, which are continually regulated to maintain tissue perfusion. Significant changes in any one of these variables result in altered function of the others as the body attempts to maintain an adequate blood pressure. For example, a drop in vasomotor tone (e.g., septic shock) is accompanied by an elevated cardiac output through increased heart rate and stroke volume; significant blood loss or dehydration causes both increased vasomotor tone and increased cardiac output. In addition, compensatory mechanisms, such as the release of endogenous catecholamines, also operate to maintain an adequate blood pressure despite compromise to one or more of these physiologic mechanisms. As shock progresses, however,

these compensatory mechanisms become inadequate, and the patient develops global deficits in oxygen and substrate delivery to vital organs, resulting in multiple organ system failure and eventually cardiopulmonary arrest.

For purposes of discussion, shock is divided into three general categories: hypovolemic, distributive, and cardiogenic. Hypovolemic shock, the most common type in the pediatric age group, is characterized by inadequate intravascular volume, resulting in a diminished stroke volume and cardiac output. Dehydration and hemorrhage are by far the most common causes, but "third-spacing" of fluids (i.e., sequestering fluids within the body but outside the cardiovascular system) can also cause hypovolemic shock. Distributive shock is characterized by peripheral vasodilatation, resulting in a drop in systemic blood pressure. The cardiac output may be normal or even elevated, but the maldistribution of blood flow causes inadequate perfusion of vital organs. This type of shock is seen in anaphylaxis, certain drug ingestions, and early sepsis. As septic shock progresses, significant intravascular fluid losses occur as well as myocardial dysfunction, and thus in the later phases of septic shock, a low cardiac output state also develops. Cardiogenic shock is characterized by myocardial dysfunction. Even though the intravascular volume and heart rate may be adequate or even increased, poor myocardial contractility results in a diminished stroke volume and diminished cardiac output. Cardiogenic shock is usually seen in patients with underlying heart disease (congenital or acquired) and metabolic derangements such as acidosis, hypoxia, hypoglycemia, and hypocalcemia.

The first scientific reports of cardiac compression were published in the late 19th and early 20th centuries. The impetus for this work was the occurrence of sudden, unexpected death of patients receiving chloroform anesthesia. Open cardiac massage was initially advocated for treating arrest patients (26,27), but this proved to be fraught with complications and required the expertise of highly trained physicians. The method of closed chest compression was initially described by Boehm in 1878 using laboratory animals (28). Further reports on this technique appeared sporadically over the next 70 years, but it was not until the work of Kouwenhoven et al., published in 1960, that closed chest cardiac compression was considered a potential intervention for arrest patients (23).

The exact mechanism by which cardiac compressions produce forward blood flow has been a point of controversy over the years (Fig. 12.2). In what has become known as the "cardiac pump theory," Kouwenhoven et al. postulated that the heart is directly compressed between the sternum and the thoracic spine, causing blood flow as the heart empties (23). Relaxation of the pressure on the chest allows the heart to refill with blood, and the cycle is continued. Although the myocardium no longer contracts, the heart nonetheless functions as a pump across which there is a pressure gradient. It was theorized that during compression, the aortic and pulmonic valves open, while retrograde flow is prevented by closure of the mitral and tricuspid valves. During the relaxation phase, the ventricles re-expand to their original size and are filled by

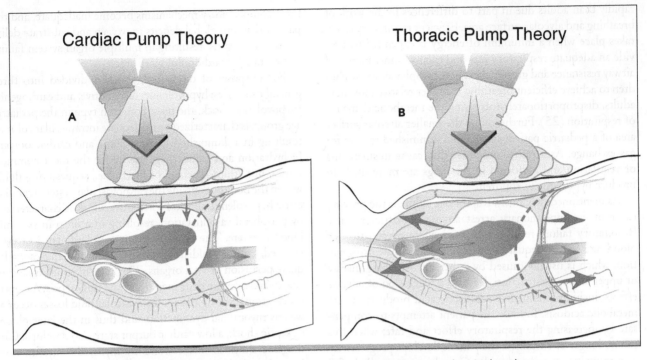

Figure 12.2 Cardiac pump theory versus thoracic pump theory. These two theories have been proposed to explain the effects of chest compressions during CPR. The cardiac pump theory postulates that direct compression of the heart causes forward flow of blood. The heart serves as a pump. The thoracic pump theory postulates that pressure generated in the entire thoracic cavity causes forward blood flow, while the heart functions more as a passive conduit.

suction effect, while arterial pressure was thought to close the aortic and pulmonic valves.

The cardiac pump theory was generally accepted until 1976, when Criley et al. (29) described a patient undergoing cardiac catheterization who developed VF. The patient began coughing in a rhythmic fashion and surprisingly remained conscious, raising questions about the mechanism of CPR. Changes in intrathoracic pressure, rather than any direct compressive effect on the heart, appeared to produce significant forward blood flow during coughing. This observation became the basis for the "thoracic pump theory." Experimental studies with large animals have shown that chest compressions produce an equal rise in pressure on all other intrathoracic structures as well as the heart (30). In other words, the heart does not function as a pump but simply as a passive conduit. During compression, an intrathoracic-to-extrathoracic pressure gradient causes forward flow through the arterial system; retrograde flow is prevented by venous valves and collapse of the veins. When the chest compression is released, the pressure gradient is reversed, and blood flows from the extrathoracic to the intrathoracic venous system (Fig. 12.2).

As might be predicted, the debate has not ended there, particularly with regard to pediatric patients. More recent studies in small animals using higher forces for chest compression have shown that intrathoracic vascular pressures are in fact much greater than pleural pressures (31). This higher than expected rise in vascular pressure would seem to be a consequence of direct cardiac compression, as originally proposed

by Kouwenhoven. Although the exact mechanism has yet to be determined, it seems likely that *both* proposed theories are applicable to pediatric patients in differing degrees. Infants and younger children, who have a relatively small, compliant chest wall, probably depend more on direct cardiac compression for forward blood flow. With older children and adolescents, overall changes in intrathoracic pressure are likely to predominate. The recommendations of the American Heart Association for the rate and duration of chest compressions are designed to have maximal effectiveness irrespective of the mechanism of flow (32).

▶ INDICATIONS

The purpose of BLS is to provide circulation of oxygenated blood to vital organs, most importantly to the heart and brain. The outcome of resuscitation depends not only on the underlying condition but also on the timeliness and effectiveness of the resuscitation effort. The most common clinical scenarios requiring BLS procedures for pediatric patients are respiratory failure and arrest, cardiopulmonary failure, and cardiopulmonary arrest.

Respiratory Failure

Respiratory failure should be suspected in any patient with significant respiratory distress manifested by increased work of breathing. The most common causes of respiratory failure among pediatric patients are lower airway diseases (e.g., pneumonia, asthma, bronchiolitis, and aspiration) and processes affecting upper airway patency (e.g., croup syndromes, foreign bodies, intrinsic mass, and laryngospasm). Ventilatory dysfunction usually occurs in patients with lung disease who can no longer sustain the increased respiratory effort necessary to adequately excrete CO_2. Pulmonary muscle fatigue leads to progressively worsening hypercarbia. Ventilatory dysfunction also can occur in patients with central nervous system depression as a result of conditions such as drug overdose, head trauma, and seizures. Hypoxemia in early respiratory failure causes a child to be agitated and difficult to console. The patient may also develop cyanosis and bradycardia. Hypercarbia generally causes lethargy, and in more severe instances it causes unconsciousness. As respiratory failure progresses, the resulting acidosis leads to worsening cardiac output, hypotension, and poor tissue perfusion (mottling, cool extremities, prolonged capillary refill). With cases of isolated respiratory failure, prompt institution of ventilatory support with either rescue breathing or positive pressure ventilation will prevent this progression of symptoms.

Respiratory Arrest

Untreated respiratory failure eventually leads to respiratory arrest. When an abrupt primary respiratory arrest occurs (e.g., from a severe opioid overdose), circulation of oxygenated blood may continue for as long as a few minutes. Because cardiac activity is still present, the brain and other vital organs receive oxygen and substrate—albeit in an increasingly abnormal and inadequate manner—and the patient initially continues to have a palpable pulse. After several minutes, however, profound hypoxemia occurs, depressing brain and cardiac function. Clinically, this is manifested by an altered level of consciousness accompanied by a weak, slow pulse and signs of poor perfusion. This relatively brief interval of time, when respirations have ceased and a pulse is still present, is a critical period. Intervention at this point usually produces a good clinical outcome without permanent neurologic injury, whereas failure to intervene almost certainly results in a progression to cardiopulmonary arrest. Once the patient develops a significant cardiac arrhythmia in this situation (e.g., pulseless electrical activity or asystole), the prognosis generally becomes much worse.

Cardiopulmonary Failure

Cardiopulmonary failure may occur in the patient with progressive respiratory failure when hypoxemia and acidosis cause myocardial dysfunction, resulting in decreased heart rate and cardiac output. It may also be seen with the patient in shock when inadequate oxygen and substrate delivery to tissue has a similar adverse effect on the heart. The patient in early or compensated shock maintains a systolic blood pressure within an age-adjusted normal range, although other signs of circulatory compromise are present. As mentioned previously, the patient commonly presents with diminished peripheral pulses,

cool distal extremities, delayed capillary refill, markedly increased pulse rate, and a widened pulse pressure. The patient may appear anxious or agitated as a result of high circulating levels of endogenous catecholamines. As the shock state progresses, compensatory mechanisms become inadequate, and frank hypotension ensues. Peripheral pulses are absent, and central pulses are diminished. The skin is mottled or cyanotic, and the patient may be diaphoretic. The coolness of the distal extremities progresses proximally. Inadequate perfusion of the brain causes worsening lethargy, leading eventually to unconsciousness.

If untreated, both respiratory and circulatory failure will lead to cardiopulmonary failure as a result of global deficits in oxygen and substrate delivery to vital organs. The patient in impending cardiopulmonary failure will usually be comatose, with weak central pulses that may be detectable only by ultrasound. The patient will often exhibit gasping or agonal respirations. Because respiratory failure is by far the most common cause of cardiopulmonary failure in children, establishing an airway and performing rescue breathing will often reverse this cascade of events. However, if the heart rate of a child remains below 60 beats per minute despite adequate airway control and ventilation, chest compressions should be initiated to provide circulatory support.

Cardiopulmonary Arrest

Untreated cardiopulmonary failure will eventually result in complete cessation of respiratory effort and blood circulation. Patients are unresponsive, apneic, and cyanotic and have no detectable central pulse. The electrocardiogram will show life-threatening arrhythmias, such as profound sinus bradycardia, asystole, an idioventricular rhythm, or VF. Although there may be some minimal cardiac output with an organized rhythm (e.g., sinus bradycardia), this will not be enough to produce a pulse (i.e., pulseless electrical activity) or perfuse vital organs. BLS must be started immediately in this situation. As soon as appropriate personnel and equipment are available, further assessment and treatment of the underlying condition that caused the arrest can be initiated.

▶ PROCEDURE

BLS requires no equipment and can be accomplished in almost any location. Outcome largely depends on the timely initiation of CPR, the skill with which the procedures are performed, and the rapidity of instituting ALS interventions.

Determining Responsiveness

The initial step in any resuscitation is a general assessment of the patient. This should always be performed in a systematic way so that no pertinent clinical data that may influence necessary actions are omitted. The child's state of consciousness and ability to breathe and the extent of any injuries should be quickly determined. Gently shaking the child (assuming there is no risk of cervical spine injury) and speaking in a loud voice are helpful in assessing the level of responsiveness. Respiratory effort and effectiveness, as well as attempts to speak, should be noted. If a head or neck injury is suspected, the cervical spine should be immobilized. The presence of significant injuries can be quickly established in most cases by looking for any deformities, bleeding, or environmental clues that indicate trauma.

Once these three quick assessments are performed, a verbal call for help is made. If there is a lone rescuer and CPR is necessary, it should be performed for five "cycles" (30 compressions and two breaths constitute a cycle for the lone rescuer) before notifying EMS. Although not the protocol for adults, this is done for children because a primary respiratory insult, the most likely etiology of a pediatric arrest, may be completely reversible with initial BLS interventions. When an arrest in a child 1 year of age or older is witnessed and sudden, as with a teenage athlete who is running and collapses, a lone provider should activate the EMS system and obtain an automatic external defibrillator (AED) device (see also Chapter 23), if available, before initiating CPR (32). If there are two rescuers, one can initiate CPR while the other notifies EMS and obtains an AED.

Airway Control

Next the airway should be assessed for patency. Using the "look, listen, feel" approach, the operator observes the patient for airway compromise, listens over the patient's nose and mouth for breathing, and/or places a hand or cheek close to the patient's face to feel any air movement (Fig. 12.3). If obstruction is suspected, the operator must act immediately to establish a patent airway. For medical arrests, the head tilt–chin lift maneuver is preferred. Any child who suffers a traumatic arrest should have full immobilization of the head and neck, and airway patency is established using the jaw thrust maneuver. With either method, the child is first placed supine on a firm, flat surface, minimizing any movement of the neck as appropriate with a trauma patient. To perform the head tilt–chin lift maneuver, the operator places one hand on the patient's forehead and one or two fingers of the other hand just lateral to the chin. The neck is then extended slightly by gently pushing the forehead while pulling upward on the mandible (Fig. 12.4). Care must be taken not to close the mouth or inadvertently compress the soft tissue under the chin, because these actions may obstruct the airway. The jaw thrust maneuver allows the operator to open the airway without significantly moving the neck. The third and/or fourth fingers of both hands are "hooked" under the angle of the mandible as both thumbs are used to provide countertraction by pressing against the forehead. The mandible is lifted upward and outward with moderate force to open the mouth and

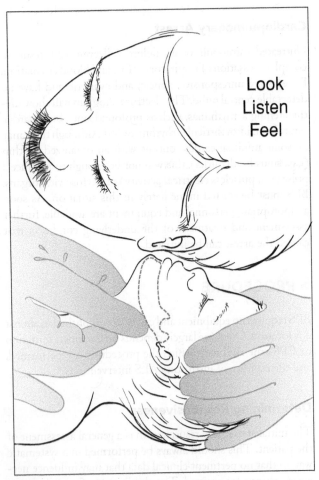

Figure 12.3 "Look, listen, feel" method of assessing air movement.

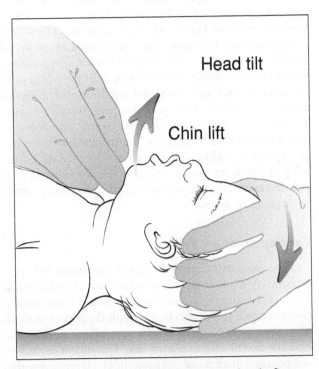

Figure 12.4 Head tilt–chin lift maneuver. Note that the fingers should not extend over the submental area, as this may produce airway obstruction.

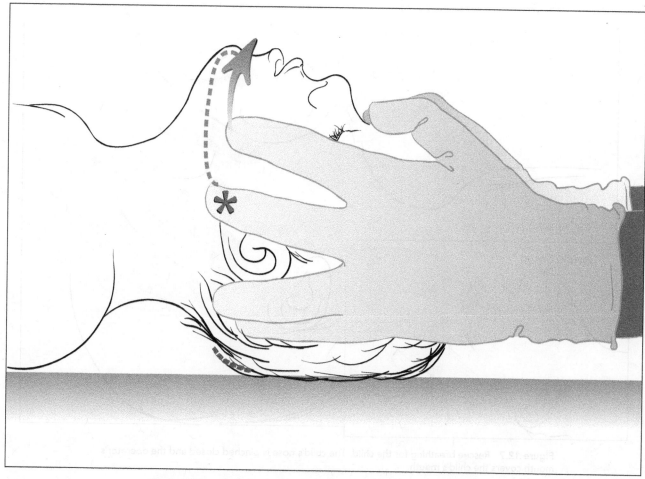

Figure 12.5 Jaw thrust maneuver with stabilization of the cervical spine.

displace the tongue anteriorly (Fig. 12.5). This maneuver is most comfortably performed with the operator's elbows resting on the surface just above the patient's head. The child with airway difficulty who is conscious should then be transported by experienced prehospital personnel to a facility where ALS and airway management can be provided.

Breathing

After airway patency has been established, the operator should assess the child's respirations. Once again, the standard "look, listen, feel" method is used. If the child is apneic or has inadequate respirations despite a patent airway, rescue breathing should be performed. With an infant, the operator places his or her mouth over the nose and mouth of the patient, creating a tight seal (Fig. 12.6). For the older child, the operator places his or her mouth over the mouth of the patient while pinching the patient's nose closed to prevent air escape (Fig. 12.7). If not already performed, the head tilt–chin lift maneuver is used to keep the airway open, as long as there is no risk of cervical spine injury.

Two breaths should be delivered slowly (over approximately 1 to 2 seconds), with a pause between breaths. Delivering the

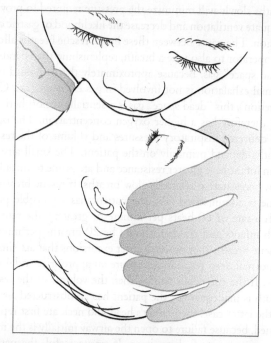

Figure 12.6 Rescue breathing for the infant. The operator's mouth covers the infant's nose and mouth.

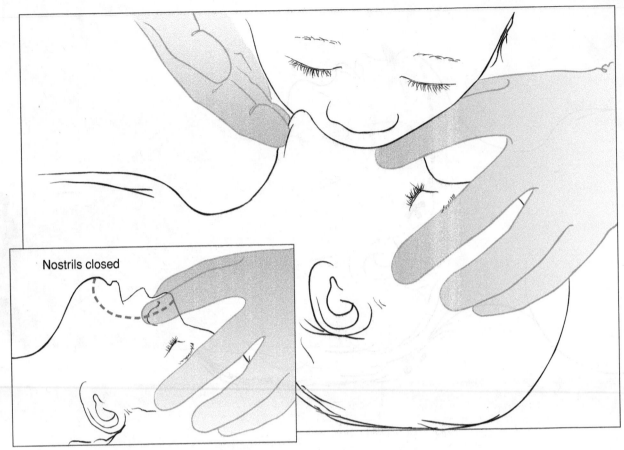

Figure 12.7   Rescue breathing for the child. The child's nose is pinched closed and the operator's mouth covers the child's mouth.

breaths slowly will minimize the pressure required to provide adequate ventilation and decrease the likelihood of gastric distension. The pause between these initial rescue breaths allows the operator to also take a breath, replenishing the operator's "dead space" gas. Because approximately the first third of a normal exhalation is not involved in gas exchange (i.e., CO_2 excretion), this "dead space" gas is essentially atmospheric air and therefore has a higher oxygen concentration. The optimal delivered inspiratory pressures and volume of the rescue breaths depend primarily on the patient. The small airways of an infant have greater resistance and are prone to turbulent flow, necessitating relatively slow breaths. If rescue breathing alone is administered (i.e., the patient has a palpable pulse with a rate of 60 beats per minute or greater), the rate for both infants and children should be 20 breaths per minute. Rescue breaths that produce chest excursions that are similar to normal deep respirations ensure an appropriate tidal volume. If the chest fails to rise, then the volume of the rescue breath is inadequate or the patient has an obstructed airway. In the latter case, the patient's head and neck are first repositioned, because failure to open the airway initially is the most common cause of obstruction. If unsuccessful, the patient may have an airway foreign body; maneuvers to identify and

alleviate this type of obstruction should then be performed (see Chapter 51).

Circulation

Checking the Pulse

After the airway has been positioned and two rescue breaths have been administered, the need for chest compressions is determined by palpating for a central pulse. In children older than 1 year, the carotid artery is the most accessible central artery for palpation. Because infants have short, chubby necks, the carotid pulse may be difficult to locate; consequently, palpating the brachial artery on the medial aspect of the upper arm is a more reliable method of checking the pulse with these patients (Fig. 12.8). Alternatively, the femoral pulse may be used. The apical impulse of the heart should not be used to verify pulselessness, because the absence of a palpable peripheral pulse does not necessarily preclude the presence of cardiac activity. If a pulse is present and the rate is greater than 60 beats per minute, then rescue breathing alone should be continued at a rate of 20 breaths per minute. If no pulse is palpable or the heart rate is less than 60 beats per minute,

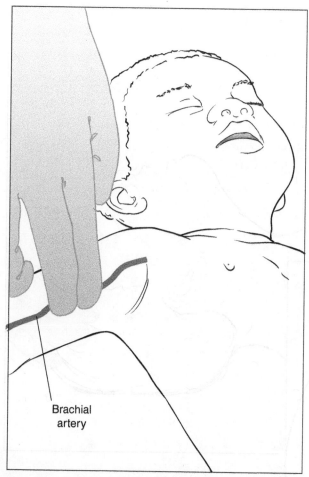

Figure 12.8 Palpating the pulse. Because infants have a short, chubby neck, palpating the brachial pulse is a more reliable method.

with signs of poor systemic perfusion, then chest compressions should be initiated and coordinated with ventilation, as described below.

Chest Compressions

The patient should be supine on a hard, flat surface in order to achieve optimal compressions. If an infant must be carried during CPR, the operator's forearm is used as a support for the infant's torso, while the head and neck are supported by the operator's hand. The other hand is used to perform compressions. The head should not be higher than the rest of the body. The compressions should be smooth and rhythmic, with equal time for compression and relaxation. The area of compression for both infants and children is the lower third of the sternum (33,34).

Infant chest compressions are performed using an imaginary line between the nipples (intermammary line) as a landmark. With the operator at the patient's side, the index finger is placed on the sternum just below the intermammary line. Sternal compressions are performed with the third and fourth fingers positioned one fingerbreadth below the intermammary line (Fig. 12.9). The depth of compression is one third to one

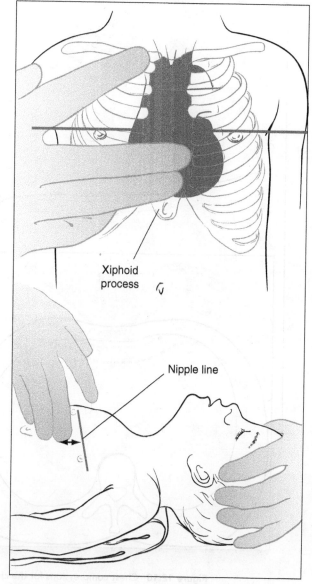

Figure 12.9 Chest compression for the infant. Compressions are performed with the fingers one fingerbreadth below the intermammary line.

half the total anteroposterior diameter of the chest, which corresponds to a compression depth of approximately half an inch to 1 inch in the infant. When there are two health care providers, the "two thumb-encircling hands" technique is recommended (32). With this method, the operator's hands encircle the patient's chest, and the two thumbs are placed together over the lower half of the patient's sternum. The operator uses both thumbs to forcefully compress the chest while using both hands to provide countertraction by squeezing the patient's thorax.

For children 1 to 8 years of age, chest compressions are performed using the heel of the hand on the lower sternum. The area of compression is located at the midline of the sternum two fingerbreadths superior to the xiphoid process (Fig. 12.10). The fingers are held away from the ribs during

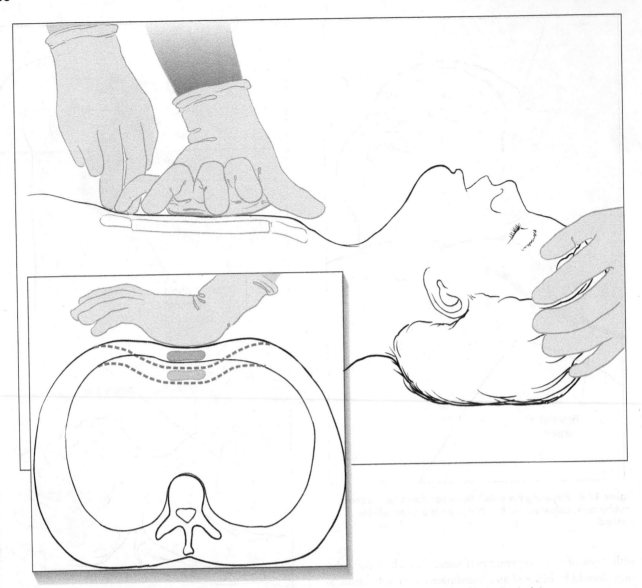

Figure 12.10 Chest compressions for the child. Compressions are performed with the heel of the hand one fingerbreadth above the xyphoid-sternal margin.

compressions to avoid injury to the ribs. Compressions should be one-third to one-half the total anteroposterior diameter of the chest, which for the child corresponds to a compression depth of approximately 1 to 1½ inches.

Recommendations from the American Hospital Association (AHA) regarding the optimal characteristics of effective chest compressions include (a) "push hard" to ensure that the chest is consistently depressed approximately one-third to one-half the anterior-posterior diameter of the chest, (b) "push fast" to ensure that compressions are consistently performed at a rate of approximately 100 per minute, (c) "release completely" to allow the chest to fully recoil and the heart to refill with blood, and (d) "minimize interruptions" so that perfusion of the vital organs is maintained at the most favorable possible level (32). The physical demands of performing chest compressions in this manner are such that rescuers should be allowed to rest or change roles frequently so that fatigue does not undermine the quality of the compressions administered.

As mentioned previously, a single rescuer should administer repeated cycles of 30 chest compressions followed by two ventilations. Pauses in chest compressions to administer ventilations (or check for pulses) should be as brief as possible. For two-rescuer CPR, the recommended ratio of chest compressions to ventilations is 15:2 (32). This approach can be used for children up to the onset of puberty, after which age the recommendations for adult patients become applicable. It should be emphasized that as the science of pediatric resuscitation advances, the best available data will undoubtedly lead to continued evolution in the preferred methods for performing BLS (compression techniques, compression-to-ventilation ratios, etc.). For this reason, it is important maintain ongoing familiarity with the most current published guidelines of the AHA and other similar organizations as they are periodically updated.

▶ COMPLICATIONS

Complications from BLS are relatively few and usually result from improper technique. For example, failure to adequately immobilize the neck with a trauma victim may result in cervical cord injury. In such cases, the jaw thrust maneuver combined with in-line immobilization should be used to maintain airway patency. In addition, the patient should be fully immobilized before any transport.

Improper positioning of the patient can also prevent effective rescue breathing. If the head tilt–chin lift maneuver is performed and adequate chest excursions are not produced, the rescuer should reposition the head until a more favorable

---

SUMMARY

1 Determine responsiveness.

    Gently shake infant or child if no injury suspected.

    Speak loudly.

2 Call out for help.

    If sudden arrest in a child (>1 yr), get AED/defibrillator.

    Apply AED immediately for sudden, witnessed arrest for child.

3 Position patient.

    Place supine on firm surface.

    Keep neck immobilized if injury suspected.

4 Assess airway patency.

    Use head tilt–chin lift maneuver.

    Use jaw thrust maneuver (if neck injury suspected).

5 Assess breathing.

    Watch for chest movement.

    Listen, feel for breaths.

6 Ventilate twice.

    Give two slow breaths.

    Watch for chest to rise.

    If no air movement, reposition and repeat.

    If still no air movement despite repositioning, perform airway obstruction maneuvers.

7 Check pulse.

    Use brachial or femoral in infant (<1 yr).

    Use carotid in child (>1 yr).

    Check for 3 to 5 seconds.

8 Perform chest compressions.

Infant (<1 yr):

    Position: One fingerbreadth below intermammary line

    Technique: Third and fourth fingers on sternum or two thumbs encircling hands technique

    Depth: One third to one half the anterior/posterior diameter of chest

    Rate: At least 100 times per minute

    Ratio: 30 compressions to 2 ventilations for one rescuer; 15 compressions to 2 ventilations for two rescuers

Child (1–8 yr):

    Position: One fingerbreadth above xyphoid-sternal margin

    Technique: Heel of hand

    Depth: One third to one half the anterior/posterior diameter of chest

    Rate: 100 times per minute

    Ratio: 30 compressions to 2 ventilations for one rescuer; 15 compressions to 2 ventilations for two rescuers

Child (>8 yr):

    Position: Lower third of sternum

    Technique: Two hands

    Depth: One third to one half the anterior/posterior diameter of chest

    Rate: 100 times per minute

    Ratio: 30 compressions to 2 ventilations for one rescuer; 15 compressions to 2 ventilations for two rescuers

9 Activate EMS.

    Call EMS after 1 minute of CPR.

10 Apply AED after five cycles of CPR for child (>1 yr).

    If shockable rhythm, give one shock and resume CPR for five cycles; repeat.

11 Reassess airway, breathing, circulation after every five cycles of CPR.

CLINICAL TIPS

▶ Whenever a cervical spine injury is suspected, the head and neck should be immobilized at all times and the jaw thrust maneuver should be used to open the airway.

▶ Pressing too hard in the submental area or hyperextending the neck when performing airway maneuvers can cause upper airway obstruction.

▶ The operator should ensure that a good seal is established and no air leak occurs when performing rescue breathing.

▶ Breaths delivered slowly (while maintaining the proper overall rate) produce better ventilation and minimize gastric distension.

▶ The head and neck should be repositioned to improve airway patency if the patient has inadequate chest wall excursions.

▶ Characteristics of good chest compressions include (a) "push hard" to ensure that the chest is consistently depressed approximately one third to one half the anterior/posterior diameter of the chest; (b) "push fast" to ensure that compressions are consistently performed at a rate of approximately 100 per minute; (c) "release completely" to allow the chest to fully recoil and the heart to refill with blood; and (d) "minimize interruptions" so that perfusion of the vital organs is maintained at the most favorable possible level

▶ When an arrest in a child 1 year of age or older is witnessed and sudden, as with a teenage athlete who is running and collapses, a lone provider should activate the EMS system and obtain an automatic external defibrillator device (AED), if available, before initiating CPR. If there are two rescuers, one can initiate CPR while the other notifies EMS and obtains an AED.

alignment of the airway is achieved and then reattempt rescue breathing. If this occurs when the jaw thrust maneuver is performed, the operator should exert greater force in displacing the mandible anteriorly, maintaining immobilization of the cervical spine as necessary. The operator can actually cause airway obstruction by pressing too firmly on the soft tissues of the submental area so that the tongue is pushed against the palate. In addition, overly aggressive extension of the neck can cause "kinking" of the airway and resulting obstruction. Maintaining a patent airway is often a matter of trial and error until the optimal position of the head and neck are established.

Failure to deliver adequate rescue breaths may be caused by leakage from an improper seal between the operator's mouth and the patient's mouth (child) or nose and mouth (infant). This also can occur when an inadequate tidal volume is delivered. In such cases, the patient may receive minimal oxygenation, increasing the risk of a poor outcome. Conversely, administering excessively high volumes or inspiratory pressures during rescue breathing will often cause gastric distension, which may lead to vomiting and aspiration. In extreme cases, pneumothorax can occur. These complications generally can be avoided if the operator delivers slow breaths and is careful to observe the patient's chest excursions.

Failure to deliver chest compressions at the recommended rate and depth will compromise blood flow to vital organs. Compressions that are too slow or too shallow must be avoided. The operator should concentrate on performing compressions in a smooth and rhythmic fashion, avoiding any abrupt or jerky movements. To maximize forward blood flow,

the chest should be allowed to fully recoil after every compression, so that the heart refills with blood before the intrathoracic pressure again rises with the next compression (32).

Two studies in adults, one assessing out-of-hospital cardiac arrests and the other assessing in-hospital cardiac arrests, suggest that the quality of CPR performed is inconsistent and often does not comply with published guidelines (35,36). In the first study, Wik et al. found that chest compressions were not delivered 38% of the time in out-of-hospital resuscitations, and most compressions were too shallow (35). In the second study, Abella et al. reported that inpatients undergoing CPR did not receive chest compressions 24% of the time, and when compressions were performed, the technique was often poor (28% inadequate rate, 37% inadequate depth). They also found that 61% of patients were hyperventilated (36). Failure to strictly adhere to recommended CPR techniques and methodologies is an important consideration in emergency medical care, as both animal and human studies have shown that "correct" CPR is associated with improved survival rates (37–39).

Injuries resulting from CPR are rare. In one study, medically significant injuries occurred in 3% of pediatric patients who received CPR (40). These included retroperitoneal hemorrhage, pneumothorax, epicardial hematoma, gastric perforation, and rib fractures. A study by Feldman and Brewer (41) failed to demonstrate rib fractures even after prolonged CPR done by health providers with variable levels of skill. Excessive force should obviously be avoided, but the greater pliability of the rib cage in most pediatric patients makes fractures less likely than with adults.

▶ SUMMARY

Although sudden respiratory and cardiac arrest are less common among infants and children than adults, BLS procedures are nonetheless commonly indicated for pediatric patients. By far the most frequent cause of a pediatric arrest is respiratory compromise. Consequently, rescue breathing is often the only initial intervention required. The overall outcome from such a respiratory insult is generally good with appropriate management. Cardiovascular compromise requiring chest compressions is usually the result of a more gradual process in pediatric patients, because ischemic heart disease, the primary cause of arrhythmia and sudden death in adults, is rare in this population. Prevention of the progression to cardiovascular collapse is therefore imperative. CPR can be performed without additional equipment by both health professionals and lay persons. The quality and "correctness" of CPR directly affect patient outcome. Consequently, all practitioners who care for children should be knowledgeable about the indications for CPR and skillful at performing the necessary procedures.

▶ ACKNOWLEDGMENT

The author would like to acknowledge the valuable contributions of Judith C. Bausher to the version of this chapter that appeared in the previous edition.

▶ REFERENCES

1. Eisenberg M, Bergner L, Hallstrom A. Epidemiology of cardiac arrest and resuscitation in children. *Ann Emerg Med.* 1983;12:672–674.

2. Torphy DE, Minter MG, Thompson BM. Cardiorespiratory arrest and resuscitation of children. *Am J Dis Child.* 1984;138:1099–1102.

3. Rosenberg NM. Pediatric cardiopulmonary arrest in the emergency department. *Am J Emerg Med.* 1984;2:497–499.

4. Zaritsky A, Nadkarni V, Getson P, et al. CPR in children. *Ann Emerg Med.* 1987;16:1107–1111.

5. Sirbaugh PE, Pepe PE, Shook JE, et al. A prospective, population-based study of the demographics, epidemiology, management, and outcome of out-of-hospital pediatric cardiopulmonary arrest. *Ann Emerg Med.* 1999;33:174–184.

6. Friesen RM, Duncan P, Tweed WA, et al. Appraisal of pediatric cardiopulmonary resuscitation. *Can Med Assoc J.* 1982;126:1055–1058.

7. Barzilay Z, Somekh E, Sagy M, et al. Pediatric cardiopulmonary resuscitation outcome. *J Med.* 1988;19:229–241.

8. Schoenfeld PS, Baker MD. Management of cardiopulmonary and trauma resuscitation in the pediatric emergency department. *Pediatrics.* 1993;91:726–729.

9. Gillis J, Dickson D, Reider D, et al. Results of inpatient pediatric resuscitation. *Crit Care Med.* 1986;14:469–471.

10. Walsh CK, Krongrad E. Terminal cardiac activity in pediatric patients. *Am J Cardiol.* 1983;51:557–561.

11. Appleton GO, Cummins RO, Larsen MP, et al. CPR and the single rescuer: at what age should you "call first" rather than "call fast"? *Ann Emerg Med.* 1995;25:492–494.

12. Mogayzel C, Quan L, Graves JR, et al. Out-of-hospital ventricular fibrillation in children and adolescents: causes and outcomes. *Ann Emerg Med.* 1995;25:484–491.

13. Lewis JK, Minter MG, Eshekman SJ, et al. Outcome of pediatric resuscitation. *Ann Emerg Med.* 1983;12:297–299.

14. O'Rourke PP. Outcome of children who are apneic and pulseless in the emergency room. *Crit Care Med.* 1986;14:466–468.

15. Hickey RW, Cohen DM, Strausbaugh S, et al. Pediatric patients requiring CPR in the prehospital setting. *Ann Emerg Med.* 1995;25:495–501.

16. Safar P. History of cardiopulmonary-cerebral resuscitation. In: Kaye W, Bircher N, eds. *Cardiopulmonary Resuscitation.* New York: Churchill Livingstone; 1989:1–36.

17. Silvester HR. A new method of resuscitating stillborn children and of restoring persons apparently dead or drowned. *Br Med J.* 1858;2:576–579.

18. Schafer EA. Description of a simple and efficient method of performing artificial respirations in the human subject. *Trans Royal Med Chirurg Soc.* 1904;87:609–623.

19. Tossach W. Man dead in appearance recovered by distending lungs with air. In: *Medical Essays and Observations.* Vol. 5, pt. 2. 5th ed. London: T. Cadell & J. Balfour; 1771:108–111.

20. Safar P, Escarraga L, Elam JO. A comparison of mouth-to-mouth and mouth-to-airway methods of artificial respiration with the chest-pressure arm-lift method. *N Engl J Med.* 1958;258:671–677.

21. Gordon AS, Frye CE, Gittleson L, et al. Mouth-to-mouth verses manual artificial respiration for children and adults. *JAMA.* 1958;167:320–328.

22. Elam JO, Brown ES, Elder JD. Artificial respiration by mouth-to-mask method: study of respiratory gas exchange of paralyzed patients ventilated by operator's expired air. *N Engl J Med.* 1954;250:749–754.

23. Kouwenhoven WB, Jude JR, Knickerbocker GC. Closed chest cardiac massage. *JAMA.* 1960;173:1064–1067.

24. Steward DJ, ed. *Manual of Pediatric Anesthesia.* New York: Churchill Livingstone; 1985:10–17.

25. Nichols DG, Rogers MC. Developmental physiology of the respiratory system. In: Rogers MC, ed. *Textbook of Pediatric Intensive Care.* Baltimore: Williams & Wilkins; 1987:83–111.

26. Keen WW. A case of total laryngectomy (unsuccessful) and a case of abdominal hysterectomy (successful) in both of which massage of the heart for chloroform collapse was employed. With notes of 25 other cases of cardiac massage. *Therap Gaz.* 1904;28:217–230.

27. Stephenson HE, Reid LC, Hinton JW. Some common denominators in 1,200 cases of cardiac arrest. *Ann Surg.* 1953;137:731–744.

28. Boehm R. Über Weiderbelebung nach Vergiftunger und Asphyxie. *Arch Exp Pathol Pharmakol.* 1878;8:68–101.

29. Criley JM, Blaufuss AN, Kissel GC. Cough-induced cardiac compression. *JAMA.* 1976;236:1246–1250.

30. Rudikoff MT, Maughan WL, Effron M, et al. Mechanisms of blood flow during cardiopulmonary resuscitation. *Circulation.* 1980;61:345–351.

31. Maier GW, Tyson GS Jr, Olsen CO, et al. The physiology of external cardiac massage: high impulse cardiopulmonary resuscitation. *Circulation.* 1984;70:86–101.

32. 2005 American Heart Association (AHA) guidelines for cardiopulmonary resuscitation (CPR) and emergency cardiovascular care (ECC) of pediatric and neonatal patients: pediatric basic life support. *Pediatrics.* 2006;117:e989–1004.

33. Orlowski JP. Optimum position for external cardiac compression in infants and young children. *Ann Emerg Med.* 1986;15:667–673.

34. Finholt DA, Kettrick RG, Wagner HR, et al. The heart is under the lower third of the sternum: implications for external cardiac massage. *Am J Dis Child.* 1986;140:646–649.

35. Wik L, Kramer-Johansen J, Myklebust H, et al. Quality of cardiopulmonary resuscitation during out-of-hospital cardiac arrest. *JAMA.* 2005;293:299–304.

36. Abella BS, Alvarado JP, Myklebust H, et al. Quality of cardiopulmonary resuscitation during in-hospital cardiac arrest. *JAMA.* 2005;293:305–310.

37. Kern KB, Hilwig RW, Berg RA, et al. Importance of continuous chest compressions during cardiopulmonary resuscitation: improved outcome during simulated single lay rescuer. *Circulation.* 2002;105:645–649.

38. Wik L, Steen PA, Bircher NG. Quality of bystander cardiopulmonary resuscitation influences after prehospital cardiac arrest. *Resuscitation.* 1994;28:195–203.

39. Gallagher EJ, Lombardi G, Gennis P. Effectiveness of bystander cardiopulmonary resuscitation survival following out-of-hospital cardiac arrest. *JAMA.* 1995;274:1922–1925.

40. Bush CM, Jones JS, Cohle SD, et al. Pediatric injuries from cardiopulmonary resuscitation. *Ann Emerg Med.* 1996;28:40–44.

41. Feldman KW, Brewer DK. Child abuse, cardiopulmonary resuscitation, and rib fractures. *Pediatrics.* 1984;73:339–342.

RICHARD J. SCARFONE

13

Oxygen Delivery, Suctioning, and Airway Adjuncts

▶ INTRODUCTION

Adults typically suffer sudden death as a result of primary cardiac events such as myocardial infarctions or dysrhythmias. In contrast, most pediatric cardiac arrests occur secondary to respiratory failure leading to hypoxemia and acidosis (1). As many as one quarter of hospitalized children experiencing cardiopulmonary arrest can be resuscitated with airway and ventilatory interventions alone (2). Status asthmaticus, bronchiolitis, pneumonia, and laryngotracheobronchitis are among the many pulmonary diseases commonly seen in children that may lead to respiratory failure. In addition, status epilepticus, medication overdoses, and sepsis are just a few of the many clinical conditions that may cause hypoventilation or apnea. It is especially important, then, for those providing emergency care to children to be skillful in the management of respiratory diseases and dysfunction.

The first step in the assessment of seriously ill or injured children is the evaluation of the patency of the airway and the adequacy of ventilation. For children who have mild to moderate respiratory distress and patent airways, simple delivery of oxygen may be the only method of support necessary. For those with airway obstruction, suctioning and/or the introduction of a pharyngeal airway may serve as a temporizing measure prior to endotracheal intubation or as a definitive treatment of the problem. This chapter describes oxygen delivery and the proper methods for performing these adjunctive airway procedures for infants and children with respiratory distress.

▶ ANATOMY AND PHYSIOLOGY

Airway Anatomy

Beginning at the nose and lips and proceeding down the airway of the infant or young child, several important anatomic differences are encountered as compared with the adult (Fig. 13.1). Many of these differences predispose the child to airway obstruction. For example, the tongue of the infant or young child is relatively large in proportion to the oral cavity. In addition, since the larynx has a more superior position in the neck of a pediatric patient compared with an adult, the tongue has a more rostral location in the hypopharynx (3). Consequently, a child lying supine may develop airway obstruction due solely to posterior displacement of the tongue, a problem that can often be alleviated with a pharyngeal airway. Infants are also obligate nasal breathers until approximately 3 to 5 months of age (3). As a result, swelling of the nasal mucosa, thick rhinorrhea, nasal foreign bodies, or choanal atresia may cause significant respiratory distress in the young infant. Perhaps the most obvious and important difference from the adult patient is that children have smaller corresponding airway luminal diameters. Because the resistance to air flow is inversely related to the fourth power of the radius (Poiseuille's law), disease states that cause further narrowing of the airways (edema, secretions, etc.) disproportionately increase the work of breathing and the resulting oxygen demand in children compared with adults (Fig. 13.2). Further discussion of pediatric airway anatomy can be found in Chapters 14 and 16.

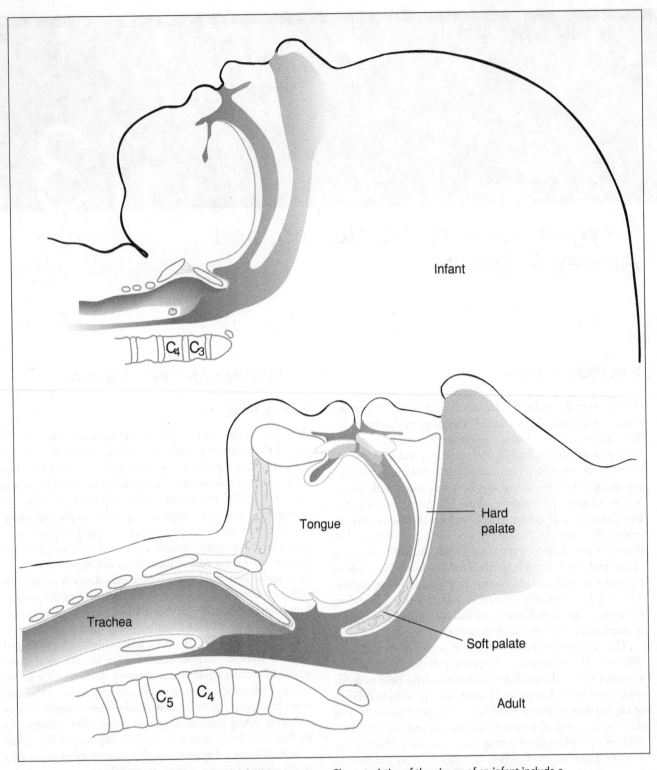

Figure 13.1 Infant versus adult airway anatomy. Characteristics of the airway of an infant include a large tongue relative to the overall size of the oropharynx and a more superior location of the tongue and larynx (opposite C3-C4) compared with the adult (opposite C4-C5). These factors produce an increased tendency for airway obstruction in the infant.

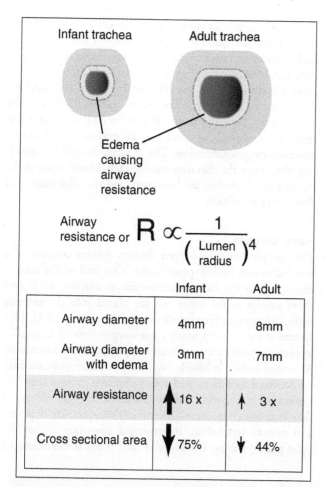

Infant trachea   Adult trachea

Edema causing airway resistance

Airway resistance or $R \propto \dfrac{1}{\left(\dfrac{\text{Lumen}}{\text{radius}}\right)^4}$

	Infant	Adult
Airway diameter	4mm	8mm
Airway diameter with edema	3mm	7mm
Airway resistance	▲ 16 x	▲ 3 x
Cross sectional area	▼ 75%	▼ 44%

Figure 13.2 Effects of airway narrowing for infants versus adults. The diameter of an infant's airway is significantly smaller than the diameter of an adult's at comparable anatomic levels. Because the resistance to gas flow is inversely proportional to the fourth power of the radius, small decreases in luminal diameter result in large increases in resistance for both infants and adults. However, this also means that with a given decrease in luminal diameter (e.g., 1 mm), the smaller lumen of the infant airway experiences a much greater increase in resistance compared with the adult. (Adapted with permission from Cote CJ, Todres ID. The pediatric airway. In: Cote CJ, Ryan JF, Todres ID, et al., eds. *A Practice of Anesthesia for Infants and Children.* 2nd ed. Philadelphia: Saunders; 1993.)

Physiology of Oxygen Utilization and Delivery

The oxygen consumption index of an infant is roughly twice that of an adult, due primarily to a higher rate of metabolism. As a result, pediatric patients develop hypoxemia more rapidly in response to inadequate oxygen delivery. Most practitioners have witnessed the precipitous decline in oxygen saturation that can occur when oxygen flow to a child in respiratory distress is briefly interrupted.

In general, the rate of oxygen flow delivered should be sufficient to maintain an oxygen saturation of 100% whenever possible. Although the concentration of oxygen delivered to the patient (F_iO_2) corresponds to the rate of flow, a linear relationship does not exist. A number of other important variables also contribute to the F_iO_2. These include the patient's

nasal and oropharyngeal resistance as well as factors that may affect the amount of atmospheric (room) air that mixes with the administered oxygen—inspiratory flow rate, minute ventilation, and tidal volume. As a rule, the greater the patient's inspiratory flow rate (which is influenced by both minute ventilation and tidal volume), the greater the mixing of relatively oxygen-poor atmospheric air with administered oxygen and therefore the lower the F_iO_2 for any given oxygen flow rate. In other words, when a patient inhales with a greater velocity than the highest possible rate of oxygen flow, atmospheric air must enter the system to make up the difference.

For example, assuming a constant oxygen flow of 3 L/min, a larger patient with a minute ventilation of 12 L/min will breathe more atmospheric air than a smaller patient with a minute ventilation of 6 L/min. Although the rate of oxygen flow is the same, the F_iO_2 is greater for the patient with a lower minute ventilation. Thus, an older child will need a higher rate of oxygen flow to achieve the same F_iO_2 as a younger child. In addition, the specific delivery system used will influence the maximal oxygen concentration delivered to the patient. At a given oxygen flow, a nonrebreathing mask will provide a higher F_iO_2 than a standard mask, because the latter system allows for greater entry of atmospheric air.

▶ OXYGEN DELIVERY

Indications

There are several diseases affecting children that may result in hypoxemia and for which the administration of oxygen is indicated. The most common of these are asthma and bronchiolitis. In these two conditions, bronchoconstriction and airway inflammation increase lower airway resistance, contribute to atelectasis and ventilation/perfusion mismatching, and increase the patient's work of breathing and oxygen consumption. The degree of hypoxemia may be exacerbated if the child has underlying chronic lung disease such as cystic fibrosis. Pneumonia and laryngotracheobronchitis (croup) also commonly affect children and may necessitate the administration of oxygen. In addition to primary pulmonary processes, other common indications for oxygen administration include status epilepticus and hypoventilation secondary to a medication overdose, such as with a sedative or narcotic. Hypercarbia and acidosis may be relatively well tolerated by a child, but even a short period of oxygen deprivation can lead to bradycardia or cardiac arrest (2). Once it is determined that the spontaneously breathing child with respiratory distress has a patent airway, oxygen should be administered empirically.

Cyanosis is the most definitive physical finding indicating hypoxemia. Typically, the perioral region and distal extremities are the first areas of the body to become cyanotic. Other signs of hypoxemia include agitation, lethargy, and bradycardia. Determination of oxygen saturation by pulse oximetry provides a means of quantifying the degree of hypoxemia (see Chapter 75). Unless adequacy of ventilation is a concern, there is

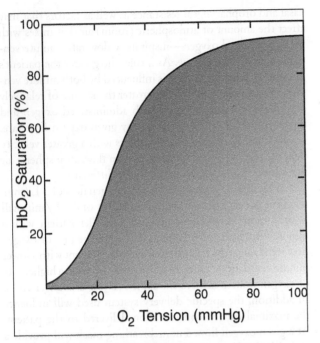

Figure 13.3 Oxyhemoglobin dissociation curve. The oxygen saturation decreases relatively gradually along the initial "flat" segment of the curve until a saturation of approximately 90%. However, when the PaO_2 falls below 60 mm Hg, the "steep" segment of the curve is reached, and the oxygen saturation falls rapidly.

usually little need to perform a painful and time-consuming arterial puncture for blood gas analysis. Pulse oximetry offers a noninvasive, "real-time" modality that rapidly gives an indirect but generally reliable indication of the partial pressure of oxygen (PaO_2). In interpreting the pulse oximeter reading, it is important to remember that the patient will maintain an oxygen saturation over 90% as long as the PaO_2 is above 60 mm Hg, even if the PaO_2 is decreasing. Physiologically, this corresponds to the initial flat segment of the oxyhemoglobin dissociation curve (Fig. 13.3). Once the PaO_2 falls below 60 mm Hg, however, oxygen saturation will drop dramatically as the patient reaches the steep segment of the curve. Therefore, oxygen saturation of 90% is only minimally acceptable in most clinical situations. If an oxygen saturation of at least 90% cannot be maintained with a given method of delivery, a system capable of administering a higher concentration should be employed. In such cases, controlled or assisted ventilation may also prove necessary.

Equipment

When administering oxygen, the clinician must first determine the concentration to be delivered and then select an appropriate delivery system. These decisions are affected by a number of patient variables, including age, degree of cooperation, respiratory effort, and extent of hypoxemia. For example, an older child in mild to moderate respiratory distress with minimal hypoxia may receive oxygen via a low-flow system such

as a nasal cannula or simple mask. However, many younger children become extremely agitated and uncooperative when such devices are used, increasing oxygen consumption and potentially exacerbating hypoxemia. In such cases, it may be more effective to use a less efficient but better tolerated delivery method, such as a hollow plastic tube held close to the child's face ("blow-by" method). For the child in greater distress, a nonrebreathing mask may be necessary to maintain adequate oxygen saturation. The clinician should be knowledgeable about the characteristics of each delivery system, the manner in which they are best used, and the advantages and disadvantages of each.

Nasal Cannula

This simple low-flow oxygen delivery system consists of a small-diameter hollow plastic tube. One end of the tube is connected to the oxygen source via an adapter, while two short prongs at the other end are placed into the anterior nares, delivering oxygen into the nasopharynx (Fig. 13.4). This system is most useful when a low oxygen flow (3 L/min or less) is adequate to maintain an acceptable oxygen saturation. As stated earlier, relatively high oxygen concentrations may be delivered to infants and young children using a low-flow system such as a nasal cannula, because the rate of oxygen flow may match or exceed the patient's inspiratory flow rate and minute ventilation. Its principal advantage is that the light plastic tubing is less bulky and often better tolerated

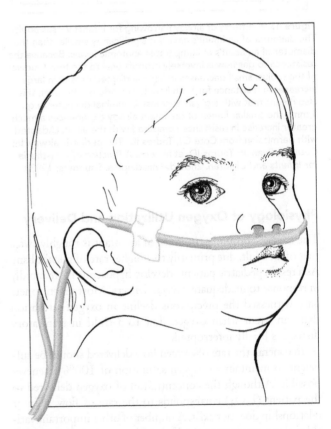

Figure 13.4 Nasal cannula for oxygen administration.

than a mask. A nasal cannula device is particularly useful for young infants who are obligate nasal breathers and for whom a properly sized mask may not be available or is poorly tolerated.

The main disadvantage of the nasal cannula system is that it is difficult to deliver oxygen in excess of 3 L/min. Higher flow rates cause irritation of the nasopharynx and are therefore not well accepted by most children. In addition, this is obviously not a "closed" system, and the F_iO_2 may vary widely if the child is mouth breathing or crying or the nares are obstructed. Consequently, a nasal cannula may not meet the oxygen demands of a patient requiring consistent delivery of a higher F_iO_2.

Simple Oxygen Mask

This delivery system consists of a clear plastic or rubber mask that fits snugly over the nose and mouth (Fig. 13.5). Centers caring for children should have a wide range of sizes available. Transparent masks allow for the visualization of vomitus, blood, or other secretions. Each side of the mask has openings that serve as exhalation ports. These openings also permit inhalation of room air if the oxygen flow rate is less than the patient's inspiratory flow rate or if the oxygen source becomes disconnected. The simple mask may be used when a relatively low oxygen flow is adequate to maintain an appropriate oxygen saturation. This system can be expected to deliver a higher F_iO_2 than can be achieved with a nasal cannula, but it may not be as well tolerated. At an oxygen flow rate of 6 to 10 L/min, a simple oxygen mask will deliver an oxygen concentration of between 35% and 60%. The principal disadvantage of this system is that the F_iO_2 is lowered by entrainment of room air through the exhalation ports. A minimum oxygen flow rate of 6 L/min must be used to maintain a higher oxygen concentration and prevent rebreathing of exhaled carbon dioxide (1).

Partial Rebreathing and Nonrebreathing Masks

A partial rebreathing mask consists of a simple face mask with a reservoir bag attached. With the simple mask, the patient's inspired air is contaminated by the inhalation of room air through the exhalation ports and the rebreathing of oxygen-poor exhaled gases. The purpose of the reservoir bag is to reduce rebreathing. The first portion of exhaled gas enters

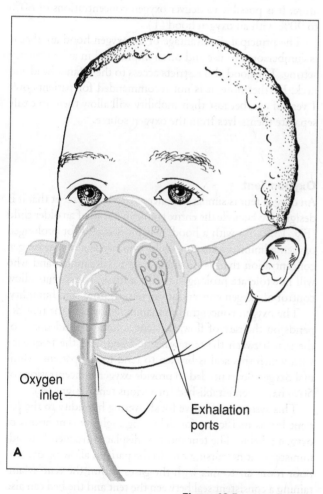

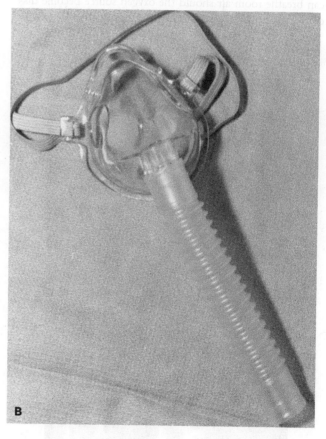

Oxygen inlet

Exhalation ports

A

B

Figure 13.5
A. Simple oxygen mask.
B. Oxygen mask with corrugated tube reservoir.

the reservoir bag, and because the source of this gas is primarily the airway rather than the lungs, it is not significantly involved with gas exchange and is therefore relatively oxygen rich (I). Remaining expired gases are vented through the exhalation ports. Assuming adequate oxygen flow into the reservoir bag (the bag should not fully deflate during inspiration), it should contain close to 100% oxygen. The patient therefore inhales oxygen flowing into the system from the oxygen source combined with the oxygen-rich gas that accumulates in the reservoir bag. However, the patient with sufficiently high inspiratory flow rates can still breathe atmospheric air that enters the system through the exhalation ports. Using a partial rebreathing mask with a flow rate of 10 to 12 L/min, an oxygen concentration of 50% to 60% can normally be achieved.

A nonrebreathing mask also contains a reservoir bag and functions in much the same manner as a simple mask but with a few important modifications. The nonrebreathing mask contains rubber seals that serve as one-way valves over the exhalation ports (Fig. 13.6). This allows egress of exhaled gases while preventing entrainment of room air into the mask during inhalation. However, safety standards mandate that only one of the two exhalation ports be sealed so that the patient can breathe room air should the oxygen source become disconnected from the reservoir bag. To further enhance oxygen

delivery, a nonrebreathing system also has a second one-way valve located between the bag and mask. This valve diverts oxygen-poor exhaled gases away from the bag and thereby further reduces rebreathing. Assuming that oxygen flow is sufficient to prevent collapse of the reservoir bag on inspiration (10 to 12 L/min) and that the mask fits properly, an inspired oxygen concentration of over 95% can usually be achieved (I). Nonrebreathing delivery systems are also available for infants, with the only modification being that a small plastic tube, rather than a bag, serves as the reservoir.

Oxygen Hood

An oxygen hood is most useful for infants who require prolonged administration of oxygen but might poorly tolerate a mask or nasal cannula. It consists of either a clear, soft plastic enclosure or a hard Plexiglas dome placed over the patient's head (Fig. 13.7). Because medical personnel have access to the infant's trunk and extremities while the hood is in use, general nursing care can be performed without lowering the F_iO_2. In addition, the administration of cool or warm humidified oxygen will not significantly affect the patient's body temperature. It is possible to deliver oxygen concentrations of 80% to 90% with an oxygen hood (I).

The principal disadvantage of an oxygen hood are that it is cumbersome to use and often impractical in an emergency setting. The hood also restricts access to the infant's head and neck. Furthermore, it is not recommended for patients over I year of age, because their mobility will allow them to easily separate themselves from the oxygen source.

Oxygen Tent

An oxygen tent is similar in concept to a hood except that it is designed to encircle the entire trunk and head of an older child (Fig. 13.8). As with a hood, it is most useful for prolonged oxygen administration to a child who needs a higher oxygen concentration than is provided by a nasal cannula and who will not tolerate prolonged use of a mask. Most tents allow control of oxygen concentration, temperature, and humidity.

The oxygen concentration maintained within the tent depends on the rate of flow, the tent volume, the adequacy of the seal between the tent walls and bed, and the frequency with which this seal is broken to tend to the patient. Minimal oxygen flows needed to provide oxygen concentrations of 50% have been established for various tent designs (4).

This system is effective for delivering humidity to the patient but is inefficient for delivering high concentrations of oxygen reliably. The tent must be displaced frequently to administer routine nursing care to the patient, allowing oxygen-poor room air to mix with the gases within the tent. Maintaining a consistent seal between the tent and the bed can also be difficult with a moving child, although placing blankets or small sand bags at the base of the tent walls may help in this

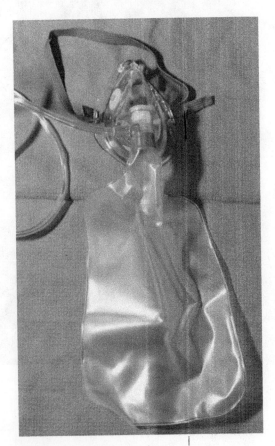

Figure 13.6 Nonrebreathing mask.

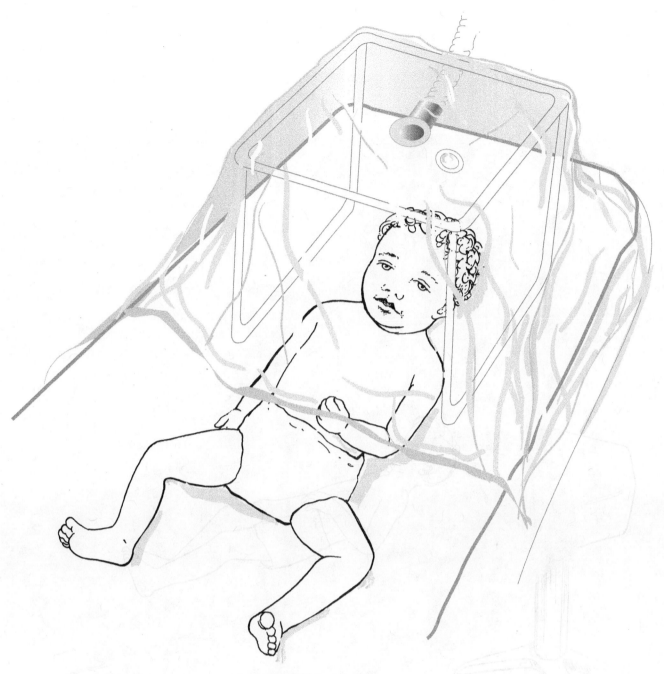

Figure 13.7 Oxygen hood.

regard. It is generally possible to maintain a reliable F_iO_2 of at least 50% within the tent.

Procedure

Oxygen administration via a nasal cannula is easily performed by inserting each short prong into the nares and draping the plastic tubing behind each ear. Taping the tubing to each cheek may help to prevent dislodgment. The child should be assessed periodically to ensure that the prongs have not become displaced. If tolerated, a mask (with or without a reservoir bag) is attached to the oxygen source via a clear

plastic tube and is held on the face with an adjustable strap placed around the occiput. It should fit snugly over the nose and mouth to decrease the amount of room air that is inspired.

When either a nasal cannula or a mask is used to deliver oxygen, the child should be allowed to assume a position of comfort. If the child is forced into the supine position, he or she may become frightened or angry and have increased oxygen consumption while struggling to remove the device. It is often prudent in such cases to allow the child to sit on a parent's lap. For the uncooperative or agitated child who will not tolerate a nasal cannula or a mask, high-flow oxygen

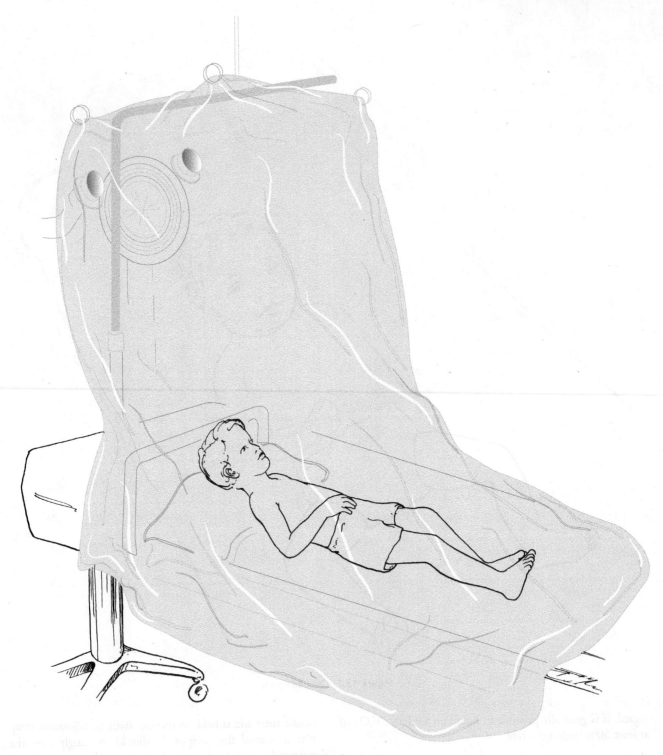

Figure 13.8 Oxygen tent.

directed at (but not touching!) the child's face using a "blow-by" setup, while not optimal, may be the only possible way of administering supplemental oxygen.

A child may be in either the prone or the supine position when placed within an oxygen hood or tent. The older child may choose to sit upright in an oxygen tent. Care should be taken to ensure that the base of the tent walls forms an adequate seal with the mattress of the bed to prevent excessive mixing of room air within the system.

Complications

For many adults with chronic respiratory disease, high concentrations of oxygen can cause a suppressed respiratory drive.

SUMMARY

Oxygen Delivery

1 Administer heated, humidified oxygen empirically once it has been established that the spontaneously breathing child with moderate respiratory distress has a patent airway.

2 Use pulse oximetry to assess oxygen saturation.

3 Maintain a minimally acceptable oxygen saturation of 90%.

4 Use a nasal cannula or a simple mask for a patient requiring only low-flow oxygen.

5 Use partial rebreathing or nonrebreathing mask for a patient requiring higher concentrations of oxygen.

6 Consider using an oxygen hood for infants or an oxygen tent for younger children when prolonged administration of oxygen and humidity is required.

For the large majority of children, however, high F_iO_2 can be delivered safely without fear of causing respiratory depression. Exceptions include children with chronic respiratory diseases such as cystic fibrosis or those with lung disease resulting from prematurity; rarely, they may experience hypoventilation with the administration of high concentrations of oxygen. For these children, respiratory effort must be monitored closely during oxygen administration, and the physician must be prepared to assist ventilation if this becomes necessary. In general, oxygen may be safely delivered to children with congenital cardiac disease, although one notable exception is the child with hypoplastic left heart syndrome. Here, oxygen will serve to dilate the pulmonary vasculature, which will increase left-to-right shunting of blood across a patent ductus arteriosus and impair peripheral perfusion.

All patients receiving supplemental oxygen should undergo serial examinations. The clinician must ensure that the delivery system has not become disconnected from the oxygen source and that the patient has not experienced a clinical deterioration requiring a change to a different oxygen delivery system or, in more severe cases, assisted or controlled ventilation.

▶ SUCTIONING

Indications

As stated earlier, the first step in the assessment of any child who is in respiratory distress is to ensure patency of the airway. Signs of airway obstruction in a child include tachypnea, stridor, snoring, cyanosis, and poor aeration despite adequate chest wall movement. In many cases, simple suctioning of the mouth and/or nose may promptly alleviate the obstruction. For example, a patient who develops respiratory distress after

sustaining oral trauma may require suctioning of teeth, blood, or vomitus from the oropharynx. A child who experiences significant blunt head trauma or who receives conscious sedation may have an altered level of consciousness followed by emesis. Here, suctioning may be required to aid in the clearance of liquid and particulate material. Alternatively, suctioning may be used in conjunction with other maneuvers to provide a patent airway. For example, airway obstruction following a seizure may be due to a combination of excessive secretions and laxity of the pharyngeal musculature, causing the tongue to fall against the posterior wall of the pharynx. In this case, manual methods of opening the airway together with suctioning of secretions, mucus, or blood from the mouth may be necessary to re-establish airway patency. Finally, suctioning is often an important step in facilitating visualization of the airway anatomy during direct laryngoscopy prior to endotracheal intubation.

Equipment

Three commonly available types of suctioning tools are the catheter tip, dental tip, and tonsil tip (Yankauer) devices (Fig. 13.9). The operator should be familiar with the features that make each of these useful in distinct clinical situations.

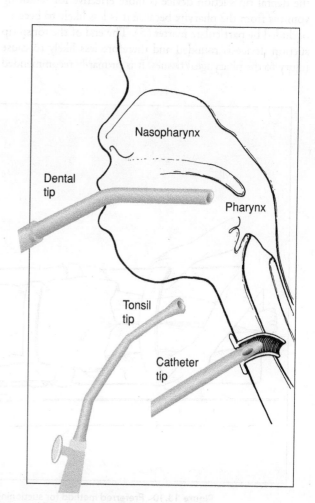

Figure 13.9 Suction devices.

Catheter Tip Suction Devices

A catheter tip suction device is simply a narrow tube made of a soft, flexible plastic. It is connected via an adapter to a longer hard plastic tube that is attached to wall suction. The catheter should be inserted gently into the patient's nasopharynx or oropharynx. Negative pressure is applied when the operator occludes the side opening on the catheter with a finger or thumb.

These devices are best suited for gentle suctioning of the nasopharynx, which can often greatly improve gas exchange and resulting oxygenation, particularly for infants. In addition, these devices are useful for suctioning thin secretions from the trachea through an endotracheal tube or tracheostomy cannula (see Chapter 79). They are not useful for suctioning thick secretions or particulate matter, because the narrow catheter lumen is likely to become occluded.

Dental Tip and Tonsil Tip Suction Devices

In most cases, airway obstruction secondary to secretions or particulate matter will most readily be alleviated with either a dental tip or tonsil tip suction device. Each consists of a wide bore catheter made of hard plastic or stainless steel. Each is attached to the wall vacuum via a hard plastic tube. Of the two, the dental tip suction device is more effective for removing vomitus from the pharynx because it is less likely to become occluded by particulate matter (5). The end of the tonsil tip suction device is rounded and therefore less likely to cause injury to the pharyngeal tissues. It is primarily recommended

for suctioning blood, as its design prevents obstruction of the tip by tissue or clot (5).

Procedure

Most devices require the operator to occlude a side hole to apply negative pressure through the lumen. In general, suctioning should be performed under direct visualization to avoid injury to the pharynx. It should also be done in brief intervals not exceeding 30 seconds to avoid prolonged hypoxemia. Supplemental oxygen should be provided in the intervals between suctioning.

Complications

Suctioning is normally a safe and well-tolerated procedure in pediatric patients. Excessively deep suctioning of any patient should be avoided to minimize the risk of vomiting, aspiration, laryngospasm, or bradycardia. Should vomiting occur, the child's head is first turned to one side, and suctioning is continued with a dental tip device until the emesis is cleared. This obviously assumes that the child is not at risk for possible cervical cord injury from movement of the neck. If such a risk exists, the child's neck should be immobilized (manually or with a cervical collar), and the entire body should be rolled to one side, preferably on a spine immobilization board (Fig. 13.10). In this way, suctioning can be effectively performed, and the child's head turned to one side, without

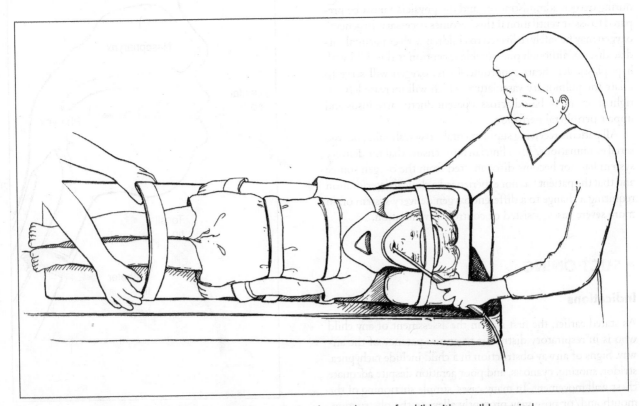

Figure 13.10 Preferred method for suctioning the oropharynx of a child with possible cervical spine injury. The patient's head is turned to the side without moving the neck.

SUMMARY

Suctioning the Airway

1 Perform suctioning under direct visualization in brief intervals not exceeding 30 seconds.

2 Provide supplemental oxygen during intervals between suctioning.

3 Use a catheter tip suction device for suctioning the nasopharynx or for suctioning through an endotracheal tube or tracheostomy cannula.

4 Use a dental tip suction device for removing vomitus or particulate matter from the pharynx.

5 Use a tonsil tip suction device for removing blood and blood clots from the pharynx.

movement of the neck. Whenever suctioning is performed, the heart rate should be monitored, since any noxious stimulus to the upper airway of a child can induce a vagal response and bradycardia.

Nasal suctioning may cause mild epistaxis, although this is not generally a significant problem if the clinician avoids excessive force. In addition, there have been several reports of nasogastric tubes and nasopharyngeal airways being inadvertently introduced into the cranium of patients with an injury to the cribriform plate (6,7). Although this complication is rare, it underscores the need for caution when inserting a suction catheter into the nasopharynx of a patient with possible head or facial injuries.

▶ USE OF ARTIFICIAL AIRWAYS

Inflammation and disease involving the soft tissues of the pharynx and supraglottic area are important causes of airway obstruction in children. In addition, the relatively large tongue and lax airway of a young child result in a greater tendency for upper airway obstruction from causes such as mental status depression or improper positioning of the head and neck. Occlusion of the airway as a result of these "fixed" processes is obviously not amenable to suctioning, but both types of conditions may be reversed with insertion of an artificial airway. An oropharyngeal or nasopharyngeal airway will often bypass the obstructing tissue, allowing the patient to resume spontaneous respirations or the operator to effectively assist ventilation with a bag-valve-mask (BVM) circuit. In such cases, proper use of an artificial airway may obviate the need for endotracheal intubation or provide a temporizing measure until intubation can be performed.

Indications

The opportunities to safely and effectively use an oropharyngeal airway are fairly limited. Ideally, the patient should be unconscious and have a diminished or absent gag reflex, with readily reversible airway obstruction resulting from laxity of the tongue or pharyngeal soft tissues. If the underlying process is transient (e.g., iatrogenic overdose with a short-acting sedative), an oral airway can often be used to maintain patency until the child regains consciousness. If the disease process is likely to result in more prolonged impairment (sepsis, head injury, etc.), an oral airway can be used to facilitate BVM ventilation before endotracheal intubation. Also, it may be used as a bite block after the patient's trachea has been intubated. Because an oropharyngeal airway directly contacts the tongue and supraglottic structures, it may induce vomiting. It is for this reason that the child who has (or regains over time) an intact gag reflex is not a good candidate for use of an oral airway, as the patient will likely gag and/or vomit repeatedly until the airway is removed. Similarly, if the child is fully awake, an oropharyngeal airway is likely to cause gagging, vomiting, soft-tissue injury, or laryngospasm and should therefore not be used (1).

A nasopharyngeal airway provides an alternative means for overcoming obstruction of the airway not alleviated with simple suctioning. It is particularly useful for a child who is conscious and not likely to tolerate an oropharyngeal airway. For example, a child who has had a prolonged seizure and is postictal may experience relaxation of the muscles of the floor of the mouth, allowing the base of the tongue to occlude the larynx. In such cases, a nasopharyngeal airway will often prevent obstruction until the child is more alert, while being much less likely than an oropharyngeal airway to induce emesis. A nasopharyngeal airway may also be useful for the patient with partial airway obstruction as a result of oral or mandibular trauma, when limited mouth opening or injury to the teeth makes use of an oropharyngeal airway inadvisable. For a child with potentially life-threatening upper airway obstruction due to severe tonsillar hypertrophy, as sometimes occurs with mononucleosis, a nasopharyngeal airway will often provide an effective conduit for gas exchange, bypassing the obstructing tissues. It should be remembered, however, that such children may also have enlarged adenoids, and special care must therefore be exercised in inserting a nasopharyngeal airway to avoid causing mucosal injury and bleeding.

Equipment

An oropharyngeal airway is a molded piece of hard plastic consisting of a curved body (stent), a short bite block, and a flange (Fig. 13.11). The flange serves as a site for taping the airway in place as well as preventing the airway from being advanced too far into the pharynx. The bite block fits between the teeth causing the mouth to remain slightly open. A central air channel is contained within the stent, providing a passage

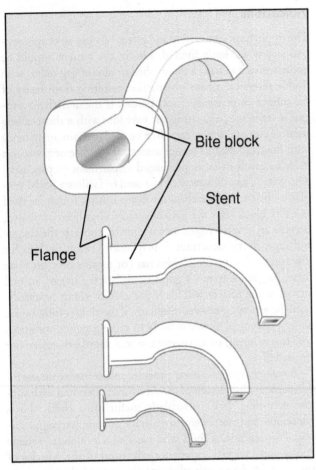

Figure 13.11 Oropharyngeal airways.

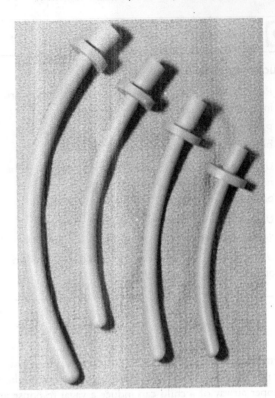

Figure 13.12 Nasopharyngeal airways.

for air exchange and allowing insertion of a suction catheter. The curved stent is designed to fit over the base of the tongue to prevent it from contacting the pharyngeal wall. A variety of pediatric oropharyngeal airway sizes are available, ranging from 4 to 10 cm in length.

Standard nasopharyngeal airways are simply rubber tubes that are narrow and flexible (Fig. 13.12). The distal end is angled to facilitate passage of the tube over the nasal turbinates. As with an oropharyngeal airway, a flange at the proximal end prevents further passage into the nose. Nasopharyngeal airways range in size from 12 to 36 French and are progressively longer as the diameter of the lumen increases. The proper size for most infants is 12 French, which is approximately the caliber of a 3-mm internal diameter (ID) endotracheal tube.

Procedure

Oropharyngeal Airway Insertion

An oropharyngeal airway of proper size is estimated by first placing it adjacent to the patient's face, with the flange at the level of the central incisors and the bite block parallel to the hard palate. Held in this position, the tip of a properly

sized airway should reach the angle of the mandible (1,8). All centers caring for children should have oropharyngeal airways in a range of sizes readily available.

Before inserting an oropharyngeal airway, the operator should ensure that the patient is appropriately monitored and receiving supplemental oxygen. A suction device and a BVM circuit should be available in case of vomiting or airway compromise. The child should be lying in the supine position. Using a tongue depressor to displace the tongue, the operator first inserts the airway into the mouth with the concave side pointing posteriorly (Fig. 13.13). The airway is then gently guided under direct visualization along the length of the soft palate until the tip is located in the posterior hypopharynx. The curved portion of the airway separates the tongue from the posterior pharyngeal wall and pulls the epiglottis slightly forward (Fig. 13.14). An alternative method of placement involves inserting the airway with the concave side pointing superiorly and then rotating it 180 degrees. This technique is not recommended for pediatric patients, because it is more likely to cause posterior displacement of the tongue and injury to the soft palate, tonsils, or teeth (9). Obviously, should a child start gagging immediately after an oropharyngeal airway is inserted, then the airway should be removed and another method of gaining airway patency should be attempted.

Once an oropharyngeal airway is in place, it may be secured to the face with tape. Assuming the obstruction was caused by occlusion of the airway by the tongue or other

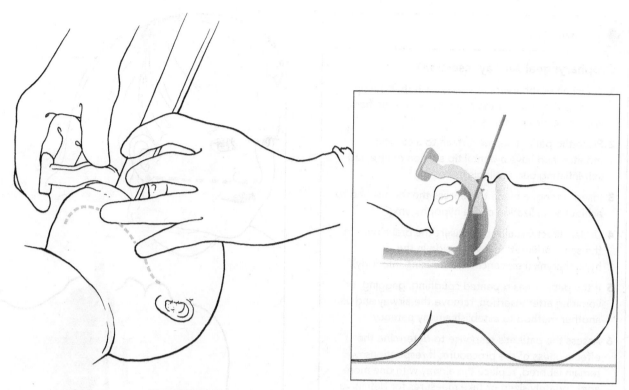

Figure 13.13 Insertion of an oropharyngeal airway using a tongue blade.

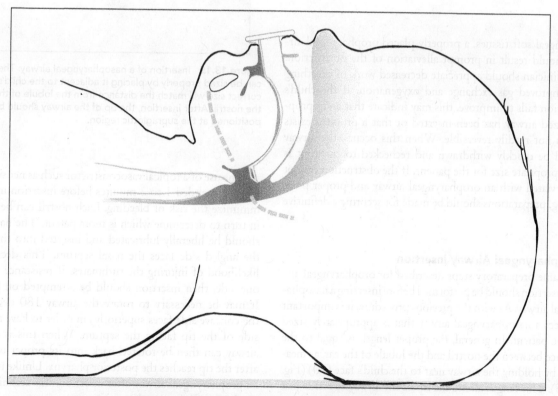

Figure 13.14 Proper position for an oropharyngeal airway.

SUMMARY

Oropharyngeal Airway Insertion

1 Select an oropharyngeal airway such that the tip reaches the angle of the mandible when the flange is at the central incisors.

2 Place the patient supine, attach to a cardiac monitor, and have a dental tip suction device and self-inflating bag available.

3 Insert a tongue blade to depress the tongue and to achieve visualization of the hypopharynx.

4 Under direct visualization, insert the oral airway in the same orientation it will reside in the hypopharynx (i.e., concave side facing inferiorly).

5 If the patient has repeated coughing, gagging, or vomiting after insertion, remove the airway and use another method to establish airway patency.

6 Assess the patient's response to determine the effectiveness of the procedure. If respirations remain labored, replace the airway with one more appropriately sized or take measures for definitive airway control.

7 If ventilation is improved and the patient is tolerating airway, tape in place.

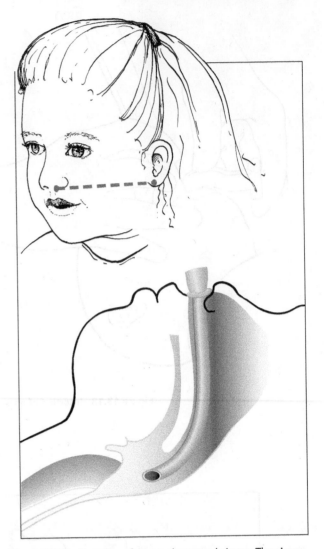

Figure 13.15 Insertion of a nasopharyngeal airway. The airway can be sized properly by placing it adjacent to the child's face. The correct size will match the distance from the lobule of the ear to the nostril. After insertion, the tip of the airway should be positioned at the supraglottic region.

pharyngeal soft tissues, a properly placed oropharyngeal airway should result in prompt alleviation of the obstruction. The clinician should appreciate decreased work of breathing and improved gas exchange and oxygenation. If the child's condition fails to improve, this may indicate that an improperly sized airway has been inserted or that a problem exists that is not readily reversible. When this occurs, the airway should be quickly withdrawn and rechecked to ensure it is the appropriate size for the patient. If the obstruction cannot be alleviated with an oropharyngeal airway and proper positioning, preparations should be made for securing a definitive airway.

Nasopharyngeal Airway Insertion

The same preparatory steps described for oropharyngeal airway insertion should be performed before inserting a nasopharyngeal airway. As with the previous procedure, it is important to select a nasopharyngeal airway that is appropriately sized for the patient. In general, the proper length is equal to the distance between the nostril and the lobule of the ear, as measured by holding the airway next to the child's face (10) (Fig. 13.15). This length allows the tip of the airway to reside just above the epiglottis.

The use of a topical vasoconstrictor such as neosynephrine is recommended 1 to 2 minutes before insertion in order to minimize the risk of bleeding. Each nostril can be occluded in turn to determine which is more patent. The nasal airway should be liberally lubricated and inserted into the naris so the angled side faces the nasal septum. This decreases the likelihood of injuring the turbinates. If resistance is met on one side, then insertion should be attempted on the other. It may be necessary to rotate the airway 180 degrees (i.e., the concave side faces superiorly) in order to have the angled side of the tip facing the septum. When this is done, the airway can then be rotated back into its proper orientation after the tip reaches the posterior pharynx. Unlike rotation of an oropharyngeal airway after insertion, this technique poses no threat of injury to the patient.

SUMMARY

Nasopharyngeal Airway Insertion

1 Select a nasopharyngeal airway such that the tip reaches the lobule of the ear when the opposite end touches the ipsilateral naris.

2 Place the patient supine, attach to a cardiac monitor, and have a dental tip suction device and self-inflating bag available.

3 Before airway insertion, apply topical vasoconstrictor such as neosynephrine to the nares and lubricate the nasal airway.

4 Occlude each nostril to determine which is more patent and use that side for insertion.

5 Insert the nasopharyngeal airway so angled side faces the nasal septum. If necessary, invert the airway 180° (i.e., with concave side facing superiorly) and then rotate it back to normal position after the tip reaches the posterior pharynx.

6 Assess the patient's response to determine the effectiveness of procedure. If respirations remain labored, replace the airway with one more appropriately sized or take measures for definitive airway control.

The patient should be reassessed following nasopharyngeal airway insertion. Ideally the clinician will see a decrease in the patient's respiratory effort and improved airflow and oxygenation if the airway has been inserted properly. As with the oropharyngeal airway, if adequate airway patency is not established more definitive measures will likely be necessary.

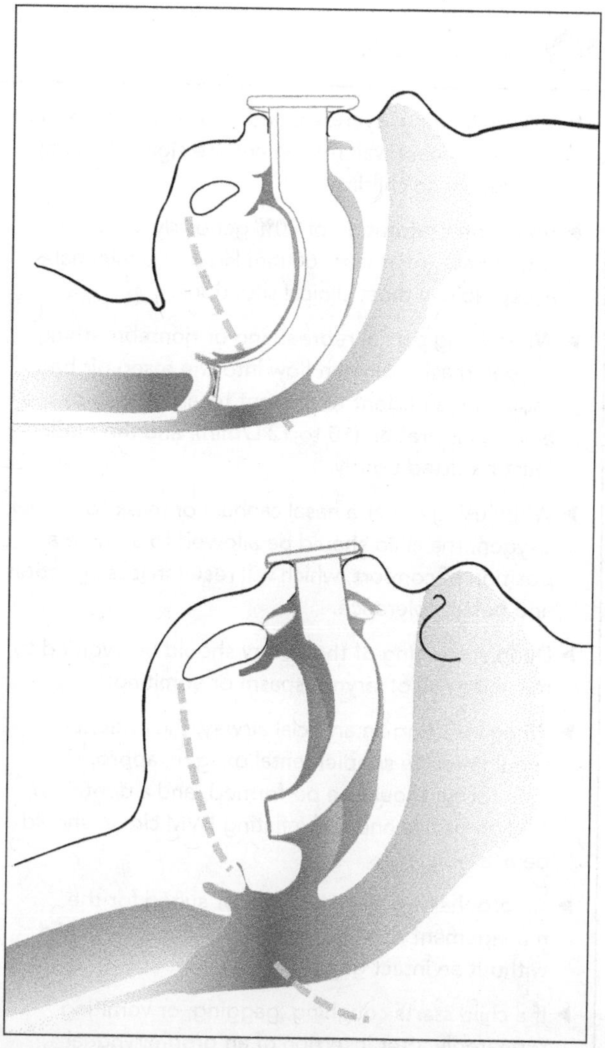

Figure 13.16 Improperly sized oropharyngeal airways. An oropharyngeal airway that is too large will displace the epiglottis inferiorly over the glottic opening. An airway that is too small will impinge on the tongue, displacing it posteriorly into the hypopharynx.

Complications

Use of an oropharyngeal airway that is either too small or too large can exacerbate airway obstruction. An airway that is too short can push the base of the tongue against the posterior pharyngeal wall, while an airway that is too long can displace the epiglottis inferiorly over the glottic opening (Fig. 13.16). Additionally, an oropharyngeal airway may induce vomiting, which can in turn can cause aspiration pneumonitis in the patient with depressed airway reflexes. If the child is awake, insertion of an oral airway can cause laryngospasm or injury of the pharyngeal soft tissues due to coughing and gagging. Such complications can usually be avoided by using an appropriately sized airway and by selecting appropriate patients for the procedure.

Few significant complications are associated with using a nasopharyngeal airway. Occasionally the airway may cause injury to nasal mucosa or adenoidal tissue, resulting in epistaxis. If the patient has a coagulopathy, such bleeding can be profuse and may cause problems with maintaining airway patency. Prolonged use of a nasopharyngeal airway has been associated with ulceration of the nasal mucosa, otitis media, and sinusitis, although these complications are not a concern during an emergent resuscitation. If the patient has a basilar skull fracture, a nasal airway may be inserted through a disruption in the cribriform plate into the anterior cranial fossa (6,7). Although this is a rare complication, a nasopharyngeal airway should not be used for any child suspected of having this injury.

CLINICAL TIPS

▶ Stridor, snoring, cyanosis, and poor aeration despite adequate chest wall movement are signs of airway obstruction in children.

▶ An oxygen saturation of 90% generally correlates with a PaO_2 of at least 60 mm Hg and is minimally acceptable in most clinical situations.

▶ When using partial rebreathing or nonrebreathing oxygen masks, oxygen flow into the reservoir bag should be sufficient to prevent total collapse of the bag on inspiration (10 to 12 L/min), and the mask must be fitted tightly.

▶ When using either a nasal cannula or mask to deliver oxygen, the child should be allowed to assume a position of comfort, which will result in less agitation and better tolerance.

▶ Deep suctioning of the airway should be avoided to minimize risk of laryngospasm or vomiting.

▶ When inserting an artificial airway, the patient should receive supplemental oxygen, appropriate monitoring should be performed, and a dental tip suction device and self-inflating BVM circuit should be available.

▶ An oropharyngeal airway is best suited for the management of a stuporous or unconscious child without an intact gag reflex.

▶ If a child starts coughing, gagging, or vomiting repeatedly after insertion of an oropharyngeal airway, the child is too alert, and another method of establishing airway patency must be employed.

▶ A nasopharyngeal airway should be used for the conscious child with partial airway obstruction.

▶ SUMMARY

Respiratory diseases are an important cause of pediatric cardiopulmonary arrest. Medical personnel must therefore be adept at providing supplemental oxygen, achieving and maintaining a patent airway, and assisting the ventilation of any critically ill child. Once it has been established that a spontaneously breathing child in respiratory distress has a patent

airway, oxygen should be provided. The clinician must be familiar with various oxygen delivery devices and select an appropriate system based on the patient's needs. In all but a few exceptional situations, an oxygen concentration should be delivered that is adequate to maintain an oxyhemoglobin saturation of 100%.

For a child with evidence of airway obstruction, suctioning of the nasopharynx or oropharynx is often beneficial. In addition, airway maneuvers may be effective in establishing patency. If these measures are unsuccessful, insertion of an artificial airway may be necessary. A nasopharyngeal airway is best suited for a more alert child, whereas an oropharyngeal airway is most appropriate for the obtunded patient with a diminished or absent gag reflex. Depending on the clinical situation, insertion of an artificial airway may serve as a definitive procedure or as a temporizing measure before endotracheal intubation. Familiarity with these adjunctive procedures and mastery of the necessary manual skills are essential for all medical personnel who care for critically ill or injured children.

▶ REFERENCES

1. Airway, ventilation, and management of respiratory distress and failure. In: Zaritsky AL, Nadkarni VN, Hickey RW, et al., eds. *Pediatric Advanced Life Support Manual.* American Heart Association, 2002;81–126.
2. Ludwig S, Kettrick RG, Parker M. Pediatric cardiopulmonary resuscitation. *Clin Pediatr* 1984;23:71–75.
3. Gerardi MJ, Sacchetti AD, Cantor, RM, et al. Rapid-sequence intubation of the pediatric patient. *Ann Emerg Med* 1996;28:55–74.
4. Gas regulation, administration, and controlling devices. In: McPhearson SP, ed. *Respiratory Therapy Equipment.* St. Louis: CV Mosby, 1990.
5. Clinton JE, McGill JW. Basic airway management and decision making. In: Roberts JR, Hedges JR, eds. *Clinical Procedures in Emergency Medicine.* 3rd ed., Philadelphia: WB Saunders Company, 1998;1–30.
6. Muzzi DA, Losasso TJ, Cucchiara RF. Complication from a nasopharyngeal airway in a patient with a basilar skull fracture. *Anesthesiology.* 1991;74:366–368.
7. Fletcher SA, Henderson LT, Minor ME, Jones JM. The successful surgical removal of intracranial nasogastric tubes. *J Trauma* 1987;27:948–952.
8. Ludwig S, Lavelle JM. Resuscitation-Pediatric basic and advanced life support. In: Fleisher G, Ludwig S, eds. *Textbook of Pediatric Emergency Medicine* 5th ed, Philadelphia: Lippincott, Williams & Wilkins, 2006;3–33.
9. Airway management and ventilation. *Advanced Trauma Life Support Manual.* Chicago: American College of Surgeons, 1994;59–86.
10. Hwang CL, Luu KC, Wu TJ, et al. Estimation of the length of nasopharyngeal airway in Chinese adults. *Anaesth Sinica* 1990;28:49–54.

CHRISTOPHER KING AND STACY L. REYNOLDS

14

Bag-Valve-Mask Ventilation

▶ INTRODUCTION

The first steps in most pediatric resuscitations are to establish a patent airway and provide adequate ventilatory support. Although definitive management of a respiratory emergency often involves endotracheal intubation, this may not be possible initially if the appropriate equipment is unavailable or properly trained personnel are not present. Even in settings where intubation can be performed rapidly, the patient may require respiratory support before the procedure. It is in such situations that bag-valve-mask (BVM) ventilation is indicated. Patients requiring assisted or controlled ventilation may be managed on an immediate basis with minimal preparation using this procedure. In most cases, BVM ventilation serves as a temporizing measure to be used before intubation and during intervals between intubation attempts. It is sometimes possible, however, to support a patient through a brief apneic episode (e.g., oversedation) with BVM ventilation alone. Furthermore, the utility of this procedure as a primary means of respiratory support for children in the prehospital setting was demonstrated in a seminal study by Gausche et al. (1). In a large, randomized trial comparing BVM ventilation alone with endotracheal intubation, these authors found no differences in survival or neurologic outcome among pediatric patients requiring transport to the hospital.

BVM ventilation is a procedure that many health care providers—including physicians, nurses, respiratory therapists, and paramedics—are called on to perform. It is undoubtedly the procedure most commonly used by medical personnel in the initial management of pediatric respiratory emergencies. But this should not be taken to mean that BVM ventilation is a simple procedure. Most practitioners who care for critically ill children can relate experiences during which performing manual ventilation proved far more difficult than endotracheal intubation. In addition, the ability of inexperi-

enced operators to effectively perform BVM ventilation with pediatric patients may be limited (2). For these reasons, as with any airway intervention, the attention of the team leader in a pediatric resuscitation should never be far from the proficiency with which BVM ventilation is being performed.

▶ ANATOMY AND PHYSIOLOGY

A number of anatomic differences exist between pediatric and adult patients that have important clinical implications regarding the use of BVM ventilation (Fig. 14.1). Not surprisingly, these differences are most apparent among infants and become less pronounced as the patient matures through older childhood and adolescence. One such characteristic is that the tongue of an infant or younger child is larger relative to the oral cavity than in the case of an adult. In addition, the tongue has a more rostral (superior) location in relation to the roof of the mouth. The larger size and "higher" position of the tongue greatly increase the likelihood of airway obstruction when the patient is lying supine. An artificial airway may therefore be necessary to maintain a conduit for gas flow when performing BVM ventilation with a pediatric patient (see Chapter 13). Infants also exhibit obligate nasal breathing until about 3 to 5 months of age as a result of obstruction of the oropharyngeal airway as the tongue rests against the roof of the mouth. Occlusion of the nares because of stenosis or choanal atresia, as well as transient causes such as blood, vomitus, or secretions, can produce profound respiratory distress and even asphyxia in an infant (3,4). In such cases, BVM ventilation is an effective means of bypassing the obstruction and providing gas exchange via the oropharynx.

The immature laryngeal cartilages of the pediatric airway are more compliant, allowing wider variation in the airway diameter in response to compressive or distending forces (5,6).

109

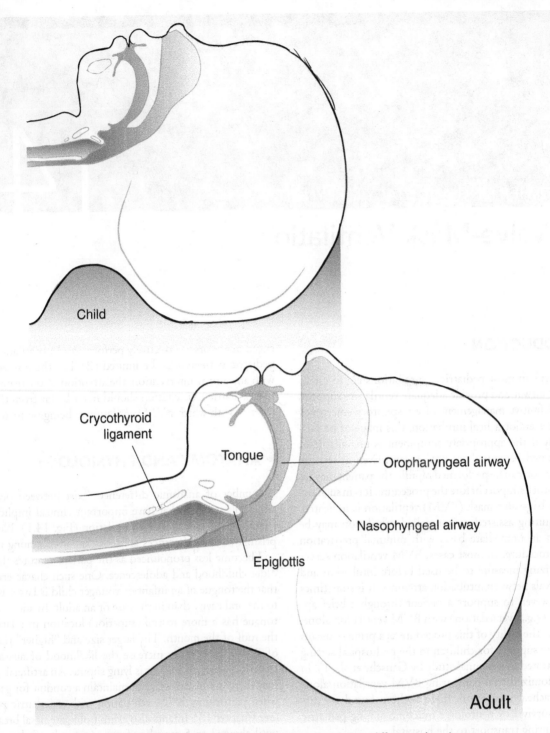

Figure 14.1 Pediatric versus adult airway. Aside from the obvious difference that airway diameters of the child are smaller at comparable anatomic levels, other important characteristics are unique to the pediatric patient. The tongue of a child is larger relative to the size of the oropharynx and has a more rostral location in the mouth compared with the adult. There is also greater laxity of the pharyngeal soft tissues. These anatomic differences all predispose the pediatric patient to the development of airway obstruction.

As a result, pediatric patients with partial airway obstruction are more prone to develop dynamic collapse of the extrathoracic airway as a result of high negative intraluminal pressures, increasing the work of breathing. Manual ventilation is often effective in such situations, because this negative pressure is reduced or eliminated (see below). Infants and children also have greater laxity of the cervical spine and neck musculature (7–9). This can lead to excessive rotation of the head during attempts to establish a patent airway, which can result in complete airway obstruction (Fig. 14.2).

As described in Chapter 16, the optimal position of the head and neck for airway patency is the so-called sniffing position. The neck is slightly flexed while the head is rotated into extension. This is said to be the position assumed when one is "sniffing the air," and it results in the most favorable alignment of the oral, pharyngeal, and tracheal axes (10) (Fig. 14.3). With adolescents and adults, it is generally necessary to place a small towel roll or pad under the head to achieve the proper degree of neck flexion. However, because infants have a relatively large occiput, such measures are not usually required (Fig. 14.4). In fact, it may be helpful to place a pad or towel roll under the shoulders to elevate the torso slightly if an infant has an especially prominent occiput.

The relative immaturity of the pediatric diaphragm, intercostal muscles, and ribs can also impact on the use of BVM ventilation. The chest wall of an infant or child is significantly

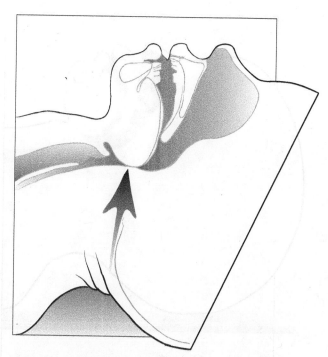

Figure 14.2 Excessive extension of the neck in an attempt to establish airway patency can actually cause or worsen obstruction.

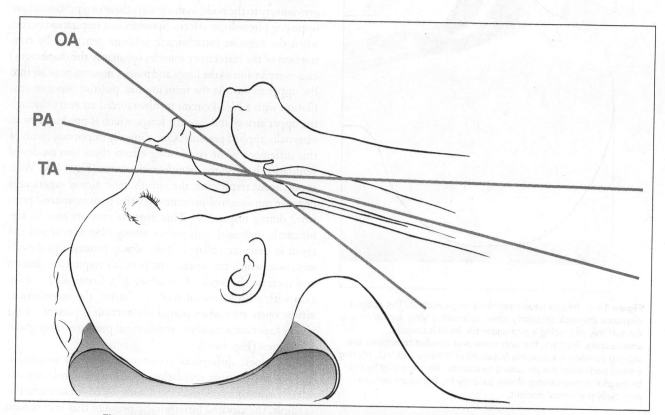

Figure 14.3 The sniffing position results in the most favorable alignment of the oral, pharyngeal, and tracheal axes for airway patency. A small pad or towel roll placed under the head may be needed to achieve the necessary flexion of the neck for an older child or adolescent (see also Fig. 16.3).

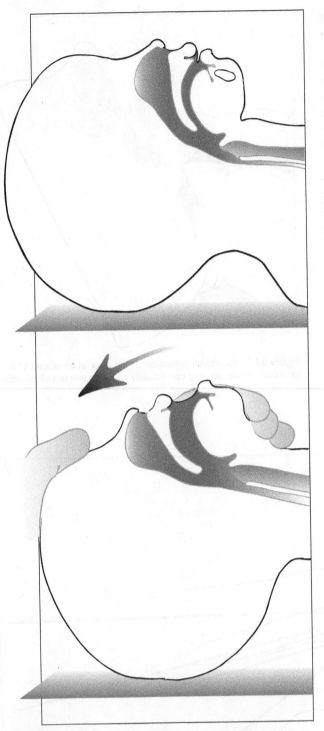

Figure 14.4 Infants have a relatively large occiput. The occiput displaces the neck anteriorly when an infant is lying supine on a flat surface, so placing a pad under the head is usually unnecessary. Typically, the only maneuver needed to achieve the sniffing position is extension (rotation) of the head. In fact, placing a small pad under the shoulders to elevate the torso slightly may be helpful in maintaining airway patency for the infant with an especially prominent occiput.

more compliant than that of an adolescent or adult (11). As a result, there is less "protective" resistance provided by the chest wall, which results in a higher incidence of barotrauma during BVM ventilation. In addition, pediatric patients have a greater tendency to develop early respiratory muscle fatigue, potentially leading to respiratory arrest. This is primarily the result of the immature diaphragm having a lower content of Type I muscle fibers (slow twitch, high oxidative capacity), which confer fatigue resistance (12). The infant's diaphragm is also more horizontal and therefore less efficient in expanding the lungs.

Certain congenital abnormalities of the face and airway can make BVM ventilation difficult or impossible to perform. For example, achieving an adequate mask seal may not be possible if the child has micrognathia or other midfacial anomalies. This is also true for patients with severe trauma to the face or mandible. In addition, administering manual ventilation may be problematic for children with macroglossia due to difficulty maintaining a patent airway. In such cases, providing positive pressure ventilation to treat respiratory failure may require immediate endotracheal intubation.

Use of BVM ventilation may be affected by several characteristics of pediatric respiratory physiology. As with endotracheal intubation, BVM ventilation is a useful means of providing respiratory support because it offers a method of delivering positive pressure ventilation. Although normal spontaneous ventilation and positive pressure ventilation both result in oxygen delivery to the body, in many ways these two processes have opposing physiologic effects. Spontaneous respiration occurs when the negative intrathoracic pressure generated by contraction of the respiratory muscles (primarily the diaphragm) causes expansion of the lungs and passive movement of air into the upper airway. As the term implies, positive pressure ventilation with a BVM circuit involves forced air entry through the upper airway and into the lungs, which is produced by an externally applied pressure. One clinically important result of this difference is the contrasting effects these two modes of ventilation have on the extrathoracic airway (Fig. 14.5). With spontaneous respiration, the extrathoracic airway experiences negative intraluminal pressures (relative to atmospheric pressure) during inspiration. This negative pressure may be significantly increased with partial airway obstruction and can result in dynamic collapse of the airway proximal to the obstruction, which can worsen the patient's respiratory distress and increase the work of breathing (5). Controlled ventilation with a BVM circuit tends to "stent" the extrathoracic airway open, even when partial obstruction is present, as the airway experiences positive intraluminal pressures throughout inspiration (Fig. 14.6).

Physiologic differences between spontaneous ventilation and positive pressure ventilation may also play a role in some adverse consequences associated with BVM ventilation. For example, the elevated intrathoracic pressure that occurs with positive pressure ventilation reduces venous return to the heart and can cause a decrease in cardiac output (13), although interestingly this may be less pronounced in children than adults

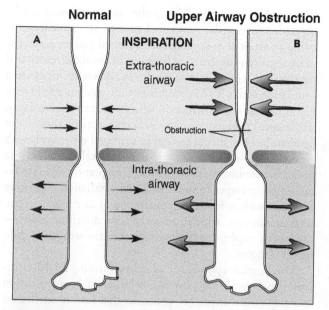

Normal   **Upper Airway Obstruction**

INSPIRATION

Extra-thoracic airway

Obstruction

Intra-thoracic airway

Figure 14.5
A. During spontaneous respiration, the extrathoracic airway experiences negative intraluminal pressure on inspiration.
B. With airway obstruction, this negative pressure increases greatly and may produce collapse of the extrathoracic airway proximal to the obstruction.

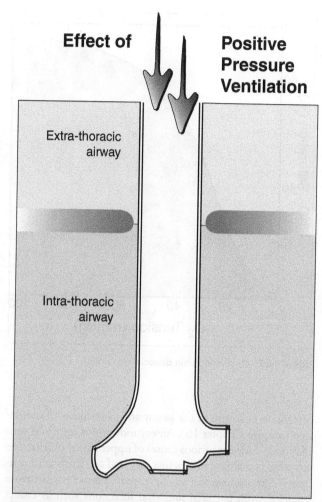

Effect of   **Positive Pressure Ventilation**

Extra-thoracic airway

Intra-thoracic airway

Figure 14.6 During BVM ventilation, the extrathoracic airway is "stented" open by the effect of positive intraluminal pressure throughout the respiratory cycle.

(14). This effect normally has clinical significance only for patients with hypovolemia or borderline cardiac function. Consequently, such patients who receive BVM ventilation may require increased intravenous fluid administration to maintain stable hemodynamics. In addition, BVM ventilation can exacerbate ventilation-perfusion (VQ) mismatching (15,16). With spontaneous ventilation, the lung bases receive the majority of both air entry and blood flow during inspiration; ventilation and perfusion are therefore well matched. When a patient receives BVM ventilation, the distribution of air entry is determined primarily by compliance of the lung parenchyma, which is greatest in the apices. As a result, while blood continues to flow preferentially to the bases, the majority of air entry now goes to the apices, resulting in VQ mismatch. This accounts for the spontaneously breathing patient who may have a decrease in oxygen saturation when assisted ventilation with a BVM circuit is initiated. For this reason, the delivered oxygen concentration should be maximized whenever manual ventilation is performed.

One of the more unwelcome events during BVM ventilation of a pediatric patient is the sudden, dramatic decline in oxygen saturation that results when oxygen delivery is inadequate. This is also related to a unique characteristic of pediatric physiology; the rate of oxygen consumption among infants and children is significantly higher than among adults. In fact, the baseline oxygen consumption of a neonate is approximately twice that of an adult (17). As a result, if the concentration of oxygen delivered by manual ventilation is insufficient for any reason (e.g., unrecognized mask leak, rebreathing of expired gases), the pO2 of a pediatric patient will

drop more rapidly than it will with an adult (18). The rapidity of the decline appears to be even more pronounced among children with upper respiratory infections (19). Because the oxygen dissociation curve has a flat segment at higher oxygen saturations, the reading of the pulse oximeter remains relatively stable initially despite the fact that the pO2 is falling (Fig. 14.7). If this problem is not recognized, oxygen saturation will suddenly decline precipitously when the pO2 reaches the steep zone of the curve. This diminished margin for error makes the timely recognition of problems leading to inadequate oxygen delivery an important priority with pediatric patients.

▶ INDICATIONS

BVM ventilation is used to provide temporary ventilatory support until definitive management can be undertaken or the patient resumes spontaneous respiration. Indications for the use of BVM ventilation can be divided into two general

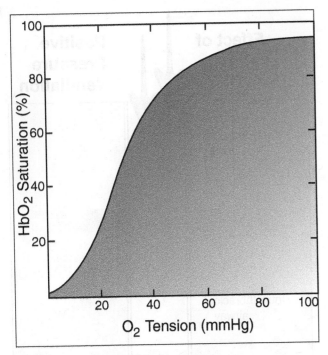

Figure 14.7 Oxyhemoglobin dissociation curve.

categories: problems of the airway and problems with ventilation (see also Chapter 16). Airway indications for BVM ventilation include the various causes of upper airway obstruction affecting pediatric patients that can lead to significant respiratory compromise. For example, partial airway obstruction resulting from bacterial and viral infections such as croup, bacterial tracheitis, and retropharyngeal abscess may serve as an indication for BVM ventilation. As mentioned previously, infants and younger children may present with frank respiratory arrest resulting solely from obstruction caused by laxity of the pharyngeal musculature and posterior displacement of the tongue. Such patients normally have other medical problems (e.g., sepsis, toxic ingestion) that are causing a profoundly depressed mental status. In this situation, the use of BVM ventilation, combined with proper positioning and insertion of an artificial airway, offers an effective initial approach to managing the respiratory component of the overall presentation. Other obstructive processes that can be addressed using BVM ventilation include hematoma, supraglottic edema, and upper airway foreign body. For the patient with a rapidly expanding hematoma of the upper airway, BVM ventilation can be used in the early stage of management, but tracheal intubation should be performed as soon as the patient is stabilized. In addition, foreign bodies should normally be removed from the airway whenever possible before initiating BVM ventilation, because smaller objects may be propelled distally by the force of ventilations (see Chapter 51).

As discussed previously, pediatric patients are prone to fatigue and may therefore develop respiratory failure or arrest from airway obstruction long before BVM ventilation would be difficult to administer. In other words, the obstruc-

tion is rarely "complete." Thus the operator should not be dissuaded from making an initial attempt at manually ventilating an arrested or severely compromised patient suspected of having airway obstruction from one of the above mentioned processes. It is important to emphasize, however, that assisted ventilation with a BVM circuit is *not* indicated for a child with high-grade airway obstruction who is, at least momentarily, stable and breathing adequately. Such a patient should not be disturbed but should instead be managed expectantly with airway equipment close at hand until surgical and anesthesia personnel are involved. Otherwise, the agitation and distress caused by attempts to perform BVM ventilation—or other measures such as forced administration of face mask oxygen, venipuncture, etc., which may not be immediately necessary—can hasten respiratory failure or arrest as the struggling child rapidly fatigues.

The ventilatory indications for performing BVM ventilation include (a) nonobstructive causes of hypoventilation and respiratory arrest, (b) processes that lead to ineffective ventilation, and (c) insults to the lungs that cause impaired gas exchange. Hypoventilation and respiratory arrest in the pediatric population can result from a wide variety of neurologic, infectious, toxicologic, and metabolic disorders. In the ED, overwhelming sepsis and traumatic brain injury are two of the most common causes. Infants are especially prone to develop apnea as the first significant manifestation of an underlying illness. BVM ventilation should be initiated during a neonatal resuscitation whenever the heart rate is below 100 or the patient has apneic spells lasting 30 seconds or longer (see Chapter 36). Transient hypoventilation resulting from iatrogenic drug overdose (e.g., benzodiazepines for status epilepticus) can sometimes be managed with BVM ventilation alone until the patient resumes spontaneous respiration. Ineffective ventilation among pediatric patients is most frequently associated with processes that affect patency of the small airways, such as asthma and bronchiolitis. Fatigue leading to hypoxia and hypercarbia usually accounts for the child's worsening condition. With these patients, BVM ventilation can be used to temporarily reduce the work of breathing, although in such situations, endotracheal intubation will usually prove necessary. The decision to initiate manual ventilation is based primarily on the clinician's assessment of the severity of the patient's respiratory compromise. Impaired alveolar gas exchange results from diverse etiologies, such as lung infection, near-drowning, and pulmonary contusion. With more severe and diffuse involvement of the lungs, the patient may manifest clinical findings consistent with respiratory distress syndrome. These children may develop profound hypoxemia and frequently require endotracheal intubation. When BVM ventilation is used in the initial management of such patients, the circuit should be configured to reliably deliver a concentration of oxygen near 100% and, if necessary, to administer positive end expiratory pressure (PEEP).

There are few contraindications to BVM ventilation. Relative contraindications include any problems that significantly undermine the effectiveness of the procedure, such as congenital or traumatic facial deformities so severe that a mask seal is impossible to maintain or a high-grade airway obstruction that prevents delivery of adequate ventilatory support. If such a process becomes apparent when BVM ventilation is attempted, an alternate procedure (e.g., immediate endotracheal intubation, percutaneous transtracheal ventilation, or a surgical airway) should be performed. In addition, BVM ventilation should not be used for any significant length of time with a patient who is suspected of having a tension pneumothorax before the appropriate interventions for this process are undertaken. Continued delivery of positive pressure ventilation can further increase the elevated intrathoracic pressure. BVM ventilation can be used for immediate stabilization if such a patient is apneic, but needle thoracostomy and/or chest tube insertion (Chapter 29) should be performed as soon as possible.

The only situations that represent absolute contraindications to BVM ventilation are (a) the initial management of a newborn suspected of having significant meconium aspiration during delivery who does not appear vigorous (20) and (b) the presence of a congenital diaphragmatic hernia in a newborn with respiratory distress, both of which require immediate endotracheal intubation. For the newborn with significant meconium aspiration, performing BVM ventilation without prior intratracheal suctioning may worsen the

TABLE 14.1	EQUIPMENT FOR BVM VENTILATION

Array of face masks
Infant, pediatric, and adult resuscitation bags
Pressure manometer (when available)
Suction devices
Oxygen source
Oropharyngeal and nasopharyngeal airways
Monitors (pulse oximetry, cardiac monitor, capnography)

resulting pneumonitis (see Chapter 37). In the case of a newborn with a congenital diaphragmatic hernia, administering positive pressure ventilation with a BVM circuit may cause air entry into the herniated segment of stomach, potentially resulting in intrathoracic tamponade and eventually cardiovascular collapse (see Chapter 39). The physiology in such circumstances is similar to that of a tension pneumothorax.

▶ EQUIPMENT

Equipment and materials used to perform BVM ventilation are listed in Table 14.1. Figure 14.8 shows a typical self-inflating BVM circuit. Appropriate sizes should be

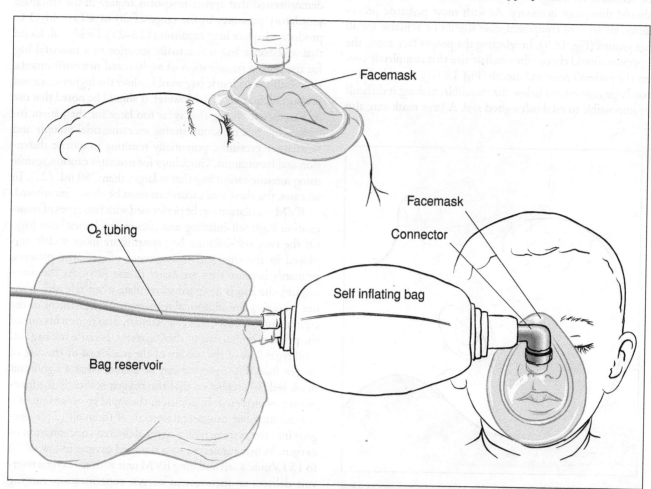

Figure 14.8 Typical self-inflating BVM circuit.

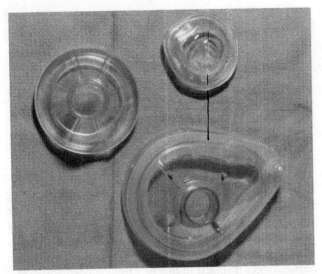

Figure 14.9 Face masks of various sizes and shapes. Premature infant through adult sizes should be available.

selected carefully, as use of the proper equipment will often determine the success or failure of the procedure. Because this is often a process of trial and error, the operator should not be reluctant to change equipment during BVM ventilation should this prove necessary. As with most pediatric procedures, an array of equipment sizes should be available for all age groups (Fig. 14.9). In selecting the proper face mask, the operator should choose the smallest size that completely covers the patient's nose and mouth (Fig. 14.10). A mask that is too large may extend below the mandible, making it difficult or impossible to establish a good seal. A large mask may also

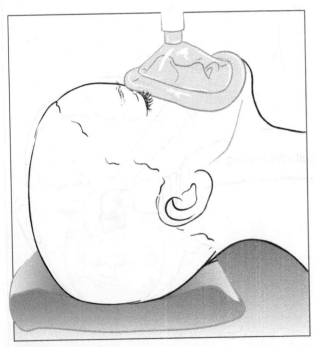

Figure 14.10 The smallest mask that completely covers the nose and mouth should be selected.

be inadvertently positioned over the eyes. Compression of the eyes can cause ocular injury or produce bradycardia as a result of vagal stimulation. Conversely, a small mask will not cover the entire mouth, causing an air leak when positive pressure ventilation is administered. It is often necessary to try more than one mask size before finding the proper fit.

A variety of different shapes and designs of pediatric face masks are available. The optimal shape of the mask depends on the size and age of the patient. For premature infants and full-term neonates, circular masks are generally most effective (21). The Laerdal pocket mask, which is often carried by prehospital personnel, is not recommended for infants, because it was found to give unacceptable results due to poor fit (22). For children and adolescents, various sizes of the traditional triangular masks are appropriate.

The most important consideration in selecting a resuscitation bag is that delivery of an adequate tidal volume must be ensured. As a general rule, a resuscitation bag one size too large will always produce better results than one that is too small, as long as the operator is careful not to deliver an excessive tidal volume. For example, a bag that would be suitable for an adolescent can normally be used effectively to administer BVM ventilation to a child. This may be particularly relevant to neonatal resuscitations. Investigators have demonstrated that apneic newborns require initial sustained ventilatory pressures in the range of 20 to 40 cm H_2O to produce adequate lung expansion (23–25). Field et al. found that a pediatric bag was actually superior to a neonatal bag for use during resuscitation of asphyxiated newborn infants, since only the pediatric bag would deliver the higher sustained pressures required (26). However, it should be noted that use of a resuscitation bag that is far too large for the patient increases the risk of administering excessive tidal volume and ventilatory pressures, potentially resulting in gastric distension and barotrauma. Guidelines for neonates caution against using a resuscitation bag that is larger than 750 mL (27). In all cases, the chest wall excursions must be closely monitored.

BVM ventilation can be performed with two types of resuscitation bags: self-inflating and conventional anesthesia bags. Of the two, self-inflating bag systems are more widely employed in the emergent management of pediatric patients, primarily because they are easier to use (28). As the name implies, the bag is designed to reinflate when released, without requiring any additional maneuvers or adjustment of the equipment. However, this characteristic also represents one of the primary limitations of these systems, because the bag will refill regardless of the quality of the mask seal or the rate of oxygen flow. The operator may be unaware that a significant mask leak is present or that the oxygen source is malfunctioning or depleted. In addition, the rapid re-expansion of a self-inflating bag causes entrainment of room air (21% oxygen) into the system, reducing the delivered concentration of oxygen. When connected to a standard oxygen inflow of 10 to 15 L/min, a self-inflating BVM unit with no oxygen reservoir delivers an inconsistent oxygen concentration, ranging from 30% to 80% (29,30). Fortunately, the widespread use

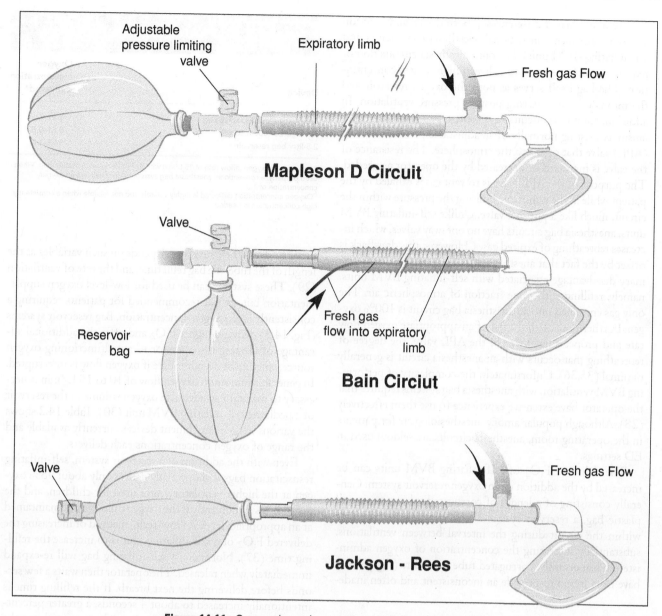

Adjustable pressure limiting valve

Expiratory limb

Fresh gas Flow

Mapleson D Circuit

Valve

Reservoir bag

Fresh gas flow into expiratory limb

Bain Circiut

Valve

Fresh gas Flow

Jackson - Rees

Figure 14.11 Commonly used conventional anesthesia bag circuits.

of reservoir devices in the design of pediatric BVM systems has largely overcome this disadvantage (see below).

The quality of the materials and the design of self-inflating BVM units have improved significantly over recent decades. Modern enhancements include nonstick one-way valves that are less susceptible to clogging with secretions, various methods for increasing the F_iO_2 delivered, in-line pressure monitors, and "pop-off" pressure valves. The purpose of a pop-off valve is to limit the ventilatory pressures generated within the circuit to a designated level (generally between 35 and 45 cm H_2O), a feature that reduces the risk of barotrauma. However, when airway resistance is high or pulmonary compliance is low, the presence of a functioning pop-off valve has been shown to significantly diminish the F_iO_2 delivered and/or prevent administration of an adequate tidal volume (30). Any BVM unit equipped with a pop-off valve should therefore have a

simple mechanism for disabling this device when necessary (31). In such cases, an in-line manometer should be used when available to prevent excessive peak inspiratory pressures and possible barotrauma (32).

In contrast to self-inflating resuscitation bags, conventional anesthesia bag circuits offer the advantage of providing a more reliable means of delivering high concentrations of oxygen. Proposed designs for a variety of these systems were originally described by Mapleson (33). The configurations most widely used for pediatric patients today are the Mapleson D circuit and two modifications of this system, the modified Mapleson D (Bain circuit) (33) and the Mapleson F (Jackson Rees circuit) (34). All three circuits share the common elements of (a) a conventional anesthesia bag, (b) an oxygen outlet, and (c) a venting mechanism. They differ with regard to where these features are positioned on the unit (Fig. 14.11).

Several important differences in both design and function are found between conventional anesthesia bag circuits and self-inflating BVM units. For one, anesthesia circuits do not require a reservoir system to deliver a high oxygen concentration. The bag itself serves as both the oxygen reservoir and the means of administering positive pressure ventilation. In addition, anesthesia circuits have some type of venting mechanism, consisting normally of an adjustable pressure limiting (APL) valve that opens to the atmosphere. The resistance of the valve is increased or decreased by the operator as needed. The purpose of the APL valve is to vent gases exhaled by the patient while at the same time limiting the pressure within the circuit, much like a pop-off valve. Unlike self-inflating BVM units, anesthesia bag circuits have no one-way valves, which increases rebreathing of expired gases. However, this drawback is offset by the fact that anesthesia circuits do not share the primary disadvantage associated with self-inflating BVM units, namely, refilling with some fraction of atmospheric air. The only gas entrained into an anesthesia bag circuit is 100% oxygen. Furthermore, with the use of an appropriate oxygen flow rate and proper adjustment of the APL valve, the degree of rebreathing that occurs with an anesthesia circuit is generally minimal (35,36). Unfortunately, the complexity of performing BVM ventilation with anesthesia bag systems requires that the operator have extensive experience to use them effectively (28). Although popular among anesthesiologists for patients in the operating room, anesthesia circuits are seldom used in ED settings.

The delivered F_iO_2 of self-inflating BVM units can be increased by the addition of an oxygen reservoir system. Generally consisting of a length of corrugated tubing or a small plastic bag, a reservoir system allows oxygen to accumulate within the circuit during the interval between ventilations, substantially increasing the concentration of oxygen administered. Importantly, corrugated tube reservoirs (Fig. 14.12) have been found to provide an inconsistent and often inade-

TABLE 14.2	OXYGEN ENRICHMENT FOR BVM VENTILATION
Device	**Oxygen concentration delivered[a]**
Oxygen line connected to bag	0.41
Corrugated tube reservoir	0.51–0.53[b]
2.5-liter bag reservoir	0.95–1.0

[a]Assumes an oxygen inflow rate of 15 L/min with self-inflating resuscitation bag. When used properly, a conventional anesthesia bag system reliably delivers an oxygen concentration of 1.0.
[b]Oxygen concentration delivered is highly variable and not reliable when a consistently high concentration is needed.

quate F_iO_2, as their function depends on such variables as the length of the tube, the bag refill time, and the rate of ventilation (29). These systems can be used for low-level oxygen supplementation but are not recommended for patients requiring a consistently high oxygen concentration. Bag reservoir systems (Fig. 14.8) deliver a higher F_iO_2 and offer the additional advantage of alerting the operator to a malfunctioning oxygen source, since most do not inflate if oxygen flow is interrupted. In general, a minimum oxygen flow of 10 to 15 L/min is necessary to maintain an adequate oxygen volume in the reservoir of a pediatric self-inflating BVM unit (30). Table 14.2 shows the various oxygen enrichment devices currently available and the range of oxygen concentrations each delivers.

Even with the addition of a reservoir system, self-inflating resuscitation bags will optimally deliver only about 95% oxygen at the higher ventilatory rates used for children, and the F_iO_2 drops significantly if the oxygen inflow is not maintained at an appropriate level. A "low-tech" method of increasing the delivered F_iO_2 of a self-inflating unit is to increase the refilling time (37). Normally, a self-inflating bag will re-expand immediately when released. The operator then waits a few seconds before delivering the next breath. If the refilling time is intentionally increased to about 4 seconds, a greater percentage of oxygen relative to ambient air will be entrained into the system. The operator accomplishes this by releasing the bag slowly, causing it to gradually reinflate over the entire interval between ventilations. This has been shown to increase the delivered F_iO_2 by as much as 40% over the traditional method. Unfortunately, this technique is only applicable to older children and adolescents, because the gradual refilling required cannot be performed effectively with ventilatory rates higher than 20 per minute (29).

▶ PROCEDURE

Management of the patient who requires BVM ventilation first involves standard basic life support assessment and intervention. A detailed discussion of this initial approach is provided in Chapter 12. The primary operator takes a position above the head of the patient at the start of the resuscitation.

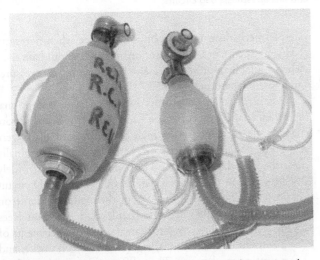

Figure 14.12 Self-inflating resuscitation bags with corrugated tube reservoir.

When possible, the height of the bed should be adjusted to an appropriate level to both improve effectiveness and reduce fatigue. As described previously, airway patency is maximized when the patient is placed in the "sniffing" position—slight flexion of the neck with extension (rotation) of the head (Figs. 14.3 and 14.4). The airway is established using either the chin lift or jaw thrust maneuvers, and the operator then assesses the patient using the "look, listen, feel" method (see Chapter 12). A useful sign indicating success in opening the airway is an audible "sighing" sound that may be heard as the patient inhales or exhales. In fact, when obstruction is solely the result of posterior displacement of the tongue, the patient may resume spontaneous respirations. If patency is not initially established, the operator should attempt to achieve a more favorable alignment of the airway by repositioning the head and neck. For example, excessive rotation of the head can actually cause airway obstruction (Fig. 14.2), and it may therefore be

necessary to reduce the degree of neck extension in performing the chin lift maneuver. Similarly, when performing the jaw thrust maneuver, it may be necessary to apply greater force in anteriorly displacing the mandible if the child has a large tongue.

Once a patent airway has been established, the operator is ready to begin performing BVM ventilation. Selection of a proper face mask and resuscitation bag is based on guidelines described previously (see "Equipment"). When the chin lift maneuver is used to maintain the airway and apply the mask, it should be performed with the nondominant hand so that the dominant hand is free to compress the resuscitation bag. The mask is held in place with the thumb and index finger (Fig. 14.13). If the jaw thrust maneuver is used, the mask is secured by the thumb and index finger of both hands (Fig. 14.14). Downward pressure on the mask also provides countertraction to facilitate displacement of the mandible anteriorly. If

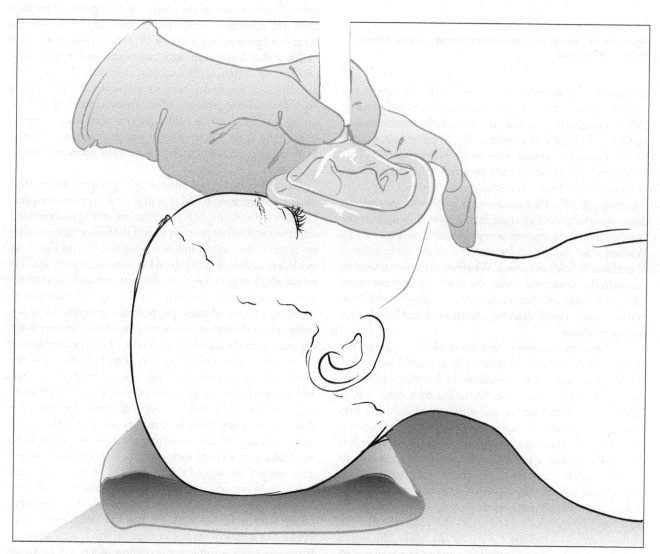

Figure 14.13 Chin lift maneuver to maintain airway patency and secure the mask. This method enhances control of the mask if the patient is moving. Otherwise, the likelihood of maintaining a good mask seal may be increased by holding the mask in place with the index finger and thumb positioned over the air-filled seal.

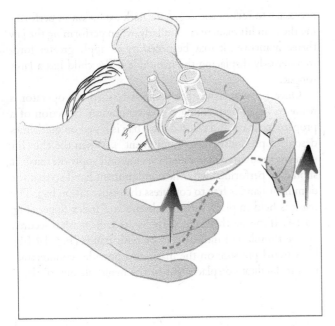

Figure 14.14 Jaw thrust maneuver to maintain airway patency and secure the mask.

TABLE 14.3	VENTILATORY RATES FOR PEDIATRIC PATIENTS
Infant	20–24 breaths/min
Child	16–20 breaths/min
Adolescent	12–16 breaths/min

the patient is an infant or younger child, the fifth finger can sometimes be used to simultaneously apply cricoid pressure (Sellick's maneuver). Cricoid pressure reduces the incidence of aspiration during BVM ventilation by (a) preventing regurgitation of stomach contents into the oropharynx and (b) limiting air entry into the stomach, preventing the accumulation of an excessively high intragastric pressure, which may cause vomiting (38,39). This maneuver is performed by pressing down over the cricoid cartilage firmly enough to occlude the esophagus without causing airway obstruction (Fig. 14.15). With an older child or adolescent, an assistant can be enlisted to perform Sellick's maneuver. Whatever maneuver is used to maintain the airway and secure the mask, the operator must take care to avoid pressing on the tissues of the submental area, as this will often result in airway obstruction, particularly with younger patients.

It is important to ensure that the mask fits snugly on the face so that no air leak can occur. The fit should be checked frequently throughout the procedure by listening and feeling around the rim of the mask. Detection of a mask leak is especially important with a self-inflating resuscitation bag, because re-expansion occurs even when there is a significant mask leak. Maintaining a good mask seal may be difficult if the child has a facial anomaly (e.g., micrognathia) or trauma to the face (mandibular or midfacial fractures, burns, etc.) or if a nasogastric tube has been inserted. In such cases, a better fit may be achieved by placing gauze pads around the rim of the mask (40). Integrity of the seal is also affected by the strength of the operator's hand and the size of the mask. Although a perfect seal may not be obtainable—and in fact may not be necessary to adequately ventilate the patient—the success or failure of the procedure will often depend on the degree to which mask leaks are minimized.

After the mask is properly applied, the operator administers positive pressure ventilation by compressing the resuscitation bag. The dominant hand is used to ensure delivery of an adequate tidal volume. Appropriate ventilatory rates for pediatric age groups are shown in Table 14.3. When a patient is simultaneously receiving chest compressions, the ratio should be two ventilations for every 15 compressions (20). To administer an appropriate tidal volume, the operator should carefully observe the patient's chest excursions during ventilation. Compression of the resuscitation bag should produce chest wall movement similar to a normal deep inspiration. As mentioned previously, patients with partial airway obstruction or diminished lung compliance may require higher ventilatory pressures to overcome the increased resistance. The operator accomplishes this by disabling the pop-off valve, performing more forceful compressions of the resuscitation bag, and ensuring that the mask is held tightly in place to prevent air leaks. Here again, observation of the chest excursions serves as the primary indicator in determining the necessary force of ventilation.

Using a conventional anesthesia bag system differs from using a self-inflating BVM unit in several important respects. Unlike a self-inflating bag, the resuscitation bag in an anesthesia circuit will inflate properly only if the following conditions are met: (a) the oxygen inflow is adequate, (b) no significant mask leak occurs, and (c) the APL valve is properly set. The rate at which oxygen flows into the system must be maintained at an appropriate level to reinflate the bag and minimize rebreathing of exhaled gases. For pediatric patients, this is generally two to three times the minute ventilation of the patient, depending on the circuit used (35,36). The operator must at all times maintain a closed system. If there is any significant mask leak, the resuscitation bag will not reinflate properly, and administration of adequate positive pressure ventilation will be impossible. Finally, the APL valve must be adjusted so that an appropriate pressure is maintained within the system. In determining the correct setting for this valve, the operator must take into account such variables as pulmonary compliance, oxygen inflow, and tidal volume. The APL valve often proves to be one of the more problematic features of an anesthesia circuit for less experienced operators. If the resistance of the valve is set too high, the bag will progressively overinflate like a balloon as the pressure in the system increases. If the resistance is too low, the outflow of gas will be greater than the oxygen inflow, and the bag will not inflate sufficiently. When all these tasks are combined with the additional responsibility of maintaining a patent airway, the high failure rate

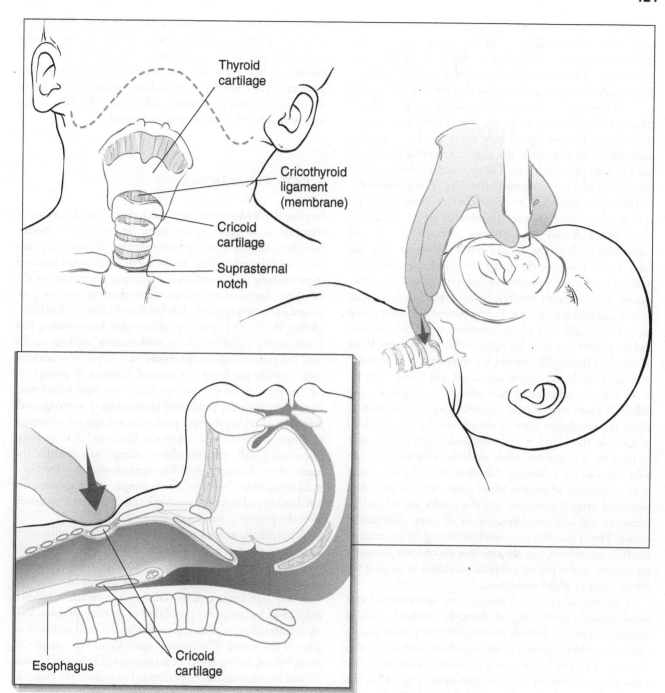

Figure 14.15 Cricoid pressure (Sellick's maneuver). With an infant or smaller child, the fifth finger can sometimes be used to apply cricoid pressure. Otherwise, the help of an assistant can be enlisted.

demonstrated by less experienced practitioners with this procedure is easy to understand (28,41).

If the operator has difficulty administering ventilations, this may be the result of one of several problems. For example, it may sometimes prove impossible to adequately compress the resuscitation bag while maintaining airway patency. This can occur if the patient requires higher ventilatory pressures, the operator has small hands, or managing the airway is particularly troublesome. In such situations, employing

the two-person technique of BVM ventilation usually provides an effective solution (see below). Assuming the airway is patent, one of the most frequent causes of inadequate ventilation is a significant air leak caused by an improper mask fit and/or poor technique. These problems can normally be avoided with careful selection of an appropriate mask size and ongoing vigilance in assessing the seal. Using a resuscitation bag that is too small for the patient can also lead to ineffective ventilation, because the tidal volume delivered will be inadequate. Poor chest wall excursions indicate that a larger bag is needed. It should be noted that a progressive increase in the amount of force necessary to deliver ventilations over a short period of time can be an ominous sign. The patient may simply have gastric distension that has reached a point of restricting expansion of the lungs, which can normally be relieved by inserting a nasogastric tube. However, if ventilations do not become significantly easier to administer after nasogastric tube placement, this may indicate that the patient has a tension pneumothorax. The approach to this especially dangerous problem is discussed below (see "Complications").

During the procedure, the operator should frequently re-evaluate the patient to ascertain whether BVM ventilation is having the desired effects. Several clinical indicators and monitoring methods can be used in this assessment. The skin color should progressively change from dusky or cyanotic to pink with adequate positive pressure ventilation. The heart rate of a patient with bradycardia as a result of hypoxemia should also return to normal. For the patient with a depressed mental status, the level of consciousness will often improve, and the patient may open his or her eyes or begin to cry. Pulse oximetry (Chapter 75) provides a noninvasive, "real-time" reading of the blood oxygen saturation and therefore serves as an indirect indicator of how effectively oxygen is being delivered. However, the pulse oximeter gives no information about the ventilatory state of the patient, because the level of CO_2 in the blood is not measured. Capnography may be used for this purpose when available (Chapter 76). The gold standard for evaluating the effect of BVM ventilation is determination of arterial blood gases, but this involves a successful arterial puncture, and the results are delayed by transport and laboratory analysis. In all cases, information obtained from the laboratory and monitoring devices must be carefully considered, but the operator should rely primarily on changes in the patient's clinical condition in judging the effectiveness of BVM ventilation.

A number of published studies have demonstrated that simultaneously performing all the tasks involved in BVM ventilation can be a difficult challenge for one person, particularly when the operator has little experience with this procedure (41–45). Jesudian et al. were the first to demonstrate that a two-person technique for BVM ventilation (Fig. 14.16) was superior based on findings from a manikin trial (46). More recently, Davidovic et al. have confirmed the effectiveness of this method (47), and it is now recommended by the American Heart Association and the American Academy of Pediatrics whenever sufficient personnel are available (48,49). The two-person technique allows one operator to use both hands to position the patient, maintain a patent airway, and hold the mask securely in place. The second operator can then use both hands if necessary to compress the resuscitation bag. This method more reliably accomplishes the two primary goals of (a) minimizing the occurrence of mask leak and problems with airway obstruction and (b) increasing the likelihood that an adequate tidal volume will be delivered. It is particularly useful with the more complicated apparatus of an anesthesia circuit. When

the available medical personnel are limited in number (e.g., in prehospital settings), the two-person technique may not be a practical alternative. Furthermore, the experienced practitioner may be capable of performing the procedure without assistance. However, for many pediatric resuscitations, initial use of the two-person technique will enhance the effectiveness with which BVM ventilation is performed.

▶ COMPLICATIONS

In general, BVM ventilation is a safe procedure. A number of relatively minor problems can occur, and only a few specific complications are typically more serious. Minor complications are primarily related to the mechanical forces involved in performing the procedure. For example, neuropraxia of the facial or trigeminal nerves can occur when excessive or prolonged pressure is applied while holding the face mask in place. During the limited course of an emergent resuscitation, this is not usually a problem. If the mask extends too high on the face, the patient may sustain injury to the eyes or periorbital area, possibly resulting in a corneal abrasion or periorbital edema. Pressure on the eyes can also cause vagal stimulation in younger patients, producing bradycardia if unrecognized. Selection of an appropriate mask size and careful adherence to proper technique will reduce the likelihood of these complications. Finally, patients who are allergic to material in the mask, or to chemicals used for sterilization, may develop a mild dermatitis of the face. These complications are generally self-limited and in most cases can be easily treated if necessary after the patient is stabilized.

A potentially serious complication of BVM ventilation is damage to the cervical cord in the patient with an unstable cervical spine injury. Although rare among pediatric patients (7,50), unstable cervical spine injuries should be suspected with any significant trauma (falls, motor vehicle accidents, etc.). In all instances, the possibility of cervical spine instability requires caution when manipulating the head and neck to control the airway. The cervical spine should be completely immobilized during BVM ventilation until radiographic and clinical assessments can be performed to exclude the possibility of cervical spine injury (see Chapter 24). To limit extension of the neck, airway patency is established using the jaw thrust maneuver. The two-person technique for BVM ventilation should be employed in this situation. This allows one operator to concentrate solely on maintaining the airway and securing the face mask and at the same time minimizes any movement of the cervical spine. It should be noted that immobilization of the cervical spine, although important, should not be given such a high priority that airway obstruction and impaired ventilation are not appropriately addressed. Published studies have indicated that morbidity in such cases is more likely to result from cerebral hypoxia, as a result of delayed or inadequate intervention for respiratory compromise, than from exacerbating a cervical spine injury (51–53).

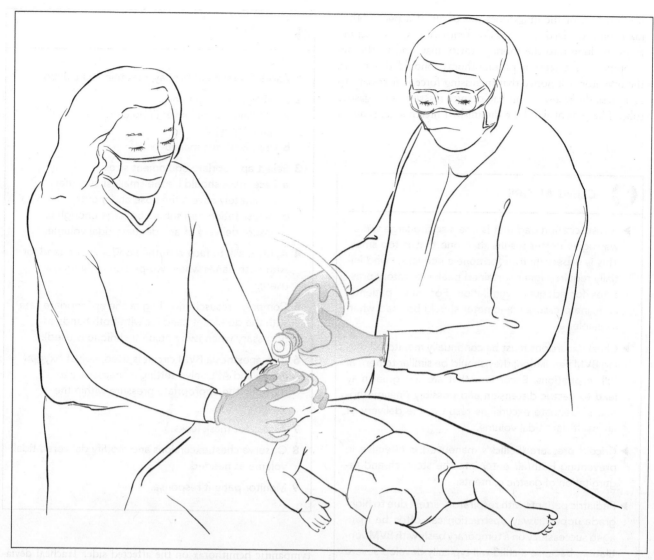

Figure 14.16 Two-person technique for BVM ventilation.

Another significant complication of BVM ventilation is aspiration pneumonitis. Patients requiring this procedure are likely to have a combination of characteristics that predispose to vomiting and aspiration (i.e., impaired mental status, a diminished or absent gag reflex, and a full stomach) (54). Aspiration pneumonitis as a consequence of BVM ventilation usually results from the following sequence of events: (a) positive pressure ventilation exceeds the opening pressure of the esophagus, resulting in air entry into the stomach; (b) the progressive increase in intragastric pressure eventually results in vomiting; and (c) regurgitated stomach contents enter the trachea and lungs due to impaired airway reflexes. Excessively elevated intragastric pressure can also impede delivery of an adequate tidal volume, as the stomach presses upward against the diaphragm and limits expansion of the lungs. The severity of the resulting pneumonitis depends on the volume and acidity of the aspirated material as well as the amount of particulate matter in the stomach contents (55). The operator can take several steps to prevent this complication. For one,

the operator or an assistant can perform Sellick's maneuver to prevent air entry into the stomach. This is particularly important when higher ventilatory pressures are necessary because of diminished lung compliance. In addition, patients who receive prolonged BVM ventilation should usually have a gastric tube inserted. This reduces the likelihood of significant aspiration by removing air and undigested food from the stomach. Finally, the operator must carefully monitor the chest wall excursions during BVM ventilation. Using the minimum force necessary to deliver an adequate tidal volume is one of the most effective means of reducing air entry into the stomach.

A final potentially serious complication of BVM ventilation is pneumothorax (56–58). As described previously, pediatric patients are more at risk for this complication than adults because of greater chest wall compliance. The risk is further increased for children with an underlying lung disease such as cystic fibrosis or congenital lobar emphysema (59). This complication can be largely prevented if the operator is careful in observing the chest wall excursions to ensure that overinflation of the lungs does not occur. If a pneumothorax is unrecognized during BVM ventilation, gases escaping from the lung into the thoracic cavity may lead to the development of a tension pneumothorax. Should this occur, the operator will notice that increasing force is necessary to compress the resuscitation bag despite insertion of a gastric tube. The patient will have diminished breath sounds and a

 CLINICAL TIPS

▶ A resuscitation bag that is one size too large will always give better results than one that is too small. This is especially true for apneic neonates, who initially require higher sustained peak inspiratory pressures for adequate ventilation. For these patients, an inline pressure manometer should be used when available.

▶ Chest excursions must be continually monitored during BVM ventilation; they should be similar to normal full respirations. Excursions that are too great may lead to gastric distension and possibly pneumothorax. Inadequate excursions result in the delivery of an insufficient tidal volume.

▶ Cricoid pressure (Sellick's maneuver) is effective in preventing both air entry into the stomach and regurgitation of gastric contents.

▶ Pediatric patients with respiratory arrest due to high-grade upper airway obstruction can often be managed successfully on a temporary basis with BVM ventilation, because a child will typically develop severe respiratory fatigue well before manual ventilation becomes impossible. In such cases, greater attention to maintaining an adequate mask seal, higher ventilatory pressures (i.e., more forceful compression of the resuscitation bag), and longer exhalation times are generally necessary.

▶ If ventilation becomes progressively more difficult to perform, the patient should be assessed for gastric distension and tension pneumothorax.

▶ For persistent airway obstruction, the following may be effective:
  ▶ Repositioning the head and neck until a more favorable alignment is achieved (note: excessive extension of the neck may actually cause obstruction)
  ▶ Insertion of an artificial airway
  ▶ Administration of higher ventilatory pressures

▶ For patients with a potential cervical spine injury, the jaw thrust maneuver should be used to open the airway and secure the mask.

 SUMMARY

1 Assess the patient (airway, breathing, circulation).

2 Establish airway patency.
  a Use chin lift maneuver (if no danger of cervical spine injury).
  b Use jaw thrust maneuver.

3 Select appropriate equipment sizes.
  a Face mask should be the smallest size that completely covers the nose and mouth.
  b Resuscitation bag should be large enough to ensure delivery of an adequate tidal volume.

4 Apply mask to face with the nondominant hand (or with both hands when two-person technique is used).

5 Compress resuscitation bag at the appropriate rate with the dominant hand (or with both hands as necessary when two-person technique is used).

6 If an anesthesia BVM circuit is used, adjust oxygen inflow and APL valve setting as necessary to maintain the appropriate pressure within the system.

7 Assess for mask leaks.

8 Observe chest excursions and modify delivered tidal volume as needed.

9 Monitor patient response.

tympanitic hemithorax on the affected side. Tracheal deviation may occur, although this is often difficult to detect in children. Eventually, the vena cava is "kinked" as the mediastinum shifts away from the tension pneumothorax, resulting in decreased venous return to the heart and a precipitous drop in systemic blood pressure. Early placement of a chest tube in any patient receiving prolonged positive pressure ventilation who develops a pneumothorax will prevent this complication. A complete discussion of the techniques used in the management of pneumothorax can be found in Chapter 29.

▶ SUMMARY

BVM ventilation is an effective method for delivering positive pressure ventilation to pediatric patients with respiratory compromise. Although a few potential complications are associated with this procedure, they can usually be avoided with careful use of proper technique. Although similar to the methods used for adult patients, BVM ventilation for infants and children requires certain specific modifications based on unique characteristics of pediatric airway anatomy and respiratory physiology. Equipment selection is an especially important aspect of this procedure, because the use of a face mask or resuscitation bag that is inappropriate for the size of the patient may result in complications or failure to provide adequate ventilatory support. BVM ventilation of a pediatric patient can sometimes challenge the abilities of even the most skillful practitioner, particularly when performed by a single operator. For this reason, the two-person technique is recommended whenever the procedure proves more difficult. In addition, the use of a conventional anesthesia circuit should only be undertaken by an experienced operator because of the complexity of the apparatus. The advantages of immediate availability, low incidence of complications, and wide clinical utility make BVM ventilation one of the most valuable tools for the health professional who provides emergent care for pediatric patients.

▶ ACKNOWLEDGMENTS

The authors would like to acknowledge the valuable contributions of Alfred T. Dorsey to the version of this chapter that appeared in the previous edition.

▶ REFERENCES

1. Gausche M, Lewis RJ, Stratton S, et al. Effect of out-of-hospital pediatric endotracheal intubation on survival and neurological outcome: a controlled clinical trial. *JAMA.* 2000;283:783–790.

2. Kitagawa KH, Nakamura NM, Yamamoto L. Retention of pediatric bag-mask ventilation efficacy skill by inexperienced medical student resuscitators using standard bag-mask ventilation masks, pocket masks, and blob masks. *Am J Emerg Med.* 2006;24;223–226.

3. Passy V, Newcron S, Snyder S. Rhinorrhea with airway obstruction. *Laryngoscope.* 1975;85:888–895.

4. Maniglia AJ, Goodwin WJ Jr. Congenital choanal atresia. *Otolaryngol Clin North Am.* 1981;14:167–173.

5. Wittenborg MH, Gyepes MT, Crocker D. Tracheal dynamics in infants with respiratory distress, stridor, and collapsing trachea. *Radiology.* 1967;88:653–662.

6. Polgar G, Kong GP. Nasal resistance in newborn infants. *J Pediatr.* 1961;67:557–567.

7. Bohn D, Armstrong D, Becker L, et al. Cervical spine injuries in children. *J Trauma.* 1990;30:463–469.

8. Rachesky I, Boyce T, Duncan B, et al. Clinical prediction of cervical spine injuries in children. *Arch Dis Child.* 1987;141:199–201.

9. Stauffer ES, Mazur JM. Cervical spine injuries in children. *Pediatr Ann.* 1982;11:502–511.

10. Morikawa S, Safar P, DeCarlo J. Influence of the head-jaw position on upper airway patency. *Anesthesiology.* 1961;22:265–279.

11. Papastamelos C, Panitch HB, England SE, et al. Developmental changes in chest wall compliance in infancy and early childhood. *J Appl Physiol.* 1995;78:179–184.

12. Keens TG, Ianuzzo CD. Development of fatigue-resistant muscle fibers in human ventilatory muscles. *Am Rev Respir Dis.* 1979;2[Suppl 119]:139–141.

13. Cournand A, Motley HL, Wesko L, et al. Physiologic studies of the effects of intermittent positive pressure breathing on cardiac output in man. *Am J Physiol.* 1948;152:162–174.

14. Clough JB, Duncan AW, Sly PD. The effect of sustained positive airway pressure on derived cardiac output in children. *Anaesth Intensive Care.* 1994;22:30–34.

15. Watson WE. Observations of physiologic deadspace during intermittent positive pressure ventilation. *Br J Anaesth.* 1962;35:502–506.

16. Kerr JH. Pulmonary oxygen transfer during positive pressure ventilation in man. *Br J Anaesth.* 1975;47:695–705.

17. Cross KW, Tizard JPM, Trythall DAH. The gaseous metabolism of the newborn infant. *Acta Paediatr.* 1957;46:265–285.

18. Patel R, Lenczyk M, Hannallah RS, et al. Age and the onset of desaturation in apnoeic children. *Can J Anaesth.* 1994;41:771–774.

19. Kinouchi K, Tanigami H, Tashiro C, et al. Duration of apnea in anesthetized infants and children required for desaturation of hemoglobin to 95%: the influence of upper respiratory infection. *Anesthesiology.* 1992;77:1105–1107.

20. 2005 American Heart Association (AHA) guidelines for cardiopulmonary resuscitation (CPR) and emergency cardiovascular care (ECC) of pediatric and neonatal patients: pediatric basic life support. *Pediatrics.* 2006;117:e989–1004.

21. Palme C, Nystrom N, Tunell R. An evaluation of the efficiency of face masks in the resuscitation of newborn infants. *Lancet.* 1985;1:207–210.

22. Terndrup TE, Kanter RK, Cherry RA. A comparison of infant ventilation methods performed by prehospital personnel. *Ann Emerg Med.* 1989;18:607–611.

23. Boon AW, Milner AD, Hopkin IE. Physiologic responses of the newborn infant to resuscitation. *Arch Dis Child.* 1979;54:492–498.

24. Milner AD, Boon AW, Hopkin IE. Lung expansion, tidal exchange and formation of the functional residual capacity during resuscitation of asphyxiated infants. *J Pediatr.* 1979;6:1031–1036.

25. Vyas H, Milner AD, Hopkin IE. Physiologic response to prolonged and slow rise inflation. *J Pediatr.* 1981;99:635–638.

26. Field D, Milner AD, Hopkin IE. Efficiency of manual resuscitators at birth. *Arch Dis Child.* 1985;61:300–302.

27. Kattwinkel J, Van Reempts P, Nadkarni V, et al. International guidelines for neonatal resuscitation: an excerpt from the guidelines 2000 for cardiopulmonary resuscitation and emergency cardiovascular care. International Consensus on Science. *Pediatrics.* 2000;106:1–34.

28. Mondolfi AA, Grenier BM, Thompson JE, et al. Comparison of self-inflating bags with anesthesia bags for bag-mask ventilation in the pediatric emergency department. *Pediatr Emerg Care.* 1997;13:312–316.

29. Campbell TP, Stewart RD, Kaplan RM, et al. Oxygen enrichment of bag-valve-mask units during positive-pressure ventilation: a comparison of various techniques. *Ann Emerg Med.* 1988;17:232–235.

30. Finer NN, Barrington KJ, Al-Fadley F, et al. Limitations of self-inflating resuscitators. *Pediatrics.* 1986;77:417–420.

31. Kauffman GW. A simple PEEP system for the Laerdal resuscitation bag. *Respir Ther.* 1981;11:3–4.

32. Kauffman GW, Hess DR. Modification of the infant Laerdal resuscitation bag to monitor airway pressure. *Crit Care Med.* 1982;10:112–113.

33. Bain JA, Speorel WE. A streamlined anaesthetic system. *Can Anaesth Soc J.* 1972;19;426–435.

34. Rees GJ. Anaesthesia in the newborn. *Brit Med J.* 1950;2:1419–1422.

35. Bain JA, Spoerel WE. Flow requirements for a modified Mapleson D system during controlled ventilation. *Can Anaesth Soc J.* 1973;20:629–636.

36. Willis BA, Pender JW, Mapleson WW. Rebreathing in a T-piece: volunteer and theoretical studies of the Jackson-Rees modification of Ayre's T-piece during spontaneous respiration. *Br J Anaesth.* 1975;47:1239–1245.

37. Priano LL, Ham J. A simple method to increase the F_DO_2 of resuscitator bags. *Crit Care Med.* 1978;6:48–49.

38. Vyas H, Milner AD, Hopkin IE. Face mask resuscitation: does it lead to gastric distension? *Arch Dis Child.* 1983;58:373–375.

39. Salem MR, Wong AY, Mani M, et al. Efficacy of cricoid pressure in preventing gastric inflation during bag-mask ventilation in pediatric patients. *Anesthesiology.* 1974;40:96–98.

40. Backofen JE, Rogers MC. Emergency management of the airway. In: Rogers MC, ed. *Textbook of Pediatric Intensive Care.* 2nd ed. Baltimore: Williams & Wilkins; 1992;75–88.

41. Kanter RK. Evaluation of mask-bag ventilation in resuscitation of infants. *Arch Dis Child.* 1987;141:761–763.

42. Harrison RR, Maull KI, Keenan RL, et al. Mouth-to-mouth ventilation: a superior method of rescue breathing. *Ann Emerg Med.* 1982;11:74–76.

43. Elling R, Politis J. An evaluation of emergency medical technicians' ability to use manual ventilation devices. *Ann Emerg Med.* 1983;12:765–768.

44. Hess D, Baran C. Ventilatory volumes using mouth-to-mouth, mouth-to-mask, and bag-valve-mask techniques. *Am J Emerg Med.* 1985;3:292–296.

45. Lawrence PJ, Navaratnam S. Ventilation during cardiopulmonary resuscitation: which method? *Med J Aust.* 1985;143:443–445.

46. Jesudian MCS, Harrison RR, Leenan RL, et al. Bag-valve-mask ventilation: two rescuers are better than one: preliminary report. *Crit Care Med.* 1985;13:122–123.

47. Davidovic L, LaCovey D, Pitetti RD. Comparison of 1- versus 2-person bag-valve-mask techniques for manikin ventilation of infants and children. *Ann Emerg Med.* 2005;46:37–42.

48. Pediatric advance life support. *JAMA.* 1992;268:2262–2275.

49. Zaritsky AL, Nadkarni V, Hickey R, et al, eds. *PALS Provider Manual.* Dallas, TX: American Heart Association.

50. Lally KP, Senac M, Hardin WD Jr, et al. Utility of the cervical spine radiograph in pediatric trauma. *Am J Surg.* 1989;158:540–542.

51. Rhee KJ, Green W, Holcroft JW, et al. Oral intubation in the multiple injured patient: the risk of exacerbating cervical spine damage. *Ann Emerg Med.* 1990;19:511–514.

52. Holley J, Jorden R. Airway management in patients with unstable cervical spine fractures. *Ann Emerg Med.* 1989;18:1237–1239.

53. Grande CM, Barton CR. Appropriate techniques for airway management of emergency patients with suspected spinal cord injury [letter]. *Anesth Analg.* 1988;67:710–718.

54. Hupp JR, Peterson LJ. Aspiration pneumonitis: etiology, therapy, and prevention. *J Oral Surg.* 1981;39:430–435.

55. Sladen A, Zanca P, Hadnott WH. Aspiration pneumonitis: the sequelae. *Chest.* 1971;59:448–450.

56. Miller RD, Hamilton WK. Pneumothorax during infant resuscitation. *JAMA.* 1969;210:1090–1092.

57. Hirschman AM, Kravath RE. Venting vs ventilating: a danger of manual resuscitation bags. *Chest.* 1982;82:369–370.

58. Dwyer ME. Pneumothorax. *Aust Paediatr J.* 1975;11:195–200.

59. Luck SR, Raffensperger JG, Sullivan HJ, et al. Management of pneumothorax in children with chronic pulmonary disease. *J Thorac Cardiovasc Surg.* 1977;74:834–839.

NOEL ZUCKERBRAUN AND RAYMOND D. PITETTI

Rapid Sequence Induction

15

▶ INTRODUCTION

A detailed discussion of the various methods for performing emergent endotracheal intubation can be found in Chapter 16. This chapter will review the techniques of pharmacologic facilitation of intubation. The standard procedure of providing sedation and inducing neuromuscular paralysis in preparation for intubation is called "rapid sequence induction" (RSI). The entire process—i.e., RSI and endotracheal intubation—is often called "rapid sequence intubation." The purpose of RSI is to allow a safe, expedient intubation while reducing the likelihood of aspiration pneumonitis. RSI minimizes or prevents many of the patient's responses to the noxious stimuli of intubation, including vomiting, coughing, breath-holding, and laryngospasm. This procedure and its modifications can also limit adverse physiologic effects of intubation, such as increased intracranial pressure (ICP), systemic hypertension and hypotension, cardiac arrhythmias, and elevated intraocular pressure. In addition, RSI facilitates laryngoscopic visualization of the airway in situations when this might otherwise be impossible, as with patients who are seizing, unable to cooperate, or combative.

Certain clinical situations require using one of several modifications of the standard RSI procedure. For example, muscle relaxants should not be administered if bag-valve-mask (BVM) ventilation and/or intubation are anticipated to be difficult for patients who are spontaneously breathing. In such cases, paralysis followed by an unsuccessful intubation produces apnea without a patent airway and therefore may be lethal. In this situation, sedation alone may be indicated to facilitate intubation without eliminating respiratory function. The various approaches that can be used in managing the potentially difficult airway are described in Chapter 17. Other modifications of RSI involve the use of alternative agents for sedation and neuromuscular blockade or the addition of ad-

junctive agents to prevent increases in ICP (e.g., with cerebral edema or a space-occupying intracranial lesion) or circulatory collapse for the patient with impending or existing shock due to hypovolemia, a low cardiac output state, etc. Agents with vasodilating or myocardial depressant effects that can exacerbate pre-existing physiologic derangements must obviously be titrated carefully or avoided. Medications can sometimes be substituted or added that may increase systemic blood pressure or decrease ICP, depending on the clinical situation. In its classic form, RSI involves preoxygenating the patient by providing 100% mask O_2 during spontaneous respiration. BVM ventilation is not performed following administration of the induction agents to reduce the likelihood of vomiting before intubation by minimizing the amount of air forced into the stomach (see also Chapter 14). However, patients with pre-existing respiratory compromise and hypoxemia may not tolerate even a brief period of apnea despite preoxygenation. These patients therefore require skilled BVM ventilation with cricoid pressure for 45 to 90 seconds with 100% O_2 until the peak effect of the muscle relaxant has been achieved and endotracheal intubation can be attempted. These and other modifications of RSI are described in this chapter.

Depending on the availability and experience of medical personnel, RSI for critically ill or injured children is generally performed by either an emergency physician or anesthesiologist. Because the potential for morbidity is high with this procedure, the physician performing RSI must be skillful with pediatric endotracheal intubation and thoroughly familiar with the risks and benefits of the medications and techniques used. Optimal settings for this procedure are the emergency department (ED), intensive care unit (ICU), and operating room. Above all, practitioners must keep in mind that RSI suppresses all respiratory effort and eliminates the ability of the patient to protect and maintain the airway. Consequently, this procedure should be performed when clinically indicated with appropriate caution and meticulous attention to proper technique.

▶ ANATOMY AND PHYSIOLOGY

Important features of pediatric airway anatomy and the physiologic effects of endotracheal intubation are described in Chapter 16. However, additional factors specifically related to the use of pharmacologic agents for facilitating intubation merit discussion. For one, the child with a suspected "difficult airway" represents a particular concern for the operator performing RSI, because the suppression of spontaneous respirations before obtaining a secure airway is especially dangerous with such patients. Identifying such patients whenever possible before initiating RSI is therefore vital. In addition, the physiology of the normal protective airway reflexes and the "full stomach" state have important consequences with regard to preventing aspiration pneumonitis, one of the primary purposes of this procedure. Finally, the operator should fully understand the pharmacologic properties and physiologic effects of the agents used in performing RSI.

Chapter 17 provides a detailed discussion of the methods used in providing respiratory support for the child with a difficult airway. In most instances, such patients can be identified before intubation is attempted. Unfortunately, this is not always possible, even when an intubation is performed on an elective basis. In the limited time available before an urgent or emergent intubation, the operator must make a rapid assessment of the patient and, to the extent possible, ascertain that BVM ventilation and endotracheal intubation will not be unduly difficult. If time permits, obtaining historical information from the parent or caretaker may be helpful in making this judgment. A known congenital abnormality, previous problems with intubation, or a history of difficulty breathing (e.g., while asleep or feeding or with upper respiratory infections) can all indicate a potentially problematic airway. A wide diversity of congenital anomalies has been associated with difficult intubation. Examples include Klippel-Feil syndrome, Down syndrome, achondroplasia, the Pierre-Robin sequence, Treacher-Collins syndrome, Marfan syndrome, Cornelia de Lange syndrome, Moebius syndrome, and familial osseous dysplasia (cherubism). The approach to such patients can only be fully tailored to the specific challenges posed by each syndrome when time is not a concern, as with an elective intubation. A complete discussion of these issues is therefore beyond the scope of this chapter. Readers interested in more information on this subject are referred to standard pediatric and anesthesiology texts. More importantly in the emergent setting, physical examination will usually reveal anatomic characteristics that would pose significant obstacles to successful laryngoscopy and/or manual ventilation, such as micrognathia (best evaluated while viewing the patient's profile), macroglossia, cleft or high arched palate, protruding upper incisors, small mouth, limited temporomandibular joint mobility, or limited cervical spine mobility (Table 15.1). Difficult

TABLE 15.1	CONGENITAL ANATOMIC ABNORMALITIES INDICATING A POTENTIALLY DIFFICULT AIRWAY

Micrognathia
Macroglossia
Cleft or high arched palate
Protruding upper incisors
Small mouth
Limited temporomandibular joint mobility
Limited cervical spine mobility

laryngoscopy should also be anticipated when the patient has any of the following acquired abnormalities: hoarseness, stridor, drooling, a preferred posture, facial burns, blunt or penetrating injury to the neck, facial bone fractures, oral trauma, epiglottitis, retropharyngeal abscess, and a foreign body in the extrathoracic airway (Table 15.2). For the patient with a potentially unstable cervical spine, laryngoscopy and intubation may be significantly hindered by in-line stabilization and use of a cervical collar, which limit neck flexion/extension and mouth opening. Indeed, this is perhaps the most common clinical scenario for a failed intubation.

It is important to remember, however, that paralysis (and, to a lesser extent, sedation) is a concern in the setting of a probable difficult airway only if the patient has some degree of adequate respiratory function prior to RSI. In other words, if there is no meaningful respiratory function to "lose" by administering a sedative or paralytic agent, then the decision to perform RSI when needed is not difficult. For example, with a spontaneously breathing child who is maintaining an acceptable oxygen saturation but who nevertheless requires urgent endotracheal intubation (e.g., a combative but otherwise stable trauma patient who needs a head CT scan), the clinician should be circumspect about eliminating respiratory function if the likelihood of a difficult airway is high. Transforming a reasonably stable situation into a "cannot bag/cannot intubate" scenario without a compelling reason for taking such a risk (e.g., rapid and potentially fatal patient deterioration) should obviously be avoided. In such cases, it is advisable to move the patient to a more stable environment (ICU, operating

TABLE 15.2	ACQUIRED ABNORMALITIES INDICATING A POTENTIALLY DIFFICULT AIRWAY

Hoarseness
Stridor
Drooling
A preferred posture
Facial burns
Blunt or penetrating injury to the neck
Facial bone fractures
Oral trauma
Epiglottitis
Retropharyngeal abscess
Foreign body in the extrathoracic airway

room) and, when available, obtain the assistance of an anesthesiologist and/or an otolaryngologist prior to performing RSI.

By contrast, a child requiring immediate endotracheal intubation who has no significant respiratory function and for whom BVM ventilation alone is inadequate (e.g., an apneic seizure patient with clenched teeth, vomiting, and worsening hypoxia), the presence of a potentially difficult airway must not inhibit the operator from performing the necessary life-saving interventions of an appropriate RSI—despite the attendant danger of a failed intubation. As described in Chapter 17, equipment for alternative methods of securing a definitive airway should be made readily available in such cases should standard endotracheal intubation and BVM ventilation prove impossible, but the RSI must be performed. In such situations, the potential hazards of RSI are outweighed by the likelihood of a patient suffering a rapid respiratory death.

Upper airway reflexes that normally serve to protect against aspiration of foreign material into the trachea and lungs can be a significant impediment to performing endotracheal intubation. Instrumentation of the airway may stimulate gagging, coughing, jaw clenching, increased production of secretions, and laryngospasm. These reflexes must often be suppressed for an intubation to be atraumatic and successful. The physiology of the various mechanisms that mediate these reflexes is complex. To briefly summarize, irritation of upper airway and digestive tract mucosa stimulates the glossopharyngeal (9th) and vagus (10th) nerves, which project to the nucleus of the solitary tract (NTS) in the medulla (1). Gagging and coughing are produced by nerve impulses relayed from the NTS back to the motor efferents of the upper airway, diaphragm, and intercostal and abdominal muscles. In addition, nerve tracts from the NTS to the medulla activate a "vomiting center," which induces emesis by coordinating such responses as contraction of the abdominal musculature, closure of the glottis, opening of the lower esophageal sphincter, and increased salivation. This medullary vomiting response can also be stimulated by the area postrema of the brainstem, which is sensitive to noxious substances circulating in the bloodstream (1). Sympathetic outflow resulting from stimulation of the NTS can cause an increase in heart rate and blood pressure, which in turn can lead to dysrhythmias and increased ICP. However, the most pronounced response to oropharyngeal manipulation in children is generally transmission from the NTS to the dorsal vagal nucleus, producing marked bradycardia. Because cardiac output in infants and younger children depends more on heart rate than changes in stroke volume, bradycardia can have a significant deleterious effect on systemic blood pressure.

Any patient undergoing emergent intubation is presumed to have a "full stomach." A full stomach may result from recent ingestion of food (within the past 8 hours) or liquid (within the past 2 hours) or delayed gastric emptying due to intestinal obstruction, trauma, pain, pregnancy, elevated ICP, or shock. Presumption of a full-stomach state means the patient is at risk for emesis and subsequent aspiration of gastric contents into the trachea and lungs. Factors increasing this risk include agitation, persistent gagging or coughing, and elevated intragastric pressure as a result of gas entry into the stomach during BVM ventilation or swallowing of air and/or blood. The normal response of gagging and possibly vomiting provoked by stimulation of the pharynx can be suppressed with pharmacologic agents, yet these same agents also reduce or eliminate closure of the epiglottis over the glottic opening that prevents aspiration should any vomiting or regurgitation of stomach contents occur. Ensuring the proper sequence of events during RSI is therefore vital when managing patients presumed to have a full stomach.

The ideal pharmacologic properties of medications used in RSI are rapid onset and short duration of effect. Anatomic and physiologic characteristics of pediatric patients can have important clinical effects on these properties. Onset and duration depend on the total body compartments of fat, muscle, and water. Total body water is 75% to 80% of body composition in a newborn, decreasing to the adult proportion of 60% at about 6 months of age. This is why infants may require a larger initial weight-based dose of water-soluble drugs than adults. In addition, agents that depend on redistribution to fat and muscle for termination of effect will have a longer duration of action in younger patients, because they have lower body fat and muscle content. With older children, the half-life of a medication will generally be shorter, because a larger proportion of the cardiac output is delivered to the liver and kidneys, causing more rapid metabolism of the drug. As a general rule, drugs have a more rapid onset of effect and a shorter duration of action in children than in adults, and a larger weight-based dose will be required to achieve the same anesthetic effect.

The primary desired effects of pharmacologic facilitation of intubation are sedation, analgesia, and muscle relaxation. Sedation is generally provided by barbiturates, benzodiazepines, and/or opioids. Barbiturates have several actions in the central nervous system (CNS) that produce sedation. Most importantly, they potentiate the neuroinhibitory actions of gamma-aminobutyric acid (GABA), which is accomplished by increasing chloride conductance and decreasing depolarization induced by glutamate. Evidence also exists of depression of the calcium-dependent action potential (2). Etomidate is a carboxylated imidazole compound that induces anesthesia by modulating GABA-mediated neurotransmission. Though not itself a barbiturate, the mode of action of etomidate is similar to that of the barbiturates. Benzodiazepines potentiate GABA-mediated inhibition as well, but little is known about their direct mechanistic effects. Neurologic inhibition by opiates is relatively complex. There are three known major categories of opioid receptors in the CNS. Analgesia is produced by endogenous and exogenous peptides that bind to the μ receptors in the brain, κ receptors in the spinal cord, and δ receptors distributed in both the brain and spinal cord. Inhibition at these sites is accomplished by a reduction in the release of neurotransmitters and inhibition of adenyl cyclase at μ and δ receptors. Evidence also exists of inhibition of calcium channels at κ receptors (2). Activation of opioid receptors causes a decrease in the sensation of pain as well as modification of the perception of a stimulus as painful. For example, the periaqueductal grey matter in the midbrain contains δ and μ receptors, and agonists at these sites inhibit the processing of nociceptive information from the spinal cord. In addition, an abundance of μ receptors are found in the locus ceruleus, which is responsible for feelings of alarm, panic, fear, and anxiety (2). Inhibition at these receptors increases the tolerance for pain and the associated psychological stress.

Muscle relaxation is produced at the motor end plate by depolarizing agents or nondepolarizing competitive agents. Normally, release of acetylcholine (ACh) from the presynaptic membrane causes summation of electrical potentials in order to form an action potential, thus stimulating muscle contraction. Depolarizing agents mimic ACh and bind directly to the postsynaptic ACh receptor, causing all skeletal muscles to depolarize. This is often evident (although more commonly in adults than children) as diffuse, random contraction of skeletal muscle fibers known as "fasciculations," followed by flaccid paralysis that remains until postsynaptic receptors again regain the ability to transmit an electrical stimulus (2). Nondepolarizing neuromuscular blocking agents competitively inhibit the nicotinic postsynaptic receptors for ACh so that depolarization cannot occur. These agents are normally metabolized over time to less active forms, which are then more easily displaced by ACh. Both types of neuromuscular blockers have no direct CNS effects and do not decrease awareness. Using these agents alone without sedation therefore leaves a patient in the terrorized state of being fully awake but unable to move or breathe.

▶ INDICATIONS

Rapid sequence induction is performed to facilitate endotracheal intubation. Consequently, the indications for RSI in the acute care setting are in part determined by the indications for emergent intubation. Yet not all patients who require intubation on an emergent basis are appropriate candidates for RSI. An algorithm illustrating the assessments and decisions involved in determining the subset of patients who should undergo RSI is presented in Figure 15.1. In general, RSI is indicated for patients with airway or ventilatory compromise who cannot be intubated without using sedatives and neuromuscular blocking agents or who would be at increased risk for complications without these drugs and techniques. Indications for one of the modifications of RSI depend on the specific clinical circumstances (see below). As mentioned previously, even in the best of situations RSI is a challenging and potentially dangerous procedure, and it should therefore be performed only when the operator presumes with reasonable certainty that the trachea can be intubated with reasonable rapidity. If intubation is delayed or impossible, subsequent positive pressure ventilation (PPV) with a BVM

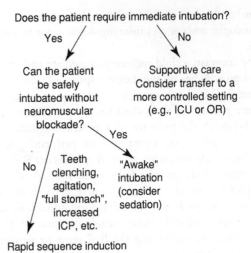

Figure 15.1 Determining indications for rapid sequence induction.

circuit may increase intragastric pressure, causing decreased total lung compliance and a greater likelihood of aspiration. In the worst-case scenario, BVM ventilation may be ineffective and therefore adequate respiratory support impossible to provide. For these reasons, RSI should be performed only after the airway has been evaluated as thoroughly as possible under the circumstances and a judgment made that endotracheal intubation, or at minimum BVM ventilation with cricoid pressure, can be successfully accomplished on a timely basis.

The first question asked in determining whether a standard RSI is indicated should be, Does the child require immediate intubation? As described in Chapter 16, there are seven primary indications for emergent intubation: (i) maintenance of the airway, (ii) protection of the airway (e.g., before gastric lavage for the obtunded patient), (iii) administration of PPV, (iv) oxygen administration, (v) delivery of resuscitation drugs through the endotracheal tube, (vi) access to the trachea for suctioning, and (vii) respiratory support when other systems are failing in the unstable patient. Numerous disease processes and injuries can cause sufficient respiratory compromise in pediatric patients to require emergent endotracheal intubation. However, in certain instances intubation will be necessary—but not immediately. Some patients with impending respiratory failure will be stable enough to transfer to a more controlled setting such as the operating room or ICU if this substantially increases the safety of an endotracheal intubation. In such cases, temporary respiratory support can be provided as necessary by assisted or controlled ventilation using a BVM circuit.

If intubation is necessary and cannot be delayed, the second question that must be asked is, Can the patient be safely intubated without sedation or neuromuscular blockade? Many intubations in the ED are performed on patients who are moribund, and therefore drugs are not needed to prevent movement or induce unconsciousness. Furthermore, many physicians prefer to make one attempt at an "awake" intubation (i.e., no muscle relaxant but possibly some degree of sedation) whenever this can be performed without additional risk to the patient. However, many situations exist in which either an awake intubation is hazardous and/or the likelihood of success with this method is clearly low from the outset. For example, when the patient is struggling forcefully and restraint is necessary or the patient's jaw is firmly clenched, an awake intubation is likely to be impossible. In such cases, attempting intubation without neuromuscular blockade may cause trauma and bleeding, which make subsequent attempts more difficult while increasing the likelihood of aspiration. Consequently, for the patient who requires immediate intubation but for whom this cannot be accomplished safely without sedation and muscle relaxation, a standard RSI is indicated.

As discussed previously, coughing, gagging, and vomiting as a result of airway manipulation are all known to cause an increase in ICP. For this reason, a modification of the RSI procedure often called a "neurologic induction" (or "neurologic intubation") should be considered with any patient, including infants, who may have elevated ICP. A neurologic induction simply refers to special measures taken to avoid further increases in ICP, which can produce cerebral hypoperfusion, cerebral swelling, and, in extreme cases, herniation. These patients present with such conditions as severe head trauma, ventriculoperitoneal (VP) shunt dysfunction, and large CNS tumors. For a neurologic induction, thiopental is usually used as the sedating agent because it is reliable in protecting the brain by preventing a rise in ICP during noxious stimulation. In addition, intravenous lidocaine can be administered because it also may attenuate the rise in ICP. Neuromuscular blockade should be provided to suppress the airway and autonomic reflexes, although the agent of choice in this situation is somewhat controversial (see "Procedure"). Prolonged apnea after administration of the muscle relaxant must be carefully avoided, as cerebral hypercarbia may exacerbate an elevated ICP, and these patients are often exquisitely sensitive to the deleterious effects of cerebral hypoxia. It should be noted that thiopental has a potent myocardial depressant effect and therefore must be administered in small, frequent doses—or avoided altogether—in patients suspected of having hypovolemia or a low cardiac output state. For the patient who is presumed to have a significantly elevated ICP and is also in a shock state, a different sedative (e.g., etomidate or midazolam) should be used.

Other indications that require special consideration relate to specific clinical presentations. For example, the patient with a possible open globe injury should not receive succinylcholine or ketamine, because both of these agents increase intraocular pressure and may cause extrusion of the vitreous. In addition, as with thiopental, other medications may induce profound hypotension in patients with cardiovascular compromise and should be avoided in such situations. For the patient with severe asthma who requires intubation, ketamine may be substituted as the sedation agent because it both supports the systemic circulation and may act as a bronchodilator. A more detailed discussion of the use of RSI with patients who require these types of specific adaptations is provided later in this chapter.

Many physicians prefer to intubate neonates without paralysis and often without sedation. This is usually more appropriate in the delivery room, where the degree of urgency and lack of intravenous access may preclude administration of intravenous medications. Although paralysis may seem unnecessary because an infant is more easily and effectively restrained, a darting tongue can sometimes prove a formidable barrier to rapid and successful laryngoscopy, and RSI should therefore be considered for patients of all ages when indicated in the ED. At the least, a sedating agent should be considered even in young infants.

Although relatively few, there are some important contraindications to RSI. For example, any child who is apneic and pulseless at presentation should undergo endotracheal intubation early in the resuscitation without undue delay. Pharmacologic agents are unnecessary in this situation. Similarly, a patient who is moribund as a result of an overwhelming disease process (e.g., sepsis) may gain no benefit from undergoing RSI. In such situations, performing RSI would add needless complexity to the management of the patient, potentially prolonging the period of inadequate oxygenation and ventilation without enhancing the safety of intubation. As mentioned previously, standard RSI is relatively contraindicated when the patient has one or more conditions associated with a potentially difficult airway and is breathing spontaneously or requires only 100% oxygen, continuous positive airway pressure, or minimal assistance with BVM ventilation. Should endotracheal intubation become necessary, an awake procedure (with judicious sedation as needed) should be attempted. In such cases, muscle relaxants should be withheld at least until effective BVM ventilation can be ensured. This is done after careful titration of sedative agents permits first assisted, and then controlled, BVM ventilation without eliminating protective airway reflexes. Additionally, nondepolarizing muscle relaxants should generally be avoided when the patient has a neuromuscular disease (e.g., Werdnig-Hoffman, myasthenia gravis, or Duchenne muscular dystrophy), because paralysis can persist for an excessively long period of time. In such cases, benzodiazepines may be used exclusively or in conjunction with an opiate. Succinylcholine, a depolarizing muscle relaxant, is absolutely contraindicated in patients with pre-existing hyperkalemia, susceptibility to malignant hyperthermia, and denervating neuromuscular diseases because of the risk of inducing an often fatal cardiac arrest. Finally, RSI is contraindicated for any spontaneously breathing patient suspected of having a tension pneumothorax, pericardial tamponade, or a mediastinal mass (e.g., lymphoma) compressing the heart, great vessels, or large airways. With such patents, sedative agents may directly or indirectly cause vasodilation and myocardial depression that could precipitate circulatory collapse. In patients with anterior mediastinal masses, neuromuscular blocking agents will also remove intrinsic muscle tone, which helps to maintain intrathoracic airway patency. Collapse of the airway resulting from compression by the mass can make endotracheal intubation ineffective for providing respiratory support because obstruction occurs below the tip of the endotracheal tube. With large masses, this catastrophic situation can be precipitated by even judicious use of sedative agents. Consequently, such children should be intubated with utmost caution and only when necessary, optimally with the patient awake and sitting in a partially upright position and given a topical anesthetic as the only medication.

▶ EQUIPMENT

The equipment necessary for performing RSI is listed in Table 15.3. Patients should have at least one reliable peripheral or central access site verified as intravenous. The appropriate pharmacologic agents should be drawn in labeled syringes. The general classifications of medications used to perform RSI are described below, with particular attention given to the most commonly used agent in each category.

Sedative Agents

Barbiturates (Thiopental)

Barbiturates are potent sedatives. From this class of drugs, thiopental is used most frequently in performing RSI. It is a rapidly acting agent, producing its peak effect in 10 to 30 seconds (2,3). The duration of effect depends on the rate of redistribution to fat and muscle but is generally between 5 and 30 minutes (3,4). Thiopental decreases the metabolic demands of the brain, thereby decreasing cerebral blood flow (3). It is therefore an excellent agent to use when the patient has a known or presumed elevated ICP (5). Thiopental also

TABLE 15.3	EQUIPMENT FOR RAPID SEQUENCE INDUCTION

Standard equipment for endotracheal intubation (see Chapter 16)
Cardiac monitor
Blood pressure monitor
Pulse oximetry
Capnography (if available)
Intravenous catheters
Tape
Benzoin
Medications:
  Atropine
  Lidocaine
Sedating agents:
  Thiopental
  Midazolam
  Propofol
  Etomidate
  Ketamine
  Fentanyl
Paralytic agents:
  Succinylcholine
  Vecuronium
  Pancuronium
  Rocuronium

has anticonvulsant effects (6). Another barbiturate used in RSI is methohexital. Methohexital has similar characteristics to thiopental (3), although one important difference is that methohexital can produce seizure activity (3,6,7).

Precautions

Thiopental is both a myocardial depressant and a peripheral vasodilator. In patients with pre-existing myocardial depression or hypovolemia, it can cause hypoperfusion associated with hypotension. Normally, baroreceptors detect a low blood pressure and compensate by producing a reflex tachycardia. However, hypovolemic patients with tachycardia may be incapable of mounting any further increase in heart rate and are therefore likely to become hypotensive. Patients with underlying cardiovascular disease may not produce adequate coronary and/or cerebral perfusion under these conditions (5,8). Consequently, any patient suspected of hypovolemia or cardiovascular disease should not receive thiopental or, if no appropriate substitute is available, should only receive it in small doses (1 to 3 mg/kg) at a decreased rate as tolerated based on blood pressure (5,6).

The physician choosing thiopental should also be aware that it has no analgesic effects (3). Patients intubated with thiopental as the sole sedative agent may have laryngospasm or cough in response to airway manipulation (9). The lack of analgesia when using thiopental alone may also allow a catecholamine response leading to systemic or intracranial hypertension in response to intubation or other noxious interventions. For these reasons, it is often beneficial for thiopental to be administered in conjunction with an analgesic, particularly when the patient is at risk for elevated ICP. In addition, extravasation or intra-arterial injection of thiopental can cause severe tissue necrosis (7). Extra care must therefore be taken to inject into an access site that recently has been verified as intravenous. It is also important to use only a dilute solution (2.5%) for injection (7).

Other precautions relate to the respiratory effects of this agent. It causes dose- and rate-dependent respiratory depression (8). Patients may have precipitous onset of apnea, particularly if there is associated hypovolemia or head trauma (7). Thiopental has minimal direct effects on bronchomotor tone, but bronchospasm may occur due to light anesthesia during noxious airway manipulation and may also result from histamine release (6). This effect is of particular concern in asthmatic patients.

How Supplied

Thiopental comes as powder for reconstitution as sodium in 250 mg, 400 mg, 500 mg, and 1 g. It is supplied with diluent for reconstitution immediately prior to use. Methohexital comes as powder for reconstitution as sodium in 500 mg, 2.5 g, and 5 g.

Dose

For normotensive patients with a normal or elevated cardiac output, the recommended dose of thiopental is 3 to 6 mg/kg given rapidly as an intravenous bolus. If the patient is hypotensive but thiopental is nonetheless the selected agent (e.g., the patient has a markedly elevated ICP), a lower dose of 1 to 3 mg/kg may be used if blood pressure remains acceptable (6). For methoxital, the recommended intravenous induction dose is 1 to 2 mg/kg.

Benzodiazepines (Midazolam, Diazepam)

The benzodiazepines produce sedation, amnesia, and hypnosis. They also have anxiolytic and anticonvulsant effects. Midazolam and diazepam are the two most commonly used benzodiazepines for RSI. However, midazolam is the preferred agent for RSI in this class due to its rapid and consistent rate of onset, shorter duration, and lack of pain with injection (6). Midazolam has a rapid onset of approximately 30 to 60 seconds and a short duration of 5 to 20 minutes, while diazepam has a variable onset of action (1 to 3 minutes) and a longer duration (10 to 30 minutes) (3,5,10). Diazepam is oil based and can cause pain and occasionally phlebitis with intravenous administration (7). Midazolam is water soluble and does not cause pain with injection (7). Both benzodiazepines have a cerebral protective effect and do not increase ICP (3).

Precautions

Although the benzodiazepines produce fewer cardiovascular side effects than the barbiturates, they are associated with a slight transient decrease in systemic blood pressure because of a decrease in systemic vascular resistance (3). Evidence suggests that an increase in venous capacitance caused by midazolam is offset by a shift of blood volume out of the splanchnic circulation and a transient increase in heart rate (11). For some patients, a small decrease in blood pressure can be beneficial in attenuating both the pressor response and the rise in ICP that can occur with laryngoscopy (12). However, the patient with increased sympathetic activity compensating for significant hypovolemia is most susceptible to the hypotensive effects of midazolam (13). For these reasons, benzodiazepines should be used with caution in cases of severe cardiovascular compromise such as septic shock or multiple trauma. However, for most patients with cardiovascular disease, cardiac output and coronary blood flow are not adversely affected by midazolam.

Similar to barbiturates, benzodiazepines have a dose- and rate-dependent respiratory depressant effect that may induce apnea (more common with diazepam) (14). This effect is potentiated by the concomitant use of narcotics (3,6). Benzodiazepines do not provide analgesia, nor will they enhance the analgesic effects of other drugs. Consequently, when used for induction, benzodiazepines are normally paired with an agent that has analgesic properties such as fentanyl or ketamine (see below).

How Supplied

Midazolam (Versed) is an injectable solution supplied in concentrations of 1 and 5 mg/mL and is stored at room temperature.

Dose

The recommended dosage range for midazolam in pediatric patients is 0.1 to 0.3 mg/kg. The lower end of the range is often chosen for use in conjunction with potent analgesics or when the patient has cardiovascular compromise, and the higher end is recommended when midazolam is used alone and/or the patient is hemodynamically stable. Attention to appropriate dosing is important, as underdosing may produce suboptimal intubation conditions (15).

Narcotics (Fentanyl and Morphine)

Narcotics such as fentanyl and morphine produce analgesia and some sedation. Fentanyl is more highly lipid soluble than morphine, and thus it crosses the blood-brain barrier more rapidly and has a more rapid redistribution time. As a result, fentanyl has a faster onset of action (about 1 to 3 minutes to peak effect) and a shorter duration (30 to 60 minutes) than morphine (onset of 5 to 6 minutes and duration of 3 to 4 hours) (5,10). The faster onset of fentanyl makes it preferable to morphine as an induction agent for RSI. At higher doses, the duration of effect of fentanyl depends not on redistribution but on hepatic clearance as the drug accumulates in the body. A more prolonged effect of fentanyl can therefore be obtained at higher doses. A second peak can also occur as a result of release from pulmonary or skeletal muscle stores (16). Fentanyl has been shown to inhibit muscle fasciculations caused by succinylcholine (17) and to blunt the hemodynamic effects of laryngoscopy (18,19). Since larger doses of fentanyl are necessary to achieve significant sedative effects, it is often combined with benzodiazepines when used for intubation.

Precautions

All opiate narcotics produce respiratory depression. This effect, which is more common in neonates and infants, is dose dependent and can be reversed with naloxone. A rare but significant additional adverse respiratory effect of opioids is chest wall rigidity, a complication that, though more widely recognized with fentanyl, can occur with all opioids (10). Chest wall rigidity can interfere with spontaneous, assisted, or controlled ventilation (5,20). The incidence of this phenomenon is thought to be dependent on the dose and rate of administration. Chest wall rigidity can be prevented by the concomitant use of muscle relaxants or by administering the medication slowly (16,20). It may also be reversible with naloxone (21).

Morphine produces varying degrees of histamine release that can cause hypotension (although this is less common among pediatric patients than adults), and this effect is not inhibited or reversed by naloxone. One advantage of fentanyl is that it does not cause histamine release (16). Another reason fentanyl is often preferred over morphine is its minimal cardiovascular effects; however, it can cause a transient reduction in heart rate (8,16). For this reason, a vagolytic such as atropine should be used in conjunction with fentanyl when bradycardia would be undesirable. As mentioned previously, narcotics are often combined with benzodiazepines when used as induction agents for RSI. However, this combination can lead to a significant drop in systemic vascular resistance and should therefore be avoided in patients with cardiovascular compromise (14).

Case reports of generalized tonic-clonic seizures after fentanyl administration have appeared in the literature (22–24). However, those undergoing simultaneous EEG during such episodes did not have identifiable seizure activity; thus, it has been suggested that the seizurelike episodes may have instead been myoclonus or severe muscular rigidity (24–26).

Historically, fentanyl had been considered to have little or no effect on ICP. Although still somewhat controversial, recent literature suggests fentanyl can cause a rise in ICP. Some investigations of adults with head trauma have found increased ICP associated with a decreased mean arterial blood pressure after fentanyl administration (27,28), while others have found no increase in ICP (29). Fentanyl is known to blunt the pressor response during intubation, which can contribute to the rise in ICP. However, it is speculated that through a separate mechanism fentanyl may cause a direct increase in ICP. The clinical significance of this effect is currently unknown, although widespread experience supports the safety of fentanyl for patients with elevated ICP (30). To date, no formal studies of the effect of fentanyl on ICP during emergent intubation of pediatric patients have been done. Fentanyl continues to be recommended for use during neurologic induction by most authorities (30). In practice, fentanyl is still used for RSI with pediatric patients suspected of having elevated ICP, especially if the patient's hemodynamic status prohibits the use of other agents. Further study is therefore warranted on this subject, particularly as it relates to infants and children.

How Supplied

Fentanyl (Sublimaze) is supplied as a 50-μg/mL injectable solution. It should be stored at room temperature away from light.

Dose

The recommended initial sedation dose for fentanyl is 2 μg/kg; however, the induction dose for RSI can range from 2 to 10 μg/kg.

Ketamine

Ketamine is a dissociative anesthetic that rapidly provides sedation, analgesia, and amnesia. Within seconds of intravenous administration, the patient is sedated and unresponsive to pain (16,31). However, the patient may appear awake because ketamine does not affect the reticular activating system; instead, it acts to interrupt the connection between thalamoneocortical tracts and the limbic system (31). Termination of the maximal sedating effects depends on redistribution and usually occurs after 10 to 20 minutes (3,32). Termination of the analgesic effect is somewhat longer (3).

Ketamine has important properties that make it a particularly valuable agent for facilitating intubation of the asthmatic patient (33). It causes the release of endogenous catecholamines, dilating bronchial smooth muscle, and stimulating β receptors in the lungs, which can increase pulmonary compliance and relieve bronchospasm (31). Ketamine also increases oropharyngeal and tracheobronchial secretions, which in some instances can reduce mucus plugging (3). However, excessive production of secretions may interfere with visualization of the larynx during direct laryngoscope, and thus administration of ketamine should always be preceded by atropine or glycopyrrolate (6).

The sympathomimetic effects of ketamine also affect the cardiovascular system. Primarily through a centrally mediated mechanism, ketamine causes an increase in heart rate, blood pressure, and cardiac output (3,31). This pressor response tends to mask its mild inherent myocardial depressant effect found in vitro (31). Consequently, ketamine is often a good choice for a patient with hypotension, particularly when caused by early endotoxic shock, hypovolemic or hemorrhagic shock, or cardiovascular compromise as seen with cardiac tamponade or restrictive pericarditis (3,31).

Precautions

The stimulatory effects of ketamine on the cardiovascular system, though beneficial to some patients, are detrimental to others. Ketamine should be avoided in patients with hypertension, unstable angina, or a recent myocardial infarction, although all of these are rare in children (7). In addition, any patient with an intracranial, thoracic, or abdominal aneurism should not receive ketamine because of the deleterious effects of increased blood pressure on these conditions. Although ketamine has beneficial effects on cardiac output in some acutely hypotensive or hypovolemic patients, there is evidence showing that it may worsen hypotension in patients who have been in shock for more prolonged periods, whose chronic low cardiac output state has been supported by endogenous catecholamines that have become depleted (31).

Ketamine produces an increase in ICP by causing cerebral vasodilation and increasing systemic blood pressure (31), although the clinical significance of this effect has not been clearly elucidated, and in fact preliminary evidence suggests that ketamine may have certain neuroprotective properties. Because of the potential negative effects associated with an increased ICP, ketamine is not currently recommended for RSI in any patient with conditions such as head injury, intracranial mass, intracranial hemorrhage, or VP shunt obstruction (3). It may also cause a slight increase in intraocular pressure and thus should be avoided in patients suspected of having an open globe injury (3).

Use of ketamine for sedation may result in so-called postemergence phenomena, which have an overall reported incidence ranging from 3% to 50% (7). In the pediatric population, the incidence is significantly less, with reports ranging from 0% to 10% (34). These reactions range from mild floating sensations and dizziness to vivid, unpleasant dreams, auditory and visual hallucinations, and frank delirium (31), although in children the reactions are generally far less dramatic than in adults. In the ED, concern about these potential effects of ketamine are more relevant to the patient who receiving procedural sedation (see Chapter 33) who will be "revived" and then discharged to home (e.g., after repair of a complex facial laceration). The child who undergoes RSI and emergent endotracheal intubation will typically receive ongoing sedation for a relatively prolonged period, and therefore postemergence phenomena of any significance are unlikely.

Ketamine does not generally cause respiratory depression and rarely causes apnea (34). Laryngeal reflexes are usually maintained with ketamine, making it advisable to use a muscle relaxant concomitantly to avoid vomiting or laryngospasm during airway manipulation. As stated above, increased production of saliva and tracheal secretions occurring with administration of ketamine may cause gagging or difficulty in visualizing the airway during laryngoscopy. For this reason, an antisialagogue (glycopyrrolate or atropine) also should be routinely administered (6).

How Supplied
Ketamine (Ketaject, Ketalar) is supplied as an injectable solution in 10-, 50-, and 100-mg/mL concentrations and is stored at room temperature.

Dose
The intravenous dose of ketamine is 1 to 2 mg/kg. When intravenous access is unobtainable, making RSI impossible, ketamine may be given as an intramuscular injection at a dose of 4 to 10 mg/kg (3,7). As described in Chapter 33, the optimal dose of IM ketamine for routine procedural sedation is 4 to 5 mg/kg (35). The onset of action and peak effect of the drug via this route will obviously be less reliable.

Propofol
Propofol is a nonopioid, nonbarbiturate sedative hypnotic agent that is unrelated to other hypnotic agents. One of the main advantages of propofol is that it is highly lipophilic. This feature allows rapid distribution within the brain and resulting fast onset (within 10 to 20 seconds) and offset (10 to 15 minutes) of action (6). Propofol also decreases cerebral metabolism and ICP (36).

Precautions
Propofol can cause decreases in systemic arterial blood pressure. A 30% decrease in blood pressure is common in healthy subjects, and in the setting of hypovolemia significant hypotension can result (36). Even at lower doses, propofol may be unsafe in these patients. Respiratory depression is also common, and apnea can occur. The concomitant use of opioids may augment these cardiorespiratory effects (36). In critically ill children with respiratory infections, continuous propofol infusion has resulted in myocardial failure and intractable metabolic acidosis (10). Additionally, propofol can cause pain at the site of administration. This effect may be attenuated by

premedication with lidocaine at a dose of 0.05 mg/kg given intravenously (37). Finally, the emulsion of propofol contains egg lecithin, and serious allergic reactions have been reported in patients with allergies to egg products (37).

How Supplied
Propofol is highly insoluble and must be kept as an emulsion to remain in solution. An injectable emulsion of 10 mg/mL is available.

Dose
The standard induction dose for propofol is 2.5 mg/kg given intravenously.

Etomidate
Etomidate is a nonbarbiturate imidazole hypnotic agent that has become a commonly used induction agent for adult RSI in the ED (38–41). Several properties make etomidate favorable in this setting. Etomidate has a reliable, short onset (5 to 15 seconds) and short duration of effect (5 to 14 minutes) (38). Another significant advantage of this agent is that it lacks the cardiovascular depression seen with other induction agents, even in patients with altered myocardial contractility (42–44). Additionally, etomidate has been shown to have a cerebral protective effect, decreasing cerebral oxygen consumption and ICP (45–47). For these reasons, it is regarded by many as the induction agent of choice in adults with hypotension and/or severe trauma. Although etomidate has become more widely used as an induction agent for RSI in pediatric patients, this is an "off-label" use of the drug, as it currently is not approved in this country for patients under 10 years of age (37). However, several studies have been published on the use of etomidate as a safe and effective intravenous anesthetic induction agent for children in the anesthesia setting (48–51) and, more recently, in the ED setting (52,53).

Precautions
The use of etomidate has been associated with both immediate and delayed side effects. Etomidate lacks analgesic properties, and consequently it does not alter the sympathetic response to endotracheal intubation. As with propofol, the administration of etomidate is also associated with pain at the site of injection. This effect has been shown to be attenuated with fentanyl and lidocaine (37). Two additional immediate side effects, myoclonus and vomiting, are uncommon when etomidate is used concurrently with paralytic agents (53,54).

Delayed side effects of etomidate include possible seizure activity and decreased adrenocortical function. Although a reported complication, the occurrence of seizures resulting from use of etomidate is based on limited and somewhat conflicting data. While etomidate has been shown to increase EEG activation with epileptiform spikes, it also has been used to induce burst suppression and as a treatment for status epilepticus (55–57). One pediatric study reported 4 of 105 patients to have seizure activity following RSI with etomidate, but all had presented with a known seizure disorder (53). Adrenocortical suppression by etomidate, especially when used as a continuous infusion, is well documented and results from inhibition of 11-beta-hydroxylase. Consequently, etomidate is not recommended for patients with suspected sepsis because of the possible adverse effect on outcome. However, the significance of adrenocortical suppression in the setting of RSI for patients who are not suspected of having sepsis (e.g., multisystem trauma), when etomidate is administered as a single dose, is not clear. Although etomidate is unlikely to cause clinically significant adrenocortical suppression in such situations, the use of even one dose for a critically ill patient has recently been questioned (58). Given the current paucity of data on this issue, and the lack of an acceptable substitute for etomidate in certain clinical scenarios, the decision to use etomidate for RSI in children should be made with appropriate caution, particularly when sepsis or pre-existing adrenocortical suppression are suspected, and consideration should be given to administering replacement corticosteroids (dexamethasone, methylprednisolone) as indicated. Clearly, further study on this subject is needed.

How Supplied

Etomidate comes as an injectable solution of 2 mg/mL.

Dose

The dose of etomidate for RSI is 0.3 to 0.5 mg/kg given intravenously.

Neuromuscular Blockade Agents

Depolarizing Agents (Succinylcholine)

Succinylcholine is the only depolarizing agent used for RSI. It acts by directly binding to the ACh receptor site at the motor end plate, causing prolonged depolarization of the muscle (fasciculations) and subsequent paralysis. Although succinylcholine is rapidly hydrolyzed by plasma pseudocholinesterase, the muscle remains refractory to further contraction until the membrane returns to the resting state. Succinylcholine is water soluble and rapidly distributed to the extracellular space (8). It has a rapid onset (20 to 60 seconds) and a short duration of effect (5 to 10 minutes) (59,60). Intraosseous administration of succinylcholine has been shown to be equally effective and to have a rate of onset comparable to that for intravenous injection (61). Succinylcholine may be given via intramuscular injection at a dose of 4 mg/kg, although the onset time is much longer (2 to 4 minutes) (8). The intraosseous route is therefore preferred over the intramuscular route for RSI when timely intravenous access cannot be established.

Precautions

Many experts believe that the rapid onset and short duration of this agent make it the muscle relaxant of choice for most standard RSI intubations. However, succinylcholine does have several side effects as well as relative and absolute contraindications. Because of its similarity to acetylcholine, succinylcholine produces varying degrees of vagal stimulation, ranging from mild to profound bradycardia and even asystole. Infants and young children are most susceptible to these vagal effects, which are augmented with repeated doses (6,60). For this reason, atropine should be routinely given before succinylcholine when performing RSI in younger patients. Administration of atropine after bradycardia is already present may be ineffective in reversing this effect.

As mentioned previously, succinylcholine may produce muscle fasciculations before paralysis because of its depolarizing action. The contraction of the diaphragm and abdominal muscles can cause an increase in intragastric pressure, which theoretically could lead to regurgitation. However, this risk is offset by the fact that succinylcholine causes a greater rise in lower esophageal sphincter pressure, which normally prevents reflux. Furthermore, since children have decreased muscle mass relative to size compared with adults, significant fasciculations are unlikely in younger patients (59,60,62–64). Regurgitation of stomach contents can usually be avoided if application of cricoid pressure is properly performed and care is taken not to administer excessive tidal volumes with BVM ventilation. A "defasciculating dose" of vecuronium or pancuronium (0.01 mg/kg) given 1 to 2 minutes before administering succinylcholine is sometimes advocated for adults to prevent fasciculations (64). Yet this practice is not routine for most standard pediatric intubations for several reasons: it is unlikely to significantly reduce the risk of aspiration pneumonitis, it increases the complexity of the procedure and adds a potential source of medical error, it can produce weakness (causing dysphoria and decreasing the patient's ability to protect the airway), and it may eliminate a useful clinical sign (fasciculations) of the onset of profound paralysis when laryngoscopy can begin. It should be noted, however, that intraocular pressure may be increased by succinylcholine as a direct result of extraocular muscle contractions during the fasciculation phase, (60) although when intubation conditions are optimized, this effect can normally be eliminated (65). For any patient with a penetrating eye injury undergoing emergent RSI, a defasciculating dose of a nondepolarizing muscle relaxant should be given (6).

Succinylcholine can cause a transient increase in serum potassium levels of approximately 0.5 mEq/L (59,60). In certain patient groups, this increase may be more pronounced and can potentially lead to ventricular arrhythmias and asystole. Patients at increased risk for this complication are those with massive tissue destruction (e.g., extensive burns or crush injuries) or muscular wasting secondary to denervating neuromuscular disorders (e.g., spinal cord injury, recent onset of multiple sclerosis, or stroke) (6,60). In patients with acute massive tissue destruction, risk of life-threatening hyperkalemia does not begin until days after the injury or onset of symptoms (60). Thus, succinylcholine is not contraindicated for burn or crush injury patients if RSI is performed within 3 days following the injury (6).

Use of succinylcholine for patients with increased ICP is controversial. Some investigators have found that it causes a transient rise in ICP, while others have found no change in ICP with this agent (66). In fact, succinylcholine has actually been shown to eliminate the increase in ICP that occurs with endotracheal suctioning, probably by suppressing the cough reflex (9). Use of an initial defasciculating dose of vecuronium or pancuronium prior to administering succinylcholine has been recommended for adults to prevent fasciculations, which may contribute to a possible rise in ICP. However, as described previously, this is not routine practice in children, even those with head injuries or other potential causes of elevated ICP, because the increased complexity and potential for error during the procedure is not warranted by the low likelihood of benefit. Furthermore, succinylcholine has a rapid onset, is highly potent, and has a short duration of effect. These properties decrease the occurrence of hypoxemia and hypercarbia, which have significant detrimental effects on cerebral blood flow and metabolism, and decrease the occurrence of aspiration pneumonitis, which necessitates higher airway pressures that independently produce a rise in ICP. These demonstrable advantages are believed by most experts to outweigh any theoretical risks associated with succinylcholine in the setting of increased ICP. Other rare adverse effects include malignant hyperthermia, which occurs in approximately 1 in 15,000 children (67), masseter spasm, and myoglobinuria, which is a more common complication among children than adults (68).

How Supplied

Succinylcholine (Anectine, Quelicin, Sucostrin) is supplied as an injectable solution in concentrations of 20 mg/mL (preferred), 50 mg/mL, and 100 mg/mL. It should be kept refrigerated to preserve potency.

Dose

For children and adolescents, the standard dose for succinylcholine is 1 to 1.5 mg/kg. Infants have a higher body composition of extracellular fluid and therefore require a higher dosage range for succinylcholine compared with older children and adolescents (62). For infants, the dose is 1.5 to 2 mg/kg.

Nondepolarizing Agents (Pancuronium, Vecuronium, Rocuronium)

Nondepolarizing agents block neuromuscular transmission by competitive inhibition of ACh at the motor end plate receptor sites. Unlike depolarizing agents, they have no neurotransmitter capability. Instead, they prevent the muscle from contracting.

Pancuronium is a long-acting agent. The onset time for good intubating conditions following a dose of 0.1 mg/kg is about 90 seconds in infants and about 3 minutes in older children and adolescents (62). Its duration of action (generally 40 to 90 minutes) initially depends on redistribution and then subsequently on renal and hepatic excretion (62,69).

The relatively long times of onset and duration have limited the use of pancuronium for RSI as newer agents have been developed.

Vecuronium is an intermediate-acting, nondepolarizing agent. At a dose of 0.1 mg/kg (the standard dose used for elective intubation), vecuronium has an onset of 1 to 3 minutes and a duration of about 75 minutes in infants and 35 to 55 minutes in older children and adolescents (60,62). Increasing the dose to 0.3 mg/kg, the usual recommendation for RSI, shortens the onset time to 40 to 60 seconds and thereby decreases the risk of hypoxia and vomiting/aspiration prior to laryngoscopy (69,70). However, at this higher dose, the duration of effect is at least 75 minutes in children.

Rocuronium, introduced in the early 1990s, is a nondepolarizing muscle relaxant with a faster onset and shorter duration of effect than vecuronium and pancuronium. Rocuronium produces favorable intubating conditions in 30 to 45 seconds. The duration of action has been reported to fall between 24 and 37 minutes, varying with dose and age (71,72). A recent Cochrane meta-analysis found succinylcholine to be superior to rocuronium in situations where there were "excellent intubation conditions"; however, where there were "clinically acceptable" intubation conditions, no statistical difference between these two drugs was discovered (73). Due to its rapid onset and short duration of effect (as compared with other nondepolarizing agents), rocuronium is the preferred paralytic for RSI when the likelihood of a failed airway is low and/or succinylcholine cannot be used (19).

How Supplied

Pancuronium (Pavulon) is supplied in injectable solutions of 1 and 2 mg/mL that must be refrigerated. Vecuronium (Norcuron) is supplied as a powder in 10-mg vials that do not require refrigeration. It must be mixed at the time of injection by adding 5 mL of normal saline to each vial to produce a 2-mg/mL solution. Rocuronium (Zemuron) is supplied as a 10-mg/mL injectable solution in 5- and 10-mL vials that must be refrigerated.

Dose

Pancuronium and vecuronium are dosed for elective intubation at 0.1 mg/kg. However, for RSI, they are dosed higher, at 0.15 mg/kg for pancuronium and 0.3 mg/kg for vecuronium. At these higher doses, the onset time is 90 seconds for pancuronium and 60 seconds for vecuronium (6). As mentioned previously, a defasciculating dose of 0.01 mg/kg of either pancuronium or vecuronium may be given if indicated 1 to 2 minutes before administering succinylcholine to suppress fasciculations.

Rocuronium is dosed at 0.6 mg/kg for elective intubations. A higher dose (1 to 1.2 mg/kg) is used for RSI in order to achieve a more rapid onset of effect (onset of 89 ± 33 seconds with 0.6 mg/kg vs. 55 ± 14 seconds with 1.2 mg/kg) (74). Rocuronium can also be given intramuscularly in the absence of intravenous access (75).

Ancillary Agents

Atropine

Atropine is a rapid-onset acetylcholine receptor antagonist that increases the heart rate for approximately 30 minutes (7). This vagolytic effect also blocks the bradycardia caused by airway manipulation and succinylcholine administration. In contrast to adults, children are more likely to respond to these stimuli with profound bradycardia and even asystole when an anticholinergic agent has not been administered. Except in rare cases (e.g., mitral stenosis, coronary artery disease, or pre-existing tachyarrhythmia), atropine should always be used during RSI for infants younger than 1 year, younger children receiving succinylcholine, and any patient with bradycardia at the time of intubation (6). In addition, atropine also reduces salivary and airway secretions, further facilitating laryngoscopy.

How Supplied

Atropine is supplied in ampules with concentrations ranging from .05- to 1-mg/mL solutions. We prefer the 0.4-mg/mL solution supplied in 1-mL vials for pediatric patients. Atropine can be stored at room temperature.

Dose

The dose for premedication before intubation is 0.02 mg/kg, with a minimum dose of 0.1 mg (about 0.4 mL of the 0.4-mg/mL solution) and a maximum dose of 0.4 mg. An infant weighing under 5 kg should not receive less than the minimum dosage, despite the weight-based guideline, as a dose of less than 0.1 mg may actually induce bradycardia.

Lidocaine

Lidocaine is an antiarrhythmic and local anesthetic agent that has been advocated for use as a premedication before intubation to blunt the rise in ICP that occurs during laryngoscopy and other noxious stimuli (e.g., airway suctioning). Although the exact mechanism of action is unclear, lidocaine is thought to attenuate the adrenergic and physiologic responses to laryngoscopy and endotracheal intubation. Intravenous and intratracheal lidocaine may also suppress the cough response. The usefulness of lidocaine in this context remains controversial (76). The utility of intravenous and intratracheal lidocaine for this purpose has been studied in patients with elevated ICP, with mixed results (9,77–79). Limited studies in children have not been able to show that it effectively blunts the catecholamine response to intubation (79). Nonetheless, many practitioners routinely administer intravenous lidocaine 2 to 3 minutes before intubation for the patient presumed to have a significantly elevated ICP. Chapter 16 provides a description of percutaneous transtracheal administration of lidocaine.

How Supplied

Lidocaine (Xylocaine) is supplied in either 10- or 20-mg/mL solutions in preservative-free, single-use 5-mL vials and is stored at room temperature.

Dose

For preintubation purposes, the intravenous dose of lidocaine is 1 to 2 mg/kg given 2 to 3 minutes before laryngoscopy.

▶ PROCEDURE

In this section, standard RSI for endotracheal intubation is described first, followed by modifications of the procedure that are indicated in specific clinical situations. The success of any RSI depends on the participation and skill of at least three qualified individuals: one person to provide 100% oxygen and perform the intubation, another to apply cricoid pressure, and a third to administer the medications. Ideally, a resuscitation team leader not involved with the procedure will have the sole task of monitoring the patient's clinical status and directing overall patient care. In this situation, individuals are assigned to perform specific duties while the team leader oversees and organizes treatment. In reality, the supervising physician will often have the responsibility of performing one or more aspects of RSI as well. When available, any additional personnel can also assist by restraining the patient as necessary and documenting the procedure.

Oxygenation and ventilation are maintained by spontaneous, assisted, or controlled ventilation during setup for the procedure. Intravenous access is obtained, and heart rate, blood pressure, and oxygen saturation monitoring are established. Preparation includes establishing maximum access to the patient around the stretcher, clearly describing assignments to assistants, verifying intravenous access, and testing all necessary equipment (e.g., suction, laryngoscopes, and endotracheal tubes).

As these preparations are finalized, the patient is preoxygenated by administering 100% F_iO_2 via face mask. In the optimal situation, this occurs as the patient spontaneously breathes oxygen from a nonrebreathing mask (see also Chapter 13). Three minutes of spontaneous respirations at a consistent F_iO_2 of 100% has been shown to allow approximately 2 minutes of apnea without desaturation in healthy children (80). When a rapid onset muscle relaxant is used, effective preoxygenation in this manner obviates the need for immediate BVM ventilation should the patient become apneic after administration of the sedative but before complete paralysis. Administration of PPV can often be delayed until after the endotracheal tube is in place and the airway is protected. This minimizes the risk of vomiting and aspiration by avoiding insufflation of air into the stomach (and higher intragastric pressure), which frequently occurs during BVM ventilation. Importantly, patients with reduced functional residual capacity (FRC) or underlying lung disease will desaturate more rapidly despite adequate preoxygenation.

For the spontaneously breathing patient, it is generally recommended that a few assisted ventilations be administered using a BVM circuit during the preoxygenation phase (see Chapter 14). As mentioned previously, this provides reasonable assurance that adequate BVM ventilation can be provided should intubation prove unsuccessful after the neuromuscular blocking agent has been administered. Adequacy of the mask seal, patency of the airway, and any difficulty with delivering PPV should be carefully assessed. Administration of a paralytic agent would obviously be inadvisable if there is significant concern that BVM ventilation may be impossible, unless the operator is confident that immediate endotracheal intubation can be accomplished. Otherwise, establishing an emergent surgical airway may become necessary. In such situations, attempting an awake intubation (with judicious use of sedating agents as necessary) may represent a more prudent approach.

The medications and dosages used for standard pediatric RSI are shown in Table 15.4. Although the sedating and neuromuscular blocking agents are given in rapid sequence immediately before intubation, atropine (0.02 mg/kg) may be administered at any time during the preoxygenation phase. Sedation for a standard RSI is provided by thiopental (3 to 6 mg/kg). This allows for induction of anesthesia in 20 to 60 seconds. Immediately following administration of thiopental, succinylcholine (1.5 mg/kg) is given to produce profound paralysis within 20 to 60 seconds. Cricoid pressure may be performed at this point to prevent regurgitation of stomach contents (see below).

In pediatric hospitals, many practitioners in the ED routinely use rocuronium (1 mg/kg) or vecuronium (0.3 mg/kg) to provide neuromuscular blockade for virtually all patients undergoing RSI, most likely because of the influence on practice of pediatric anesthesiology. For elective intubations in the operating room, the risk of a failed airway may be deemed less likely than the risk from complications associated with the use of succinylcholine (hyperkalemia, malignant hyperthermia), and therefore the longer duration of action of the nondepolarizing agents is considered less dangerous. As mentioned previously, however, unless contraindicated, succinylcholine may be preferred for RSI in the ED due to its potency, faster onset, and shorter duration of effect. This is especially true

in settings where infants and children constitute a minority of ED patients, and thus experience with pediatric intubation (not to mention availability of backup by pediatric anesthesiology) is comparatively limited. The rapid onset of succinylcholine normally allows the operator to safely avoid BVM ventilation after induction agents are administered, since the time to complete paralysis is brief, thereby decreasing the likelihood of vomiting during the procedure. More importantly, the spontaneously breathing patient will resume respirations within a few minutes after administration of succinylcholine should attempts at endotracheal intubation and BVM ventilation prove unsuccessful.

Whatever agent is selected, laryngoscopy should begin as soon as fasciculations occur or apnea and hypotonia are observed. These signs indicate the patient is sufficiently paralyzed to insert the endotracheal tube without eliciting coughing or gagging. When succinylcholine is used for neuromuscular blockade and preoxygenation is completed with 100% oxygen, the operator generally has at least 1 to 2 minutes of "safe" time to insert the endotracheal tube (i.e., before desaturation occurs and before return of normal muscle tone). Once the endotracheal tube has been placed, the lung fields should be auscultated and capnography used to confirm proper tube position (see Chapter 16). Cricoid pressure should be maintained until tube placement is confirmed. The patient should be ventilated manually or by mechanical ventilation and the tube should be taped in place. A nasogastric tube should be placed and a chest radiograph obtained to verify tube position. The operator may consider giving longer-acting sedative and paralytic agents to facilitate mechanical ventilation and/or transport.

Modifications

The ideal circumstances for performing an endotracheal intubation using RSI are unfortunately not always present in an emergent situation. Often one or more problems exist that require a modification of RSI. As previously described, the optimal method of preoxygenating the patient is to apply a nonrebreathing face mask delivering 100% oxygen for 2 to 5 minutes before intubation while the patient breathes spontaneously. When succinylcholine is used for RSI in this situation, its rapid effect often allows the operator to avoid performing BVM ventilation during the brief interval between the onset of apnea (caused by the sedative) and complete paralysis. However, the patient with significant respiratory compromise may require assisted or controlled ventilation with a BVM circuit and a modified preoxygenation phase. The risk of aspiration is already high when the patient is acutely ill and is likely to have a full stomach. PPV before intubation adds to this risk to the extent that air enters the stomach and increases the intragastric pressure. When the patient is receiving BVM ventilation before intubation, the rapid onset of succinylcholine is less of an advantage. In addition, there is a theoretical possibility that regurgitation of stomach contents may be produced by fasciculations as a result of

TABLE 15.4	MEDICATIONS AND DOSAGES FOR STANDARD RAPID SEQUENCE INDUCTION

Vagolytic
  Atropine 0.02 mg/kg (minimum dose 0.1 mg, maximum dose 0.4 mg)
Sedation
  Thiopental 3–6 mg/kg
  If patient is hypotensive, use
    Ketamine 1–2 mg/kg
    OR
    Midazolam 0.1–0.3 mg/kg
    OR
    Etomidate 0.3–0.5 mg/kg
Neuromuscular blockade
  Succinylcholine 1.5 mg/kg
  If succinylcholine contraindicated, use
    Vecuronium 0.3 mg/kg
    OR
    Rocuronium 1 mg/kg

succinylcholine, further increasing the risk of aspiration. In this situation, a nondepolarizing agent such as rocuronium or vecuronium may therefore be preferred.

For the patient requiring ongoing assisted or controlled ventilation, cricoid pressure (Sellick's maneuver) should be performed by an assistant from the time BVM ventilation is initiated until verification has been obtained that the trachea is successfully intubated (e.g., using an end-tidal CO_2 detector). This prevents the accumulation of excessive intragastric pressure and possible regurgitation of stomach contents or vomiting (81–86). The technique for performing Sellick's maneuver is shown in Figure 16.16. The cricoid cartilage can be palpated inferior to the thyroid cartilage as a firm ring-shaped structure. With the patient supine, pressure is applied directly downward over the cricoid cartilage to compress the esophagus. Notably, excessive pressure that compresses the airway must be avoided, as this can make laryngoscopy and passage of the endotracheal tube more difficult. In addition, cricoid pressure should be discontinued if the patient vomits, because extreme pressures generated in this situation may result in gastric or esophageal rupture. Above all, the operator managing the airway must take particular care to administer "gentle" BVM ventilation so that chest excursions are adequate to maintain good oxygenation but not so forceful that excessive inspiratory pressures cause air entry into the stomach. PPV must continue until the patient is fully paralyzed, at which point the operator may proceed with laryngoscopy. The remainder of the procedure is the same as with standard RSI.

As mentioned previously, another modification of RSI (neurologic induction/intubation) is designed to prevent increases in ICP when the patient is suspected of having pre-existing, clinically significant elevation in ICP. In this situation, it is particularly important to avoid hypoxemia, hypercarbia, systemic hypertension or hypotension, excessive positive airway pressure, and noxious stimulation with inadequate anesthesia. Examples of the medications and dosages for pediatric neurologic induction are listed in Table 15.5. This method includes two additional agents in the premedication phase while the patient is receiving 100% oxygen. After the atropine has been given, intravenous fentanyl (1 μg/mg) can be administered. Fentanyl has been shown to decrease the pressor response and the rise in ICP that occurs with laryngoscopy among both children and adults (18). It should be given at least 30 to 60 seconds before intubation during the preoxygenation phase. Because it acts as a respiratory and CNS depressant, immediate elimination of soft-tissue obstruction, initiation of PPV, and suctioning may become necessary. As an adjunct, intravenous lidocaine (1 to 1.5 mg/kg) can then be given immediately before administering the sedative. Lidocaine may attenuate the rise in ICP during intubation with little myocardial depressant effect. Thiopental (3 to 6 mg/kg) is the primary sedative agent in this situation because of its protective effect on the brain. As discussed previously, the patient at risk for increased ICP who has low cardiac output may be given small, frequent 1- to 3-mg/kg doses

TABLE 15.5	MEDICATIONS AND DOSAGES FOR NEUROLOGIC INDUCTION

Premedications
  Atropine 0.02 mg/kg (minimum dose 0.1 mg, maximum dose 0.4 mg)
  Fentanyl 1 μg/kg
  Vecuronium 0.01 mg/kg (may be given as a "defasciculating dose" if desired
    when succinylcholine is used for muscle relaxation)
  Lidocaine 1 mg/kg
Sedation
  Thiopental 3–6 mg/kg
  If patient is hypotensive, use
    Midazolam 0.2–0.3 mg/kg.
    OR
    Fentanyl 1–5 μg/kg
    OR
    Etomidate 0.3–0.5 mg/kg
    OR
    Thiopental 1–3 mg/kg
Neuromuscular blockade
  Succinylcholine 1.5 mg/kg
  If succinylcholine contraindicated, use
    Vecuroniam 0.3 mg/kg
    OR
    Rocuronium 1 mg/kg

of thiopental every 20 to 60 seconds, titrated to sedative effect and hemodynamic stability. Alternatively, midazolam (0.1 to 0.3 mg/kg) or etomidate (0.3 to 0.5 mg/kg) may be used.

Either succinylcholine or a potent nondepolarizing drug used at a high dose is an acceptable part of a neurologic RSI. Of the neuromuscular blockers, succinylcholine provides the fastest onset of paralysis, and many prefer it to minimize the likelihood of hypoxemia, hypercarbia, and aspiration. However, some animal evidence suggests that succinylcholine can cause a transient increase in ICP as a result of muscle fasciculations. If desired, a defasciculating dose of vecuronium or pancuronium (0.01 mg/kg) can be given 2 to 3 minutes before succinylcholine to prevent muscle fasciculations. As described previously, most experts believe this is unnecessary for pediatric patients and adds needless complexity and risk to the procedure. An alternative approach is to use a competitive blocker such as vecuronium (0.3 mg/kg) or rocuronium (1 mg/kg) rather than succinylcholine. At the higher doses used for RSI, the time to complete paralysis with these agents is closer to that of succinylcholine. However, it may be necessary to administer gentle PPV from the time the peak effect of thiopental occurs (about 15 to 40 seconds) until complete paralysis is observed (60 to 90 seconds with vecuronium or rocuronium) to prevent hypercarbia. Even with cricoid pressure, this approach may increase the likelihood of vomiting and aspiration due to air entry into the stomach during BVM ventilation. It should also be remembered that use of the higher doses of the nondepolarizing agents significantly prolongs the time that the patient will be paralyzed. As long as intubation is accomplished rapidly, this longer duration poses no problem. In fact, it will often be desirable because paralysis will facilitate head imaging studies that require the patient to be motionless. But for the rare patient who proves unexpectedly difficult to both intubate and manually ventilate, such a prolonged period of paralysis can lead to significant morbidity or mortality. Many practitioners, primarily for these reasons, prefer succinylcholine in such emergency circumstances with spontaneously breathing patients.

For the patient requiring RSI who is hypotensive but not at risk for increased ICP, ketamine (1 to 2 mg/kg) is preferred for induction over thiopental. Ketamine causes the release of endogenous catecholamines that maintain or even raise the systemic blood pressure, unlike thiopental, which has a potent myocardial depressant effect. A secondary option in this situation would be etomidate (0.3 to 0.5 mg/kg) or midazolam (0.1 to 0.3 mg/kg), which have minimal (etomidate) to mild (midazolam) cardiovascular effects.

Ketamine is also an excellent choice for induction of the asthmatic patient who requires intubation. Unlike thiopental and midazolam, ketamine is a potent bronchodilator. Ketamine also increases airway and salivary secretions. As mentioned previously, although this may have some beneficial effect in relieving mucus plugging, it can significantly hinder laryngoscopy, and therefore the use of ketamine should be preceded by the use of atropine or glycopyrrolate.

A final modification of RSI relates to patients with glaucoma or possible open globe injury. These patients should not receive succinylcholine for neuromuscular blockade unless preceded by a defasciculating dose of a nondepolarizing agent. Fasciculations caused by succinylcholine increase the intraocular pressure, and in patients with an eye injury, extrusion of the ocular contents can occur. The preference in this situation is to use vecuronium (0.3 mg/kg) or rocuronium (1 mg/kg) to produce muscle relaxation. In addition, these patients should not receive ketamine as an induction agent, as the use of ketamine can result in an increase in intraocular pressure.

 SUMMARY

Standard Rapid Sequence Induction

Note: this method is used when there is no risk of increased ICP. Patients suspected of having increased ICP should undergo the "neurologic induction" method.

1 Establish appropriate monitoring (EKG, blood pressure cuff, pulse oximeter).

2 Establish intravenous access.

3 Maintain a patent airway and an effective seal of the face mask.

4 Preoxygenate with 100% F_iO_2 for 2 to 3 minutes if FRC is normal or up to 5 minutes if FRC is very high or very low. If respiratory insufficiency exists, assist or control ventilation with a BVM circuit while applying cricoid pressure.

5 Administer atropine (0.02 mg/kg, minimum dose 0.1 mg, maximum dose 0.4 mg).

6 Administer sedation:

Use thiopental (3 to 6 mg/kg) unless contraindicated.

If systemic blood pressure is decreased, use midazolam (0.1 to 0.3 mg/kg), ketamine (1 to 2 mg/kg), etomidate (0.3 to 0.5 mg/kg), or fentanyl (1 to 5 mg/kg).

If the patient has status asthmaticus, use ketamine (1 to 2 mg/kg).

If the patient has diminished sensorium, sedation may be unnecessary.

7 Administer muscle relaxant (unless contraindicated):

Use succinylcholine (1.5 mg/kg) unless contraindicated.

If succinylcholine is contraindicated, use vecuronium (0.3 mg/kg) or rocuronium (1 mg/kg).

8 Apply cricoid pressure (if not already performed).

9 Provide gentle controlled BVM ventilation only if necessary from the time the sedative causes apnea until the muscle relaxant produces complete paralysis.

10 Perform laryngoscopy, visualize the tube entering the trachea, and begin PPV.

11 Auscultate both lung fields under each axilla to check tube placement.

12 If available, use a CO_2 detector to verify tracheal placement.

13 Release cricoid pressure once the tube is verified to be in the trachea.

14 Secure the tube at midtracheal position.

15 Insert orogastric or nasogastric tube to suction gastric contents.

16 Obtain a chest radiograph to confirm tube position.

17 Consider additional sedation with narcotics, which can be completely antagonized with naloxone if necessary.

▶ COMPLICATIONS

Aspiration is a serious potential complication of RSI because the technique is performed with patients presumed to have a full stomach (87,88). Cricoid pressure, avoidance of BVM ventilation, and proper use of pharmacologic agents will decrease the likelihood of aspiration. If BVM ventilation is required, it should be performed using the minimum necessary inspiratory pressures so that excessive air entry into the stomach is avoided. Complete elimination of soft-tissue obstruction with an effective jaw thrust and avoidance of excessive tidal volumes, with peak inflating pressures ideally below 15 to 20 cm H_2O, will reduce the risk of elevated intragastric pressure.

Sympathetic stimulation associated with laryngoscopy and intubation can lead to cardiovascular collapse, particularly when the patient presents with hypoxemia, myocardial ischemia, or a low cardiac output state. In addition, vagotonic effects of laryngoscopy often predominate in infants and younger children (88,89), potentially leading to significant bradycardia and asystole. Both complications can normally be avoided with careful selection of induction agents tailored to the patient's clinical status. Hypotensive patients should receive an agent that does not further depress myocardial function and systemic blood pressure. In many cases, there will be sufficient time to perform volume resuscitation while temporizing with BVM ventilation. Many believe that atropine should always be given to children

---

 SUMMARY

Neurologic Induction

Note: this method should be used for patients with head trauma, intracranial mass lesion, CNS infection, VP shunt dysfunction, or another CNS process potentially causing elevated ICP.

1 Establish appropriate monitoring (ECG, blood pressure cuff, pulse oximeter).

2 Establish intravenous access.

3 Maintain patent airway and effective seal of the face mask.

4 Preoxygenate with 100% F_IO_2 for 2 to 3 minutes if FRC is normal or up to 5 minutes if FRC is very high or very low. If respiratory insufficiency exists, assist or control ventilation with BVM circuit while applying cricoid pressure.

5 Administer premedication:

Atropine (0.02 mg/kg, minimum dose 0.1 mg, maximum dose 0.4 mg)

Fentanyl (1 μg/kg) (optional)

Vecuronium (0.01 mg/kg) (optional)

Lidocaine (1 mg/kg)

6 If necessary, remove front piece of cervical collar and provide in-line stabilization.

7 Administer sedation:

Use thiopental (3 to 6 mg/kg) unless contraindicated.

If systemic blood pressure is decreased, use midazolam (0.1 to 0.3 mg/kg), fentanyl (1 to

5 μg/kg), etomidate (0.3 to 0.5 mg/kg), or lower doses of thiopental (1 to 3 mg/kg, titrate doses).

8 Administer muscle relaxant (unless contraindicated):

Use succinylcholine (1.5 mg/kg) unless contraindicated.

If succinylcholine is contraindicated, use vecuronium (0.3 mg/kg) or rocuronium (1 mg/kg).

9 Apply cricoid pressure (if not already performed).

10 Provide gentle controlled BVM ventilation only if necessary from the time the sedative causes apnea until the muscle relaxant produces complete paralysis.

11 Perform laryngoscopy, visualize tube entering the trachea, and begin PPV.

12 Auscultate both lung fields under each axilla to check tube placement.

13 If available, verify tracheal placement with CO_2 detector.

14 Release cricoid pressure once tube is verified to be in trachea.

15 Secure tube at midtracheal position.

16 Insert orogastric or nasogastric tube to suction gastric contents.

17 Obtain chest radiograph to confirm tube position.

18 Consider additional sedation with narcotics, which can be completely antagonized with naloxone if necessary.

CLINICAL TIPS

▶ Materials and setup should be properly organized and assignments precisely communicated to assistants before any drug is administered.

▶ A muscle relaxant should not be used unless both BVM ventilation and endotracheal intubation are very likely to be achieved without undue difficulty.

▶ Intravenous placement of the peripheral access catheter should be verified and all tubing connections should be checked before administering medications.

▶ An effective mask seal should be ensured at all times during preoxygenation.

▶ Drugs should be administered through an access port close to the patient, preferably through a T-connector attached to the intravenous catheter.

▶ Laryngoscopy should begin at the moment of full muscle relaxation. Premature instrumentation may cause trauma or vomiting. Delayed instrumentation reduces the time available for intubation before the onset of desaturation.

▶ Cricoid pressure should not be released until correct tube position is confirmed unless the patient vomits. Continued cricoid pressure during vomiting can cause gastric or esophageal rupture.

▶ For the hypotensive patient, thiopental should be avoided or administered in low doses of 1 to 3 mg/kg and titrated to adequate sedation and hemodynamic stability. Midazolam, fentanyl, or etomidate may be substituted.

▶ Ketamine supports the circulation and acts as a bronchodilator, which are both indications for its use in the asthmatic patient requiring intubation. Ketamine should not be used when the patient has an open globe injury or is at risk for increased ICP.

▶ Succinylcholine should never be administered to patients with glaucoma or possible open globe injury unless preceded by a defasciculating dose of a nondepolarizing muscle relaxant. Succinylcholine is contraindicated in patients with denervating neuromuscular diseases, susceptibility to malignant hyperthermia, and thermal and crush injuries beginning days after the traumatic event.

before intubation to both avoid bradycardia and reduce airway secretions.

Exacerbation of an elevated ICP may occur during intubation if an inappropriate or poorly executed RSI regimen is used. Most patients suspected of having increased ICP—

such as those with space occupying lesions and/or cerebral edema—should undergo a neurologic induction. Although this modification of RSI will likely minimize the effect of laryngoscopy and endotracheal intubation on ICP, the most important priorities remain the prevention of hypoxemia and aspiration.

Inadequate sedation during RSI can lead to systemic hypertension, dysrhythmias, and myocardial ischemia. Furthermore, the patient can have the terrifying experience of being awake but paralyzed even before a painful stimulus is applied. Proper sedation, as a bolus or titrated in small, frequent increments, can be safely achieved in almost all patients who require neuromuscular blocking agents.

If laryngoscopy is performed before complete sedation and paralysis, the patient may cough, vomit, or have adverse cardiovascular changes. Conversely, if the period of apnea before intubation is prolonged, profound hypoxemia may result. The operator must therefore wait an appropriate length of time before initiating intubation, but then act immediately once paralysis is complete. Clearly, timing is a critical element in the success of RSI.

Finally, failure to accomplish intubation in a paralyzed patient creates an immediate dependency on BVM ventilation as the life-saving means of gas exchange. If intubation is unsuccessful after RSI has been performed, BVM ventilation should be administered with effective cricoid pressure until the effects of the neuromuscular blocking agent have subsided or another airway intervention can be performed. It cannot be overemphasized that before choosing to administer a muscle relaxant, the operator must ensure to the best extent possible that both intubation and manual ventilation can be accomplished without undue difficulty. Otherwise, spontaneous ventilation must be preserved, with intubation performed using little or no sedation and no muscle relaxant.

▶ SUMMARY

The purpose of RSI is to facilitate a safe endotracheal intubation. It is intended to protect the patient from several potentially adverse effects of intubation. Patients presenting acutely who require emergent intubation are presumed to have a full stomach and are therefore at risk for aspiration of gastric contents. RSI is designed to minimize this risk. In addition, modifications of this procedure include methods that are intended to attenuate the rise in ICP associated with intubation, to avoid exacerbating systemic hypotension, and to facilitate intubation of the asthmatic patient. Familiarity with the necessary induction agents and muscle relaxants is essential to successful RSI. The operator must also understand the indications, limitations, and potential hazards of this procedure. When used appropriately, RSI significantly enhances the capabilities of those who provide emergency airway management for pediatric patients.

▶ ACKNOWLEDGMENTS

The authors would like to acknowledge the valuable contributions of Joanne M. Decker and David A. Lowe to the version of this chapter that appeared in the previous edition.

▶ REFERENCES

1. *Best and Taylor's physiological basis of medical practice.* 12th ed. Baltimore: Williams & Wilkins; 1991.

2. Evers AS, Crowder M. General anesthetics. In: Hardman JG, Limbird LE, eds. *Goodman and Gilman's The Pharmacological Basis of Therapeutics.* New York: McGraw-Hill; 2001:343.

3. Reves JG, Glass PSA Lubarsky DA, et al. Intravenous nonopioid anesthetics. In: Miller RD, ed. *Miller's Anesthesia.* 6th ed. New York: Churchill Livingstone, 2005:317–378.

4. Sorbo S, Hudson RJ, Loomis JC. The pharmacokinetics of thiopental in pediatric surgical patients. *Anesthesiology.* 1984;61:666–670.

5. Yamamoto LG, Yim GK, Britten AG. Rapid sequence anesthesia induction for emergency intubation. *Pediatr Emerg Care.* 1990;6:200–213.

6. Gerardi MJ, Sacchetti AD, Cantor RM, et al. Rapid-sequence intubation of the pediatric patient. Pediatric Emergency Medicine Committee of the American College of Emergency Physicians. *Ann Emerg Med.* 1996;28:55–74.

7. General anesthetics. In: *Drug Evaluations Annual 1995.* Chicago: American Medical Association; 1995.

8. Cote CJ. Pediatric anesthesia. In: Miller RD, ed. *Miller's Anesthesia* 6th ed. New York: Churchill Livingston; 2005:60.

9. White PF, Schlobohm RM, Pitts LH, et al. A randomized study of drugs for preventing increases in intracranial pressure during endotracheal suctioning. *Anesthesiology.* 1982;57:242–244.

10. Hollman GA. Analgesia and sedation in pediatric critical care. In: Fuhrman BP, Zimmerman JS, eds. *Pediatric Critical Care.* 2nd ed. St. Louis: Mosby-Year Book; 1998:1363–1379.

11. Gelman S, Reves JG, Harris D. Circulatory responses to midazolam anesthesia: emphasis on canine splanchnic circulation. *Anesth Analg.* 1983;62:135–139.

12. Chraemmer-Jorgensen B, Hertel S, Strom J, et al. Catecholamine response to laryngoscopy and intubation: the influence of three different drug combinations commonly used for induction of anaesthesia. *Anaesthesia.* 1992;47:750–756.

13. Adams P, Gelman S, Reves JG, et al. Midazolam pharmacodynamics and pharmacokinetics during acute hypovolemia. *Anesthesiology.* 1985;63:140–146.

14. Bledsoe GH, Schexnayder SM. Pediatric rapid sequence intubation: a review. *Pediatr Emerg Care.* 2004;20:339–344.

15. Sivilotti ML, Filbin MR, Murray HE, et al. Does the sedative agent facilitate emergency rapid sequence intubation? *Acad Emerg Med.* 2003;10:612–620.

16. Fackler JC, Arnold JH. Anesthetic principles and operating room anesthesia regimens. In: Fuhrman BP, Zimmerman JS, eds. *Pediatric Critical Care.* St. Louis: Mosby-Year Book; 1992:1265–1273.

17. Lindgren L, Saarnivaara L. Effect of competitive myoneural blockade and fentanyl on muscle fasciculation caused by suxamethonium in children. *Br J Anaesth.* 1983;55:747–751.

18. Sims CH, Splinter WM. Fentanyl blunts the haemodynamic response of children to laryngoscopy. *Can J Anaesth.* 1990;37:S91.

19. Sullivan KJ, Kissoon N. Securing the child's airway in the emergency department. *Pediatr Emerg Care.* 2002;18:108–121.

20. Hill AB, Nahrwold ML, de Rosayro AM, et al. Prevention of rigidity during fentanyl-oxygen induction of anesthesia. *Anesthesiology.* 1981;55:452–454.

21. Fahnenstich H, Steffan J, Kau N, et al. Fentanyl-induced chest wall rigidity and laryngospasm in preterm and term infants. *Crit Care Med.* 2000;28:836–839.

22. Hoien AO. Another case of grand mal seizure after fentanyl administration. *Anesthesiology.* 1984;60:387–388.

23. Safwat AM, Daniel D. Grand mal seizure after fentanyl administration. *Anesthesiology.* 1983;59:78.

24. Sprung J, Schedewie HK. Apparent focal motor seizure with a jacksonian march induced by fentanyl: a case report and review of the literature. *J Clin Anesth.* 1992;4:139–143.

25. Scott JC, Sarnquist FH. Seizure-like movements during a fentanyl infusion with absence of seizure activity in a simultaneous EEG recording. *Anesthesiology.* 1985;62:812–814.

26. Sebel PS, Bovill JG. Fentanyl and convulsions. *Anesth Analg.* 1983;62:858–859.

27. Sperry RJ, Bailey PL, Reichman MV, et al. Fentanyl and sufentanil increase intracranial pressure in head trauma patients. *Anesthesiology.* 1992;77:416–420.

28. Albanese J, Viviand X, Potie F, et al. Sufentanil, fentanyl, and alfentanil in head trauma patients: a study on cerebral hemodynamics. *Crit Care Med.* 1999;27:407–411.

29. Lauer KK, Connolly LA, Schmeling WT. Opioid sedation does not alter intracranial pressure in head injured patients. *Can J Anaesth.* 1997;44:929–933.

30. Fukuda K. Intravenous Opiod Anesthetics. In: Miller RD, ed. *Miller's Anesthesia.* New York: Churchill Livingstone; 2005:437.

31. White PF, Way WL, Trevor AJ. Ketamine: its pharmacology and therapeutic uses. *Anesthesiology.* 1982;56:119–136.

32. Fackler JC, Arnold JH. Anesthetic principles and operating room anesthesia regimens. In: Fuhrman BP, Zimmerman JS, eds. *Pediatric Critical Care.* 2nd ed. St. Louis: Mosby-Year Book; 1998:1353–1362.

33. DeNicola LK, Gayle MO, Blake KV. Drug therapy approaches in the treatment of acute severe asthma in hospitalised children. *Paediatr Drugs.* 2001;3:509–537.

34. Howes MC. Ketamine for paediatric sedation/analgesia in the emergency department. *Emerg Med J.* 2004;21:275–280.

35. Green SM, Hummel CB, Wittlake WA, et al. What is the optimal dose of intramuscular ketamine for pediatric sedation? *Acad Emerg Med.* 1999;6:21–26.

36. Hartmannsgruber MW, Gabrielli A, Layon AJ, et al. The traumatic airway: the anesthesiologist's role in the emergency room. *Int Anesthesiol Clin.* 2000;38:87–104.

37. Rothermel LK. Newer pharmacologic agents for procedural sedation of children in the emergency department: etomidate and propofol. *Curr Opin Pediatr.* 2003;15:200–203.

38. Bergen JM, Smith DC. A review of etomidate for rapid sequence intubation in the emergency department. *J Emerg Med.* 1997;15:221–230.

39. Tayal VS, Riggs RW, Marx JA, et al. Rapid-sequence intubation at an emergency medicine residency: success rate and adverse events during a two-year period. *Acad Emerg Med.* 1999;6:31–37.

40. Sakles JC, Laurin EG, Rantapaa AA, et al. Airway management in the emergency department: a one-year study of 610 tracheal intubations. *Ann Emerg Med.* 1998;31:325–332.

41. Plewa MC, King R, Johnson D, et al. Etomidate use during emergency intubation of trauma patients. *Am J Emerg Med.* 1997;15:98–100.

42. Latson TW, McCarroll SM, Mirhej MA, et al. Effects of three anesthetic induction techniques on heart rate variability. *J Clin Anesth.* 1992;4:265–276.

43. Giese JL, Stockham RJ, Stanley TH, et al. Etomidate versus thiopental for induction of anesthesia. *Anesth Analg.* 1985;64:871–876.

44. Gooding JM, Weng JT, Smith RA, et al. Cardiovascular and pulmonary responses following etomidate induction of anesthesia in patients with demonstrated cardiac disease. *Anesth Analg.* 1979;58:40–41.

45. Moss E, Powell D, Gibson RM, et al. Effect of etomidate on intracranial pressure and cerebral perfusion pressure. *Br J Anaesth.* 1979;51:347–352.

46. Bergen JM, Smith DC. A review of etomidate for rapid sequence intubation in the emergency department. *J Emerg Med.* 1997;15:221–230.

47. Modica PA, Tempelhoff R. Intracranial pressure during induction of anaesthesia and tracheal intubation with etomidate-induced EEG burst suppression. *Can J Anaesth.* 1992;39:236–241.

48. Kay B. A clinical assessment of the use of etomidate in children. *Br J Anaesth.* 1976;48:207–211.

49. Kay B. Total intravenous anesthesia with etomidate, II: evaluation of a practical technique for children. *Acta Anaesthesiol Belg.* 1977;28:115–121.

50. Scheiber G, Ribeiro FC, Marichal A, et al. Intubating conditions and onset of action after rocuronium, vecuronium, and atracurium in young children. *Anesth Analg.* 1996;83:320–324.

51. Ribeiro FC, Scheiber G, Marichal A. Comparison of time course of neuromuscular blockade in young children following rocuronium and atracurium. *Eur J Anaesthesiol.* 1998;15:310–313.

52. Sokolove PE, Price DD, Okada P. The safety of etomidate for emergency rapid sequence intubation of pediatric patients. *Pediatr Emerg Care.* 2000;16:18–21.

53. Guldner G, Schultz J, Sexton P, et al. Etomidate for rapid-sequence intubation in young children: hemodynamic effects and adverse events. *Acad Emerg Med.* 2003;10:134–139.

54. Smith DC, Bergen JM, Smithline H, et al. A trial of etomidate for rapid sequence intubation in the emergency department. *J Emerg Med.* 2000;18:13–16.

55. Tobias JD. Etomidate: applications in pediatric critical care and pediatric anesthesiology. *Pediatr Crit Care Med.* 2000;1:100–106.

56. Modica PA, Tempelhoff R. Intracranial pressure during induction of anaesthesia and tracheal intubation with etomidate-induced EEG burst suppression. *Can J Anaesth.* 1992;39:236–241.

57. Modica PA, Tempelhoff R, White PF. Pro- and anticonvulsant effects of anesthetics. Pt 2. *Anesth Analg.* 1990;70:433–444.

58. Jackson WL Jr. Should we use etomidate as an induction agent for endotracheal intubation in patients with septic shock? A critical appraisal. *Chest.* 2005;127:1031–1038.

59. DeGarmo BH, Dronen S. Pharmacology and clinical use of neuromuscular blocking agents. *Ann Emerg Med.* 1983;12:48–55.

60. Cook DR. Neuromuscular blocking agents. In: Fuhrman BP, Zimmerman JS, eds. *Pediatric Critical Care.* St. Louis: Mosby-Year Book; 1992:1251–1263.

61. Tobias JD, Nichols DG. Intraosseous succinylcholine for orotracheal intubation. *Pediatr Emerg Care.* 1990;6:108–109.

62. Meretoja OA. Neuromuscular blocking agents in paediatric patients: influence of age on the response. *Anaesth Intensive Care.* 1990;18:440–448.

63. Salem MR, Wong AY, Lin YH. The effect of suxamethonium on the intragastric pressure in infants and children. *Br J Anaesth.* 1972;44:166–170.

64. Nugent SK, Laravuso R, Rogers MC. Pharmacology and use of muscle relaxants in infants and children. *J Pediatr.* 1979;94:481–487.

65. Vinik HR. Intraocular pressure changes during rapid sequence induction and intubation: a comparison of rocuronium, atracurium, and succinylcholine. *J Clin Anesth.* 1999;11:95–100.

66. Clancy M, Halford S, Walls R, et al. In patients with head injuries who undergo rapid sequence intubation using succinylcholine, does pretreatment with a competitive neuromuscular blocking agent improve outcome? A literature review. *Emerg Med J.* 2001;18:373–375.

67. Tsang HS, Schoenfeld FG. Malignant hyperthermia. *IMJ Ill Med J.* 1976;149:471–473.

68. Cook DR. Neuromuscular blocking agents. In: Fuhrman BP, Zimmerman JS, eds. *Pediatric Critical Care.* 2nd ed. St. Louis: Mosby-Year Book; 1998:1334–1351.

69. Sloan MH, Lerman J, Bissonnette B. Pharmacodynamics of high-dose vecuronium in children during balanced anesthesia. *Anesthesiology.* 1991;74:656–659.

70. Koller ME, Husby P. High-dose vecuronium may be an alternative to suxamethonium for rapid-sequence intubation. *Acta Anaesthesiol Scand.* 1993;37:465–468.

71. Huizinga AC, Vandenbrom RH, Wierda JM, et al. Intubating conditions and onset of neuromuscular block of rocuronium (Org 9426): a comparison with suxamethonium. *Acta Anaesthesiol Scand.* 1992;36:463–468.

72. Vuksanaj D, Fisher DM. Pharmacokinetics of rocuronium in children aged 4–11 years. *Anesthesiology.* 1995;82:1104–1110.

73. Perry J, Lee J, Wells G. Rocuronium versus succinylcholine for rapid sequence induction intubation. *Cochrane Database Syst Rev.* 2003;No. 1:CD002788.

74. Naguib M, Lien C. Pharmacology of muscle relaxants and their antagonists. In: Miller RD, ed. *Miller's Anesthesia.* 6th ed. New York: Churchill Livingstone; 2005:481–572.

75. Reynolds LM, Lau M, Brown R, et al. Bioavailability of intramuscular rocuronium in infants and children. *Anesthesiology.* 1997;87:1096–1105.

76. Lev R, Rosen P. Prophylactic lidocaine use preintubation: a review. *J Emerg Med.* 1994;12:499–506.

77. Yano M, Nishiyama H, Yokota H, et al. Effect of lidocaine on ICP response to endotracheal suctioning. *Anesthesiology.* 1986;64:651–653.

78. Hamill JF, Bedford RF, Weaver DC, et al. Lidocaine before endotracheal intubation: intravenous or laryngotracheal? *Anesthesiology.* 1981;55:578–581.

79. Splinter WM. Intravenous lidocaine does not attenuate the haemodynamic response of children to laryngoscopy and tracheal intubation. *Can J Anaesth.* 1990;37(4 pt 1):440–443.

80. Sellick BA. Cricoid pressure to control regurgitation of stomach contents during induction of anaesthesia. *Lancet.* 1961;2:404–406.

81. Salem MR, Wong AY, Mani M, et al. Efficacy of cricoid pressure in preventing gastric inflation during bag-mask ventilation in pediatric patients. *Anesthesiology.* 1974;40:96–98.

82. Admani M, Yeh TF, Jain R, et al. Prevention of gastric inflation during mask ventilation in newborn infants. *Crit Care Med.* 1985;13:592–593.

83. Moynihan RJ, Brock-Utne JG, Archer JH, et al. The effect of cricoid pressure on preventing gastric insufflation in infants and children. *Anesthesiology.* 1993;78:652–656.

84. Fanning GL. The efficacy of cricoid pressure in preventing regurgitation of gastric contents. *Anesthesiology.* 1970;32:553–555.

85. Salem MR, Wong AY, Fizzotti GF. Efficacy of cricoid pressure in preventing aspiration of gastric contents in paediatric patients. *Br J Anaesth.* 1972;44:401–404.

86. Hupp JR, Peterson LJ. Aspiration pneumonitis: etiology, therapy, and prevention. *J Oral Surg.* 1981;39:430–435.

87. Sladen A, Zanca P, Hadnott WH. Aspiration pneumonitis: the sequelae. *Chest.* 1971;59:448–450.

88. Cordero L Jr, Hon EH. Neonatal bradycardia following nasopharyngeal stimulation. *J Pediatr.* 1971;78:441–447.

89. Marshall TA, Deeder R, Pai S, et al. Physiologic changes associated with endotracheal intubation in preterm infants. *Crit Care Med.* 1984;12:501–503.

16

CHRISTOPHER KING AND LARA DAVIDOVIC RAPPAPORT

Emergent Endotracheal Intubation

▶ INTRODUCTION

Few procedures have the same degree of potential impact on the care of a critically ill infant or child as endotracheal intubation. It represents one of the central elements of pediatric resuscitation. Yet the term obviously does not specify a single procedure. It encompasses a variety of techniques that, when successful, lead to the same outcome: insertion of a tube into the trachea for the purpose of delivering positive pressure ventilation to the lungs. By far the most commonly used approach for this procedure is conventional orotracheal intubation via direct laryngoscopy. Mastery of this technique is essential for any practitioner who provides emergency care to children. Blind nasotracheal intubation is a popular choice in the management of adult respiratory emergencies; however, for a variety of reasons discussed later in this chapter, its use is much more restricted among pediatric patients.

The focus of this chapter is emergent intubation, which differs in several respects from elective intubation. The most obvious difference is the importance of time as a constraint during an emergent intubation, because the patient's condition may be rapidly deteriorating. Furthermore, the patient must always be assumed to have a full stomach, which significantly increases the risk of vomiting and aspiration of gastric contents into the lungs. Depending on the presentation, sedative and paralytic medications may be contraindicated, adding the movements of a struggling child to the list of potential challenges. Finally, compromise due to trauma or an underlying disease process may make the patient more susceptible to adverse physiologic effects of the procedure. These and other factors combine to increase both the complexity and the potential morbidity of emergent endotracheal intubation.

Although it is a skill that requires considerable technical expertise, pediatric intubation is performed by a diverse group of health professionals, including emergency physicians, anesthesiologists, pediatricians, nurse anesthetists, and paramedics. The complexity of this procedure can vary greatly depending on the clinical circumstances. As discussed in Chapter 14, endotracheal intubation can at times prove to be less difficult than properly performed bag-valve-mask (BVM) ventilation. Although the prospect of intubating an apneic child can be a source of anxiety for those who primarily treat adults, certain aspects of pediatric anatomy (e.g., a supple neck, absence of teeth in infants) may make intubating an child less of a challenge. However, all of this is not to say that emergent endotracheal intubation of a pediatric patient can ever be approached casually, because a host of potential hazards must be carefully avoided. This procedure is best performed with an appropriate mixture of confidence and caution to ensure the greatest likelihood for success.

Management of the difficult airway has become an area of intensive study and education and for that reason is the subject of a detailed description in Chapter 17. Nontraditional intubation methods, such as retrograde intubation and tactile intubation, can be effective when used on patients with a known or suspected difficult airway. In addition, improvements in fiberoptic technology have added lighted stylet intubation and flexible fiberoptic intubation to the options available for pediatric patients. Although the majority of endotracheal intubations are managed routinely with orotracheal intubation, proficiency with one or more of the alternative techniques discussed in Chapter 17 can prove invaluable when dealing with the more challenging situations.

▶ ANATOMY AND PHYSIOLOGY

The most obvious anatomic difference between the airway of an infant or child and that of an adult is size. However, differences also are found in the shape, orientation, and relative positions of structures. These anatomic characteristics change progressively from infancy through adolescence as a result of growth and continuing maturation of the head and neck (Fig. 16.1). Proceeding along the airway from the nose and mouth, several unique features of pediatric anatomy can be identified that have clinical importance in performing endotracheal intubation. Adenoid hypertrophy is common among pediatric patients and may contribute to nasal airway obstruction during manual ventilation. Enlarged adenoids also are more likely to be injured when an endotracheal tube is passed through the nasopharynx, even when gentle pressure is used. Tooth eruption typically begins between 4 and 6 months of age. The emerging teeth of a younger child can potentially be damaged from excessive force applied during direct laryngoscopy. Although infants lack dentition, injury to the alveolar ridge can occur in a similar manner, potentially resulting in abnormalities in subsequent dental development. Primary teeth are shed between 5 and 10 years of age. Accidental dislodgment of one or more primary teeth is not generally harmful to the developing dentition, but an avulsed tooth can be aspirated into the tracheobronchial tree (see "Complications").

The tongue of a pediatric patient is large in proportion to the rest of the oral cavity (1). With most adults, the mouth will open wide enough to permit the operator to insert a large laryngoscope blade, making retraction of the tongue less difficult. For infants and children, the combination of a small mouth opening and a relatively large tongue frequently requires using a laryngoscope blade that may not easily displace the tongue. Although an often repeated axiom, the pediatric larynx is not anterior but is actually rostral (superior) when compared with an adult's larynx (2). For example, the larynx of an infant is opposite the C3-C4 interspace, while the larynx of an adult is opposite the C4-C5 interspace (Fig. 16.1). This more superior location of the larynx makes direct visualization of airway landmarks difficult, because the angulation between the base of the tongue and the glottic opening is more acute.

The epiglottis of an adult is broad and has a longitudinal axis that is essentially parallel to that of the trachea. The epiglottis of an infant or young child is relatively narrow, is omega shaped, and has a more acute angle in relation to the axis of the trachea (Fig. 16.2) (3). This angled orientation causes the epiglottis to cover more of the glottic opening and makes retraction with a laryngoscope blade more difficult. Furthermore, the hyoepiglottic ligament, which connects the hyoid bone to the epiglottis, is relatively lax in pediatric patients. In adults, placement of the tip of a curved laryngoscope blade in the vallecula (the space between the base of the tongue and the epiglottis), followed by anterior traction, displaces the hyoid bone anteriorly, which in turn typically retracts the epiglottis because of tension produced in the hyoepiglottic ligament. Laxity in the hyoepiglottic ligament of a child frequently causes this maneuver to be ineffective, requiring direct instrumentation of the epiglottis with the tip of a straight laryngoscope blade to reveal the vocal cords.

When considering the anatomical structures involved with direct laryngoscopy, it is useful to conceptualize the airway as forming 3 axes—the oral axis, the pharyngeal axis, and the laryngeal (or tracheal) axis (Fig. 16.3). Direct visualization of the anatomic landmarks is greatly facilitated by achieving the most favorable alignment possible of these axes. This is best accomplished by placing the child in the so-called sniffing position, that is, with slight anterior displacement of the neck and extension (rotation) of the head. This is said to be the position normally assumed when a person is "sniffing the air." With adolescents and older children, achieving the necessary anterior displacement of the neck often requires placing a pad or small towel roll under the head. Because infants and younger children have a relatively large occiput, the neck is already displaced anteriorly when the patient is lying supine, making such additional measures unnecessary. With these younger patients, extension of the head is generally the only maneuver required to achieve the sniffing position. If the occiput is especially pronounced, it may necessary to place a small pad or towel roll under the shoulders to prevent excessive neck flexion.

The major cartilaginous skeleton of the larynx is formed by the thyroid cartilage anteriorly, the cricoid cartilage circumferentially, and the arytenoids posteriorly. The overall shape of the airway formed by these cartilages is different in infants than in adults. Because of an underdeveloped cricoid cartilage, the airway of an infant is shaped like a cone, whereas the airway of an adult has a more cylindrical shape (Fig. 16.4). The arytenoids are the cartilaginous attachments of the true vocal cords. During a difficult laryngoscopy, the arytenoids (which appear white compared with the surrounding tissues) may be the only structures of the larynx visualized. In such cases, the endotracheal tube can be guided into the larynx by directing it along the midline anterior to the arytenoid cartilages and thereby through the glottic opening. Additionally, an infant's vocal cords have a lower attachment anteriorly than posteriorly so that the cords slant "away from" the laryngoscopist, whereas the vocal cords of an adult are essentially perpendicular to the trachea (Fig. 16.2) (3). This angled orientation of the cords increases the likelihood that an endotracheal tube will be held up at the anterior commissure during nasal intubation of an infant or younger child.

The trachea of a newborn is 4 to 5 cm in length and grows to 7 cm by around 18 months of age. The adult trachea is approximately 12 cm long (4). Consequently, movement of the endotracheal tube of only 2 cm within the trachea of an infant may result in endobronchial intubation or tracheal extubation. It is therefore crucial to confirm midtracheal placement of the tube and to properly secure the tube so that minimal movement can occur. The narrowest segment of the larynx in an infant or younger child is at the level of the cricoid cartilage,

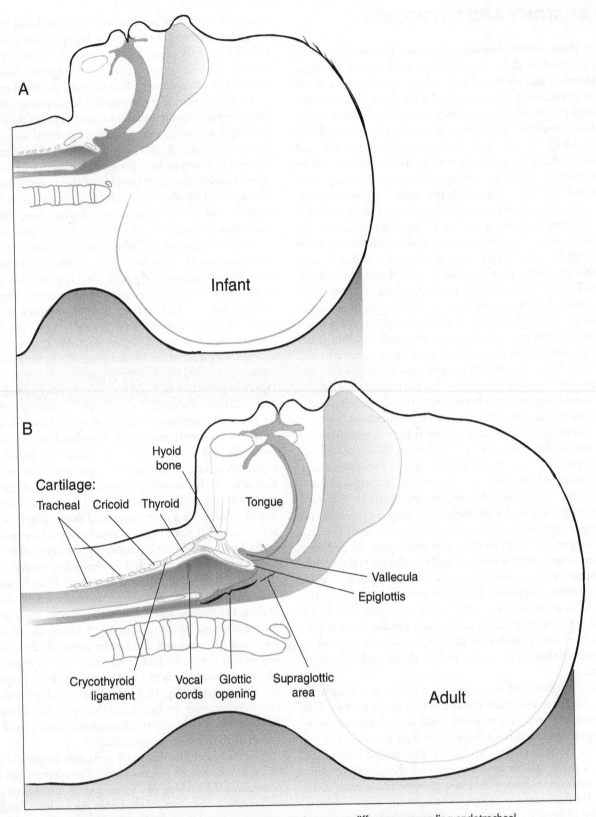

Figure 16.1 Infant versus adult airway anatomy. Important differences regarding endotracheal intubation include the following: (a) the tongue of infant is more rostral and larger relative to the size of the oropharynx, increasing the likelihood of obstruction and making retraction with a laryngoscope blade more difficult; (b) the epiglottis of an infant is more acutely angled over the glottic opening (see also Fig. 16.2); and (c) the larynx of an infant is more rostral (opposite C3-C4) compared with an adult larynx (opposite C4-C5), making the angle of entry into the trachea for tube insertion more acute.

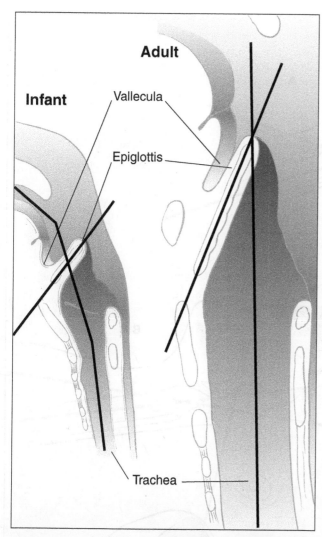

Figure 16.2 The epiglottis of an infant has a greater angle relative to the axis of the trachea, so it covers more of the glottic opening. The epiglottis of an adult has a more parallel orientation. In addition, an infant's vocal cords have a lower attachment anteriorly than posteriorly, whereas the vocal cords of an adult are perpendicular to the trachea. This "slanted" position of the cords increases the likelihood that an endotracheal tube will be caught in the anterior commissure. (Adapted with permission from Cote CJ, Todres ID. The pediatric airway. In: Cote CJ, Ryan JF, Todres ID, et al., eds. *A Practice of Anesthesia for Infants and Children.* 2nd ed. Philadelphia: WB Saunders; 1993.)

whereas the adult extrathoracic airway is narrowest at the vocal cords (5). An endotracheal tube that passes through the glottis of an adult fits loosely in the trachea, because the airway beyond has a larger diameter. However, an endotracheal tube that passes easily through the vocal cords of a young infant may fit tightly in the subglottic region, possibly leading to injury over time. By approximately 10 to 12 years of age, the cricoid and thyroid cartilages have matured sufficiently that both the angulation of the vocal cords and the narrowed subglottic area are no longer present.

After birth, the number of alveoli in the lungs increases rapidly. Approximately 20 million alveolar saccules are present at birth (6), increasing to approximately 300 million alveoli by 8 years of age (7). The alveoli grow in both size and number as the child matures, which in turn increases the gas-exchanging surface area of the lung. Therefore, the alveolar surface area of an infant is only one third to one half that of an adult when normalized for body surface. The adult lung also contains small channels that allow ventilation distal to an obstructed bronchus; these pathways are not present in infancy, developing subsequently between the first and second year of life (8). The smaller size of the alveolus and the absence of channels for collateral ventilation combine to increase the risk of developing atelectasis among infants.

To understand pulmonary ventilation and the pathophysiologic processes that lead to respiratory failure in children, it is useful to review the functional subdivisions of the lungs (Fig. 16.5). The relative size of the lung compartments is approximately constant from infancy through adulthood. The total lung capacity (TLC) is the maximum lung volume that can be achieved during inspiration. The residual volume (RV) is the amount of air remaining in the lung after maximum expiration and equals approximately one fourth of TLC. The functional residual capacity (FRC) is the lung volume at the completion of normal, unforced exhalation. FRC is determined by the balance between the outward stretch of the thorax versus the inward recoil of the lung and normally equals about one half of TLC. As gas is exhaled and lung volumes decrease, the terminal bronchioles are no longer supported by the elastic recoil of the lung and eventually collapse. The lung volume at which this occurs is the closing volume (CV). When CV is reached, alveolar units distal to the collapsed bronchioles do not participate in gas exchange. Lungs of infants and younger children are extremely compliant (i.e., have a low elastic recoil), probably because the elastic fibers are insufficiently developed. This characteristic resembles that of geriatric, emphysematous lungs in which the closing volume is greater than FRC. Consequently, some lung segments will not be ventilated during normal tidal breathing when younger patients lie supine (9,10). This results in an intrapulmonary shunt, which contributes to the rapid desaturation that occurs when ventilation is interrupted.

One of the most important physiologic concepts with regard to airway management of a pediatric patient is Poiseuille's law, which states that the resistance to gas flowing through an airway is inversely proportional to the fourth power of the radius of the airway. In other words, a small decrease in the diameter of an airway results in a large increase in resistance. This can have a profound impact on the work of breathing. Because the airway of a child is smaller to begin with, a decrease in the internal diameter by a given amount (due to edema, obstruction, etc.) results in a greater increase in resistance for pediatric patients than for adults (Fig. 16.6). Furthermore, disease processes that lead to the narrowing of small airways disproportionately increase the work of breathing in infants and children, which accounts for the greater incidence of lower airway obstructive disease seen in this age group.

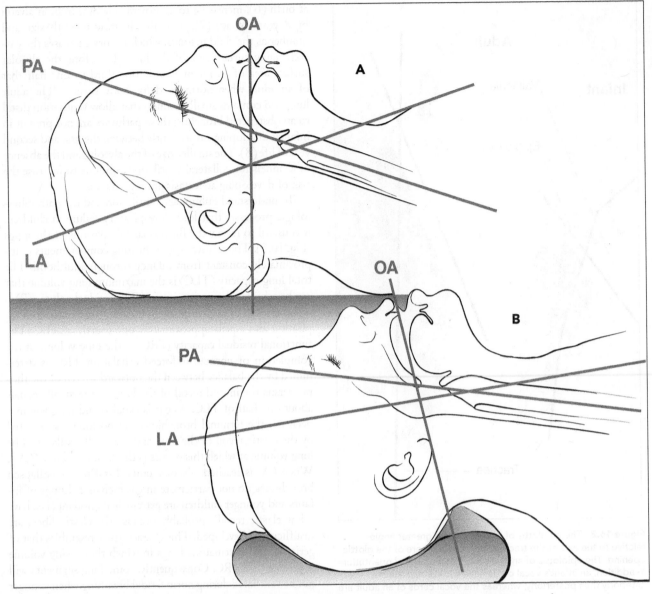

Figure 16.3 "Sniffing position." The most favorable position for airway patency and insertion of an endotracheal tube is achieved when the oral axis (OA), pharyngeal axis (PA), and laryngeal (or tracheal) axis (LA) are optimally aligned. This is the position naturally assumed by a child with airway compromise when sitting upright, because resistance to gas flow is minimized. **A.** When the patient is lying supine on a flat surface, the axes are poorly aligned. **B.** Placing a small pad or towel roll under the head better aligns the pharyngeal and tracheal axes. *(continued)*.

Because infants and younger children have a highly compliant chest wall and horizontally positioned ribs, thoracic ventilation is relatively inefficient. These patients therefore rely predominately on diaphragmatic breathing (11,12). For this reason, increases in abdominal pressure will significantly compromise ventilation, because movement of the diaphragm is impeded. In addition, infants are predisposed to ventilatory muscle fatigue because they have a lower percentage of slow-twitch, fatigue-resistant muscle fibers in the diaphragm (13–15).

Respiratory failure may be defined as the inability of the respiratory system to meet the metabolic demands of the body for the uptake of oxygen and CO_2 excretion. Respiratory failure is caused by one of two processes—either failure of the lungs to exchange gas or failure of the respiratory pump to ventilate the lungs. Gas exchange involves conduction of gas through airways, diffusion of gas across the alveoli, and distribution of gas from the pulmonary circulation to the body. Disease processes that affect any of these physiologic mechanisms will impair the gas-exchanging capability of the lungs.

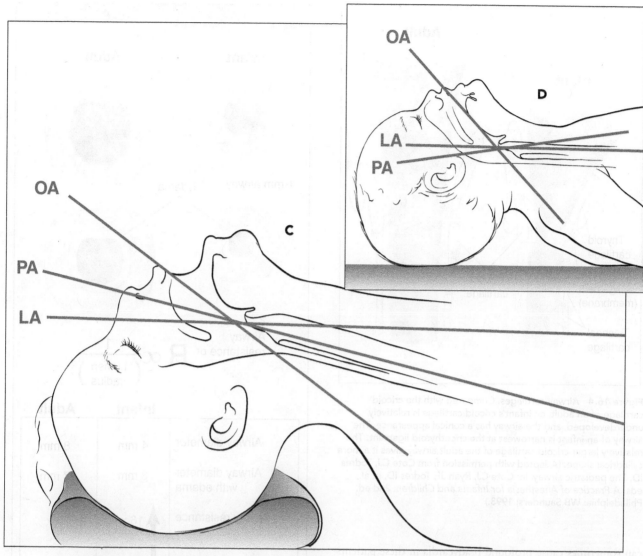

Figure 16.3 (*Continued*)
C. Extension of the neck then aligns all three axes.
D. Because infants have a relatively large occiput, making the use of a towel roll unnecessary, extension of the neck is the only maneuver needed to achieve the sniffing position. (Adapted with permission from Cote CJ, Todres ID. The pediatric airway. In: Cote CJ, Ryan JF, Todres ID, et al., eds. *A Practice of Anesthesia for Infants and Children.* 2nd ed. Philadelphia: WB Saunders; 1993.)

In the majority of patients, the primary disturbance is an alteration in the normal ventilation (V) and perfusion (Q) in the lung, resulting in hypoxemia. The term "respiratory pump" is used when referring to those structures and mechanisms that control ventilation of the lungs (i.e., the nervous system, respiratory musculature, and thoracic cage). In response to changes in pCO_2 and pO_2, respiratory centers in the brainstem send a signal via the phrenic and intercostal nerves to the respiratory muscles. The resulting contraction of these muscles causes expansion of the thorax and the development of negative pressure within the pleural space. The pressure gradient produced causes gas flow into the lungs. Exhalation occurs passively through elastic recoil of the lungs and

chest wall. Failure of gas exchange, through VQ mismatch or intrapulmonary shunting, primarily impairs oxygenation. By contrast, disorders that affect ventilation manifest predominately with hypercarbia as a result of inadequate excretion of CO_2. Mild hypoxia also may be present with ventilatory insufficiency, because increased CO_2 in the alveolus dilutes available O_2.

Physiologic characteristics of the pediatric cardiovascular system also can have important clinical consequences during endotracheal intubation. For example, infants (and particularly neonates) have an exaggerated response to vagotonic stimuli, due primarily to a relative lack of sympathetic development in the heart (16,17). Consequently, vagal stimulation

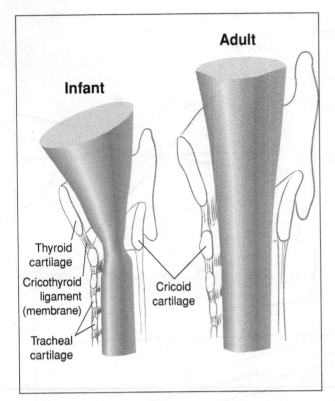

Figure 16.4 Airway cartilages. Compared with the cricoid cartilage of an adult, an infant's cricoid cartilage is relatively underdeveloped, and the airway has a conical appearance. The airway of an infant is narrowest at the cricothyroid ligament. The relatively larger cricoid cartilage of the adult airway gives it a more cylindrical shape. (Adapted with permission from Cote CJ, Todres ID. The pediatric airway. In: Cote CJ, Ryan JF, Todres ID, et al., eds. *A Practice of Anesthesia for Infants and Children*. 2nd ed. Philadelphia: WB Saunders; 1993.)

can sometimes cause profound bradycardia in these patients (18,19). Furthermore, neonatal lamb studies suggest that immature myocardium has a limited ability to increase stroke volume, and therefore cardiac output primarily depends on heart rate (20,21). The combination of these two factors accounts

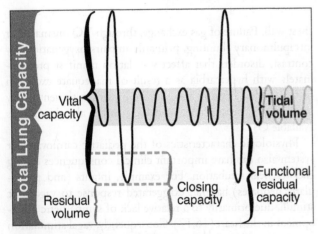

Figure 16.5 Physiologic subdivisions of the lungs.

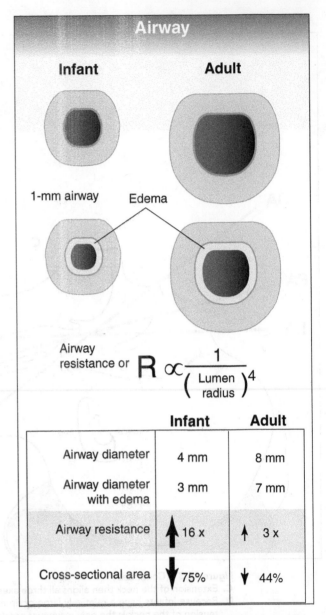

$$R \propto \frac{1}{\left(\dfrac{\text{Lumen}}{\text{radius}}\right)^4}$$

	Infant	Adult
Airway diameter	4 mm	8 mm
Airway diameter with edema	3 mm	7 mm
Airway resistance	↑ 16 x	↑ 3 x
Cross-sectional area	↓ 75%	↓ 44%

Figure 16.6 Effects of airway narrowing. Resistance to gas flow is inversely proportional to the fourth power of the radius of the airway lumen, meaning that small decreases in luminal diameter result in large increases in airway resistance. Because infants and children have smaller airways than adults at comparable levels, the same amount of airway narrowing (e.g., 1 mm) results in a disproportionate increase in resistance for these patients. This problem is compounded by the fact that the immature respiratory musculature of a pediatric patient is less efficient and therefore more prone to fatigue than that of an adult. (Adapted with permission from Cote CJ, Todres ID. The pediatric airway. In: Cote CJ, Ryan JF, Todres ID, et al., eds. *A Practice of Anesthesia for Infants and Children*. 2nd ed. Philadelphia: WB Saunders; 1993.)

for the fact that vagal stimuli have a much greater negative impact on cardiac output in younger patients, potentially resulting in significant hypotension. Laryngoscopy can have a wide range of physiologic effects on the cardiovascular system (Table 16.1). Catecholamine release during laryngoscopy can lead to an increase in heart rate and systemic blood pressure,

TABLE 16.1	PHYSIOLOGIC EFFECTS OF LARYNGOSCOPY

Pain
Anxiety
Hypertension
Tachycardia (catecholamine release)
Bradycardia (vagal stimulation)
Hypoxemia
Hypercarbia
Increased intracranial pressure
Increased intraocular pressure

TABLE 16.2	INDICATIONS FOR EMERGENT ENDOTRACHEAL INTUBATION OF PEDIATIRC PATIENTS

Airway obstruction
  Congenital anomalies
  Acquired airway lesions
    Infection
      Retropharyngeal abscess
      Ludwig angina
      Penonsllar abscess
      Laryngotracheal bronchitis (croup)
      Bacterial tracheitis
      Epiglottitis
  Airway trauma
  Burns (chemical or thermal)
  Foreign body aspiration
Respiratory failure
  Impaired gas exchange
    Obstructive lung disease
      Bronchopulmonary dysplasia
      Bronchiolitis
      Asthma
    Pneumonitis and pneumonia
    Pulmonary edema (cardiogenic and ARDS)
    Thoracic trauma
    Near drowning
  Respiratory pump failure
    Apnea
    Spinal cord trauma
    Neuromuscular diseases
      Tetanus
      Poliomyelitis
      Guillain-Barré syndrome
      Myasthenia gravis
      Botulism
Common clinical scenarios
  Cardiopulmonary resuscitation
  Drug administration via endotracheal tube
  Facilitate hypocapnic ventilation
  Decrease intracranial pressure
  Eliminate work of breathing for patient in circulatory failure
  Suction tracheobronchial debris
  Protect lungs from aspiration pneumonitis in patient with absent protective airway reflexes

although this is more common among adults; with pediatric patients, the vagal effects of upper airway instrumentation tend to predominate. Another potential adverse consequence of tracheal intubation relates to the institution of positive pressure ventilation, which may produce hypotension when venous return is diminished as a result of elevated intrathoracic pressure. During spontaneous ventilation, the negative intrathoracic pressure generated favors venous return to the heart. In a hypovolemic patient, a significant fall in cardiac output and blood pressure may occur when spontaneous ventilation is converted to controlled ventilation.

▶ INDICATIONS

Disease processes and patient presentations that serve as indications for emergent endotracheal intubation are so numerous that it would be beyond the scope of this chapter to discuss all possibilities in detail. Instead, an overview of the most clinically important topics is given. In general, the two main indications for emergent endotracheal intubation are airway obstruction and respiratory failure. There are also specific clinical scenarios that necessitate this procedure. Primary indications for emergent endotracheal intubation of the pediatric patient are listed in Table 16.2.

Airway Obstruction

Partial or complete airway obstruction is most likely to be life-threatening, and therefore to require emergent endotracheal intubation, when the anatomic site of the obstruction is within the trachea superior to the carina. With a more inferior obstruction, only one of the lungs will be involved, and the patient is less likely to have an acutely dangerous respiratory insult, although the process may become more serious with the passage of time. Obstruction that involves the entire trachea is often referred to as "upper airway" obstruction and represents one of the most rapidly evolving potential causes of death in a patient. This is why, as described in Chapter 12, the first step in the "ABCs" of basic life support is to establish a patent airway through proper positioning of the head and neck. When necessary, endotracheal intubation provides

a means of securing a "definitive" airway that ensures a reliable conduit for gas exchange.

When the airway is partially obstructed, airflow becomes turbulent, and noisy respirations or stridor can be heard as air passes through the narrowed portion of the airway. Observation of the timing of stridor can aid in diagnosing the location of airway obstruction (22). Inspiratory stridor is common when airway narrowing is located at the supraglottic or glottic airway. Expiratory stridor is more often noted with airway compression below the level of the thoracic inlet. Both inspiratory and expiratory stridor will be heard with fixed lesions, such as subglottic stenosis, that do not change airway diameter with respirations (23). A barking cough is frequently described with subglottic narrowing, as with croup.

The extent of airway obstruction will determine which clinical signs are present. Children with mild obstruction may have stridor but only with increased airflow, as with crying.

Moderate airway obstruction usually causes retractions, tachypnea, tachycardia, restlessness, and confusion. As airway obstruction progresses, small children will manifest paradoxical chest wall movement: with attempted inspiration against the obstructed airway, the diaphragm distends as the abdomen protrudes, and the compliant chest wall retracts. Cyanosis is a late sign of airway obstruction and necessitates emergency intervention. Appropriate treatment for the child with airway obstruction is based on diagnosis, rate of progression of symptoms, and initial response to therapy. Presence of fever suggests an infection. Patients with congenital anatomic abnormalities (e.g., vocal cord paralysis, laryngomalacia, vascular ring, congenital subglottic stenosis, laryngeal web, or laryngeal cyst) will usually manifest stridor at birth.

A child with severe airway obstruction rapidly develops pronounced fatigue and becomes unable to continue adequate respiration, so respiratory failure is quickly followed by respiratory arrest. This progression is accelerated by energy-consuming activities such as crying and agitated movements. The operator must therefore make every effort to calm a child who has severe airway obstruction and to avoid actions that increase agitation (forcing an oxygen mask on the child, restraining the child in a supine position on a bed, etc.) However, it should be emphasized that sedatives or narcotics should not be used for this purpose before securing a definitive airway. Using these drugs can lead to suppression of respiratory drive, resulting in hypoventilation or apnea. In fact, obtaining intravenous access may not be appropriate until the patient is moved to a more controlled setting such as the operating room or intensive care unit (ICU). Parents can be enlisted to distract and comfort the patient (3). The child should be maintained in a comfortable position, humidified oxygen delivered via face mask (or simply using "blow-by" tubing if a face mask causes agitation), and protective airway reflexes maintained until the diagnosis is made and any appropriate treatment can be initiated (e.g., nebulized racemic epinephrine).

For any child who presents with airway obstruction and severe respiratory distress, emergency preparations should be made to secure the airway. Since routine direct laryngoscopy may be difficult or impossible because of altered anatomy, assistance should be sought from a qualified anesthesiologist or otolaryngologist when available. The course of action should be carefully planned, including the primary approach (usually conventional orotracheal intubation) and one or more backup approaches (e.g., fiberoptic laryngoscopy or retrograde intubation) (see also Chapter 17). Preparations also should be made for emergency tracheotomy or cricothyroidotomy if personnel capable of performing these procedures are present (see also Chapter 26). A variety of endotracheal tube sizes should be available in case the initially estimated size does not pass through the narrowed airway. Because a surgical procedure may become necessary in this situation, optimal management of the patient would take place in the operating room, assuming that the child's clinical condition allows sufficient time for transport.

Acquired Airway Lesions

Infection

Acute laryngotracheobronchitis (croup) usually occurs between the ages of 6 months and 3 years. It is characterized by a preceding upper respiratory tract infection; gradual onset of a hoarse, barking cough; stridor; and thin, copious secretions (23). Diagnosis is generally made on clinical grounds but can be confirmed by a funnel-shaped appearance of the glottic and subglottic area on a frontal radiograph of the neck. Inhaled racemic epinephrine usually reverses airway obstruction. Indications for establishment of an artificial airway include cyanosis, fatigue, and frequent need for racemic epinephrine (more often than every 30 minutes). Establishment of the airway is best accomplished in the operating room, where facilities for bronchoscopy and tracheostomy are readily available (23).

Bacterial tracheitis occurs most commonly in infants and toddlers (24). Many patients will initially have croup, followed by the acute onset of stridor, fever, hoarseness, dysphasia, and a brassy cough. The child generally appears quite ill. Suctioning through an artificial airway is frequently necessary because of significant obstruction from the purulent tracheal exudate (25).

Patients with retropharyngeal cellulitis or abscess typically present with one or more of the following: a history of preceding upper respiratory infection or sore throat, dysphasia, drooling, stridor, meningismus, and a toxic appearance. This process usually affects younger children. On a lateral neck radiograph, a widening of the soft tissues between the air column and cervical vertebrae is evident (23), and an air-fluid level associated with an abscess also may be seen. Caution must be exercised with intubation because the normal anatomy of the larynx may be distorted and abscess rupture can occur.

Blunt Trauma

Potential causes of airway obstruction resulting from orofacial trauma include (a) foreign body (e.g., dislodged teeth), (b) laryngeal or tracheal disruption, and (c) external compression of the airway by an enlarging hematoma. Mandibular fractures are commonly associated with trismus, which will impede mouth opening during intubation. Patients may present with hemoptysis, stridor, subcutaneous emphysema, pneumomediastinum, or pneumothorax when an airway injury has occurred (26–30). Evaluation and appropriate management of potential cervical spine injury must always be considered in patients who have significant orofacial trauma.

Burns

Thermal burns in the airway occur from direct flame injury, explosion products, hot gases, and steam. Patients who present with burns of the face or singed facial hair have been exposed to high-temperature gas that should be assumed to have caused a respiratory burn. Thermal injury usually affects the nasopharynx and larynx, but a burn injury below the vocal cords occurs only infrequently because the temperature of dry gas decreases rapidly in the extrathoracic airway. Patients who have been exposed to high-temperature gases should be observed for evidence of respiratory obstruction or distress (31,32). If progressive respiratory distress develops, intubation is indicated to clear secretions and carbonaceous sputum and to bypass an edematous larynx. It is important to have available smaller-sized endotracheal tubes than the one estimated for age because of the possibility of airway narrowing as a result of laryngeal and tracheal edema.

Chemical burns of the airway usually occur in children after ingestion of caustic substances, particularly following emesis and aspiration. The glottis and subglottic regions are most commonly affected, typically exhibiting inflammation, ulceration, and edema. Tracheal intubation is indicated for patients presenting with respiratory distress (23).

Foreign Body Aspiration

Aspiration of a foreign body usually occurs in toddlers from 1 to 3 years of age. Although virtually any small household article may be aspirated (marbles, toys, etc.), the most commonly retrieved object is a peanut. The most likely cause of life-threatening airway obstruction in a child is a piece of hot dog (33,34). If the patient is unable to speak or otherwise phonate, complete tracheal obstruction should be presumed, and emergent laryngoscopy is indicated for foreign body removal and/or possible intubation. A stable patient with partial airway obstruction should not undergo direct laryngoscopy in the emergency department (ED). A foreign body in a mainstem bronchus may produce a ball-valve effect with positive pressure ventilation. An already hyperinflated lung may become further distended, shifting the mediastinum and leading to cardiovascular collapse. Importantly, attempts at endotracheal intubation in a stable child with partial airway obstruction may further advance a foreign body, causing complete obstruction, and the object may not be retrievable. A patient with partial airway obstruction from a foreign body should therefore be given supportive therapy until the object can be removed endoscopically in the operating room. Only when severe dyspnea and cyanosis occur as a result of airway obstruction and respiratory fatigue should immediate laryngoscopy for removal or intubation be attempted in the ED. A complete discussion of the management of airway foreign bodies can be found in Chapter 51.

Respiratory Failure

Respiratory failure is a common indication for endotracheal intubation and mechanical ventilation. As described previously, disease processes that lead to respiratory failure affect either gas exchange in the lungs or the normal function of the respiratory pump (see "Anatomy and Physiology"). Children with respiratory failure resulting from poor gas exchange demonstrate obvious signs of respiratory distress: tachypnea, nasal flaring, intercostal and suprasternal retractions, and use

of accessory muscles of respiration. Arterial blood gases or pulse oximetry will reveal hypoxemia well before the onset of hypercarbia. Persistent hypoxemia causes the patient to be tachypneic and agitated. The decision to intubate is based on the presence of physical findings suggesting excessive work of breathing, severe hypoxemia that is unresponsive to supplemental oxygen, and/or an inadequate response of the patient to initial therapeutic interventions. By comparison, patients with respiratory pump failure may not appear greatly distressed. Arterial blood gas analysis will reveal CO_2 retention reflecting the degree of ventilatory insufficiency. For these patients, endotracheal intubation should be performed when it is apparent that ventilatory efforts are inadequate or the clinical condition deteriorates.

Impaired Gas Exchange

Obstructive Lung Disease

Bronchiolitis, asthma, and bronchopulmonary dysplasia primarily affect gas flow through the small airways in the lung and are common causes of respiratory failure in children. Bronchopulmonary dysplasia results from unresolved neonatal lung injury, which causes diffuse fibrosis and a decreased number of alveolar units. These patients also have increased small airway resistance, which can often be partially corrected with bronchodilators (35,36). Bronchiolitis is an acute inflammatory disease of the lower respiratory tract that results in obstruction of small airways. Infants who develop bronchiolitis initially manifest symptoms of an upper respiratory tract infection, which may progress to marked respiratory distress characterized by tachypnea, nasal flaring, chest wall retractions, audible wheezing, and irritability. Lungs are hyperinflated, and auscultation reveals wheezing, prolonged expiration, and rales (37). Asthma is a diffuse obstructive pulmonary disease associated with generalized narrowing of the lower airways from mucosal edema, pulmonary secretions, and constriction of bronchial smooth muscle. Patients with status asthmaticus (i.e., asthma that is unresponsive to standard therapy) present with persistent dyspnea, prolonged expiratory wheezing, tachycardia, use of accessory respiratory muscles, and eventually cyanosis. The only absolute indication for emergent intubation of patients with status asthmaticus, bronchiolitis, or bronchopulmonary dysplasia is frank respiratory failure. Aggressive medical management is preferable to endotracheal intubation and mechanical ventilation when feasible, because such patients may be difficult to ventilate and are prone to problems from air trapping (e.g., pneumothorax). However, emergent intubation should be considered whenever the patient has any of the following: (a) a decreased respiratory effort as a result of progressively severe fatigue (38,39), (b) deterioration in mental status (38,40), (c) absence of both breath sounds and wheezing (suggesting minimal gas exchange) (41), (d) cyanosis despite receiving 40% oxygen (41), (e) hypoxemia with a pO_2 less than 60 while receiving 6 L/min of O_2 (41,42), and (f) hypercapnia with a pCO_2

TABLE 16.3	CONDITIONS PREDISPOSING TO A REDUCTION IN FUNCTIONAL RESIDUAL CAPACITY

Supine position
Abdominal distention
Thoracic or abdominal surgery
Atelectasis
Thoracic trauma
Pulmonary edema
ARDS
Near drowning
Diffuse pneumonitis
  Aspiration
  Idiopathic interstitial
  Bacterial
  Viral
  Opportunistic organisms
  Radiation

over 65 torr and increasing by more than 5 torr per hour (41). Even with successful intubation, patients may develop reflex bronchospasm, which can lead to worsened hypoxemia and cardiac arrest. The patient's blood pressure, cardiac rhythm, and oxygen saturation must be carefully monitored during and after this procedure.

Diffuse Pneumonitis

Pneumonitis is one of several conditions that can lead to a reduction in FRC, causing severe impairment of gas exchange, and it is characterized by inflammation of the lung parenchyma (Table 16.3). Infectious pneumonitis may be caused by bacterial, viral, or fungal illness. A chemical pneumonitis may be caused by aspiration, inhalation, or ingestion of toxins (43). These processes result in terminal closure of gas-exchanging units as alveoli collapse (or become fluid filled), producing a large intrapulmonary shunt. Shunting of desaturated blood through the lung causes the patient to manifest significant hypoxemia. Lung compliance is also reduced, leading to an increase in the work of breathing. The decision to perform endotracheal intubation in this situation is based on the response to supplemental oxygen therapy and the degree of respiratory compromise. Patients who are receiving face mask oxygen of 60% or greater but have persistent cyanosis or an oxygen saturation of less than 90% require intubation and positive pressure ventilation. Intubation also should be performed when the patient has an altered mental status or shows signs suggesting excessive work of breathing (e.g., respiratory rate greater than twice normal or accessory respiratory muscle use).

Pulmonary Edema

Pulmonary edema occurs when extravascular fluid accumulates in the lungs. Cardiogenic (hydrostatic) pulmonary edema is caused by impaired left ventricular function as a result of congenital or acquired cardiac disease. Therapy should be directed toward improving cardiac function with pharmacologic or surgical therapies. Noncardiogenic pulmonary edema or respiratory distress syndrome (RDS) occurs following primary lung injury (pneumonia, hydrocarbon aspiration, smoke inhalation, near drowning) or an insult not directly involving the lungs (shock, trauma, sepsis). In this case, pulmonary edema develops from increased permeability of the alveolar-capillary membrane (44). Patients with pulmonary edema exhibit agitation, tachypnea, and hypoxemia from intrapulmonary shunting of venous blood. Hypoxemia may be particularly profound with patients who have noncardiogenic pulmonary edema. The need for endotracheal intubation is based on the patient's clinical condition and the response to initial therapy for the underlying disease.

Thoracic Trauma

The incidence of acute respiratory failure after chest trauma is approximately 10%, with motor vehicle crashes accounting for the majority of cases (45). Two primary causes of impaired gas exchange in this situation are pulmonary contusion and flail chest. Pulmonary contusion occurs when the lung experiences significant force from blunt trauma to the chest wall. Children are particularly susceptible to this injury because they have increased chest wall compliance and reduced protection from the ribs. Hypoxemia occurs with pulmonary contusion when alveoli collapse and fill with fluid and/or blood. Flail chest, a less common injury among children as compared with adults results from multiple rib fractures and causes a disruption in chest wall integrity. A free-floating portion of the chest wall (the flail segment) moves paradoxically with respiration (i.e., inward with inspiration and outward with expiration). This paradoxical movement leads to atelectasis and VQ mismatching of the underlying lung parenchyma, which often results in significant hypoxemia. Patients with a flail chest frequently have a coexisting pulmonary contusion.

Respiratory Pump Failure

As described previously, the respiratory pump refers to the bellows function of the chest and muscles which moves gas through the conducting airways (see "Anatomy and Physiology"). The brain, spinal cord, peripheral nerves, neuromuscular junction, and muscles make up the five anatomic components necessary for normal function of the respiratory pump. The pump is primarily controlled in the brainstem through the input of chemoreceptors sensitive to $PaCO_2$, PaO_2, and pH and through input from the lung regarding airway irritation and stretch applied to the intercostal muscles. Respiratory pump failure may result from muscle weakness or lack of respiratory drive. Endotracheal intubation should be considered whenever a patient manifests the following: (a) frequent episodes of apnea that resolve only with significant stimulation or are associated with hypoxemia and/or bradycardia, (b) a pCO_2 increasing at greater than 5 torr per hour, (c) arterial pH less than 7.25, and (d) insufficient strength to generate a cough or gag.

Apnea

Apnea is one of the most common forms of respiratory pump failure among pediatric patients. Risk factors include

TABLE 16.4	DIFFERENTIAL DIAGNOSIS OF APNEA	
	Neonate, infant	**Older child**
Central nervous system	Infection (meningitis, encephalitis)	Infection
	Seizures	Toxin
	Prematurity	Tumor
	Intraventricular hemorrhage	Seizure
	Increased ICP	Increase ICP (trauma, hydrocephalus)
	Congenital anomaly (Arnold Chiari)	Obstructive sleep apnea
		Breath-holding spell
Upper airway	Laryngospasm (gastroesophageal reflux)	Infection (epiglottitis, croup)
	Infection (croup)	Foreign body
	Congenital anomaly (Down syndrome)	
Lower airway	Infection (pneumonia, bronchiolitis)	Infection
	Infant botulism	Asthma
	Congenital anomaly	Guillain-Barré syndrome
	Spinal cord injury	
	Flail chest	
Other	Hypocalcemia, hypoglycemia	Arrhythmia
	Anemia	
	Sepsis	
	Arrhythmia	
	Sudden infant death syndrome	

prematurity, cardiac or pulmonary disease, respiratory infection, brain injury, gastroesophageal reflux, sepsis, and drug ingestion (Table 16.4). Newborn or premature infants do not display the same increased ventilatory drive from hypoxemia or hypercarbia as adults (46–48), and they commonly develop apnea in response to an increased respiratory load (see "Anatomy and Physiology"). Viral infections, particularly infection with a respiratory syncytial virus, can cause central apnea in infants. Infants with cyanotic congenital heart disease have chronic hypoxemia and do not express the normal increased ventilatory drive in response to lower oxygen tension (49). Patients with underlying chronic pulmonary disease (e.g., bronchopulmonary dysplasia) may have chronic CO_2 retention and an abnormal sensitivity to increasing CO_2 (50). The brain-injured patient most often develops hyperventilation or abnormal respiratory patterns that lower arterial CO_2, such as Cheyne-Stokes respiration, although apnea also commonly occurs with injury to the brainstem. Indications for emergent intubation of these patients include (a) impairment or loss of protective airway reflexes, (b) prolonged seizures, and (c) progression of the brain injury to the point of causing abrupt onset of hypoventilation or apnea.

Patients with systemic infection have stress-related release of catecholamines, glucagon, and cortisol, which contribute to a hypermetabolic state. The normal response to infection is hyperventilation, although overwhelming sepsis usually leads to respiratory depression (51). When a child with sepsis fails to hyperventilate, incipient respiratory failure should be suspected. Temperature has a direct effect on ventilatory drive. Hyperventilation usually accompanies both heat and cold stress, but deep accidental hypothermia can profoundly depress ventilatory drive. Infants are particularly prone to develop apnea in response to hypothermia. Finally, numerous

drugs administered therapeutically or ingested accidentally may suppress normal respiratory efforts. These include opioids and other analgesics, benzodiazepines, and barbiturates. When even small doses of these medications are administered to an acutely ill patient, the effects on respiratory drive may cause hypoventilation or apnea.

Spinal Cord Trauma

Respiratory motor deficits are directly related to the level of spinal injury. High cervical cord injuries (C1-C2), which children are especially prone to sustain, result in apnea and early death without respiratory support. Injury to the middle cervical cord (C3-C5) results in loss of diaphragmatic, intercostal, and abdominal muscle function (52). Accessory muscles of inspiration in the neck and shoulders remain intact, but respiratory insufficiency rapidly develops because these accessory muscles are inadequate to maintain gas exchange. Injury to the spinal cord below the level of C5 may lead to respiratory failure through the development of neurogenic pulmonary edema, but respiratory muscle function is usually adequate to maintain ventilation. Although spinal cord injuries are rare in children, a high index of suspicion should be maintained for all patients with severe head and neck trauma, especially those manifesting coma, flaccidity, hypotension, or hypoventilation.

Neuromuscular Diseases

Many peripheral neuromuscular diseases are complicated by respiratory failure: tetanus, poliomyelitis, Guillain-Barré syndrome, myasthenia gravis, botulism, and myopathies involving the skeletal muscles. Tetanus is now rare because of widespread immunization. Cases of neonatal tetanus, which usually result from contamination and infection of the umbilicus, are still seen occasionally. Laryngospasm and/or spasm of the respiratory muscles may lead to inadequate ventilation (53,54). Poliomyelitis is caused by an acute viral infection of the CNS, which, in severe cases, results in muscle paralysis and associated respiratory failure. In the United States, sporadic cases are seen among immunocompromised patients exposed to live attenuated virus used for active immunization (55). Guillain-Barré syndrome is an acute inflammatory peripheral neuropathy of unknown etiology that affects both adults and children. Patients typically develop progressive muscle weakness, which is most severe in the lower extremities. Approximately 20% of children with Guillain-Barré syndrome ultimately develop respiratory failure (56). Myasthenia gravis results from the production of antibodies to the acetylcholine receptor, leading to dysfunction of signal transmission at the neuromuscular junction. The disease takes several forms in the pediatric population, each with a unique pathogenesis and clinical picture. Weakness is apparent soon after birth with both the congenital and the neonatal forms of myasthenia and develops later in childhood with juvenile myasthenia (57). Botulism is an acute paralytic disorder caused by ingestion of neurotoxin released by *Clostridium botulinum*. The toxin is found in food that is contaminated with the organism and processed under anaerobic conditions (58). Patients who ingest the toxin manifest generalized muscle weakness within 36 hours. Infant botulism is a form of the disease unique to children under 9 months of age. The organism is ingested in vivo and colonizes the gastrointestinal tract of the infant, leading to a slow release of toxin. These patients most commonly present between 2 and 4 months of age and manifest poor feeding, constipation, lethargy, and generalized hypotonia. In severe cases, these infants may require emergent intubation and mechanical ventilation (59–61).

Common Clinical Scenarios

Cardiopulmonary Resuscitation

The most frequent cause of cardiac arrest in pediatric patients is a preceding respiratory arrest. In a review of the causes of cardiac arrest in 119 patients younger than 18 years of age, the most common presentation was SIDS (32%), followed by drowning (22%), other respiratory causes (9%), congenital cardiac problems (4%), cancer (3%), other cardiac causes (3%), drug overdose (3%), and smoke inhalation (2%) (62). Initial attempts to restore oxygenation and ventilation should first be performed with BVM ventilation. If no spontaneous respirations return, the practitioner should proceed with endotracheal intubation. During cardiopulmonary resuscitation, certain medications (atropine, epinephrine, lidocaine, and naloxone) may be delivered via the endotracheal tube and absorbed into the systemic circulation (63).

Airway Protection

Patients with a depressed mental status and absent cough and gag reflexes should undergo endotracheal intubation to prevent aspiration of oropharyngeal secretions and/or gastric contents. Potential causes for this type of presentation include drug ingestion, trauma, metabolic encephalopathy, and intracranial mass lesion. Intubation is particularly important for such patients if gastric lavage will be performed for a suspected ingestion.

Facilitating Hypocapnic Ventilation

Lowering the $PaCO_2$ will decrease cerebral arterial blood flow and lower intracranial pressure. Patients suspected of having an intracranial mass lesion with impending brain herniation should undergo emergent endotracheal intubation to protect the airway and reduce intracranial pressure using hypocapnic ventilation before an imaging study is obtained. Performing a "neurologic induction" to minimize any rise in intracranial pressure during intubation may also be indicated in such cases (see Chapter 15).

Ventilatory Support during Circulatory Failure

The child with circulatory failure may have compromised oxygen delivery from both poor circulation and respiratory dysfunction. In addition, decreased respiratory pump function may result from diminished respiratory muscle perfusion, acidosis, hypoxia, and electrolyte abnormalities (64). In this situation, endotracheal intubation and mechanical ventilatory support may improve cardiac output and oxygen delivery while decreasing the work of breathing. Cautious use of sedatives and preparation for rapid administration of intravenous fluids should be established before attempting intubation of patients in circulatory failure because the procedure itself may precipitate hypotension.

Facilitating Tracheobronchial Suctioning

Patients with thick, tenacious secretions due to respiratory infection or mucociliary abnormalities (cystic fibrosis, Kartagener syndrome) may be unable to adequately clear airway secretions. Such patients will present with respiratory distress and hypoxemia. Tracheal intubation will provide access to the airway below the vocal cords, allowing suctioning with saline lavage and improved pulmonary toilet (see Chapter 79). Newborns delivered in the ED suspected of having significant meconium aspiration may also require intubation and tracheal suctioning (see Chapter 36).

Use of Specific Approaches

Adults are commonly intubated awake, either orally or nasally, when they have an increased risk for complications with the use of anesthetic agents or muscle relaxants. Awake intubations are normally performed after the application of topical anesthesia and administration of a sedative or analgesic. However, even with excellent topical anesthesia and sedation, it is usually difficult or impossible to talk a child through an awake procedure. In children less than 4 to 6 months of age, awake intubation is frequently used to avoid both the risks associated with anesthetic agents and the loss of protective airway reflexes. Rarely does harm come from an attempt at awake intubation, and many authorities recommend this approach in appropriate circumstances. Indications for awake intubation include (a) known anatomic abnormality of the airway, (b) inexperience with pediatric intubation, (c) circulatory instability, and (d) severe hypoxemia. Even a short disruption in ventilation may significantly worsen pre-existing hypoxemia, and the hemodynamically unstable patient often will not tolerate the circulatory effects of sedatives or analgesics.

By far the majority of emergent and urgent tracheal intubations in children are performed via the oral route using direct laryngoscopy. Blind nasotracheal intubation is rarely successful in patients younger than 8 years of age because (a) it requires a substantial degree of patient cooperation; (b) the larynx is in a more superior position; and (c) the vocal cords are angled, resulting in poor alignment of the nasopharyngeal airway and glottic opening. Additionally, children commonly have enlarged adenoids that may be traumatized during passage of a nasotracheal tube, often causing significant bleeding. Consequently, nasal intubation should not be performed for urgent or emergent airway control for young children, although this approach may be considered for older children or adolescents. As mentioned previously, several alternative techniques for endotracheal intubation have been developed for the "known difficult airway" and "failed airway" situations. These methods are described in Chapter 17.

Contraindications

No absolute contraindications exist for securing the airway. Because inadequate oxygenation rapidly leads to brain injury and death, control of the airway takes precedence over other considerations in the severely compromised patient. However, one circumstance does exist in which endotracheal intubation should not be the primary method of securing the airway—an unstable patient with blunt or penetrating injury to the larynx should undergo emergency cricothyrotomy or tracheotomy without attempted direct laryngoscopy. When the larynx is fractured or disrupted, an endotracheal tube passed through the vocal cords may dissect into the soft tissues of the neck, creating a traumatic false passage. When positive pressure ventilation is then attempted, gas will be forced into the soft tissues, further distorting the anatomic structures of the neck and making attempted tracheotomy difficult or impossible.

Situations occur in which endotracheal intubation should be delayed if possible until additional interventions can be performed, additional personnel are available (e.g., an anesthesiologist or otolaryngologist), and/or the patient can be moved to a more controlled setting (Table 16.5). The decision to delay intubation obviously depends on the degree of respiratory compromise and how rapidly the patient's clinical condition is deteriorating. A problematic intubation should be anticipated

TABLE 16.5	SITUATIONS IN WHICH INCREASED RISK OF COMPLICATIONS FROM ENDOTRACHEAL INTUBATION OCCUR

Anatomic abnormalities of the airway
Increased risk of aspiration
Unstable cervical spine
Elevated intracranial pressure
Hypovolemia or shock
Open globe injury
Pre-existing hypoxemia

whenever the patient has a prior history of either difficult intubation or episodes of airway obstruction that suggest an anatomic abnormality. Clearly, obtaining a detailed history in this regard may not be possible with a critically ill patient. However, a brief physical examination will often reveal findings that may make both manual ventilation and visualization of the larynx difficult (e.g., macroglossia, micrognathia, facial clefts, midface hypoplasia, facial asymmetry, small mouth, or short neck). Limited mobility of the temporomandibular joint or cervical spine also increases the difficulty of visualizing the larynx by direct laryngoscopy. Patients with head and neck trauma may have midfacial instability, airway bleeding, edema, masses, or foreign bodies that distort or obscure normal airway anatomy. The operator should carefully plan the approach to intubation for these patients, ideally having available the items necessary for at least one backup method as well as the standard intubation equipment (see Chapter 17). Whenever the patient's clinical condition allows, it is prudent in these situations to delay intubation until the patient can be transferred to the ICU or operating room, where procedures such as fiberoptic bronchoscopy or emergent tracheostomy can be more easily performed if necessary.

Contraindications to awake intubation with a pediatric patient include raised intracranial pressure and an unstable cervical spine. As mentioned previously, elevation of intracranial pressure associated with laryngoscopy and intubation should be suppressed using appropriate medications for patients suspected of having a process such as intracranial hemorrhage, severe traumatic brain injury, or intracranial mass lesion (see Chapter 15). In addition, head and neck movement by a struggling patient with an unstable cervical spine can potentially exacerbate a cord injury. When endotracheal intubation is immediately necessary in this situation, many authorities recommend that the clinician (a) immobilize the neck with in-line stabilization, (b) perform a rapid sequence induction, and (c) intubate the patient using the method that is least likely to produce movement of the neck and that the operator is capable of performing.

In many cases, the likelihood of complications as a result of an endotracheal intubation may be minimized if, instead of being performed immediately, the procedure is momentarily delayed until after intravenous access is obtained and medications are given or other therapy is implemented. For example, most patients who require emergent intubation are at increased risk for aspiration of gastric contents. When time allows, intravenous administration of the medications used for rapid sequence induction can often significantly diminish this risk. Patients with pre-existing hypovolemia or shock should ideally receive a bolus of intravenous fluid before intubation, because positive pressure ventilation can exacerbate hypotension. It is important to remember that these are only relative contraindications to immediate intubation. Securing control of the airway is always the first priority, and the operator must not wait until fluids or medications can be administered if the patient is rapidly deteriorating because of inadequate oxygenation. However, when the airway can be appropriately managed on a temporary basis using manual ventilation, such interventions can significantly reduce the incidence of morbidity associated with emergent intubation.

▶ EQUIPMENT

An important goal that must be accomplished before endotracheal intubation is to ensure that all necessary equipment is readily available. Reaching a crucial step only to find that a needed piece of equipment is not at hand can force the operator to abort the procedure and start over from the beginning. In many instances, emergent intubation must be performed with little warning or time to prepare. Therefore, it is highly important that all equipment necessary for intubation be assembled and checked before a patient with respiratory failure arrives in the ED. Preparing a cart that contains all the items needed to intubate any patient from neonate to adult is one method of organizing the necessary materials. One drawer may contain all the endotracheal tubes, ranging in size from 2.5- to cuffed 8.0-mm tubes. Another drawer can be used to hold an array of laryngoscope blades and extra laryngoscope handles. A third drawer may contain useful adjuncts for BVM ventilation and endotracheal intubation, such as Yankauer and flexible suction catheters, stylets of different sizes, oral airways from size 50 to 100 mm, nasopharyngeal airways, tincture of benzoin, and tape. A lockable drawer can hold syringes and medications. Other such systems can be devised based on the needs of each individual facility. Whatever method is used, adequate stocking with functional equipment should be checked at each shift, and materials must be cleaned and replaced immediately after they are used. A helpful memory aid in going through the mental checklist of equipment needed for an endotracheal intubation is SOAPIM (a variation on the "SOAP" mnemonic)—suction, oxygen, airway equipment, pharmacologic agents, intravenous access, and monitors (Table 16.6).

Suction

A large-bore (14 French) flexible suction catheter is preferred when intubating children under 1 year of age. The catheter should be multi-orifice and without a control port (i.e., it

TABLE 16.6	EQUIPMENT CHECKLIST: SOAPIM MNEMONIC

Suction. Flexible catheter (for infants and children under 1 year) and/or Yankauer suction device (for older children and adolescents); suction tubing: functioning wall suction set on full (200 cm H_2O).

Oxygen and positive pressure delivery system. Face masks: oxygen tubing; high-flow oxygen source (wall mounted or tank oxygen); resuscitation bags.

Airway equipment. Laryngoscope handles and blades; endotracheal tubes; stylets; nasopharyngeal and oropharyngeal airways.

Pharmacologic agents. Sedatives: analgesics: neuromuscular blocking agents: atropine.

Intravenous access. Peripheral and/or central venous catheters; intravenous tubing; intravenous fluids.

Monitors, Cardiac monitor; pulse oximetry: capnography.

should provide continuous suction). These catheters are easily directed in the mouth of an infant and are less cumbersome than a Yankauer-style suction device when mouth opening is limited. The vacuum source should always be on full (200 cm H_2O). For older children who consume solid foods, a Yankauer suction device is superior because of its large-diameter suction orifice and rigid design, allowing the operator greater ease in removing particulate matter (see also Chapter 13).

Oxygen and Positive Pressure Delivery System

A wall oxygen source with flow meter that permits 10 L/min or greater flow should be used whenever possible. An oxygen tank is less desirable, because there is a risk of emptying the tank. Oxygen delivery systems are further discussed in Chapter 13. Two types of positive pressure resuscitation bags are available—self-inflating systems and conventional anesthesia systems. Self-inflating systems are used most commonly in the ED because of the simplicity of the apparatus. Primary drawbacks to self-inflating systems are that they generally deliver a lower concentration of oxygen and provide a lack of tactile feedback to the operator. Disadvantages of anesthesia delivery systems are that they are more difficult for a single person to operate and may lead to rebreathing of CO_2. Oxygen flow into the system must exceed the patient's minute ventilation by at least 2.5 to 3 times; otherwise, exhaled CO_2 will be redelivered to the patient by the anesthesia bag (65). A detailed description of positive pressure delivery systems can be found in Chapter 14.

Airway Equipment

Airway equipment includes everything used in manipulating the airway during an intubation (i.e., endotracheal tubes, stylet, laryngoscope, and artificial airways). Disposable, sterile, implant-tested endotracheal tubes are used exclusively in the United States. Most endotracheal tubes designed for pediatric use have length markers starting at the tip to aid the operator

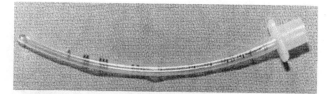

Figure 16.7 Mallinckrodt oral endotracheal tube.

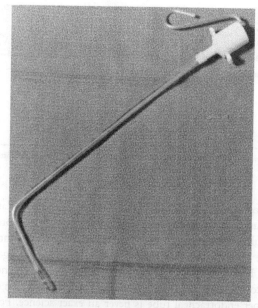

Figure 16.9 Styleted endotracheal tube molded into "hockey stick" configuration.

in ensuring the proper depth of insertion. A Mallinckrodt oral tube (Fig. 16.7) is relatively short and therefore cannot be used for nasal intubation. Endotracheal tubes manufactured by Portex are slightly longer, allowing them to be used as either oral or nasal tubes (Fig. 16.8). Most tubes have single, double, and triple circumferential line markers at the distal tip approximately 1 cm apart. Positioning the double line marking at the glottis usually ensures the proper depth of insertion.

Many experts recommend using a stylet for all conventional orotracheal intubations, although practitioners with significant experience performing intubations in neonates often prefer not to use a stylet for those patients. The advantage of a stylet is that it confers stiffness to an otherwise floppy endotracheal tube, allowing the operator to more precisely direct the tube in the confined space of a small airway. Furthermore, the tube and stylet can be molded into a so-called hockey stick configuration so that an acute angle of entry into the trachea is more easily negotiated (Fig. 16.9). If intubation proves to be uncomplicated, the presence of a stylet in the tube does not hinder the procedure in any way, even though it may not have been needed. However, if the trachea has a particularly superior location and intubation is more difficult, no time will be lost removing the tube and inserting a stylet. To avoid injury to the airway soft tissues, the stylet should not extend beyond the tip of the endotracheal tube. In addition, the stylet should be lubricated with a water-soluble jelly so that it can be easily removed after intubation without dislodging the tube.

As mentioned previously, the narrowest portion of the airway in most children younger than 8 years of age is at the cricoid cartilage, which is where the tip of the endotracheal

tube will lie. Because the tip fits snugly within the airway at this level, inflating a cuff may be unnecessary to achieve an adequate seal. For this reason, uncuffed endotracheal tubes were previously recommended for these patients. However, inadvertent use of an uncuffed tube that is too small often results in a large air leak around the tube that may make delivery of adequate tidal volumes difficult or impossible. This is especially true for children with diminished lung compliance (e.g., those with submersion injuries), who require higher inspiratory pressures to achieve adequate ventilation. In such cases, the tube must be removed and replaced with a larger size, posing a risk of losing the airway.

The primary concern about using cuffed tubes in young children was that increased pressure would cause a greater likelihood of mucosal inflammation, leading to possible subglottic injury and resulting stenosis (66). Yet the risk of laryngeal mucosal inflammation has been reported with both cuffed and uncuffed endotracheal tubes in settings of prolonged intubation (67–69). Moreover, the presence of a poorly fitted endotracheal tube in the airway is a risk factor for laryngeal mucosal inflammation whether the tube is cuffed or uncuffed (70). When used properly, the advantages of a modern (low-pressure, high-volume) cuffed endotracheal tube that is appropriately sized, positioned, and inflated—i.e., better control of air leakage and a lower risk of aspiration and infection—likely outweigh the risks of airway injury (71). For this reason, recent guidelines from the American Heart Association suggest that a cuffed endotracheal tube may be used in the ED for any pediatric patient (excluding newborns) as long as the cuff inflation pressure is maintained at less than 20 cm H_2O (72).

If a cuffed tube is used, the cuff should be inflated before intubation and tested to ensure that there is no leak. After a

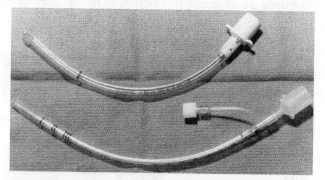

Figure 16.8 Portex endotracheal tubes may be used for oral or nasal intubation.

TABLE 16.7	FORMULAS FOR CALCULATING ENDOTRACHEAL TUBE SIZES IN CHILDREN*

Internal diameter (mm) $= [16 + age\ (yr)]/4$

OR

$= [age\ (yr)]/4 + 4$

OR

$= [height\ (cm)]/20$

*The internal diameter is also approximately equal to the size of the patient's fifth finger.

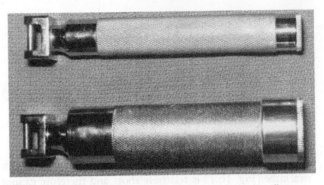

Figure 16.10 Standard and pediatric laryngoscope handles.

cuffed tube is passed into the trachea, it should be inflated to a "just seal" pressure, and if possible, the inflation pressure should be measured. The appropriate cuffed and uncuffed tube sizes can be estimated based on the patient's age (Tables 16.7 and 16.8). Unfortunately, as a result of the normal anatomic variation among pediatric patients, selection of the proper endotracheal tube is never an exact science. For this reason, it is generally advisable to have available at least two additional tubes (one 0.5 mm larger and one 0.5 mm smaller) in case the initial estimation proves incorrect.

Laryngoscope handles of standard length are suitable for pediatric use, although those of smaller diameter are much easier to manipulate and are recommended when available (Fig. 16.10). The operator should always have at least one backup laryngoscope handle available in case the first one fails (typically from a battery that "dies") during the procedure. A straight blade is generally more suitable than a curved blade for infants and young children, because it facilitates lifting the base of the tongue and exposing the glottic opening. The selected blade size and type depend on the size of the patient and the preference of the laryngoscopist (Table 16.9).

Several differences exist among the various straight laryngoscope blades available. The curved tip of the Miller straight blade (Fig. 16.11) allows the operator to make an initial attempt at retracting the epiglottis indirectly by advancing the

tip into the vallecula and applying tension to the hyoepiglottic ligament. Should this fail to reveal the vocal cords, the epiglottis can then be instrumented directly. If the patient is an infant, the wider bore of the Wisconsin and Flagg blades generally provides a better view and allows easier passage of the endotracheal tube than does the flattened profile of a Miller blade. A Wis-Hipple 1.5 blade, which has a light source very near the tip and a low profile, is a good choice for children aged 2 to 4 years. For older children, the Miller blade is preferred since it is less likely to chip large new incisors. As mentioned previously, children older than 8 to 10 years are normally intubated with a cuffed tube. For these patients, a Macintosh (curved) blade (Fig. 16.12) may prove easier to use because it allows more room for passage of the bulky cuff, although many practitioners prefer to use a straight blade for all pediatric patients. Predicting which laryngoscope blade will work best before performing an intubation may not be possible, and therefore it is always advisable to have available an array of blades in various sizes and styles.

When testing a laryngoscope blade, the clinician should first ensure that the light bulb is functional by snapping the blade into the proper position on the handle. An acceptable bulb will produce a high-intensity light. A dim, yellow light denotes a failing battery and may not provide adequate illumination of the airway. Newer laryngoscopes have a high-intensity, gas-filled bulb housed in the handle rather than on the blade itself. They emit a cool, bright light through a fiberoptic glass filament that extends to the tip, eliminating

TABLE 16.8	PEDIATRIC ENDOTRACHEAL TUBE SIZES

Weight/Age	Internal Diameter (mm)*	Tube Marking at Lips (cm)
Under 1,500 g	2.5 uncuffed	Wt in kg + 6.0 cm
1,500–5,000 g	3.0 uncuffed	Wt in kg + 6.0 cm
>5,000 g–6 mo	3.5 cuffed or uncuffed	12.0–13.0
6–18 mo	3.5–4.0 cuffed or uncuffed	13.0–14.0
18 mo–3 y	4.0–4.5 cuffed or uncuffed	13.5–14.5
3–5 y	4.5 cuffed or uncuffed	14.5–15.5
5–6 y	5.0 cuffed or uncuffed	15.5–17.0
6–8 y	5.5–6.0 cuffed or uncuffed	17.0–19.0
8–10 y	5.5–6.0 cuffed	19.0–20.0
10–12 y	6.0–6.5 cuffed	20.0–21.0
12–14 y	6.5–7.0 cuffed	21.0–22.0
14–16 y	7.0–7.5 cuffed	22.0–23.0

*Two additional endotracheal tubes (one half size larger and smaller) should also be readily available in case the initial estimation proves incorrect.

TABLE 16.9	PEDIATRIC LARYNGOSCOPE BLADE SIZES

Age/Weight	Size (Type)
2.5 kg	0 (straight)
0–3 mo	1.0 (straight)
3 mo–3 y	1.5 (straight)
3–12 y	2.0 (straight or curved)*
12–18 y	3.0 (straight or curved)

*A curved blade may be used for older children, but a straight blade is generally preferred.

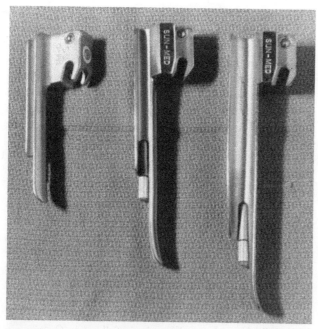

Figure 16.11 Miller (straight) blades.

the problems associated with electrical connections that can occur with traditional laryngoscopes.

An artificial airway is often an effective adjunct to manual ventilation before intubation. As mentioned previously, a child's tongue is relatively large in proportion to the oropharynx and is therefore prone to obstruct the airway. Pharyngeal hypotonia is also a relatively common cause of partial airway obstruction in the pediatric patient. Inserting an oral or nasopharyngeal airway will displace the tongue and airway

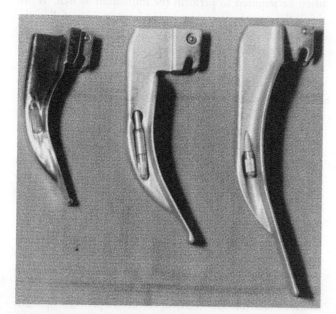

Figure 16.12 Macintosh (curved) blades.

soft tissues, thereby providing a passage for unobstructed gas exchange (see also Chapter 13).

Pharmacologic Agents

Although drug-free intubation is certainly possible and sometimes even required, physiologic and psychological benefits associated with sedatives, analgesics, and paralytic agents often outweigh their potential disadvantages. However, excellent airway skills are an important prerequisite to using pharmacologic agents during an intubation, because loss of airway control in this situation invites catastrophe. A thorough discussion of the use of medications to facilitate endotracheal intubation is presented in Chapter 15.

Intravenous Access

An intravenous line, either central or peripheral, should be inserted before intubation whenever possible (see Chapters 19 and 73). Intravenous access allows the administration of medications and intravenous fluids both to facilitate intubation and to treat the hemodynamic effects of intubation and positive pressure ventilation.

Monitors

Patients who undergo intubation generally have significant cardiovascular or respiratory dysfunction. Furthermore, profound physiologic changes often occur as a direct result of intubation or medications administered during the procedure. For these reasons, patients must be adequately monitored at all times. The minimum necessary modalities for any intubation in the ED include cardiac monitoring (Chapter 5), blood pressure monitoring (Chapter 5), and pulse oximetry (Chapter 75). Capnography should also be used when available, because this modality is the most rapid and reliable method of avoiding inadvertent esophageal intubation (73, 75–77) (Chapter 76). Additional personnel should be enlisted to assess changes in heart rate, blood pressure, and oxygen saturation and to alert the laryngoscopist about the need to perform BVM ventilation.

Importantly, the operator must understand the limitations of pulse oximetry to use this modality correctly during endotracheal intubation. The pulse oximeter measures oxygen saturation, not PaO_2. Oxygen saturation is maintained at greater than 90% as the PaO_2 falls from over 500 to approximately 60 along the flat portion of the oxyhemoglobin dissociation curve (Fig. 16.13). This decrease occurs especially rapidly in pediatric patients, because they have a higher metabolic rate and consequently a higher rate of oxygen consumption. Not until the PaO_2 falls below 60 will there be a similarly rapid decrease in oxygen saturation reflected by the pulse oximeter reading. Furthermore, a pulse oximetry transducer applied to the digit of an extremity has a delay of approximately 30 seconds in response time compared to measurements of arterial blood (74). For these reasons, efforts to intubate a patient

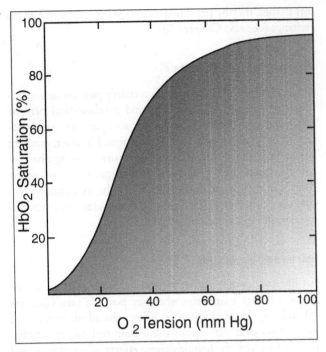

Figure 16.13 Oxyhemoglobin dissociation curve.

should be aborted as soon as the oxygen saturation reading reaches 90%, assuming that the patient had a normal saturation at the beginning of the procedure. Even with prompt restoration of ventilation at this point, true arterial saturation will frequently fall below 70%.

▶ PROCEDURE

Overview

As with all technically complex tasks, one of the most important keys to performing a successful endotracheal intubation is to work in an unhurried, methodical manner. Sudden or rushed movements increase the likelihood of injuring the patient and do not generally result in accomplishing intubation more rapidly. The operator should proceed from one stage of the procedure to the next with deliberate and efficient actions. In addition, endotracheal intubation is greatly facilitated by focusing attention solely on the goal at hand and, to the extent possible, ignoring all distractions. Obviously, this can be difficult in the frequently loud and eventful setting of a pediatric resuscitation. Yet the skillful operator often appears virtually oblivious of the noisy surroundings while performing this procedure.

Although sometimes overlooked in the rush of events, the role of an experienced assistant who aids the primary operator can also be extremely important. This person may be a physician, nurse, or other health care professional. A good assistant will make the proper piece of equipment available at precisely the right moment so that the operator's attention

need not be diverted from the patient. The assistant also can perform other necessary maneuvers (e.g., neck extension or flexion, cricoid pressure, retraction of the cheek or lip) at critical points in the procedure. Finally, the assistant can make the operator aware of important information, such as rate or rhythm changes on the cardiac monitor, a declining oxygen saturation on the pulse oximeter, or the time interval since initiation of an intubation attempt. Such assistance can be invaluable in ensuring a smooth and successful intubation.

Monitoring

As discussed previously, monitoring modalities used during an endotracheal intubation will vary depending on the status of the patient and the setting for the procedure (see "Equipment"). When an intubation is performed outside the hospital (e.g., in a prehospital intervention or during an interhospital transport), cardiac monitoring may be the only available method. Patients who undergo emergent intubation in the hospital should have at least cardiac monitoring and pulse oximetry, although pulse oximetry is not likely to be useful initially for patients who arrive in full arrest. Continuous capnography continues to gain wider availability for emergent intubation. The value of these monitoring techniques is that the operator has continuous, "real-time" information about the cardiovascular and respiratory status of the patient during the invasive and potentially compromising maneuvers of intubation.

Although it is certainly important to concentrate on the technical aspects of an endotracheal intubation, the operator should nevertheless maintain ongoing awareness of the monitor readings. Ideally, the team leader will be someone other than the person performing the intubation so that the primary responsibility for following the monitor readings can be assumed by an individual not directly involved in the procedure. In reality, the person who leads the resuscitation will often be required to perform the intubation as well. When this is the case, the operator can ideally continue to follow the readings while managing the airway by listening to the audible tones produced by the monitors. If pulse oximetry is not available, the heart rate can be used as an approximate indicator of the oxygenation status of the patient, because infants and children rapidly develop bradycardia as oxygen saturation decreases. When no monitoring modality is available, each intubation attempt should be continued for no longer than 30 to 45 seconds before the patient again receives positive pressure ventilation with a BVM circuit. As mentioned, an assistant can be enlisted to call out appropriate time intervals during the procedure.

Preoxygenation

One primary factor contributing to the difficulty of an emergent endotracheal intubation is the time limitation. The patient's overall clinical status may be deteriorating to the extent that securing a definitive airway must take place rapidly. In addition, each intubation attempt involves a period of apnea or hypoventilation during which the procedure is performed, and the patient's oxygen saturation often begins to decline within a short period. This is a particular problem with younger patients, because a linear relationship exists between the onset of desaturation and age (78). However, one way to offset this limitation is to "preload" the patient with oxygen, which will significantly increase the time available to perform the procedure (79–81). Preoxygenation of the spontaneously breathing patient may be accomplished simply by administering 100% oxygen via face mask for 2 to 3 minutes before attempting intubation. It is essential that a tight mask seal is maintained so that oxygen delivery is optimized. If the child is struggling, one hand may be used to properly position the head while the other hand secures the mask. For the hemodynamically stable patient receiving assisted or controlled ventilation with a BVM circuit, adequate preoxygenation can be achieved by delivering 100% oxygen over approximately 2 minutes (see Chapter 14). For most children, this will provide at least 2 minutes of "safe" apnea during which direct laryngoscopy can be performed (81). When a rapid sequence induction is performed, preoxygenation should take place during spontaneous ventilation whenever possible (i.e., before the paralytic agent is administered) because positive pressure ventilation after paralysis greatly increases the risk of vomiting and aspiration (see Chapter 15). Preoxygenation is less effective for the patient in full arrest, because the benefits are greatly diminished in the low-flow state that results with chest compressions. In this situation, intubation should be accomplished as rapidly as possible.

Selecting an Approach

The clinical condition of the patient, the nature of the underlying illness, and the skill of the operator with a given technique should all be considered in selecting the approach to be used for endotracheal intubation. The need for sedatives or neuromuscular relaxants also will be an important factor in making this decision. Clearly, a procedure that the operator does not feel confident in performing should not be the method of choice, regardless of how appropriate it might otherwise be given the clinical situation. Above all, it is important to have a well-formulated plan of action in the event that intubation is initially unsuccessful. In addition to the primary approach selected, the operator must be prepared to perform one or more backup procedures for providing respiratory support should this become necessary. Secondary techniques include percutaneous transtracheal ventilation (see Chapter 18), alternative methods of endotracheal intubation (e.g., retrograde or lighted stylet intubation) (see chapter 17), and a surgical airway (see Chapter 26). Equipment for these secondary methods should be readily accessible, ideally in a prepackaged kit.

Preparation and Testing of Equipment

Before initiating the procedure, the operator must ensure that all necessary equipment is functional and readily available. It is

potentially dangerous to reach a critical step only to find that a piece of equipment does not work properly or is not at hand. The operator should develop a standard routine for gathering the appropriate equipment (such as the SOAPIM mnemonic described previously) and for performing necessary testing. This should be consistently practiced with every intubation. The equipment is logically arranged within easy reach, and medications are drawn up in the appropriate dosages, with the syringes labeled. As mentioned previously, estimating the size of the tracheal diameter can sometimes be difficult with pediatric patients, and therefore at least three endotracheal tubes should be available—the size that will be used on the initial attempt as well as the next larger and smaller sizes. When an assistant is available, the operator should review specific points during the procedure when that person will be needed to provide a particular piece of equipment.

Gastric Tube Insertion and Cricoid Pressure

Regurgitation and aspiration of gastric contents during endotracheal intubation can result in pneumonitis and pulmonary edema (see "Complications"). Inserting a gastric tube and using cricoid pressure are two measures that may reduce the incidence of these complications. Primary factors that lead to aspiration pneumonitis are the presence of undigested food and gastric acid in the stomach, lack of protective airway reflexes, and elevated intragastric pressure as a result of air swallowing and/or forced entry of gases into the stomach during manual ventilation (82,83). When appropriate, insertion of a gastric tube before endotracheal intubation allows evacuation of stomach contents, which reduces intragastric pressure (see Chapter 84). Gastric tube placement should only be performed when the patient has an intact gag reflex or after the airway is protected, because inserting the tube may itself induce vomiting.

Cricoid pressure (Sellick's maneuver) is a simple technique that can be highly beneficial both before and during an intubation. Before the procedure, cricoid pressure limits the amount of gas entering the stomach during BVM ventilation (84–86). During an intubation, cricoid pressure prevents reflux of gastric contents into the oropharynx (87,88), reducing the likelihood of aspiration pneumonitis and facilitating visualization of the larynx during direct laryngoscopy. The maneuver is performed by placing the thumb and index finger over the superior cricoid cartilage and applying downward pressure (Fig. 16.14). The stiff rings of cartilage maintain patency of the tracheal lumen while the more compliant esophagus is occluded. For older children and adolescents, firm pressure may be necessary to collapse the esophagus, but it should be remembered that with infants even relatively gentle cricoid pressure may actually induce airway obstruction. Cricoid pressure also provides an effective method for displacing the glottic opening posteriorly when the view of the trachea appears to be anterior (superior). Although generally a safe maneuver, cricoid pressure should not be continued if the patient is forcefully vomiting, because this may result

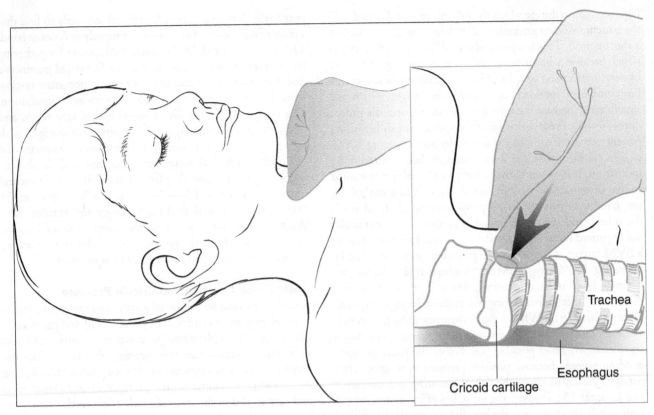

Figure 16.14 Cricoid pressure (Sellick's maneuver). Posterior displacement of the airway cartilages occludes the compliant esophagus without impairing airway patency.

in excessive pressure in the stomach and esophagus, potentially leading to rupture. Furthermore, excessive pressure may distort the airway, increasing the difficulty of visualizing the larynx or passing the endotracheal tube.

Conventional Orotracheal Intubation

As discussed previously, this is by far the most commonly used method for emergent pediatric intubation. Practitioners who must care for critically ill children should be thoroughly familiar and skillful with this procedure.

Positioning

While standing above the head of the bed, the operator places the patient in the sniffing position (Fig. 16.3). As described previously, this position results in the most favorable alignment of the pharyngeal and laryngeal axes for airway patency (see "Anatomy and Physiology"). The neck is extended by placing the palm of the right hand on the patient's forehead (with the fingers on the patient's scalp) and applying pressure posteriorly (Fig. 16.15). This maneuver also causes the patient's mouth to open, allowing insertion of the laryngoscope blade. It should be emphasized that excessive neck extension must be avoided with any patient who may have an unstable cervical spine injury. If conventional orotracheal intubation is the approach selected in this situation, in-line stabiliza-

tion should be performed and movement of the neck must be minimized.

Direct Laryngoscopy

Perhaps the most important aspect of orotracheal intubation is obtaining an adequate view of the airway anatomy during direct laryngoscopy. Once this is accomplished, insertion of the endotracheal tube is relatively straightforward. As with any complex task, the likelihood of success with laryngoscopy is increased when a given series of actions is systematically reproduced each time the procedure is performed. If this standardized approach fails, the operator must be prepared to perform alternate maneuvers designed to overcome any problems encountered.

The techniques for direct laryngoscopy differ significantly depending on the type of laryngoscope blade used (i.e., straight vs. curved). As discussed previously, a straight blade should be used for infants and most children. A curved blade may be used for some older children and adolescents, although the method preferred by many is to use a straight blade for all pediatric patients. The handle of the laryngoscope is held in the left hand, as shown in Figure 16.16, leaving the right hand free to position the patient and to insert the endotracheal tube. All laryngoscopes, except specially ordered equipment, are designed to be held in the left hand regardless of whether the operator is right- or left-hand dominant. If the mouth

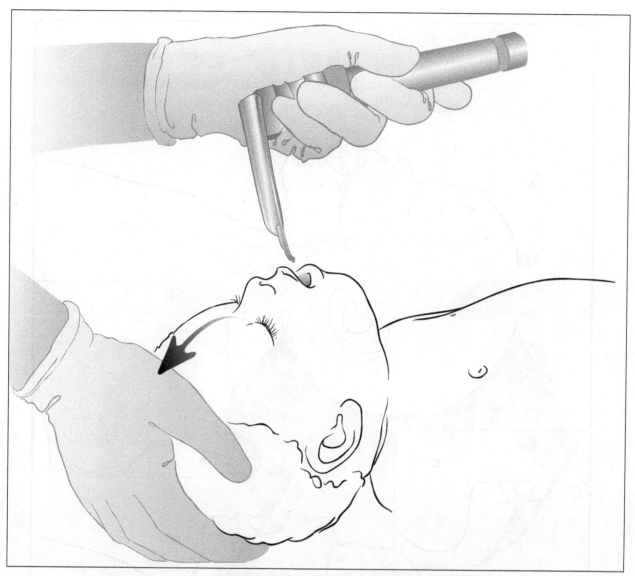

Figure 16.15 Positioning the head and neck for insertion of the laryngoscope blade. Posterior pressure on the forehead extends the neck and usually causes the mouth to open.

must be opened further to allow insertion of the laryngoscope blade, this can be accomplished with younger patients by pressing down on the patient's chin with the fifth finger of the left hand (Fig. 16.16A). When neuromuscular blockade is not administered to a child with a tendency to clench the teeth, a "scissor" technique using the thumb and forefinger of the right hand may be necessary (Fig. 16.16B).

The large flange of a Macintosh (curved) blade facilitates displacement of the tongue, and the curve allows easy insertion into the vallecula. A straight blade has the advantage of not retracting the larynx into a more anterior (angulated) position as well as allowing the operator to directly lift the epiglottis to expose the glottic opening. Although direct laryngoscopy with a straight blade additionally requires maneuvers not necessary with a curved blade, the ability to retract the epiglottis and thus provide a better view of the larynx offsets this diffi-

culty. Traditionally, the novice practitioner is taught to insert a straight laryngoscope blade into the patient's mouth from the right side and "sweep" the tongue to the left (Fig. 16.17). However, inserting a straight blade just to the right of the midline is equally effective and generally a simpler technique. When inserting the blade, the operator must always make certain that the patient's lower lip is not caught against the teeth to avoid causing a laceration. An assistant can be enlisted to retract the lip if necessary.

As described previously, the operator should use the largest straight blade that will readily fit into the patient's mouth. A common mistake made with pediatric intubations is to select a blade that is inappropriately small for the patient, making adequate retraction of the tongue and soft tissues difficult or impossible. After the laryngoscope blade has been inserted into the vallecula, the handle is then pulled upward at an angle

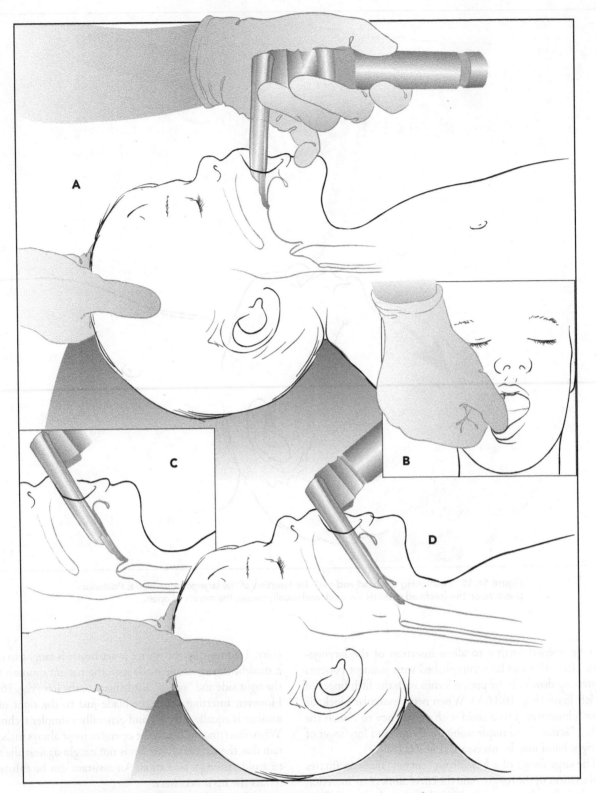

Figure 16.16   Direct laryngoscopy using a straight blade.
A. The head is positioned with the right hand, and the mouth is opened using the fifth finger of the left hand (if necessary).
B. Alternatively, the mouth may be opened with the thumb and index finger of the right hand using a "scissor" technique.
C. The laryngoscope blade is inserted under direct vision over the tongue and into the vallecula. One attempt may be made at this point to elevate the epiglottis by lifting upward on the laryngoscope handle at a 45-degree angle.
D. If unsuccessful, the tip of the blade is used to directly retract the epiglottis, revealing the vocal cords and glottic opening.

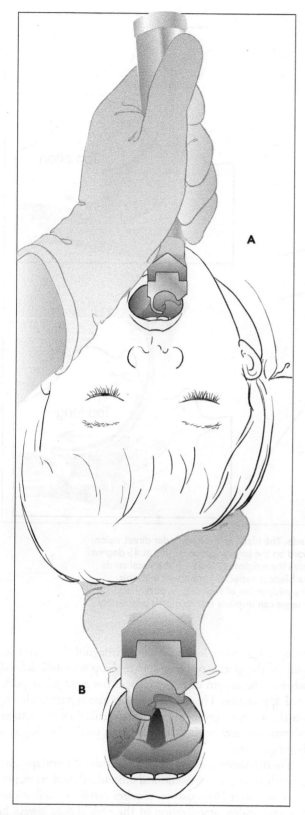

Figure 16.17
A. Inserting the straight laryngoscope blade from the right.
B. "Sweeping" the tongue to the left.

of approximately 45 degrees relative to the patient (Fig. 16.16C). The operator must take care to avoid levering the laryngoscope blade on the maxillary teeth or alveolar ridge, as this may result in tooth avulsion or gingival injury. Moreover, even though levering the blade may sometimes marginally improve the view of the larynx, the patient's mouth opening will be compromised, making it more difficult to pass the endotracheal tube. These problems are best avoided by always pulling along the axis of the handle and minimizing any rotation of the wrist.

Once the tongue and soft tissues are retracted, the important structures of the extrathoracic airway must be identified. When using a straight blade, the next step is to elevate the epiglottis so that the glottic opening can be visualized. This can be accomplished using one of two methods. The technique used most commonly is to insert the tip of the blade below (or posterior to) the epiglottis and then lifting it directly (Fig. 16.16D). Because the epiglottis is relatively large and floppy, and airway secretions make it prone to slip off the blade, this is generally the most difficult aspect of direct laryngoscopy with a straight blade. A superior approach is to make one attempt to elevate the epiglottis by advancing the tip of the blade into the vallecula and lifting upward, much in the same way that a curved blade is used (see next paragraph). In addition to being easier to perform, this method has the advantage of minimizing trauma to the epiglottis, which is not directly instrumented. Unfortunately, the operator will not always obtain an adequate view of the glottic opening, because the relatively large, floppy epiglottis of a child may not be sufficiently retracted. In such cases, the standard method of lifting the epiglottis with the tip of the blade is then performed.

As mentioned previously, a curved laryngoscope blade is inserted in the mouth just to the right of the midline following the contour of the tongue. The blade is advanced under direct visualization down the base of the tongue into the vallecula (Fig. 16.18). Estimating the proper size of a curved blade to be used for a pediatric patient is crucial to successful laryngoscopy. If the laryngoscope blade is too large, the tip will force the epiglottis down, obscuring the glottic opening; if the blade is too small, the tongue and epiglottis may not be adequately retracted. Once the laryngoscope blade is inserted, the operator pulls upward on the handle at a 45-degree angle relative to the patient to retract the tongue. This is done in exactly the same manner performed when using a straight blade. However, in this case upward tension on the hyoepiglottic ligament displaces the epiglottis so that the glottic opening can be visualized. The additional step of directly lifting the epiglottis with the tip of the blade is unnecessary. Although this method is almost always effective for older adolescents and adults, the large epiglottis and lax airway soft tissues of infants and children frequently make it impossible to adequately elevate the epiglottis using a curved blade. Even when proper technique is used, the operator will often pull upward on the laryngoscope handle only to find the epiglottis completely covering the glottic opening. For this reason, attempting

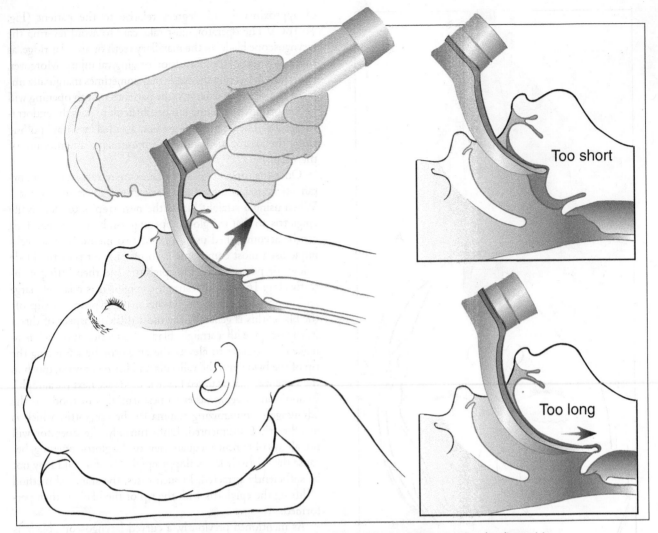

Figure 16.18 Direct laryngoscopy using a curved blade. The blade is inserted under direct vision until the tip is positioned in the vallecula. Pulling upward on the laryngoscope handle at 45-degree angle retracts the tongue and at the same time elevates the epiglottis, revealing the vocal cords and glottis. Selection of the appropriate laryngoscope blade is especially important with this technique. A blade that is too small will impinge on the midportion of the tongue, potentially obscuring the landmarks, whereas a blade that is too large can displace the epiglottis posteriorly over the glottic opening.

direct laryngoscopy using a curved blade is not recommended for younger patients.

Anatomic landmarks to be identified during direct laryngoscopy are shown in Figure 16.19. The epiglottis is a flat, elongated structure with an anterior attachment that drapes over the glottis like a hood. It appears omega-shaped in infants and younger children. Perhaps the most easily recognizable landmarks are the arytenoid cartilages, which are white structures on either side of and posterior to the glottic opening. In some cases, the arytenoids may not be visible until the epiglottis is retracted. The vocal cords are upright, slightly tilted structures that are separated by the dark midline space of the glottis. They can often be seen to move rhythmically with respirations if the patient is breathing. The most posterior structure seen during direct laryngoscopy is the esophagus. Although the esophagus is sometimes confused with the glot-

tic opening, certain features make it distinguishable. The margins of the glottic opening appear sharp and well defined, whereas the margin of the esophagus has a ridged or puckered appearance. The glottic opening also is surrounded by the characteristic geometric shapes of cartilaginous structures, whereas the area immediately adjacent to the esophagus is homogeneous.

For the patient with a potentially unstable cervical spine injury who undergoes conventional orotracheal intubation, performing direct laryngoscopy requires certain modifications. For one, in-line stabilization of the neck should always be provided by assistants (Fig. 16.20) (89–91). Because it may impede displacement of the chin and mandible, the front piece of the cervical collar is normally removed (or a one-piece collar is opened) before direct laryngoscopy and then subsequently replaced. In-line stabilization should be performed during

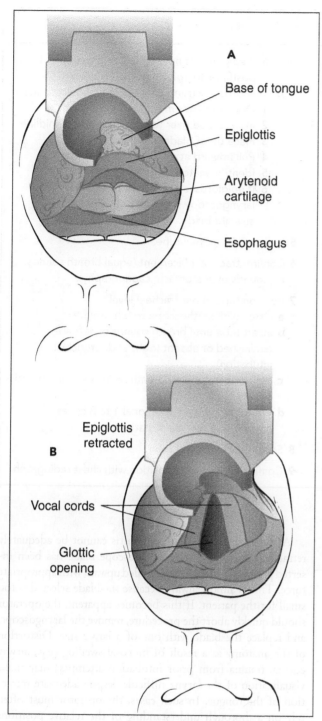

Figure 16.19 Anatomic landmarks for direct laryngoscopy.
A. After initial retraction of the tongue with a straight blade, the epiglottis may remain draped posteriorly, partially or completely covering the glottic opening.
B. Retraction of the epiglottis with the tip of the blade allows visualization of the glottis and surrounding structures.

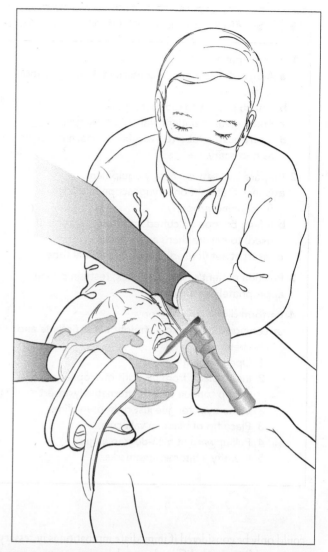

Figure 16.20 In-line stabilization of the head and neck. A second assistant should hold the shoulders in place against the stretcher to prevent movement of the torso.

this entire time, both to prevent any voluntary movements by an awake patient and to limit movement of the neck during direct laryngoscopy. To perform in-line stabilization, the assistant places his or her hands firmly on either side of the patient's head and maintains the neck in a neutral position.

To avoid interfering with the actions of the laryngoscopist, the assistant should kneel until his or her head is at or below the level of the patient. This technique must be explicitly distinguished from in-line traction, which involves pulling back on the patient's head along the axis of the body. Although previously recommended by many sources, in-line traction has been shown in cadaver models to increase subluxation of an unstable cervical spine and should not be performed (90). A second assistant should hold the patient's shoulders down against the stretcher to prevent movement of the upper torso (see also Fig. 24.7). As mentioned previously, another modification is that the operator must attempt to perform direct laryngoscopy causing as little movement of the patient's head and neck as possible. Maneuvers that involve significant flexion or extension of the neck, although sometimes necessary during a standard intubation, should be avoided when the patient has a potentially unstable cervical spine. Such maneuvers

SUMMARY: CONVENTIONAL OROTRACHEAL INTUBATION

1 Prepare patient.
  a Administer assisted or controlled BVM ventilation as needed.
  b Attach patient to monitoring devices.
  c Preoxygenate patient with 100% oxygen.
  d Insert gastric tube to evacuate stomach contents as necessary.

2 Prepare and test necessary equipment.
  a Check that light on laryngoscope blade is functioning properly.
  b Inflate balloon on cuffed endotracheal tube (if used) to ensure there are no leaks.
  c Insert stylet (if used) into endotracheal tube.

3 Position patient's head and neck; restrain patient appropriately as needed.

4 Perform direct laryngoscopy.
  a Laryngoscopy using a straight blade (infants and children):
    1 Open patient's mouth.
    2 Insert blade from far right of oropharynx and sweep tongue to left; alternatively, insert blade over tongue just right of midline.
    3 Place tip of blade in vallecula.
    4 Pull upward at a 45-degree angle.
    5 Identify anatomic landmarks.
    6 If epiglottis is not retracted, insert tip of blade posterior to epiglottis and lift upward.
  b Laryngoscopy using curved blade (adolescents):
    1 Open patient's mouth.
    2 Insert blade over tongue just right of midline.
    3 Place tip of blade in vallecula.
    4 Pull upward at a 45-degree angle.
    5 Identify anatomic landmarks.
    6 If epiglottis is not retracted, direct laryngoscopy should be attempted using straight blade.

5 Insert endotracheal tube.

6 Confirm tracheal placement (equal breath sounds, no sounds over stomach, capnography).

7 Position tube at midtracheal level.
  a Listen with stethoscope to left axilla.
  b Insert tube until breath sounds on left are diminished or absent (right endobronchial intubation).
  c Withdraw tube until breath sounds are first heard on left (tip at carina).
  d Withdraw tube an additional 1 to 3 cm as appropriate for age of patient.

8 Secure endotracheal tube.

9 Confirm proper tube position with chest radiograph.

---

could only be considered if immediate intubation is necessary to save the patient's life and no other airway intervention can be performed. In most cases, adequate oxygenation and ventilation can be achieved temporarily using a BVM circuit until an alternative method of securing the airway becomes possible.

A number of potential obstacles may be encountered during direct laryngoscopy that can limit the view of the larynx. Some of the more common problems include the presence of vomitus or secretions in the hypopharynx, difficulty in retracting the tongue and epiglottis, and anatomic variations or abnormalities. When copious secretions impair visualization, properly suctioning the oropharynx can be an important key to successful laryngoscopy (see also Chapter 13). Taking the time to obtain a clear field in the posterior hypopharynx can greatly facilitate identification of anatomic landmarks. A Yankauer or tonsil-tip suction device is usually most effective for older children and adolescents, although with children under 2 years, these larger devices may be too bulky. A 14 F multi-orifice, flexible suction catheter without a control valve (i.e., one that provides continuous suction) is therefore recommended for younger patients. Whatever device is used, the vacuum should be set at the maximum level of 200 cm H_2O.

At times the tongue and epiglottis cannot be adequately retracted even though the laryngoscope blade has been inserted properly and the handle pulled upward with appropriate force. This is almost always because the blade selected is too small for the patient. If this becomes apparent, the operator should quickly abort the procedure, remove the laryngoscope, and replace the blade with one of a larger size. Distortion of the anatomy as a result of mucosal swelling (e.g., airway edema, trauma from prior intubation attempts) may make visualization of the larynx difficult despite adequate retraction of the tongue. In such cases, the operator must often rely on a thorough understanding of the relative positions of the anatomic structures. For example, even if the vocal cords are not visible, the bright reflection of the arytenoids can be recognized in most instances. Once these landmarks are located, the operator then looks anteriorly along the midline to find the darkened silhouette of the glottic opening. If the difficulty is in locating the epiglottis, it may be helpful to intentionally insert the laryngoscope blade into the esophagus and then slowly remove it. As the blade is withdrawn, the epiglottis will fall into view. Although often effective, this technique should only be used when other methods have failed, because abrasion of the epiglottis may cause

CLINICAL TIPS: CONVENTIONAL OROTRACHEAL INTUBATION

1 A straight laryngoscope blade should be used for infants and children. A curved blade may be used for adolescents.

2 Using the teeth or alveolar ridge as a "lever" for the laryngoscope blade must be carefully avoided, because this may cause tooth avulsion or gingival injury.

3 Inserting the tip of a straight blade into the vallecula of an infant or younger child and then lifting upward will often expose the glottic opening without causing trauma to the epiglottis. Making one such attempt with each intubation is recommended. If this fails, the standard method of directly retracting the epiglottis with the tip of the blade can then be used.

4 In-line stabilization of the head and neck is necessary whenever conventional orotracheal intubation is performed on the patient who has a potentially unstable cervical spine.

5 If the vocal cords are not visible during direct laryngoscopy, the bright white reflection of the arytenoid cartilages may be used as a landmark. The glottic opening is anterior to these structures in the midline.

6 To identify the epiglottis during a difficult laryngoscopy, the operator may intentionally insert the laryngoscope blade into the esophagus and then gradually withdraw it until the epiglottis falls into view. However, this should not be performed routinely, because abrasion of the epiglottis can lead to swelling.

7 The endotracheal tube should be inserted so that the concavity is in a somewhat horizontal plane rather than perfectly upright. The tube also should be inserted from the right side of the oropharynx (an assistant can be enlisted to retract the cheek as necessary). These maneuvers will prevent the tube from obscuring the operator's view of the glottic opening.

8 The operator should make certain to use both eyes when inserting the endotracheal tube to preserve binocular vision and depth perception.

9 A plan should always be formulated for using an alternative intubation approach if conventional orotracheal intubation is unsuccessful.

swelling and make subsequent laryngoscopy attempts more difficult.

If the angle of entry into the trachea is especially severe, any attempts at visualizing the larynx may be obstructed by the base of the tongue. In this situation, further extension of the neck, well beyond the normal position achieved during laryngoscopy, may bring the desired structures into view. Simultaneous cricoid pressure also may be effective in displacing the trachea posteriorly so that the glottic opening can be seen. If these measures fail, it may be necessary to use more resourceful methods. One approach is to insert the laryngoscope blade and retract the tongue in the normal fashion with the left hand while using the right hand to manipulate the anterior neck to achieve a favorable position of the larynx. The operator may apply cricoid pressure or shift the laryngeal structures to the right or left as necessary. Once the glottic opening is in view, an assistant can be instructed to position the larynx in the exact same manner while the operator continues to retract the patient's tongue with the laryngoscope. When the glottis is again visualized, the operator can then insert the endotracheal tube.

Inserting the Endotracheal Tube

After the operator has successfully performed direct laryngoscopy, the next task is to insert the endotracheal tube through the glottic opening and into the trachea. Ideally, once the anatomic landmarks are visualized, the operator will not have to shift his or her gaze or concentration from these structures until the patient is intubated. Losing a clear view of the vocal cords because of a distraction requires the operator to readjust the laryngoscope and prolong the period of apnea. Once again, the aid of an assistant can be very helpful. When the glottis is visualized, the operator holds out his or her right hand, without diverting attention from the patient, and receives the endotracheal tube from the assistant. If no assistant is available, the tube should be placed in a nearby position where it can be easily retrieved "by feel."

As mentioned previously, we recommend using a stylet for all conventional orotracheal intubations. The endotracheal tube is held between the thumb and first two fingers of the right hand (Fig. 16.21). If the natural arc of the tube is imagined as occupying a single plane, one common error is to insert the tube so that this plane is perfectly vertical (i.e., with the tube concave directly upward). In the small opening of a pediatric airway, this often results in having both the tube and the operator's hand obstruct the line of vision. A superior method is to insert the tube in a more horizontal plane, which allows the operator to keep the cords in constant view while watching the tip enter the glottic opening. The tube can then be rotated into the vertical plane after intubation is accomplished. Another technique that will aid the operator in maintaining visualization of the vocal cords is to introduce the endotracheal tube into the patient's mouth somewhat right of the midline. This also keeps the tip of the tube from blocking the operator's view. Although this may sometimes be difficult with a younger patient because of the small size of the mouth,

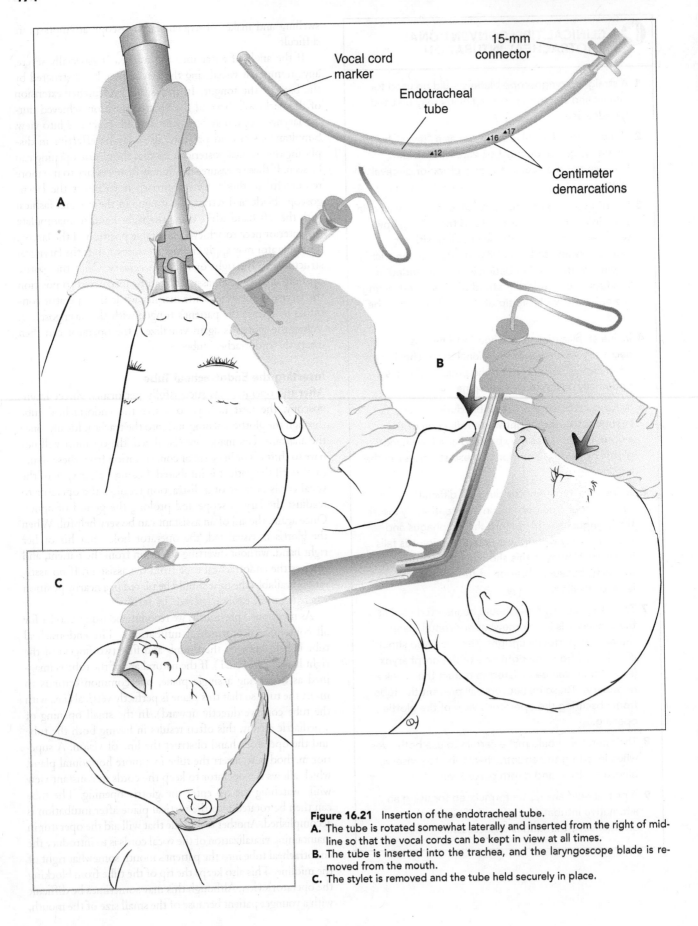

Figure 16.21 Insertion of the endotracheal tube.
A. The tube is rotated somewhat laterally and inserted from the right of midline so that the vocal cords can be kept in view at all times.
B. The tube is inserted into the trachea, and the laryngoscope blade is removed from the mouth.
C. The stylet is removed and the tube held securely in place.

enlisting the aid of an assistant to retract the right cheek will generally provide the additional space needed.

While inserting the endotracheal tube, the operator should always stay far enough back from the patient to preserve binocular vision. Getting so close that both eyes are not used (or closing one eye to "aim") causes the operator to lose valuable depth perception. As with threading a needle, inserting an endotracheal tube is greatly facilitated by using both eyes. Occasionally the angled tip of a styleted endotracheal tube will impinge on the anterior wall of the trachea after insertion, preventing further entry of the tube. If this happens, the tube should be advanced as the stylet is carefully removed, in much the same manner that an intravenous catheter is advanced off the needle into a vein.

Another potential problem occurs when the vocal cords are tightly constricted during a prolonged cough or a mild episode of laryngospasm, temporarily making insertion of the endotracheal tube impossible. In most cases, the operator need only wait a few seconds until the patient takes a breath, at which time the vocal cords will abduct, allowing the tube to pass. If this does not happen after 15 to 20 seconds, the patient may be experiencing a more significant episode of laryngospasm that will not resolve spontaneously, requiring the administration of a rapid-onset muscle relaxant (see Chapter 15).

Although relatively uncommon, occasional instances will occur in which the glottic opening cannot be identified despite appropriate laryngoscopy technique. In such cases, it may be necessary to insert the endotracheal tube without direct visualization. If the epiglottis is the only recognizable structure, the operator uses a styleted endotracheal tube that has a 90-degree angle 2 to 3 cm from the tip. The tube is slipped under the epiglottis and advanced in the most anterior trajectory possible along the midline. This will normally result in successful intubation of the trachea. It should be emphasized that inserting an endotracheal tube in this manner without direct visualization significantly increases the likelihood of esophageal intubation. Confirmation of proper tube position is therefore especially important. If no alternative technique of intubation can be immediately performed, however, this method is worth a single attempt before undertaking an emergent surgical airway. Because of the risks associated with this method, it should only be performed by the most experienced available operator. In all cases, the most effective and reliable way of avoiding an esophageal intubation is to directly observe the tube as it passes between the vocal cords into the trachea.

Once the patient is intubated, the tube should be held securely in place at all times with the thumb and index finger while the other three fingers rest against the patient's face (Fig. 16.21C). Maintaining contact in this way ensures that the operator's hand will follow any unexpected movements of the patient's head so that the tube does not become accidentally dislodged. Confirmation of the appropriate depth of insertion and securing the tube in place are performed as described below (see "Postintubation Care").

 SUMMARY: BLIND NASOTRACHEAL INTUBATION

1 Prepare patient.
  a Attach patient to monitoring devices.
  b Apply topical anesthetic and topical vasoconstrictor to nasal mucosa.
  c Administer mild sedative as needed.
  d Position patient sitting upright with hands gently restrained as necessary.
  e Preoxygenate patient with 100% oxygen.

2 Select an endotracheal tube and test balloon for any leaks.

3 Check nares for patency by occluding each one in turn.

4 If right nostril is patent, insert the tube on this side (concave downward) so that bevel faces nasal septum. If right nostril is not patent, insert the tube on left side by inverting it (concave upward). Once tip reaches posterior pharynx, rotate the tube back to normal position.

5 Insert tube until tip reaches supraglottic region; listen for breath sounds through tube and observe for fogging of tube with respirations.

6 Advance tube until breath sounds are lost (esophageal placement) and withdraw it a few centimeters so that tip is just proximal to glottis (optional).

7 Listen to breath sounds for a few seconds to get a sense of their rhythm.

8 Advance tube briskly at moment patient starts inspiration.

9 Any recognizable vocalizations (talking, moaning, etc.) indicate esophageal placement.

10 Confirm tracheal placement (equal breath sounds, no sounds over stomach, capnography).

11 After successful intubation, inflate balloon and secure tube.

12 Confirm proper tube placement with chest radiograph.

Blind Nasotracheal Intubation

As discussed in the "Indications" section, this approach is only rarely used with pediatric patients. The more cephalad position of the larynx in younger patients does not allow the glottic opening to align with the nasopharyngeal air passage. Consequently, blind passage of the tube is virtually impossible with infants and children. Furthermore, a significant degree of

CLINICAL TIPS: BLIND NASOTRACHEAL INTUBATION

▶ If blind nasotracheal intubation is unsuccessful after three or four attempts, an alternative method should be used.

▶ This procedure is best suited for adolescents. Children are rarely if ever good candidates for blind nasotracheal intubation.

▶ If the tip of the endotracheal tube gets caught in one of the pyriform sinuses, the operator will appreciate a bulge lateral to the midline on either side of the neck. In such cases, the tube should be rotated back to a midline position before the next attempt at passage.

▶ If the tip of the tube gets caught in the vallecula or anterior commissure of the vocal cords, the operator will appreciate a bulge in the submental region of the neck. In such cases, the patient's neck should be flexed somewhat before the next attempt at passage.

▶ If the tube persistently enters the esophagus, the following may be effective: (a) using an Endotrol tube and pulling the ring to deflect the tip anteriorly, (b) applying cricoid pressure during insertion, and (c) extending the patient's neck.

▶ If the ring of an Endotrol tube sits tightly against the nose after insertion, the ligature should be cut and the ring removed. Otherwise, tension on the ligature will cause the tube to exert continuous anterior pressure on the trachea.

patient cooperation is required to perform this procedure successfully. A crying, struggling child is not a candidate for blind nasotracheal intubation. Finally, the likelihood of passing the tube through the vocal cords is substantially increased when the patient is making strong respiratory efforts. An adult patient with an exacerbation of emphysema or congestive heart failure normally has a deep, prolonged inspiratory phase during which the vocal cords are widely abducted. This greatly facilitates blind insertion of the tube. Conditions requiring emergent intubation that cause a similar increased respiratory effort among children are relatively uncommon. Thus the most likely pediatric patient for whom blind nasotracheal intubation might prove useful would be a cooperative adolescent with status asthmaticus or, in rare cases, severe congestive heart failure or RDS. Although it is sometimes advocated for pediatric trauma patients requiring cervical spine immobilization, experience has shown that blind nasotracheal intubation is extremely difficult to perform successfully even in the most

favorable circumstances. It is contraindicated for the child with a bleeding tumor or abscess above the glottis due to the risk of hemorrhage and further encroachment of the airway (92).

With those caveats in mind, it is worth reviewing the potential benefits of blind nasotracheal intubation. The most important advantage is that the patient is awake and maintains spontaneous respirations and intact airway reflexes at all times, eliminating risks associated with the administration of anesthetic agents or neuromuscular blockade. Aspiration of gastric contents is rare, and if the procedure is unsuccessful, the patient is still conscious and breathing ("no bridges are burned"). An adolescent patient with airway anomalies who is suspected of having a potentially difficult airway or for whom manual ventilation may be problematic might well be considered for this approach. The second major advantage is that many of the potential complications associated with direct laryngoscopy are avoided (tooth avulsion, lip or tongue laceration, etc.). Used in the appropriate circumstances, blind nasotracheal intubation offers a safe, controlled method for securing the airway (93–96). Nasotracheal intubation under direct laryngoscopic visualization is rarely performed on an emergent basis and is therefore not discussed here. Readers interested in information on this approach are referred to standard pediatric anesthesiology texts.

Before performing a blind nasotracheal intubation, the operator should take steps to minimize any discomfort experienced by the patient. This not only makes the procedure as humane as possible, but because patient cooperation is so essential, it also increases the likelihood of success. Enhancement of patient tolerance is best achieved by the application of topical anesthesia to the airway mucosa. Because a few minutes must pass before the full anesthetic effect is achieved, this should be one of the first steps performed. For most patients, spraying the hypopharynx with a topical anesthetic (e.g., Cetacaine) and instilling a small amount of lidocaine jelly into the nares are sufficient to produce adequate anesthesia. Both nares are anesthetized so that if one side does not permit insertion of the tube, passage can be attempted on the other side without delay. Transtracheal instillation of 1% (10 mg/mL) lidocaine solution also can be performed to provide a greater degree of anesthesia (Fig. 16.22), although this is not generally required to successfully perform a blind nasotracheal intubation. Whatever methods are used, the operator must make certain that the maximum allowable dosage of lidocaine (approximately 5 to 7 mg/kg) is not exceeded. Another possible option for enhancing patient cooperation is to administer a small dose of an intravenous sedative such as midazolam (0.1 mg/kg). Although judicious doses of a sedative may facilitate the procedure, deep sedation is obviously not appropriate, because the primary aim with this approach is to maintain airway reflexes. With a mature adolescent who is fully cooperative, sedation is usually unnecessary.

Preparation of the nasal mucosa also includes application of a topical vasoconstrictor to decrease mucosal edema and limit potential bleeding. Significant epistaxis often will force

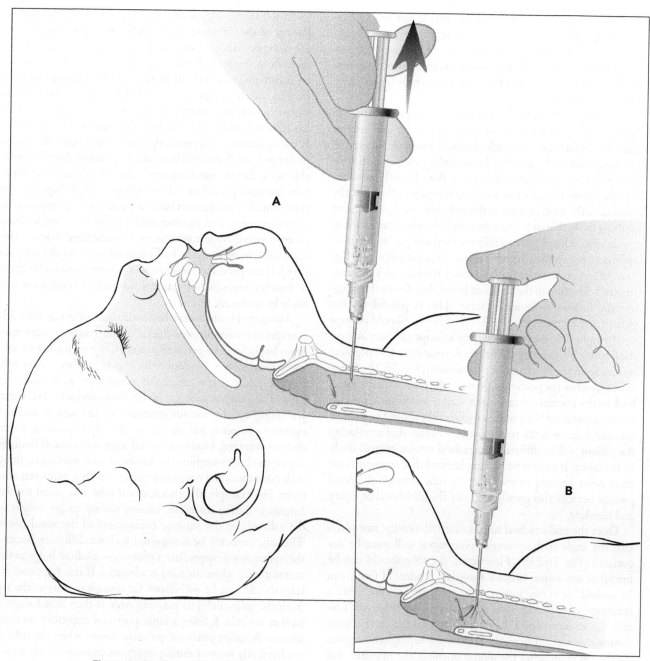

Figure 16.22 Transtracheal anesthesia.
A. The needle is advanced through the cricothyroid membrane with negative pressure on the syringe. Entry into the trachea is indicated by the appearance of bubbles in the syringe.
B. Lidocaine is injected into the trachea, and the needle is rapidly removed to avoid injury to the vocal cords when the patient coughs.

the operator to abort this approach. Phenylephrine spray (0.25%) can be used if it is the only available agent, but oxymetazoline spray (0.05%) is preferred because it has no potential for causing systemic hypertension. For adolescent patients, topical phenylephrine should be diluted to 0.1% and the total dose limited to 2 to 3 mL. As with application of the topical anesthesia, the vasoconstrictor should be applied 2 to 4 minutes before performing the procedure so that the full effect is obtained.

Unfortunately, no simple formulas are available for determining the proper tube size for a blind nasotracheal intubation. Because this procedure will rarely be performed with a child younger than 8 years, a cuffed tube will virtually always be necessary. In general, the internal diameter of the tube used with this approach should be 0.5 to 1 mm smaller than one that would be appropriate for a conventional orotracheal intubation. For example, if a patient is estimated to require a 7.0-mm internal diameter (ID) tube for an oral intubation, a reasonable first choice for a nasal intubation would be a 6.5- or 6.0-mm ID tube. The tube must be large enough to adequately ventilate the patient without being so large that the nasal mucosa is injured during insertion. In addition, pressure on the nasal mucosa from a tube that fits too tightly may cause ulceration and necrosis over time.

The patient should be positioned sitting upright with the hands gently restrained as necessary to prevent grabbing at the tube. Before the endotracheal tube is inserted, patency of the nares should be assessed by occluding each one in turn and observing any obstruction to air flow. If both nares are equally patent, the tube is inserted on the right side so that the bevel faces the nasal septum, as this will decrease the chances of injuring the turbinates. The tube is held concave downward in the dominant hand and carefully inserted using a "straight in" approach, perpendicular to the plane of the patient's face (Fig. 16.23A). A common error is to insert the tube in a superior (rostral) direction in the mistaken belief that the nasal passage initially follows an upward course. This is painful for the patient and increases the likelihood of injury. Should passage on the right side prove difficult, an attempt can be made on the left side by inverting the tube (i.e., rotating it 180 degrees) so that again the bevel will face the septum (Fig. 16.24). Once the tip reaches the posterior pharynx, the tube is then rotated back to the normal concave downward orientation. If passage is unsuccessful on both sides, a smaller tube should be used. If this also fails, or if the tube must be so small that ventilating the patient will be difficult, orotracheal intubation will likely be necessary. It cannot be overemphasized that excessive force must never be used in inserting the tube through the nasal passage because this greatly increases the likelihood of injury and bleeding.

Once the endotracheal tube is inserted into the nasopharynx, the angle at the posterior pharyngeal wall must be negotiated (Fig. 16.23B). Here again, the tube should not be forced at any point, because tonsillar or adenoid tissue can be avulsed, or in rare instances the tube can actually create a traumatic false passage into the posterior hypopharynx. Ideally, the endotracheal tube should be inserted in one easy, continuous motion from the nose to the supraglottic region. As the tip approaches the glottic opening, the operator will begin to see fogging of the tube with each expiration and hear breath sounds transmitted through the tube. Slowly advancing the endotracheal tube until these signs are lost and then withdrawing slightly ensures that the tip is positioned just superior to the glottic opening (Fig. 16.23C). If breath sounds are difficult to appreciate through the tube because of a noisy environment or the patient's poor respiratory effort, using a BAAM (Beck airway airflow monitor) may assist the operator in positioning the tube (97,98). This simple and inexpensive device, which fits on the proximal opening of an endotracheal tube, has a small aperture that makes a distinctive whistling sound even when the patient has diminished respirations. Location of the tip of the endotracheal tube at the proper level is indicated when this whistling sound is most prominent.

At this point, the operator is ready to intubate the trachea. Passage of the tube must be carefully timed with the patient's respirations so that the vocal cords will be fully abducted when the tube is inserted. A useful practice is to spend a few seconds listening to the respirations to get a good sense of their rhythm. At the moment the patient first begins inspiration, when exposure and patency of the glottic opening are greatest, the tube is briskly advanced into the trachea (Fig. 16.23D). If the operator is successful, the patient will normally have a prolonged cough and will be unable to phonate. Any recognizable vocalization (speaking, moaning, etc.) indicates that the tube has been passed into the esophagus. If this happens, the tube should be withdrawn back to a point just superior to the glottic opening, and another attempt should be made using an appropriate corrective maneuver as described below. After successful intubation, the balloon is inflated and the tube secured. If the procedure has not been accomplished after three to four attempts, a conventional orotracheal intubation will likely be necessary.

Although blind nasotracheal intubation offers distinct advantages in the appropriate clinical circumstances, it can sometimes be difficult to perform successfully even for the experienced practitioner. Undoubtedly, this is another reason why this procedure is not commonly performed on an emergent basis. The primary problem is that the endotracheal tube can get "hung up" by various structures in the airway, and the operator obviously has no way of directly visualizing where this has occurred. However, several suggestive clinical findings can be used to determine the nature of such problems, along with corresponding corrective maneuvers that may overcome them. For example, the endotracheal tube may travel too far anteriorly during insertion, causing the tip to get caught in the vallecula or the anterior commissure of the vocal cords. This can normally be recognized without difficulty because the operator will appreciate a prominent midline bulge in the anterior neck when the tube is advanced. If this happens, the tube should first be withdrawn far enough to remove the tip from the vallecula. The patient's neck is then flexed slightly so that the tube follows a more posterior trajectory on reinsertion. Another potential problem occurs when the tube is inadvertently rotated during insertion, causing the tip to get caught in one of the piriform sinuses. This also can be identified based on the presence of a bulge in the neck, although in this case it will be somewhat lateral to the midline on either side. To reposition the tip in the midline, the operator rotates the proximal end of the tube away from the involved piriform sinus. In other words, if the tip is caught in the left piriform sinus, the tube is rotated in a clockwise direction; if the tip is caught in the right piriform sinus, the tube is rotated counterclockwise.

As mentioned, one of the most common problems with blind nasotracheal intubation occurs when the angle of entry into the trachea is so acute that the tube persistently passes into the esophagus. In most instances, this results from a particularly cephalad location of the trachea, which makes negotiating the turn at the base of the tongue more difficult

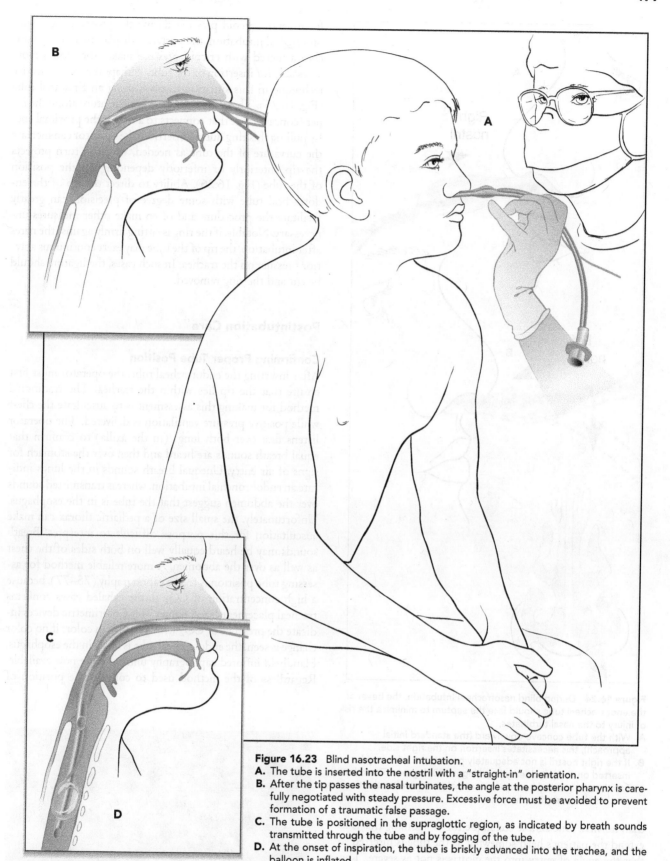

Figure 16.23 Blind nasotracheal intubation.
A. The tube is inserted into the nostril with a "straight-in" orientation.
B. After the tip passes the nasal turbinates, the angle at the posterior pharynx is carefully negotiated with steady pressure. Excessive force must be avoided to prevent formation of a traumatic false passage.
C. The tube is positioned in the supraglottic region, as indicated by breath sounds transmitted through the tube and by fogging of the tube.
D. At the onset of inspiration, the tube is briskly advanced into the trachea, and the balloon is inflated.

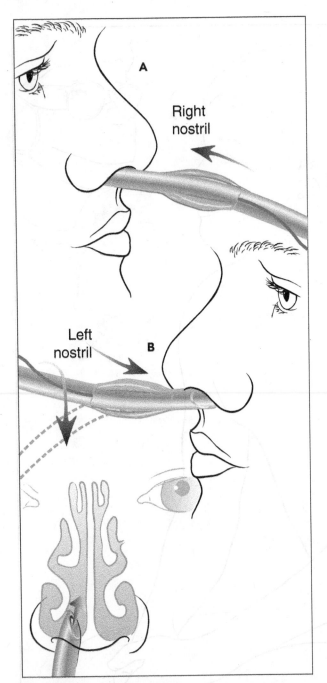

Figure 16.24 During blind nasotracheal intubation, the bevel of the endotracheal tube should face the septum to minimize the risk of injury to the nasal turbinates.

A. With the tube concave downward (the standard initial approach), this necessitates insertion on the right side.

B. If the right nostril is not adequately patent, the tube may be inserted on the left side by inverting it 180 degrees. The tube can then be rotated back to the normal position after the tip reaches the posterior pharynx.

than normal. One simple technique for overcoming this is to extend the patient's head somewhat as the tube is inserted so that the angle of entry into the glottis is not as severe. This often allows the normal curvature of the tube to project the tip far enough anteriorly that it will enter the glottic opening. Another method is to enlist the aid of an assistant to per-

form gentle cricoid pressure during the procedure. As with orotracheal intubation, the posterior displacement of the trachea achieved with cricoid pressure makes the glottis more accessible for insertion of the tube. Perhaps the most effective technique in this situation involves using an Endotrol tube (Fig. 16.25). These tubes have a plastic ligature along the inner (concave) side that connects to a ring at the proximal end. By pulling this ring during insertion, the operator can increase the curvature of the tube as needed, which in turn projects the tip anteriorly or inferiorly depending on the position of the tube (Fig. 16.26). Ability to direct the tip of the endotracheal tube with some degree of precision can greatly facilitate the procedure and often make other measures unnecessary. Notably, if the ring is sitting firmly against the nares after intubation, the tip of the tube may exert continuous anterior pressure on the trachea. In such cases, the ligature should be cut and the ring removed.

Postintubation Care

Confirming Proper Tube Position

After inserting the endotracheal tube, the operator must first ensure that the tip lies within the trachea. The traditional method for making this assessment is to auscultate the chest while positive pressure ventilation is delivered. The operator listens first over both lungs (in the axilla) to confirm that equal breath sounds are heard and then over the stomach for signs of air entry. Unequal breath sounds in the lungs indicate an endobronchial intubation, whereas transmitted sounds over the abdomen suggest that the tube is in the esophagus. Unfortunately, the small size of a pediatric thorax can make auscultation for this purpose difficult to interpret. Breath sounds may be heard equally well on both sides of the chest as well as over the abdomen. A more reliable method for assessing tube position is to use capnography (75–77), because a high concentration of CO_2 in the exhaled gases confirms tracheal placement (see Chapter 76). Colorimetric devices indicate the presence of CO_2 with a change in color; if no color change is seen, the endotracheal tube is likely in the esophagus. Handheld infrared capnography units also are now available. Regardless of the method used to confirm the position of

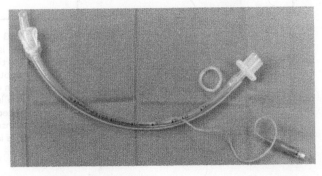

Figure 16.25 Endotrol tube.

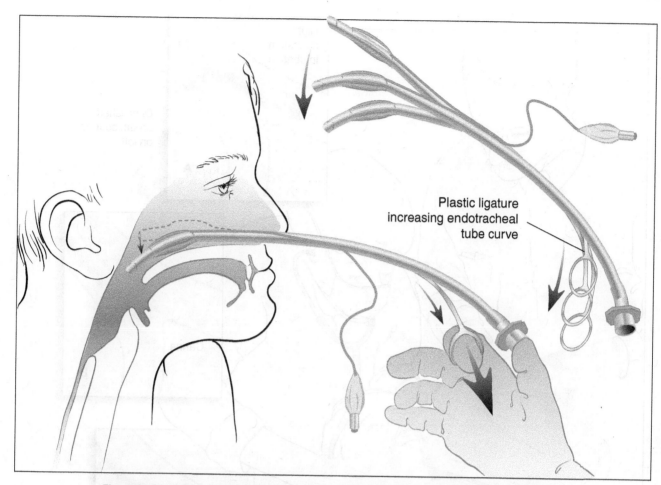

Figure 16.26 Pulling the ring of an Endotrol tube exerts tension on the plastic ligature, which in turn increases the curvature of the tube. In this way, the operator can direct the tip to some extent during insertion. This facilitates passage of the tube at the posterior pharynx by deflecting the tip inferiorly. In addition, persistent passage of the tube into the esophagus when the patient has a more superiorly positioned trachea also may be overcome using this technique.

Plastic ligature increasing endotracheal tube curve

the endotracheal tube, the importance of this step cannot be overstated, because an unrecognized esophageal intubation is associated with significant potential morbidity or mortality. Additional findings that may be useful in distinguishing tracheal versus esophageal intubation are listed in Table 16.10.

TABLE 16.10	SIGNS INDICATING TUBE PLACEMENT IN THE TRACHEA

Most reliable
  Capnography
  Direct visualization of tube insertion through vocal cords
Less reliable
  Equal breath sounds in both lungs
  No breath sounds over stomach
  Symmetric rise of chest wall
  "Fogging" of endotracheal tube with expiration
  No gastric distension
  Consistently high oxygen saturation by pulse oximetry

The operator must next position the tube at the proper depth of insertion within the trachea. The ideal location for the tip of the endotracheal tube is at the midpoint between the thoracic inlet and the carina. If the tip is too high (rostral), it may become dislodged from the trachea with any movement of the patient. If the tip is too low (caudal), it increases the risk of endobronchial intubation with changes in head position. For infants and young children, the proper position will normally be 1 to 2 cm above the carina. For children over the age of 5 to 6 years, this distance may be increased to 3 cm (99). With adults, positioning the endotracheal tube correctly can generally be ensured by placing a given external demarcation on the tube at the incisors. Unfortunately, no such single measurement applies to the various sizes of infants and children. Age- and weight-dependent formulas have been devised for this purpose, but these can be difficult to recall or calculate during a resuscitation. One favored method is shown in Figure 16.27. After the endotracheal tube is inserted into the trachea, the operator first confirms that equal breath sounds are heard on both sides of the chest as positive pressure ventilation is

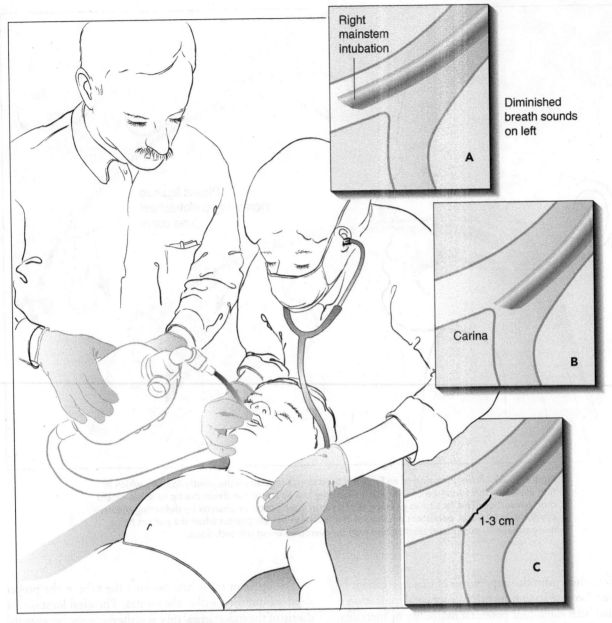

Figure 16.27 Confirming the proper depth of the tube insertion.
A. While auscultating the left chest, the operator advances the endotracheal tube until breath sounds are diminished or absent (right mainstem intubation).
B. The tube is then withdrawn until breath sounds are first heard again normally on the left, indicating the tip is just proximal to the carina.
C. The tube is then withdrawn an additional 1 to 3 cm (depending on the age and size of the patient) to achieve proper midtracheal positioning of the tip.

delivered. While listening continuously with the stethoscope to the left chest at the axilla, the operator then advances the tube until a decrease in the breath sounds is heard (right endobronchial intubation). Because the breath sounds are so well transmitted in the chest of a child, it is not necessary to advance the tube until breath sounds disappear entirely, as this usually indicates that the tube has passed several branches in the airway. At this point, the tube is slowly withdrawn to the point where breath sounds are first well heard again on the left, indicating that the tip is at the level of the carina. Finally, the operator withdraws the tube an additional 1 to 3 cm so that the tip is located at the midtracheal position. Aside from being relatively simple to perform, primary advantages of this method are that it is applicable to any age group, it provides consistently reliable results, and it does not involve memorized formulas (99). Definitive confirmation of proper tube position should always be obtained with a chest radiograph.

Positive Pressure Ventilation

Immediately after intubation, the patient should receive positive pressure ventilation delivered using a resuscitation bag attached to the endotracheal tube. A thorough description of the various features of self-inflating bags and conventional anesthesia circuits is given in Chapter 14. The patient should always initially receive the highest concentration of oxygen the circuit is capable of administering; the concentration can later be adjusted as appropriate. Because the exact tidal volume delivered with a resuscitation bag cannot be easily measured, the operator should squeeze the bag with sufficient force to produce chest excursions similar to normal spontaneous respirations. Consistently inadequate tidal volumes will result in the retention of CO_2, whereas excessive tidal volumes can cause a pneumothorax. Occasionally, the proper size of an uncuffed endotracheal tube is significantly underestimated, resulting in an excessive air leak during positive pressure ventilation. So much air may escape that delivering an adequate tidal volume is impossible. If this is the case, it will be necessary to remove the endotracheal tube and replace it with a larger size and/or use a cuffed tube. As discussed previously, this is one reason that cuffed endotracheal tubes are now recommended as an acceptable option for all pediatric patients except neonates (72). Once the operator has established that the endotracheal tube is in the correct position and positive pressure ventilation can be properly administered, mechanical ventilation can be safely initiated (see Chapter 82).

Securing the Tube

The final step of an intubation is to secure the endotracheal tube in such a way that it will not be accidentally dislodged from the trachea or further advanced into a mainstem bronchus. Before securing the tube, the operator should note mentally (and later document in the chart) the external centimeter marking on the tube that corresponds with the level of the central incisors or alveolar ridge. This should then be rechecked after the tube is secured to ensure that it has not been inadvertently advanced or withdrawn.

The most common method for securing an endotracheal tube is with standard adhesive tape, as shown in Figure 16.28. Applying tincture of benzoin to the face and tube before taping enhances adhesion. It is important to remember that with patients who are not paralyzed, securing the tube may also involve appropriately restraining the hands. For increased stability (e.g., before transport), the tape may be extended around the back of the patient's head, and then the tube is taped on both sides. Tracheotomy tapes may be used in a similar manner. Synthetic straps that have attachment devices, rather than adhesive, to hold the tube in place also are available commercially. The primary advantage of the synthetic straps is that the need for frequent retaping is eliminated, because there is no problem with decreased adhesion as a result of traction and contact with saliva. The disadvantage of tracheotomy tapes is that they must be tied tightly to limit movement of the tube to less than 1 cm. This can lead to pressure necrosis

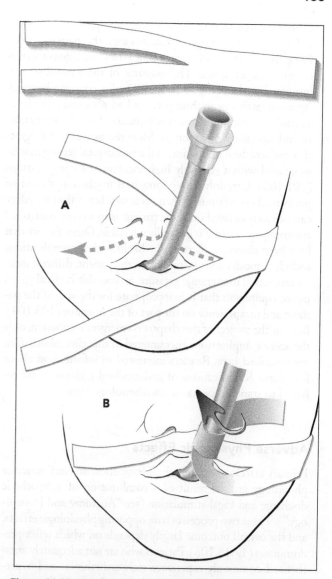

Figure 16.28 Securing the endotracheal tube.
A. The tape is split into a Y and the base is applied to the cheek.
B. One strip of tape is then applied to the skin above or below the lips while the other secures the tube. A second piece of tape may be applied from the other side in a similar manner for greater stability. Tincture of benzoin also may be used to increase adhesion.

of the skin under the ties over time. Placing gauze padding under the ties reduces the likelihood of this problem.

▶ COMPLICATIONS

Several potential complications can occur during an emergent endotracheal intubation. Clearly the most effective way to avoid any possible risk of such complications is to refrain from attempting the procedure in the first place. This raises the question of when *not* to perform an emergent intubation. In a review of complications associated with endotracheal intubation of pediatric trauma patients, Nakayama et al. (100)

contended that in over 30% of cases the procedure was not indicated on an emergent basis because the patients had a Glasgow coma score of greater than 10 and no signs of airway compromise or apnea. The majority of these patients were intubated at the scene or in the ED of a referring hospital. Approximately one in three patients had what was considered a significant complication, which included vocal cord paralysis and aspiration pneumonitis. More recent evidence suggests that endotracheal intubation in the prehospital setting may be associated with a relatively high incidence of complications (101,102). Certainly, an endotracheal intubation should be performed expeditiously when necessary, but if the procedure can be safely delayed until the patient is in a more controlled environment, waiting is generally advisable. Other factors that have been shown to increase the likelihood of complications include hemodynamic instability of the patient, difficult intubation, raised intracranial pressure, an unstable cervical spine, use of equipment that is inappropriate for the size of the patient, and inexperience on the part of the operator (103,104). Because the subject of this chapter is emergent intubation, only the acute complications encountered in this clinical situation are described here. Readers interested in information about long-term complications of endotracheal intubation are referred to standard pediatric anesthesiology texts.

Adverse Physiologic Effects

Primary effects of endotracheal intubation on cardiovascular physiology are the result of a combination of sympathetic discharge and vagal stimulation (see "Anatomy and Physiology"). These two processes have opposing physiologic effects, and the overall outcome largely depends on which reflex predominates (17,18,105). Patients who are not adequately anesthetized commonly experience tachyarrhythmias and hypertension from sympathetic stimulation. Occasionally patients develop profound bradycardia and hypotension because of vagal effects. Infants and younger children may be particularly susceptible to this response (17). Bradycardia also can be the result of hypoxemia during an excessively prolonged intubation attempt. The likelihood of significant bradycardia can be decreased by administering atropine before the procedure (see Chapter 15).

Another immediate adverse physiologic effect of endotracheal intubation is increased intracranial pressure. Exactly why this occurs is not well understood, although it is likely due in part to a combination of elevated cerebral venous pressure (coughing, straining, changes in head position) and increased cerebral arterial pressure from the systemic hypertension that occurs during laryngoscopy (106–108). This effect normally has clinical significance only when pre-existing elevated intracranial pressure is exacerbated (ruptured cerebral aneurysm, epidural hematoma, etc.). In extreme cases, development of a cerebral herniation syndrome is possible. When the patient is at risk for these complications, pharmacologic agents that blunt the rise in intracranial pressure should be administered (see Chapter 15).

Inadequate Oxygenation

One of the most significant complications of endotracheal intubation is ischemic brain injury due to inadequate oxygenation. This can result from any of the following causes: (a) inability to provide adequate bag-valve-mask ventilatory support, (b) excessively prolonged laryngoscopy, (c) unrecognized esophageal intubation, (d) endobronchial intubation, (e) obstruction of the endotracheal tube, and (f) pneumothorax. Although a persistent episode of laryngospasm also can prevent oxygenation during laryngoscopy, this complication is rare. In most cases, laryngospasm is transient and subsides spontaneously after several seconds. As mentioned previously, a prolonged episode of laryngospasm requires administration of a rapid onset muscle relaxant. Esophageal intubation can result either from inadvertent insertion of the endotracheal tube into the esophagus or from subsequent movement of the patient's head that dislodges the tube from the trachea. This can normally be recognized through the use of pulse oximetry (Chapter 75) and capnography (Chapter 76) before any injury to the patient occurs. Capnography is the superior modality for identifying esophageal intubation because the capnograph will immediately display an abnormally low or absent CO_2 level (73,75–77).

Another potential cause of inadequate oxygenation is insertion of the endotracheal tube into a mainstem bronchus. This can result from advancing the tube too far into the trachea during intubation, from inadequately securing the tube, or from movement of the patient's head (109–112). After endotracheal intubation is performed, a chest radiograph should always be obtained to assess the location of the tube within the trachea. The tip of the endotracheal tube should lie halfway between the thoracic inlet and the carina. Should an endobronchial intubation occur, the patient will normally have a persistently low oxygen saturation measured by the pulse oximeter. A sudden rise in inspiratory pressures also may be necessary to expand the chest, as evidenced by greater difficulty performing manual ventilation or the necessity for higher peak inflating pressures from a mechanical ventilator. This complication is best avoided by performing serial auscultatory examinations of the chest to ensure that equal breath sounds are heard. Simple observation of the patient is not sufficient because chest excursion may appear symmetric despite endobronchial intubation. If this problem is suspected, the patient's head should be repositioned or the endotracheal tube withdrawn until equal breath sounds are heard in both lungs.

Impaired oxygenation also occurs when the endotracheal tube becomes partially obstructed. With infants, this may occur acutely when the tip of the tube abuts against the tracheal wall. The likelihood of this complication is increased when the infant's head is turned to one side and the bevel of the tube faces the opposite direction (113). Obstruction of the endotracheal tube from airway secretions is far more common, although this usually occurs after longer periods of intubation. Humidification of inspired gases is likely the most effective measure for avoiding this complication (114). Suctioning the endotracheal tube after instilling saline is normally sufficient to relieve a partial obstruction resulting from airway secretions. However, if the patient continues to have increased pulmonary resistance that cannot be explained by other factors, the endotracheal tube should be replaced.

Barotrauma

Pediatric patients are at greater risk than adults for sustaining barotrauma to the lungs from positive pressure ventilation primarily because infants and children have greater compliance of the ribs and chest wall musculature (115–117). The relatively diminished protective effects of chest wall resistance result in a greater likelihood of pulmonary overinflation and lung injury. Risk is further increased for children with an underlying lung disease such as cystic fibrosis or congenital lobar emphysema (118). Complications from barotrauma that are normally minor include pneumomediastinum, subcutaneous emphysema, and pneumopericardium. These are usually self-limited processes that typically do not require intervention. In rare cases, pneumopericardium can cause cardiac tamponade, necessitating emergent decompression. Complications from barotrauma more commonly associated with significant morbidity are pneumothorax and tension pneumothorax. Tube thoracostomy should be performed whenever a patient receiving positive pressure ventilations develops a pneumothorax. If a pneumothorax is not promptly recognized and treated appropriately in this setting, the patient is at increased risk for developing a tension pneumothorax, a potentially life-threatening complication. Characteristic findings of a tension pneumothorax include a tympanitic hemithorax with diminished breath sounds, hypotension, and deviation of the trachea. Management of pneumothorax and tension pneumothorax is described fully in Chapter 29.

Mechanical Trauma

The most common type of complication resulting from endotracheal intubation is mechanical trauma. Because the procedure involves relatively forceful manipulation and instrumentation of various structures of the head and neck, a wide array of injuries can occur, ranging from minor abrasions to potentially life-threatening hemorrhage. Although sometimes unavoidable, this type of complication can normally be minimized if the operator maintains a high degree of awareness and employs careful technique.

A relatively minor injury that can result during an intubation is corneal abrasion. Even such seemingly trivial actions as leaning a forearm against the patient's brow to steady the hand or inadvertently sweeping a sleeve over the patient's face can cause a corneal abrasion. Vigilance regarding the possibility of this complication is generally the most effective way of avoiding it. The teeth of older children (or the alveolar ridge of infants) also may be injured during an intubation. This usually results when the laryngoscope blade is used to lever the mouth open, with the teeth or gingiva serving as a fulcrum. This practice must be carefully avoided. Significant trauma to the gingiva of an infant can lead to abnormal tooth eruption or dental development (119). If a tooth is accidentally avulsed during intubation, it should be immediately retrieved to prevent aspiration of the tooth into the trachea. A "lost" tooth may well be found later on chest radiograph, located in a bronchus.

A potentially serious complication resulting from mechanical forces is airway bleeding, which usually results from injury to the nasal turbinates, adenoids, or palatine tonsils (104). Mucosal surfaces of these structures may be abraded by the laryngoscope blade or endotracheal tube, and if subjected to sufficient force, adenoids and palatine tonsils can be partially or completely avulsed. Such tissue avulsions can result in airway obstruction and bleeding. Direct laryngoscopy during an orotracheal intubation may result in injury to the tonsils, and significant epistaxis can occur with blind nasotracheal intubation (93–95). Percutaneous puncture of the cricothyroid membrane to perform transtracheal anesthesia also can cause bleeding in the airway. Although in most cases these are minor problems, representing more of a temporary impediment to the procedure than a danger to the patient, a child with hemophilia or an acquired coagulopathy can develop extensive and potentially life-threatening airway bleeding or obstruction due to a hematoma (120,121). Clearly, any child with a clinically significant bleeding disorder should undergo intubation in the least traumatic manner possible. If bleeding is extensive and persistent, the airway should be secured as rapidly as possible, and an otolaryngologist should be urgently consulted to evaluate the patient.

Other soft-tissue injuries resulting from the mechanical effects of endotracheal intubation may involve the lips, tongue, retropharynx, epiglottis, arytenoids, trachea, and esophagus (104,122–125). Indeed, virtually any airway structure above the bronchi can be traumatized. The epiglottis and arytenoid cartilages can be abraded by the laryngoscope blade, particularly if the blade is first inserted into the esophagus and then withdrawn. Insertion of the endotracheal tube has been associated with a wide variety of complications, including dislocation of the arytenoids and perforation of the retropharynx, trachea, and epiglottis. Laceration injuries are particularly common when the tip of a stylet improperly extends beyond the end of the tube.

Aspiration Pneumonitis

Pediatric patients who undergo emergent endotracheal intubation should always be considered to have the primary risk factors for aspiration of gastric contents into the lungs: a decreased level of consciousness, a diminished or absent gag reflex, and a full stomach. A full-stomach state exists when the patient has had a recent meal, has an intestinal obstruction, or has some process causing decreased gastric motility (increased intracranial pressure, extreme pain, pregnancy, etc.). The severity of the resulting lung injury is related to the acidity and volume of the aspirate and the amount of particulate matter aspirated (101). Clinical consequences of aspiration can have a wide range of manifestations, including no detectable effect, a self-limited pneumonitis, significant hypoxemia, bacterial pneumonia, and, in more severe cases, lung abscess formation and the development of RDS (83). Although possible after intubation is successfully accomplished, aspiration is far more likely to occur during the actual procedure, when instrumentation causes vomiting before the airway is protected (126).

Several steps can be taken to reduce the incidence of aspiration during an emergent intubation. Prior insertion of a gastric tube evacuates much of the stomach contents, and therefore the likelihood that the patient will vomit during the procedure is decreased. However, this procedure may not be possible if the patient has severe respiratory distress, and as it may induce vomiting, it should not be performed in the patient who may have a diminished gag reflex. If a rapid sequence induction is performed, the patient with spontaneous respirations should not receive manual ventilation until after successful intubation (whenever this is possible) so that vomiting does not result from elevated intragastric pressure caused by forced air entry into the stomach. Ideally, preoxygenation is performed by allowing the patient to breath 100% oxygen by mask before administration of neuromuscular blocking agents (see Chapter 15). Aspiration also is less likely to occur when cricoid pressure is performed (83–88). Salem et al. (88) demonstrated in a study of postmortem infants that cricoid pressure was effective in preventing reflux of gastric contents even in the presence of elevated intragastric and intraesophageal pressures. Unless contraindicated, this technique is recommended for all children with an impaired or absent gag reflex who undergo emergent endotracheal intubation.

Pulmonary Edema

A relatively unusual but physiologically interesting complication of endotracheal intubation in pediatric patients is acute pulmonary edema that occurs after relief of extrathoracic airway obstruction (127–131). Children with severe croup, epiglottitis, or other causes of airway obstruction who undergo intubation may develop the typical clinical signs of pulmonary edema—frothy secretions, diffuse alveolar densities on chest radiograph, and hypoxemia. This complication also can occur when a child bites down on an endotracheal tube already in place. The pathogenesis of this process remains poorly understood, although it is likely due in part to increased hydrostatic pressure in the lungs during labored respirations, which causes a rapid influx of interstitial fluid. If a child is intubated without using a paralytic agent, the operator should insert a bite block when appropriate to prevent occlusion of the endotracheal tube. Furthermore, any pediatric patient with a known cause of significant airway obstruction who requires intubation should be considered at risk for developing acute pulmonary edema. In most cases, manifestations of this complication are relatively mild, and basic supportive measures (e.g., increased supplemental oxygen delivery and positive end-expiratory pressure) are generally the only interventions necessary.

Cervical Cord Injury

Perhaps the most intensively studied complication of endotracheal intubation is exacerbation of spinal cord trauma in the patient with an unstable cervical spine (132–140). The best approach to airway management for these patients remains highly controversial. Some practitioners believe that orotracheal intubation has proven to be a safe procedure even in the presence of a cervical spine injury. They cite the experience with thousands of patients managed at major trauma centers and the lack of demonstrable evidence of worsened neurologic outcome among patients with cervical spine injuries after orotracheal intubation (141). Many authorities contend that the most important source of morbidity for such patients is ischemic brain injury due to inadequate airway intervention resulting from an overemphasis on protecting the cervical cord. Others believe that the maneuvers involved with an orotracheal intubation represent a significant risk for causing neurologic injury in the patient with a potentially unstable cervical spine. This view is based primarily on cadaver studies that show that even with in-line stabilization, distraction, and subluxation at the site of injury can occur. Some practitioners recommend using airway interventions that minimize movement of the neck, such as blind nasotracheal intubation, awake fiberoptic intubation, digital intubation, retrograde intubation, or a surgical airway.

The possibility of exacerbating a cord injury during intubation is fortunately less of a concern with pediatric patients than with adults, because the incidence of unstable cervical spine fractures among infants and children is low (142,143). Nevertheless, the relative rarity of cervical spine injuries among pediatric patients does not make the question of how best to manage this presentation easier to decide. In the absence of any definitive case series on the safety of conventional orotracheal intubation for the patient with an unstable cervical spine injury, it would seem most prudent to intubate the patient using the least traumatic approach that the operator is capable of performing. If the operator is proficient with an alternative intubation technique that minimizes movement of the patient's neck, then making an attempt using that method would be a logical approach. Conversely, if a patient with a potentially unstable cervical spine requires immediate intubation, and the operator is competent only with conventional orotracheal intubation, then this method should be used with appropriate caution. In this case, an assistant should maintain in-line stabilization, as described previously, and movement of the neck should be minimized. Above all, the perceived threat of injury to the cervical cord in a pediatric trauma patient must not take precedence over the very real need to provide adequate airway and ventilatory support.

▶ SUMMARY

Emergent endotracheal intubation of pediatric patients presents a unique set of challenges and rewards. Unlike adults, children are often unable to cooperate with the procedure out of fear or lack of understanding. The confined spaces, relatively large tongue, and small mandible of a pediatric patient can test the skill of even the most experienced practitioner. Furthermore, an emergent intubation allows the operator much less time for preparation than an elective intubation because respiratory decompensation (or, for that matter, the arrival of the patient at the hospital) may occur with very little warning. This leads to a greater degree of urgency and more restrictive time constraints. However, despite these obstacles, few accomplishments are more gratifying in medical practice than a successful intubation that preserves the life of a child.

Emergent endotracheal intubation is an invasive procedure associated with several potential complications. The operator must be knowledgeable about appropriate indications for emergent intubation because the best way to avoid complications is to perform the procedure only when truly necessary. Optimal management may involve transferring the patient to a more controlled environment before intubation is attempted. Unfortunately, relatively few easily defined rules are available for deciding when an emergent intubation should be performed. Laboratory tests and imaging techniques consume valuable time and seldom provide a definitive answer. The most important determining factor generally proves to be the experience and judgment of the practitioner in evaluating the condition of the patient. Considering the number and potential severity of the complications associated with this procedure, it is in fact surprising that they are not encountered more frequently in clinical practice. In reality, when endotracheal intubation is performed in an appropriate setting using proper technique, significant complications can normally be avoided.

Certainly the most dreaded circumstance occurs when the patient cannot be intubated and BVM ventilation is not adequately effective. This represents a worst-case scenario in which a surgical airway, with all the attendant risks of that procedure, must then be attempted. The most effective way to avoid such an unwelcome situation is to develop skills in performing at least one other intubation technique so that failure with one approach can be quickly followed by success with another. Although conventional orotracheal intubation is by far the most commonly used method, alternative approaches such as those described in Chapter 17 may prove invaluable in a difficult situation. Although it is by no means necessary to become adept at all these additional techniques,

the resourceful practitioner will always have another "arrow in the quiver" when orotracheal intubation is unsuccessful.

▶ ACKNOWLEDGMENT

The authors would like to acknowledge the valuable contributions of Stephen A. Stayer to the version of this chapter that appeared in the previous edition.

▶ REFERENCES

1. Motoyama EK. Endotracheal intubation. In: Motoyama EK, Davis PJ, eds. *Smith's Anesthesia for Infants and Children.* 5th ed. St. Louis: Mosby; 1990:269–275.
2. Sasaki CT, Levine PA, Laitman JT, et al. Postnatal descent of the epiglottis in man. *Arch Otolaryngol.* 1977;103:169–171.
3. Cote CJ, Todres ID. The pediatric airway. In: Cote CJ, Ryan JF, Todres ID, et al., eds. *A Practice of Anesthesia for Infants and Children.* 2nd ed. Philadelphia: Saunders; 1993:122.
4. Morgan GA, Steward DJ. Linear airway dimensions in children, including those with cleft palate. *Can Anaesth Soc J.* 1982;29:1–8.
5. Eckenhoff J. Some anatomic considerations of the infant's larynx, influencing endotracheal anesthesia. *Anesthesiology.* 1951;12:401–410.
6. Boyden EA, Tompsett DH. The changing patterns in the developing lungs of infants. *Acta Anat (Basel).* 1965;61:164–192.
7. Dunnill MS. Postnatal growth of the lung. *Thorax.* 1962;17:329–333.
8. Macklem PT. Airway obstruction and collateral ventilation. *Physiol Rev.* 1971;51:368–436.
9. Mansell A, Bryan C, Levinson H. Airway closure in children. *J Appl Physiol.* 1972;33:711–714.
10. Anthonisen NR, Danson J, Robertson PC, et al. Airway closure as a function of age. *Respir Physiol.* 1969;8:58–65.
11. Bryan AC, Mansell AL, Levison H. Development of the mechanical properties of the respiratory system. In: Hodson WA, ed. *Development of the Lung.* New York: Marcel Dekker; 1976:445.
12. Guslits BG, Gaston SE, Bryan MH, et al. Diaphragmatic work of breathing in premature human infants. *J Appl Physiol.* 1987;62:1410–1415.
13. Keens TG, Bryan AC, Levison H, et al. Developmental pattern of muscle fiber types in human ventilatory muscles. *J Appl Physiol.* 1978;44:909–913.
14. Keens TG, Lanuzzo CD. Development of fatigue-resistant muscle fibers in human ventilatory muscles. *Am Rev Respir Dis.* 1979;2[Suppl 119]:139–141.
15. Keens TG, Chen V, Patel P, et al. Cellular adaptations of the ventilatory muscles to a chronic increased respiratory load. *J Appl Physiol.* 1978;44:905–908.
16. Unna KR, Glaser K, Lipton EL, et al. Dosage of drugs in infants and children, I: atropine. *Pediatrics.* 1950;6:197–207.
17. Lipton EL, Steinschneider A, Richmond JB. The autonomic nervous system in early life. *N Eng J Med.* 1965;273:147–153.
18. Cordero L Jr, Hon EH. Neonatal bradycardia following nasopharyngeal stimulation. *J Pediatr.* 1971;78:441–447.
19. Marshall TA, Deeder R, Pai S, et al. Physiologic changes associated with endotracheal intubation in preterm infants. *Crit Care Med.* 1984;12:501–503.
20. Hawkins J, Van Hare GF, Schmidt KG, et al. Effects of increasing afterload on left ventricular output in fetal lambs. *Circ Res.* 1989;65:127–134.

21. Van Hare GF, Jawkins JA, Schmidt KG, et al. The effects of increasing mean arterial pressure on left ventricular output in newborn lambs. *Circ Res.* 1990;67:78–83.

22. Holinger LD. Etiology of stridor in the neonate, infant, and child. *Ann Otol Rhinol Laryngol.* 1980;89:397–400.

23. Backofen JE, Rogers MC. Upper airway disease. In: Rogers MC, ed. *Textbook of Pediatric Intensive Care.* 2nd ed. Baltimore: Williams & Wilkins; 1992:234.

24. Jones R, Santos JI, Overall JC. Bacterial tracheitis. *JAMA.* 1979;242:721–726.

25. Kasian GF, Bingham WT, Steinberg J, et al. Bacterial tracheitis in children. *Can Med Assoc J.* 1989;140:46–50.

26. Bryce DP. Current management of laryngotracheal injury. *Adv Otorhinolaryngol.* 1983;29:27–38.

27. Cohn AM, Larson DL. Laryngeal injury. *Arch Otolaryngol.* 1976;102:166–170.

28. Dalal FY, Schmidt GB, Bennett EJ, et al. Fractures of the larynx in children. *Can Anaesth Soc J.* 1974;21:376–378.

29. Mahour GH, Lynn HB, Sanderson DR. Rupture of the bronchus. *J Pediatr Surg.* 1967;2:263–267.

30. Nakayama DK, Rowe MI. Intrathoracic tracheobronchial injuries in childhood. *Int Anesthesiol Clin.* 1988;26:42–49.

31. Fein A, Leff A, Hopewell PC. Pathophysiology and management of the complications resulting from fire and the inhaled products of combustion: review of the literature. *Crit Care Med.* 1980;8:94–98.

32. Vivori E, Cudmore RE. Management of airway complications of burns in children. *Br Med J.* 1977;2:1462–1464.

33. Kosloske AM. Bronchoscopic extraction of aspirated foreign bodies in children. *Am J Dis Child.* 1982;136:924–927.

34. Rothmann BF, Boeckman CR. Foreign bodies in the larynx and tracheobronchial tree in children: a review of 225 cases. *Ann Otol Rhinol Laryngol.* 1980;89:434–436.

35. Brudno DS, Parker DH, Slaton G. Response of pulmonary mechanics to terbutaline in patients with bronchopulmonary dysplasia. *Am J Med Sci.* 1989;297:166–168.

36. Wilkie RA, Bryan MH. Effect of bronchodilators on airway resistance in ventilator-dependent neonates with chronic lung disease. *J Pediatr.* 1987;111:278–282.

37. Helfaer MA, Nichols DG, Chantarojanasiri T, et al. Lower airway disease: bronchiolitis and asthma. In: Rogers MC, ed. *Textbook of Pediatric Intensive Care.* 2nd ed. Baltimore: Williams & Wilkins; 1992:258.

38. Stempel DA, Mellon M. Management of acute severe asthma. *Ped Clin North Am.* 1984;31:879–890.

39. Bierman CW, Pierson WE, Shapiro GG. Treatment of status asthmaticus in children. *South Med J.* 1975;68:1556–1560.

40. Wood DW, Downes JJ, Lecks HI. The management of respiratory failure in childhood status asthmaticus: experience with 30 episodes and evolution of a technique. *J Allergy.* 1968;42:261–267.

41. Schulaner FA, Mattikow MS. Treatment of status asthmaticus: bronchial asthma. Pt 3. *J Med Soc N J.* 1980;77:501–505.

42. Petty TL. Oxygen and mechanical ventilation in status asthmaticus. In: Weiss EB, ed. *Status Asthmaticus.* Baltimore: University Park Press; 1978:285.

43. Rice TB, Torres A Jr. Pneumonitis and interstitial disease. In: Fuhrman BP, Zimmerman JJ, eds. *Pediatric Critical Care.* St. Louis: Mosby; 1992:465.

44. Riordan JF, Walters G. Pulmonary edema in bacterial shock. *Lancet.* 1968;1:719–721.

45. Klein JJ, Haeringen JR, Slinter HJ, et al. Pulmonary function after recovery from adult respiratory distress syndrome. *Chest.* 1976;69:350–355.

46. Rigatto H, Kalapesi Z, Leahy FN, et al. Ventilatory response to 100% and 15% O_2 during wakefulness and sleep in preterm infants. *Early Hum Dev.* 1982;7:1–10.

47. Frantz ID III, Adler SM, Thach BT, et al. Maturational effects on respiratory responses to carbon dioxide in premature infants. *J Appl Physiol.* 1976;41:634.

48. Brady JP, Ceruit E. Chemoreceptor reflexes in the newborn infant: effects of varying degrees of hypoxia on heart rate and ventilation in a warm environment. *J Physiol.* 1966;184:631–645.

49. Blesa MI, Lahiri S, Rashkind WJ, et al. Normalization of the blunted ventilatory response to acute hypoxia in congenital cyanotic heart disease. *N Engl J Med.* 1977;296:237–241.

50. Garg M, Kurzner SI, Bautista D, et al. Hypoxic arousal responses in infants with bronchopulmonary dysplasia. *Pediatrics.* 1988;82:59–63.

51. Kanter RK. Control of breathing and acute respiratory failure. In: Fuhrman BP, Zimmerman JJ, eds. *Pediatric Critical Care.* St. Louis: Mosby, 1992:515.

52. Kewalramani LS, Tori JA. Spinal cord trauma in children: neurologic patterns, radiologic features, and pathomechanics of injury. *Spine.* 1980;5:11–18.

53. Weinstein L. Tetanus. *N Engl J Med.* 1973;289:1293–1296.

54. Alfrey D, Rauscher A. Tetanus: a review. *Crit Care Med.* 1979;7:176.

55. Feigin RD, Guggenheim MA, Johnsen SD. Vaccine-related paralytic poliomyelitis in an immunodeficient child. *J Pediatr.* 1971;79:642–647.

56. Moore P, James O. Guillain-Barré syndrome: incidence, management and outcome of major complications. *Crit Care Med.* 1981;9:549–555.

57. Menkes JH. Diseases of the motor unit. In: Menkes JH. *Textbook of Child Neurology.* Philadelphia: Lea & Febiger; 1975:463.

58. Sellin LC. The action of botulism toxin at the neuromuscular junction. *Med Biol.* 1981;59:11–20.

59. Johnson RO, Clay SA, Arnon SS. Diagnosis and management of infant botulism. *Am J Dis Child.* 1979;133:586–593.

60. Long SS, Gajewski JL, Brown LW, et al. Clinical, laboratory and environmental features of infant botulism in southeastern Pennsylvania. *Pediatrics.* 1985;75:935–941.

61. Thompson JA, Glasgow LA, Warpinski JR, et al. Infant botulism: clinical spectrum and epidemiology. *Pediatrics.* 1980;66:936–942.

62. Eisenberg M, Berginer L, Hallstrom A. Epidemiology of cardiac arrest and resuscitation in children. *Ann Emerg Med.* 1983;12:672–674.

63. Ward JT Jr. Endotracheal drug therapy. *Am J Emerg Med.* 1983;1:71–82.

64. Ward ME, Roussos C. The respiratory muscles in shock: service or disservice? *Int Crit Care Diag.* 1985;4:3–5.

65. Rose DK, Byrick RJ, Froese AB. Carbon dioxide elimination during spontaneous ventilation with a modified Mapleson D system: studies in a lung model. *Can Anaesth Soc J.* 1978;25:353–360.

66. Bishop MJ, Wegmeller EA, Fink BR. Laryngeal effects of prolonged intubation. *Anesth Analg.* 1984;63:335–342.

67. Joshi VV, Mandavia SG, Stern L, et al. Acute lesions induced by endotracheal intubation. *Am J Dis Child.* 1972;124:646–649.

68. Strong RM, Passy V. Endotracheal intubation: complications in neonates. *Arch Otolaryngol.* 1977;103:329–335.

69. Windsor HM, Shanahan MX, Cherian K, et al. Tracheal injury following prolonged intubation. *Aust N Z J Surg.* 1976;46:18–25.

70. Stamm D, Floret D, Stamm C, et al. Subglottic stenosis following intubation in children. *Arch Fr Pediatr.* 1993;50:21–25.

71. Fine G, Borland L. The future of the cuffed endotracheal tube. *Paediatr Anaesth.* 2004;14:38–42.

72. 2005 American Heart Association (AHA) guidelines for cardiopulmonary resuscitation (CPR) and emergency cardiovascular care

(ECC) of pediatric and neonatal patients: pediatric basic life support. *Pediatrics.* 2006;117:e989–1004.

73. Linko K, Paloheimo M, Tammisto T. Capnography for detection of accidental oesophageal intubation. *Acta Anaesthesiol Scand.* 1983;27:199–202.

74. Kagle DM, Alexander CM, Berko RS, et al. Evaluation of the Ohmeda Biox 3700 pulse oximeter: steady state and transient response characteristics. *Anesthesiology.* 1987;66:376–380.

75. Rosenberg M, Block CS. A simple, disposable end-tidal carbon dioxide detector. *Anesth Prog.* 1991;38:24–26.

76. Ko FY, Hsieh KS, Yu CK. Detection of airway CO_2 partial pressure to avoid esophageal intubation. *Acta Paediatr Sin.* 1993;34:91–97.

77. White RD, Asplin BR. Out-of-hospital quantitative monitoring of end-tidal carbon dioxide pressure during CPR. *Ann Emerg Med.* 1994;23:25–30.

78. Patel R, Lenczyk M, Hannallah RS, et al. Age and the onset of desaturation in apnoeic children. *Can J Anaesth.* 1994;41:771–774.

79. Videira RL, Neto PP, do Amaral RV, et al. Preoxygenation in children: for how long? *Acta Anaesthesiol Scand.* 1992;36:109–111.

80. Khoo ST, Woo M, Kumar A. An assessment of preoxygenation techniques using the pulse oximeter. *Ann Acad Med.* 1992;21:705–707.

81. Xue FS, Tong SY, Wang XL, et al. Study of the optimal duration of preoxygenation in children. *J Clin Anesth.* 1995;7:93–96.

82. Hupp JR, Peterson LJ. Aspiration pneumonitis: etiology, therapy, and prevention. *J Oral Surg.* 1981;39:430–435.

83. Sladen A, Zanca P, Hadnott WH. Aspiration pneumonitis: the sequelae. *Chest.* 1971;59:448–450.

84. Salem MR, Wong AY, Mani M, et al. Efficacy of cricoid pressure in preventing gastric inflation during bag-mask ventilation in pediatric patients. *Anesthesiology.* 1974;40:96–98.

85. Admani M, Yeh TF, Jain R, et al. Prevention of gastric inflation during mask ventilation in newborn infants. *Crit Care Med.* 1985;13:592–593.

86. Moynihan RJ, Brock-Utne JG, Archer JH, et al. The effect of cricoid pressure on preventing gastric insufflation in infants and children. *Anesthesiology.* 1993;78:652–656.

87. Fanning GL. The efficacy of cricoid pressure in preventing regurgitation of gastric contents. *Anesthesiology.* 1970;32:553–555.

88. Salem MR, Wong AY, Fizzotti GF. Efficacy of cricoid pressure in preventing aspiration of gastric contents in paediatric patients. *Br J Anaesth.* 1972;44:401–404.

89. Criswell JC, Parr MJ, Nolan JP. Emergency airway management in patients with cervical spine injuries. *Anaesthesia.* 1994;49:900–903.

90. Bivins HG, Ford S, Bezmalinovic Z, et al. The effect of axial traction during orotracheal intubation of the trauma victim with an unstable cervical spine. *Ann Emerg Med.* 1988;17:25–29.

91. Majernick T, Bieniek R, Houston J, et al. Cervical spine movement during orotracheal intubation. *Ann Emerg Med.* 1986;15:417–420.

92. Backofen JE, Rogers MC. Emergency management of the airway. In: Rogers MC, ed. *Textbook of Pediatric Intensive Care.* 2nd ed. Baltimore: William & Wilkins; 1992.

93. Dauphinee K. Nasotracheal intubation. *Emerg Med Clin North Am.* 1988;6:715–723.

94. Walker WE, Bender HW Jr. Blind nasotracheal intubation. *Surg Gynecol Obstet.* 1981;152:87–88.

95. Iserson KV. Blind nasotracheal intubation. *Ann Emerg Med.* 1981;10:468–471.

96. Danzl DF, Thomas DM. Nasotracheal intubations in the emergency department. *Crit Care Med.* 1980;8:677–682.

97. Jantzen JP. Tracheal intubation: blind but not mute [letter]. *Anesth Analg.* 1985;64:646.

98. Krishel S, Jackimczyk K, Balazs K. Endotracheal tube whistle: an adjunct to blind nasotracheal intubation. *Ann Emerg Med.* 1992;21:33–36.

99. Bloch EC, Ossey K, Ginsberg B. Tracheal intubation in children: a new method for ensuring correct depth of tube placement. *Anesth Analg.* 1988;67:590–592.

100. Nakayama DK, Gardner MJ, Rowe MI. Emergency endotracheal intubation in pediatric trauma. *Ann Surg.* 1990;211:218–223.

101. Ehrlich PF, Seidman PS, Attallah O, et al. Endotracheal intubation in rural pediatric trauma patients. *J Pediatr Surg.* 2004;39:1376–1380.

102. Gausche M, Lewis RJ, Stratton SJ, et al. Effect of out-of-hospital pediatric endotracheal intubation on survival and neurologic outcome: a controlled clinical trial. *JAMA.* 2000;283:783–790.

103. Adriani J, Naraghi M, Ward M. Complications of endotracheal intubation. *South Med J.* 1988;81:739–744.

104. Blanc VF, Tremblay NAG. The complications of tracheal intubation: a new classification with a review of the literature. *Anesth Analg.* 1974;53:202–213.

105. Lindgren L, Saarnivaara L. Cardiovascular responses to tracheal intubation in small children. *Br J Anaesth.* 1985;57:1183–1187.

106. Burney RG, Winn R. Increased cerebrospinal fluid pressure during laryngoscopy and intubation for induction of anesthesia. *Anesth Analg.* 1975;54:687–690.

107. Raju TN, Vidyasagar D, Torres C, et al. Intracranial pressure during intubation and anesthesia in infants. *J Pediatr.* 1980;96:860–862.

108. Durand M, Bikramjit S, Cabal LA, et al. Cardiopulmonary and intracranial pressure changes related to endotracheal suctioning in preterm infants. *Crit Care Med.* 1989;17:506–510.

109. Owen RL, Cheney FW. Endobronchial intubation: a preventable complication. *Anesthesiology.* 1987;67:255–257.

110. Conrardy PA, Goodman LR, Lainge F, et al. Alteration of endotracheal tube position: flexion and extension of the neck. *Crit Care Med.* 1976;4(1):7–12.

111. Todres ID, deBros F, Kramer SS, et al. Endotracheal tube position in the newborn infant. *J Pediatr.* 1976;89:126–127.

112. Toung TJ, Grayson R, Saklad J, et al. Movement of the distal end of the endotracheal tube during flexion and extension of the neck [letter]. *Anesth Analg.* 1985;64:1029.

113. Brasch RC, Heldt GP, Hecht ST. Endotracheal tube orifice abutting the tracheal wall: a cause of infant airway obstruction. *Radiology.* 1981;141:387–391.

114. Redding GJ, Fan L, Cotton EK, et al. Partial obstruction of endotracheal tubes in children: incidence, etiology, significance. *Crit Care Med.* 1979;7:227–231.

115. Miller RD, Hamilton WK. Pneumothorax during infant resuscitation. *JAMA.* 1969;210:1090–1091.

116. Hirschman AM, Kravath RE. Venting vs. ventilating: a danger of manual resuscitation bags. *Chest.* 1982;82:369–370.

117. Dwyer ME: Pneumothorax. *Aust Paediatr J.* 1975;11:195–200.

118. Luck SR, Raffensperger JG, Sullivan HJ, et al. Management of pneumothorax in children with chronic pulmonary disease. *J Thorac Cardiovasc Surg.* 1977;74:834–839.

119. Moylan FMB, Seldin EB, Shannon DC, et al. Defective primary dentition in survivors of neonatal mechanical ventilation. *J Pediatr.* 1980;96:106–108.

120. Stanievich JF, Marshak G, Stool SE. Airway obstruction in a hemophiliac child. *Ann Otol Rhinol Laryngol.* 1980;89:572–573.

121. Lewis JH. Causes of death in hemophilia. *JAMA.* 1970;214:1707.

122. Othersen HB Jr. Intubation injuries of the trachea in children: management and prevention. *Ann Surg.* 1979;189:601–606.

123. Fan LL, Flynn JW, Pathak DR. Risk factors predicting laryngeal injury in intubated neonates. *Crit Care Med.* 1983;11:431–433.

124. Serlin SP, Daily WJR. Tracheal perforation in the neonate: a complication of endotracheal intubation. *J Pediatr.* 1975;86:596–597.

125. Ducharme JC, Bertrand MR, Debie J. Perforation of the pharynx in the newborn: a condition of mimicking esophageal atresia. *Can Med Assoc J.* 1971;104:785–787.

126. Goitein KJ, Rein AJ, Gornstein A. Incidence of aspiration in endotracheally intubated infants and children. *Crit Care Med.* 1984;12:19–21.

127. Galvis AG, Stool SE, Bluestone CK. Pulmonary edema following relief of acute upper airway obstruction. *Ann Otol Rhinol Laryngol.* 1980;89:124–128.

128. Sofer S, Bar-Ziv J, Scharf SM. Pulmonary edema following relief of upper airway obstruction. *Chest.* 1984;86:401–403.

129. Barin ES, Stevenson IF, Donnelly GL. Pulmonary edema following acute upper airway obstruction. *Anaesth Intensive Care.* 1986;14:54–57.

130. Warner LO, Beach TP, Martino JD. Negative pressure pulmonary oedema secondary to airway obstruction in an intubated infant. *Can J Anaesth.* 1988;35:507–510.

131. Kanter RK, Watchko JF. Pulmonary edema associated with upper airway obstruction. *Am J Dis Child.* 1984;138:356–358.

132. Grande CM, Barton CR. Appropriate techniques for airway management of emergency patients with suspected spinal cord injury [letter]. *Anesth Analg.* 1988;67:710.

133. Doolan LA, O'Brien JF. Safe intubation in cervical spine injury. *Anaesth Intensive Care.* 1985;13:319–324.

134. Wright SW, Robinson GG, Wright MB. Cervical spine injuries in blunt trauma patients requiring emergent endotracheal intubation. *Am J Emerg Med.* 1992;10:104–109.

135. Hastings RH, Marks JD. Airway management for trauma patients with potential cervical spine injuries. *Anesth Analg.* 1991;73:471–482.

136. Wood PR, Lawler PGP. Managing the airway in cervical spine injury: a review of the Advanced Trauma Life Support protocol. *Anaesthesia.* 1992;47:792–797.

137. Joyce SM. Cervical immobilization during orotracheal intubation in trauma victims [editorial]. *Ann Emerg Med.* 1988;17:88.

138. Knopp RK. The safety of orotracheal intubation in patients with suspected cervical spine injury [editorial]. *Ann Emerg Med.* 1990;19:603–604.

139. Rhee KJ, Green W, Holcroft JW, et al. Oral intubation in the multiply injured patient: the risk of exacerbating cervical spine damage. *Ann Emerg Med.* 1990;19:511–514.

140. Holley J, Jorden R. Airway management in patients with unstable cervical spine fractures. *Ann Emerg Med.* 1989;18:1237–1239.

141. Shatney CH, Brunner RD, Nguyen TQ. The safety of orotracheal intubation in patients with unstable cervical spine fracture or high spinal cord injury. *Am J Surg.* 1995;170:676–679.

142. Lally KP, Senac M, Hardin WE, et al. Utility of the cervical spine radiograph in pediatric trauma. *Am J Surg.* 1989;158:540–541.

143. Rachesky I, Boyce T, Duncan B, et al. Clinical prediction of cervical spine injuries in children. *Am J Dis Child.* 1987;141:199–201.

BRENT R. KING AND CARIN A. HAGBERG

Management of the Difficult Airway

17

▶ INTRODUCTION

One of the most challenging tasks facing caregivers is maintaining the technical skills necessary for the management of the difficult airway. This is especially true for those providing care to pediatric patients. Data for anesthesiologists regarding closed malpractice claims show a higher frequency of adverse respiratory events in the pediatric population (1,2). The majority of these events were related to inadequate ventilation, airway obstruction, and complications of endotracheal intubation. Although corollary data from the emergency department (ED) have not been reported, it seems likely that if such adverse events are a significant problem in the controlled environment of the operating room, they are even more frequent in the ED.

Fortunately, the vast majority of children who require airway management for respiratory failure or airway protection in the ED are successfully managed using standard techniques such as bag-valve-mask ventilation (see Chapter 14) and endotracheal intubation (see Chapter 16). However, in some cases these methods fail, whether because of unique anatomic characteristics of the pediatric airway, acquired or congenital abnormalities, operator inexperience, or some combination of these factors. When failure occurs, an alternative technique must be quickly employed or the child may suffer irreversible hypoxemic injury. This chapter describes many of the alternatives to standard airway management, along with the rationale for their use. It is not intended to provide an exhaustive list of every available tool or device. Furthermore, certain techniques that might be used to manage a difficult airway are covered elsewhere within this text and therefore will not be described in this chapter, including blind nasotracheal intubation (see Chapter 16), percutaneous transtracheal ventilation (see Chapter 18), and surgical cricothyrotomy (see Chapter 26). Finally, the reader must understand that, like all types

of medical technology, the tools and techniques used for managing the difficult airway are constantly evolving.

▶ DEFINITIONS

Several important definitions are vital to a thorough understanding of the information that follows. Caregivers who manage the airway are often confronted with the responsibility of determining whether or not a patient will present increased difficulty for airway management.

Predicted Difficult Airway

Based on certain physical characteristics, some patients can be predicted to have a problematic airway. Such difficulty arises in regard to five different techniques of airway management: (a) bag-valve-mask (BVM) ventilation, (b) laryngoscopy, (c) orotracheal and/or nasotracheal intubation, (d) supraglottic airway placement, and (e) surgical airway. Since a given patient might require any one or more of these techniques, every patient should be evaluated for possible problems regarding all of them. Many patients will have more than one area of potential difficulty, and such considerations should dictate the type of airway management utilized (see below).

Known Difficult Airway

Patients who have had previous difficult or failed attempts at airway management are said to have a known difficult airway. Whenever possible, family members should be specifically questioned about any history the patient might have of prior problems with airway management. Likewise, those who have undergone a difficult or failed airway attempt should be advised to purchase and wear medical identification jewelry indicating this (e.g., Medic-Alert bracelets), and if time permits, emergency providers should always look for such identifying jewelry when a patient requires airway management.

Failed Airway

Although failed intubation—or the inability to place the endotracheal tube after multiple attempts—is a clear endpoint, there is no single accepted definition of a "failed airway." The American Society for Anesthesiology (ASA) defines a failed airway as the inability to obtain a definitive airway after three attempts by an experienced laryngoscopist. Others describe a failed airway as any attempt in which the patient becomes hypoxemic. Critical to all definitions, however, is the concept that it is unwise for the same operator to continue using the same unsuccessful technique repeatedly while the condition of the patient deteriorates. Although simple, this can be a difficult concept to acknowledge in the heat of a resuscitation that is going poorly. Above all, each operator should approach every intubation with a planned primary technique and at least one alternative technique in mind.

Emergent Airway

When the patient requires immediate airway management, with little or no time for stabilization and assessment, a true emergency exists. In such cases, the operator's options for management may be limited.

Urgent Airway

Many patients have impending respiratory failure or a waning level of consciousness and will require that their airway be secured. However, they are stable enough to allow the operator the opportunity to perform a somewhat more thorough assessment in order to determine the most appropriate course of action.

Elective Airway

Patients undergoing elective airway management are those who require endotracheal intubation, but not on an urgent or emergent basis. Airway management of such patients should be held to the same standards of care as patients electively intubated in the operating room.

▶ ANATOMY AND PHYSIOLOGY

Detailed descriptions of the key anatomic features of the pediatric airway and important differences from the adult airway, as well as clinically relevant aspects of pediatric respiratory physiology, can be found in Chapters 12, 14, and 16. This section will therefore focus on anatomic and physiologic principles related to the difficult pediatric airway, with an emphasis on congenital and acquired abnormalities that pose the primary obstacles to successful airway management. Knowledge of syndromes that may adversely affect the operator's ability to secure a definitive airway is crucial in caring for children with severe respiratory problems. Moreover, the presence of one anomaly mandates the search for others. Considerations regarding pediatric airway anatomy and respiratory physiology are described as they pertain to the five types of airway management.

Difficult Bag-Valve-Mask Ventilation

Inability to provide adequate BVM ventilation generally results from one or more of the following problems: inadequate mask seal, excessive gas leak, and excessive resistance to the ingress or egress of gas (3). While failure to intubate does not necessarily lead to hypoxia, since BVM ventilation can be often be continued temporarily as an effective means of respiratory support, failure to intubate *and* provide adequate BVM ventilation can quickly result in profound and life-threatening hypoxia. Interestingly, there is a paucity of literature describing the prediction of difficult BVM ventilation.

Problems with maintaining a mask seal during BVM ventilation can be anticipated in children with midfacial abnormalities. The most common congenital abnormality of the midface with the potential to affect the quality of the mask seal is cleft lip. Additionally, certain children have abnormal facial shapes (e.g., mandibular hypoplasia) that make it difficult or impossible to provide an adequate mask seal. The mask seal can also be adversely affected by severe trauma to the face. Of note, it may not be possible to properly apply a face mask with children who have dental appliances and other medical hardware that involve the oral cavity or the area between the nose and chin.

Obstruction can occur at any level from the oral cavity to the lower airway. For example, children with Beckwith-Wiedemann syndrome have an excessively large tongue, which can obstruct the airway. Angioedema can also cause a dramatically enlarged tongue. Congenital and acquired conditions involving the glottis and adjacent structures that produce airway obstruction (croup, bacterial tracheitis, foreign body, thermal injuries, etc.) can make BVM ventilation impossible. Finally, as described in Chapter 14, effective manual ventilation requires proper positioning of the head and neck to maximize airflow. Obstruction can occur even in a child with a relatively normal airway when the neck is immobilized in a cervical collar and cannot be adequately positioned. Neck mobility may also be limited in patients with certain congenital syndromes and obesity (4).

Difficult Laryngoscopy

Difficult laryngoscopy is defined as the inability to visualize any portion of the vocal cords by conventional laryngoscopy. Many investigators include grades III (visualization of the epiglottis but not the vocal cords) and IV (visualization of only the tongue or the tongue and the soft palate) or grade IV alone, according to the Cormack-Lehane original grading of the rigid laryngoscopic view (5) (Fig. 17.1). Difficulty in performing endotracheal intubation is the end result of difficult laryngoscopy and is dependent on the operator's level of expertise, patient characteristics, and clinical circumstances. Thus it has been suggested that the definition of difficult intubation be based on a uniform understanding of the best attempt at performing laryngoscopy/intubation and should use the number of attempts and time as boundaries only (6). The best attempt should incorporate the effect of changing the patient's position; the effect of changing the length or type of laryngoscope blade; and the effect of simple airway manipulations, such as conventional cricoid pressure, backwards, upwards, rightward pressure (BURP), and optimal external laryngeal manipulation (OELM) (see Chapter 16).

Difficult Endotracheal Intubation

Difficult endotracheal intubation is described as intubation that requires multiple attempts in the presence or absence of tracheal pathology. Endotracheal intubation primarily depends on an adequate laryngoscopic view of the airway. Problems that affect the operator's ability to visualize the airway would be expected to negatively affect endotracheal intubation. Although rarely encountered in clinical practice, there are several of these potential problems.

Any patient with serious midface trauma or instability may prove difficult to intubate. Likewise, certain medical appliances or impaled objects involving the lower face may impede the passage of the laryngoscope blade. Facial abnormalities, such as an excessively long or short mandible or neck, will change the position of the airway as compared with normal patients and can make adequate visualization of the airway difficult or impossible. A classic example of such an abnormality is Pierre-Robin syndrome, a congenital disorder that includes severe micrognathia. Many patients have problems with the oral cavity itself, such as impaired mouth opening secondary to medical appliances, facial scars, or abnormalities of the temporomandibular joint; the large tongue of Beckwith-Wiedemann syndrome; and cleft palate. With cleft palate, the laryngoscope can slide into a cleft, impairing visualization and potentially causing trauma. Also, significant trauma to the structures within the oral cavity or to the extrathoracic airway can distort the normal anatomy and make laryngoscopic visualization impossible. Additionally, blood and other secretions may prevent the operator from obtaining an acceptable view of the airway.

It may be possible to predict difficulty with endotracheal intubation based on the extent to which the palate, uvula, and tonsils can be visualized with the patient's mouth open and tongue extended or depressed with a tongue depressor. Several investigators, most notably Cormack and Lehane (5) and Mallampati et al. (7), have demonstrated the relationship between this view of the airway and later difficulty with endotracheal intubation (Fig. 17.2). If the posterior palate is easily visualized, the patient is unlikely to have a difficult intubation,

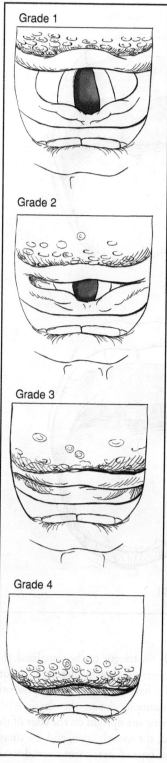

Figure 17.1 Cormack-Lehane laryngoscopic grading system. Grade 1 is visualization of the entire glottic aperture. Grade 2 is visualization of just the arytenoid cartilages or the posterior portion of the glottic aperture. Grade 3 is visualization of only the epiglottis. Grade 4 is visualization of only the tongue or the tongue and soft palate.

Figure 17.2 The Mallampati scale.

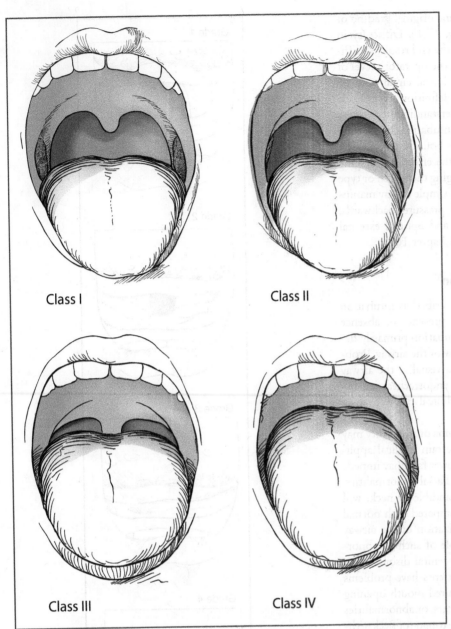

Class I

Class II

Class III

Class IV

whereas if only the tongue can be visualized, the likelihood of a difficult intubation is greatly increased. Unfortunately, most of these studies have involved patients presenting for elective surgery. For example, during the classic Mallampati evaluation, the patient sits upright on the edge of the bed with the neck extended, the mouth open, and the tongue protruding. Obviously, this type of assessment is not directly applicable to most emergency intubations. Yet in many cases, the emergency physician will be able to make at least a reasonable estimate of the patient's Mallampati/Cormack-Lehane score. For the unconscious patient, it may be possible to briefly inspect the mouth by simply using a tongue depressor. Likewise, many patients with respiratory distress will nonetheless be able to cooperate with voluntary mouth opening. For crying infants and children, this inspection may in fact be relatively easy,

although there is some evidence suggesting that these predictive scoring systems may be less accurate in younger patients.

Airway obstruction can also prevent successful endotracheal intubation, so a critical part of airway assessment is the identification of possible obstruction. The characteristic signs of this condition are familiar to most emergency physicians. Patients with stridulous breathing, dysphonia, aphonia, drooling, and/or so-called tripod positioning are likely to have obstruction of the extrathoracic airway. In some cases, the cause of the obstruction (e.g., a foreign body) can be identified and corrected promptly so that intubation can be performed without undue delay. However, many causes of severe airway obstruction are not amenable to immediate correction, and an alternative technique may be required. As with BVM ventilation, decreased mobility of the neck can be a significant impediment, especially for the patient with airway obstruction, and it often greatly decreases the likelihood that intubation will be accomplished.

Difficult Supraglottic Airway Placement

With some notable exceptions, the devices used to "rescue" the airway when standard techniques have failed are placed in the supraglottic region with or without occlusion of the esophagus. Their effectiveness relies on lower airway resistance distal to the glottic opening. Consequently, in patients with significant airway obstruction or with obstructive lung disease, these devices may not provide effective ventilation, because the resistance to airflow is actually lower in the proximal portion of the upper airway (i.e., the oral cavity) than in the distal airway. Likewise, such devices may be difficult to insert when mouth opening is significantly restricted or there is distorted airway anatomy.

Difficult Surgical Airway

The term "surgical airway" is often used to describe several potentially life-saving methods of securing the airway by creating an external air passage into the trachea. However, all of these techniques share similar potential drawbacks of vital consideration for proper patient selection. For example, any method for securing a surgical airway requires the identification of external anatomic landmarks. If these structures cannot be readily identified (e.g., the patient is morbidly obese or has severe edema involving the neck), the likelihood of success on a timely basis decreases significantly. Furthermore, patients who have undergone prior airway surgery may have scar tissue or anatomic variation that adds another layer of complexity to an already difficult task. Finally, frank disruption of the airway may require direct surgical intervention, and therefore certain invasive airway techniques, such as retrograde intubation or cricothyrotomy, may not be effective.

▶ AIRWAY MANAGEMENT ALGORITHMS

Airway Assessment

For anesthesiologists, preoperative evaluation is important in the identification of patients at risk for airway management problems, as any anatomical features and clinical factors associated with a difficult airway can be carefully evaluated (5,8–13). Unfortunately, emergency physicians rarely have the opportunity to perform such a detailed assessment.

It should be noted that many of the evaluations used for predicting a difficult airway in adults have not been extrapolated to the pediatric population. Patient cooperation cannot be assured, and therefore the airway exam is often limited. Even under the best of circumstances, some characteristics predisposing to a difficult airway will only be discovered after the patient has undergone a rapid sequence induction. Thus

the emergency physician must rely on the most thorough assessment that can be performed given the time constraints imposed by the patient's condition and should always be prepared with alternative techniques for the possibility of an unanticipated difficult airway. Clinicians should also be familiar with one or more of the published airway management algorithms (Figs. 17.3 and 17.4).

Anatomic features that can negatively affect airway management have been discussed previously (see "Anatomy and Physiology"). What follows is a brief description of a rapid, systematic assessment aimed at identifying patients at risk for the five types of difficult airway (Table 17.1). If, based on this evaluation, problems can be anticipated with intubation and/or the alternative techniques described below, then the operator should consider securing the airway without the use of paralytic agents.

The ED airway evaluation should begin with a brief external examination, the purpose of which is to identify features that might adversely affect airway management. These may include obvious characteristics like severe trauma, congenital facial abnormalities, and medical appliances, as well as more commonplace traits like obesity and the presence of facial hair. The operator should then (a) look for any problems the patient might have with opening the mouth; (b) estimate the patient's Mallampati/Cormack-Lehane score; (c) assess the relative length of the mandible; and (d) determine the location of the hyoid bone, which serves as a landmark for the most caudal portion of the airway. Limited mouth opening, an excessively long or short mandible, and a more rostrally or caudally located hyoid bone all suggest that an optimal laryngoscopic view of the airway might be difficult to obtain. While guidelines for determining these proportions are well described for adult patients, the development of pediatric guidelines has lagged far behind. As mentioned, preliminary data indicate that the Mallampati classification may be an insensitive predictor of difficult intubation in the pediatric population (14). Also, Berry has suggested that the appropriate thyromental distance in infants should be one fingerbreadth (1.5 cm) (15).

During this evaluation, the operator should also be alert for clues suggesting airway obstruction and the degree to which the problems can be corrected by simple maneuvers designed to reposition the airway. Signs like snoring and noisy breathing, symptoms of upper respiratory tract infection, or a history of recurrent croup or problems with breathing while feeding suggests that the child has or is prone to extrathoracic airway obstruction. Such children may be difficult to ventilate with a BVM circuit or a supraglottic device.

Finally, the operator must determine whether there will be any significant impediment to moving the patient's neck, as this can be an important factor in both obtaining an adequate laryngoscopic view of the airway and performing effective BVM ventilation. Patients with a suspected unstable cervical spine fracture whose head, neck, and torso are fully immobilized or those with congenital abnormalities that severely restrict neck mobility may be difficult to intubate and/or

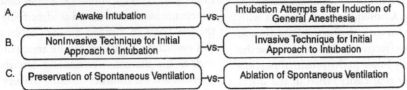

DIFFICULT AIRWAY ALGORITHM

1. Assess the likelihood and clinical impact of basic management problems:
   A. Difficult Ventilation
   B. Difficult Intubation
   C. Difficulty with Patient Cooperation or Consent
   D. Difficult Tracheostomy

2. Actively pursue opportunities to deliver supplemental oxygen throughout the process of difficult airway management

3. Consider the relative merits and feasibility of basic management choices:

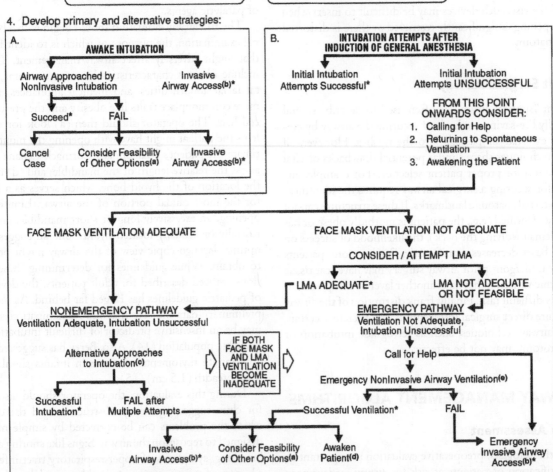

4. Develop primary and alternative strategies:

* Confirm ventilation, tracheal intubation, or LMA placement with exhaled CO_2

a. Other options include (but are not limited to): surgery utilizing face mask or LMA anesthesia, local anesthesia infiltration or regional nerve blockade. Pursuit of these options usually implies that mask ventilation will not be problematic. Therefore, these options may be of limited value if this step in the algorithm has been reached via the Emergency Pathway.

b. Invasive airway access includes surgical or percutaneous tracheostomy or cricothyrotomy.

c. Alternative noninvasive approaches to difficult intubation include (but are not limited to): use of different laryngoscope blades, LMA as an intubation conduit (with or without fiberoptic guidance), fiberoptic intubation, intubating stylet or tube changer, light wand, retrograde intubation, and blind oral or nasal intubation.

d. Consider repreparation of the patient for awake intubation or canceling surgery.

e. Options for emergency noninvasive airway ventilation include (but are not limited to): rigid bronchoscope, esophageal-tracheal Combitube ventilation, or transtracheal jet ventilation.

Figure 17.3 Difficult airway algorithm. (Reproduced with permission from Practice Guidelines for the management of the difficult airway: an updated report by the American Society of Anesthesiologists Task Force on Management of the Difficult Airway. *Anesthesiology.* 2003;98:1269–1277.)

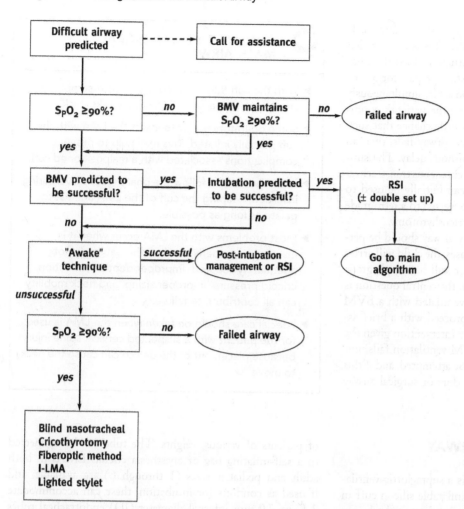

Figure 17.4 The emergency difficult airway algorithm. (Reproduced with permission from Walls RM. The emergency airway algorithms. In: Walls RM, Murphy MF, Luten RC, et al., eds. *Manual of Emergency Airway Management.* 2nd ed. Philadelphia: Lippincott Williams & Wilkins; 2004:9.)

manually ventilate, especially if another airway problem is present (large tongue, extreme rostral location of the glottis, etc.)

When a patient is suspected of having a difficult airway, the operator should consider whether the procedure can proceed as planned or whether an alternative technique should be chosen. As mentioned previously, one of the most important questions is whether a paralytic agent should be used. If the airway exam suggests potential difficulty in more than one of the areas discussed (especially BVM ventilation), then intubation should be delayed whenever possible until equipment

TABLE 17.1	RAPID AIRWAY ASSESSMENT

1. Look for obvious injuries or abnormalities that might affect ventilation, intubation, placement of a supraglottic device, or performance of a surgical airway procedure.
2. Evaluate the size of the mouth opening, the length of the mandible, and the distance between the thyroid cartilage and the floor of the mouth.
3. If possible, look into the mouth and determine an approximate Mallampati score.
4. Determine whether the neck can be safely moved to facilitate laryngoscopy.
5. Look and listen for signs of airway obstruction.

and personnel are available for an alternative technique, such as awake fiberoptic intubation with judicious use of sedation. Unfortunately, this is not always an option in the ED. The condition of the patient often mandates that a definitive airway be secured immediately. Consequently, many authorities recommend a so-called double setup approach to the patient with a potentially difficult airway. To perform a double setup, the operator or an assistant prepares the materials for orotracheal intubation (and/or alternative techniques) as well as those for a surgical airway. Prior to the administration of paralytic agents, the patient's cricothyroid membrane is identified and the skin is cleaned with aseptic solution so that a surgical airway can be performed quickly should other methods fail.

Unanticipated Versus Anticipated Difficult Airway

In the case of an unanticipated difficult airway, it is assumed in most algorithms that the patient who cannot be intubated has already received a paralytic agent as part of a rapid sequence induction regimen. In such cases, the first question is whether the patient can be ventilated with a BVM device. If so, then ventilation should proceed pending an alternative technique or an intubation attempt by another clinician. If not, then the operator must act rapidly. This is the dreaded "cannot intubate–cannot ventilate" situation. In such situations, the operator should have an assistant prepare for one of the invasive airway techniques and, if possible, simultaneously attempt to place a rescue airway, unless the patient's condition or anatomy suggests that there is little chance that such an airway would succeed. If the rescue airway fails, then an invasive airway must be established without delay. The simplest technique for most children is percutaneous transtracheal ventilation (see Chapter 18), which can initially be used to provide ventilation and then can be converted to a retrograde intubation or a wire-guided surgical cricothyrotomy.

Management of the true emergency airway should be performed in a similar fashion. In most cases, the child will arrive in the ED unconscious and apneic or will have high-grade upper airway obstruction. Once again, the central question is whether the child can be effectively ventilated with a BVM device. If so, then the operator can proceed with a brief assessment, followed by the appropriate intervention given the specific clinical circumstances. If BVM ventilation fails, immediate endotracheal intubation can be attempted, and if this is unsuccessful, a rescue airway procedure or surgical airway must be expeditiously performed.

 CLINICAL TIPS: LARYNGEAL MASK AIRWAY

▶ With the cuff fully deflated, the LMA resembles a small boat with a curved mast or smokestack.

▶ Some operators prefer to insert the LMA with the cuff partially inflated. This may help to prevent complications associated with a malpositioned cuff.

▶ It is important to follow the pharyngeal curve during insertion, keeping the cuff of the LMA against the palate as long as possible.

▶ Most problems with the LMA occur when it is inserted improperly or when the patient is not adequately sedated. Improper depth of insertion, cricoid pressure, improper sizing, and neck mobility can all contribute to failure.

▶ Special care should be taken when the LMA is used for the patient with a suspected cervical spine injury because placement of the device can cause the neck to move.

▶ LARYNGEAL MASK AIRWAY

The laryngeal mask airway (LMA) is a supraglottic ventilatory device that consists of an oval inflatable silicon cuff in continuity with a wide-bore tube designed to fit the larynx

 SUMMARY: LARYNGEAL MASK AIRWAY

1 Select an appropriately sized LMA.

2 Remove the LMA from its packaging and inspect the cuff for leaks.

3 Completely deflate the cuff (a) using a commercial deflator or (b) by pressing the ventilating side against a flat surface and placing the fingers of the nondominant hand around the cuff while deflating the cuff with the dominant hand.

4 Lubricate the cuff using a water-soluble lubricant.

5 Open the patient's mouth and, holding the LMA like a pen or pencil, guide the cuff along the palate and over the tongue. Continue with insertion until the LMA cannot be advanced further.

6 Inflate the cuff and connect the LMA to a bag and attempt to ventilate the patient.

7 If ventilation is not successful, check for an air leak or malpositioning of the cuff.

of patients of various weights. The tube can be connected to a self-inflating bag or anesthesia circuit. LMAs in both adult and pediatric sizes (1 through 6) are available, and if used as conduits for intubation, these can accommodate 3.5- to 7.0-mm internal diameter (ID) endotracheal tubes (Fig. 17.5).

Indications

Although originally developed for airway management of routine cases with spontaneous ventilation, the LMA is now listed in the ASA difficult airway algorithm as an airway ventilatory device or a conduit for endotracheal intubation (3,16). It can be used in both pediatric and adult patients for whom BVM ventilation and intubation are difficult or impossible.

The LMA is unlikely to be effective in cases of upper airway obstruction or significant airway disruption. Additionally, the

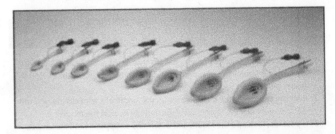

Figure 17.5 The LMA Classic. (Reproduced with permission from LMA North America, Inc., http://www.lmana.com/prod/components/products/ lma_classic.html.)

TABLE 17.2	SIZING CHART FOR THE LARYNGEAL MASK AIRWAY (LMA CLASSIC)
Size	**Patient Selection Guidelines**
1	Neonates/infants up to 5 kg
1½	Infants 5–10 kg
2	Infants/children 10–20 kg
2½	Children 20–30 kg
3	Children 30–50 kg
4	Adults 50–70 kg
5	Adults 70–100 kg
6	Large adults over 100 kg

Source: Adapted with permission from a table on the LMA North America, Inc., website: http://www.lmana.com/prod/components/products/lma_classic.html.

LMA does not provide complete occlusion of the esophagus and therefore offers less protection against aspiration than other alternative devices or techniques. However, in many cases the benefits to be gained by effective ventilation outweigh such risks.

Equipment

An array of pediatric and adult sizes are commercially available (LMA North America, Inc., San Diego, CA). An LMA of the appropriate size, a water-soluble lubricant, and a syringe to inflate the cuff are the only pieces of equipment required. The suggested weight for each size of LMA is listed on the side of the ventilating tube, along with the volume required to inflate the cuff (Table 17.2).

Procedure

After the LMA is removed from its package, the cuff should be inspected for damage. An essential component of LMA placement is the complete and proper deflation of the cuff. Although there is a special tool for this purpose, the cuff can be deflated without this tool, as follows. The anterior portion of the LMA cuff is placed against a firm, flat surface such as a table or countertop. The index and middle fingers of the operator's nondominant hand are placed on either side of the cuff to compress it while a syringe in the operator's dominant hand is used to remove all air until the cuff is completely empty. When properly deflated, the cuff has the appearance of a small boat with a long, curved mast or smokestack. After deflation, the LMA cuff should be lubricated with a water-soluble lubricant along its tip and posterior surface.

Two techniques for the use of an LMA are most commonly employed. To perform the first technique, the operator stands above the patient at the head of the bed in a position similar to that for a standard orotracheal intubation. The LMA is initially placed in the oropharynx with the ventilating portion facing the tongue. Holding the LMA like a pen or pencil (Fig. 17.6A), the operator uses the index finger of the dominant hand to guide the LMA along the patient's palate until it cannot be advanced any further (Fig. 17.6B–E). At this point, the operator releases the shaft of the LMA, and the cuff is then inflated. Inflation of the cuff often helps the LMA to "seat" itself in the proper position. Once the LMA is in place, a resuscitation bag is attached, and the patient can be ventilated. The operator should then check for a leak. If a leak occurs at less than 15 cm H_2O, the LMA may require repositioning or possibly removal and reinsertion. The second technique involves using the operator's thumb to insert the device. With this method, the operator stands at the side of the bed facing the patient. Other methods have also been described in the literature, including insertion of the device with the ventilating portion facing the hard palate (17) and insertion with partial cuff inflation (18).

Complications

The most common complication associated with the placement of an LMA is lack of effective ventilation. This is usually dependent on the user's skill and experience, the patient's level of consciousness, and patient-specific anatomic or physiologic abnormalities (19). Placing the LMA correctly can be difficult in some patients. The mask may fold on itself either under or over its main axis. The incidence of failed placement is 1% to 5%, although the incidence tends to decrease with increasing operator experience (20). Failure to insert the LMA most often results from inadequate anesthesia, suboptimal head and neck position, incorrect mask deflation, failure to follow the palatopharyngeal curve during insertion, inadequate depth of insertion, cricoid pressure, and oral pathology such as large tonsils.

Laryngospasm and coughing may result from inadequate anesthesia, tip impaction against the glottis, or aspiration. Some operators prefer to insert the LMA with the cuff partially inflated in an attempt to avoid these problems. Complete epiglottis downfolding can increase the work of breathing and cause coughing and laryngospasm as well as complete airway obstruction (21).

Mask leaks or the inability to ventilate the lungs may also result from inadequate anesthesia, malpositioning of mask, inappropriate mask size, and high airway pressures. Hypoventilation due to coma or complete paralysis may lead to high end-tidal carbon dioxide concentration. Effects of pharyngolaryngeal reflexes like laryngospasm, coughing, gagging, bronchospasm, breath-holding, and retching may be associated with use of an LMA. Displacement of the LMA after insertion may be caused by inadequate anesthetic depth, a pulled or twisted tube, and an inadequately sized LMA. Patients who awaken with an LMA in place may have tube occlusion from biting. Additionally, cuff deflation and tube removal at an inadequate depth of anesthesia can cause vomiting, severe coughing, and laryngospasm.

Several other complications of varying severity have been reported with use of an LMA. A known disadvantage of the device is the inability to protect against regurgitation

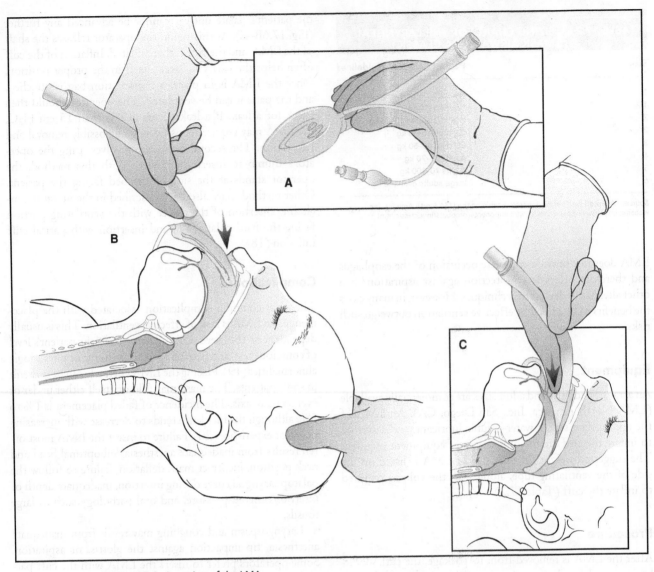

Figure 17.6 Insertion of the LMA.
A. The LMA is held in the operator's dominant hand like a pen or pencil, with the index finger at the cuff as shown.
B. The patient's mouth is opened, and the LMA is pressed against the patient's hard palate. The wrist of the operator should remain flexed. If neck movement is not prohibited, placement of the operator's nondominant hand as shown can increase leverage and facilitate placement.
C. The LMA mask is pressed inward by extension of the index finger. Contact with the palate is maintained.

of gastric contents and pulmonary aspiration. Because the LMA does not isolate the trachea from the esophagus, the patient who has a full stomach or requires high airway pressures for adequate positive pressure ventilation is at greater risk for aspiration pneumonitis. However, when the indications and contraindications for the procedure are strictly observed, the likelihood of this complication is comparable to the likelihood with endotracheal intubation (22). In the ED, where every patient is assumed to have a full stomach, the potential risk of aspiration pneumonitis must be weighed against the advantages of the LMA in cases of difficult in-

tubation and ventilation, when use of this device may be life-saving.

▶ INTUBATING LARYNGEAL MASK AIRWAY (FASTRACH)

The Fastrach (LMA North America, Inc, San Diego, CA) is a special type of LMA that allows the patient to be ventilated in a manner similar to the standard LMA but also serves as a conduit for intubation. The Fastrach looks distinctly

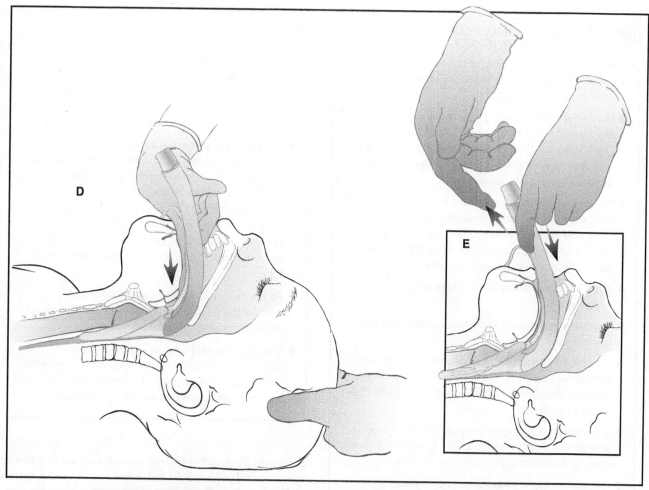

Figure 17.6 *(Continued)*
D. The index finger is pressed toward the nondominant hand to exert counterpressure.
E. The LMA cuff is advanced into the hypopharynx until resistance is felt. The operator maintains gentle downward pressure on the tube while removing the index finger from the patient's mouth. (Adapted with permission from *The LMA Airway Instruction Manual*. The Laryngeal Mask Company Limited; 2004. http://www.lmana.com/prod/content/education/LMA_Airways_Manual.pdf.)

different from the standard LMA and its other variations. It consists of a mask attached to a rigid stainless steel tube curved to align the barrel aperture to the glottic vestibule. The set includes an LMA with a stainless steel shaft covered with silicon (reusable version), a tracheal tube stabilizer (tube pusher), and a silicon-reinforced tracheal tube (Fig. 17.7). Whereas the standard LMA has a flexible tube resembling an endotracheal tube, the Fastrach has a rigid metal tube that is curved into a U shape. The Fastrach also has a large spatula-like handle near its distal end. Finally, within the cuff of the Fastrach is located a tiny lever that is designed to lift the epiglottis when the endotracheal tube passes through the metal tube.

Indications

The Fastrach is indicated for patients with existing or impending respiratory failure who require artificial ventilation and who do not have obstruction of the extrathoracic airway. Although designed for blind orotracheal intubation, it can be

used in conjunction with lighted stylets, a fiberoptic bronchoscope, or the Flexible Airway Scope Tool (FAST, Clarus Medical, MN).

The Fastrach is contraindicated in patients with upper airway obstruction. Since the endotracheal tube is usually placed blindly, it is less likely to be successful when the patient's anatomy is abnormal. The first-pass success rate is 93% to 97%, although the rate increases to 100% when the Fastrach is used in conjunction with a fiberoptic bronchoscope (23–25). Additionally, when used for ventilation, the Fastrach has the same disadvantage as a standard LMA in offering less protection of the airway than an endotracheal tube from aspiration of stomach contents into the lungs if reflux or regurgitation occurs.

Equipment

The Fastrach is available in three sizes (3 through 5) and can accommodate 6- to 8-mm ID endotracheal tubes. Although

SUMMARY: INTUBATING LARYNGEAL MASK AIRWAY (FASTRACH)

1 Prepare the Fastrach in a manner similar to that used for a standard LMA.

2 Guide the Fastrach into position using the fingers of the nondominant hand, as described for a standard LMA; however, the rigid structure of the Fastrach dictates the path it will follow (the metal handle can facilitate correct placement).

3 When the Fastrach cannot be advanced further, inflate the cuff, attach a resuscitation bag to the tube, and attempt to ventilate the patient; if ventilation is successful, proceed to the next step; if not, replace or reposition the device.

4 Make sure that the patient is adequately oxygenated.

5 Lubricate the silicone endotracheal tube and inspect the cuff for leaks.

6 Pass the endotracheal tube into the Fastrach while simultaneously lifting the handle gently upward (an assistant should apply moderate pressure over the thyroid cartilage).

7 If resistance is felt, gently reposition the device; slightly more or less lifting of the handle or slightly more or less cricoid pressure may be effective.

8 Once the tube has been successfully passed, confirm its position with an end-tidal CO_2 detector.

9 Inflate the cuff of the endotracheal tube, ventilate the patient a few times, then remove the adapter from the endotracheal tube and deflate the cuff of the Fastrach.

10 Begin removing the Fastrach; as the device approaches the top of the endotracheal tube, attach the rubber stabilizing bar to the endotracheal tube; continue to pass the Fastrach over the rubber stabilizing bar until it is completely out of the patient's mouth; during this process, maintain control of the endotracheal tube.

11 After the Fastrach and the stabilizing bar have been removed, replace the adapter on the endotracheal tube and resume ventilation.

12 Secure the endotracheal tube using standard methods.

CLINICAL TIPS: INTUBATING LARYNGEAL MASK AIRWAY (FASTRACH)

▶ The Fastrach may not be perfectly aligned with the glottic opening. Just as in a standard intubation attempt, it may be necessary to manipulate external structures in order to pass the endotracheal tube.

▶ The Fastrach can be used as a conduit through which a flexible fiberoptic scope or an airway guide is passed. The former method allows for direct visualization of the airway, while the latter provides tactile feedback confirming that the airway guide has passed into the trachea. Additionally, a lighted stylet can be passed into the Fastrach and used as a guide for proper placement of the endotracheal tube.

▶ As the Fastrach is being passed over the endotracheal tube, special care should be taken to avoid dislodging the tube.

▶ The endotracheal tube designed for use with the Fastrach is made of flexible silicone and reinforced with wire. It can be damaged very easily. When this tube is used, a bite block is recommended.

the special silicon tubes are recommended for use with this device, standard polyvinyl chloride tubes may be used if warmed and softened or if used in conjunction with a fiberoptic bronchoscope.

Procedure

As with the standard LMA, proper use of the Fastrach requires that the cuff be inspected for damage and correctly deflated. The Fastrach is then placed into the oropharynx and guided along the palate into position (Fig. 17.8A,B). Unlike in the case of the standard LMA, the rigid nature of the Fastrach dictates the path that it follows; care should be taken to guide the device along the middle of the palate (Fig. 17.8C). The handle facilitates this process to some extent. Once resistance is met, no further advancement of the device is made, and the cuff is inflated (Fig. 17.8D). A standard resuscitation bag is attached, and ventilation is attempted (Fig. 17.8E). If ventilation is effective, then the operator can proceed with insertion of an endotracheal tube. The patient should first be adequately preoxygenated so that a brief period of apnea will be tolerated as the tube is inserted. The resuscitation bag is disconnected, and the special silicon endotracheal tube is inserted into the Fastrach and advanced (Fig. 17.8F). During advancement, the Fastrach should be lifted upward, and a slight amount of pressure should be applied over the thyroid cartilage (Fig. 17.8G,H). If resistance is met, the tube should be removed and reinserted.

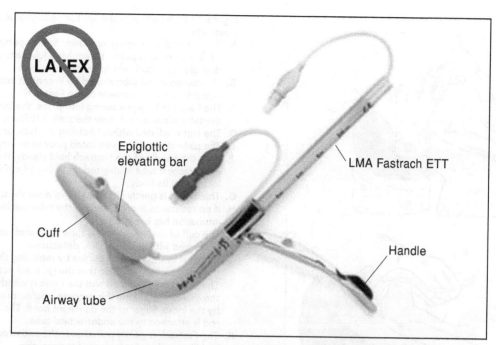

Figure 17.7 The intubating laryngeal mask airway (Fastrach). (Reproduced with permission from LMA North American, Inc., http://www.lmana.com/prod/components/products/lma_fastrach.html.)

Once successfully placed, the endotracheal tube cuff is inflated (Fig. 17.8I). Proper placement should be confirmed by a colorimetric device or capnography (see Chapter 76). The cuff of the Fastrach can then be deflated (Fig. 17.8J). The tube connector is removed, and the stabilizing device is placed through the Fastrach and used to advance the endotracheal tube while the Fastrach is carefully passed over the flexible endotracheal tube and removed from the patient's mouth (Fig. 17.8K,L). The stabilizing device is then removed so the pilot balloon can be passed through the shaft of the Fastrach (Fig. 17.8M). At this point, the tube connector is reattached to accommodate a resuscitation bag or ventilator (Fig. 17.8N), and the endotracheal tube is secured using standard methods. If a silicon endotracheal tube is used, insertion of a bite block is recommended, because these soft, wire-reinforced tubes are easily damaged and will not re-expand.

Complications

In addition to the previously described complications associated with the standard LMA, the Fastrach has its own potential complications, the most important of which is failure to pass the endotracheal tube into the trachea. In some cases, the Fastrach can be repositioned in order to facilitate passage; alternatively, the operator may attempt external manipulation of the airway as described above. Other solutions include the use of a fiberoptic bronchoscope, a lighted stylet, or an airway guide to direct the tube into the trachea. As with any form of endotracheal intubation, capnography should always be used to confirm that the tube is located within the trachea to avoid the potentially catastrophic complication of an unrecognized esophageal intubation.

▶ COMBITUBE

The Esophageal Tracheal Combitube (Tyco-Kendall, Mansfield, MA) is another supraglottic ventilatory device that can be used emergently as a rescue airway and is included in the ASA Difficult Airway Algorithm (3). The Combitube is a disposable double-lumen tube that combines features of a conventional endotracheal tube with an esophageal obturator airway. It has a large proximal latex oropharyngeal balloon, eight ventilatory holes, and a distal esophageal low-pressure cuff. It comes in two adult sizes based on height: a standard size (41 F) for adults taller than 5 feet and a small adult size (37 F) for those 4 to 5½ feet in height. Because the Combitube has a distal cuff which occludes the esophagus when inflated, it may offer a greater degree of airway protection than the LMA. The proximal balloon on the standard adult Combitube is inflated with up to 100 cc of air while that on the small adult Combitube is inflated with up to 85 cc of air. The smaller balloons require approximately 15 cc and 12 cc of air, respectively. Once placed, ventilation is possible with either tracheal or esophageal intubation. The operator must simply determine which lumen should be used for ventilation—the esophageal lumen (labeled "1") for esophageal intubation versus the tracheal lumen (labeled "2") for tracheal intubation.

Indications

The Combitube is indicated for patients without extrathoracic airway obstruction who require artificial ventilation and who cannot be intubated or ventilated using standard techniques.

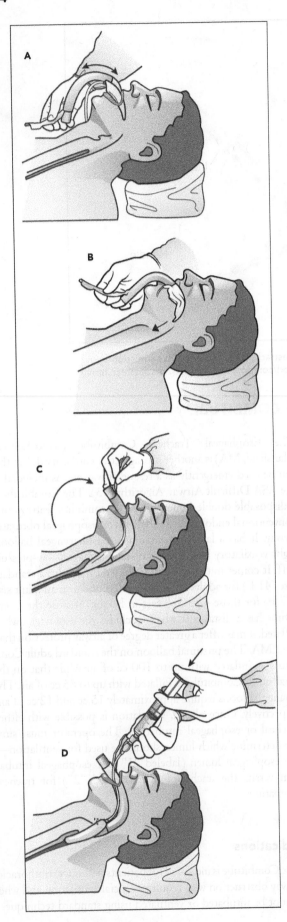

Figure 17.8 Insertion of the intubating laryngeal mask airway (Fastrach).

A. The Fastrach is inserted as shown. Some operators elect to lubricate the hard palate by applying lubricant to the LMA and then sliding it back and forth after insertion.

B. The curved metal tube should be in contact with the patient's chin prior to advancement of the Fastrach.

C. The Fastrach is gently swung into place, the curved body of the tube allowed to dictate the path it follows.

D. The cuff is inflated without holding the tube or handle.

E. The patient should be ventilated prior to attempted intubation.

F. With the handle of the Fastrach held steady, the special endotracheal tube is inserted up to the 15-cm depth marker located on its body.

G. The handle is gently lifted as shown while the tube is advanced.

H. If no resistance is encountered, the tube can be advanced until intubation has been achieved.

I. The cuff of the endotracheal tube is inflated, and its position is confirmed with end-tidal CO_2 detection.

J. Removal of the Fastrach begins by removing the connector of the endotracheal tube, so that the tube will not be dislodged. The cuff is then deflated and the mask is withdrawn back into the oral cavity. During this process, counterpressure is applied by the index finger of the dominant hand. The rubber stabilizer rod is attached to the endotracheal tube.

K. The Fastrach is gently pulled over the endotracheal tube and stabilizer rod until it is clear of the mouth.

L. The stabilizer rod is removed, and the endotracheal tube is held securely at the level of the incisors.

M. The Fastrach can then be separated from the endotracheal tube. Care must be taken to gently unthread the inflation line and pilot balloon.

N. The endotracheal tube connector is reattached.

(Adapted with permission from *LMA Fastrach Single Use and Reusable Manual*, LMA North America, Inc., San Diego, CA.)

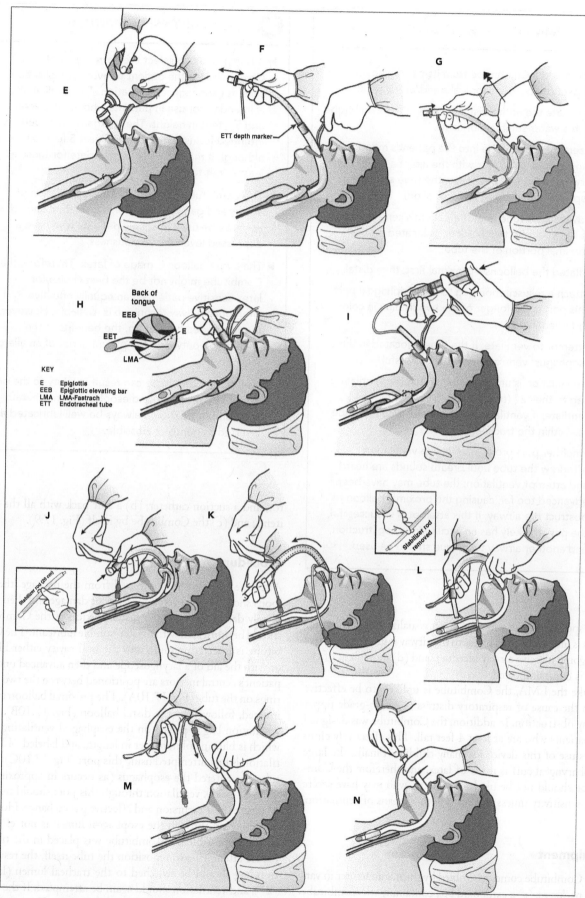

Figure 17.8 (Continued)

SUMMARY: COMBITUBE

1 Remove the Combitube from its packaging and inspect the balloons for leaks and/or damage.

2 Lubricate the entire distal portion of the Combitube with a water-soluble lubricant.

3 Insert the Combitube into the patient's mouth; this can be done blindly or with the aid of a laryngoscope (in either case, the tube should be kept in the midline as it is advanced).

4 Advance the tube until the patient's central incisors lie between the two black rings located on the proximal portion of the tube.

5 Inflated the balloons—proximal first, then distal.

6 Attach a resuscitation bag to the esophageal port (this port is the longer of the two, is blue in color, and is labeled "1").

7 Attempt to ventilate; if the tube is located in the esophagus, ventilation will be successful.

8 If ventilation is unsuccessful, switch the ventilating bag to the "2" (tracheal) port and attempt to ventilate; if ventilation is successful, then the tube lies within the trachea.

9 If neither port provides effective ventilation, withdraw the tube until breath sounds are heard and attempt ventilation; the tube may have been advanced too far, causing the proximal balloon to obstruct the airway; if this attempt is unsuccessful, the patient likely has an occult airway obstruction, and another airway technique should be used.

CLINICAL TIPS: COMBITUBE

▶ It is important to select the correct size of Combitube for the patient to avoid complications such as esophageal perforation. The small adult size is intended for use in patients who are between 4 and 5½ feet in height. The standard Combitube is intended for use in persons at least 5 feet tall, although it may be more appropriate for those at least 6 feet tall.

▶ The Combitube causes extensive stimulation of airway and gag reflexes. Consequently, it should normally be used in apneic patients who have a depressed level of consciousness.

▶ The larger balloon is made of latex. Therefore, the Combitube might not be the best choice for latex-sensitive patients if an equally effective alternative airway technique is available. However, in a life-or-death situation, the benefits of the Combitube outweigh the potential risk of an allergic reaction.

▶ Use of the Combitube can result in injury to the oral cavity, upper airway, and esophagus, and therefore the Combitube should always be well lubricated and inserted as gently as possible.

tor, and a suction catheter; (b) a soft pack with all the same items; and (c) the Combitube by itself (Fig. 17.9).

It is especially useful when (a) direct visualization of the vocal cords is impossible, (b) access to the airway is limited, (c) there is ongoing massive airway bleeding, and (d) movement of the neck is contraindicated.

Like the LMA, the Combitube is unlikely to be effective when the cause of respiratory distress is a high-grade upper airway obstruction. In addition, the Combitube was designed for patients who are at least 4 feet tall. This effectively eliminates use of this device for many children. Finally, the large oropharyngeal cuff is made of latex, and therefore the Combitube should not be used for patients who may have severe latex sensitivity unless there is no other means of ventilation.

Equipment

The Combitube comes assembled by the manufacturer in various packages: (a) a cardboard box containing the Combitube enclosed in a hard pack, two syringes, a plastic elbow connec-

Procedure

After the Combitube is removed from the package, the balloons should be inspected for leaks or damage and then completely deflated. The entire distal portion of the Combitube should be lubricated with a water-soluble lubricant. The Combitube is inserted midline into the oral cavity either blindly or with the aid of a laryngoscope and then advanced until the patient's central incisors are positioned between the two black rings on the tube (Fig. 17.10A). The proximal balloon is then inflated, followed by the distal balloon (Fig. 17.10B). A resuscitation bag is placed on the esophageal ventilating port, which is blue in color, longer in length, and labeled "1." Ventilation is first attempted using this port (Fig. 17.10C). If the tube has entered the esophagus (as occurs in approximately 98% of cases), ventilation through this port should result in adequate chest excursion and effective gas exchange. However, if ventilation through the esophageal lumen is not effective, then it is possible the Combitube was placed in the trachea. Before attempting to reposition the tube itself, the resuscitation bag should be switched to the tracheal lumen (labeled "2"), and ventilation should again be attempted. If the Combitube is indeed located within the trachea, then ventilation

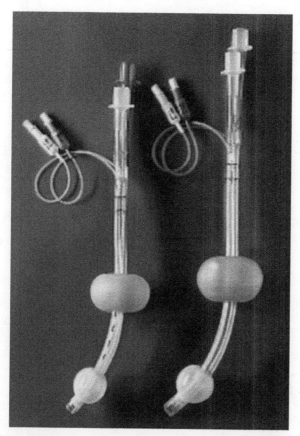

Figure 17.9 The Combitube. (Reproduced with permission from Nellcor, Pleasanton, CA, http://www.nellcor.com/prod/Product.aspx?id=259.)

through the tracheal lumen will be effective (Fig. 17.10D). If ventilation cannot be accomplished through either lumen, the operator should consider occult airway obstruction or the possibility that the tube was advanced too deeply and the proximal balloon is obstructing the glottis.

Complications

Few complications have been reported with use of the Combitube. Sore throat has been reported in 16% to 48% of patients (26–28). In two patients, the device was inserted too deeply, causing the large pharyngeal cuff to lie directly over the glottis and obstruct the upper airway (26). Consequently, neither lumen provided effective ventilation. This problem was easily resolved by partially withdrawing the Combitube until breath sounds were heard. Although tongue discoloration during inflation of the pharyngeal cuff has been reported, it usually resolves immediately without further adverse sequelae once the cuff is deflated. Subcutaneous emphysema, pneumomediastinum, and pneumoperitoneum during resuscitations have been reported (27).

Two esophageal lacerations were reported by Vezina et al., but in both cases the distal cuff was overinflated with 20 to 40 mL instead of the recommended 12 mL, and the larger Combitube (F 41) was used in a small patient (29). Klein et al. reported a case of iatrogenic esophageal perforation

during Combitube use in a patient with a hiatal hernia (30). They proposed that the rupture resulted from direct trauma by the Combitube or from increased intraluminal pressure distal to the tube, with poor patient selection as a contributing factor. Nonetheless, esophageal trauma is a rare potential complication of Combitube use, and its incidence may further be reduced by (a) using the small adult Combitube for any patient 4 to 6 feet tall, (b) inserting it under direct vision and with an adequate depth of anesthesia, (c) assuring that cuff overinflation does not occur, and (d) avoiding its use in patients with any suspicion of esophageal pathology (30). As previously mentioned, the Combitube does contain latex, and latex-sensitive individuals can experience severe allergic reactions, including anaphylaxis.

▶ LIGHTED STYLET

The lighted stylet, also called a "lightwand," is a device that allows blind insertion of an endotracheal tube into the trachea using an intense light to guide the tube into the proper position. The Trachlight (Laerdal Medical Corporation, Stavanger, Norway) is considered by many to be the best of the lightwands and is the device discussed in this section. It consists of a reusable handle, a flexible wand, and a stiff, retractable stylet, and it is available in three sizes (adult, child, and infant), accommodating 2.5- to 10-mm ID endotracheal tubes. Lighted stylet intubation is a blind technique that can be used alone or in conjunction with other devices, including traditional laryngoscopes.

Indications

The lighted stylet is most useful as an alternative to standard techniques of orotracheal intubation when adequate visualization of the airway with direct laryngoscopy proves impossible. Such situations can occur if neck mobility or mouth opening is severely limited or when there is excessive blood or debris in the airway. The lighted stylet can also be employed when a fiberoptic bronchoscope or an operator skilled in the use of this device is unavailable (e.g., in the ED or an ambulance) or when bronchoscopy is difficult to perform (e.g., when the airway is obscured by blood, vomit, or secretions). It should be noted that like all procedures performed blindly, success with the lightwand often depends on whether the patient has normal airway anatomy. In those with distorted anatomy (severe trauma, mass lesion, etc.) attempted intubation with a lighted stylet may fail.

Equipment

There are several types of lighted stylets, but all share certain features, including a light source, which is generally powered by batteries contained in the handle, and a malleable stylet with a light bulb at its tip. The stylet can be permanently attached to the handle, in which case multiple handle-stylet combinations are needed for patients of various sizes, or it can be

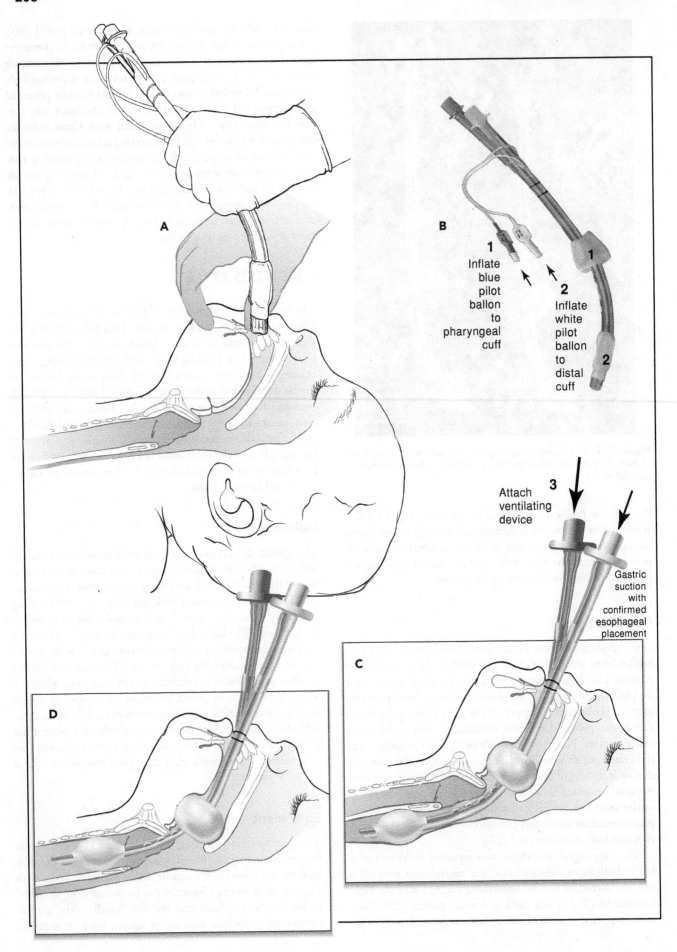

A

B

1
Inflate
blue
pilot
ballon
to
pharyngeal
cuff

2
Inflate
white
pilot
ballon
to
distal
cuff

3
Attach
ventilating
device

Gastric
suction
with
confirmed
esophageal
placement

C

D

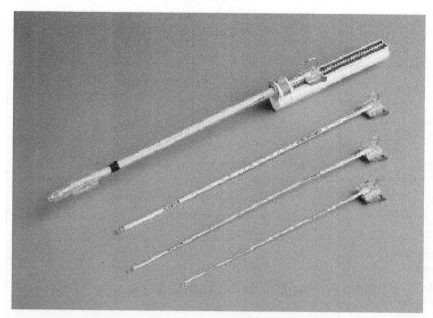

Figure 17.11 Laerdal Trachlight handle and three sizes of wands: adult, pediatric, and infant. The wand and rigid internal stylet combination has been attached to the handle, and an endotracheal tube loaded onto the wand. Note the point of connection between the endotracheal tube and the handle. (Reproduced with permission from Murphy MF, Huang OR. Lighted stylet intubation. In: Walls RM, Murphy MF, Luten RC, et al., eds. *Manual of Emergency Airway Management.* 2nd ed. Philadelphia: Lippincott Williams & Wilkins; 2004:121.)

removable, which allows the same handle to be used with stylets of all sizes. As mentioned above, this chapter discusses the use of the Trachlight, a device that employs a detachable rigid stylet that fits within the flexible lightwand (Fig. 17.11). In addition to the lighted stylet itself, the operator should prepare an appropriately sized endotracheal tube and have lubricant available. Since most lighted stylets are battery powered, it is prudent to always test the light source prior to use, as is common practice with laryngoscopes, to ensure that the device is functioning properly.

Procedure

The operator should select the correct stylet based on the patient's size and attach it to the handle according to manufacturer instructions. The light should be tested to confirm that it is bright and continuous, and both the stylet and tip of the endotracheal tube should be lubricated with a small amount of water-soluble lubricant.

The endotracheal tube is then passed over the stylet and adjusted so that the light bulb is at the level of the Murphy eyehole. (The Trachlight has a clamp that serves to lock the adapter of the endotracheal tube in this position.) The operator then bends the stylet and endotracheal tube so that the tip of the tube will enter the glottic opening. The stylet may

have a mark indicating where it should be bent for a "normal patient." The actual point at which to bend the stylet-endotracheal tube combination is the same distance from the tip of the tube as the distance from the patient's mentum to the thyroid notch. If the patient has abnormal anatomy, this distance should be measured. The next consideration is the angle of the bend. When the patient's head and neck are in a neutral position, the bend should roughly form a 90-degree angle. If the head is flexed, the angle should be decreased, and if the head is extended, the angle should be increased.

Although not essential, dimming the ambient lights often provides optimal transillumination. The light on the lighted stylet is turned on by a switch on the handle. Using the dominant hand, the operator inserts the lighted stylet and endotracheal tube into the patient's oral cavity while lifting the mandible with the nondominant hand. With the stylet-endotracheal tube in the midline, the tip of the tube is progressively advanced as the operator uses the handle to produce a back-and-forth rocking motion along the long axis of the tube. Passage of the tube through the vocal cords is often felt as the tip "pops" into place, but the principal indication of successful intubation is an intense glow concentrated at the patient's thyroid cartilage. A more diffuse glow, or one that is not in the midline, suggests that the glottis has not been entered. If the light disappears, the tube has likely entered

Figure 17.10 Insertion of the Combitube.
A. The Combitube is inserted blindly into the patient's mouth and advanced until the teeth are aligned between the two black rings.
B. The line labeled "1" (blue pilot balloon) is inflated (100 mL for large adult Combitube, 85 mL for small adult Combitube), and then the other line (labeled "2") is inflated (15 mL for large adult Combitube, 12 mL for small adult Combitube).
C. Ventilation is first attempted through the port labeled "1" (blue). Auscultation should confirm the presence of breath sounds.
D. If breath sounds are not heard with ventilation through port 1, then the Combitube may have been inserted into the trachea, and ventilation should be attempted through port 2. (Adapted with permission from Nellcor, Pleasanton, CA, http://www.nellcor.com/_Catalog/PDF/Product/combitube.pdf.)

SUMMARY: LIGHTED STYLET (TRACHLIGHT)

1 Select an appropriately sized stylet.

2 Remove the Trachlight handle and stylet from the packaging, attach the stylet to the handle, and confirm that the light is functioning properly.

3 Remove the stylet from the handle.

4 Select an appropriately sized endotracheal tube.

5 Lubricate the stylet well and guide it onto the handle from the base of the handle through the locking ring.

6 Guide the endotracheal tube onto the stylet and adjust the position of the stylet so that the light is level with the Murphy eye of the tube. Lock the adapter of the endotracheal tube onto the locking ring.

7 Bend the stylet and tube using the indicator mark on the side of the stylet as a guide to the location of the bend. If the patient's head is in the neutral position, the bend should be approximately 90 degrees.

8 While holding the Trachlight in the dominant hand, activate the light (although not essential, some operators prefer to dim the room lights before proceeding).

9 Using the nondominant hand, open the patient's mouth; grasp the patient's mandible and gently lift upward.

10 Using the dominant hand, insert the Trachlight into the patient's mouth; following the midline of the tongue, direct the tube into the airway (this is best accomplished with a gentle rocking motion, tilting the device back and forth along its long axis until the endotracheal tube passes into the trachea).

11 When the desired light pattern is visible on the anterior neck, withdraw the metal stylet approximately 10 cm and advance the flexible stylet and endotracheal tube until the glow is seen at the level of the sternal notch.

12 While maintaining the position of the endotracheal tube, remove the stylet and confirm proper placement of the tube.

13 Secure the endotracheal tube using standard methods.

CLINICAL TIPS: LIGHTED STYLET (TRACHLIGHT)

▶ A slight "pop" or give may be felt as the endotracheal tube enters the glottic opening, but the primary indication that the tube is in the correct location is an intense, concentrated glowing of the thyroid cartilage.

▶ The bend of the stylet should correlate with the patient's head position. If the patient's head is flexed, the bend should be less than 90 degrees; if the patient's head is extended, it should be greater than 90 degrees.

▶ Keeping the lighted stylet in the midline during insertion maximizes the likelihood of success.

▶ Because this is blind procedure, lighted stylet intubation may be difficult or impossible with abnormal or distorted airway anatomy.

▶ If difficulty is encountered, it may be helpful to insert a standard laryngoscope to aid in visualizing the epiglottis so that the lighted stylet can be directed beneath it.

▶ The lighted stylet should not simply be "pushed" into the pharynx. Instead, it is useful to think of the bend as a fulcrum. The lighted stylet should be gently rocked back and forth around this fulcrum as it is inserted.

▶ The lighted stylet can be used effectively for most patients without darkening the room. However, in some cases it may be prudent to test the effect of ambient lighting prior to the intubation attempt. This can be accomplished by first inserting the lighted stylet into the right pyriform recess. The intensity of the light visible through the skin of the lateral neck is roughly equivalent to that seen at the thyroid cartilage. If this test demonstrates that the light cannot be seen adequately, then the room lights should be dimmed before intubation is attempted.

the esophagus. Once a well-circumscribed light glow is visualized, the operator should advance the lighted stylet while at the same time retracting the rigid internal stylet until the glow appears in the suprasternal notch. This indicates that the tip of the endotracheal tube is now in good position. The operator then withdraws the lighted stylet while holding the endotracheal tube in place. Tracheal position is confirmed by using a colorimetric device or capnography and listening for bilateral breath sounds (Fig. 17.12).

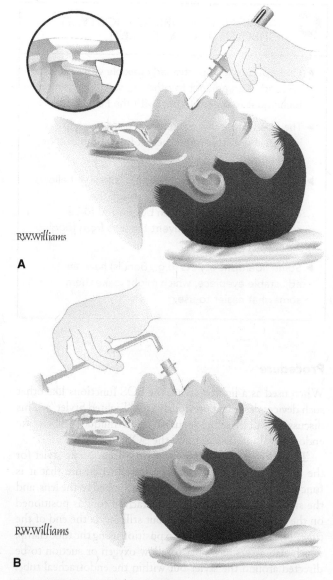

R.W.Williams

A

R.W.Williams

B

Figure 17.12 Trachlight intubation.
A. The operator is holding the device by the handle rather than holding the endotracheal tube–Trachlight unit, a technical detail that most prefer. In this figure, the head is rather more extended than ordinarily recommended. A neutral position is preferred.
B. Once the endotracheal tube–Trachlight unit has been placed in the trachea, the Trachlight is removed. (Reproduced with permission from Murphy MF, Huang OR. Lighted stylet intubation. In: Walls RM, Murphy MF, Luten RC, et al., eds. *Manual of Emergency Airway Management.* 2nd ed. Philadelphia: Lippincott Williams & Wilkins; 2004:124.)

Complications

The primary complication resulting from use of a lighted stylet is failure of the intubation attempt. Success with this technique requires practice. The epiglottis must be lifted out of the way to allow successful passage of the lighted stylet. If difficulty occurs during the procedure, a laryngoscope may be used to facilitate the intubation.

Several complications have been reported with the use of this device. Although unusual, the patient's airway or oropharynx can be injured with the lighted stylet. Sore throat, hoarseness, and mucosal damage are possible (31). Cases have been reported in which the light became dislodged from the end of the stylet (32–34). In another instance, the protective tubing was not removed from the stylet and thus had the potential to become dislodged within the trachea (35). Several cases of arytenoid subluxation have also been reported with the use of this device (36,37). Heat damage to the tracheal mucosa during prolonged intubation attempts is a potential risk with inappropriate handling (38). The bulb on the Trachlight flashes on and off after 30 seconds to remind the operator of the duration of the intubation attempt. It is important to ensure that the stylet is always positioned within the endotracheal tube to avoid exposing airway tissue to the heat of the light source.

▶ SHIKANI OPTICAL STYLET

The Shikani Optical Stylet (SOS) (Clarus Medical, Minneapolis, MN) combines many of the features of the lighted stylet and a fiberoptic laryngoscope. It allows blind or visually guided insertion of an endotracheal tube without direct laryngoscopy. It is a high-resolution, stainless steel, rigid fiberoptic stylet that comes in a preformed J shape, yet is malleable. It has an adjustable tube stop and an integral oxygen port. It comes in two sizes: an adult size, which fits endotracheal tubes greater than 5.5 mm ID, and a pediatric size, which fits endotracheal tubes greater than 3.5 mm ID. The fiberoptic light allows it to be used much like a standard lighted stylet, while the optical component allows for indirect visualization of the airway (39). It can be used alone or as an adjunct to laryngoscopy and is especially useful for those unable to maintain skills with a bronchoscope. This combined tool allows the operator to overcome many of the limitations of standard techniques; however, trauma to the airway resulting in tissue distortion and significant bleeding may limit the utility of the optical stylet.

Indications

The SOS can be used as an alternative to standard laryngoscopic intubation. It is especially useful in cases where poor neck or jaw mobility, facial abnormalities, or an abnormal airway (e.g., small mouth, large tongue) make standard laryngoscopy difficult or impossible. If there is a significant amount of blood or debris in the airway, the SOS can be used as a lighted stylet. The SOS is available in both semirigid and flexible versions. The latter tool can be used in combination with other devices such as the Fastrach to visualize the airway and facilitate placement of an endotracheal tube. It can also be used for quick confirmation of endotracheal tube or Combitube placement.

The SOS has the advantages of two airway management tools combined into one, but it also shares some of the

SUMMARY: FIBEROPTIC STYLET (SHIKANI OPTICAL STYLET)

1 Select an appropriately sized fiberoptic stylet and endotracheal tube for the patient.

2 Confirm that the light is functioning properly.

3 Apply a water-soluble lubricant to the stylet and antifog liquid to its lens.

4 Insert the stylet into the endotracheal tube with the tube extending slightly beyond the end of the stylet and lock the tube into position using the locking device; if desired, attach an oxygen or air source to the port on the side of the tube lock.

5 If a malleable stylet is used, bend the stylet and tube into the desired position.

6 Suction the oropharynx well (when time permits, consider administration of an antisialagogue) and, using the nondominant hand, lift the mandible anteriorly.

7 Insert the stylet in the midline below the tongue and attempt to visualize the epiglottis and/or glottis through the eyepiece; alternatively, insert the stylet laterally and guide it between the tongue and posterior pharyngeal wall and then into the airway (with the second technique, turn the patient's head to facilitate passage of the endotracheal tube if desired, provided there is no contraindication to neck movement).

8 Once the vocal cords are seen, insert the stylet and then advance the endotracheal tube into position.

9 Confirm proper tube placement.

 CLINICAL TIPS: FIBEROPTIC STYLET (SHIKANI OPTICAL STYLET)

▶ Fiberoptic stylets, particularly flexible versions, can be used as an adjunct to other airway management techniques (e.g., intubation with the Fastrach).

▶ The fiberoptic stylet can also be used much like a lighted stylet. This might be useful when blood or secretions obscure the airway.

▶ The air/oxygen port on the side of the stylet allows oxygen or air to be directed through the endotracheal tube. This can be used to force secretions aside and prevent the lens from fogging during the procedure.

▶ Some fiberoptic stylets (e.g., Bonfils) have an adjustable eyepiece, which might make them somewhat easier to use.

Procedure

When used as a lighted stylet, the SOS functions like other such devices described previously (see "Lighted Stylet"). This discussion will therefore focus on the technique of fiberoptic endotracheal intubation using the SOS.

The operator should first select the appropriate stylet for the patient. The light should be tested to ensure that it is functioning properly. Antifog liquid is applied to the lens, and the stylet is lubricated. The endotracheal tube is positioned on the stylet with the lens near but still inside the end of the tube. The tube is then fixed into position using the tube clamp, which also serves as a port to allow oxygen or suction to be directed around the stylet but within the endotracheal tube.

weaknesses of both. The fiberoptic lens is subject to fogging and should be treated with antifog solution prior to its use. Likewise, blood or debris in the airway may make visualization through the lens difficult. In such circumstances, the operator should have adequate suction available or use the device as a lighted stylet. When employed in this fashion, the SOS has the same potential drawbacks as standard lightwands.

Equipment

The SOS requires a light source to power the fiberoptic light, which can be either a battery pack in the handle or an external fiberoptic light source. A water-soluble lubricant, a proper size endotracheal tube, and suction are also required (Fig. 17.13).

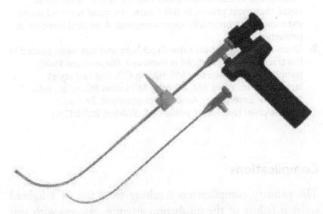

Figure 17.13 Adult and pediatric Shikani Optical Stylet. (Reproduced with permission from Murphy MF, Law JA. Rigid and semirigid fiberoptic intubation. In: Walls RM, Murphy MF, Luten RC, et al., eds. *Manual of Emergency Airway Management.* 2nd ed. Philadelphia: Lippincott Williams & Wilkins; 2004:144.)

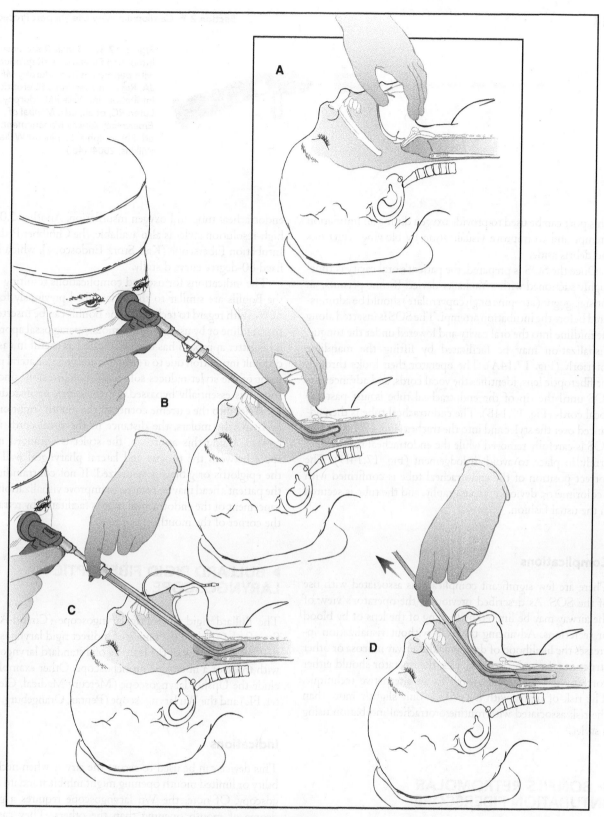

Figure 17.14 Intubation using the Shikani Optical Stylet.

A. The patient's mandible and tongue are retracted anteriorly with the nondominant hand. Using the dominant hand, the operator inserts the scope and endotracheal tube into the center of the patient's mouth and advances them over the tongue.

B. While looking through the eyepiece, the operator advances the stylet and endotracheal tube beneath the epiglottis and into the glottic opening.

C. The endotracheal tube is released from the adjustable stop and passed over the stylet into the proper position.

D. The stylet is carefully removed, with care taken not to dislodge the endotracheal tube.

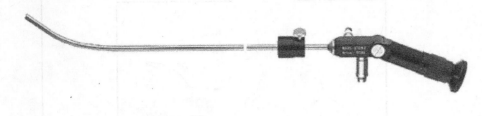

Figure 17.15 Bonfils Retromolar Intubation Fiberscope. (Reproduced with permission from Murphy MF, Law JA. Rigid and semirigid fiberoptic intubation. In: Walls RM, Murphy MF, Luten RC, et al., eds. *Manual of Emergency Airway Management*. 2nd ed. Philadelphia: Lippincott Williams & Wilkins; 2004:146.)

This port can be used to provide oxygen during an intubation attempt and to improve visualization by blowing secretions and debris aside.

Once the SOS is prepared, the patient's oral cavity is thoroughly suctioned with a Yankauer device. If time permits, an antisialagogue (atropine or glycopyrrolate) should be administered before the intubation attempt. The SOS is inserted along the midline into the oral cavity and lowered under the tongue. Visualization may be facilitated by lifting the mandible anteriorly (Fig. 17.14A). The operator then looks through the fiberoptic lens, identifies the vocal cords, and advances the SOS until the tip of the endotracheal tube is just past the vocal cords (Fig. 17.14B). The endotracheal tube is then advanced over the stylet and into the trachea (Fig. 17.14C). The SOS is carefully removed while the endotracheal tube is held firmly in place to avoid dislodgement (Fig. 17.14D). The correct position of the endotracheal tube is confirmed with a colorimetric device or capnography, and the tube is secured in the usual fashion.

Complications

There are few significant complications associated with use of the SOS. As described previously, the operator's view of the airway may be limited by fogging of the lens or by blood or secretions. Advancing the SOS without visualization increases the likelihood of damaging the airway mucosa or other structures. In such circumstances, the operator should either correct the problem or switch to an alternative technique. The risk of injury with the SOS is only slightly more than the risk associated with routine orotracheal intubation using a stylet.

▶ BONFILS RETROMOLAR INTUBATION FIBERSCOPE

The Bonfils Retromolar Intubation Fiberscope (Karl Storz Endoscopy, Tuttlingen, Germany, and Culver City, CA) is a high-resolution, rigid fiberoptic stylet that has a fixed 40-degree curve distally and is available in both adult and pediatric sizes (5.0 mm and 2.0 mm, respectively) (Fig. 17.15). The device has a moveable eyepiece, which allows ergonomic movement during intubation, and an adapter for fixation of an

endotracheal tube and oxygen insufflation. Another 2.0-mm high-resolution stylet is also available, the Chhibber Pediatric Intubation Fiberscope (Karl Storz Endoscopy), which has a fixed 80-degree curve distally.

The indications for use and complications resulting from the Bonfils are similar to those described previously for the SOS. With regard to technique, the Bonfils can be inserted either midline or by using the retromolar/paraglossal approach. This latter approach has been advocated as useful in cases of difficult intubation due to a small mandible (3). Lateral placement of the stylet reduces soft-tissue compression, since the tongue is essentially bypassed. Furthermore, by introducing the stylet into the extreme corner of the mouth (right or left) overlying the molars, the distance to the vocal cords is decreased. Using this approach, the stylet is advanced in the space between the tongue and lateral pharyngeal wall until the epiglottis or glottis is visualized. If not contraindicated, the patient's head may be rotated to improve visualization. Advancement of the endotracheal tube is facilitated by retracting the corner of the mouth.

▶ BULLARD RIGID FIBEROPTIC LARYNGOSCOPE

The Bullard rigid fiberoptic laryngoscope (Circon-ACMI, Stamford, CT) is in the family of indirect rigid laryngoscopes that combine many of the features of a standard laryngoscope with those of a fiberoptic bronchoscope. Other examples include the Upsher laryngoscope (Mercury Medical, Clearwater, FL) and the Wu laryngoscope (Pentax, Orangeburg, NY).

Indications

This device can be used to secure the airway when neck mobility or limited mouth opening might inhibit standard laryngoscopy. Of note, the Wu laryngoscope requires a greater degree of mouth opening than the others. They can also be used in patients who have anatomic abnormalities or Mallampati/Cormack-Lehane class III and IV airways and for whom standard laryngoscopy is predicted to be difficult or impossible (40).

Like all fiberoptic scopes, the Bullard's optical port may be obscured by excessive blood or secretions. In such cases, it is generally prudent to choose an alternative method. Effective

SUMMARY: BULLARD RIGID FIBEROPTIC LARYNGOSCOPE

1 Based on the patient's size, select the appropriate Bullard and an appropriately sized endotracheal tube.

2 Confirm that the light is functioning properly; if a standard laryngoscope handle is used, make sure that the batteries have sufficient power.

3 Assemble the Bullard laryngoscope (if the stylet is used, it should be well lubricated with a water-soluble lubricant, and the endotracheal tube should be placed onto the stylet such that the tip of the stylet extends just beyond the end of the tube); then attach the stylet to the laryngoscope (if the tip extender is required, it should be attached with the open notch down and pressed into position).

4 Apply antifog solution to the lens and adjust the focus using the focus ring on the eyepiece.

5 Hold the Bullard in the nondominant hand so that it is parallel with the patient's body, with the tip of the blade just above the patient's mouth.

6 Open the patient's mouth with the dominant hand and insert the Bullard in the midline; smoothly rotate the handle 90 degrees while advancing the Bullard below the patient's tongue.

7 Without tilting the Bullard significantly in any direction, lift up on the handle and look through the eyepiece.

8 If the vocal cords are seen, advance the endotracheal tube under direct visualization.

9 If the vocal cords are not seen, allow the blade of the Bullard to drop into the posterior pharynx, then lift the handle upward once more to lift the epiglottis.

10 Confirm the position of the endotracheal tube and secure it using standard methods.

 CLINICAL TIPS: BULLARD RIGID FIBEROPTIC LARYNGOSCOPE

▶ The tip extender must be firmly attached; otherwise, it may become dislodged in the hypopharynx or upper airway.

▶ The hollow stylet allows the Bullard to be used in conjunction with a flexible fiberoptic laryngoscope, airway guide, or guidewire.

▶ Some operators prefer to attach a three-way stopcock to the suction port so that the port can be used either for suction or to force air/oxygen into the airway, which helps prevent fogging of the lens during the procedure.

▶ When using the Bullard in conjunction with the stylet, some operators prefer to position it so that the vocal cords appear in the right side of the eyepiece. This roughly aligns the stylet with the glottic opening.

use of the Bullard requires training and practice, and an inexperienced operator should obviously not attempt to use the Bullard for the first time in a critical situation.

Equipment

The Bullard rigid fiberoptic laryngoscope (see Fig. 17.16) is available in three sizes: adult, pediatric, and infant. All three are configured identically. The lower portion of the Bullard is a long metal blade with a distinct curve near its end. Several ports run behind the blade and terminate just proximal to its

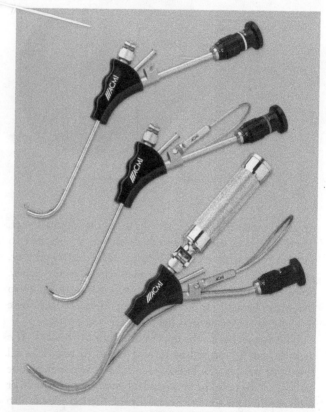

Figure 17.16 Bullard rigid fiberoptic laryngoscope. (Reproduced with permission from ACMI Stamford Division, Stamford, CT, http://www.acmicorp.com/acmi/images/products/2283_fm.jpg.)

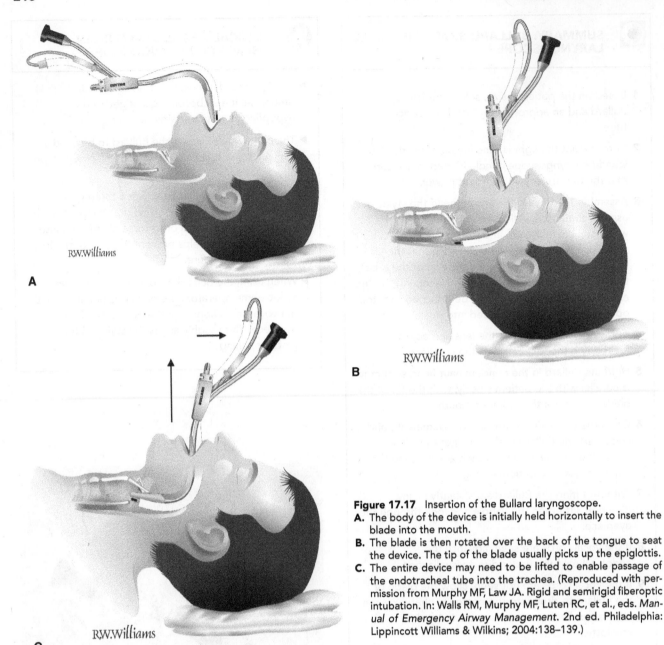

Figure 17.17 Insertion of the Bullard laryngoscope.
A. The body of the device is initially held horizontally to insert the blade into the mouth.
B. The blade is then rotated over the back of the tongue to seat the device. The tip of the blade usually picks up the epiglottis.
C. The entire device may need to be lifted to enable passage of the endotracheal tube into the trachea. (Reproduced with permission from Murphy MF, Law JA. Rigid and semirigid fiberoptic intubation. In: Walls RM, Murphy MF, Luten RC, et al., eds. *Manual of Emergency Airway Management*. 2nd ed. Philadelphia: Lippincott Williams & Wilkins; 2004:138–139.)

tip, the most important of which is the optical port. There is also a suction port that can be (a) attached to vacuum to provide suction, (b) used to deliver oxygen/air, or (c) used to administer topical anesthetics into the airway. Some operators attach a three-way stopcock to this port so that it can be used for more than one purpose. Finally, there is a light port that projects light into the oral cavity.

The eyepiece is on the upper portion of the Bullard. The eyepiece can be focused by turning the focus ring. Like all fiberoptic devices, the Bullard requires a power source. The Bullard can be powered by a standard laryngoscope handle or a fiberoptic light source. Access for the suction port is also located on the upper portion of the Bullard.

There are two optional pieces of equipment that can be attached to the Bullard laryngoscope. The first is a stylet that allows the endotracheal tube to be mounted along and

slightly beneath the right-hand side of the blade. This stylet is available in two styles: a semirigid, nonmalleable, solid stylet and a hollow stylet that can accommodate a 4-mm fiberoptic bronchoscope, a similarly sized airway guide, or a guidewire. The other piece of optional equipment is a disposable plastic tip extender, which is recommended when the Bullard is being used in very large patients. This device might be necessary when the Bullard is used to intubate a large adolescent.

Procedure

The Bullard laryngoscope should be prepared for use in advance if possible, as the device requires some assembly. First, the operator should check the light source, focus the eyepiece, and apply antifog solution to the fiberoptic lens. If the stylet is used, it should be lubricated and inserted into an appropriately sized endotracheal tube so that the tip of the stylet extends very slightly beyond the tip of the endotracheal tube. The stylet is then mounted along the right side of the Bullard and connected to the appropriate slot, which is located between the eyepiece and the attachment for the laryngoscope handle. The operator should slide the tube back and forth a few times to be certain that it will slide off the stylet smoothly during intubation. If the blade extender is used, it should be attached with the open notch down and pressed into position so that a distinct snap is heard and/or felt. The operator should then test the blade extender to ensure that it is firmly attached and will not accidentally come off the blade during an intubation attempt (41).

To insert the Bullard laryngoscope, the operator stands at the head of the bed, as with a standard oropharyngeal intubation. Using the nondominant hand, the operator holds the Bullard laryngoscope parallel to the patient's body with the tip of the blade level with the patient's mouth (Fig. 17.17A). The operator then opens the patient's mouth and inserts the Bullard so that the blade is centered over the tongue. Of note, the Bullard can be inserted into the mouth of a patient with an inter-incisor distance as small as 0.6 cm; however, when intubating with a large endotracheal tube, a larger mouth opening may be required. Following the curve of the tongue, the Bullard is then rotated 90 degrees so that it is upright and the eyepiece is in a functional position (Fig. 17.17B). Ideally, the tip of the Bullard should lie beneath the epiglottis. The operator then gently lifts the Bullard upward (toward the ceiling) while looking through the viewing port (Fig. 17.17C). The cords should be visible, and the endotracheal tube can simply be advanced over the stylet and through the glottic opening. Because the endotracheal tube is attached slightly to the right of the fiberoptic port, some operators prefer to gently reposition the Bullard so that the cords are visualized on the right side of the viewing port and therefore roughly aligned with the endotracheal tube. Alternatively, the operator may elect not to use the stylet at all, instead using the Bullard as a laryngoscope and passing the tube in a manner similar to standard laryngoscopy. As with any fiberoptic device, the operator is more likely to be successful with a Bullard if the device is moved smoothly and deliberately, because quick or jerky movements often cause disorientation.

If blood or secretions obscure the operator's view, then the suction port or an external suction device (e.g., a Yankauer) can be used to improve visualization. If, in the absence of blood or secretions, the cords cannot be visualized, then the operator should reposition the device by allowing the blade to drop toward the posterior pharynx and then lifting the device back into position.

Complications

Like a standard laryngoscope, the Bullard has a metal blade as well as a metal stylet. Both of these can cause lacerations or abrasions. Other potential complications associated with the Bullard are similar to those encountered with any intubation

attempt (e.g., hypoxia from prolonged apnea). Incorrect use of the Bullard can also result in excessive neck movement.

▶ FLEXIBLE FIBEROPTIC INTUBATION

The utility of flexible fiberoptic intubation in the emergent setting has been demonstrated in several case series (42–49). Important general principles of fiberoptic laryngoscopy are described in detail in Chapter 61. Endotracheal intubation using this technique involves a few relatively straightforward modifications of these principles. Fiberoptic intubation can be performed orally or nasally, although the nasal approach is usually easier for novices, since there is not as much room for the scope to migrate. The disadvantage of using the nasal approach is that a smaller endotracheal tube is often necessary and there is a higher risk of epistaxis, which causes difficulty in visualization.

Indications

The flexible fiberoptic laryngoscope-bronchoscope is primarily indicated for selected patients with predicted difficult airways. Examples include patients with (a) supraglottic lesions or abnormalities (e.g., angioedema), (b) impaired neck mobility (e.g., immobilization for suspected unstable cervical spine fracture), or (c) limited mouth opening. It can also be used to manage patients with certain anatomic abnormalities that make other forms of airway management difficult or impossible. The flexible fiberoptic scope is used to manage patients who are difficult to intubate but who *can* be ventilated.

Fiberoptic intubation requires a high degree of skill to be used effectively and should therefore only be performed by practitioners with appropriate training and experience. Likewise, even under the best of circumstances this procedure is somewhat time consuming and should not be used to manage patients who can be neither intubated nor ventilated. Furthermore, it may be dangerous to attempt this technique in patients with certain types of airway obstruction. Significant blood or secretions in the airway are likely to greatly limit visualization, and if these cannot be effectively controlled, flexible fiberoptic intubation should not be attempted. Finally, patient cooperation is critical to the success of this procedure if performed in the awake patient. In some cases, this problem can be overcome with the judicious use of sedation. However, if the patient cannot reasonably be expected to cooperate, an alternative technique should be chosen.

Equipment

Fiberoptic laryngoscopes and bronchoscopes are composed of a flexible fiberoptic bundle attached to a viewing port. The tip of the fiberoptic bundle can be moved upward or downward using a toggle switch on the side of the scope; side-to-side motion is controlled by rotating the scope. Most fiberoptic scopes attach to a standard fiberoptic light source,

SUMMARY: FLEXIBLE FIBEROPTIC LARYNGOSCOPE

1 Prepare the patient for the procedure:
  a Explain the procedure to the patient.
  b Administer an antisialagogue and/or a topical vasoconstrictor as needed, depending on the approach (i.e., nasal vs. oral).
  c Administer a topical anesthetic to the airway (anesthetic spray, nebulized lidocaine, and/or transtracheal anesthetic).
  d Administer sedation as needed.

2 Prepare the equipment:
  a Assemble the necessary equipment.
  b Inspect the fiberoptic laryngoscope to ensure that the light source is functioning, the tip moves through its full range of motion, and the eyepiece is focused properly.
  c Attach the suction port to wall suction or to air/oxygen, depending on operator preference.
  d Apply antifog solution to the lens.
  e Lubricate the fiberoptic bundle with a water-soluble lubricant and check that the endotracheal tube slides easily along its length (if the endotracheal tube will be threaded entirely onto the fiberoptic laryngoscope, it may be necessary to remove the connector from the endotracheal tube when using a smaller scope).

3 Starting the procedure using the nasal approach:
  a If the topical vasoconstrictor has been administered in advance of the procedure, consider passing the endotracheal tube into the nose first; if not, or if the risk of bleeding is very high, place the tube on the fiberoptic laryngoscope and insert the fiberoptic scope into the nose first (the risk of trauma can be reduced

by softening the tip of the endotracheal tube in warm water when time permits).
  b Using the eyepiece or a monitor, advance the fiberoptic laryngoscope along the floor of the nose and into the posterior pharynx. Inferior deflection of the tip of the endotracheal tube facilitates passage.

4 Starting the procedure using the oral approach:
  a Place a bite block or a pharyngeal airway into the patient's mouth (with some pharyngeal airways, it may be possible to insert the endotracheal tube into the pharyngeal airway first and then advance the scope through the tube).
  b Maintenance of midline position is critical to success (some operators place the middle finger of their nondominant hand on the patient's lip, aligned with the space between the central incisors, to serve as a guide).
  c Advance the fiberoptic scope over the tongue and, directing the tip inferiorly, into the posterior pharynx.

5 Advance the fiberoptic scope toward the glottis (it is easy to become disoriented at this stage; if this happens, withdraw the scope until familiar structures are seen and then readvance it).

6 Once the glottic opening has been identified, advance the scope through the vocal cords and down to the level of the carina.

7 Advance the endotracheal tube into position and remove the fiberoptic laryngoscope.

8 Confirm the position of the tube and secure the tube using standard methods.

although some can also be powered by a battery pack. Many fiberoptic scopes can be attached to overhead monitors, which allows both a larger image and an enhanced ability to teach. Many fiberoptic scopes have suction ports and instrumentation ports. Improving fiberoptic technology has resulted in the manufacture of progressively smaller flexible fiberoptic scopes. Currently, pediatric sizes are available that offer good illumination and high-quality image resolution, although these smaller scopes often lack auxiliary ports.

In addition to an appropriately sized fiberoptic scope, several other pieces of equipment are necessary. These include an endotracheal tube, a light source, and a lubricant. Topical anesthetic should be liberally applied to the airway if an awake intubation is performed. For the nasal approach, a topical vasoconstrictor must be used for preparation of the nasopharynx. For the oral approach, the operator should have

a bite block or a special adjunct such as the Berman intubating/pharyngeal airway.

Procedure

Perhaps more than any other intubation approach, fiberoptic endotracheal intubation requires a high degree of cooperation from the patient. Proper patient selection is therefore especially important. In general, emergent fiberoptic endotracheal intubation should be performed with a spontaneously breathing patient. A mild sedative may be administered to the awake patient to facilitate the procedure. Although it is possible to perform this procedure on an unconscious, apneic patient, this should only be attempted by a practitioner with extensive experience, as the time available to accomplish intubation is greatly diminished.

CLINICAL TIPS TABLE: FLEXIBLE FIBEROPTIC LARYNGOSCOPE

▶ Administration of a nasal vasoconstrictor (nasal approach) and/or an antisialagogue (oral approach) will greatly facilitate successful intubation. Excessive blood and/or oral secretions often make this procedure difficult or impossible to complete.

▶ Mild sedation may be necessary, although spontaneous respirations and normal protective airway reflexes should be preserved.

▶ The suction port may be connected to high-flow oxygen/air. This port can then be used to "blow" secretions from the field of view, administer oxygen, and/or prevent fogging of the lens.

▶ The laryngoscope should always be advanced gently and under direct vision.

▶ If the procedure has not been successful within 3 minutes, the likelihood of success is greatly diminished, and an alternative procedure should be considered.

Because the awake technique relies on patient cooperation, adequate airway anesthesia is essential. Although the right naris is usually chosen when the nasal approach is planned, both nares should be prepared. With either approach, the posterior pharynx should be sprayed with a topical anesthetic such as Cetacaine. Alternatively, if time permits, preoxygenation can be combined with administration of atomized or nebulized lidocaine (2% to 4% lidocaine). The operator also may choose to perform transtracheal anesthesia (described below in "Retrograde Intubation"). In addition, when using the nasal approach, a topical vasoconstrictor should always be applied to the nasal mucosa 2 to 4 minutes before the procedure. Significant epistaxis is one of the most common causes of failure with fiberoptic nasotracheal intubation, because obtaining an adequate view of the larynx becomes impossible. This is less likely to occur with generous use of a vasoconstrictor sprayed in the nares. It is also advisable to administer an antisialagogue (atropine or glycopyrrolate) well in advance of the procedure before attempting any type of fiberoptic intubation, because excessive secretions can obscure the operator's view.

Next, the necessary equipment should be prepared. The fiberoptic scope should be tested to ensure that the tip can be easily manipulated throughout its full range of positions and that a good image is seen through the eyepiece. If the fiberoptic scope has a suction port, this should be connected to wall suction. Alternatively, many practitioners prefer using low-flow oxygen (3 L/min) through the suction port. This can serve as an effective method for dispersing secretions or blood in the airway while at the same time delivering 100% oxygen and helping to prevent the lens from fogging. If adequate time is available during a nasal fiberoptic procedure, the operator can immerse the tip of the endotracheal tube in warm water for a few minutes to soften it. This decreases the chances of injuring the nasal mucosa.

Because the bevel of the endotracheal tube is less likely to lacerate or avulse the turbinates if inserted in the right naris (i.e., bevel facing the septum), this is the preferred site of entry. If the right naris is not patent, the tube can be inverted 180 degrees (concave upward), inserted in the left naris, and advanced until the tip passes beyond the turbinates, then "flipped" back into the normal concave downward position. This technique is shown in Chapter 16 as it applies to blind nasotracheal intubation (see Fig. 16.24).

The endotracheal tube is next passed as far as possible up the fiberoptic scope. With smaller fiberoptic scopes, the 15-mm connector can be removed if necessary so that the scope extends beyond the tip of the endotracheal tube. The fiberoptic scope and endotracheal tube are then generously lubricated, both to facilitate passage and to allow easy removal of the scope at the appropriate time. When the orotracheal route is chosen, the operator should place a bite block into the patient's mouth to facilitate passage of the fiberoptic scope and prevent inadvertent damage to the fiberoptic bundles caused by a patient's teeth. Alternatively, a piece of gauze may be utilized to gently retract the tongue, thus facilitating the procedure and also preventing the patient from biting down on the fiberoptic bundle.

Depending on individual preference, the operator can stand to one side of the bed (facing superiorly toward the patient's head) or in the traditional position used for direct laryngoscopy (above the head of the bed). It should be noted that the images seen through the eyepiece from one of these two positions will be inverted 180 degrees when compared with those obtained in the other position. The patient's head and neck are maintained in a neutral position during fiberoptic laryngoscopy. When attempting fiberoptic nasotracheal intubation, one of two methods may be used for insertion of the scope and endotracheal tube. If a topical vasoconstrictor has been applied to the nasal mucosa for a sufficient length of time, the endotracheal tube may be first passed through the most patent nostril until it reaches the hypopharynx in a manner similar to a blind nasotracheal intubation. The fiberoptic scope is then inserted through the tube and easily passed into the supraglottic region (Fig. 17.18). This method allows the endotracheal tube to serve as a guide for the scope and also facilitates subsequent insertion of the tube into the trachea. However, if the topical vasoconstrictor has not been applied for a sufficient length of time or previous intubation attempts have caused bleeding, the laryngoscopic view may be hindered. In this situation, the fiberoptic bundle should be inserted into the trachea first, and only then is the endotracheal tube passed. To perform this technique, the operator first slides the endotracheal tube as far as possible up the fiberoptic bundle. The operator then inserts the fiberoptic bundle into the patient's nose until it reaches the posterior pharynx, taking care not to injure the turbinates or nasal mucosa (Fig. 17.19A).

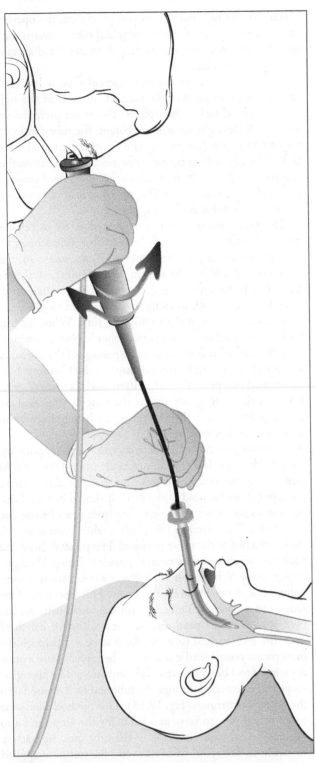

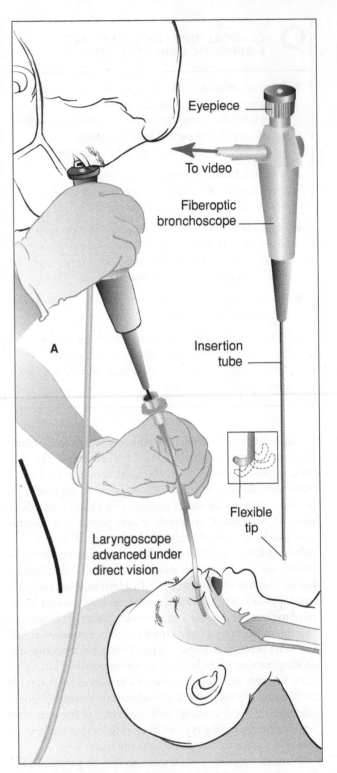

Figure 17.18 Using this method of fiberoptic nasotracheal intubation, the endotracheal tube is first inserted until the tip reaches the supraglottic area. The fiberoptic laryngoscope is then inserted through the tube until the appropriate landmarks can be seen through the eyepiece. The trachea is then intubated as shown in Figure 17.19. This method should only be used when the nasal mucosa has been adequately prepared with a vasoconstrictor, because prior insertion of the tube will otherwise cause bleeding that may obscure visualization.

Figure 17.19 Fiberoptic intubation.
A. Using this method, the endotracheal tube is first threaded up the entire length of the fiberoptic strand. The fiberoptic laryngoscope is then inserted into the nose under visualization through the eyepiece.

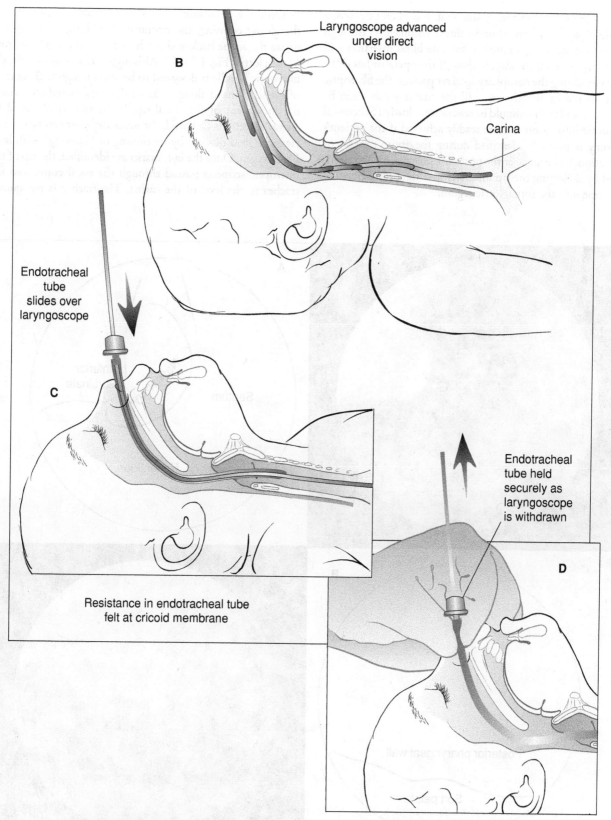

Figure 17.19 *(Continued)*

B. The fiberoptic laryngoscope is advanced beyond the angle at the posterior pharynx into the supraglottic area until the appropriate landmarks can be seen. Once the glottis is identified, the fiberoptic laryngoscope is further advanced into the trachea to the level of the carina.

C. Using the fiberoptic laryngoscope as a guide, the endotracheal tube is inserted through the nose into the hypopharynx and through the glottic opening into the trachea.

D. The laryngoscope is then carefully removed while the endotracheal tube is held securely in place.

It is important to emphasize that the fiberoptic scope should always be advanced under direct vision either through the eyepiece or using a monitor, because blind insertion will lead to mucosal injury and bleeding. If the operator has difficulty visualizing the nasopharyngeal air passage, the fiberoptic scope should be withdrawn until the anatomy can again be identified, and then it should be readvanced slowly. (Successful fiberoptic intubation is more readily achieved if the patient's anatomy is properly identified during the entire process of intubation.) The angle at the posterior pharynx is then negotiated by deflecting the tip inferiorly and carefully advancing the scope into the supraglottic region.

Once the fiberoptic scope is positioned just proximal to the glottic opening, the operator should angle the tip and rotate the scope back and forth to center the scope in front of the glottis (Fig. 17.19B). Although remarkably flexible, the fiberoptic bundle is designed to be stiff enough that rotation of the scope head along its axis will be translated into a similar movement of the distal tip. If the view is obscured by airway secretions or blood, the accessory port can be used to clear the field of view by suctioning or "blowing" with low-flow oxygen. Once the landmarks are identified, the tip of the fiberoptic scope is passed through the vocal cords into the trachea to the level of the carina. The trachea is recognized

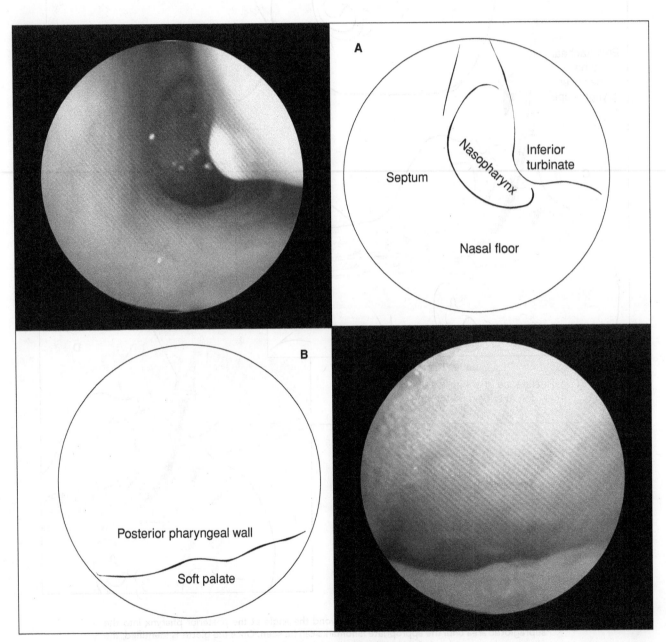

Figure 17.20 Laryngoscopic views at various levels of the airway.
A. Nasal cavity.
B. Posterior nasopharynx.

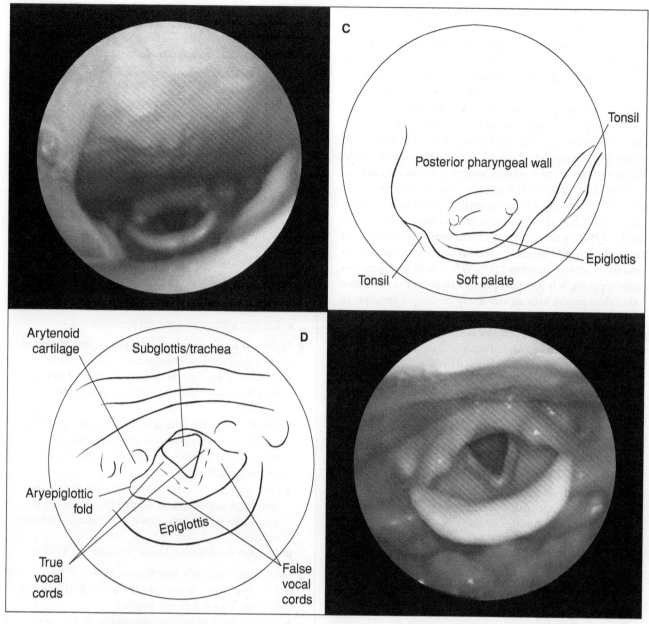

Figure 17.20 *(Continued)*
C. Proximal oropharynx.
D. Supraglottic region.
(Photographs courtesy of Dr. Clark Rosen, University of Pittsburgh School of Medicine.)

by its characteristic cartilaginous rings. Maintaining the position of the scope, the operator slides the endotracheal tube along the fiberoptic bundle through the glottic opening until the carina is visualized (Fig. 17.19C). The fiberoptic scope is then carefully withdrawn while the tube is held securely in place (Fig. 17.19D). Figure 17.20 shows the various levels of the airway as seen during fiberoptic laryngoscopy. These images were obtained during laryngoscopy performed at the patient's side, with the operator facing superiorly toward the patient's head. They are therefore the standard anatomic views seen with an upright patient, rather than the "upside down" views of the airway seen during fiberoptic laryngoscopy per-

formed with the operator standing above the head of the bed.

Orotracheal intubation using the fiberoptic scope is very similar to nasotracheal intubation but is somewhat more challenging. As described previously, the principle difficulty lies in maintaining the scope in the midline position. Some operators choose to place the long finger of the nondominant hand in the middle of the patient's upper lip, aligned with the space between the central incisors, to serve as reference point. The patient's tongue can occlude the oral cavity, so it may be useful to have an assistant grasp the tongue with a piece of gauge and gently retract it. Commercially produced adjuncts like the Berman intubating/pharyngeal airway can solve the problem of both maintaining midline position and controlling the tongue. As described with the nasal technique, the endotracheal tube can be inserted into the Berman airway, and the scope can be passed through the endotracheal tube.

One of the greatest potential obstacles to successfully performing this procedure is inadequate patient cooperation. Even with optimal conditions, fiberoptic endotracheal intubation requires considerable skill on the part of the primary operator; with a struggling child, it becomes virtually impossible. When necessary, intravenous sedation may be used to facilitate the procedure, although this must be done judiciously so that the patient continues to have normal respirations and airway reflexes (see Chapter 33). Another pitfall that may be encountered is difficulty in identifying the anatomic landmarks. This can be the result of bleeding, excessive secretions, vomitus, or variants in airway anatomy (50). When such problems become apparent, it is generally prudent to abort the procedure rather than persist with an excessively prolonged attempt. In fact, investigators have recommended that if the patient is not intubated within the first 3 minutes after initiating a fiberoptic intubation, the likelihood of success decreases significantly and another approach should be used (46).

Complications

Because the procedure is performed under direct visualization, intubation using the fiberoptic scope is remarkably free of significant complications. The greatest risk of injury is to the scope itself, which can be easily damaged by an uncooperative patient or an unskilled operator. In order to minimize damage to the scope, force should never be utilized during the procedure, and the top of the scope should always be in a straight orientation when it is removed from the endotracheal tube following intubation. As described previously, nasotracheal intubation can cause epistaxis. The most important caveat is that this technique should be used by skilled operators in well-selected patients.

▶ AIRWAY GUIDES AND TUBE EXCHANGERS

A wide variety of devices, ranging from flexible solid plastic rods to hollow conduits, can be used to guide an endotracheal tube into the glottis or to replace a properly positioned but improperly sized or damaged endotracheal tube. Tube replacement can be especially important when the intubation attempt has been difficult and failure may occur with a second attempt.

Indications

These devices are used for the following indications: (a) to guide an endotracheal tube into proper position when only the epiglottis or a partial view of the glottis can be obtained

SUMMARY: AIRWAY GUIDES AND TUBE EXCHANGERS

1 Facilitation of endotracheal intubation:
   a Select an appropriate airway guide or tube exchanger and lubricate it with a water-soluble lubricant, if necessary.
   b Begin the intubation attempt as described in Chapter 16.
   c If only part of the airway (e.g., the epiglottis) can be visualized, advance the airway guide underneath the epiglottis and toward the point where the glottic opening should be located; tracheal placement will be felt as the airway guide touches the tracheal rings.
   d Once the airway guide is located within the trachea, advance the endotracheal tube along the airway guide and into the trachea.
   e Confirm endotracheal tube position.

2 Exchange of a properly placed but improperly sized or damaged endotracheal tube:
   a Pass the airway guide or tube exchanger through the original endotracheal tube and into the trachea.
   b Deflate the cuff of the original tube and guide it out of the airway over the airway exchange catheter; take care not to dislodge the airway exchange catheter.
   c Pass the new endotracheal tube over the airway exchange catheter, and using a laryngoscope to guide placement, advance it into the appropriate position.
   d Confirm endotracheal tube position.

3 Intubation through a supraglottic device:
   a Pass the airway guide into the supraglottic device and advance it into the trachea.
   b Deflate the cuff of the supraglottic device, and taking care not to dislodge the airway guide, remove it from the airway.
   c Using a laryngoscope to guide placement, advance an endotracheal tube down the supraglottic device and into the trachea.
   d Confirm endotracheal tube position.

(51), (b) to safely exchange an improperly sized or damaged endotracheal tube, or (c) to replace a supraglottic airway with an endotracheal tube. Disruption, laceration, or perforation of the trachea is a relative contraindication to the use of these devices, because they can slide through the site of injury and cause the endotracheal tube to perforate the trachea. If necessary, they can be placed blindly by directing them to the

CLINICAL TIPS: AIRWAY GUIDES AND TUBE EXCHANGERS

▶ Tracheal location of the airway guide should be confirmed by a distinct tactile sensation similar to running a finger along a regularly uneven surface. If this sensation is not felt, then the airway guide is not located within the trachea.

▶ Even though the airway guide is located within the trachea, it may still be difficult to pass an endotracheal tube. Most often the tube will encounter resistance from the epiglottis or the arytenoids. Using a laryngoscope (either standard or rigid fiberoptic) may facilitate placement.

▶ Some airway guides come equipped with special adapters that can be used to provide oxygen or jet ventilation.

▶ Some supraglottic devices (e.g., the LMA and Fastrach) provide better conduits for passage of an airway guide than others.

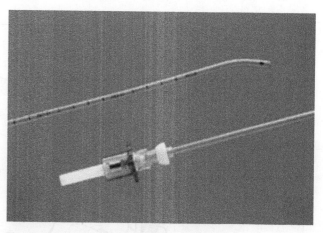

Figure 17.21 The Frova Intubating Introducer. (Reproduced with permission from Cook Critical Care, Bloomington, IN, http://www.cookcriticalcare.com/discip/em_med/2_09/2_09_08.html.)

point where the glottic opening is thought to be located. However, when these devices are used in this way, an abnormally positioned airway can make proper placement difficult or impossible. Aside from tracheal injury, there are no true contraindications to the use of these tools for exchange of an improperly sized or damaged endotracheal tube. When using an airway guide/tube exchanger to replace a supraglottic airway, the operator must weigh the risks associated with loss of the supraglottic airway with the benefits of endotracheal intubation, especially when the patient is being adequately ventilated and replacement of the supraglottic airway might be difficult.

Equipment

The simplest airway guides/tube exchangers are flexible or semirigid plastic or rubber rods. In most cases, the distal 1.5 to 2 cm are angled slightly upward, so that when the device is placed under the epiglottis, it is more likely to enter the trachea. More complex hollow versions, such as the Frova Intubating Introducer (Cook Critical Care, Bloomington, IN), are also available (Fig. 17.21). The major advantage of the hollow tubes is that they can be used to oxygenate the patient during intubation attempts. The Frova devices come with Rapi-Fit adapters that allow them to be connected to jet ventilators, resuscitation bags, and mechanical ventilators. In addition to the airway guide/tube exchanger itself, a properly sized endotracheal tube and all of the other equipment needed for standard orotracheal intubation (see Chapter 16) should be available.

Procedure

Facilitation of Endotracheal Intubation

When using a tube exchanger to facilitate endotracheal intubation, the intubation attempt proceeds as described in Chapter 16. However, if only a partial laryngoscopic view of the airway can be obtained (e.g., the tip of the epiglottis), then the airway guide is advanced toward the likely location of the glottis. Entry into the trachea is indicated by the tactile sensation of the tip of the airway guide/tube exchanger bouncing off of the tracheal rings. This sensation is readily distinguishable from the lack of resistance associated with entry into the esophagus. When the operator has placed the airway guide/tube exchanger into the trachea, an appropriately sized endotracheal tube is then advanced over the airway guide into proper position (Fig. 17.22). Visualization with direct or fiberoptic laryngoscopy should be maintained during the procedure, because the endotracheal tube will often encounter resistance from the epiglottis or arytenoids. Tube position is confirmed using standard methods.

Exchange of an Endotracheal Tube

Sometimes endotracheal intubation is successful but ventilation ineffective because the endotracheal tube chosen is too small (e.g., a large air leak with an uncuffed tube) or the cuff was damaged during the process of intubation. Of course, the operator has the option of replacing the original endotracheal tube by again performing direct laryngoscopy, but in many cases the outcome of a subsequent intubation attempt is uncertain. This is especially true when intubation was initially accomplished with difficulty. A safer alternative is to use an airway guide/tube exchanger. Using this method, the operator simply passes the airway guide/tube exchanger through the original endotracheal tube and into the trachea. As previously described, the tracheal position of the tube may be confirmed by the tactile sensation of the airway guide/tube exchanger encountering the tracheal rings. Once the guide is

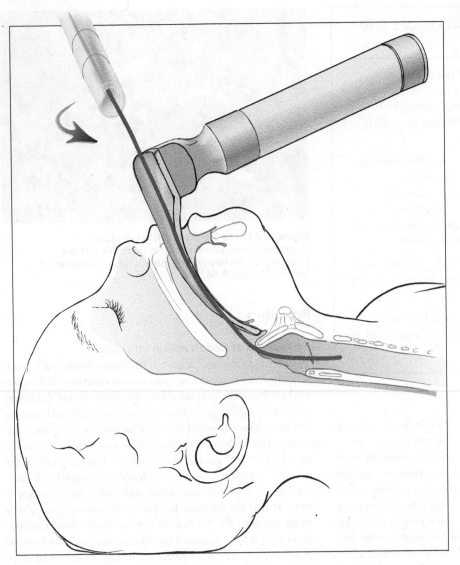

Figure 17.22 Intubation using an airway guide.

in position, the original tube is removed and the new tube is advanced over the airway guide/tube exchange catheter, as described above.

Exchange of a Supraglottic Ventilatory Device

Under certain circumstances (e.g., a failed intubation), insertion of a supraglottic ventilatory device may be necessary to achieve or maintain effective ventilation. However, most critically ill patients will ultimately require placement of a definitive airway. One option is to advance an airway guide/tube exchange catheter into the trachea through the supraglottic device and then use the airway guide/tube exchange catheter to insert an endotracheal tube. It should be noted that some supraglottic devices (e.g., the LMA) are better suited for this purpose than others, and therefore the likelihood of success with this approach may depend on the type of device in place (52).

The actual technique of insertion is nearly identical to that used for an endotracheal tube exchange. In this case, however, the airway guide/tube exchanger is advanced through the adapter of the supraglottic device, and the catheter is moved back and forth until the operator is certain that the airway guide/tube exchanger lies within the trachea. Once the operator has tactile confirmation that the airway guide/tube exchanger is located within the trachea, the supraglottic device can be removed. An endotracheal tube is then advanced over the airway guide/tube exchanger into the trachea. As described above, placement of the endotracheal tube should be aided by direct or fiberoptic laryngoscopy.

A new intubation catheter, the Aintree (Cook Critical Care, Bloomington, IN), is designed specifically for exchange of an LMA or endotracheal tube using a fiberoptic bronchoscope. Its hollow lumen allows insertion of a fiberoptic bronchoscope directly through the catheter so that the airway can be indirectly visualized. To date, a pediatric version has not been manufactured. The smallest endotracheal tube that can fit over this catheter is a 7.0-mm ID endotracheal tube, so it may be considered for use in adolescents.

Complications

The most significant complication associated with the use of airway guides/tube exchange catheters is failure to place the device into the trachea. As previously mentioned, proper placement is indicated by the tactile sensation of the airway guide/tube exchange catheter encountering the tracheal rings as it moves. This is a vibratory feeling, similar to running one's finger along a regularly uneven surface. The feeling should be both distinct and obvious. If this is not felt, the operator should assume that the airway guide/tube exchanger is not located within the trachea and should not proceed with attempts to advance an endotracheal tube. If the Aintree catheter is used, the tracheal rings may be visualized rather than felt.

Use of airway guides/tube exchangers is associated with a minimal risk of injury to the trachea but can, as described above, exacerbate existing injuries. These devices should therefore be used with caution if there are tracheal injuries.

▶ TACTILE INTUBATION

Indications

This is an old procedure that has gone in and out of favor multiple times over the years. More recently, it has been well documented as an effective method for adults (53–56). However, as pointed out by Hancock and Peterson (57), neonates and young infants may be the ideal candidates for this approach for two reasons: (a) they are edentulous, eliminating the risk of bite injuries to the operator, and (b) they have a relatively small extrathoracic airway, making it easier to reach the supraglottic structures even for those not endowed with large hands. Tactile intubation has the additional advantages of potentially decreasing neck movement for the patient with a possible cervical spine injury and of requiring a minimum of equipment to perform. Although not widely used for pediatric patients, the benefits offered by this technique for emergent intubation may increase its popularity once again. This technique may be especially useful in the prehospital setting when the patient cannot be appropriately positioned and/or adjunctive airway equipment is unavailable.

Tactile intubation is generally contraindicated when other means of definitive airway management are available and are likely to be successful. Because the operator's fingers can be easily injured, tactile intubation should only be used for infants or unconscious patients. Additionally, because one of the primary considerations of this technique is the relationship between the length of the operator's fingers and the depth of

---

SUMMARY: TACTILE INTUBATION

1 Select an appropriately sized endotracheal tube, and if desired, insert a stylet; if a stylet is used, the endotracheal tube/stylet should be shaped into a gentle arc rather than a "hockey stick" configuration.

2 Apply a small amount of water-soluble lubricant or sterile water to the end of the endotracheal tube.

3 Stand to the patient's side (right-handed operators should stand on the patient's left side).

4 Open the patient's mouth; using the nondominant hand, slide the index finger down the midline surface of the patient's tongue until the epiglottis and the arytenoids can be palpated (gently lifting the epiglottis may facilitate palpation of the arytenoids).

5 Using the nondominant index finger to keep the endotracheal tube in the midline, advance the tube using the dominant hand; use the thumb of the nondominant hand to apply cricoid pressure if needed.

6 Position the endotracheal tube within the trachea, confirm its location, and secure it using standard methods.

---

the patient's airway, some operators may be physically unable to perform tactile intubation with certain patients.

Procedure

Depending on individual preference, this procedure may be performed with or without using a stylet. Although a stylet is sometimes recommended to facilitate insertion of the endotracheal tube, many practitioners who are experienced with tactile intubation do not find using a stylet to be necessary. If the operator elects to use a stylet, the endotracheal tube should be molded into a gentle arc rather than the "hockey stick" configuration used for orotracheal intubation (Fig. 17.23). As always, the tip of the stylet should not extend beyond the end of the tube to prevent injury to the airway soft tissues.

The tip of the endotracheal tube should be lightly lubricated or moistened with sterile water so that it will slide more easily into the glottic opening. This procedure is best performed with the operator standing to one side of the patient (a right-handed operator to the patient's left). Following appropriate preoxygenation, the operator's nondominant index finger is inserted into the patient's mouth along the midline

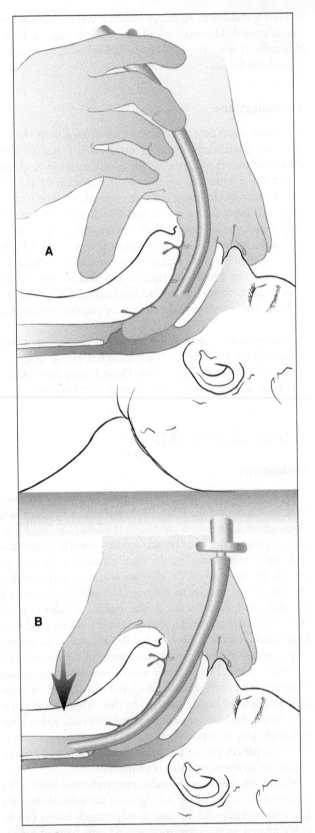

of the tongue until the epiglottis and arytenoid cartilages are felt (Fig. 17.23A). If necessary, the epiglottis should be gently lifted so that the arytenoids can be palpated. The endotracheal tube is then inserted into the mouth with the dominant hand while the index finger of the nondominant hand is used to direct the tube along the midline (Fig. 17.23B). The thumb of the nondominant hand may also be used to apply cricoid pressure, which steadies the trachea and displaces it posteriorly to facilitate insertion of the tube. As the tube is advanced, the index finger of the nondominant hand guides the tip into the glottic opening. The tube is then further advanced to the appropriate depth of insertion, and the stylet (if used) is removed. Proper midtracheal position of the endotracheal tube is confirmed using the methods described in Chapter 16.

Complications

Like most airway management techniques, this method of intubation carries with it the risks of injury to the airway and esophageal intubation. Additionally, the operator can suffer a significant bite wound and body fluid exposure.

▶ RETROGRADE INTUBATION

Retrograde intubation is an excellent technique for securing a difficult airway either alone or in conjunction with other airway techniques (58–63). All practitioners involved in airway management should be skilled in performing this simple, straightforward technique. Recent advancements in this technique include the addition of the Arndt Airway Exchange

Figure 17.23 Tactile (digital) intubation.
A. The index finger of the nondominant hand is used to palpate the arytenoids and retract the epiglottis.
B. The tube is inserted using the index finger to guide the tip into the trachea. The thumb may be used to apply simultaneous cricoid pressure.

SUMMARY TABLE: RETROGRADE INTUBATION

1 If the patient is awake, explain the procedure.

2 Assemble all necessary equipment and check to make sure that the endotracheal balloon is undamaged and that the laryngoscope light is functioning properly.

3 Administer a sedative or anxiolytic.

4 Identify the cricothyroid membrane and apply antiseptic solution to the site. If possible, apply sterile drapes (although this may be difficult if the procedure is being performed with the patient seated).

5 Using a 25- or 27-gauge needle, infiltrate the skin overlying the cricothyroid membrane with lidocaine; then puncture the membrane, aspirate to confirm intratracheal position, and administer transtracheal anesthesia (optional but recommended for the conscious patient).

6 Anesthetize the oral cavity and hypopharynx well with topical anesthetic spray or nebulized lidocaine if the patient is conscious (preparation with nebulized lidocaine can be performed in conjunction with preoxygenation while other tasks are being performed).

7 Using an 18-gauge needle or intravenous catheter attached to a syringe, puncture the cricothyroid membrane while stabilizing the trachea with the nondominant hand (the needle should be inserted perpendicular to the membrane, with the bevel facing superiorly).

8 Advance the needle while aspirating (tracheal entry is indicated by return of air into the syringe); advance the needle or catheter until it is located well within the trachea; if a catheter is being used, remove the needle at this point.

9 Remove the syringe and angle the catheter or needle cranially so that the guidewire is directed toward the nose and mouth.

10 Advance the guidewire through the needle or catheter (in most cases, the guidewire will, without intervention, enter the nose); if an orotracheal intubation is desired, identify the guidewire in the posterior pharynx using a laryngoscope or flashlight and retrieve it through the mouth with a hemostat or forceps.

11 Withdraw a sufficient length of guidewire from the nose or mouth; at this point, an introducer (contained in many commercial retrograde intubation kits) can be threaded over the guidewire and advanced it until it meets resistance; tenting of the skin in the area of the cricothyroid membrane indicates that the introducer is pressing on its posterior surface.

12 Advance the endotracheal tube over the guidewire or introducer and into the hypopharynx (in the case of orotracheal intubation, it may be necessary to use a laryngoscope to guide the endotracheal tube under the epiglottis and past the arytenoids).

13 Advance the endotracheal tube below the vocal cords until it meets resistance; as with an introducer, skin tenting may be observed at the level of the cricoid membrane.

14 While maintaining gentle caudal pressure on the endotracheal tube, withdraw the guidewire or the guidewire and introducer from the mouth or nose and then advance the tube into the desired intratracheal location.

15 Confirm that the tube is within the trachea and secure it using standard methods.

Catheter and needle holder to the pre-existing retrograde intubation kit (Cook Critical Care, Bloomington, IN).

Indications

The principal indications for these techniques is failure (or anticipated failure) of standard airway management, especially in those cases when a supraglottic device is also likely to fail. Unless the practitioner is highly skilled in the performance of retrograde intubation, this technique should not be used in "cannot intubate, cannot ventilate" situations. Although not an absolute contraindication, this situation requires caution, because the time required for successful placement may leave the patient without adequate oxygenation for a signif-

icant length of time. It is used most often when the patient can maintain spontaneous ventilation or be manually ventilated during all or most intubation attempts. It is particularly useful for patients with limited neck mobility associated with cervical spine pathology or patients who have suffered airway trauma. Retrograde intubation is not likely to be successful when there is significant mechanical obstruction of the extrathoracic airway, simply because the obstruction will impede advancement of the endotracheal tube into the airway. Although the thin guidewire passes easily, it may prove impossible to insert the larger endotracheal tube. This technique can also fail when the patient has a perforated or transected airway. In such cases, the clinical picture will dictate whether or not it is prudent to attempt retrograde intubation.

CLINICAL TIPS: RETROGRADE INTUBATION

▶ The cricothyroid membrane is most easily found in adolescents and older children by identifying the laryngeal prominence of the thyroid cartilage ("Adam's apple"), then palpating inferiorly in the midline until a second, smaller prominence is felt. This is the superior border of the cricoid cartilage. The membrane lies just rostral to this landmark.

▶ In infants, the thyroid prominence is not well developed and may be difficult to identify. While some have recommended identifying the prominent hyoid bone and palpating caudally, it is safer to identify the trachea and palpate rostrally.

▶ The syringe used to advance the needle or catheter should be fluid filled so that entry into the trachea is indicated by the appearance of bubbles in the fluid.

▶ If the tube cannot be passed easily into the trachea over the wire, the tube should be withdrawn somewhat as the tension in the wire is diminished. The wire should then be pulled taut again, and another attempt made. In such instances, it may be necessary to rotate the tube 90 degrees before reinsertion or to use a smaller tube.

▶ Retrograde intubation can be combined with other techniques, and this may improve the chances of success. For example, the guidewire can be inserted through the suction or instrumentation port of a fiberoptic laryngoscope or through the hollow stylet of the Bullard laryngoscope and guided into the airway under direct vision.

▶ Failure to intubate the trachea after two or three attempts with the retrograde technique generally indicates that another method should be chosen.

Equipment

The minimum required equipment for retrograde intubation consists of a properly sized endotracheal tube, antiseptic solution, a guidewire, a syringe, and a needle or catheter through which the guidewire will pass. The guidewire must be of sufficient length that it can be passed from the neck through the entire airway and extend out of the patient's mouth far enough to easily accommodate the length of an endotracheal tube. There should be ample length at both the insertion site in the neck and beyond the end of the endotracheal tube to allow the operator to readily control the guidewire for the duration of the procedure. Retrieval of the guidewire from the mouth is facilitated by hemostats or forceps. All of these items are contained in the new retrograde intubation kits manufactured by Cook Critical Care. Performing this procedure with an awake or sedated patient also requires local anesthetic for infiltration at the insertion site and topical anesthetic for the airway.

Procedure

Initial steps of a retrograde intubation are exactly the same as those performed for percutaneous transtracheal ventilation (see Chapter 18). As the patient continues to receive manual ventilation, the skin of the anterior neck overlying the trachea is thoroughly cleansed with an antiseptic solution and a sterile field is established. Standing to one side of the patient (a right-handed operator at the patient's right), the operator identifies the relevant external anatomic landmarks (see Fig. 18.1). This is done by first palpating the laryngeal prominence (thyroid cartilage) and then moving down along the midline until a small "bump" is felt at the superior aspect of the cricoid cartilage. The cricothyroid membrane is just cephalad to this point. With younger patients who do not have a well-developed laryngeal prominence, it may be necessary to proceed upward from the tracheal rings until the bulge at the cricoid cartilage is appreciated.

If retrograde intubation is being performed in an awake patient, the operator should first administer adequate sedation (see Chapter 33). In patients with respiratory distress, some or all of this technique can be performed with the patient seated. After or coincident with sedation, the operator should anesthetize the airway. First, a topical anesthetic can be administered using a commercial anesthetic spray or by having the patient breathe a nebulized solution of 2% to 4% lidocaine. Next, the skin overlying the puncture site is anesthetized with local anesthetic. Then without removing the syringe, the operator should puncture the cricothyroid membrane, confirm its location by aspirating air, and anesthetize the trachea by instilling the remaining local anesthetic (2 to 3 mL of 2% lidocaine). The awake patient will often cough during this process, and the operator should be prepared for this. The technique of transtracheal anesthesia is illustrated in Chapter 16 (see Fig. 16.22).

At this point, a needle or (preferably) an over-the-needle catheter of sufficient caliber to accommodate the guidewire is passed through the cricothyroid membrane, and again air should be aspirated into the syringe to confirm position within the trachea (Fig. 17.24A). The needle or catheter is directed in a superior (rostral) orientation to ensure that the guidewire travels in the proper direction. The guidewire is inserted into the needle or catheter and advanced (Fig. 17.24B). The patient's mouth is opened and, with use of a laryngoscope or other light source, the guidewire is identified in the patient's mouth and retrieved either by hand or using a hemostat or forceps. It should be noted that the guidewire may enter the nose and that the procedure can be completed as a nasotracheal intubation. However, this increases the complexity of the procedure, limits the size of the endotracheal tube that can be inserted, and increases the risk of bleeding.

When a sufficient length of guidewire has been advanced through the mouth or nose, the operator can proceed with advancing an endotracheal tube over the guidewire. Alternatively, the optional step of placing an introducer sheath over the guidewire can be performed. The introducer sheath is threaded over the guidewire and advanced until its distal tip encounters the site at which the wire enters the cricothyroid membrane. At this point, the operator will be unable to easily advance the introducer further, and the introducer may visibly "tent" the skin as an additional sign that it has been inserted as far as possible. If the guidewire alone is used, it can be threaded either entirely through the lumen of the endotracheal tube or initially through the Murphy eye and then through the lumen. If the introducer-guidewire combination is used, it should be threaded entirely through the lumen of the tube. The endotracheal tube is then advanced into the airway (Fig. 17.24C). Although this can be done blindly, direct laryngoscopy may facilitate tube passage through the glottis. When the tube is passed as far as it can easily be advanced, the operator may again see tenting of the skin and/or movement of local structures, indicating that the tip has reached the proper position. The guidewire or guidewire/introducer are then removed through the oral or nasal cavity (Fig. 17.24D). During this process, the operator should maintain pressure on the endotracheal tube to further advance it into the airway. This helps to prevent the endotracheal tube from becoming dislodged as the guidewire or guidewire-introducer are removed.

As a modification of the procedure, the endotracheal tube can be mounted onto a fiberoptic bronchoscope and the guidewire passed through its suction port. Then, while an assistant maintains control of the guidewire, the operator advances the fiberoptic scope until it is below the vocal cords and abuts the cricothyroid membrane. The guidewire is then removed from above and the endotracheal tube is directly advanced into the trachea. Once the tube is in place, its position should be confirmed with a colorimetric device or capnography, and it should be secured in the usual fashion. This combined technique has been successfully used in management of the difficult pediatric airway (64).

Complications

Although simple in concept, retrograde intubation is associated with several problems and potential complications. The procedure takes some time to perform and should not be considered in emergency circumstances unless the practitioner is very experienced. Furthermore, the tip of the endotracheal tube may become entrapped in the glottic structures and fail to enter the larynx. The likelihood of this problem may be decreased by using a tapered dilator inside the endotracheal tube or by using an epidural catheter as the guidewire to assist

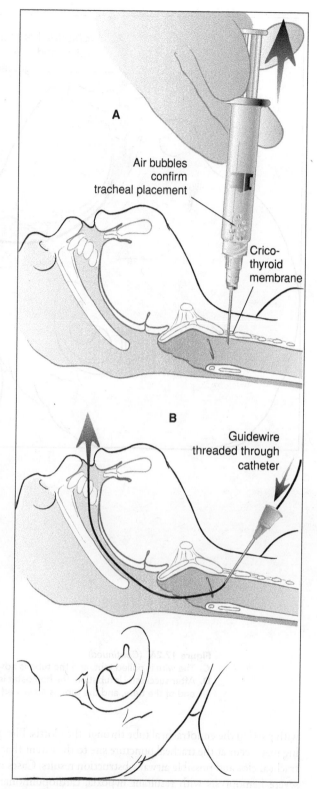

Figure 17.24 Retrograde intubation.
A. The needle is inserted through the cricothyroid membrane with negative pressure on the fluid-filled syringe. Entry into the trachea is indicated by the appearance of bubbles in the fluid.
B. The needle is directed superiorly, and the needle and syringe are removed as the catheter is advanced to its hub. The guidewire is inserted through the catheter until it can be retrieved from the nose or mouth.

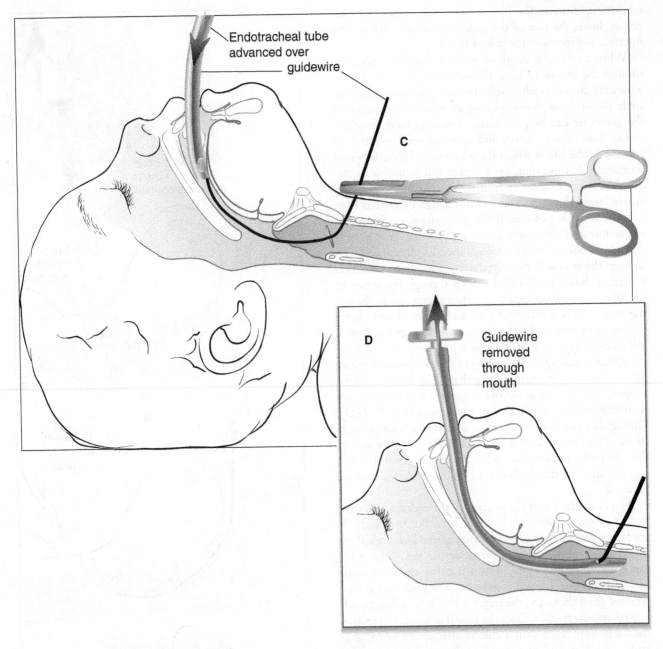

Figure 17.24 (*Continued*)
C. The wire is pulled taut, and the tube is advanced into the trachea over the wire.
D. After successful intubation, the hemostat is removed, the wire is withdrawn through the proximal end of the tube, and the tube is advanced to the appropriate depth of insertion.

with passing the endotracheal tube through the glottis. Bleeding may occur at the tracheal puncture site to the extent that a tracheal clot and possible airway obstruction results. Cases of severe hemoptysis with resultant hypoxia, cardiopulmonary arrest, dysrhythmias, and death following retrograde intubation have been reported (65–68). Subcutaneous emphysema localized to the area of the transtracheal needle puncture is common but generally self-limiting. In severe cases, the air can track through the fascial planes of the neck, leading to tracheal compression with resultant airway compromise as

well as pneumomediastinum and pneumothorax (69,70). Laryngospasm may result from irritation by the retrograde wire unless the vocal cords are sufficiently anesthetized. Other less common complications include esophageal perforation, tracheal hematoma, laryngeal edema, infection, tracheitis, tracheal fistula, trigeminal nerve injury, and vocal cord damage (71,72). Severe complications reported with retrograde intubation are usually associated with multiple attempts, large-gauge needles, and untrained personnel in emergency settings (73).

▶ SURGICAL AIRWAY

A surgical airway typically becomes necessary when impending airway loss cannot be averted with BVM ventilation or endotracheal intubation. Such situations include airway compromise from severe maxillofacial, pharyngeal, or laryngeal trauma; airway anomalies; a lack of oral access because of intermaxillary fixation; and masticatory space infection and consequent limitation of temporomandibular joint motion. Early identification of these patients affords practitioners the opportunity to prepare for potential airway loss prior to attempting intubation. The decision to abandon traditional intubation methods and attempt one of the surgical airway procedures is difficult, especially for those unaccustomed to performing these invasive techniques. This is compounded by the unfavorable convergence of circumstances and the lack of time for deliberation or consultation with colleagues.

Three surgical airway procedures qualify for consideration in the emergent setting: percutaneous transtracheal ventilation, surgical cricothyrotomy, and emergency tracheostomy. Percutaneous transtracheal ventilation is described in Chapter 18, and surgical cricothyrotomy (including wire-guided cricothyroidotomy) is described in Chapter 26. Although rarely performed in the ED, emergency tracheostomy is described here because it is the only procedure indicated for surgical airway access in the newborn period. In this population, there is insufficient space between the cricoid and thyroid cartilages—both of which are positioned high in the neck—to perform other procedures.

Emergent Tracheostomy

Emergent tracheostomy establishes transcutaneous access to the trachea below the level of the cricoid cartilage (74,75). Three procedures are included in this category: percutaneous dilational tracheostomy, translaryngeal tracheostomy, and surgical tracheostomy. Unless a practitioner is very experienced, performing an emergency tracheostomy should be a rare occurrence, because the depth of the trachea in the neck and the presence of significant overlying vascular structures lead to frequent complications.

Indications

Emergent tracheostomy may be necessary when (a) percutaneous transtracheal ventilation is contraindicated or fails in a child younger than 6 years, (b) a child's cricothyroid space is considered too small for cannulation (58), or (c) the laryngeal anatomy of a child has been distorted by the presence of pathologic lesions or infection. Nonemergent tracheostomies are performed for a number of reasons, including in patients with stable airways who cannot be intubated through a transoral or transnasal route, patients in whom prolonged intubation (e.g., longer than 2 weeks) is anticipated, and patients who have been intubated translaryngeally for more than 3 days.

SUMMARY: EMERGENT TRACHEOSTOMY

1 Position the patient with a towel under the back to hyperextend the neck unless neck or spine movement is contraindicated.

2 Rapidly apply antiseptic solution to the anterior neck.

3 If possible, identify the cricoid cartilage, and use a scalpel or electrocautery device to make a vertical incision caudally to the sternal notch (this incision should extend through the skin and subcutaneous tissue).

4 While an assistant retracts the skin, quickly palpate the trachea with the nondominant hand, stabilize the trachea, and then incise the remaining soft tissue and the trachea itself (this should be a vertical incision that is large enough to accommodate the endotracheal tube or tracheostomy tube selected).

5 Using the back of the scalpel, a tracheostomy hook, or hemostats, open the incision and insert the tube.

6 Advance the tube into the desired position, confirm that it is located within the trachea, and begin positive pressure ventilation.

7 Secure the tube with suture, tape, or tracheostomy ties.

Absolute contraindications to an emergent tracheostomy do not exist, since this is a life-saving procedure. Relative contraindications include coagulopathy, infections involving the fascial planes of the neck and paratracheal regions, cervical injuries, and severe limitation of neck extension.

Equipment

Although this technique is not usually recommended for emergency use, it may be appropriate in skilled hands, and many preassembled kits are now available. At a minimum, a scalpel, materials for establishing a sterile field, retractors, sponges, and an endotracheal tube or tracheostomy tube and will be needed. The use of electrocautery is generally preferred over a scalpel to minimize bleeding, but this may not be available in the ED. The help of an assistant should always be enlisted.

Procedure

Emergent tracheostomy should always be performed by the most skilled practitioner available, ideally, a trained surgeon. The patient is placed supine with a roll under the shoulders to hyperextend the neck unless cervical injuries preclude this

CLINICAL TIPS: EMERGENT TRACHEOSTOMY

▶ This is a high risk procedure that should only be attempted as a last resort by inexperienced personnel. Even then, the most experienced provider available should perform the procedure.

▶ An important key to success is the ability to identify and maintain control of the trachea. Passage of hemostats or forceps into the tracheal incision may allow the incision to be gently held open while the endotracheal tube is inserted. However this should be done gently so as not to disrupt the tracheal tissue.

▶ The need to perform this procedure means that the patient has been without effective ventilation for at least a few minutes. Positive pressure ventilation should therefore be administered as quickly as possible after the tube has been placed in the trachea.

▶ While the endotracheal tube or tracheostomy tube is being secured and positive pressure ventilation is being administered, it is imperative that someone maintain constant control of the tube because it can be easily dislodged during this process.

▶ One of the most common reasons for performing this procedure is the presence of complete airway obstruction. Often this problem can be resolved (e.g., by removal of the foreign body) once the airway is secured. Therefore, if the endotracheal tube or tracheostomy tube becomes dislodged after the procedure and the resolution of the underlying problem, the most appropriate airway management technique is generally standard orotracheal intubation rather than attempted replacement of the tube into the tracheostomy. The tracheostomy site is often difficult or impossible to locate and cannulate in such situations.

position. A midline vertical incision extending from the inferior border of the cricoid cartilage to the sternal notch is made through the skin and subcutaneous tissue. The position of the trachea is confirmed by palpation through the skin incision with the nondominant index finger before the remaining soft tissues overlying the trachea are incised. An incision in the trachea large enough to allow insertion of an endotracheal tube or tracheostomy tube should then be made below the first tracheal ring. Once the tube is inserted, positive pressure ventilation is administered. When performed by a skilled practitioner, this procedure can usually be accomplished in less than 1 minute.

Complications

Bleeding, subcutaneous and mediastinal emphysema, pneumothorax, airway obstruction, aspiration, infection, and death are early complications of emergent tracheostomy. Accidental extubation is a serious event, as replacement of the cannula may be impossible. In this situation, orotracheal intubation or translaryngeal oxygenation is required (76). Delayed complications include hoarseness, tracheoesophageal and tracheocutaneous fistulas, tracheal stenosis, and neck scarring. The incidence of complications associated with percutaneous dilatational tracheostomy is approximately 2% (77), which is lower than the incidence associated with a formal tracheostomy.

As with any surgical procedure, hemorrhage can occur with an emergent tracheostomy. Minitracheostomy occasionally results in severe bleeding into the airway, necessitating progression to a full surgical tracheostomy. The inflated cuff of the formal tracheostomy prevents pulmonary aspiration of blood. In rare cases, excessive pressure from the tracheostomy tube can cause the innominate artery to rupture into the trachea, resulting in massive airway hemorrhage. Air embolism during the operative procedure is another possible complication.

If an air leak occurs and the skin has healed around the tracheostomy tube, air can escape into the subcutaneous spaces of the neck, resulting in subcutaneous emphysema. If the condition goes unrecognized and the patient is maintained on high-pressure mechanical ventilation, the air may track into other locations. Air escaping into the paratracheal spaces can result in a pneumomediastinum, and air released into the pleural cavity can result in a tension pneumothorax.

A tracheostomy tube can cause tracheal erosion, particularly into the esophagus (tracheoesophageal fistula) or the brachiocephalic artery. These tubes typically reside low in the trachea and are designed with a fixed curve. Furthermore, tube pressure can damage the skin at the insertion site.

Accidental extubation and dislodgement of the cannula occurs occasionally, most commonly in the early postoperative period. If the cannula is inadvertently removed from a fresh tracheostomy, it should be replaced as quickly as possible. Infection, mediastinal sepsis, tracheal stenosis, and tracheomalacia are rare late complications.

▶ SUMMARY

Most airway problems can be solved with relatively simple devices and techniques, but clinical judgment born of experience is crucial to their application. As with any intubation technique, practice and routine use will improve performance and may reduce the likelihood of complications. Each airway device has unique properties that may be advantageous in certain situations yet limiting in others. Specific airway management techniques are greatly influenced by individual disease processes and the anatomy of the patient, and successful management may require combinations of multiple devices and techniques.

▶ ACKNOWLEDGMENTS

The authors are grateful to Drs. C. Christopher King and Stephen Stayer for their contributions to the first edition of this textbook and to Dr. King for his advice and contributions to this chapter. We are likewise grateful to our friend and colleague Dr. Michael Murphy for his advice and suggestions.

▶ REFERENCES

1. Morray JP, Geiduscheck JM, Caplan RA, et al. A comparison of adult and pediatric anesthesia closed malpractice claims. *Anesthesiology.* 1993;78:461–467.

2. Morray JP, Geiduschel JM, Ramamoorthy C, et al. Anesthesia-related cardiac arrest in children. *Anesthesiology.* 2000;93:6–14.

3. Practice guidelines for management of the difficult airway: an updated report by the American Society of Anesthesiologists Task Force on Management of the Difficult Airway. *Anesthesiology.* 2003;98:1269–1277.

4. Langeron O, Mazzo E, Huraux C, et al. Prediction of difficult mask ventilation. *Anesthesiology.* 2000;92:1229–1236.

5. Cormack RS, Lehane J. Difficult tracheal intubation in obstetrics. *Anaesthesia.* 1984;39:1105–1111.

6. Klock PA, Benumof JL. Definition and incidence of the difficult airway. In: Hagberg CA, ed. *Benumont's Airway Management. Principles and Practice.* Mosby Elsevier. 2007:215–220.

7. Mallampati SR, Gatt SP, Gugino LD, et al. A clinical sign to predict difficult intubation: a prospective study. *Can Anaesth Soc J.* 1985;32:429–434.

8. Turkan S, Ates Y, Cuhruk H, et al. Should we reevaluate the variables for predicting the airway in anesthesiology? *Anesth Analg.* 2002;94:1340–1344.

9. Rocke DA, Murray WB, Rout CC, et al. Relative risk analysis of factors associated with difficult intubation in obstetric anesthesia. *Anesthesiology.* 1992;77:67–73.

10. Arne J, Descoins P, Fusciardi J, et al. Preoperative assessment for difficult intubation in general and ENT surgery: predictive value of a clinical multivariate risk index. *Br J Anaesth.* 1998;80:140–146.

11. Cattano D, Pescini A, Paolicchi A, et al. Difficult intubation: an overview on a cohort of 1327 consecutive patients. *Minerva Anestesiol.* 2001;67:45.

12. Rose DK, Cohen MM. The airway: problems and prediction in 18,500 patients. *Can J Anaesth.* 1994;41:372–383.

13. Crosby ET, Cooper RM, Douglas MJ, et al. The unanticipated difficult airway with recommendation for management. *Can J Anaesth.* 1998;45:757–776.

14. Kopp VJ, Bailey A, Valley RD, et al. Utility of the Mallampati classification for predicting difficult intubation in pediatric patients. *Anesthesiology.* 1995;83:A1147.

15. Berry FA. Anesthesia for the child with a difficult airway. In: Berry FA, ed. *Anesthetic Management of Difficult and Routine Pediatric Patients.* 2nd ed. New York: Churchill-Livingston; 1990:167–198.

16. Benumof JL. Laryngeal mask airway and the ASA difficult airway algorithm. *Anesthesiology.* 1996;84:686–699.

17. Tsujimura Y. Downfolding of the epiglottis induced by the laryngeal mask airway in children: a comparison between two insertion techniques. *Anaesthesia.* 2003;58:390–391.

18. O'Neill B, Templeton JJ, Caramico L, et al. The laryngeal mask airway in pediatric patients: factors affecting ease of use during insertion and emergence. *Anesth Analg.* 1994;78:659–662.

19. Krier C, Georgi R. *Airway* management. Stuttgart: Thieme; 2001:36, 193–194.

20. Brimacombe JR, Brain AIJ. Problems and complications. In: Brimacombe JR, Brian AIJ, eds. *The Laryngeal Mask Airway: A Review and Practice Guide.* Philadelphia: WB Saunders; 1997:117–133.

21. Brain AIJ. *The Intravent Laryngeal Mask Instruction Manual.* 2nd ed. Berkshire, England: Brain Medical; 1992.

22. Verghese C, Smith TG, Young E. Prospective survey of the use of the laryngeal mask in 2,359 patients. *Anaesthesia.* 1993;48:58–60.

23. Ferson DZ, Rosenblatt WH, Johansen MJ, et al. Use of the intubating LMA-Fastrach in 254 patients with difficult-to-manage airways. *Anesthesiology.* 2001;95:1175–1181.

24. Fukutome T, Amaha K, Nakazawa K, et al. Tracheal intubation through the intubating laryngeal mask airway (LMA-Fastrach) in patients with difficult airways. *Anaesth Intensive Care.* 1998;26:387–391.

25. Kapila A, Addy EV, Verghese C, et al. The intubating laryngeal mask airway: an initial assessment of performance. *Br J Anaesth.* 1997;79:710–713.

26. Oczenski W, Krenn H, Dahaba AA, et al. Complications following the use of the Combitube, tracheal tube and laryngeal mask airway. *Anaesthesia.* 1999;54:1161–1165.

27. Gaitini LA, Vaida SJ, Mostafa S, et al. The Combitube in elective surgery. *Anesthesiology.* 2001;94:79–82.

28. Hartmann T, Hoerauf KH, Benumof JL, et al. The esophageal-tracheal Combitube small adult: an alternative airway for ventilatory support during gynaecological laparoscopy. *Anaesthesia.* 2000;55:670–675.

29. Venzina D, Lessard MR, Bussieres J, et al. Complications associated with the use of the esophageal-tracheal Combitube. *Can J Anaesth.* 1998;45:75–80.

30. Klein H, Williamsom M, Sue-Ling HM, et al. Esophageal rupture associated with the use of the Combitube. *Anesth Analg.* 1997;85:973–979.

31. Hung OR, Pytka S, Morris I, et al. Clinical trial of a new light-wand device (Trachlight) to intubate the trachea. *Anesthesiology.* 1995;83:509–514.

32. Ellis DG, Jakymec A, Kaplan RM, et al. Guided orotracheal intubation in the operating room using a lighted stylet: a comparison with direct laryngoscopic technique. *Anesthesiology.* 1986;64:823–826.

33. Stone DJ, Stirt JA, Kaplan MJ, et al. A complication of lightwand-guided nasotracheal intubation. *Anesthesiology.* 1984;61:780–781.

34. Williams RT, Stewart RD. Transillumination of the trachea with a lighted stylet [letter]. *Anesth Analg.* 1986;65:542–543.

35. Moukabary K, Peterson CJ, Kingsley CP. A potential complication with the lightwand [letter]. *Anesthesiology.* 1994;81:523–524.

36. Szigeti CL, Baeuerle JJ, Mongan PD, et al. Arytenoid dislocation with lighted stylet intubation: case report and retrospective review. *Anesth Analg.* 1994;78:185–186.

37. Davis L, Cook-Sather SD, Schreiner MS. Lighted stylet tracheal intubation: a review. *Anesth Analg.* 2000;90:745–756.

38. Henderson JJ. The use of paraglossal straight blade laryngoscopy in difficult tracheal intubation. *Anaesthesia.* 1997;51:552–560.

39. Pfitzner L, Cooper MG, Ho D. The Shikani Seeing Optical Stylet for difficult intubation in children: initial experience. *Anaesth Intensive Care.* 2002;30:462–466.

40. Gorback MS. Management of the challenging airway with the Bullard laryngoscope. *J Clin Anesth.* 1991;3:473–477.

41. Marshall KA, James CF. Complication of Bullard laryngoscope: dislodgement of blade-extender resulting in an upper airway foreign body. *Anesthesiology.* 1998;89:1604–1605.

42. Audenaert SM, Montgomery CL, Stone B, et al. Retrograde-assisted fiberoptic tracheal intubation in children with difficult airways. *Anesth Analg.* 1991;73:660–664.

43. Gupta B, McDonald JS, Brooks JHJ, et al. Oral fiberoptic intubation over a retrograde guide wire. *Anesth Analg.* 1989;68:517–519.

44. Afilalo M, Guttman A, Stern E, et al. Fiberoptic intubation in the emergency department: a case series. *J Emerg Med.* 1993;11:387–391.

45. Delaney KA, Hessler R. Emergency flexible fiberoptic nasotracheal intubation: a report of 60 cases. *Ann Emerg Med.* 1988;17:919–926.

46. Minik EJ Jr, Clinton JE, Plummer D, et al. Fiberoptic intubation in the emergency department. *Ann Emerg Med.* 1990;19:359–362.

47. Mulder DS, Wallace DH, Woolhouse FM. The use of the fiberoptic bronchoscope to facilitate endotracheal intubation following head and neck trauma. *J Trauma.* 1975;15:638–640.

48. Vauthy PA, Reddy R. Acute upper airway obstruction in infants and children: evaluation by the fiberoptic bronchoscope. *Ann Otol Rhinol Laryngol.* 1980;89:417–418.

49. Berthelsen P, Prytz S, Jacobsen E. Two-stage fiberoptic nasotracheal intubation in infants: a new approach to difficult pediatric intubation. *Anesthesiology.* 1985;63:457–458.

50. Ovassapian A, Yelich SF, Dykes MHM, et al. Fiberoptic nasotracheal intubation: incidence and causes of failure. *Anesth Analg.* 1983;62:692–695.

51. Hagberg CA. Current concepts in the management of the difficult airway. In: *ASA Refresher Courses in Anesthesiology.* Vol. 29. Baltimore: Lippincott Williams & Wilkins; 2001:135–146.

52. Inada T, Fujise K, Tachiban K, et al. Orotracheal intubation through the laryngeal mask airway in patients with Treacher Collins syndrome. *Paediatr Anaesth.* 1995;5:129–132.

53. Stewart RD. Tactile orotracheal intubation. *Ann Emerg Med.* 1984;13:175–178.

54. Wijesundera CD. Digital intubation of the trachea [letter]. *Ceylon Med J.* 1990;35:81–82.

55. Hardwick WC, Bluhm D. Digital intubation. *J Emerg Med.* 1984;1:317–320.

56. Siddall WJW. Tactile orotracheal intubation. *Anaesthesia.* 1966;21:221–222.

57. Hancock PJ, Peterson G. Finger intubation of the trachea in newborns. *Pediatrics.* 1992;89:325–327.

58. Audenaert SM, Montgomery CL, Stone B, et al. Retrograde-assisted fiberoptic tracheal intubation in children with difficult airways. *Anesth Analg.* 1991;73:660–664.

59. McNamara RM. Retrograde intubation of the trachea. *Ann Emerg Med.* 1987;16:680–682.

60. Cooper CMS, Murray-Wilson A. Retrograde intubation: management of a 4.8 kg, 5-month infant. *Anaesthesia.* 1987;42:1197–1200.

61. Borland LM, Swan DM, Leff S. Difficult pediatric endotracheal intubation: a new approach to the retrograde technique. *Anesthesiology.* 1981;55:577–578.

62. Audenaert SM, Montgomery CL, Stone B, et al. Retrograde-assisted fiberoptic tracheal intubation in children with difficult airways. *Anesth Analg.* 1991;73:660–664.

63. Barriot P, Riou B. Retrograde technique for tracheal intubation in trauma patients. *Crit Care Med.* 1988;16:712–713.

64. Diaz JH, Guarisco JL, LeJeune FE Jr. Perioperative management of pediatric microstomia. *Can J Anaesth.* 1991;38:217–221.

65. Schillaci CR, Iacovoni VF, Conte RS, et al. Transtracheal aspiration complicated by fatal endotracheal hemorrhage. *N Engl J Med.* 1976;295:488–490.

66. Spencer CD, Beaty HN. Complications of transtracheal aspiration. *N Engl J Med.* 1972;286:304–306.

67. Unger KM, Moser KM. Fatal complication of transtracheal aspiration: a report of two cases. *Arch Intern Med.* 1973;132:437–439.

68. Kalinske RW, Parker RH, Brandt D. Diagnostic usefulness and safety of transtracheal aspiration. *N Engl J Med.* 1967;276:604–608.

69. Marty-Ane C, Picard E, Jonquet O, et al. Membranous tracheal rupture after endotracheal intubation. *Ann Thorac Surg.* 1995;60:1367–1371.

70. Poon YK. Case history number 89: a life-threatening complication of cricothyroid membrane puncture. *Anesth Analg.* 1976;55:298–301.

71. Faithfull NS. Injury to terminal branches of the trigeminal nerve following tracheal intubation. *Br J Anaesth.* 1985;57:535–537.

72. Sanchez A. Retrograde intubation technique. In: Hagberg CA, ed. *Airway Management: Principles and Practice.* Philadelphia: Mosby Elsevier; 2007:439–462.

73. Parmet JL, Metz S. Anesthesiology issues in general surgery: retrograde endotracheal intubation: an underutilized tool for management of the difficult airway. *Contemp Surg.* 1996;49:300–306.

74. Granholm T, Farmer DL. The surgical airway. *Respir Care Clin N Am.* 2001;7:13–23.

75. Isaacs JH, Pedersen AD. Emergency cricothyroidotomy. *Am Surg.* 1997;63:346–349.

76. Wong EK, Bradrick JP. Surgical approaches to airway management for anesthesia practitioners. In: Hagberg CA, ed. *Handbook of Difficult Airway Management.* Philadelphia: Churchill Livingstone; 2000:209–210.

77. Berrouschot J, Oeken J, Steiniger L, et al. Perioperative complications of percutaneous dilational tracheostomy. *Laryngoscope.* 1997;107:1538–1544.

MANOJ K. MITTAL AND JILL M. BAREN

18

Percutaneous Transtracheal Ventilation

▶ INTRODUCTION

The importance of maintaining adequate oxygenation and ventilation for the critically ill child cannot be overstated. In most cases, standard airway interventions, such as bag-valve-mask (BVM) ventilation and endotracheal intubation, can be performed successfully without incident. However, physicians responsible for managing critically ill children must also be prepared for those situations in which standard methods unexpectedly fail. Such circumstances require knowledge of alternative techniques for providing respiratory support (see also Chapter 17). Percutaneous transtracheal ventilation (PTV), also called "translaryngeal ventilation," is one such technique. Although sometimes a point of confusion, PTV should not be mistaken for high-frequency transtracheal jet ventilation, which involves delivering very small volumes of oxygen at extremely high rates. High-frequency transtracheal jet ventilation requires special equipment not generally found in the emergency department (ED).

Initial animal studies in the development of PTV dealt with passive transtracheal oxygenation (1). This method, however, was abandoned in favor of intermittent administration of compressed air via a transtracheal catheter, since this provides both ventilation and oxygenation (2). Successful human studies and various modifications of this technique followed, as well as data showing that transtracheal gas exchange could sustain life for prolonged periods of time (3–5). Smith and Ravussin subsequently published reports documenting the successful use of PTV in children aged 4 months to 11 years (6,7). Considering the potential complications associated with surgical cricothyrotomy and tracheotomy in young children, PTV should be considered the invasive (surgical airway) rescue modality of choice in this age group. The advantages of needle cricothyrotomy with PTV over surgical cricothyrotomy include faster performance, easier technique, less equipment required, no need for an assistant, smaller scar

formation, decreased bleeding, and less frequent subglottic or glottic stenosis. The disadvantages of PTV include incomplete control of the airway, greater potential for aspiration, increased likelihood of barotrauma, and inability to perform adequate tracheal suctioning (8).

▶ ANATOMY AND PHYSIOLOGY

The cricothyroid membrane is bound superiorly by the thyroid cartilage and inferiorly by the cricoid cartilage. Bennett et al. studied the anatomy of the cricothyroid membrane in 13 adult fresh cadavers (9). The vertical measurement was 8 to 19 mm (mean, 13.7 mm), and the transverse measurement was 9 to 19 mm (mean, 12.4 mm). Similar information for pediatric patients has not been published. The cricothyroid arteries typically course through the apical portion of the membrane, although aberrant vessels may rarely complicate procedures in this area (10). For young infants, performing PTV can be difficult due to the small size of the cricothyroid membrane. However, this is also true of other invasive airway techniques, and PTV can often be performed more rapidly and with fewer complications. Furthermore, if the cricothyroid membrane of a younger patient cannot be located, the procedure can be performed by introducing the needle through the tracheal cartilage without additional risk to the patient (see below).

The operator must be thoroughly familiar with the anatomy of the anterior neck in order to perform this procedure successfully (Fig. 18.1). Five specific landmarks should be identified: the hyoid bone, the laryngeal prominence of the thyroid cartilage, the cricothyroid membrane, the cricoid cartilage, and the remaining tracheal rings. The laryngeal prominence develops during adolescence and is easily palpable in most adults, whereas the most readily identifiable landmarks

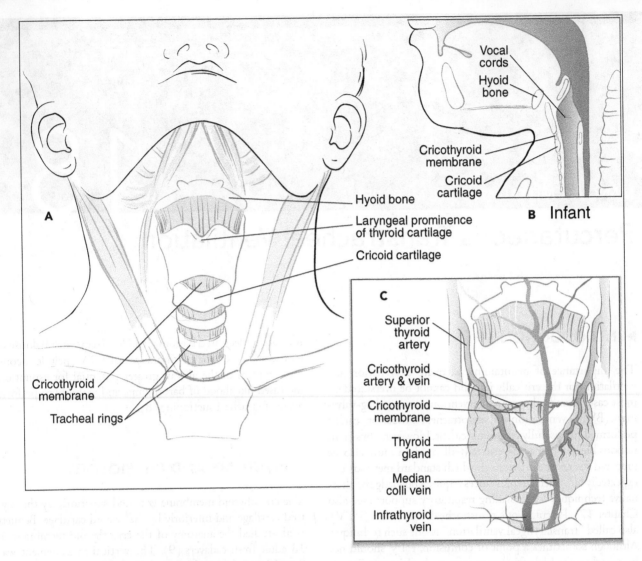

Figure 18.1 Anatomic landmarks for PTV.
A. Cartilaginous skeleton of the extrathoracic airway. With older children and adolescents, the laryngeal prominence at the superior border of the thyroid cartilage can usually be palpated. The thyroid cartilage is followed inferiorly to locate the cricothyroid membrane.
B. With infants and younger children, the laryngeal prominence is not developed. The rings of the tracheal cartilage are followed superiorly to locate the prominence of the cricoid cartilage. The cricothyroid membrane is just superior to the cricoid cartilage.
C. A midline approach will avoid the normal position of the cricothyroid artery.

in infants and young children are the hyoid bone and cricoid cartilage.

Delivered tidal volume during PTV is affected by a number of factors, including lung compliance, airway resistance, size of catheter, inspiratory pressure, and duration of inspiration (11). Jacobs estimated that a maximum 70% of the volume of oxygen delivered to the catheter tip reaches the lower respiratory tract of adults with normal lung compliance (12). The remainder passes up through the glottic opening and out the nose and mouth, decreasing the efficiency of gas exchange when compared with endotracheal intubation (4,12–14). Because of the relatively small size of the airways, pediatric patients generally have significantly greater airway resistance than

adults. Thus even with a small child, it is important to use a catheter with an adequate luminal diameter and a high-pressure oxygen source to perform this procedure effectively. When used with a low-pressure oxygen delivery system, PTV provides adequate oxygenation but may not provide adequate ventilation, causing retention of CO_2 over time. An example of such a system would be a self-inflating bag-valve-mask circuit connected to the catheter via a 3.0-mm internal diameter (ID) endotracheal tube adapter (see "Equipment"). It has been suggested that use of a large-diameter catheter will largely overcome the problem of increasing hypercarbia with a low-pressure system (15), but Marr and Yamamoto recently showed that catheter size does not substantially affect gas flow rates (16). They found that Poiseuille's law is not applicable in this situation, because it applies to laminar flow rather than gas flowing in a turbulent fashion, which is what occurs when oxygen is forced at high pressure through a narrow tube. Consequently, these authors recommend use of high-pressure oxygen from a wall source, although they contend that "if a device to perform this is not available, then a self-inflating bag-valve-mask circuit may still be sufficient" for PTV (16).

PTV provides oxygen via intermittent bulk flow of gas under high pressure. Exhalation is achieved passively through the elastic recoil of the chest, with gases being expelled through the mouth and nose. The "ball-valve" effect of most partial laryngeal obstructions permits adequate exhalation during PTV, but complete obstruction prevents any egress of gas and may result in a dangerously rapid rise in intrapulmonary pressure (17). With a 50-psi oxygen source, volumes of 950 mL/sec, 1,200 mL/sec, and 1,300 mL/sec can be delivered through 16-gauge, 14-gauge, and 13-gauge catheters, respectively (18). These flow rates are more than adequate for maintaining ventilation and oxygenation in adults. Actual peak inspiratory pressures and intratracheal pressures are relatively low, even with a driving pressure of 50 psi; however, smaller catheters (16- to 18-gauge) and lower driving pressures (25 to 35 psi) must be used for pediatric patients in order to prevent barotrauma. Tran et al. compared the efficacy of PTV in the unparalyzed and paralyzed states using a canine model and showed that gas exchange and lung mechanics were similar. This suggests that it may be unnecessary to induce paralysis when using PTV for emergency ventilation of a sedated patient (19).

The primary drawback to long-term use of PTV is CO_2 retention. For this reason, PTV previously has been viewed only as a temporizing procedure. However, when adequate oxygenation is maintained, even relatively high levels of hypercarbia may not be as deleterious as once believed (20,21). In fact, PTV has been shown to be safe for hours at a time, limited only by the ability of the system used to deliver humidified gases. Only in the setting of increased intracranial pressure or complete airway obstruction should PTV be considered solely as a temporizing measure.

▶ INDICATIONS

Indications for the emergent use of PTV are similar to those for surgical cricothyrotomy; that is, any patient whose airway cannot be maintained with standard interventions or a "nonsurgical rescue" procedure (such as insertion of a laryngeal mask airway) should be considered a possible candidate. Potential clinical scenarios include severe blunt or penetrating maxillofacial trauma; laryngeal foreign bodies that cannot readily be removed; severe swelling of the upper airway from infection (e.g., epiglottitis), an allergic process (e.g., hereditary angioedema, snakebite), or local trauma (e.g., airway thermal or chemical burns); and congenital anomalies such as Treacher Collins syndrome or Pierre Robin syndrome (22–24). PTV

has also been used to provide oxygenation and ventilation before potentially difficult intubations as well as for elective procedures such as head and neck surgery (6–7,13,25–26). With younger children, PTV should always be considered before surgical cricothyrotomy because it is associated with far fewer complications and can be completed in a much shorter period of time (see also Chapter 26). PTV should not be performed when there is known damage to the cricoid cartilage or in the setting of tracheal rupture (8). These situations represent the only absolute contraindications for this procedure. Relative contraindications, such as mild to moderate local swelling of the anterior neck or the presence of a hematoma, should be balanced against the potentially devastating complications of failing to provide adequate airway intervention.

Controversy surrounds the use of PTV in the setting of complete upper airway obstruction. A blockage cephalad to the catheter will prevent passive exhalation of delivered gases through the mouth and nose. In a study of animals subjected to total airway obstruction, Jorden et al. reported that standard PTV caused massive distention of the lungs, severe barotrauma, and subsequent death (27). However, additional studies have challenged the dogma that PTV is absolutely contraindicated in the presence of complete upper airway obstruction (28–32). Successful application of PTV in animals with complete airway obstruction using prolonged exhalation times and large-ID catheters has been reported (30). Frame et al. reported a feline study of total airway obstruction using low flow rates (3 to 5 L/min) in which adequate oxygenation and ventilation were maintained without complication (32); they hypothesized that these data might be extrapolated to infants. Without the benefit of further studies to settle this issue, it seems reasonable to use PTV as a temporizing measure for infants and younger children when complete upper airway obstruction is present and other methods have been unsuccessful. In such a situation, prolonged exhalation times, lower oxygen delivery pressures, and the use of larger than normal catheters would all be required. For older children and adolescents, surgical cricothyrotomy remains the procedure of choice for emergent airway management in the presence of complete upper airway obstruction.

▶ EQUIPMENT

Because of the lack of controlled data on the use of PTV for children, no definitive standards exist regarding appropriate equipment. However, multiple models have been advocated in the adult literature, and many of these are applicable to pediatric patients. Equipment setups used to perform PTV range from those employing standard materials readily available in any ED to relatively sophisticated, commercially available devices (Fig. 18.2). Universal requirements include (a) a high-pressure oxygen source (up to 50 psi), (b) tubing capable of withstanding high pressures, (c) a manual in-line valve to control the intermittent flow of oxygen to the patient, and (d) a large-bore catheter (Table 18.1).

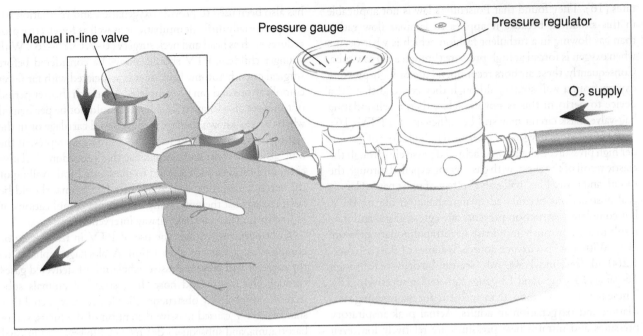

Figure 18.2 Permanent in-line valve PTV system.

Oxygen delivered at 50 psi can be obtained directly from a hospital wall outlet (without a regulator), from the flush valve of a mechanical ventilator, or by attaching the tubing directly to an oxygen tank line (without using a flow valve). Although high pressures are necessary to provide adequate ventilation for older adolescents and adults, lower pressures (between 25 and 35 psi) should be used for children so that the likelihood of complications from barotrauma is minimized. Such lower pressures can be obtained by using a standard wall outlet with a regulator set at 10 to 12 L/min. Tubing designed for gas delivery under high pressure must be used throughout the system.

If a permanent valve system is not available for performing PTV, a makeshift in-line valve must be fabricated using materials in the ED (Fig. 18.3). This can be easily accomplished by cutting a small hole in the distal end of the tubing to create a side port. The operator can then control the flow of gas by intermittently occluding the port with a finger or thumb. Alternatively, a plastic Y-connector or three-way stopcock (Fig. 18.4) interposed between two pieces of high-pressure tubing also permits control of gas flow. Occlusion of the open end of the connector or stopcock results in gas delivery to the trachea, while removal of the fingertip allows for exhalation.

Many creative models for performing PTV have been described. Multiple studies have employed mechanical ventilators as the high-pressure oxygen source (33–35). Suction tubing, an endotracheal tube connector, and a syringe with the plunger removed have been interposed between the catheter and oxygen source (Fig. 18.5) (33,36,37). Syringes have also been placed in series with endotracheal tube adapters, inflated endotracheal tubes, and disposable ventilator tubing (36,38,39). One commercially produced setup (Instrumentation Industries, Inc., Bethel Park, PA) comes complete with high-pressure tubing, a permanent in-line on/off valve, a pressure regulator, and disposable tubing with Luer-Lok to provide more secure catheter attachment.

Most studies concerning adult PTV have employed 12- and 16-gauge catheters, that is, catheters with an ID ranging from 1.5 to 2.8 mm (40). However, Hauswald et al. showed in a canine model that flow rates achievable with 18- to 20-gauge catheters and standard oxygen sources may be adequate for PTV in adults when the upper airway is repetitively obstructed to mimic a normal respiratory cycle (41). One commercially available PTV catheter (Acutronic USA Inc., Pittsburgh, PA) is curved for easier placement and has distal side holes that spray the delivered volume of gas over a wider area. Teflon catheters offer the advantage of being kink-resistant. Smaller catheters, in the range of 16- to 18-gauge, should be used for children. A Luer-Lok, mentioned above, can be used to securely attach the distal end of the catheter to the high-pressure tubing.

Prepackaged kits that can be used to obtain tracheal access via a modified Seldinger technique are also now widely available. The Pertrach (Pertrach Inc., Bridgeport, WV) is

TABLE 18.1	EQUIPMENT

1. High pressure oxygen source: 50 psi can be obtain directly from hospital wall outlet (used for adolescents and adults); 25 to 35 psi safely delivered through a standard regulator set at 10 to 12 L/min (used for younger children)
2. High pressure tubing
3. Inline valve (permanent, side hole cut in distal end of tubing, Y-connector, or 3-way stopcock)
4. Syringe containing 2 to 3 mL of saline or lidocain
5. 16- or 18-gauge catheter

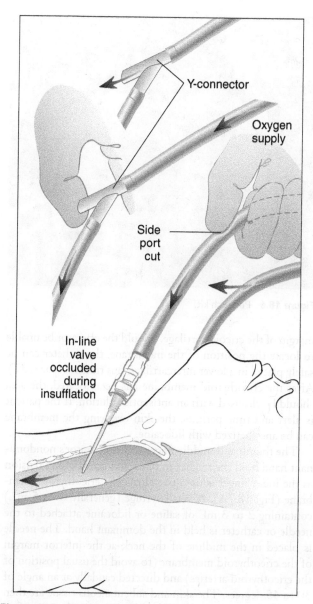

Figure 18.3 PTV setups utilizing a Y-connector and oxygen tubing with a cut side port.

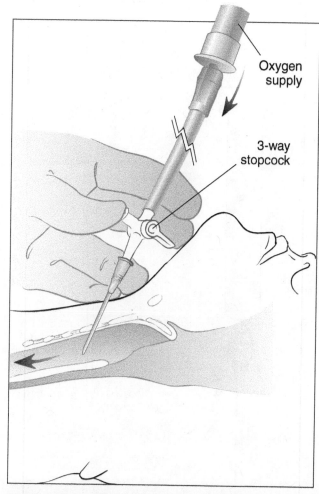

Figure 18.4 PTV setup utilizing a three-way stopcock.

one such kit; it includes three uncuffed tubes with IDs ranging from 3.0 to 4.0 mm for use with infants and children up to 10 years of age (Fig. 18.6). Craven and Vanner used an experimental model to compare the effectiveness of four devices: the Ravussin 13-gauge cannula (VBM Medical, Noblesville, IN), the Quicktrach 4 mm ID cannula (VBM Medical), the Melker 6 mm ID cannula (Cook Critical Care, Bloomington, IN), and a 6.0 mm ID cuffed endotracheal tube (42). These authors concluded that the Melker cannula was the best choice for emergency respiratory support of the four devices evaluated because it was easy to insert, had a low rate of complications compared with surgical cricothyrotomy, and could be used with a standard anesthetic circuit. Additionally, Chan et al. reported that cricothyrotomy using the modified Seldinger technique could be performed with a ra-

pidity and an effectiveness comparable to those of standard surgical cricothyrotomy (43).

Regardless of the equipment selected, a preassembled system for PTV should be readily available if this procedure is to be used as a potential option for airway management. The policy statement regarding preparedness for care of pediatric patients in the ED issued by the American College of Emergency Physicians and the American Academy of Pediatrics states that a PTV tray with appropriate cannula sizes should be available in any ED where care is provided for children (44). In their description of the "model of the clinical practice of emergency medicine," Hockberger et al. recommend that emergency physicians should be familiar with the technique of performing PTV (45). Other medical personnel who will be involved with this procedure should also be fully trained in the proper use of the equipment.

▶ PROCEDURE

The operator can most easily locate the cricothyroid membrane in older adolescents and adults by running a finger in a

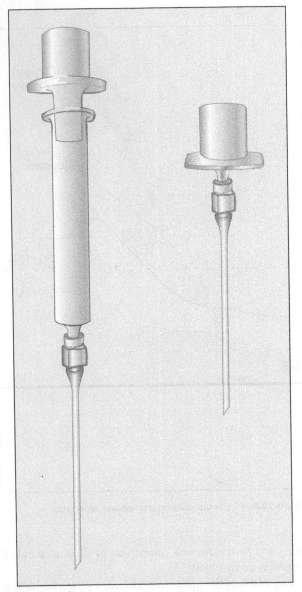

Figure 18.5 A 3-mL syringe with the plunger removed may be used as an adapter between the catheter and a 7.5 mm ID endotracheal tube. Alternatively, a 3.0 mm ID endotracheal tube connector can be inserted directly into the catheter hub. Both methods can be used to connect the catheter to a standard self-inflating resuscitation bag.

caudal direction from the laryngeal prominence until a small bump is felt (see Fig. 18.1), which is the cricoid cartilage. The cricothyroid membrane is appreciated as a subtle depression with slightly more "give" or "bounce" just superior to the cricoid cartilage. However, because the laryngeal prominence does not develop fully until adolescence, this method may not be useful for infants and children. For these patients, the operator's most reliable method for locating the membrane is to run a finger in a cephalad direction along the tracheal rings until a more prominent bulge is felt, representing the cricoid cartilage. Even if the cricothyroid membrane is not palpable, its location can be assumed as just cephalad to the superior

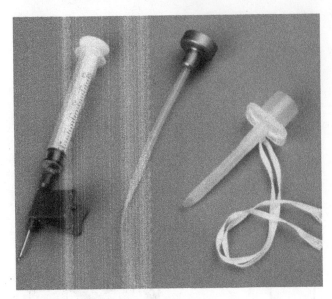

Figure 18.6 Pertrach kit.

margin of the cricoid cartilage. Should the operator be unable to locate the position of the membrane, the catheter can be safely placed in a lower intercartilaginous tracheal space (37). After the cricothyroid membrane has been located, the area should be cleansed with an antiseptic solution. If the patient is alert and time permits, the skin overlying the membrane can be anesthetized with lidocaine.

The thumb and middle finger of the operator's nondominant hand hold the trachea in place and provide skin tension as the index finger is used to palpate the cricothyroid membrane (Fig. 18.7A). A small syringe (generally 3 or 5 mL) containing 2 to 3 mL of saline or lidocaine attached to the needle or catheter is held in the dominant hand. The needle is placed in the midline of the neck at the inferior margin of the cricothyroid membrane (to avoid the usual position of the cricothyroid arteries) and directed caudally at an angle of 30 to 45 degrees. The skin and subcutaneous tissue are then punctured with the needle. The operator may choose to first make a small nick in the skin with a scalpel blade to facilitate insertion of the needle (18). While applying continuous negative pressure on the syringe, the operator advances the needle through the membrane until air bubbles are seen in the syringe, confirming intratracheal placement.

Capnography (monitoring of CO_2 level) during needle advancement into the trachea can serve as an additional safety measure to ensure the intratracheal location of the needle or catheter (see also Chapter 76). This can be done by interposing a stopcock between the needle and syringe. The stopcock is left open in all three directions, and the side port is attached to small-bore tubing connected to the capnometer (46). The catheter is then advanced forward off the needle until its hub rests at the skin surface. The needle and syringe are then removed (Fig. 18.7B). To reduce the likelihood of causing subcutaneous emphysema, the operator (or an assistant) should hold the catheter firmly in place at all times until it can be secured with a suture. The high-pressure

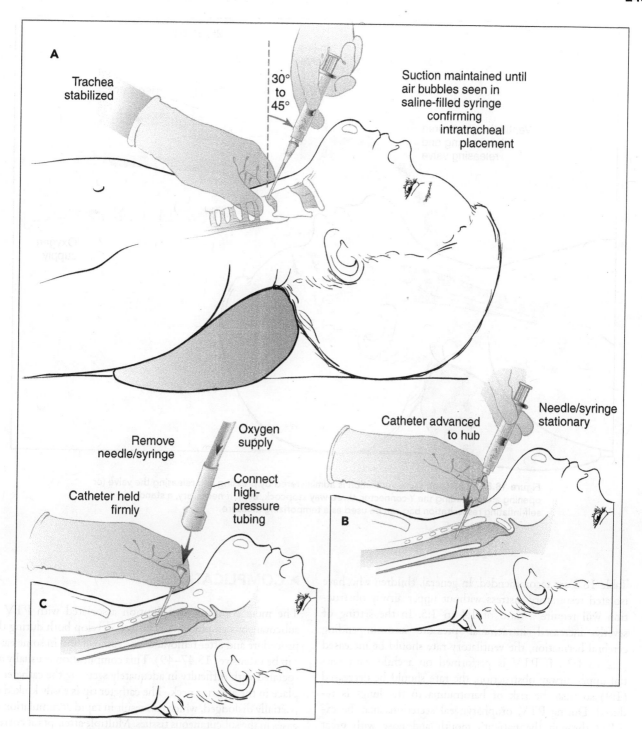

Figure 18.7 Performing PTV.
A. The needle is angled caudally at 30 to 45 degrees and inserted through the cricothyroid membrane until bubbles are seen in the fluid-filled syringe, indicating puncture of the trachea.
B. The catheter is advanced to the hub as the needle and syringe are removed.
C. The catheter is secured in place and connected to the oxygen delivery system.

tubing and 100% oxygen source are then connected to the catheter (Fig. 18.7C), and a few short bursts of gas are delivered, both to reconfirm placement and ensure that the equipment is functioning properly. At this point, the patient can be ventilated by opening and closing the in-line valve apparatus, if such a system is used, or by intermit-

tently occluding the side port, Y-connector, or stopcock (Fig. 18.8).

To date, no controlled studies have been performed to determine the optimal I:E (inspiratory to expiratory) ratio for children when performing PTV. Based on published experience in the available literature, the ratios listed in

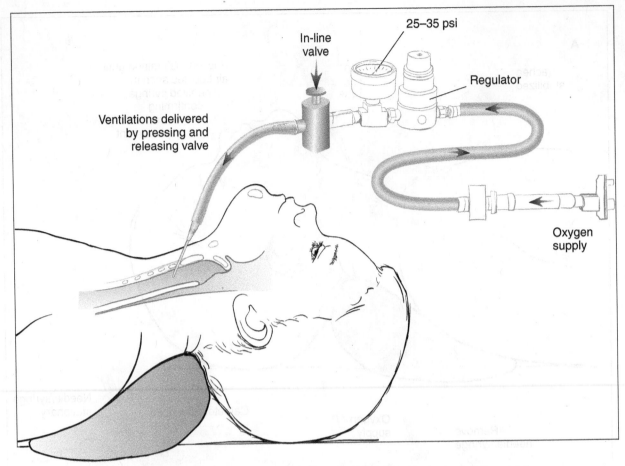

Figure 18.8 Positive pressure ventilation is administered by pressing and releasing the valve (or opening and occluding the Y-connector, three-way stopcock, etc.). If necessary, a standard self-inflating resuscitation bag can be used as a temporizing measure.

Table 18.2 are recommended. In general, children who have isolated respiratory distress without upper airway obstruction will require a ratio of 1:4 to 1:5. In the setting of severly increased intracranial pressure and impending cerebral herniation, the ventilatory rate should be increased (1:2 to 1:3). If PTV is performed on a child with partial upper airway obstruction, the rate should be decreased (1:9) so that the risk of barotrauma to the lungs is reduced. During PTV, oropharyngeal secretions may be expelled through the patient's mouth and nose with great force. Operators should stand clear and observe universal precautions.

TABLE 18.2	RECOMMENDED I:E RATIOS FOR PTV
Standard	1:4 to 1:5
Cerebral herniation	1:2
Airway obstruction	1:9

▶ COMPLICATIONS

The most common complication associated with PTV is subcutaneous emphysema. This can develop both during the procedure and after removal of the catheter and in some cases can be extensive (18,47–49). This complication is usually associated with difficulty in adequately securing the catheter in place in the anterior neck. The catheter tip is easily kinked or partially dislodged, which can result in rapid accumulation of gases in the subcutaneous tissues. Multiple attempts at correct placement of the catheter can also result in localized subcutaneous emphysema as gas escapes through previous puncture sites and enters the soft tissue (48). The likelihood of subcutaneous emphysema can be reduced by (a) using kink-resistant Teflon catheters, (b) assigning one individual to be responsible for holding the catheter hub in place at all times, (c) using one of the commercially available PTV catheters with attached flanges for securing the catheter, and (d) minimizing attempts at catheter placement. On removal of the catheter, a fingertip should be placed firmly over the puncture site and held for a few minutes to prevent air entry into the subcutaneous tissue.

Allowing insufficient time for passive exhalation (i.e., a ventilatory rate that is too rapid) can lead to barotrauma to the lungs, with resulting pneumomediastinum and pneumothorax (14,22,27,37,48,49). This is more likely if PTV is performed when complete upper airway obstruction is present. Although there have been no reports of perforation of the posterior trachea, this complication would seem more likely with children, resulting from increased compliance of the tracheal cartilages, and should be carefully avoided.

Other reported complications associated with using PTV include minor bleeding from arterial perforation, pneumatocele formation, prevertebral cellulitis and cervical osteomyelitis, and fire in conjunction with electrocautery use (50–52). It is important to remember that PTV does not provide complete control of the airway, and therefore aspiration is still a possibility. However, at least one animal study has suggested that PTV may provide some protection from aspiration (53).

CLINICAL TIPS

▸ The laryngeal prominence does not fully develop until adolescence; the important landmarks are the hyoid bone and cricoid cartilage in young children.

▸ If the cricothyroid membrane cannot be located, the catheter may be safely inserted in a lower intercartilaginous tracheal space.

▸ The cricothyroid membrane should be punctured in the lower third to avoid the cricothyroid vessels.

▸ One person should be assigned to hold the hub of catheter in place until it is secured in order to prevent subcutaneous emphysema.

▸ Regular performance of "mock resuscitation" scenarios using the equipment will increase the likelihood of successful performance of the technique in emergency situations.

SUMMARY

1 Attach a 3- to 5-mL syringe with a few milliliters of saline or lidocaine to the needle and catheter.

2 Locate the cricothyroid membrane, bound by the thyroid cartilage superiorly and the cricoid cartilage inferiorly.

3 Hold the trachea in place and provide skin tension with the thumb and middle finger of the nondominant hand.

4 Place the tip of needle at the inferior midline of membrane, directing the needle caudally at a 30- to 45-degree angle.

5 Advance the needle while pulling back on the plunger of the syringe. The appearance of air bubbles within the syringe confirms intratracheal placement.

6 Slide the catheter over the needle until the hub rests securely on the skin surface.

7 Remove the needle and the syringe as a unit.

8 Connect high-pressure tubing and an oxygen source to the catheter.

9 Confirm correct placement with a few short bursts of oxygen.

10 Ventilate at the appropriate rate by opening and closing the permanent valve or occluding the side port, stopcock, or Y-connector.

11 Assess patient response.

12 Suture the catheter securely in place.

▸ SUMMARY

Percutaneous transtracheal ventilation is an underutilized technique for the management of the difficult pediatric airway. The indications for PTV are essentially the same as for surgical cricothyrotomy, although cricothyrotomy remains the procedure of choice for establishing a surgical airway with older children and adults in the setting of complete airway obstruction. PTV requires no special surgical skills and can be initiated within a matter of moments. Familiarity with alternative methods of airway management such as PTV can often provide the temporary respiratory support needed for a critically ill child until more definitive measures can be performed.

▸ ACKNOWLEDGMENT

The authors would like to acknowledge the valuable contributions of Russell H. Greenfield to the version of this chapter that appeared in the previous edition.

▸ REFERENCES

1. Jacoby JJ, Hamelberg W, Reed JP, et al. A simple technique for artificial respiration. *Am J Physiol.* 1951;167:798–799.
2. Reed JP, Kemph JP, Hamelberg W, et al. Studies with transtracheal artificial respiration. *Anesthesiology.* 1954;15:28–41.
3. Spoerel WE, Narayanan PS, Singh NP. Transtracheal ventilation. *Br J Anaesth.* 1971;43:932–939.
4. Jacobs HB. Emergency percutaneous transtracheal catheter and ventilator. *J Trauma.* 1972;12:50–55.
5. Slutsky AS, Watson J, Leith DE, et al. Tracheal insufflation of O_2 (TRIO) at low flow rates sustains life for several hours. *Anesthesiology.* 1985;63:278–286.

6. Smith RB, Myers N, Sherman H. Transtracheal ventilation in paediatric patients: case reports. *Br J Anaesth.* 1974;46:313–314.

7. Ravussin P, Bayer-Berger M, Monnier P, et al. Percutaneous transtracheal ventilation for laser endoscopic procedures infants and small children with laryngeal obstruction: report of two cases. *Can J Anaesth.* 1987;34:83–86.

8. Percutaneous translaryngeal jet ventilation (needle cricothyrotomy). In: Roberts JR, Hedges JR, eds. *Clinical Procedures in Emergency Medicine.* Philadelphia: WB Saunders; 2004:125–132.

9. Bennett JD, Guha SC, Sankar AB. Cricothyrotomy: the anatomical basis. *J R Coll Surg Edinb.* 1996;41:57–60.

10. Little CM, Parker MG, Tarnopolsky R. The incidence of vasculature at risk during cricothyroidostomy. *Ann Emerg Med.* 1986;15:805–807.

11. Yealy DM, Plewa MC, Stewart RD. An evaluation of cannulae and oxygen sources for pediatric jet ventilation. *Am J Emerg Med.* 1991;9:20–23.

12. Jacobs HB, Smyth NPD, Witorsch P. Transtracheal catheter ventilation: clinical experience in 36 patients. *Chest.* 1974;65:36–40.

13. Wagner DJ, Coombs DW, Doyle SC. Percutaneous transtracheal ventilation for emergency dental appliance removal. *Anesthesiology.* 1985;62:664–666.

14. Ward KR, Menegazzi JJ, Yealy DM, et al. Translaryngeal jet ventilation and end-tidal pCO$_2$ monitoring during varying degrees of upper airway obstruction. *Ann Emerg Med.* 1991;20:1193–1197.

15. Yealy DM, Stewart RD, Kaplan RM. Clarifications on translaryngeal ventilation [letter]. *Ann Emerg Med.* 1988;17:1130.

16. Marr JK, Yamamoto LG. Gas flow rates through transtracheal ventilation catheters. *Am J Emerg Med.* 2004;22:264–266.

17. Zornow MH, Thomas TC, Scheller MS. The efficacy of three different methods of transtracheal ventilation. *Can J Anaesth.* 1989;36:624–628.

18. Stewart RD. Manual translaryngeal jet ventilation. *Emerg Med Clin North Am.* 1989;7:155–164.

19. Tran TP, Rhee KJ, Schultz HD, et al. Gas exchange and lung mechanics during percutaneous transtracheal ventilation in an unparalyzed canine model. *Acad Emerg Med.* 1998;5:320–324.

20. Cote CJ, Eavey RD, Todres ID, et al. Cricothyroid membrane puncture: oxygenation and ventilation in a dog model using an intravenous catheter. *Crit Care Med.* 1988;16:615–619.

21. Goldstein B, Shannon DC, Todres ID. Supercarbia in children: clinical course and outcome. *Crit Care Med.* 1990;18:166–168.

22. Levinson MM, Scuderi PE, Gibson RL, et al. Emergency percutaneous transtracheal ventilation. *JACEP.* 1979;8:396–400.

23. Konrad B, Siedlecki K, Bosch S, et al. Asphyxiation by laryngeal edema in patients with hereditary angioedema. *Mayo Clin Proc.* 2000;75:349–354.

24. Hinze JD, Barker JA, Jones TR, et al. Life-threatening upper airway edema caused by a distal rattlesnake bite. *Ann Emerg Med.* 2001;38:79–82.

25. Benumof JL, Scheller MS. The importance of transtracheal jet ventilation in the management of the difficult airway. *Anesthesiology.* 1989;71:769–778.

26. Weymuller EA, Paugh D, Pavlin EG, et al. Management of difficult airway problems with percutaneous transtracheal ventilation. *Ann Otol Rhinol Laryngol.* 1987;96:34–37.

27. Jorden RC, Moore EE, Marx JA, et al. A comparison of PTV and endotracheal ventilation in an acute trauma model. *J Trauma.* 1985;25:978–983.

28. Frame SB, Simon JM, Kerstein MD, et al. Percutaneous transtracheal catheter ventilation (PTCV) in complete airway obstruction: a canine model. *J Trauma.* 1989;29:774–781.

29. Neff CC, Pfister RC, van Sonnenberg E. Percutaneous transtracheal ventilation: experimental and practical aspects. *J Trauma.* 1983;23:84–90.

30. Stothert JC, Stout MJ, Lewis LM, et al. High pressure percutaneous transtracheal ventilation: the use of large gauge intravenous-type catheters in the totally obstructed airway. *Am J Emerg Med.* 1990;8:184–189.

31. Campbell CT, Harris RC, Cook MH, et al. A new device for emergency percutaneous transtracheal ventilation in partial and complete airway obstruction. *Ann Emerg Med.* 1988;17:927–931.

32. Frame SB, Timberlake GA, Kerstein MD, et al. Transtracheal needle catheter ventilation in complete airway obstruction: an animal model. *Ann Emerg Med.* 1989;18:127–133.

33. Zucker-Pinchoff B, Ramani T. A simple device for transtracheal ventilation. *J Clin Anesth.* 1992;4:342–343.

34. Delaney WA, Kaiser RE. Percutaneous transtracheal jet ventilation made easy. *Anesthesiology.* 1991;74:952.

35. Scuderi PE, McLeskey CH, Comer PB. Emergency percutaneous transtracheal ventilation during anesthesia using readily available equipment. *Anesth Analg.* 1982;61:867–870.

36. Patel R. Systems for transtracheal ventilation. *Anesthesiology.* 1983;59:165.

37. Attia RR, Battit GE, Murphy JD. Transtracheal ventilation. *JAMA.* 1975;234:1152–1153.

38. Gildar JS. A simple system for transtracheal ventilation. *Anesthesiology.* 1983;58:106.

39. Aye LS. Percutaneous transtracheal ventilation. *Anesth Analg.* 1983;62:619.

40. Yealy DM, Stewart RD, Kaplan RM. Myths and pitfalls in emergency translaryngeal ventilation: correcting misimpressions. *Ann Emerg Med.* 1988;17:690–692.

41. Hauswald M, Ong G, Yeoh E. Percutaneous needle cricothyroidotomy with repetitive airway obstruction. *Am J Emerg Med.* 1995;13:623–625.

42. Craven RM, Vanner RG. Ventilation of a model lung using various cricothyrotomy devices. *Anaesthesia.* 2004;59:595–599.

43. Chan TC, Bramwell KJ, Davis DP, et al. Comparison of wire-guided cricothyrotomy versus standard surgical cricothyrotomy technique. *J Emerg Med.* 1999;17:957–962.

44. Policy statement. Care of children in the emergency department: guidelines for preparedness. *Ann Emerg Med.* 2001;37:423–427.

45. Hockberger RS, Binder LS, Graber MA, et al. The model of the clinical practice of emergency medicine. *Ann Emerg Med.* 2001;37:745–770.

46. Tobias J, Higgins M. Capnography during transtracheal needle cricothyrotomy. *Anesth Analg.* 1995;81:1077–1078.

47. Koch E, Benumof JL. Percutaneous transtracheal jet ventilation: an important airway adjunct. *AANA J.* 1990;58:337–339.

48. Jorden RC. Percutaneous transtracheal ventilation. *Emerg Med Clin North Am.* 1988;6:745–752.

49. Craig DB. Transtracheal ventilation [letter]. *JAMA.* 1976;235:2082.

50. Carden E, Calcaterra TC, Lechtman A. Pneumatocele of the larynx: a complication of percutaneous transtracheal ventilation. *Anesth Analg.* 1976;55:600–601.

51. Newlands SD, Makielski KH. Cervical osteomyelitis after percutaneous transtracheal ventilation and tracheotomy. *Head Neck.* 1996;18:295–298.

52. Bowdle TA, Glenn M, Colston L, et al. Fire following use of electrocautery during emergency percutaneous transtracheal ventilation. *Anesthesiology.* 1987;66:697–698.

53. Yealy DM, Plewa MC, Reed JJ, et al. Manual translaryngeal jet ventilation and the risk of aspiration in a canine model. *Ann Emerg Med.* 1990;19:1238–1241.

JANE M. LAVELLE AND ANDREW T. COSTARINO

19

Central Venous Cannulation

▶ INTRODUCTION

Central venous cannulation (CVC) involves percutaneous placement of a vascular catheter so that its tip is within the lumen of a major, high-flow vein of the abdomen or thorax. CVC is a crucial skill for any clinician who regularly participates in resuscitation and stabilization of critically ill infants and children in an emergency department (ED).

Placing a catheter into the central circulation became a theoretical possibility once Harvey made the revolutionary discovery of the circulation and function of the heart in 1628. Development of vascular access came as the result of the need to understand the clinical function of the circulation and the need to administer intravenous fluids, blood products, and medications. The first record of central venous catheterization was made in England by Stephen Hales in 1733. As part of his investigation of the circulation, he inserted a glass tube into the jugular vein of a horse to measure the central venous pressure. Later the value of intravenous fluid administration was recognized. In 1833, W. B. O'Shaughnessy described the treatment of cholera victims to replace the lost "neutral saline ingredients" of serum. Intravenous saline solutions were first used to treat shock associated with surgery by Rudolph Matas in 1891. Following the identification of the blood types by Landsteiner in 1901 and the development of a method to prevent coagulation in stored blood in 1914, blood transfusion became another important clinical application of intravenous infusion therapy. By the mid-1900s, intravenous fluids, blood products, and medications were a regular part of clinical practice.

When Seldinger described a practical technique for percutaneous entry to central vessels in 1953, the stage was set for CVC to become a standard therapeutic option. By the late 1960s, CVC use had gained widespread clinical acceptance. Today CVC is performed for a broad range of clinical purposes in adults and children of all ages (1,2). Percutaneous

CVC is often employed as an emergency procedure during initial patient stabilization, but it is also used as a definitive procedure for long-term patient management. This chapter reviews percutaneous CVC using the Seldinger method and similar techniques via the femoral, brachial, jugular, and subclavian veins as well as the basilic and median veins of the forearm.

▶ ANATOMY AND PHYSIOLOGY

General Anatomic Considerations

Major sites for percutaneous cannulation of the central veins include the internal and external jugular veins as well as the brachial, subclavian, and femoral veins. Figure 19.1 shows these vessels and their relation to the abdominal and thoracic vena cava and the heart. While vascular anatomy is similar in all age groups, some subtle and important differences exist, particularly in young infants. General differences, including small body size, tissue softness, and compressibility (particularly of the chest), make the body surface landmarks used in locating deep veins less apparent and more easily distorted in younger patients.

More specific considerations also exist for some of the common CVC sites. For example, in infants less than 1 year of age, anatomic factors make subclavian vein entry less attractive than entry at other sites. In this age group, the subclavian vein arches more superiorly as it courses toward the atrium, resulting in acute angles that may obstruct catheter placement. The subclavian arch takes on the more typical horizontal position within the chest only after 1 year of age. Additionally, in young infants, the notch on the inferior aspect of the first rib, a landmark commonly employed to identify the percutaneous entry site for the subclavian vein, is difficult to identify. Finally, the diameter of the subclavian vein is smaller than that of the

247

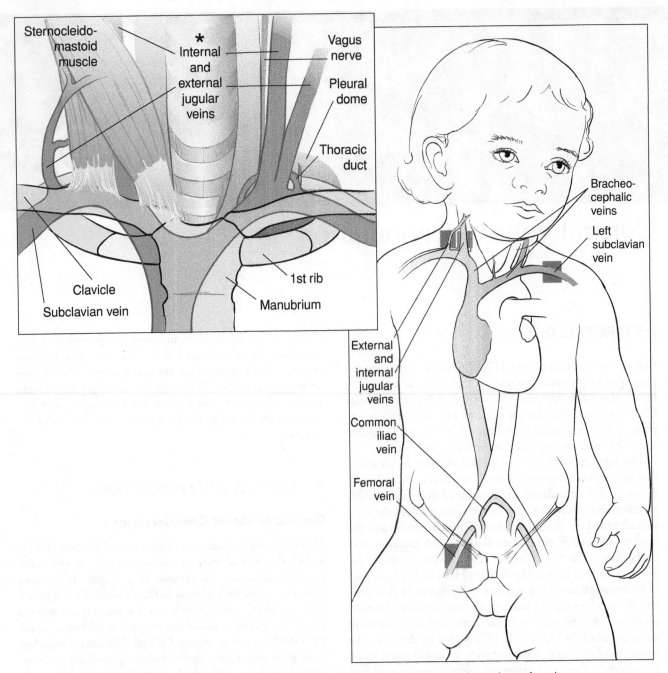

Figure 19.1 Anatomy of the central venous circulation. The shaded areas indicate the preferred sites for cannulation.

internal jugular vein in this population, and for this reason many clinicians prefer the jugular site (3–6).

A general anatomic consideration for both children and adults relates to the choice of the internal jugular vein (IJV) or subclavian vein (SV) for catheter placement: these vessels are more easily cannulated on the right side rather than the left. On the right, the IJV assumes a straight course and joins the right SV to form the brachiocephalic (or innominate), which continues on into the superior vena cava (SVC). The left IJV joins the SV at a more acute angle; moreover, the left brachiocephalic forms a sharp angle with the superior

vena cava. Adding to the difficulties associated with left side approaches are problems that arise due to the lymphatic communications with these veins. The larger left thoracic duct enters the left SV at its junction with the IJV. The right lymphatic duct is a much smaller structure and frequently is congenitally absent. Finally, the left pleural dome is higher than the right, increasing the likelihood of a pneumothorax during the procedure. Although specific clinical situations such as right-sided neck or chest trauma may preclude use of the right-sided vessels, they are preferred whenever possible (3–6).

Anatomy of Specific Sites

Femoral Vein

The femoral vein (FV) travels superficially in the anterior thigh, then passes beneath the inguinal ligament, coursing deep into the pelvis to become the external iliac vein. In the proximal thigh (distal to the inguinal ligament), the FV lies within the femoral sheath, where it is medial to the femoral artery, which in turn is medial to the femoral nerve. The mnemonic NAVL (pronounced "navel") is often used to remember this orientation from lateral to medial: nerve, artery, vein, lymphatic. Thus, the FV can be identified 1 to 2 cm medial to the femoral artery pulse when palpated 1 to 2 cm below the inguinal ligament (4).

Jugular Veins

Internal Jugular Vein

The IJV exits the skull via the jugular foramina and follows a relatively straight course through the neck before emptying into the SV. As mentioned, the right IJV joins the right SV just lateral to the sternoclavicular joint, forming the brachiocephalic (innominate) vein, which continues on in a straight path to the SVC. On the left side, the IJV joins the SV vein at an almost perpendicular angle. Similarly, the left innominate then joins the SVC at a sharp angle (see Fig. 19.1). As the IJV moves caudal in the neck, it becomes more superficial and larger in diameter.

In the cephalad portion of its course on either side of the neck, the IJV is medial to the sternal (medial) head of the sternocleidomastoid muscles. In the midportion of the neck, it is located beneath the line that bisects the angle formed by the sternal and clavicular (lateral) heads of the sternocleidomastoid. In the caudad portion of the neck, it lies just medial to (or sometimes beneath) the clavicular head of the sternocleidomastoid.

Other important structures are in close proximity to the IJV. Within the carotid sheaths, the carotid arteries are medial, posterior and deep to the vein, while the vagus nerve is between the carotid artery and IJV. The cervical sympathetic chain and stellate ganglion are deep and medial to the IJV, and the brachial plexus is found deep to all these structures. The phrenic nerve is lateral and the laryngeal nerve is medial to the carotid-jugular vascular bundle. Lymphatic ducts enter the SV near the junction of the IJV with the SV. The right IJV is preferred for cannulation whenever possible (5,7–9) for the reasons mentioned previously.

External Jugular Vein

The external jugular vein (EJV) drains the structures of the exterior of the cranium and the deep face. It begins within the parotid gland at the level of the angle of the mandible and travels obliquely across the sternocleidomastoid muscle from the angle of the mandible to the middle of the clavicle. Below the clavicle at the level of the posterior border of the sternocleidomastoid muscle, the EJV empties into the subclavian vein at virtually a right angle (5,7–9).

Subclavian Vein

The SV arises from the axillary vein as it passes over the first rib. It continues superiorly, passing anterior to the scalenus anterior muscle, before descending slightly as it joins the IJV to form the brachiocephalic vein behind the sternoclavicular joint. The brachiocephalic vein then empties into the SVC. The SV lies anterior to the subclavian artery and the brachial plexus; it is separated from these structures by the thin scalenus anterior muscle. Ventral to the scalenus anterior muscle at this point, the thoracic duct crosses to terminate at the junction of the IJV and the SV. As with the IJV, the right-sided SV is preferred for cannulation for the reasons listed previously (6,10).

Veins of the Forearm

The superficial veins of the forearm are increasingly being used to access the central venous system (Fig. 19.2). The basilic vein, which is used most commonly for this purpose, arises from the ulnar (medial) side of the dorsal venous network of the hand. The network drainage then curves around the medial side of the forearm, joining to form the large basilic vein. The cephalic vein arises on the radial (lateral) border of the dorsal venous drainage of the hand. It passes upward anterior to the elbow along the lateral side of the arm and empties into the upper part of the axillary vein. The basilic vein communicates with the cephalic vein via the median cubital vein. Proximal to the elbow, the basilic vein passes more deeply up the medial side of the arm to join the axillary vein. In most cases, advancing a catheter from the superficial veins of the forearm into the SV or SVC requires passage through the basilic vein rather than the cephalic vein, because the cephalic system is usually too tortuous at the upper shoulder and has a narrow and acute junction with the axillary vein and SVC in the anterior chest.

▶ INDICATIONS

General Considerations

CVC in children is almost always performed by a physician, usually an emergency medicine specialist, intensivist, anesthesiologist, radiologist, or surgeon. The operator should be skilled in the technique and familiar with the indications, anatomy, and potential complications of the procedure so that the balance of benefit versus risk can be appropriately judged. As shown in Table 19.1, indications for percutaneous CVC include (a) the need to obtain access to the vascular space in patients with circulatory failure when vasoconstriction, vascular depletion, or other factors preclude access via superficial veins; (b) providing a means for placement of other devices such as a Swan-Ganz catheter or transvenous pacemaker; (c) the administration of vasoactive substances,

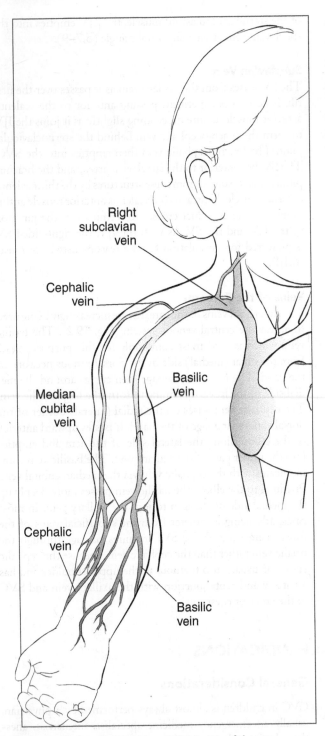

Figure 19.2 Anatomy of the superficial veins of the arm.

TABLE 19.1	INDICATIONS FOR CENTRAL VENOUS CANNULATION

Administration of fluids or medications to treat circulatory failure
Administration of vasoactive medications
Administration of hypertonic fluids (TPN, chemotherapy, etc.)
Measurement of venous vascular pressures
Measurement of mixed venous blood gases
Access for Swan-Ganz catheter or pacemaker placement
Long-term vascular access

administration of medications that may injure a peripheral vein or for repeated blood sampling.

The only absolute contraindications for this procedure are vascular disease in the involved extremity and congenital or acquired vascular abnormality. Relative contraindications include acute inflammation or injury to the skin over the planned entry site and the presence of a hypercoagulable state or bleeding diathesis. Relative contraindications for specific anatomic sites are described below.

Site-Specific Considerations

Femoral Vein
The femoral site has become the first choice for emergent CVC in children for several reasons. First, access at the femoral site does not interfere with airway management or chest compressions. It also has clearly identifiable anatomic landmarks and can be easily compressed to stop bleeding. Unlike the cervical and thoracic sites, where pneumothorax and other serious acute complications can occur, the femoral site is relatively free of such hazards (4,10–12). Relative contraindications for CVC at the femoral site include abnormal vascular status of the lower extremity, congenital malformation of the lower extremity, femoral hernia, abdominal tumor or trauma, abdominal ascites, and anticipated cardiac catheterization.

Jugular Veins
General patient care, movement, and entry site dressing care are less problematic if the catheter is not near an extremity. In addition, an entry site for a central venous cannula near the chest ensures that the tip will lie within the thorax, allowing for accurate central venous pressure measurement should this prove necessary. These are the primary advantages that have made the neck and upper chest entry sites popular for CVC, especially in adult patients.

Internal Jugular Vein
The anatomic landmarks for CVC using the IJV are similar in infants, small children, and adolescents. Compared to the EJV, this site has a much higher rate of success for accessing the central circulation. Compared to the SV, the IJV approach has a lower risk of causing pneumothorax but has a higher risk of inadvertent puncture of the carotid artery or stellate ganglion. The proximity of the IJV to the carotid artery and other

thrombogenic therapies, or other medications in order to allow more rapid distribution and onset of these therapies; (d) providing a means for safe administration of hypertonic fluids or highly concentrated medications into a large-volume, high-flow body space; (e) assessment of cardiac function and tissue oxygen delivery through central venous pressure measurement and/or mixed venous blood gas measurement; and (f) providing long-term access to the circulation for repeated

important structures make this site relatively contraindicated in children with a coagulopathy (5).

External Jugular Vein

The EJV is occasionally used for access to the central circulation but is more commonly used for peripheral access. The primary advantage of this site is that the vessel is located superficially, which reduces the likelihood of pneumothorax, carotid puncture, or injury to the sympathetic chain. The major disadvantage of the EJV is that successful CVC occurs significantly less frequently than with the other sites. Difficulty in passing catheters into the superior vena cava from an EJV entry site is due to the sharp turn made by the vein as it courses under the clavicle and to its virtually perpendicular angle of entry into the SV (5).

Subclavian Vein

The SV is the least common site used for percutaneous CVC in children. As mentioned previously, specific anatomic characteristics of infants and children make this approach disadvantageous, which is the reason the site is usually avoided. The size and softness of the chest and clavicles make the landmarks for CVC at the SV site more difficult to identify, and the curvature of the anterior chest in the infant reduces the space available for entering the vein without puncturing the lung or artery. Skill and experience are required to perform this procedure without complications.

As with jugular venous cannulation, the right-sided SV cannulation is favored over the left due primarily to anatomic considerations. The cupola of the lung, which lies inferior to the junction of the IJV and SV and posterior to the subclavian artery, is higher in relation to these vascular structures on the left side as compared with the right. Additionally, the left thoracic duct is large and may be injured during cannulation. Finally, the acute angle of entry by the left-sided subclavian/innominate into the SVC places the patient at greater risk for intimal damage and vascular perforation (6).

Veins of the Forearm

The basilic or medial veins of the forearm are the sites commonly chosen for so-called peripherally inserted central catheters (often referred to as "PICC lines"). These catheters enter the skin at a peripheral site and are then advanced through the vessel so that the tip of the catheter lies in a large central vein. The advantages of a PICC include (a) there is a reduced incidence of infection compared with a catheter that directly enters a central vessel, and (b) there is a lower risk of vascular injury, arterial puncture, and other complications (e.g., pneumothorax) during placement. The disadvantages compared with direct central venous placement include (a) limited sites exist that provide for successful entry to the central circulation; (b) PICC lines are smaller caliber and are usually limited to single- or double-lumen catheters; and (c) peripheral entry also means longer catheter length, which, combined with the smaller caliber, greatly increases resistance to flow. Consequently, PICC placement is not the method of choice for rapid volume resuscitation. As mentioned previously, advancing a PICC into the SV or SVC is less likely to be successful via the lateral cephalic system because the vessels are tortuous at the shoulder and have a narrow caliber and acute angle of entry at the junction with the SV in the chest. Other sites of entry in the neck and leg have been used but pose greater difficulty in advancing the catheter to a large central vein. Additionally, as the site of skin entry moves closer to the point of entry of the catheter tip into the central circulation, many of the advantages of the PICC technique are lost, and a more traditional method of CVC often becomes a better choice.

▶ EQUIPMENT

As shown in Table 19.2, the equipment necessary for performing CVC can be grouped in four general categories: (a) equipment necessary for establishing an aseptic field and maintenance of sterile technique during the procedure; (b) the various catheters, needles, and wires, along with any other equipment needed for placing, securing, and dressing the catheter; (c) monitoring and other equipment necessary to ensure patient safety during the procedure and after the catheter is in place (see Chapter 5); and (d) medications and other equipment necessary to ensure patient comfort and cooperation during the procedure (see Chapter 33).

Ensuring that all the proper equipment for CVC is available is now relatively easy because of the many commercially produced kits available (e.g., Cooke, Abbott, Arrow, and Viggo-Spectramed) (Fig. 19.3). These kits contain most of the equipment included in the first two categories, including antiseptic solution and drapes. Organizing any additional

TABLE 19.2	EQUIPMENT CHECKLIST

I. Aseptic technique
    Povidone-iodine or chlorhexidine solution
    Sterile 4″ × 4″ gauze
    Sterile towels, drapes
    Sterile gloves
    Sterile gowns, masks
II. Catheter kit, suturing material
    Intravascular catheters (have an extra on hand)
    Finder needle (usually 20–22 gauge, 1.5 inches)
    Flexible guidewire (straight or J-tip; make sure it fits the catheter)
    Heparinized saline solution
    Syringes, 3 or 5 mL
    Silk suture (3.0 or 4.0)
    Needle holder
III. Monitoring and other equipment
    Pulse oximeter
    Cardiac monitor
    Blood pressure monitor
    Capnometer
    Handheld ultrasound device
IV. Medications
    Lidocaine 1% (without epinephrine)
    Midazolam 0.1 mg/kg
    Morphine sulfate 0.1 to 0.15 mg/kg

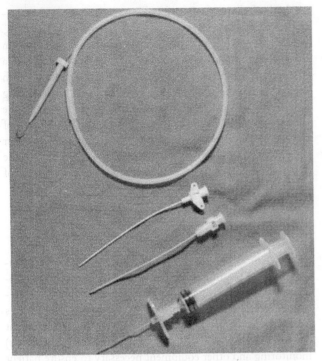

Figure 19.3 Items in a commercially produced pediatric central venous catheter tray (available from various manufacturers).

desired ancillary equipment into prepackaged trays or packets for performing CVC will also improve efficiency and reduce the likelihood of errors.

Types of Catheters

The two catheter types used most commonly reflect the two most popular methods of percutaneous CVC, one involving passage of the catheter over a guidewire (Seldinger technique) and the other involving passage of the catheter through an introducer (PICC technique). A third type, the "catheter-over-the-needle" system commonly employed for superficial venous access (Fig. 19.4), is often included in central venous access kits. These catheters are sometimes used to begin the process but are not the primary tool for performing CVC.

Seldinger Technique

The most popular method for CVC in both children and adults is the Seldinger technique (Fig. 19.5). Described by Sven Ivar Seldinger in 1953 for placement of vascular catheters, this technique has been so successful that its basic principles have now been extended to other procedures, such as emergency tracheostomy placement and nonoperative gastrostomy tube placement. It utilizes a small-gauge entry needle, which punctures the skin and enters the blood vessel lumen. A guidewire is threaded through the entry needle into the blood vessel, and the entry needle is removed while the wire is left in place. A larger-caliber vascular catheter is then advanced over the wire into the blood vessel. The entire procedure may be repeated with increasing sizes of wires and catheters to achieve the desired catheter size, even when starting with a small entry needle.

The guidewires used for the Seldinger technique have both a flexible end and a rigid end. The flexible tip is designed to enter a blood vessel and negotiate its twists and turns while minimizing the likelihood of puncturing the vessel wall. Often the tip is made in a J configuration (Fig. 19.3) and comes with a plastic sleeve used to straighten the J while threading the wire into the entry needle hub. J-wires are particularly useful for situations in which acute angles or sharp turns are encountered within the cannulated blood vessel (see the external jugular

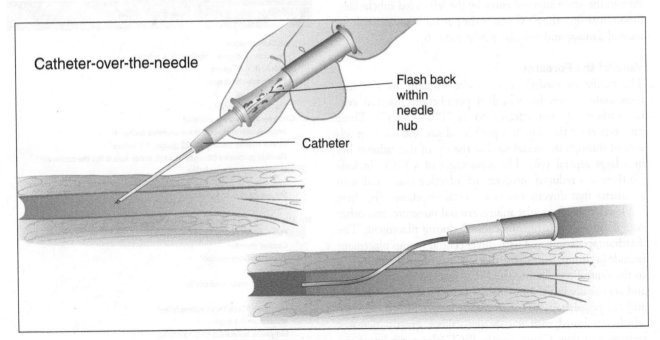

Figure 19.4 Catheter-over-the-needle technique.

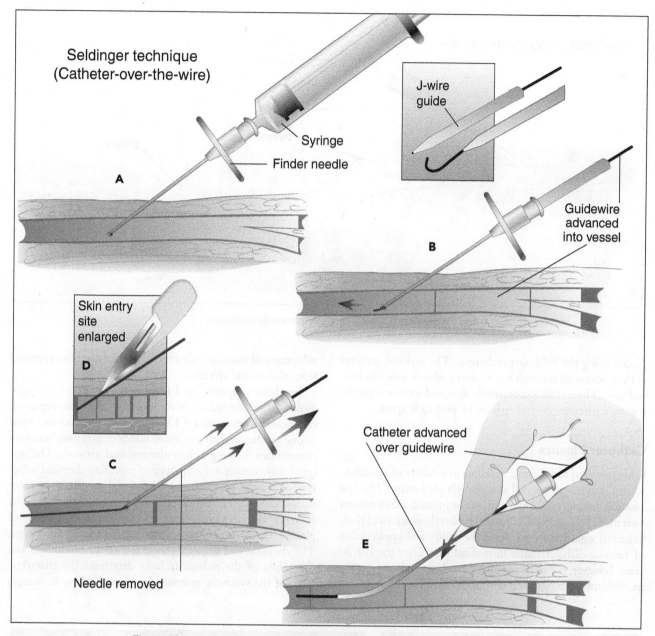

Figure 19.5 Catheter-over-the-wire (Seldinger) technique.
A. The central vein is first punctured using a needle and syringe.
B. The syringe is removed and the guidewire is inserted through the needle into the vein.
C. The needle is removed and the wire is left in place.
D. A small incision is made at the entry site to facilitate insertion of the catheter.
E. The catheter is inserted over the guidewire and the wire is removed.

vein approach below). The rigid end of the wire is designed to facilitate threading of the stiff catheter over the guidewire.

Peripherally Inserted Central Catheter

The introducer technique for inserting a catheter is most commonly employed in the placement of PICC lines. The skin is punctured with a relatively large hollow needle, and after blood return is observed, a catheter is then passed through the needle lumen and advanced into the vein. The needle is removed from the skin once the catheter is in the proper position. In older systems using this technique, the needle remained in place surrounding the catheter, often housed in a plastic shield to prevent it from injuring the patient or cutting the catheter wall (Fig. 19.6). More recently, this technique employs needles that can be peeled apart and completely removed from the catheter (Fig. 19.7). In the various kits for this method, the catheter usually contains a wire stylet that provides added rigidity to facilitate advancement within the lumen of the vein. The stylet is then removed before the catheter is used. In a common variation of this method, a soft, short introducer catheter is first

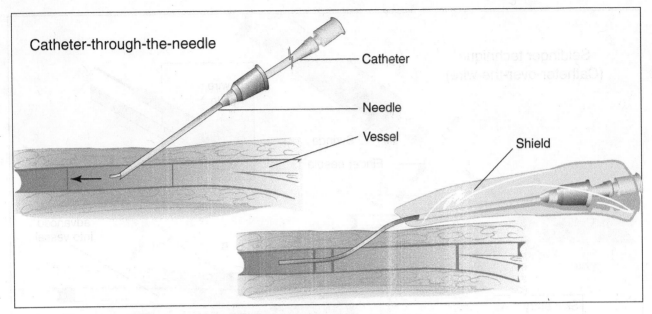

Figure 19.6   Catheter-through-the-needle technique.

placed using the Seldinger technique. The styleted catheter is then advanced through the shorter catheter into the central vein. The introducer is usually designed so that it can be removed from the central catheter by peeling it apart.

Catheter Plastics

Catheters used today for CVC come in a variety of materials, widths, and lengths as well as with multiple lumens. The first vascular catheters used for infusions or pressure measurement were made of glass, steel, or natural rubber; limitations of these materials significantly restricted the utility and applicability of vascular catheterization in medical care. Over the last 30 years, however, the introduction of synthetic polymers in the manufacture of biomedical devices has been crucial in the de-

velopment of vascular catheters that are relatively inexpensive, safe, reliable, and effective.

Synthetic polymers used in biomedical devices are high-molecular-weight materials composed of a simple, repeating chemical unit (monomer) (13). The monomers may be linked to one another in chains of linear bonds or may have branched connections forming a three-dimensional network. The material may contain only one type of repeating chemical structure or may be composed of a combination of two or more chemically different copolymers. The most popular material currently used in vascular catheter manufacture is a family of plastics, the polyurethanes, composed of various copolymers. The chemical and physical properties of the monomers and the nature of the polymeric links determine the characteristics of the synthetic polymer, for example, how it changes

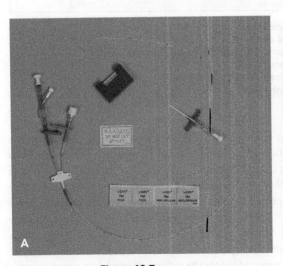
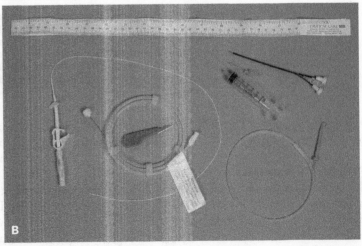

Figure 19.7
A. PICC catheter kit with breakaway butterfly entry catheter.
B. PICC catheter kit with soft peel-away catheter initially placed using the Seldinger technique.

in relation to temperature, how it interacts with the blood and other tissues, and whether it is hard or soft, brittle or flexible, etc. In turn, these features determine how suited the materials are for use in the manufacture of vascular catheters and what specific purposes the resulting catheters can be employed for.

Teflon was the first popular material in the manufacture of central venous catheters. Teflon is strong, which allows for a large internal diameter–external diameter ratio and thus maximal lumen size; this also makes the catheter stiff, for improved percutaneous insertion. In addition, Teflon can be made radiopaque because it can be readily mixed with radiocontrast material. The primary disadvantage of Teflon is that catheters made of this material kink easily (14). In addition, although the surface of Teflon is smooth, which reduces thrombus formation in the lumen or at the tip of the catheter, the stiffness of a Teflon catheter can lead to endothelial injury and vascular mural thrombi.

Polyvinylchloride is another plastic used in many biomedical devices, including vascular catheters. Polyvinylchloride has not remained popular for use in long-term vascular catheters for two reasons. First, the material is associated with high thrombogenicity. Although pulmonary artery (Swan-Ganz) catheters are still often made of polyvinylchloride, they are almost always manufactured with a heparin coating to reduce thrombus formation during the relatively short length of time these catheters are designed to be used. The other problem limiting the use of polyvinylchloride for vascular catheters is that drugs infused through these catheters adsorb to the plastic.

Silicone rubber (Silastic) is polymerized polydimethylsiloxane, which confers a flexible rubberlike quality, mixed with silica powder to increase its hardness. Hickman and later Broviac described techniques for providing long-term vascular access using catheters subcutaneously tunneled proximal to their entry into the vein. This remains the primary use of such catheters today. Silicone is smooth and soft, giving catheters made of this material a remarkable record of low infection and clotting rates and a low incidence of injury to vascular and cardiac structures. However, the softness of silicone catheters means that surgical incision and dissection (15–17) is needed for placement and predisposes them to fracture or rupture. Kits designed to overcome the need for surgical placement and allow percutaneous placement have been designed, but this technique is not practical for emergency catheter placement. The accuracy of vascular pressure measurements obtained through silicone catheters also has been questioned, although published data do not support this contention (18).

In recent years, catheters made of polyurethane have proven to be the most popular. This is because the various polyurethanes currently available provide the best combination of biocompatibility, stiffness (to ease percutaneous placement), softness and smoothness (to reduce vascular injury, thrombosis, and infectious complications), low tendency to kink, the ability to incorporate radiocontrast, and low manufacturing cost (19).

Catheter Diameter and Flow Characteristics

The diameter of vascular catheters are designated in one of two measurement systems: gauge or French. In the French measurement scale, each unit is equivalent to 0.33 mm in outer diameter (OD). For example, a 5 French catheter has an OD of 1.65 mm. The gauge system developed in a more empiric fashion but is now standardized. The ODs in millimeters for commonly used pediatric catheters are as follows: 14 gauge = 2.1 mm, 16 gauge = 1.6 mm, 18 gauge = 1.3 mm, 20 gauge = 1.1 mm, and 22 gauge = 0.7 mm. Guidelines for the selection of catheters based on age, weight, and height are presented in Tables 19.3 and 19.4.

The French or gauge designations always refer to the OD of the catheter, but with the plastics used in the manufacture of catheters today, one can assume that the luminal diameter is about 40% to 50% of the OD. In multiple-lumen catheters, the equivalent OD is often marked on each lumen port. If all ports are of equal size, a reasonable assumption is to divide the diameter by the number of lumens to estimate the size of each lumen.

Catheter diameter and length have a great impact on medical utility. The appeal of central venous cannulae for the treatment of circulatory failure include the ability to (a) bypass local venous constriction present in hypovolemic states, (b) remain relatively unimpeded by patient movement that might otherwise result in altered infusion rates or loss of access, and (c) avoid extravascular infiltration of fluid. It should be remembered, however, that the necessary length and diameter of these catheters may reduce the infusate flow rate. Factors that determine flow rate through a catheter are expressed in Poiseuille's law:

$$\text{Flow rate} = \frac{\pi(P_1 - P_2)}{8vL}$$

where π is the constant Pi, P_1 is the hydrostatic pressure driving the fluid into the catheter, P_2 is hydrostatic pressure in the blood vessel outside the catheter tip, R is the radius of the catheter lumen, v is the viscosity of the infused fluid, and L is the length of the catheter. Flow therefore increases in proportion to the fourth power of the lumen radius but decreases in proportion to the length of the catheter. In addition, the rate of flow is inversely proportional to the viscosity of the fluid, and so saline and other crystalloid solutions will flow more rapidly than blood products. Increasing the hydrostatic pressure driving the fluid into the catheter will increase the flow rate, whereas high vascular hydrostatic pressure outside the tip of the catheter will reduce the flow rate.

Theoretic considerations determined by Poiseuille's law can have important clinical implications. For example, when a 16-gauge catheter (1.6 mm OD) is used rather than a 14-gauge catheter (2.1 mm OD) during a resuscitation, the operator should be aware that while the catheter diameter is only reduced by 24%, the rate of flow will be decreased by 66%, assuming all other factors are constant. Similarly, the number of lumens within a catheter must be considered. A 14-gauge double-lumen catheter with one lumen 16 gauge (1.6 mm)

TABLE 19.3	CATHETER SIZES FOR PEDIATRIC PATIENTS				
			Average Catheter Length (cm)		
Age	Average Weight (kg)	Average Height (cm)	IJ	SC	Fem
1 mo	4.2	55	6.0	5.5	15.7
3 mo	5.8	61	6.6	6.0	17.3
6 mo	7.8	68	7.3	6.6	19.1
9 mo	9.2	72	7.6	6.9	20.1
1 y	10.2	76	8.0	7.3	21.1
1.5 y	11.5	83	8.7	7.9	22.9
2 y	12.8	88	9.2	8.3	24.2
4 y	16.5	103	10.6	9.6	28.1
6 y	20.5	116	11.8	10.7	31.4
8 y	26	127	12.9	11.7	34.2
10 y	31	137	13.8	12.5	36.8
12 y	39	149	15.0	13.5	39.9
14 y	50	165	16.5	14.9	44.0
16 y	62.5	174	17.3	15.7	46.3

Fem, femoral; IJ, internal jugular; SC, subclavian.

and the other 20 gauge (1.1 mm OD) will have a 66% reduction in flow rate if the 16-gauge lumen is used and a 90% reduction in flow rate if the 20-gauge lumen is used compared with a 14-gauge single-lumen catheter.

While the theoretic considerations described above are qualitatively true, actual flow measurements in studies of pediatric catheters have demonstrated slightly greater flow rates than are predicted by Poiseuille's law. Changes in length have a linear effect on flow rate; thus, if other factors remain constant, a catheter of one half the length will have twice the maximum flow rate. Although this consideration suggests that large-caliber, short peripheral catheters may better serve patients in need of rapid fluid replacement than longer central circulation catheters, experimental data indicate that in children this may not always hold true. Hydrostatic pressure in a tortuous or compressed peripheral vein may explain why comparable flow rates are achieved with longer central venous catheters and shorter peripheral catheters in these studies.

The driving pressure forcing fluid through the catheter is another important component determining flow rate through catheters. A 500-mL bag of saline attached to standard 200-cm intravenous tubing exerts approximately 85 mm Hg pressure when held 100 cm above the catheter connector. Manually inflated pressure bags generally increase driving pressure to about 300 or 400 mm Hg and in some cases to as high as 700 mm Hg. Pneumatically driven automatic pressure bags achieve pressures above 400 mm Hg, while a handheld syringe can achieve pressures as high as 2,000 mm Hg (although this is highly variable because the individual pushing the syringe fatigues quickly). Syringe infusion pumps available for clinical use have safety limits preventing them from generating pressures in excess of 500 to 1,200 mm Hg.

In order to put these driving pressure numbers in perspective, the theoretic calculations derived from Poiseuille's equation should be considered in light of experimental data from studies on this subject. For example, the total blood volume of a briskly hemorrhaging 40-kg child is approximately 2,600 mL. If this patient has a 25-cm, 14-gauge-lumen central venous catheter in place, it would take approximately 50 minutes to replace the total blood volume if the bag is simply raised 100 cm above the entry site of the catheter. If a manual pressure bag is applied at 300 mm Hg, the replacement time would be reduced to 15 minutes. To replace an ongoing loss of 500 mL/minute with the same catheter, 900 mm Hg of pressure would be required continuously to transfuse the patient (20–25).

Monitoring Equipment

Frequent heart rate, blood pressure, and pulse oximetry measurements are mandatory when performing CVC (see Chapters 5 and 75). Routine ECG monitoring is desirable in most cases, but it is required if the catheter tip or guidewire is likely to touch the endocardium. For intubated, mechanically ventilated patients, end-tidal CO_2 monitoring is also advantageous (see Chapter 76). These monitoring recommendations are based on considerations related to the patient's underlying disease, the sedative or analgesic medicines used to

TABLE 19.4	CATHETER DIAMETERS FOR PEDIATRIC PATIENTS		
	Catheter Diameter (French)		
Age	IJ	SC[a]	Fem
0–6 mo	3	3	3
6 mo–2 y	3	3	3–4
3–6 y	4	4	4
7–12 y	4–5	4–5	4–5

Fem, femoral; IJ, internal jugular; SC, subclavian.
[a]For infants and younger children, the subclavian approach should only be performed by highly experienced operators.

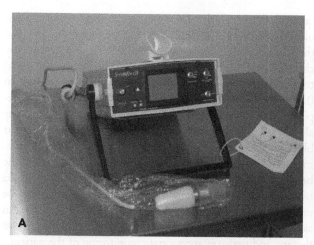
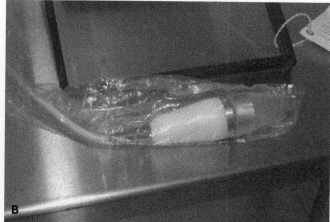

Figure 19.8
A. Handheld ultrasound device.
B. Ultrasound probe head with sterile covering.

facilitate the procedure, and the likelihood that a good portion of the patient's body will be draped, obscuring observation during the procedure. Additionally, if the physician primarily responsible for the patient's treatment is also the individual performing CVC, his or her attention may be focused on the procedure. In these circumstances, the aid of an assistant, in addition to the electronic monitors, is imperative to ensure patient safety.

Ultrasound Guidance

Ultrasound devices have been developed that can be easily used at the bedside in the ED to identify the location of vessels during vascular cannulation (Fig. 19.8) (26,27). A detailed description of the use of ultrasound guidance for obtaining vascular access can be found in Chapter 137. The ultrasound probe is first applied to the area of the patient's body where CVC will be performed to confirm the proposed skin entry site (i.e., a patent vessel in the expected location). The probe can also be placed just proximal to the insertion site to directly observe needle placement into the blood vessel lumen. As with most medical procedures, practice is necessary for successful use of these tools. Over time, however, regular use of ultrasound guidance has been shown to increase success rates and reduce complications with CVC. These devices give the operator a better understanding of the anatomy of the various sites, including the anterior-posterior relationships of the arterial, venous, and nonvascular structures (26,27).

Ensuring Patient Comfort and Cooperation

Medications and equipment required to ensure patient comfort and cooperation during the procedure include local anesthetic, intravenous sedatives and analgesics, neuromuscular blocking agents, and physical restraints. Obviously, neuromuscular blockade would only be considered for the child who has a definitive airway already in place. Which of these adjuncts are selected and how they are used will vary significantly from patient to patient, but careful preparation of these items is necessary for successfully performing CVC (see Chapters 3, 33, and 35).

▶ PROCEDURE

Successful CVC requires careful preparation and attention to the patient and environment before, during, and immediately after the procedure. As with most complex procedures, meticulously attending to all the important details is the best way of ensuring that events will proceed smoothly and safely. Some of the more generic issues regarding CVC, as well as a description of the steps involved in standard Seldinger technique and PICC placement, are described first. Then important points related to the specific entry sites that may be used are presented.

Obtaining Consent

When possible, obtaining consent is always desirable prior to performing any medical procedure (see Chapter 9). Patients and parents usually appreciate a brief discussion of the steps involved in the procedure, including patient positioning, the use of monitoring devices, sterile draping that may cover the child's face, the use of sedation and analgesia, and potential complications. A note in the chart describing this interaction or (depending on institutional policy) a signed consent form is often helpful to other professionals involved in the patient's care and may protect the physician and hospital at a later time. The details of these practices vary, but the general principals are applicable to all settings. However, while obtaining consent is always preferable, CVC is often performed on an emergent basis, when time and circumstances do not permit this step. In such cases, a brief retrospective discussion of the procedure provided for the patient and/or family members is often very helpful.

Preparing the Environment

The assistants, medications, equipment, and monitors used to ensure patient comfort and safety during the procedure should all be ready (e.g., the medications and equipment should be conveniently available to the operator and the equipment should be functioning properly) prior to positioning or medicating the patient. As discussed above, it is recommended that heart rate, blood pressure, and pulse oximetry be measured and recorded frequently (every 1 to 2 minutes) or displayed continuously during the procedure. Whenever stimulation of the endocardium is anticipated, a continuous electrocardiogram is also required. Finally, it should be emphasized that all the sophisticated electronic monitors available today cannot substitute for human observation. Since the physician operator will be concentrating on the procedure, it is important to have one or more experienced assistants who are practiced in the assessment of critically ill children and familiar with the procedure.

Preparing the Patient

Once the personnel, medications, equipment, and monitors are in place, the next step is to properly position the patient. Details of positioning are addressed below in the discussion of each specific approach, but one general principle is that ensuring patient comfort is a key to success. Medications for analgesia and sedation are helpful in meeting this goal, but their use must be individualized to each patient's needs. Any underlying medical problems, particularly those related to circulatory and respiratory function, must be carefully considered in the decision to use these adjuncts.

Most patients will benefit from a local anesthetic applied to the site of the skin puncture. This is most often a 1% lidocaine solution (10 mg/mL) without epinephrine, which will adequately anesthetize the site without exceeding a toxic threshold dose of approximately 7 mg/kg (see Chapter 35). For the anxious patient with stable circulation, the operator may choose to use intravenous sedatives and/or analgesics titrated to the desired effect. An effective combination is 0.05 to 0.1 mg/kg of midazolam and 0.05 to 0.1 mg/kg of morphine sulfate (see Chapter 33), although other regimens may also be used. Restraints used judiciously—or neuromuscular blockade in mechanically ventilated patients capable of moving suddenly—may also be valuable adjuncts. As always, the benefit of a soothing voice or gentle hand in helping the child tolerate and cooperate with these procedures should not be underestimated. Whenever moderate sedation is provided, an assistant qualified in sedation practice should administer that therapy and perform appropriate monitoring of the patient.

Preparing the Site

After the patient is properly positioned, comfortable, and cooperative, the cannulation site can be prepared using aseptic technique (see Chapter 7). The use of sterile gowns, masks, and hats is recommended during placement, although few data exist to prove these adjuncts decrease infection. These additional precautions are helpful particularly when placing long catheters or when instructing another physician, as in these situations equipment has a tendency to accidentally touch the operator's chest or arms.

When cleansing the anatomic site with the antiseptic solution of choice, it is important to clean an area large enough to allow observation and palpation of anatomic landmarks adjacent to the site of entry without contaminating the sterile field. Trimming hair with scissors rather than shaving the area prevents abrading and inflaming the skin, which can lead to an increased incidence of infection. The area should be adequately

---

 SUMMARY: SELDINGER TECHNIQUE FOR CENTRAL VENOUS CATHETER PLACEMENT

1 Obtain consent, as appropriate

2 Gather necessary equipment (Table 18.2)

3 Attach monitors: cardiograph, pulse oximetery, blood pressure

4 Select approach and position patient accordingly

5 Prepare sterile field

6 Infiltrate local anesthetic, as necessary

7 Attach entry needle to small (3 or 5 mL) syringe and rinse with heparin

8 Insert entry needle through skin and eject small volume of fluid to clear any skin plugs

9 While applying negative pressure to syringe, insert needle until blood is aspirated from vein

10 Advance needle an additional 1 to 2 mm, so tip is well within vessel lumen

11 Carefully remove syringe from needle

12 Insert guide wire, making sure proximal end is always secured

13 Remove needle, leaving wire in place

14 Enlarge skin puncture site by inserting No. 11 scalpel blade to its hub along wire

15 Insert dilator to enlarge entry site (optional)

16 Insert venous catheter and aspirate blood to ensure proper placement

17 Secure catheter in place with suture and apply dressing

18 Obtain radiograph to confirm proper placement of catheter

19 Document procedure in medical record

draped with sterile towels to provide a sterile workspace large enough to prevent accidental contamination of the catheter, wire, or other equipment.

Once the area is properly draped and the landmarks re-examined, the skin is infiltrated with a local anesthetic. A generous skin wheal is first made using a short 25-gauge needle. The subcutaneous tissues may then be infiltrated using a slightly longer 21- or 22-gauge needle. In small infants, the cutaneous and subcutaneous injections are easily accomplished in one step using the smaller needle. The syringe should always be aspirated before infiltrating the skin to avoid inadvertent intravascular administration of the local anesthetic.

Inserting the Catheter

Seldinger Technique

After the anatomic landmarks appropriate for the specific entry site are identified, the cleaned and draped skin puncture site is well anesthetized. The entry needle is attached to a small 3- or 5-mL syringe rinsed with a heparinized saline solution. The small syringe prevents air embolism, and the heparin reduces clot formation in the needle. It is generally useful to eject a small volume (less than 0.5 mL) of fluid out of the needle just after making the skin puncture to flush out any skin plug that may be caught in the beveled needle tip. Otherwise, blood may not be aspirated even though the needle has entered the vessel lumen. Once through the skin, a small amount of negative pressure is applied to aid blood return as the needle is advanced. When blood return is apparent, the needle should be inserted an additional 1 to 2 mm until a free flow of blood is obtained to ensure that the beveled tip of the needle lies well within the blood vessel lumen.

A few helpful techniques for this part of the procedure deserve emphasis. First, the use of a small syringe with gentle suction while locating the vein will prevent its collapse even in a small hypovolemic child. Second, if blood flow is not obtained after deeply advancing the needle, the needle should be slowly withdrawn to a depth just beneath the surface of the skin while gentle negative pressure is maintained. In this way, if the vessel lumen was inadvertently passed completely through during needle entry, it can be identified during needle withdrawal. If blood return into the needle is not noted during this withdrawal procedure, the needle tip is redirected and advanced again. By this slow, careful advance and withdrawal, multiple vein lacerations and hematoma formation are avoided. Finally, use of a non-Luer-Lok syringe on the entry needle prevents accidental dislodgement of the needle from the vessel as the syringe is removed for the next stage of the procedure. Most commercially available kits provide these.

After successful entry into the vessel with the needle, the syringe is carefully detached in order to place the flexible tip of the guidewire into the hub of the entry needle. After the syringe is removed, and before the wire inserted, the needle lumen is occluded with the thumb of the operating hand. If the needle hub or catheter is left unoccluded, air embolus or significant blood loss may result. The guidewire is then inserted a short distance beyond the tip of the entry needle.

The rigid (proximal) end of the wire must always be visible protruding from the hub of the entry needle. Accidental loss of the guidewire in the central circulation is prevented by this method.

If the wire does not pass with minimal resistance, it should be removed. When a guidewire does not pass easily, reconfirmation of the needle position within the vessel should be attempted by observing for free flow of blood. Strategies that are helpful on subsequent attempts include redirection or rotation of the needle bevel or manipulation of the J-wire. The J-wire should be gently rolled between the operator's thumb and forefinger during advancement. These maneuvers may help the wire pass. If resistance is ever encountered during wire removal from the entry needle, the needle and wire must be removed together to prevent shearing of the wire by the beveled tip of the needle.

After the wire is successfully placed in the vein, the entry needle is removed, and a scalpel blade (No. 11) is used to enlarge the skin puncture. The blade is placed perpendicular to the skin (with the sharp edge pointed away from the wire) and advanced along the path of the guidewire through the skin and subcutaneous tissue. This incision allows easier passage of the larger-caliber catheter into the blood vessel and protects the catheter tip from fraying. Before advancing the catheter into the vessel, the wire should be observed to emerge from the proximal end of the catheter. During catheter advancement, the operator places his or her fingertips close to the catheter tip and applies steady, gentle pressure with a slow twisting motion. This facilitates controlled insertion of the catheter through the subcutaneous tissues and into the lumen of the vein.

If resistance is met at this stage of the procedure, a few additional techniques may be helpful. First, the catheter should be removed so that the tip can be examined. Fraying of the tip will prevent its smooth entry into the vessel. If fraying is present, the catheter must be replaced. Before attempting insertion with the new catheter, the operator should repeat the scalpel incision but this time extend it slightly deeper into the subcutaneous tissue. Alternatively, a stiff single-lumen dilator may be used to create a tract through which the softer permanent vascular catheter can pass. Many commercially available catheters are now packaged with a dilator that is tightly fit within the lumen of the permanent catheter (Fig. 19.9). When using one of these kits, the technique for placement is the same, except that the combined venodilator-catheter is passed over the wire in a single step. The dilator and wire are then removed together, leaving the catheter in place. In addition to performing standard CVC, methods used for the Seldinger technique can be used to replace an existing catheter with a new one using a guidewire, place an introducer through which a Swan-Ganz catheter or transvenous pacemaker may be inserted, and perform other maneuvers.

Peripherally Inserted Central Catheter Placement

The first step in PICC placement is to measure the distance from the anticipated site of entry to the surface landmark associated with the desired location of the catheter tip within the central venous circulation. For the usual forearm entry site,

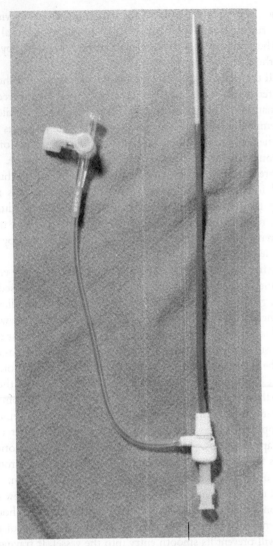

Figure 19.9 Central venous catheter with dilator suitable for an older adolescent or adult.

the appropriate length of the catheter will be the summation of the distances from the insertion site to the shoulder, from the shoulder to the sternal notch, and from the sternal notch to the proximal third of the sternum. A tourniquet is placed on the extremity proximal to the point of entry, and the area is cleaned and draped as described previously. An assistant should have easy access to the tourniquet under the drapes so that it can be removed after successful venipuncture.

The PICC catheter is then taken by the operator from the kit using sterile technique and, based on the previous measurement of the patient, trimmed to the proper length. The wire stylet must be removed from the catheter to allow the catheter to be cut. It is important to remember that the stylet should not be advanced beyond the end of the shortened catheter; it should always stay completely within the catheter when the PICC is advanced through the vasculature. Local anesthetic is then infiltrated at the entry site in preparation for catheter insertion.

Depending on whether the introducer needle technique or the introducer sheath has been selected, one of two meth-

ods of insertion is utilized at this point. With the introducer needle technique (Fig. 19.7A), the vein is punctured using a peel-away butterfly needle. When free flow of blood is observed, the tourniquet is removed, and the PICC is advanced into the vein to the desired length. The stylet is then removed, and the catheter is aspirated for blood. When the PICC is properly positioned, the introducer butterfly catheter should be carefully removed from the patient's arm, peeled in half, removed, and discarded. Care must be taken during this process not to damage the PICC. If an introducer sheath is used, the operator simply performs a modification of the Seldinger technique. The vein is punctured using a straight needle or standard peripheral intravenous catheter. A guidewire is then advanced 6 to 10 cm into the vein, and the tourniquet is removed. The thin peel-away introducer sheath is advanced into the vessel over the wire. The introducer sheath comes in the kit with a stiff, tapered catheter that fits within the sheath lumen (Fig. 19.7B). This allows the sheath to be easily advanced over the wire into the vein. As with any use of the Seldinger technique, control of the wire must always be maintained to prevent it from being lost into the vessel. After the sheath-catheter system is advance into the vein, the wire and stiff introducer catheter are removed, leaving the peel-away sheath in the vein ready to accept the PICC catheter. The precut PICC is advanced through the sheath and into the vein to the desired distance. Once a good blood return is confirmed, the sheath is withdrawn, peeled from the PICC, and discarded. The operator must be careful not to inadvertently withdraw the PICC when removing the introducer sheath.

The last step for both techniques prior to dressing the catheter is to ensure that the tip is properly positioned. The appearance of the blood, blood gas tensions, and vascular pressure measurement can be used to confirm venous rather than arterial position. For catheters placed in the FV, such methods alone are adequate. For all other catheters, a portable chest x-ray and/or abdominal x-ray is also necessary to confirm proper placement. The catheter should be oriented within the blood vessel so that the tip is parallel to the vascular wall; this prevents inadvertent vessel laceration or endothelium injury with movement of the catheter or patient. When accessing the central circulation from sites cephalad to the heart, the best position for the catheter is in the vena cava just outside the right atrium—vena cava junction. This position ensures that (a) infusions are entering a high-volume, high-flow space, (b) vascular pressure measurements reflect the intrathoracic pressure, and (c) myocardial injury does not occur. More proximal catheter tip positions are acceptable as long as the tip-wall orientation remains parallel. Central venous pressure measurements from the infradiaphragmatic tip position (femoral venous entry site) have been shown to correlate with intrathoracic tip measurements as long as a pressure wave form is observed on the monitor. Of note, it is important to ensure that the catheter has not been advanced retrograde to the direction of blood flow into any of the veins draining major organs (e.g., renal, hepatic, or jugular veins). Furthermore, at no time should a catheter tip be allowed to remain within the right atrium. Atrial wall perforation with hemopericardium is a rare but catastrophic CVC complication that is avoided by keeping the catheter tip out of the heart.

Securing and Dressing the Catheter

After the catheter is properly positioned it should be sutured in place at the entry site, and the entry wound is then dressed. Infection is the most common complication of CVC, and the incidence of this complication is influenced by the type and care of the catheter wound dressing. Some experts have recommended abandoning the conventional dressing technique of sterile gauze held in place with tape and instead using a transparent polyurethane sheet (Tegaderm, Opsite) placed over the catheter at the skin entry site (28,29). Advocates for these polyurethane dressing systems note that they allow for continuous inspection of the site while reliably securing the catheter and allowing the patient to more easily bathe. A meta-analysis of studies comparing this technique with the older methods suggest that the polyurethane covering is associated with a higher risk of catheter tip infection, bacteremia, and sepsis (30); however, this remains controversial, and a comparison study in children did not demonstrate a difference (31). Moreover, the newest transparent dressings are semipermeable to moisture and may be superior to the original versions in relation to infection. The Centers for Disease Control (CDC) consensus recommendations (Table 19.5) suggest that both clear polyurethane and more traditional dry gauze dressings are acceptable, but if the site is likely to be bloody or have tissue breakdown for other reasons, a dry dressing may be preferable (32–35).

With regard to longer-term care, it is helpful to place a label on the catheter dressing documenting the date and time of insertion and the last dressing change. Dressing changes are performed at least three times per week or more often if necessary. During the dressing change, the site is inspected for signs of inflammation and then cleansed with povidone-iodine solution following strict sterile technique. The intravenous tubing is changed every 48 hours unless hyperalimentation solutions are being infused through the catheter, in which case the tubing is changed every 24 hours. The tubing extending from the hub of each lumen of a multiple-lumen catheter is secured to the patient's skin with silk tape or Steri-strips. This will prevent accidental dislodgment of the catheter and kinking of the tubing. It is useful to interpose a stopcock-tubing attachment between the catheter hub and the intravenous tubing to allow access for multiple medication infusions or the addition of intermittent bolus medications through each lumen (28,36–41).

Documentation

Whenever CVC is performed, a note should be entered in the patient's chart that includes the following information: date and time of catheter insertion; type, gauge, and length of catheter placed; any complications encountered; method of catheter placement confirmation; and the patient's condition after completion of the procedure.

Selecting the Site

As described previously, the most common sites used for percutaneous CVC are, in order of preference, the femoral vein, the jugular veins (internal and external), and the subclavian vein. Site selection for CVC is influenced by operator experience, pre-existing medical conditions of the patient, equipment considerations, the purpose or indication for placing the catheter, and the urgency of the procedure. Advantages and disadvantages of the potential sites are listed in Table 19.6.

The femoral site is so popular for pediatric CVC that it might well be considered the site of first choice. Its primary advantage is that it is farthest away from the head and

TABLE 19.5	CDC RECOMMENDATIONS REGARDING CATHETER DRESSING		
CDC Recommendation		**Level of Support**	**Ref.**
Use either sterile gauze or sterile, transparent, semipermeable dressing to cover the catheter site.		Category IA	33,34,35
Tunneled CVC sites that are well healed might not require dressings.		Category II	
If the patient is diaphoretic or if the site is bleeding or oozing, a gauze dressing is preferable to a transparent, semipermeable dressing.		Category II	29,33,34,35
Replace catheter site dressing if the dressing becomes damp, loosened, or visibly soiled.		Category IB	33,35
Change dressings at least weekly for adult and adolescent patients depending on the circumstances of the individual patient.		Category II	34
Do not use topical antibiotic ointment or creams on insertion sites (except when using dialysis catheters) because of their potential to promote fungal infections and antimicrobial resistance.		Category IA	67,68
Do not submerge the catheter under water. Showering should be permitted if precautions can be taken to reduce the likelihood of introducing organisms into the catheter (e.g., if the catheter and connecting device are protected with an impermeable cover during the shower).		Category II	69,70

Source: O'Grady NP, Alexander M, Dellinger EP, et al. *Guidelines for the Prevention of Intravascular Catheter-Related Infections.* www.cdc.gov/mmwr/preview/mmwrhtml/rr5110a1.htm. Accessed June 7, 2005.

TABLE 19.6	**ADVANTAGES AND DISADVANTAGES OF SPECIFIC SITES**				
Site	Landmarks	Advantages	Disadvantages	Complications	Ref.
FV	Femoral triangle	Requires least operator experience; fastest; out of the way of resuscitation; anatomy exposed; available for direct compression	Risk of contamination; may be harder to secure; may be more uncomfortable for the pt difficult in obese pts need fluoroscopy to place Swan-Ganz catheter	Infection; bleeding; thrombosis	4,42,44,71
IJV	Angle formed by the 2 heads of the SCM m	Right side offers direct route to SVC, out of resuscitation field, anatomy exposed, available for direct compression	Requires operator experience; generally takes longer; more difficult in pts <1 year with short, fat necks; more difficult in pts with tracheostomy and pts who are not intubated	Carotid artery puncture; PTX; on left side, risk of thoracic duct injury; cardiac tamponade; multiple neuropathies; thrombosis; infection	6,7,46,47
EJV	Visible in the neck crossing posteriorly over SCM m	Visible; superficial; available for direct compression; fewest complications	Difficult to cannulate central circulation from this site; if not visible, cannot use this site	Hematoma	5,7
SV	Supraclavicular: Lateral to clavicular SVC, head of SCM m, above the clavicle Infraclavicular: Just beneath junction of middle and lateral thirds of the clavicle	Right side offers direct route to SVC; vein may be less collapsible	Requires operator experience; difficult in pts. <1 y; no access to control bleeding	PTX; bleeding; tamponade; dysrhythmias; thoracic duct injury; catheter malposition; air embolism; neuropathies	4,6
Arm veins	Palpable on the medial aspect of the arm at or just below or above the antecubital fossa	Low incidence of complications; ease of dressing and care	May be difficult to advance the catheter through the peripheral vein into the central circulation; long length results in high resistance to flow through catheter	Catheter can advance upward into neck and head; infection	

FV, femoral vein; IJV, internal jugular vein; EJV, external jugular vein; SV, subclavian vein; AV, axillary vein; SVC, superior vena cava; CA, carotid artery; PTX , pneumothorax; SCM, sternocleidomastoid.

chest and does not interfere with the evaluation or treatment of the critically ill child (e.g., endotracheal intubation, chest compressions). It also requires less technical expertise than the jugular or subclavian sites and allows for relatively easy hemostasis should bleeding occur at the insertion site. For most practitioners, the jugular sites would be considered a secondary choice. As discussed previously, the subclavian site is used infrequently in children because it requires the highest degree of expertise and is associated with the greatest incidence of serious complications, such as significant hemorrhage and pneumothorax. Methods for identifying appropriate sites for catheter insertion based on surface landmarks are described here, but it should be remembered that there can be significant variation in the underlying venous anatomy. Bedside ultrasound to facilitate the performance of CVC can be a valuable adjunct for this reason (26,27).

Femoral Vein

Although once thought to be associated with a high rate of complications, CVC at the femoral site has proven to be safe and effective in pediatric patients. Swanson et al. reported an 89% success rate of percutaneously placed femoral catheters in critically ill ED patients, with the only reported complication being an arterial puncture that caused a groin hematoma in one patient (12). Failure was due to inability to locate the vein or to thread the catheter. Similarly, Kanter et al. found that pediatric residents demonstrated an 86% success rate (11).

Remarkably, this physician group, with relatively little previous experience, achieved this success rate with a median time to placement of only 5 minutes in a critically ill pediatric population, with 48% of patients demonstrating signs of shock. Furthermore, in this 33-month survey, femoral catheters had a complication rate that was no different from the rate for central lines placed at other sites.

Although the femoral approach has several advantages, a few relative contraindications exist. These include abnormal vascular anatomy or congenital malformation of the lower extremity, femoral hernia, abdominal tumor or trauma, abdominal ascites, and future plans for cardiac catheterization.

Identification of Landmarks

The FV can be identified 1 to 2 cm medial to the femoral artery pulse (when palpable) 1 to 2 cm below the inguinal ligament. When the child has weak or absent pulses, the position of the FV can be located by identifying the point halfway between the pubic tubercle and the anterior iliac spine and 1 to 2 cm below the inguinal ligament. On cross-sectional ultrasound imaging, the more easily compressed FV is medial and superficial to the smaller and pulsatile femoral artery (Figs. 19.10 and 19.11).

Procedure

When cannulating the FV, optimal patient positioning requires abduction and external rotation at the hip. A folded

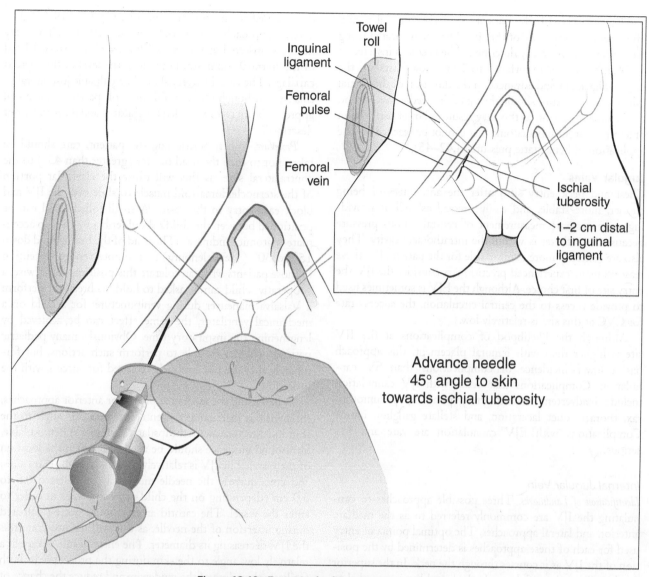

Towel roll

Inguinal ligament

Femoral pulse

Femoral vein

Ischial tuberosity

1–2 cm distal to inguinal ligament

Advance needle 45° angle to skin towards ischial tuberosity

Figure 19.10 Entry site for femoral vein cannulation.

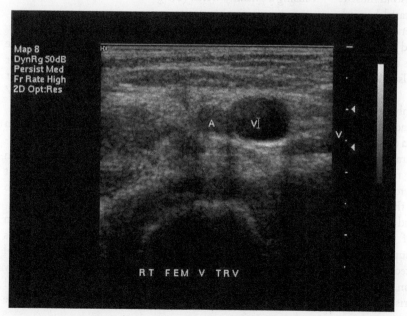

Map 8
DynRg 50dB
Persist Med
Fr Rate High
2D Opt:Res

RT FEM V TRV

Figure 19.11 Cross-sectional ultrasound image of femoral vein and artery.

towel placed beneath the patient's ipsilateral gluteal region often improves exposure of the site. The site is located using the landmarks previously described. The needle is inserted at a 45° angle to the skin surface 1 to 2 cm below (distal to) the inguinal ligament and advanced in the direction of the ischial tuberosity. At no time should the tip of the needle pass beyond the inguinal ligament, as this may result in bowel perforation or a retroperitoneal hematoma that cannot be reached for the application of hemostatic pressure (4,42–45).

Jugular Veins

Chest and neck entry sites offer the advantages of being cleaner, more stable, and easily dressed as well as providing more accurate measurement of central venous pressure because the catheter is within the intrathoracic cavity. They also are generally more comfortable for the patient. For these reasons, many experienced practitioners consider the IJV the entry site of first choice. Although the EJV is sometimes used to provide access to the central circulation, the success rate for CVC at this site is relatively low.

Although the likelihood of complications at the IJV site is higher than with femoral placement, this approach has a lower incidence of complications than SV cannulation. Complications that occur with IJV cannulation include inadvertent carotid artery puncture, pneumothorax, thoracic duct laceration, and stellate ganglion injury. Complications with EJV cannulation are rare and less serious.

Internal Jugular Vein

Identification of Landmarks. Three possible approaches to cannulating the IJV are commonly referred to as the median, anterior, and lateral approaches. The optimal points of entry used for each of these approaches is determined by the position of the IJV as it courses through the neck. In the superior (cephalad) portion of the neck, the vessel lies just medial to the sternal (medial) head of the sternocleidomastoid muscle. In the midportion of the neck, the IJV is located beneath the junction of the sternal and clavicular (lateral) heads of the sternocleidomastoid. In the inferior (caudad) portion of the neck, the IJV lies just medial to (or sometimes beneath) the clavicular head of the sternocleidomastoid (see also "Anatomy and Physiology").

The median approach is the most commonly used (Fig. 19.12). For all approaches, the patient's head is turned approximately 30° away from the side of planned entry. To locate the median entry site, an imaginary line is drawn between the sternal notch and the mastoid process. The middle third of this line should be directly lateral to the thyroid cartilage and cross over the apex of the triangle formed by the two heads of the sternocleidomastoid muscle laterally and the clavicle inferiorly. The IJV is just below the apex of the triangle between the two segments of the muscle. It is superficial and lateral to the carotid artery, which can be palpated just medial to this triangle. Using ultrasound visualization, the IJV is superficial, lateral, and compressible in comparison with the

deeper, smaller, and pulsatile carotid artery (Fig. 19.13). The anterior approach is less popular but also effective. The entry needle is inserted at the medial border of the sternal head of the sternocleidomastoid muscle at the level of the thyroid cartilage. The carotid artery should be palpable just lateral to this site. Although often useful for adult patients, the lateral approach is not recommended for children and is therefore not described.

Procedure. When positioning the patient, care should be taken not to turn the head too far (greater than 45°) to the contralateral side, as this will cause the clavicular portion of the sternocleidomastoid muscle to slide over the IJV and block easy entry to the vessel. A small rolled towel can be positioned between the child's shoulder blades to help accentuate anatomic landmarks. The head of the bed is tilted down 15° to 30° (Trendelenburg) to promote venous distention in those patients who can tolerate this position. Otherwise, a cooperative child can be asked to hold his breath or perform a Valsalva maneuver during venipuncture; for a child on a mechanical ventilator, the same effect can be achieved by lengthening the inspiratory time. Obviously, many pediatric patients will not be able to perform such actions, but fortunately they are not routinely required for success with the procedure.

When using the median approach or anterior approaches, the needle is inserted at the entry site at a 30° angle to the skin and directed toward the ipsilateral nipple. When available, ultrasound guidance should be used to confirm the location of the vessel. The IJV is relatively superficial at the entry sites, and consequently the needle must only be inserted 0.5 to 3.0 cm (depending on the child's age and size) in order to enter the vessel. The carotid artery should not be palpated during insertion of the needle, as this will tend to compress the IJV, decreasing its diameter. The entry needle is kept at a relatively low angle to the skin during the procedure to both facilitate threading of the guidewire and reduce the chance of causing a pneumothorax (5,7).

External Jugular Vein

As described previously, advantages of the EJV site include a low risk of pneumothorax, hematoma, carotid puncture, or injury to the sympathetic chain. However, successful vascular cannulation occurs significantly less frequently via the EJV than with the other sites.

Identification of Landmarks. When the patient is positioned in the supine position with the head turned 45° to the contralateral side, the EJV vein should be identifiable by inspection of the lateral neck (Fig. 19.14). If the vein is not visible as it crosses the sternocleidomastoid muscle, it is probably best to choose another site of entry.

Procedure. If possible, the patient should be positioned in 15° to 30° Trendelenburg to promote venous distention; this is one situation when such positioning can be very helpful for locating the vessel. The operator stabilizes the vein by applying gentle traction to the skin cephalad to the point of entry using the nondominant hand. The vein is entered at the

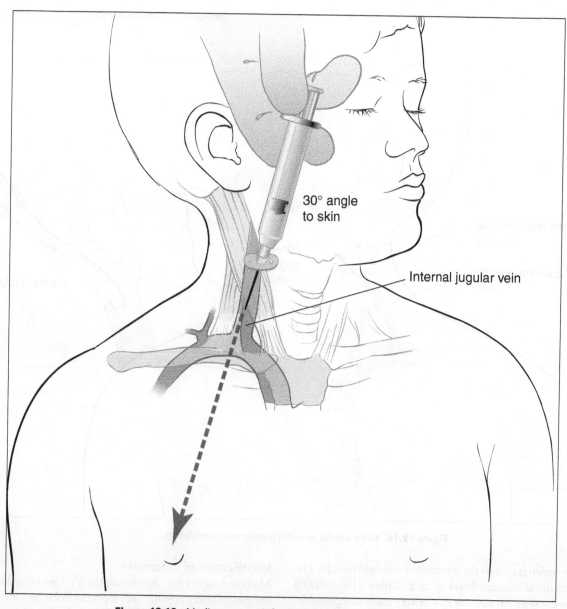

30° angle
to skin

Internal jugular vein

Figure 19.12 Median approach for internal jugular vein cannulation.

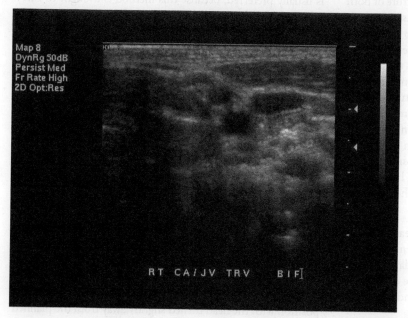

Map 8
DynRg 50dB
Persist Med
Fr Rate High
2D Opt:Res

RT CA/JV TRV   BIF

Figure 19.13 Cross-sectional ultrasound image of internal jugular vein and carotid artery.

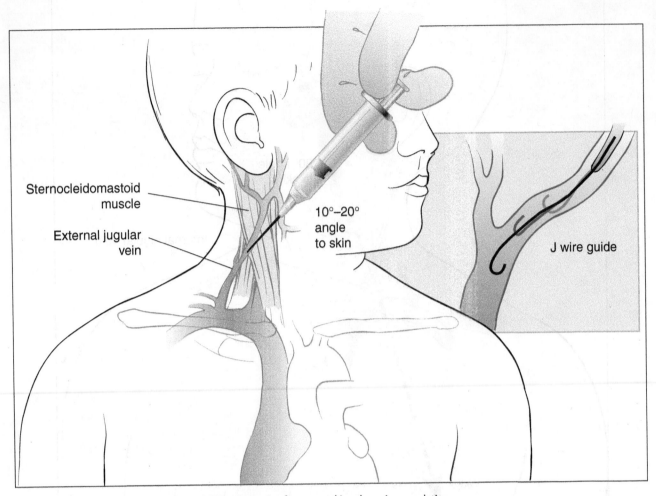

Figure 19.14 Entry site for external jugular vein cannulation.

point at which it crosses the sternocleidomastoid muscle. The entry needle is inserted bevel up at a shallow (10° to 20°) angle to the skin. Because the EJV is very easily compressible, relatively superficial, and highly mobile in the subcutaneous tissue, inserting a needle alone often leads to puncture of both walls of the vessel, resulting in a hematoma. Consequently, it is generally advisable to use a short catheter (3 to 4 cm) over the needle, which is advanced into the vessel after insertion. Once in place, the short, flexible catheter serves as the conduit for the guidewire. The J-wire is used when cannulating the EJV because it is more likely to negotiate the tortuous course of the vessel into the central circulation. The wire is steadily advanced using a gentle twisting motion. Insertion of the wire may also be facilitated by medial or lateral flexion of the neck and/or abduction with lateral rotation of the ipsilateral arm at the shoulder. If the central circulation cannot be accessed, the catheter can be left in place to provide peripheral access.

Subclavian Vein

For reasons previously mentioned, the SV is the least common site used for percutaneous CVC in young children. The small size and increased compliance of the chest and clavicles make identification of the appropriate landmarks more difficult. In addition, a higher incidence of pneumothorax and subclavian artery puncture have been reported.

Identification of Landmarks

Many techniques for cannulating the SV have been described, but two primary approaches (supraclavicular and infraclavicular) are most commonly used. The infraclavicular approach is usually preferred, because this method is thought to carry a lower risk of pneumothorax and other complications. In theory, movement of the needle is limited by the rib and the clavicle, as opposed to the supraclavicular approach, which requires the operator to more directly maintain control of the needle. However, studies of SV cannulation have not confirmed this hypothesis.

With the patient's head turned to the contralateral side, the entry site for the supraclavicular approach is identified by locating the lateral border of the clavicular head of the sternocleidomastoid muscle and the superior border of the clavicle. The site of skin entry is approximately one fingerbreadth lateral to the muscle just above the clavicle. The infraclavicular entry site is found by identifying the clavicle and the suprasternal notch. The skin entry site is located at or just lateral to the midclavicular line below the clavicle (Fig. 19.15).

Procedure

The patient is placed in a supine 10° to 25° Trendelenburg position with the head turned slightly away from the planned

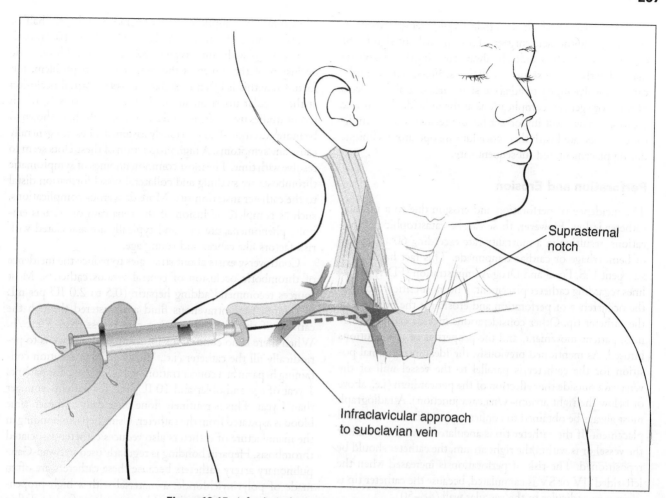

Figure 19.15 Infraclavicular approach for subclavian vein cannulation.

cannulation site. A rolled towel can be positioned longitudinally between the shoulder blades so that the child's shoulders
fall posteriorly away from the chest. The ipsilateral arm should
be at the child's side; gentle downward traction of the ipsilateral arm may also be helpful. The operator is positioned at
the patient's side when using the infraclavicular approach or at
the head of the bed when using the supraclavicular approach.

For the supraclavicular approach, the entry site is first identified as stated above, and the finder needle is then directed so
that it bisects the angle formed by the clavicle and the sternocleidomastoid muscle when aimed toward the contralateral
nipple. The needle should be angled 10° to 15° above the
coronal plane. The catheter is slowly advanced to a distance
equal to two to three times the width of the clavicle. If the
operator is unsuccessful with the first pass, the needle is redirected 5° to 10° in the coronal plane.

When using the infraclavicular approach, the patient is
positioned in the same manner as used for the supraclavicular
approach, and the entry site is located as described above. The
needle is advanced slowly just beneath the inferior surface
of the clavicle 2 to 4 cm, aimed toward the sternal notch
and kept as nearly parallel to the horizontal plane of the
chest as possible. If the first pass is unsuccessful, the needle is
withdrawn and only minimally redirected inferiorly. Keeping
the initial orientation of the needle near the horizontal plane

just under the clavicle and then making small realignments
on subsequent passes minimizes the likelihood of subclavian
artery puncture or pneumothorax (6,10,46,47).

Veins of the Forearm

As mentioned previously, the basilic vein is most commonly
used for central venous access. It is usually readily visible or
palpable when a tourniquet is placed on the arm proximal to
the entry site. The vein arises from the ulnar (medial) side of
the dorsal venous network of the hand. The network drainage
then curves around the medial side of the forearm, joining to
form the large basilic vein. The basilic vein communicates
with the cephalic vein via the median cubital vein. Proximal
to the elbow the basilic passes more deeply up the medial side
of the arm to join the axillary vein. The vein can be entered at
this location, but skill with ultrasound-guided venipuncture
is usually necessary for this approach.

▸ COMPLICATIONS

Thrombosis, vascular/cardiac perforation, cardiac arrhythmia, air embolism, catheter fragment embolism, and infection can occur with any method of performing CVC. A rare
complication is accidental entry of the guidewire into the

central circulation, which potentially requires removal by a vascular or cardiothoracic surgeon. This unusual but significant complication can be avoided by always ensuring that the proximal end of the wire is secured at all times. Site-specific complications involve injury to adjacent structures or unique effects of the more general complications at the individual anatomic locations. The most important factors related to all complications associated with this procedure are operator technique during placement and subsequent care.

Perforation and Erosion

The incidence of perforation and erosion due to a vascular catheter is low. However, these can be catastrophic complications, resulting in a mortality rate exceeding 60% because of hemorrhage or cardiac tamponade. This fact has lead to stringent U.S. Food and Drug Administration (FDA) guidelines regarding catheter placement. The most critical factor in the occurrence of perforation and erosion is the position of the catheter tip. Other considerations include catheter stiffness, patient movement, and the properties of the solutions infused. As mentioned previously, the ideal intraluminal position for the catheter is parallel to the vessel wall of the vena cava outside the reflection of the pericardium (i.e., above or below the right atrium–vena cava junction). A radiograph must always be obtained to confirm appropriate intraluminal placement. If the catheter tip is angulated toward the wall of the vessel or is within the right atrium, the catheter should be repositioned. The risk of perforation is increased when the left-sided IJV or SV is cannulated, because the catheter tip is often perpendicular to the vascular wall (48–50).

In a prospective evaluation of catheter tip placement in adult patients, McGee et al. found that almost half of the time the tip was positioned in the right atrium (51). Neck flexion has been shown to cause migration of up to 3 cm with SV and IJV catheters in adults, and even greater migration can occur with arm movement when cephalic or axillary sites are used. Careful attention to the confirmation of proper catheter tip position and orientation within the vessel is therefore an essential aspect of minimizing the potential for complications related to perforation and erosion (49,52,53).

Thrombosis

Catheter-related thrombosis is a common occurrence and encompasses a wide range of potential consequences. These include minute fibrin deposition around the catheter tip, thrombotic occlusion of the catheter lumen, thrombosis of the vessel at the insertion site, varying sizes of central vascular wall thrombi, major thrombosis in the central venous system or atrium, complete vascular obstruction and collateral vessel formation, and thrombosis with symptomatic embolic signs and symptoms. The frequency of thrombotic complications caused by vascular catheters is difficult to infer from available studies due to the great differences in study design, the methods of thrombus detection, the various study definitions, and the underlying disease states of study subjects. However, if all thrombotic complications are included, well over half of central venous catheters left in place longer than a 10 days will be associated with some type of adverse event. Thrombotic occlusion of the lumen is the most common problem, but fortunately this is often treatable (48–60). Partial occlusion at the vascular insertion site or in the central vessels, which recent studies using ultrasound and venography have shown to be more common than previously assumed, does not generally cause any symptoms. A high proportion of these clots seem to resolve with time. The most common findings of symptomatic thrombosis are swelling and collateral vessel formation distal to the catheter insertion site. More dangerous complications, such as complete occlusion of the vena cava or serious embolic phenomena, are rare and typically are associated with risk factors like cancer and young age.

Controversy exists about strategies to reduce the incidence of thrombotic occlusion of central venous catheters. Most sources recommend adding heparin (0.5 to 2.0 IU per mL of solution) to intravenous fluid administered through the catheter if the planned infusion rate is less than 3 mL/h. When there is no continuous infusion, our practice is to periodically fill the catheter (i.e., "flush") with a solution containing heparin at a concentration of 100 IU/mL for patients 1 year of age and older and 10 IU/mL for patients younger than 1 year. This is routinely done once daily and each time blood is aspirated from the catheter. Using heparin bonding in the manufacture of catheters also reduces catheter-associated thrombosis. Heparin bonding is regularly used in Swan-Ganz pulmonary artery catheters because these catheters are often made of polyvinylchloride, a material with a high propensity for thrombus formation. The smooth surface of Teflon catheters allows little thrombus attachment, but the inherent stiffness of this material increases the incidence of vascular wall injury and mural thrombosis.

Thrombolytic agents can often be used to salvage catheters that become occluded by thrombosis. In the past, urokinase was widely used for this purpose, but in the late 1990s concerns about infectious disease transmission lead to the removal of this product from the market. More recently, recombinant tissue plasminogen activator (tPA) has proved effective for this purpose. When dealing with an occluded central venous catheter, adhering to a specific protocol will usually optimize results. Important points include these:

1 Kinking, twisting, and unrecognized clamping or displacement of the catheter should be carefully ruled out.
2 Occlusion is confirmed with alternating gentle aspiration and infusion ("push/pull") of 3 to 5 mL of saline.
3 Catheter lumen volume should be determined from manufacturer documentation (if possible) or estimated as follows:
   - <5.0 French catheter ≈ 0.5 mL
   - >5.0 French catheter ≈ 1.0 mL
   - Pediatric infusaport ≈ 1.0 mL
   - Adult infusaport ≈ 1.5 mL
   - PICC line ≈ 1.0 mL

4 A volume of tPa (2.0 mg/mL) equal to the volume of the lumen (plus 0.2 mL overfill) is gently instilled. The medication is allowed to dwell in the clamped catheter for 30 to 60 minutes.

5 For completely occluded catheters, partial instillation with release after 10 to 15 minutes, followed by reinstillation of progressively increasing volumes up to the appropriate amount, may be successful in opening the lumen.

Infection

Vascular catheters, like other prosthetic devices, are prone to bacterial colonization, which in some cases leads to a true infection. Infectious complications include cellulitis at the entry site, thrombophlebitis of the peripheral veins, bacteremia, sepsis, and metastatic infections (endocarditis, abscess, etc.). These nosocomial infections are an important cause of morbidity and mortality and greatly increase the cost of care in hospitalized adults and children (61–64). It is likely that over 250,000 catheter-associated infections occur in the United States each year, with about 80,000 occurring in ICU settings (32,62). Mortality estimates vary but range from 12% to 25%, making this a major problem of modern health care (64,65). The overall annual cost of these infections may be

as much as $2.3 billion, or approximately $50,000 per occurrence (66). In our multidisciplinary PICU, we observed an incremental cost of $50,383 per infection and a median cost for PICU hospitalization among patients who had this complication that was almost double the cost for those who did not (63).

The CDC recommends that the incidence of catheter infections be expressed as infections per catheter days. Using this metric, the overall incidence of catheter-related bloodstream infection is approximately one infection per 5.3 catheter days in ICU patients (62), although this rate can vary greatly depending on the patient population and use of the catheter. When duration of catheter placement is considered, there is a steep increase in infection rate for catheters in place longer than 7 days.

Mechanisms of catheter infection include (a) migration or pathogenic organisms colonizing the skin down the catheter from the insertion site, (b) contamination of the hub during catheter access, and, infrequently, (c) catheter colonization caused by hematogenous spread from a distant site. Not surprisingly, the organisms most commonly associated with catheter infection are those that colonize the skin of the patient and the care providers. Coagulase-negative staphylococci, *Staphylococcus aureus*, and enterocci are the most common agents, although Gram-negative organisms (e.g., *Klebsiella,*

 CLINICAL TIPS

▶ Ejecting a small volume of fluid from the entry needle after initial insertion through the skin will clear any skin plugs and facilitate aspiration of blood.

▶ The use of a small (3 to 5 mL) syringe to initially locate the vein will prevent collapse of the vessel, even with a small, hypovolemic child.

▶ If blood flow is not obtained after deep insertion of the entry needle, the needle should be slowly withdrawn while maintaining negative pressure on the syringe. If the vessel was inadvertently passed through, blood may be aspirated as the needle is withdrawn.

▶ In locating the central vessel, the entry needle should be inserted and withdrawn in a slow, methodical pattern in order to prevent multiple vein lacerations.

▶ Bright red blood and/or pulsatile flow indicate arterial puncture, although these findings may not be readily apparent when cardiac output is severely compromised. If there is any remaining question about whether the blood aspirated has a venous or arterial source, a specimen can be sent to the laboratory for blood gas analysis.

▶ Use of a non-Luer-Lok syringe prevents accidental dislodgment of the needle on removal of the syringe before insertion of the guide wire.

▶ After the syringe is removed from the entry needle, but before the guide wire is inserted, the hub of the needle should be occluded by a finger to prevent air embolus and/or blood loss.

▶ The operator must always ensure that the proximal end of the guide wire is secured at all times to prevent entry of the wire into the central circulation.

▶ If resistance is felt with removal of the guide wire through the needle, the wire and needle should be removed together in order to prevent shearing of the wire by the beveled tip of the needle.

▶ The catheter tip should not lie within the right atrium, since this may result in erosion and perforation of the atrial wall.

▶ To obtain an accurate reading using a central venous pressure monitor, the transducer reference point must first be set by zeroing to the midaxillary line with the patient supine (i.e., zeroing to the level of the heart).

Pseudomonas) and *Candida* also occur regularly. Each hospital should have a surveillance program to help track local common organisms and antibiotic sensitivities. Colonizing bacteria attach to the thin layer of fibrin that covers the surface of all vascular catheters shortly after placement. While this fibrin layer allows the patient's system to tolerate the foreign material, it may also inhibit immunologic defenses. Some bacteria have the ability to generate a protective covering of slime that can impede immunologic recognition and attack by host

defenses and provides a barrier to antibiotics. The presence or absence of mural thrombosis also affects the incidence of infection.

The site of catheter placement appears to be a significant determinant in the occurrence of infection among adult patients, with femoral catheters having the highest likelihood of infection. However, the importance of this factor with regard to children is less clear. Currently, the CDC guidelines recommend that the preferred order for site selection when

TABLE 19.7	CDC GUIDELINES FOR MINIMIZING THE RISK OF CVC INFECTION
Quality assurance and continuing education	A balance between patient safety and cost-effectiveness.
	The risk for infection declines following standardization of aseptic care.
	Insertion and maintenance of intravascular catheters by inexperienced staff increase the risk for catheter colonization and CRBSI.
	Specialized "I.V. teams" reduce the incidence of catheter-related infections.
	Infection risk increases when nurse-patient ratio is reduced.
Site of catheter insertion	The influence of site on the risk for catheter infections is related to the risk for thrombophlebitis and density of local skin flora, but no randomized trial has satisfactorily compared infection rates for catheters placed in jugular, subclavian, and femoral sites. In adults, femoral catheters have been demonstrated to have relatively high colonization rates, and catheters are associated with a higher risk for deep venous thrombosis than are internal jugular or subclavian catheters. Thus there is a presumption that such catheters are more likely to become infected. Studies in pediatric patients have demonstrated that femoral catheters have a low incidence of mechanical complications and might have an infection rate equivalent to that of nonfemoral catheters.
	Current best evidence for adult patients suggests that CVCs should be placed in a subclavian site instead of a jugular or femoral site to reduce the risk of infection. No order of preference exists for infants and young children.
Type of catheter material	Teflon or polyurethane catheters have been associated with fewer infectious complications than catheters made of polyvinyl chloride or polyethylene.
Hand hygiene and aseptic technique	Maximal sterile barrier precautions (e.g., cap, mask, sterile gown, sterile gloves, and large sterile drapes) during the insertion of CVCs substantially reduces the incidence of CRBSI compared with standard precautions (e.g., sterile gloves and small drapes).
Skin antisepsis	Acceptable antiseptic cleansing solutions include povidone-iodine, chlorhexidine gluconate, and 70% alcohol. Povidone-iodine is the most widely used antiseptic for cleaning arterial catheter and CVC-insertion sites. Recent evidence suggests that 2% chlorhexidine gluconate (but not other preparations of chlorhexidine) may be superior to povidone-iodine and 70% alcohol.
Catheter site dressing regimens	Acceptable dressings include transparent polyurethane adhesive dressings and standard gauze and tape dressings. The transparent dressings help secure the device, permit continuous visual inspection of the catheter site, permit careful bathing, and require less frequent changes than do gauze and tape.
	If blood is oozing from the catheter insertion site, gauze dressing might be preferred.
	Chlorhexidine-impregnated sponge (Biopatch) placed over the site of short-term arterial and central venous cannulation may reduce the risk for catheter colonization and CRBSI.
Catheter securement devices	Securement with sutures or sutureless devices is acceptable. Data are inadequate to recommend one system over the other in relation to infection risk.
In-line filters	In-line filters reduce the incidence of infusion-related phlebitis, but no data support their efficacy in preventing infections associated with intravascular catheters and infusion systems.
Antimicrobial- or antiseptic-impregnated catheters and cuffs	Limited data suggest some value in but also some risks from antimicrobial-impregnated catheters. All of the studies have been conducted in adults; however, these catheters have been approved by the FDA for use in patients weighing ≥ 3 kg.
	Chlorhexidine/silver sulfadiazine. Current evidence suggests surface covering with chlorhexidine/silver sulfadiazine reduces the risk of CRBSI compared with standard noncoated catheters. The benefit for the patients who receive these catheters will be realized within the first 14 days.
	Minocycline/rifampin. CVCs impregnated on both the external and internal surfaces with minocycline/rifampin are available, and limited data suggest use is associated with lower rates of CRBSI. The beneficial effect began after day 6 of catheterization. However, in vitro data indicate that these impregnated catheters could increase the incidence of minocycline and rifampin resistance among pathogens, especially staphylococci. The half-life of antimicrobial activity against *Staphylococcus epidermidis* is 25 days with catheters coated with minocycline/rifampin, compared with 3 days for the first-generation catheters coated with chlorhexidine/silver sulfadiazine in vitro.
	Platinum/silver. Recently approved by the FDA for use in the United States, but no published studies have been presented to support an antimicrobial effect.
Antimicrobial ointments at the dressing site	Mupirocin ointment applied at the insertion sites of CVCs may reduce the incidence of CRBSI but may increase mupirocin-resistant organisms and may reduce the integrity of polyurethane catheters.
	Other antibiotic ointments applied to the catheter insertion site also have been studied and have yielded conflicting results.
	Any ointment that is applied to the catheter insertion site should be checked against the catheter and ointment manufacturers' recommendations regarding compatibility.
Antibiotic lock prophylaxis	This practice has been studied in immunocompromised patients with conflicting results. Current evidence does not support this practice for routine application.
Anticoagulants	Anticoagulant flush solutions are used widely to prevent catheter thrombosis and thrombi, and fibrin deposits on catheters might serve as a nidus for microbial colonization of intravascular catheters. However, current evidence does not suggest the incidence of CRBSI is reduced through the use of heparin flush solution or the treatment of the patient with warfarin.

CRBSI, catheter-related bloodstream infection.

performing CVC to minimize catheter infection is (a) sub-clavian, (b) jugular, and (c) femoral. Yet studies that compare infection rate with insertion site in children do not demonstrate differences that support preferential site selection (32). Clinical judgment may indicate that other factors (acuity of illness, likelihood of success, etc.) may take precedence over this consideration in the management of a critically ill pediatric patient. Strategies to reduce infection are multifactorial and include aspects related to catheter materials, site selection, placement procedure, and catheter dressing and care. A summary of recent CDC consensus recommendations is provided in Table 19.7.

▶ SUMMARY

Although CVC is more commonly performed in adult patients, obtaining access to the central circulation for the purpose of administering fluids, medications, blood products, etc., can be a life-saving intervention for pediatric patients in the ED and other acute care settings. Multiple potential anatomic locations are available for performing CVC, but the site used most commonly for younger children remains the proximal femoral vein at the groin. For "adult-sized" adolescents, infectious concerns may prompt the operator to choose the subclavian or jugular entry sites instead. Knowledge of the anatomy, placement technique, catheter materials, and complications associated with this procedure, as well as the risk-benefit balance, is imperative for the physician performing CVC in this population. Clinical experience, coupled with the efforts of manufacturers and researchers, continues to advance the technology underlying the use of these procedures. The ongoing development of new catheter systems and materials will likely enhance both the safety and clinical application of CVC for pediatric patients.

▶ REFERENCES

1. Smith RA, Mallory DL, Wilson GI, et al. Vascular access: past, present, and future. *Probl Crit Care.* 1988;2:199–216.
2. Kalso E. A short history of central venous catheterization. *Acta Anaesthesiol Scand.* 1985;81(suppl):7–10.
3. Cobb LM, Vincour CD, Wagner CW, et al. The central venous anatomy in infants. *Surg Gynecol Obstet.* 1987;165:230–234.
4. Tribett D, Brenner M. Peripheral and femoral vein cannulation. *Probl Crit Care.* 1988;2:266–285.
5. McGee WT, Mallory DL. Cannulations of the internal and external jugular veins. *Probl Crit Care.* 1988;2:217–241.
6. Novak RA, Venus B. Clavicular approaches for central vein cannulation. *Probl Crit Care.* 1988;2:242–265.
7. Nicolson SC, Sweeney MF, Moore RA, et al. Comparison of internal and external jugular cannulation of the central circulation in the pediatric patient. *Crit Care Med.* 1985;13:747–749.
8. Belani KG, Buckley JJ, Gordon JR, et al. Percutaneous cervical central venous line placement: a comparison of the internal and external jugular vein routes. *Anesth Analg.* 1980;59:40–44.
9. Cote CJ, Jobes DR, Schwartz AJ, et al. Two approaches to cannulation of a child's internal jugular vein. *Anaesthesia.* 1979;50:371–373.
10. Venkataraman ST, Orr RA, Thompson AW. Percutaneous infraclavicular subclavian vein catheterization in critically ill infants and children. *J Pediatr.* 1988;112:480–485.
11. Kant RK, Zimmerman JJ, Strauss RH. Central venous catheter insertion by femoral vein: safety and effectiveness for the pediatric patient. *Pediatrics.* 1986;77:842–847.
12. Swanson RS, Uhlig PN, Gross PL, et al. Emergency intravenous access through the femoral vein. *Ann Emerg Med.* 1984;13:243–247.
13. Habal M. The biologic basis for the clinical application of the silicones. *Arch Surg.* 1984;119:843–848.
14. Gingles B. Personal communication. Cooke Critical Care, Bloomington, IN; 1994.
15. DiCostanzo J, Sastre B, Choux R, et al. Mechanism of thrombogenesis during total parenteral nutrition: role of catheter composition. *J Parenter Enteral Nutr.* 1988;12:190–194.
16. Welch GW, McKeel DW Jr, Silverstein P, et al. The role of catheter composition in the development of thrombophlebitis. *Surg Gynecol Obstet.* 1974;138:421–424.
17. Larm O, Lins LE, Olsson P. An approach to antithrombosis by surface modification. *Prog Artif Organs.* 1985;2:313–318.
18. Hutyra J, Bunegin L, Albin MS. Evaluation of pressure recording characteristics of silicone elastomer polyurethane, and polyethylene catheters [abstract]. *Crit Care Med.* 1987;15:384.
19. Linder LE, Curelaru I, Gustavsson B, et al. Material thrombogenicity in central venous catheterization: a comparison between soft, antebrachial catheters of silicone elastomer and polyurethane. *J Parenter Enteral Nutr.* 1984;8:399–406.
20. Idris AH, Melker RJ. High-flow sheaths for pediatric fluid resuscitation: a comparison of flow rates with standard pediatric catheters. *Pediatr Emerg Care.* 1992;8:119–122.
21. Hodge D, Fleisher G. Pediatric catheter flow rates. *Am J Emerg Med.* 1985;3:403–407.
22. Hodge D, Delgado-Paredes C, Fleisher G. Central and peripheral catheter flow rates in "pediatric" dogs. *Ann Emerg Med.* 1986;15:1151–1154.
23. Mateer JR, Thompson BM, Aprahamian C, et al. Rapid fluid resuscitation with central venous catheters. *Ann Emerg Med.* 1983;12:149–152.
24. Rosen KR, Rosen DA. Comparative flow rates for small bore peripheral intravenous catheters. *Pediatr Emerg Care.* 1986;2:153–156.
25. Spivey WH, Lather CM, Malone DR, et al. Comparison of intraosseous, central, and peripheral routes of sodium bicarbonate administration during CPR in pigs. *Ann Emerg Med.* 1985;14:1135–1140.
26. Lin BS, Kong CW, Tarng DC, et al. Anatomical variation of the internal jugular vein and its impact on temporary haemodialysis vascular access: an ultrasonographic survey in uraemic patients. *Nephrol Dial Transplant.* 1998;47:134–138.
27. Caridi JG, Hawkins IF Jr, Wiechmann BN, et al. Sonographic guidance when using the right internal jugular vein for central vein access. *AJR Am J Roentgenol.* 1998;171:1259–1263.
28. Hoffman KK, Weber DJ, Samsa GP, et al. Transparent polyurethane film as an intravenous catheter dressing. *JAMA.* 1992;267:2072–2076.
29. Madeo M, Martin CR, Turner C, et al. A randomized trial comparing Arglaes (a transparent dressing containing silver ions) to Tegaderm (a transparent polyurethane dressing) for dressing peripheral arterial catheters and central vascular catheters. *Intensive Crit Care Nurs.* 1998;14:187–191.
30. Maki DG, Ringer M. Evaluation of dressing regimens for prevention of infection and peripheral intravenous catheters. *JAMA.* 1987;258:2396–2403.
31. Freiberger D, Bryant J, Marino B. The effect of different central venous line dressing changes on bacterial growth in a pediatric oncology population. *J Pediatr Oncol Nurs.* 1992;9:3–7.

32. O'Grady NP, Alexander M, Dellinger EP, et al. Guidelines for the prevention of intravascular catheter-related infections. Centers for Disease Control and Prevention. *MMWR Recomm Rep.* 2002;51(RR10):1–26. www.cdc.gov/mmwr/preview/mmwrhtml/rr5110a1.htm. Accessed June 7, 2005.

33. Bijma R, Girbes AR, Kleijer DJ, et al. Preventing central venous catheter-related infection in a surgical intensive-care unit. *Infect Control Hosp Epidemiol.* 1999;20:618–620.

34. Rasero L, Degl'Innocenti M, Mocali M, et al. Comparison of two different time interval protocols for central venous catheter dressing in bone marrow transplant patients: results of a randomized, multicenter study. *Haematologica.* 2000;85:275–279.

35. Maki DG, Stolz SS, Wheeler S, et al. A prospective, randomized trial of gauze and two polyurethane dressings for site care of pulmonary artery catheters: implications for catheter management. *Crit Care Med.* 1994;22:1729–1737.

36. Vicari M, Sweeker M. Care of venous cannulas. *Problems Crit Care.* 1988;2:314–323.

37. Maki DG, Ringer M. Evaluation of dressing regimens for prevention of infection with peripheral intravenous catheters: gauze, a transparent polyurethane dressing, and an iodophor-transparent dressing. *JAMA.* 1987;258:2396–2403.

38. Sitges-Serra A, Linares J, Perez JL, et al. Hub colonization as the initial step in an outbreak of catheter-treated sepsis due to coagulase-negative staphylococci during parenteral nutrition. *J Parenter Enteral Nutr.* 1984;8:668–672.

39. Maki DG, Ringer M. Evaluations of dressing regimens for prevention of infection with peripheral intravenous catheters. *JAMA.* 1987;258:2396–2403.

40. Viall CD. Your complete guide to central venous catheters. *Nursing.* 1990;2:35–41.

41. Hoffman KK, Weber DJ, Sama GP, et al. Transparent polyurethane film as an intravenous catheter dressing. *JAMA.* 1992;267:2072–2076.

42. Williams JF, Seneff MG, Friedman BC, et al. Use of femoral venous catheters in critically ill adults: prospective study. *Crit Care Med.* 1991;19:550–553.

43. Kanter RK, Zimmerman JJ, Strauss RH, et al. Central venous catheter insertion by femoral vein: safety and effectiveness for the pediatric patient. *Pediatrics.* 1986;77:842–847.

44. Swansons RS, Uhlig PN, Gross PL, et al. Emergency intravenous access through the femoral vein. *Ann Emerg Med.* 1984;77:842–847.

45. Kanter RK, Zimmerman JJ, Strauss RH, et al. Pediatric emergency intravenous access. *Am J Dis Child.* 1986;140:132–134.

46. Groff DB, Ahmen N. Subclavian vein catheterization in the infant. *J Pediatr Surg.* 1974;9:171–174.

47. Irwin G, Fifield G, Clinton J. Emergency catheterization of the superior vena cava in pediatric patients. *Am J Emerg Med.* 1984;2:494–496.

48. Scott WL. Complications associated with central venous catheters. *Chest.* 1988;94:1221–1224.

49. Langston CS. The aberrant central venous catheter and its complications. *Radiology.* 1971;10:55–59.

50. Walters MB, Stanger HA, Rotem CE. Complications with percutaneous central venous catheters. *JAMA.* 1972;220:1455–1457.

51. McGee WT, Ackerman BL, Rouben LR, et al. Accurate placement of central venous catheters: a prospective, randomized, multicenter trial. *Crit Care Med.* 1993;21:1118–1123.

52. Sheep RE, Guiney WB. Fatal cardiac tamponade. *JAMA.* 1982;258:1632–1635.

53. Grisoni ER, Mehta SK, Connors AF, Thrombosis and infection complicating central venous catheterization in neonates. *J Pediatr Surg.* 1986;21:772–776.

54. Sitzman JV, Townsend TR, Siler MC, et al. Septic and technical complications of central venous catheterization: a prospective study of 200 consecutive patients. *Ann Surg.* 1985;202:766–770.

55. Torramade JR, Cienfuegos JA, Hernandez JL, et al. The complications of central venous access systems: a study of 218 patients. *Eur J Surg.* 1993;159:323–327.

56. Stenzel JP, Green TP, Fuhrman BP, et al. Percutaneous central venous catheterization in a pediatric intensive care unit: a survival analysis of complications. *Crit Care Med.* 1989;17:984–988.

57. Scott WL. *Central Venous Catheter Complications.* Rockville, MD: U.S. Food and Drug Administration, Center for Devices and Radiologic Health, Office of Training and Assistance; 1994. Publication HFZ-250.

58. Goutail-Flaud MP, Sfez M, Berg A, et al. Central venous catheter-related complications in newborns and infants: a 587 case survey. *J Pediatr Surg.* 1991;26:645–650.

59. Eisenhauer ED, Derveloy RJ, Hatings PR. Prospective evaluation of central venous pressure (CVP) catheters in a large city-county hospital. *Ann Surg.* 1982:196:560–564.

60. Ross P, Ehrenkranz R, Kleinman CS, et al. Thrombus associated with central venous catheters in infants and children. *J Pediatr Surg.* 1989;24:253–256.

61. Centers for Disease Control Working Group. Guidelines for prevention of intravenous therapy-related infections. *Infect Control.* 1982;4:472–473.

62. CDC. National Nosocomial Infections Surveillance (NNIS) System report, data summary from October 1986–April 1998, issued June 1998. *Am J Infect Control.* 1998;26:522–533.

63. Dominguez T, Chalom R, Costarino A. The impact of adverse patient occurrences on hospital costs. *Crit Care Med.* 2001;29:169–175.

64. Rello J, Ochagavia A, Sabanes E, et al. Evaluation of outcome of intravenous catheter-related infections in critically ill patients. *Am J Respir Crit Care Med.* 2000;162:1027–1030.

65. Soufir L, Timsit JF, Mahe C, et al. Attributable morbidity and mortality of catheter-related septicemia in critically ill patients: a matched, risk-adjusted, cohort study. *Infect Control Hosp Epidemiol.* 1999;20:396–401.

66. Digiovine B, Chenoweth C, Watts C, et al. The attributable mortality and costs of primary nosocomial bloodstream infections in the intensive care unit. *Am J Respir Crit Care Med.* 1999;160:976–981.

67. Zakrzewska-Bode A, Muytjens HL, Liem KD, et al. Mupirocin resistance in coagulase-negative staphylococci, after topical prophylaxis for the reduction of colonization of central venous catheters. *J Hosp Infect.* 1995;31:189–193.

68. Flowers RH, Schwenzer KJ, Kopel RF, et al. Efficacy of an attachable subcutaneous cuff for the prevention of intravascular catheter-related infection: a randomized, controlled trial. *JAMA.* 1989;261:878–883.

69. Robbins J, Cromwell P, Korones DN. Swimming and central venous catheter-related infections in the child with cancer. *J Pediatr Oncol Nurs.* 1999;16:51–56.

70. Howell PB, Walters PE, Donowitz GR, et al. Risk factors for infection of adult patients with cancer who have tunneled central venous catheters. *Cancer.* 1995;75:1367–1375.

71. Stenzel JP, Green TP, Fuhrman BP, et al. Percutaneous femoral venous catheterizations: a prospective study of complications. *J Pediatr.* 1989;114:411–415.

ROBERT J. VINCI

20

Venous Cutdown Catheterization

▶ INTRODUCTION

Obtaining vascular access is an integral component of pediatric resuscitation. It allows for the emergency administration of fluids, blood products, and pharmacologic agents required for treatment and stabilization of the acutely ill patient. In 1945, Kirkham first described the technique for saphenous vein cutdown, and through the years other anatomic locations have been demonstrated as possible sites for performing emergency venous cutdown (1,2). Although recent advances such as percutaneous central venous cannulation (see Chapter 19) and intraosseous infusion (see Chapter 21) have diminished the role of venous cutdown, it remains an important option for emergency vascular access in the critically ill or injured pediatric patient (3).

Venous cutdown catheterization is most often indicated for infants and young children, especially in the face of hypovolemia. Clinicians can take advantage of a number of possible anatomic sites, although once the vein is identified, the technique for performing a venous cutdown is similar regardless of which site is used. A venous cutdown is best reserved for the hospital setting because of the time required and the expertise needed to perform the procedure. This procedure is generally performed by emergency physicians, critical care specialists, and surgeons.

▶ ANATOMY AND PHYSIOLOGY

Venous Anatomy and External Landmarks

Distal Saphenous Vein at the Ankle

The distal saphenous vein is the most common site for a venous cutdown. Located just anterior and superior to the medial malleolus, the saphenous vein courses adjacent to the periosteum along the medial aspect of the ankle (Fig. 20.1). After the initial skin incision, blunt dissection is usually all that is necessary to locate the saphenous vein (see "Procedure"). The saphenous nerve travels adjacent to the vein and can be confused with the vein, especially when the vein is constricted due to hypovolemia. While the position of the saphenous vein remains constant regardless of age, the diameter of the vessel varies greatly, which has implications for the size of the catheter chosen for vascular access.

Proximal Saphenous Vein at the Groin

In its proximal location, the saphenous vein lies medial to the femoral vein as it courses toward the inguinal region. It passes through the fascia lata of the thigh, where it enters the femoral vein approximately 2 to 3 cm distal to the inguinal ligament. In its proximal location, the saphenous vein can be isolated by using the landmark demarcated by the junction of the thigh with the lateral margin of the labial or scrotal folds (Fig. 20.2). The operator must be careful not to enter the femoral sheath during the procedure so that injury to the adjacent neurovascular structures is avoided. The advantage of the saphenous cutdown at the groin is that the increased diameter of the vessel allows for a larger-bore catheter than does the saphenous vein at the ankle. This is especially useful when rapid infusion of intravenous fluid is required (4,5).

Basilic Vein

The basilic vein is a superficial vessel located just proximal to the flexor crease of the elbow (Fig. 20.3). While the distal portion of the basilic vein originates in the medial aspect of the hand, the vessel diameter is too small in this distal location to be clinically useful for cutdown. However, above the elbow the basilic vein is joined by the median cubital vein and is accessible to dissection and subsequent venotomy. It can be isolated as it courses between the tendons of the biceps and

273

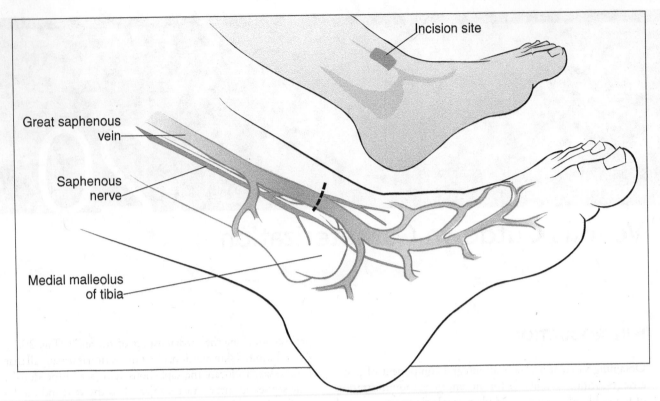

Figure 20.1 Distal saphenous vein cutdown site.

pronator muscle groups. The median cutaneous nerve of the forearm is often found adjacent to the basilic vein; it should be identified in order to avoid injury to this nerve and potential impairment of sensation over the medial forearm.

Axillary Vein

Isolation of the axillary vein has been described in newborns as another site for venous cutdown (6). The axillary vein of the proximal arm is situated within the axillary sheath as it traverses the inferior surface of the axilla. To localize the axillary vein, a transverse incision can be performed along the midaxillary line in the deepest skin fold of the axilla. Blunt dissection is then performed to extend the incision to the axillary sheath (Fig. 20.4). The axillary sheath encloses the axillary artery and vein as well as the roots of the brachial plexus. Because of these contiguous major neurovascular structures, a cutdown of the axillary vein is associated with a high complication rate and should only be attempted by experienced clinicians.

Circulatory Physiology

A detailed description of the physiologic effects of the shock state on pediatric patients can be found in Chapter 12. Hypovolemia, tissue hypoxia, and metabolic acidosis are commonly seen in the acutely ill or traumatized pediatric patient. Compensatory mechanisms maintain cardiac output by shunting blood away from nonvital organs, producing counter-regulatory hormones, and buffering lactic acid resulting from cellular anaerobic metabolism. Profound vasocon-

striction, particularly when combined with volume depletion (e.g., dehydration, blood loss), can make timely percutaneous vascular access difficult or impossible for the pediatric patient in shock. A properly performed venous cutdown will allow for the rapid volume expansion required to restore vascular tone. It also provides entry into the venous circulation for the pharmacologic treatment of the critically ill child.

▶ INDICATIONS

Percutaneous peripheral venous cannulation (see Chapter 73) is normally the procedure of choice when venous access is needed in a pediatric patient. However, acute hypovolemia and acidosis can produce extreme peripheral vasoconstriction, which may make it impossible to cannulate a peripheral vein during a resuscitation. Although an array of vascular procedures (including central venous cannulation and insertion of an intraosseous line) may be initially attempted, performing a venous cutdown remains a viable therapeutic option. This is especially true when other methods are unsuccessful or contraindicated. For example, venous cutdown catheterization is superior to intraosseous infusion with regard to rapid administration of intravenous volume, and a venous cutdown catheterization may prove easier to accomplish than central venous cannulation in certain cases. Consequently, it is imperative to develop clear written guidelines that delineate the protocol and sequence of vascular procedures during a pediatric

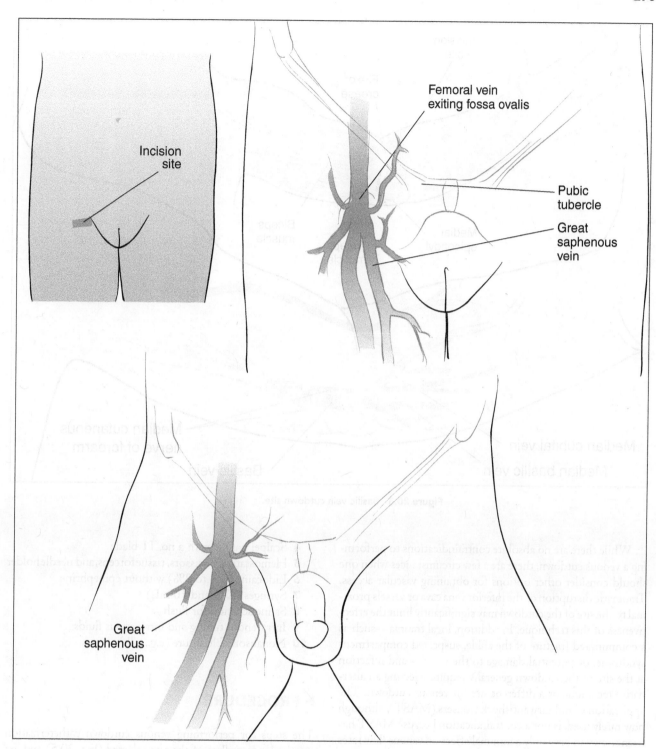

Figure 20.2 Proximal saphenous vein cutdown site.

resuscitation to ensure that a venous cutdown is properly utilized for the patient requiring emergent vascular access (5).

Peripheral vein cutdown is warranted in any situation that requires rapid volume expansion or treatment of metabolic derangements commonly seen in the acutely ill child. Hypovolemic shock from severe gastroenteritis, thermal burns, or metabolic disorders such as diabetes mellitus require prompt restoration of circulating blood volume. Additionally, acute

blood loss from blunt or penetrating trauma and acute hemorrhage secondary to bleeding diathesis, gastric ulcer, and inflammatory bowel disease may warrant emergency vascular access. Patients with overwhelming infection, sepsis, and cardiopulmonary failure may also require a venous cutdown for emergency treatment. Finally, in selected situations a venous cutdown may be indicated for the ongoing stabilization of a patient or in preparation for interfacility transport.

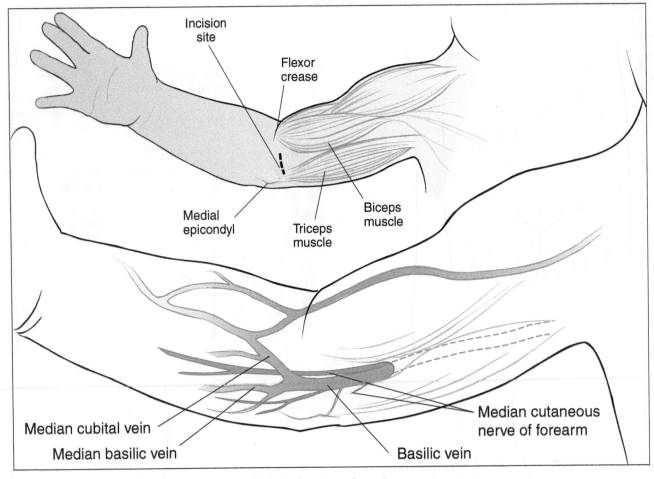

Figure 20.3 Basilic vein cutdown site.

While there are no absolute contraindications to performing a venous cutdown, there are a few circumstances when one should consider other options for obtaining vascular access. Traumatic disruption of the inferior vena cava or vessels proximal to the site of the cutdown may significantly limit the effectiveness of this technique. In addition, local trauma—such as a comminuted fracture of the ankle, suspected compartment syndrome, or potential damage to the vessel—and infection at the site of the cutdown generally require selecting an alternative technique or a different site for venous cutdown. The application of military antishock trousers (MAST), although now rarely used, is not a contraindication because MAST has been shown to have only a minimal effect on venous flow rates from a distal saphenous cutdown.

▶ EQUIPMENT

1 Sterile drapes, dressings, gloves, face shields, and 4″ × 4″ sponges
2 1% Betadine solution or surgical scrub
3 Intravenous catheters (14 to 22 gauge) or CVP catheters (3.0 to 8.0 French)

4 Scalpel handle with a no. 11 blade
5 Hemostats, iris scissors, tissue forceps, and needle holder
6 Lidocaine (1% to 2%) without epinephrine
7 Syringes (3, 5, and 10 mL)
8 Saline solution for flush
9 Intravenous tubing and intravenous fluids
10 Nonabsorbable suture (e.g., silk)

▶ PROCEDURE

The steps for performing venous cutdown catheterization are similar regardless of the site selected (Fig. 20.5) and are summarized in the following description of the procedure at the most commonly used site, the saphenous vein at the ankle. Specific aspects of the procedure relevant to all the individual approaches are also described in this section.

Saphenous Vein at the Ankle

The ankle should be positioned with lateral deviation of the foot to provide maximum exposure of the medial malleolus.

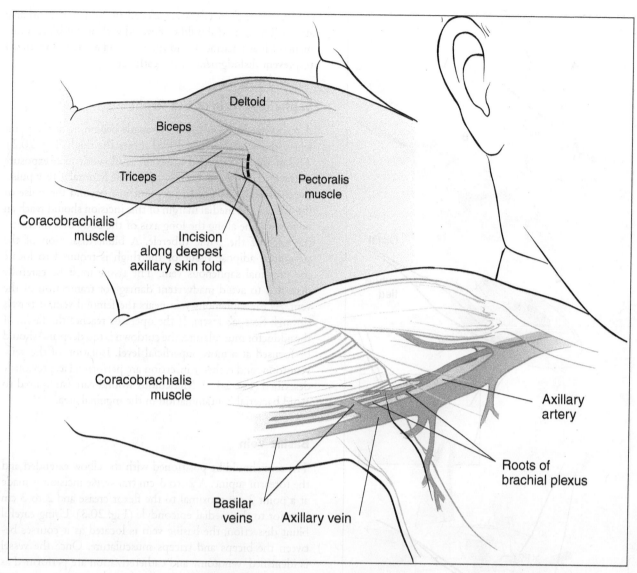

Figure 20.4 Axillary vein cutdown site.

In the awake patient, the foot and lower leg should be restrained to prevent movement. Care must be taken to avoid constricting dressings that may inhibit venous flow. The area is scrubbed with 1% Betadine solution or surgical scrub, and the field is surrounded with sterile drapes. The site for the skin incision is identified by drawing a line 1 cm superior and anterior to the medial malleolus (Fig. 20.1). A 1- to 2-cm transverse incision should be made beginning 1 cm superior to the medial malleolus just posterior to the anterior margin of the bone (Fig. 20.5A). For the child under 1 year of age, a 1-cm incision is often sufficient to locate the vein. The subcutaneous tissue and fat should be separated with a pair of curved forceps (Fig. 20.5B). While keeping the forceps parallel to the incision with the curved edge facing upward (toward the skin edge), the operator advances the forceps until contact is made with the tibia. The tissue is elevated and separated from the anterior tibia until the saphenous vein is located. Blunt dissection is continued until the vein is isolated and sepa-

rated from the surrounding tissue and the saphenous nerve. A nonabsorbable suture (e.g., silk) is placed beneath the vein, and the loop of the suture is grasped with a pair of forceps. After pulling the suture beneath the vein, the operator cuts the loop to form two ligatures extending around the vessel. The distal suture is then tied (Fig. 20.5C). Using the proximal suture to elevate the vessel, the operator makes a small nick (venotomy) in the vessel, through which the catheter is inserted (Figs. 20.5D and 20.5E). Alternatively, the operator may choose to insert a catheter over a needle without incising the vessel in a manner similar to placing a standard percutaneous intravenous line. A syringe attached to the catheter is aspirated to determine proper placement within the vessel. With infants or small children, the operator may not see significant blood return with aspiration. If this is the case, he or she can attempt infusion of fluid and check for any leakage or soft-tissue swelling. The catheter is secured in place by tying the proximal suture around the vessel and catheter

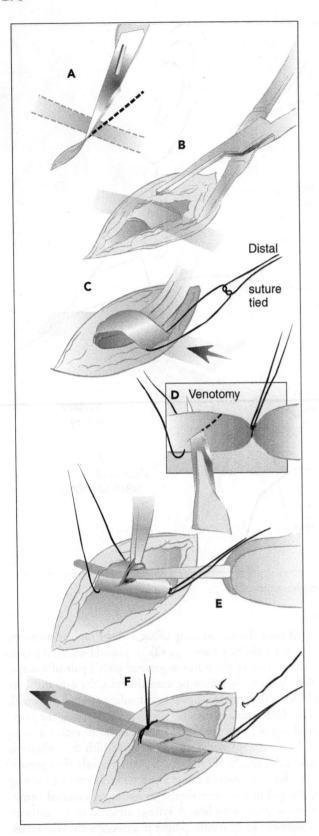

(Fig. 20.5F). Skin edges are closed using a nonabsorbable suture. The wound should be covered with an antibiotic ointment such as bacitracin, and the foot and ankle immobilized to prevent dislodgment of the catheter.

Saphenous Vein at the Groin

A transverse incision should be made beginning at the point where the scrotal or labial fold meets the thigh (Fig. 20.2). This incision is extended 4 to 6 cm to allow adequate exposure of the area. If the patient has a palpable femoral artery pulse, the incision is extended to a point just beyond the pulse of the artery. The medial margin of this incision should reach an imaginary line along the long axis of the body that intersects the edge of the pubic tubercle. A blunt dissection of the superficial adipose tissue of the thigh is required to locate the proximal saphenous vein. The tissue must be carefully dissected to avoid inadvertent damage or transection of the vein. As the saphenous vein nears the femoral vein, it travels through Scarpa's fascia. If the operator reaches the fascia of the adductor musculature, the cutdown is too deep and should be focused at a more superficial level. Isolation of the vein, venotomy, and catheter insertion are performed as previously described (Fig. 20.5). Meticulous wound care is required to avoid bacterial contamination in the inguinal area.

Basilic Vein

The arm should be positioned with the elbow extended and the forearm supine. A 2- to 3-cm transverse incision is made at a point 2 cm proximal to the flexor crease and 2 to 3 cm anterior to the medial epicondyle (Fig. 20.3). Using careful blunt dissection, the basilic vein is located as it courses between the biceps and triceps musculature. Once the vessel is identified, venotomy and catheterization are performed as described previously (Fig. 20.5).

Axillary Vein

The arm should be extended and abducted, with care taken to provide proper restraint. For the awake patient, local anesthetic

---

Figure 20.5 Procedure for venous cutdown catheterization.
A. A transverse incision is made at the appropriate site. The incision should extend into the subcutaneous tissue but not deep enough to potentially lacerate the vein.
B. The vein is isolated using blunt dissection. A suture is passed around the vein and cut to give two ligatures.
C. The distal suture is tied and used to stabilize the vessel.
D. Venotomy is performed to allow insertion of the catheter. Alternatively, the operator may choose to insert the catheter over a needle without performing a venotomy, in a manner similar to percutaneous catheterization.
E. The catheter is inserted into the vein. Placement within the vessel is confirmed by aspirating blood or infusing fluid.
F. The proximal suture is tied and the wound is closed and dressed.

SUMMARY: VENOUS CUTDOWN CATHETERIZATION AT THE DISTAL SAPHENOUS VEIN

1 Scrub the medial malleolus and surrounding area with aseptic solution.

2 Make 1- to 2-cm skin incision beginning 1 cm superior to the medial malleolus and just posterior to the anterior margin of the bone.

3 Bluntly dissect the subcutaneous tissue and fat with a curved forceps.

4 Identify the saphenous vein and gently separate it from the surrounding tissue.

5 Insert the loop of nonabsorbable suture around vessel and then cut the loop so two ligatures are formed.

6 Tie off the distal portion of the vessel.

7 Lift the proximal suture to elevate the vessel and make a small venotomy incision.

8 Cannulate the vessel.

9 Tie a proximal suture around the catheter and vessel.

10 Close the skin with a nonabsorbable suture.

11 Stabilize cutdown site.

should be infiltrated along the midaxillary line in the deepest skin fold of the axilla. A small transverse incision should be made at this site, and gentle blunt dissection is utilized to identify the axillary sheath (Fig. 20.4). The axillary sheath is a neurovascular bundle that contains the great nerves and vessels of the arm. The axillary artery is the deepest structure within the axillary sheath, and its pulsation can be used to help locate the axillary vein.

SUMMARY: VENOUS CUTDOWN CATHETERIZATION AT THE PROXIMAL SAPHENOUS VEIN

1 Begin a 4- to 6-cm transverse incision at the point where the scrotal or labial fold meets the thigh.

2 Use blunt dissection of the adipose tissue to locate the proximal saphenous vein just distal to its junction with the femoral vein.

3 Isolate the vein and perform venotomy and catheter insertion as described for distal saphenous vein cutdown.

SUMMARY: VENOUS CUTDOWN CATHETERIZATION AT THE BASILIC VEIN

1 Position the arm so the elbow is extended and the forearm lies supine.

2 Make a 2- to 3-cm transverse incision just proximal to the flexor crease and anterior to the medial epicondyle.

3 Using careful blunt dissection, locate the basilic vein between the biceps and triceps muscles.

4 Isolate the vessel and perform venotomy and catheter insertion as described for distal saphenous vein cutdown.

The axillary sheath is released from its attachments and entered using a hemostat to perform blunt dissection so that the contents can be identified. The axillary vein is the most superficial and inferior structure and should be separated with blunt dissection to allow placement of sutures around the vessel. A venotomy is performed as described previously, although the distal end of the axillary vein is usually not ligated with a suture. Catheterization is performed as described (Fig. 20.5).

CLINICAL TIPS

▶ The most commonly used (and probably easiest) site for performing emergency venous cutdown catheterization is the distal saphenous vein at the ankle.

▶ After making the initial skin incision, the remainder of the cutdown should normally be performed using blunt dissection to avoid injury to nerves and vessels.

▶ Slipping a loop of nonabsorbable suture (e.g., silk) around the vessel and then cutting the loop forms both ligatures needed to perform the procedure in a single step.

▶ Once the ligatures are extended around the vessel, they can be used to more easily manipulate the vessel during venotomy and catheterization.

▶ A larger-diameter catheter (16 gauge or 18 gauge) should be used to maximize intravenous infusion.

SUMMARY: VENOUS CUTDOWN CATHETERIZATION AT THE AXILLARY VEIN

1 Extend and abduct the arm using restraint methods as necessary.

2 Make a small transverse incision along the deepest skin fold of the axilla and identify the axillary sheath with blunt dissection.

3 After isolating the axillary sheath, use blunt dissection with hemostat to enter the sheath and isolate the axillary vein

4 Separate the axillary vein by encircling it with a suture and perform venotomy and catheter insertion as described for distal saphenous vein cutdown (*note*: the distal end of the axillary vein is usually not ligated).

▶ COMPLICATIONS

Complications, although uncommon, can occur after any invasive vascular procedure such as a venous cutdown. Important safety measures to avoid complications are meticulous sterile technique and wound care as well as careful monitoring of the cutdown site over time. Common complications include such consequences of failed cannulation as hemorrhage, hematoma, and extravasation of intravenous fluids (3,7). Phlebitis may be associated with a venous cutdown, but this occurs most commonly after prolonged use of the site. Infection can present both as a localized soft-tissue infection (cellulitis) or as a suppurative phlebitis. Local injury to a contiguous structure such as an artery or a peripheral nerve can also occur, but this can generally be avoided with proper technique. Finally,

catheter-related sepsis, although less frequent than sepsis associated with a central venous line, has been reported as a complication of venous cutdown catheterization (8).

▶ SUMMARY

Emergency intravenous access is required for acute management and stabilization during medical or trauma resuscitation of pediatric patients. Venous cutdown catheterization at the saphenous vein in the ankle or groin, as well as the axillary and basilic veins, can be utilized to provide access to administer life-saving intravenous fluids, blood products, and medications. Clinicians responsible for the care of critically ill children should be familiar with at least one method of performing this procedure.

▶ REFERENCES

1. Kirkham JH. Infusion into the internal saphenous vein at the ankle. *Lancet.* 1945;2:815.
2. Wax PM, Talan DA. Advances in cutdown techniques. *Emerg Med Clin North Am.* 1989;7:65–82.
3. Stovroff M, Teague GW. Intravenous access in infants and children. *Pediatr Clin North Am.* 1998;45;6;1373–1393.
4. Rogers FB. Technical note: a quick and simple method of obtaining venous access in traumatic exsanguination. *J Trauma.* 1993;34:142–143.
5. *Advanced Trauma Life Support.* 7th ed. Chicago: American College of Surgeons; 2004.
6. Stephens BL, Lelli JL, Allen D. Silastic catheterization of the axillary vein in neonates: an alternative to the internal jugular vein. *J Pediatr Surg.* 1993;28:31–35.
7. McIntosh BB, Dulchavsky SA. Peripheral vascular cutdown. *Crit Care Clin.* 1992;8:807–818.
8. O'Grady NP, Alexander M, Dellinger EP, et al. Guidelines for the prevention of intravascular catheter-related infections. Centers for Disease Control and Prevention. *MMWR Recomm Rep.* 2002;51(RR10):1–26.

DEE HODGE, III

Intraosseous Infusion

21

▶ INTRODUCTION

After ensuring an adequate airway and providing adequate ventilation, assessing circulation and establishing vascular access are the next priorities in pediatric resuscitation. Traditional approaches to vascular access in children (peripheral catheters, central catheters, and cutdowns) may be difficult under any circumstances and may be almost impossible when vascular collapse is present. In one study of pediatric arrests, 24% of the patients required more than 10 minutes before vascular access was achieved (1). Intraosseous infusion is a rapid method of obtaining vascular access during critical situations. Intraosseous lines can be placed quickly and fluids and/or medications given rapidly via this route.

Intraosseous infusion is an old technique first developed during the 1930s as the preferred route of vascular access in children (2–4). With the advent of butterfly needles and plastic catheters during the 1950s and 1960s, the technique fell out of favor and was rarely if ever performed. The development of advanced pediatric life support interventions brought the need for a rapid, reliable method of vascular access. Intraosseous infusion has filled that need.

The technique is used in the prehospital, emergency department (ED), and hospital settings where critical intravenous access is necessary. The procedure is relatively straightforward and can be effectively performed by physicians, physician assistants, nurses, and paramedics (5–7). Intraosseous lines are most commonly placed in children under 3 years of age because this group usually represents the greatest challenge in obtaining vascular access; however, the technique may be used in any age group (8,9).

▶ ANATOMY AND PHYSIOLOGY

The marrow space of the long bones functions essentially as a noncollapsible vein (10). Blood flows from the venous sinusoids of the medullary cavity of the long bones to drain into a central venous canal. From the central canal, blood drains by nutrient or emissary veins into the central circulation (Fig. 21.1). Absorption from the medullary cavity of a long bone into the systemic circulation is rapid, although obviously slower than occurs with peripheral or central intravenous lines (3,11,12). Intraosseous flow rates are influenced by venous valves, venous tortuosity, venous pressure, and blood flow through the marrow cavity. The tibia and femur are the preferred sites, because the marrow cavity is well developed even in the neonatal period, and the limbs are readily accessible (13–15). Insertion at the proximal and distal tibia is generally easier than at the distal femur because there is less subcutaneous tissue overlying the bone (Fig. 21.2). To enter the distal femur, the needle must pass through the relatively bulky quadriceps femoris muscle. In addition, the bony cortex is thinner and more easily penetrated at the tibial sites.

Obtaining vascular access is generally more problematic for children than adults because of the small size of the vessels and the abundance of subcutaneous fat, both of which make identification of veins by palpation more difficult. With cardiopulmonary failure and other shock states, blood flow is shunted away from the periphery to supply vital organs. In the early stages of shock due to hypovolemia or pump failure, the blood pressure of a child is maintained by an increased heart rate and a marked increase in the peripheral vascular resistance (compensated shock). This is largely the result of sympathetic nervous system stimulation and circulating catecholamines. Preload is also enhanced by contraction of capacitance veins.

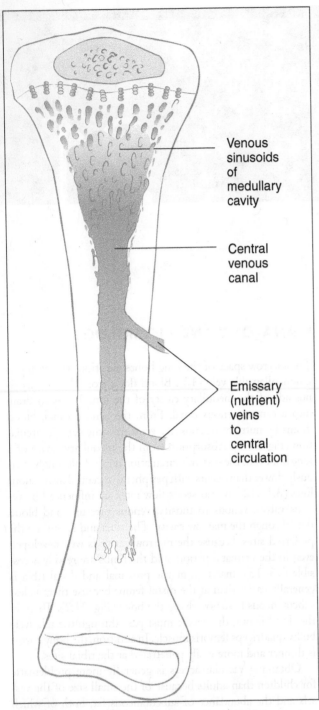

Figure 21.1 Venous drainage from the medullary cavity.

For the child in shock, this resulting vasoconstriction can sometimes make it impossible to obtain either peripheral or central vascular access within an acceptable time interval.

▶ INDICATIONS

Intraosseous infusion is indicated for those situations in which immediate vascular access is required, most often cardiopul-

monary arrest and shock (see also Chapters 19 and 73). Unlike the administration of medications, many of which can be given through the endotracheal tube or rectally, fluid volume can only be given via vascular access. Because the flow rates achieved are not sufficient to fully treat severe hypovolemic shock, this technique should not be considered to provide "definitive" access. Intraosseous access should therefore be attempted simultaneously with attempts at peripheral and central access. However, often after an initial bolus of fluid has been administered via an intraosseous line, the vessels are more prominent, and establishing peripheral or central access then becomes possible. The few absolute contraindications to this procedure include recent fractures in the bone to be used, osteogenesis imperfecta, and osteopetrosis. Cellulitis or an infected burn at the site of insertion are relative contraindications (11,13,16–18).

▶ EQUIPMENT

The equipment necessary for performing intraosseous infusion is listed in Table 21.1. Intraosseous needles are manufactured by several companies, with multiple designs incorporating the main desired features. It is useful to have regular in-service training sessions or "mock codes" during which the intraosseous needle is used so that ED personnel can become familiar with these features. Needles used for the procedure should have a trocar or some method to prevent bone from occluding the needle, a short shaft to prevent bending or displacement, and a hub to fit in the palm of the operator's hand during placement. A protective flange or a method to adjust the depth of penetration of the needle also affords some advantage (Jamshidi, Cook-Sussmane-Raszynski models). Some experts believe threaded needles (Cook-Sur-Fast model) that screw into the bone offer no significant advantage and have the potential drawback of not providing the "feel" of entering the marrow cavity (19). Newer pediatric devices include a "bone injection gun" (WaisMed, Caesarea, Israel), which employs a spring-loaded needle that is injected into the bone, as well as the EZ-IO (Vidacare, San Antonio, TX), a compact battery-powered drill with a threaded intraosseous needle. Povidone-iodine (Betadine) is needed for skin preparation, and gloves should be worn in observance of universal precautions (see Chapters 7 and 8). Lidocaine should be used for local anesthesia in awake patients.

▶ PROCEDURE

The most common sites used for insertion are the proximal tibia, the distal tibia, and the distal femur. The proximal tibia may be used in patients up to age 3 to 4 years. After this age, the patient's proximal tibia is more difficult to penetrate, and therefore the distal tibia should generally be used. To locate the proximal tibia site, the operator first identifies the anterior medial surface of the tibia and palpates the tibial tuberosity. The entry site is halfway between the

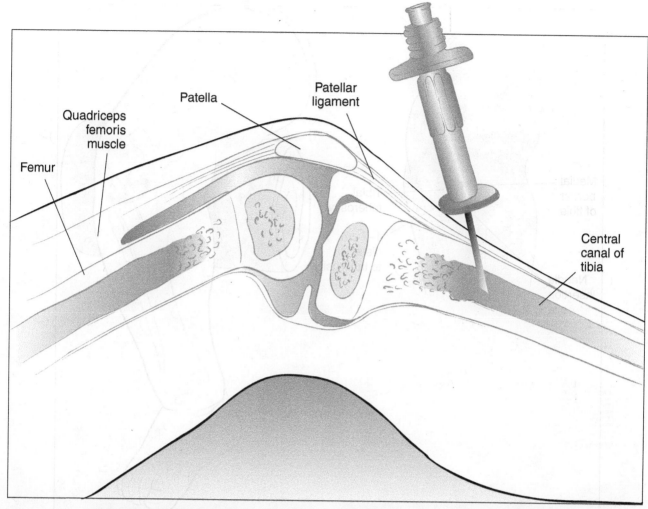

Figure 21.2 The proximal tibia is a preferred site for intraosseous needle insertion because there is little overlying soft tissue.

anterior and posterior border of the tibia and 1 to 2 cm distal to the tibial tuberosity (20) (Fig. 21.3). At the distal tibia, the site of insertion is located just proximal to the medial malleolus halfway between the anterior and posterior borders of the bone (Fig. 21.4). The distal femur is used as a secondary site in infants or when the operator fails to enter the tibia. The location of insertion is approximately 1 cm proximal to the femoral plateau (Fig. 21.5).

If the patient is alert, 1 to 2 mL of a local anesthetic should be injected into the skin and periosteum. After prep-

ping the skin with povidone-iodine, the operator stabilizes the leg and/or foot using the nondominant hand. The needle is oriented perpendicular to the bone or angled slightly away from the joint space during insertion. It is best to hold the intraosseous device so that the hub rests in the palm while the thumb and index finger are 1 to 2 cm from the tip of the needle (Fig. 21.6A). Gradually increasing pressure is applied with a back-and-forth rotational motion until the operator feels a sudden decrease in resistance ("trap-door effect") (Fig. 21.6B). The operator must take care not to insert the needle with the tip angled into the joint space, as this may injure physeal (growth plate) structures. The operator should also avoid rocking the needle from side to side because this will enlarge the entrance hole and allow for extravasation of administered fluid into the soft tissues. Excessive or sudden force should be avoided at all times because this will often result in puncture of both cortices. Once the marrow space is entered, the needle need not be advanced further; usually 1 cm beyond the bony cortex is sufficient in infants and small children. The trocar is then removed, with the hollow needle left in place. To confirm proper needle position, a syringe is attached and blood

TABLE 21.1	EQUIPMENT FOR INTRAOSSEOUS INFUSION

Lidocaine 1% to 2% (without epinephrine)
Syringe/needle (25 gauge)
Antiseptic prep solution (e.g., Betadine)
Intraosseous or bone marrow aspiration needle or 20-gauge spinal needle
10-cc syringe
Saline/heparinized saline

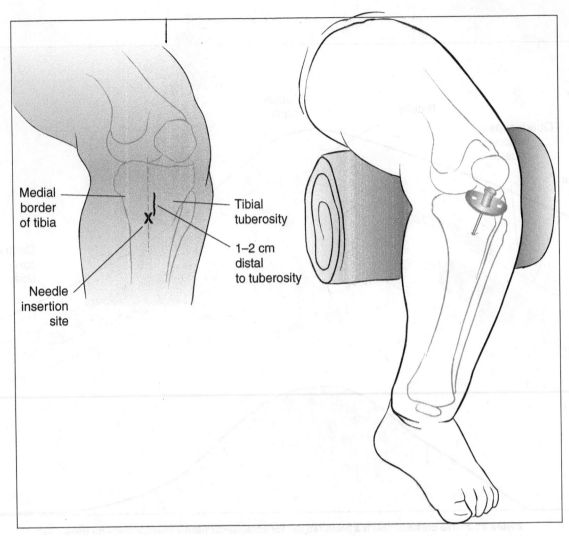

Medial border of tibia

Tibial tuberosity

1–2 cm distal to tuberosity

Needle insertion site

Figure 21.3   Entry site at the proximal tibia.

or marrow is aspirated (Fig. 21.6C). If marrow contents are not aspirated, 2 to 3 mL of sterile plain or heparinized saline is injected. The saline should infuse easily without evidence of extravasation. Alternatively, the operator may choose to reaspirate the injected fluid. If the fluid is pink-tinged, the tip of the needle is likely in the marrow cavity.

Once the correct position has been confirmed, the hub is attached to an intravenous infusion system. Failure to place the needle in the marrow cavity results in a failure to infuse. If the needle punctures both cortices, fluid will extravasate into the soft tissues. In this situation, continued infusion of fluid under pressure can potentially result in compartment syndrome. These problems can generally be avoided by ensuring proper needle placement and closely monitoring the insertion site and surrounding soft tissue for increasing firmness or swelling (6,7,21). Infusion should obviously be discontinued if extravasation is suspected. The line may then be secured in a manner similar to taping an umbilical line (Fig. 21.7). The line should not be dressed with a bulky dressing or taped in a way that obscures visualization of the insertion site.

The success rate of this procedure is high (5,6,21); how-ever, reasons for failure include improper placement, bending of the needle, dense marrow, and an underlying process that re-sults in replacement of marrow by fat or fibrous tissue (6–8, 11,21). The flow rates achieved with intraosseous infusion vary from 11 to 45 mL/min (12,22). In addition to volume replacement, all current drugs used in pediatric advanced life support can be given via the intraosseous route at the usual doses (23–29). Blood aspirated from the marrow may be used for laboratory tests such as electrolytes, glucose, BUN, and creatinine but not for a complete blood count. Marrow aspirate may also be used for type and cross-match (30,31).

▶ COMPLICATIONS

Based on current and historical data, this technique is safe and associated with a low complication rate (1,4). Most compli-cations are related to the length of time the needle is left in place, and therefore intraosseous lines should be removed as

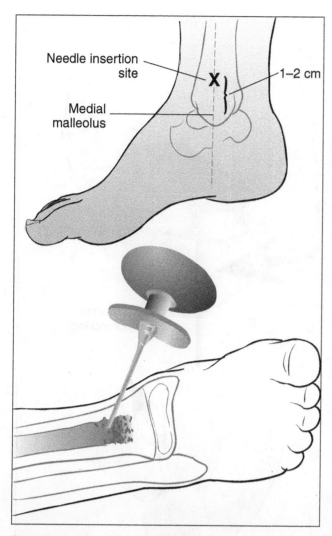

Figure 21.4   Entry site at the distal tibia.

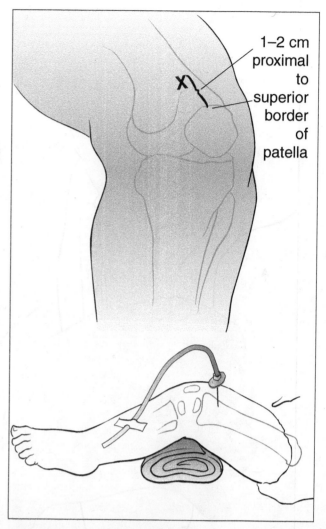

Figure 21.5   Entry site at the distal femur.

soon as other stable vascular access is obtained. Whenever possible, lines should be removed within 12 hours. Furunculosis and osteochondritis are complications that are rarely seen but are described in the literature (18). Other reported complications are listed below.

Osteomyelitis

Osteomyelitis is the most often discussed complication, but the published rate in the early literature and for more recent experience is less than 1% (1,4,32). As with other infectious complications, the likelihood of osteomyelitis is minimized by performing proper aseptic skin preparation and by using sterile gloves during needle placement (see also Chapters 7 and 8). Furthermore, the rate of osteomyelitis primarily depends on the length of time the intraosseous needle is left in place; lines left in for over 24 hours have a higher incidence of osteomyelitis. For this reason, most experts advise removing the intraosseous line as soon as another route of vascular access has been established.

Cellulitis and Subcutaneous Abscess

Both cellulitis and subcutaneous abscess, though rare, are typically associated with extravasation of fluid at the insertion site as well as inadequate skin preparation. As with osteomyelitis, the incidence primarily depends on the length of time the intraosseous needle is left in place.

Compartment Syndrome

Compartment syndrome can occur when fluid extravasates or leaks around the insertion site. This may be avoided by proper needle placement and close monitoring of the surrounding tissues. As mentioned previously, the operator should be careful to use a rotational ("screwing") motion, rather than a side-to-side "rocking" motion, with increasing downward pressure when inserting an intraosseous needle (see "Procedure"). In addition, the calf or lower thigh should be serially examined for the development of any tension, firmness, or swelling (33,34). If extravasation of fluid is suspected, use of the line should be discontinued.

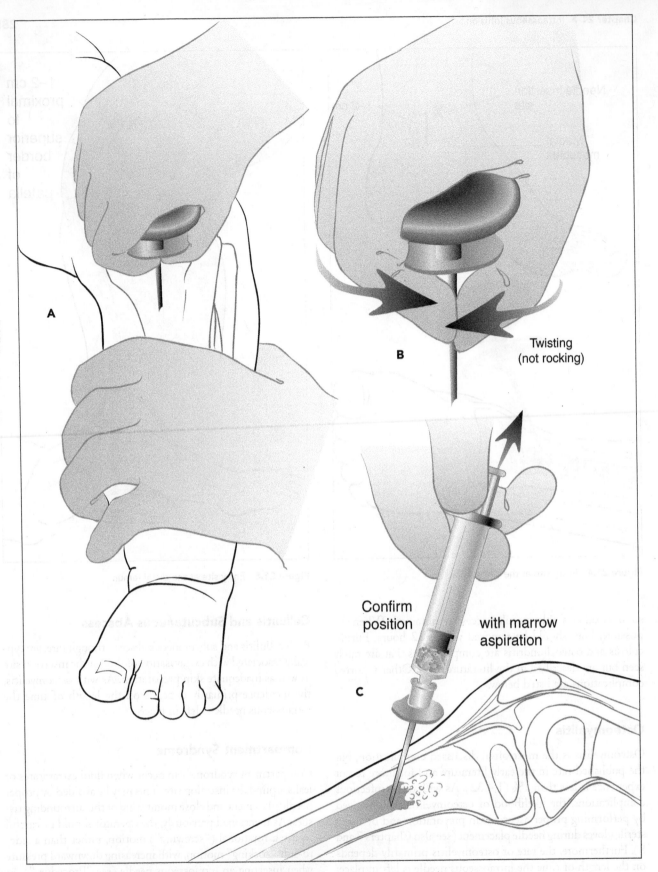

Figure 21.6 Procedure for intraosseous infusion.
A. The needle is angled slightly away from the joint space or, as some more recent sources have recommended, perpendicular to the bone.
B. A back-and-forth "screwing" motion is used to insert the needle. "Rocking" the needle from side to side results in enlargement of the puncture site and extravasation of infused fluid.
C. Intramedullary placement is confirmed by aspirating marrow.

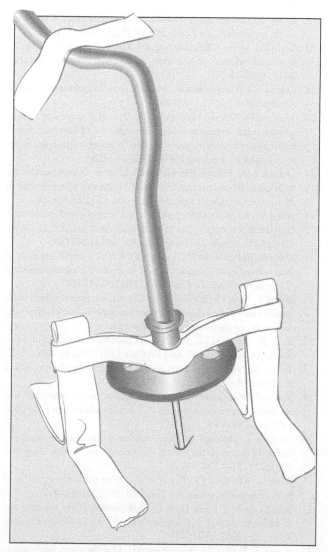

Figure 21.7 Securing an intraosseous line.

Fat Embolus

Although a theoretical complication, no cases of fat embolus have been reported in humans. One study using animals showed no ventilation-perfusion mismatch (35).

Fracture and Damage to the Growth Plate

Fracture and damage to the growth plate may occur if the patient has osteopetrosis or osteoporosis. Fractures also may occur if too large a needle is used relative to the size of the bone. Additionally, if the extremity is not properly stabilized at the time of insertion, fractures may occur (36,37). Needle insertion through the growth plate should be avoided to prevent damage that may affect normal bone growth. Although a theoretical problem, no cases have been reported in humans, and a study using animals showed no growth impairment (38–40).

SUMMARY

1 Restrain the patient appropriately.

2 Prepare an aseptic field.

3 Provide local anesthesia for the awake patient.

4 Choose an appropriate insertion site: the proximal tibia for patients younger than 3 years, the distal tibia for patients older than 3 years, or the distal femur if insertion in the tibia fails.

5 Insert needle perpendicular to the bony cortex or angled slightly away from the joint space.

6 Use a steady back-and-forth rotational movement rather than "rocking" the needle from side to side.

7 Aspirate marrow to confirm needle placement or infuse a small amount of saline and aspirate, looking for pink fluid.

8 Attach to intravenous infusion setup and secure line.

9 Monitor for extravasation and swelling of tissues.

Septicemia and Bacteremia

While potential complications, septicemia and bacteremia are often seen in patients who were septic as part of their underlying condition. As with other possible infectious complications, this is primarily a risk when intraosseous lines are left in place longer than 12 to 24 hours.

CLINICAL TIPS

▶ The needle should not be angled into the joint space in order to avoid injuring the growth plate of the bone.

▶ Excessive or sudden force should not be used because this will often result in the puncture of both cortices.

▶ If marrow or blood are not aspirated, it may be helpful to insert a few milliliters of saline and reaspirate; obtaining pink-tinged fluid indicates likely placement in the marrow cavity.

▶ All standard life-support medications can be safely injected through an intraosseous line.

▶ SUMMARY

Intraosseous infusion is a rapid method of obtaining vascular access during critical life-support situations involving infants and young children. Intraosseous lines can be placed quickly and fluids and medications given rapidly via this route. The most common sites used for insertion are the proximal tibia, the distal tibia, and the distal femur. The procedure is easy to learn and the success rate is high. The technique has been demonstrated to be safe and to have a low complication rate.

▶ REFERENCES

1. Rosetti VA, Thompson BM, Aprahamian C. Difficulty and delay in intravenous access in pediatric arrests. *Ann Emerg Med.* 1984;13:406.

2. Josefson A. A new method of treatment: intraosseous injection. *Acta Med Scand.* 1934;81:550–564.

3. Tocantins LM, O'Neil JF. Infusion of blood and other fluids into circulation via the bone marrow. *Proc Soc Exp Bio Med.* 1940;45:782–783.

4. Heinild S, Soderguard T, Tudvad F. Bone marrow infusion in childhood: experiences from a thousand infusions. *J Pediatr.* 1947;30:400–411.

5. Seigler RS, Tecklenburg FW, Shealy R. Prehospital intraosseous infusion by emergency medical services personnel: a prospective study. *Pediatrics.* 1989;84:173–177.

6. Glaeser PW, Hellmich TR, Szewczuga D. Five-year experience in prehospital intraosseous infusions in children and adults. *Ann Emerg Med.* 1993;22:1119–1124.

7. Smith RJ, Keseg DP, Manley LK, et al. Intraosseous infusions by prehospital personnel in critically ill pediatric patients. *Ann Emerg Med.* 1988;17:491–495.

8. Valdes MM. Intraosseous fluid administration in emergencies. *Lancet.* 1977;1:1235–1236.

9. Calkins MD, Fitzgerald G, Bently TB, et al. Intraosseous infusion devices: a comparison for potential use in special operations. *J Trauma.* 2000;48:1068–1074.

10. Drinker CK, Drinker KR, Lund CC. The circulation in the mammalian bone marrow. *Am J Physiol.* 1922;62:1–92.

11. Spivey WH. Intraosseous infusions. *J Pediatr.* 1987;111:639–643.

12. Hodge D III, Delgado-Paredes C, Fleisher G. Intraosseous infusion flow rates in hypovolemic "pediatric" dogs. *Ann Emerg Med.* 1987;16:305–307.

13. Tocantins LM, O'Neil JF. Complications of intraosseous therapy. *Ann Surg.* 1945;122:266–277.

14. Ellemunter H, Simma B, Trawoger R, et al. Intraosseous lines in preterm and full term neonates. *Arch Dis Child.* 1999;80:74F–75F.

15. Keith KA, Blum GT, Yamamoto LG. Intraosseous is faster and easier than umbilical venous catheterization in newborn emergency vascular access models. *Am J Emerg Med.* 2000;18:126–129.

16. Fiser DH. Intraosseous infusions. *N Engl J Med.* 1990;322:1579–1581.

17. Hodge D III. Intraosseous infusions: a review. *Pediatr Emerg Care.* 1985;1:215–218.

18. Kanter RK, Zimmerman JJ, Straus RH, et al. Pediatric emergency intravenous access: evaluation of a protocol. *Am J Dis Child.* 1986;140:132–134.

19. Jun H, Haruyama AZ, Chang KSG, et al. Comparison of a new screw-tipped intraosseous needle versus a standard bone marrow aspiration needle for infusion. *Am J Emerg Med.* 2000;18:135–139.

20. Boon JM, Gorry DLA, Meiring JH. Finding an ideal site for intraosseous infusion of the tibia: an anatomical study. *Clin Anat.* 2003;16:15–18.

21. Rosetti VA, Thompson BM, Miller J, et al. Intraosseous infusions. *Ann Emerg Med.* 1985;14:885–887.

22. Warren DW, Kissoon N, Sommerauer JF, et al. Comparison of fluid infusion rates among peripheral intravenous and humerus, femur, malleolus, and tibial intraosseous sites in normovolemic and hypovolemic piglets. *Ann Emerg Med.* 1993;22:183–186.

23. Dubeck MA, Pfeiffer JW, Clifford CB, et al. Comparison of intraosseous and intravenous delivery of hypertonic saline/dextran in anesthetized, euvolemic pigs. *Ann Emerg Med.* 1992;21:498–503.

24. Spivey WH, Malone D, Unger HD, et al. Comparison of intraosseous, central and peripheral routes of administration of sodium bicarbonate during CPR in pigs. *Ann Emerg Med.* 1985;14:1135–1140.

25. Orlowski JP, Porembka DT, Gallagher JM, et al. Comparison study of intraosseous, central intravenous, and peripheral intravenous infusions of emergency drugs. *Am J Dis Child.* 1990;144:112–117.

26. Sapien R, Stein H, Padbury JF, et al. Intraosseous versus intravenous epinephrine infusions in lambs: pharmacokinetics and pharmacodynamics. *Pediatr Emerg Care.* 1992;8:179–183.

27. Biello JF, O'Hair KC, Kirby WC, et al. Intraosseous infusion of dobutamine and isoproterenol. *Am J Dis Child.* 1991:145;165–167.

28. Tobias JD, Nichols DG. Intraosseous succinylcholine for orotracheal intubation. *Pediatr Emerg Care.* 1990;6:108–109.

29. Jaimovich DG, Kumar A, Francom S. Evaluation of intraosseous versus intravenous antibiotic levels in a porcine model. *Am J Dis Child.* 1991;145:946–949.

30. Grisham J, Hastings C. Bone marrow aspirate as an accessible and reliable source for critical laboratory studies. *Ann Emerg Med.* 1991;20:1121–1124.

31. Brickman KR, Krupp K, Rega P, et al. Typing and screening of blood from intraosseous access. *Ann Emerg Med.* 1992;21:414–417.

32. Stoll E, Golej J, Burda G, et al. Osteomyelitis at the injection site of adrenalin through an intraosseous needle in a 3-month-old infant. *Resuscitation.* 2002;53:315–318.

33. Rimar S, Westry JA, Rodriguez RL. Compartment syndrome in an infant following emergency intraosseous infusion. *Clin Pediatr.* 1988;27:259–260.

34. Vidal R, Kissoon N, Gayle M. Compartment syndrome following intraosseous infusion. *Pediatrics.* 1993;91:1201–1202.

35. Orlowski JP, Julius CJ, Petras RE, et al. The safety of intraosseous infusions: risks of fat and bone marrow emboli to the lungs. *Ann Emerg Med.* 1989;18:1062–1067.

36. LaFleche FR, Slepin JM, Vargas J, et al. Iatrogenic bilateral tibial fractures after intraosseous infusion attempts in a 3-month-old infant. *Ann Emerg Med.* 1989;18:1099–1101.

37. Bowley DMG, Loveland J, Pitcher GJ. Tibial fracture as a complication of intraosseous infusion during pediatric resuscitation. *J Trauma.* 2003;55:786–787.

38. Dedrick DK, Mase C, Ranger W, et al. The effects of intraosseous infusion on the growth plate in a nestling rabbit model. *Ann Emerg Med.* 1992;21:494–497.

39. Claudet I, Baunin C, Laporte-Turpin E, et al. Long-term effects on tibial growth after intraosseous infusion: a prospective, radiographic analysis. *Pediatr Emerg Care.* 2003;19:397–401.

40. Fiser RT, Walker WM, Siebert JJ, et al. Tibial length following intraosseous infection: a prospective radiographic analysis. *Pediatr Emerg Care.* 1997;13:186–188.

KATHLEEN P. KELLY AND MICHAEL ALTIERI

22

Cardiac Pacing

▶ INTRODUCTION

Emergency cardiac pacing is rarely performed in children but in selected cases can prove life-saving. With the increasing prevalence of cardiac surgery among pediatric patients with congenital heart disease, the likelihood of encountering children with arrhythmias in the emergency department (ED) has increased. Emergency cardiac pacing enables the physician to initiate and sustain a cardiac rhythm that will provide perfusion of the vital organs in a patient with symptomatic bradyarrhythmia. Clinicians who care for critically ill infants and children should be familiar with the unique aspects of performing cardiac pacing for these patients. Two methods used in the emergency setting are the transvenous approach and the transcutaneous approach. Transvenous cardiac pacing involves placement of a pacing wire in direct contact with the myocardium via the central venous circulation. Transcutaneous pacing, which can be performed far more rapidly, utilizes electrodes incorporated into adhesive pads that are applied directly to the external chest wall. Although easier, this method yields less reliable results and is most commonly used as a temporizing measure until transvenous pacing can be performed. Emergency transvenous pacers are inserted by physicians in the ED, intensive care unit (ICU), or operating room. Transcutaneous pacers are technically easier to use and may be applied and operated by physicians, nurses, or paramedics.

The ability to electrically depolarize muscle was first noted over a century ago; however, it was not until 1952 that the clinical utility of cardiac pacing for humans was demonstrated

by Zoll. Pacemaker technology advanced from the original devices, which consisted of wires passing through the skin into the myocardium, to a more modern endocardial transvenous pacer introduced in 1959 by Furman and Schwedel. The first implantable permanent pacemaker also was developed in 1959. With the creation of the balloon-tipped central venous catheter by Swann in 1970 came the flow-directed transvenous pacers used today. The most recent development in pacing technology is the transcutaneous pacer. Although the initial experiments with transcutaneous pacing actually predated transvenous pacing, this technique was all but abandoned because of the pain caused by severe muscle contractions. This problem now has been overcome primarily with the use of decreased delivered current, an electrode with a larger surface area, and an electrical impulse with a longer duration. Consequently, it is now feasible in many instances to perform cardiac pacing effectively without using an invasive procedure.

▶ ANATOMY AND PHYSIOLOGY

Sites used for transvenous pacer insertion are the femoral, right internal jugular, and left subclavian veins (Fig. 22.1). In adolescents, the right internal jugular vein site and, if necessary, the left subclavian vein site may be used. Whenever possible, the right internal jugular access site should be used so that the left subclavian vein is preserved for possible long-term pacemaker placement. When inserted through the right internal jugular vein, the pacer wire has a more or less straight-in approach to the right atrium via the superior vena cava. Disadvantages of this approach include possible carotid artery puncture, dislodgment of the catheter with movement of the head, and an increase risk of thrombophlebitis of the internal jugular vein. When inserted through the left subclavian vein, the angle of entry into the superior vena cava is less

---

Dr. Michael Altieri passed away in January 2004. It has been a great loss to me and to pediatric emergency medicine. He and I originally wrote this chapter together, with Mike writing the entire beginning part of the chapter and me writing the second half. As his portion is essentially unaltered from the first edition, he remains an author of the chapter.

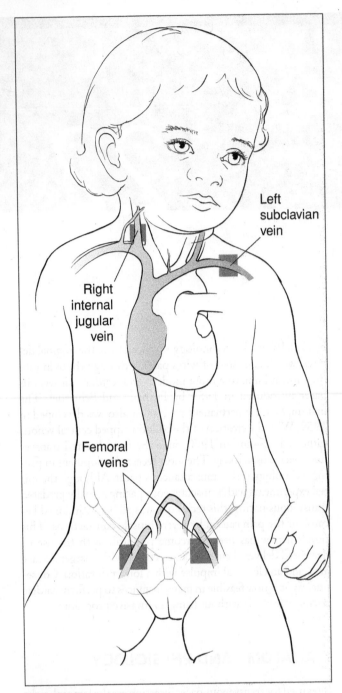

Figure 22.1 Preferred sites for transvenous pacemaker placement. (Note: the left subclavian vein site is recommended only for adolescents.)

acute than is encountered with the right subclavian approach. The main disadvantage of subclavian placement is possible pneumothorax.

Because infants and younger children have a relatively short neck and a subclavian vein that is less accessible behind the clavicle, the femoral approach is preferred. Many clinicians use the femoral approach for all pediatric patients. The pacer wire passes along the length of the femoral vein into the inferior vena cava and ultimately enters the right atrium. The

principle disadvantages of this route are an increased risk of thrombophlebitis, a higher incidence of infection, and restricted patient mobility because the catheter is easily dislodged with movement. In addition, the increased distance to the heart from a femoral access site often requires the use of fluoroscopic guidance in a child with poor cardiac output (i.e., when flow-directed catheters are less effective). An alternative approach is via the brachial vein, although this method is seldom used because of the smaller size of the vein and the relative difficulty of this technique. A cutdown is often necessary when using the brachial vein approach. The pacer wire passes along the brachial vein into the subclavian vein and finally through the inferior vena cava into the right atrium. Further discussion of these central venous access approaches is provided in Chapter 19.

Unlike transvenous pacing, transcutaneous pacing is easy to perform with pediatric patients and is often more effective for children than for adults. This is primarily because children have decreased density and thickness of the chest wall (ribs and muscle), which results in a lower transthoracic resistance, and a smaller chest diameter. Transcutaneous pacing can even be used with small children, as there are pediatric size electrodes as small as 6 × 7 cm.

Before discussing the applications of cardiac pacing, it is useful to briefly review the conduction system of the heart (Fig. 22.2). Electrical activity is initiated by the sinoatrial

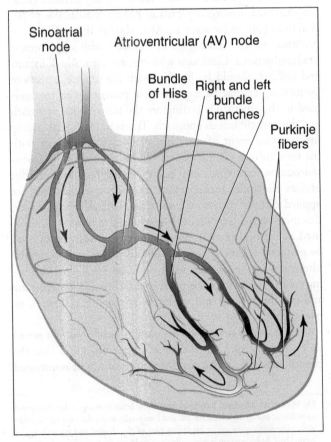

Figure 22.2 Anatomy of the cardiac conduction system.

node, located at the junction of the superior vena cava and the right atrium. The stimulus is then spread throughout the atria and terminates at the atrioventricular (AV) node in the lower part of the right atrium. From there, the electrical impulse is conducted through the bundle of His, which divides to form the right and left bundle branches of the ventricles. The bundle branches further divide into the Purkinje fibers, which penetrate the myocardium, allowing rapid conduction of the impulse throughout the ventricles, with resulting contraction.

Most life-threatening arrhythmias in children are bradyarrhythmias. Asystole is also a common terminal rhythm in children, although not amenable to pacing. For infants and younger children, cardiac output directly depends on heart rate, and therefore bradyarrhythmias produce a fall in cardiac output and resulting circulatory compromise. Sinus bradycardia (a rate less than 60 bpm) resulting from a primary cardiac abnormality is relatively uncommon in the pediatric age group and generally indicates markedly increased vagal tone. Failure of impulse formation or transmission from the sinus node is referred to as "sinoatrial block" and may manifest as a nodal rhythm. Complete AV block is usually a congenital condition but can also be seen with digitalis intoxication and rheumatic carditis.

▶ INDICATIONS

Conditions that lead to arrhythmias that require cardiac pacing are relatively uncommon in children. Consequently, this procedure will be indicated only in rare instances. However, in those circumstances where cardiac pacing is necessary, the procedure can be life-saving. In general, the indications for cardiac pacing can be divided into two categories: urgent and emergent. Situations requiring urgent cardiac pacing are those in which a child has a persistent arrhythmia that is refractory to drug therapy. Although minor associated symptoms may exist (e.g., mild dizziness, orthostasis), the cardiovascular status of the patient is otherwise stable. Potential arrhythmias include supraventricular tachycardia (SVT), which may require overdrive pacing in the ICU, or stable AV dissociation, which may require eventual surgical implantation of a permanent pacemaker. For these patients, transcutaneous pacing should be available in the ED, but transvenous pacing is generally unnecessary as part of the initial management. If transvenous pacing proves to be necessary, this procedure can normally be performed on a semi-elective basis in the radiology suite with the aid of fluoroscopic guidance, because any clinical deterioration in the patient is typically gradual. In such cases, echocardiography is an alternative means of visualizing placement of the pacer wire.

Emergent cardiac pacing is the procedure that will be indicated for children in the ED. These patients have significant hypotension associated with a refractory bradyarrhythmia, most commonly AV dissociation. Transcutaneous pacing can be attempted in such cases, but because the presenting rhythms are often difficult to abort, this should occur while

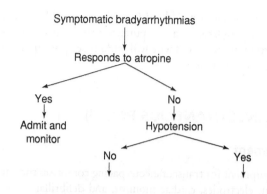

Figure 22.3 Indications for cardiac pacing.

the equipment required for transvenous pacing is being assembled and appropriate central venous access is obtained. An algorithm showing the indications for cardiac pacing is presented in Figure 22.3.

The young child with a significant bradyarrhythmia typically shows signs of poor perfusion. The patient may be pale and/or mottled. The extremities are often cool and cyanotic, and capillary refill time may be prolonged. Urine output is decreased or absent, and the child will often be lethargic or, in more extreme cases, unconscious.

Congenital heart defects are associated with a variety of clinically significant arrhythmias, including the bradyasystolic rhythms. Such defects include Ebstein anomaly, transposition of the great vessels, and congenital mitral stenosis. Among neonates, congenital complete heart block is associated with maternal systemic lupus erythematosus. Pediatric patients who have undergone cardiac surgery for repair of a congenital anomaly (e.g., tetralogy of Fallot, atrial and ventricular septal defects, endocardial cushion defects) are also at risk for arrhythmias. Additionally, acquired processes may be associated with an increased incidence of bradyarrhythmias, such as rheumatic heart disease, myocarditis, cardiac tumors, and certain metabolic and electrolyte disturbances.

In general, infants and younger children requiring emergent transvenous pacing should have the wire inserted via a catheter in the femoral vein, using fluoroscopic guidance as indicated. Older children and adolescents may be managed similarly to the adult patient, using the right internal jugular vein or subclavian vein. Although the left subclavian vein provides a more reliable approach for insertion of a transvenous pacer, it should only be used when absolutely necessary, because the left subclavian is also the preferred site for a permanent pacemaker. A balloon-tipped flexible catheter should be used to avoid cardiac perforation. A rigid wire is indicated only in an arrest state with no significant blood flow. Because children rarely suffer a full bradycardic arrest purely on the basis of cardiac dysfunction, using a rigid wire will seldom be appropriate for this patient population.

▶ TRANSCUTANEOUS PACING

Equipment

The equipment for transcutaneous pacing comprises the pacing unit, electrodes, cardiac monitor, and defibrillator. Several transcutaneous pacing models are available that perform only pacing (e.g., Zoll, NTP, ZMI Corp., Cambridge, MA). However, many practitioners prefer to use a unit that combines external pacing with cardiac monitoring and defibrillator capabilities (e.g., Lifepak 20, Medtronic Physio-Control, Redmond, WA) (Fig. 22.4). These units are equipped with digital display and buttons to control the delivered current and to select either demand or asynchronous modes. The Lifepak 20 has a variable rate control ranging from 40 to 170 bpm. This is an improvement for use in children over earlier models, which had maximum rates of 90 bpm.

The electrodes for transcutaneous pacing are now available in adult and pediatric sizes (Fig. 22.5). They are silver/silver chloride pads measuring 13 × 15 cm for older children and adults and 6 × 7 cm for smaller children and infants. The electrodes have been shown to be safe for both the patient and medical personnel. Clinicians can perform CPR with their hands directly over them if necessary.

Procedure

Transcutaneous pacing electrodes are easily applied to the anterior and posterior chest walls with the adhesive. The normal location of the V3 lead of the ECG is an ideal anterior position, while the posterior lead should be placed on the upper back between the scapulae (Fig. 22.6). If capture does not occur in these positions, the posterior lead can be moved to

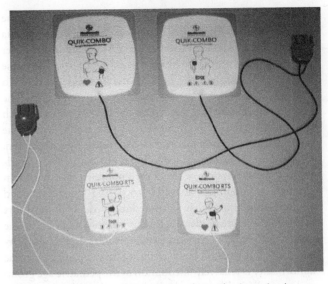

Figure 22.5 Transcutaneous pacing electrodes (two sizes).

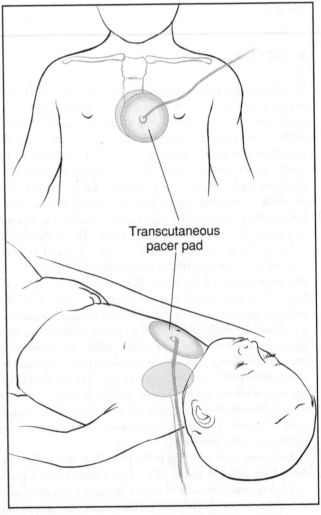

Transcutaneous pacer pad

Figure 22.6 Proper placement of transcutaneous pacing electrodes.

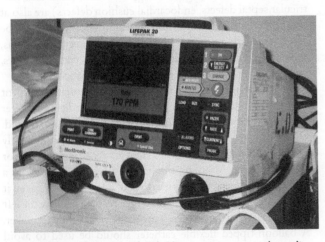

Figure 22.4 Medtronic LifePak 20 transcutaneous pacing unit.

SUMMARY: TRANSCUTANEOUS PACING

1 Sedate patient as indicated.

2 Apply adhesive electrodes to anterior and posterior chest walls.

3 Connect patient to monitoring system of pacing module.

4 Set rate just above patient's rate.

5 Set system on demand mode if patient has an intermittently acceptable intrinsic rate; otherwise set system on asynchronous mode.

6 Set output to lowest value.

7 Turn on pacer.

8 Gradually increase output until capture is noted.

9 Set output just above pacer threshold.

10 Set rate to minimum desired rate.

11 Make plans for transvenous pacing.

a more lateral or even axillary location. If possible, the leads should not be placed over bony structures such as a scapula.

The patient should be monitored using the cardiac-monitoring capabilities of the transcutaneous pacer. In general, pediatric patients should be sedated before transcutaneous pacing (see Chapter 33). The rate should be set appropriately based on the age of the child. Assuming there is an intrinsic rate, the pacemaker is set on demand mode so that pacing will occur only when the patient's own ventricular rate is inadequate. The monitor is turned on with the output at the lowest level, and the output is gradually increased until capture is obtained. The rate is then set to a minimum acceptable heart rate for the patient, and the output is set just above the pacing threshold. At this point, immediate plans should be made for transvenous pacing as needed on an urgent (stable patient) or emergent (unstable patient) basis.

CLINICAL TIPS: TRANSCUTANEOUS PACING

▶ If possible, the pacer electrodes should not be placed over bony structures such as the scapula.

▶ The two pacer electrodes should be prevented from touching one another to prevent a short circuit, which could result in the loss of delivered current.

Complications

No significant complications are associated with transcutaneous pacing. Muscle damage, burns, and other injuries associated with cardioversion do not occur, because the energy of the delivery currents is low. Medical personnel are at no risk. The most common difficulty is sedation.

▶ TRANSVENOUS PACING

Equipment

Pacemakers operate by delivering a small amount of electrical energy to the myocardium, thus stimulating contraction. Some are equipped to sense the patient's cardiac rhythm so that pacing occurs when a slow or absent rhythm is sensed and is inhibited when a normal rhythm is present. Stimulation of the heart muscle results when the positive pole (anode) and the negative pole (cathode) of the pacemaker battery are briefly connected, allowing current to flow. If the energy delivered exceeds the minimum amount required for cardiac muscle stimulation, a contraction occurs. The completed circuit therefore is composed of the two poles of the battery, pacing lead wires, and electrodes as well as the intervening cardiac and body tissues. The pacing system employs one of two possible electrode configurations: unipolar or bipolar. Unipolar pacing has a single electrode at the cardiac end of the pacing lead, and the pulse generator serves as an "indifferent" electrode. During a paced impulse, current flows through the large circuit formed by the components of the pacing system and the body tissue. Bipolar pacing has an additional small ring electrode located on the pacing lead just proximal to the tip of the electrode; current flows between these two electrodes.

Because transvenous pacing can be technically challenging, prior preparation is crucial for this procedure. It is advisable to have available in the ED at all times a pediatric central venous access tray as well as an introducer sheath with a rubber diaphragm, which can be easily used for pacer wire placement (see Chapter 19). The pacemaker and a spare 9-volt battery should be kept on the pediatric code cart, and battery function should be checked initially as well as on a routine basis. Pacing wires also should be stored with the pacemaker and should include both the rigid type and the flexible type (floating or semifloating). Because most children can be paced with a 3 or 4 French pacer wire through a 5 or 6 French sheath, a prepared pediatric pacing tray can be assembled that includes these items as well as necessary equipment for central venous access (Table 22.1). Medtronic has recently introduced a 2 French pacer wire for infants with a screw-type distal tip that has a lower risk of dislodgement, although it is currently used primarily in cardiology suites and is placed fluoroscopically.

Medical personnel involved with pacer insertion should be knowledgeable about the specific characteristics of the pacing equipment at their institution, as a cardiac emergency obviously does not allow time to become familiar with these items. Pacemakers are available from a variety of manufactures, but

TABLE 22.1	EQUIPMENT FOR TRANSVENOUS PACING

9-volt battery

A central venous access tray, including introducer sheath with rubber diaphragm suitable for pacer wire placement (see Chapter 19)[a]

Rigid and flexible (floating or semifloating) pacer wires[a]

Cardiac monitor

Pulse oximeter

Supplemental oxygen

[a]Most children can be paced with a 3 or 4 French pacer wire through a 5 or 6 French sheath.

the general design features are similar. Newer models, such as the Medtronic 5385 (Fig. 22.7), have digital displays. While they share the same basic functions as the older models, these newer models have the added functionality of multiple screen menus.

A typical model of pacemaker with representative design characteristics is the Medtronic 5375 (Fig. 22.8). This device has an on/off switch that when put in the "on" position releases a spring-loaded button that acts as a safety lock to prevent accidental pacer interruption. It also has an output

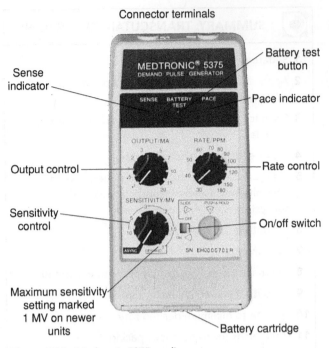

Figure 22.8 Medtronic 5375 cardiac pacer.

control that allows for adjustment of the stimulus current amplitude from 0.1 to 20 mA. The rate control dial can be varied from 20 to 180 bpm, which is an adequate range for ventricular pacing in all adults and children. It does not achieve the high rates needed for atrial overdrive pacing in some children, but this procedure would rarely be performed in the ED. The device also is equipped with a sensitivity control that sets the magnitude of the R-wave signal required to suppress the pulse generator. In the full counterclockwise position, the pacer does not sense at all and is in asynchronous mode. It also has two signal lights that indicate sensing and pacing. The sensing indicator flashes when a cardiac impulse is sensed. The pacer indicator flashes when a pacing stimulus is generated (although this does not necessarily indicate capture). Finally, the battery test button provides a battery voltage check. When the test button is depressed, both the sensing and the pacing indicators flash simultaneously, indicating sufficient voltage for use (1).

Pacemaker wires used for emergency transvenous pacing are also available in prepackaged kits from several manufacturers (e.g., Balectrode, Medtronic). These wires come in a wide variety of sizes, but a 3 or 4 French wire should generally suffice for most infants and children. The wires are approximately 100 cm in length and are marked at 10-cm intervals to aid with positioning. Many pediatric cardiologists prefer the rigid wire rather than the floating or semifloating type, due to the controlled setting in which they normally insert pacemakers. It should be pointed out, however, that the rigid wires carry more danger of cardiac perforation (2–4). Without the benefit of visual guidance, the semifloating balloon-tipped wires may be easiest to use in low-flow states (5). The balloon is inflated with 1.5 mL of air and "floats" the catheter into

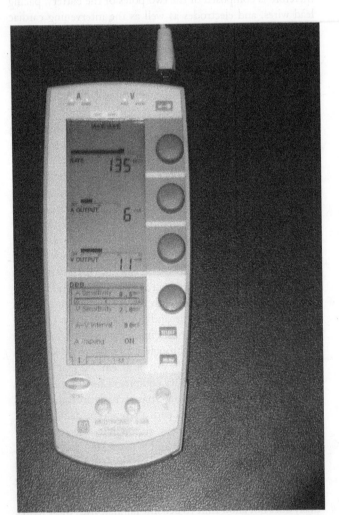

Figure 22.7 Medtronic 5385 digital display cardiac pacer.

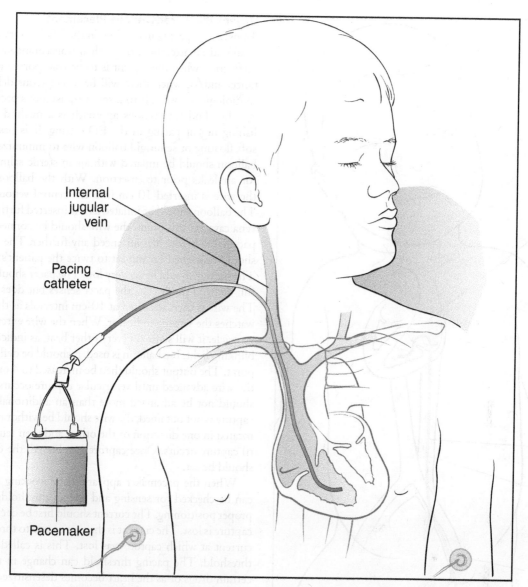

Figure 22.9 Transvenous pacemaker placement via the right internal jugular vein.

the heart if some circulation is present (6,7). The balloon is checked initially for leaks by inflating it while it is immersed in sterile water. If the patient has no forward blood flow, the balloon is of no use, and the rigid catheter should be used. In adult patients and adolescents, the pacemaker may be inserted using electrocardiographic guidance. However, this technique is difficult and impractical for infants and children due to the small heart size and short distances between chambers (7,8).

All patients undergoing pacemaker insertion will require cardiac monitoring, supplemental oxygen, and pulse oximetry monitoring. Pulse oximetry is particularly important if sedation is used (see Chapter 33). When personnel and equipment for performing bedside echocardiography are available, this can be a highly useful tool for rapid replacement of the transvenous pacemaker. The ideal modality to assist placement is fluoroscopy, particularly when the femoral access site is used. However, patients undergoing fluoroscopic pacemaker insertion away from the ED require careful cardiac monitoring and close observation, as the incidence of dysrhythmias is high.

Procedure

Pacemakers are placed into the central venous circulation using the internal jugular, femoral, and subclavian approaches. The right internal jugular is a direct approach used primarily with older children and adolescents (Fig. 22.9). For most younger children, the femoral vein is the easiest and safest approach (Fig. 22.10). This is particularly true when chest compressions or airway control must be performed, because the femoral approach does not interfere with these actions. As stated previously, it is best to leave the left subclavian vein available for permanent pacer insertion should that prove necessary (Fig. 22.11).

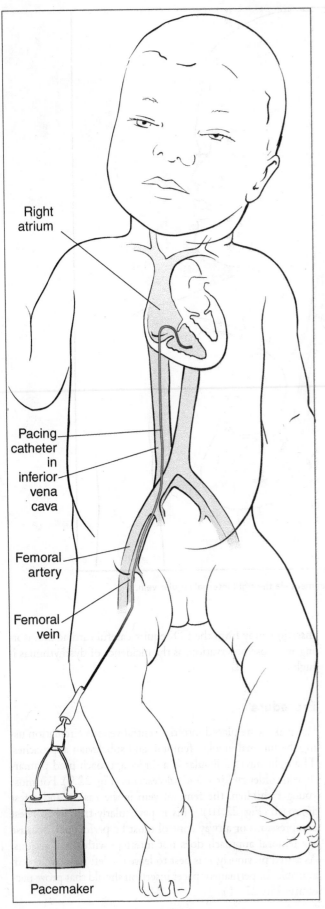

Right atrium

Pacing catheter in inferior vena cava

Femoral artery

Femoral vein

Pacemaker

Urgent Blind Transvenous Placement

Transvenous pacing in children in the ED is a very rare event. It should be attempted only when transcutaneous pacing is ineffective, when the patient is to be transported a long distance, and/or when there will be a dangerous delay until a cardiologist is available to insert a transvenous pacer.

The blind transvenous approach is a method for establishing urgent pacing in the ED setting. It is best to use a soft floating or semirigid balloon wire to minimize risk. The balloon should be inflated with air in sterile saline to check for air leaks prior to insertion. With the balloon deflated, the wire is inserted 10 cm into the central venous catheter. The balloon should be inflated as it is inserted further into the vena cava. At this point, the wire should be connected to the pacemaker before it is advanced any further. The pacemaker should be turned on and set to twice the patient's heart rate. The output should be set very low. The pacer should be in the full demand mode (i.e., the pacer senses but does not pace). The wire is then advanced at 10-cm intervals as the operator watches the sensing indicator. When the wire enters the right ventricle, it will sense on every other beat, as indicated by the blinking light. If a balloon is used, it should be deflated at this point. The output should then be increased to 4 or 5 mA and the wire advanced until ventricular capture occurs. The wire should not be advanced more than an additional 10 cm. If capture is not obtained, the wire should be withdrawn slightly, rotated in one direction or the other, and then reinserted until capture occurs. Once capture is achieved, the desired rate should be set.

When the pacemaker appears to be working properly, it can be checked for sensing and pacing thresholds as well as proper positioning. The current should first be decreased until capture is lost. The current is then set to two to three times the current at which capture was lost. This is called the pacing threshold. The pacing threshold can change in response to certain drugs or as the heart becomes desensitized over time. To check the pacer for appropriate sensing, the rate should be decreased while in full demand mode until the patient's intrinsic rhythm suppresses the pacer. This ensures that the sensor is working. The rate should then be reset to the desired minimal level (7–13).

Emergent Blind Transvenous Placement

Emergent blind transvenous placement is indicated in absent cardiac flow states when there is no time to place the pacemaker by other means (i.e., fluoroscopic or ultrasound-guided methods). The risks of this procedure are significant, but it is

Figure 22.10 Transvenous pacemaker placement via the femoral vein. In patients with severe impairment of cardiac output, fluoroscopic guidance may be required to successfully transverse the greater distance from the femoral site to the right ventricle. For blind pacer insertion at the groin, flow-directed catheters are usually necessary, but in a low-flow state such catheters are often ineffective.

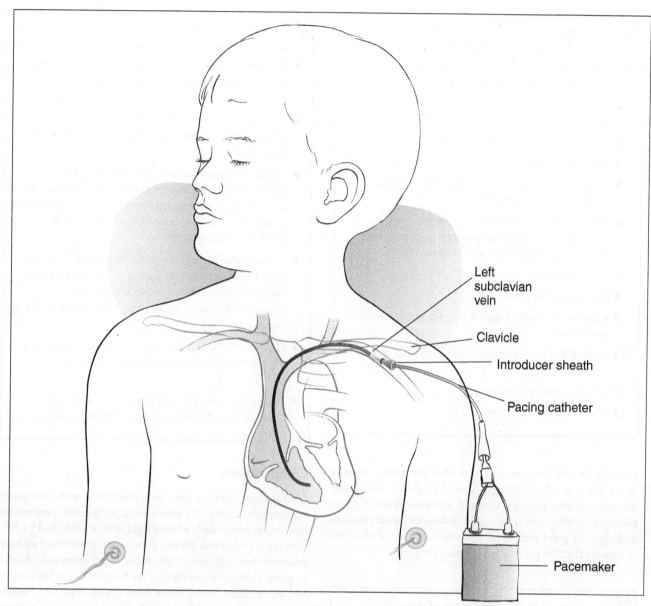

Figure 22.11 Transvenous pacemaker placement via the left subclavian vein. (Note: this site should be reserved for later permanent pacemaker placement, if feasible.)

used in situations when the likely alternative for the patient is death. A rigid wire is used without a balloon, because the balloon will be ineffective with no blood flow. The wire is introduced into the central circulation and attached to the pacemaker. The settings for the pacemaker should be asynchronous mode, maximal output, and an appropriate rate for the age of the patient. The wire is advanced until capture occurs. A reasonable estimate of the length of wire needed can be obtained before insertion by measuring the distance that must be traversed from the point of insertion to the approximate position of the right ventricle. For this approach, the left subclavian provides the most direct route of insertion (9,14). Using the femoral access site with this technique is usually impossible, since the distance from the groin to the heart is much greater, and the pathway through the vessels is more

tortuous. For this reason, all pediatric patients (even infants and younger children) should generally have pacer insertion via the internal jugular vein or left subclavian vein in such situations. The risk of cardiac perforation is high with this method because it is performed blindly using a rigid catheter.

Postpacemaker Assessment

A chest radiograph must be obtained immediately after placement to assess proper positioning of the pacer wire in the right ventricle. An electrocardiogram should also be performed to identify the characteristic left bundle branch block pattern during paced beats. A right bundle branch block pattern indicates that (a) the wire may be in the coronary sinus, (b) the wire is positioned too close to the septum in the right

SUMMARY: URGENT BLIND TRANSVENOUS PACING

1 Establish central venous access.

2 Advance pacer wire 10 cm into central venous sheath and inflate balloon.

3 Attach pacer wire to pacer source.

4 Turn pacemaker on.

5 Set pacemaker to lowest output, full demand mode, and twice patient's rate.

6 Advance pacer wire at 10-cm intervals until blinking sensor light corresponds to every other beat, indicating placement in right ventricle.

7 Deflate balloon.

8 Turn output to 5 mA.

9 Advance wire until capture takes place (no more than 10 cm).

10 Once 100% capture occurs, set threshold and check sensing.

11 Suture pacer wire in place.

12 Check chest radiograph and ECG.

CLINICAL TIPS: TRANSVENOUS PACING

▶ The natural curve of the pacer wire should be used to aid in positioning the tip in the right ventricle (i.e., curving toward the left side of the chest).

▶ The operator should ensure that the catheter sheath is larger than the pacer wire before beginning the procedure.

▶ If no evidence of capture exists or if capture is intermittent, the pacemaker should be turned off and the pacer wire repositioned. Often a clockwise or counterclockwise twist of the catheter will be helpful in this situation.

▶ If ventricular ectopy develops, the catheter should be withdrawn until this ceases. If ectopy is frequent, administration of intravenous lidocaine or amiodarone may be necessary before continuing the procedure.

▶ The pacer wire should be coiled at the skin surface after suturing to decrease the likelihood of dislodgement.

▶ The on/off switch on the pacemaker should be covered at all times to avoid accidental power loss.

---

ventricle, or (c) the wire has perforated the septum and is in the left ventricle. Vital signs should be closely monitored immediately after pacing is initiated, as the incidence of complications at this time is increased. Adequate blood pressure and signs of good peripheral perfusion are two of the best indicators that the pacer is functioning properly.

SUMMARY: EMERGENT BLIND TRANSVENOUS PACING

1 Establish central venous access.

2 Measure approximate length of wire needed to reach right ventricle externally before beginning.

3 Advance pacer wire into catheter sheath 10 cm.

4 Attach wire to pacemaker and set on asynchronous mode, maximum output, and average rate for age.

5 Advance until capture takes place.

6 Withdraw and reposition if unsuccessful.

7 If capture takes place, set threshold and check sensing.

8 Suture pacer wire in place.

9 Check chest radiograph and ECG.

Complications

Several complications have been associated with emergency transvenous pacing. As mentioned, ventricular perforation may occur, particularly when a rigid wire is used (2–4). Children are at higher risk for this complication because they have relatively thin right ventricular walls. Rigid wires only should be passed blindly when there is no discernible cardiac output and when direct visualization with fluoroscopy or echocardiography is impossible. Air embolism secondary to rupture of the balloon in the floating pacer wires has also occurred (15,16). Checking the balloon for leaks before insertion will decrease the likelihood of this problem. Care should also be taken not to overinflate the balloon.

Transvenous pacing wires have also been known to cause venous thrombosis in small children. In the past, narrow vein size has limited transvenous pacing in children under 10 kg. Newer technologies, allowing lead diameters as small as 2 French, are making transvenous pacing an increasingly viable therapeutic option in these younger patients (16).

▶ REFERENCES

1. *Medtronic Model 5375 Technical Manual: External Demand Pulse Generator and Accessories.* Minneapolis, MN: Medtronic Inc; 1990:10–12.
2. Goswani M, Gould L, Gomprecht RF, et al. Perforation of the heart by flexible transvenous pacemaker. *JAMA.* 1971;216(12):2013–2014.

3. Anielson GK, Shabetai R, Bryant LR. Failure of endocardial pacemaker due to myocardial perforation. *J Thorac Cardiovasc Surg*. 1967;54(1): 42–48.

4. Kalloor GJ. Cardiac tamponade: report of a case after insertion of transvenous endocardial electrode. *Am Heart J*. 1974;88(1):88–89.

5. Lang R, David D, Klein HO, et al. The use of the balloon-tipped floating catheter in temporary transvenous cardiac pacing. *Pacing Clin Electrophysiol*. 1981;4(5):491–496.

6. Swan HJ, Ganz W, Forrester J, et al. Catheterization of the heart in man with use of a flow-directed, balloon-tipped catheter. *N Engl J Med*. 1970;283:447–451.

7. Schnitzler RN, Caracta RA, Damato AN. "Floating" catheter for temporary transvenous ventricular pacing. *Am J Cardiol*. 1973;31: 351–354.

8. Kimball JT, Killip T. A simple bedside method for transvenous intracardiac pacing. *Am Heart J*. 1965;70:35–39.

9. Harris CW, Hurlburt JC, Floyd WL, et al. Percutaneous technique for cardiac pacing with a platinum-tipped electrode catheter. *Am J Cardiol*. 1965;15:48–50.

10. Escher DJ, Furman S. Emergency treatment of cardiac arrhythmias: emphasis on use of electrical pacing. *JAMA*. 1970;214(11): 2028–2034.

11. Hazard PB, Benton C, Milnor JP. Transvenous cardiac pacing in cardiopulmonary resuscitation. *Crit Care Med*. 1981;9: 666–668.

12. Goldberger E. Temporary cardiac pacing. In: Goldberger E, ed. *Treatment of Cardiac Emergencies*. 4th ed. St. Louis: Mosby; 1985: 272–274.

13. Benjamin GC. Emergency transvenous cardiac pacing. In: Roberts JR, Hedges JR, eds. *Clinical Procedures in Emergency Medicine*. 2nd ed. Philadelphia: WB Saunders; 1985:170–191.

14. Rosenberg AS, Grossman JI, Escher DJ, et al. Bedside transvenous cardiac pacing. *Am Heart J*. 1969;77:697–703.

15. Foote GA, Schabel SI, Hodges M. Pulmonary complications of the flow-directed, balloon-tipped catheter. *N Engl J Med*. 1974;290: 927–931.

16. Berul CL, Cecchin F. Indications and techniques of pediatric cardiac pacing. *Expert Rev Cardiovasc Ther*. 2003;1:165–176.

23

RICHARD J. SCARFONE AND CHRISTINE S. CHO

Cardioversion and Defibrillation

▶ INTRODUCTION

Synchronized cardioversion is the application of direct current electricity to terminate dysrhythmias. Current is timed (synchronized) so that it is delivered outside the vulnerable phase of the cardiac cycle to minimize the risk of precipitating ventricular fibrillation (VF). Types of dysrhythmias seen in children that may require synchronized cardioversion include supraventricular tachycardia (SVT), atrial fibrillation, atrial flutter, and stable ventricular tachycardia (VT). Defibrillation is the application of a high initial dose of direct current electricity that is not timed to the cardiac cycle (asynchronous). A large segment of the myocardium is depolarized, rendering it refractory to further disorganized cardiac conduction. Defibrillation is used in the treatment of VF or pulseless VT (1). The development of the automatic external defibrillator (AED) is an important recent advancement in defibrillator technology. AED use for pediatric patients is discussed later in this chapter, after standard cardioversion and defibrillation techniques.

Because the most common cause of cardiopulmonary arrest in children is respiratory failure leading to hypoxemia and asystole rather than primary cardiac dysfunction with dysrhythmias, cardioversion and defibrillation are not frequently performed in this patient population. However, recent advances in pediatric cardiothoracic surgery have led to substantially higher survival rates among children with congenital heart disease, and these patients are at increased risk for dysrhythmias. In addition, children who accidentally or intentionally ingest excessive amounts of medications such as tricyclic antidepressants or sympathomimetics may also develop atrial and ventricular dysrhythmias. These drugs have become more prevalent in society as ever-increasing numbers of adolescents and adults are treated with antidepressant medications. For those children who present with cardiac dysrhythmias and hemodynamic compromise, cardioversion and defibrillation represent life-saving interventions that must be performed in a timely and appropriate manner.

▶ ANATOMY AND PHYSIOLOGY

Under normal circumstances, the sinoatrial (SA) node, located in the right atrium, serves as the primary source of cardiac impulses (Fig. 23.1). A depolarization wave travels through the atria to the atrioventricular (AV) node at the lower portion of the right atrium. Here conduction of the current is slowed, allowing sufficient time for completion of atrial contraction. The impulse is then conducted along the bundle of His through the right and left bundle branches to the Purkinje fibers, resulting in an organized ventricular depolarization and contraction.

Tachyarrhythmias commonly occur as a result of re-entrant conduction (2). As shown in Figure 23.2, during re-entry the usual conduction route for an electrical impulse (path A) is in a state of depressed excitability. While the current travels a more slowly conducted secondary path (path B), path A repolarizes. The current is then conducted along path A, but in a retrograde direction. The resulting pattern of rapidly cycling current (down path B and up path A) produces repetitive depolarizations leading to tachyarrhythmias. Re-entry may result in a rapid atrial and/or ventricular rate, depending on the extent of conduction from the atria to the ventricles and the location of the re-entrant circuit within the myocardium.

With cardioversion, an externally applied electrical current depolarizes a segment of the myocardium, rendering it refractory to continued depolarization by the re-entry impulse. This often allows the SA node to resume its role as pacemaker, because it normally has the greatest intrinsic automaticity. A synchronized cardioversion impulse is timed so that it is not given during the vulnerable period of the cardiac cycle in the

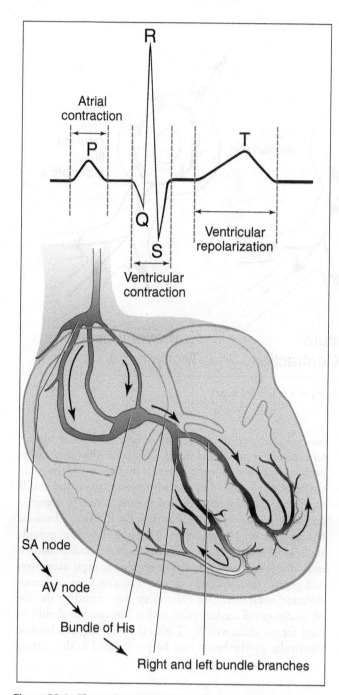

Figure 23.1 The cardiac cycle and cardiac conduction system.

phase of early repolarization, represented on the ECG tracing by the beginning of the T wave. An electric shock delivered at this time (the so-called R on T phenomenon) may produce VF (3).

The physiology of fibrillation is not well understood. Factors such as ischemia and acidosis are believed to decrease the refractory period that myocardial cells normally enter following depolarization (4). Numerous depolarization wavefronts that arise outside of the sinus node may then be conducted, beginning a series of re-entry circuits leading to asynchronous activity. Fibrillation may occur in both the atria and the ven-

tricles. In most instances, atrial fibrillation is not a serious dysrhythmia, as long as the resulting ventricular rate maintains a stable blood pressure. Therefore, emergent therapy is usually unnecessary. In contrast, VF is extremely dangerous if untreated. The ventricles contract in an ineffective and disorganized manner, leading to a rapid progression of minimal to nonexistent cardiac output, inadequate tissue perfusion, hypoxemia, and death. The heart is said to resemble a "bag of worms" during the chaotic depolarizations of VF. Electrical defibrillation is often the only intervention that will reverse this lethal cascade of events. Defibrillation involves an externally applied asynchronous electrical impulse that results in the depolarization of a large segment of ventricular tissue. After depolarization, these cells are refractory to ectopic impulses. As with direct cardioversion, the SA node can then take over the function of generating cardiac depolarizations, ideally resulting in a resumption of normal sinus rhythm.

▶ INDICATIONS

The decision to apply electrical current to the heart depends on the specific dysrhythmia present and the extent of hemodynamic instability. Signs of hemodynamic compromise among children include hypotension, agitation or lethargy, weak pulses, mottling, and delayed capillary refill. With children, proper assessment of blood pressure must be based on the normal range for each age group in question. A listing of normal blood pressure ranges for pediatric patients is presented in Table 4.3.

Supraventricular Tachycardia

SVT is the most common significant dysrhythmia in children (5). It most often occurs as a result of re-entry as described previously, although a non–re-entrant ectopic atrial focus may be the cause. Distinguishing SVT from sinus tachycardia can be difficult in children, although the degree of tachycardia with SVT is typically more extreme. In infants, the rate of SVT ranges from 220 to 320 bpm, and in older children from 150 to 250 bpm. Fever, anxiety, pain, and respiratory distress are a few conditions that may contribute to sinus tachycardia, but the heart rate rarely exceeds 210 bpm, even in young infants. In addition to extreme tachycardia, ECG findings consistent with SVT include a regular RR interval that does not vary with respiratory pattern, narrow QRS complexes, and dysmorphic or absent P waves (Fig. 23.3). Causes of SVT in children include congenital heart disease, Wolff-Parkinson-White syndrome, fever, and medications such as sympathomimetics. One case report described a child with albuterol-induced SVT, which was terminated with adenosine (6). Among infants, 50% of cases are classified as idiopathic (7).

Severe tachycardia associated with this condition results in decreased diastolic filling time, eventually leading to congestive heart failure. Older children with SVT typically come to

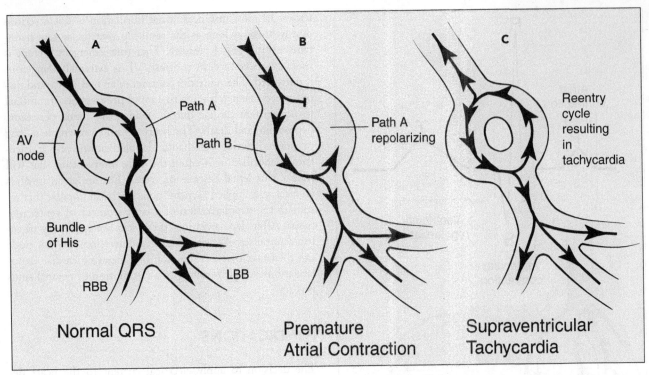

Figure 23.2 Schematic anatomy of a re-entrant focus.

medical attention relatively early in their clinical course when they complain of palpitations or chest pain. Consequently, they may not have significant hemodynamic compromise at presentation. In contrast, infants and young children with SVT will often have signs of significant cardiac decompensation (congestive heart failure, inadequate peripheral perfusion) when diagnosed. Thus, children with SVT will have a variable clinical presentation ranging from tachycardia alone to cardiogenic shock, depending on the duration of the dysrhythmia.

For children with stable hemodynamics, maneuvers designed to increase vagal stimulation to the heart may be both diagnostic and therapeutic in the management of SVT (see Chapter 70). For those with SVT, vagal maneuvers either will have no effect on the heart rate or will result in an abrupt termination of the dysrhythmia. For those with sinus tachycardia, vagal stimulation may result in a gradual decrease in the heart rate, followed by a steady return to the initial rate. If vagal maneuvers are unsuccessful, the next step is to administer intravenous medication. For the past 15 years, adenosine has been the drug of choice in treating the hemodynamically stable child with SVT (8–17). Synchronized cardioversion is indicated for patients who fail to respond to vagal maneuvers and pharmacologic agents or who manifest signs of hemodynamic instability. One cautionary note regarding the use of synchronized cardioversion is that low energies should be used for the child with SVT who is taking digoxin, because ventricular dysrhythmias may be precipitated in this setting

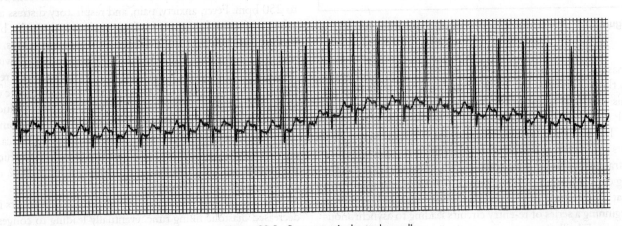

Figure 23.3 Supraventricular tachycardia.

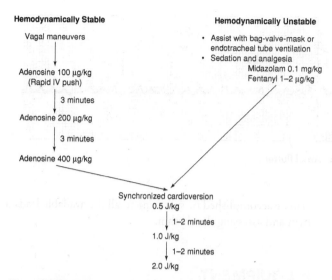

Figure 23.4 Treatment of supraventricular tachycardia.

(3). The recommended management approach is shown in Figure 23.4.

Atrial Fibrillation and Atrial Flutter

Although relatively uncommon in children, atrial fibrillation and atrial flutter should be recognized and treated appropriately. Atrial fibrillation appears on the ECG tracing as fine oscillating waves between QRS complexes without definable P waves. The hallmark of atrial fibrillation is an irregular ventricular response (Fig. 23.5). Atrial flutter is characterized by a regular ventricular rhythm with "sawtooth" waves between each QRS complex (Fig. 23.6). Atrial rates may exceed 400 bpm with either atrial fibrillation or atrial flutter, but since typically not all of the impulses are conducted to the ventricles, the ventricular rate will be considerably less. The clinical state of the patient depends on the rate of the ventricular response, the effects of any underlying heart disease, and the duration of the dysrhythmia. With a very rapid ventricular rate, diastolic filling time is diminished, resulting in decreased cardiac output.

With atrial fibrillation, ample time is usually available to initiate drug therapy in an attempt to terminate the dysrhythmia. If the patient fails to respond to drug therapy or becomes hemodynamically unstable, however, synchronized cardiover-

sion is indicated. Success rates as high as 90% have been reported for adults with no underlying heart disease who were treated with direct cardioversion for atrial fibrillation (3). For atrial flutter, on the other hand, synchronized cardioversion is now considered the treatment of choice, even when the patient is stable (3). This is true because atrial flutter is notoriously difficult to convert with drug therapy, and successful treatment with cardioversion has been reported in 72% to 100% of cases (3).

Ventricular Tachycardia

VT is also an uncommon dysrhythmia in the pediatric population. Conditions that may predispose to VT in children include underlying heart disease, a tricyclic antidepressant overdose, and disease processes leading to hyperkalemia such as renal failure or congenital adrenal hyperplasia.

As with SVT, VT may occur either as the result of re-entry or an ectopic focus, although here the abnormality is obviously ventricular in origin. On the ECG, the characteristic feature of VT is wide QRS complexes (greater than 0.12 seconds) with a bundle branch morphology (Fig. 23.7). The rate may vary from 120 to 400 bpm but is typically 200 to 300 bpm. P waves may be absent, retrograde (i.e., inverted and appearing after the QRS complex), or unrelated to the QRS complex (AV dissociation). SVT with aberrant conduction can be difficult or impossible to distinguish from VT based on ECG alone. However, because fewer than 10% of children with SVT have aberrant conduction, the clinician must assume the presence of VT when treating a child with a wide complex tachycardia (1).

Children with VT decompensate far more rapidly than those with SVT. As with SVT, tachycardia can result in a decreased ventricular filling time, which in turn leads to diminished stroke volume and cardiac output. Prolonged VT may also degenerate into VF. For patients who are hemodynamically stable, intravenous amiodarone is the treatment of choice (1). If the patient fails amiodarone therapy or shows signs of hemodynamic decompensation while still having a palpable pulse, synchronized cardioversion is indicated. For patients with pulseless VT, the most recent American Heart Association (AHA) guidelines recommend immediate asynchronous defibrillation (1). Studies with adults show that cardioversion is successful in converting VT in over 95% of cases (3).

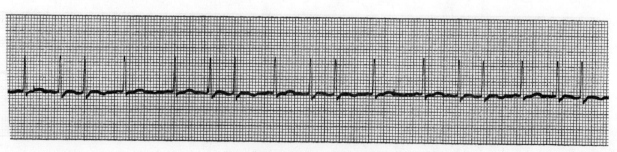

Figure 23.5 Atrial fibrillation.

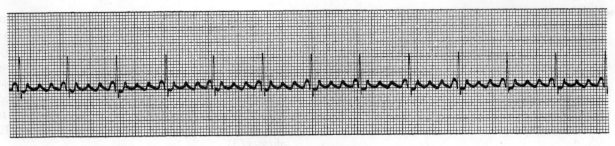

Figure 23.6 Atrial flutter.

Ventricular Fibrillation

Myocardial ischemia, a rare condition in children, is the most important factor in lowering the heart's fibrillation threshold (4). VF, when present in children, usually results from congenital heart disease, electrolyte disturbances, myocarditis, or drug toxicity. For adults, VF is the primary cause of sudden cardiac death (3), whereas the most common terminal dysrhythmias in children are asystole and bradycardia (18). VF appears on the ECG as a coarse or fine oscillating baseline without discernable QRS complexes (Fig. 23.8). The ventricles contract ineffectively, resulting in the absence of any significant cardiac output and consequent pulselessness. If electrical activity consistent with VF is noted on the monitor, the clinician should confirm this finding by examining the patient for palpable pulses, because a disconnected lead or a malfunctioning monitor can sometimes mimic this dysrhythmia. If no pulses are present, defibrillation should be performed immediately. The clinician should not delay defibrillation until an airway or intravenous access is established. To treat VF, one shock (2 J/kg) should be given, followed by 5 cycles of CPR, and then followed by a second shock (4 J/kg) if VF persists (1). In one study of hospitalized children who developed VF and were promptly treated with defibrillation, 89% were successfully resuscitated (19).

Defibrillation is not effective in the management of children with asystole and is therefore not indicated for this purpose (20). However, fine VF oscillations with amplitude of 1 mm or less may be mistaken for asystole. When using the paddles as "quick look" monitor leads, the operator should rotate the paddles 90 degrees to assess the rhythm in a different plane before assuming the dysrhythmia is asystole. If the child is connected to a standard cardiac monitor, this can also be accomplished by switching to all the available leads in turn and assessing the rhythm.

▶ EQUIPMENT

The source of the electrical current for all cardioversion devices in clinical use today is a direct current depolarizer. Units available in most hospitals can be used for both cardioversion and defibrillation. Cardioversion is performed in synchronous mode, and defibrillation is performed in asynchronous mode. The synchronizer allows discharge of current only after a repetitive series of R waves to ensure that energy is delivered outside of the vulnerable period of the cardiac cycle. Many machines have separate on/off switches for the defibrillator and the oscilloscope screen or monitor. In addition, all devices have a control to select the energy level, a control to initiate charging of the machine, and a light to indicate the machine is fully charged (Fig. 23.9).

The depolarizer delivers energy to the patient via two electrode paddles (Fig. 23.10). Typically, the controls allowing discharge of current are present on the paddle handles, but in some cases they are on a separate panel located on the machine. The most recent AHA guidelines recommend paddles with a 4.5-cm diameter for infants and children weighing less than 10 kg and 8-cm (adult) paddles for children over 10 kg (1). The goal is to choose the largest paddle that allows chest wall contact over its entire surface area. The larger the paddle, the lower the impedance and the greater the amount of cardiac muscle depolarized (4). In addition, larger paddles will produce less myocardial injury by allowing the energy to be dissipated over a greater surface area (3). However, if the

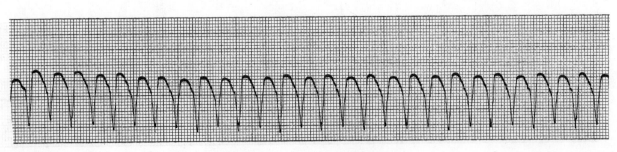

Figure 23.7 Ventricular tachycardia.

SUMMARY: SYNCHRONIZED CARDIOVERSION

1 Assess patient:
   a For patients who are hemodynamically unstable, perform cardioversion before establishing intravenous access or securing definitive airway.
   b For patients who are stable, administer supplemental oxygen and intravenous sedation/analgesia before performing cardioversion.

2 Turn cardioverter on.

3 Attach ECG leads to patient (if stable).

4 Select lead that displays tallest R wave.

5 Set machine on synchronous mode.

6 Apply electrode paste or gel to paddles.

7 Select energy and charge unit.

8 Place paddles firmly on chest in appropriate positions.

9 Ensure that operator is not contacting patient and that patient is not contacting any metal parts of stretcher.

10 Clear area ("All clear!").

11 Apply current by depressing discharge buttons simultaneously and holding paddles in place for several moments.

12 If dysrhythmia persists, double energy level, recharge unit, and apply current immediately.

13 If patient develops postcardioversion dysrhythmia, treat appropriately.

14 After patient is stabilized, address other management issues (administration of antiarrhythmic agents, correction of metabolic abnormalities, etc.).

 SUMMARY: DEFIBRILLATION

1 Perform defibrillation when indicated before establishing intravenous access or securing definitive airway.

2 Apply electrode paste or gel to paddles.

3 Turn machine on.

4 Select "quick look" paddle leads to assess rhythm.

5 Apply paddles firmly to appropriate positions on chest.

6 If monitor waveform appears to be asystole, rotate paddles 90 degrees to assess rhythm in another plane, since true rhythm may be fine VF.

7 Select energy and charge unit.

8 Ensure that operator is not contacting patient and that patient is not contacting any metal parts of stretcher.

9 Clear area ("All clear!").

10 Apply current by depressing discharge buttons simultaneously.

11 If dysrhythmia persists, double energy level, recharge unit, and reapply current immediately.

12 After three unsuccessful attempts, focus on correcting underlying process that is lowering fibrillation threshold.

prompts to provide instructions on the correct sequence of actions.

Procedure

Because of the high incidence of primary respiratory failure leading to cardiac arrest in children, it is recommended that a lone rescuer administer 1 minute of cardiopulmonary resuscitation (CPR) prior to using an AED (22). If the patient remains pulseless, the user turns on the AED and applies the two adhesive electrode pads to the patient's chest. One electrode is applied to the right upper sternal border and the other to the left anterior axillary line at the level of the nipple. Adult-sized pads may be used for pediatric patients who are older than 8 years of age or who weigh over 25 kg. Pediatric attenuated electrodes should be used for patients between 1 and 8 years of age to decrease the amount of electrical current administered (23). The patient is cleared while the AED analyzes the rhythm. If the device identifies a rhythm that is appropriate for treatment with electricity, the user is then instructed by a voice prompt when to deliver a shock by pressing a button.

concluded in 2003 that AED use is indicated for patients 1 year of age and older without signs of circulation (24).

Equipment

The greatest advantage of AEDs is the simplicity of their operation. They automate most of the steps involved with defibrillation based on internal programming and are designed to be used by members of the lay public when necessary. The user merely applies two electrodes to the chest of the patient, and the device automatically evaluates the cardiac rhythm, charges to an appropriate dose of electricity, and uses voice

CLINICAL TIPS

▶ Hemodynamic instability is indicated by hypotension, signs of inadequate cerebral or peripheral perfusion (lethargy, agitation, weak pulses, mottling, etc.), and heart failure.

▶ Before assuming that a dysrhythmia is asystole rather than fine VF, the operator must turn to another lead on the unit or rotate the monitoring electrode paddles 90 degrees.

▶ For infants and younger children weighing less than 10 kg, paddles with a 4.5-cm diameter are recommended. For children over 10 kg, 8-cm (adult) paddles should be used.

▶ Commercial pastes and gels lower the transthoracic impedance more than saline pads; alcohol pads and sonographic gel are contraindicated as a paddle-chest interface material.

▶ The synchronous mode must be set for direct cardioversion. The asynchronous mode must be set for defibrillation.

▶ With extreme tachycardia, the cardioverter may not be able to deliver a synchronous shock. Depending on the patient's condition, it may be necessary to set the machine on asynchronous mode in order to administer an electrical discharge.

▶ If pediatric paddles are unavailable, adult-size paddles can generally be used effectively for infants and younger children with the anteroposterior placement method.

▶ Defibrillation is not indicated for the treatment of asystole.

▶ Precautions during synchronized cardioversion that minimize the risk of injury to operator and patient include the following:
  ▶ Administration of sedation/analgesia (when appropriate)
  ▶ Selection of proper paddle size
  ▶ Liberal application of electrode paste or gel
  ▶ Use of the lowest recommended energy level initially

Complications

Complications associated with AED use are similar to those encountered with standard cardioversion and defibrillation. Additionally, motion artifact can sometimes lead to false interpretation of the cardiac rhythm by the device (4). If an AED incorrectly identifies a rhythm, a shock may be delivered

when not indicated, but this problem is relatively uncommon (24). The higher baseline heart rates of children can also decrease specificity in rhythm identification by adult-calibrated machines, but reports have indicated comparatively good sensitivity and specificity in this regard for pediatric patients (25,26).

▶ SUMMARY

With direct current cardioversion and defibrillation, electricity is administered to patients to terminate dysrhythmias. These procedures are indicated for patients exhibiting signs or symptoms of cardiovascular compromise resulting from dysrhythmias or for patients who fail to respond to pharmacologic therapy. Although attention should be given to other aspects of patient care, such as respiratory and metabolic abnormalities, delay in administering electrical current when indicated for the unstable patient must be avoided. Medical personnel caring for critically ill children should be knowledgeable about all aspects of cardioversion and defibrillation, including sedation methods, selection of correct energy dosage and paddle sizes, and standard operation of the equipment. When properly performed, cardioversion and defibrillation provide a means of terminating potentially life-threatening dysrhythmias with a relatively low incidence of complications.

▶ REFERENCES

1. 2005 American Heart Association (AHA) guidelines for cardiopulmonary resuscitation (CPR) and emergency cardiovascular care (ECC) of pediatric and neonatal patients: Pediatric Advanced Life Support. *Pediatrics* 117(5);e1005–e1028.
2. Suddaby EC, Riker SL. Defibrillation and cardioversion in children. *Pediatric Nurs.* 1991;17(5):477–481.
3. Hedges JR, Greenberg MI. Defibrillation. In: Roberts JR, Hedges J, eds. *Clinical procedures in emergency medicine.* 3rd ed., Philadelphia: WB Saunders Company, 1998, 186–196.
4. Ventriglia WJ, Hamilton GC. Electrical interventions in cardiopulmonary resuscitation: defibrillation. *Emerg Med Clin North Am.* 1983;1(3):515–534.
5. Wylie TW, Sharieff GQ. Cardiac disorders in the pediatric patient. *Pediatric Emergency Medicine Reports.* 2005;10(1):1–12.
6. Cook P, Scarfone RJ, Cook RT. Adenosine in the termination of albuterol-induced supraventricular tachycardia. *Ann Emerg Med.* 1994;24:316–318.
7. Gewitz MH, Woolf PK. Cardiac emergencies. In: Fleisher GR, Ludwig S, eds. *Textbook of pediatric emergency medicine.* 5th ed. Philadelphia, PA: Lippincott, Williams & Wilkins, 2006, 717–759.
8. DiMarco JP, Miles W, Akhtar M, et al. Adenosine for paroxysmal supraventricular tachycardia: dose ranging and comparison with verapamil. *Ann Int Med.* 1990;113:104–110.
9. Pinski SL, Maloney JD. Adenosine: a new drug for acute termination of supraventricular tachycardia. *Cleveland J Med.* 1990;57(4):383–388.
10. Owens M, Zellers-Jacobs L. Adenosine: the newest drug for PSVT. *RN.* 1992;55(12):38–41.
11. Cairns CB, Niemann JT. Intravenous adenosine in the emergency department management of paroxysmal supraventricular tachycardia. *Ann Emerg Med.* 1991;20:717–721.

12. Till J, Shinebourne EA, Rigby ML, et al. Efficacy and safety of adenosine in the treatment of supraventricular tachycardia in infants and children. *Br Heart J.* 1989;62:204–211.

13. Ros SP, Fisher EA, Bell TJ. Adenosine in the emergency management of supraventricular tachycardia. *Ped Emerg Care.* 1991;7(4): 222–223.

14. Reyes G, et al. Adenosine in the treatment of paroxysmal supraventricular tachycardia in children. *Ann Emerg Med.* 1992;12: 119–121.

15. Litman RS, et al. Termination of supraventricular tachycardia with adenosine in a healthy child undergoing anesthesia. *Anaesth Analg.* 1991;73:665–667.

16. Rossi AF, Burton DA: Adenosine in altering short- and long-term treatment of supraventricular tachycardia in infants. *Am J Cardiol.* 1989;9(64):685–686.

17. Overholt ED, Rheuban KS, Gutgesell HP, et al. Usefulness of adenosine for arrhythmias in infants and children. *Am J Cardiol.* 1988; 61:336–340.

18. Seidel J. Pediatric cardiopulmonary resuscitation: an update based on the new American Heart Association guidelines. *Ped Emerg Care.* 1993;9(2):98–103.

19. Gutgesell HP, Tacker WA, Geddes LA, et al. Energy dose for ventricular defibrillation of children. *Pediatrics.* 1976;58(6):898–901.

20. Losek JD, Hennes H, Glaeser PW, et al. Prehospital countershock treatment of pediatric asystole. *Am J Emerg Med.* 1980;7:571–575.

21. Young KD, Seidel JS. Pediatric cardiopulmonary resuscitation: A collective review. *Ann Emerg Med.* 1999;33(2):195–205.

22. Sampson RA, Berg RA, Bingham R. Use of automated external defibrillators for children: an update-an advisory statement for the pediatric advanced life support task force, International Liaison Committee on Resuscitation. *Pediatrics.* 2003;112(1):163–168.

23. Jorgensen D, Morgan C, Snyder D, et al. Energy attenuator for pediatric application of an automated external defibrillator. *Crit Care Med.* 2002;30(4):S145–147.

24. Liddle R, Davies CS, Colquhoun M, Handley AJ. The automated external defibrillator. *BMJ* 2003;327:1216–1218.

25. Cecchin F, Jorgenson DB, Berul CI, et al. Is arrhythmia detection by automatic external defibrillator accurate for children? *Circulation.* 2001;103:2483–2488.

26. Atkinson E, Mikysa B, Conway JA, et al. Specificity and sensitivity of automated external defibrillator rhythm analysis in infants and children. *Ann Emerg Med.* 2003;42:185–196.

SECTION 3 ▶ TRAUMA LIFE SUPPORT PROCEDURES

SECTION EDITOR: BRENT R. KING

GEORGE A. WOODWARD AND NANETTE C. DUDLEY

24

Cervical Spine Immobilization and Imaging

▶ INTRODUCTION

Cervical spine injuries, fortunately, are uncommon in the pediatric population. It has been estimated that cervical spine injuries occur in only 1% to 2% of pediatric patients with multiple trauma (1). However, the potentially devastating consequences of a cervical spine injury mandate proper immobilization and evaluation of all children who might have sustained such injuries. The purpose of cervical spine immobilization is to prevent the occurrence or exacerbation of spinal cord injury in the child with an unstable cervical spine. A variety of techniques may be used to attempt cervical spine immobilization, although some of these are more effective than others.

Mechanisms of injury most often associated with cervical spine damage in children include motor vehicle collisions, sports (contact, high-force activities), falls, diving accidents, and difficult newborn deliveries (breech, forceps) (2) (Table 24.1). All multiple trauma victims and those who have experienced a high-risk mechanism of injury should have cervical spine immobilization and evaluation.

To be effective and prevent secondary or ongoing injury, proper immobilization and care of the cervical spine should be started as soon as possible and continued until significant cervical spine injury has been excluded. Although cervical spine injuries can be devastating, necessary airway management and stabilization should not be delayed while awaiting formal cervical spine evaluation. Furthermore, there are at least two types of cervical spine immobilization, immobilization pending formal cervical spine evaluation and immobilization used for procedures like airway management. This chapter addresses these and other methods of cervical spine immobilization.

▶ ANATOMY AND PHYSIOLOGY

The pediatric cervical spine is similar to the adult's in that it can be anatomically divided into two sections (3). The anterior cervical spine is bordered by the anterior and posterior longitudinal ligaments and contains the bodies of the cervical vertebrae as well as the intervertebral disks. The posterior cervical spine includes the pedicles, lamina, spinous processes, and facet joints and the remainder of the cervical ligaments. Disruption of bony or ligamentous elements can potentially lead to an unstable cervical spine.

The child's cervical spine differs in many ways from that of the adult (2,4,5) (Table 24.2). The infant's large head and relatively weak neck muscles cause the fulcrum of the neck to be at C2-3, compared with C5-6 in the adult. Therefore, younger children tend to have upper cervical spine fractures whereas older children and adolescents have fractures in lower cervical

TABLE 24.1	HIGH-RISK MECHANISMS OF INJURY

Motor vehicle accident
Sports injury
Falls
Dives
Difficult delivery

spine regions, similar to adults (6). The large amount of cartilage in the pediatric cervical spine cushions direct vertical forces and limits the occurrence of bursting or compression-type fractures. The radiolucent cartilaginous component of the pediatric cervical spine, however, can make radiographic evaluation challenging. Children have more horizontal facet joints and increased ligamentous laxity, allowing for increased anterior and posterior motion of the cervical spine. This flexibility allows for significant spine distortion during the traumatic event, and the spine can subsequently appear normal when evaluated radiographically.

Children have relatively large occiputs in comparison to their chest circumference, which leads to relative kyphosis of the neck in a supine position (7). Immobilization of an adult with a long spine board leaves his or her neck in a neutral (30-degree lordosis) position. A similarly immobilized young child, however, will have his or her neck forced into relative kyphosis (Fig. 24.1). By age 8, many of these differences have diminished, and the patient can be immobilized and evaluated as an adult.

▶ INDICATIONS AND RADIOGRAPHIC EVALUATION

As described in the introduction, most pediatric cervical spine injuries are the result of high-force blunt trauma or specific mechanisms of injury like traction or axial loading. In children who are victims of these and many other types of trauma, prudence dictates cervical spine immobilization pending further evaluation. It should also be noted that, as compared with their adult counterparts, pediatric trauma victims can be dif-

TABLE 24.2	PEDIATRIC CERVICAL SPINE DIFFERENCES

Higher fulcrum of neck motion
  Large occiput
  Weaker neck muscles
Increased anterior/posterior motion
  Horizontal facet joints
  Increased ligamentous laxity
  Pseudosubluxation
Large carrilage component
  Growth plates
  Tapered anterior vertebrae
  Radiologic artifact
Lack of lordosis until age 6
Soft-tissue variability with breathing, vocalization
Congenital abnormalities (clefts, accessory ossicles)

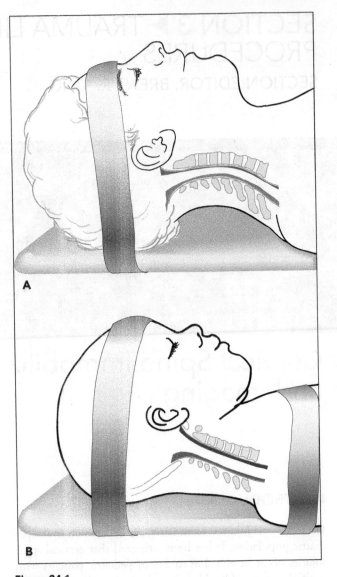

Figure 24.1
A. Adult's neck in neutral position on spine board.
B. Child's neck in kyphotic position on spine board.

ficult to evaluate. As is often the case with adult patients, the physician may be hampered by lack of patient cooperation and the absence of reliable witnesses, but young children present further problems because fear, pain, or lack of language skills may prevent them from relaying the symptoms (weakness, sensory changes) indicative of a cervical spine injury.

Physical findings suggestive of cervical spine or cord injury include cervical pain (especially pain in the midline), traumatic torticollis, limitation of cervical motion, motor weakness, sensory changes, diaphragmatic breathing without retractions, hypotension without tachycardia, bowel or bladder dysfunction, and priapism (5). These patients may or may not have cervical spine immobilization in place on presentation to the emergency department (ED).

Full cervical spine immobilization (hard cervical collar, spine board, spacers, and straps) should be applied to any patient with an unwitnessed or unclear mechanism of injury, a high-risk mechanism of injury, or a head injury involving loss of consciousness or altered mental status and whenever neurologic deficit or symptoms suggest a cervical cord injury. When the patient requires airway manipulation or intervention, in-line stabilization should be used. Although this can be accomplished from above or below the patient, immobilization from below may allow the airway to be managed in a less impeded manner.

Although cervical spine protection is important, immobilization should not delay airway assessment or intervention. Gentle airway maneuvers such as the jaw thrust, suctioning, and cricoid pressure can be performed without worsening an existing cervical injury. Vigorous airway maneuvers can, however, be detrimental to a patient with an unstable cervical spine (8).

Once a cervical spine injury has been diagnosed or is suspected, neurosurgical consultation may be necessary for further evaluation and definitive therapy. Transport of a patient with an unstable cervical spine over a long distance may require semipermanent immobilization (tongs, traction), and if the equipment and expertise does not exist at the referring hospital, a neurosurgeon may be included with the transport team.

Radiographic options for cervical spine evaluation include routine radiographs, tomograms, computerized tomography (CT), and magnetic resonance imaging (MRI) (5,6) (Fig. 24.2). The most useful radiograph for cervical spine assessment is a lateral view, often performed at the bedside

during trauma evaluation using portable equipment (9). This view should show any persistent dislocation or distraction but has an injury identification sensitivity of only 80% to 95%. The lateral cervical spine radiograph should be evaluated with regard to the alignment of the vertebral bodies, the integrity of the bones and cartilage, and the status of the soft tissues. The addition of at least two anterior views, C1-2 (odontoid view) and C3 through C7, increases the fracture identification sensitivity of the radiographic evaluation to 94% or greater (10). The odontoid view can be difficult to obtain on younger children (less than 5 years) and is not always done routinely in this age group (11). If a specific concern exists, a CT scan through C1 and C2 with reconstruction can replace the odontoid view (5). Oblique (pillar) views will provide further information about the posterior cervical column (pedicles, lamina, articulating and spinal processes) but rarely add significant information (12). Oblique views are potentially dangerous if performed with the standard 15-degree cranial angulation and neck rotation. CT scanning, when available, has replaced oblique views and tomograms if fractures are suspected on the initial radiographic film or series. Flexion and extension radiographs can be added for the awake patient who has a normal neurologic examination and three-view trauma series but for whom a persistent concern about possible column or ligamentous injury exists. Flexion and extension are performed by the patient, not by the radiology technician, and only to the point of mild discomfort. Clearly any initial radiographic evaluation should not involve neck motion if a cervical fracture is suspected. If an abnormality is identified, a search for other injuries that may not be contiguous is still necessary. Further radiographic views of an identified fracture, however, usually are not helpful in the acute evaluation. Importantly, cartilage fractures and ligamentous injuries will not be directly visible on the cervical radiograph. These might only be suspected if the patient presents with an abnormal neurologic examination or if radiographs demonstrate increased soft-tissue swelling.

A CT scan of the neck can be helpful to assess areas of the spine not adequately visualized with routine films, to delineate fractures suspected on radiographs, and to further elucidate an identified injury. A CT scan can be performed quickly and efficiently without neck motion. CT scans done properly can be reconstructed to avoid missing fractures in the horizontal plane.

MRI is useful acutely in the identification of spinal cord injury when neurologic deficits are present. MRI is excellent for the detection of blood accumulation (epidural hematoma), ligamentous injury, and cord damage. Although CT technology is still superior for fracture identification, newer technology has improved the MRI with regards to the identification of cortical bone injury (13). The difficulties associated with managing acutely ill patients during an MRI scan and the requirement that the patient not move during image acquisition limit its usefulness for acute injury evaluation. MRI has, however, been used in children with altered mental status to facilitate early removal of cervical immobilization (13,14).

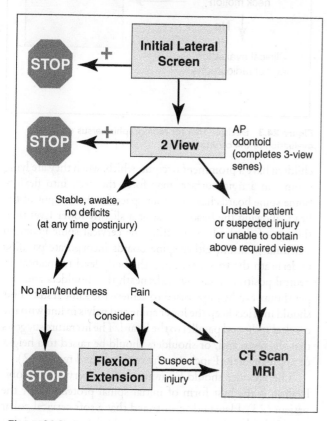

Figure 24.2 Radiographic scheme for cervical spine evaluation.

The syndrome of spinal cord injury without radiographic abnormality (SCIWORA) is more common in children less than 8 years of age (2,15,16). When applied to a child's spine, forces that would result in fracture or dislocation in an adult might not result in an abnormality on radiograph or CT scan because of the child's ability to realign the flexible cervical spine. The patient may, however, have had significant neurologic compromise. SCIWORA was first identified before MRI, and many SCIWORA patients have identifiable injury with MRI (17). Any patient suspected of having SCIWORA should remain immobilized pending evaluation by a neurosurgeon and, if necessary, further imaging studies.

Medical personnel should consider exclusion of significant injury upon clinical grounds, so-called "clearing" of the cervical spine, without radiographs if the patient has not been involved in a high-risk mode of injury, is awake and alert, has normal mental status (i.e., has no head injury or shock and is not under the influence of drugs or alcohol), and has no other painful injuries that might mask perception or appreciation of neck pain. Additionally, the child must have no evidence of neck pain, no tenderness to palpation of the cervical spine, full range of motion of the neck, a normal neurologic examination (motor, sensory, mental status), and no history of transient neurologic symptoms (18,19) (Fig. 24.3). Older, verbal children (e.g., those at least 4 to 5 years old) are more easily evaluated because they should be able to have a meaningful conversation. The cervical spine should not be cleared, regardless of radiographic findings, in the patient with altered mental status. Only when the patient is alert and awake and demonstrates normal neurologic status in concert with normal radiographs should the cervical spine be cleared. If questions arise during the assessment of a child's cervical spine, consultation with a radiologist or neurosurgeon may be helpful.

A difficult scenario arises when a child presents hours or days after the injury with neck pain. The type and extent of immobilization that should be placed while awaiting the radiographic evaluation of such patients is controversial. Some authors recommend placement of a hard cervical collar and limitation of patient movement during evaluation to help minimize potential risk to the patient and the provider.

▶ EQUIPMENT

Optimal immobilization of the cervical spine requires a spine board, a hard cervical collar, soft spacing or padding devices, and straps and wide tape to help secure the patient to the spine board (20) (Fig. 24.4). Optional equipment may include head cushions from a cervical immobilization device, a commercial pediatric immobilization device, and a vest-type immobilization device (21). A long, rigid spine board is used to immobilize the child's entire body. Vacuum mattresses or spilt scoop stretchers, if available, may be more appropriate for transfer than the rigid rescue boards. The head and neck must be kept in a neutral position or in slight extension. Young

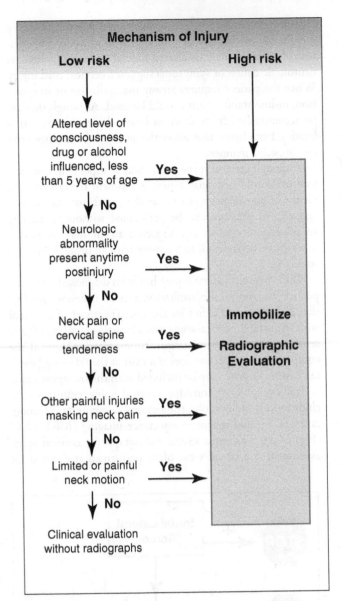

Figure 24.3 Decision tree for radiographic versus clinical evaluation of the cervical spine.

children have a prominent occiput, which, when they are lying supine on a rigid surface, may force the neck into flexion. Some spine boards have a cutout space for the occiput of the head, allowing the head to rest at a slightly lower level than the rest of the body and letting the cervical spine maintain a neutral position. Other spine boards incorporate padding underneath the torso, elevating the body level to maintain a neutral position. Padding underneath the shoulders and upper thorax can be improvised to achieve the same result. This should in effect keep the lower spine and pelvis in line with the cervical spine and parallel to the board. The literature suggests that the torso and/or shoulders should be raised to a height of approximately 1 inch to achieve the desired result (22).

The provider should be aware that full cervical immobilization is the best form of initial spinal protection for the patient (23). Heurta demonstrated that a soft cervical collar provided no protection against cervical spine motion and that

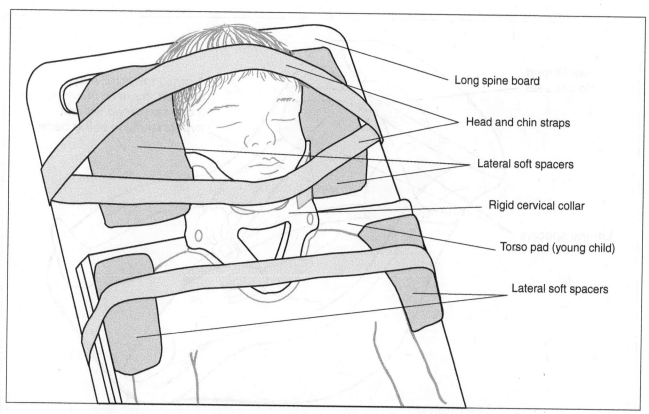

Figure 24.4 Ideal immobilization, including long spine board, pad to elevate torso, hard collar, soft lateral spacers, and forehead and chin straps.

the hard cervical collars, when used alone, were little better (24). A soft cervical collar provides inadequate immobilization and should not be used in the emergency setting. A hard cervical collar (Stifneck, Philadelphia, or other), when used in combination with a spine board and spacing devices, provides effective immobilization that is easy to implement. These collars are made of a hard foam or flexible plastic and have a foam lining and Velcro attachments (25,26). They are available in various sizes and do not interfere with radiographs or resuscitative efforts. With caution, the clinician can proceed with endotracheal intubation while a child is immobilized in a cervical collar, although partial removal or opening may facilitate airway interventions. Furthermore, most collars have a cutout area in front that allows the stabilization and visualization of a surgical airway.

After a cervical collar is applied, the child must be secured to a long spine board. The spine board serves to immobilize the joints above and below the suspected injury site, an important concept in the splinting of any suspected bony injury. Spine boards may be the traditional adult length or smaller specialized pediatric boards. The length chosen should ensure that the board can accommodate the child's entire body.

Many techniques for securing the patient to the spine board are used. Recently, disposable devices consisting of foam pads placed beside the head or cardboard barriers to lateral head movement have been developed. If these are not available, towel rolls or i.v. bags placed beside the patient's head can achieve

a similar result. Soft spacers are better than heavy sandbags, which can cause patient injury if they shift during logrolling. In all cases, the child's forehead and the chin area of the hard collar should be secured to these spacing devices and to the spine board. Although commercial immobilization straps may be purchased and are often included with spine boards, surgical tape can also be used. Placement of the strap (or tape) on the chin rather than on the cervical collar should be avoided because it might cause hyperextension of the neck and further injury. The chin strap should be secured to the cervical collar to effectively immobilize both the collar and the patient. In addition to immobilization of the child's head, the rest of the body must be secured to the spine board. Straps immobilizing the bony prominences of the shoulders and pelvis are most effective. Conversely, straps that are incorrectly or too tightly placed around the chest and abdomen can restrict chest wall movement and diaphragmatic excursion, leading to significant respiratory compromise (27). Soft padding should be used to fill in gaps along the patient's sides to help prevent lateral movement.

Young infants are often difficult to immobilize by traditional means. An infant in a car seat may be partially immobilized using towel rolls and the car seat's own seatbelt along with additional tape to secure the infant's head to the car seat (Fig. 24.5). This technique should not be used in an infant who has multiple injuries, has airway compromise, or is unstable.

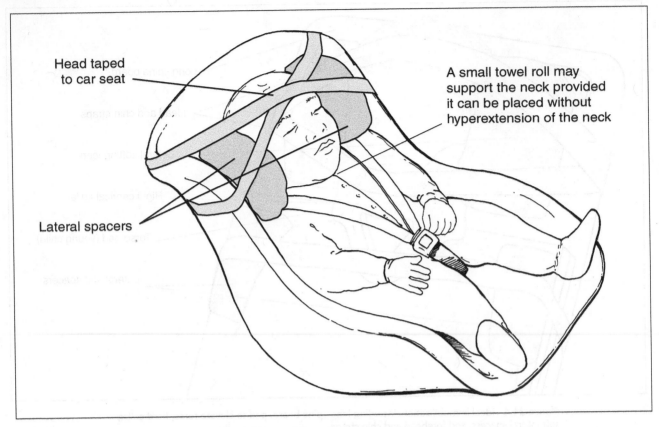

Figure 24.5 Infant immobilized in a car seat.

Immobilized children require constant observation. Suction should always be available. The potential need to logroll a patient who is vomiting must be anticipated. As mentioned previously, chest and abdominal straps can restrict respiration, and even properly placed straps can shift, causing problems. Children should have cardiorespiratory and oxygen saturation monitors in place as well as constant observation during immobilization.

If an unstable cervical spine injury is documented or highly suspected, neurosurgical consultation is recommended. The injury may necessitate further immobilization and/or fracture reduction in the ED to avoid worsening of the injury. Cervical tongs can be applied in the ED, providing weighted skeletal traction, which allows for bony reduction and maintenance of neutral alignment of the cervical spine (28,29). Problems with skeletal traction include difficulties with transport, patient movement, radiographic evaluation, airway intervention (as a result of the traction apparatus), and the need for the patient to remain supine. Other types of immobilization include halos and halo vests, which maintain alignment between the head, thorax, and cervical spine (30,31).

▶ PROCEDURE

Assessing Prior Immobilization

A patient who arrives with cervical spine immobilization in place should have an immediate assessment of that im-

mobilization. The ED personnel should ask the following questions:

- Are all the components of full immobilization present?
- Is the cervical collar of the correct type and size for the patient?
- Is the patient's neck in the neutral position?
- Is the patient securely strapped to a long spine board?
- Has the patient or the immobilization shifted during transport, making it less effective or causing hyperflexion or hyperextension of the cervical spine or compromise excursion of the chest with respiration?
- Is the immobilization in any way interfering with necessary assessment or management of the patient?

If these or any other immobilization difficulties are identified, they should be immediately addressed.

Application of Full Cervical Immobilization

The initial stage of cervical spine stabilization is in-line immobilization. In-line immobilization (not traction) is applied by placing hands on both sides of the patient's head and holding the head and neck in a neutral position. Cervical collars help to maintain this neutral position. Application of a cervical collar is best accomplished as a two-person procedure. This helps to avoid sudden movements of the neck and potential injury.

Selection of a collar of the correct size is important. A short collar may allow the neck to flex, a tall collar may result in hyperextension. The tallest collar that does not hyperextend the neck is the correct selection. A rapid examination of the neck for signs of injury (e.g., open wounds, expanding hematomas, subcutaneous air, anatomic distortion, shifted trachea) should precede placement of the collar (Fig. 24.6).

The Stifneck collar is a one-piece device that lies flat for storage and is assembled for use by moving the end of the chin piece and pushing the black fastener through the small hole on the collar, which forms the chin support at the front of the collar (32). The correct size is chosen by measuring the distance between the top of the shoulders and the bottom of the chin. If the child is supine, the back portion of the collar then slides behind the neck. It is helpful to fold the Velcro before applying the collar to avoid it becoming caught on hair or debris. Once the back of the collar is visible on the other side of the neck, the chin piece is fitted by sliding the collar up the chest wall. The chin should be well supported by the collar and should cover the central fastener on the collar. The collar can then be fastened with the Velcro and adjusted to obtain proper chin support. If tightening the collar causes hyperextension of the neck, then a smaller size should be selected. If the patient is sitting, the chin support is fitted first, as just described, then the back portion of the collar slides behind the patient's neck.

The Philadelphia collar is a two-piece, preformed cervical collar. Again, the proper size is selected to provide adequate

chin support, avoiding flexion or hyperextension of the neck. The back portion of the collar slides behind the patient's neck. The front portion of the collar moves up the chest wall until the chin support meets the chin. If the chin appears to be well supported, without flexion or hyperextension of the neck, then the Velcro attachments are fastened.

Neutral alignment must be maintained manually throughout application of any cervical collar. If the patient is wearing a helmet at the time of injury, it should be removed before applying the cervical collar (see Chapter 25).

Once the cervical collar is applied, the supine child is logrolled (or lifted) as a unit, maintaining in-line manual immobilization of the head and neck (20). An ideal logroll requires four people, one to hold the head and three to roll the chest, pelvis, and limbs. A specific rescuer may need to restrain the patient's limbs to reduce motion during this step. A long spine board, padded if necessary, is placed behind the patient. A vacuum mattress may also be used for immobilization at this point. When air is withdrawn from a vacuum mattress, it becomes a form-fitting mold to help secure the patient. The child is rolled (or lifted) as a unit onto the long board. If the child is seated, a short spine board is positioned behind the patient, who is then secured to that board. Next, a long spine board is placed beside the child. The child (and the short immobilization board, if used) is then pivoted and lowered onto the long board, keeping the knees and hips bent at right angles until the child is completely on the board. The child's legs are then lowered and secured to the board.

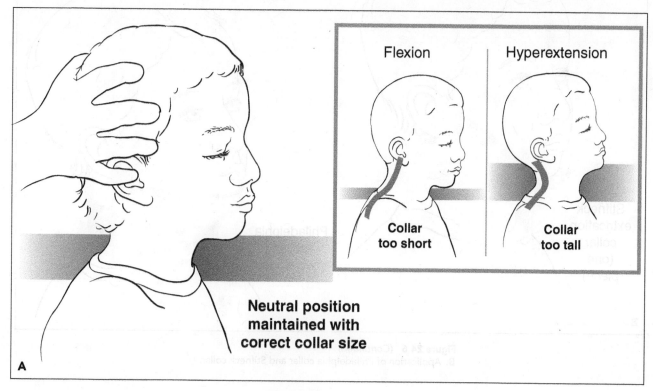

Figure 24.6
A. Appropriate sizing and (continued)

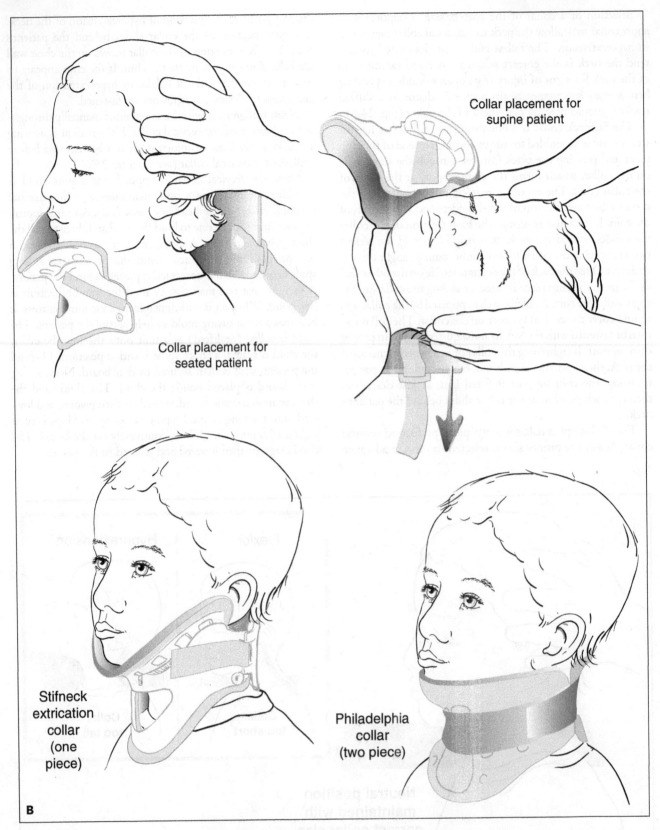

Collar placement for supine patient

Collar placement for seated patient

Stifneck extrication collar (one piece)

Philadelphia collar (two piece)

B

Figure 24.6 (Continued)
B. Application of Philadelphia collar and Stifneck collar.

To secure the child to the spine board, soft spacing devices are placed on both sides of the head and neck as well as in open spaces under the patient. The forehead strap or tape is then applied, originating on one side of the board and traveling over the spacers, across the forehead (using a non-sticky surface if placed over the eyebrows), and down the opposite side. The chin support strap (tape) should originate from the same location on the spine board, but it should travel over the spacers, across the chin support of the cervical collar, and down the opposite side to meet the forehead strap on that side. After padding is applied to the sides of the patient, the shoulder and pelvis straps are then applied. If proper equipment is unavailable, any adequately sized, rigid surface can substitute for a spine board, and towel rolls, i.v. bags, or other soft items such as pillows can be used as spacing devices, with tape substituting for straps. The manual immobilization of the cervical spine should be maintained until the entire spine is properly and securely immobilized.

Assessment of Cervical Spine Immobilization

Once a child is immobilized, the effectiveness of the procedure must be evaluated. The head and neck must be in a neutral position (slight extension). Airway, breathing, and circulation should be reassessed for potential compromise caused by the procedure. Effective ventilation should not be impaired by the straps or tape. The child may be crying and upset but should not be able to move significantly. Flexion, extension, or lateral movement of the head and neck should be prohibited. Finally, the child's neurologic state should be reassessed and should ideally be unchanged or improved after immobilization has been placed.

Semipermanent Cervical Spine Immobilization

If the child has evidence of cervical spine injury (e.g., an abnormal radiograph or physical examination or suggestive symptoms), neurosurgical consultation is required for possible external or semipermanent cervical spine immobilization. Successful skeletal traction relies more on the principle of application than on using a particular instrument. Contraindications to application of cervical tongs include bony disease leading to brittle or fragile bones and loss of skeletal integrity due to multiple skull fractures or patent sutures. Concerns with cervical traction in children include the relatively thin skull (more likelihood of inner table penetration), lighter body weight (less counterforce for traction), and more elastic ligaments and less developed musculature (risk of overdistraction) (33). Longer-term issues may be more common in children and include pin loosening, purulent site infections, dural penetration, and supraorbital nerve injury (33).

Cervical tongs are applied to the scalp in a coronal plane that passes through the mastoid processes (28,29). Hair should be shaved at the tong insertion points, the skin prepped with an antiseptic solution, and local anesthesia injected. The tips of the tongs point toward the top of the skull so that increased pressure will direct them inward and avoid slippage of the tongs from the skull. The screws of the tongs (Gardner) are tightened until approximately 30 pounds of pressure is exerted, indicated by protrusion of the distal spring-loaded points.

Once the tongs are in place, gradual cervical realignment and reduction of the fracture is begun with weights attached to a pulley system and the tongs. Although there is some debate about the ideal rate at which reduction should take place, no attempt should be made to immediately reduce the fracture, as the force necessary to do this may cause further spinal cord injury. Frequent neurologic examinations and cervical spine radiographs are necessary to evaluate the effects of the traction. If at any time further symptoms or evidence of neurologic abnormality occurs, traction should be reduced and radiographs retaken. Once satisfactory alignment is attained, the traction weight is reduced to the minimum required to hold the correct position, which will allow the spinal ligaments to heal. Neurosurgical consultation for the application of skeletal traction should be obtained before its use and continued until final disposition or transport of the patient. Cervical halo–vest combinations are also useful for immobilization of the cervical spine and offer an advantage in that free weights are not needed for reduction (30,31). This may be important in the patient who needs transport or frequent position changes.

In-line Stabilization for Airway Control

If intubation is required, the orotracheal route is preferred in children. This can be accomplished by having an experienced clinician immobilize the head and neck from above or below (most efficient) to prevent neck flexion or extension during intubation (Fig. 24.7). Excessive force causing neck movement must be carefully avoided. The patient's neck must always remain in a neutral position while airway or other interventions are ongoing (see also Fig. 16.25). Although intubation can be performed with the cervical collar in place, it is usually more efficient to open the collar anteriorly to facilitate mandibular motion and visualization of the anterior and cephalad larynx. Nasal intubation can be performed on adults or adolescents but should not be attempted in children. If surgical airway placement is indicated, active neck immobilization must again be performed by an experienced clinician. In addition, the operator performing a surgical airway must be vigilant to avoid applying excessive downward pressure on the neck while making incisions or inserting airway devices.

▶ COMPLICATIONS

A patient with cervical spine immobilization is at risk for several potential complications and for iatrogenic injury (Table 24.3). Incorrect or inadequate stabilization or a lack of vigilance also could lead to an adverse outcome for the patient.

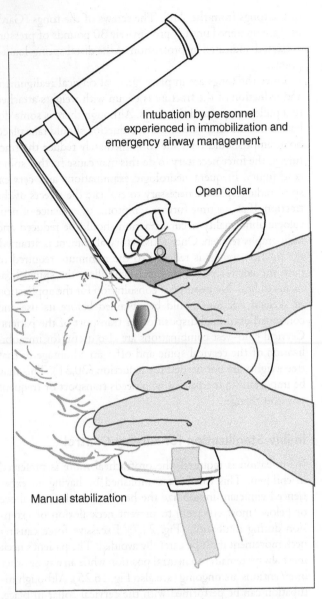

Intubation by personnel experienced in immobilization and emergency airway management

Open collar

Manual stabilization

Figure 24.7 Manual immobilization from below, with open cervical collar, during intubation attempt.

TABLE 24.3	POTENTIAL COMPLICATIONS OF CERVICAL IMMOBILIZATION

TABLE 24.3	POTENTIAL COMPLICATIONS OF CERVICAL IMMOBILIZATION

Inadequate immobilization with potential neck mobility
   Use of soft collar for immobilization
   Reliance of hard collar alone for immobilization
Innapropriate immobilization with respiratory restriction
   Initial incorrect immobilization
   Shifted patient/immobilization during transport
Incorrect immobilization with hyperflexion/extension
   Incorrect size collar
   Child on hard spine board without torso elevation
   Resistant patient forced into immobilization
Restricted access to immobilized child
   Inability to physically examine/assess neck with collar in place
   Difficult airway intervention (intubation, surgical airway)
   Difficult venous access (external/internal jugulars)
   Airway compromise with vomiting, bleeding, aspiration; when secured in supine position

Incorrect sizing of the cervical collar can lead to hyperextension or flexion of the neck and worsen the underlying injury. Ensuring that the cervical collar is correctly sized is imperative in order to prevent this complication.

The cervical collar, while protecting the cervical spine, may limit visualization of a shifted trachea, expanding neck hematoma, or subcutaneous emphysema. Although not a complication of the immobilization, cervical spine stabilization also limits the accessibility of external or internal jugular vein catheterization because the clinician cannot manipulate the neck in a lateral or anteroposterior direction to facilitate venous access. These procedures are best avoided in a patient suspected of having a cervical spine or cord injury.

Inappropriate securing of the patient to the spine board can complicate immobilization. Straps connecting the patient to the spine board that cross the chest, abdomen, neck, or chin may cause problems with ventilation or exacerbate the spinal injury. This is also true of immobilization that has shifted during transport. Frequent reassessments of the patient and the immobilization should help to alleviate these difficulties. Clinicians should also be aware that even a patient in a hard cervical collar on a long spine board with appropriate spacer devices and properly attached straps has the potential for neck motion and worsening of an existing injury.

The patient should be firmly secured to the long cervical spine board so that when logrolling is needed (e.g., in response to emesis), the cervical spine is not subjected to increased lateral forces or motion. Soft spacing devices should be used to avoid adding stress to the neck during the logrolling procedure. Large-bore suction should be immediately available to avoid aspiration.

As mentioned, manual immobilization is sometimes required for airway management. Incorrect manual stabilization or a lack of vigilance could also lead to an undesirable outcome for the patient. Replacement of a hard spine board with a padded rigid surface should be considered once the patient is evaluated in the ED setting to avoid pressure injuries.

Airway compromise with vomiting, bleeding, or aspiration can occur while the patient is supine. The child could easily choke, aspirate, or have a respiratory arrest if the airway is not kept free of debris. Children with vomiting may need to be suctioned and/or logrolled while still immobilized to prevent aspiration (see Fig. 13.10). As mentioned previously, cervical spine immobilization may have to be partially removed for airway management. When this is necessary, manual stabilization of the cervical spine must be maintained.

Attempts at placing a cervical collar on a struggling patient may worsen the underlying injury due to patient exertion. In most instances, a patient is better off without formal immobilization if he or she vigorously resists cervical collar application but is otherwise calm.

SUMMARY

1 Assess any prior immobilization and correct or modify as necessary.

2 Stabilize head and neck in neutral position using in-line immobilization.

3 Apply cervical collar (best as two-person procedure):
 a Check collar size.
 b Assemble collar (if necessary).
 c Slide collar behind neck.
 d Slide chin piece up chest wall (for two-piece collar).
 e Fasten Velcro on collar.
 f Recheck neutral alignment.

4 Position patient on spine board or vacuum mattress. If patient is supine:
 a Logroll (or lift) child while maintaining in-line manual immobilization.
 b Place long spine board under child or lift child onto board or vacuum mattress.
 c Roll (or lift) child as a unit onto board or vacuum mattress.
 If patient is seated:
 a Position short spine board behind child.
 b Secure child to short board.
 c Place long spine board alongside child.
 d Pivot and lower child onto long board (knees and hips bent).
 e Lower child's legs to long board.

5 Secure patient to spine board:
 a Place soft spacing devices on both sides of head and neck.
 b Pad open spaces between patient and spine boards.
 c Apply forehead strap.
 d Apply chin support strap.
 e Pad alongside patient to help prevent lateral movement.
 f Apply shoulder and pelvis straps.

6 Evaluate effectiveness of procedure:
 a Assess for respiratory or airway compromise.
 b Maintain head and neck in neutral position.
 c Ensure immobilization prevents any significant movement of head and neck of patient.

7 Reassess ABCs.

8 Repeat neurologic exam.

 CLINICAL TIPS

▶ Cervical injury should always be suspected.

▶ The most important initial goals in a trauma resuscitation are to stabilize the primary injury and to prevent secondary injury.

▶ Adequate cervical immobilization will only be achieved if the appropriate equipment and proper sizes are used.

▶ The effectiveness of cervical immobilization should be reassessed frequently.

▶ Neurosurgical consultation should be sought early when indicated.

▶ Cervical immobilization should not be removed until clinical and (if necessary) radiographic "clearing" and a normal neurologic examination are completed.

Because of the possibility of SCIWORA in children, radiographs alone are insufficient to exclude cervical spine injury when documentation of a normal neurologic examination is not possible. An unconscious or multiply injured patient with normal cervical spine radiographs should have immobilization maintained until his or her mental status allows for complete neurologic examination. In such cases, cervical spine immobilization should not be removed until a complete normal neurologic examination has been documented. It is vitally important to provide constant attention to the patient's cervical spine immobilization and to continue to assess the patient for changes in status, shifting of immobilization, and other clues to ongoing injury.

▶ SUMMARY

All patients who have a suspected cervical spine injury, neurologic abnormality, altered level of consciousness, mental status changes, or other painful injuries, who experienced a high-risk mechanism of injury or multiple trauma, or who cannot be assessed because they are young should be immobilized. It is important to realize that immobilization must be complete to be effective. Incomplete or improper immobilization can predispose the patient to secondary injury. Although the incidence of cervical spine injury in children is low, the devastating consequences demand that if an injury is suspected, correct immobilization and evaluation be performed. As with any emergency procedure, a complete evaluation, along with proper documentation, before and after any intervention is important.

▶ REFERENCES

1. Wilberger J. *Spinal Cord Injuries in Children*. New York: Futura; 1986.
2. Dickman C, Rekate H, Sonntag V, et al. Pediatric spine trauma: vertebral column and spinal cord injuries in children. *Pediatr Neurosci*. 1989;15:237–256.
3. Doris P, Wilson R. The next logical step in the emergency radiographic evaluation of cervical spine trauma: the five-view trauma series. *J Emerg Med*. 1985;3:371–385.
4. Roche C, Carty H. Spinal trauma in children. *Pediatr Radiol*. 2001;31:677–700.
5. Woodward GA. Neck trauma. In: Fleisher GR, Ludwig S, Henretig FM, eds. *Textbook of Pediatric Emergency Medicine*. 5th ed. Philadelphia: Lippincott Williams & Wilkins; 2006:1389–1432.
6. Swischuk LE. *Imaging of the Cervical Spine in Children*. New York: Springer-Verlag; 2002.
7. Herzenberg JE, Hensinger RN, Dedrick DK, et al. Emergency transport and positioning of young children who have an injury of the cervical spine. *J Bone Joint Surg Am*. 1989;71:15–22.
8. Bivins H, Ford S, Bezmalinovic Z, et al. The effects of axial traction during orotracheal intubation of the trauma victim with an unstable cervical spine. *Ann Emerg Med*. 1988;17:53–57.
9. Swischuk LE. *Emergency Imaging of the Acutely Ill or Injured Child*. 4th ed. Philadelphia: Lippincott Williams & Wilkins; 2000:532–535.
10. Baker C, Kadish H, Schunk JE. Evaluation of pediatric cervical spine injuries. *Am J Emerg Med*. 1999:17;230–234.
11. Swischuk LE, John SD, Hendrick EP. Is the open-mouth odontoid view necessary in children under 5 years? *Pediatr Radiol*. 2000;30:186–189.
12. Ralston ME, Ecklund K, Emans JB, et al. Role of oblique radiographs in blunt pediatric cervical spine injury. *Pediatr Emerg Care*. 2003:19;68–72.
13. Frank JB, Lim CK, Flynn JM, et al. The efficacy of magnetic resonance imaging in pediatric cervical spine clearance. *Spine*. 2002;27:1176–1179.
14. Flynn JM, Closkey RF, Mahboubi S, et al. Role of magnetic resonance imaging in the assessment of pediatric cervical spine injuries. *J Pediatr Orthop*. 2002;22:573–577.
15. Pang D, Pollack I. Spinal cord injury without radiographic abnormality in children: the SCIWORA syndrome. *J Trauma*. 1989;29:654–664.
16. Grabb PA, Oyesiku NM, Przybylski GJ, et al. *Guidelines for the Management of Acute Cervical Spine and Spinal Cord Injuries: Spinal Cord Injury without Radiographic Abnormalities (SCIWORA) Recommendations*. Section on Disorders of the Spine and Peripheral Nerves of the American Association of Neurologic Surgeons and the Congress of Neurologic Surgeons; August 2001:281–295. http://www.spineuniverse.com/pdf/traumaguide/finished1116.pdf.
17. Grabb PA, Pang D. Magnetic resonance imaging in the evaluation of spinal cord injury without radiographic abnormality in children. *Neurosurgery*. 1994;35:406–414.
18. Jaffe DM, Binns H, Radkowski MA, et al. Developing a clinical algorithm for early management of cervical spine injury in child trauma victims. *Ann Emerg Med*. 1987;16:270–276.
19. Viccellio P, Simon H, Pressman BD, et al. A prospective multicenter study of cervical spine injury in children. *Pediatrics*. 2001;108:2/e20.
20. Spine and spinal cord trauma. In: *Manual of Advanced Trauma Life Support*, 7th ed. Chicago: American College of Surgeons; 2004:177–204.
21. Diekmann R, Brownstein D, Gausche-Hill M, eds. *Pediatric Education for Prehospital Professionals*. Sudbury: Jones and Bartlett; 2006;362–366.
22. Nypaver M, Treloar DJ. Neutral cervical spine positioning in children. *Ann Emerg Med*. 1994;23:208–211.
23. Podolsky S, Baraff LJ, Simon RR, et al. Efficacy of cervical spine immobilization methods. *J Trauma*. 1983;3:461–464.
24. Huerta C, Griffith R, Joyce S. Cervical spine stabilization in pediatric patients: evaluation of current techniques. *Ann Emerg Med*. 1987;16:55–60.
25. McCabe JB, Nolan DJ. Comparison of the effectiveness of different cervical immobilization collars. *Ann Emerg Med*. 1986;15:50–53.
26. Dick T. Prehospital splinting. In: Roberts JR, Hedges JR, eds. *Clinical Procedures in Emergency Medicine*. Philadelphia: WB Saunders; 1985.
27. Schafermeyer RW, Ribbeck BM, Gaskins J, et al. Respiratory effects of spinal immobilization in children. *Ann Emerg Med*. 1991;20:1017–1019.
28. Gardner WJ. The principle of spring-loaded points for cervical traction. *J Neurosurg*. 1973;39:543–544.
29. Crutchfield WG. Skeletal traction in treatment of injuries to the cervical spine. *JAMA*. 1954;155:29–32.
30. Heary RF, Hunt CD, Krieger AJ, et al. Acute stabilization of the cervical spine by halo/vest application facilitates evaluation and treatment of multiple trauma patients. *J Trauma*. 1992;33:445–451.
31. Chandler DR, Nemejic C, Adkins RH, et al. Emergency cervical spine immobilization. *Ann Emerg Med*. 1992;21:1185–1188.
32. Stifneck package insert. Sacramento, CA: California Medical Products, Inc; 1989.
33. Grabb PA, Oyesiku NM, Przybylski GJ, et al. *Guidelines for the Management of Acute Cervical Spine and Spinal Cord Injuries: Management of Pediatric Cervical Spine and Spinal Cord Injuries*. Section on Disorders of the Spine and Peripheral Nerves of the American Association of Neurologic Surgeons and the Congress of Neurologic Surgeons; August 2001:237–280. http://www.spineuniverse.com/pdf/traumaguide/finished1116.pdf.

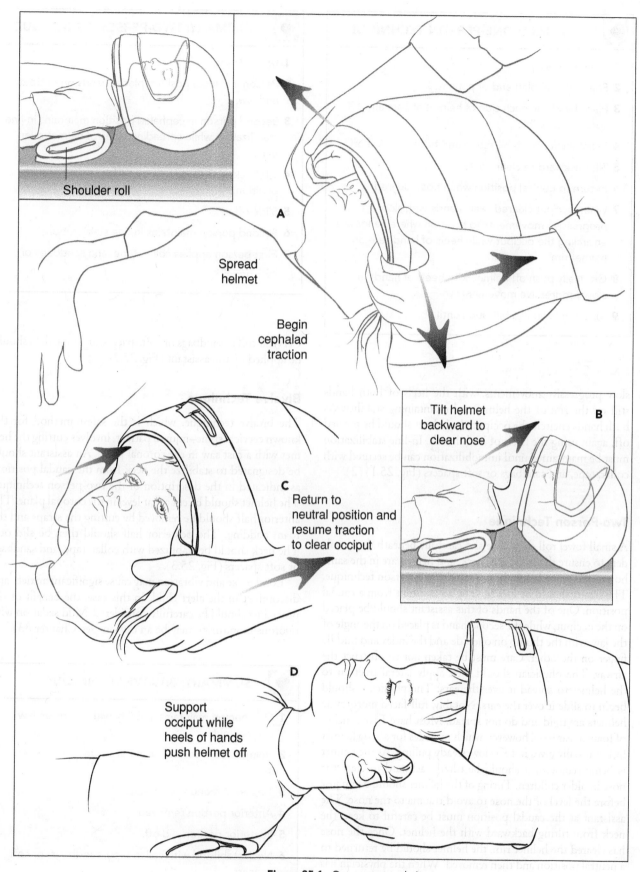

Shoulder roll

A

Spread
helmet

Begin
cephalad
traction

Tilt helmet
backward to
clear nose

B

C

Return to
neutral position and
resume traction
to clear occiput

D

Support
occiput while
heels of hands
push helmet off

Figure 25.1 One-person technique.

SUMMARY: ONE-PERSON TECHNIQUE

1 Untie straps.

2 Stand at cephalad end of patient.

3 Place hands on each side of helmet at ears and spread if possible.

4 Maintain in-line stabilization and begin to slide off.

5 Tilt backward to clear nose.

6 Return to neutral position when nose cleared.

7 When occiput cleared, walk hands with slow progressive movements to position where hands are encircling the occiput while heels of hands are on helmet rim.

8 Gradually push off helmet with heels of hands in slow progressive movements.

9 Maintain in-line stabilization until able to stabilize.

SUMMARY: TWO-PERSON TECHNIQUE

1 Untie straps.

2 Person in caudal position places hands on occiput and jaw.

3 Second person in cephalad position maintains in-line stabilization while spreading sides of helmet over ears.

4 Tilt backward to clear nose and return to neutral position.

5 Slide off.

6 Second person maintains in-line stabilization.

7 First person applies collar, tape, and sandbags or soft spacers.

slow progressive movements, with the heels of both hands still on the rim of the helmet and maintaining stability. As both hands encircle the occiput, the helmet should be pushed off, again using the heels of both hands. In-line stabilization must be maintained until immobilization can be secured with collar, tape, and sandbags or soft spacers (Fig. 25.1) (2).

Two-Person Technique

A small towel roll should be slid carefully beneath the shoulders to ensure that the body, neck, and helmet are in the same horizontal plane before beginning the two-person technique. The straps should be loosened by an assistant from a caudal position. One of the hands of this assistant should be placed on the occiput, while the second hand is placed on the angle of the jaw, with the thumb on one side and the index and middle finger on the other. Care must be taken not to obstruct the airway. The physician should then apply lateral traction to the helmet to spread it over the ears. The physician should begin to slide it over the ears. Notably, full-faced motorcycle helmets are rigid and do not spread. Most have 1 to 2 inches of foam at ear level, however, which provides for a snug helmet fit but usually gives in to a slow, steady pulling. As the helmet is being removed, it should be tilted backward to clear the nose in older children. Tilting of the helmet should begin just before the level of the nose to avoid trauma to the nose. The assistant at the caudal position must be careful to keep the neck from tilting backward with the helmet. Once the nose has cleared the helmet rim, the helmet should be returned to a neutral position and then removed. When the physician has removed the helmet, his or her hands should be placed on the occiput, and in-line stabilization should be maintained.

Cervical collar, sandbags or soft spacers, and tape then should be applied by the assistant (Fig. 25.2) (4).

Bivalve Technique

The bivalve technique, which is the safest method for the known cervical spine–injured patient, involves cutting the helmet with a cast saw in the coronal plane. An assistant should be designated to stabilize the neck from the caudal position, as indicated in the description of the two-person technique. The helmet should be cut at ear level in the coronal plane. The anterior half should be removed by cutting the straps and the foam padding. The posterior half should then be slid out. The neck should be stabilized with collar, tape, and sandbags or soft spacers (Fig. 25.3).

Loud noise and vibration may cause significant anxiety and discomfort in the alert child. In this case, the benefit of the procedure should be carefully considered. Mild sedation with rigorous monitoring may be an option (see Chapter 33).

SUMMARY: BIVALVE TECHNIQUE

1 One person maintains stability with hands on jaw and occiput.

2 Helmet cut in coronal plane at ear level using cast saw.

3 Ties are cut and foam is cut.

4 Anterior portion removed.

5 Posterior portion slid off.

6 Neck stabilized with collar, tape, sandbags, or soft spacers.

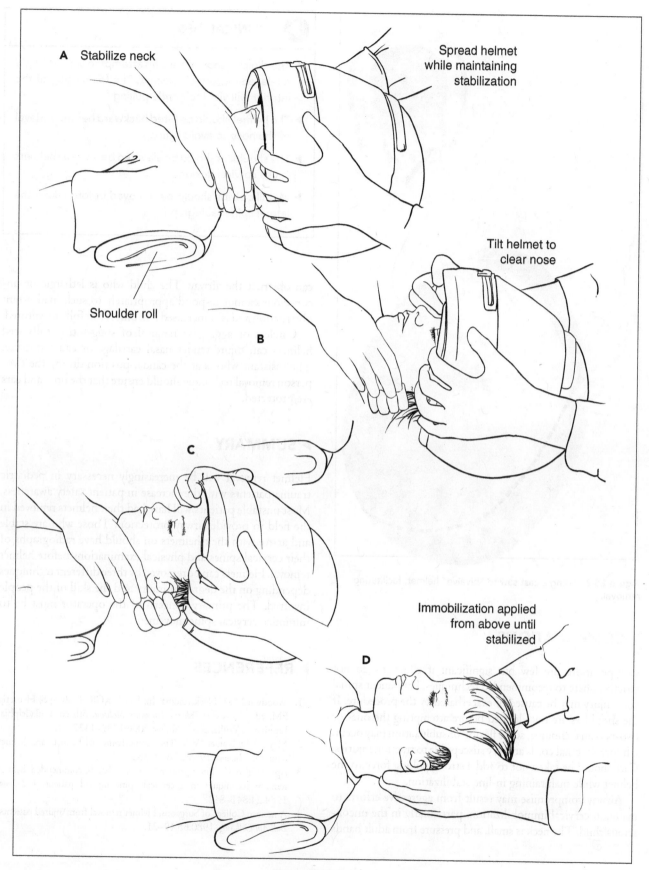

A Stabilize neck

Spread helmet while maintaining stabilization

Shoulder roll

B Tilt helmet to clear nose

C

D Immobilization applied from above until stabilized

Figure 25.2 Two-person technique.

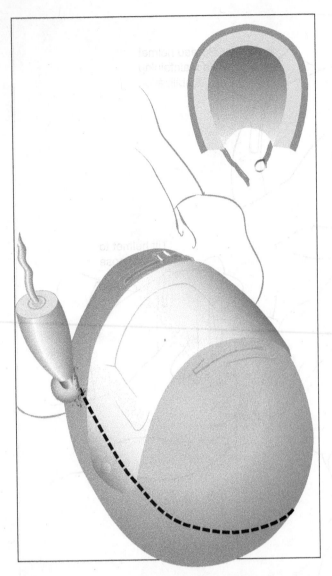

Figure 25.3 Using a cast saw to "bivalve" helmet, facilitating removal.

▶ COMPLICATIONS

Complications are few but significant if clinicians do not strictly adhere to recommended techniques. Permanent spinal cord injury may be caused or exacerbated by the procedure. If the shoulders are not elevated before attempting the one- or two-person technique, some flexion or subluxation may occur. Children's spinal cords are very susceptible to traction injuries. Care should be taken not to add a strong pulling force to the helmet while maintaining in-line stabilization.

Airway compromise may result from aggressive efforts to maintain cervical immobilization, particularly in the unconscious child. The neck is small, and pressure from adult hands

 CLINICAL TIPS

▶ The clinician should make no attempt to spread a rigid full-faced motorcycle helmet. The foam lining of the interior will yield to gentle pulling.

▶ The helmet should be tilted backward before the level of the nose to avoid injury.

▶ The shoulders should be elevated because all helmets cause cervical flexion.

▶ Metallic strips should be removed before taking the lateral spine radiograph.

can obstruct the airway. The child who is lethargic or unconscious cannot respond appropriately to such inadvertent obstruction and is at increased risk unless carefully monitored.

Careless or aggressive removal of snug-fitting full-faced helmets can injure tender nasal cartilage or cause fracture. The assistant who is at the caudal position during the two-person removal technique should ensure that the nose and ears are protected.

▶ SUMMARY

Helmet removal will be increasingly necessary in pediatric trauma patients with the increase in patient safety awareness. Most unstable patients will have had their helmets removed in the field to provide airway protection. Those who are stable and arrive with their helmets on should have radiographs of their cervical spines and physical examinations before helmet removal. Helmets can be removed by three different techniques depending on the degree of injury and the skill of the people involved. The primary concern of the operator must be to minimize cervical spine movement.

▶ REFERENCES

1. Woodward GA. Neck trauma. In: Fleisher GR, Ludwig S, Henretig FM, eds. *Textbook of Pediatric Emergency Medicine.* 5th ed. Philadelphia: Lippincott Williams & Wilkins; 2006:1389–1432.

2. Meyer RD, Daniel WW. The biomechanics of helmets and helmet removal. *J Trauma.* 1985;25:329–332.

3. Aprahamian C, Thompson BM, Darin JC. Recommended helmet removal techniques in a cervical spine injured patient. *J Trauma.* 1984;24:841–842.

4. American College of Surgeons. Helmet removal from injured patients. *Bull Am Coll Surg.* 1980;65:19–21.

GARY R. STRANGE AND LEO G. NIEDERMAN

26

Surgical Cricothyrotomy

▶ INTRODUCTION

The majority of children who require airway control or assisted ventilation can be managed with standard means such as bag-valve-mask (BVM) ventilation or tracheal intubation. However, occasionally these techniques fail or cannot be performed. In these cases, alternative means of airway control must be employed. Three common alternatives to standard airway techniques are surgical cricothyrotomy, percutaneous needle cricothyroidotomy with transtracheal ventilation, and retrograde intubation. This chapter discusses the technique of surgical cricothyrotomy; the other two techniques are discussed in Chapters 17 and 18.

Surgical cricothyrotomy involves dissection of the anterior neck and visualized incision of the cricothyroid membrane or, alternatively, wire-guided insertion of a special catheter or tracheal tube. The technique has been well described in the adult population, but experience in young children is anecdotal or limited. Furthermore, surgical cricothyrotomy has received little description in standard pediatric emergency medicine texts, and ideal training for this procedure in children has not been developed or evaluated.

▶ ANATOMY AND PHYSIOLOGY

Important to understanding any invasive airway procedure is knowledge of the anatomy of the anterior neck, larynx, and trachea (Fig. 26.1). The larynx, which consists of the thyroid cartilage, the cricothyroid membrane, and the cricoid cartilage, lies in the anterior neck, deep to the skin, subcutaneous tissues, and sternohyoid muscle. The thyroid cartilage is cephalad to the cricothyroid membrane, and the cricoid cartilage is caudad to it. The fibroelastic cricothyroid membrane can be palpated as an indentation between the two more prominent cartilage structures.

The cricoid cartilage attaches inferiorly to the tracheal rings. At approximately the same level of the junction of the cricoid membrane and the trachea is the isthmus of the thyroid gland. Care must be taken during dissection to avoid this structure. Additionally, although the cricothyroid membrane is relatively avascular, the superior thyroid artery crosses the superior portion of the membrane and can be damaged during dissection or incision.

In adolescents and adults, the cricothyroid membrane is approximately 20 to 30 mm in width and 9 to 10 mm in superior-to-inferior length. In infants and children, the larynx is smaller and positioned more rostrally, making the topical landmarks of the thyroid and cricoid cartilage more difficult to identify. Furthermore, in this population, the hyoid bone may be more easily felt than the thyroid cartilage. In infants, the cricothyroid membrane is only about 3 mm in rostrocaudal length. For this reason, some medical personnel recommend that alternative techniques be employed in young children (1) (see "Indications").

▶ INDICATIONS

The primary indication for surgical cricothyrotomy is to achieve airway control when less invasive techniques are unsuccessful or contraindicated. In infants and children, this will occur most often when an upper airway obstruction results from an irremovable foreign body or massive edema (such as epiglottitis or Ludwig angina) or when significant maxillofacial, mandibular, oropharyngeal, or laryngeal trauma has occurred and caused significant edema or severe anatomic distortion. Usually, masseter spasm or laryngeal spasm in children can be managed by other means, such as pharmacologic

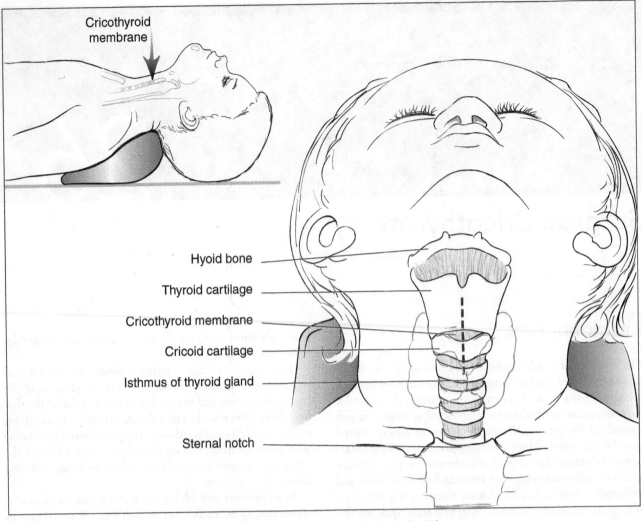

Figure 26.1 Anatomical landmarks for surgical cricothyroidotomy.

paralysis and endotracheal intubation. The use of surgical cricothyrotomy in children with known or suspected cervical spine injury is controversial. It is an option when BVM ventilation or controlled orotracheal intubation with in-line stabilization of the head and neck cannot be safely accomplished in the apneic or hypoxemic child.

The major contraindication to this technique is the ability to provide adequate oxygenation and ventilation by more standard, less invasive means (see Chapters 13 to 18). Massive trauma to the larynx or the trachea, particularly transecting injury, is also a relative contraindication to surgical or needle cricothyrotomy; these techniques should be attempted under these circumstances only when other means of airway control are impossible and death is imminent. Additionally, because of the small size of the cricothyroid membrane in young children, some medical personnel suggest that this technique not be employed in children less than 5 years of age (1). Needle cricothyrotomy is preferred in younger children.

Other relative contraindications include neck trauma or edema that hinders surgical dissection or landmark identification. Known bleeding diathesis also may increase the risk of

failure to obtain airway control rapidly and increase the risk of other complications as well.

Surgical cricothyrotomy most often will be performed by physicians; however, in many situations airway control must be accomplished in the field. It is therefore vital that prehospital providers be familiar with this technique or with one of the alternatives discussed in Section 2.

▶ EQUIPMENT

The equipment necessary to perform surgical cricothyrotomy is listed in Table 26.1. As is the problem with other procedures, this technique is rarely employed in children, and the equipment available on a surgical airway tray may be inappropriate for use in children. Valuable time may be lost in an attempt to gather the proper equipment when the need for it arises. Therefore, it is important to include pediatric equipment on such trays or to develop a pediatric surgical airway tray. It is particularly important to have the proper size tracheal tubes and/or tracheostomy tubes, and a range of tube

TABLE 26.1	EQUIPMENT

Standard Cricothyroidotomy

1. Scalpels with No. 15 and No. 11 blades loaded
2. Trachea hook(s)
3. Trousseau dilator (trachea dilator; note that this device may be too large for young children)
4. Curved Mayo scissors
5. Curved hemostats (2)
6. Small vascular clamps (2)
7. Needle holder
8. Suture or circumferential tie for tracheostomy tubes
9. Syringe with 25-gauge needle for infiltration of lidocaine
10. 1% or 2% lidocaine (with epinephrine)
11. Sterile gauze pads
12. Sterile drapes
13. Appropriately sided tubes (listed in order of desirability)
    a. Cricothyroidotomy tubes
    b. Endotracheal tubes (2.5 to 7.0 mm internal diameter)
    c. Tracheostomy tubes (Shiley 0 to 6)

Additional Equipment for Wire-Guided Cricothyroidotomy
Wire-guided cricothyroidotomy kit OR

1. Guidewire
2. Needle sized appropriately to accommodate the guidewire
3. 10-cc syringe
4. Dilator/introducer designed to fit within the cricothyroidotomy tube (optional)

sizes should be immediately available. Equipment necessary to perform wire-guided cricothyroidotomy can be purchased in a kit. Many facilities choose this option because it is convenient and ensures that all necessary tools will be available when the need arises. One piece of equipment should be used with caution: Standard tracheostomy tubes are designed such that the intratracheal portion has a more acute angle with the flange than does the cricothyroidotomy catheter (see Fig. 26.3D). They are, therefore, more difficult to fully insert than cricothyroidotomy catheters.

▶ PROCEDURE

Surgical Cricothyrotomy: Standard Technique

The cricothyroid membrane should be identified below the tip or notch of the thyroid cartilage and above the cricoid cartilage. As stated previously, these structures can be difficult to palpate in young children, but the thyroid cartilage is large enough to be felt in most children. Once this structure is identified, its anterior surface should be palpated in a rostrocaudal fashion. The palpating finger should drop into the notch below the thyroid cartilage; this is the location of the cricothyroid membrane. When the thyroid cartilage cannot be identified by palpation, an alternative is to identify the hyoid bone and to then palpate caudally. Either the thyroid cartilage or the cricoid cartilage (or both) can be identified by this method.

If time permits, adequate surgical preparation and local anesthetic infiltration using lidocaine with epinephrine should be done. A vertical midline incision is made over the entire cricothyroid membrane (Fig. 26.2A). The midline incision should protect most of the major neck vessels, which are located laterally, but some venous bleeding should be anticipated. Limiting the caudad extension of the incision is necessary to avoid the highly vascular thyroid gland. The skin and subcutaneous tissue should be incised and then held open with retractors (Fig. 26.2B). After this incision, the cricothyroid membrane should be quickly palpated a second time to confirm its position. The sternohyoid muscle then should be carefully incised or separated by blunt dissection, exposing the cricothyroid membrane (Fig. 26.2C). The trachea is stabilized with either a tracheal hook or the fingers of the nonsurgical hand, and a short horizontal incision is made with the point of a No. 11 scalpel blade. The incision is made in the lower half of the membrane, near the cricoid cartilage (Fig. 26.2D). Care must be taken to direct the scalpel blade perpendicular to the frontal plane of the membrane and not to enter too deeply into the trachea, because this could result in injury to the posterior wall of the trachea and the esophagus behind it. Curved Mayo scissors or a curved hemostat is inserted into the incision, turned, and spread to widen the opening. While the blades of the scissors or hemostat are used to maintain the opening, the trachea is stabilized and lifted anteriorly, and an appropriate size tracheostomy tube or endotracheal tube is inserted between the scissor or hemostat blades and into the trachea (Fig. 26.2E). Alternatively, a tracheal hook can be inserted into the caudal portion of the incision and used to elevate the cricoid cartilage and trachea. The tube can be passed below the hook and into the trachea. The tube is secured and attached to a bag-valve device, and ventilation is assessed (Fig. 26.2F).

Finally, the above describes the procedure as performed under ideal circumstances. Occasionally, the technique may have to be modified. For example, if bleeding prevents visualization of the cricothyroid membrane, it can be identified using palpation. The membrane has an elastic feel compared to the more rigid cartilage above and below it. Likewise, if the membrane, after being opened, is lost from view, the operator may be able to find it again using escaping air bubbles. In the spontaneously breathing patient, these will occur with each exhalation. In the apneic patient, pressure should be applied to the chest to force air from the incision (2,3).

Surgical Cricothyroidotomy: Wire-Guided Technique

Wire-guided cricothyroidotomy requires a needle or catheter (18 gauge) and a syringe. The guidewire required for this procedure is significantly shorter than that required for retrograde intubation. However, one needs a guidewire long enough to extend well into the trachea while leaving room for the introducer ventilating tube. A scalpel is also necessary to perforate the cricothyroid membrane. Sterile prep material and drapes are usually recommended but can be omitted when time is not sufficient. The same holds true for local anesthetic. Many commercial kits also include a dilator/introducer that serves

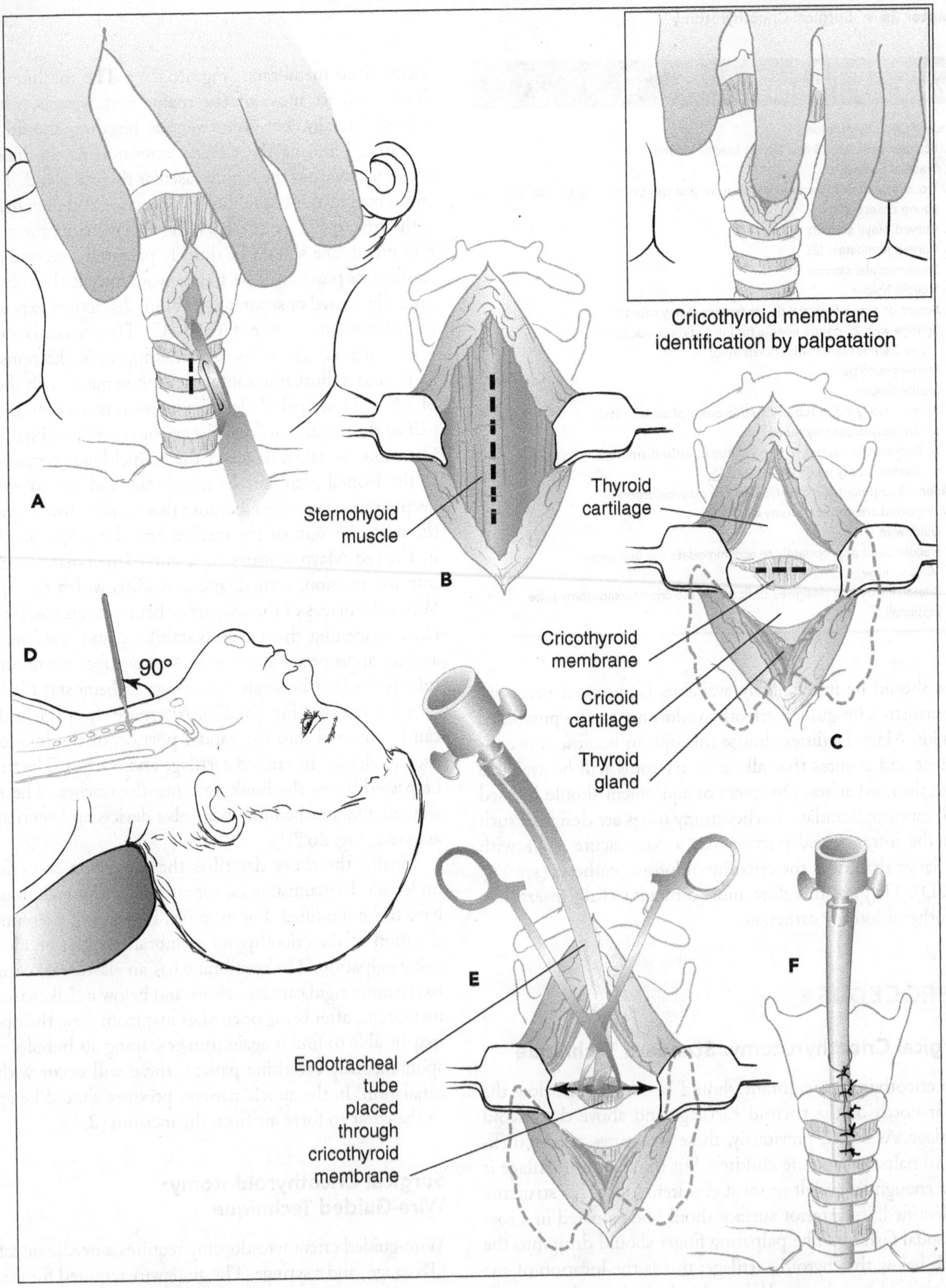

Cricothyroid membrane
identification by palpatation

Sternohyoid
muscle

Thyroid
cartilage

Cricothyroid
membrane

Cricoid
cartilage

Thyroid
gland

90°

Endotracheal
tube
placed
through
cricothyroid
membrane

Figure 26.2
A. Initial vertical incision with manual stabilization of the trachea.
B. Skin retraction and exposure of the sternohyoid muscle.
C. Retraction of the sternohyoid muscle and exposure of the cricothyroid membrane (note that the location of the incision is indicated).
D. Horizontal incision through the cricothyroid membrane with the scalpel perpendicular to the membrane.
E. Hemostats or scissors used to maintain the opening in the membrane while a tracheal tube is passed through the incision and into the trachea.
F. Tracheal tube secured in place.

SUMMARY: STANDARD CRICOTHYROIDOTOMY

1 Identify landmarks in anterior neck by palpating hyoid bone, thyroid cartilage, and cricoid cartilage.

2 When time permits, prepare skin with antiseptic solution and administer local infiltrative anesthesia.

3 Stabilize trachea with nonoperating hand.

4 Make vertical midline incision over cricoid membrane, attempting to avoid isthmus of thyroid gland.

5 While an assistant retracts skin and subcutaneous tissue, bluntly dissect through sternohyoid muscle until cricothyroid membrane is visualized.

6 Using No. 11 scalpel blade, make small horizontal incision near inferior border of membrane.

7 Insert pair of curved Mayo scissors or small curved hemostat into incision and spread jaws of scissors or hemostat to enlarge incision.

8 Maintain patency of incision either by keeping scissors or hemostats in place or by inserting trachea hook into inferior margin and gently lifting edge of incision anteriorly.

9 Insert appropriate size endotracheal tube or tracheostomy tube into incision and secure.

10 Assess adequacy of ventilation.

CLINICAL TIPS: STANDARD CRICOTHYROIDOTOMY

▶ Alternative means of airway control, such as needle cricothyroidotomy or retrograde intubation, should always be considered first, particularly if the patient is a young child.

▶ The initial incision is made vertical and in the midline. This reduces the risk of damage to vascular structures.

▶ In some cases, the cricothyroid membrane may not be easily visualized. In these instances, the membrane should be palpated with a fingertip. "Blind" incision is a technique of last resort because of the risk of damage to vascular structures in the area.

▶ A tracheal hook or the blades of the scissors or hemostats should be used to keep the incision open and to maintain location of the incision.

▶ If the incision is "lost," bubbles of exhaled air will often identify its location. In the apneic patient, these may be produced by pressure on the anterior chest wall.

▶ Even a small airway is better than none. If a small endotracheal or tracheostomy tube is all that will pass through the incision, then it should be used until more effective airway control can be established.

the same function as the similar device in many Seldinger central line kits (4,5). While this facilitates placement of the cricothyroidotomy catheter, the procedure can be performed without such a device.

Like standard surgical cricothyroidotomy, the wire-guided technique begins with identification of the cricothyroid membrane and with sterile preparation of the puncture site. The next step is similar to retrograde intubation in that the cricothyroid membrane is punctured with a catheter or needle large enough to accommodate the guidewire (Fig. 26.3A). However, since this technique is often being performed under emergency circumstances and on unconscious patients, it may not be necessary to anesthetize the overlying skin or the trachea itself. Also, in this case the catheter or needle is directed caudally to facilitate passage of the guidewire distally (Fig. 26.3B). Finally, unlike retrograde intubation, the guidewire used in wire-guided cricothyroidotomy need only be long enough to accommodate the cricothyroidotomy tube and its introducer.

After the guidewire has been inserted, the introducer needle or catheter can be removed (Fig. 26.3C). Then a scalpel is used to incise the skin and the cricothyroid membrane. Some bleeding might occur at this point. Then the cricothyroidotomy tube and, if one is used, the introducer are advanced over the wire and into position (Fig. 26.3D). Use of the introducer is strongly recommended because it not only facilitates advancement of the tube but helps to prevent placement of the tube into a "false lumen" created by tissue planes. Also, care must be taken with this step since, as is the case with Seldinger vascular procedures, the guidewire can be inadvertently fully advanced into the trachea. Therefore, the operator should maintain control of the wire at all times (Fig. 26.3E).

Once the tube and introducer have been advanced as far as possible, the introducer and guidewire are removed (Fig. 26.3F). If the tube is cuffed, the cuff should be inflated, and the tube's position should be confirmed by end-tidal CO_2 detection. The tube may then be secured with standard tracheostomy ties or skin sutures (4).

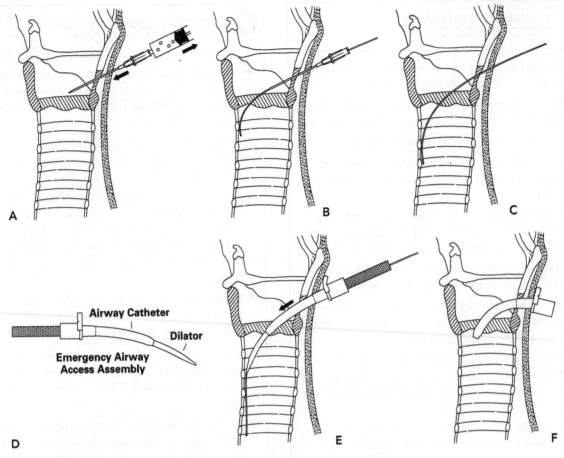

Figure 26.3

A. Insert needle into cricothyroid membrane and aspirate air.

B. An over-the-needle catheter may be used in place of the needle. If this option is chosen, the needle portion should be removed, leaving the plastic catheter in place.

C. Direct the needle or catheter toward the distal airway and advance the guidewire into the airway distally.

D. The optional dilator may be loaded into the cricothyroidotomy catheter.

E. Incise the skin and membrane with a scalpel, then advance the cricothyroidotomy catheter, endotracheal tube, or tracheostomy down the guidewire and into the airway.

F. Remove the guidewire, and dilator, if used, and confirm that the catheter is in the airway using an end-tidal CO_2 detector.

(Adapted from Melker JS, Gabriella A. Melker cricothyrotomy kit: an alternative to the surgical technique. *Ann Otol Rhinol Laryngol.* 2005;114:525–528.)

▶ COMPLICATIONS

In adults, complication rates for this procedure have been reported to be as high as 40% (6,7). Complications include incorrect site of incision or tube placement, prolonged procedure time, hemorrhage, and failure of the procedure to access the airway. Less commonly, esophageal and mediastinal perforation, subcutaneous emphysema, pneumothorax, pneumomediastinum, and laryngeal injury may occur (2,3,6,7). Traditional teaching has emphasized the risk of subglottic stenosis after this procedure. However, more recent literature suggests that this complication may occur less frequently than was previously thought (8,9). Furthermore, some risks that are unacceptable for an elective procedure become quite acceptable in an emergency situation for which the alternative to

a relatively high risk procedure may be death. Unfortunately, there are no reports of large series of surgical cricothyrotomy in children, but complication rates would be expected to exceed those seen in adult series as a result of the increased technical difficulties involved in working with small structures.

The risk of occurrence of some of the previously mentioned complications can be minimized with careful attention to proper technique. A vertical midline incision above the level of the thyroid isthmus reduces the chance of inadvertent injury to vascular structures because most of the major vessels lie lateral to the midline. Likewise, when possible, puncture of the cricothyroid cartilage should be performed in the inferior section of the membrane because a portion of the superior thyroid artery sometimes crosses the membrane along its rostral border. The incision should be made

SUMMARY: WIRE GUIDED CRICOTHYROIDOTOMY

1 Identify landmarks in anterior neck by palpating hyoid bone, thyroid cartilage, and cricoid cartilage.

2 When time permits, prepare skin with antiseptic solution and administer local infiltrative anesthesia.

3 Stabilize trachea with nonoperating hand.

4 Load an 18-gauge needle or over-the-needle catheter onto a 10-cc syringe.

5 Puncture the cricothyroid membrane in its inferior portion, and confirm that the needle or catheter is located within the trachea by aspiration of air.

6 If an over-the-needle catheter has been used, remove the needle, leaving the plastic catheter in place.

7 Direct the needle or catheter distally and advance the guidewire into the distal airway, taking care to leave sufficient guidewire to advance the cricothyroidotomy tube, endotracheal tube, or tracheostomy tube.

8 Incise the skin and cricothyroid membrane using a No. 11 or No. 15 scalpel.

9 If an introducer is being used, load this into the cricothyroidotomy tube (note: this step can be accomplished earlier).

10 Advance the cricothyroidotomy tube, endotracheal tube, or tracheostomy tube over the guidewire and into the trachea.

11 If an introducer was used, remove it.

12 Confirm that the tube lies within the trachea using end-tidal CO_2.

13 Secure the tube using, tape, suture, and/or tracheostomy ties.

 CLINICAL TIPS: WIRE GUIDED CRICOTHYROIDOTOMY

▶ Equipment for wire-guided cricothyroidotomy should be a part of every difficult airway cart or tray.

▶ Kits that include all necessary equipment are available and should be considered.

▶ The needle should be angled inferiorly and with the bevel anterior.

▶ As in any Seldinger line technique, control of the guidewire is critical.

▶ Cricothyroidotomy catheters, particularly those with introducers, function better than tracheostomy tubes.

▶ In older or larger patients, cuffed tubes are preferred.

is made caudal to the cricothyroid membrane, in the trachea. The result is an unintended tracheostomy. This is a moderately serious complication, but given that this procedure will most likely be attempted only when the patient's life is at risk, as long as the result is adequate ventilation the potential consequences of the tracheostomy are of less concern and can be managed once the patient is stable. Of greater concern is a needle puncture that is made too rostrally. In this case, the procedure might be performed above the vocal cords, resulting in failure. As described above, many recommend that surgical cricothyroidotomy be performed in the lower or caudal portion of the membrane because the cricothyroid artery and vein tend to be located in the upper portion. Because the wire-guided technique is not preformed under direct vision, it may be more difficult for the operator to place the needle in the desired location, and the artery or vein might be injured. In some cases, the bleeding is significant and requires operative intervention. In emergency settings, however, this procedure is typically being performed under life-and-death circumstances in which the potential benefits justify the risks.

▶ SUMMARY

Surgical cricothyrotomy is a potentially life-saving technique that can be used to obtain necessary airway control when circumstances prevent the effective use of more traditional and less invasive techniques. This procedure is closely related to needle cricothyroidotomy with transtracheal ventilation and to retrograde tracheal intubation, both of which are discussed in Section 2. For some patients, particularly young children, one of these techniques may be preferred.

under direct vision whenever possible and should be just large enough to permit scissors or vascular clamps to be inserted. The scalpel also should be kept perpendicular to the membrane and not allowed to penetrate too deeply into the larynx. These two precautions help to avoid damage to the vocal cords, which lie above the cricothyroid membrane, and to the posterior trachea and esophagus, which lie posterior to it.

In addition to the potential complications described above, wire-guided cricothyroidotomy poses some unique risks. When attempting wire-guided cricothyroidotomy, the operator may not correctly identify the cricothyroid membrane and may puncture another site. In most cases, the puncture

▶ REFERENCES

1. Tucker JA. Obstruction of the major pediatric airway. *Otolaryngol Clin North Am.* 1979;12:329–341.
2. Mace SE. Cricothyrotomy. *J Emerg Med.* 1988;6:309–319.
3. Walls RM. Cricothyroidotomy. *Emerg Med Clin North Am.* 1988;6: 725–736.
4. Corke C, Cranswick P. A Seldinger technique for mini-tracheostomy insertion. *Anaesth Intensive Care.* 1988;16:206–207.
5. Melker JS, Gabriella A. Melker cricothyrotomy kit: an alternative to the surgical technique. *Ann Otol Rhinol Laryngol.* 2005;114:525–528.
6. McGill J, Clinton JE, Ruiz E. Cricothyrotomy in the emergency department. *Ann Emerg Med.* 1982;11:361–364.
7. Kress TD, Balsubramaniam S. Cricothyrotomy. *Ann Emerg Med.* 1982;11:197–201.
8. Brautigan CO, Grow JB. Cricothyroidotomy revisited again. *Ear Nose Throat J.* 1980;59:289–295.
9. Brautigan CO, Grow JB. Subglottic stenosis after cricothyroidotomy. *Surgery.* 1982;91:217–221.

DEBORAH M. FERNON AND BRENT R. KING

Diagnostic Peritoneal Lavage

27

▶ INTRODUCTION

When assessing children who have sustained abdominal trauma, the emergency physician or surgeon must quickly determine if these children have sustained a serious injury necessitating emergency surgery. In some cases, this determination can be made on clinical grounds alone, but often a diagnostic procedure is required. Diagnostic peritoneal lavage (DPL) is one method by which abdominal injuries can be identified. Shortly after being introduced by Dr. Root in 1964, DPL became the primary means of evaluating the abdomen after blunt trauma (1). Peritoneal lavage is also used as a therapeutic tool in hypothermia (2). DPL involves two separate components, peritoneal aspiration and peritoneal lavage, if the aspiration is not successful in obtaining free peritoneal blood. DPL is a very sensitive modality for the detection of intraperitoneal blood but does not identify the injured organ or the need for exploratory laparotomy. In this era of new imaging modalities, noninvasive testing, and conservative management of the trauma victim, DPL is rarely performed (3–5). Today, DPL's main utility lies in the evaluation of the hemodynamically unstable patient when bedside ultrasound is not available or provides equivocal results. For this reason, recommended techniques and applications of DPL are presented with particular emphasis on those aspects that specifically relate to children.

▶ ANATOMY AND PHYSIOLOGY

Because DPL is in many ways a "blind" procedure, it is important to understand the anatomy of the abdomen and especially how the abdominal anatomy of infants and young children differs from that of adults. The abdominal cavity is continuous with the pelvic cavity. It is bordered superiorly by the muscular thoracoabdominal diaphragm and inferiorly by the pelvic diaphragm. The anterior abdominal wall consists of skin, fat, and several layers of underlying muscles whose tendinous sheaths fuse together in the midline to form the linea alba. This relatively avascular area is the site for needle insertion into the abdominal cavity. In infants and young children, the muscles of the anterior abdominal wall are relatively weak when compared to those of adolescents and adults, providing less protection for the abdominal organs. The pliable bones of the child's chest wall gives relative protection from rib fractures while allowing greater forces to be transmitted within the thoracic cavity, making these patients more susceptible to pulmonary contusions and injury to the intrathoracic abdominal organs—the diaphragm, liver, spleen, and stomach.

The intra-abdominal organs in children occupy a relatively larger portion of the abdominal cavity than these organs do in adults. The bladder is of particular concern, because in young children the bladder is more an abdominal than a pelvic organ. The stomach, when distended, may extend far into the abdominal cavity. Because young, crying children may ingest large quantities of air, a large, distended stomach should be anticipated. The combination of a relatively large liver and spleen and weak anterior abdominal muscles predisposes the child to splenic and/or hepatic hemorrhage after significant blunt abdominal trauma (5). Additionally, under certain circumstances, such as when a young child is involved in a motor vehicle accident while wearing a standard automobile lap belt, a hollow viscus injury can occur (6,7). Other important mechanisms for blunt abdominal injury in children include automobile verses pedestrian accidents and child abuse (8–10).

▶ INDICATIONS

Clearly, all children who sustain an injury involving the abdomen are not candidates for DPL. On one end of the spectrum are the children who are determined to require urgent

339

laparotomy on clinical grounds alone. This group includes those who have (a) sustained gunshot wounds that clearly penetrate the peritoneum, (b) abdominal distension (which is persistent after gastric tube placement), (c) peritonitis, (d) hypotension (which does not respond to fluid resuscitation), (e) free peritoneal air, or (f) bleeding into the gastrointestinal tract. On the other end of the spectrum are those children in whom a significant injury can be reasonably excluded without further testing. This procedure should instead be reserved for patients who do not have a clear indication for laparotomy when close observation, serial examinations, and computed tomography (CT) are not an option. In trauma patients who require immediate nonabdominal surgery (e.g., craniotomy for the evacuation of an epidural hematoma), DPL may be performed in the operating room.

When DPL was introduced, management of suspected intra-abdominal injury was by emergency laparotomy. Although DPL certainly reduced the number of exploratory laparotomies for abdominal trauma, patients who had a positive DPL were still managed surgically. Since that time, however, two important changes have occurred that have had a profound effect on the evaluation and management of the potentially injured abdomen. First, advances in imaging technology have provided sophisticated and accurate forms of noninvasive imaging. Second, the overall trend in management of children with solid organ injury has changed from surgical management to nonsurgical management (11–13).

Ultrasonography (US) performed by a surgeon or emergency physician has largely replaced DPL in many trauma centers. In addition to detecting peritoneal fluid, US can identify pericardial fluid and hemothorax (14). It also has the advantages of being noninvasive, requiring no sedation and, because it is a bedside procedure, no patient transportation. It is extremely sensitive in identifying abnormal intraperitoneal fluid collections but less accurate in identifying the specific organ injured (15–17). This technique has not proved to be as useful as CT scanning in detecting the exact location and extent of injury, but in several studies it has been shown to compare favorably to DPL in detecting the presence of injury (15,18,19) (see also Chapter 137).

CT has become the imaging modality of choice in hemodynamically stable patients with blunt abdominal trauma because it has been shown to be accurate in defining solid and hollow visceral injury as well as visualizing retroperitoneal structures (pancreas, kidneys, aorta, vena cava, and retroperitoneal portions of the duodenum and colon) and the vertebral column. The accuracy of CT for bowel and mesenteric injury has improved in the last decade as faster CT detectors that produce fewer artifacts and thinner slices have been developed (20,21). A number of authors have reported using the latest generation of CT to identify active abdominal hemorrhage possibly requiring immediate surgical intervention (22). CT offers valuable information in a time when nonoperative management is used in greater than 80% of solid organ injury in children with blunt trauma (23,24). For these reasons, in many medical centers CT scanning has all but eclipsed DPL in the evaluation of children who are victims of abdominal trauma (25,26).

CT scanning, however, is not universally available on an emergent basis and has its limitations, visualizing solid organ injury better than hollow visceral and diaphragm injury. CT scanning requires transportation of the patient from the resuscitation area and, in many centers, completely out of the emergency department (ED). Once the patient is on the CT scanner table, the management of emergent problems becomes more difficult. For these reasons, some patients are too unstable to undergo this procedure.

Because DPL, CT scanning, and US may provide different types of information, they may be considered complementary (27,28). Notably, before any imaging technique or DPL is undertaken, the surgeon who will be responsible for the patient should be contacted and offered the opportunity to participate in the initial evaluation of the patient.

▶ BLUNT TRAUMA

In the case of blunt trauma, DPL has traditionally been used to detect intra-abdominal bleeding in the hemodynamically unstable child unresponsive to appropriate resuscitation. It is most useful in the hypotensive child who is going to the operating room for urgent nonabdominal surgery when US is not available or produces equivocal results. Some have advocated using DPL in detecting bowel and mesenteric injuries, which are uncommon in blunt trauma but difficult to detect by CT scanning. DPL has been used traditionally to detect free hemorrhage or intestinal contents as evidence of potential bowel or mesenteric injury and is considered by some to be diagnostically superior to evaluation by CT (29).

▶ PENETRATING TRAUMA

DPL is used in the evaluation of penetrating thoracoabdominal and abdominal trauma to detect peritoneal penetration and serves as an adjunct to local wound exploration. DPL has an accuracy rate of 90% for diagnosing injury when using the cell counts as described for blunt abdominal trauma (30). With the increased incidence of hollow viscus and diaphragm injury from stab wounds, some authors have recommended using lower RBC counts ($5,000/mm^3$ for low chest and $20,000/mm^3$ for anterior abdomen) because there is less blood loss with these injuries (31). If DPL lavage fluid does not exit the wound and contains fewer cells than the previously described thresholds, the child can be observed. Laparotomy is no longer considered mandatory for all abdominal stab wounds (32).

Gunshot wounds to the abdomen usually require exploration; the destructive force of firearms places the patient at great risk for significant injury. However, in some cases the bullet pathway is tangential to the abdomen, and peritoneal penetration is not apparent. Local wound exploration of gunshot wounds is rarely conclusive. In such situations, DPL may be helpful in making this determination (33).

▶ CONTRAINDICATIONS

The only absolute contraindication to DPL exists when its performance would delay surgical management of a patient for whom such intervention is clearly indicated. Relative contraindications are severe obesity, infection, previous abdominal surgery, coagulopathies, and second- or third-trimester pregnancy. Adhesions from prior abdominal surgery can compartmentalize the peritoneal cavity, leading to iatrogenic bowel perforation or inability to recover an adequate volume of fluid for interpretation. If DPL must be done, the physician should choose the abdominal position (supraumbilical versus infraumbilical) farthest from the previous incision using an open technique. If the physician feels that DPL is necessary in a pregnant adolescent, the supraumbilical approach is recommended. Ultrasound has obvious advantages for the pregnant patient because it allows evaluation of the fetus and involves no radiation exposure. The patient with a pelvic fracture should have the procedure using the open technique 1 to 2 cm above the umbilicus to avoid the hematoma commonly associated with this injury.

▶ EQUIPMENT

Most equipment required for diagnostic peritoneal lavage is readily available in the ED. In fact, many EDs have prepackaged equipment trays designed for this procedure. Although these trays are mainly designed for use in adult patients, they can be adapted for pediatric use with the addition of selected equipment. Table 27.1 lists the equipment necessary for the performance of this procedure. When performing DPL using the open or semiopen technique, the following additional equipment is needed: a No. 10 scalpel, abdomi-

TABLE 27.1	EQUIPMENT FOR DIAGNOSTIC PERITONEAL LAVAGE

Povidine solution
1% or 2% lidocaine with epinephrine
Sterile drapes
Introducer needle or angiocatheter—18 or 19 gauge
Guide wire with soft J end
No. 11 scalpel blade
Lavage catheter
Normal saline or Ringer lactate
Syringes

nal skin retractors, two tissue forceps, two Allis clamps, four hemostats, a needle driver, and absorbable and nonabsorbable sutures.

▶ PROCEDURE

When the physician decides to perform DPL, he or she must determine which of the several described variations is best suited for the clinical situation and his or her skills. These variations are open, semiopen, and closed. The original DPL was essentially a "minilaparotomy." This procedure, referred to as the open technique, has some distinct disadvantages. It is somewhat time consuming and involves a midline incision (albeit small). The most popular alternative to the classic diagnostic peritoneal lavage is the so-called closed technique, in which a guidewire passed through a needle is used to direct the lavage catheter (34). Because DPL will rarely be performed in children, the clinician is better served to learn and use one approach.

In preparation for DPL, sedation may be administered as needed (see Chapter 33). The stomach is decompressed using a nasogastric or orogastric tube (see Chapter 84), and the bladder is emptied using a bladder catheter (see Chapter 95). These procedures decrease the risk of inadvertent puncture of these organs.

The child is then placed in the supine position with full exposure from the xiphoid to the symphysis pubis. The abdomen is prepared with povidone-iodine solution, and sterile drapes are applied (see Chapter 7). The physician should don mask, sterile gown, and gloves for the procedure. The usual site for needle insertion is in the midline below the umbilicus approximately one third of the distance from the umbilicus to the symphysis pubis (Fig. 27.1). In adults, this distance is usually approximately 3 cm but will be less in a small child (usually 1 to 2 cm). This infraumbilical approach is generally used unless the patient is pregnant or has a pelvic fracture, an abdominal wall hematoma, or local skin infection at the infraumbilical site. The supraumbilical approach is recommended for these patients, and the needle is inserted 1 to 3 cm above the umbilicus. Using the midline location allows the needle to pass through the relatively avascular linea alba. This helps to prevent bleeding and therefore a false-positive result. Once the patient is prepared and the site of insertion chosen, local anesthetic (see Chapter 35) is administered into the skin and down to the fascia. Use of local anesthetic containing epinephrine is recommended to reduce the amount of local bleeding.

Closed (Seldinger) Technique

The closed (Seldinger) technique is the preferred method because it is faster but has the same complication rates and accuracy as the open technique (34). An 18-gauge introducer needle is inserted through the linea alba 1 to 2 cm below

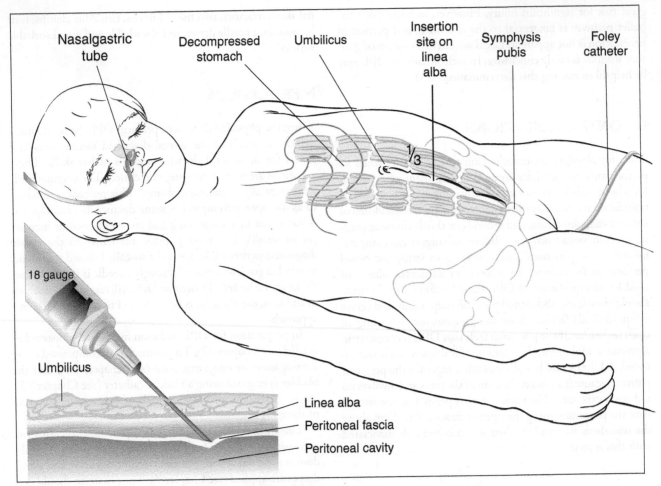

Figure 27.1 Anatomical landmarks for diagnostic peritoneal lavage.

the umbilicus. The needle is directed toward the pelvis at a 45-degree angle while constant negative pressure is applied to the attached syringe. The needle is advanced through the skin and soft tissue until resistance is felt at the fascial level. At this point, additional gentle pressure should be applied in order to penetrate the fascia. Fascial penetration is often accompanied by one or two distinct "pops." The needle is then advanced 2 to 3 mm into the peritoneal cavity. If blood is aspirated into the syringe, indicating a hemoperitoneum, the procedure is terminated at this time.

If no blood is aspirated into the syringe, the introducer needle is stabilized using the operator's nondominant hand, and he or she uses the other hand to remove the syringe. The guidewire is passed through the insertion needle and advanced until resistance is felt or until 10 cm of the wire remains outside the needle (Fig. 27.2A) (the guidewire in a commercially available peritoneal lavage kit is 45 cm in length). In the case of small children and infants, more of the wire will be left outside the needle hub. The needle is then removed from the abdominal cavity, leaving the guidewire in place. A No. 11 blade scalpel is used to make a small incision through the skin and subcutaneous tissue alongside the guidewire (Fig 27.2B). The peritoneal lavage catheter is passed over the guidewire into the

peritoneal cavity, and the guidewire is removed (Fig. 27.2C). A syringe is then attached to the catheter, and aspiration is attempted. If gross blood is aspirated, the procedure is terminated, although some controversy exists as to whether this constitutes a "positive tap" mandating laparotomy (35).

If no blood is aspirated, an assistant should attach the proximal end of i.v. tubing into a bag of warmed i.v. fluid (normal saline or Ringer lactate) and prime the tubing. The distal portion of the i.v. tubing is then attached to the lavage catheter; the clamp is opened and 10 to 15 mL/kg (up to 1 liter) is infused into the peritoneal cavity (Fig. 27.2E). The volume of fluid infused must be limited to 10 to 15 mL/kg because infusion of large amounts of fluid into the child's peritoneum may affect diaphragmatic excursion and therefore breathing. Once the fluid is fully infused, if the patient's condition permits, he or she should be gently rolled onto the right and left sides to allow the fluid to "wash" over the peritoneal cavity. Any fluid remaining within the bag should be removed. The bag is then dropped to a level below that of the patient's abdomen, and the fluid allowed to return to the bag by gravity (Fig. 27.2F). Although most of the fluid should return to the bag, it is not necessary to recover more than 3 to 5 mL/kg (about 20% of the instilled fluid) to

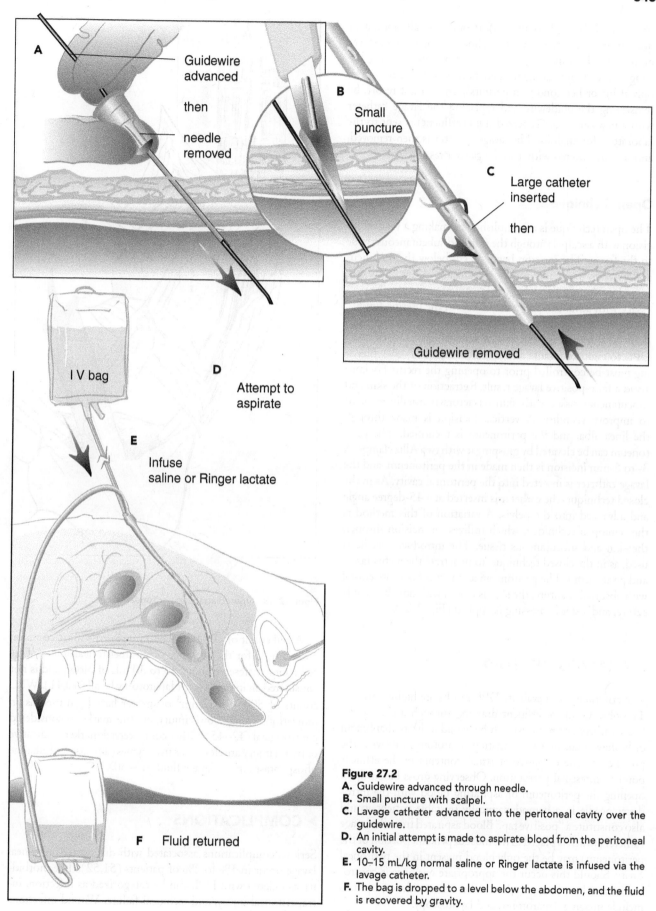

Figure 27.2
A. Guidewire advanced through needle.
B. Small puncture with scalpel.
C. Lavage catheter advanced into the peritoneal cavity over the guidewire.
D. An initial attempt is made to aspirate blood from the peritoneal cavity.
E. 10–15 mL/kg normal saline or Ringer lactate is infused via the lavage catheter.
F. The bag is dropped to a level below the abdomen, and the fluid is recovered by gravity.

obtain a reliable cell count (36). If only a small amount of fluid returns, however, an effort should be made to recover more fluid. This may be accomplished by repositioning the lavage catheter, by rotating the patient from side to side (again, only if his or her condition permits), or, as a last resort, by reinserting the guidewire and replacing the lavage catheter with a new one. The recovered fluid (effluent) is sent to the laboratory for analysis. The lavage catheter is then removed, and the site covered with a sterile gauze dressing.

Open Technique

The open technique is accomplished by making a vertical incision with a scalpel through the skin and subcutaneous tissue to the fascia. The incision begins 2 cm below the umbilicus and extends 4 cm inferiorly or 2 cm above the umbilicus, extending 4 cm superiorly. A more superior site may be necessary with advanced pregnancy to avoid the uterine fundus. An open infraumbilical site is used when there are upper abdominal scars and is preferred by some surgeons when using DPL to evaluate infants and small children (37–39). Bleeding must be controlled prior to opening the rectus fascia to avoid a false-positive lavage result. Retraction of the skin and subcutaneous tissue with skin retractors is usually required to improve visibility. A vertical incision is made through the linea alba, and the peritoneum is identified. The peritoneum can be elevated by grasping it with two Allis clamps. A 3- to 5-mm incision is then made in the peritoneum, and the lavage catheter is inserted into the peritoneal cavity. As in the closed technique, the catheter is inserted at a 45-degree angle and advanced into the pelvis. A variation of this method is the semiopen technique, which utilizes an incision through the skin and subcutaneous tissue. The introducer needle is used, as in the closed technique, to penetrate the rectus fascia and peritoneum. The peritoneum and rectus fascia are closed with absorbable suture, the skin is closed with nonabsorbable suture, and a sterile dressing is applied (Fig. 27.3).

▶ ANALYSIS OF FLUID

The criteria used to evaluate DPL results are highly variable. The observation of effluent draining through a chest tube, Foley catheter, or nasogastric tube would indicate diaphragm or hollow viscus injury, mandating laparotomy. Likewise, the presence of bile or gastrointestinal contents in the effluent point to intestinal perforation. Observing gross blood upon opening the peritoneum or aspirating blood with the introducer needle in a hemodynamically unstable patient would also constitute a "positive tap." Blood aspirated from the lavage catheter (which is placed in the most dependant portion of the peritoneum) may be the only blood present in the peritoneal cavity. Should this occur the appropriate response is controversial and based on anecdote rather than evidence; options include imaging, laparotomy, and laparoscopy.

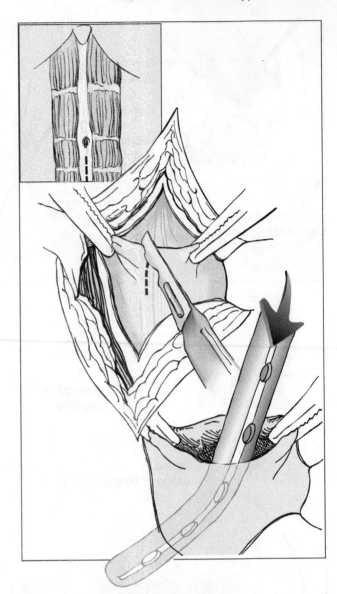

Figure 27.3 Open diagnostic peritoneal lavage.

A cell count of 100,000 RBC/mm^3 is the most common criteria used for the presence of intraperitoneal injury. This cell count represents about 20 to 30 mL of blood and is not considered an indication for laparotomy by all (40,41). WBC counts of 500 WBC/mm^3 or greater have been used as an indication of small bowel injury, but this marker is considered controversial (42–45). Other controversial markers indicative of bowel injury are elevations in enzymes (amylase and alkaline phosphatase) in the lavage fluid (46–50).

▶ COMPLICATIONS

Serious complications associated with diagnostic peritoneal lavage occur in 1% to 2% of patients (51,52). The morbidity associated with DPL can be categorized as infection, intraperitoneal injury, and technical failure. Wound infections

SUMMARY

1 Prepare patient by using sedation and restraint as necessary; insert nasogastric or orogastric tube and bladder catheter.

2 Sterilely prep abdomen and apply sterile drapes, exposing approximately 4 cm around umbilicus.

3 Select infraumbilical or supraumbilical approach as indicated (see text), then infiltrate selected site with lidocaine with epinephrine.

4 Using 18-gauge introducer needle, or equipment provided in a commercial kit, enter peritoneal cavity.

5 Pass guidewire through catheter or needle into peritoneal cavity.

6 Using a No. 11 scalpel blade, incise skin where guidewire enters, enlarging hole.

7 Thread lavage catheter onto wire and then direct it caudally into peritoneal cavity.

8 Attempt to aspirate fluid from peritoneal cavity; if any frank blood is recovered in a young child, this is deemed to be a positive result, and the procedure can be terminated.

9 If no frank blood is recovered, then instill 10 to 15 mL/kg of normal saline or Ringer lactate rapidly by gravity.

10 When all fluid is in peritoneal cavity, patient may be rocked from side to side; bag is then dropped to a level below abdomen.

11 Fluid recovered in bag should be sent to laboratory for analysis.

 CLINICAL TIPS

▶ Alternative imaging techniques should be considered based on availability and patient condition.

▶ Surgical consultation should be obtained early in the management of the patient.

▶ Adequate restraint and conscious sedation should be used as needed to minimize risk of injury.

▶ A gastric tube and bladder catheter should be inserted to reduce risk of inadvertent puncture of the stomach or bladder.

▶ Local anesthetic containing epinephrine should be used to decrease bleeding around the site of insertion of the lavage catheter. This helps to reduce the possibility of a false-positive result.

▶ The supraumbilical approach should be used for patients who are pregnant, have pelvic fractures, or have local irritation or skin infection in the infraumbilical area. For patients who have had previous abdominal surgeries, the site farthest from the previous incision is used. The infraumbilical approach is indicated for all others.

▶ The needle should be directed slightly caudad. A lateral trajectory of the needle (off the midline) must always be avoided.

▶ The guidewire should advance very smoothly. If it does not, then both the wire and the insertion needle should be removed together as a unit. Do not withdraw the guidewire through the needle because the tip may shear off.

▶ The lavage catheter should be directed caudally during insertion.

▶ Infusion of saline or Ringer lactate into the peritoneal cavity should be limited to 10 to 15 mL/kg to avoid interference with respiratory function.

▶ If the clinical condition permits, the patient should be rolled from side to side to allow the lavage fluid to wash over the peritoneal cavity.

▶ It is only necessary to recover 3 to 5 mL/kg of fluid. If less fluid is recovered, the patient can be rolled from side to side or the blunt lavage catheter can be repositioned or replaced.

and hematomas are rare complications; adherence to sterile technique and careful hemostasis should alleviate these problems.

The most important complications involve direct injury to an intra-abdominal structure. Of all the intra-abdominal organs, the liver and spleen are the least likely to be injured; however, if the needle is directed laterally, needle puncture of these organs is possible. Even in the unlikely case that one of these organs is penetrated by the needle, no serious injury is likely to occur.

A potentially more serious situation is perforation of bowel by the needle. Although normal intestine should be somewhat resistant to penetration because it is in essence floating and should simply move aside, it is still possible for the needle to enter the bowel lumen. This risk is increased when adhesions have caused the bowel to be relatively fixed in place or to become adherent to the peritoneal lining.

The two organs at greatest risk during DPL are the stomach and the bladder. Nasogastric or orogastric decompression should be used to minimize the size of the stomach. Furthermore, the catheter should not be directed laterally. Although the stomach may reseal itself after penetration with the needle (as does the bowel), penetration of the stomach may allow gastric contents into the peritoneal cavity, causing potentially serious peritonitis. As previously stated, the bladder in infants and young children can extend quite far into the abdomen, placing it at risk for penetration. This is a less serious situation because the relative muscular bladder wall reseals itself readily. In fact, aspiration of urine from the bladder is one means by which sterile urine samples are sometimes obtained in infants. Penetration of the bladder, however, can be avoided by decompressing the bladder with a urinary catheter.

The other potentially serious complication from DPL is injury to vascular structures within the abdominal wall or peritoneal cavity. Such injury rarely leads to significant hemorrhage into the peritoneal cavity but is often the cause of a false-positive DPL, which could result in the child undergoing an unnecessary laparotomy. Using a midline location for needle placement and avoiding lateral direction of the needle are the best ways to avoid this complication. If doubt exists about whether blood recovered from the peritoneal cavity represents an actual injury, and if the patient's condition permits, CT or US should be used. If the patient's condition does not permit, the blood must be assumed to represent a significant injury.

Technical failures may give inaccurate results, leading to missed injuries or unnecessary laparotomies. Inability to retrieve an adequate amount of effluent may cause low cell counts in the effluent. This can occur if the fluid is infused into the preperitoneal space or compartmentalized by adhesions. Falsely elevated cell counts can occur with inadequate hemostasis or insertion of the needle through an abdominal wall hematoma.

▶ SUMMARY

Diagnostic peritoneal lavage is a time-tested method of determining the presence of significant intra-abdominal injury after abdominal trauma. It offers the advantage of being a low-cost bedside procedure that can be performed with readily available equipment. It does not require transportation of the patient from the resuscitation area, and the samples of fluid obtained can be easily analyzed by most laboratories. DPL is an invasive procedure, however, and the results offer no information about the location and extent of injury. Furthermore, DPL yields no information about retroperitoneal structures. DPL is highly sensitive but lacks specificity and may lead to unnecessary laparotomies. With the advent of accurate noninvasive imaging techniques and conservative management of children with intra-abdominal injuries, indications for DPL in the pediatric population have become fewer. As more EDs obtain ultrasound equipment and more emergency physicians and surgeons become facile in its use, DPL is likely to become a rare

procedure. At present, however, emergency physicians should remain familiar with the technique of DPL and its indications.

▶ ACKNOWLEDGMENT

The authors would like to acknowledge the valuable contributions of Patricia L. Van Devander and David K. Wagner to the version of this chapter that appeared in the previous edition.

▶ REFERENCES

1. Root HD, Hawser CW, McKinley CR, et al. Diagnostic peritoneal lavage. *Surgery.* 1965;57:633–637.
2. Weinberg AD. Hypothermia. *Ann Emerg Med.* 1993;22(2 Pt 2):370–377.
3. Fakhry SM, Watts DD, Michetti C, et al. The resident experience on trauma: declining surgical opportunities and career incentives? Analysis of data from a large multi-institutional study. *J Trauma.* 2003;54:1–7; discussion 7–8.
4. Maxwell-Armstrong C, Brooks A, Field M, et al. Diagnostic peritoneal lavage analysis: should trauma guidelines be revised? *Emerg Med J.* 2002;19:524–525.
5. Richardson JD, Belin RP, Griffen WO Jr. Blunt abdominal trauma in children. *Ann Surg.* 1972;176:213–216.
6. Newman KD, Bowman LW, Eichelberger MR, et al. The lap belt complex: intestinal and lumbar spine injury in children. *J Trauma.* 1990;30:1133–1138; discussion 1138–1140.
7. Statter MB, Coran AG. Appendiceal transection in a child associated with a lap belt restraint: case report. *J Trauma.* 1992;33:765–766.
8. Hood JM, Smyth BT. Nonpenetrating intraabdominal injuries in children. *J Pediatr Surg.* 1974;9:69–77.
9. Levy JL Jr, Linder LH. Major abdominal trauma in children. *Am J Surg.* 1970;120:55–58.
10. Sivit CJ, Taylor GA, Eichelberger MR. Visceral injury in battered children: a changing perspective. *Radiology.* 1989;173:659–661.
11. Schiffman MA. Nonoperative management of blunt abdominal trauma in pediatrics. *Emerg Med Clin North Am.* 1989;7:519–535.
12. Delius RE, Frankel W, Coran AG. A comparison between operative and nonoperative management of blunt injuries to the liver and spleen in adult and pediatric patients. *Surgery.* 1989;106:788–792; discussion 792–793.
13. Partrick DA, Moore EE, Bensard DD, et al. Operative management of injured children at an adult level I trauma center. *J Trauma.* 2000;48:894–901.
14. MA OJ, Mateer JR. Trauma. In: Seils A, Panton N, eds. *Emergency Ultrasound.* New York: McGraw-Hill; 2003:67–88.
15. Akgur FM, Tanyel FC, Ahkan O, et al. The place of ultrasonographic examination in the initial evaluation of children sustaining blunt abdominal trauma. *J Pediatr Surg.* 1993;28:78–81.
16. Luks FI, Lemire A, St-Vil D, et al. Blunt abdominal trauma in children: the practical value of ultrasonography. *J Trauma.* 1993;34:607–610; discussion 610–611.
17. Richards JR, Knopf NA, Wang L, et al. Blunt abdominal trauma in children: evaluation with emergency US. *Radiology.* 2002;222:749–754.
18. Chambers JA, Pilbrow WJ. Ultrasound in abdominal trauma: an alternative to peritoneal lavage. *Arch Emerg Med.* 1988;5:26–33.
19. Boulanger BR, Brenneman FD, McLellan BA, et al. A prospective study of emergent abdominal sonography after blunt trauma. *J Trauma.* 1995;39:325–330.

20. Malhotra AK, Fabian TC, Katsis SB, et al. Blunt bowel and mesenteric injuries: the role of screening computed tomography. *J Trauma.* 2000;48:991–998; discussion 998–1000.

21. Killeen KL, Shanmuganathan K, Poletti PA, et al. Helical computed tomography of bowel and mesenteric injuries. *J Trauma.* 2001;51:26–36.

22. Willmann JK, Roos JE, Platz A, et al. Multidetector CT: detection of active hemorrhage in patients with blunt abdominal trauma. *AJR Am J Roentgenol.* 2002;179:437–444.

23. Bensard DD, Beaver BL, Besner GE, et al. Small bowel injury in children after blunt abdominal trauma: is diagnostic delay important? *J Trauma.* 1996;41:476–483.

24. Peterson MD, Henderson B. Thoracoabdominal trauma. In: Hall JK, Berman JM, eds. *Pediatric Trauma Anesthesia and Critical Care.* Armonk, NY: Futura; 1996:245–275.

25. Karp MP, Cooney DR, Berger PE, et al. The role of computed tomography in the evaluation of blunt abdominal trauma in children. *J Pediatr Surg.* 1981;16:316–323.

26. Goldstein AS, Sclafani SJ, Kupferstein NH, et al. The diagnostic superiority of computerized tomography. *J Trauma.* 1985;25:938–946.

27. Sorkey AJ, Farnell MB, Williams HJ, et al. The complementary roles of diagnostic peritoneal lavage and computed tomography in the evaluation of blunt abdominal trauma. *Surgery.* 1989;106:794–800; discussion 800–801.

28. Thal ER, Meyer DM. The evaluation of blunt abdominal trauma: computed tomography scan, lavage, or sonography? *Adv Surg.* 1991;24:201–228.

29. Fang JF, Chen RJ, Lin BC, et al. Small bowel perforation: is urgent surgery necessary? *J Trauma.* 1999;47:515–520.

30. American College of Surgeons, Committee on Trauma. *Advanced Life Support Course: Student Manual.* Chicago: American College of Surgeons; 1993.

31. Nagy KK, Roberts RR, Joseph KT, et al. Experience with over 2,500 diagnostic peritoneal lavages. *Injury.* 2000;31:479–482.

32. Renz BM, Feliciano DV. Unnecessary laparotomies for trauma: a prospective study of morbidity. *J Trauma.* 1995;38:350–356.

33. Kelemen JJ 3rd, Martin RR, Obney JA, et al. Evaluation of diagnostic peritoneal lavage in stable patients with gunshot wounds to the abdomen. *Arch Surg.* 1997;132:909–913.

34. Howdieshell TR, Osler TM, Demarest GB. Open versus closed peritoneal lavage with particular attention to time, accuracy, and cost. *Am J Emerg Med.* 1989;7:367–371.

35. Nagy KK, Fildes JJ, Sloan EP, et al. Aspiration of free blood from the peritoneal cavity does not mandate immediate laparotomy. *Am Surg.* 1995;61:790–795.

36. Sweeney JF, Albrink MH, Bischof E, et al. Diagnostic peritoneal lavage: volume of lavage effluent needed for accurate determination of a negative lavage. *Injury.* 1994;25:659–661.

37. Halow KD, Ford EG. Abdominal injury. In: Ford EG, Andrassy RJ, eds. *Pediatric Trauma: Initial Assessment and Management.* Philadelphia: WB Saunders Company; 1994:201–213.

38. Magnuson DK, Eichelberger MR. Approach to pediatric trauma patients. In: Oldham KT, Colombani PM, Foglia RP, eds. *Surgery of Infants and Children: Scientific Principles and Practice.* Philadelphia: Lippincott-Raven; 1997:391–410.

39. Eichelberger MR. Procedures. In: Eichelberger MR, ed. *Pediatric Trauma: Prevention, Acute Care, Rehabilitation.* St. Louis: Mosby Year-Book; 1993:637.

40. Otomo Y, Henmi H, Mashiko K, et al. New diagnostic peritoneal lavage criteria for diagnosis of intestinal injury. *J Trauma.* 1998;44:991–997; discussion 997–999.

41. Bain IM, Kirby RM, Tiwari P, et al. Survey of abdominal ultrasound and diagnostic peritoneal lavage for suspected intra-abdominal injury following blunt trauma. *Injury.* 1998;29:65–71.

42. Fang JF, Chen RJ, Lin BC. Cell count ratio: new criterion of diagnostic peritoneal lavage for detection of hollow organ perforation. *J Trauma.* 1998;45:540–544.

43. D'Amelio LF, Rhodes M. A reassessment of the peritoneal lavage leukocyte count in blunt abdominal trauma. *J Trauma.* 1990;30:1291–1293.

44. Jacobs DG, Angus L, Rodriguez A, et al. Peritoneal lavage white count: a reassessment. *J Trauma.* 1990;30:607–612.

45. Soyka JM, Martin M, Sloan EP, et al. Diagnostic peritoneal lavage: is an isolated WBC count greater than or equal to 500/mm^3 predictive of intra-abdominal injury requiring celiotomy in blunt trauma patients? *J Trauma.* 1990;30:874–879.

46. McAnena OJ, Marx JA, Moore EE. Contributions of peritoneal lavage enzyme determinations to the management of isolated hollow visceral abdominal injuries. *Ann Emerg Med.* 1991;20:834–837.

47. Marx JA, Bar-Or D, Moore EE, et al. Utility of lavage alkaline phosphatase in detection of isolated small intestinal injury. *Ann Emerg Med.* 1985;14:10–14.

48. Megison SM, Weigelt JA. The value of alkaline phosphatase in peritoneal lavage. *Ann Emerg Med.* 1990;19:503–505.

49. Alyono D, Perry JF Jr. Value of quantitative cell count and amylase activity of peritoneal lavage fluid. *J Trauma.* 1981;21:345–348.

50. Jaffin JH, Ochsner MG, Cole FJ, et al. Alkaline phosphatase levels in diagnostic peritoneal lavage fluid as a predictor of hollow visceral injury. *J Trauma.* 1993;34:829–833.

51. Henneman PL, Marx JA, Moore EE, et al. Diagnostic peritoneal lavage: accuracy in predicting necessary laparotomy following blunt and penetrating trauma. *J Trauma.* 1990;30:1345–1355.

52. Falcone RE, Thomas B, Hrutkay L. Safety and efficacy of diagnostic peritoneal lavage performed by supervised surgical and emergency medicine residents. *Eur J Emerg Med.* 1997;4:150–155.

28

WILLIAM TSAI AND KATHLEEN BROWN

Control of Exsanguinating External Hemorrhage

▶ INTRODUCTION

The control of exsanguinating external hemorrhage is an important skill needed in the treatment of childhood injuries. While most injuries to children involve minimal blood loss, significant injuries to soft tissues and vascular structures may result in rapid exsanguination, multisystem organ failure, and death. In addition, because of anatomical and physiologic differences between children and adults, significant blood loss may be unrecognized, and blood loss that might be considered inconsequential in an adult may threaten the life of a child. Therefore, it is essential that all personnel who care for injured children be adept at using techniques designed to stop or limit hemorrhage.

▶ ANATOMY AND PHYSIOLOGY

Injuries that result in exsanguination involve damage to blood vessels in two general anatomic locations. The peripheral vessels lie in the tissues above the fascia. These vessels are usually small, are rarely a source of significant bleeding, and respond well to basic methods of hemorrhage control. Central vessels lie deep to the fascia and are at risk in penetrating trauma, significant blunt trauma, and fractures. Injury to these vessels may result in significant external hemorrhage. Bleeding from peripheral and central veins is manifested by continuous flow of dark-colored blood. On the other hand, arterial hemorrhage is seen as bright red, pulsatile blood.

Important differences in anatomy and physiology between adults and children should be noted. First, because children have a smaller body mass than adults, trauma results in greater force applied per unit body area (1). Second, this greater force is applied to a body with less subcutaneous fat and protective connective tissue and results in a relative increased exposure of vital structures (1). Third, children have an enhanced ability to maintain blood pressure in the face of significant blood loss. Tachycardia and decreased skin perfusion may be the only signs of significant hemorrhagic shock and may only occur with at least a 25% diminution in blood volume (1). A drop in blood pressure is a late sign of shock in children and may signal imminent cardiac arrest (2).

▶ INDICATIONS

Lacerations, puncture wounds, gunshot wounds, soft-tissue injuries, and traumatic amputations are all indications for immediate control of hemorrhage. In general, the basic procedures of hemorrhage control should first be employed. The clinician should then proceed to the advanced procedures when these basic procedures have failed.

▶ PROCEDURES

Basic Procedures

Manual Pressure

Direct pressure controls most bleeding as soon as it is initiated (Fig. 28.1). Using a gloved hand and sterile gauze, direct and constant pressure over the bleeding site should be applied. Care should be taken to determine that pressure is being applied to the proper site of bleeding because dressings and the confusion associated with other interventions may obscure the bleeding site and cause pressure to be directed in the vicinity

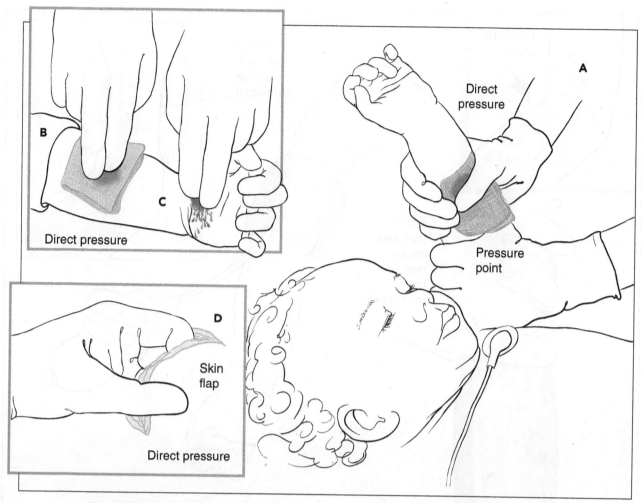

Figure 28.1
A. Direct pressure applied to the site of bleeding is the initial maneuver in attempts to control external hemorrhage. Direct pressure may be augmented by applying pressure to a proximal "pressure point."
B. Direct pressure at the site of the injury with a sterile gauze pad used to cover the bleeding site.
C. Direct pressure at the site of injury using sterile gloved fingers.
D. Pinching a bleeding skin flap between the thumb and forefingers to control hemorrhage.

of but not directly on the source of bleeding. An acceptable alternative is to apply direct pressure with a gloved finger (3,4). Bleeding from the edge of a large tissue flap may be controlled by pinching the bleeding site between the thumb and forefinger. Ideally, when either of these methods is used, pressure should be applied for a specific period of time, usually at least 10 to 15 minutes. Time passes slowly when performing a monotonous activity such as holding pressure, so it is best to use a timepiece to ensure that pressure is maintained for the desired duration.

Control of high-pressure arterial bleeding may be facilitated by applying pressure proximal to the site of bleeding. The pressure point is identified by locating the arterial pulse proximal to the site of bleeding, then compressing the artery with the fingers. Pressure exerted at these areas serves to reduce blood flow at the site of hemorrhage. The ideal pressure point is an area where the artery passes in close proximity to a bone or other firm anatomic structure against which it may be

compressed. It may be necessary for the clinician to palpate along the course of the artery to identify the best site at which to apply pressure (Fig. 28.2).

Elevation of the Bleeding Area
When possible, elevation of the injured area may reduce hemorrhage. In optimal circumstances, the area should be elevated to a height above the level of the heart. If this is not possible, the bleeding site should be kept level with the rest of the body and not allowed to become dependent.

Pressure Bandages
Pressure bandages may be used as a temporary alternative to direct pressure when the patient has other, more severe injuries that require the attention of all available personnel. The procedure is performed by first placing a stack of gauze pads approximately 1 inch thick directly over the site of bleeding. An elastic bandage is then wrapped over the gauze pads tight

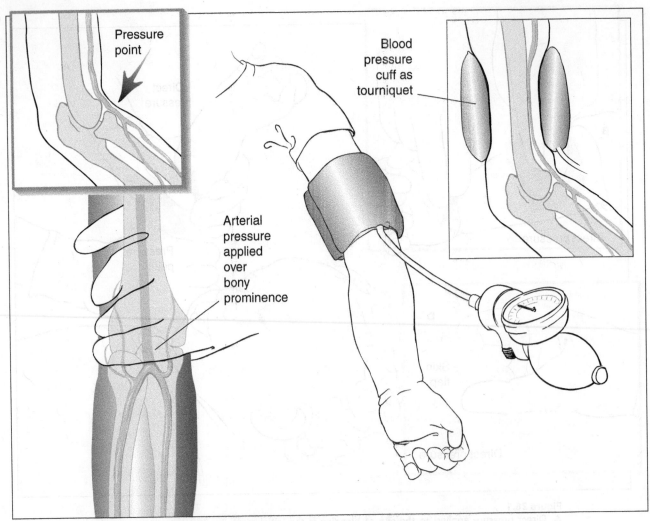

Pressure point

Blood pressure cuff as tourniquet

Arterial pressure applied over bony prominence

Figure 28.2 Pressure may be applied proximal to a site of bleeding using either manual pressure applied at a pressure point or, in more severe cases, an inflated blood pressure cuff.

enough to provide adequate hemostasis. Some commercial variations of pressure bandages employ a semirigid styrene block placed directly over the site of bleeding, which is first covered by a gauze pad. The block is then pressed and molded into the wound by an elastic overwrap (5).

Pressure bandages do have potential complications. If wrapped too tightly, they can lead to distal ischemia; therefore, distal perfusion should be monitored frequently, every 30 minutes at a minimum, while the pressure bandage is in place. If wrapped too loosely, the pressure bandage will not stop the bleeding but will instead obscure it, and the child may exsanguinate.

Topical Vasoconstrictors
Epinephrine solution (1:1000) can be diluted in saline and applied to gauze pads that are then placed over the wound. This solution works well to control areas of persistent low-pressure bleeding, particularly when a tissue bed continues to ooze blood. Care must be taken to avoid injection of this solution into a vessel, and large volumes should not be administered, as epinephrine can be absorbed by the tissues and can cause clinical effects. Epinephrine should not be used on fingers, toes, the penis, ears, or the tip of the nose because of the risk of vasoconstriction that may result in tissue necrosis. An additional mode of topical therapy involves direct application of fibrin or gel-foam to the site of bleeding.

Suturing
In general, suturing the wound closed is very effective for halting minor bleeding. This strategy is often very effective in controlling significant scalp bleeding. This procedure may provide enough tissue pressure from hematoma formation to tamponade bleeding. An alternative is to use a "figure-of-eight" stitch. Absorbable suture is used, and the stitch is placed proximal to the site of bleeding by one of the methods shown (Fig. 28.3). This stitch compresses the tissue surrounding the bleeding vessel and tamponades the hemorrhage.

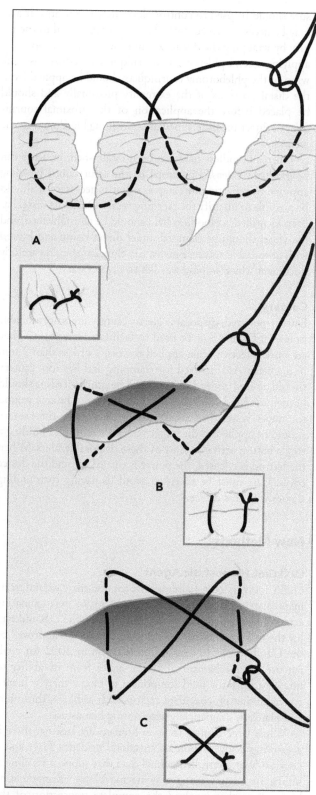

Figure 28.3 A "figure-of-eight" stitch may be used to tamponade a bleeding vessel.
A. A vertical figure-of-eight stitch.
B–C. Two types of horizontal figure-of-eight stitches.

Advanced Procedures

Tourniquets

A tourniquet may be used in extreme cases of uncontrolled hemorrhage. This technique should be reserved for those cases in which it may be acceptable to sacrifice the injured limb in order to save the child's life. A manual blood pressure cuff may be employed for this purpose (Fig. 28.2). An appropriately sized blood pressure cuff is placed on the injured extremity proximal to the site of bleeding and inflated until the bleeding stops. This usually occurs at a pressure just higher than the child's systolic blood pressure (6). Once hemostasis has been achieved, the tubing must be occluded to prevent leakage of air from the cuff. Occlusion is most easily accomplished by cross-clamping the tubing with a hemostat.

Some commercially available tourniquets are air inflated and have valves that control air ingress and egress. Because these devices are built for this purpose, they leak less frequently than do blood pressure cuffs. Commercial tourniquets may be available in hospital operating rooms, where they are used to maintain a bloodless field for extremity surgery. In field situations, any device (e.g., belt, necktie, purse strap) that can be placed circumferentially around the injured extremity and tightened to interrupt blood flow may be used as a temporary tourniquet.

Application of a tourniquet for control of hemorrhage (other than to facilitate wound exploration) implies that the medical team has recognized that the injured limb may be sacrificed to prevent death from exsanguination. This decision should be documented in the medical record along with the time when the tourniquet was placed. This time should also be prominently displayed on the bed sheets or on a sticker placed on the patient. Displaying the time is particularly important for patients who will be transferred, but it should be done for every patient on whom a tourniquet is placed. Furthermore, the condition of the extremity distal to the tourniquet should be carefully monitored and documented. When the tourniquet must be left in place for a protracted period of time, it should be loosened after 30 minutes and occasionally thereafter to ensure that it is still required. In an ED setting, it is very unlikely that a tourniquet would be required, and in no case should a tourniquet be used in the ED for more than 1 hour.

Significant bleeding from a finger injury may be controlled by a Penrose drain or a phlebotomy tourniquet clamped tightly at the base of the finger (7). A wide tourniquet should be used because narrow bands may allow too much pressure to be applied over a small surface area, causing pressure necrosis at the site of application. A large clamp should be used so that everyone notes the presence of a tourniquet. As stated, the time of tourniquet application should be prominently displayed on the patient or on the bed, and the reasons for tourniquet use should be clearly documented in the patient's medical record. A finger tourniquet should not be left in place for more than 20 minutes except in exceptional circumstances.

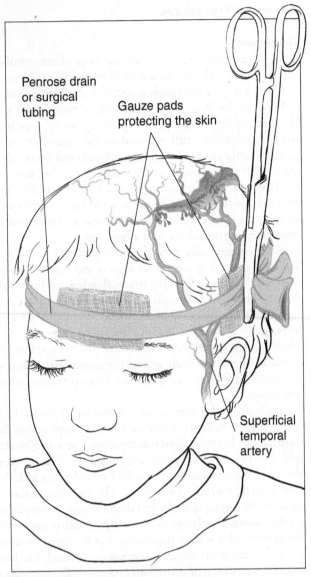

Penrose drain
or surgical
tubing

Gauze pads
protecting the skin

Superficial
temporal
artery

Figure 28.4 A Penrose drain used to control hemorrhage from a scalp laceration.

When direct pressure fails to control hemorrhage from a scalp wound, hemostasis may be attempted with the application of a Penrose drain applied as a snug headband at the level of the forehead and the occiput. This device should compress the scalp vasculature enough to help provide hemostasis (8,9) (Fig. 28.4).

Clamping Bleeding Vessels

Clamping bleeding vessels should be avoided if at all possible. Veins, arteries, and nerves are usually found together, and blind clamping of a bleeding vessel may result in irreversible damage to the adjacent nerve. If the clinician feels that clamping is necessary, then the following method should be employed. First, a tourniquet or some other source of pres-

sure should be used to control blood flow to the area. It also may be necessary to control venous bleeding distal to the injury by wrapping the distal extremity with elastic wrap or by applying several phlebotomy tourniquets. In either case, the wrap or the phlebotomy tourniquets should be applied from the distal portions of the extremity proximally and should be placed before the application of the proximal tourniquet or direct pressure aimed at controlling bleeding into the wound.

Once a bloodless field has been established, pressure can be gradually released proximal to the injury until bleeding appears. By repeating this step as often as necessary, it should be possible to identify the bleeding vessel. Once this vessel has been identified, a bloodless field should be re-established, and the vessel should be clamped under direct vision and ligated with absorbable suture. Finally, the clinician should carefully document why clamping was felt to be necessary.

Cautery

Battery-powered, disposable electrocautery units are available in most EDs and may be used to facilitate hemostasis. They are most effective when applied to vessels of less than 2 mm in diameter. As discussed for clamping and ligation, cautery should be used under direct vision. The site of bleeding should be identified and a bloodless field established. The area around the target vessel then should be dried. Finally, the cautery should be applied to the target vessel. Pressing and holding a single button activates most of these disposable units. When the button is released, the power is turned off and the device cools. Care must be taken to avoid damaging surrounding tissues with this device.

New Methods

QuikClot Hemostatic Agent

QuikClot is an inert, highly adsorbent traumatic wound treatment material that can quickly arrest major exsanguinating external hemorrhage. It is currently used by the U.S. military for the treatment of battlefield wounds and was approved by the U.S. Food and Drug Administration in 2002 for civilian use. Its mechanism of action arises from its ability to quickly adsorb the fluid component of blood, thereby hemoconcentrating procoagulant factors such as fibrin, thrombin, and platelets, dramatically accelerating hemostasis.

While large clinical trials in humans are lacking, there is a growing body of human anecdotal evidence (10) and a large body of controlled animal data that support its clinical utility. In a study using a swine model for exsanguinating hemorrhage that involved the complete transection of the femoral artery and vein, the application of QuikClot resulted in 100% survival, versus 35% survival with the use of standard thrombostatic dressings (11).

The material is packaged in individual 3.5-oz packets as a granular powder and is available without prescription. When used in cases where moderate to severe bleeding persists despite application of standard measures, previously applied dressings should be removed, excess blood and fluid should be wiped away, and the agent should be gradually poured onto the source of bleeding in a back-and-forth motion. As the agent adsorbs moisture, it changes from light beige to a dark color. Pouring should cease when a dry layer is noted. Direct pressure should be applied for 1 to 2 minutes, and the area should then be wrapped with a compression bandage. To remove the agent prior to more definitive wound treatment, dry granules should be removed from the wound surface, and the area can then be irrigated with standard irrigation solutions.

While potential side effects for this very promising agent have not been fully elucidated, one known side effect is a highly exothermic reaction that occurs as the result of rapid fluid adsorption. Local temperatures as high as 80°C to 90°C may last for a few seconds but have not been associated with any long-term untoward effects. In addition, the long-term effects of unremoved granules are not known.

▶ COMPLICATIONS

Direct pressure, pressure bandages, and tourniquets all carry the risk of ischemia distal to the wound. Areas distal to the injury should be monitored carefully during the application of pressure, particularly when tourniquets are applied. Tourniquets should be loosened after 30 minutes to determine whether they have been effective and to allow the distal tissues to receive some blood. Pressure (particularly pressure from a tourniquet) also carries the risk of nerve compression and permanent injury. A carefully documented neurosensory examination and documentation of the need for the tourniquet and ongoing monitoring may be useful later should a child be found to have sustained nerve damage after an injury.

Both direct clamping of vessels and use of electrocautery may cause injury to other nearby structures. Nerves are particularly vulnerable because of their close proximity to blood vessels. Additionally, clamps can cause crush injury, which leads to devitalization of tissues, and electrocautery devices may cause burns.

Solutions containing epinephrine can cause vasoconstriction of blood vessels distal to the site of injection and result in distal ischemia. Care should be taken when epinephrine is employed near areas that are supplied by distal arterial branches and have no collateral blood supply.

Any method involving direct contact with an open wound places the patient at risk for a wound infection and medical personnel at risk for contact with infected blood. Aseptic technique (Chapter 7) and universal precautions (Chapter 8) should be used at all times.

 SUMMARY

1 Perform an initial screening examination aimed at identifying sources of bleeding, detecting early evidence of hypovolemia, and documenting the neurovascular status of the involved area.

2 Use sterile technique and universal precautions to protect both the patient and the staff.

3 Apply direct pressure to the site of bleeding with either gloved fingers or a gauze pad. This may be augmented by simultaneous application of pressure at a pressure point. Hold pressure for at least 10 to 15 minutes by the clock.

4 While pressure is being applied, elevate the involved area to a higher level than the heart, if possible.

5 If direct pressure and elevation fail or if all available personnel are required to address other injuries, then apply a pressure bandage to the area. Use a commercial pressure dressing or stack of gauze pads approximately 1 inch thick surrounded by an elastic wrap to provide pressure. Check the neurovascular status of the area distal to the dressing frequently after it is applied.

6 In situations with moderate to severe hemorrhage despite basic procedures, consider the use of QuikClot hemostatic agent if available.

7 In extreme situations when a choice must be made between life and limb, a tourniquet may be used. Apply a blood pressure cuff or commercial tourniquet to an area proximal to the site of bleeding and inflate the device until bleeding stops. Record the time that the tourniquet was placed and mark it in a prominent location on the bed or patient. Carefully monitor the neurovascular status of the distal extremity subsequent to tourniquet inflation. Carefully document the reasons for tourniquet use, the time of inflation, and the results of ongoing monitoring in the medical record.

8 Under certain circumstances and in certain anatomic locations (e.g., the scalp), bleeding vessels may be clamped under direct vision and then ligated or cauterized. These procedures have the potential to injure nerves and other tissues and should be used judiciously if at all.

9 Persistent low-pressure bleeding may be controlled by using epinephrine-soaked pads (1:1000 epinephrine) or injecting lidocaine with epinephrine (1:100,000 epinephrine) and by applying agents such as QuikClot, fibrin, or gel-foam directly to the site of bleeding.

CLINICAL TIPS

▶ Some significant bleeding sites may not be initially obvious. It must be remembered that the "E" in the "ABCDE" mnemonic stands for "expose." All areas of bleeding should be inspected and pressure should be applied until the injury can be definitively addressed.

▶ Scalp lacerations may be lethal in young children. Every attempt should be made to stop bleeding from these areas promptly. If the patient has to wait before wound closure, then a pressure dressing must be applied.

▶ If gauze pads are used to cover the site of bleeding while applying pressure, they can obscure the actual site of bleeding and prevent adequate pressure from being directed at the correct site. An excellent alternative is to use one or two fingers covered by a sterile glove to achieve hemostasis.

▶ Tourniquets may be useful to facilitate exploration of wounds. Using tourniquets to control hemorrhage is almost never necessary in the ED.

▶ Clamping of bleeding vessels in an attempt to achieve hemostasis is dangerous. Blind clamping should be used only on the scalp. In all other areas, clamping should be done under direct vision. An alternative to clamping is almost always available.

▶ If hemorrhage persists despite basic procedures, consider using QuikClot hemostatic agent.

▶ SUMMARY

Control of significant hemorrhage is of primary importance in the resuscitation of trauma victims. Fortunately, simple techniques such as the application of direct pressure can readily control most hemorrhages. QuikClot seems to be a very promising agent for the control of moderate to significant hemorrhage. When bleeding is refractory to minimally invasive measures, however, health care personnel should not hesitate to employ more aggressive means of hemostasis. When these more invasive techniques are used, the reasons for use should be clearly documented. Certain special types of injuries (e.g., flaps) may be best managed using methods specifically designed for their treatment.

▶ ACKNOWLEDGMENT

The authors acknowledge with gratitude the contributions of Dr. John J. Kelly to the version of this chapter in the first edition of this text.

▶ REFERENCES

1. American College of Surgeons. Pediatric trauma. In: *Advanced Trauma Life Support.* 6th ed. Chicago: American College of Surgeons; 1997:289–311.
2. American Academy of Pediatrics. Recognition of respiratory failure and shock. In: *PALS Provider Manual.* Dallas, TX: American Heart Association; 2002:23–40.
3. Boericke PH. Emergency! II: first aid for open wounds, severe bleeding, shock, and closed wounds. *Nursing.* 1975;5:40–46.
4. Borja AR, Lansing AM. Immediate control of intermediate vascular bleeding. *Surg Gynecol Obstet.* 1971;132:494–496.
5. Safar P, Bircher NG, Yealy D. Basic and advanced life support. In: Schwartz GR, Cayten CA, Mangelsen MA, et al., eds. *Principles and Practice of Emergency Medicine.* Philadelphia: Lea & Febiger; 1992:89–214.
6. Edlich RF, Rodeheaver GT. Scientific basis for wound management. *Emerg Med Ann.* 1983;2:1.
7. Lubah JD, Koeneman J, Kosar K. The digital hand tourniquet: how safe is it? *J Hand Surg.* 1985;10(A):664–669.
8. Lammers RL. Principles of wound management. In: Roberts JR, Hedges JR, eds. *Clinical Procedures in Emergency Medicine.* Philadelphia: WB Saunders; 1991:515–564.
9. Barst HH. Hemostasis for head injuries [letter]. *Lancet.* 1968;153:1204.
10. Wright FL, Hua HT, Velhamos G, et al. Intracorporeal use of the hemostatic agent QuikClot in a coagulopathic patient with combined thoracoabdominal penetrating trauma. *J Trauma.* 2004;56:205–208.
11. Alam HB, Chen Z, Jaskille A, et al. Application of a zeolite hemostatic agent achieves 100% survival in a lethal model of complex groin injury in swine. *J Trauma.* 2004;56:974–983.

STEVEN BALDWIN AND THOMAS E. TERNDRUP

29

Thoracostomy and Related Procedures

SECTION A: THORACOSTOMY PROCEDURES

▶ INTRODUCTION

This chapter is divided into two sections. The first section describes the issues and procedural details relevant to needle, catheter and tube thoracostomies. The second section describes open (sucking) chest wounds.

Hippocrates was the first to describe entering the pleural space with a metal tube to drain "bad humors" (1). Playfair, in 1875, and Hewitt, in 1876, described closed chest tube drainage with a tube and an underwater seal (2,3). The technique of tube thoracostomy, however, was not widely used until 1917 when it became useful in treating post influenza empyema (4). During World War II, tube thoracostomy gained widespread use for the treatment of traumatic hemopneumothorax and empyema. It is now commonly used to treat many types of pleural collections.

Various types of thoracostomy procedures have been described. These include needle thoracostomy, catheter thoracostomy (Seldinger technique or catheter over needle technique), and tube thoracostomy. In most cases, each can be performed at the bedside. Other variations exist but are not relevant to the emergency physician and will not be discussed.

Thoracostomy procedures are primarily used to treat a few specific clinical problems that involve the pleural space(s). Some of these problems are life-threatening and require immediate intervention, but most can be successfully stabilized or even definitively treated by performing a thoracostomy procedure. Other problems are less emergent and able to be managed by a thoracostomy procedure performed urgently or semi-electively. The ability to perform thoracostomy procedures emergently is a critical resuscitative skill for all physicians who provide emergency care.

Emergent thoracostomy procedures are rarely needed in children. They are most commonly needed to treat pneumothoraces complicating mechanical ventilation of preterm and term neonates. In most emergency department settings, the majority of emergent thoracostomy procedures are performed for conditions resulting from blunt thoracic trauma, but they may also be required to manage complications related to positive pressure mechanical ventilation, vascular access, or other procedures and to manage problems related to inadequacy, failure, or dislodgement of an existing thoracostomy drainage device. Thoracostomy procedures performed for other, nonsurgical indications are rare and most commonly performed for various infectious or inflammatory conditions causing fluid collections in the pleural space, for spontaneous pneumothoraces, and for other very rare reasons that are not pertinent to emergency care.

▶ ANATOMY AND PHYSIOLOGY

Proper performance of thoracostomy procedures requires an appropriate understanding of thoracic anatomy and respiratory physiology (5–9). This knowledge allows for the early identification of potential thoracic pathology and the determination of the need for intervention. After a thoracostomy procedure is ordered, the operator must be able to apply additional specific anatomic and physiologic knowledge to optimally perform the procedure and to appropriately manage the patient afterward. In particular, the operator needs sufficient understanding of relevant anatomy and physiology to properly select an appropriate operative site, adapt the procedure to the patient's condition, manage the expected clinical consequences of the procedure, and recognize significant complications related to the procedure.

The thorax consists of the thoracic wall and its associated internal contents. The thoracic wall is formed by the sternum, the ribs and their associated cartilages, the spine, the musculature attached to the skeletal elements, and the covering skin. The ribs articulate with the thoracic vertebrae to allow the excursion necessary for breathing movements. This respiratory pump action is also partially subsumed by the action of the diaphragm.

The thoracic cavity is delimited by the chest wall and the diaphragm. There are several important structures contained within this area: the lower trachea, bronchi, lungs, heart and pericardium, great vessels, esophagus, phrenic nerves, thoracic duct, and several lesser structures.

A serous pleural membrane covers the inner surface of the chest wall; the outer surface of the lungs, including the lobar fissures; the thoracic surface of the portions of the diaphragm in direct contact with the lungs; and the lateral aspects of the mediastinum. This arrangement creates a pleural space in each hemithorax. Each pleural space is normally only a potential space containing a trivial amount of serous fluid. Introduction of a significant volume of air, fluid, or blood will cause the pleural space to expand and occupy a portion of the intrathoracic volume with a consequent impact on respiratory function.

In addition to understanding thoracic anatomy well enough to recognize when thoracostomy might be indicated, operators must also understand several additional anatomic relationships that are relevant to the performance of the procedure. Understanding these issues is especially important to

the proper placement of thoracostomy drainage devices and to the avoidance of several serious procedure-related complications.

Bedside thoracostomy procedures invariably must traverse the soft tissues of an intercostal space to reach the pleural space. Understanding the anatomy of the intercostal space is important to reduce the risk of nerve or vascular injury. Each intercostal space is bounded by ribs superiorly and inferiorly. A neurovascular bundle resides along the inferior border of each rib. Therefore, instrumentation should occur only along the superior rib margin and dissection or procedure related trauma near the inferior border should be avoided. Inadvertent injury to the neurovascular bundle can result in the loss of intercostal nerve function or serious intercostal artery bleeding. Bleeding from an intercostal artery can be very difficult to control because there is often no easy way to apply direct pressure to the vessel. In some instances, iatrogenic injury to an intercostal artery may necessitate operative intervention to control the bleeding. The risk of neurovascular bundle injury in small babies is significantly greater than it is for larger children, adolescents, and adults because the intercostal space is much narrower.

In addition to understanding the anatomy of the intercostal space, the operator must also be able to correlate external thoracic landmarks with the position of certain internal structures (Fig. 29.1). This knowledge is important to assure proper placement of drainage devices and to avoid injury

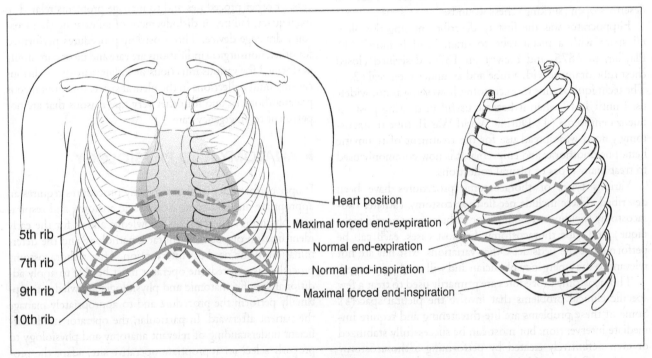

5th rib
7th rib
9th rib
10th rib

Heart position
Maximal forced end-expiration
Normal end-expiration
Normal end-inspiration
Maximal forced end-inspiration

Figure 29.1 The relationship between the position of the diaphragm, heart and external thoracic landmarks. During normal tidal volume breathing, excursions of the dome of the diaphragm normally range between approximately the level of the seventh rib at normal end-expiration and approximately the level of the ninth rib at normal end-inspiration. Maximal forced end-expiration can elevate the dome of the diaphragm to the level of the fourth to fifth rib. Maximal forced end-inspiration can depress the dome of the diaphragm to the level of the 10th to 11th rib.

to internal organs or structures. Perhaps the most critical issue is the location of the diaphragm, which normally extends significantly above the bottom of the rib cage. A significant portion of the upper abdomen is enclosed by the lower ribs. Hence, care must be taken during the procedure to ensure that the device is placed within the pleural space and not through the diaphragm into the abdomen. Entry to the abdomen has serious risks and a life-threatening injury to the liver, spleen, stomach, intestine, and other abdominal structures is possible. Patient position can affect the location of the diaphragm. Patient positions (e.g., fetal position) or conditions (e.g., pregnancy) that increase intra-abdominal pressure will tend to push the diaphragm higher into the thoracic cavity. Positions that place the abdomen at or above the level of the thorax (e.g., Trendelenburg position) also can displace the diaphragm cephalad due to abdominal contents pushing up against the diaphragm. Patient positions that reduce abdominal pressure and/or put the abdomen below the level of the thorax (e.g., sitting, semi-upright, or upright positions) will tend to lower the level of the diaphragm.

The level of the diaphragm is also affected by the phases of breathing. It is usually highest at end-expiration and lowest at end-inspiration. At forced end-expiration, the diaphragm may elevate as high as the fourth interspace in some patients. If the patient is able to cooperate and control his breathing according to the operator's commands, then he may be able to help the operator by holding his breath at end-inspiration as the operator enters the pleural space. The operator should also consider the possibility that the diaphragm may lie in an abnormal position when the patient has abdominal distention, increased abdominal pressure, paralysis of a portion of the diaphragm, severe scoliosis or other major chest wall deformities, or other suggestive findings. Rarely, diaphragmatic hernias, either congenital or traumatic, may allow unintended entry into the abdominal cavity during a thoracostomy procedure. Even worse, a diaphragmatic hernia may allow abdominal contents to enter the thorax placing them at risk for injury.

The operator must also understand the normal relative position of the mediastinum with respect to external thoracic landmarks in order to avoid entering or injuring the mediastinum. The mediastinum does not normally communicate with the pleural space of either hemithorax directly. Therefore, thoracostomy drainage devices that are unintentionally placed in the mediastinum are likely to be ineffectual for pleural drainage. Additionally, mediastinal structures, especially the heart, are put at risk for injury. The mediastinum normally occupies much of the central portion of the thoracic cavity. It extends laterally further into the left hemithorax because of the leftward projection of the heart. It contains the thymus, heart and pericardium, portions of the great vessels, trachea and esophagus. The pleurae reflect and cover both sides of the mediastinum laterally. Perforation of the lateral membrane of the mediastinum may allow communication with the pleural space on the affected side. The pleural space on each side of the chest extends close to the midline along the

undersurface of the anterior chest wall and in front of the heart and pericardium. Prior to performing a thoracostomy procedure, the clinician should try to anticipate conditions that may alter the size or location of the mediastinum. In particular, history, examination, imaging, or other findings suggesting extreme cardiomegaly, abnormal situs, or other issues should be recognized. The heart wall may be nearly or even immediately adjacent to the lateral chest wall in patients with marked cardiomegaly. Unintended placement of a drainage device in a heart chamber is a catastrophic event. Rarely, patients with mediastinal tumors will require thoracostomy procedures. Such tumors can significantly increase the size of the mediastinum and distort its position. The greatest concern regarding massive mediastinal tumors is, however, their tendency to compromise the patient's airway. Therefore, careful attention should be paid to sedation, analgesia, patient positioning, and contingency planning in the event of deterioration or complications when performing a thoracostomy procedure.

For cosmetic reasons, breast tissue should be avoided during thoracostomy procedures. It is particularly important to avoid the breast bud tissue in prepubertal females to avoid any risk of abnormal breast development during puberty. The operator should leave a significant distance between any palpable breast tissue and the operative site. If there is no palpable breast tissue, the operator should choose an operative site that is at least several centimeters away from the outer edge of the areola. Subcutaneous dissection should assiduously avoid the breast bud and areolar areas as well.

In rare cases, the clinician may need to perform a thoracostomy procedure for a patient with another medical device in place near the intended operative site. Examples of medical devices in the thoracic area that may impact the selection of an operative site include indwelling central venous catheter ports and tubing, pacemakers or implanted defibrillators and their associated leads, CSF shunt tubing, implanted infusion pumps, and vagal nerve stimulators with their associated leads. The operator may also encounter patients with postsurgical drains, transthoracic pacing wires, monitoring catheters, and other devices. The clinician performing a thoracostomy should be aware of these devices and avoid them, if possible. Coordination with consultants should be undertaken when necessary or appropriate.

Sometimes, a patient will require a thoracostomy procedure prior to another surgical procedure involving the chest. If it is anticipated or known that a patient will soon undergo placement of a medical device and/or a major surgical procedure affecting the thorax, then the clinician performing the thoracostomy procedure should avoid, whenever possible, the areas of the chest that will be used for the future surgical procedure(s). Such consideration may facilitate the upcoming surgery and reduce the risk of infection or other complications. When possible, care should be coordinated with the surgical team.

Prior surgery, infectious or inflammatory processes, neoplastic diseases, or other conditions involving the pleural space sometimes can impact the performance of a thoracostomy procedure. This is primarily due to pleural adhesions and scars. If pleural adhesions or scars are disrupted, significant bleeding may arise from associated blood vessels. When bleeding is persistent or severe, operative intervention may be required. Breaking apart pleural adhesions may also risk lung injury or disruption of prior surgical sites with resultant bleeding, air leaks, or other consequences. Attempting to pass thoracostomy drainage devices across thick pleural adhesions, such as those that may arise at an old thoracotomy incision site, can be particularly risky. Performing a thoracostomy procedure at a site that might contain major pleural adhesions also increases the risk that the drainage device will not freely communicate with all parts of the pleural space and may not function properly. Imaging studies often help to identify a procedure site that will allow effective drainage of intrapleural air or fluid but avoids the prior surgical site.

The ability to appropriately select a surgical site and perform the steps of a thoracostomy procedure is largely related to an understanding of the pertinent anatomy. However, the ability to determine that an individual patient actually requires a thoracostomy procedure, that a thoracostomy procedure needs to be adapted to meet some specific patient need, or that a complication has occurred is usually related to an understanding of physiology.

Thoracostomy procedures are primarily designed to ameliorate various conditions that cause physiologic derangements involving the thorax or thoracic structures. The most common conditions that can be corrected by thoracostomy procedures are those caused by abnormal accumulations of air and/or fluid in the pleural space (Fig. 29.2).

An abnormal air collection in the pleural space is termed a pneumothorax. Pneumothoraces can be caused by a traumatic injury to the lung or bronchi or from wounds that fully traverse the chest wall. Pneumothoraces can also result from positive pressure applied to the lungs during assisted ventilation, a forceful Valsalva maneuver, or scuba diving. Lung blebs can predispose the patient to the development of pneumothoraces. Iatrogenically induced pneumothoraces can complicate catheterization of subclavian or jugular vessels, and other procedures. In rare cases, a pneumomediastinum or a pneumopericardium will extend to create a concomitant pneumothorax. Air in the pleural space can also rarely result from free air tracking into the pleural space from the abdomen or from an esophageal rupture or injury.

There are several types of fluid that may collect in the pleural space. Blood in the pleural space is termed a "hemothorax" and most commonly results from blunt or penetrating thoracic trauma. Less common causes of bleeding into the pleural space include: bleeding due to iatrogenic mishaps or complications related to catheterization of a subclavian, jugular, or other vessel; bleeding related to other types of surgical procedures (including thoracostomies) in or around the chest area; bleeding caused by erosion of blood vessels related to an adjacent disease process; and bleeding associated with other rare conditions. In very rare cases, transfused blood can en-

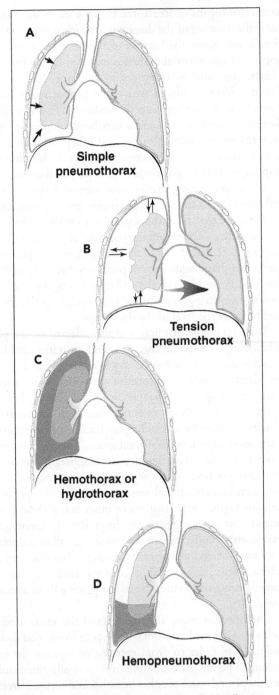

Figure 29.2 Types of intrapleural air and/or fluid collections.
A. Simple pneumothorax.
B. Tension pneumothorax.
C. Hemothorax or hydrothorax.
D. Hemopneumothorax.

ter the pleural space via a malpositioned or eroded vascular catheter. Coagulopathy greatly increases the risk of a significant hemothorax.

Other than blood, various fluids can also collect in the pleural space and produce a pleural effusion (hydrothorax). The Starling equation explains many of the possible pathophysiologic mechanisms that can promote the accumulation of fluid in the pleural space. (The Starling equation indicates that transmembrane fluid flux gradients are related to the net difference between a hydrostatic pressure term which is calculated as a permeability coefficient times the net hydrostatic pressure across the membrane and an oncotic pressure term, which is calculated as a selectivity/activity coefficient times the net oncotic pressure across the membrane.) Net accumulation of pleural fluid occurs whenever the factors in the Starling equation promote pleural fluid production faster than pleural lymphatic function can remove it. Therefore, primary pleural fluid collections can arise due to changes in net hydrostatic pressure and/or net oncotic pressure favoring fluid transudation into the pleural space, changes in endothelial permeability or integrity (selectivity) favoring fluid exudation into the pleural space, or decreased lymphatic function causing impaired ability to reabsorb fluid from the pleural space or other extravascular compartments (see also Fig. 81.1).

Many conditions can cause a pleural effusion via one or more of these pathophysiologic mechanisms. Examples include congestive heart failure, nephrotic syndrome and other hypoalbuminemic states, infectious diseases, inflammatory diseases, neoplasms, and others. Secondary pleural fluid collections can result from ascites, fistula drainage, or other abdominal fluids directly extending from the abdomen into the pleural space. They can also result from iatrogenic administration of fluid into the pleural space as can occur with certain CSF shunts and with mishaps involving administration of crystalloid, colloid, or intravenous alimentation fluids via faulty vascular access. Other extrathoracic circumstances are very rare causes of secondary effusions. Empyema is a collection of pus that usually results from extension of a pneumonia or lung abscess into the pleural space or from a pleural effusion that subsequently becomes directly infected. Chylothorax, due to injury or other problems related to the thoracic duct, is an uncommon type of pleural fluid collection. It is also possible to have a mixture of air and/or fluid and/or blood accumulate in the pleural space due to combinations of the various aforementioned mechanisms.

The thorax normally performs several important physiologic functions that may be adversely impacted by a pleural collection of air and/or fluid. The thorax acts like a pump to produce gas exchange via the lungs. Inspiratory excursions of the diaphragm and chest wall generate net negative intrathoracic pressures with respect to the ambient atmosphere and, thereby, achieve normal lung expansion during inspiration. The juxtaposition of the visceral pleural membrane covering the outer lung and the parietal pleural membrane covering the intrathoracic surfaces of the thoracic wall, diaphragm, and mediastinum is maintained by the viscoelastic force generated by the trivial amount of lubricating fluid normally contained in the pleural space. Without this viscoelastic effect, the lung would tend to elastically recoil, lose contact with the chest wall and diaphragm, and not inflate well during inspiration. The viscoelastic effect of the pleura also is very important for normal exhalation function. The expiratory phase of breathing is normally mostly passive due to elastic recoil forces in the chest wall and lungs. The apposition of the visceral and the

parietal pleural membranes counteracts the residual elastic recoil force of the lungs once the chest wall and diaphragm have reached their end-expiratory position. This protects against further lung collapse at end-expiration. As a result, the lungs remain partially inflated and in contact with the chest wall, diaphragm, and mediastinum at end-expiration. The serous nature of the pleural membrane, along with the scant amount of lubricating pleural fluid that is normally present, also allows the visceral and parietal pleurae to slide against each other throughout the phases of breathing without significant friction or irritation.

Progressive filling of the pleural space with air, fluid, and/or blood causes a gradual loss of effectiveness of the respiratory pump function of the thorax. Abnormal increases in pleural volume directly impinge on lung volume. In addition, loss of the normal viscoelastic approximation between the visceral pleura and the parietal pleural predisposes to subtotal or even total collapse below the usual end-expiratory volume of affected areas of the lung. Once an area of lung collapses, substantial additional inspiratory force (pressure) must be supplied to restore the collapsed lung to normal end-expiratory volume. When atelectasis is present, discordant lung inflation may occur because the normal lung requires less pressure to achieve inflation and may be preferentially inflated and even hyperinflated compared to the collapsed lung. Atelectatic areas of lung also have a significantly lower pulmonary vascular resistance compared to inflated lung. This results in shunting of blood through collapsed portions of lung. Atelectasis-associated shunting can result in significant hypoxemia. Patients who have significant amounts of collapsed lung can also be more sensitive to intravascular volume deficits. Infusing fluid intravascularly will often improve hemodynamics in such cases.

The impaired respiratory pump function accompanying significant pleural air and/or fluid collections results in a compensatory increase in work of breathing to maintain satisfactory ventilation. Normally, work of breathing represents about 5 percent of total body oxygen consumption. Supranormal work of breathing requires increased perfusion of respiratory muscle to meet their increased oxygen needs. The respiratory muscles of patients with severely increased work of breathing can consume up to 8 to 10 times more oxygen than those of normally breathing individuals. Patients who are seriously ill or injured may not be able to meet or sustain the oxygen delivery needs of their respiratory muscles when intrapleural air or fluid causes their work of breathing to increase. Decreasing the work of breathing by draining an abnormal pleural air or fluid collection may be very beneficial in such cases.

In addition to deleterious effects on lung ventilation, perfusion, and mechanics, intrapleural air and/or fluid collections can significantly affect the cardiovascular system. Air and/or fluid in the pleural space not only occupy intrapleural volume, but also may increase the relative pressure inside the thorax and sometimes shift the position of the mediastinum. This affects the circulation in several ways. First, indirect compression and/or altered transmural pressures affecting the heart results in decreased cardiac output. Second, altered transmural pressure also compresses the great veins, causing decreased venous return to the heart. Third, increases in intrathoracic pressure may significantly reduce the transthoracic pressure gradient that normally favors venous return into the thorax. These effects on venous return can seriously decrease cardiac output and are analogous to the effects produced by positive pressure ventilation. Cardiac output diminishes further if the pressure becomes great enough to shift the mediastinal position, distorting and obstructing vessels. Pressure alterations within the thorax from pleural air and/or fluid collections also can affect ECG tracings and invasive hemodynamic monitoring values and waveforms.

Simple pneumothoraces and hydrothoraces can produce near-atmospheric pressure in the affected pleural space (Fig. 29.2 A,C). Either can impair normal physiology through one or more of the aforementioned mechanisms. Patients who are otherwise healthy generally tolerate the impaired ventilation that results from partial or even total collapse of a single lung such as might occur with moderate to severe instances of either of these conditions. Cardiovascular embarrassment is generally mild to moderate and satisfactorily tolerated in otherwise healthy and euvolemic individuals. Serial physiologic assessment is very important to assure maintenance of pulmonary and cardiovascular function whenever a significant pleural air or fluid collection is present. Significant tachypnea, dyspnea, tachycardia, hypoxemia, hypotension, or changing mental status should raise concerns that pulmonary or cardiovascular compromise is not being adequately tolerated or is worsening. Maintenance of adequate intravascular volume is particularly important to compensate for the abnormal venous return when larger air or fluid collections are present. Because simple pneumothoraces and hydrothoraces are generally adequately tolerated by healthy patients, therapeutic thoracostomy can usually be performed semi-electively or urgently in such cases. Rarely, severely affected patients and those with significant co-morbid conditions may require an emergency thoracostomy procedure.

The potential cardiovascular consequences of hemothoraces and tension pneumothoraces are much more significant than those associated with simple pneumothoraces and simple pleural effusions. Hemothoraces cause the same volume and pressure impacts on intrathoracic structures that occur with other intrapleural air or fluid collections but often cause additional direct and serious cardiovascular compromise due to the intravascular blood loss that they represent. Because hemothoraces result in loss of red blood cells from the intravascular compartment, there is decreased oxygen delivery to tissues. In other words, blood loss associated with hemothoraces impacts physiologic functioning in three ways; it produces hypoxemia, hypovolemia, and anemia. Restoration of intravascular volume with crystalloid solutions is usually satisfactory for small hemothoraces. Blood replacement with packed red blood cells or autotransfused blood recovered from the hemothorax may be necessary when a larger hemothorax is present (see

Chapter 30). In this type of situation, hemoglobin levels must be restored to overcome anemic cardiac dysfunction and hypoxemia.

The severity of a hemothorax can be influenced by several factors. The vascular pressure head of the pulmonary circulation is usually significantly less than that of the systemic circulation. Therefore, bleeding from a site supplied by the pulmonary circulation tends to be less severe and more likely to cease spontaneously than bleeding from a site supplied by the systemic circulation. Coagulation status also influences severity. Blood contained in a hemothorax can play a role in controlling further intrathoracic bleeding. The hemothorax can help produce a covering clot or occasionally help tamponade a bleeding site. As a consequence, thoracostomy drainage of a hemothorax can occasionally cause resumption or worsening of intrathoracic bleeding by removing blood and clots that are helping to control hemorrhage. This should not prevent the performance of a thoracostomy procedure that is clearly indicated to treat a hemothorax. Thoracostomy drainage of a significant hemothorax provides the clinician with the ability to directly measure the amount and rate of blood loss into the pleural space. This can be invaluable for guiding fluid and blood replacement as well as contributing to a determination that a thoracotomy or other operative intervention is likely to be necessary. There is often no effective way to apply direct pressure to an intrathoracic bleeding site, so surgical intervention is indicated for persistent, significant bleeding. Tube thoracostomy also enables autotransfusion of blood contained in a hemothorax.

Tension pneumothoraces are the most dangerous of all pleural conditions. Tension pneumothoraces result when the pressure exerted by air contained in the pleural space becomes supra-atmospheric. They can be life-threatening even in very healthy individuals when the pleural pressure becomes high enough to seriously impede venous return into the chest, compress cardiovascular structures, or obstruct intrathoracic blood vessels (Fig. 29.2B). The cardiovascular compromise resulting from a tension pneumothorax is often the clinical finding that suggests the diagnosis. Acute changes in end-tidal CO_2 concentration or capnography waveform may, however, suggest the diagnosis even before cardiovascular compromise develops because these monitors detect acute changes in ventilation and pulmonary blood flow within a few breaths of their onset. Declining oxygen saturation as determined by a pulse oximeter may also be an early sign of deterioration in cardiopulmonary function due to a pneumothorax. Death from a tension pneumothorax is usually due to the cardiovascular pathophysiology just described. Increasing intravascular volume and cardiac inotropy may help offset some of these deleterious effects. However, in all but the mildest cases, such interventions are inadequate to restore cardiovascular function. Therefore, thoracostomy drainage of tension pneumothoraces should be viewed as the initial and most important therapeutic intervention for such cases. By performing a thoracostomy procedure, the supra-atmospheric pressure can be relieved and the tension pneumothorax can be effectively converted to a simple pneumothorax with non-life-threatening cardiovascular consequences. After satisfactory thoracostomy drainage of a tension pneumothorax is achieved, additional cardiovascular support measures can be considered and implemented as warranted.

Many patients maintain spontaneous respiration before and after a thoracostomy procedure is performed. However, some patients require positive pressure ventilation. It is important to understand the impact of positive pressure ventilation on chest physiology in general and on thoracostomy management in particular.

During spontaneous breathing, intrathoracic pressure is subatmospheric during the inspiratory portions of the breathing cycle. This is important for promoting venous return into the thorax and the heart. When positive pressure ventilation is administered, the inspiratory phase of the breathing cycle becomes supra-atmospheric and thus impedes venous return to the heart. This effect can be particularly important in patients requiring high mean airway pressures to achieve adequate ventilation, in patients with intravascular volume deficits (e.g., hypovolemic shock) and in patients with conditions that cause inappropriate vasodilatation or distribution of perfusion (e.g., septic shock, neurogenic shock, anaphylactic shock). The cardiovascular consequences of positive pressure ventilation are further aggravated whenever a significant air and/or fluid collection are present in the pleural space. The clinician should, therefore, anticipate a sudden worsening of the patient's hemodynamic status at the initiation of positive pressure ventilation in such cases. Intravascular fluid infusion to augment intravascular volume and/or cardiotonic medication to improve cardiac performance and/or vasoactive medication to favorably improve vascular tone may be required. Emergent thoracostomy drainage of a significant pleural air and/or fluid collection may provide substantial additional cardiovascular benefit. Apart from the usual effects of positive pressure ventilation on venous return, induction of a tension pneumothorax also should be considered when a patient undergoes cardiovascular deterioration after the initiation of positive pressure ventilation.

Another important physiologic consideration arises whenever a patient with a pneumothorax will experience significant changes in ambient atmospheric pressure over a relatively short period of time as can occur during transportation via aircraft, travel across widely changing elevations, or administration of hyperbaric therapy. Pneumothoraces that do not readily communicate with the ambient atmosphere are unable to equilibrate with changing atmospheric pressure except very slowly by diffusion of gas across the pleural membrane. Because gas does not flow rapidly into nor out of a noncommunicating pneumothorax, it approximates a closed system and the usual gas laws of physics apply (e.g., $P_I V_I = P_2 V_2$). Therefore, if ambient atmospheric pressure becomes significantly less than the pressure in the pneumothorax, the pressure in the pneumothorax acutely becomes relatively supra-atmospheric, creating in effect a tension pneumothorax. Conversely, if the ambient atmospheric pressure acutely becomes significantly

greater than the pressure in a noncommunicating pneumothorax, then the pressure in the pneumothorax will become relatively subatmospheric and the pneumothorax will decrease in size acutely. If extrathoracic air pressure remains relatively higher than the pressure in the pneumothorax over a period of time, then the air in the pleural space and the ambient atmosphere will begin to approach equilibrium. When, after significant equilibration occurs, the patient acutely transitions to a lower atmospheric pressure, the intrapleural air pressure acutely will become relatively supra-atmospheric and behave as a tension pneumothorax. Almost all pneumothoraces can act this way because they are caused by a relatively small hole in the lung parenchyma or a bronchus that does not allow quick equilibration of pleural space pressure. Performing a thoracostomy protects against the effects of rapid changes in atmospheric pressure because the communication created through the chest wall allows constant rapid and free airflow to maintain pressure equilibrium between the pleural space and the atmosphere. The pneumothorax thus is converted to an open system that will not develop supra-atmospheric pressure. Instead, when ambient atmospheric pressure changes acutely the necessary amount of air flows immediately across the thoracostomy drainage device until the pressure in the pleural space equals the new barometric pressure. (Typically, a one-way valve is interposed in the drainage system between the pleural space and the atmosphere. This arrangement allows air to escape the pleural space whenever intrapleural pressure becomes supra-atmospheric and prevents air from entering the pleural space whenever the intrapleural pressure becomes subatmospheric. Although not a totally free communication, such an arrangement does effectively prevent the unwanted development of a tension pneumothorax.)

An analogous situation can occur when the partial pressure of a gas that is being breathed changes significantly with respect to the air contained within a pneumothorax. This is an important consideration when an inhaled anesthetic agent is administered to a patient with a pneumothorax. Administered anesthetic gases will accumulate in the pneumothorax as long as the partial pressure of the anesthetic gas in the lung (and, hence, the circulating blood) is higher than in the pneumothorax. After anesthetic gas administration is discontinued, residual anesthetic gas in the circulating blood is cleared by the lungs and exhaled. However, the pneumothorax will also contain residual anesthetic gases that are not so readily mobilized. Anesthetic gas in the pneumothorax may take some time to diffuse back into the blood. As anesthetic gas diffuses out of the pneumothorax and into the circulation, systemic anesthetic effects may persist or recur. These same principles are used to the patient's benefit when a clinician administers air with a higher than normal concentration of oxygen (and correspondingly lower than normal concentration of nitrogen) to hasten the resolution of a pneumothorax. This generates a partial pressure gradient favoring diffusion of nitrogen out of the pneumothorax. Oxygen contained in the pneumothorax is reabsorbed readily because oxygen that diffuses into nearby tissues is used for aerobic metabolism and because the high affinity of hemoglobin and low partial pressure of oxygen in nearby capillaries favors reabsorption of oxygen from the pneumothorax. Placing a thoracostomy drainage device essentially eliminates issues related to partial pressure differentials across the pleural membrane.

Some patients develop pulmonary edema upon re-expansion of compressed or atelectatic portions of a lung following drainage of a pleural air or fluid collection. The physiologic mechanism for this is not clear. The development of dyspnea or hypoxemia, auscultatory findings, and radiographic evidence usually establish the diagnosis. Therapy is supportive until spontaneous resolution occurs.

Extrathoracic structures may be indirectly but severely impacted by the effects of intrathoracic volume or pressure changes. For example, intracranial pressure may rise if increased intrathoracic pressure interferes with venous blood flow from the head into the thorax. In the setting of head trauma or other conditions in which intracranial pressure is already elevated, a further rise in intracranial pressure might be devastating. Pleural air or fluid accumulations can also affect intracranial pressure if they interfere with ventilation and thereby cause an increase in pCO_2 or a decrease in pH. Likewise, serious and even fatal exacerbations of other conditions that are critically related to acid-base status (e.g., pulmonary hypertension, certain poisonings, metabolic disorders, respiratory failure, vasopressor therapy, shock) may occur whenever pleural space problems decrease pulmonary ventilation with a resultant increased pCO_2 or decreased pH.

Occasionally, the physiologic impact of a pneumothorax, hydrothorax, or hemothorax can be ameliorated by changing the position of the patient. In general, gravity causes the dependent lung to receive relatively more blood flow and to ventilate less effectively than the other lung. Positioning the patient on one side versus the other, or even using the prone position may take advantage of gravity to produce a more favorable situation. The effect of such maneuvers is usually small but can be significant.

▶ INDICATIONS

Thoracostomy procedures are most commonly indicated to drain air, blood, or other fluid from the pleural space. The patient's history or exam will often provide the initial clue to the presence of one of these conditions. For example, the patient may have a history of trauma, recent surgery, pain, dyspnea, or disease involving the chest. Typical examination findings may include: abnormalities or changes in vital signs measurements reflecting respiratory function, cardiac function, or both; signs of trauma; abnormal auscultatory findings, abnormal percussion findings; signs of prior surgery; the presence of certain medical devices; and signs of disease states affecting the chest. Imaging studies or other interventions may occasionally serve to initially identify pleural space problems and are often used to confirm the presence of abnormal contents in the pleural space (10–25).

Once it is suspected that air and/or fluid is present in the pleural space, the clinician can perform additional physical examination. Careful percussion and auscultation of the chest are especially useful to help confirm these suspicions and to clarify the severity of the situation. Imaging studies, such as frontal and lateral view plain chest radiographs, may further help elucidate the nature, location, and degree of the problem(s). More specialized imaging studies, such as decubitus view chest radiographs or computerized tomography imaging of the chest, can provide additional useful information in selected cases. In particular, special imaging can help the operator determine whether or not intrapleural fluid is free flowing and drainable with a thoracostomy catheter or tube.

Progressive filling of the pleural space with air, fluid, and/or blood usually causes progressive physiologic deterioration and compensatory physiologic responses are often the earliest clinically recognizable warning signs of these conditions. As the disorder progresses, more dire warning signs of organ dysfunction appear. An individual patient may present at any point along this spectrum of worsening physiologic impact from essentially asymptomatic to extremis depending on his/her individual circumstances.

The pulmonary and/or the cardiovascular systems are most commonly and most significantly impacted by serious pleural space problems. Therefore, findings of abnormal pulmonary function (ventilation, oxygenation, work of breathing, or pulmonary mechanics) or abnormal cardiovascular function (heart rate, rhythm, blood pressure, perfusion, or oxygenation) are the most important warning signs of significant intrapleural air and/or fluid collections. Local pain, findings associated with significant blood loss, the presence of blunt or penetrating chest trauma, or additional manifestations of disease processes affecting the chest are other clues to the presence of air and/or fluid in the pleural space.

Once a pleural air and/or fluid collection is confirmed, the clinician must determine its physiologic importance. By understanding the physiologic impact and the anticipated course of a pleural air and/or fluid collection, the need for and relative timing of a thoracostomy procedure can be properly determined. An appreciation of the potential impact of other coexisting conditions or other planned interventions will sometimes affect these decisions.

Pneumothoraces, hydrothoraces, and/or hemothoraces that are very small, well-tolerated, and not expected to worsen, can often be monitored without intervention unless worsening or complications occur. Aspiration of fluid solely for diagnostic purposes may or may not be desirable in some of these cases. Therapeutic thoracostomy becomes clearly indicated if significant physiologic embarrassment is present, awaiting spontaneous resolution poses unacceptable risk, or serious worsening is anticipated.

Pulmonary and/or cardiovascular compromise is the primary indication for a thoracostomy procedure. Rarely, other indications arise. Perhaps the most significant of these is the problem of achieving good antibiotic concentrations in pleural fluid. Infected pleural fluid collections are akin to abscesses elsewhere. Because there are no vascular beds within the pleural fluid collection itself, drug concentrations in pleural effusions depend on diffusion of the drug from nearby vascular beds, resulting in lower antimicrobial concentrations. Therefore, better and faster resolution of some types of infections may result when infected fluid or blood is removed. Often, knowledge of the properties of the infecting organism(s) and the specific antimicrobial agent(s) will help determine when drainage of an infected pleural effusion is indicated. This issue can become more complicated if one or more loculated intrapleural fluid collections are present. In such cases, the risk of a poorly responding or persistent infection may increase. The difficulty associated with achieving good thoracostomy drainage also increases. Failure to drain infected pleural fluid when indicated can result in significant complications. However, these are more often a concern for the physician managing the patient in the hospital than for the emergency physician.

Pleural air or fluid collections related to certain conditions are associated with long resolution times, greater complication risks or less favorable outcomes if allowed to spontaneously resolve. In particular, drainage is beneficial, even in the absence of physiological embarrassment for pleural effusions caused by certain infectious diseases, inflammatory processes, or other types of conditions that tend to produce scarring or adhesions involving intrathoracic structures. Analysis of drained pleural fluid using culture, serology, chemical analysis, or other diagnostic tests can often facilitate diagnosis of many of these conditions. Usually thoracentesis is preferred when pleural fluid is to be removed for diagnostic purposes only (see Chapter 81).

Patients with pneumothoraces are at significant risk for worsening whenever positive pressure ventilation is administered. As a rule, a therapeutic intrapleural drainage device should be placed in all such cases to prevent the development of a devastating tension pneumothorax. Likewise, certain circumstances, such as a need for interhospital aeromedical transportation, a requirement for major surgery, a lack of an available appropriate inpatient bed, or other situations that will sufficiently impair or preclude the ability to monitor a patient effectively and/or perform a thoracostomy if it becomes needed, should be construed as strong general indications to perform an antecedent therapeutic thoracostomy.

Occasionally, patients who have significant amounts of air, blood, or fluid in their pleural space will have pre-existing or concomitant conditions that additionally impact their pulmonary or cardiovascular physiology beyond that due to their pleural space pathology. Pre-existing conditions that can be of additive physiologic significance may include congenital or acquired heart disease, asthma or chronic lung diseases, and anemia. Patients with trauma-related pleural air or blood collections frequently have associated lung injuries and occasionally have cardiac or great vessel injuries. They also may have significant derangements due to blood losses in the chest or elsewhere. Patients with pleural effusions due to infectious or inflammatory disorders may also have co-existing direct involvement of their lungs or heart due to their primary condition or indirect involvement of these organs due to circulating mediators or toxins. Additionally, pre-existing or concomitant conditions or therapeutic interventions may interfere with the patient's ability to compensate for the physiologic effects of pleural air or fluid collections. The patient therefore should be assessed for conditions and medications that might impact his/her ability to compensate for physiologic compromise.

Thoracostomy procedures are occasionally needed to facilitate other interventional procedures or to manage their complications. For example, a thoracostomy procedure may be needed to manage a pneumothorax complicating subclavian vein catheterization. When a patient already has a thoracostomy tube in place, procedures such as subclavian vein catheterization, which may induce a pneumothorax or hemothorax, should be performed on the same side as the pre-existing chest tube in order to avoid further complications.

Rarely, a pneumothorax can arise from a large rupture or tear of the trachea or a major bronchus. The resistance to airflow through a tracheobronchial hole lessens as the hole becomes larger. So, air will preferentially flow into the pleural space rather than the lung through a large defect. This will produce serious hypoventilation and resultant hypoxemia. The presence of a large tracheobronchial disruption is suggested by significant airflow out of the thoracostomy tube with each inspiration. Positive pressure ventilation using a rapid rate, low inspired and mean airway pressures, and a high concentration of inspired oxygen will improve lung ventilation and oxygenation. A functioning thoracostomy drainage device will prevent development of a tension pneumothorax. In this circumstance, suction should not be applied to the drainage device in order to minimize the pressure gradient favoring airflow across the tracheobronchial rent.

Different sizes of thoracostomy catheters and tubes are available to accommodate the spectrum of patient sizes from preterm neonate to obese adult. The criteria for selecting an appropriately sized catheter or tube for an individual patient are described in the following section. Beyond choosing a catheter or tube that is appropriate for the patient's size, it is also necessary to consider the type and volume of material that must be drained from the pleural space. Generally, air and freely flowing serous fluid can be very effectively drained with a modestly sized catheter. However, blood, pus, or other viscid fluid should be drained with a large bore chest tube. If autotransfusion of blood from a hemothorax is contemplated, then an autotransfusion apparatus is needed (Chapter 30).

When formulating a risk-benefit analysis regarding the performance of a thoracostomy procedure, the operator should consider not only the direct risks of the thoracostomy procedure itself but also the associated risks of periprocedural sedation and of coexisting conditions. (See the Complications section below.)

There are a few other potential indications for a thoracostomy procedure; all are rare and generally not emergent occurrences. They include administration of drugs, sclerosants, or other agents into the pleural space, measurement of intrapleural pressure, and induction of lung collapse.

▶ PROCEDURES

Other than issues related to the sizing of equipment, essentially no significant modifications are required when performing thoracostomy procedures in children versus adults. However, the practitioner must choose the most appropriate management strategy for each clinical situation. These management strategies and their attendant advantages and disadvantages are described below (8,13–15,17,23, 26–32).

Conservative Management

In some cases, small, unilateral pneumothoraces can be managed conservatively. This option can be considered for stable older children and adolescents who have no evidence of respiratory distress, who will not undergo surgery, be placed in a hyperbaric chamber, or be transported by aircraft. However, there is some debate as to what constitutes a "small" pneumothorax. Many have suggested that pneumothoraces as large as 20 percent of the pleural space might be managed conservatively. But, there are few methods by which the clinician can accurately estimate the size of a pneumothorax using the results of imaging studies. Perhaps the most simple and accurate of these methods was developed by Rhea (18) who developed an (adult-based) nomogram based upon the average intrapleural distance (Fig. 29.3).

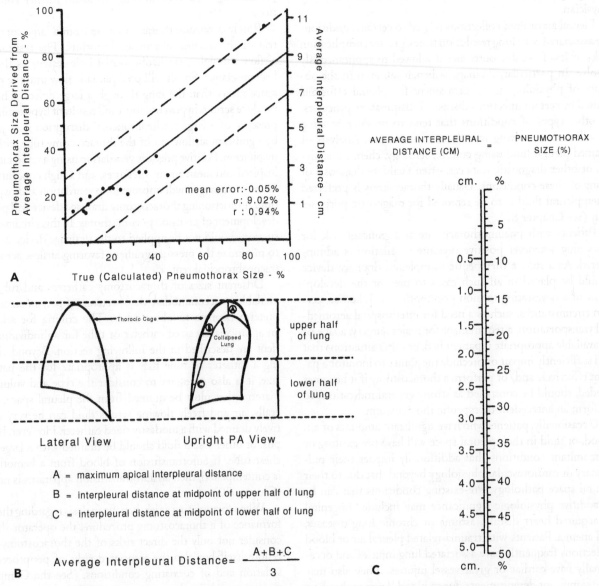

Figure 29.3 Calculation of percent pneumothorax (based on adults), using the average interpleural distance method. The number obtained from the calculation on the left (**B**) can be used to obtain a percentage from the nomogram on the right (**C**). (From Rhea JT, Deluca SA, Greene RE. Determining the size of pneumothorax in the upright patient. *Radiology.* 1982;144:733, with permission.)

Needle Thoracostomy

Indications

Although a needle thoracostomy can temporarily relieve most pneumothoraces, the primary indication for this procedure is the emergent palliative decompression of a tension pneumothorax pending the placement of a larger thoracostomy tube. Needle thoracostomy can also assist in the diagnosis of tension pneumothorax. Needle thoracostomy can occasionally serve as the definitive procedure for neonates and small children but even in these cases there is often ongoing air leak into the pleural space which requires treatment with a thoracostomy catheter.

Equipment

Angiocath (catheter over needle device) or butterfly type needle (neonates)
Sterile prep solution
Sterile gloves

Procedure

The operator should select an insertion site on a nondependent area of the chest wall on the affected side(s). If the patient is supine then the 2nd or 3rd intercostal space in the midclavicular line is typically chosen (Fig. 29.4). However, other interspaces may be used if potential complications make the infraclavicular site undesirable. If the patient is not supine,

SUMMARY

Needle Thoracostomy

1 Assemble all equipment and assign duties to personnel.

2 Explain the procedure and obtain consent (as indicated).

3 Position the patient, and prepare and anesthetize (as time allows) the skin and subcutaneous structures.

4 Advance the over-the-needle catheter device over superior aspect of rib while maintaining negative pressure in syringe.

5 When air returns, remove the needle while leaving catheter in place.

6 Evacuate the pneumothorax.

7 Obtain a chest radiograph.

then an antidependent area of an intercostal space can be used. The proposed site for the procedure should be chosen specifically to avoid entering the heart, traversing the diaphragm into the abdomen, and to minimize other risks. The insertion site should be sterilely prepped with antibacterial solution. A syringe is then partially filled with a small amount of sterile saline and attached to the angiocath device. Using sterile technique, the angiocath device is inserted perpendicularly just through the skin at the intended site on the chest wall (Fig. 29.5). The syringe should be left in place during insertion. The angiocath is then advanced through the intercostal muscles and the pleura. Some operators prefer to grasp the shaft of the angiocath firmly between the thumb and fingers of their free hand at a distance above the skin about equal to the anticipated thickness of the patient's chest wall so that their fingers will act as a stop during advancement of the angiocath device. This helps to avoid unintentional, overly deep penetration of the angiocath into the thorax. The angiocath should be advanced immediately over the superior aspect of the rib that forms the inferior margin of the intercostal space. This avoids injury to the neurovascular bundle that courses along the inferior border of each rib. Some operators prefer to intentionally touch the outer surface of the rib with the angiocath needle, 'walk' the needle over the superior aspect of that rib, and then advance the needle into the pleural space in an attempt to further minimize the risk of injury to the neurovascular bundle. Upon entering the pleural space, the operator should perceive a modest decrease in resistance to further advancement of the angiocath. Once the pleural space is entered, the angiocath should not be advanced further. The operator should assess for air return from the pleural space. This helps determine the presence or absence of tension or simple pneumothorax.

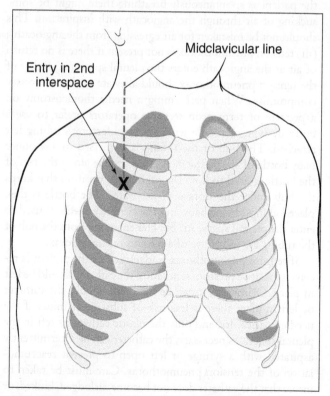

Figure 29.4 Site for needle thoracostomy evacuation of a tension pneumothorax: 2nd interspace, midclavicular line.

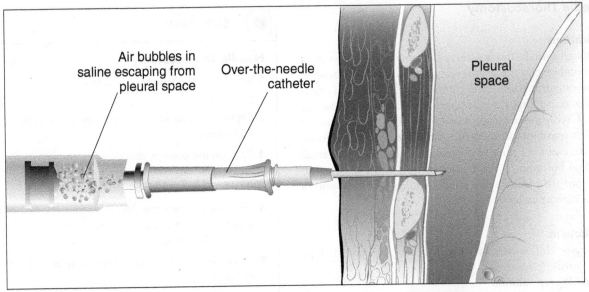

Figure 29.5 Needle thoracostomy. An angiocath attached to a syringe partially filled with saline is advanced over the rib, and air is aspirated when the needle enters the pleural space.

If a tension pneumothorax is present then immediately upon entering the pleural space, air bubbles will often be noted in the fluid-filled syringe. Depending on the initial volume of the tension pneumothorax and the ongoing rate of air leakage, further aspiration may be required to fully relieve the tension physiology. When larger air leaks are present, then removal of the syringe from the angiocath will facilitate more rapid drainage of intrapleural air. Rarely, an additional needle thoracostomy may be needed to achieve satisfactory decompression of a tension pneumothorax while preparations for a more definitive procedure are undertaken. Relief of the tension associated with a pneumothorax will relieve cardiopulmonary compromise. Persistent, severe cardiopulmonary compromise following a needle thoracostomy suggests that either the tension pneumothorax has not been adequately decompressed or the patient has another coexisting condition.

If a simple pneumothorax is present, then air return into the syringe will not occur spontaneously but will occur with aspiration. If neither a tension pneumothorax nor a simple pneumothorax is present, then there will be no significant return of air into the syringe either spontaneously or with aspiration. Occasionally, the angiocath will enter the surface of the lung and a tiny amount of air will be aspirated with each breathing cycle. Some operators prefer not to attach a syringe partially filled with saline to the angiocath when advancing the device into the pleural space. This option may be less desirable because spontaneously breathing patients may suck air into their pleural space during inspiration via the uncovered angiocath hub thus creating a pneumothorax. If a procedure-related pneumothorax occurs, it may cause confusion because the clinician may have difficulty determining whether the pneumothorax is due to the procedure or to another cause. Patients who are receiving positive pressure ventilation and are not spontaneously breathing do not have this problem because intrathoracic pressure never becomes

subatmospheric. When a needle thoracostomy is performed without a syringe attached to the angiocath, the presence or absence of a tension pneumothorax can generally be inferred by the following criteria: (i) tension pneumothorax is present when a return of air occurs via the angiocath needle as the pleural space is entered; (ii) air flowing out of the hub of the angiocath can be felt against an area of the operator's skin or, often heard as a hissing or whistling type of sound. (If the patient is spontaneously breathing there might be some sucking of air through the angiocath with inspiration. This should not be mistaken for air egressing from the angiocath); (iii) tension pneumothorax is not present if there is no return of air as the angiocath enters the pleural space. (iv) Relief of the tension pneumothorax should alleviate cardiopulmonary compromise. When performing a needle thoracostomy on a preterm or term neonate some operators prefer to use a butterfly type of needle with the manufacturer's tubing left attached. The hub of the tubing is immersed in a 4 ounce baby bottle of sterile water. A piece of tape along the rim of the bottle is used to hold the tubing in a position that keeps the hub under the surface of the water. The bottle is then placed alongside the baby and the butterfly needle is used to enter the pleural space. Air bubbles emerging from the hub of the tubing are indicative of a tension pneumothorax.

If tension pneumothorax is identified or the patient is receiving positive pressure ventilation the catheter should be left in place. Otherwise, it can be removed. Should the catheter be left in place there is less risk of subsequent injury if the needle is discarded and only the plastic catheter is left in the pleural space. As necessary, the catheter can be intermittently aspirated with a syringe or left open to prevent reaccumulation of the tension pneumothorax. Care must be taken to insure that the catheter does not become dislodged, kinked, or obstructed. If the patient is receiving positive pressure ventilation and findings associated with a tension pneumothorax are not present, then it is still reasonable to leave the catheter in place temporarily while the operator completes his/her evaluation. Leaving the catheter in place helps to guard against development of a tension pneumothorax. As long as the patient is receiving positive pressure ventilation, there is little risk that the needle thoracostomy catheter itself will create or worsen a simple pneumothorax. If a significant pneumothorax or a tension pneumothorax is found, then a catheter or tube thoracostomy procedure must be performed for definitive management.

Complications/Cautions

Even with needle thoracostomy, there is a small risk of injury to the neurovascular bundle or to intrathoracic structures. This can be minimized by attention to a few simple guidelines. Once the angiocath enters the pleural space, the operator should withdraw the needle portion of the angiocath so that the needle no longer extends beyond the tip of the plastic catheter or discard the needle altogether. In order to minimize the risk of lung injury, he/she should avoid to and fro movements of the angiocath while the needle remains in the pleural space. Likewise, standard needles should not be substituted for angiocaths unless an immediately life-threatening tension pneumothorax is suspected and no angiocath is immediately available. Generally, an angiocath that is 2 to 3 inches in length is sufficiently long to reach the pleural space, even in adolescents. Obese adolescent patients often require a longer angiocath. Shorter angiocaths may be satisfactory for smaller children. In most cases, a size #16, #18, or possibly a #20 angiocath is adequate for adolescent patients. A stiffer catheter is preferable to minimize the risk of catheter obstruction due to kinking or compression. Similarly sized catheters can be used for all pediatric patients, except the smallest of babies.

Patients with serious coagulopathies can undergo needle thoracostomy for life-threatening tension pneumothoraces. In fact, it may be preferable to begin with a needle thoracostomy rather than a large chest tube. If the patient's condition can be stabilized with a needle thoracostomy, then this can be left in place until the patient's coagulopathy can be sufficiently ameliorated to allow a more invasive procedure.

Infrequently, an intrathoracic air leak is so large that a single catheter cannot drain the air quickly enough to relieve a tension pneumothorax. In such cases, additional needle thoracostomies can be performed. Better yet, placing a chest tube or even making the incision prior to chest tube insertion will allow air to be vented from the pleural space more adequately.

Positive pressure ventilation can convert simple pneumothoraces to tension pneumothoraces. Therefore, simple pneumothoraces should be vented with a thoracostomy catheter or tube whenever positive pressure ventilation is administered. Similarly, patients with simple pneumothoraces who require transportation that will involve significant changes of altitude, are also at risk for the development of tension pneumothoraces. Therefore, simple pneumothoraces generally should be vented prior to transport. A chest catheter or chest tube is preferred over a needle thoracostomy in this situation because,

as previously described, the angiocath can too easily become kinked or dislodged.

Patients who have undergone prior thoracic surgery, especially large or multiple lateral thoracotomies may not have continuity of the entire pleural space on the affected side. In such cases, a tension pneumothorax may be compartmentalized to one portion of the pleural space by pleural scars or adhesions. It may be necessary to perform needle thoracostomy above and/or below old surgical incisions in order to successfully reach the portion of the pleural space containing the tension pneumothorax. Analogous issues apply to patients with pleural scars from prior infectious, inflammatory, or neoplastic disorders.

The insertion site must be selected carefully for patients with massive cardiomegaly, abnormal cardiac situs, or abdominal distention because the normal relationships between external landmarks and underlying organs may be distorted leading to inadvertent organ injury or entry into the abdomen. Although such injuries may be well tolerated, angiocath placement in the traditional infraclavicular site generally avoids this problem. Care should be taken to avoid damaging medical devices, shunts, and lines that may be near the operative site.

Catheter Thoracostomy—Seldinger Method

Indications

Wire guided (Seldinger) thoracostomy is indicated for the drainage of air, blood, or fluid from the pleural space. Because the catheters used are smaller in diameter than standard thoracostomy tubes, they may not provide effective treatment of hemothoraces or empyemas. On the other hand, they are nearly ideal for the management of simple pneumothoraces because they are effective and yet minimize both scar formation and patient discomfort.

Equipment

Sterile gloves
Sterile mask
Sterile gown
Surgical hat
Sterile prep solution
Sterile towels
Scalpel
Seldinger thoracostomy catheter kit
    Needle or angiocath
    Syringe
    Guidewire
    Dilator catheter
    Thoracostomy catheter
Local anesthetic
Heavy suture
Heimlich valve or drainage/suction assembly with adaptor connectors and tubing
Sterile gauze or semipermeable membrane dressing
Tape

SUMMARY

Catheter Thoracostomy—Seldinger Method

1–3 Same as for a needle thoracostomy.

4 Advance syringe/needle over superior aspect of rib (consider Z-track method, Fig. 29.6) while maintaining negative pressure in syringe.

5 When air returns, remove the syringe while leaving the needle in place and advance the guide wire through the needle.

6 Remove the needle while leaving guide wire in place.

7 Make a small incision at the guide wire skin entry site.

8 Use dilators over the guide wire as needed.

9 Advance catheter over the guide wire.

10 Remove the guide wire and secure catheter in place.

11 Evacuate the pneumothorax.

12 Obtain a chest radiograph.

Procedure

After obtaining informed consent when appropriate, a Seldinger thoracostomy catheter of the appropriate size is selected. All Seldinger thoracostomy catheters have end holes and some have side holes. Straight and pigtail configurations are also available. The most important consideration, however, is the position of the side holes. All must be completely inside the chest when the catheter is in proper position. The Seldinger thoracostomy catheter kit should be checked to be sure that the guidewire is capable of freely sliding through the needle, the dilator catheter, and the thoracostomy catheter.

An appropriate insertion site is then selected. The site should be selected according to the guidelines previously described. Most commonly the lateral aspect of an intercostal space between the third and the seventh ribs (usually safely above the top of the dome of the diaphragm) is used and most catheters are placed in the fourth, fifth, or sixth intercostal interspace. After selecting the intercostal space that will be used to access the pleural space the operator needs to identify a concordant site to puncture the skin. It is often desirable to "Z-track" the catheter under the skin a short distance before entering the intercostal space to reduce the risk of leakage around the catheter and of persistent leakage through the skin tract after the catheter is removed (Fig. 29.6). Depending upon its intended use, the operator may wish to control the positioning of the intrathoracic portion of the chest tube. For supine patients, catheters that are placed to drain air are sometimes more effective when placed in the anterior chest

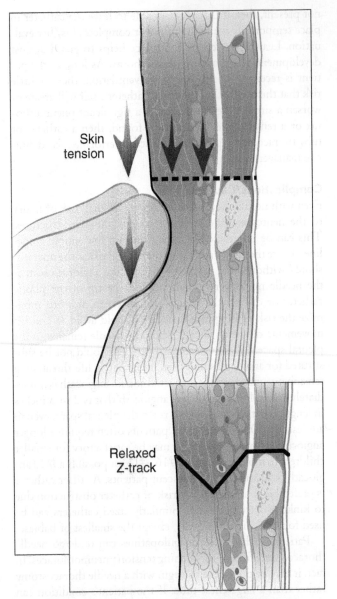

Figure 29.6 Z-track method for insertion of a needle or catheter. Before the catheter is advanced, the patient's skin and subcutaneous tissues are stretched 1 to 2 cm inferior to the proposed point of insertion. This tension is maintained while the needle or catheter is inserted and advanced. Once the tension is released and the needle or catheter is removed, the tract will be discontinuous through the tissue planes.

while those intended to drain fluid are better positioned in the posterior chest. The direction that the operator tunnels the catheter under the skin will largely determine whether the tip resides anteriorly or posteriorly. In order to direct a catheter anteriorly, the operator should tunnel under the skin in an anterior and cephalad manner, while tunneling in a posterior and cephalad manner will cause the catheter to be directed posteriorly. Catheters inadvertently placed in an anterior position when a posterior position was intended or vice versa should be replaced only if they do not function well. Catheters that function poorly should be withdrawn and replaced with a new catheter redirected into the desired position. Alternatively, placement of the patient in a lateral decubitus or prone position may allow the malpositioned catheter to function as intended.

Once the puncture site is selected, the patient can be placed in the desired position. In most cases, the patient should be placed with the unaffected side slightly dependent. This can be accomplished by placing folded linen under the affected hemithorax. The ipsilateral arm should be abducted and placed above the patient's head. Assistants may be needed to maintain the patient in proper position.

The operator should wear appropriate sterile attire. The operative site should be sterilely prepped and a sterile surgical field placed around the site. Catheter thoracostomy is a painful procedure and analgesia is essential. Local anesthetic (Chapter 35) should be administered at the skin puncture site and along the anticipated path of the catheter. Topical anesthetic gel, ethyl chloride spray, or other techniques may help to minimize the discomfort associated with local anesthetic infiltration. Patients who are unable to cooperate during the procedure may be candidates for sedation and restraint. Hypnosis and/or administration of anxiolytics may also be helpful for some patients (Chapter 33).

After infiltration of local anesthetic, a syringe should be attached to the needle that will be used to introduce the guidewire into the pleural space. Some operators prefer to partially fill the syringe with saline to facilitate visualization of returned air or fluid as the needle is advanced. The skin is then punctured at the desired site and the needle is guided over the superior margin of the rib forming the lower border of the interspace into the pleural space. Some operators prefer to first contact the body of the rib and then "walk" the needle over its superior margin; the needle should remain perpendicular to the chest wall. It may be necessary to make a 2 to 3 mm skin incision to facilitate passage of larger bore needles through the skin. Once the needle enters the pleural space, there is often a modest decrease in resistance to further advancement. Pleural space contents (i.e., air or fluid) may be returned, further confirming that the needle is properly positioned (Fig. 29.7A). Holding the needle firmly in place, the syringe is removed, and the soft or "J-tip" end of the guidewire is advanced into the hub of the needle (Fig. 29.7B). This process should be accomplished quickly for spontaneously breathing patients because respiratory efforts can draw air into the pleural space and enlarge the pneumothorax. The guidewire should be inserted a sufficient distance into the pleural space so that its end extends a few centimeters beyond the tip of the needle. The needle is then removed while the operator controls the guidewire to prevent inadvertent backward or forward movement. The needle can be returned to the equipment tray. A scalpel is used to make a tiny incision where the guidewire enters the skin (Fig. 29.7C). Care must be taken to avoid cutting the guidewire. This can be most safely done by abutting the superior (dull) surface of the scalpel against the guidewire just above the point where it enters the skin and then sliding the scalpel blade down perpendicularly into the skin a sufficient distance to make a 3 to 4 millimeter incision. Next, the semirigid dilator is threaded over the guidewire and ad-

vanced down to the skin surface (Fig. 29.7D). As previously discussed, care must be taken to avoid accidentally advancing the guidewire into the chest or removing it altogether. Once the dilator catheter is positioned at the surface of the skin, the operator should stabilize the guidewire by grasping its free end firmly just above the hub of the dilator catheter. With the other hand, he/she should grasp the body of the dilator catheter and advance it through the skin with a rotating motion. Rotating the catheter facilitates advancement and avoids damage to the tip as it passes through the skin. If resistance from the skin is excessive, it may be necessary to enlarge the incision. The dilator should be advanced through the intercostal muscles and into the pleural space. There may be significant resistance when the dilator bends to pass over the superior rib margin and into the pleural cavity. Rotating the dilator while advancing it will facilitate its passage through the intercostal tissues. After the dilator has been passed into the pleural space, it can be withdrawn using a technique identical to that used for the needle. As previously described, the operator must take care to avoid a mishap related to unintended movement of the guidewire. Next, the thoracostomy catheter is threaded over the guidewire and advanced into the pleural space (Fig. 29.7E). Like advancement of the dilator, rotation of the catheter as it advances through the tissues facilitates proper passage. Once the thoracostomy catheter is in place, the guidewire can be removed from its lumen and returned to the equipment tray or discarded. Proper location of the catheter should, of course be confirmed by x-ray, but before the catheter is secured with suture, the operator should be reasonably certain that the catheter is in the pleural space. In most cases, airflow or pleural fluid drainage can be detected at the hub of the catheter. Clear catheters may also "fog" with water vapor. The catheter should then be secured with heavy suture. A variety of techniques have been described but many practitioners choose to use a purse string technique because it helps to prevent air leak around the catheter. Alternatively, some catheters have fixed or removable flanges for securing sutures. Otherwise, the suture can be secured around the hub of the catheter or the catheter itself as long as care is taken to avoid kinking or obstructing the catheter by tying the suture too tight. Once the catheter is secured, a sterile Heimlich valve or drainage/suction apparatus may be attached to the hub of the catheter using appropriate adaptors. Suction can be applied as appropriate. One or two pieces of tape should be used to secure a section of the proximal portion of the drainage tubing to the patient's side. A dressing comprised of sterile gauze and/or a sterile semipermeable plastic dressing should be applied to the operative site. Petrolatum gauze also can be used but it tends to lubricate the catheter so that it may slide through the securing suture and become malpositioned more easily. Air that enters the chest along the tract around the thoracostomy catheter is readily drained via the catheter as long as it is in place. Therefore, it is not necessary to create a completely air tight seal with petrolatum gauze. Only when the catheter is removed from the chest does it become necessary to assure that there is no air leakage through the catheter tract so that a pneumothorax does not ensue.

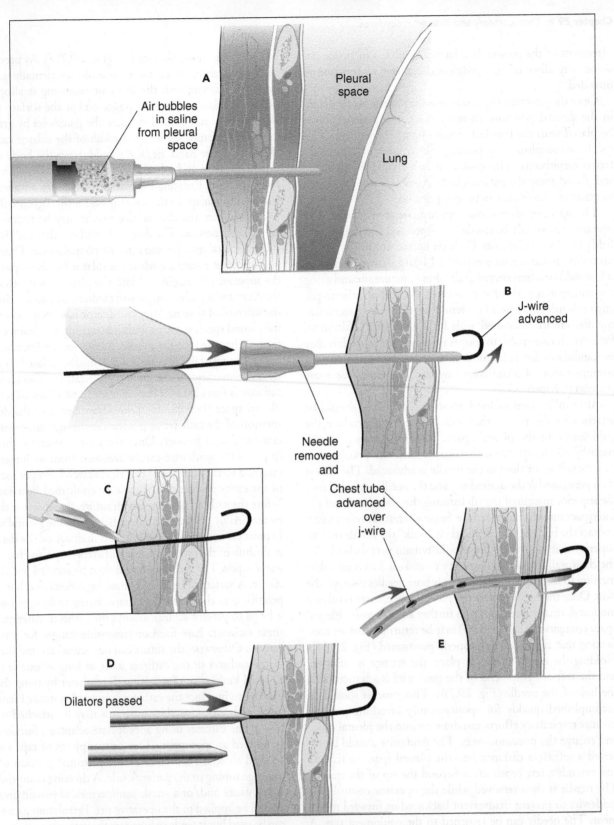

Figure 29.7 Modified Seldinger technique for catheter thoracostomy.
A. A needle attached to a partially filled syringe of saline is advanced over the rib at the proposed site of insertion. Air or fluid is aspirated when the needle is in the pleural space.
B. A guide wire is advanced through the needle into the pleural space.
C. The needle is removed leaving the guidewire in place. A small incision is made where the guidewire enters the skin.
D. If needed, a dilator may be advanced into the pleural space over the guidewire. The dilator is removed leaving the guidewire in place.
E. The thoracostomy catheter is passed into the pleural space over the guidewire. (The guidewire is then removed, and the catheter is secured in place).

A chest x-ray is generally indicated following placement of a thoracostomy catheter. The chest x-ray will confirm proper positioning of the catheter within the chest, assess the effectiveness of the catheter with respect to drainage of pneumothoraces or pleural fluid collections, and assist with recognition of procedure related complications.

Catheter Thoracostomy—Catheter Over Needle Method

Indications

The indications for this technique are similar to those described above for wire guided catheter thoracostomy.

Equipment

Sterile gloves
Sterile mask
Sterile gown
Surgical hat
Sterile prep solution
Sterile towels
Scalpel
Catheter over needle thoracostomy kit
   Catheter over needle thoracostomy device
   Syringe
Local anesthetic
Heavy suture
Heimlich valve or drainage/suction assembly with adaptor connectors and tubing
Sterile gauze or semipermeable membrane dressing
Tape

Procedure

The device used for this technique resembles a large over-the-needle intravenous catheter that has been specially adapted for placement into the pleural space. The procedure for insertion of this device is initially very similar to that detailed in the above description for Catheter Thoracostomy—Seldinger Method.

 SUMMARY

Catheter Thoracostomy—Catheter Over Needle Method

1–3 Same as for a needle thoracostomy.

4 Make a small nick in the skin at insertion site.

5 Using the catheter over needle device, advance needle over superior aspect of rib while maintaining negative pressure in syringe.

6 When air returns, advance the catheter over needle device into the pleural space.

7 Evacuate the pneumothorax.

8 Obtain a chest radiograph.

An insertion site is selected and the needle and catheter assembly is passed through the skin and directed into the pleural cavity. As with the Seldinger technique, making a 2- to 3-mm incision will facilitate passage of the device through the skin. Holding the needle at a 30- to 45- degree angle to the chest wall, the operator should guide the needle through the skin. The operator should make contact with the body of the rib forming the caudal margin of the chosen interspace. While maintaining contact with the rib, the operator should elevate the device so that it is perpendicular to the chest wall. Then, the needle is "walked" rostrally until the needle and catheter can be advanced through the intercostal muscles and into the pleural cavity. Entry into the pleural space is often accompanied by decreased resistance to further advancement of the needle and by return of pleural contents (i.e., air or fluid). Once inside the pleural cavity, the catheter and needle apparatus can be angled to help control the direction that the catheter will follow when it is advanced off the needle. Care should be taken to avoid inserting the needle too deeply and to avoid uncontrolled to and fro movements that may injure lung or other intrathoracic structures. While the operator holds the needle firmly, the catheter is advanced off the needle so that the desired length is introduced into the pleural space. Finally, the operator holds the catheter firmly in place while fully withdrawing the needle. As described in the previous section, the hub of the catheter should not be left open to room air for a protracted period of time because patients who are spontaneously breathing can draw air into their pleural space with each inspiration and cause worsening of the pneumothorax. Once the needle has been even partially removed, under no circumstances should it be advanced back into the catheter because the catheter may be damaged or a portion may be sheared off. As previously described, the catheter should be secured into place with suture. Some catheters have fixed or removable flanges for securing sutures. Otherwise, the suture can be tied around the hub of the catheter or the catheter itself as long as care is taken to avoid kinking or obstructing the catheter by tying the suture too tight. Once the catheter is secured, a sterile Heimlich valve or drainage/suction apparatus is attached to the hub of the catheter using appropriate adaptors. Suction can be applied as appropriate. One or two pieces of tape should be used to secure a section of the proximal portion of the drainage tubing securely to the patient's side. A dressing comprised of sterile gauze and/or a sterile semipermeable plastic dressing can then be applied to the incision site as previously described. For reasons previously stated, a chest x-ray should be obtained following placement of a thoracostomy catheter.

Tube Thoracostomy

Indications

Tube thoracostomy is indicated for the drainage of air, fluid, or blood from the pleural space. This procedure may be the only effective method of relieving a hemothorax or empyema. Because this technique is somewhat more invasive than catheter

SUMMARY

Tube Thoracostomy

1–3 Same as for a needle thoracostomy, but don sterile attire and prepare a sterile surgical field.

4 Anesthetize skin incision site and along dissection path.

5 Incise skin over rib below interspace of intended tube placement.

6 Bluntly dissect subcutaneously and superiorly.

7 Enter the pleural space with clamp tips closed and confirm location by exploration with finger, if patient size allows.

8 Insert a chest tube while directing it superiorly and posteriorly.

9 Attach the tube to a water seal and suction.

10 Secure with chest tube with sutures, gauze, and tape.

11 Obtain a chest radiograph.

thoracostomy, the practitioner may wish to consider the former technique when managing simple pneumothoraces and pleural effusions. Occasionally, a thoracostomy tube is placed for the instillation of material into the pleural space. This may include drugs, sclerosants, or other materials. However, this procedure is not often performed in the emergency department.

Equipment

Chest tube (appropriately sized)
Scalpel
Large hemostat (2)
Heavy suture
Local anesthetic
Syringe
Needle
Sterile prep solution
Sterile towels to create a surgical field
Sterile surgical gloves
Surgical mask
Surgical hat
Surgical gown
Sterile drainage/suction system or Heimlich valve
Sterile gauze dressing supplies
Dissecting scissors
Small hemostat (2)
Other surgical instruments per the preference of the operator (optional)

Procedure

When appropriate, informed consent should be obtained. The operator must select an appropriate chest tube. Chest tubes are generally sized according to their diameter using French units. All have end holes and all but the smallest sizes have side holes. Larger diameter chest tubes have both larger and more side holes. Smaller chest tubes are used for babies and infants, intermediate sizes for children, and larger sizes for adolescents. Guidelines for selecting an appropriately sized chest tube may be found in Table 29.1. Alternatively, some operators use other adjuncts such as the Broselow-Luten (length based) tape to help select an appropriately sized chest tube (see Chapter 6). Most importantly, the operator must make sure that all of the side holes on the chest tube will lie completely within the chest cavity after insertion. This can usually be satisfactorily gauged by overlying the chest tube across the hemithorax according to its anticipated final position and noting whether all side holes are likely to be contained in the chest cavity. If perchance a side hole lies outside of the thorax after a chest tube is properly inserted, then the tube must be removed and replaced with a smaller or differently configured tube.

An appropriate operative site must be selected using the guidelines presented above. Although the chest tube can be placed either anteriorly or laterally, most operators prefer the lateral approach with the tube being inserted in the 4th, 5th, or 6th intercostal space on the affected side (Fig. 29.8). As previously described, once the insertion site has been selected the operator should plan a skin incision site one to two interspaces caudal to that location to allow the tube to be tunneled under the skin.

The operator should don appropriate sterile attire. The operative site should be sterilely prepped and a sterile surgical field should be created around the site. As described for catheter thoracostomy, tube thoracostomy is painful. In addition to local anesthetic many patients, especially young children, will require a combination of intravenous sedation and analgesia and restraint. Topical anesthetic agents and local vapocoolants may be useful adjuncts as may hypnosis and guided imagery (Chapter 33). Local anesthetic (Chapter 35) should be administered at the anticipated incision site and along the planned dissection path through the subcutaneous and intercostal tissues (Fig. 29.9A–B). It should be noted that

TABLE 29.1	GUIDE FOR SELECTING CHEST TUBE SIZES	
Patient age	**Approximate chest tube size (French)**
Neonate (<5 kg)	8–12
0–1 years (5–10 kg)	10–14
1–2 years (10–15 kg)	14–20
2–5 years (15–20 kg)	20–24
5–10 years (20–30 kg)	20–28
>10 years (30–50 kg)	28–40
Adult (>50 kg)	32–40

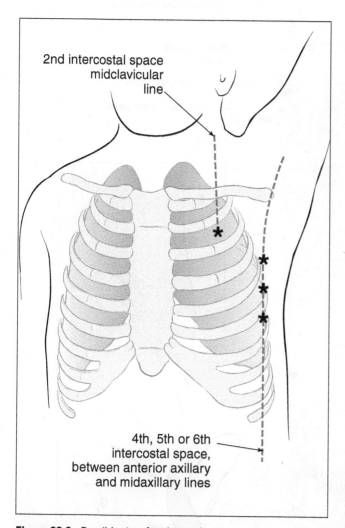

Figure 29.8 Possible sites for chest tube placement.

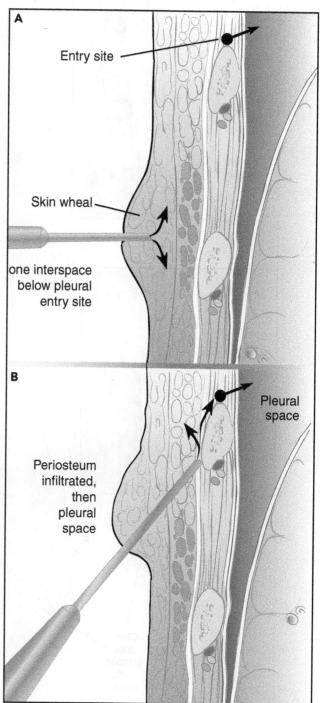

Figure 29.9 Local anesthesia for catheter/tube thoracostomy procedures.

the path of the chest tube will be largely determined by its purpose. Tubes that are placed to drain air should be directed anteriorly and, therefore, the operator should tunnel under the skin such that the tube is angled in a cephalad and anterior direction. Conversely, tubes intended to drain fluid may work best when placed posteriorly so the skin tract should be directed rostrally and toward the patient's back. Once satisfactory local anesthesia is achieved, a small skin incision should be made parallel to the intercostal space (Fig. 29.10A). The length of the incision should be approximately 2 to 3 times the diameter of the chest tube that will be placed. The incision should be long enough to allow simultaneous presence of the chest tube and a hemostat in the wound. A hemostat, finger, or blunt-tipped dissecting scissors should be used to tunnel under the skin using a blunt dissection technique (Fig. 29.10B). If a hemostat or blunt-tipped scissors are used to perform the tunneling, then the tips should be opened in a spreading maneuver as the instrument is advanced. The tunnel is then extended under the skin until it reaches the point where the intercostal space will be penetrated by the chest tube. A hemostat or dissecting scissors are then used to enter the desired point in the intercostal space. Using the tip of the hemostat

or the scissors to 'palpate' the rib forming the inferior aspect of the desired intercostal space, the scissors or hemostats are kept in contact with the rib and advanced over its superior margin. There are three accepted methods for entering the pleural space. Some operators prefer to simply push the tip of a closed hemostat through the muscle attachments and the pleura in a controlled manner using firm steady pressure and a secure grip on the hemostat so that his/her fingers will act as a stop to prevent the hemostat from penetrating the chest

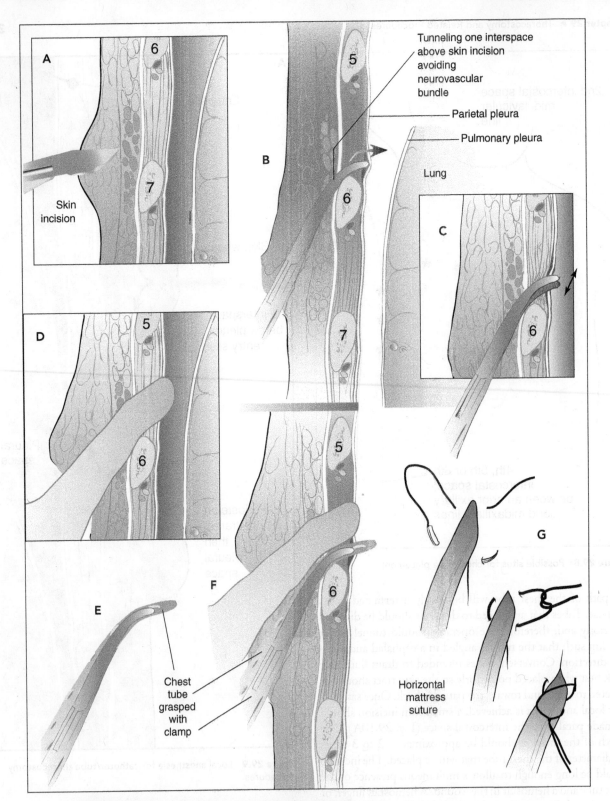

Figure 29.10 Blunt dissection technique for thoracostomy.
  A. An incision is made one to two interspaces inferior to proposed point of thoracostomy tube insertion.
  B. Blunt dissection through the subcutaneous tissue is performed using a clamp.
  C. The clamp is spread after entering the pleural space.
  D. If patient size allows, probing finger is inserted to confirm entry into the pleural space and to identify the diaphragm and any adhesions.
  E–F. The chest tube is gripped with a clamp and inserted (using a finger as a guide if patient size allows).
  G. The chest tube is sutured securely in place.

Labels in figure: Skin incision; Tunneling one interspace above skin incision avoiding neurovascular bundle; Parietal pleura; Pulmonary pleura; Lung; Chest tube grasped with clamp; Horizontal mattress suture

cavity too deeply. Once the tip of the hemostat is through the intercostal muscles and pleura, the blades are forcefully spread to enlarge the hole enough to accommodate the chest tube (Fig. 29.10C). Other operators prefer to use a sharp dissection technique. If this technique is chosen, the operator should dissect the intercostal muscle attachments free from the superior aspect of the rib. Dissecting only along the superior aspect of the rib avoids injury to the neurovascular bundle that lies along the inferior border of each rib. The third technique uses a sharp pointed trocar inserted into the chest tube so that its tip extends a short distance beyond the end of the chest tube. Rather than dissect through the intercostal tissue, the operator grasps the chest tube and trocar and directs its tip above the superior margin of the appropriate rib and exerts firm, steady pressure until the trocar and tube penetrate the pleural space. This technique is the most dangerous of the three because resistance to advancement of the trocar and chest tube diminishes dramatically once the pleural cavity is entered. This places intrathoracic organs at risk for injury. The operator must maintain control of the trocar in order to avoid complications. One method that can be used to prevent unintended advancement of the trocar is to tightly grasp the chest tube/trocar combination using the operator's free hand at a position $1/2$ to 1 centimeter proximal to the distance from the trocar tip that is anticipated to be required to just fully penetrate the intercostal muscles and pleura. However, even this method will not prevent all injuries because the chest tube and trocar assembly can sometimes slip through the operator's grip and advance further than was intended. Alternatively, a large hemostat can be clamped on the chest tube/trocar assembly so that the tip can just penetrate the pleural space. As an additional safety measure, the operator should grip the tube and trocar tightly, as described above. During advancement, the trocar often tends to slide back into the chest tube so the operator also needs to control the trocar position with respect to the chest tube during advancement.

In babies and young children, the chest wall is very flexible because the ribs are cartilaginous. When trying to enter the intercostal space, the operator may note substantial deformity of the chest wall as pressure is applied with the tip of the instrument or trocar. This is to be anticipated. The operator should be prepared, however, for a dramatic decrease in resistance to further advancement once the instrument or trocar dissects through the intercostal tissue. Unintended advancement of the dissecting instrument or trocar deep into the thorax is a significant risk unless the operator maintains control by using one hand to grip the instrument or trocar device near its tip and simultaneously brace against the chest wall.

Once the intercostal muscles and pleura are penetrated, there may be a return of pleural contents (i.e., air, fluid, or blood). This confirms that the pleural space has been entered. After entry, some operators prefer to insert a finger into the intercostal defect to ascertain whether or not there are nearby pleural adhesions (Fig. 29.10D). The chest tube is inserted by guiding it along the tunnel under the skin, through the

intercostal defect, and into the pleural cavity. Typically, this is done by clamping a hemostat onto the tip of the chest tube so that the blades of the hemostat are parallel to the long axis of the chest tube. The hemostat is used to guide the tip of the chest tube along the dissected path into the pleural space (Fig. 29.10E–F). Once the tip of the chest tube is inside the pleural space, the hemostat is unclamped and withdrawn. The chest tube is then advanced the correct distance into the chest. After the chest tube has been inserted, heavy suture should be used to secure it (Fig. 29.10G). Some operators prefer to place the suture using a purse string stitch in the skin then use the suture tails to wrap tightly around the circumference of the chest tube several times so that it will not slide through the suture. Other operators prefer to use a two suture technique. An initial skin suture is placed on one end of the skin incision then the tails are wrapped around the chest tube several times prior to tying a knot. A second skin suture is then placed at the other end of the skin incision and the tails of the suture are again wrapped around the chest tube several times and then knotted.

A sterile gauze dressing or a sterile semipermeable membrane dressing should be applied to cover the skin incision site. One or two pieces of tape should be used to tape the middle of the external portion of the chest tube securely to the patient's side. A sterile Heimlich valve (Fig. 29.11) or a sterile closed fluid collection/suction apparatus (Fig. 29.12) should

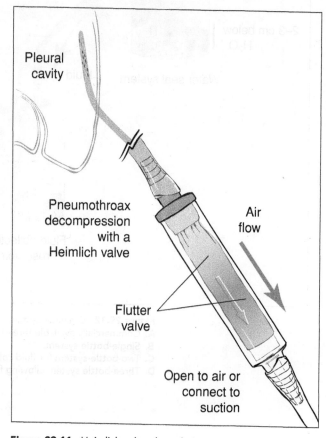

Figure 29.11 Heimlich valve chest drainage system.

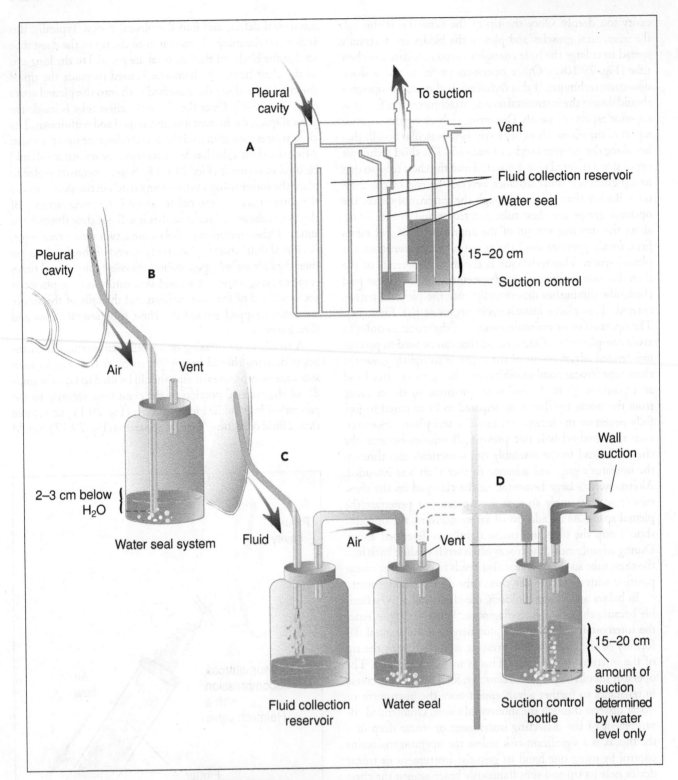

Figure 29.12 Drainage systems.
A. Commercially available three-bottle system.
B. Single-bottle system.
C. Two-bottle-system for fluid collection.
D. Three-bottle system allowing fluid collection and regulated suction.

be securely attached to the end of the chest tube. Suction can be applied as appropriate.

A chest x-ray is generally indicated following placement of a chest tube. The chest x-ray will confirm proper positioning of the chest tube, assess its effectiveness, and assist with recognition of procedure-related complications. Should the chest radiograph demonstrate that the tip of the chest tube is impinging upon or distorting the mediastinum, the side holes are not fully in the pleural cavity, the tube is kinked or lies anterior instead of posterior or vice versa, or is unintentionally positioned in the interlobar fissure of the lung, the operator may wish to consider repositioning the tube or removing it and replacing it with another tube. An anteroposterior and a lateral view may be needed to determine with certainty that the chest tube is in the intended position. Additional chest radiographs should be obtained each time that a chest tube is repositioned.

Drainage Devices

Some form of drainage device should be attached to a thoracostomy catheter/tube after it is placed. The drainage device generally serves to maintain sterility of the lumen of the thoracostomy catheter/tube, to provide a one-way valve allowing only egress of pleural space contents from the chest, to collect and measure drained fluid or blood, to allow clinical recognition of air draining out of the thorax, and to apply suction to the thoracostomy catheter/tube to facilitate drainage (Fig. 29.12) (33–35).

The internal surfaces of thoracostomy drainage systems and their connectors should remain sterile. All tubing, connectors, and drainage devices should be connected in a sterile fashion when initially deployed. Any subsequent manipulation or replacement of tubing, connectors or devices requires prepping with antiseptic solution and sterile technique. Drainage system tubing and connection adaptors must also be tightly and securely connected. It is not unusual for connection points to become loose and develop leaks or even become fully disconnected. They can also become pinched or otherwise occluded. Whenever a patient with a thoracostomy catheter/tube in place undergoes clinical deterioration, the clinician should always make a rapid but rigorous assessment of the thoracostomy catheter/tube and the associated drainage device. This is usually most effectively and efficiently accomplished by evaluating the integrity and functioning of the system beginning with the patient's pleural space and continuing distally.

Suction is commonly applied to drainage devices to improve drainage from the pleural cavity. It may also facilitate re-expansion of a collapsed lung. Applied suction should be regulated. In most cases, the drainage device itself will allow the amount of applied suction to be controlled but sometimes the amount of suction must be controlled with a suction regulator on the wall outlet or by other means. Excessive suction can damage the lung or other tissues so it is usually limited to 15 to 25 cm of water pressure or less. For preterm and

term neonates, the lowest effective suction setting should be chosen. Although suction within the safe range is generally harmless, there is one possible exception. When a large tracheobronchial disruption is present, the application of suction may increase air flow through the tracheobronchial defect and, thereby, reduce effective ventilation of the lungs.

Occasionally, patients will require multiple thoracostomy catheters/tubes. In such circumstances, it is generally best to avoid the practice of using 'Y' connectors to connect more than one catheter/tube to a single drainage device. By using a separate drainage device for each catheter/tube, the clinician can fully monitor the performance of every catheter/tube. Furthermore, if a single catheter/tube becomes dysfunctional, the others will generally be unaffected if each has its own dedicated drainage system. If a 'Y' connection is used, then only catheters/tubes from the same hemithorax should share a single drainage device. Connecting devices from both sides of the chest to a single drainage device makes it difficult to rapidly determine which side of the chest may be the source of the problem should the patient suddenly deteriorate.

Thoracostomy catheters, tubes, or drainage tubing sometimes become obstructed with drained material or clots. Percussing the chest catheter/tube with a solid object and milking the drainage tubing are commonly used to restore patency. "Stripping" of chest drainage tubing refers to the practice of completely occluding the drainage tubing just distal to its connection to the thoracostomy catheter/tube by tightly compressing or pinching it together with one hand and then sliding the other hand distally along the length of the remaining tubing to fully collapse its lumen. This stripping maneuver initially milks fluid and clots from the lumen of the drainage tubing. When the grips of both hands are quickly released, the rapid re-expansion of the collapsed lumen of the drainage tubing applies additional brief suction to the thoracostomy catheter/tube and promotes evacuation and passage of obstructing material. This practice is generally safe and is commonly used to maintain the patency of chest tubes. Some clinicians believe that the additional suction created by stripping may on occasion cause lung or other tissue injury. However, this assertion remains unsubstantiated. If such injury does occur, the most likely victims are small infants and preterm neonates. Rarely, a chest catheter, chest tube, or associated drainage tubing will become completely and irreversibly occluded. If the device in question is a chest catheter, strong consideration should be given to replacing it with a large bore chest tube. For chest tubes, sterile extraction or irrigation to remove the obstructing material can be considered prior to replacement of the chest tube.

Heimlich Valve Device

Heimlich valve devices are comprised of a rubber or plastic flutter valve encased in a transparent plastic cylinder with a proximal port which allows connection to chest tubes or catheter drainage systems (Fig. 29.11). The flutter valve functions as a one-way valve that permits only egress of air or fluid from the thoracostomy catheter/tube. Because the flutter valve is a one-way valve, it is necessary to ensure that the Heimlich valve is correctly oriented when it is connected. Heimlich valves are not preferred for hydrothoraces or hemothoraces, but they effectively drain simple and tension pneumothoraces and have, in fact, been used for this purpose on an outpatient basis.

Observation of the flutter valve provides useful diagnostic information. One should see phasic movements of the proximal portion of the flutter valve because the phasic pressure fluctuations within the pleural space during the breathing cycle are transmitted to the flutter valve via the thoracostomy catheter/tube. These phasic breathing fluctuations are present with spontaneous, assisted, or mechanical ventilation. If these movements are not seen, then either the patient is apneic or a part of the thoracostomy drainage system is not functioning properly. If air is draining from the pleural space via the Heimlich valve, then the distal portion of the valve will open periodically. Often, the Heimlich device is used without suction, but suction can be applied using the second (distal) connection port on the device. The distal port can also be used to attach tubing to a drainage reservoir for collecting drained fluid or blood. Many clinicians choose to use a drainage reservoir—water seal—suction apparatus instead of a Heimlich device when treating pleural fluid collections or hemothoraces. (See the subsection on drainage reservoir—water seal—suction drainage devices below.)

Drainage Reservoir—Water Seal—Suction Devices

These devices use a reservoir to collect drained fluid, a reservoir to form a one-way valve (water seal), and a reservoir to control suction. Each reservoir is connected in series and in the order noted (Fig. 29.12).

Most institutions use commercially made disposable integrated units (Fig. 29.12A). Large diameter tubing and adaptor connectors are used to interconnect the thoracostomy catheter/tube and the drainage device. The drainage reservoir section of the unit contains a transparent window that is marked with graduated volume units. These allow the clinician to quantify fluid or blood output volumes and rates. Another section of the unit performs the one-way valve (water seal) function. Water with a depth of about 2 to 3 cm is interposed between the thoracostomy catheter and the ambient atmosphere. Another transparent window allows viewing of the water seal chamber. Pleural air bubbles through the water behind the water seal section window whenever air in the pleural space exerts a pressure greater than that of the water within the chamber (i.e., 2 to 3 cm H_2O). The unit is designed so that air distal to the water seal is vented to the atmosphere or to suction. Therefore, the air pressure on the distal side of the water seal can never become great enough to bubble backward through the water seal even when intrapleural pressure is negative with respect to the atmosphere. The distal venting

allows re-equilibration of pressure across the water seal before backflow of air can occur. Analogous to the Heimlich valve device, there should normally be a small phasic movement of the water behind the water seal window corresponding to the intrapleural pressure changes during respiration. If this to and fro movement is absent then the thoracostomy catheter/tube or the drainage unit is dislodged, disconnected or obstructed. If air bubbles are seen passing through the water in the water seal compartment, then drainage of pleural air is occurring. The third section of the integrated device allows regulation of the suction applied to the thoracostomy catheter/device. This section contains a transparent window with graduated markings corresponding to different amounts of suction. Water is poured into this section until the depth of water rises to the mark corresponding to the desired level of suction. The height of the water column in this compartment determines the amount of suction applied to the pleural space. Tubing from the device is then connected to wall suction or another source of continuous vacuum that is greater than or equal to the desired amount of suction. If the suction level must be changed, then water can be added to the reservoir to increase the amount of suction or water can be drained to lower it. Some systems use a valve to allow adjustment of the water level that controls the degree of suction.

Improvised Devices

Improvised drainage devices are primarily intended to solve the need for a temporary one-way valve between the thoracostomy catheter/tube and the ambient atmosphere. The one-way valve prevents patients who are making spontaneous breathing efforts (or receiving negative pressure ventilation) from drawing atmospheric air into their pleural space during inspiration when intrapleural pressure is subatmospheric. Patients who are receiving positive pressure ventilation are not significantly impacted by leaving the end of a thoracostomy catheter/tube without an attached one-way valve device because positive pressure ventilation produces supraatmospheric pressure in the pleural space during a significant portion of the breathing cycle. This induced pressure gradient causes air to flow out of the pleural space and prevents the accumulation of a significant amount of air in the pleural space.

If a commercial drainage device is not immediately available, the clinician can improvise a satisfactory substitute. The simplest option is to create an improvised flutter valve by attaching a sterile surgeon's glove to the end of the chest catheter/tube. The base of the glove is attached to the chest catheter/tube by tying it around the end of the tube or by securing it with a suture ligature or tape. A small piece of one finger of the glove is then cut away to create the one-way flutter valve. A finger cot or other analogous item can be similarly used. Latex should be avoided in patients who are latex sensitive and in those who are at risk for latex sensitivity.

A simple temporary drainage system can also be created by attaching a piece of tubing to the end of the thoracostomy catheter/tube and then placing the end of the tubing 2 to 3 cm under water in an uncapped bottle placed well below the level of the patient's chest. (Fig. 29.12B). The water bottle must be set low enough to prevent siphoning or sucking of water from the bottle into the patient's chest during breathing. Immersing the end of the extension tubing under the water surface in the bottle provides an effective one-way valve. Filling the bottle to the brim with water will keep the end of the tubing at a constant distance (pressure) under the surface of the water despite any quantity of pleural fluid or blood that subsequently drains into the bottle. A basin placed underneath the water bottle will collect and contain water displaced by fluid or blood draining from the chest.

An improvised drainage reservoir—water seal—suction device is also relatively easy to construct but requires several items and some time (Fig. 29.12C–D). This type of device is termed the three bottle system. It was the standard method of chest tube drainage prior to the development of disposable integrated units.

Removing Devices

A functioning angiocath or needle used to perform an emergent needle thoracostomy should be left in place until a thoracostomy catheter or tube is successfully placed and satisfactorily functioning. The angiocath or needle can be simply withdrawn once its function is subsumed by a thoracostomy catheter or tube. The soft tissue of the chest wall will seal the needle tract immediately.

Thoracostomy catheters and tubes that are no longer needed should be removed to reduce the risk of complications. It is generally safe to remove thoracostomy drainage devices when no further air drainage and only a negligible amount of fluid or blood drainage is detected during a reasonable period of observation. The absence of air drainage is confirmed by the lack of air bubbling through a water seal (or fluctuations caused by air passing through the flutter valve of a Heimlich device) during an observation period of at least 1 to 2 minutes. Fluid or blood output from the thoracostomy catheter can be measured directly. For spontaneously breathing patients there should be no air drainage and negligible fluid or blood output for at least 12 to 24 hours before one should consider removing a thoracostomy catheter or tube. Clinicians are often more conservative when deciding whether to remove a chest catheter or tube from patients receiving positive pressure ventilation. Many require that there be no air output for at least 24 to 48 hours prior to removal of tubes placed for the treatment of pneumothoraces. However, even in mechanically ventilated patients, tubes or catheters placed primarily to drain blood or fluid can be removed after 12 to 24 hours. Chest radiographs prior to removal help to confirm that the chest tube or catheter has served its intended purpose. If multiple catheters or tubes are present, then it may be best to remove them one at a time with a period of observation prior to removing the next one. This approach minimizes the risk that a device will have to be reinserted.

Once the criteria for device removal have been met, small catheters can be simply withdrawn. The soft tissue around the catheter tract will seal off the tract in most cases. However, the tract associated with a chest tube is often large enough to place the patient at risk for the development of a secondary pneumothorax after the tube is removed. Therefore, the following technique is recommended when removing chest tubes.

The process should be explained to the patient when appropriate. The operator may wish to consider premedication of the patient with analgesics (or local anesthetic). All necessary equipment should be assembled. At a minimum this includes: several sterile 4 × 4 gauze sponges, 2-inch wide tape, and a sterile piece of petrolatum gauze that is big enough to cover the skin entrance site and at least 2 cm of the surrounding skin on all sides of the wound.

The operator should insure that he/she and the staff are protected from blood and body fluid exposure. The tape and the dressings covering the insertion site should then be removed. With the catheter held firmly in place, the securing sutures should be cut. If a purse string suture with preserved suture tails is present, some operators prefer to cut or undo the suture so that the purse string and the tails are preserved. This allows the suture to be cinched and tied to help close the wound as the chest tube is withdrawn. The petrolatum gauze should then be placed over the skin entrance site and covered with the stack of 4 × 4 gauze pads prior to withdrawing the chest tube. If the patient is spontaneously breathing, the operator should ask him/her to hold his/her breath at the point of maximum forced inspiration. (For mechanically ventilated patients, the operator should wait until the beginning of inspiration or induce and sustain an inspiratory pause with the ventilator.) At the point of full inspiration, the catheter or tube is quickly pulled completely out of the chest while the operator applies steady firm pressure on the stack of gauze. The goal is to remove the device during the exhalation portion of the breathing cycle so that intrathoracic pressure remains above atmospheric pressure as the chest tube is removed. This way no air is drawn into the pleural space while the device is being removed. The stack of gauze and underlying petrolatum sheet must be kept in firm contact with the chest wall and then taped firmly in place. A chest x-ray should be obtained to check for postremoval pneumothorax and other complications.

▶ COMPLICATIONS

There are numerous potential complications associated with thoracostomy procedures. Preprocedural, intraprocedural, and postprocedural complications are well recognized. However, neither the relative risk nor the incidence of specific complications is well defined. Based on the authors' personal experiences, it is likely that specific patient issues, as well as operator experience, technique and skill significantly, affect the risk and the incidence of various complications. Furthermore, emergency thoracostomy procedures may pose more risk of complications than nonemergent procedures. But greater risks are often justified when one is managing a life-threatening condition (36–45).

Because the operator's skill is critical to the prevention of complications, all of those who practice in acute care settings should be familiar with one or more of the above procedures. Furthermore, if they cannot be assured of adequate exposure to these techniques in their practice providers should arrange for frequent skill-maintenance sessions using animals, cadavers, or manikins. Even the best prepared clinician may, however, encounter a situation that requires skills beyond his/her own and in such cases prudence dictates consultation with an appropriate specialist.

Table 29.2 lists many of the potential complications that may be associated with thoracostomy procedures. The list cannot completely anticipate all circumstances so clinicians may need to consider special or unusual situations beyond those that are listed. Many of these potential complications can be avoided or minimized by attention to details. Patients should be properly identified and the operator(s) should insure that the procedure is being performed on the correct side of the body. Likewise, they must consider relevant anatomic and physiologic issues, provide necessary analgesia/sedation, perform a thorough preprocedure assessment, and insure proper patient monitoring, procedural technique, and consultant utilization. Even when everything has been done correctly, complications will occasionally occur. Patients and family should understand the pertinent risks and benefits of the procedure as part of the informed consent process.

In the authors' personal experience, cognitive and technical problems are occasional sources of errors or complications. This may relate in part to the relative paucity of children requiring thoracostomy procedures, the diversity of underlying conditions that may necessitate the procedure, and the number of concomitant associated or confounding conditions that may be present. Problems also occur because, to some extent, decision making related to chest catheters/tubes is semisubjective and experiential. Although several of the major potential complications related to the various thoracostomy procedures were covered in the sections detailing each technique, what follows is a brief recapitulation of the most significant of these.

Potential complications include improper device placement, injury to the chest wall or internal structures, infection, bleeding, and others. An often underappreciated risk relates to potential scarring or anatomical distortions such as pleural adhesions from prior infectious, inflammatory conditions, or prior procedural interventions. Performing invasive procedures that may disrupt an adhesion or impact an internal structure can risk life-threatening bleeding or organ injury. Thoracostomy procedures are painful and require patient cooperation. Judicious use of analgesia and sedation can facilitate performance of the procedure. However, some patients may be at increased risk for complications related to sedation because they have pulmonary or cardiac disease or hypovolemia or risk factors related to their pleural air or fluid collection. Risks from serious coexisting conditions, such as bleeding disorders, should be minimized whenever possible by deferring the thoracostomy procedure until the coexisting condition can be improved. Sometimes this is not possible, but the risk can often be reduced by adapting the thoracostomy procedure. For example, using a small caliber catheter instead of a large bore chest tube to drain a pneumothorax may substantially reduce the risk of bleeding in a thrombocytopenic patient. Although no technique is completely safe, it is important to re-emphasize that catheter thoracostomy procedures are generally safer than tube thoracostomies. However, chest tubes may be required for drainage of hemothoraces and thick empyemas. When performing a tube thoracostomy, the use of blunt dissection and the insertion of an exploratory finger into the pleural cavity (when the patient is large enough) is generally considered to be the safest technique while the use of trocar devices is generally considered to be the least safe.

Tube thoracostomy is a significant surgical procedure with a low but not negligible risk of infection. Some operators believe that empirical perioperative or extended antibiotics may reduce this risk; however, there is no definitive evidence for this practice. Most practitioners reserve antibiotics for cases with clinical signs or laboratory evidence of infection. If periprocedural antibiotics are given, then they should be directed against staphylococcus and streptococcus and administered shortly before the skin incision is made. If a procedure related infection develops, then antibiotic therapy should be guided by culture and sensitivity testing when possible.

CLINICAL TIPS: NEEDLE AND TUBE THORACOSTOMY

▶ All necessary equipment should be assembled and tube size(s) should be checked before starting.

▶ Adequate sedation and analgesia must be provided for the conscious patient.

▶ For tube thoracostomy, the incision should be made directly over a rib.

▶ Passage of the chest tube should not be attempted through an incision that is too small.

▶ A probing finger should be used whenever possible to verify that the pleural space has been entered and to identify the diaphragm and any adhesions.

▶ For needle decompression of a pneumothorax, a saline-filled syringe is used to detect bubbles.

| TABLE 29.2 | POTENTIAL COMPLICATIONS ASSOCIATED WITH THORACOSTOMY PROCEDURES |

Preprocedural

Improper patient identification.

Lack of informed consent.

Failure to recognize an indication for procedure.

Misdiagnosis/misunderstanding of indications for procedure.

Failure to recognize other patient conditions that will affect the procedure.

Failure to anticipate or recognize analgesia/sedation risks properly. (See Chapter 33.)

Failure to anticipate worsening associated with mechanical ventilation, aeromedical transport, or other issues.

Failure to perform thoracostomy procedure when indicated leading to death or worsened hypoventilation, hypoxemia, acid-base problems, hypotension, intracranial hypertension, pulmonary hypertension, or other physiologic derangements.

Procedural

Death or further morbidity due to bleeding, hypoxia, analgesia/sedation, or inability to rapidly perform the procedure.

Analgesia/sedation related complications. (See Chapter 33.)

Injury to chest wall structure(s).
    Rib
    Intercostal neurovascular bundle
    Skin
    Internal mammary artery
    Breast or breast bud

Injury to intrathoracic structure(s).
    Lung
    Trachea/major bronchus
    Diaphragm
    Pericardium
    Heart
    Esophagus
    Phrenic nerve
    Thoracic duct
    Great vessels
    Thymus
    Mediastinum

Injury to extrathoracic structures.
    Neck
    Abdomen
        Liver
        Spleen
        Intestine
        Stomach

Infection.
    Skin
    Chest wall
    Pleural space/empyema
    Blood/sepsis
    Others

Bleeding.
    Skin

    Chest wall/intercostal vessel/internal mammary vessel
    Lung
    Pleural adhesions
    Other sites
    Risks of blood product administration (if required for the bleeding)

Peripheral nerve injury (intercostal nerve, phrenic nerve, thoracic nerve, other).

Drug/allergic reaction (latex, anesthetic, prep solution, analgesics, sedatives, antibiotics, others).

Procedure performed on wrong side/location.

Error in use of drainage/suction system.

Inadequate analgesia/sedation/restraint.

Improper extrathoracic position of catheter/tube (subcutaneous, muscular, or abdominal position).

Catheter/tube leak due to side port outside of the thorax or faulty drainage device connections.

Failure to properly secure the catheter/tube in place.

Failure to check postprocedure chest x-ray or adjust catheter/tube position based on x-ray.

Inability to perform procedure in a timely manner for a patient in extremis.

Misinterpretation of needle thoracostomy findings.

Failure to use appropriate size catheter/tube that requires repeat procedure.

Dysrhythmia.

Improper skin incision that causes unnecessary cosmetic impact.

Damage to another medical device near the operative site.

Connecting a Heimlich valve in the wrong direction.

Improper set-up of a water seal–drainage reservoir–suction apparatus.

Hemoptysis.

Postprocedural

Death or further morbidity due to infection, bleeding, or failure to correct a dysfunctional device.

Kinked, obstructed, or dislodged catheter/tube.

Inadequate monitoring/serial assessment after device placement.

Failure to recognize catheter/tube or drainage/suction device malfunction.

Late injury or erosion of an anatomic structure due to the catheter/tube.

Dysfunction of an anatomic structure due to impingement by the catheter/tube.

Premature removal of a device that necessitates an additional procedure.

Failure to remove device when it is no longer needed.

Late infection.
    Blood
    Skin
    Chest wall
    Pleural space/empyema
    Others

Inadequate analgesia/sedation/restraint during device use or removal.

Pneumothorax upon catheter/tube removal that requires intervention.

Pleural fistula.

Failure to place additional catheters/tubes when drainage by a single catheter/tube is inadequate to restore satisfactory physiologic status.

Injury to lung or other tissues due to excessive suction.

Failure to maintain sterile technique during manipulation of device or drainage system.

SECTION B: OPEN CHEST WOUNDS

▶ INTRODUCTION

Although many of the issues pertaining to thoracostomy procedures are also relevant to open chest wounds, there are also some unique considerations (46,47). This section emphasizes the evaluation and management of open chest wounds. Reference to the preceding section of this chapter is recommended for detailed discussion of thoracostomy procedures.

Open chest wounds are wounds that fully traverse the chest wall. Although there are a few other causes, the vast majority are caused by penetrating trauma and most of the rest by blunt trauma. Surgical procedures involving the thorax, such as thoracostomy or thoracotomy, also produce open chest wounds, but these wounds are created and managed in a controlled setting, so they rarely require emergency evaluation and intervention. Occasionally, however, an inpatient will require emergency evaluation and intervention when a surgically created chest wall wound dehisces or a pleural drainage device comes out unexpectedly. Open chest wounds are relatively rare among pediatric patients but may be more frequently seen in areas with a high incidence of penetrating trauma.

Because open chest wounds are the result of significant thoracic trauma, the clinician must consider the physiologic consequences of the open wound itself and those related to associated injuries which can involve virtually any thoracic structure with resultant cardiac and/or pulmonary compromise. The circumstances must dictate the clinician's approach to an individual case and a complete review of the management of thoracic trauma is beyond the scope of this chapter. What follows, therefore, details only the management of the open chest wound itself. More general information regarding the management of thoracic trauma may be found elsewhere, and the clinician is encouraged to consult these sources (47). Finally, it should be noted that all personnel responsible for the treatment of injured children should be familiar with the management of open chest wounds. In particular, EMS providers should understand the procedures described below because most of these procedures are intended only as temporary measures prior to the placement of a thoracostomy tube or catheter.

▶ ANATOMY AND PHYSIOLOGY

Anatomy

The relevant anatomy of the thorax is discussed in the section above which details the anatomic considerations in the placement of thoracostomy tubes and drainage devices. It will not be repeated here. However, the clinician treating a patient with an open chest wound may have to address bleeding and/or issues related to air flow through the chest wall defect.

Significant bleeding from an open chest wound may represent hemorrhage from soft tissue, a blood vessel, a fractured bone, or an injured internal organ. Wounds affecting the rib cage may lead to bleeding from one or more injured intercostal arteries or veins. Rarely, chest wall trauma results in bleeding from an internal mammary, axillary or subclavian vessel. At times, a bleeding site may be directly visualized. In such cases, direct pressure with a gloved finger may control the hemorrhage until further surgical intervention can be accomplished. Sometimes, the site(s) causing bleeding from an open chest wound cannot be easily determined. Surgical consultation may be needed when the bleeding site is internal, indeterminate, or uncontrollable.

The consequences of an open chest wound are largely determined by its size, relative patency and location. Wounds may be trivial, self-approximating, and self-sealing or large enough to be intermittently or continuously patent with some degree of on-going airflow through the chest wall defect. The location of the open chest wound largely determines which, if any, underlying structures may have been damaged. Attention must be given to the evaluation and management of these injuries as well as the open chest wound itself.

Almost all open chest wounds that produce significant physiologic compromise ultimately require a thoracostomy procedure for definitive stabilization. The anatomical concerns related to performing a thoracostomy procedure therefore become relevant when managing an open chest wound. (See also the first section of this chapter, which discusses tube thoracostomy procedures.)

Rarely, a chest wall wound is sufficiently large or complex to require surgical intervention to achieve satisfactory repair or closure of the defect.

Physiology

Open chest wounds always are associated with two independent but additive acute physiologic concerns. The first relates to the physiologic impact of the wound itself. The second relates to the physiologic impact of coexisting injuries due to the causative event. The magnitude of the physiologic consequences due to the wound and those due to the coexisting injuries each can range from insignificant to profound. Beyond these two concerns, some patients have pre-existing conditions or secondary complications which cause additional physiologic compromise. Like all significant injuries, open chest wounds can be associated with hypovolemia and anemia related to persistent or severe bleeding from the wound itself. Control of hemorrhage, restoration of blood volume and/or replacement of red blood cells can be important in such cases.

The unique physiology of open chest wounds centers on the movement of air across the thoracic wall defect. These types of wounds can behave in three distinct ways. There are wounds with no airflow through them, wounds with unidirectional (inspiratory) restricted airflow through them, and wounds with continuous bidirectional (inspiratory and expiratory) airflow through them (Fig. 29.13).

The first and simplest pathophysiology relates to wounds that traverse the chest wall fully but are self-sealing and thus do not allow air to pass through them (Fig. 29.13A). A small amount of air may enter the pleural space or mediastinum when this type of wound is created. However, soon thereafter, the soft tissues of the chest wall become approximated and prevent any further passage of air into the thorax. The physiologic impact of such a wound is usually negligible. Some impairment of breathing efforts due to pain may occur but this is often modest and well tolerated by the patient. When appropriate, a simple surgical repair of the wound may promote healing and reduce the risk of the wound subsequently gaping during activity and allowing air to enter the thorax. Other surgical interventions, including thoracostomy or thoracotomy, may be necessary for management of serious wound-related bleeding or additional coexisting internal injuries.

The second type of wounds are those that allow mainly unidirectional (inspiratory) airflow through the wound (Fig. 29.13B). A wound of this type is not physiologically benign because it allows progressive accumulation of air in the pleural space. Inspiratory movement of the chest wall causes traction on the soft tissues around the wound such that the wound

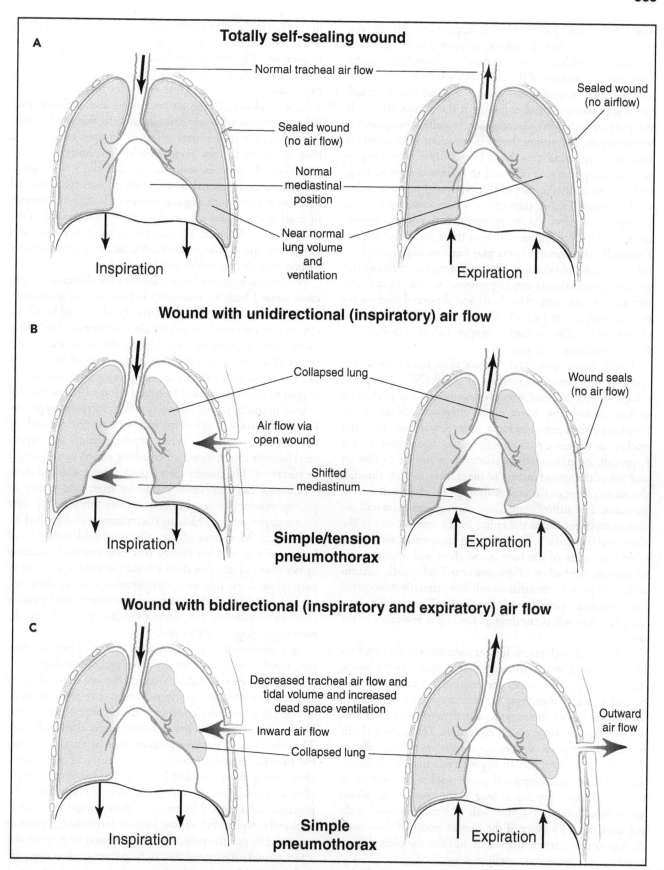

A **Totally self-sealing wound**

Normal tracheal air flow

Sealed wound (no airflow)

Sealed wound (no air flow)

Normal mediastinal position

Near normal lung volume and ventilation

Inspiration

Expiration

B **Wound with unidirectional (inspiratory) air flow**

Collapsed lung

Air flow via open wound

Wound seals (no air flow)

Shifted mediastinum

Inspiration

Simple/tension pneumothorax

Expiration

C **Wound with bidirectional (inspiratory and expiratory) air flow**

Decreased tracheal air flow and tidal volume and increased dead space ventilation

Inward air flow

Collapsed lung

Outward air flow

Inspiration

Simple pneumothorax

Expiration

Figure 29.13 Potential pathophysiologic effects of open chest wounds.
A. Open chest wounds that are fully self-sealing.
B. Open chest wounds with unidirectional (inspiratory) airflow.
C. Open chest wounds with bidirectional (inspiratory and expiratory) airflow.

tends to become patent. During inspiration, intrathoracic pressure is also relatively negative compared to extrathoracic pressure so outside air flows into the chest through the wound. Expiratory movement of the chest wall relaxes tension on the soft tissues surrounding the wound. This allows better soft tissue approximation and occlusion of the wound, effectively trapping air within the pleural space. Initially, a progressively worsening simple pneumothorax is produced. This results in increasing hypoventilation due to lung collapse, worsening intrapulmonary shunting of blood in collapsed areas of lung, and progressive inefficiency of the respiratory pump function of the thorax. This in turn causes a compensatory increase in respiratory effort. As the pneumothorax worsens, hypoxemia develops and increases due to these combined effects. Eventually, the pneumothorax may become large enough to exhibit tension physiology. The cardiovascular effects of the tension pneumothorax can be profound and can include decreased venous return to the heart and abnormal traction on the mediastinum and associated major vessels. Both of these effects reduce effective cardiac output and, if untreated, can lead to circulatory collapse.

Finally, some open chest wounds allow bidirectional (inspiratory and expiratory) airflow (Fig. 29.13C). The physiologic impact of these wounds depends on the physics of airflow through the defect in the chest wall. Spontaneous breathing efforts normally cause air to flow in and out of the trachea. But when a continuously patent open chest wound is present, breathing efforts also cause some air to flow in and out of the wound instead of the trachea. Airflow through the trachea decreases as airflow through the chest wall wound increases. The airflow component through the chest wall increases exponentially as the radius of the open wound in the chest wall increases. Life-threatening hypoventilation occurs when the radius of the hole in the chest wall approximates or exceeds the radius of the trachea. Under such circumstances, physics dictates that air will flow primarily through the lower resistance path through the chest wall wound. Dramatically less flow will occur through the higher resistance of the trachea.

Additional mechanisms further contribute to the hypoventilation caused by continuously patent open chest wounds. An obligatory open simple pneumothorax accompanies this type of wound. Air entering the pleural space on the affected side causes loss of the normal pleural viscoelastic force that opposes lung collapse at end-expiration. The normal elastic recoil of the lung becomes unopposed leading to lung collapse. This further contributes to hypoventilation. The pneumothorax and associated lung collapse persist but a tension pneumothorax cannot develop as long as the open wound allows air to flow through the chest wall in both directions without restriction. However, if the characteristics of the wound change so that restricted egress of air from the pleural space occurs then tension can rapidly develop.

Dead space ventilation effects further compound the hypoventilation produced by open chest wounds. Anatomic dead space ventilation refers to the oxygen-poor air that remains in the pharynx and tracheobronchial system at end-expiration and is re-inspired into the alveoli at the beginning of the next inspiration. The volume of dead space air must be inhaled back into the lung before any fresh air can reach the alveoli. Normally dead space air represents a fraction of usual tidal volume so plenty of fresh air reaches the alveoli. Dead space volume remains relatively constant as tidal volume becomes subnormal due to the 'steal' effect of an open chest wound that allows air to flow preferentially via a lower resistance path through the chest wall instead of through the trachea. Therefore, the fractional contribution of dead space to tidal volume becomes much larger. In other words, the same amount of dead space air but a lesser amount of fresh air enters the alveoli with each breath. This dead space effect essentially acts to decrease the net oxygen concentration and increase the net carbon dioxide concentration of inspired air.

Worsening hypoventilation caused by the effects of an open chest wound leads to worsening hypoxemia and a compensatory increase in respiratory efforts. The increased breathing efforts may improve lung ventilation in some cases but if they cause only increased airflow through the chest wall defect rather than the trachea they are likely to be of little benefit. The respiratory muscles require supranormal amounts of oxygen to sustain increased breathing efforts. Hypoxemia will worsen unless increased breathing efforts increase oxygen delivery sufficiently to offset the increased oxygen demands of the respiratory muscles. When hypoventilation and hypoxemia become severe, increased breathing efforts can no longer be sustained. The patient then rapidly deteriorates and dies.

Patients can sometimes transition from one variety of pathophysiology to another one or more times during their course depending on changing circumstances and applied interventions. Movement of the spine or shoulder, changes of body position or other factors that may promote widening or occlusion of an open chest wound can induce a change of pathophysiology. Likewise, interventions such as dressings, wound exploration, thoracostomy procedures, and positive pressure ventilation, can affect the patency and hence the pathophysiology of the wound.

It is important to understand the effects of positive pressure ventilation on each of the three pathophysiologic varieties of open chest wounds. Wounds that are self-sealing are generally not specifically affected by positive pressure ventilation. Of course, the usual physiologic alterations directly attributable to positive pressure ventilation alone still exist. The initiation of positive pressure ventilation also reverses the pressure gradient favoring further entry of air into the chest during inspiration and limits accumulation of air in the pleural space. This may reduce the size or progression of a pneumothorax caused by an open chest wound with unidirectional (inspiratory) airflow. Positive intrathoracic pressure produced by positive pressure ventilation may or may not also affect wound patency and thereby help force some of the accumulated intrathoracic air back through the open chest wound. When unrestricted to and fro airflow is occurring across an open chest wound positive pressure ventilation allows total control of tracheal airflow and tidal volume and can restore both to satisfactory levels.

Positive pressure ventilation can have negative or positive effects on coexisting conditions. In particular, the use of positive pressure ventilation may create or increase air leakage from coexisting lung injuries. If the associated open chest wound is not functionally patent then a tension pneumothorax will develop unless a thoracostomy drainage device is in place. Administration of positive pressure ventilation has positive therapeutic benefits for patients with lung contusions, hypoventilation, increased work of breathing, major traumatic brain injuries, apnea, and several other types of coexisting conditions. Further discussion of the potential consequences of ventilator associated issues is beyond the scope of this chapter (see also Chapter 82).

The physiologic consequences of coexisting thoracic and nonthoracic injuries associated with an open chest wound are often additive to those of the open chest wound itself. Analysis and synthesis of the physiologic impact and interrelationships of pre-existing and/or coexisting conditions may be complex. Determining whether or not physiologic compromise is due to an open chest wound or another concomitant condition may be difficult. Observing the response to interventions for the open chest wound versus the response following interventions for the other conditions will often provide insight and help to guide further treatment. In particular, continuing physiologic compromise following emergency stabilization of an open chest wound is suggestive of a significant coexisting condition.

▶ INDICATIONS

Approach to Open Chest Wounds

An individual patient with an open chest wound may present at any point along a spectrum of worsening physiologic compromise from essentially asymptomatic to extremis. Compensatory physiologic responses are usually the earliest sign of physiologic embarrassment due to an open chest wound and/or a coexisting injury. With progressive worsening, more profound signs of cardiopulmonary collapse appear.

The pulmonary and/or the cardiovascular systems are most commonly and significantly impacted by open chest wounds. Findings of abnormal pulmonary function, particularly dyspnea, hypoventilation and hypoxemia, or abnormal cardiovascular function, particularly tachycardia, hypotension, and hypoperfusion are characteristically the most important warning signs of significant pathophysiology. Local pain, findings due to significant blood loss and/or signs of other injuries due to blunt or penetrating chest trauma may be other significant features associated with serious open chest wounds or concomitant associated injuries.

The focused evaluation and management of an open chest wound begins with the identification of a wound that involves the chest wall. Initial patient information obtained prior to arrival or upon arrival may provide a history of penetrating or blunt chest trauma. Confirmation of the presence of a nontrivial chest wound by examination of the chest should prompt further rapid evaluation of the wound to determine its clinical significance.

Much of the relevant clinical evaluation of an open chest wound requires only brief observation of the wound. Direct inspection of the wound identifies the presence of serious bleeding. If serious bleeding is noted then direct digital pressure can be applied to any obvious and accessible bleeding site. Surgical consultation should be rapidly obtained for significant bleeding from a deeper site or uncontrollable bleeding from a chest wall site. If substantial amounts of intrathoracic blood appear to be draining through the wound then a tube thoracostomy procedure at a site remote from the open chest wound and/or possibly emergency operative intervention is indicated.

When examining a spontaneously breathing patient with an open chest wound brief observation of the wound usually identifies whether or not air is flowing through it and therefore the likely associated pathophysiologic consequences.

If the examination reveals a nongaping wound with no apparent airflow then the wound either does not fully traverse the chest wall or is self-sealing. In either case, the wound is unlikely to be physiologically significant and subsequent management mainly consists of further evaluation for coexisting injuries, close observation for signs of deterioration, appropriate wound management, and analgesic medication, as necessary.

A wound with unidirectional airflow into the chest with each inspiration (a so called "sucking chest wound") indicates the concomitant presence of at least a pneumothorax and possibly a tension pneumothorax. A tension pneumothorax may develop at any time without treatment. Wounds with unidirectional (inspiratory) airflow are best managed with an emergent thoracostomy procedure. A temporizing occlusive/flutter valve dressing can be used until a thoracostomy procedure can be performed. The temporary occlusive/flutter valve dressing should be configured to function as a one-way valve so that air can no longer flow into the thorax and intrathoracic air under tension can escape through the wound.

A wound with bidirectional airflow during each breath or a large gaping wound with continuously visible intrathoracic contents both signify a wound that is competing with the trachea for airflow. Hypoventilation due to 'stealing' of airflow from the trachea and a collapsed lung are obligatorily present. Correction of the 'tracheal' hypoventilation is the critical intervention that is needed most urgently. This can be most rapidly and effective achieved by initiating positive pressure ventilation with a bag-valve-mask device or via an endotracheal tube. After the 'tracheal' hypoventilation is managed a catheter or tube thoracostomy procedure should be performed at a location separated from the open chest wound. The chest wound can be occluded and if appropriate repaired after the thoracostomy drainage device is placed. An occlusive/flutter valve dressing that functions as a one-way valve to prevent inspiratory inflow of air and to allow drainage of any air under tension from the affected hemithorax can be used as a temporizing measure while awaiting positive pressure ventilation and/or tube thoracostomy.

As previously described, patient positioning may affect the pathophysiologic characteristics of an open chest wound. For example, if the patient lies on a wound it may become totally occluded while postures that place traction on the wound may cause it to open.

Finally, it must be remembered that coexisting thoracic injuries commonly accompany open chest wounds. Thorough evaluation should be undertaken to identify such conditions. Further discussion of the evaluation and management of trauma patients is beyond the scope of this chapter. Reference to other appropriate texts and consultation with appropriate specialists should be performed when indicated (45–47).

Procedures for Managing Open Chest Wounds

Procedures that may help manage the direct physiologic consequences of an open chest wound include administration of high concentration oxygen (Chapter 13), positive pressure ventilation (Chapters 14, 16), creation of a temporizing occlusive/flutter valve dressing, and thoracostomy procedures as discussed earlier in Section A of this chapter. Supplemental oxygen should be administered when possible to all patients with signs of physiologic compromise associated with an open chest wound. Endotracheal intubation to facilitate positive pressure ventilation is often beneficial. The role of positive pressure ventilation is to primarily improve ventilation and administer high concentrations of oxygen. It restores tracheal airflow and tidal volume, promotes reinflation of atelectatic lung and reverses the direction of the pressure gradient that draws air into the chest during inspiration. Coexisting injuries may also benefit from endotracheal intubation with positive pressure ventilation. A temporizing occlusive/flutter valve dressing can be used to safely create a one-way valve over the wound that prevents further accumulation of air in the pleural space and may permit egress of some of the already accumulated pleural air. The potential uses for thoracostomy procedures include needle thoracostomy to permit temporary emergency drainage of a tension pneumothorax and catheter or tube thoracostomy to permit definitive emergency drainage of a pneumothorax or tension pneumothorax due to an open chest wound. Most operators prefer to perform thoracostomy procedures at a site somewhat removed from the site of the open chest wound. Occasionally, however, some operators will place a thoracostomy catheter or tube through an open chest wound. The relative risk of doing this is not clear. Certainly, there is the possibility that this procedure will create or exacerbate bleeding, injure underlying structures, or enter into a false lumen or missile tract. Cardiorespiratory and pulse oximeter monitoring should be used whenever a significant open chest wound is present to continuously assess physiologic parameters and to help detect deterioration.

A patient with an open chest wound will occasionally present in extremis with a totally occlusive dressing in place over the wound. The cause of the patient's condition may be due, in part, to the dressing itself, which has prevented the egress of intrapleural air and created a tension pneumothorax. In such cases, simply removing the dressing may allow sufficient venting of accumulated pleural air to relieve the symptoms.

The definitive indications and the order of prioritization for the various procedures that may benefit a patient with an open chest wound combined with other associated conditions are somewhat subjective, experiential, and circumstantial. However it is generally true that when multiple critical emergency interventions are needed, one should follow the familiar "A-B-C" algorithm and address airway management first. Once the airway has been secured, the operator can then support breathing and circulation. It is possible that some critically ill patients may undergo endotracheal intubation and the administration of positive pressure ventilation with high concentrations of oxygen before the chest is fully examined and an open chest wound is identified. Open chest wounds with on-going unidirectional or bidirectional airflow across them pose a particularly high risk of physiologic compromise and intervention should occur as soon as possible after such an injury is recognized.

An occasional inpatient may develop an iatrogenic open chest wound when a surgical incision dehisces, when a thoracostomy catheter or tube develops an air leak around it or becomes dislodged unexpectedly, when a drainage system becomes loose or disconnected, or the tract of a thoracostomy catheter or tube is not properly occluded after the device is removed. Often, the sound of air moving through the chest wound is the first sign of a wound dehiscence or a dislodged thoracostomy catheter or tube. If there is no thoracostomy catheter or tube in place, then the open chest wound should be evaluated and managed as previously described. When needed, a thoracostomy catheter or tube may be placed at a site remote from the wound. If there is a thoracostomy catheter or tube still in place, then the operator should insure that the device is correctly positioned and functioning while applying an occlusive dressing around the site of the air leak. If the thoracostomy catheter or tube has come out, replacing it may be the best strategy for emergency management. Some operators simply reinsert a catheter or tube through the existing tract. Others prefer to insert a new catheter or tube at a site somewhat removed from the first site and then occlude the original site. The relative risk-benefit difference between these two approaches is not known. When suction is being applied to a thoracostomy drainage system, a sudden increase in the amount of air flowing through a Heimlich valve or a water seal device usually indicates a leak or a loose connection somewhere in the drainage system. When no suction is being applied to the thoracostomy drainage system, a large leak or disconnection will abolish the normal tidal fluctuations of the Heimlich valve or the water seal device. Simply repairing the leak with tape or correcting the loose or disconnected portion in the thoracostomy drainage system will solve problems of this type.

▶ PROCEDURE

The procedural details related to configuring a temporizing occlusive dressing to function as a one-way flutter valve are described below. Thoracostomy procedures are described in the preceding section of this chapter. Details related to endotracheal intubation and positive pressure ventilation are described in Chapters 14 and 16.

Occlusive/Flutter Valve Dressings

Indications
Occlusive dressings are indicated for the temporary emergency stabilization of an intermittently or continuously patent open chest wound

Equipment
See Table 29.3.

Procedure
The operator should wear gloves, a protective gown, a mask, and an eye shield to protect him/her from direct contact with the patient's body fluids. This procedure can be done in a sterile or nonsterile fashion with little, if any increased risk of infection to the patient. Sterile technique may consume precious time in critical cases. If sterile technique is employed the wound and surrounding tissues should be washed with povidone/iodine solution or an alternative antiseptic solution.

The occlusive dressing material is then prepared. Improvisation often is required when selecting the material. Important considerations include insuring that the material is nearly or completely impervious to air, thin and flexible enough to conform to the shape of the chest wall, unlikely to tightly adhere to the skin around the wound, pliable enough to allow air and blood to flow underneath when applied over the wound, and large enough to cover the entire chest wound with at least 1- to 2-inch margins beyond the edge of the wound on all sides. The material should also be inert and nonsensitizing if possible. Various materials at hand may be used. These may include a piece of lightweight flexible plastic or cellophane such as that used for packaging sterile items,

TABLE 29.3	EQUIPMENT NEEDED FOR TEMPORIZING OCCLUSIVE/FLUTTER VALVE DRESSING

Personal protection gear
  Gloves
  Mask
  Eye shield
  Gown
Surgical antiseptic prep solution (optional)
Piece of impermeable material of sufficient size
Adhesive tape
Tincture of benzoin (optional)

a piece of nonabsorbent paper such as that used for packaging gauze or gloves or wrapping sterile trays, two or three 4 × 4 gauze sponges with an overlying outer covering of petrolatum gauze, a single semipermeable plastic dressing with the nonadhesive side over the wound, two semipermeable plastic dressings stuck together adhesive side to adhesive side, a piece of plastic cut from a clean trash bag, or some other alternative option. If the piece of material is too big, then it can be trimmed to fit. The occlusive dressing material is then applied over the open chest wound. As noted above there should be 1- to 2-inch margins beyond all wound edges. The operator then securely tapes three sides of the occlusive dressing to the adjacent skin of the chest (Fig. 29.14). The nondependent edge of the occlusive dressing should remain untaped. Some operators prefer to use benzoin to promote adhesion of the tape to the skin. If benzoin is used, then the operator should be careful that the benzoin is not applied around the entire circumference of the wound and does not run under the occlusive dressing. Otherwise, the occlusive dressing may adhere to the skin in a complete circle around the wound forming a seal rather than a flutter valve. Benzoin tincture that contacts exposed tissue in the wound may cause pain. When there is bleeding from the wound it may be necessary to create or leave an additional modest opening along the most dependent margin of the occlusive/flutter valve dressing to allow drainage of blood under the device. An alternative method of creating a occlusive dressing that allows air to exit the chest is to place a piece of impermeable material over the entire wound and seal it in place with tape on all sides then pierce the occlusive material with an angiocath or thoracostomy catheter that is then secured in place and attached to a Heimlich valve, a water seal suction apparatus, or an improvised flutter valve. (See the section on drainage devices in the first section of this chapter.) While this method is theoretically attractive for a variety of reasons, it is rarely used in practice because it requires more time and equipment than the usual occlusive/flutter valve dressing technique. Once the dressing is in place, its functioning should be assessed. If there is still inspiratory airflow through the wound, then the taped edges should be examined to insure that they are secure. If inspiratory airflow via the wound still persists, then the flutter valve dressing should be removed and replaced with a new one with wider margins. Once in place, the free edge of the dressing must remain patent at all times. This is best assured by leaving the dressing and the area surrounding it uncovered and by maintaining the patient in a position that does not put pressure or tension on the dressing. If the patient deteriorates following application of an occlusive/flutter valve dressing, then the operator should be suspicious that progression of a simple pneumothorax or development of a tension pneumothorax has occurred. When one of these things occurs, there are two possible mechanisms. The patient may have an on-going air leak from the injured lung that is leading to further air accumulation in the pleural space because the open chest wound tract has become obstructed by the application of the occlusive/flutter valve dressing and/or because the dressing is not

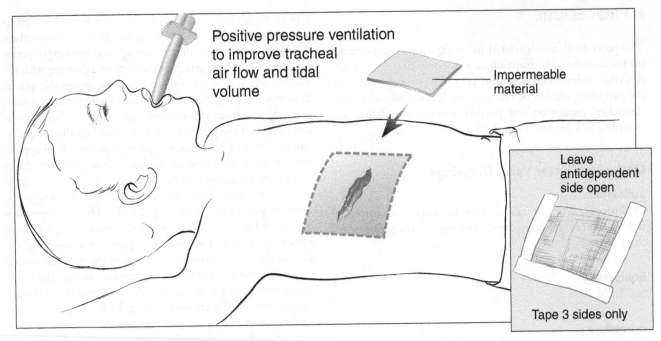

Positive pressure ventilation to improve tracheal air flow and tidal volume

Impermeable material

Leave antidependent side open

Tape 3 sides only

Figure 29.14 Application of a temporizing occlusive flutter valve dressing.

properly functioning to allow egress of air from the pleural space. Alternatively, the occlusive/flutter valve dressing may have become dislodged or is otherwise not satisfactorily occluding the open chest wound during the patient's inspiratory efforts and thereby allowing additional air into the chest. If a large pneumothorax or a tension pneumothorax is suspected, then the occlusive/flutter valve dressing can be quickly manipulated or removed in an attempt to vent pleural air. In addition to manipulation of the dressing, the operator may wish to consider initiation of positive pressure ventilation, placement of a needle thoracostomy, and/or placement of an emergency tube or catheter thoracostomy. Continued instability after the initiation of the above maneuvers should prompt a search for a coexisting condition.

▶ COMPLICATIONS

The procedure-related complications that occur during the management of open chest wounds are mainly the concatenation of the complications of each of the individual procedures applied to the patient. The procedures likely to be performed alone or in variable combinations to a patient with an open chest wound include temporizing occlusive/flutter valve dressing, endotracheal intubation, positive pressure ventilation, needle thoracostomy, and catheter/tube thoracostomy. Many of the potential complications related to temporizing occlusive/flutter valve dressing devices are listed in Table 29.4. The list in this table cannot completely anticipate all circumstances so clinicians rarely may need to consider special, unusual contexts other than those listed. The

TABLE 29.4	POTENTIAL COMPLICATIONS RELATED TO TEMPORARY OCCLUSIVE/FLUTTER VALVE DRESSINGS

Preprocedure complications
Failure to recognize and intervene for severe simple/tension pneumothorax that has already developed
Misdiagnosis of chest wound that does not fully traverse chest wall
Misdiagnosis of chest wound that passes into an extrathoracic space
Failure to recognize additional open chest wounds
Delay in performing procedure
Improper prioritization of multiple procedures, particularly endotracheal intubation, and/or positive pressure ventilation

Procedure related complications
Failure due to improper size/configuration/type of material used
Pneumothorax or tension pneumothorax if chest wall dressing is inadvertently sealed on all four sides with complete occlusion of the defect
Failure to perform timely subsequent catheter or tube thoracostomy when appropriate

Postprocedure complications
Dressing becomes dysfunctional or dislodged
Interference with other procedures (e.g., defibrillation)
Infection
Allergy/sensitivity to materials used
Improper monitoring/recognition of developing complications (e.g., tension pneumothorax)
Failure to leave area uncovered/exposed for proper monitoring and functioning
Failure to properly manage/repair wound after device is no longer needed
Foreign body introduction into the wound (e.g., dressing material)
Failure to restrain patient when necessary to protect device
Turning patient on the affected side or other positioning that interferes with device functioning
Interference with drainage of blood from the wound or thorax

CLINICAL TIPS

▶ Assess chest wounds for serious bleeding. Obtain surgical consultation if present.

▶ Assess chest wounds for airflow across the wound.

  ▶ If no airflow is present assess for other coexisting injuries, especially pneumothorax and hemothorax. Manage coexisting injuries with the appropriate priority and interventions.

  ▶ If unidirectional (inspiratory) airflow is present then perform an emergent tube thoracostomy. A temporizing occlusive/flutter valve dressing can be applied while awaiting completion of tube thoracostomy. A temporizing needle thoracostomy may relieve a tension pneumothorax until a chest tube is in place. Endotracheal intubation and positive pressure ventilation also may be indicated.

  ▶ If bidirectional (inspiratory and expiratory) airflow is present then positive pressure ventilation and a tube thoracostomy procedure should be performed emergently. A temporizing occlusive/flutter valve dressing can be applied while initiating positive pressure ventilation and completing tube thoracostomy.

▶ Administer high concentration oxygen and monitor with cardiorespiratory and pulse oximeter monitors and frequent close serial observation.

SUMMARY

1 Wear appropriate personal protective gear.

2 Improvise a piece of impermeable material of sufficient size to provide at least 1- to 2-inch margins around all edges of the wound.

3 Secure the impermeable material over the open chest wound by taping on three sides only. (Leave the antidependent margin free and unencumbered.)

4 Leave the dressing open to full view.

5 Do not let the patient lie on the dressing.

6 Frequently monitor the device to be sure it is properly functioning.

7 Perform emergent tube thoracostomy. Endotracheal intubation and positive pressure ventilation may also be indicated. Needle thoracostomy can be used as a temporizing measure for a tension pneumothorax.

potential complications of endotracheal intubation and positive pressure ventilation are discussed elsewhere in this book. (See Chapters 14, 16, 17, and 81.) The potential complications of needle thoracostomy, catheter thoracostomy and tube thoracostomy are listed in Table 29.2 in the first section of this chapter. Only the potential complications associated with occlusive/flutter valve dressings are discussed below.

Although, preprocedural, intraprocedural, and postprocedural complications related to the use of an occlusive/flutter valve dressing can be anticipated, the most significant risk is complete occlusion of the chest wall defect with the subsequent development of a pneumothorax or tension pneumothorax as described above. Care must, therefore, be taken to insure that the dressing is sealed against the skin on only three sides so that it indeed functions as a one-way valve. Furthermore, it must be remembered that the dressing is only a temporizing measure. A thoracostomy tube or catheter should be placed as soon as possible after the dressing is applied. Ongoing patient monitoring during this process is mandatory.

▶ SUMMARY

Management of an open chest wound is a rarely used but vital skill required of clinicians performing or supporting resuscitation services. Appreciation of the physics and physiology of open chest wounds should allow appropriate emergent interventions. Emergent application of a temporizing occlusive/flutter valve dressing over the "sucking chest wound" while awaiting positive pressure ventilation and/or a catheter or tube thoracostomy may be beneficial. Tube thoracostomy and possibly positive pressure ventilation in conjunction with wound management is the definitive emergency stabilization needed for most significant open chest wounds. Hemorrhage may be an additional concern in some cases. Coexisting intrathoracic and/or extrathoracic injuries are commonly associated with open chest wounds. Concomitant injuries should be rigorously sought and managed in a prioritized and appropriate manner.

▶ ACKNOWLEDGMENT

The authors would like to acknowledge the valuable contributions of Richard M. Cantor and Kathleen M. Connors to the version of this chapter that appeared in the previous edition.

▶ REFERENCES

1. Hippocrates. *Genuine Works*. Vol. 2 (translated by Francis Adams). New York: William Wood and Company; 1886:226.

2. Playfair GE. Case of empyema treated by aspiration and subsequently by drainage: recovery. *Br Med J*. 1875;1:45.

3. Hewett FC. Drainage for empyema. *Br Med J*. 1876;1:1317.

4. Graham EA, Bell RD. Open pneumothorax: its relation to the treatment of empyema: war medicine. *Am J Med Sci*. 1918;156:839.

5. Beaver BL, Laschinger JC. Pediatric thoracic trauma. *Sem Thor Card Surg.* 1992;4:255–262.

6. Helafer MA, Nichols DG, Rogers MC. Development physiology of the respiratory system. In: Rogers MC, ed. *Textbook of Pediatric Intensive Care.* 2nd ed. Baltimore: Williams & Wilkins; 1992:104–133.

7. Yu VY, Lieu SW, Robertson NR. Pneumothorax in the newborn: changing patterns. *Arch Dis Child.* 1975;50:449.

8. Monin P, Vert P. Pneumothorax. *Clin Perinatol.* 1978;5:535.

9. Wiggllesworth JS. Pathology of the lung in the fetus and neonate, with particular reference to problems of growth and maturation. *Histopathology.* 1987;11(7):671–689.

10. Plaus WJ. Delayed pneumothorax after subclavian vein catheterization. *J Parent Enteral Nutr.* 1990;14:414–415.

11. Collins JC, Levine G, Waxman K. Occult traumatic pneumothorax: immediate tube thoracostomy versus expectant management. *Am Surg.* 1992;58:743–746.

12. Wolfman NT, Gilpin JW, Bechtold RE, et al. Occult pneumothorax in patients with abdominal trauma: CT studies. *J Comput Assist Tomagr.* 1993;17:56–59.

13. Frumkin K, Wright SW. Tube thoracostomy. In: Roberts JR, Hedges JR, eds. *Clinical Procedures in Emergency Medicine.* 2nd ed. Philadelphia: WB Saunders; 1985:128–149.

14. Iberti TJ, Stern PM. Chest tube thoracostomy. *Crit Care Clin.* 1992;8:879–894.

15. Silver M, Bone RC. Techniques for chest tube insertion and pleurodesis. *J Crit Ill.* 1993;8:631–637.

16. Vukick DJ. Diseases of the pleural space. *Emerg Med Clin North Am.* 1989;7(2):309–324.

17. Templeton JM. Thoracic trauma. In: Fleischer GR, Ludwig S, eds. *Textbook of Pediatric Emergency Medicine.* 3rd ed. Baltimore: Williams & Wilkins; 1993:1336–1360.

18. Rhea JT, Deluca SA, Greene RE. Determining the size of pneumothorax in the upright patient. *Radiology.* 1982;144:733.

19. Garramore JR, Jacobs LM, Sahdev P. An objective method to measure and manage occult pneumothorax. *Surg Syn Obstet.* 1991;173:257–261.

20. Minami H, Saka H, Senda K, et al. Small catheter drainage for spontaneous pneumothorax. *Am J Med Sci.* 1992;304:345–347.

21. Conces DJ, Tarver RD, Gray WC, et al. Treatment of pneumothoraces utilizing small caliber chest tubes. *Chest.* 1988;94:55–57.

22. Bone RC. The technique of small catheter pleural aspiration. *J Crit Ill.* 1993;8:827–883.

23. Vallee P, Sullivan M, Richardson H, et al. Sequential treatment of a simple pneumothorax. *Ann Emerg Med.* 1988;19:936.

24. Delius RE, Obeid FN, Horst HM, et al. Catheter aspiration for simple pneumothorax. Experience with 114 patients. *Arch Surg.* 1989;124(7):833–836.

25. Bayne CG. Pulmonary complications of the McSwain dart. *Ann Emerg Med.* 1982;11:136.

26. Kircher LT, Swartzel RL. Spontaneous pneumothorax and its treatment. *JAMA.* 1954;155:24.

27. Northfield TC. Oxygen therapy for spontaneous pneumothorax. *Br Med J.* 1971;4:86.

28. Symbas PN. Chest drainage tubes. *Surg Clin North Am.* 1989;69:41–46.

29. Miller KS, Sahn SA. Chest tubes: indications, technique, management and complications. *Chest.* 1987;91:258–264.

30. Barkin RM, Rosen P, eds. *Emergency Pediatrics: A Guide to Ambulatory Care.* 3rd ed. St. Louis: CV Mosby Co; 1990.

31. Buhrman BP, Landrum BG, Ferrara TB, et al. Pleural drainage using modified pigtail catheters. *Crit Care Med.* 1986;14:575.

32. Lawless S, Orr R, Killian A, et al. New pigtail catheter for pleural drainage in pediatric patients. *Crit Care Med.* 1989;17:173.

33. Bernstein A, et al. Management of a spontaneous pneumothorax using a Heimlich flutter valve. *Thorax.* 1973;28:386–389.

34. Obeid FN, Shapiro MJ, Richardson HH, et al. Catheter aspiration for simple pneumothorax (CASP) in the outpatient management of a simple traumatic pneumothorax. *J Trauma.* 1985;25:882–886.

35. Hamilton AD, Archer GJ. Treatment of pneumothorax by simple aspiration. *Thorax.* 1983;38:934–936.

36. Moore HV. Complications of thoracentesis and thoracostomy. In: Cordell AR, Ellison RG, eds. *Complications of Intrathoracic Surgery.* Boston: Little, Brown; 1979:142.

37. Daly RC, Mucha P, Pairolero PC, Farrell M. The risk of percutaneous chest tube thoracostomy for blunt thoracic trauma. *Ann Emerg Med.* 1985;14:865–870.

38. Fraser RS. Lung perforation complicating tube thoracostomy: pathological description of three cases. *Human Pathol.* 1988;19:518–523.

39. Foresti V, Villa A, Casati O, et al. Abdominal placement of tube thoracostomy due to lack of recognition of paralysis of hemidiaphragm. *Chest.* 1992;102:29.

40. Kolleff MH, Dothager DW. Reversible cardiogenic shock due to chest tube compression of the right ventricle. *Chest.* 1991;99(4):976–980.

41. Mahfood S, Hix WR, Aaron BL, et al. Reexpansion pulmonary edema. *Ann Thorac Surg.* 1988;45:340.

42. Cook T, Kietzman L, Leibold R. "Pneumo-ptosis" in the emergency department. *Am J Emerg Med.* 1992;10:431–434.

43. Bertino RE, Wesbey GE, Johnson R. Horner syndrome occurring as a complication of chest tube placement. *Radiology.* 1987;164:745.

44. Cefolio RJ. Advances in thoracostomy tube management. *Surg Clin North Amer.* 2002;82: 833.

45. Bliss D. Pediatric thoracic trauma. *Crit Care Med.* 2002;30:S409.

46. Beaver BL. Pediatric thoracic trauma. *Sem Thor Card Surg.* 1992;4:255–262.

47. Livingston DH, Hauser CJ. Trauma to the chest wall and lung. In: Moore EE, Feliciano DV, Mattox KL, eds. *Trauma.* 5th ed. New York: McGraw-Hill; 2004:507–538.

ELLIOTT M. HARRIS AND JAMES D'AGOSTINO

30

Autotransfusion

▶ INTRODUCTION

Autotransfusion or autologous blood transfusion is the collection of blood from a hemorrhaging trauma victim, its preparation, and its reinfusion. Autotransfusion was first used by Blundell in 1818 in women with postpartum hemorrhage (1). Reports on the use of autotransfusion for thoracic trauma date to 1917 (2) and for abdominal trauma to 1927 (3). The development of blood banking cooled the enthusiasm for autotransfusion; however, shortages of homologous blood and concerns about infectious complications renewed interest in the procedure in the 1970s. Collection of blood for autotransfusion can be performed by physicians, nurses, and trained technicians in emergency departments, operating rooms, and intensive care units.

Autotransfusion offers several advantages over transfusion of homologous blood. The patient is not exposed to blood-borne infectious disease, there is no risk of transfusion reaction, and the blood is immediately available. The advantages of recycling fresh, warm, autologous blood outweigh the potential disadvantages of clotting abnormalities, renal and pulmonary complications, and the inadvertent infusion of blood contaminated with bacteria.

The equipment needed to perform autotransfusion can be assembled quickly, and the process of collection, preparation, and reinfusion of blood can be easily performed even in the traumatized pediatric patient. Autotransfusion may offer the advantage of being lower in cost than transfusion of banked blood, but this depends on the relative costs of the equipment for autotransfusion compared with those for the transfusion of banked blood. When smaller volumes of blood are transfused, autotransfusion may be slightly more expensive. The physician will have to weigh the potentially higher cost of autotransfusion against the risks associated with the transfusion of banked blood (3).

▶ ANATOMY AND PHYSIOLOGY

In children, as in adults, the torso is often the target of both intentional and accidental trauma. Traumatic hemorrhage into the thoracic cavity is most often the result of bleeding from the lung parenchyma, the intercostal vessels, or the internal mammary arteries (4). However, the source of the bleeding may be the heart or great vessels or, in cases of diaphragmatic injury, the abdominal organs. Bleeding into the abdominal cavity can be the result of injury to solid organs such as the spleen and liver or injury to intra-abdominal vessels.

Hemothorax and hemoperitoneum can result in exsanguinating hemorrhage. Additionally, hemothorax may result in raised intrathoracic pressures, which in turn cause impaired venous return to the heart. Hemothorax may also cause impaired gas exchange secondary to compression of the ipsilateral lung.

The shed blood recovered from the peritoneal and thoracic cavities behaves somewhat differently than blood that is lost to external hemorrhage in that it does not clot as readily (5). It is felt that this is due to defibrination from contact with a serosal surface, especially with hemothorax. This fact favors using intracavitary blood for autotransfusion. Additionally, autotransfused blood has higher levels of 2,3-diphosphoglycerate than banked, homologous blood (6), which makes it more effective for tissue oxygen delivery.

▶ INDICATIONS

In addition to patients who are in shock as a result of hemorrhage and have had minimal if any response to crystalloid therapy, blood replacement should be considered for those patients who are deemed to have lost 30% or more of their

TABLE 30.1	INDICATIONS AND CONTRAINDICATIONS FOR AUTOTRANSFUSION

Indications
- Hemothorax with shock unresponsive to crystalloid therapy
- Hemothorax with loss of at least 30% of the circulating blood volume
- Loss of less than 30% of the circulating blood volume but with ongoing blood loss
- Open thoracotomy to relieve ongoing intrathoracic bleeding

Contraindications (absolute)
- Blood more than 4 hours old
- Presence of large blood clots
- Patient with known malignant neoplasm or coagulopathy
- Sepsis or pulmonary, mediastinal, or pericardial infection
- Blood known or strongly suspected to be contaminated by bacteria (e.g., gross fecal contamination)

Contraindications (relative)
- Blood recovered from the peritoneal cavity (note: this blood should be used in the ED only when the benefit clearly outweighs the risk of inadvertent infusion of blood contaminated with bacteria)

circulating blood volume as well as those who have lost lesser amounts of blood but have evidence of ongoing hemorrhage (6) (Table 30.1). In adults, 30% of the circulating blood volume is approximately 1,500 mL. In children, the amount of blood loss necessary to cause significant hemorrhage varies with both age and size. Circulating blood volume is about 8% to 9% of body weight in young children, as opposed to 7% in adults. This typically amounts to 80 mL per kilogram of body weight.

In the traumatized adult patient, hemothorax is the most common cause of shock. The major indication for autotransfusion is hypotension associated with hemothorax, especially when there is ongoing blood loss. Other potential indications include a stable hemothorax, emergency thoracotomy, and intra-abdominal injury from hepatic, splenic, or vascular injury without hollow viscous injury.

Autotransfusion is contraindicated when the blood is collected from injuries that are more than 4 hours old or in the presence of large clots. Likewise, contamination of the blood with intestinal contents or a communication between the abdomen and the chest represent contraindications to ED autotransfusion (6,7). Other conditions that are contraindications to autotransfusion are known coagulopathy or disseminated intravascular coagulation (DIC); sepsis; pulmonary, pericardial, and mediastinal infections; and malignant neoplasms. Blood containing wound irrigants, such as Betadine, or topical hemostatic agents, such as thrombin, should not be salvaged (8). Using blood recovered from traumatic hemoperitoneum is controversial. In most cases, this blood should not be used in the ED setting because it is impossible for the resuscitation team to determine whether the blood is contaminated with bowel contents. However, in some circumstances this may be the only blood available for the patient. In such cases, the potential benefits of transfusion clearly outweigh the risks (9). Blood recovered from a hemoperitoneum may be used for intraoperative transfusion.

▶ PROCEDURE

Several autotransfusion devices are commercially available. The following procedure describes the Atrium 2450 system; however, with some minor differences, most systems function similarly. Clinicians should become familiar with the equipment used in their institution. Other systems include the Sorensen device, the Bently device, the Baylor Rapid System, and the Haemonics Cell Saver unit. The Baylor system has a cell-washing step, and the Haemonics unit has both washing and concentrating abilities. The necessity for the cell-washing step, at least in the ED setting, has been questioned, and many health care centers do not use this step. Cell washing removes free hemoglobin, particulate debris, activated clotting factors, and bacteria but creates some delay before reinfusion of the blood and adds to the cost of the procedure. Although felt to be advantageous, there are few data to support the routine use of cell washing (10).

Monitoring is important during autotransfusion. Vital signs should be recorded at frequent intervals during the procedure, and continuous cardiorespiratory monitoring and pulse oximetry should be performed. Additionally, depending on the volume of blood infused and whether anticoagulant is used, CBC, PT/PTT, calcium, and electrolytes may need to be monitored (see "Complications").

The first step in the procedure is the insertion of a large-bore chest tube such as might be used to treat any hemothorax (see Chapter 29). As the tube is being inserted, the Atrium 2450 (or another appropriate blood recovery unit) is prepared. This procedure is similar to that employed when a chest tube drainage system is prepared. When the equipment is assembled, the citrate phosphate dextrose (CPD) solution is added to the anticoagulant port of the recovery unit. The manufacturer recommends adding 14 mL of CPD solution to each 100 mL of recovered autologous blood. Many health care centers do not routinely add anticoagulant to the autologous blood because, as previously stated, blood recovered from body cavities does not clot quickly, and forgoing the addition of anticoagulant simplifies the process.

The chest tube is attached to the chest drainage port of the recovery unit. The autotransfusion system (ATS) blood recovery bag is then attached to the ATS access line located in the inferior section of the chest drainage unit. The two clamps are opened, and the self-filling ATS blood recovery bag is activated by gently bending it upward where indicated.

When the ATS bag is full, it should be removed and connected to a blood filter and infusion tubing. A cell-washing step may be added before infusion into the patient. The ATS recovery bag and filter are then connected to IV tubing and air is carefully purged from the tubing. The autologous blood may then be infused through the blood filter (preferably with a pore size of 20 to 40 μM) (5,6,11) (Fig. 30.1). In general, the entire volume of salvaged blood should be reinfused.

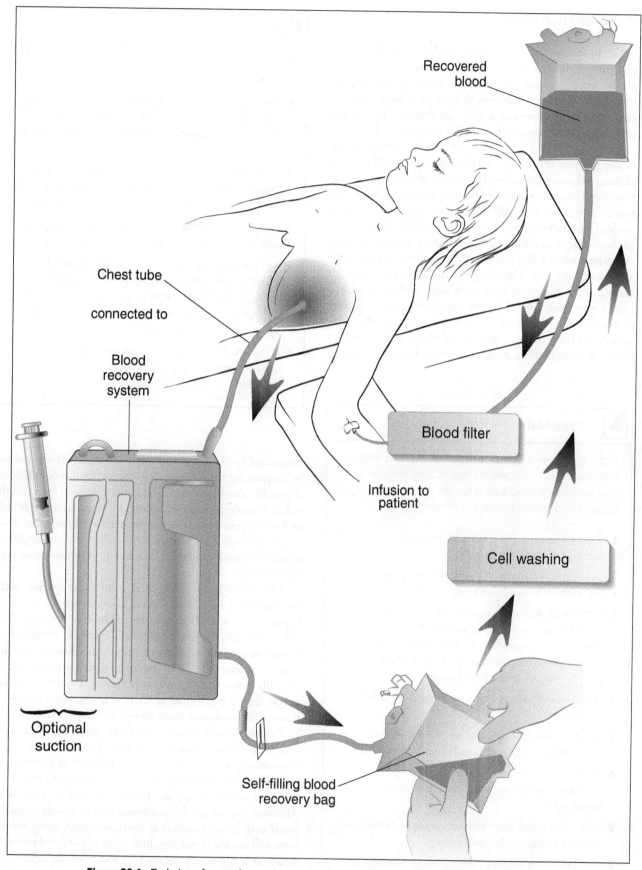

Figure 30.1 Technique for autologous blood transfusion using blood from a hemothorax.

▶ COMPLICATIONS

Autotransfusion is relatively free of complications. Most complications and potential complications discussed in this chapter are remarkably rare or have never been reported but are theoretically possible. However, this can be a dangerous procedure, and it is important for the physician to have an understanding of the potential complications involved.

Coagulopathies due to decreased platelets, fibrinogen, or clotting factors may occur, and the risk is increased with increasing volumes of transfused blood. To avoid this complication, it has been recommended that the amount of autotransfused blood not exceed 2,000 mL; however, reports have been made of autotransfusion of larger volumes (10). Air embolism has been described during cardiopulmonary bypass and intraoperatively when roller pump–type units have been used for autotransfusion (6). This complication has never been described when gravity infusion units such as those described herein have been used. However, prudent practice dictates that air be purged from the system before transfusion. Hyperkalemia from the hemolysis of red blood cells is another potential complication. Risk of excessive hemolysis may be

CLINICAL TIPS

▶ Autotransfusion is primarily indicated in cases of hemothorax with shock or significant blood loss.

▶ Regular in-service sessions for physicians, nurses, and other involved personnel to familiarize them with the appropriate autotransfusion equipment are highly valuable.

▶ Hemolysis is avoided when recovering blood by maintaining low suction pressure (5 to 15 mm Hg) and by avoiding the suctioning of air with blood.

▶ If the recovered blood is to be used immediately, adding anticoagulant is probably unnecessary.

▶ Cell washing may be used to minimize risk of infection when the transfused blood may be contaminated with bacteria; however, such blood should be used only when the potential benefits outweigh the potential risks.

▶ If potentially contaminated blood is used, broad-spectrum antibiotic therapy to cover enteric organisms should be instituted.

SUMMARY

Note: Clinicians should familiarize themselves with autotransfusion equipment used at their institution. (The procedure described is for the Atrium system, but most systems function in a similar fashion.)

1 Insert large-bore chest tube for evacuation of the hemothorax (see Chapter 29).

2 Connect suction port of blood recovery unit to low wall suction (5 to 15 mm Hg).

3 If citrate phosphate dextrose (CDP) solution, an anticoagulant, is added to system, it should be added at this point; for the Atrium system, the manufacturer recommends adding 14 mL of CDP to each 100 mL of autologous blood.

4 Attach chest tube to chest drainage port of blood recovery unit.

5 Attach blood recovery bag to ATS access line located on inferior section of chest drainage unit.

6 Open two clamps and activate self-filling blood recovery bag by gently bending it upward where indicated.

7 When bag is full, remove from recovery system and connect to blood filter and tubing.

8 A cell-washing step may be introduced before infusion of recovered blood.

minimized by using low wall suction to recover the blood and by keeping the suction tip below the surface of pooled blood, if possible. Air-blood interfacing during suction increases the risk of hemolysis. Some authorities recommend using as little as 5 to 15 mm Hg of suction pressure to recover the blood (6). Hemolysis leads to increased levels of free hemoglobin, which may result in renal failure, but no such cases have been reported (6).

The citrate buffer CDP used as an anticoagulant in the preparation of the recovered blood places the patient at risk for hypocalcemia when large amounts of blood are transfused. To reduce this risk, the volume of transfused blood should be the minimum amount needed to ensure hemodynamic stability, and the amount of CDP added to the recovery unit should be carefully monitored. As previously discussed, many authorities believe that the addition of CDP is unnecessary, and some newer autotransfusion units do not include this step (6).

Bacteremia is a concern, and the physician must avoid collecting blood contaminated with intestinal contents. A cell-washing step may decrease the incidence of infection, although this has not been proven (10). Fortunately, even when infection occurs, it appears to respond well to antibiotics. Although use of autologous blood that is grossly contaminated with bowel contents is contraindicated, many institutions will use the blood even in the face of potential intestinal injury as a life-saving measure in the critically injured patient. In such cases, broad-spectrum antibiotics are routinely administered. Finally, pulmonary and renal complications of autotransfusion have been described, and a cell-washing step could potentially remove the unknown factors responsible for this condition (6,10).

▶ SUMMARY

Autotransfusion offers a relatively safe alternative to homologous blood transfusion in the hemorrhaging trauma victim. Because this technique is fairly simple and free from complications, it should be considered for use in pediatric trauma victims.

▶ REFERENCES

1. Blundell J. Experiments in the transfusion of blood. *Medico-Chir Trans.* 1818;9:56.
2. Anderson CB. Autotransfusion in traumatic hemothorax. *Missouri Med.* 1975;72:541–544.
3. Smith LA, Barker DE, Burns RP. Autotransfusion utilization in abdominal trauma. *Am Surg.* 1997;63:47–49.
4. Kadish H. Thoracic trauma. In: Ludwig S, Fleisher GR, Henretig FM, eds. *Textbook of Pediatric Emergency Medicine.* 5th ed. Baltimore: Lippincott Williams & Wilkins; 2006:1433–1452.
5. McGhee A, Swinton S, Watt M. Use of autologous transfusion in the management of acute traumatic haemothorax in the accident and emergency department. *J Accid Emerg Med.* 1999;16:451–452.
6. Kharasch SJ, Millham F, Vinci RJ. The use of autotransfusion in pediatric chest trauma. *Pediatr Emerg Care.* 1994;10:109–112.
7. American Association of Blood Banks. *Guidelines for Blood Salvage and Reinfusion in Surgery and Trauma.* Arlington, VA: American Association of Blood Banks; 1990.
8. Stehling L, Zauder HL. Autologous blood salvage procedures. *Biotechnology.* 1991;19:47–73.
9. Timberlake GA, McSwain NE Jr. Autotransfusion of blood contaminated by enteric contents: a potentially life-saving measure in the massively hemorrhaging trauma patient? *J Trauma.* 1988;28:855–857.
10. Plaisier BR, McCarthy MC, Canal DF, et al. Autotransfusion in trauma: a comparison of two systems. *Am Surg.* 1992;58:562–566.
11. *Atrium 2450 Blood Recovery System: instructions for use.* Hudson, NH: Atrium Medical Corp; 2003.

31

CHRISTINE E. KOERNER AND BRENT R. KING

Emergency Thoracotomy

▶ INTRODUCTION

Few procedures are as dramatic as open emergency thoracotomy. This technique can save a child from otherwise certain death when performed for the appropriate indications. However, this procedure must be used selectively, because only a small subset of patients will benefit (1–14). This chapter discusses both the indications for and the technique of open thoracotomy as performed in the emergency department (ED).

Although emergency thoracotomy is most successful when used to relieve pericardial tamponade (1–3,5,9,10,15–23), which is usually the result of penetrating injury to the heart, other purposes for this procedure include control of exsanguinating hemorrhage within the thoracic or abdominal cavity, redistribution of limited blood volume to the myocardium and brain, correction of an air embolism, and performance of open cardiac massage (9,13,15,24). One should focus on these objectives when performing the procedure, as the goal for the ED team is stabilization rather than definitive repair (5,8,25).

The concept of thoracotomy as a method of resuscitation is not new. Original descriptions of the procedure occurred in the late 1800s (12,13,26,27). In the years before the development of closed chest cardiopulmonary compressions, in-hospital arrests were sometimes managed by direct open chest cardiac compressions (8). Since the development of closed chest compressions as a means to perform resuscitation, open thoracotomy has been employed almost exclusively in the resuscitation of trauma victims who are in extremis. It has long been recognized that victims of trauma who succumb during the initial phase of resuscitation have often sustained significant injury to the heart or great vessels (28). In such cases, blood can collect between the heart and the pericardium, leading to pericardial tamponade, or the patient can experience exsanguinating hemorrhage into the thoracic cavity. In this sit-

uation, immediate thoracotomy to identify and repair injuries may be life saving. Occasionally, emergency pericardiocentesis (Chapter 71) may provide temporary relief and allow for thoracotomy under more controlled circumstances.

▶ ANATOMY AND PHYSIOLOGY

In terms of anatomy relevant to this procedure, a few differences exist between children and adults. For all patients, the wall of the thorax is composed of the muscles of the anterior and posterior chest wall, the ribs, and three sets of intercostal muscles—the external intercostal muscles, the internal intercostal muscles, and the innermost intercostal muscles. The external intercostal muscle exists as a membrane anterior to the midclavicular line, and the internal intercostal muscle is a membrane posterior to the midaxillary line. The neurovascular bundles containing the veins, arteries, and nerves lie along the lower margins of the ribs. The ribs themselves are very pliable in infants and young children, but in older children and adolescents the ribs are more like those of adults. Deep to the ribs is the parietal pleura, which is adherent to the interior of the thoracic wall, and deep to the parietal pleura is the mediastinum, which contains the heart surrounded by the pericardium and the origins of the great vessels.

Viewed from the standpoint of a thoracotomy, the right ventricle lies anterior, just beneath the sternum, with the left ventricle posterior and slightly lateral to the right ventricle. The left phrenic nerve lies on the pericardium on the lateral aspect of the left ventricle, placing it at risk during the procedure. Between the superficial tissues and the left ventricle is the left lung, which is invaginated by the ventricle. When the standard left lateral thoracotomy is used, the anterior and lateral walls of the left ventricle are visible once the left lung is retracted. Situated in a position cephalad to the heart itself lie the great vessels; lateral and slightly posterior to these are the structures of the pulmonary hili. One distinct, if obvious, difference between adults and children is the size of the structures involved. This procedure can be much more difficult in a small child simply because everything is smaller (29,30).

The physiologic considerations involved in pediatric thoracotomy are likewise similar to those in the adult procedure. Direct trauma to the heart often allows blood to accumulate between the heart and the pericardial sac, particularly if the hole in the pericardium is small, because the pericardial defect will often partially or fully seal itself. Even a small amount of blood in the space between the heart and the pericardium can restrict cardiac function. In a small child, this can be a few milliliters. Fortunately, removal of even a portion of this fluid often results in dramatic improvement in cardiac output. Conversely, if the hole is large or fails to seal, then the blood exits the heart into the mediastinum or the thorax. The child can exsanguinate rapidly in this circumstance.

It is for relief of pericardial tamponade and correction of a direct penetrating injury to the heart that thoracotomy is most likely to be successful, but it also may be used in cases of direct injury to the great vessels, to highly vascular abdominal structures, or to the pulmonary hilar structures. In the aforementioned situations, thoracotomy is done to halt exsanguinating hemorrhage into the thoracic or abdominal cavities. In cases of intra-abdominal hemorrhage, thoracotomy allows the interruption of blood flow to the abdomen (by clamping the aorta) and selective perfusion of the brain and the cardiopulmonary system. Experimentally, direct (open) cardiac compressions result in better cardiac output than do indirect (closed) cardiac compressions (31), maintaining homodynamic variables almost in a normal physiologic range (32).

▶ INDICATIONS

Historically, emergency thoracotomy had its inception as part of the resuscitation of trauma victims in the 1960s and 1970s, and since then indications for performance of this procedure have been the subject of intense investigation. Initially, virtually any victim of trauma who arrived in full cardiopulmonary arrest, who arrested in the resuscitation area, or who failed to respond to maximal resuscitation efforts was considered a candidate for this procedure. However, with experience, indications for thoracotomy have become clearer (7,33–44). In virtually all studies of resuscitative thoracotomy, victims of blunt trauma have fared far worse than victims of penetrating trauma. This difference almost certainly reflects both the high incidence of head trauma associated with blunt trauma and the fact that injury in blunt trauma often involves multiple organs (4). In any case, survivorship with good neurologic outcome is rare for blunt trauma victims who arrest during the prehospital phase of resuscitation (4,14).

Victims of penetrating trauma can be further subdivided into victims of shooting and victims of stabbing. While penetrating trauma carries a better prognosis overall, shooting victims are less likely to survive than are victims of stabbing (2,11,16,24,45). The most reasonable explanation for this difference in survivorship is that stabbing is a relatively low velocity injury that often results in damage to a single organ, while shooting, primarily because of the higher velocity, often involves multiple organs and far more tissue destruction. In the case of penetrating trauma, survivorship appears to be determined by the time elapsed between the event and the institution of definitive treatment. Most large studies have few survivors who had undetectable vital signs for more than a few minutes (1,2,11–13,16).

Unfortunately, little information is found in the medical literature dealing specifically with children (1,14,22,23,46). To date, only four studies of resuscitative thoracotomy have been restricted to patients <18 years of age. These studies demonstrate a similar outcome pattern to those involving adults, with survivorship being rare in blunt trauma victims. A total of 142 patients in the four studies underwent emergency thoracotomy; 85 sustained blunt trauma and 57 penetrating trauma. Of the 85 victims of blunt trauma, 2 survived, whereas 7 children who had a penetrating injury survived to hospital discharge. Of the three studies that specifically list the ages of the involved children, no patient younger than 15 years of age survived. This reflects both the high incidence of blunt trauma in young children and the little appreciated fact that although children may be better able to resist full cardiopulmonary arrest than adults, once arrested they are unlikely to recover (4,47,48). Additionally, these results demonstrate the level of interpersonal violence among teenagers that ultimately leads to penetrating injuries (23,25).

Although some might argue that an injured child should be given every possible chance to recover and that thoracotomy should be used liberally despite the dismal statistics, there are three compelling reasons to limit the application of this technique in children, just as the literature suggests that it be limited in adults. First, this is a highly invasive technique that is often performed under less than ideal circumstances. This combination makes thoracotomy very risky to medical personnel from the standpoint of blood exposure (7,20,49). Second, whether successful or not, thoracotomy is costly in financial, emotional, and operational terms (3,14,21,50). Finally, this procedure may produce a limited period of spontaneous circulation in a patient after a period of protracted arrest. In such circumstances, the outcome will almost certainly be either a protracted death from multiorgan system failure or survival with neurologic devastation (1,9,12).

With this information in mind, some recommendations can be made for patient selection:

- Victims of blunt trauma who arrest during the prehospital phase of care and who are without detectable vital signs for more than 5 minutes have virtually no chance for intact survival and should not be considered candidates for this procedure (4,20,25).

- Victims of either penetrating or blunt trauma who have no pulse, no detectable blood pressure, and no organized electrical activity on a cardiac monitor will benefit from thoracotomy only if the procedure is performed promptly. If thoracotomy cannot be undertaken within 5 minutes of the time of arrest, or if the victim of penetrating trauma is in asystole with injuries not isolated to the thorax, then thoracotomy is unlikely to be successful and should not be performed (14,12,31).
- Victims of penetrating trauma, particularly those with penetrating trauma to the chest and upper abdomen, who have short arrest times or arrest en route to the ED and those who fail to respond to initial resuscitation should be considered candidates for this procedure (45).
- Rarely, a victim of nontraumatic arrest may be considered a candidate for thoracotomy. Medical personnel should consider this technique in cases of severe chest wall abnormality and other situations that make traditional closed chest compressions impossible or ineffective (32).

▶ FAST (FOCUSED ASSESSMENT WITH SONOGRAPHY IN TRAUMA)

The focused assessment with sonography for trauma (FAST) examination was initially developed to evaluate patients with blunt abdominal trauma; however, it has also proven useful in evaluating isolated penetrating cardiac injury. When faced with a hypotensive patient with a pericardial effusion following a penetrating chest or back wound, the treating clinician must intercede expeditiously, since cardiac injuries have a high incidence of mortality. The FAST examination has been found to be both sensitive and specific in the determination of traumatic pericardial effusion indicative of injury and may be used as an adjunct to effectively guide emergency surgical decision making (51,52).

▶ EQUIPMENT

The list of necessary equipment for thoracotomy is limited. The procedure can be performed with a scalpel and some sort of chest wall retractor. Several other pieces of equipment are useful, however, and these are listed in Table 32.1. The equipment listed in Part I of Table 32.1 represents a standard thoracotomy tray, which may be used for large children, adolescents, and adults. Part 2 lists equipment that is useful for small children and infants. Notably, this procedure is rarely performed in most EDs, but the likely candidates for this procedure would be adolescents or adults. It is, therefore, reasonable to maintain a single thoracotomy tray in the ED that contains some equipment for infant and small child resuscitation as well as the more standard equipment for adults and adolescents.

TABLE 31.1	EQUIPMENT

I. Equipment for Standard Thoracotomy Tray
Scalpel—No. 20 blade
Mayo scissors
Chest wall retractor ("rib spreaders")—Finichetto or other type
Tissue forceps—10 inch
Vascular (Satinsky) clamps—2 to 4
Needle holder—10 inch
Suture—2.0 silk, curved needle
4.0 silk, vascular needle
Teflon pledgets
Aortic tamponade instrument
Vascular tape
Metzenbaum scissors
Curved hemostats—4 to 10
Right-angle clamps—2 to 4
Lebsche knife/sternal osteotome with hammer/sternal saw
Chest tubes—sizes 20 through 40
Foley catheters—16 through 24 French
Sponges
Drapes/towels
Sterile suction equipment
Sterile internal defibrillator paddles—6 inch

II. Additional Equipment for Child/Infant Resuscitation
Scalpel—No. 15 Blade
Foley catheters—5 through 12 French
Chest tubes—10 through 20 French
Internal defibrillator paddles—2 inch and 4 inch
Small chest wall retractor

▶ PROCEDURE

Performing an emergency thoracotomy is not as awesome a task as it might seem. The technique employed is a logical sequence of steps involving relatively straightforward manual skills. It is important for the emergency physician to be thoroughly familiar with the technique and with the equipment prior to performing the procedure. Adequate assistance is also important for success.

As with all resuscitation efforts, the upper airway should be secured and artificial ventilation begun before the circulatory status of the patient is addressed (Chapters 14 to 17). If enough skilled personnel are available, airway control can be accomplished simultaneously with the initiation of resuscitative thoracotomy. Consideration must always be given to the possibility of lower airway obstruction with concomitant circulatory compromise (i.e., tension pneumothorax), in which case needle decompression of the chest (Chapter 29) should be performed either in advance of or concomitantly with upper airway control measures.

Exposure

In the ED, the left anterolateral thoracotomy is the preferred incision of urgent access for resuscitation of the acutely injured patient in extremis (8,20,24,27,32). With the patient positioned supine, an antiseptic such as povidone-iodine should rapidly be applied to the chest wall. An incision is made at the left fourth or fifth intercostal space from the sternal border to

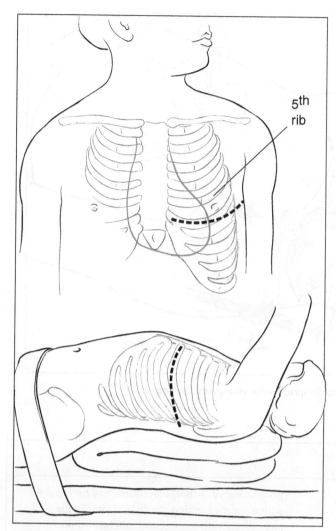

Figure 31.1 Anatomical landmarks for performance of emergency department thoracotomy.

the posterior axillary line using one large stroke. The correct line of incision usually passes just below the left nipple and follows the curve of the rib (Fig. 31.1). In females, breast tissue should be spared by manually retracting the breast superiorly, if necessary. In the young female, the clinician should avoid cutting the breast bud. If the correct interspace cannot be identified, then the incision can be started at the posterior axillary line even with the inferior tip of the scapular wing and completed at the sternal border. Once the skin incision has been completed, the intercostal tissue is cut using the Mayo scissors along the upper border of the rib so as not to damage the neurovascular bundle that runs along the lower rib margin (5).

Once the chest wall is open, the chest wall retractor ("rib spreader") is placed into the incision. Although several types of chest wall retractors are available, the Finichetto device is the most commonly used in adults and adolescents. The placement of the Finichetto retractor is critical to the success of the procedure. The bar and ratchet handle should be placed so that they are perpendicular to the base of the incision,

with the bar extending into the axilla as shown in Figure 31.2. This is opposite to the position of the retractor in the usual operating room thoracotomy (8). Insertion in this fashion allows extension of the incision into the right chest, if necessary. Once the chest wall retractor is in place, the rachet handle is used to open the ribs wide.

Exploration

After the ribs are retracted open, the next task is to control obvious hemorrhage. If an obvious site of bleeding can be readily identified, then direct pressure should be used to stop it, if possible. The source of bleeding may not be obvious, in which case blood should be evacuated from the chest to allow for better visualization. A cell saver can be used to collect the blood for use in autotransfusion (Chapter 30). If, on opening the chest, no bleeding occurs, then the pericardium should be examined and in most cases opened.

Of the several methods described for opening the pericardium, none can be considered absolutely correct; however, the two methods to be described offer advantages over the others. The pericardium should be opened by an initial incision made anterior to the phrenic nerve. This incision can be made by picking up the pericardium with a pair of forceps or a hemostat and then cutting with scissors or a scalpel. When pericardial tamponade is present, the pericardial sac may be so tense that it cannot be grasped. In this case, it can be trapped between the blades of a pair of Mayo scissors and incised in this fashion (Fig. 31.3). Once the pericardium is open, the incision should be extended widely, which allows for easy exploration of the myocardium and prevents herniation of the heart through a small opening. Such herniation can inhibit myocardial function by constricting the inflow and outflow tracts of the heart and can be very difficult to relieve.

The next stage of the procedure depends somewhat on the findings after the pericardium is incised. If opening the pericardium relieves a tamponade, then all clots should be removed from the pericardial space, and the myocardium should be quickly explored to identify the source of bleeding, usually an atrial or ventricular laceration. When such a laceration is found, it should be occluded so as to stop the hemorrhage. For a ventricular injury, the first method to use is to place a fingertip over the bleeding site and apply direct pressure. More protracted occlusion of a ventricular laceration can be accomplished by passing a sterile Foley catheter through the hole, inflating the balloon, and then placing traction on the catheter, which in turn pulls the balloon against the hole. Additionally, the lumen of the catheter may be used to rapidly infuse large quantities of fluid. In the case of an atrial laceration, a vascular (Satinsky) clamp may be used to temporarily close the defect. These techniques are shown in Figure 31.4.

Once the defect has been occluded and resuscitation efforts are well underway, the injury to the heart should be definitively closed with suture material. For atrial lacerations, a simple running stitch using 3.0 nonabsorbable suture can be used. Most ventricular lacerations can be closed with

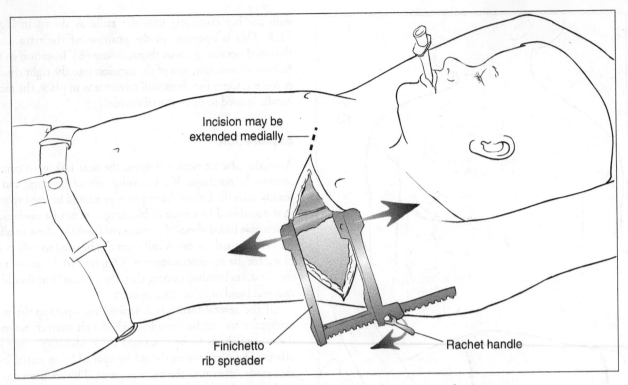

Figure 31.2 Correct placement of the Finichetto rib spreader for emergency thoracotomy.

 SUMMARY

1 Rapidly apply sterile povidone-iodine solution to chest wall.

2 Make incision at fourth or fifth costal interspace from sternum along rib margin to posterior axillary line, cutting through skin and muscles of chest wall.

3 Cut through intercostal muscles with heavy scissors along upper rib margin.

4 Insert Finichetto chest wall retractor with bar extending into axilla and use ratchet handle to open ribs.

5 Using suction, remove any blood obstructing a clear view of heart. Remember that blood can be saved for autotransfusion.

6 Open pericardium anterior to phrenic nerve. Remove any blood or clots and explore myocardium for injuries. Remember to keep heart as warm as possible through use of warm saline and/or heat lamps.

7 Apply direct pressure to any sites of hemorrhage from heart; pressure should be maintained until injury can be definitively repaired.

8 Repair any myocardial injuries, if possible. Be careful to avoid damage to coronary arteries or phrenic nerve. Atrial lacerations may be repaired with a simple running stitch, and ventricular lacerations with interrupted stitches reinforced with Teflon pledgets.

9 If no myocardial injury is found, retract left lung out of chest anteriorly and superiorly. Identify aorta, separate it from esophagus and prevertebral fascia, and occlude it using fingers, a vascular clamp, vascular tape, or an aortic tamponade device.

10 Extend incision into right chest by making a right-sided thoracotomy incision identical to left-sided one and then cutting sternum with a sternal saw or a Lebsche knife. Ligate internal mammary arteries, if possible.

11 Explore thoracic cavity for other sources of bleeding and apply pressure to any bleeding site identified. Vessels that can be exposed may be cross-clamped.

12 If heart is beating spontaneously, continue resuscitation with fluids and blood. If not, begin open cardiac massage and then defibrillate using internal paddles.

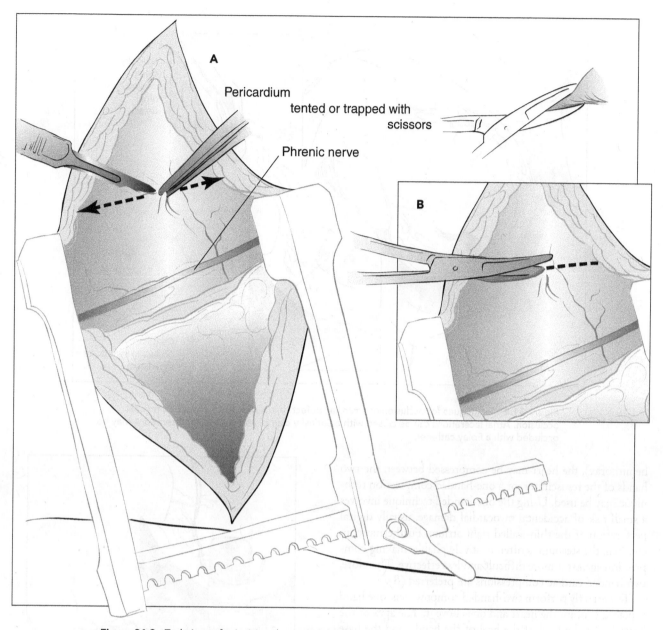

Figure 31.3 Techniques for incising the pericardium.
A. The pericardium may be grasped with a pair of forceps and then nicked with a scalpel.
B. The pericardium may be trapped between the blades of a pair of scissors, then cut.

simple interrupted sutures (2.0 or 3.0). Nonabsorbable sutures should be used. The suture material is passed beneath the occluding finger or about the Foley catheter and then tied (Fig. 31.5). If a Foley catheter has been used as a temporizing measure, care must be taken to avoid pulling the catheter through the heart wound or puncturing the catheter balloon with the needle. Ventricular wall, like all muscle tissue, separates easily, making suturing somewhat difficult. Some of this difficulty can be overcome by placing Teflon pledgets on either side of the laceration to reinforce the tissues. If the laceration is in close proximity to a coronary artery or to the phrenic nerve, then a mattress stitch (Fig. 31.5) should be used to prevent ligation of the artery or nerve. Finally, if the heart

is beating, the repairs previously described may be difficult or impossible to accomplish. If this proves to be the case, then the temporizing maneuvers should be continued until the patient can be taken to the operating room and placed on cardiopulmonary bypass.

Once pericardial tamponade has been relieved, the heart may resume spontaneous activity. If not, then after identifying and closing lacerations as previously described, direct cardiac massage should be started and preparations for internal defibrillation should begin. Internal massage may be correctly performed in three ways (Fig. 31.6). The heart may be compressed from below against the sternum (unless the incision has been extended through the sternum into the right

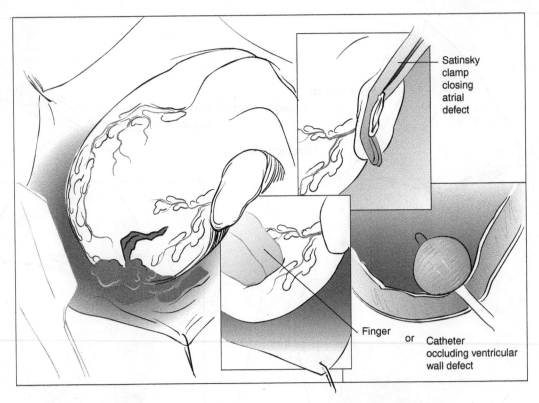

Figure 31.4 Techniques for occlusion of a cardiac defect. Initial maneuver should be manual occlusion. Atrial lacerations can be closed with a Satinsky clamp, and ventricular lacerations may be occluded with a Foley catheter.

hemithorax), the heart may be compressed between the two hands of the resuscitator, or a one-handed compression technique may be used. Using the one-handed technique involves a small risk of accidental myocardial damage, usually digital perforation of the thin-walled right atrium. Furthermore, in children, the sternum is often relatively pliable, making compression against it more difficult and less effective. Therefore, two-handed cardiac compressions are preferred (8).

To correctly perform two-handed compressions, one hand is placed beneath the heart and one above it. The apex of the heart lies at the level of the heel of the hands, and the base of the heart lies between the fingertips. The heart is compressed between the hands. Starting at the heels of the hands, pressure is progressively applied through the palm and to the fingertips. As in closed chest cardiac compression, the rate should be maintained at 100 beats per minute, if possible. During cardiac compressions with the chest open, the heart can become hypothermic relatively quickly. This hypothermia makes the myocardium resistant to defibrillation. Hypothermia can be minimized by intermittently bathing the heart in a direct stream of warm saline and by using some external warming source, such as heat lamps (5,8).

If the heart does not resume beating, then internal defibrillator paddles should be used. The paddle size for an adolescent is 6 cm, for a child 4 cm, and for an infant 2 cm. The paddles are placed in the chest as shown in Figure 31.7. Using saline-soaked pads as conductive material, one paddle

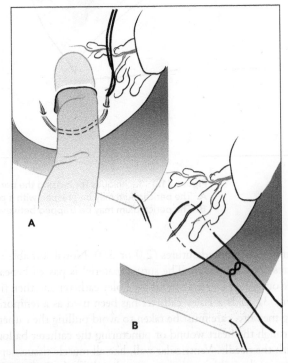

Figure 31.5
A. Definitive closure of ventricular defects may be accomplished using a simple nonabsorbable suture.
B. In cases where the laceration is in proximity to one of the coronary arteries or the phrenic nerve, a mattress stitch should be used.

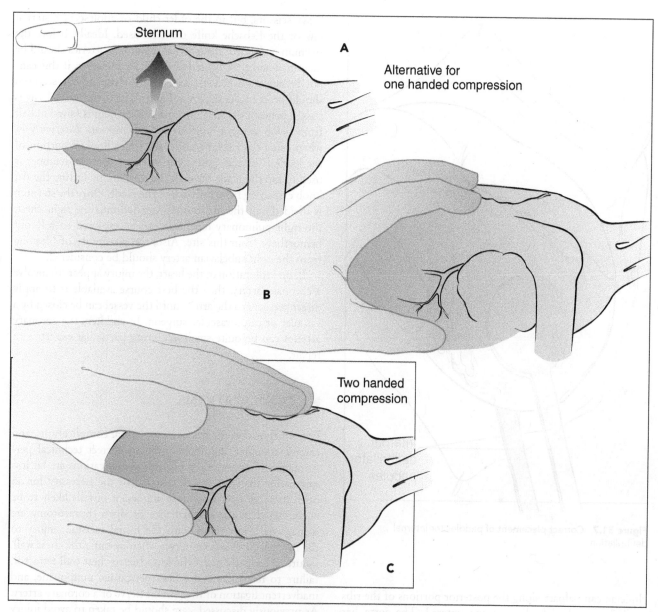

Figure 31.6 Techniques for open cardiac compressions.
A. The heart is compressed against the sternum.
B. One-handed compressions.
C. Two-handed compressions (the recommended technique).

is placed posteriorly, usually behind the left ventricle, and the other is placed anteriorly, over the right ventricle. The ideal defibrillator charge for a child in these circumstances is unknown; however, it has been suggested that starting doses should be in the range of 5 J and proceed up to 20 J. The starting dose of electricity for an adolescent is 20 J, followed by subsequent doses of 40 and 60 J, if necessary.

If no pericardial tamponade is present and no cardiac laceration can be identified, then the source of bleeding is either elsewhere in the chest or within the abdominal cavity. Bleeding elsewhere in the chest may be obvious, but if not, then the in-

cision should be extended into the right chest (see below). For suspected bleeding occurring primarily within the abdomen, as well as to improve perfusion to the brain and myocardium, the aorta should be identified and occluded. This is best accomplished by rotating the left lung anteriorly and superiorly out of the chest so that the aorta can be directly visualized or at least easily identified.

After the aorta is visualized, the mediastinal pleura is incised, and by the use of blunt dissection, the aorta is freed from its anterior attachment to the esophagus and its posterior attachment to the prevertebral fascia. Alternatively, the

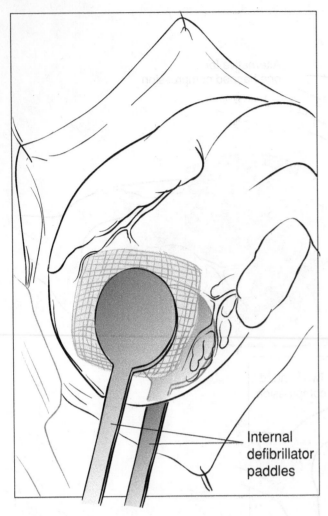

Figure 31.7　Correct placement of paddles for internal defibrillation.

clinician can palpate along the posterior portions of the ribs until the vertebral bodies are encountered. The aorta lies just anterior to the vertebral bodies. Once this has been accomplished, the aorta can be occluded without risk of damage to the aorta or to the esophagus. The initial technique for aortic occlusion is to trap the aorta between two fingers. If an extended period of aortic occlusion is anticipated, however, the aorta should be either cross-clamped using a vascular clamp, tamponaded using a specially designed instrument, or encircled with vascular tape (Fig. 31.8). Aortic occlusion to control suspected intra-abdominal hemorrhage should be a prelude to immediate transfer of the patient to the operating room for definitive exploration of the abdomen.

If, on opening the chest, the source of bleeding appears to be from the right chest, then the incision should be extended across the sternum. The right-sided incision is made in exactly the same fashion as the left-sided one. Dividing the sternum in a small child can be accomplished using a pair of heavy scissors, but in the older child or adolescent a sternal saw or the Lebsche knife must be used. Ideally, before the sternum is divided, the internal mammary arteries should be identified and then ligated (Fig. 31.9). However, if this cannot be accomplished quickly, then division of the sternum should proceed. As shown in Figure 31.10, the sternal saw is passed beneath the sternum, and the sternum is sawed in half from below using a rapid to-and-fro motion. Alternatively, when using the Lebsche knife, the sharp hooked portion of the blade is placed against the sternum, and the hammer is used to tap the blade through the sternum by hitting the flat knob extending from the back of the blade. Once the sternum is divided and the incision is extended into the right chest, the right pulmonary hilar area can be explored to rule out hemorrhage from this site. Also, the possibility of bleeding from the right subclavian artery should be considered.

If, on exploration of the heart, the injury appears to involve a coronary artery, then the best course available is to apply direct pressure to the artery until the vessel can be closed by a vascular or cardiovascular surgeon. In children, the coronary arteries can be quite small, requiring particular expertise to repair.

▶ COMPLICATIONS

Exigent thoracotomy has many potential complications, and careful attention should be given to correct technical performance. However, most of these complications are far less worrisome than the injury that led to the necessity for an open thoracotomy. The most important pitfalls likely to be encountered in the performance of open thoracotomy are damage to breast tissue with the initial incision, injury to the intercostal vessels or nerves when opening the chest wall, failure to properly insert the Finochietto chest wall retractor, failure to recognize and relieve pericardial tamponade, and inadvertent ligation of the phrenic nerve or a coronary artery. As previously discussed, care should be taken to avoid injury to the breast tissue in female patients. In young children, the incision should be made so as to avoid cutting the breast bud, and in adolescents the breast should be retracted superiorly out of the line of the incision (8).

The neurovascular bundles of the ribs lie along the lower rib margins. When opening the chest wall, the intercostal tissues should be cut near the upper border of the rib to avoid injury to these structures. Intercostal arteries, if damaged, are a potential source of significant bleeding.

The Finochietto retractor should be inserted so that the bar and ratchet handle are at the base of the incision, with the bar extending into the patient's axilla. This allows the incision to be extended into the right chest if necessary. Placement of this device in the more traditional thoracotomy position, with the bar at the top (anterior portion) of the incision, prevents extension because the bar blocks any attempt to cut through the sternum.

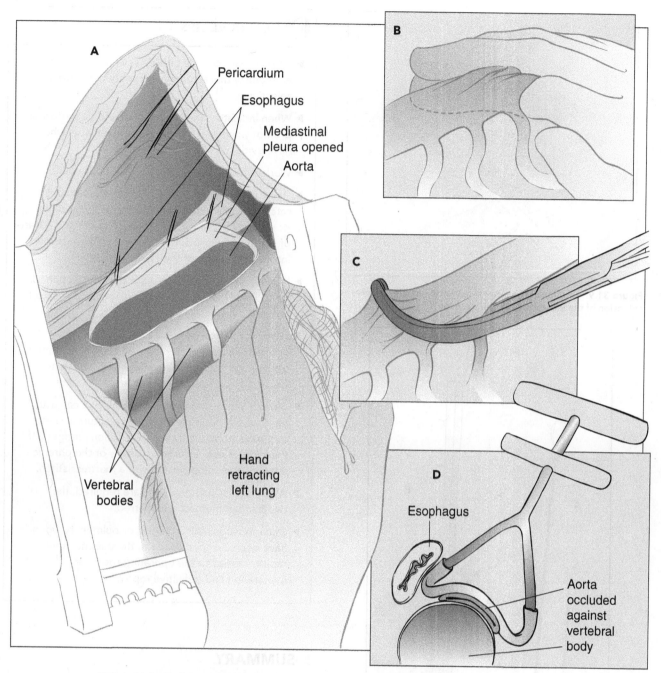

Figure 31.8 Occlusion of the aorta.
A. Anatomical landmarks visible after the left lung is manually retracted.
B. Manual occlusion of the aorta.
C. Aortic occlusion using a vascular clamp.
D. Aortic occlusion by compression against the vertebral bodies using a compression-type aortic occlusion device.

Pericardial tamponade can be difficult to recognize on inspection alone. Most authorities recommend opening the pericardium in every case so as not to miss this very treatable entity. Once the pericardium is incised, the incision should be extended widely to avoid herniation of the myocardium through the incision, with subsequent restriction of myocardial function.

When an injury to the myocardium is near one of the coronary arteries or the phrenic nerve, it must be repaired carefully to avoid accidental ligation of either of these structures. Lacerations should be repaired using a mattress-type stitch, as shown in Figure 31.5. The suture material is passed beneath the structure and tied parallel to it. Notably, even in the best of circumstances, the child's survival is far from ensured.

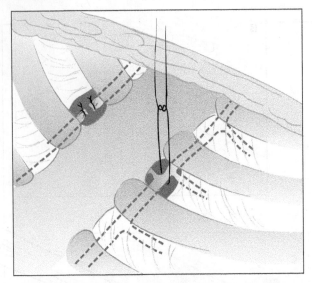

Figure 31.9 Ligation of the internal mammary arteries before extension of the incision across the sternum.

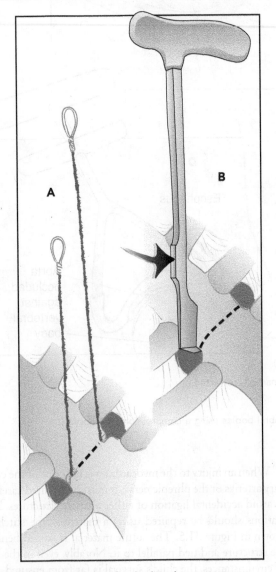

Figure 31.10 Techniques for dividing the sternum.
A. Use of a sternal saw.
B. Use of a Lebsche knife.

CLINICAL TIPS

▶ The clinician must be familiar with the indications for emergency thoracotomy and apply this technique selectively.

▶ When indicated, thoracotomy should be performed promptly. Survival is more likely in patients who have evidence of cardiac activity.

▶ Work quickly—in this situation, seconds count.

▶ Insert the Finichetto retractor with the bar and ratchet handle extending into the axilla (upside down and backward). This places the bar at the base of the incision, allowing extension of the incision into the right side of the chest, if needed.

▶ In most cases, the pericardium should be opened. Tamponade can be difficult to diagnose on clinical grounds alone.

▶ When the pericardium is opened, it should be opened widely. This prevents accidental herniation of the heart through a small opening, which may result in further restriction of cardiac function.

▶ When a ventricular injury is identified, it can usually be closed with simple interrupted sutures. These may have to be reinforced with Teflon pledgets. If the injury is near a coronary artery or the phrenic nerve, it should be closed with a mattress stitch.

▶ When cardiac compressions are required, the two-handed method is preferred.

▶ Once exsanguinating cardiac or pulmonary wounds have been clamped or sewn, the patient should be rapidly moved to the operating room for exploration and definitive repair.

▶ SUMMARY

Open resuscitative thoracotomy has the potential to be life saving if employed promptly in properly selected patients. However, the success of this technique relies upon rapid exposure of the intrathoracic organs and equally rapid control of hemorrhage. Because correction of cardiac tamponade and direct injury to the heart offers the best chance of survival, exploration of these areas should be undertaken first. If no cardiac injury is present, then the search for another source of intrathoracic bleeding should begin. Cross-clamping of the aorta may provide for temporary control of intra-abdominal hemorrhage pending laparotomy. While there are many potential complications of this procedure, even a perfectly performed open thoracotomy offers only a slim chance for long-term survival.

▶ ACKNOWLEDGMENT

The authors would like to thank Dr. David Wagner for his contribution as coauthor of the version of this chapter published in the first edition of this text.

▶ REFERENCES

1. Beaver BL, Colombani PM, Buck JR, et al. Efficacy of emergency room thoracotomy in pediatric trauma. *J Pediatr Surg.* 1987;22:19–23.
2. Boyd M, Vanek VW, Bourguet CC. Emergency room resuscitative thoracotomy: when is it indicated? *J Trauma.* 1992;33:714–721.
3. Brown SE, Gomez GA. Penetrating chest trauma: should indications for emergency thoracotomy be limited? *Am Surg.* 1996;62:530–533; discussion 533–534.
4. Calkins CM, Bensard DD, Partrick DA, et al. A critical analysis of outcome for children sustaining cardiac arrest after blunt trauma. *J Pediatr Surg.* 2002;37:180–184.
5. Durham LA III, Richardson RJ, Wall MJ Jr, et al. Emergency center thoracotomy: impact of prehospital resuscitation. *J Trauma.* 1992;32:775–779.
6. Eckstein M. Termination of resuscitative efforts: medical futility for the trauma patient. *Curr Opin Crit Care.* 2001;7:450–454.
7. Esposito TJ, Jurkovich GJ, Rice CL, et al. Reappraisal of emergency room thoracotomy in a changing environment. *J Trauma.* 1991;31:881–885; discussion 885–887.
8. Feliciano DV, Mattox KL. Indications, technique and pitfalls of emergency center thoracotomy. *Surg Rounds.* 1981;32–37:40.
9. Grove CA, Lemmon G, Anderson G, et al. Emergency thoracotomy: appropriate use in the resuscitation of trauma patients. *Am Surg.* 2002;68:313–316; discussion 316–317.
10. Ivatury RR, Kazigo J, Rohman M, et al. "Directed" emergency room thoracotomy: a prognostic prerequisite for survival. *J Trauma.* 1991;31:1076–1081; discussion 1081–1082.
11. Kavolius J, Golocovsky M, Champion HR. Predictors of outcomes in patients who have sustained trauma and who undergo emergency thoracotomy. *Arch Surg.* 1993;128:1158–1162.
12. Millham FH, Grindlinger GA. Survival determinants in patients undergoing emergency room thoracotomy for penetrating chest injury. *J Trauma.* 1993;34:332–336.
13. Rhee PM, Acosta J, Bridgeman A, et al. Survival after emergency department thoracotomy: review of published data from the past 25 years. *J Am Coll Surg.* 2000;190:288–298.
14. Sheikh AA, Culbertson CB. Emergency department thoracotomy in children: rationale for selective application. *J Trauma.* 1993;34:323–328.
15. Hoth JJ, Scott MJ, Bullock TK, et al. Thoracotomy for blunt trauma: traditional indications may not apply. *Am Surg.* 2003;69:1108–1111.
16. Inci I, Ozcelik C, Nizam O, et al. Penetrating chest injuries in children: a review of 94 cases. *J Pediatr Surg.* 1996;31:673–676.
17. Jahangiri M, Hyde J, Griffin S, et al. Emergency thoracotomy for thoracic trauma in the accident and emergency department: indications and outcome. *Ann R Coll Surg Engl.* 1996;78(3 Pt. 1):221–224.
18. Keogh SP, Wilson AW. Survival following pre-hospital arrest with on-scene thoracotomy for a stabbed heart. *Injury.* 1996;27:525–527.
19. Kuisma M, Suominen P, Korpela R. Pediatric out-of-hospital cardiac arrests: epidemiology and outcome. *Resuscitation.* 1995;30:141–150.
20. Lorenz HP, Steinmetz B, Lieberman J, et al. Emergency thoracotomy: survival correlates with physiologic status. *J Trauma.* 1992;32:780–785; discussion 785–788.
21. Mazzorana V, Smith RS, Morabito DJ, et al. Limited utility of emergency department thoracotomy. *Am Surg.* 1994;60:516–522.
22. Powell RW, Gill EA, Jurkovich GJ, et al. Resuscitative thoracotomy in children and adolescents. *Am Surg.* 1988;54:188–191.
23. Reilly JP, Brandt ML, Mattox KL, et al. Thoracic trauma in children. *J Trauma.* 1993;34:329–331.
24. Karmy-Jones R, Nathens A, Jurkovich GJ, et al. Urgent and emergent thoracotomy for penetrating chest trauma. *J Trauma.* 2004;56:664–668; discussion 668–669.
25. Polhgeers A, Ruddy RM. An update on pediatric trauma. *Emerg Med Clin North Am.* 1995;13:267–289.
26. Rehn L. Veber penetriren den herzwunden und hertnacht. *Arch Clin Chir.* 1896;55:315.
27. von Oppell UO, Bautz P, DeGroot M. Penetrating thoracic injuries: what we have learnt. *Thorac Cardiovasc Surg.* 2000;48:55–61.
28. Brewer LA. Wounds of the chest in war and peace. *Ann Thorac Surg.* 1969;7:387–408.
29. Moore KL. The thorax. In: Moore KL, ed. *Clinically Oriented Anatomy.* 2nd ed. Baltimore: Williams & Wilkins; 1985.
30. Woodburne RT, ed. *The Chest in Essentials of Human Anatomy.* 6th ed. New York: Oxford University Press; 1978.
31. Bircher N, Safar P. Manual open-chest cardiopulmonary resuscitation. *Ann Emerg Med.* 1984;13(9 Pt. 2):770–773.
32. Alzaga-Fernandez AG, Varon, J. Open-chest cardiopulmonary resuscitation: past, present, and future. *Resuscitation.* 2005;64:149–156.
33. Mattox KL, Espada R, Beall AC, et al. Performing thoracotomy in the emergency center. *JACEP.* 1974;3:13–17.
34. Siemens R, Polk HC, Gray LA, et al. Indications for thoracotomy following penetrating thoracic injury. *J Trauma.* 1977;17:493–500.
35. MacDonald JR, McDowell RM. Emergency department thoracotomies in a community hospital. *JACEP.* 1978;7:423–428.
36. Moore EE, Moore JB, Galloway AC, et al. Postinjury thoracotomy in the emergency department: a critical evaluation. *Surgery.* 1979;6:590–598.
37. Baker CC, Thomas AN, Trunkey DD. The role of emergency department thoracotomy in trauma. *J Trauma.* 1980;20:848–855.
38. Harnar TJ, Oreskovich MD, Copass MK, et al. Role of emergency thoracotomy in the resuscitation of moribund trauma victims: 100 consecutive cases. *Am J Surg.* 1981;142:96–99.
39. Cogbill TH, Moore EE, Millikan JS, et al. Rationale for selective application of emergency department thoracotomy in trauma. *J Trauma.* 1983;23:453–460.
40. Shimazu S, Shatney CH. Outcomes of trauma patients with no vital signs on hospital admission. *J Trauma.* 1983;23:213–216.
41. Hoyt DB, Shackford SR, Davis JW, et al. Thoracotomy during trauma resuscitations: an appraisal by board certified general surgeons. *J Trauma.* 1989;29:1318–1321.
42. Lorenz HP, Steinmetz B, Lieberman J, et al. Emergency thoracotomy: survival correlates with physiologic status. *J Trauma.* 1992;32:780–788.
43. Bodai BL, Smith JP, Blaisdell FW. The role of emergency thoracotomy in blunt trauma. *J Trauma.* 1982;22:487–491.
44. Mansour MA, Moore EE, Moore FA. Exigent postinjury thoracotomy: analysis of blunt vs. penetrating trauma. *Surg Gynecol Obstet.* 1992;175:97–101.
45. Tyburski JG, Astra L, Wilson RF, et al. Factors affecting prognosis with penetrating wounds of the heart. *J Trauma.* 2000;48:587–591.
46. Rothenberg SS, Moore EE, Moore FA, et al. Emergency department thoracotomy in children: a critical analysis. *J Trauma.* 1989;29:1322–1324.
47. Torphy DE, Minter MG, Thompson GM. Cardiorespiratory arrest and resuscitation of children. *Am J Dis Child.* 1984;138:1099–1102.
48. Ludwig S, Fleisher G. Pediatric cardiopulmonary resuscitation: a review and a proposal. *Pediatr Emerg Care.* 1985;1:40–44.

49. McCray E. Occupational risk of acquired immuno-deficiency syndrome among health care workers. *N Engl J Med*. 1986;314:1127.

50. Perron AD, Sing RF, Branas CC, et al. Predicting survival in pediatric trauma patients receiving cardiopulmonary resuscitation in the prehospital setting. *Prehosp Emerg Care*. 2001;5:6–9.

51. Tayal VS, Beatty MA, Marz JA, et al. FAST (focused assessment with sonography in trauma) accurate for cardiac and intraperitoneal injury in penetrating anterior chest trauma. *J Ultrasound Med*. 2004;23:467–472.

52. Rozycki GS, Feliciano DV, Oschner MG, et al. The role of ultrasound in patients with possible penetrating cardiac wounds: a perspective multicenter study. *J Trauma*. 1999;46:543–551; discussion 551–552.

FLOYD S. OTA

32

Retrograde Urethrography and Cystography

▶ INTRODUCTION

Early recognition and treatment of injury to the pediatric lower genitourinary tract following trauma can prevent significant morbidity. Pediatric bladder and urethral injuries are most commonly seen in association with pelvic fractures from blunt motor vehicle trauma. Other injury mechanisms include straddle injury, penetrating trauma, and iatrogenic injury (e.g., during bladder catheterization) (1,2). The incidence of lower genitourinary tract injuries is reported to range from 7% to 28% among adult patients with pelvic fractures (3,4). In similarly injured children, this incidence appears to be much lower, ranging from 0.9% to 8% (5–9).

Retrograde urethrography and cystography are diagnostic procedures that have been used to evaluate the lower genitourinary tract following traumatic injury. The history of retrograde cystography dates back to the early 20th century. In 1905, the techniques of retrograde cystography and pyelography using Kollargol, a silver-containing preparation, were introduced by Volecker and Von Lichentberg (10). Since their introduction, these techniques have become widely available, aided, in part, by the development of newer and safer iodinated contrast agents (10).

The popularity and diagnostic utility of computed tomography (CT) in the evaluation of the patient with trauma is increasing. However, CT alone cannot replace retrograde urethrography and/or cystography in the complete evaluation of lower genitourinary tract injuries (4,8,11). For example, contrast-enhanced abdominal and pelvic CT cannot completely examine the urethra, differentiate intra-abdominal urine from blood, or determine the location of a bladder injury, and it may fail to detect small tears if the bladder is not fully distended by contrast during the study (8,11)

(Fig. 32.1). Retrograde urethrography and cystography remain two readily available procedures that can provide important structural and functional information during emergency department evaluation.

▶ ANATOMY AND PHYSIOLOGY

The urogenital diaphragm divides the male urethra into two portions, anterior and posterior. The penile urethra and bulbous urethra make up the anterior portion. The membranous urethra and prostatic urethra make up the posterior portion. The anterior urethra is more commonly injured by blunt trauma (straddle injury) or penetrating trauma, whereas posterior urethral injury is often associated with pelvic fractures.

Bladder injuries include bladder contusions and ruptures (intraperitoneal or extraperitoneal). Extraperitoneal rupture is more common and is often seen with pelvic fractures. Intraperitoneal ruptures generally occur at the dome of the bladder as the result of blunt lower abdominal trauma when the bladder is full of urine. Finally, it should be noted that there are other possible causes of hematuria. Hematuria in a child following relatively minor trauma may be the first sign of an occult renal anomaly or kidney disease (e.g., glomerulonephritis, hydronephrosis, Wilms tumor).

▶ RETROGRADE URETHROGRAPHY AND CYSTOGRAPHY

Indications

Retrograde urethrography and cystography may be emergently indicated in the evaluation of blunt or penetrating trauma to

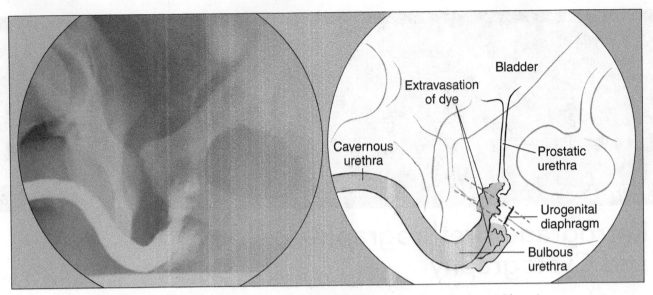

Figure 32.1 Retrograde urethrogram demonstrating extravasation of contrast material from the proximal urethra.

the perineum, penis, or pelvis to evaluate the integrity of the urethra and bladder (1,2,4,8,9,12). Urethral tears and bladder injuries should be suspected whenever there is the finding of blood at the urethral meatus, gross hematuria, an inability to void, or an abnormal genital examination (scrotal hematoma or direct trauma to the penis) (1,2,4,9). An injured child with a pelvic fracture and isolated microscopic hematuria (less than 50 RBC per high-powered field) does not require imaging of the lower genitourinary tract (9,11). The evidence suggests that in the pediatric population there is a low incidence of urethral injuries associated with pelvic fractures (7–9). Furthermore, in the absence of gross hematuria, no clinically significant injuries were found in one study of 212 children with pelvic fractures (9).

In the setting of an injured child with pelvic arterial bleeding, pelvic angiography takes precedence over urethrography, even if there is a clinical suspicion of a urethral disruption, because extravasated contrast material from the lower genitourinary tract may obscure areas of bleeding from small pelvic vessels (10). Furthermore, retrograde urethrography should always be performed prior to cystography because a known urethral injury is a contraindication to transurethral bladder catheterization. Thus, when difficulty is encountered passing a urethral catheter following lower abdominal trauma, no further attempts should be made. Additional attempts at catheterization may convert a partial urethral tear into a complete tear, increasing morbidity and the complexity of management (1,4). In the presence of a complete urethral injury, prompt consultation with a pediatric surgical specialist for possible suprapubic cystostomy and/or surgical repair is indicated.

▶ PROCEDURE

Retrograde Urethrography

Before the procedure begins, the equipment should be checked, and if a Foley catheter is being used, the balloon should be tested with normal saline. Patient size and equipment availability may dictate whether a Foley catheter or feeding tube is used. In infants, a small feeding tube may be all that is available (see Table 32.1 for approximate sizes based on patient age). The catheter is then moistened with normal saline. In general, lubricant should not be used because it may cause the catheter to fall out with injection of the contrast. The feeding tube or Foley catheter should be filled with contrast media prior to insertion. With the patient in a supine position and the penis sterilely draped and cleansed, the feeding tube or Foley catheter should then be placed into the distal penile urethra and advanced to the level of the base of the

TABLE 32.1	ESTIMATED URETHRAL CATHETER SIZE
Age	**Catheter size**
Newborn	5 French (feeding tube)
3 mo	8 French
1 y	8–10 French
3 y	10 French
6 y	10 French
8 y	10–12 French
10 y	12 French
12 y	12–14 French
Teen/adult	16+ French

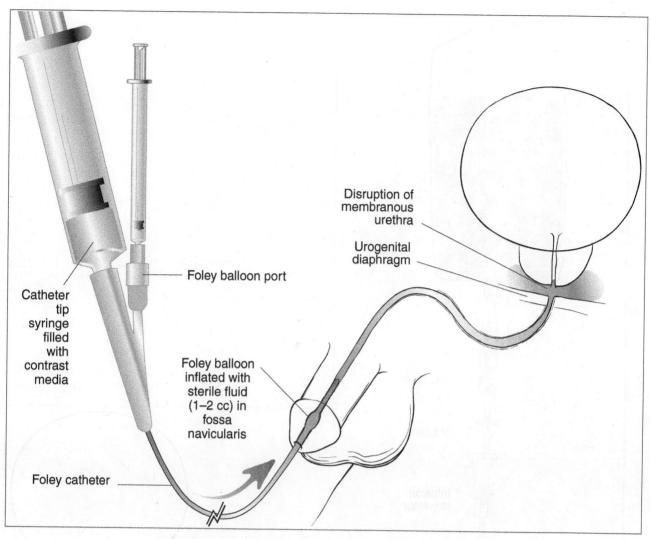

Figure 32.2 The Foley catheter technique for retrograde urethrography.

glans penis or slightly beyond. The catheter should fill the urethral lumen so that contrast is less likely to flow distally with injection. In the adolescent or adult patient, some authorities recommend inflating the Foley balloon in the fossa navicularis with 1 to 2 mL of saline to secure the position of the catheter and prevent leakage of the contrast back out of the meatus. If this advice is followed, extreme caution should be exercised in order to prevent traumatizing the urethra. If the Foley technique is used, a 30- or 60-mL catheter-tipped syringe containing contrast media may be connected to the distal port of the catheter (Fig. 32.2). If a feeding tube is used as the urethral catheter, it may be connected to i.v. tubing, the proximal end of which is inserted into a bottle of contrast media or simply attached to a syringe filled with media.

Regardless of the method chosen, care should be taken to prime the tubing and catheters so that a significant volume of air is not injected into the urethra and bladder. A scout film should be obtained after catheter insertion. The urethra

should be filled using 15 to 30 mL of contrast media (less is necessary in younger patients), while films of the penis and lower pelvis are obtained with the radiograph beam at a 30- or 40-degree oblique projection. Once the integrity of the urethra has been confirmed radiographically, the catheter may be advanced to the level of the bladder for the cystography portion of the study. If the Foley balloon had been inflated, it should be deflated before advancement.

Retrograde Cystography

Once the bladder has been catheterized, its contents should be drained, and an anteroposterior (AP) film of the pelvis should be obtained as a scout film. Contrast media is then instilled by gravity from a hanging bottle of contrast media connected to i.v. tubing (Fig. 32.3) or by slow injection (Foley technique) until the patient experiences discomfort or the predicted volume has been instilled (Table 32.2 lists

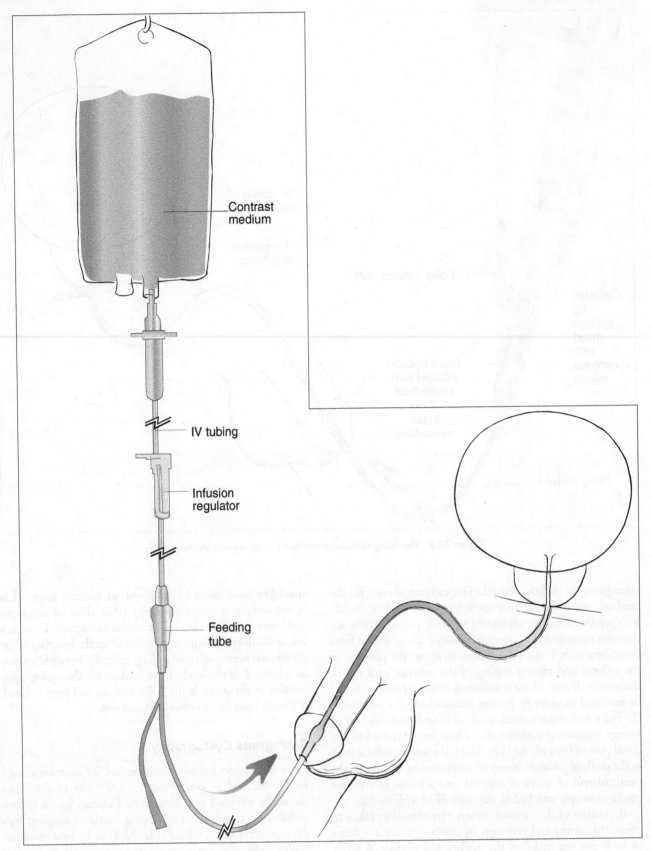

Contrast medium

IV tubing

Infusion regulator

Feeding tube

Figure 32.3 Technique for retrograde cystography.

TABLE 32.2	FORMULA FOR PREDICTING BLADDER CAPACITY
Age	**Bladder capacity**
<1 y	wt (kg) × 10 = mL
>1 y	(age + 2) × 30 = mL*

*Maximum volume = 400 mL.

the formula for calculating predicted bladder capacity based on age). If fluoroscopy is used, radiation exposure should be brief and intermittent to minimize gonadal irradiation. AP and oblique radiographs of the pelvis should be obtained in an attempt to identify intraperitoneal or extraperitoneal extravasation from bladder rupture. Once adequate films have been obtained with a contrast-filled bladder, the bladder is drained and postdrainage films are obtained to avoid missing extravasated contrast material that might have been hidden by the contrast-filled bladder.

▶ COMPLICATIONS

Complications related to retrograde urethrography and cystourethrography include bleeding and catheter-related trauma to the urethra and/or bladder. Iatrogenic trauma to the urethra can result in the development of urethral strictures.

Adverse reactions to intravenous contrast agents occur in approximately 3.8% to 12% of patients receiving the higher osmolality agents and in 0.7% to 3.1% of patients receiving nonionic contrast material (13). Adverse reactions to contrast applied in a retrograde fashion, through the lower urogenital tract, are rare but still reported in the literature, presumably because a small amount of contrast is absorbed into the blood stream when injected into the bladder (14,15). Hypersensitivity reactions to intravenous contrast can be divided in to two categories, immediate (less than 1 hour) and nonimmediate (more than 1 hour) (13,16). The most significant risk factor for immediate sensitivity reaction is a previous immediate reaction (13,16). Other risk factors are severe allergies, cardiac disease, and bronchial asthma. Risk factors for nonimmediate reactions are a previous nonimmediate reaction, serum creatinine greater than 2.0, interleukin-2 treatment, and severe allergies (13,16). Manifestations of an immediate reaction may range from pruritus and urticaria to severe anaphylaxis and shock (13). Nonimmediate reactions are more insidious and may present with a macular or papular rash, angioedema, and, in severe cases, Stevens-Johnson syndrome, toxic epidermal necrolysis, or a cutaneous vasculitis (13). In adult patients,

---

SUMMARY: RETROGRADE URETHROCYSTOGRAPHY

1 Prime Foley catheter or feeding tube and i.v. tubing or syringe with contrast agent.

2 Sterilely drape and prep penis for catheter insertion.

3 Insert Foley or feeding tube into distal penile urethra with tip at base of glans (no lubricant).

4 Obtain a scout film of penis and/or lower pelvis.

5 Inject 15 to 30 mL contrast into penile urethra and obtain a spot film with radiograph beam at a 30- to 40-degree oblique angle to penis.

6 Once urethral integrity is confirmed radiographically, advance catheter to level of bladder.

7 Drain bladder of its contents and again obtain AP scout film of pelvis.

8 Instill or inject contrast into bladder until patient feels discomfort or predicted amount of contrast has been given (Table 32.2).

9 Obtain oblique and AP films of bladder and pelvis.

10 Empty bladder and obtain repeat films postdrainage.

CLINICAL TIPS

▶ Injury to the urethra and bladder must be considered in the evaluation of the injured male with blood at the urethral meatus, gross hematuria, an inability to void, or an abnormal genital examination (scrotal hematoma or direct trauma to the penis).

▶ If a urethral injury is suspected on the basis of history or clinical findings, then the penis should NOT be catheterized until urethral injury has been ruled out.

▶ The use of CT should always be considered for more serious trauma, particularly when the patient may have sustained injuries to other intra-abdominal or retroperitoneal structures. Evaluation of the urethra and bladder may need to be postponed until the patient is clinically stable.

▶ The patient (or parents) should be asked about previous exposure to contrast material and allergic reactions. The health care provider should be prepared to emergently treat a contrast reaction.

▶ Gross hematuria in a child following relatively minor trauma may be the first sign of an underlying occult renal anomaly or kidney disease (e.g., glomerulonephritis, hydronephrosis, or Wilm tumor).

corticosteroids are routinely administered to high-risk patients prior to receiving intravenous contrast. However, it is unclear if this practice applies to children who are undergoing a retrograde urethrogram or cystogram. Regardless, drugs to treat anaphylaxis and advanced airway equipment should be available during the procedure in case of an adverse reaction.

▶ SUMMARY

Injury to the penile urethra and bladder must be considered in the evaluation of the injured patient. The techniques described are important adjuncts to the evaluation and stabilization of many pediatric trauma victims. Retrograde urethrography must be performed prior to instrumentation or catheterization of the urethra in all males suspected of having sustained an injury to the urethra. Failure to identify such injuries may result in significant morbidity.

▶ ACKNOWLEDGMENT

The authors would like to acknowledge the valuable contributions of Cynthia C. Hoecker and Richard M. Ruddy to the version of this chapter that appeared in the previous edition.

▶ REFERENCES

1. Sandler CM, Corriere JN. Urethrography in the diagnosis of acute urethral injuries. *Urol Clin North Am.* 1989;16:283–289.
2. Holland AJ, Cohen RC, McKertich KM, et al. Urethral trauma in children. *Pediatr Surg Int.* 2001;17:58–61.
3. Koraitim MM, Marzouk ME, Atta MA, et al. Risk factors and mechanism of urethral injury in pelvic fractures. *Brit J Urol.* 1996;77:876–880.
4. Chan L, Nade S, Brooks A, et al. Experience with lower urinary tract disruptions associated with pelvic fractures: implications for emergency room management. *Aust N Z J Surg.* 1994;64:395–399.
5. Reichard SA, Helikson MA, Shorter N, et al. Pelvic fractures in children: review of 120 patients with a new look at general management. *J Pediatr Surg.* 1980;15:727–734.
6. Musemeche CA, Fischer RP, Cotler HB, et al. Selective management of pediatric pelvic fractures: a conservative approach. *J Pediatr Surg.* 1987;22:538–540.
7. Torode I, Zieg D. Pelvic fractures in children. *J Pediatr Orthop.* 1985;5:76–84.
8. McAleer IM, Kaplan GW, Scherz HC, et al. Genitourinary trauma in the pediatric patient. *Urology.* 1993;42:563–568.
9. Tarman GJ, Kaplan GW, Lerman SL, et al. Lower genitourinary injury and pelvic fractures in pediatric patients. *Pediatr Urol.* 2002;59:123–126.
10. Dunnick NR, Sandler CM, Newhouse JH, et al. *Textbook of Uroradiology.* 3rd ed. Philadelphia: Lippincott Williams & Wilkins; 2001.
11. Rehm C. Blunt traumatic bladder rupture: the role of retrograde cystogram. *Ann Emerg Med.* 1991;20:845–847.
12. Sandler CM, Phillips JM, Harris JD, et al. Radiology of the bladder and urethra in blunt pelvic trauma. *Radiol Clin North Am.* 1981;19:195–211.
13. Brockow K, Kanny G, Bircher A, et al. Management of hypersensitivity reactions in iodinated contrast media. *Allergy.* 2005;60:150–158.
14. Weese DL, Greenberg HM, Zimmern PE. Contrast media reactions during voiding cystourethrography or retrograde pyelography. *Urology.* 1993;41:81–84.
15. Currarino G, Weinberg A, Putnam R. Resorption of contrast material from the bladder during cystourethrography causing an excretory urethrogram. *Radiology.* 1977;123:149–150.
16. Christiansen C. X-ray contrast media: an overview. *Toxicology.* 2005;209:185–187.

SECTION 4 ▶ ANESTHESIA AND SEDATION PROCEDURES

SECTION EDITOR: BRENT R. KING

33

SANDRA J. CUNNINGHAM AND WASEEM HAFEEZ

Procedural Sedation and Pain Management Techniques

A second of pain lasts as long as a day of pleasure.
—Proverb

▶ INTRODUCTION

Pain can be defined as an unpleasant sensory and emotional experience arising from actual or potential tissue damage (1,2). Managing pain is a large part of emergency care, both diagnostic and therapeutic, and an assessment of pain is now considered by many as the "fifth vital sign." Most injuries are associated with pain, and it is often a marker for serious illness.

Pain is multifactorial and subjective (3). In the emergency setting, several factors affect the nature and degree of pain a child experiences. These factors are related to the child, the provider, and the procedure. Child-related factors include any underlying medical conditions, previous painful events, the culture and environment in which the child is reared, and his or her developmental, cognitive, and emotional level. Provider factors include the attitude, experience, and competence of the physician. In addition, the type of procedure, the part of the body involved, the duration of manipulation, the degree of immobility required, and the type of medication used will affect the child's perception of pain.

It is important to understand the terminology used in describing pain control. *Anesthesia* is the medically induced loss of all sensation. When sensory loss is restricted to one anatomic area, it is termed *local anesthesia*, whereas *general anesthesia* refers to a state in which the patient is completely insensate. *Analgesia* is the reduction or elimination of pain sensation (4). Lidocaine is an excellent local anesthetic because infiltration eliminates the ability to perceive pain in the area involved. Acetaminophen and ibuprofen are appropriate analgesics because they reduce the general feeling of pain. *Sedation* is the act of calming that can be achieved by pharmacologic or psychological interventions, such as distraction, cognitive behavior therapy, and hypnosis (4). Sedation can help a child cope with a painful procedure but does not by itself alleviate pain. *Procedural sedation and analgesia* refers to the technique of administering sedatives or dissociative agents with or without analgesics to induce a state that allows the patient to tolerate unpleasant procedures while maintaining independent cardiorespiratory function (5).

As shown in Table 33.1, the American Society of Anesthesiologists (ASA) has described the different levels of sedation and analgesia by taking into account the patient's response to commands as well as airway, ventilation, and cardiovascular functions (6). *Light (or minimal) sedation* is a pharmacologically induced state in which the patient can respond to verbal stimulation, albeit more slowly than normal, and should be able to follow commands. Lightly sedated patients maintain airway protective reflexes and generally experience minimal, if any, effects on the cardiovascular system. The *moderately sedated*

415

TABLE 33.1	CONTINUUM OF DEPTH OF SEDATION: DEFINITION OF ANESTHESIA			
Levels of sedation/ analgesia	Minimal sedation (anxiolysis)	Moderate sedation/analgesia	Deep sedation/analgesia	General anesthesia
Responsiveness	Normal response to verbal stimulation	Purposeful response to verbal or tactile stimulation	Purposeful response after repeated or painful stimulation	Unarousable, even with painful stimulus
Airway	Unaffected	No intervention required	Intervention may be required	Intervention often required
Spontaneous ventilation	Unaffected	Adequate	May be inadequate	Frequently inadequate
Cardiovascular function	Unaffected	Usually maintained	Usually maintained	May be impaired

Source: Adapted from Practice guidelines for sedation and analgesia by non-anesthesiologists: a report by the American Society of Anesthesiologists Task Force on Sedation and Analgesia by Non-Anesthesiologists. *Anesthesiology.* 2002;96:1005.

patient responds to verbal stimulation or light tactile stimulation but may not be able to follow commands. Airway protective reflexes are intact, and spontaneous ventilation is usually adequate. Cardiovascular function is generally not affected. Finally, the *deeply sedated* patient may experience ventilatory compromise, and airway protective reflexes are suppressed and may be lost. The patient generally requires more vigorous stimulation to elicit a response and is unlikely to be able to follow verbal commands, although cardiovascular function is typically normal. By contrast, with true general anesthesia, the normal protective airway reflexes (most importantly, closure of the epiglottis over the glottic opening with vomiting or regurgitation of stomach contents) are absent, putting the patient at risk for aspiration pneumonitis. Self-maintenance of airway patency is also much less likely (1). Sedation producing this state should only be induced in an operating room by an anesthesiologist or during rapid sequence intubation in the emergency department (ED).

Although the specific terminology just presented is now preferred over the more generic term *conscious sedation* used previously, it is important that the physician and support staff understand that these definitions are merely (somewhat arbitrary) points along a continuum that begins with full alertness and ends with general anesthesia. Any patient can be more or less sedated than was originally intended and can move in either direction along this spectrum as a result of changes in the degree of stimulation, the passage of time, or the administration of additional medication.

The physician caring for young children is faced with the challenging additional task of separating pain from anxiety and discerning which is the predominant contributor to the child's state. In the ED, there is often a need for both pain reduction and alleviation of anxiety. Some drug classes, such as benzodiazepines, do not provide analgesia but offer a significant sedative effect; other agents, like nonsteroidal anti-inflammatory drugs (NSAIDs), can relieve pain but not anxiety; while still other agents, most notably the opioids, have both effects, although their analgesic effect is predominant. It is the important responsibility of the physician to strike a balance between safety and symptom relief by choosing appropriate agents and ensuring adequate monitoring. In many cases, it is prudent to administer an anxiolytic initially, because the operator can perform a more accurate examination and

thus better assess the need for analgesia once the child is calm. Furthermore, the psychological development, pain threshold, and anxiety level of the individual must be considered on a case-by-case basis (Table 33.2). A younger child may require sedation for a painless procedure like a computed tomography (CT) scan, while an older child may need nothing more than a local anesthetic for repair of a large wound.

Common Myths

It is no longer a matter of debate that all children, including neonates, experience pain (7). However, several myths and misunderstandings about pain relating to children persist and must be dispelled. Following are some of the more common of these (8).

Myth No. 1: Compared to adults, infants experience less pain because their nervous system is immature. Neuroanatomical studies have shown that by 29 weeks of gestation the neurological pathways for the transmission and modulation of painful sensations and the cortical and subcortical centers involved in the perception of pain are well developed (9).

Myth No. 2: Infants and young children have no memory of painful experiences. Recent studies suggest that early experiences of pain, such as those associated with circumcision, may produce permanent structural and functional reorganization of developing nociceptive neural pathways that can endure in memory. This

TABLE 33.2	DEVELOPMENTAL SEQUENCE OF UNDERSTANDING PAIN
Age	**Understanding of pain**
0–3 mo	No obvious understanding; memory of pain likely but not proven; pain responses are dominated perceptually
3–6 mo	Infantile pain response persists; initiation of toddler anger response
6–18 mo	Fear response develops; words for pain appear: "ouchie," "boo-boo," etc.; localization of some pain occurs
18 mo–6 y	Prelogical thinking: concrete, egocentric, transductive logic
7–10 y	Concrete operational thinking: ability to distinguish self from environment; behavioral coping strategies
11 + y	Formal logical thinking: abstraction, introspection; cognitive coping strategies

Source: Adapted from McGrath PJ, Craig KD. Developmental and psychological factors in children's pain. *Pediatr Clin North Am.* 1989;36:826.

can cause disturbances of feeding and sleeping and can affect future experiences of pain (10).

Myth No. 3: Children need less pain medication than adults. Physicians often have an exaggerated fear of complications when using pain medication for pediatric patients, resulting in the use of less potent regimens or underdosing of medication. Oligoanalgesia is particularly prevalent in younger children, who are significantly less likely to receive analgesics, particularly opioid analgesics (11). Of note, children receiving care at a community ED are at greater risk for oligoanalgesia than those receiving care at an academic pediatric emergency center (12).

Myth No. 4: Infants and children are more sensitive to the respiratory depressant effects of narcotics. The potential for these complications is not disputed, yet there are no data to support the belief that children are more susceptible than adults to the risk of narcotic-induced respiratory depression. In fact, because of their increased metabolic rate, children often tolerate proportionally larger and more frequent doses of analgesics than adults. With an understanding of drug pharmacology, proper use of monitoring equipment, and the availability of reversal agents, clinicians can safely administer opioid analgesics to children in the ED (8).

Myth No. 5: Children are at increased risk for addiction. Despite fears to the contrary, there are no known physiologic or psychological characteristics of children that make them more vulnerable to addiction than adults (13,14).

Myth No. 6: Narcotic use may mask symptoms of intra-abdominal pathology. Morphine provides significant pain reduction to children with acute abdominal pain without adversely affecting the examination (15). The use of analgesics makes children more comfortable and facilitates both abdominal examination and diagnostic testing (e.g., ultrasound).

▶ ANATOMY AND PHYSIOLOGY

The pathway by which pain is transmitted from the skin or other organs to the brain is multifaceted and can be modulated in several ways. A peripheral stimulus for pain is detected by specialized sets of peripheral nerve endings in the skin. One set of these pain receptors, or nociceptors, is composed of thinly myelinated Aδ fibers, which conduct impulses rapidly and are responsible for the initial feeling of sharp or pricking pain. The other set of nociceptors contains unmyelinated C fibers, which conduct impulses more slowly and are responsible for longer-lasting burning or dull pain sensations (16). Because the fibers of these nociceptors are unmyelinated, they are more amenable to the effects of local anesthesia (17). Aδ fibers are located in the skin and mucous membranes; C fibers are widely distributed in deep tissues and the skin. In addition to nociceptors, thermoreceptors and mechanoreceptors are composed of Aα or Aβ fibers, which are responsible for the perception of touch and light pressure. All these receptors convert a stimulus to electrical activity, which is then transmitted through various routes in the spinal cord to the brain.

The initial cortical response is probably reflexive, but the subsequent response may be altered by cortical activity, including inputs from the frontal lobes and the limbic system (18).

Several theories have been offered to explain why other cutaneous stimuli and emotional stress can alter the quality and intensity of pain. For example, the gate control theory, hypothesized by Melzack and Wall (19), suggests that input from the Aβ touch fibers and input from the Aδ and C fibers have antagonistic effects on so-called "gate cells" in the substantia gelatinosa in the spinal cord (16). This would explain why a person who suffers a blow to the arm instinctively rubs the affected area—that is, to stimulate the touch fibers that antagonize the pain receptors—or why a cream that causes a mild burning sensation in the skin alleviates underlying muscle pain. This principle can be applied when attempting venipuncture by rubbing or slapping the skin before inserting the needle.

A variety of developmental and psychological factors, combined with responses conditioned by the environment, interact to influence a child's perception of and response to pain (20). Appreciation for the child's cognitive developmental level is mandatory for appropriate pain management. The explanation of a procedure must be age appropriate and address the fears of the patient. A developmental sequence of understanding pain is shown in Table 33.2 (21).

An understanding of some general pharmacologic principles and metabolic differences in the pediatric age group will help determine the most appropriate type of drug, the proper dosage, and the route of administration. As always with pediatric patients, one of the most challenging issues is the major age-related variations that exist from infancy through adolescence, the most obvious being body size. Although body surface area represents a highly reliable reference measurement for medication dosing in children, the child's weight in kilograms is a reasonable and more accessible alternative for clinical management. Drug dosage is determined on a per-kilogram basis throughout the early pediatric years. However, the calculated dose should serve only as a starting point. In many cases, it will be necessary to administer additional medication in a titrated fashion to achieve the desired effect. No single agent or dosage is appropriate for all children. Therefore, the medication used and the dosing regimen should be determined by the nature of the procedure and the child's psychological and physiologic makeup.

The speed of onset, peak effect, and duration of action of a given drug are determined largely by its rate of absorption and clearance. The rate of absorption is influenced by drug solubility, rate of dissolution, concentration, absorbing surface, circulation to the site of absorption, and route of administration (22). Six common routes of administration of sedative and analgesic medications used in the ED are oral, intramuscular, intravenous, subcutaneous, intranasal, and rectal. Each route has characteristic absorption patterns that may provide specific advantages depending on the clinical setting. For example, when careful titration of medication is necessary, the intravenous route is preferred.

The clinician must be aware of drug metabolism when choosing a route of administration. Alkaline drugs, such as opiates and benzodiazepines, cross cell membranes more easily than acidic drugs, because the intracellular pH is more acidic than the extracellular pH. Acidic drugs, such as barbiturates, do not enter cells as readily. The elimination half-life of alkaline drugs is usually longer, because the drugs are more widely distributed (23). Both the medication chosen and the route of administration will determine the level of sedation. Wide variation in the clinical effects of medications given in similar doses by the same route is the rule, not the exception. An understanding of physiology and pharmacokinetics does not replace careful dosing and meticulous monitoring.

Oral administration of medications is convenient and economical, but absorption may be variable and incomplete. Factors that limit or delay absorption by the oral route include a full stomach, decreased gastric emptying, and reduced small bowel surface area. Many oral medications undergo a "first pass effect" by the liver whereby they are metabolized before reaching the systemic circulation. Furthermore, many pediatric patients cannot or will not take medication orally. Nevertheless, for management of postprocedural pain, especially on an outpatient basis, the oral route is preferred.

When it is impossible or inappropriate to give oral medication, acceptable alternatives include intranasal and rectal administration. The intranasal route has been shown to be effective for certain medications such as midazolam. Midazolam is rapidly absorbed from the nasal mucosa. However, it is difficult to deliver large volumes, especially in small children, by the intranasal route, and this might make it difficult to provide an adequate dose of medication. Some medications, particularly those that are lipophilic, are well absorbed through the rectal mucosa. However, absorption can be delayed by stool in the rectum, and introduction of the medication might stimulate the urge to defecate, causing some medication to be expelled. Oral, intranasal, and rectal agents are useful for less painful procedures such as routine laceration repair, for which a local anesthetic will also be given. Additionally, these routes are often preferred when sedating a child for nonpainful diagnostic studies such as magnetic resonance imaging (MRI) or CT scans. However, as noted previously, the onset, depth, and duration of sedation are less predictable than with parenterally administered drugs.

Nitrous oxide, an inhalational agent, is appropriate for adolescents and cooperative children who are able to follow directions (see Chapter 34). When administered with a local anesthetic, it is useful for brief procedures involving mild to moderate pain. It may also be used for procedures that are merely anxiety provoking.

In most cases, subcutaneous and intramuscular administration can provide prompt and sustained absorption of the drug resulting in a smoother induction of analgesia. However, drugs given in this manner cannot be titrated. In addition, when circulation to the site of injection is poor (e.g., impaired perfusion of an extremity, large burns), absorption may be erratic. In these cases, intramuscular and subcutaneous routes

may be ineffective for the prompt delivery of pain medications. While these routes are generally associated with fewer complications at a given dose, the pain of injection to some degree defeats the purpose of the sedation and analgesia, and a child may refrain from requesting pain medications for fear of the injection.

For the management of acute pain in the ED, the intravenous route allows the most rapid and reliable delivery of medication. Intravenous analgesia usually provides immediate pain relief. Intravenous sedation should be considered for any child undergoing a very painful procedure, such as closed reduction of a fracture or incision and drainage of a large abscess. In general, the intravenous route allows the operator to safely induce a deeper and more controlled level of sedation, which not only maximizes patient comfort but also facilitates procedures requiring meticulous care by ensuring that the patient remains motionless. Precise titration of sedation and/or analgesia using incremental doses of intravenous medication prevents "overshooting" to a level of sedation that is deeper than intended. A final advantage of the intravenous route is the ability to rapidly administer reversal agents such as naloxone or flumazenil if needed. Yet the physician must also be aware of the drawbacks of intravenous administration. For example, drugs given by this route escape the first pass effect in the liver, which increases the risk of complications, because high concentrations of the drugs are achieved rapidly and overdosing may occur. Intravenous medications should therefore be administered slowly at the T connector site by an experienced provider, with constant monitoring of the patient (Fig. 33.1).

▶ INDICATIONS

Pain Management

Because pain is a subjective experience, management must be directed toward the child's perception rather than the parent's or physician's perception. Pain management techniques should be used any time a child complains of pain. Unfortunately, attentiveness to pain control in children is usually inadequate (9,11,13). Although children, including neonates, exhibit significant stress responses (24), the responses often are not well appreciated by the provider. As opposed to adult patients who clearly verbalize their discomfort, a child's cry is nonspecific and often misinterpreted. This is particularly true in nonverbal children.

Difficulty in pediatric pain assessment results from the inability of the young child to clearly articulate the extent of discomfort. Assessment techniques include patient self-reports, behavioral observation, and physiologic measures. Accurate evaluation utilizes components of all three parameters. In the older child with well-developed verbal skills, self-reported pain assessment is an effective guide to pain management. Many have found objective instruments to be the most effective means of performing this assessment, because they allow for comparison at various time points. Similar scales are also

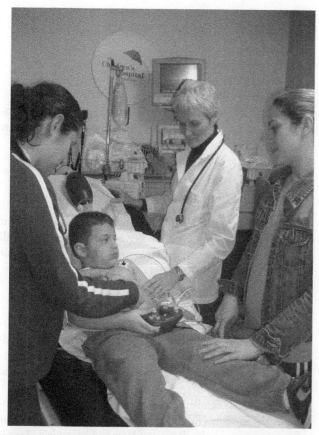

Figure 33.1 Procedure for moderate sedation and analgesia. Procedural sedation and analgesia are being administered to patient by adequate personnel with concurrent monitoring of vital signs and pulse oximetry. Patient is being distracted by playing a video game with parental presence to calm him.

TABLE 33.3	AMERICAN SOCIETY OF ANESTHESIOLOGISTS RISK CLASSIFICATIONS
ASA Class I	Healthy patient
ASA Class II	Mild systemic disease: no functional limitations or well-controlled disease
ASA Class III	Severe systemic disease: definite functional limitations or disease not well controlled
ASA Class IV	Severe systemic disease: constant threat to life
ASA Class V	Moribund patient: unlikely to survive 24 hours

available for younger children. Commonly used instruments include (1) the linear analogue scale (a horizontal line with no pain and severe pain at each end; the child marks the line at any point to indicate pain intensity) (25), the "Oucher scale" (a photographic scale of six facial expressions with a numerical 0 to 10 scale) (26), and the "Faces scale" (cartoon drawings of faces from no pain to crying) (27). Objective evaluation is more difficult in infants, but a combination of behavioral and physiological measures—such as facial expression, body movement, crying, eye squeeze, tachycardia, and hypertension—have been demonstrated as indicative of pain (28,29).

Despite concerns on the part of some physicians that pain medications might "mask" symptoms and thereby impede the diagnostic evaluation, it is generally acceptable to provide analgesia to children with abdominal pain, headache after head trauma, and other such conditions. In fact, there is some evidence that pain medications can aid in the diagnostic evaluation by causing diffuse pain to become more localized. Furthermore, it is worth noting that the proscription against administration of pain medications in these situations came about in a bygone era, one that lacked the advanced diagnostic and monitoring technology that we enjoy today. Certainly,

once a diagnosis is confirmed (e.g., deciding to operate on a child with appendicitis) or excluded (e.g., a negative head CT scan in a child with head trauma), there is usually no compelling reason to withhold analgesics.

Sedation

The goals of sedation should be to ensure the patient's safety, minimize pain and discomfort, diminish negative psychological responses, maximize any amnesic effects, and provide a rapid return to a baseline state of functioning. The method of sedation chosen must always be tailored to the clinical situation. In many cases, a combination of medications and techniques will be required to achieve the desired goals. Relaxation and behavior therapy should be tried in most children. The decision to use physical restraints or pharmacologic therapy is based on the child's cognitive development and general temperament, combined with the actual or anticipated pain of the event.

Proper patient selection is critical to the safe administration of sedation. For the emergency physician, there are three important considerations. First is the patient's general state of health. Some patients, by virtue of comorbidities or underlying medical conditions, are not suitable candidates for sedation in the ED. The ASA classifies patients into five risk categories based on health status (Table 33.3). As a general rule, only patients in classes 1 and 2 are appropriate for sedation outside of an operating room or intensive care unit (see "Presedation Assessment"). The second consideration is the nature of the problem requiring sedation. An extensive or highly complex laceration in an otherwise healthy child might require more sedation, local anesthetic, and/or time than it is wise to give in the ED. Such patients should be managed in an operating room. Finally, the emergency physician must consider resource issues in the ED at the time. On a busy night in an understaffed ED, there may be insufficient personnel available to safely manage even a relatively minor procedure.

▶ EQUIPMENT

The equipment required for administration of pain medications depends on the agent administered or the technique used.

Nonpharmacologic techniques and common oral analgesics (acetaminophen, ibuprofen, concentrated sucrose solution for infants) can generally be administered without risk of serious side effects and require no special monitoring equipment. The more potent analgesics and sedatives, including narcotics and benzodiazepines, should be given by a physician who has experience using these medications and is familiar with the management of potential associated complications. Both a physician and a nurse must assume responsibility for monitoring the child when these medications are used. Nonpharmacologic means of sedation and local anesthetics have no risk for respiratory depression or cardiovascular compromise and therefore require little, if any, monitoring, although the clinician must be alert to the risk of allergic reaction when using local anesthetics. However, administration of agents with potentially untoward physiologic effects requires continuous electronic monitoring of cardiac rate and rhythm, respiratory rate, and pulse oximetry as well as visual and/or auscultatory assessment of respiratory effort and an assessment of mental status and response to stimulation.

Patient monitoring should be recorded on a sedation or pain-control flow sheet in the medical record. Vital signs, pulse oximeter reading, level of consciousness, response to stimulation, and color should be noted at premedication and at regular intervals (5 to 15 minutes) thereafter. The following equipment and medications should be available at the bedside:

- Monitoring equipment
  - Pulse oximeter
  - Cardiorespiratory monitor
- Resuscitation equipment
  - Intravenous line setup
  - Suction (Yankauer)
  - Oxygen source

- Bag-valve-mask circuit
- Nonrebreather face mask and nasal canula
- Oral and nasopharyngeal airway
- Laryngoscope
- Endotracheal tubes and stylets
- Pediatric defibrillator
- Resuscitation medications (including atropine, amiodarone, epinephrine, diphenhydramine, dexamethasone, lidocaine, lorazepam and vasopressin)
- Reversal agents (including naloxone and flumazenil)

Agents for Pain Management and Sedation

A variety of medications are available for pain management and sedation in the ED. The choice of a particular agent will depend on a number of factors, as previously noted. Some of the more commonly used agents are listed in Table 33.4.

Management of Mild to Moderate Pain

Medications such as aspirin, acetaminophen, and those classified as NSAIDs can be used for acute pain of mild or moderate severity in the ED. Indications include headache, superficial burns or abrasions, arthralgias, soft-tissue injuries, and dysmenorrhea.

Aspirin is an excellent anti-inflammatory drug that is infrequently used in children under 16 years of age because of its association with Reye syndrome. The aspirin dose is 10 mg/kg given every 4 to 6 hours up to six times a day. Aspirin may cause gastrointestinal irritation and interferes with hemostasis by irreversibly inhibiting platelet function for the life of the platelet. Acetaminophen is better tolerated and has fewer side effects than aspirin. Although acetaminophen is as potent an analgesic as aspirin, it does not have any anti-inflammatory properties and therefore may be less useful for

TABLE 33.4	COMMONLY USED SEDATIVE/ANALGESIC AGENTS				
Drug	**Dose**	**Route**	**Duration**	**Comments**	
Aspirin	10 mg/kg	PO	4 h	Association with Reyes syndrome	
Acetaminophen	15 mg/kg	PO/PR	4 h	No anti-inflammatory effects	
Ibuprofen	10 mg/kg	PO	6 h	Beware in ASA allergic	
Ketorolac	0.5 mg/kg	IM/IV	6 h	Max to 30 mg q6h	
Morphine	0.1–0.2 mg/kg	IM/SC/IV	2–4 h	Max 15 mg/dose	
Fentanyl	1–4 μg/kg	IV	0.5–1 h	Chest wall rigidity with rapid bolus	
Midazolam	0.1–0.3 mg/kg	IM/IV	0.5 h	Titrate	
	0.2–0.6 mg/kg	IN/PO	0.5–1.0 h	Mild sedation	
Methohexital	25 mg/kg	PR	1.0–1.5 h	Max dose 1 g	
Pentobarbital	1–3 mg/kg	IV	1–4 h	Rapid onset	
	2–6 mg/kg	IM/PO/PR	2–4 h	Onset up to 1 h	
Chloral hydrate	25–100 mg/kg	PO/PR	2–6 h	Infants: max to 1 g	
				Children: max to 2 g	
Ketamine	3 mg/kg	IM	0.5–1.5 h	Give with atropine	
	1–2 mg/kg	IV	1–2 h	Max to 50 mg	
Propofol	1.5 mg/kg	IV	<15 min	Additional dose of 0.5 mg/kg may be necessary	
Etomidate	0.15–0.2 mg/kg	IV	<15 min	Myoclonus frequent	

IM, intramuscular; IN, intranasal; IV, intravenous; PO, per os; PR, per rectum; SC, subcutaneous.

the management of generalized myalgias and inflammatory arthritides. The acetaminophen dose is 15 mg/kg given every 4 to 6 hours up to six times a day.

Nonselective NSAIDs are propionic acid derivatives that have aspirin-like properties. The most widely used NSAIDs are ibuprofen and naproxen. NSAIDs have excellent anti-inflammatory, analgesic, and antipyretic activities. They are particularly useful in the management of arthritic pain seen with inflammatory diseases. In addition, NSAIDs have become prime drugs in the management of pain associated with viral syndromes, dysmenorrhea, and soft-tissue injuries. Although the patient may have some gastrointestinal side effects, NSAIDs are generally better tolerated than aspirin. Furthermore, the longer half-life of NSAIDs allows a longer dosing interval. The ibuprofen dose is 10 mg/kg every 6 hours up to four times a day. Naproxen can be used in children older than 2 years of age. The dose is 5 to 7 mg/kg every 8 to 12 hours. It should be noted that, at the aforementioned doses, the analgesic effect predominates, and higher doses are required to achieve maximal anti-inflammatory action.

Because these medications are given orally, the analgesic effect may not be appreciated for 30 to 90 minutes after administration. Therefore, in the management of acute pain, it may be preferable to administer the drug at regular intervals to provide continuous analgesia rather than waiting for the child to complain of pain. Both aspirin and nonselective NSAIDs can precipitate asthma attacks in aspirin-sensitive individuals.

Ketorolac is an injectable NSAID with analgesic properties comparable to morphine (30). The dose of ketorolac is 0.5 mg/kg administered intravenously or intramuscularly for children 2 years of age and older. It has been shown to be efficacious in children with headache, sickle cell crisis, and renal colic (31,32). However, in children able to tolerate oral medication, it is no more effective than equipotent doses of other nonsteroidal anti-inflammatory agents and is much more expensive.

Sedation and Management of Moderate to Severe Pain

Opioids

Opioids provide strong analgesia for painful procedures, elevating the pain threshold and altering mood. These drugs act at various receptor sites throughout the central nervous system (CNS) designated μ, δ, κ, and σ. It is at the μ-receptor sites that the classic effects of opioids are seen—analgesia, respiratory depression, and euphoria. Animal studies indicate that the number and sensitivity of receptor sites are age related (7); respiratory depression is more profound in the newborn. An advantageous property of opioids is that the effects are reversible with naloxone, a pure opioid antagonist. Naloxone reverses all effects of opioids, including analgesia, respiratory depression, sedation, and gastrointestinal effects. Reversal is almost immediate when naloxone is administered intravenously.

Morphine   Morphine is the principle alkaloid of opium and is the drug by which the potency of other narcotics is measured (7). It is a potent analgesic that works via opioid receptors in the CNS. Morphine exhibits less protein-binding in newborns than adults, resulting in higher "free" morphine levels and greater penetration into the CNS. Clearance of morphine is decreased in infants younger than 2 months of age. Higher peak levels and decreased clearance justify restriction of morphine use in young infants to carefully monitored settings. Morphine is an appropriate agent for treatment of moderate or severe pain, and it is well suited for use during prolonged, painful procedures where its longer elimination half-life is beneficial.

Given intravenously, the onset of morphine is almost immediate, but the peak effect is not reached until 15 to 20 minutes. Morphine is less useful for intravenous titration than fentanyl or midazolam, which reach peak effect more rapidly. Additional doses can be safely given after 20 to 30 minutes if the child is still in pain and there have been no adverse reactions. The elimination half-life for morphine is approximately 2 to 3 hours. Intravenous morphine is given at the T-connector site as a slow intravenous infusion. The dose is 0.1 to 0.2 mg/kg up to a maximum of 10 mg. It can also be given as an intramuscular or subcutaneous injection, but these routes of administration are less useful for procedural sedation than for analgesia alone.

With proper dosing and monitoring, clinical complications associated with use of morphine are uncommon. Administration of morphine alone does not usually require the intensive monitoring needed when using more potent opioids such as fentanyl, although the clinician should always be prepared to intervene if necessary. Furthermore, when morphine is combined with a benzodiazepine, the patient should be fully monitored. Morphine causes peripheral vasodilation, but hemodynamic effects are generally minimal if the patient is euvolemic and has a normal blood pressure. Miosis is an expected side effect. Adverse events include respiratory depression, vasodilation leading to hypotension in the hypovolemic patient, nausea or vomiting, urticaria, and, at very high doses, seizures.

As mentioned previously, untoward effects of morphine are reversible with naloxone. For complete reversal, the intravenous dose of naloxone is 0.1 mg/kg up to a maximum of 2.0 mg. A smaller dose of naloxone (0.01 mg/kg) can reverse respiratory depression while maintaining some analgesia. When intravenous access is not available, naloxone may be given subcutaneously or intramuscularly. However, these routes of administration are less desirable, because the onset of effect can be delayed, and titration is not possible. Because naloxone has a serum half-life of approximately 60 minutes, patients must be monitored carefully for return of CNS and respiratory depression.

Fentanyl   Fentanyl is a synthetic opioid that is 100 times more potent than morphine. Fentanyl alone or in combination with a benzodiazepine provides predictable sedation and analgesia for painful procedures. Similar to morphine, it is reversible with naloxone, but it is less likely than morphine to cause hypotension when administered to hypovolemic patients.

Fentanyl has a rapid onset of action and reaches its peak effect in 2 to 3 minutes because it rapidly enters the CNS (7). Fentanyl also has a short duration of effect, with most patients recovering completely in approximately 30 minutes (31). These features make it ideal for brief, painful procedures. The dose of fentanyl is 1 to 4 μg/kg. Unlike most other agents, the dose given per unit of time is as important as the maximum dose administered. Most authorities recommend that fentanyl be infused at a rate of 0.5 μg/kg/min to a maximum of 25 μg/min, since rapid infusion of even an appropriate dose can induce apnea. Because of its potency, fentanyl should always be administered through a T connector. Instilling the drug at a point on a line more distant from the intravenous catheter may decrease the physician's control of the infusion rate and potentially cause the administration of boluses rather than a slow, steady infusion. Patients receiving fentanyl must be closely monitored. A pulse oximeter and cardiorespiratory monitor are required. A physician or nurse responsible for monitoring the patient should remain in close visual contact until the sedative effects begin to subside.

Fentanyl frequently causes facial pruritus. Children undergoing repair of facial lacerations may contaminate the sterile field as they attempt to rub their face. As with all opioids, respiratory depression is the major complication of fentanyl, even at appropriate doses. Respiratory depression can last up to 30 minutes. Most patients who hypoventilate do not, however, need naloxone. They can often be aroused with verbal or physical stimulation and will breathe deeply on command. Chest wall rigidity ("wooden chest") is a rare but serious complication that makes adequate ventilation difficult or impossible. It typically occurs after a rapid bolus of a high dose of fentanyl and is reversible with naloxone, although reversal may require higher naloxone doses than normally used. Use of a paralytic agent is also effective in this situation, but the patient will obviously require controlled ventilation until the effect of the paralytic subsides. Other reported complications of fentanyl include hypotension, bradycardia, nausea, and vomiting.

Fentanyl combined with midazolam provides excellent sedation and analgesia for painful procedures (33). When the drugs are used together, midazolam can be administered first at a dose of 0.1 mg/kg over 1 to 2 minutes to a maximum dose of 5 mg, followed by fentanyl as previously described. Generally, a lower dose of fentanyl (approximately 50% of the usual dose) is recommended when it is used in combination with midazolam. Alternatively, fentanyl can be administered first to provide an objectively determined (e.g., visual analogue scale) degree of analgesia, and then a lower dose of midazolam can be infused to achieve the necessary level of sedation. Because both drugs are potential respiratory depressants, the patient must be carefully monitored until their effects have subsided.

Benzodiazepines

Benzodiazepines are used for their sedative-hypnotic, anxiolytic, and amnestic effects (32). Although these drugs have no analgesic effects, they nonetheless often create amnesia for the pain experienced during a procedure, an obviously desirable property. Drugs in this class that are commonly used for outpatient sedation include diazepam, lorazepam, and midazolam. Benzodiazepines can be administered alone to manage the anxiety associated with diagnostic testing (e.g., MRI) or combined with a narcotic or local anesthetic to facilitate the performance of moderately painful procedures in anxious children.

Midazolam   Midazolam is a short-acting benzodiazepine. It provides anxiolysis, sedation, and antegrade amnesia. It is often used in combination with a narcotic (e.g., fentanyl, morphine) or as premedication for procedures that will be performed under local anesthesia. Several studies assessing the use of midazolam in children have shown this agent to be safe and effective (34). The onset of action for intravenous midazolam is 2 to 3 minutes, and the duration of effect is 30 minutes. The plasma half-life is approximately 2 hours. Given these properties, midazolam is an excellent sedative and anxiolytic for brief procedures and is the preferred agent for use in the ED.

When administered alone, the intravenous dose of midazolam is 0.1 mg/kg, with a maximum recommended sedation dose of 0.3 mg/kg. Children should receive 0.05 to 0.1 mg/kg as a first dose (maximum of 5 mg) given as a slow infusion over 1 to 2 minutes. Dosing may be repeated at 5-minute intervals until the desired level of sedation has been achieved, unless respiratory depression or other untoward side effects occur. Unlike diazepam, the same initial dose of midazolam (0.05 to 0.1 mg/kg) can also be given as an intramuscular injection. However, intramuscular injection is painful, does not allow for effective titration of the medication, and has been associated with respiratory depression (6). When using intravenous midazolam in conjunction with fentanyl, one of the two agents should be given first as previously described. The initial dose of the second medication should be reduced and then titrated to achieve the desired effect.

Midazolam is rapidly absorbed into the systemic circulation from the nasal mucosa, making intranasal administration an effective route of drug delivery (6). Intranasal midazolam is useful as an anxiolytic for nonpainful procedures (e.g., CT scan, MRI) or when additional analgesia will be provided. The concentrated solution (5 mg/mL) must be used to minimize the volume of fluid instilled into the nostrils. The dose is 0.2 to 0.6 mg/kg up to a maximum of 6 mg. One-half of the total dose is placed in each nostril. Patients with nasal secretions (e.g., an upper respiratory tract infection) may not be able to absorb the drug adequately. When midazolam is administered by the intranasal route, the onset of clinically effective sedation is typically 5 to 10 minutes. Oral midazolam is also effective as an anxiolytic premedication with indications similar to those for intranasal midazolam. However, it is most effective when administered to a child with an empty stomach. Absorption may be erratic in those who have recently eaten, leading to an unpredictable onset of action and depth of sedation. The usual dose is 0.2 to 0.6 mg/kg, and the maximum clinical effect may not occur for 25 to 40 minutes.

The major complication of benzodiazepines is respiratory depression, which is almost exclusively associated with intravenous administration although is occasionally reported with intramuscular injections. Complications are minimal when benzodiazepines are used as a single agent or when they are administered by the oral or nasal route. However, because benzodiazepines act synergistically with narcotics and barbiturates, their effects—and potential complications—are increased when they are used in conjunction with these other agents. In addition, some children who receive benzodiazepines experience a so-called "paradoxical" reaction. Rather than being sedated, these patients become more anxious and agitated after administration of the medication. In such cases, it appears that the child predominately experiences the disinhibitory effect of the drug instead of the sedative effect. Although paradoxical reactions can be reversed with flumazenil, they may also respond favorably to administration of additional benzodiazepine.

Flumazenil is a benzodiazepine antagonist that blocks the activity of benzodiazepines at CNS receptor sites (35). Its use in the pediatric population has not been widely studied. It may be appropriate in iatrogenic overdose or when adverse side effects are experienced but is not recommended for routine use to reduce the duration of benzodiazepine-induced sedation. The pediatric dose of flumazenil is 0.02 mg/kg, given by slow intravenous infusion, up to a maximum of 1 mg. The onset of action is within 1 to 3 minutes. Patients must be monitored closely for resedation because the effects of flumazenil subside before the sedative effects of the benzodiazepine. Additionally, flumazenil itself has some potential untoward effects. Most are minor and include crying, agitation, headache, and dizziness. However, it has rarely been associated with seizures.

Barbiturates

Barbiturates are sedative-hypnotics that act as general depressants of the central and peripheral nervous systems and of skeletal, smooth, and cardiac muscles. Their clinical effects are dose dependent and vary widely from mild sedation to coma. Barbiturates can be divided into four groups: ultrashort-acting (thiopental and methohexital), short-acting (pentobarbital), intermediate (butabarbital), and long-acting (phenobarbital). Generally, the ultrashort-acting and short-acting barbiturates are utilized for procedural sedation. When used alone at the proper sedative dose, adverse side effects are rare. Higher doses (e.g., a preintubation dose of methohexital) can, however, cause apnea, transient hypotension, and bradycardia. Barbiturates have no analgesic qualities when used at sedative doses; analgesia is only provided when high anesthetic doses are administered. Thus, when the patient is anticipated to experience pain, an additional analgesic (parenteral or local) must be used.

Methohexital Methohexital is an ultrashort-acting barbiturate that can be given rectally for brief, painless procedures or procedures with which local anesthetic will be used. The onset of action is approximately 8 minutes. When used as a sedative for painless procedures (e.g., CT scan, MRI), it is 95% effective (36). The methohexital dose is 25 mg/kg per rectum, up to a maximum dose of 1 g. Adverse events include hypoventilation and oxygen desaturation, hiccups, cough, and hypersalivation. Although methohexital can also be given by intravenous injection, there are few data regarding this route of administration for pediatric procedural sedation. Furthermore, safer alternative agents are available.

Pentobarbital Pentobarbital is a short-acting barbiturate that is useful for longer procedures or as a preoperative sedative. It can be used in conjunction with an analgesic for painful procedures and may be given parenterally, orally, or rectally. When administered as an intravenous injection, onset of action for pentobarbital occurs in approximately 6 minutes, and the duration of effect is approximately 60 minutes. Oral administration and rectal administration are associated with a delayed onset of sedation (up to 45 minutes). Successful sedation occurs in approximately 99% of patients, but the best sedation results are seen in children younger than 8 years of age (33,37). The oral, rectal, or intramuscular dose of pentobarbital is 2 to 6 mg/kg, up to a maximum dose of 150 mg. The intravenous dose of pentobarbital is 1 to 3 mg/kg. Adverse events associated with pentobarbital administration include respiratory depression, emergence reactions, and paradoxical hyperactivity.

Chloral Hydrate

Chloral hydrate is a sedative-hypnotic CNS depressant used in children as a sedative for procedures which are painless but require cooperation, such as a CT scan, MRI, or electroencephalogram (EEG). It can also be used in conjunction with a local anesthetic for mildly painful procedures such as minor dental work or wound repair (31,38). The drug is readily absorbed through the gastrointestinal tract and may be administered orally or rectally. The dose is 25 to 100 mg/kg, up to a maximum of 1 g in infants and 2 g in children. Peak therapeutic levels occur in approximately 30 to 60 minutes. Chloral hydrate is metabolized in the liver to its active metabolite, trichloroethanol. The elimination half-life of this metabolite is 8 to 12 hours.

When chloral hydrate is administered in low doses (e.g., 25 mg/kg) for light sedation, monitoring beyond the initial period of sedation need only consist of periodic assessment of vital signs. Patients given higher doses of the drug (50 to 100 mg/kg) should be monitored with continuous pulse oximetry. Adverse side effects include excessive somnolence and paradoxical excitation. Major disadvantages of chloral hydrate use include lack of a reversal agent, unpredictable onset and degree of sedation, and a long half-life that requires a protracted period of monitoring.

Ketamine

Ketamine is a phencyclidine derivative that acts as a dissociative anesthetic. It produces pronounced sedation and uncouples cortical pain perception (33). Ketamine is essentially unique among powerful sedative and analgesic agents in that it rarely causes respiratory depression or circulatory compromise. In fact, it is often associated with mild elevations in both heart rate and blood pressure (39,40). Many experienced clinicians view ketamine as offering the most favorable combination of safety and effectiveness among the sedative-analgesics routinely used for pediatric patients.

Ketamine is useful as a sedative-analgesic for painful procedures of short or intermediate duration, such as closed fracture reduction, incision and drainage of an abscess, and wound repair. Ketamine causes increased levels of epinephrine and norepinephrine, which results in increased heart rate, blood pressure, cardiac output, myocardial oxygen consumption, and ocular pressure. It is therefore contraindicated for patients with certain cardiovascular diseases (e.g., severe hypertension) and for those who may be harmed by an elevation in intraocular pressure (e.g., open globe injury). Ketamine also causes bronchodilation, making it a good choice for rapid sequence intubation of an asthmatic patient, as well as increased oral and airway secretions. While the most significant result of this latter effect is generally mild drooling, many opt to administer an antisialagogue (e.g., atropine or glycopyrrolate) when using ketamine.

Ketamine is a cerebral vasodilator and can cause increased cerebral blood flow, cerebral spinal fluid pressure, and intracranial pressure. Consequently, it has traditionally been considered inadvisable to administer ketamine to children with significant head injury or other potential causes of raised intracranial pressure (e.g., brain tumor). However, more recent data suggest that ketamine may actually be neuroprotective (41), and the time may come when ketamine is the preferred sedative for patients with possible brain injury. Yet until this issue is resolved, prudence dictates that alternative agents be used for sedation of children with conditions that may be exacerbated by an increase in intracranial pressure.

Occasionally, ketamine causes mild "laryngospasm," manifested as stridor and coughing, which, while disconcerting in appearance, has proved over long clinical experience to be essentially harmless. The symptoms are transient, and unlike in the case of true laryngospasm, patients do not require any type of advance airway intervention. The condition might be more appropriately described as "pharmacologic croup." Repositioning the airway and administering humidified oxygen are generally the only measures necessary. It should be noted, however, that excessively high doses of ketamine can produce profound respiratory depression, and it is therefore mandatory that equipment for airway support be immediately available whenever ketamine is administered. Both laryngospasm and respiratory depression are more common in infants receiving ketamine, and consequently it should not be administered to patients under 3 months of age.

Episodes of myoclonus, random movements, and/or unusual postures are sometimes seen in conjunction with ketamine but are of no clinical consequence unless the procedure in question requires that the patient remain motionless. Although many patients report hallucinations and vivid dream experiences while under the effects of ketamine, so-called "emergence reactions" are a widely described but uncommon side effect. When they occur, they can include visual hallucinations, anxiety, agitation, and unpleasant dreams. Emergence reactions appear to be more prevalent in older children and adults. Additionally, they occur more frequently in noisy, chaotic settings (e.g., an ED) and seem to be related to preprocedure agitation. There is no evidence that the addition of a benzodiazepine decreases the occurrence of emergence reactions and may be associated with more episodes of oxygen desaturation (42,43). Finally, vomiting during the recovery phase is common after sedation with ketamine.

Ketamine can be given as either an intravenous or intramuscular injection. It can also be given orally or rectally, although first-pass metabolism makes these routes less reliable, and considerably higher doses must be used. When administered as an intravenous or intramuscular injection, the onset and duration of action for ketamine are route and dose dependent. The intramuscular route appears to be safe and effective and obviates the need for intravenous access. The dose of ketamine for intramuscular injection is 3 to 4 mg/kg. If desired, atropine can be administered in the same syringe at a dose of 0.01 mg/kg, up to a maximum of 0.3 mg. It should be noted that the time to onset of ketamine is considerably shorter than that of atropine, and the patient may experience some increase in oral secretions before the atropine takes effect. The intravenous dose of ketamine is 1 to 2 mg/kg, up to a maximum of 50 mg. The dose should be pushed slowly over 1 to 2 minutes, as rapid infusion can cause apnea. With longer procedures, it may be appropriate to administer up to two additional doses of 1 mg/kg if the child begins to awaken and remains stable from a cardiorespiratory standpoint. Although there is no reversal agent for ketamine, this drug offers the advantages of potent sedation and analgesia, ease of administration, and, when used properly, a low complication rate.

Propofol

Propofol is an ultrashort-acting sedative-hypnotic that causes rapid and deep sedation at therapeutic doses. It has no amnestic or analgesic effects. Propofol has been used extensively for surgical anesthesia, and more recently it has gained popularity as a sedative for brief procedures in the ED. It provides predictable sedation for procedures such as fracture reduction, incision and drainage, foreign body removal, and shoulder reduction (44,45). Propofol can be combined with a short-acting opiate or local anesthetic for painful procedures but often is used alone because of its potent sedative properties. In addition to a rapid onset of action and very brief duration of effect, propofol offers another advantage over other sedatives: it has intrinsic antiemetic properties, thus reducing the risk of aspiration (46). It is not appropriate for patients requiring ongoing pain management or sedation because continuous infusion results in excessive accumulation of the drug in tissue (47). Infusions for longer than 48 hours have been associated with severe lactic acidemia and bradyarrhythmias (48).

The onset of action for propofol is almost immediate, and its effect lasts for approximately 8 minutes. It is given as an intravenous bolus at an initial dose of 1.5 mg/kg. Additional bolus doses of 0.5 mg/kg may be necessary to achieve sedation for the duration of the procedure (49). Adverse events include pain at the site of administration, vomiting (although less than most other agents), hypotension, respiratory depression, hypoxia, and apnea. Pain at the site of injection can be managed by concomitant administration of lidocaine or by pretreatment with lidocaine. Pretreatment seems to be more effective. This is done by first applying a tourniquet to the patient's arm at a site proximal to the intravenous catheter and leaving it in place. A 0.5-mg/kg dose of lidocaine is then administered through the intravenous catheter. After 1 to 2 minutes, the tourniquet is removed and the propofol is given (46). Many patients receiving propofol will reach a state of general anesthesia at some point during administration of the drug. For this reason, equipment for advanced cardiorespiratory support must be readily available, and fasting guidelines should always be followed (46).

Etomidate

Etomidate is a nonbarbiturate sedative hypnotic that has been used in operating rooms for more than 25 years. It induces sedation by acting on GABA receptors in the CNS and is structurally unrelated to any other compound. Etomidate lowers cerebral metabolism, cerebral blood flow, and intracranial pressure. Additionally, it lacks the adverse hemodynamic effects of many other sedative agents, and it does not negatively impact mean arterial pressure, cardiac output, or systemic vascular resistance. Because of these properties, etomidate is often used in the ED as an induction agent for endotracheal intubation, particularly for head-injured patients and for those with underlying cardiac disease. More recently, it has gained favor as a sedative for brief ED procedures.

Etomidate has a rapid onset of action (less than 1 minute) and a short duration of effect (less than 12 minutes). It has no analgesic properties but produces amnesia for the event in the majority of patients. Indications for use include procedures of short duration, such as CT scan, reduction of dislocations, fracture reduction, incision and drainage of an abscess, limited wound débridement, and foreign body removal (50). Because it has a short duration of action and may cause adrenal suppression with multiple doses (see below), this agent is not the best choice as a sedative for prolonged procedures. Additionally, as it causes relatively frequent postsedation vomiting, the risks and benefits of etomidate should be carefully assessed in the patient with recent food intake.

The dose of etomidate for procedural sedation is 0.15 to 0.2 mg/kg administered as a slow intravenous push over 1 minute to decrease the potential for respiratory depression or apnea. Since etomidate has no analgesic properties, the patient will usually require addition of an analgesic medication for more painful procedures. It is often appropriate to initially "preload" the patient who has a painful injury and will require a procedure (e.g., shoulder dislocation, angulated fracture) with one or more doses of an analgesic (morphine, fentanyl) prior to formal sedation with etomidate.

Adverse side effects of etomidate include pain at the injection site, vomiting (both during and after sedation), respiratory depression and oxygen desaturation (especially when etomidate is used in combination with opioids), and myoclonus (51,52). Myoclonus is a relatively frequent occurrence and may last up to 1 minute. These movements are not associated with seizure activity on EEG but may limit the utility of etomidate for certain procedures that require the patient to remain immobile. Additionally, clinically significant adrenal insufficiency has been reported with etomidate when given by continuous infusion or in multiple doses. This results from direct inhibition of 11-beta hydroxylase, which disrupts conversion of 11-deoxy cortisol to cortisol. Although cortisol depression has been demonstrated after a single dose of etomidate (the most likely mode of use in the ED), serum cortisol levels remain within the normal range, and there are no sequelae (53). Some preliminary data suggest that etomidate may also have a negative effect on white blood cell activity. However, both cortisol suppression and impaired white blood cell function are problems that are more likely to limit the use of etomidate for prolonged sedation of children with serious medical conditions (e.g., in an intensive care unit) rather than for procedural sedation of otherwise healthy children in the ED.

▶ PROCEDURE

Appropriate procedural sedation and anesthesia involves the following: (a) preparation and relaxation, (b) presedation assessment, (c) administration of medications, (d) monitoring during sedation, and (e) postprocedure recovery and patient discharge guidelines.

Preparation and Relaxation

With appreciation of the child's fears and concerns, the clinician should create as relaxed an environment as can be provided. When possible, a quiet examination room should be used; it will obviously be more difficult for a child to relax if other children can be heard screaming and crying. After the initial examination, overhead lights should be dimmed if possible. A gooseneck or operating room light can be used for illumination. Once the child has been told of an impending painful procedure, long delays should be avoided. All necessary equipment (suture kit, needles, etc.) should be prepared in advance and away from the child's direct sight. Opening needles and unfamiliar equipment in front of the child will only heighten anxiety.

Having a Child Life specialist as a part of the team can greatly facilitate both preparing for and performing the procedure. Child Life specialists based in the ED have been shown to (a) decrease children's anxiety and perception of pain, (b) teach the children and staff simple distraction techniques, and (c) support family involvement (54–56). Ideally, they should be involved as soon as possible to prepare a child who will require a painful or anxiety-provoking procedure. Unfortunately, these professionals are unlikely to be available outside of children's hospitals and those community hospitals with a large pediatric service.

In many cases, having a parent present for a painful or frightening procedure will both comfort the child and facilitate relaxation (Fig. 33.1) (57). Furthermore, parents can often accurately predict their child's degree of distress to the painful stimulus and thus guide the staff in their preparations (58). However, the decision about whether parents should remain in the room during a procedure is affected by several factors, such as the child's age and emotional needs as well as the parents' ability to tolerate seeing the child in a sedated state and/or undergoing potentially upsetting procedures (fracture reduction, wound closure, etc.). The parent who does not feel capable of witnessing such events should be allowed to leave, without feelings of guilt, once the child is sedated.

Behavior Therapy

The provider should never lie or downplay a child's perception of pain with flippant remarks such as "This won't hurt" or "Oh, come on, that didn't really hurt you." These remarks only serve to erode the trust between the child and the provider. Words should be chosen carefully and communicated in an empathetic tone, with consistent positive reinforcements. Children should be encouraged to express their feelings and not be made to feel they must prove how brave or "grown up" they are by internalizing their emotions (59). Stoicism should not be an expectation of a child. Younger children think in concrete terms, making cognitive and behavioral techniques less applicable. They may not understand that an intravenous line will help them but may believe that a Band-Aid or a parent's kiss can relieve pain.

Distraction

Different techniques can be used to distract the child, depending on age. Preschool children can play with popup toys, look through a kaleidoscope, or blow bubbles. Older children can play video games, watch movies, or listen to music through headphones (Fig. 33.1).

Guided Imagery

Many children can be further relaxed through guided imagery. The child's favorite doll or television character in an adventure story can be used, with the hope of focusing the child on the fantasy. These stories should be age appropriate and incorporate the child's interests (e.g., Sesame Street or fairytales for young children, beach scenes or sporting events for the older child).

Hypnosis

Rather than trying to distract the child, hypnosis uses guided imagery to facilitate pain control (60). This approach seems to work best with children who have a vivid imagination and those who are "hypersuggestible." The child's developmental level will largely determine the most effective hypnotic approach. Various types of hypnotic suggestions have been reported as effective (61), including (a) direct suggestion ("Pretend you are painting numbing medicine on the part of your body that hurts"), (b) distancing suggestions ("Imagine you are in your favorite place"), and (c) suggestions for feeling that are antithetical to pain ("Think of the funniest movie you ever saw"). Hypnotic techniques are most effective when used in a quiet, comfortable environment, which is sometimes difficult to provide in a hectic ED. Furthermore, although hypnosis can often be a valuable adjunct in pain control, the operator should not refrain from also using pharmacologic agents when needed.

Restraint

Despite even the best attempts at relaxation, physical restraints may be needed for certain procedures. It is often better to perform appropriate restraint techniques before beginning a procedure than to take a chance that the child will lay still, only to find that three people are needed to restrain the patient at a critical moment. However, restraints should be used in conjunction with relaxation techniques and pharmacologic therapy. Furthermore, an explanation of the restraint technique should be given to the child. Specific types of restraints and their uses are described in Chapter 3.

Presedation Assessment

Current guidelines from the American Academy of Pediatrics (AAP), the American Society of Anesthesiologists (ASA), and the American College of Emergency Physicians (ACEP) all recommend a structured evaluation of children that allows risk stratification before beginning sedation (6,56,62,63).

Safety precautions must be observed when using any anxiolytic or analgesic agent. A systematic risk assessment involves a directed history and focused physical evaluation. Patients (or legal guardians in the case of minors) should be informed of and agree to the administration of sedation or analgesia. Appropriate informed consent for sedation must cover its benefits, risks, and limitations as well as possible alternatives.

A presedation assessment should be completed and recorded for every patient. At a minimum, this should include an evaluation of the child's physical and mental status, current clinical condition, significant past medical history (previous adverse experience with sedation or analgesia, allergies, medication use, etc.), and last oral intake of solids. Every patient requiring sedation or analgesia should also undergo a focused physical examination that includes evaluation of the vital signs, auscultation of the heart and lungs, and examination of the airway. According to ASA guidelines, children are appropriate candidates for procedural sedation if they can be categorized as Class I (a normal healthy patient) or Class II (a patient with mild systemic disease that does not interfere with daily routines, such as well-controlled asthma or diabetes) (62) (Table 33.3).

One of the most common serious complications of sedation is respiratory depression. Should this occur, the patient's life may literally depend on the operator's ability to provide effective assisted or controlled ventilation. Consequently, an evaluation of the patient's airway should be a part of every presedation assessment. It is particularly important for the operator to identify those children who are predicted to have a so-called "difficult airway," because this knowledge is likely to significantly influence the choice of a sedation regimen. A complete discussion of assessing the potentially difficult airway can be found in Chapter 17.

For elective operative procedures, the ASA recommends restriction of clear liquids for 2 hours, breast milk for 4 hours, and infant formula or solids for 6 hours (64). In the ED, however, where urgent or emergent procedures are often performed, the potential for pulmonary aspiration of gastric contents must be considered and weighed against the need for the procedure. For the child with recent oral intake, the clinician must determine (a) the target level of sedation, (b) whether the procedure should (or can) be delayed, and (c) whether the trachea must be protected by intubation prior to the initiation of sedation (6).

Finally, several regulatory agencies, including the Joint Commission for Accreditation of Healthcare Organizations (JCAHO), have begun to focus on patient safety. One recent initiative is the inclusion of a pause or "timeout" before the start of any procedure so that the staff can confirm that the procedure is being performed on the right patient and at the correct anatomic location. Although "wrong site" and "wrong patient" errors are probably less likely in the ED than the operating room, this precaution is strongly recommended for any patient undergoing procedural sedation.

Administration of Medications

As described above, prior to the sedation the operator must consider several factors, including the patient's age, current and underlying medical problems, and psychological state, as well as the nature of the procedure, the capabilities of the facility and its staff, and the operator's own level of experience. However, once the method of sedation has been chosen, the best chance of success lies with an organized approach that emphasizes both the safety and the comfort of the patient.

In most cases, the procedure should begin with the child being placed in a quiet room and relaxation techniques such as behavior therapy or hypnosis being attempted. Appropriate monitoring techniques should then be instituted. Some-

times an extremely agitated child may require restraint or even premedication prior to the initiation of monitoring. The room chosen should be equipped to support resuscitation should the need arise. Suction, oxygen, an appropriately sized bag-valve-mask circuit, and airway equipment should be readily available. All medications should be drawn up and labeled and the doses double-checked prior to administration. Antagonist medications, such as naloxone or flumazenil, should also be on hand. One member of the care team, whether a physician or nurse, should be assigned to monitor the patient. This individual should not have other duties.

For a patient receiving intravenous medications, vascular access should be maintained throughout the procedure and until the patient is ready to be discharged. For a patient who has received sedation or analgesia by nonintravenous routes, an individual with the skills to establish rapid intravenous access should be immediately available. Alternatively, an intravenous line can be established while the child is sedated so that it is available for emergency use.

Medications should be administered only after all of the previously described preparations are completed and the operator is ready to begin the procedure. The process of medication administration should be tailored to the medication(s) being used. Intravenous sedatives and narcotic analgesics should be administered slowly. Agents with a rapid onset of action (e.g., fentanyl, midazolam) should be titrated to the desired effect. This is done by administering an initial dose at the lower end of the dosage range, followed by an assessment of the child's level of sedation approximately 2 to 5 minutes later. If needed, an additional dose of medication is then administered. This process can be repeated at intervals until the patient is deemed to have reached the necessary level of sedation. A word of caution about this process is warranted, however. It is possible to give doses of medication so close together that the peak effects of each dose coincide. This is known as "stacking" medication doses. Dose stacking is most likely to occur when two different medications are being simultaneously given. Thus, when two drugs are being used for procedural sedation, it is often advisable to titrate one of them to a desired level before administering the second. For example, an analgesic can be administered such that a specific degree of pain relief is achieved, and then an anxiolytic medication can be added to further enhance sedation. In most cases, when the patient's eyelids are at "half mast," adequate sedation has been achieved. During prolonged procedures, serial reassessment is necessary to determine when additional doses of medication are needed.

Monitoring during Sedation

Effective monitoring is essential to the safe conduct of procedural sedation. The most effective monitoring combines repeated clinical evaluations with continuous electronic measurements. Clinical monitoring includes assessments of the patient's level of consciousness, quality of peripheral pulses, and effectiveness of respiratory efforts. Blood pressure monitoring can be performed manually or electronically. In addition, a cardiorespiratory monitor and pulse oximeter should be used to monitor patients at increased risk for developing hypoxemia (e.g., patients given multiple drugs and/or high doses, patients with significant comorbidity, etc.) (Fig. 33.1). Bispectral index (BIS) monitoring is a new modality that is becoming commonly used in operating rooms. It uses a single lead EEG applied to the forehead to assess the depth of sedation, although the extent of analgesia is not measured. While there is much interest in the use of BIS monitoring to more precisely control procedural sedation, there is currently insufficient evidence to support its routine use in the ED (65).

Results of monitoring should be recorded at regular intervals, both to enhance patient safety and to provide a clear record of appropriate care in the event of an adverse outcome. Recordings should be made as follows: (a) at the beginning of the procedure; (b) after administration of sedative or analgesic agents; (c) at regular intervals during the procedure, typically every 5 to 15 minutes, depending on the depth of sedation; (d) during recovery; and (e) just prior to discharge. If recording is performed automatically, device alarms should be set to alert the care team to clinically significant changes in the patient's status (6).

Personnel responsible for patient monitoring should be able to recognize the complications commonly associated with sedation. If experienced personnel who are comfortable with basic life support and monitoring are not available, then procedural sedation should not be undertaken. Attending to the ABCs of basic life support—airway, breathing, and circulation—throughout a procedure and until the patient has recovered from the effects of the medication will allow the physician to recognize and respond to potentially life-threatening complications. If the respiratory rate or oxygen saturation drops, the child should be given a clear command to take a deep breath, and supplemental oxygen should be administered. If respiratory depression or desaturation continues, bag-valve-mask ventilation with 100% oxygen should be initiated, and if no improvement is seen, an appropriate reversal agent (naloxone and/or flumazenil) should be administered. In rare cases, endotracheal intubation may be necessary. This is most likely to occur when bag-valve-mask ventilation is ineffective and there is no effective reversal agent for the medication used for sedation (e.g., ketamine). As mentioned previously, reversal agents should not be used simply to awaken a child after an uncomplicated sedation, since this may induce severe agitation, and the effect of the reversal agent may subside before the effects of the sedative(s).

After the procedure for which sedation was performed is completed, monitoring must continue until the child has fully recovered. Sedation-related complications are most likely to occur (a) within 5 to 20 minutes after receipt of intravenous medications and (b) during the postprocedure period, when the sedative effects are still quite profound and the child no longer is stimulated by the pain of the procedure (66). The physician responsible for managing the sedation should remain at the bedside during the recovery phase until the child has awakened enough that there is little risk of rapid deterioration. The period of sedation may be considered complete when the child returns to a pretreatment level of awareness, can recognize caregivers, and shows purposeful movement.

Discharge Criteria

The decision to discharge a child after procedural sedation should be made by someone aware of the details of the individual case. Each facility where procedural sedation and analgesia are administered to children should establish policies and procedures for recovery and discharge similar to the recommendations published by ACEP and AAP. Presedation status, medications and route of administration, time since administration, level of alertness, ability to take oral fluids, and ability to ambulate should be considered before discharge (62,63). The AAP guidelines for discharge include these:

- Airway patency and cardiovascular status are stable, and vital signs are within acceptable limits.
- Airway protective reflexes are intact.
- Patients are easily arousable and can talk at baseline ability.
- Hydration status is adequate.
- Very young or developmentally delayed child must be:
  - Close to the presedation level of responsiveness or baseline activity.
  - Able to follow age-appropriate commands and able to sit up unaided (if a baseline capability).

Additional observation may be indicated if any of the following are true:

- The patient has received reversal agents (naloxone or flumazenil). Such patients should be monitored for at least 2 hours after the last dose of these drugs to assess for resedation.
- The patient received a sedative medication with a long half-life.
- There is evidence of ongoing significant blood or fluid loss (e.g., the wound dressing is becoming saturated with blood or other fluids).
- The patient is dizzy or lightheaded when supine.
- The patient has persistent nausea or vomiting.

Prior to discharge, patients and parents should be given written instructions regarding diet, medications, and activities, and a phone number to be called in case of an emergency should also be provided. Instructions should, when possible, be tailored to

SUMMARY

1 Explain purpose, type, and anticipated depth of sedation to patient and parent.

2 Administer medications under supervision of personnel experienced in sedation and airway management.

3 Select appropriate medication(s), route(s) of administration, and dose(s) based on the specific patient and procedure.

4 Have the following equipment readily available in procedure room:
  ▶ Cardiorespiratory monitor
  ▶ Pulse oximeter
  ▶ Suction
  ▶ Oxygen
  ▶ Nonrebreather face mask
  ▶ Bag-valve-mask
  ▶ Advanced airway equipment

5 Prepare all equipment and medications in advance and out of sight of the patient.

6 Place the patient in a quiet room with lights dimmed if possible.

7 Allow parents to remain with their child during induction if desired.

8 Relax the child with guided imagery, behavior therapy, and/or hypnosis.

9 Place the cardiac monitor leads and pulse oximeter probe after child is relaxed.

10 Record vital signs before, during, and after the period of sedation.

11 Place an intravenous line if needed.

12 Titrate medications by the intravenous route whenever possible.

13 Administer local anesthetic when appropriate for painful procedures.

14 Administer supplemental oxygen and instruct child to breathe deeply if respiratory rate decreases or oxygen saturation falls.

15 Ventilate with a bag-valve-mask device if significant respiratory depression occurs and patient does not respond to verbal or tactile stimuli.

16 Give naloxone and/or flumazenil to patient if he or she has received opioids or benzodiazepines and has developed respiratory depression or circulatory compromise.

17 Continue monitoring until the patient recovers, leaving the room only when the patient awakens to the extent that there is no further likelihood of rapid deterioration.

18 Discharge the child when he or she is alert, taking oral fluids, and ambulating without difficulty.

19 Give the patient's family appropriate instructions regarding diet and activity as well as emergency contact information prior to discharge.

the substances administered, but general instructions should include these:

- Restrict walking or crawling in the first few hours.
- Allow only clear fluids until nausea resolves, and then advance the diet gradually as tolerated.
- Prohibit high-risk activities for 12 hours (e.g., bicycling, in-line skating).
- Prohibit the operation of motorized equipment for at least 6 hours.
- Closely supervise the child for the next 12 hours.
- Return to the ED if the child experiences any difficulty breathing or persistent nausea and vomiting.

▶ COMPLICATIONS

Complications associated with the use of pain medications and sedative agents occur in four major areas: nausea and vomiting, airway compromise with or without respiratory depression, paradoxical drug reactions (e.g., agitation, hallucinations), and abnormal CNS activity (e.g., seizures). Initial management of any complication begins with the standard basic life support assessment of airway, breathing, and circulation. Keen awareness of these basic life support measures will avert much of the morbidity that occurs when measures to ensure ventilation, oxygenation, and perfusion are overlooked. Detailed descriptions of basic life support measures and management of airway compromise in pediatric patients are provided in Section 2 of this textbook. After appropriate assessment and, if necessary, stabilization of any problems related to airway, breathing, and circulation, children with paradoxical hyperactivity and/or agitation can be given intravenous benzodiazepines (e.g., diazepam or midazolam 0.1 mg/kg). However, the clinician should be certain that the agitation is secondary to a drug reaction and not a sign of hypoxia or inadequate ventilation. Similarly, basic life support measures should precede intravenous benzodiazepines (diazepam 0.1 mg/kg or lorazepam 0.05 mg/kg) in the management of seizures.

CLINICAL TIPS

▶ Moderate sedation of pediatric patients should not be undertaken unless the facility is appropriately equipped and staff have adequate experience with this procedure.

▶ Extra caution is required when sedating children with underlying illness, especially those with neurologic disease.

▶ Children may cry or move while under sedation, and therefore personnel should be prepared to apply physical restraint if necessary.

▶ The safest approach to procedural sedation is to titrate medications in a stepwise fashion to a desired level of sedation, starting with the lowest effective dose. More medication can always be given, but excessive medication already administered cannot be withdrawn.

▶ If deep sedation or anesthesia is necessary, the procedure should likely be performed in the operating room. Any procedure should be stopped if it becomes clear that a different setting would be more appropriate or safer for the patient.

▶ Physician supervision of procedural sedation should not end simply because the procedure is finished. This is in fact one of the most dangerous times for the patient. The highest risk of complications—especially respiratory depression and apnea—occurs at the beginning of sedation (when medications have just been administered) and during the immediate postprocedure period (when painful stimuli are removed).

▶ A child should always be carefully evaluated before discharge, and the clinician should not be unduly influenced by pressure to discharge the patient too early.

▶ SUMMARY

Many children presenting to the ED will require pain management, sedation to facilitate a specific procedure, or both. Sensitivity to the needs of the child and appreciation of the child's fears and apprehensions are of paramount importance. The clinician must assess a variety of patient and environmental factors, enlist the aid of experienced personnel, be familiar with basic nonpharmacologic techniques, and use medications correctly. With meticulous attention to clinical preassessment, medication dosing, and patient monitoring, untoward effects of sedation and analgesia can be minimized, and intervention to prevent complications can be prompt and effective.

▶ ACKNOWLEDGMENT

The authors would like to acknowledge the valuable contributions of Jeffrey Avner and Ellen Crain to the version of this chapter that appeared in the previous edition.

▶ REFERENCES

1. International Association for the Study of Pain. Pain terms: a list with definitions and notes on usage. *Pain.* 1979;6:249.
2. Merskey H. An investigation of pain in psychological illness [D.M. thesis]. Oxford: Oxford University; 1964.
3. Goodman J, McGrath PJ. The epidemiology of pain in children and adolescents: a review. *Pain.* 1991;46:247–264.
4. *Stedman's Medical Dictionary.* 21st ed. S.v. "analgesia."
5. American College of Emergency Physicians. Clinical policy for procedural sedation and analgesia in the emergency department. *Ann Emerg Med.* 1998;31:663–677.
6. Practice guidelines for sedation and analgesia by non-anesthesiologists: a report by the American Society of Anesthesiologists Task Force on Sedation and Analgesia by Non-Anesthesiologists. *Anesthesiology.* 2002;96:1004–1017.
7. Yaster M, Deshpande JK. Medical progress: management of pediatric pain with opioid analgesics. *J Pediatr.* 1988;113:421–429.
8. Walco GA, Cassidy RC, Schechter NL. Pain, hurt, and harm: the ethics of pain control in infants and children. *N Engl J Med.* 1994;331:541–544.
9. Anand KJS, Hickey PR. Pain and its effects in the human neonate and fetus. *N Engl J Med.* 1987;317:1321–1329.
10. Fitzgerald M, Anand KJS. Developmental neuroanatomy and neurophysiology of pain. In: Schechter NL, Berde CB, Yaster M, eds. *Pain in Infants, Children, and Adolescents.* Baltimore: Williams & Wilkins; 1993:11–31.
11. Selbst SM, Clark M. Analgesic use in the emergency department. *Ann Emerg Med.* 1990;19:1010–1013.
12. Rupp T, Delaney KA. Inadequate analgesia in emergency medicine. *Ann Emerg Med.* 2004;43:494–503.
13. Schechter NL, Allan DA. Physicians' attitudes toward pain in children. *J Dev Behav Pediatr.* 1986;7:350–354.
14. McCaffery M, Ferrell BR. Opioid analgesics: nurses' knowledge of doses and psychological dependence. *J Nurs Staff Dev.* 1992;8:77–84.
15. Kim MK, Strait RT, Sato T. A randomized clinical trial of analgesia in children with acute abdominal pain. *Acad Emerg Med.* 2002;9:281–287.
16. Kelly DD. Central representations of pain and analgesia. In: Kandel ER, Schwartz JH, eds. *Principles of Neural Science.* New York: Elsevier North Holland; 1981:200–212.
17. Hendler N. The anatomy and psychopharmacology of chronic pain. *J Clin Psych.* 1982;43:5–20.
18. Schechter NL. Pain and pain control in children. *Curr Probl Pediatr.* 1985;15:6–67.
19. Melzack R, Wall PD. Pain mechanism: a new theory. *Science.* 1965;150:971–979.
20. Schechter NC, Berde CB, Yaster M. Pain in infants, children and adolescents: an overview. In: Schechter NC, Bende CB, Yaster M, eds. *Pain in Infants, Children, and Adolescents.* Baltimore: Williams & Wilkins; 1993:3–10.
21. McGrath PJ, Craig KD. Developmental and psychological factors in children's pain. *Pediatr Clin North Am.* 1989;36:823–835.
22. Mayer SE, Melmon KL, Gilman AG. Introduction: the dynamics of drug absorption, distribution, and elimination. In: Gilman AG, Goodman LS, Gilman A, eds. *The Pharmacologic Basis of Therapeutics.* 6th ed. New York: Macmillian; 1980:1–27.

23. Ellenhorn MJ, Barceloux DG. *Medical Toxicology: Diagnosis and Treatment of Human Poisoning*. New York: Elsevier; 1988.

24. Arand K. The biology of pain perception in newborn infants. In: Tyler D, Krane E, eds. *Advances in Pain Research and Therapy: Pediatric Pain*. New York: Raven Press; 1990:113–122.

25. Broadman L, Rice L, Hannallah R. Evaluation of an objective pain scale for infants and children. *Reg Anesth*. 1988;13:45.

26. Beyer J. *The Oucher: a user's manual and technical report*. Denver: University of Colorado Health Sciences Center; 1988.

27. LeBaron S, Zeltzer L. Assessment of acute pain and anxiety in children and adolescents by self-reports, observer reports, and behavioral checklist. *J Consult Clin Psychol*. 1984;52:729–738.

28. Johnston CC, Stranda ME. Acute pain response in infants: a multidimensional description. *Pain*. 1986;24:373–382.

29. Granau RVE, Craig KD. Pain expression in neonates: facial action and cry. *Pain*. 1984;28:395–410.

30. *Drugs of Choice from the Medical Letter*. 14th ed. New Rochelle, NY: The Medical Letter; 2001:138–150.

31. Flood RG, Krauss B, Procedural sedation and analgesia for children in the emergency department. *Emerg Med Clin North Am*. 2003;21:121–139.

32. Qureshi F, Lewis D Managing headache in the pediatric emergency department. *Clin Pediatr Emerg Med*. 2003;4:159–170.

33. Clinical policy: evidence-based approach to pharmacologic agents used in pediatric sedation and analgesia in the emergency department. *Ann Emerg Med*. 2004;44:342–377.

34. Sievers TD, Yee JD, Foley ME, et al. Midazolam for conscious sedation during pediatric oncology procedures: safety and recovery parameters. *Pediatrics*. 1991;88:1172–1179.

35. Jones RD, Lawson AD, Andrew LJ, et al. Antagonism of the hypnotic effect of midazolam in children: a randomized, double-blind study of placebo and flumazenil administered after midazolam-induced anesthesia. *Br J Anaesth*. 1991;66:660–666.

36. Pomeranz ES, Chudnofsky CR, Deegan TJ, et al. Rectal methohexital sedation for computed tomography imaging of stable pediatric emergency department patients. *Pediatrics*. 2000;105:1110–1114.

37. Mason KP, Zurakowski D, Karian VE, et al. Sedatives used in pediatric imaging: comparison of IV pentobarbital with IV pentobarbital with midazolam added. *AJR Am J Roentgenol*. 2001;177:427–430.

38. Committee on Drugs and Committee on Environmental Health. Use of chloral hydrate for sedation in children. *Pediatrics*. 1993;92:471–473.

39. Green SM, Nakamura R, Johnson NE. Ketamine sedation for pediatric procedures, I: a prospective series. *Ann Emerg Med*. 1990;19:1024–1032.

40. Green SM, Johnson NE. Ketamine sedation for pediatric procedures, II: review and implications. *Ann Emerg Med*. 1990;19:1033–1046.

41. Raeder JC, Stenseth LB. Ketamine: a new look at an old drug. *Curr Opin Anesthesiol*. 2000;113:463–468.

42. Sherwin TS. Does adjunctive midazolam reduce recovery agitation after ketamine sedation for pediatric procedures? A randomized, double-blind, placebo-controlled trial. *Ann Emerg Med*. 2000;35:297–299.

43. Walthen JE, Roback MG, Mackenzie T, et al. Does midazolam alter the clinical effects of intravenous ketamine sedation in children? A double-blind, randomized, controlled, emergency department trial. *Ann Emerg Med*. 2000;36:579–588.

44. Bassett KE, Anderson JL, Pribble CG, et al. Propofol for procedural sedation in children in the emergency department. *Ann Emerg Med*. 2003;42:773–782.

45. Taylor DM, O'Brien D, Ritchie P, et al. Propofol versus midazolam/fentanyl for reduction of anterior shoulder dislocation. *Acad Emerg Med*. 2005;12:13–19.

46. Barnett P. Propofol for pediatric sedation. *Pediatr Emerg Care*. 2005;21:111–117.

47. Zuppa AF, Helfaer MA, Adamson PC. Propofol pharmacokinetics. *Pediatr Crit Care Med*. 2003;4:124–125.

48. Cray SH, Robinson BH, Cox PN. Lactic acidemia and bradyarrhythmia in a child sedated with propofol. *Crit Care Med*. 1998;26:2087–2092.

49. Klein SM, Hauser GJ, Anderson BD, et al. Comparison of intermittent versus continuous infusion of propofol for elective oncology procedures in children. *Pediatr Crit Care Med*. 2003;4:78–82.

50. Dickinson R, Singer A, Wessley C. Etomidate for pediatric sedation prior to fracture reduction. *Acad Emerg Med*. 2001;8:74–77.

51. Ruth W, Burton J, Bock A. Intravenous etomidate for procedural sedation in the emergency department. *Acad Emerg Med*. 2001;8:13–18.

52. McDowell RH, Scher CS, Brast SM. Total intravenous anesthesia for children undergoing brief diagnostic or therapeutic procedures. *J Clin Anesth*. 1995;7:273–280.

53. Scheart C, Burton J, Riker R. Adrenocortical dysfunction following etomidate induction in emergency department patients. *Acad Emerg Med*. 2001;8:1–7.

54. Alcock DS, Feldman W, Goodman JT, et al. Evaluation of child life intervention in emergency department suturing. *Pediatr Emerg Care*. 1985;1:111–115.

55. American Academy of Pediatrics, Committee on Hospital Care. Child life services. *Pediatrics*. 2000;106:1156–1159.

56. Zempsky WT, Cravero JP. Relief of pain and anxiety in pediatric patients in emergency medical systems. *Pediatrics*. 2004;114:1348–1356.

57. Bauchner H, Waring C, Vinci R. Parental presence during procedures in an emergency room: results from 50 observations. *Pediatrics*. 1991;87:544–548.

58. Schecter NL, Bernstein BA, Beck A, et al. Individual differences in children's response to pain: role of temperament and parental characteristics. *Pediatrics*. 1991;87:171–177.

59. LeBaron S, Zeltzer L. Assessment of acute pain and anxiety in children and adolescents by self-reports, observer reports, and behavioral checklist. *J Consult Clin Psych*. 1984;52:729–738.

60. Zeltzer L, LeBaron S. Hypnosis and nonhypnotic techniques for reduction of pain and anxiety during painful procedures in children and adolescents with cancer. *J Pediatr*. 1982;101:1032–1035.

61. Gardner GG, Olness K. *Hypnosis and Hypnotherapy in Children*. New York: Grune & Stratton; 1981.

62. American Academy of Pediatrics, Committee on Drugs. Guidelines for monitoring and management of pediatric patients during and after sedation for diagnostic and therapeutic procedures. *Pediatrics*. 1992;89:1110–1115.

63. American Academy of Pediatrics, Committee on Drugs. Guidelines for monitoring and management of pediatric patients during and after sedation for diagnostic and therapeutic procedures: addendum. *Pediatrics*. 2002;110:836–838.

64. Practice guidelines for preoperative fasting and the use of pharmacologic agents to reduce the risk of pulmonary aspiration: application to healthy patients undergoing elective procedures. A report by the American Society of Anesthesiologist Task Force on Preoperative Fasting. *Anesthesiology*. 1999;90:896–905.

65. American College of Emergency Physicians. Clinical policy: procedural sedation and analgesia in the emergency department. *Ann Emerg Med*. 2005;45:177–196.

66. Bailey PL, Pace NL, Ashburn MA. Frequent hypoxemia and apnea after sedation with midazolam and fentanyl. *Anesthesiology*. 1990;73:826–830.

34

JOHN H. BURTON AND CHRISTOPHER KING

Nitrous Oxide Administration

▶ INTRODUCTION

Nitrous oxide has a long history of utilization and experimentation over the last 2 centuries. The first documented medical application of a nitrous oxide–oxygen combination was to facilitate a dental extraction in 1840 (I). Nitrous oxide is now widely used for sedation in a variety of clinical settings.

The advantages offered by nitrous oxide are a quick onset of action, a low incidence of complications, and the rapid return of the patient's baseline level of consciousness. For the pediatric population, perhaps the greatest advantage is that nitrous oxide can be administered without inflicting the pain of an intravenous line insertion or intramuscular injection. The primary disadvantage of nitrous oxide administration is that its clinical effects are somewhat unpredictable; that is, the degree of anxiolysis and analgesia experienced can be variable. Furthermore, effective delivery of the gas is predicated on the patient's acceptance of the mask and willingness to inhale the gas mixture. Lack of interest and/or cooperation often results in inadequate administration of nitrous oxide and a poor clinical response.

Several investigations have described nitrous oxide utilization for procedural sedation and analgesia in pediatric patients (2–12). At least two relatively large studies in children have shown good efficacy and a low rate of complications when nitrous oxide is used to facilitate minor procedures (2,3). In most reports, nitrous oxide concentrations of 33% to 60% delivered by mask have led to clinically important relief of pain and anxiety in pediatric patients. While vomiting and respiratory events (e.g., desaturation, apnea) are typically cited as the most serious complications encountered, both are infrequent (less than 1% for respiratory complications) and resolve with cessation of nitrous oxide administration. Among the procedures that nitrous oxide has been used to facilitate in children are laceration repair, venous cannulation, incision and débridement of wounds, and fracture reduction.

Although most published studies have focused on the self-administered delivery of nitrous oxide, physician-assisted delivery of gas to pediatric patients also has proven to be safe and effective (2–9). As described below, this method allows the operator to provide sedation and analgesia to younger children, typically between the ages of 2 and 5 years, who might not otherwise understand or cooperate with self-administration. Using nitrous oxide sedation for children under 2 years of age is uncommon, primarily because it is often difficult or impossible to convince a younger child to accept the mask apparatus. Administration of a nitrous oxide–oxygen mixture to pediatric patients requires skill and experience with airway management procedures and a thorough familiarity with the delivery apparatus and the physiologic effects of the gas.

▶ ANATOMY AND PHYSIOLOGY

The unique aspect of nitrous oxide that distinguishes it from other agents used for procedural sedation and analgesia outside the operating room is that it is a gas. Although a daily activity for the anesthesiologist, the use of gaseous agents by most other practitioners is less common. Consequently, an understanding of the physiologic mechanisms governing the uptake, distribution, and excretion of an administered gas is important when using nitrous oxide.

Inhaled medications must be transferred from a respiratory circuit to the patient's lungs, taken up by the pulmonary vasculature, and distributed to the tissues where it will have an effect, primarily the central nervous system. Several qualities of both the gas and the patient will govern the uptake and elimination of an inhaled medication. The most important physical property of the gas is its solubility. An insoluble gas is taken up in the lungs much more rapidly than a highly soluble gas. Nitrous oxide is the most insoluble gas used in anesthesia; as a result, a high concentration develops in the alveoli, favoring a large concentration gradient to the blood, which in turn causes rapid uptake. A more soluble agent is continually washed out of the lung and therefore produces a lower concentration gradient.

Once the gas is in the lung, the patient's minute ventilation will determine the rate of delivery of the gas to the blood. The cardiac output will determine the rate of uptake of the gas. A high minute ventilation (which is normal in children) increases the uptake of the gas. However, this effect is partially offset by a high cardiac output, which will delay gas uptake. This occurs because the gas is washed out of the lung, producing a lower concentration gradient from the alveoli to the blood. Despite these competing effects, the nitrous oxide onset of action for a pediatric patient is rapid (2 to 3 minutes) as a result of the low solubility of the gas and a high minute ventilation.

Elimination of a gas (off-loading) occurs in a manner that is essentially the reverse of uptake. Off-loading occurs as a concentration gradient develops from the blood to the alveoli when gas delivery is discontinued and the agent is excreted each time the patient exhales. Several factors contribute to the rapid off-loading of nitrous oxide, which normally takes 2 to 5 minutes (13). For one thing, nitrous oxide is not metabolized before excretion, so elimination begins immediately. Nitrous oxide also is lipid insoluble, and therefore uptake by the muscle, fat, and solid organs is minimal. This lowers the total body stores and makes the gas rapidly available for excretion. Finally, nitrous oxide is not significantly protein bound, which enhances the diffusion of the gas from the blood to the alveoli.

The mechanism of action of nitrous oxide is poorly understood, although it does appear to act directly on the endogenous opioid system (14,15). This finding in part accounts for its analgesic properties. Nitrous oxide also acts as an anxiolytic, but the mechanism of this effect is unknown. Despite being a potent CNS depressant, nitrous oxide has been shown to have minimal effects on the normal protective airway reflexes in children (16). As mentioned previously, patients can have a wide range of clinical responses using this agent. Anxiolysis, a sense of detachment, and euphoria are most commonly observed. In addition, the patient is usually amnestic after the procedure. This profile of sedation, analgesia, and amnesia is one of the primary reasons that nitrous oxide is an excellent choice in selected cases for pediatric conscious sedation.

▶ INDICATIONS

The typical pediatric candidate for nitrous oxide use is the child who requires a short duration of sedation and/or analgesia during a painful or anxiety-provoking procedure. Nitrous oxide provides a low to moderate depth of sedation in the majority of patients. Specific clinical circumstances in which nitrous oxide might be chosen include foreign body removal, intravenous access with an anxious child, laceration repair, fracture reduction, minor joint relocation, incision and

drainage of an abscess, and burn débridement. However, almost any minor pediatric procedure can be facilitated by nitrous oxide administration.

As with any procedure, if the level of procedural sedation and analgesia proves to be inadequate, another method should be used. One point worth emphasizing is that nitrous oxide should not be used as a replacement for local anesthesia during painful wound management procedures. As with virtually all forms of procedural sedation and analgesia, a local anesthetic should be administered intradermally or topically whenever possible. Otherwise, the goal of using nitrous oxide becomes not only sedation and analgesia but the complete elimination of any perception of pain—an unrealistic expectation that makes a successful sedation far less likely.

Contraindications to using a nitrous oxide–oxygen mixture are relatively few. One important concern with this agent is the property of expansion within closed spaces. Nitrous oxide readily diffuses across biologic membranes. This diffusion theoretically continues until equilibrium is reached for the gases contained within any space. Consequently, the volume of gas within a closed space will increase as diffusion of nitrous oxide continues, eventually leading to excessively high pressures. Any known or suspected gaseous pocket in the body has the potential for expansion during the use of nitrous oxide. Nitrous oxide is therefore contraindicated in patients with suspected pneumothorax, bowel obstruction, or otitis media, a particularly common pediatric problem. Examining the ears and eliciting any history of otalgia is therefore especially important before using nitrous oxide with children. Potential adverse consequences include tension pneumothorax, bowel perforation, and tympanic membrane rupture (see also "Complications").

Another contraindication to using nitrous oxide is impairment of the patient's level of consciousness. Because safe and effective use of this agent requires significant cooperation, the patient with mental status changes who requires sedation would likely be better managed with an intravenous regimen. For example, the child with a minor head injury who has postconcussive agitation or lethargy would not be an appropriate candidate for nitrous oxide sedation (e.g., to repair a complex facial laceration or to reduce a displaced fracture). In such situations, the patient is unlikely to provide the degree of cooperation necessary to use nitrous oxide appropriately.

▶ EQUIPMENT

The equipment used for nitrous oxide delivery is commercially available from a number of suppliers. Although the specific characteristics of delivery systems vary by manufacturer, the units can be divided into two general categories based on the number of tanks required: single-tank systems and multiple-tank systems. Overall, the characteristics of these two types of nitrous oxide delivery systems are similar regardless of the brand.

Single-Tank Systems

These systems normally consist of a tank containing a 50:50 mixture of nitrous oxide and oxygen, a regulator valve apparatus, and a scavenging device (Fig. 34.1). The concentration of nitrous oxide delivered is fixed at 50%. Once the supply of the gas mixture is exhausted, a new premixed tank must be obtained. This type of system is especially popular among prehospital and emergency medical services (EMS) personnel because of its simplicity, compactness, and light weight. One drawback of a single-tank system is that the operator does not have the ability to increase or decrease the nitrous oxide concentration administered, potentially making the level of sedation somewhat more difficult to control. In the outpatient setting, titration can usually be carried out effectively by varying the amount of time that the patient is breathing the nitrous oxide–oxygen mixture. With increased pain, the child is assisted in maintaining a tight mask seal while breathing the gas; when the child becomes too sleepy, the mask is removed. If a pediatric patient is likely to have the desired response to nitrous oxide, a 50% concentration will usually be adequate to provide sedation.

A potential disadvantage of single-tank systems with more serious implications relates to the fact that nitrous oxide is heavier than oxygen, which in a cold environment can cause settling and fractionation of the agents within the tank. It is therefore theoretically possible for the patient to receive a higher concentration of oxygen until the tank is almost empty and then receive almost pure nitrous oxide, resulting in profound hypoxemia (see "Complications"). Although this is only likely with a tank that is both stored and used in cold temperatures (e.g., a prehospital field setting), it is generally a good practice to invert the tank before use to ensure adequate mixing of the agents.

Multiple-Tank Systems

These systems offer the ability to titrate the concentration of nitrous oxide delivered (usually 0% to 70%). Multiple-tank

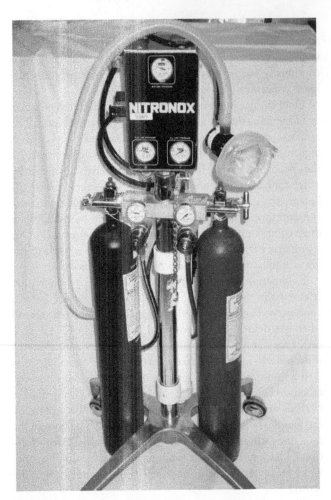

Figure 34.2 Multiple-tank apparatus.

setups typically utilize the same D cylinders of nitrous oxide and oxygen commonly found in most hospitals and operating rooms (Fig. 34.2). Although titration of gases may offer the advantage of providing a more gradual induction, evidence suggests that exceeding a 50% concentration of nitrous oxide increases the incidence of complications (e.g., emesis) without significantly enhancing clinical response (2,3,9). All systems should have one or more safeguards to prevent delivery of an excessive nitrous oxide concentration. This typically consists of a valve system that will allow a maximum nitrous oxide concentration of 70% and/or a shutoff device that is triggered if the F_iO_2 is lower than 30%. Alternative systems also are now available that combine elements of both the single- and multiple-tank setups. Utilizing a single tank of nitrous oxide, these devices mix an appropriate concentration of oxygen supplied from a standard wall-mounted valve, eliminating the need for tank oxygen.

Most commercially available delivery systems incorporate some type of scavenger system, which provides a means of removing nitrous oxide from the environment (17,18). Once connected to standard wall suction, the scavenger system will exhaust the gases exhaled by the patient, preventing accumulation of excessive ambient concentrations of nitrous oxide.

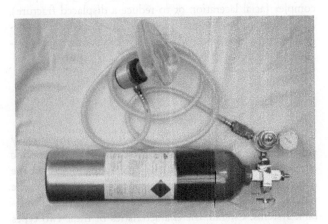

Figure 34.1 Single-tank apparatus for delivering a fixed nitrous oxide–oxygen concentration.

1. Commercially available single- or multiple-tank delivery apparatus
2. Variety of pediatric face masks and/or nasal masks
3. Spare cylinders of nitrous oxide and oxygen or premixed single tank
4. Scavenger device (usually included with delivery apparatus)
5. Flavored scents (Chapstick) with several options from which the patient can choose
6. Patient monitoring and resuscitation equipment: pulse oximeter, cardiac and blood pressure monitors, suction, bag-valve-mask, etc.

Prolonged exposure to high levels of nitrous oxide by medical personnel has been associated with adverse health effects (see "Complications").

A variety of standard pediatric nasal or face masks may be used to administer nitrous oxide. The operator should carefully assess the fit and seal of the mask to ensure proper gas delivery. If a nondisposable mask is used, it should be thoroughly cleaned or sterilized between uses. Applying flavored scents (e.g., Chapstick) to the inner lining of the mask will often enhance acceptance by the pediatric patient (4).

As with all methods of pediatric procedural sedation and analgesia, the minimum necessary monitoring modalities include cardiac monitoring and pulse oximetry. Equipment necessary for basic and advanced airway management also must be readily available (Table 34.1). These precautions should be taken even though airway and ventilatory compromise are less likely to occur with nitrous oxide than with other sedation regimens (see also Chapter 33).

▶ PROCEDURE

Administration of nitrous oxide sedation begins with a discussion between the physician and the patient and parents about the procedure, the equipment, and the likely effects of the agent. A favorable outcome is directly related to the degree of cooperation by the patient. Therefore, time taken to enhance the interest of the child and calm any anxieties experienced by the parents is well invested as it increases the likelihood of success.

Preparation of the delivery apparatus should be routinely performed before each use; this includes checking the function of the tank system and ensuring the availability of the proper volume of gas needed for the procedure. A mask should be selected that is appropriate for the size of the patient. Allowing the child to hold and investigate the mask while the procedure is explained often will alleviate any concerns about the equipment. Pointing out the similarity of the mask to a "space mask" or another familiar object also may enhance the child's desire to participate. To give the patient a sense of control with respect to the procedure, he or she should select the flavored scent applied to the inside of the mask (orange, cherry, bubblegum, etc.).

Proper positioning should be based on the nature of the procedure and the patient's wishes. A child may initially be fearful of lying supine and should therefore be allowed to remain sitting upright. After the nitrous oxide has been administered for a few moments, the patient will often begin to feel somewhat dizzy or lightheaded and wish to lie down. Acceptance of the gas mixture should be controlled by the patient. Delivery is always optimal with the patient holding the mask and breathing the nitrous oxide as necessary during the procedure (Fig. 34.3). However, younger children often prefer a parent to hold the mask, and this should be allowed as long as the parent has a clear understanding that the mask must not be forced on the patient and that it should be temporarily removed whenever the patient falls asleep.

Individual features of the tank setups vary, but the first step to initiating gas flow is usually to open one or more valves. If the unit has a security system, a key may be required to open the primary regulator valve. The operator should check any gauges on the tanks to ensure that they are reading in the appropriate range for proper gas flow. The dial may be color-coded to indicate the correct range. When available, the scavenger device should be connected to wall suction. Because flow is governed by a demand system, gas is only administered in response to the negative pressure exerted when the patient inspires; otherwise, no gas flow occurs. With a single-tank setup, a uniform concentration of nitrous oxide and oxygen is delivered, depending on the fraction of each gas within the tank. As mentioned previously, this is normally a 50:50 mixture. With a multiple-tank setup, the relative concentrations of nitrous oxide and oxygen can be adjusted by the operator using the primary regulator valve. For example, if oxygen is flowing at 4 L/min and nitrous oxide is flowing at 6 L/min, this constitutes a 60% nitrous oxide concentration delivered. With most systems, the highest allowable concentration of nitrous oxide is 70%, since the minimum flow of oxygen is 3 L/min and the maximum flow of nitrous oxide is 7 L/min. Because of the risk of hypoxemia with inadequate oxygen flow, nitrous oxide concentrations higher than 70% should not be used for conscious sedation.

When effects of the gas are apparent, the concentration of nitrous oxide may then be titrated (if the system has this option) to the desired clinical response. Titration is necessary most commonly when the child becomes overly sedated during the procedure. Should this occur, the concentration can be decreased until the desired level of sedation is obtained. If the tank system does not offer titration as an option, the seal of the mask can be modified to allow entrainment of air into the mask, decreasing the inhaled nitrous oxide concentration. The mask can also be intermittently removed altogether, as needed. As mentioned previously, nitrous oxide can have a relatively wide range of clinical effects, from inducement of quiet sleep throughout the procedure to hysterical, uncontrollable giggling. However, most children will lapse into a detached yet alert state within a few minutes of inhalation.

After the gas has been administered for a few moments and the child observed to demonstrate adequate sedation,

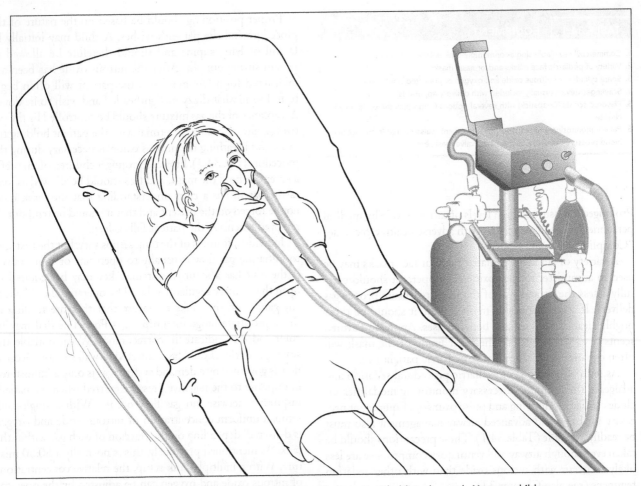

Figure 34.3 Nitrous oxide delivery is optimal with the patient holding the mask. Younger children may prefer that a parent or the physician hold the mask.

painful procedures can be performed. Although the degree to which the child will feel pain will depend on the response to the nitrous oxide administration, anxiety is frequently minimized and cooperation greatly enhanced by the administration.

A calm, reassuring voice is very effective in facilitating sedation with nitrous oxide. Guided imagery techniques (telling a story, talking about favorite places, etc.) may be used by a parent or by the operator. Questions directed to the child regarding the sensations felt are helpful in assessing the level of anxiolysis and analgesia attained. The patient may experience dizziness, lightheadedness, or a sensation of floating. Reassurance that these are normal effects of the gas is generally the only measure necessary to alleviate any discomfort. Refusal of the nitrous oxide should be allowed at any time during the procedure. However, the patient's interest in the flavored mask scent or the sensation experienced will usually be adequate to maintain cooperation throughout the procedure. If the patient does not respond to the gas in a manner conducive to completion of the procedure, the mask should be removed and an alternate method of sedation used.

Once administration of the nitrous oxide is terminated, the patient should remain in a sitting or supine position for approximately 3 to 5 minutes. Oxygen may be administered during this time, but with healthy children (i.e., children with no underlying lung disease) this is unnecessary. Patients who rise and attempt to walk will often experience increased vertigo and are at risk for falling. After the effects of the gas subside and the patient's level of consciousness returns essentially to baseline (which generally takes about 20 to 40 minutes), normal activities may be resumed.

▶ COMPLICATIONS

When used appropriately, nitrous oxide has been associated with relatively few complications. A screening physical examination and history will normally identify any patients at risk for gaseous expansion within a closed space (otitis media, pneumothorax, intestinal obstruction, etc.). As mentioned previously, such patients are at risk for exacerbation of the underlying condition, potentially resulting in tympanic membrane perforation, tension pneumothorax, or bowel perforation (19,20). Less severe complications such as dizziness or emesis can generally be managed with routine supportive care.

SUMMARY

1 Discuss with the patient and parents typical gas effects and the use of the delivery apparatus.

2 Ensure that the nitrous oxide and oxygen supplies are adequate for the planned intervention.

3 Select proper nasal or face mask for inhalation.

4 Position patient for optimum comfort and delivery of gas.

5 Start flow of nitrous oxide–oxygen mixture and check that gauges are reading correctly.

6 Allow patient to hold mask and titrate gas inhalation whenever possible. If necessary, physician-assisted administration may be performed with younger patients.

7 Titrate nitrous oxide concentration (if delivery apparatus allows) or occasionally remove or adjust mask seal to provide the appropriate level of sedation.

8 On completing procedure, remove mask and have patient remain in supine or sitting position until effects subside. When needed, administer oxygen during first few minutes of recovery.

Hypoxemia as a result of improper gas concentrations and/or nitrous oxide delivery is a potential danger that must be avoided. Patient-titrated administration and, when necessary, physician-assisted administration are the only acceptable methods of delivery. Periodic checks of the delivery apparatus should be made to ensure that safety features designed to prevent this complication are functional. In addition, although clinically significant depression of protective airway reflexes is uncommon with nitrous oxide administration, the response of the patient must be carefully monitored during the procedure. If at any time the patient appears too deeply sedated, administration of the gas mixture should be immediately terminated, which will normally cause the patient to quickly return to a baseline mental status. Appropriate resuscitation equipment should always be readily available whenever conscious sedation is administered to a pediatric patient.

An often repeated concern regarding the use of nitrous oxide–oxygen mixtures is the phenomenon of "diffusion hypoxia." First described by Fink in 1955 (21), diffusion hypoxia occurs when high concentrations of nitrous oxide in the body rapidly diffuse out of the tissues back into the alveoli on termination of gas administration, potentially displacing oxygen and thereby causing hypoxemia. A number of more recent studies have demonstrated that with the concentration of oxygen and nitrous oxide most commonly used for sedation (i.e., a 50:50 mixture), diffusion hypoxia does not occur

in healthy patients (22–25). This represents a potential risk only for patients with significant underlying lung diseases or with higher nitrous oxide concentrations. Any risk of this complication can be eliminated if the patient receives 100% oxygen for a few minutes after the procedure.

As mentioned previously, nitrous oxide is heavier than oxygen. If a single-tank system is exposed to cold temperatures (less than 5°C) for prolonged periods of time, the nitrous oxide will settle to the bottom, resulting in fractionation of the agents. Obviously, this is only likely to be a concern when the tank system is used in a field setting. Furthermore, this problem should be recognized quickly, because a high concentration of oxygen will be administered initially, making sedation impossible. However, in the unlikely event that the oxygen is completely vented, the patient could theoretically receive pure nitrous oxide, causing profound hypoxemia. This complication can easily be avoided if the tank is inverted each time before use to adequately mix the agents.

Recurrent exposure of health care providers to nitrous oxide has been associated with a number of potential health problems, including hepatic dysfunction, neurologic disorders, and reproductive abnormalities (26–28). However, studies on this subject have dealt with exposure to high ambient levels of nitrous oxide over long periods of time. With the intermittent use of nitrous oxide that occurs in most acute care settings, such prolonged and frequent exposures are extremely unlikely. Furthermore, no such risks have been demonstrated for patients who undergo an isolated nitrous oxide sedation.

 CLINICAL TIPS

▶ The equipment and typical effects of nitrous oxide should be thoroughly explained to parents and patient before the procedure.

▶ A comparison of the mask to a "space mask" or other familiar object may increase the understanding and interest of the child.

▶ Flavored scents (bubble gum, orange, cherry, etc.) can be used to increase interest in gas inhalation and minimize gas odor.

▶ Three to 5 minutes of inhalation should be allowed in order for the complete effects of the nitrous oxide to take place.

▶ Reassurance with a calm, soothing voice, and use of guided imagery techniques are highly effective in facilitating conscious sedation of pediatric patients.

▶ The mask must never be forced on the patient because oversedation may occur. Furthermore, insistence on the part of the operator or parent is usually met with refusal by the patient.

Nevertheless, to reduce any potential risk to medical personnel, nitrous oxide–oxygen mixtures should only be administered in an adequately ventilated room. In addition, it is recommended that all delivery systems used on a regular basis should have a functional scavenging device.

▶ SUMMARY

Nitrous oxide–oxygen mixtures have been shown to be safe and effective when administered to pediatric patients. Subjects generally experience pain relief, anxiolysis, and amnesia. The rapid onset, short duration of action, and ease of use make nitrous oxide sedation an attractive option for the acute care setting. It is particularly suited for children, since administration is painless. Potential side effects with this agent are few, although the patient may experience nausea, vomiting, dizziness, and increased excitability. More serious problems, such as oversedation and hypoxemia, are uncommon, resolve with cessation of administration, and can usually be avoided with proper technique.

▶ REFERENCES

1. American Dental Association Horace Wells Centenary Committee. *Horace Wells, Dentist, Father of Surgical Anesthesia.* Hartford, CT: Connecticut Printers; 1948.
2. Griffin G, Campbell V, Jones R. Nitrous oxide–oxygen sedation for minor surgery: experience in a pediatric setting. *JAMA.* 1981;245:2411–2413.
3. Gall O, Annequin D, Benoit G, et al. Adverse events of premixed nitrous oxide and oxygen for procedural sedation in children. *Lancet.* 2001;358:1514–1515.
4. Burton JH, Auble TE, Fuchs SM. Effectiveness of 50% nitrous oxide/50% oxygen during laceration repair in children. *Acad Emerg Med.* 1998;5:112–117.
5. Kanagasundaram SA, Lane LJ, Cavalletto BP, et al. Efficacy and safety of nitrous oxide in alleviating pain and anxiety during painful procedures. *Arch Dis Child.* 2001;84:492–495.
6. Luhmann JD, Kennedy RM, Porter FL, et al. A randomized clinical trial of continuous-flow nitrous oxide and midazolam for sedation of young children during laceration repair. *Ann Emerg Med.* 2001;37:20–27.
7. Luhmann JD, Kennedy RM, Jaffe DM, et al. Continuous-flow delivery of nitrous oxide and oxygen: a safe and cost-effective technique for inhalation analgesia and sedation of pediatric patients. *Pediatr Emerg Care.* 1999;15:388–392.
8. Gamis AS, Knapp JF, Glenski JA. Nitrous oxide analgesia in a pediatric emergency department. *Ann Emerg Med.* 1989;18:177–181.
9. Henderson JM, Spence DG, Komocar LM, et al. Administration of nitrous oxide to pediatric patients provides analgesia for venous cannulation. *Anesthesiology.* 1990;72:269–271.
10. Wattenmaker I, Kasser JR, McGravey A. Self-administered nitrous oxide for fracture reduction in children in an emergency room setting. *J Orthop Trauma.* 1990;4:35–38.
11. Evans JK, Buckley MD, Alexander AH, et al. Analgesia for the reduction of fractures in children: a comparison of nitrous oxide with intramuscular sedation. *J Pediatr Orthop.* 1995;15:73–77.
12. Hennrikus WJ, Simpson RB, Klingelberger CE, et al. Self-administered nitrous oxide analgesia for pediatric fracture reductions. *J Pediatr Orthop.* 1995;14:538–542.
13. Stewart RD. Nitrous oxide sedation/analgesia in emergency medicine. *Ann Emerg Med.* 1985;4:139–148.
14. Gillman MA. Analgesic (subanesthetic) nitrous oxide interacts with the endogenous opioid system: review of the evidence. *Life Sci.* 1986;39:1209–1211.
15. Gilman MA. Opioid action of analgesic nitrous oxide [letter]. *Ann Emerg Med.* 1990;19:843.
16. Roberts GJ, Wignall BK. Efficacy of the laryngeal reflex during oxygen–nitrous oxide sedation. *Br J Anaesth.* 1982;54:1277–1281.
17. Dula DJ, Skiendzielewski JJ, Royko M. The scavenger device for nitrous oxide administration. *Ann Emerg Med.* 1981;10:575–578.
18. Dula DJ, Skiendzielewski JJ, Snover SW. The scavenger device for nitrous oxide administration. *Ann Emerg Med.* 1983;12:759–761.
19. Eger EJ, Saidman LT. Hazards of nitrous oxide anesthesia in bowel obstruction and pneumothorax. *Anesthesiology.* 1965;26:61–64.
20. Perreault L, Normandin N, Plamondon L, et al. Tympanic membrane rupture after anesthesia with nitrous oxide. *Anesthesiology.* 1982;57:325–326.
21. Fink BR. Diffusion anoxia. *Anesthesiology.* 1955;16:511–519.
22. Stewart RD, Gorayeb MJ, Pelton GH. Determination of arterial blood gases before, during and after nitrous oxide: oxygen administration. *Ann Emerg Med.* 1986;15:1177–1180.
23. Murphy IL, Splinter WM. The clinical significance of diffusion hypoxia in children. *Can J Anaesth.* 1990;37:S40.
24. Dunn-Russell T, Adair SM, Sams DR, et al. Oxygen saturation and diffusion hypoxia in children following nitrous oxide sedation. *Pediatr Dent.* 1993;16:88–92.
25. Quarnstrom FC, Milgrom P, Bishop MJ, et al. Clinical study of diffusion hypoxia after nitrous oxide analgesia. *Anesth Prog.* 1991;38:21–23.
26. Rowland A, Baird D, Weinberg C, et al. Reduced fertility among women employed as dental assistants exposed to high levels of nitrous oxide. *N Engl J Med.* 1992;327:993–997.
27. Yagiela JA. Health hazards and nitrous oxide: a time for reappraisal. *Anesth Prog.* 1991;38(1):1–11.
28. Donaldson D, Meechan JG. The hazards of chronic exposure to nitrous oxide: an update. *Br Dent J.* 1995;178:95–100.

AUDRA McCREIGHT AND MARIA STEPHAN

35

Local and Regional Anesthesia

▶ INTRODUCTION

Local anesthesia is a useful adjunct in the treatment of pediatric patients with a variety of injuries and illnesses. Local anesthetics can be administered by tissue infiltration, by topical application, and/or for regional (nerve block) anesthesia. The unique properties of these agents allow physicians and other health care providers to safely and effectively reduce the patient's discomfort, often without the complications associated with the more time-consuming process of sedation. However, successful administration of local anesthetics is dependent on a basic understanding of their pharmacology and, in the case of regional anesthesia, familiarity with the local anatomy of the nerve and its associated landmarks (1). For the sake of clarity, certain types of nerve blocks are discussed elsewhere in this text. The auricular block of the external ear is described in Chapter 55, and nerve blocks of the oral and facial areas are described in Chapter 62.

▶ GENERAL CONCEPTS

Anesthetic Structure

Local anesthetics are classified by their chemical structure and linkage. This basic chemical structure is: aromatic segment–intermediate chain–hydrophilic segment (2–5).

The most commonly used anesthetics are aminoesters and aminoamides (2,3,5,6). In common parlance, these agents are often referred to as simply "esters" and "amides," and these terms are used to denote aminoesters and aminoamides throughout the remainder of this chapter. Procaine, cocaine, chloroprocaine, and tetracaine are examples of esters, and lidocaine, bupivacaine, prilocaine, mepivacaine, and etidocaine are amides. Drugs from the amide group are used more frequently for pediatric patients. The ester and amide local anesthetics differ in their chemical stability, locus of biotransformation, and antigenic potential. Amides are extremely stable, whereas esters are relatively unstable in solution.

The aromatic moiety of the anesthetic molecule contributes to its lipid solubility: 2-6-dimethylanaline for amides and p-aminobenzoic acid for esters. Changes in the structure of the aromatic portion have effects on lipid solubility and pK_a (5,7). Combining them with hydrogen chloride to form the salt of a weak acid solubilizes local anesthetics. The proportion of local anesthetic in the ionized form is determined by its pK_a and the pH of the solution. Neutral or alkaline pH favors the nonionized form, which is more lipid soluble and therefore better able to penetrate nerve membranes. Differences in the intermediate chain of the local anesthetic molecule determine its metabolism and clearance (2,3,5,7).

Ester and amide local anesthetics also differ in their allergic potential. Ester-linked local anesthetics (e.g., cocaine, tetracaine) are quickly hydrolyzed by plasma pseudocholinesterase and are excreted in the urine. Patients with pseudocholinesterase deficiency—those sensitive to succinylcholine, those taking cholinesterase inhibitors, and those with myasthenia gravis—are therefore more susceptible to toxic overdose of ester anesthetics (8). Cocaine, an ester, is an exception in that it is also metabolized by hepatic carboxylesterase (9). Esters also undergo degradation to the metabolite para-aminobenzoic acid, which is often responsible for producing allergic reactions (10). Amide-linked local anesthetics (e.g., lidocaine, mepivacaine, bupivacaine, ropivacaine) are conjugated in the liver by microsomal enzymes and are excreted in the urine. Unlike ester agents, the amide anesthetics rarely are associated with allergic reactions (11).

Molecular Action

When placed in proximity to nerve membranes, local anesthetic agents produce a transient and reversible blockade of neural impulses (12). Recent data show that local anesthetics act to displace calcium ions at an internal receptor site of the sodium channel in the nerve cell membrane. This displacement of calcium ions stabilizes cell membrane permeability to the flow of sodium ions into the cell, slowing the rate of depolarization such that the threshold potential is not reached (13). By inhibiting the influx of sodium ions through selective ion channels, local anesthetics prevent the initiation and propagation of an action potential (10). Inhibition of nerve conduction in the region of local anesthetic injection causes a temporary loss of sensation that dissipates with time as the local anesthetic molecules are released from the sodium channel (14).

The sodium channel plays a central role in the mechanism by which local anesthetics block action potentials along the nerve axons. The nerve axon is surrounded by a membrane consisting of lipid and protein molecules (15), which control the passage of small ions such as potassium and sodium. An electrostatic gradient (16,17) is generated by the sodium-potassium ATPase pump, with high concentrations of intracellular potassium and extracellular sodium and chloride. A resting potential of between ∼70 to ∼90 mV is thereby maintained.

When a nerve impulse is generated, depolarization occurs through a complex process in which membrane proteins ("gates") become permeable to sodium and potassium. As sodium enters the cell, the transmembrane potential reaches a threshold, and an action potential is propagated (2,15,18,19). Repolarization occurs as sodium and potassium ions are actively transported by the sodium ATPase pump, reestablishing the resting potential. Local anesthetics interact with the membrane protein gates and prevent sodium entry into the cell, although the precise mechanism of this interaction is not currently known. Without an influx of sodium, the electrochemical gradient does not reach the threshold potential, and no action potential is generated. This effectively blocks transmission of impulses from sensory receptors to the central nervous system (CNS).

Nerve Structure

A nerve fiber is composed of the axon and its surrounding Schwann cell sheath. A single Schwann cell may surround several unmyelinated nerve fibers (15). Myelinated nerve fibers often have one Schwann cell wrapped around a single axon. Myelin greatly increases the speed of nerve conduction by insulating the axolemma from the surrounding conducting salt medium and forcing the action current to flow through the axoplasm to the nodes of Ranvier, which are junctions between the sheaths along the axon (20). These myelin-deficient junctions are the sites where sodium channels necessary for depolarization are located. The nodes are more excitable than the rest of the membrane, allowing the impulse to skip from node to node and increasing conduction velocity. As the diameter of the axon increases, the nodes of Ranvier are spaced farther apart.

Nerve fibers can be classified into three types: A, B, and C fibers (3,7,15,17,21). The diameter and degree of myeli-nation of the nerve predict its sensitivity to local anesthetics (21). With subcutaneous infiltration of local anesthetic, the smallest, unmyelinated fibers are affected first, and the larger, myelinated fibers are affected last. Consequently, thick, myelinated type A nerve fibers (motor, proprioception, reflex, pressure, and touch) are less readily blocked than thin, unmyelinated type C fibers (pain and temperature) (3,4,22). Because pain sensation typically is conveyed on smaller, unmyelinated nerves, and motor impulses are carried on larger, myelinated nerves, a predictable pattern of loss of function occurs. The sensation of pain disappears first, followed by the ability to sense temperature, touch, proprioception, and, finally, skeletal muscle tone (12). By using an appropriate dose of anesthetic, it is therefore possible to completely block pain sensation while preserving full motor function. This can be advantageous, as with the repair of facial lacerations, because the patient can follow motor commands despite anesthesia to sensory stimuli. Anxious patients may interpret any sensation as failure of the anesthetic; therefore, the physician should prepare the patient by explaining that the sensation of pressure may remain but not pain (8). The recovery of function occurs in reverse as the local anesthetic dissipates (i.e., motor function returns before pain sensation). A variety of factors determine the final concentration of anesthetic presented to the nerve membrane, including dilution of the anesthetic by tissue fluid, fibrous tissue barriers, uptake by surrounding fatty areas, and systemic absorption (2,3,17).

Anesthetic Effectiveness

The effectiveness of a local anesthetic is influenced by various aspects of the physiologic environment and by its inherent chemical activity, which largely determines its onset of action, potency, and duration. Diffusion of local anesthetics (and therefore, their potency) depends primarily on lipid solubility. Local anesthetics with greater inherent lipid solubility are generally more potent. Hydrophobic effects are also important, because the anesthetic molecule must penetrate the nerve membrane and bind at a partially hydrophobic site on the Na^+ channel (23,24). The nonionized form is more lipid soluble. The ratio of ionized to nonionized forms depends on both the pK_a of the parent molecule and the pH of the solution, as described by the Henderson-Hasselbach equation (1):

$$pH = pK_a \log(\text{ionized form}/\text{nonionized form})$$

Local anesthetics are commercially available as water-soluble salts in an acidic solution, which primarily contains the cationic form of the drug (21,25,26). Raising the pH by adding sodium bicarbonate before administration increases the proportion of molecules in the nonionized, more lipid-soluble form, which speeds the onset of action (2,21,27). The rate and extent of diffusion also depend on molecular weight and concentration (2,4,5). Additionally, the site of administration plays an important role. As the amount of surrounding tissue or the size of the nerve sheath increases, the onset is delayed because of the greater distance the drug must travel to reach its receptor (2,4,7).

Protein binding of the anesthetic is an important factor in determining the duration of action. Binding reduces the amount of free drug available to diffuse into nerves directly (2,5,7,16,21). Agents that bind more tightly to the protein receptor remain in the sodium channel longer (18). Vasodilation produced by local anesthetics inversely influences the potency and duration of action (4,5). Local blood flow can remove the drug from the area before it is bound in nerve tissue and other binding sites. Vasoconstriction decreases this "washout" effect, allowing more molecules to remain at the peripheral nerve. In this way, epinephrine added to the local anesthetic solution can significantly increase the potency and duration of anesthesia (4,8,21,28,29). The duration also varies with the mode of administration and the dose. Topical application usually produces a shorter period of anesthesia than tissue infiltration. Increasing the concentration of anesthetic, while being cautious to avoid any toxic effects, can prolong the duration of action.

Important differences exist in the distribution and metabolism of local anesthetics in pediatric patients compared with adults. Infants have a larger volume of distribution, more rapid absorption, and lower plasma levels of albumin and α_1-glycoprotein (which binds lidocaine) (2,30). The activity of plasma pseudocholinesterase and microsomal enzyme systems in the liver is also low in this age group, resulting in a longer half-life of local anesthetics (30,31). Furthermore, the relatively increased cardiac output in young children leads to a more rapid peak plasma concentration. Because of the differences in pharmacokinetics, the toxic threshold in infants and toddlers is approximately one half that of children older than 5 years of age and adults (32). Special caution and reduced dosages are therefore warranted when using local anesthetics for these younger patients.

After the first few months of life, children have a greater clearance of local anesthetics than adults (30). Myelination is not complete until age 8 to 12 years. In laboratory studies, young animals are more sensitive to lidocaine, because they possess fewer myelinated type A fibers (17). The difference in the myelination of nerve fibers may account for the effectiveness of lower concentrations of local anesthetics in children.

Adverse Reactions

Systemic toxicity may occur by inadvertent intravascular injection or by using excessively large doses of local agents. After injection, peak blood levels are reached in 10 to 60 minutes. The more potent agents also are more toxic. Those with high lipid solubility and protein binding tend to become sequestered in tissue and have a slower rate of absorption, which produces a lower blood concentration. Esters are difficult to measure in blood due to their rapid hydrolysis by pseudocholinesterase. Toxic effects usually involve the CNS or the cardiovascular system. Local anesthetics are administered to inhibit conduction in the peripheral nerves, but any excitable nerve membrane (e.g., heart, brain, neuromuscular junction) may be affected if a higher drug concentration is reached (33).

Local anesthetics are lipophilic and cross the blood-brain barrier. As serum concentrations increase, patients initially complain of numbness of the lips and a metallic taste in the mouth. Nystagmus may follow, progressing to muscle twitching, tremors, seizures, and ultimately CNS depression and respiratory arrest at excessive concentrations (2,3,24,33–36). The blood-brain barrier is more permeable in infants than in adults, resulting in greater CNS concentrations of local anesthetic and therefore increased potential for complications (2). The cardiovascular system seems to be more resistant to toxic effects than the CNS. A decrease in blood pressure, however, may be observed secondary to the negative inotropic action of these agents, which can lead to a diminished cardiac output and stroke volume (2,3,21,33,34,37). Cocaine, which is rarely used now for topical anesthesia, produces its toxic effects on the cardiovascular system by inhibiting reuptake of catecholamines (epinephrine and norepinephrine) at adrenergic nerve endings, leading to increased blood pressure and/or ventricular dysrhythmias.

Allergic reactions to local anesthetics are uncommon. Most reports involve the esters which have a para-aminobenzoic acid nucleus (33,34). Reactions to amide anesthetics are rare. More often, methylparaben, a common preservative found in commercial preparations, causes allergic reactions that are subsequently (and often inappropriately) attributed the anesthetic agents themselves (33,38). Local anesthetics are available in a preservative-free preparation that avoids the aforementioned problems. Allergic reactions manifest as dermatitis, urticaria, anaphylaxis, pruritus, and bronchospasm. Small lacerations in allergic individuals may be repaired without local anesthesia or with normal saline infiltration. Diphenhydramine has also been used as a local anesthetic in a 1% solution (50 mg/mL diluted with 4 mL of normal saline to produce a 1% solution).

Tissue injury can result from the injection of anesthetic into a nerve or from passage of the needle. Neuropathy has been reported, especially with direct intraneuronal injection (39). In addition, inflammatory changes in muscle have been observed, but wound healing does not seem to be impaired (40,41). Tissue ischemia may result when epinephrine-containing solutions are injected in areas perfused by end arteries. Epinephrine administration is therefore contraindicated for use in digits, penis, nasal alae, and pinna of the ear. Local anesthetics do not affect the incidence of wound infection (42,43). Lidocaine has some antiseptic properties, but its presence has little effect on wound infection rates. If a wound is to be cultured, however, the swab should be obtained before local infiltration with lidocaine. Vasoconstrictors such as epinephrine have been associated with increased potential for infection in animal studies, but clinical studies in humans show no difference in actual rates of infection. Methemoglobinemia has been described with large doses of prilocaine and benzocaine (2). Toxicity is decreased by using an appropriate dose and route of administration as well as by administering vasoconstrictor-containing solutions (to prevent bolus absorption of large quantities of anesthetic) when not contraindicated. Contraindications to the use of regional anesthesia include (a) allergy to anesthetic agent, (b) infection

| TABLE 35.1 | CHARACTERISTICS OF COMMONLY USED LOCAL ANESTHETICS |

Infiltration anesthetic	Concentration	Physiochemical properties				Maximum allowable dose	
		Lipid solubility	Relative potency	Onset of action (min)	Duration (min)	mg/kg	mL/kg
Procaine (Novocaine)	1%	0.6	1	5–10	60–90	7–10	0.7–1
Lidocaine (Xylocaine)							
—Without epinephrine	1%	2.9	2	2–5	50–120	4–5	0.4–0.5
—With epinephrine (1: 200,000)	1%	2.9	2	2–5	60–180	5–7	0.5–0.7
Mepivacaine (Carbacaine)	1%	0.8	2	2–5	90–180	5	0.5
Bupivacaine* (Marcaine)	0.25%	27.5	8	5–10	240–480	2	0.8

*Some authorities do not recommend bupivacaine for use in children under 12 years of age.

at injection site, (c) poor patient acceptance or cooperation, (d) coagulopathy, and (e) inadequate skill or knowledge on the part of the clinician (1).

Selecting a Local Anesthetic

Although no local anesthetic is perfect in all respects, ideally a local anesthetic should (a) have a rapid onset of action and a long duration of action, (b) be nonirritating and nontoxic to tissues, (c) be effective both topically and by injection, (d) have a high therapeutic index and minimal undesirable side effects, (e) be stable in solution, (f) be water soluble, and (g) be heat stable for sterilization (1). The agents used for children that most closely approximate this optimal profile are lidocaine (Xylocaine) and procaine (Novocain), which account for approximately 90% of the use of local anesthetics. Plain lidocaine may be administered in doses up to 5 mg/kg, whereas the addition of epinephrine allows for a maximum dose of 7 mg/kg. Bupivacaine, a long-acting local anesthetic, is not approved by the U.S. Food and Drug Administration (FDA) for children under 12 years of age. Table 35.1 summarizes information on the most commonly used local anesthetics (3,21,34,38).

For increased safety in the use of local anesthetics for younger patients (less than 8 years of age), the following guidelines are recommended (44): (a) the dosage should be reduced to 80% of the maximal allowable dose; (b) the anesthetic should be administered slowly, in divided doses when possible; and (c) epinephrine (1:100,000 to 1:400,000) should be added if not contraindicated. As mentioned previously, the addition of epinephrine delays absorption but is contraindicated in areas where end arteries exist. For most procedures, it is unnecessary to choose a local anesthetic based on its onset of action. Simply waiting 5 to 10 minutes will generally obviate the need for additional local anesthetic.

Minimizing Pain with Injection

Rapid infiltration of an acidic solution of local anesthetic is painful. Decreasing the speed of infiltration can significantly reduce pain during injection (45–47). In addition, warming the local anesthetic to 40°C and using sodium bicarbonate as a buffer not only improves potency but also reduces the pain

associated with infiltration (47–49). To buffer a local anesthetic solution, 1 part sodium bicarbonate is mixed with 10 parts anesthetic (by volume) in a syringe. Buffering an entire bottle reduces the shelf life and is not generally recommended (38). Likewise, because a precipitate is created, buffering of bupivacaine with sodium bicarbonate is contraindicated.

▶ INFILTRATION ANESTHESIA

Wound infiltration is a safe, rapid, and easy method for providing anesthesia and hemostasis to a localized area. It is used for the majority of minor procedures (e.g., laceration repair, wound débridement, foreign body removal, abscess drainage). The two primary methods of infiltration of anesthetics are direct infiltration and parallel margin infiltration.

Direct infiltration involves the injection of an anesthetic agent directly into the tissues, and it results in the production of localized analgesia at the site of infiltration. Individual nerves are not specifically blocked but become anesthetized in the tissue planes surrounding the wound. The region is rendered painless by altering the perception of pain, although the sensation of touch may persist. Direct infiltration is the most commonly used technique for the administration of local anesthetic for laceration repair.

Parallel margin infiltration (field block) involves injecting adjacent tracts of anesthesia parallel to the wounded edge or surgical field. This results in the interruption of nerve impulses from the site to the CNS. As with direct infiltration, individual nerves are not sought specifically; they are anesthetized in the tissue plane in which they lie. The technique for this procedure is essentially the same as the technique for local infiltration except that the local anesthetic is injected circumferentially at a distance from the wound rather than into the wound margins. Field blocks are preferred for procedures in areas of inflammation or gross contamination. This method allows for the instillation of anesthetic away from acidic, infected areas, where local anesthetic is likely to have decreased effectiveness. Parallel margin infiltration also prevents the needle from carrying debris or bacteria from the wound into uncontaminated surrounding tissues. In addition, this method does not distort tissue planes that must be accurately reapproximated to optimize the cosmetic result of laceration repair. It is therefore preferred over direct wound infiltration when preservation of the wound architecture is desired.

Anatomy and Physiology

The skin is composed of the epidermis, dermis, and superficial fascia. Free nerve endings that generate impulses from painful stimuli are plentiful in the dermis and epidermis. The preferred plane of injection is into the superficial fascia, immediately below the dermis, where nerve fibers transmitting painful stimuli are easily blocked by infiltration of local anesthetic. Insertion of the needle through the margin of the wound beneath the majority of free nerve endings is less painful than insertion through intact, densely innervated epidermis. Tissue resistance and pain from the instillation of anesthetic are also less in the subdermal tissue plane than in the epidermis or dermis (50).

As in direct wound infiltration, the plane of injection for a field block is the superficial fascia, just beneath the dermis. Proximal to the laceration, nerves (bundles of nerve fibers) can be blocked, producing a field of anesthesia distally. With parallel margin infiltration, the superficial fascial layer is approached through intact skin parallel to the wound or field edge. As a result, needle insertion with this technique is more painful than direct wound infiltration, because it passes through intact skin.

Indications

Direct wound infiltration is indicated for most wounds and lacerations. In highly contaminated wounds, injection through intact skin may be preferred as a means of preventing the introduction of organisms from the wound margin into the surrounding tissues.

Some tissues, such as the sole of the foot, are difficult to infiltrate because of the fibrous, septated subcutaneous tissue structure. In other areas, swelling and distortion of the anatomy with infiltration make it more difficult to accurately reapproximate tissue planes and optimize the cosmetic result. Nerve blocks described later in this chapter are often superior to infiltration anesthesia in such cases.

Indications for field blocks are (a) local anesthesia for procedures in areas of inflammation or infection (grossly contaminated lacerations, incision and drainage of abscesses, etc.) or (b) local anesthesia with preservation of the wound architecture.

Equipment

10% povidone-iodine solution
Sterile gauze
Sterile gloves
1% lidocaine (with or without epinephrine, depending on location) and 8.4% sodium bicarbonate (1 mEq/mL)
3-, 5-, or 10-mL syringe
27- or 30-gauge, 1.5-inch hypodermic needle

Procedure

Direct Infiltration

The region is checked for perfusion, sensation, motor function, and associated injuries before anesthetic injection. To minimize patient anxiety, the syringe is filled with warmed, buffered lidocaine out of view of the child or before the child enters the treatment room. Whenever possible, the child should not be allowed to see the needle. All materials should be ready to use before the start of the procedure. After an appropriate explanation of the procedure, infiltration should begin without delay. A sensitive, calm, and soothing approach that engages the child in conversation or distracts the child may avoid the need for sedation. The young child should be immobilized by either an assistant, a papoose restraint, or both (see Chapter 3).

The area surrounding the wound is cleansed with povidone-iodine solution and dried with sterile gauze. A few drops of anesthetic are instilled directly into the wound. A 27- or 30-gauge, 1.5-inch needle is inserted through the wounding opening into the subcutaneous tissue exposed by the laceration. Anesthetic solution is slowly injected as the needle is

---

 SUMMARY: DIRECT INFILTRATION

1. Check region for perfusion, sensation, motor function, and associated injuries before anesthetic injection.

2. Explain procedure to parents and (as appropriate) to child, and keep needle out of view of child.

3. Restrain child if necessary.

4. Cleanse surrounding area with povidone-iodine solution and dry with sterile gauze.

5. If an open wound, instill a few drops of anesthetic directly into wound; then insert needle through margin of exposed subcutaneous tissue (rather than intact skin).

6. If not an open wound (e.g., foreign body removal) insert needle through adjacent intact skin into subcutaneous tissue.

7. Slowly inject anesthetic solution as needle is advanced, or insert needle completely and inject as it is withdrawn.

8. Remove needle and, if necessary, reinsert it into adjacent tissue through an area that has already been anesthetized.

9. Continue injecting tissue until entire area requiring anesthesia has been infiltrated.

10. After a few minutes, lightly apply needle to test for adequate anesthesia.

advanced. Alternatively, the needle may be fully inserted and slow injection performed on withdrawal. Aspiration is generally necessary only in the vicinity of major vessels, as only a small amount of anesthetic is injected at any given point while the needle is continually advancing. The needle is removed and then reinserted into adjacent tissue through the previously anesthetized subdermis. Reinsertion and slow injection of anesthetic continues sequentially until the entire perimeter of the wound has been infiltrated. Optimal anesthetic effect is reached in less than 5 minutes. The needle can be lightly applied to the skin around the wound site to test for adequate wound anesthesia.

Parallel Margin Infiltration (Field Block)

Preparation for this technique up to the point of needle insertion is the same as for direct infiltration. Because this technique involves the injection of anesthetic through intact skin, the operator may choose to administer topical anesthesia (see below) prior to parallel margin infiltration. A 27- or 30-gauge, 1.5-inch needle is first inserted through the skin to the subcutaneous tissue 1 to 2 cm proximal to the laceration. Small amounts of anesthetic are injected as the needle is advanced to at least two thirds its entire length. Slow injection is continued as the needle is withdrawn from the insertion site. The needle is then reinserted at the end of the first wheal where the skin is anesthetized. In similar fashion, the injection is repeated until

CLINICAL TIPS: INFILTRATION ANESTHESIA

▶ A longer needle allows for fewer needlesticks.

▶ Slower injection minimizes pain.

▶ Nerve blocks or general anesthesia, rather than infiltration anesthesia, prevents systemic lidocaine toxicity if lacerations are large.

▶ Stabilizing the ends of a wound with the nondominant hand and bracing the syringe against the nondominant thumb helps control the injection with a struggling patient.

▶ Aspiration is generally necessary only in the vicinity of major vessels, as only a small amount of anesthetic is injected while the needle is advancing.

complete infiltration of the circumference has been achieved. Optimal local anesthesia is achieved in about 5 minutes.

Complications

Direct wound infiltration and parallel margin infiltration are generally safe procedures, as long as correct medication dosages are administered and careful technique is practiced. Complications of both techniques include infection, bleeding, and intravascular injection of anesthetic.

▶ TOPICAL ANESTHESIA

Topical anesthesia is an alternative to local infiltrative anesthesia. It is used to anesthetize certain small wounds and intact skin for simple procedures. Topical agents are often advantageous because they are easier and less painful to apply, they do not distort wound margins, and they can decrease the need for sedation and physical restraint of pediatric patients. There are, however, some important limitations to the use of topical anesthetics: they have a relatively slow onset of action, they will not provide adequate anesthesia in many cases, and the agents are somewhat costly. Finally, occasional local and systemic adverse reactions are associated with the use of topical medications.

Tetracaine-Adrenaline-Cocaine

Tetracaine-adrenaline-cocaine (TAC) is a clear solution of 0.5% tetracaine, 1:2000 epinephrine, and 11.8% cocaine. Its anesthetic efficacy was first described by Pryor et al. in 1980 (51). The use of TAC has decreased dramatically in recent years due to the development of other topical anesthetics that carry fewer adverse side effects, cost less, and do not have

SUMMARY: PARALLEL MARGIN INFILTRATION

1 Check region for perfusion, sensation, motor function, and associated injuries before anesthetic injection.

2 Explain procedure to parents and (as appropriate) to child, and keep needle out of view of child.

3 Restrain child if necessary.

4 Cleanse surrounding area with povidone-iodine solution and dry with sterile gauze.

5 Insert needle into skin proximal to laceration to level of subcutaneous tissue.

6 Inject small amounts of anesthetic as needle is advanced to at least two thirds its entire length.

7 Slowly inject anesthetic as needle is withdrawn.

8 Reinsert needle at end of first wheal where skin is anesthetized and inject anesthetic.

9 Continue injections until complete infiltration around circumference has been achieved.

10 After a few minutes, lightly apply needle to test for adequate anesthesia.

appreciable abuse potential. Significant blood levels of cocaine have been detected and cocaine toxicity reported with its use (52). For the sake of completeness, however, its uses will be briefly described.

TAC topical anesthesia is about as effective as lidocaine infiltration for anesthetizing pediatric facial and scalp lacerations. It is less effective on trunk and extremity lacerations and in adult patients (53,54). Topical application of TAC is advantageous because it is easy and painless and has been shown to improve patient compliance with the subsequent wound repair procedure (51,53,55). The psychological trauma associated with restraint and painful procedures is reduced because of the relative absence of pain. Additionally, topical application avoids the swelling and distortion of wound margins caused by infiltrative anesthesia. This may enhance accurate tissue approximation and cosmetic outcome. TAC does not appear to increase bacterial proliferation or wound infection rates when compared with lidocaine (56).

The major disadvantage of TAC is that its use is limited to highly vascularized, non-mucous-membrane regions. Even when applied to selected wounds, adequate anesthesia may not be achieved. However, if additional local anesthetic is required, subsequent lidocaine infiltration is often less painful after TAC administration. Another disadvantage is that TAC costs significantly more per patient dose than lidocaine and also incurs the additional indirect costs associated with using a Schedule II agent (54,57). Finally, the time required to achieve effective anesthesia is considerably longer than that for lidocaine infiltration.

Anatomy and Physiology

TAC causes local anesthesia by the diffusion of the topical anesthetic combination through the margins of lacerated tissues. Tetracaine hydrochloride is a long-acting ester group local anesthetic. It acts on the neuronal membrane, interacting with the sodium channel to prevent the generation and conduction of nerve impulses in axons of the peripheral nervous system (54). Cocaine hydrochloride, which is derived from the leaves of the *Erythroxylon coca* plant, is an ester group local anesthetic with vasoconstrictive properties. Cocaine induces anesthesia by preventing impulse generation and conduction in sensory nerves, and it also blocks the presynaptic reuptake of norepinephrine and other catecholamines. This process results in excess norepinephrine concentrations in the synaptic cleft and is responsible for the vasoconstrictive properties (54). Epinephrine, an endogenous catecholamine with vasoconstrictive effects, prolongs the duration of action of locally infiltrated anesthetics by retarding drug removal and limiting systemic absorption.

Indications

TAC is used for the repair of wounds less than 4 cm in length that are located in well-vascularized, non-mucous-membrane regions. Typically, these are facial and scalp lacerations. TAC is contraindicated in areas of end-arteriolar supply (pinna of the ear, nasal alae, penis, digits), because vasoconstriction with-

out collateral circulation can result in tissue ischemia. TAC should not be used on mucosal surfaces or on areas of extensively burned or abraded skin, as excessive uptake into the systemic circulation may cause toxicity. In addition, TAC use in or around the eye may result in corneal injury. Other contraindications include an allergy to any of the components of TAC, cholinesterase deficiency, and significant hepatic disease. TAC should be used with caution in children with underlying seizures or cardiac dysrhythmias, as systemic absorption of the cocaine and tetracaine may exacerbate these conditions.

Equipment

TAC solution/gel (0.5% tetracaine, 1:2000 epinephrine, 11.8% cocaine)
Sterile 3-mL syringe
Sterile cotton ball or gauze
Protective gloves

Procedure

TAC should always be administered with gloved hands, as the compound may cause vasoconstriction of normal skin. To maximize TAC penetration, debris, blood clots, and devitalized tissue are removed from the wound surface. TAC solution is applied directly to the wound surface by dripping it onto the laceration or by "painting" it on with a sterile cotton swab. If TAC gel is used, an occlusive dressing is applied following application. A portion of the TAC dose can be placed on a sterile cotton ball or gauze and applied to the wound with firm continuous pressure for at least 10 to 20 minutes. As a safety precaution, a health professional may apply the TAC or carefully supervise parental application. TAC must not inadvertently come in contact with the eyes or mucous membranes, where it is more likely to produce complications. Blanching of the skin that surrounds the wound from the vasoconstrictor effect indicates that anesthesia should be adequate. Anesthesia generally persists for up to 1 hour.

Lidocaine-Epinephrine-Tetracaine

Lidocaine-epinephrine-tetracaine (LET) is a safer, more cost-effective alternative to TAC solution (58,59). LET, a combination of 4% lidocaine (substituted for cocaine) mixed with 1% epinephrine and 0.5% tetracaine, is not available commercially but must be compounded by a pharmacist. It is generally used on nonmucosal, lacerated skin surfaces. LET is available in a solution or gel formulation (60). LET gel is at least as effective as LET solution and often more convenient to use for the repair of uncomplicated facial and scalp lacerations (61). LET has been found to have anesthetic efficacy comparable to that of TAC in the repair of pediatric facial and scalp lacerations, although it is less effective when applied to extremity lacerations. No adverse side effects due to systemic adsorption have been reported with the use of LET (60). Because it has fewer complications, is considerably less expensive, and does not include a controlled substance in its formulation, LET has almost completely supplanted TAC for use in children (62). Another formulation, lidocaine-adrenaline-tetracaine (LAT), is also available. LAT is prepared as a gel and is often used interchangeably with LET. The information provided here is applicable to both LET and LAT.

Indications

LET is generally indicated for the repair of lacerations less than 4 cm in length. It is approved for the use on nonmucosal surfaces. LET should be avoided on areas of end-arteriolar supply or areas of extensive burn or abrasion. Contact of LET with the eye area should also be avoided because this risks corneal injury (60).

Equipment

    LET gel/solution
    Sterile 3-mL syringe
    Sterile cotton ball or gauze
    Protective gloves
    Adhesive bandage or other dressing

Procedure

LET should be administered with a gloved hand to avoid vaso-constriction of normal tissue. Any debris or blood clot should be removed from the wound before application to maximize effectiveness. LET is applied directly to the wound (gel) or to a sterile cotton ball or gauze (solution) that is then applied to the wound. Constant pressure should be maintained for 20 to 30 minutes; this can usually be accomplished using an adhesive bandage or other dressing. Eyes and mucus membranes should be avoided due to systemic adsorption of the component agents, although, as mentioned, this has not been reported to cause significant side effects with LET.

Eutectic Mixture of Local Anesthetics

Eutectic mixture of local anesthetics (EMLA) is a topical anesthetic formulation developed for use on intact skin (60). The term "eutectic" refers to the phenomenon whereby the melting point of the combination of agents is lower after mixing than that of any of the agents alone. The active ingredients of the EMLA mixture are the local anesthetics lidocaine and prilocaine.

EMLA 5% cream produces reliable anesthesia after a 60 to 120 minutes when applied under an occlusive dressing. Anesthesia has been reported to reach a depth of 3 mm below the surface of the skin following a 60-minute application and 5 mm following a 120-minute application. In addition, analgesia continues and may in fact increase for up to 60 minutes following removal of the cream. Rates of percutaneous absorption vary according to the location of application and the condition of the skin. Absorption occurs faster on diseased skin, facial skin, and Caucasian skin than on normal intact skin, extremity skin, and African-American skin, respectively (63,64). After typical application, the duration of topical anesthesia is approximately 2 hours (62). The maximal depth of analgesia to needle insertion is about 5 mm (65).

Use of eutectic lidocaine-prilocaine cream to relieve the pain associated with a variety of medical and surgical procedures is well established. EMLA has been demonstrated to have analgesic efficacy similar to that of lidocaine infiltration and ethyl chloride spray in children undergoing venipuncture and intravenous cannulation (66–71). In children undergoing lumbar puncture, the analgesic efficacy of EMLA was significantly better than placebo in double-blind trials (72,73). Its usefulness in providing anesthesia for repair of extremity lacerations has been demonstrated, and it allows a large percentage of these to be closed without additional infiltrative anesthesia prior to suturing (74,75). Although EMLA is currently not indicated for application to mucous membranes, its beneficial effect is evident for a variety of ocular, oral, and genitourinary procedures (60).

The major limitation of EMLA cream as an emergency department (ED) anesthetic is its slow onset of analgesic action. The time to onset of effective analgesia is approximately 45 to 60 minutes (62). Although pain was adequately relieved when EMLA was used before venous cannulation, there is no evidence that its use improved patient cooperation (67,71). Other shortcomings of topical anesthesia with EMLA include the limited total dose that can be applied, the fact that it often provides inadequate skin depth of analgesia, and the limited number of current indications for ED procedures. It is possible, however, that increased experience and further study will lead to a wider range of future applications.

ELA-Max, an over-the-counter combination of 4% lidocaine cream in a liposomal matrix, has recently been approved by the FDA for temporary relief of pain caused by minor cuts or abrasions. The liposomal quality of the matrix (lipid layers surrounded by aqueous layers) allows this mixture to penetrate the stratum corneum due to its resemblance to the lipid bilayers of the cell membrane. It is applied to intact skin for 15 to 40 minutes and does not require an occlusive dressing. The popularity of ELA-Max has increased despite a lack of data demonstrating its superiority to EMLA (60,76).

Anatomy and Physiology

EMLA results in dermal analgesia through the diffusion of the amide anesthetics (lidocaine and prilocaine) into the epidermal and dermal layers of the skin. The resultant accumulation of anesthetics stabilizes neuronal membranes by inhibiting the ionic fluxes required for impulse conduction.

The amount of lidocaine and prilocaine systemically absorbed from the eutectic mixture is directly related to the area and duration of contact as well as the region over which it is applied. Pharmacokinetic studies have demonstrated that the maximum plasma concentrations of lidocaine and prilocaine after topical application are 10- to 100-fold less than those considered to be potentially toxic (63).

Indications

Eutectic lidocaine-prilocaine cream is currently approved for topical analgesia only on normal intact skin. The cream has proved useful for venipuncture, intravenous cannulation, superficial surgery, and lumbar punctures in children.

EMLA is contraindicated in patients who have a history of sensitivity to local amide anesthetics or who have congenital or idiopathic methemoglobinemia. The cream is not recommended for use in infants less than 3 months of age (because of immaturity of the NADH reductase enzyme) and in those under 12 months old who are receiving treatment with methemoglobin-inducing agents (60). However, applications of 1 g or less may be safely administered to infants less than 3 months old without an appreciable increase in serum methemoglobin levels (66).

Equipment

EMLA cream

Occlusive dressing (adhesive bandage, plastic wrap, or Duoderm)

Procedure

A thick layer of 5% EMLA cream is applied to intact skin and covered with an occlusive dressing. Dermal anesthesia will increase during the initial 3 hours after application and lasts for 1 to 2 hours after the cream is removed. Application time should not exceed 4 hours in children less than 1 year of age (63).

For minor dermal procedures such as venipuncture and intravenous cannulation, 2.5 g (i.e., one-half of the 5-g tube) of EMLA 5% cream is applied over 20 to 25 cm^2 of skin surface for at least 1 hour before the procedure. For superficial surgeries or procedures that involve a larger surface area of dermis, approximately 1.5 to 2.0 g per 10 cm^2 is applied at least 2 hours before the procedure.

Ethyl Chloride

Ethyl chloride (chloroethane) is a sterile, colorless, flammable liquid used as a topical analgesic for superficial procedures. A spray bottle is used to direct pressurized liquid to cool the skin and produce instantaneous anesthesia.

Ethyl chloride has been demonstrated to significantly reduce the pain of venipuncture and lumbar puncture (77,78). When compared with intradermal lidocaine for venipuncture, there was no difference between the agents in terms of the perceived pain of application, but ethyl chloride was less effective in producing skin anesthesia (77). Nevertheless, ethyl chloride does not cause tissue distortion or vasoconstriction and results in less interference with venous cannulation than lidocaine (77).

Ethyl chloride is quick and easy to use, readily accessible, and dependable. The cost is approximately five dollars per multidose bottle (78). However, cooling only results in brief superficial anesthesia, and ethyl chloride should not be used for deeper pain, which is better managed with local infiltration or nerve blockade. Appropriate room ventilation is essential, and its use is prohibited near ignition sources.

Anatomy and Physiology

Ethyl chloride is a vapocoolant. The liquid has a boiling point of 12°C to 13°C. On contact with skin, it vaporizes and cools the surrounding area to ~20°C, thereby freezing any water vapor present, which crystallizes as a white precipitate. The anesthetic action of ethyl chloride may be sustained for as long as 1 minute but usually lasts no longer than a few seconds.

Indications

The application of ethyl chloride for topical anesthesia is indicated for minor surgical procedures (e.g., incision and drainage of a small superficial abscess) and before needlesticks for phlebotomy, venous cannulation, injections, and arthrocentesis. Ethyl chloride is contraindicated in individuals with a history of ethyl chloride or cold hypersensitivity.

Equipment

Bottle or metal tube of ethyl chloride with metal spray trigger

Procedure

Petrolatum can be applied to areas adjacent to the skin to be anesthetized to limit the area exposed to ethyl chloride. Appropriate patient restraint and control of the spray will prevent inadvertent eye exposure. All necessary equipment should be readily available before beginning the procedure.

In a well-ventilated room, the bottle of ethyl chloride should be inverted and held 6 to 12 inches from the application site. The spring cap should be depressed completely to allow for a steady stream of ethyl chloride to flow from the bottle. The spray is directed at the site selected for the procedure for a few seconds. Frost formation on the skin indicates that the area has been cooled and that maximal anesthesia is likely achieved. Because the duration of anesthesia is brief, the procedure should be performed promptly.

Iontophoresis

Iontophoresis is a method of obtaining topical anesthesia via a small electric current. Lidocaine-impregnated sponges are applied to the skin, and electrodes are placed on top of the anesthetic. A DC current is then applied to the circuit. Onset of effective anesthesia is approximately 10 minutes, and the duration of action is 10 to 20 minutes. When used for minor procedures involving a small area of skin, iontophoresis compares favorably with EMLA and offers the advantages of a more rapid onset of action and a greater tissue depth of effective anesthesia. The major limitation to the use of iontophoresis is the cumbersome nature of the equipment. In addition, some patients do not tolerate the tingling sensation produced by higher currents (60).

Other Methods

Additional topical formulations, including prilocaine-phenylephrine and bupivacaine-phenylephrine, are being investigated as alternatives to TAC and lidocaine. Both prilocaine-phenylephrine and bupivacaine-phenylephrine have shown equal if not superior effectiveness for laceration repair and may represent viable alternatives for local anesthesia (79,80). Additional approaches to topical anesthesia are currently under investigation. These include the uses of amethocaine, a gel similar to tetracaine but with a shorter onset of action, and a novel product called the S-caine patch. This patch utilizes a heat delivery system that increases skin temperature at the site of application to shorten the onset of local anesthesia.

Complications

TAC

Appropriate use of TAC is relatively safe. Patients and their families should be advised that with routine use blood and urine samples may become positive for cocaine and its metabolites, even without clinical signs of toxicity (81–83). However, misuse of TAC can lead to serious complications. Most such problems have occurred when TAC has been inappropriately applied on or in close proximity to mucosal surfaces, resulting in increased absorption. Complications may also occur with application of excessive amounts (more than 5 mL or repeated dosing) or when TAC is used on large areas of burned or abraded skin. Relatively minor reactions include pupillary dilation, agitation, and tachycardia; the major complications are seizures, apnea, and death (84–90). These systemic toxicities result from cocaine or tetracaine poisoning or possibly from the combined toxicities of all three component drugs (54). As mentioned previously, the risk of such serious complications is one of the major reasons that the use of TAC for children has been largely abandoned in favor of LET and other similar formulations. Corneal abrasions also may result when TAC contacts the eye (87). Complications of TAC can be minimized by strict adherence to correct application procedures and through restriction of its use to non-mucous-membrane, non-end-arteriolar regions. Additionally, using half-strength TAC may decrease the risk of side effects while maintaining adequate analgesia (91).

EMLA

The most frequent adverse effects of topical EMLA cream are mild local cutaneous reactions. Pallor (37%), erythema (30%), altered temperature sensation (7%), edema (6%), itching (2%), and rash (less than 1%) were noted in 56% of over 1,300 patients (60). The effects are transient and resolve within 1 to 2 hours after cream removal.

Metabolites of prilocaine are capable of inducing methemoglobinemia, and this complication has occurred after the application of EMLA cream (92). Infants under 3 months of age and children receiving other methemoglobin-producing agents appear to be at particular risk; EMLA should therefore be avoided in these individuals. The methemoglobinemia probably develops through the overloading of methemoglobin

reductase (93). Studies in children 3 months to 6 years of age have demonstrated a twofold increase in methemoglobin levels after treatment with EMLA. However, the methemoglobin levels of these patients remained within the normal range, and the elevations were not considered clinically significant (93–95).

SUMMARY: TOPICAL ANESTHESIA

1 Apply anesthetic (e.g., LET) directly to wound (gel) or to cotton ball or gauze placed on the wound, or as appropriate, apply to intact skin (e.g., EMLA).

2 Apply adhesive bandage or other dressing over wound to keep anesthetic in place.

3 Allow 15 to 60 minutes for anesthetic to take effect.

4 Lightly apply needle to wound margin to test for adequate anesthesia.

CLINICAL TIPS: TOPICAL ANESTHESIA

▶ Topical anesthetics are primarily useful for wounds of the face and scalp and often fail to provide effective anesthesia for trunk or extremity wounds. However, applying a topical anesthetic to a trunk or extremity wound may decrease pain associated with subsequent infiltration anesthesia.

▶ Blanching of surrounding skin usually indicates onset of anesthesia with a topical agent.

▶ Contact with eyes, mucous membranes, and end-arteriolar locations must be avoided when using topical agents to anesthetize wounds.

▶ When EMLA is used for venipuncture or venous cannulation, an additional site (or sites) should be prepared in case the initial attempt is unsuccessful.

▶ To be effective, EMLA must be applied at least 1 hour before the painful procedure.

▶ When using EMLA with a young child, care must be taken to ensure that the child does not loosen the occlusive dressing and ingest the EMLA or place it on a mucous membrane.

▶ When using ethyl chloride, prior application of petrolatum to the skin surrounding the desired area of anesthesia will limit skin exposure.

▶ Maximal anesthesia with ethyl chloride is usually indicated by frost formation on the skin.

Ingestion and ocular and airway instillation of EMLA cream have occurred through disruption of the occlusive dressing (96). Precautionary measures should be taken to ensure that the young child does not remove the dressing. Although rare, allergic reactions also may occur (62).

Ethyl Chloride

Prolonged spraying with ethyl chloride may result in chemical frostbite, skin ulceration, and muscle damage (97). Rarely, contact dermatitis may occur after topical spray application (98). Ethyl chloride must always be sprayed in a well-ventilated room, as inhalation may produce narcotic and general anesthetic effects. The solution is highly volatile and should never be used near an open flame or electrical cautery equipment.

▶ NERVE BLOCK ANESTHESIA

In certain cases, local infiltrative anesthesia is impractical or would likely be excessively painful. Examples include repair of a nailbed laceration, incision and drainage of a paronychia, manipulation of the foreskin when it is tightly entrapped in a zipper, excision of an ingrown toenail, and repair of a large laceration on the palm of the hand or sole of the foot. It may be difficult or impossible to achieve adequate local anesthesia of the fingertip, nailbed, or penis, and infiltration of the highly innervated palm and sole is usually extremely painful. In such cases, regional anesthesia using an appropriate nerve block might be the best (or only) method for providing effective anesthesia.

Upper Extremity Nerve Blocks

Nerves of the upper extremity most amenable to regional anesthesia in the acute care setting are the median, ulnar, radial, and digital nerves. These nerves innervate the highly pain-sensitive areas of the fingers and hand. Administering one or more nerve blocks before performing painful procedures in these areas often provides excellent anesthesia while minimizing discomfort for the patient.

Median Nerve Block

Anatomy

At the wrist, the median nerve enters the palm through the carpal tunnel and lies deep to the palmaris longus tendon, between the tendons of the flexor digitorum superficialis and flexor carpi radialis. At the proximal end of the tunnel, the location of the nerve is easily identified between the palmaris longus and flexor carpi radialis tendons where the nerve is bridged by the retinaculum (Fig. 35.1A).

Indications

The median nerve block is used to provide anesthesia for procedures involving specific areas of the thumb, index, middle, and fourth fingers (Fig. 35.1B). Median nerve blocks can be combined with radial and ulnar nerve blocks for procedures involving more extensive areas of the hand. Carpal tunnel syndrome is a relative contraindication to performing a median nerve block at the wrist (99).

Equipment

- 1% lidocaine solution
- 25- or 27-gauge, 0.5- or 1-inch hypodermic needle
- 5-mL syringe
- 10% povidone-iodine or other antiseptic solution
- Sterile gauze

Procedure

The area requiring anesthesia is carefully identified. The hand and digits are checked for perfusion, sensation, and motor nerve function before injecting the anesthetic agent. Apposition of the thumb and fifth finger with flexion of the wrist against some resistance will easily identify the tendon of the palmaris longus, which protrudes along the volar aspect of the wrist. The overlying skin is prepared with povidone-iodine or alcohol.

A 25- or 27-gauge, 0.5-inch needle is inserted perpendicularly, just radial to the palmaris longus tendon at the level of the proximal flexor wrist crease (Fig. 35.1C). A "pop" may be felt as the retinaculum is pierced (100). Paresthesias (i.e., tingling sensations or jolts in the distribution of the nerve) occur when the needle mechanically stimulates nerve fibers. It may be difficult for a child to cooperate with the physician and distinguish between the pain of needle insertion and the sensation of paresthesia. If a paresthesia is elicited, the needle tip is certain to be in close proximity to the nerve. The needle is withdrawn slightly to avoid intraneuronal injection, and 2 to 3 mL of anesthetic is injected. If a paresthesia is not elicited, a larger volume of anesthetic (about 3 to 5 mL) is injected to increase the likelihood that the nerve will blocked by diffusion of the medication. Optimal anesthetic effect is usually achieved after 10 to 20 minutes.

Ulnar Nerve Block

Anatomy

At the level of the elbow, the ulnar nerve lies in the groove between the medial epicondyle and the olecranon (Fig. 35.2). As it approaches the middle of the forearm, the ulnar nerve lies between the flexor digitorum profundus and the flexor carpi ulnaris (Fig. 35.2A). In the distal forearm, it divides about 0.5 cm proximal to the wrist, giving off two cutaneous branches—the palmar cutaneous branch, which provides some sensation to the ulnar side of the wrist and hand, and the dorsal cutaneous branch, supplying the ulnar side of the hand and the ulnar half of the fourth finger and the dorsum of the fifth finger. At the wrist, the ulnar nerve passes between the tendon of the flexor carpi ulnaris and ulnar artery, deep to the artery. Its superficial terminal branch supplies the skin of the anterior fifth finger and ulnar half of the fourth finger. If local anesthesia is needed throughout the entire ulnar

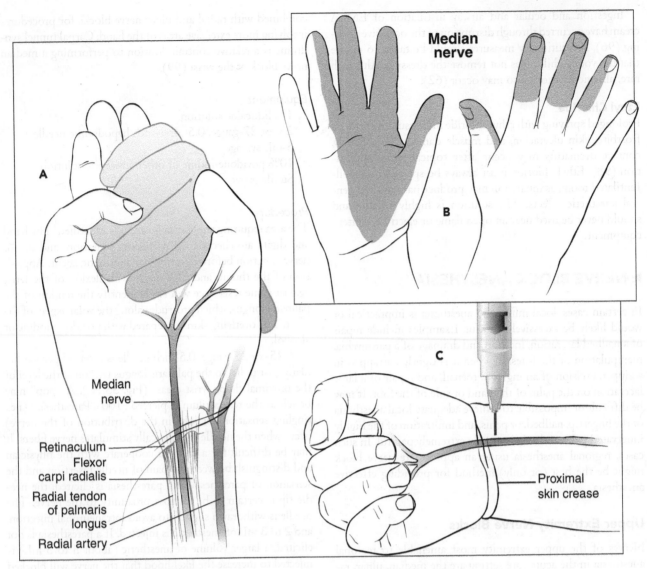

Figure 35.1
A. The median nerve is located just radial to the palmaris longus tendon at the wrist.
B. Sensory innervation of the median nerve.
C. Median nerve block.

distribution, it is preferable to block at the elbow (before the nerve subdivides) instead of at the wrist (101).

Indications

The ulnar nerve block should be used to provide anesthesia of the dorsal and palmar aspects of the ulnar side of the hand, fifth finger, and ulnar side of the fourth finger (Fig. 35.2B). As with other nerve blocks, this technique is used for painful procedures such as laceration repair, reduction of hand fractures, and removal of a foreign body. It is often used in combination with median and/or radial nerve blocks to achieve a larger field of anesthesia.

Equipment

- 1% lidocaine solution
- 25- or 27-gauge, 0.5- or 1-inch hypodermic needle
- 5-mL syringe (for block at wrist)
- 10-mL syringe (for block at elbow)
- 10% povidone-iodine or other antiseptic solution
- Sterile gauze

Procedure

Ulnar Nerve Block at the Wrist. The area requiring anesthetic is carefully identified. The hand and digits are checked for perfusion, sensation, and motor nerve function before injecting the anesthetic agent. A modified Allen test may be used to verify collateral arterial supply to the hand, although this test is not always reliable. The tendon of the flexor carpi ulnaris is located by having the patient flex the wrist against mild resistance. The skin of the lateral wrist is prepared with povidone-iodine or alcohol.

The palmar cutaneous branch of the ulnar nerve is anesthetized by raising a skin wheal at the level of the proximal wrist crease (ulnar styloid), between the tendon of the flexor

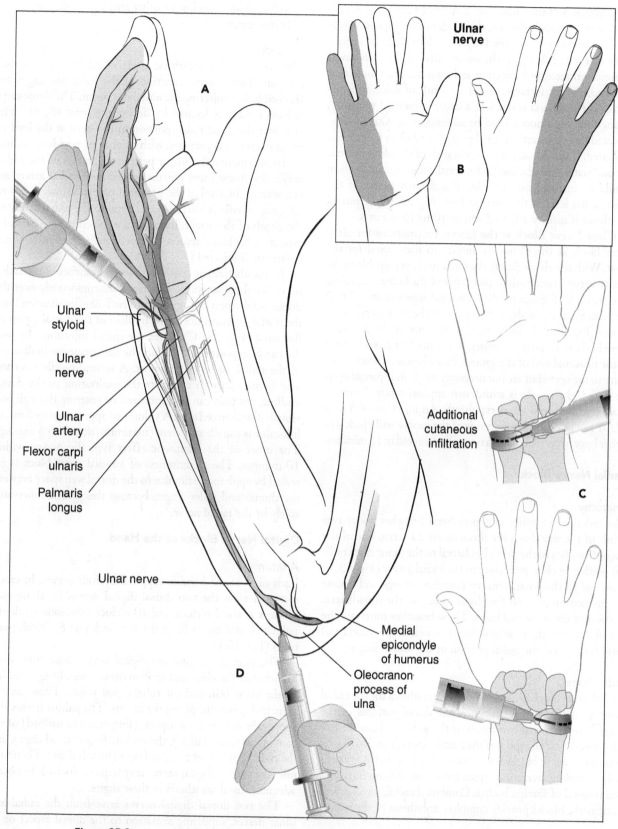

Figure 35.2
A. The ulnar nerve at the wrist runs beneath the ulnar artery and flexor carpi ulnaris tendon.
B. Sensory innervation of the ulnar nerve.
C. Cutaneous branches are anesthetized with a subcutaneous injection from the flexor carpi ulnaris
tendon around to the dorsum of the wrist.
D. Ulnar nerve block at the elbow.

carpi ulnaris and the ulnar artery. A 25- to 27-gauge needle is advanced through the wheal to a depth of approximately 0.5 cm (just deep to the tendon). Paresthesia indicates proximity of the needle tip to the nerve. After slight withdrawal to avoid intraneuronal injection and aspiration to ensure that the needle is not intravascular, 1 to 3 mL of solution is injected. If paresthesia is not felt, a larger volume (3 to 5 mL) of anesthetic solution should be administered. Alternatively, repeated fanned insertions can be done until ulnar paresthesia is elicited. If the dorsal cutaneous branch of the ulnar nerve is not adequately anesthetized, additional cutaneous infiltration should be instilled over the dorsal and ulnar aspect of the wrist, at the level of the ulnar styloid (Fig. 35.2C). Optimal anesthesia is usually achieved within 10 to 15 minutes.

Ulnar Nerve Block at the Elbow. Preparations for ulnar nerve block at the elbow are similar to those used for the wrist. With the elbow flexed, the ulnar nerve is palpable in the groove between the medial epicondyle of the humerus and the olecranon. A 25-gauge needle is inserted approximately 1 to 2 cm proximal and parallel to the course of the ulnar nerve in the groove (Fig. 35.2D). Blocking the nerve within the groove is more likely to cause nerve injury, so the needle tip is advanced to the proximal end of the groove. Paresthesias indicate proximity to the nerve but are not necessary to elicit. If paresthesias are noted, the needle is withdrawn approximately 2 mm to avoid injection into the nerve sheath. An injection of 3 to 5 mL of 1% lidocaine on each side of the groove will block this rather large nerve. Anesthesia is usually achieved in 15 minutes.

Radial Nerve Block

Anatomy

The radial nerve splits into peripheral branches about two thirds of the way down the forearm. At the wrist, one of the major branches of the nerve lies lateral to the flexor carpi radialis tendon in close proximity to the radial artery (Fig. 35.3). Proximal to the wrist, sensory branches emerge and course subcutaneously around the distal radius to the dorsolateral portion of the wrist and hand. These branches innervate the dorsal aspect of the proximal thumb as well as the second and third fingers and the radial portion of the fourth finger.

Indications

Radial nerve block is used to provide anesthesia for the radial portion of the thenar eminence, the dorsal surfaces of the thumb, the proximal two thirds of the index and middle fingers, and the radial aspect of the fourth finger (Fig. 35.3B). As with other nerve blocks, radial nerve block is useful for procedures such as laceration repair, reduction of hand fractures, and removal of foreign bodies. Combined radial, median, and ulnar nerve blocks provide complete anesthesia of the hand.

Equipment

1% lidocaine solution
25- or 27-gauge, 1-inch hypodermic needle
10-mL syringe

10% povidone-iodine or other antiseptic solution
Sterile gauze

Procedure

The area requiring anesthetic is identified. Perfusion, sensation, and motor nerve function of the hand and digits are checked before injecting the anesthetic agent. The flexor carpi radialis tendon is located by flexing the wrist slightly. The skin over the distal radial portion of the wrist at the level of the skin creases is prepared with alcohol or povidone-iodine.

To anesthetize the major peripheral branch of the radial nerve, the flexor carpi radialis tendon and radial artery are palpated at the level of the proximal palmar crease. A 25- to 27-gauge needle is inserted just lateral to the radial artery to the depth of the artery. Intravascular injection is avoided by aspirating for blood return. Approximately 2 to 4 mL of local anesthetic is injected (Fig. 35.3A).

To anesthetize the dorsal cutaneous branches of the radial nerve, local anesthetic is infiltrated subcutaneously over the dorsoradial aspect of the wrist in a cuff-like distribution from the initial injection site to the midline of the dorsal aspect of the wrist (Fig. 35.3C). After the initial injection, the needle can be repositioned to start the subcutaneous infiltration of the radial aspect of the wrist. A second needle insertion may be necessary to complete the infiltration to the dorsal midline, but pain can be minimized by entering through previously anesthetized skin. A volume of approximately 5 mL of lidocaine is usually sufficient (maximum dose 3 to 5 mg/kg). The onset of the anesthetic effect typically occurs within 10 minutes. The effectiveness of a radial nerve block is assessed by applying a stimulus to the dorsal web space between the thumb and index finger, because this area is innervated solely by the radial nerve.

Digital Nerve Blocks of the Hand

Anatomy

Each digit of the hand is supplied by four nerves. In cross-sectional view, the two dorsal digital nerves lie along each phalanx at the 2 o'clock and 10 o'clock positions, while the palmar digital nerves lie at the 4 o'clock and 8 o'clock positions (Fig. 35.4).

The palmar or common digital nerves arise from deep branches of the ulnar and median nerves, supplying sensation to the volar skin and interphalangeal joints. These are the principal nerves supplying the fingers. The palmar nerves also supply the dorsal distal aspects (fingertip and nailbed) of the forefinger (second digit), the middle finger (third digit), and the radial portion of the ring finger (fourth digit). Therefore, only the palmar digital nerves may require blockade to obtain adequate distal anesthesia in these digits.

The two dorsal digital nerves arise from the radial and ulnar nerves, supplying sensation to the dorsal aspect of all five fingers to the level of the distal interphalangeal joints. The dorsal nerves also supply the dorsal distal aspects (fingertip and nailbed) of the thumb and fifth digit and the ulnar aspect of the fourth finger. In these digits, therefore, all four nerves

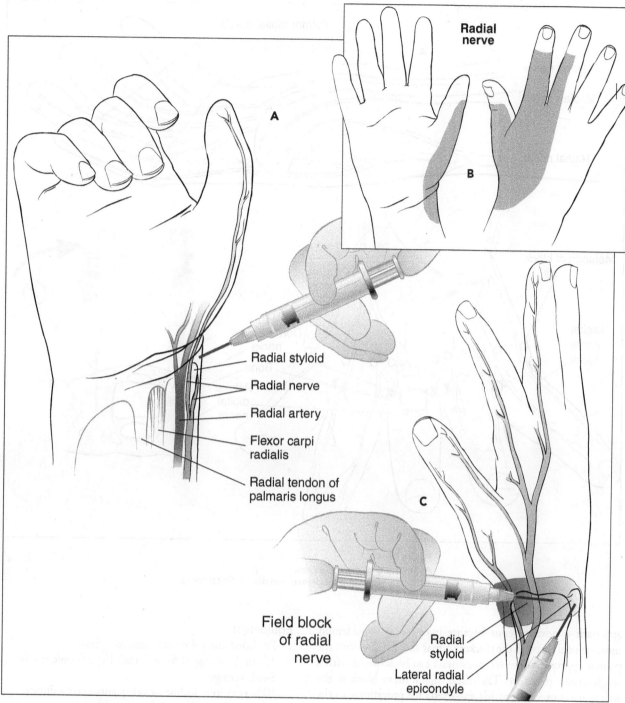

Figure 35.3
A. The radial nerve at the wrist is blocked just lateral to the radial artery.
B. Sensory innervation of the radial nerve.
C. Cutaneous branches are anesthetized with subcutaneous injection in a cuff-like distribution around to the dorsal midline.

must always be blocked to obtain adequate anesthesia for distal repairs.

Indications

Digital nerve blocks are used to provide anesthesia of the fingers for procedures such as finger laceration and nailbed repair, drainage of a paronychia, and reduction of fractures and dislocations. The digital nerve block is the most common nerve block used by ED physicians for minor wound care (100).

The common digital nerve block can be performed from either the dorsal or the palmar aspects of the finger. The dorsal

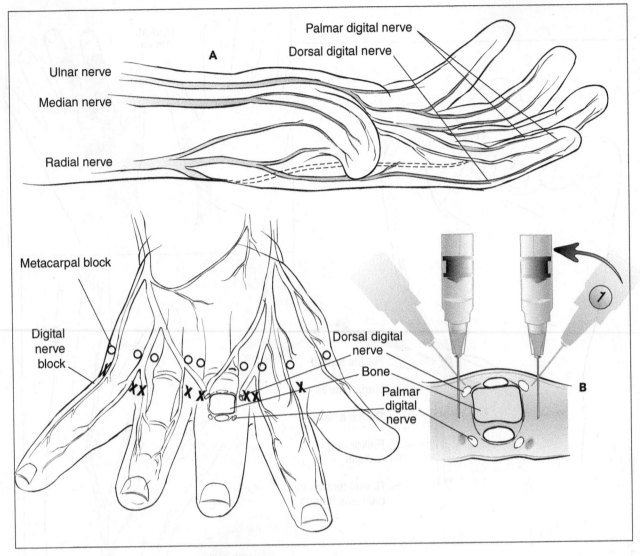

Figure 35.4
A. Anatomy of digital nerves.
B. Dorsal technique for palmar and dorsal digital nerve.

approach is advantageous because injection is considerably more painful through the thicker palmar skin (102). With the palmar approach, however, anesthesia can be achieved with a single needle puncture. The distal digital nerve block at the web space is used to provide anesthesia for procedures to the distal two thirds of the fingers. Effective distal digital nerve blockade can be achieved with a small volume of local anesthetic. Large volumes are unnecessary and pose the additional risks of vascular compression and patient discomfort. A proximal block at the level of the distal metacarpal may be preferred over the distal digital nerve block, because it reduces the risk of vascular compromise by compression of the arterial supply. It also anesthetizes the entire length of the finger. Only the palmar digital nerves need to be blocked in the middle three fingers to achieve complete anesthesia of the fingertip (100). The thumb and fifth digit require both palmar and dorsal digital nerve blockade.

Equipment

1% lidocaine solution *without epinephrine*
25- or 27-gauge, 0.5- or 1-inch hypodermic needle
5-mL syringe
10% povidone-iodine or other antiseptic solution
Sterile gauze

Procedure

Preparations for each of the digital nerve blocks are similar. The area requiring anesthetic is first identified. The distal fingers are assessed for perfusion, sensation, and motor nerve function before injection. Because the digital nerve may have been damaged by the initial finger injury, it is important to determine and document digital nerve function in the affected finger before nerve blockade. Sterile injection technique after preparation of the skin with alcohol or povidone-iodine is necessary, but sterile gloves and drapes are not required.

Distal Digital Nerve Block. The interdigital web space skin is prepared with povidone-iodine solution. A 25- or 27-gauge needle is inserted into the dorsal aspect of the web space distal to the metacarpal-phalangeal joint. The needle is advanced toward the bone of the affected finger. If no blood return occurs with aspiration, 0.5 to 1.0 mL of local anesthetic is injected to block the dorsal digital nerves (Fig. 35.4B). Next the needle is redirected toward the palmar surface of the digit, and an additional 0.5 to 1.0 mL of solution is deposited to anesthetize the palmar digital nerve. The procedure is repeated on the opposite side of the digit to achieve complete anesthesia of all four digital nerves. The anesthetic effect is usually adequate in 5 to 10 minutes.

Proximal (Common) Digital Nerve Block or Metacarpal Block. To perform the dorsal technique for the proximal digital nerve block, the skin over the dorsal surface of the metacarpals is first prepared with alcohol or povidone-iodine. A subcutaneous skin wheal is raised between the metacarpal bones on the dorsum of the hand approximately 1 to 2 cm proximal to the web space. With a 25-gauge, 1-inch needle, the skin is entered through the wheal, and the needle is slowly advanced until its tip rests just below the palmar skin surface. Aspiration prior to infiltration prevents intravascular injection. Local anesthetic (2 to 3 mL) is deposited. Because the common digital nerve lies just above the flexor retinaculum of the hand, most of the local anesthetic should be delivered close to the palmar surface. The procedure is repeated on the opposite side of the metacarpal to ensure that both sides of the involved digit are anesthetized (Fig. 35.4B). The block takes effect in 10 to 15 minutes.

To perform the palmar technique of the proximal digital nerve block, the palmar skin over the metacarpal heads is first prepared with alcohol or povidone-iodine. A 25- or 27-gauge, 1-inch needle is inserted at the level of the distal palmar crease, over the center of the metacarpal head (Fig. 35.4B). Anesthetic solution is injected as the needle is advanced to the bone. The needle is withdrawn slightly, redirected toward the radial aspect of the metacarpal head, and advanced a few millimeters. Aspiration to ensure no blood return prevents intravascular injection. Approximately 1.0 to 1.5 mL of local anesthetic is deposited. The needle is withdrawn a few millimeters, angled toward the ulnar aspect of the metacarpal head, and advanced slightly. An additional 1.0 to 1.5 mL is injected after aspiration (Fig. 35.4B). The block usually takes effect in 10 to 15 minutes.

Lower Extremity Nerve Blocks

Ankle Blocks

Sensory innervation of the foot involves five nerves that course through the ankle. Considerable overlap is evident in the sensory distribution, frequently necessitating more than one nerve block at the ankle for complete anesthesia. Nerve blocks of the deep peroneal, posterior tibial, saphenous, superficial peroneal, and sural nerves can be used alone or in combination

for procedures involving the foot. They are often preferable to infiltrative anesthesia because in many areas the skin of the foot is more sensitive than the skin at the ankle, and the dense, septated subcutaneous connective tissue of the foot is not easily infiltrated (103).

The saphenous nerve provides sensation to the medial aspect of the ankle and instep. The superficial peroneal nerve innervates the central dorsum of the foot. Because local infiltrative anesthesia is generally quite successful for lacerations and wound repair in these areas, saphenous and superficial peroneal nerve blocks will not be described.

Anatomy

The posterior tibial and sural nerves supply sensory innervation to the entire sole of the foot (Fig. 35.5). When both nerves are blocked simultaneously, this is often referred to as a "posterior ankle block." The posterior tibial nerve is a branch of the sciatic nerve, and at the ankle it runs behind the medial malleolus just posterior to the easily palpated posterior tibial artery. The posterior tibial nerve provides sensation to the medial portion of the sole of the foot anteriorly and the plantar surfaces of the hallux and the second and third toes and the medial side of the fourth toe. The sural nerve courses with the short saphenous vein behind the fibula and lateral malleolus. It provides sensation to the heel and the lateral portion of the sole of the foot anteriorly and the plantar surface of the lateral aspect of the fourth toe and the entire fifth toe.

The deep peroneal nerve arises from the bifurcation of the common peroneal nerve and is located anteriorly (Fig. 35.6). In the ankle, it lies under the extensor hallucis longus tendon continuing to the dorsum of the foot. It innervates the short extensors to the toes as well as the skin on the lateral side of the hallux and on the medial side of the second toe.

Indications

Ankle blocks are used for performing any painful procedures involving the foot, such as laceration repair, drainage of infections, and foreign body removal. The sural and posterior tibial nerve blocks provide anesthesia of the heel and sole of the foot (Fig. 35.5A,B). The deep peroneal nerve block provides anesthesia of the distal foot at the web space between the great and second toes and is often combined with other ankle blocks (Fig. 35.6A).

Equipment

1% lidocaine solution
25- or 27-gauge, 1.0- or 1.5-inch hypodermic needle
10-mL syringe
10% povidone-iodine or other antiseptic solution
Sterile gauze

Procedure

Initial preparation for each of the ankle blocks to be described is identical. The area requiring anesthesia is first identified, and perfusion and sensation are assessed before injection of

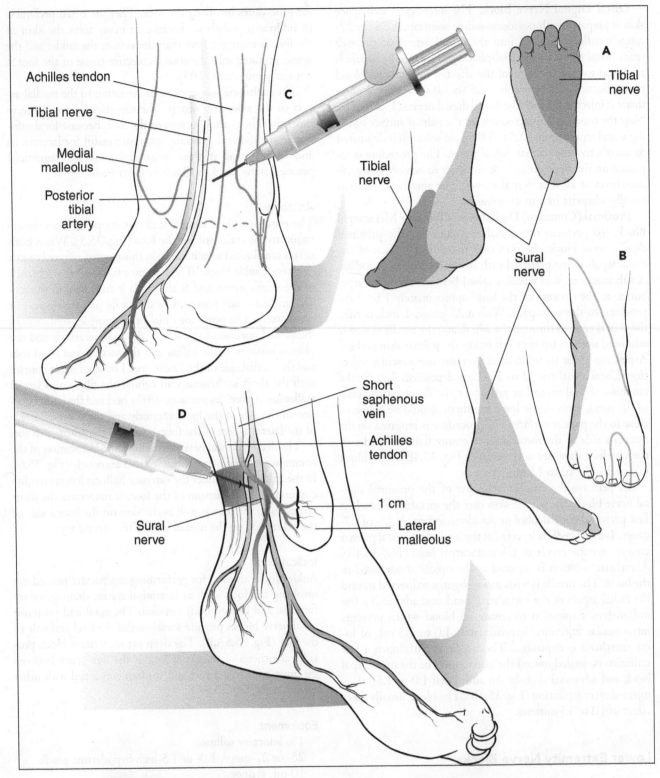

Figure 35.5
A. Distribution of sensory innervation of posterior tibial and sural nerves (medial and plantar aspects).
B. Distribution of sensory innervation of posterior tibial and sural nerves (lateral and dorsal aspects).
C. Posterior tibial nerve block.
D. Sural nerve block.

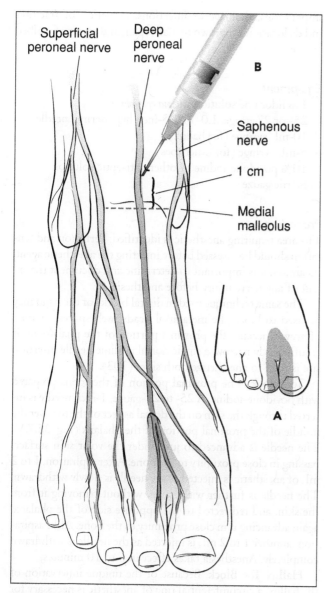

Figure 35.6
A. Distribution of sensory innervation of deep peroneal (anterior tibial) nerve.
B. Deep peroneal nerve block.

is advanced to a position approximately 1 mm from the underlying tibia. Paresthesias along the sole of the foot may be elicited with movement of the tip of the needle. When this occurs, the needle should be withdrawn 1 to 2 mm to prevent intraneuronal injection. After aspiration to prevent intravascular injection, 3 to 4 mL of anesthetic solution is injected. If no paresthesia is elicited, 5 mL of anesthetic is injected as the needle is slowly withdrawn. The anesthetic effect may be tested in 5 to 10 minutes. A successful block may cause an increase in the skin temperature of the foot due to vasodilation (100,105).

Sural Nerve Block. The patient should be positioned as previously described for the posterior tibial nerve block. The skin over the lateral malleolus extending posteriorly to the Achilles tendon is prepared with povidone-iodine. A 25- or 27-gauge, 1.0- to 1.5-inch needle is inserted just lateral to the Achilles tendon about 1 cm superior to the lateral malleolus. The needle is advanced subcutaneously toward the lateral malleolus (Fig. 35.5D). After aspiration, the branches of the sural nerve are blocked by creating a subcutaneous band of anesthetic (3 to 5 mL) extending from the posterior aspect of the lateral malleolus to the anterior margin of the Achilles tendon. The anesthetic effect is usually adequate in 5 to 10 minutes. As with the posterior tibial nerve block, the patient may experience an increase in the skin temperature of the foot due to vasodilation.

Deep Peroneal (Anterior Tibial) Nerve Block. The deep peroneal nerve is blocked anteriorly beneath the extensor hallucis longus and anterior tibial tendons. The patient is placed in the supine position. Dorsiflexion of the great toe can help locate the tendon of the extensor hallucis longus 1 cm above the superior aspect of the medial malleolus (Fig. 35.5B). The area is prepared with povidone-iodine. With a 1.0- or 1.5-inch 27-gauge needle, a wheal is raised just medial to the tendon of the extensor hallucis longus. The needle is directed 30 degrees laterally, beneath the tendon, and advanced 0.5 to 1.0 cm until it strikes the tibia. After withdrawal of the needle about 1 mm and aspiration, 3 to 5 mL of local anesthetic is deposited. Anesthesia of the web space between the hallux and second toe should be achieved within 15 minutes.

Digital Nerve Blocks of the Foot

As with the fingers, local infiltration of the toes is generally quite painful and may not provide adequate anesthesia. This is particularly true of the volar aspect of the toes and the nailbed. For this reason, a digital nerve block is often superior to local anesthesia for performing painful procedures involving the toes.

Anatomy

Each toe is supplied by four nerves. In cross-sectional view, the two dorsal digital nerves lie along each phalanx at the 2 o'clock and 10 o'clock positions, while the volar digital nerves lie at the 4 o'clock and 8 o'clock positions (Fig. 35.7). The dorsal digital nerves arise from branches of the deep and superficial peroneal nerves, supplying sensation to the dorsal skin and

the anesthetic agent. Evaluation for nerve or tendon injury must be performed before nerve blockade.

Posterior Tibial Nerve Block. The patient should be placed in the prone position, with the foot extending beyond the end of the stretcher and held in slight dorsiflexion (104). The skin over the medial malleolus extending posteriorly to the Achilles tendon is prepared with povidone-iodine. The posterior tibial artery is palpated just posterior to the medial malleolus. A 25- or 27-gauge, 1.0- or 1.5-inch needle is inserted perpendicular to the skin, at the level of the top of the medial malleolus just posterior to the pulse of the artery. If the arterial pulse is not palpable, the insertion site is located between the superior border of the medial malleolus and the Achilles tendon (Fig. 35.5C). The tip of the needle

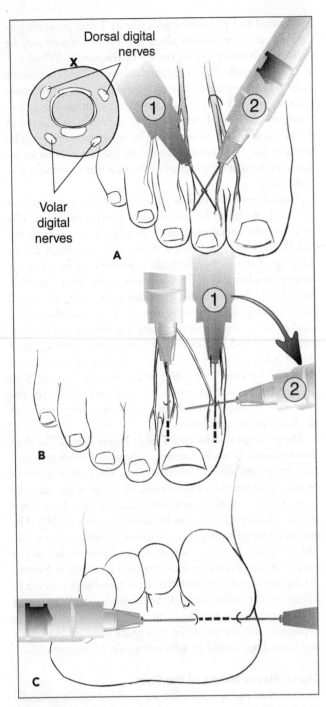

Figure 35.7
A. Digital block of toe.
B,C. Digital block of the hallux is achieved with a circumferential ring of anesthetic.

amputations, drainage of infections, reduction of fractures and dislocations, ingrown toenail repair, and repair of nailbed injuries.

Equipment
1% lidocaine solution *without epinephrine*
25- or 27-gauge, 1.0- or 1.5-inch hypodermic needle
10-mL syringe (for hallux)
5-mL syringe (for other toes)
10% povidone-iodine or other antiseptic solution
Sterile gauze

Procedure
The area requiring anesthetic is identified. Perfusion and sensation should be assessed before injecting the anesthetic agent. As always, it is important to determine and document the extent of any nerve injury before anesthesia.

The same technique used in digital blocks of the hand may be used to block the metatarsal heads, web spaces, or toes. However, because the proximal portion of the phalanx itself is sufficiently narrow, a single dorsal midline needle insertion site is used to anesthetize both sides (103).

Toe Block. The proximal portion of the toe is prepared with povidone-iodine. A 25- to 27-gauge, 1-inch needle is inserted through the skin on the dorsal aspect of the toe over the middle of the proximal portion of the phalanx (Fig. 35.7A). The needle is advanced to just under the volar skin surface, passing in close proximity to the bone. After aspiration, 1 to 2 mL of anesthetic is injected as the needle is slowly withdrawn. The needle is further withdrawn, without removing it from the skin, and redirected to the opposite side of the phalanx, again advancing it in close proximity to the bone. After aspiration, another 1 to 2 mL is injected as the needle is withdrawn completely. Anesthesia takes effect in 5 to 10 minutes.

Hallux Toe Block. Because of the unique innervation of the hallux, a circumferential ring of anesthetic is necessary for a complete nerve block. The dorsal surface of the great toe is prepared with povidone-iodine. A 25- to 27-gauge, 1-inch needle is inserted in the dorsomedial aspect of the proximal portion of the great toe, extending to the plantar surface (Fig. 35.7B). After aspiration, 1 to 2 mL of anesthetic is deposited as the needle is withdrawn. Without removal of the needle, it is redirected across the dorsal surface of the proximal phalanx laterally, and 1 to 2 mL of solution is injected as the needle is withdrawn completely. The needle is then inserted through the dorsolateral aspect of the proximal portion the great toe (which was infiltrated with anesthetic with the first injection). The needle is advanced to the plantar surface, and 1 to 2 mL of anesthetic solution is injected as the needle is removed. To complete a circumferential block of the hallux, the needle is inserted in a medial-to-lateral direction along the plantar surface of the great toe, at the proximal portion of the phalanx. After aspiration, 1 to 2 mL of solution is injected as the needle is removed. Full anesthesia is achieved in 5 to 10 minutes (Fig. 35.7C).

interphalangeal joints of all five toes. The volar nerves, which are branches of the posterior tibial and sural nerves, supply the distal volar aspects of the toes.

Indications
Digital nerve block is used to provide anesthesia of the toes for painful procedures such as toe laceration and repair of partial

Penile Nerve Blocks

Anatomy

The second, third, and fourth sacral nerve roots join to form the sacral plexus. The pudendal nerve arises from this sacral plexus, and a deep terminal branch (the dorsal nerve of the penis) furnishes most of the somatosensory innervation of the glans and shaft of the penis. The dorsal nerves of the penis lie just lateral to the midline, adjacent to the dorsal veins and arteries beneath the Buck fascia (Fig. 35.8).

Indications

Penile nerve block is used to provide anesthesia for minor procedures of the penis. In the emergency setting, this block is useful for a dorsal slit, removal of a zipper that has entrapped the foreskin, and paraphimosis reduction.

Equipment

1% lidocaine solution *without epinephrine*
25- to 27-gauge, 1.0- or 1.5-inch hypodermic needle
1- or 5-mL syringe
10% povidone-iodine or other antiseptic solution
Sterile gauze

Procedure

Using aseptic technique, the skin at the base of the penis is prepared with povidone-iodine solution. Local anesthetic is drawn into a syringe. In the neonate, 0.8 mL of 1% lidocaine is traditionally used, whereas 1 to 5 mL of lidocaine is used for older children. For the child over 12 years, 1 to 5 mL of 0.25% bupivacaine is preferred to provide longer-lasting anesthetic effect. Because the neighboring dorsal penile arteries are end arteries, it is imperative that only local anesthetic without epinephrine be used.

A 25- to 27-gauge needle attached to the syringe is inserted at the junction of the penile base and suprapubic skin. The anesthetic should be injected just inside the Buck fascia, which lies approximately 3 to 5 mm beneath the skin surface. A "pop" is usually felt as the needle pierces the Buck fascia. Aspiration is necessary to avoid intravascular injection in this highly vascular region. Half of the anesthetic is deposited at the 10 o'clock position. The needle is reinserted at the 2 o'clock position (Fig. 35.8B), and the remaining anesthetic is injected. No significant resistance should be felt as the lidocaine is injected.

Alternative methods include injecting a subcutaneous ring of anesthetic around the base of the shaft of the penis. To avoid two needle insertions, a single midline injection technique can be used. The needle is inserted in the midline and advanced perpendicularly through the skin at the lower surface of the symphysis pubis into the Buck fascia. A "pop" is again felt as the needle traverses the Buck fascia. After aspirating to confirm that the needle does not lie within a blood vessel, approximately 1 to 4 mL of local anesthetic is deposited. Diffusion of the anesthetic through the Buck fascia to both

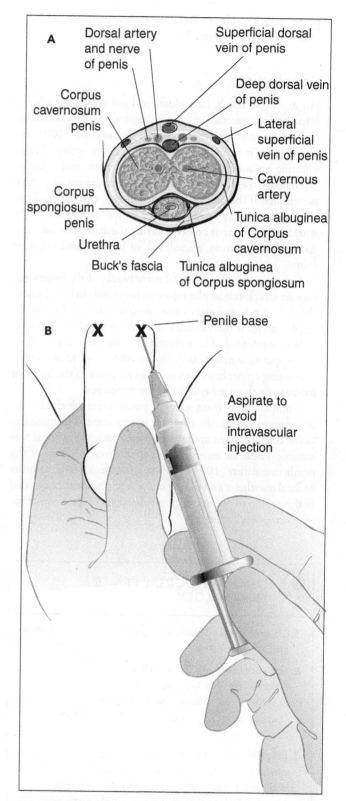

Figure 35.8
A. The dorsal penile nerves are located beneath the Buck fascia at the 2 o'clock and 10 o'clock positions.
B. Dorsal penile nerve block.

penile nerves results in local anesthesia. Optimal anesthetic effect is generally achieved in 5 minutes.

Complications

For any nerve block, large doses of local anesthetic injected into the intravascular space can cause systemic toxicity, including seizures and cardiovascular dysfunction (100). For this reason, it is important to aspirate the syringe before injecting an anesthetic. In addition, intraneuronal injection can damage the nerve, resulting in either transient or permanent injury. If the patient feels paresthesias, this may indicate that the nerve has been pierced, and the needle should be withdrawn somewhat before injecting the anesthetic solution. As with any injection, a small risk of bleeding and infection exists.

Complications from digital nerve blocks of the fingers and toes are rare. Intravascular injection may result in blanching of the digit due to ischemia from vasospasm or capillary blood displacement. If this occurs, the injection should be immediately discontinued. The ischemia is usually transient and resolves spontaneously (100). Inadvertent use of an anesthetic containing epinephrine can result in ischemia of the finger or toe because these are end-arteriolar structures.

Complications from a dorsal penile nerve block also are uncommon and usually clinically insignificant. The most frequent complications are bruising and (rarely) hematoma formation. These are most likely to result from puncture of the penile vasculature (106). As with digital blocks, large volumes of local anesthetic and the use of epinephrine must be avoided in this region to prevent ischemia through compression or vasospasm of end arteries.

SUMMARY: DORSAL PENILE NERVE BLOCK

1 Cleanse base of penis with povidone-iodine or other antiseptic solution.

2 For neonates, use 0.8 mL 1% lidocaine *without epinephrine* in a 1-mL syringe. For older children, use 1 to 5 mL of lidocaine *without epinephrine*. For children over 12 years, use 1 to 5 mL of 0.25% bupivacaine *without epinephrine*.

3 Insert needle 3 to 5 mm beneath skin at the junction of the penile base and suprapubic skin at the 10 o'clock position; after a negative aspiration for blood, infiltrate half of the anesthetic dose.

4 Repeat step 3 at the 2 o'clock position and inject remaining anesthetic.

5 Wait 5 minutes and test for anesthetic effect before performing procedure.

CLINICAL TIPS: NERVE BLOCK ANESTHESIA

▶ An anesthetic solution containing epinephrine should never be used for nerve blocks of the fingers, toes, or penis.

▶ Nerve blocks are often preferred over local infiltration anesthesia for procedures involving the hands or feet because insertion of the needle at the appropriate sites for a nerve block is generally much less painful than through the highly innervated skin of the palm of the hand or sole of the foot.

▶ For certain procedures (e.g., nailbed repairs, replacing a minor fingertip avulsion, ingrown toenail repair, and incision and drainage of a paronychia), a digital block of the finger or toe is virtually always the anesthetic method of choice.

▶ When repairing injuries, the sensory and motor function of distal structures should be tested if possible (depending on the child's age) so that no confusion occurs about whether any neurologic damage resulted from the initial injury or the nerve block.

▶ To obtain adequate anesthesia of the hand or foot, it is sometimes necessary to combine two or more nerve blocks.

▶ Unlike in the case of infiltration anesthesia, when performing a nerve block it is generally necessary to wait at least 10 to 20 minutes after injection to obtain the full anesthetic effect.

▶ If the patient reports numbness and tingling (paresthesias) on insertion of the needle, the needle should be withdrawn 1 to 2 mm before injecting the anesthetic solution so that intraneuronal injection does not occur. With younger children, the occurrence of paresthesias may be difficult to distinguish from the pain of the injection.

▶ Aspiration for blood should always be performed before injecting the anesthetic solution to prevent intravascular injection.

▶ INTRAVENOUS REGIONAL ANESTHESIA (BIER AND "MINIDOSE" BIER BLOCKS)

The desire for a rapid, safe, effective, and easy-to-perform technique to anesthetize extremities for orthopedic reduction or minor procedures led to the development of intravenous regional anesthesia by Bier in 1908 (107). This procedure involves exsanguination of an affected extremity through elevation and the application of a tourniquet, followed by distal instillation of intravenous local anesthetic (lidocaine, prilocaine). This results in rapid anesthesia and a relatively bloodless field. Although prilocaine and lidocaine are effective for forearm fracture reductions in children, lidocaine appears to provide superior analgesia for this procedure (108). A 20-year review comparing prilocaine and lidocaine for intravenous regional anesthesia for forearm fracture reduction in children involving 1,900 patients demonstrated no mortality or major morbidity. Only 1.6% of patients experienced minor events, such as temporary dizziness, tinnitus, or mild bradycardia (109). A "minidose" Bier block uses half the usual dose of lidocaine used in the traditional Bier block, and its safety and efficacy in the ED have been demonstrated (110). This lower dose may decrease the incidence of CNS side effects and is therefore preferred in the emergency setting.

The Bier and minidose Bier blocks provide satisfactory anesthesia and muscle relaxation of the hand and forearm in 95% to 98% of patients (111,112). This procedure may be used alone or may be supplemented by light sedation. The technique is easily mastered and has a very low failure rate. Although most often performed in the operating room, intravenous regional anesthesia can be used effectively in the ED for fracture reduction, repositioning of dislocations, and repair of multiple or large lacerations. Although most of the literature relates to this technique as it is performed on the upper extremity, it also may be used successfully in the lower extremity for procedures below the knee.

Regional anesthesia such as the minidose Bier block has several advantages over general anesthesia. For one, it is often preferable for an emergency procedure in the patient with a presumed full stomach, because the airway reflexes are obviously not affected. In addition, regional anesthesia is cost-effective; the cost of this procedure is less than 20% of the cost of performing general anesthesia (113). Intravenous regional anesthesia also can be accomplished rapidly. For example, the total time from beginning the minidose Bier block to orthopedic reduction and casting is usually less than 30 minutes (110).

Anatomy and Physiology

The site and mechanisms of action of intravenous regional anesthesia are not completely understood (114–118). The three most probable sites of action are at the sensory nerve endings, the neuromuscular junction, and the nerve trunks. It is likely that a combination of theories pointing to these sites may best explain the clinical findings (119). The anesthetic does not diffuse throughout the extremity distal to the tourniquet, even though anesthesia of the arm or leg is complete. The effects begin distally, suggesting the central portions of the nerve trunks are blocked first. The transient ischemia of the extremity produced by the pneumatic tourniquet also may contribute to the anesthetic effect.

Indications

The Bier and minidose Bier blocks may be used to achieve regional anesthesia, muscle relaxation, and/or a bloodless field. This type of anesthesia is effective for procedures of the arm (at or below the elbow) or of the leg (below the midcalf). As mentioned previously, such procedures include reduction of fractures and dislocations, laceration repair, removal of foreign bodies, débridement of burns, and drainage of infection. Intravenous regional anesthesia has been widely used in the outpatient setting for children with upper extremity injuries (112,113,120,121).

Contraindications to these procedures include significant underlying cardiac disease and any allergies to local anesthetics. This method cannot be used for manipulations in which the pulse must be monitored as a guide to reduction (e.g., supracondylar humeral fractures) because the pulse cannot be palpated while the pneumatic tourniquet is inflated. It should also be used with caution for patients with sickle cell disease, as the effects of the ischemic tourniquet on red blood cells have yet to be clarified. Because the minidose Bier block is generally safer than the traditional Bier block, using only the minidose Bier block for children in the outpatient setting is recommended.

Equipment

Resuscitation cart (with benzodiazepine anticonvulsants) at bedside
Cardiac and blood pressure monitors
Pulse oximeter
Intravenous catheters
Normal saline solution and intravenous extension tubing
Esmarch rubber or Ace elastic bandage
Two single pneumatic tourniquets or a double-cuff pneumatic tourniquet (Note: standard blood pressure cuffs are not recommended because they often leak or rupture and may fail to sustain high pressures for a prolonged period of time)
Lidocaine 0.5% *without epinephrine* (may dilute 1% lidocaine with sterile saline to form 0.5% solution)
50-mL infusion syringe
18-gauge needle

Procedure

Informed consent is first obtained. Younger children and those who are overly anxious may benefit from light sedation before performance of the procedure (see Chapter 33). Leads for the cardiac monitor and pulse oximeter are placed on the child. Resuscitation equipment, including anticonvulsant medications, should be readily available. Since this discussion will be limited to intravenous regional anesthesia for pediatric patients, only the minidose Bier block is described.

For a procedure of the arm, intravenous access is obtained in both upper extremities. A large-bore intravenous catheter with normal saline solution infusing is established in the

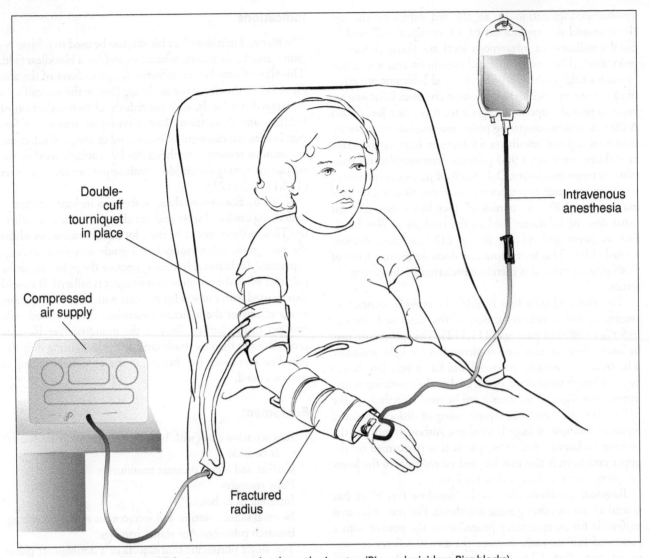

Figure 35.9 Intravenous regional anesthesia setup (Bier and minidose Bier blocks).

unaffected extremity for administration of resuscitation medications should they be needed. The intravenous line in the affected limb is used for lidocaine infusion. This is usually inserted at the dorsum of the hand rather than the antecubital space because evidence suggests that the procedure is more likely to be successful when the anesthetic is injected distally (122).

A double pneumatic tourniquet or two single pneumatic tourniquets are placed above the elbow (Fig. 35.9). The affected limb is exsanguinated either by elevation for a few minutes or by elevation and wrapping the extremity with an Esmarch rubber or Ace elastic bandage in a distal-to-proximal fashion. With the extremity still elevated, the upper or proximal pneumatic cuff is inflated to 50 mm Hg above the systolic blood pressure to occlude the arterial blood supply. The bandage is removed, and the extremity is lowered back onto the stretcher.

As described by Farrell (110), a minidose Bier block is performed by first infusing 0.5% lidocaine intravenously into the affected extremity at a dose of 1.5 mg/kg (maximum

100 mg) over 60 to 90 seconds. Using alkalinized lidocaine during intravenous regional anesthesia offers no advantage (103). Tourniquet pressure must be maintained at all times throughout the procedure. In addition, injection of local anesthetic into the limb should be performed slowly to avoid generating supra-arterial pressure in the venous system, leading to escape of drug under the tourniquet. Following injection, the skin will often blanch and become erythematous in patches as residual blood is displaced from the vascular compartment. This is not a toxic manifestation and usually signifies success of the procedure.

Over the next several minutes, the patient will experience paresthesias or warmth, beginning distally and spreading proximally. At this point, the lower or distal cuff is inflated to 50 mm Hg above systolic pressure, and the proximal cuff is then deflated. In this way, the tourniquet pressure is now over an area that is already anesthetized, eliminating the pain caused by the proximal tourniquet. Anesthesia, which is usually satisfactory in about 10 minutes, is followed by muscle relaxation. Gentle manipulation of the painful site should be used to test for adequate anesthesia. Although pain is eliminated, the patient may still have tactile and proprioceptive sensation and may retain some motor function (110).

An additional 0.5 mg/kg of lidocaine may be used with the minidose Bier block if anesthesia is still inadequate after 15 minutes. However, the overall maximum dose of 100 mg of lidocaine should not be exceeded. Additional lidocaine infusion is required in about 7% of cases (110).

Once adequate analgesia has been reached, the infusion catheter is removed and the site adequately bandaged to prevent extravasation of the anesthetic. The procedure should be performed promptly. For fracture reduction, portable postreduction radiographs should be obtained while the tourniquet is still inflated. This allows for repeat reduction under the same anesthetic if necessary.

With the minidose Bier block, the tourniquet should be left in place a minimum of 15 to 20 minutes and a maximum of 60 to 90 minutes after the infusion of lidocaine, because peak blood levels are related to the duration of vascular occlusion (123,124). To prevent a bolus of lidocaine from entering the intravascular compartment, the cuff is slowly deflated through a series of cycles. The cuff should be deflated for 5 seconds, then reinflated for 1 to 2 minutes. This cycle is repeated several times until distal perfusion is restored, as indicated by capillary refill. After the tourniquet is removed, sensation returns in 5 to 10 minutes. The child should be observed for at least 1 hour after the procedure before discharge (102).

Complications

Although infrequent, complications can occur if strict adherence to proper technique and meticulous attention to the functioning of the equipment are lacking. The most common complication relating to anesthetic is a rapid systemic vascular infusion. This may occur with rapid intravascular infusion at pressures surpassing tourniquet cuff pressure, tourniquet leakage, blood pressure cuff malfunction, early release of the tourniquet, medication error (i.e., an excessively high dose), or intravenous lines placed in close proximity to the tourniquet. Although the consequences of an inadvertent lidocaine bolus are potentially serious, the minidose technique has been shown to be very safe, because the dosages are similar to therapeutic intravenous boluses given to patients with cardiac dysrhythmias. The extremely low incidence of airway compromise (as compared with conscious sedation) also contributes to the relative safety of this procedure.

A lidocaine bolus into the systemic circulation may result in dizziness, headache, lethargy, and blurred vision. This is reported in 2% to 3% of patients and requires no additional treatment (125). Seizures are quite rare, having been reported in 0.2% of patients (126). Seizures should be managed with standard supportive care and anticonvulsant medications. With massive overdoses of intravenous lidocaine, bradycardia, vasomotor collapse, and cardiac depression or arrest can occur. Seven deaths have been reported in the United Kingdom using this technique. The deaths were felt to be due to equip-

SUMMARY: MINIDOSE BIER BLOCK

1. Prepare all items (including resuscitation equipment at bedside) that may be needed during procedure.

2. Place monitor and pulse oximetry leads appropriately on patient.

3. Obtain large-bore intravenous access in uninvolved extremity and distal intravenous access in involved extremity.

4. Position double tourniquet (just above elbow for upper extremity; no higher than midcalf for lower extremity).

5. Elevate and exsanguinate extremity (optional: wrap extremity with Esmarch rubber or Ace elastic bandage in a distal-to-proximal fashion to speed exsanguination).

6. Inflate proximal tourniquet to 50 mm Hg above systemic blood pressure and place extremity back on stretcher.

7. Gradually infuse 1.5 mg/kg (maximum 100 mg) of 0.5% lidocaine solution (a 1:1 mixture of 1% lidocaine and sterile saline) over 60 to 90 seconds.

8. Inflate distal tourniquet to 50 mm Hg above systemic blood pressure, and when secure, deflate proximal tourniquet.

9. Check for adequate anesthesia.

10. Perform procedure for which anesthesia has been administered.

11. Deflate tourniquet after a minimum of 20 to 30 minutes and a maximum of 60 to 90 minutes via a series of several deflation cycles; each cycle should consist of 5 seconds of deflation alternating with 1 to 2 minutes of reinflation.

12. When patient has normal distal capillary refill, remove tourniquet.

13. Observe patient for 1 hour for possible reaction.

ment failure (not maintaining adequate pressure in the cuff), use of bupivacaine, and operator inexperience (127).

Other complications include tissue extravasation of the anesthetic from an infiltrated intravenous catheter and intra-arterial injection resulting in distal limb necrosis. If any doubt exists about venous versus arterial placement of the catheter, another catheter should be inserted. Alternatively, a blood gas analysis can be performed to determine the source of the blood. Allergy to lidocaine is rare. Any history of significant allergic reactions to local anesthetics should cause the operator to consider using another method of anesthesia. Pain at the

CLINICAL TIPS: INTRAVENOUS REGIONAL ANESTHESIA

▶ Because it is safer than the traditional Bier block owing to the lower dosage of lidocaine, the minidose Bier block should be used for children in the ED.

▶ Rapid administration of lidocaine can cause venous pressures to exceed the pressure of the pneumatic tourniquet, resulting in leakage of the lidocaine under the cuff and into the systemic circulation.

▶ Intravenous regional anesthesia should not be used for any procedure that requires the pulse to be monitored (e.g., reduction of a supracondylar fracture) because the pulse will be lost when the tourniquet is inflated.

▶ Because of the slight possibility of delivering a large bolus of lidocaine to the systemic circulation, resuscitation equipment (including anticonvulsant medications) should always be at the bedside during this procedure.

▶ Two reliable intravenous lines should be started before performing intravenous regional anesthesia, one distally in the affected limb and one in another limb. In this way, resuscitation medications can be administered if necessary without deflating the pneumatic tourniquet.

▶ A double pneumatic tourniquet or two single pneumatic tourniquets are ideal for this procedure. A standard blood pressure cuff is not recommended because it may leak or rupture.

▶ By using two tourniquets, the physician can minimize the pain associated with prolonged pressure on the extremity. The proximal tourniquet is inflated first, and the lidocaine is administered. When the anesthesia begins to take effect, the distal tourniquet is inflated and the proximal tourniquet is deflated. In this way, the tourniquet that remains inflated throughout the procedure is positioned over an area of the extremity that is already anesthetized.

▶ Children who undergo intravenous regional anesthesia should be observed for 1 hour after the pneumatic tourniquet is deflated so that any adverse reactions can be appropriately managed.

tourniquet site may also occur. This is more frequent when using a single pneumatic cuff or with prolonged tourniquet times. When regional anesthesia is used in the lower extremity, the patient may develop phlebitis. In addition, tourniquets

must be placed no higher than midcalf to avoid peroneal nerve damage.

▶ SUMMARY

Infiltration anesthesia is by far the most commonly used method of providing local anesthesia in the ED. Ideally, the needle should be inserted through exposed subcutaneous tissue in a wound rather than through intact skin, and the anesthetic solution should be slowly injected around the entire wound margin. It is a straightforward procedure that achieves a high rate of success. Parallel margin anesthesia is similar to infiltration anesthesia, although in this case the needle is inserted in a circumferential fashion through intact skin 1 to 2 cm from the site of the procedure. The primary advantage of this technique is that the wound edges of a laceration are not distorted.

In appropriate clinical situations, topical anesthesia is an excellent technique for pediatric patients. Currently, the most popular topical anesthetic for wound repair is LET (lidocaine-epinephrine-tetracaine). It can be used alone or in combination with supplemental lidocaine infiltration if necessary. Careful adherence to proper usage will minimize the likelihood of complications. LET is painless, easily applied, and does not distort the margins of a wound. EMLA (eutectic mixture of local anesthetics) contains lidocaine and prilocaine and is a safe, easy, and effective method for dermal anesthesia of intact skin. The slow onset of action, however, limits its widespread applicability in the emergency setting. The approval of ELA-Max may reduce the time needed to obtain dermal anesthesia, and this agent is beginning to gain widespread acceptance. Ethyl chloride provides reliable, convenient, and effective dermal analgesia, but this agent has been used less frequently since the introduction of more effective methods.

Performing a nerve block or use of intravenous regional anesthesia eliminates pain sensation over an entire area of the body. Nerve blocks can provide effective anesthesia of especially pain-sensitive structures, primarily the fingers, toes, palm of the hand, and sole of the foot. Injection of anesthetic solution at a more proximal site is generally much less painful. More than one nerve block may be performed to anesthetize a larger area. Intravenous regional anesthesia results in safe and effective analgesia for selected extremity procedures. For pediatric patients, the minidose Bier block is recommended for use in the ED because it is generally as effective as a standard Bier block and uses a lower dose of lidocaine.

▶ ACKNOWLEDGMENT

The authors would like to acknowledge the valuable contributions of Lisa S. Lewis to the version of this chapter that appeared in the previous edition.

▶ **REFERENCES**

1. Gohara S. Regional anesthesia for office procedures, I: head and neck surgeries. *Am Fam Physician.* 2004;69:585–590.
2. Denson D, Mazoit J. Physiology, pharmacology, and toxicity of local anesthetics: adult and pediatric consideration. In: Prithviraj P, ed. *Clinical Practice of Regional Anesthesia.* New York: Churchill Livingstone; 1991:73–105.
3. Goth A. Pharmacology of local anesthesia. In: Clark WG, Brater DC, Johnson AR, ed. *Medical Pharmacology: Principles and Concepts.* St. Louis: CV Mosby; 1988:407–415.
4. Covino B. Pharmacology of local anesthetic agents. *Br J Anaesth.* 1986;58:701–716.
5. Mulroy M. Local anesthetics. In: Little J, Brown A, ed. *Regional Anesthesia.* Boston: 1989:1–12.
6. Wildsmith JAN, Armitage G, Edward N. Pharmacology of local anesthetics. In: *Principles and Practice of Regional Anesthesia.* New York: Churchill Livingstone; 1993:29–46.
7. Tucker G. Pharmacokinetics of local anesthesias. *Br J Anaesth.* 1986;58:717–731.
8. Ehlert TK, Arnold DE. Local anesthesia for soft-tissue surgery. *Otolaryngol Clin North Am.* 1990;23:831.
9. Strichartz G, Berde C. Local anesthetics. In: Fleisher LA, Johns RA, Savarese JJ, et al. *Miller's Anesthesia.* 6th ed. San Francisco: Churchill Livingstone; 2005:573–599.
10. Feinstein R, Nielsen Helge C. Local anesthetics. In: Thomas JR, Holt, ed. *Facial Scars: Incision, Revision and Camouflage.* St. Louis: CV Mosby; 1989:33–47.
11. Graham HD III, Duplechain G. Anesthesia in facial plastic surgery. In: Willett JM, ed. *Facial Plastic Surgery.* Stamford, CT: Appleton & Lange: 1997:5–26.
12. Gordon HL. The selection of drugs in office surgery. *Clin Plast Surg.* 1983;10:277.
13. Ahlstrom K, Frodel J. Local anesthetics for facial plastic procedures. *Otolaryngol Clin North Am.* 2002;35:29–53.
14. de Jong RH. Local anesthetics in clinical practice. In: Waldman SD, Winnie AP, eds. *Interventional Pain Management.* Philadelphia: WB Saunders; 1996:51–74.
15. Wildsmith J. Peripheral nerve and local anesthetic drugs. *Br J Anaesth.* 1986;58:692–700.
16. Heavner J. Molecular action of local anesthetics. In: Prithviraj P, ed. *Clinical Practice of Regional Anesthesia.* New York: Churchill Livingstone; 1991:67–71.
17. Benzon HT, Strichartz GR, Glissen AJ. Developmental neurophysiology of mammalian peripheral nerves and age-related differential sensitivity to local anesthetics. *Br J Anaesth.* 1988;61:754–760.
18. Butterworth J, Strichantz G. Molecular mechanisms of local anesthesia: a review. *Anesthesiology.* 1990;72:711–734.
19. Hille B. Common mode of action of three agents that decrease the transient change in sodium permeability in nerves. *Nature.* 1966;216:1220–1221.
20. Ritchie JM, Rogart RB. Density of sodium channels in mammalian myelinated nerve fibers and nature of the axonal membrane under the myelin sheath. *Proc Nat Acad Sci U S A.* 1977;74:211–215.
21. Mather L, Cousins M. Local anesthetics and their clinical use. *Drugs.* 1979;18:185–205.
22. Tetslaff JE. The pharmacology of local anesthetics. *Anesth Clin North Am.* 2000;18:217–233.
23. Courtney KR. Structure-activity relations for frequency-dependent sodium channel block in nerve by local anesthetics. *J Phamacol Exp Ther.* 1980;213:114–119.
24. Bokesch PM, Post C, Strichartz G. Structure-activity relationship of lidocaine homologs producing tonic and frequency-

25. Moore D. The pH of local anesthetic solutions. *Anesth Analg.* 1981;60:833–834.
26. Frazier DT, Narahashi T, Yamada M. The site of action and active form of local anesthetics, II: experiment with quaternary compounds. *J Pharm Exp Ther.* 1970;171:45–51.
27. Narahashi T, Frazier DT, Yamada M. The site of action and active form of local anesthetics, I: theory and pH experiments with tertiary compounds. *J Pharm Exp Ther.* 1970;171:32–44.
28. Mulroy M. Clinical characteristics of local anesthetics. In: *Regional Anesthesia.* 3rd ed. Philadelphia: Lippincott Williams and Wilkins, 2002;12–28.
29. Swerdlow M, Jones R. The duration of action of bupivacaine, prilocaine, and lignocaine. *Br J Anaesth.* 1970;42:335–339.
30. Arthur D, McNicol L. Local anesthetic techniques in pediatric surgery. *Br J Anaesth.* 1986;58:760–778.
31. Ecoffey C, Desparmet J, Berdeaux A. Pharmokinetics of lignocaine in children following caudal anesthesia. *Br J Anaesth.* 1984;56:1399–1401.
32. Lin YC, Krane EJ. Regional anesthesia and pain management in ambulatory pediatric patients. *Anesth Clin North Am.* 1996;14:803–816.
33. de Jong R. Toxic effects of local anesthesia. *JAMA.* 1978;239:1166–1168.
34. Mulroy M. Complications of regional anesthesia. In: *Regional Anesthesia. An Illustrated Procedural Guide,* 3rd ed. Philadelphia: Lippincott Williams and Wilkins, 2002;29–41.
35. Munson E, Embrow PW. Central nervous system toxicity of local anesthetic mixtures in monkeys. *Anesthesiology.* 1977;46:179.
36. Scott D. Toxic effects of local anesthetic agents on the central nervous system. *Br J Anaesth.* 1986;58:732–735.
37. Reiz S, Nath S. Cardiotoxicity of local anesthetic agents. *Br J Anaesth.* 1986;58:736–746.
38. Trott A. Infiltration and nerve block anesthesia. In: *Wounds and Lacerations: Emergency Care and Closure.* St. Louis: CV Mosby; 1991:30–36.
39. Born G. Neuropathy after bupivacaine wrist and metacarpal nerve blocks. *J Hand Surg.* 1984;9A:109–112.
40. Benoit P, Beit WD. Some effects of local anesthetic agents on skeletal muscle. *Exp Neurol.* 1972;34:264–278.
41. Chvapil M, Haneroff S, O'Dea K. Local anesthetics and wound healing. *J Surg Res.* 1979;27:267.
42. Fariss B, Foresman P, Rodeheaver G, et al. Anesthetic properties and toxicity of bupivacaine and lidocaine for infiltration anesthesia. *J Emerg Med.* 1987;5:275–282.
43. Barker W, Rodeheaver GT, Edgerton MT. Damage to tissue defenses by a topical anesthetic agent. *Ann Emerg Med.* 1982;11:307–310.
44. Smith RM. Local and regional anesthesia. In: *Anesthesia for Infants and Children.* St. Louis: CV Mosby; 1980:229–233.
45. Rund DA. *Essentials of Emergency Medicine.* Aghababian RV, Allison EJ, Boyet GR, et al., eds. East Norwalk, CT: Appleton-Lange; 1986:274.
46. Wrightman M, Vaughn R. Comparison of compounds used for intradermal anesthesia. *Anesthesiology.* 1976;45:687–689.
47. Christoph R, Buchanan L, Begalla K, et al. Pain reduction in local anesthetic administration through pH buffering. *Ann Emerg Med.* 1988;17:117–120.
48. McKay W, Morris R, Mushlin P. Sodium bicarbonate attenuates pain on skin infiltration with lidocaine, with or without epinephrine. *Anesth Analg.* 1987;66:572–574.
49. Morris R, Mckay W, Mushlin P. Comparison of pain associated with intradermal and subcutaneous infiltration with various local anesthetic solutions. *Anesth Analg.* 1988;66:1180–1182.

50. Arndt KA, Burton C, Noe JM. Minimizing the pain of local anesthesia. *Plast Reconstr Surg.* 1983;72:676–679.

51. Pryor GJ, Kilpatrick WR, Opp AR. Local anesthesia in minor lacerations: topical TAC versus lidocaine infiltration. *Ann Emerg Med.* 1980;9:568–571.

52. Schilling CG, Bank DE, Borchert BA, et al. Tetracaine, epinephrine (adrenalin), and cocaine (TAC) versus lidocaine, epinephrine, and tetracaine (LET) for anesthesia of laceration in children. *Ann Emerg Med.* 1995;25:203–208.

53. Hegenbarth MA, Altieri MF, Hawk WH, et al. Comparison of tetracaine, adrenaline, and cocaine with cocaine alone for topical anesthesia. *Ann Emerg Med.* 1990;19:63–67.

54. Grant SAD, Hoffman RS. Use of tetracaine, epinephrine, and cocaine as a topical anesthetic in the emergency department. *Ann Emerg Med.* 1992;21:987–997.

55. Anderson AB, Colecchi C, Baronoski R, et al. Local anesthesia in pediatric patients: topical TAC versus lidocaine. *Ann Emerg Med.* 1990;19:519–522.

56. Martin JR, Doezema D, Tandberg D, et al. The effect of local anesthetics on bacterial proliferation: TAC versus lidocaine. *Ann Emerg Med.* 1990;19:987–990.

57. Schaffer DJ. Clinical comparison of TAC anesthetic solutions with and without cocaine. *Ann Emerg Med.* 1985;14:1077–1080.

58. Ernst AA, Marvez E, Nick TG, et al. Lidocaine, adrenaline, tetracaine gel versus tetracaine, adrenaline, cocaine gel for topical anesthesia in linear scalp and facial lacerations in children aged 5 to 17 years. *Pediatrics.* 1995;95:255–258.

59. Schilling CG, Band DE, Borchert BA, et al. Tetracaine, epinephrine (adrenaline), and cocaine (TAC) versus lidocaine, epinephrine, and tetracaine (LET) for anesthesia of lacerations in children. *Ann Emerg Med.* 1995;25:203–208.

60. Kundu S. Principles of office anesthesia, II: topical anesthesia. *Am Fam Physician.* 2002;66:124–128.

61. Resch K, Shilling C, Borchert BD, et al. topical anesthesia for pediatric lacerations: a randomized trial of lidocaine-epinephrine-tetracaine solution vs. gel. *Ann Emerg Med.* 1998;32:693–697.

62. Lycka BA. EMLA: a new and effective topical anesthetic. *J Dermatol Surg Oncol.* 1992;18:859–862.

63. Buckley MM, Benfield P. Eutectic lidocaine/prilocaine cream: a review of the topical anaesthetic/analgesic efficacy of a eutectic mixture of local anaesthetics (EMLA). *Drugs.* 1993;46:126–151.

64. Juhlin L, Evers H. EMLA: a new topical anesthetic. *Adv Dermatol.* 1990;5:75–92.

65. Bjerring P, Arendt-Nielsen L. Depth and duration of skin analgesia to needle insertion after topical application of EMLA cream. *Br J Anaesth.* 1990;64:173–177.

66. Cooper CM, Gerrish DP, Hardwick M, et al. EMLA cream reduces the pain of venipuncture in children. *Eur J Anaesth.* 1987;4:441–448.

67. de Jong PC, Verburg MP, Lillieborg S. EMLA cream versus ethylchloride spray: a comparison of the analgesic efficacy in children. *Eur J Anaesth.* 1990;7:473–481.

68. Hopkins CS, Buckley CJ, Bush GH. Pain-free injection in infants: use of a lidocaine-prilocaine cream to prevent pain at intravenous induction of general anesthesia in 1- to 5-year-old children. *Anaesthesia.* 1988;43:198–201.

69. Joyce TH, Skjonsby BS, Taylor BD, et al. Dermal anesthesia using a eutectic mixture of lidocaine and prilocaine (EMLA) for venipuncture in children. *Pain Digest.* 1992;2:137–141.

70. Robieux I, Kumar R, Radhakrishnan S, et al. Assessing pain and analgesia with a lidocaine-prilocaine emulsion in infants and toddlers during venipuncture. *J Pediatr.* 1991;118:971–973.

71. Soliman IE, Broadman LM, Hannallah RS, et al. Comparison of the analgesic effects of EMLA (eutectic mixture of local anesthetics)

to intradermal lidocaine infiltration prior to venous cannulation in unpremedicated children. *Anesthesiology.* 1988;68:804–806.

72. Halperin DL, Koren G, Attias D, et al. Topical skin anesthesia for venous, subcutaneous drug reservoir and lumbar punctures in children. *Pediatrics.* 1989;84:281–284.

73. Kapelushnik J, Koren G, Solh H, et al. Evaluating the efficacy of EMLA in alleviating pain associated with lumbar puncture: comparison of open and double-blinded protocols in children. *Pain.* 1990;42:31–34.

74. Rylander E, Sjoberg I, Lillieborg S, et al. Local anesthesia of the genital mucosa with a lidocaine/prilocaine cream (EMLA) for laser treatment of condylomata acuminata: a placebo-controlled trial. *Obstet Gynecol.* 1990;75:302–306.

75. Brisman M, Ljung BM, Otterborn I, et al. Methemoglobin formation after the use of EMLA cream in neonates. *Acta Paediatr.* 1998;87:1191–1194.

76. Luhmann J, Hurt S, Shootman M, et al. A comparison of buffered lidocaine versus ELA-Max before peripheral intravenous catheter insertions in children. *Pediatrics.* 2004;113:217–220.

77. Armstrong P, Young C, McKeown D. Ethyl chloride and venipuncture pain: a comparison with intradermal lidocaine. *Can J Anaesth.* 1990;37:656–658.

78. Azppa SC, Nabors SB. Use of ethyl chloride topical anesthetic to reduce procedural pain in pediatric oncology patients. *Cancer Nurs.* 1992;15:130–136.

79. Smith GA, Strausbaugh SD, Harbeck-Weber C, et al. Prilocaine-phenylephrine and bupivacaine-phenylephrine topical anesthetics compared with tetracaine-adrenaline-cocaine during repair of lacerations. *Am J Emerg Med.* 1998;16:121–124.

80. Smith GA, Strausbaugh SD, Harbeck-Weber C, et al. Prilocaine-phenylephrine topical anesthesia for repair of mucous membrane lacerations. *Pediatr Emerg Care.* 1998;14:324–328.

81. Altieri M, Bogema S, Schwartz RH. TAC topical anesthesia produces positive urine tests for cocaine. *Ann Emerg Med.* 1990;19:577–579.

82. Fitzmaurice LS, Wasserman GS, Knapp JF, et al. TAC use and absorption of cocaine in a pediatric emergency department. *Ann Emerg Med.* 1990;19:515–518.

83. Terndrup TE, Walls HC, Mariani PJ, et al. Plasma cocaine and tetracaine levels following application of topical anesthesia in children. *Ann Emerg Med.* 1992;21:162–166.

84. Dailey RH. Fatality secondary to misuse of TAC solution. *Ann Emerg Med.* 1988;17:159–160.

85. Daya MR, Burton BT, Schleiss MR, et al. Recurrent seizures following mucosal application of TAC. *Ann Emerg Med.* 1988;17:646–648.

86. Dronen SC. Complications of TAC [letter]. *Ann Emerg Med.* 1983;12:333.

87. Jacobsen S. Errors in emergency practice. *Emerg Med.* 1987;19:109.

88. Tipton GA, DeWitt GW, Eisenstein SJ. Topical TAC (tetracaine, adrenaline, cocaine) solution for local anesthesia in children: prescribing inconsistency and acute toxicity. *South Med J.* 1989;82:1344–1346.

89. Tripp M, Dowd DD, Eitel DR. TAC toxicity in the emergency department. *Ann Emerg Med.* 1991;20:106–107.

90. Wehner D, Hamilton GD. Seizures following topical application of local anesthetics to burn patients. *Ann Emerg Med.* 1984;13:456–458.

91. Bonadio WA, Wagner V. Half–strength TAC topical anesthetic. *Clin Pediatr.* 1988;27:495–498.

92. Jakobson B, Nilsson A. Methemoglobinemia associated with a prilocaine-lidocaine cream and trimethoprim-sulfamethoxazole: a case report. *Acta Anaesth Scand.* 1985;29:253–255.

93. Nilsson A, Engberg G, Henneberg S, et al. Inverse relationship between age-dependent erythrocyte activity of methaemoglobin reduc-

tase and prilocaine-induced methaemoglobinaemia during infancy. *Br J Anaesth.* 1990;64:72–76.

94. Engberg G, Danielson K, Henneberg S, et al. Plasma concentrations of prilocaine and lidocaine and methaemoglobin formation in infants after epicutaneous application of 5% lidocaine-prilocaine cream (EMLA). *Acta Anaesth Scand.* 1987;31:624–628.

95. Frayling IM, Addison GM, Chattergee K, et al. Methaemoglobinaemia in children treated with prilocaine-lignocaine cream. *Brit Med J.* 1990;301:153–154.

96. Norman J, Jones PL. Complications of the use of EMLA [letter]. *Br J Anaesth.* 1990;64:403–406.

97. Nielsen AJ. Precautions about ethyl chloride. *Phys Ther.* 1980;60:474–475.

98. Aberer W. Local anaesthesia with chloride freezing: problems despite proper application. *Br J Dermatol.* 1991;124:113–114.

99. Murphy M. Regional anesthesia in the emergency department. *Emerg Med Clin North Am.* 1988;6:783–809.

100. Orlinsky M, Dean E. Local and topical anesthesia and nerve blocks of the thorax and extremities. In: Roberts J, Hedges J, eds. *Clinical Procedures in Emergency Medicine.* Philadelphia: WB Saunders; 1991:450–486.

101. Katz J. Sections on head, upper and lower extremities. In: *Atlas of Regional Anesthesia.* East Norwalk, CT: Appleton-Lange; 1994:1–36, 61–92, 149–174.

102. Stewart S. Local anesthesia. In: Paris P, Stewart S, eds. *Pain Management in Emergency Medicine.* East Norwalk, CT: Appleton-Lange; 1988:77.

103. Trott A. Infiltration and nerve block anesthesia. In: *Wounds and Lacerations: Emergency Care and Closure.* St. Louis: CV Mosby; 1991: 30–54.

104. Simon R, Brenner B. Anesthesia and regional blocks. In: Simon R, Brenner B, eds. *Procedures and Techniques in Emergency Medicine.* Baltimore: Williams & Wilkins; 1982:87–122.

105. Locke RK. Nerve blocks of the foot. *JACEP.* 1976;5:698.

106. Snellman LW, Stang HJ. Prospective evaluation of complications of dorsal penile nerve block for neonatal circumcision. *Pediatrics.* 1995;95:705.

107. Bier A. Uber einen neuen Weg Lokalanaesthesia an den Gliedmasses zu erzeugen. *Arch Klin Chir.* 1908;86:1007.

108. Davidson. AJ. A Comparison of prilocaine and lidocaine for intravenous regional anesthesia for forearm fracture reduction in children. *Paediatr Anaesth.* 2001;12:146–150.

109. Brown M, McGriff JT, Malinowski RW. Intravenous regional anesthesia: review of twenty years experience. *Can J Anaesth.* 1989;136:307–310.

110. Farrell RG, Swanson SL, Walter JK. Safe and effective i.v. regional anesthesia for use in the emergency department. *Ann Emerg Med.* 1985;14:288–292.

111. Chambers WA, Wildsmith JA. Upper limb. In: Nimmo WS, Smith G, eds. *Anesthesia.* Oxford: Blackwell Scientific Publications; 1989:1071–1073.

112. Juliano PJ, Mazur JM, Cummings RJ, et al. Low-dose lidocaine intravenous regional anesthesia for forearm fractures in children. *J Pediatr Orthop.* 1992;12:633–635.

113. Barnes CL, Blasier RD, Dodge BM. Intravenous regional anesthesia: a safe and cost-effective outpatient anesthetic for upper extremity fracture treatment in children. *J Pediatr Orthop.* 1991;11:717–720.

114. Miles DW, James JL, Clark DE, et al. Site of action of intravenous regional anesthesia. *J Neurol Neurosurg Psychiatry.* 1964;27:574–576.

115. Fleming SA, Veiga-Pires JA, McCutcheon RM, et al. A demonstration of the site of action of intravenous lignocaine. *Can Anaesth Soc J.* 1966;13:21–27.

116. Raj PP, Garcia CE, Burleson JW, et al. The site of action of intravenous regional anesthesia. *Anesth Analg.* 1972;51:776–786.

117. Raj PP. Site of action of intravenous regional anesthesia. *Reg Anaesth.* 1979;4:8.

118. Lillie PE, Glynn CJ, Fenwick DG. Site of action of intravenous regional anesthesia. *Anesthesiology.* 1984;61:507–510.

119. Rosenberg PH, Heavner JE. Multiple and complementary mechanisms produce analgesia during intravenous regional anesthesia. *Anesthesiology.* 1985;62:840–842.

120. Olney BW, Lugg PC, Turner PL, et al. Outpatient treatment of upper extremity injuries in childhood using intravenous regional anesthesia. *J Pediatr Orthop.* 1988;8:576–579.

121. Colizza WA, Said E. Intravenous regional anesthesia in the treatment of forearm and wrist fractures and dislocations in children. *Can J Surg.* 1993;36:225–228.

122. Sorbie C, Chacho PB. Regional anesthesia by the intravenous route. *Br Med J.* 1965;1:957–960.

123. Covino BG. Pharmacokinetics of intravenous regional anesthesia. *Reg Anaesth.* 1979;4:5.

124. Tucker GT, Boas RA. Pharmacokinetic aspects of intravenous regional anesthesia. *Anesthesiology.* 1971;34:538–549.

125. Dunbar RW, Mazze RI. Intravenous regional anesthesia experience with 779 cases. *Anesth Analg.* 1967;46:806–813.

126. Van Niekerk JP, Tonkin PA. Intravenous regional analgesia. *S Afr Med J.* 1966;40:165–169.

127. Heath M. Deaths after intravenous regional anesthesia. *Br Med J.* 1982;285:913–914.

SECTION 5 ▶ SPECIAL PROCEDURES FOR NEONATES

SECTION EDITOR: JOHN M. LOISELLE

36

ALAN FUJII AND ROBERT J. VINCI

Neonatal Resuscitation Procedures

▶ INTRODUCTION

Neonates require cardiopulmonary resuscitation more commonly than any other age group. It is estimated that 10% of newborn deliveries will require some degree of resuscitation by a skilled clinical team (1). While newborn deliveries are an uncommon event in the emergency department (ED), those that occur in the prehospital setting or in the ED are frequently from high-risk groups (i.e., lack of prenatal care, trauma-induced labor, drug abuse) and may be more prone to complications. Newborn deliveries that occur outside of a hospital obstetrical unit place the neonate at risk for complications such as hypothermia, acute blood loss, hypoglycemia, and asphyxia. Therefore, it is imperative for the ED physician to be skilled in resuscitation techniques in order to minimize these complications. Neonatal asphyxia, the most serious of all neonatal complications, must be treated efficiently and aggressively to avoid devastating neurological injury to the newborn infant. For this reason, current recommendations state that "every birth should be attended by at least one person skilled in neonatal resuscitation whose sole responsibility is management of the newborn" (2). Standardized courses such as the Neonatal Resuscitation Program (NRP) provide a teaching format and curriculum for improving the resuscitation skills of all appropriate practitioners. Precipitous deliveries can occur anywhere in the prehospital setting, including in the home, in an office practice, or during a prehospital transport. Therefore, it is incumbent upon all practitioners, including nurses,

physicians, midwives, and prehospital personnel, to be familiar with the techniques described in this chapter.

▶ ANATOMY AND PHYSIOLOGY

Fetal Transition

Transition from fetal to neonatal life involves a series of rapid anatomic and physiologic adaptations. In fetal circulation, blood flow to the lungs is minimal as a result of high pulmonary vascular resistance, a patent ductus arteriosus, and low resistance of the systemic (placental) circulation. At birth, the fetus must establish the lungs as the site of gas exchange. Inherent in this process are the physiologic mechanisms that clear the airway of fetal lung fluid. Thoracic compression during labor, catecholamine stimulation of lymphatic drainage of alveolar fluid, and the newborn's initial respiratory effort contribute to this process. The circulation, which previously shunted blood away from the lungs, must now fully perfuse the pulmonary vasculature, thus enabling adequate gas exchange at the alveoli-capillary unit.

Although surfactant production begins at approximately 24 weeks gestation, adequate amounts of surfactant to open alveoli may not be present until 36 weeks. A combination of events at birth act to initiate respiration. These events include the interruption of umbilical circulation, stimulation of peripheral and central chemoreceptors, and tactile and thermal

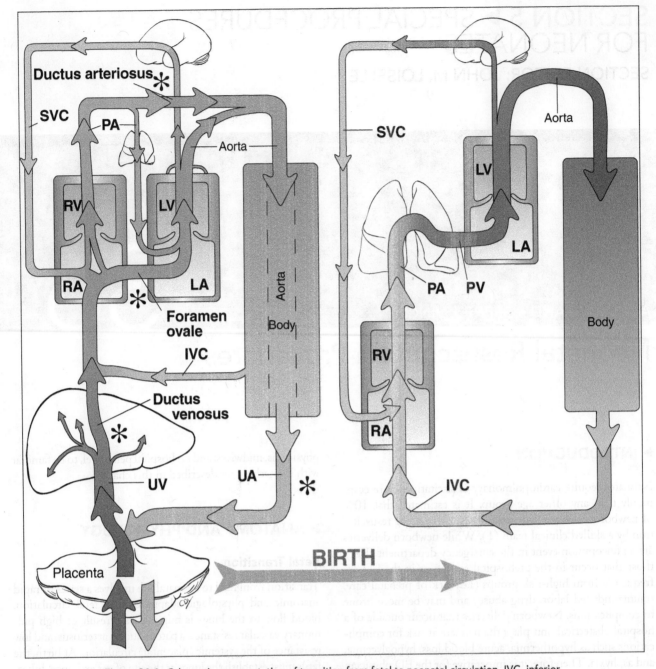

Figure 36.1 Schematic representation of transition from fetal to neonatal circulation. IVC, inferior vena cava; LA, left atrium; LV, left ventricle; PA, pulmonary arteries; PV, pulmonary veins; RA, right atrium; RV, right ventricle; SVC, superior vena cava; UA, umbilical arteries; UV, umbilical vein. Shading represents relative oxygen saturation. Structures marked with an asterisk (*) close soon after birth. See Figure 38.1 for a more detailed depiction of the umbilical vessels and their connections.

stimulation. The first few breaths must clear amniotic fluid from the lungs and establish a functional residual capacity. With the onset of respirations, the increase in oxygenation leads to the production of prostaglandins, which in turn reduces pulmonary vascular resistance. A fall in pulmonary vascular resistance decreases the right-to-left shunt through the ductus arteriosus, and the increase in left atrial pressure leads to subsequent closure of the foramen ovale. Fetal circulation now assumes the adult pattern (Fig. 36.1) (3).

Asphyxia

Birth asphyxia accounts for almost 20% of neonatal deaths (4). Neonatal asphyxia can result from multiple maternal and neonatal factors (Table 36.1). Asphyxia is the initial event that produces pulmonary vasoconstriction and delays closure of the ductus arteriosus. Fetal circulation is therefore maintained with a suboptimal increase in pulmonary blood flow. The goal with any asphyxiated newborn is to reverse the asphyxia as soon as possible before permanent injury occurs. In an asystolic newborn, if adequate cardiac output is not established within the first 10 to 15 minutes of resuscitation, survival or survival without severe disability is unlikely (5,6).

When asphyxia occurs (either in utero or following delivery), an initial period of hyperpnea develops with sinus tachycardia. If hypoxia continues, respiratory effort ceases and bradycardia ensues (primary apnea). Providing oxygen and stimulation during this period in many cases will induce spontaneous respirations. If asphyxia continues, the newborn develops gasping respirations, the heart rate continues to decrease, and blood pressure falls. With the cessation of gasping respirations, secondary apnea develops, the newborn becomes unresponsive to stimulation, and neonatal asphyxial injury may develop. Positive pressure ventilation (PPV) must be initiated rapidly. The clinician must realize that when he or she evaluates a newborn in distress or full arrest, the asphyxiating event may have begun in utero; therefore, apnea at birth should be treated as secondary apnea, and resuscitation with positive pressure ventilation should begin immediately.

The Environment

Because of a large surface area to mass ratio, the neonate is susceptible to significant heat loss, and because many ED deliveries involve the birth of a premature newborn, heat loss may be a significant problem. Newborns, especially premature newborns, may be unable to effectively modulate their own temperature control and have limited capacity to generate heat. Without appropriate attention to thermal management, hypothermia may occur. Hypothermic stress in the newborn may contribute to acidosis, hypoglycemia, and respiratory depression (7). Hyperthermia should also be avoided, as it may lead to perinatal respiratory depression (8).

▶ INDICATIONS

Basic techniques involved in neonatal resuscitation are applicable to the delivery of all newborns. While the delivery of a depressed or asphyxiated newborn can be anticipated in many cases based on antepartum or intrapartum history (Table 36.1), it may not always be possible to elicit these factors in the ED. Many asphyxiated newborns will have no risk factors and are only recognized at the time of birth. Resuscitation is required for about 80% of newborns with birthweights less than 1,500 g. Approximately 5% to 10% of term newborns require resuscitation beyond suctioning, drying, and stimulation. Preparation for high-risk situations in the ED requires proper equipment and personnel trained in the techniques of neonatal resuscitation. Because of the difficulty in accurately assessing gestational age in unanticipated deliveries, initiation of resuscitation is indicated unless it can be reliably determined that the newborn is less than 23 weeks gestation or less (9). Neonatology consultation in questionable circumstances should be obtained when possible.

TABLE 36.1	FACTORS ASSOCIATED WITH NEONATAL ASPHYXIA

Antepartum factors
  Maternal diabetes
  Pregnancy-induced hypertension
  Chronic hypertension
  Chronic maternal illness
  Previous Rh sensitization
  Previous fetal or neonatal death
  Bleeding in second or third trimester
  Maternal infection
  Polyhydramnios
  Oligohydramnios
  Premature rupture of membranes
  Postterm gestation
  Multiple gestation
  Size-date discrepancy
  Drug therapy (lithium carbonate, magnesium, adrenergic blocking agents)
  Maternal substance abuse
  Fetal malformation
  Absent prenatal care
  Age <16 or >35 years

Intrapartum risk factors
  Emergency cesarean section
  Abnormal presentation (breech, footling breech)
  Forceps- or vacuum-assisted delivery
  Premature labor
  Prolonged rupture of membranes (>18 hours before delivery)
  Prolonged labor (>24 hours before delivery)
  Precipitous delivery
  Chorioamnionitis
  Prolonged second stage of labor (>2 hours)
  Non-reassuring fetal heart rate patterns
  Use of general anesthesia
  Uterine tetany
  Narcotic administration to mother within 4 hours of delivery
  Meconium-stained amniotic fluid
  Prolapsed cord
  Abruptio placentae
  Placenta previa

Note: Techniques involved in neonatal resuscitation are applicable to the delivery of all newborns. More aggressive resuscitation and evaluation of the depressed or asphyxiated newborn can be anticipated in many cases based on information found in the antepartum and intrapartum histories.
Source: Modified from Kattwinkel J. *Textbook of Neonatal Resuscitation.* 4th edition. Elk Grove Village, IL: American Heart Association, American Academy of Pediatrics; 2000.

▶ EQUIPMENT

Equipment requirements for more extensive resuscitations can be found in the chapters noted.

Suction Equipment

  Bulb syringe
  Mechanical suction with regulator
  Suction catheter (6, 8, and 10 French)
  Meconium aspirator (Chapter 37)

Warming Equipment

  Radiant warmer
  Warm, dry blankets

Stockinette hat

Chemical warming blankets (extremely premature infants less than 1,000 g birthweight)

Bag-Mask Equipment

See Chapter 14.

Intubation Equipment

See Chapter 16.

Medications

Epinephrine (1:10,000): 3- or 10-mL ampules

Sodium bicarbonate: 4.2% (5 mEq/10 mL) 10-mL ampules

Dextrose: 10% 250 mL

Naloxone hydrochloride: 0.4 mg/mL in 1-mL ampules or 1 mg/mL in 2-mL ampules

Surfactant (multiple preparations available)

Normal saline

Volume expander

Additional Equipment

Sterile gloves

Stethoscope

Cardiac monitor

Umbilical vessel catheterization tray (Chapter 38)

Luer-Lok syringes (1, 3, 5, 10, 20, and 50 mL)

Blood gas syringes (1 mL)

Needles (25, 21, and 18 gauge)

Butterfly needles (25 and 23 gauge)

Needles (intraosseous)

Intravenous catheters (24, 22, 20, and 18 gauge)

End-tidal or chemical CO_2 detector

Adhesive tape

Alcohol pads

Chest tube kit

Umbilical vessel cannulation kit

▶ PROCEDURE

A summary of the resuscitation process is presented in Figure 36.2. All newborn infants undergo the initial steps of resuscitation, including thermal management, clearing of the airway, and tactile stimulation. These first steps can generally be completed within 20 seconds.

Preventing Heat Loss

Immediate drying of the newborn with removal of amniotic fluid will prevent evaporative heat loss. All wet blankets should then be removed. An overhead warmer is necessary to

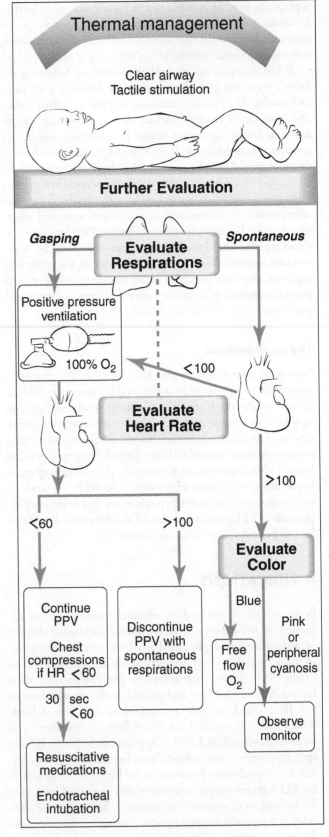

Figure 36.2 A summary of the resuscitation process.

minimize radiant and convective heat loss. Initially, the unit should be set to the manual mode at the maximum temperature setting. This will allow for an immediate warm environment for the newborn. Eventually the servo mode can be used to allow for the temperature to be modulated by the newborn's own body temperature. A targeted body temperature (37°C) is selected by adjusting the skin temperature control point setting. With the newborn in the supine position, a skin temperature probe is placed on the abdomen between the xiphoid process and the umbilicus so that exposed skin surrounding the probe is in direct line with radiation from the warmer. Ideally the resuscitation area should be kept as warm as possible to minimize the newborn's heat loss to the environment.

Adjunctive measures such as wrapping the newborn in warm, dry blankets and covering the newborn's head with a stockinette hat can be used to prevent evaporative heat loss. Exothermic chemical warming blankets are useful to maintain extremely low birthweight infants in a thermal-neutral range.

Clearing the Airway

Establishing an open airway is accomplished by positioning the newborn correctly and suctioning the mouth and then the nose. The newborn should be placed supine in slight Trendelenburg position with the neck slightly extended (Fig. 36.3). Care should be taken not to hyperextend or hyperflex the neck because either position may result in decreased air entry. The airway can be cleared with a suction catheter (10 French) or bulb syringe (Fig. 36.4). The mouth should be suctioned first to prevent aspiration should the newborn gasp while suctioning the nose. Suctioning of the deep oropharynx or stomach is not routinely recommended because of the likelihood of vagal stimulation. The negative pressure of the suction apparatus should not exceed 100 mm Hg (136 cm H_2O) (10). Meconium-stained amniotic fluid should be managed according to current guidelines (Chapter 37).

Tactile Stimulation

Usually drying and suctioning the newborn infant provides enough tactile stimulation to initiate respirations. If not, stimulating the soles of the feet either by slapping or flicking the feet may initiate respirations in the mildly depressed newborn (Fig. 36.5). Firmly rubbing the newborn's back also is an acceptable method of tactile stimulation in an attempt to initiate respirations. Methods of stimulation used in the past, which include slapping the newborn's back, squeezing the rib cage, and forcing the thighs onto the abdomen, can be harmful to the newborn and should not be used. If the newborn remains apneic after appropriate techniques are attempted once or twice, tactile stimulation should stop and PPV must be instituted immediately.

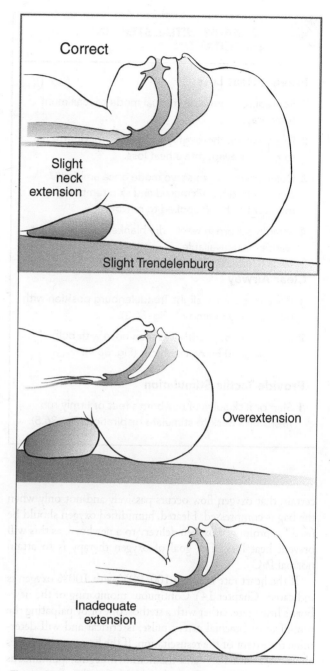

Figure 36.3 Positioning the neonatal airway.

Further Evaluation

After completing the initial steps in resuscitation, further action will depend on the evaluation of respiratory effort, heart rate, and color (Fig. 36.2). If the newborn has spontaneous respirations and the heart rate is above 100, the newborn's color should be evaluated. If central cyanosis is present, oxygen should be administered via a free flow system. A flow of 5 L/min, with either an oxygen tube held one-half inch from the newborn's nose or an oxygen mask, will provide an oxygen concentration of approximately 80%. When providing oxygen therapy through a self-inflating bag, clinicians must be

SUMMARY: INITIAL STEPS IN RESUSCITATION

Prevent Heat Loss

1 Set radiant warmer in manual mode to maximum temperature.

2 Dry newborn thoroughly and place stockinette hat to prevent evaporative heat loss.

3 Convert warmer to servo mode once ambient temperature has increased and skin temperature monitor has been applied to newborn.

4 Wrap newborn in warm, dry blankets when radiant warmer is unavailable.

Clear Airway

1 Place newborn in slight Trendelenburg position with neck slightly extended (Fig. 36.3).

2 Gently suction mouth and then nose with bulb syringe or 10 French catheter (Fig. 36.4).

Provide Tactile Stimulation

1 Slap or flick soles of newborn's feet or firmly rub newborn's back to stimulate respiration (Fig. 36.5).

certain that oxygen flow occurs passively and not only when the bag is compressed. Heated, humidified oxygen should be used for prolonged oxygen delivery to a newborn, as this will prevent heat loss. The goal of oxygen therapy is to attain normal PaO_2.

If the heart rate is below 100, PPV with 100% oxygen is indicated (Chapter 14). Continuous monitoring of the newborn's heart rate, either with a stethoscope or by palpating the umbilical or brachial artery pulse, is critical and will determine the extent of the resuscitation. If the heart rate increases above 100 with PPV and the newborn begins spontaneous respirations, PPV can be replaced with free flow oxygen.

If the heart rate is between 60 and 100 and appears to be increasing, PPV should continue until the heart rate is greater than 100 and spontaneous respirations develop. Newborns who fail to improve despite adequate ventilation (i.e., sufficient chest movement and good breath sounds) should continue to receive PPV. Chest compressions should be instituted if the heart rate falls below 60 despite adequate PPV with 100% oxygen (Chapter 12). Chest compressions should be coordinated with newborn ventilation at a 3:1 ratio, with a rate of approximately 90 compressions and 30 breaths per minute. If the newborn's condition continues to deteriorate or fails to improve despite assisted ventilation and chest compressions, endotracheal intubation (Chapter 16) and administration of resuscitation medications may be required.

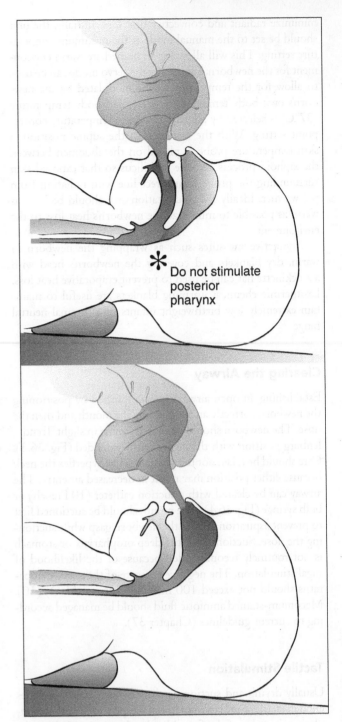

Figure 36.4 Suctioning the mouth and nose.

Resuscitation Medications

Clinicians involved in the resuscitation of newborn infants must be familiar with the pharmacologic agents routinely used in the management of the distressed newborn. The resuscitation area must be stocked and have easy access to the agents commonly used to enhance cardiac output and to treat neonatal asphyxia. These agents can only be used after the clinician has obtained vascular access (Chapter 38) or has

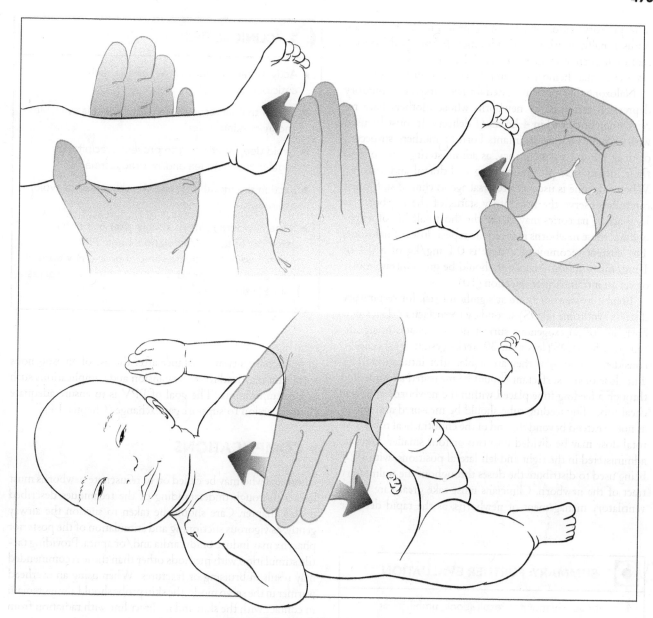

Figure 36.5 Tactile stimulation of the newborn.

secured an endotracheal tube (Chapter 16). Bradycardia is the most common rhythm disturbance in newborn infants and is most likely due to inadequate ventilation. Therefore, the resuscitation team must ensure adequate ventilation and a stable airway before proceeding to pharmacologic management of the newborn.

After oxygen, epinephrine is the pharmacologic agent most commonly used in the neonate. It is indicated for persistent bradycardia (greater than 30 seconds despite adequate ventilation) and asystole. Current guidelines recommend a dose of 0.01 to 0.03 mg/kg (0.1 to 0.3 mL/kg of 1:10,000 solution) administered via intravenous catheter. Endotracheal epinephrine (1 mL/kg, 0.1 mg/kg) may be considered until IV access is obtained.

Volume expansion with normal saline is indicated in any neonate who demonstrates shock secondary to acute blood loss, asphyxia, metabolic acidosis, or severe anemia. An initial bolus of 10 mL/kg should be given intravenously over 5 to 10 minutes. Repeat fluid boluses may be indicated in the setting of severe shock; however, care must be taken to avoid volume overload, which has been associated with intraventricular hemorrhage in asphyxiated newborn infants (11). Albumin-containing solutions are no longer considered first-line therapy for fluid resuscitation because of the risk of infectious disease and an association with increased mortality (12).

The use of sodium bicarbonate therapy is controversial in newborn resuscitations (13). Volume expansion coupled with efficient management of the newborn's airway may be sufficient to treat metabolic acidosis. In newborns with severe, persistent metabolic acidosis, sodium bicarbonate may be indicated, but careful attention must be paid to the newborn's respiratory status, as bicarbonate use in the setting of respiratory acidosis may worsen the intracellular acid base status. Finally, bicarbonate therapy must be used with extreme caution in premature newborns, as it has been associated with intraventricular hemorrhage in preterm newborns (14).

Naloxone therapy is indicated for reversing the respiratory depression exhibited by newborns whose mothers have received narcotics within 4 hours of delivery. It must be used with extreme caution in infants born to mothers suspected of drug use during pregnancy, as administering naloxone to these infants may precipitate drug withdrawal and seizures. When naloxone is used as a reversal agent, clinical staff must carefully observe the respiratory status of the newborn, as long-acting narcotics may exceed the short half-life of naloxone and these newborns may require repeat doses of naloxone. The current recommended dose is 0.1 mg/kg of a 0.4 or 1 mg/mL solution. Naloxone should be given intravenously or via an intramuscular injection (10).

Premature newborns are at significant risk for respiratory distress syndrome (RDS) secondary to surfactant deficiency. Early use of an exogenous surfactant in neonates at significant risk for RDS (less than 30 weeks gestation) should be considered as soon as they are stable, after intubation (15). The dose of the surfactant should be measured and instilled through a feeding tube placed within the newborn's endotracheal tube. The feeding tube should be measured and cut so as not to extend beyond the end of the endotracheal tube. The total dose may be divided into two or four smaller aliquots, administered in the right and left lateral positions, with PPV being used to distribute the doses throughout the pulmonary tract of the newborn. Clinicians must take great care in the ventilatory management of newborns, as the rapid decrease

CLINICAL TIPS

▶ Activate radiant warmer as soon as delivery is anticipated.

▶ Ensure that all resuscitation equipment is available and in working order.

▶ Avoid deep suctioning to prevent precipitating vagal-induced apnea and/or bradycardia.

▶ Suction the mouth first and then the nose to avoid aspiration.

▶ If the newborn remains apneic after one or two attempts of tactile stimulation, begin PPV. Continued use of tactile stimulation in a newborn who does not respond is not warranted and wastes valuable time.

in pulmonary airway resistance after the use of an exogenous surfactant may lead to overexpansion and complications such as a pneumothorax. The goal of PPV is to ensure adequate chest excursion to support gas exchange (Chapter 14).

▶ COMPLICATIONS

Clinicians who may be called on to resuscitate newborns must have a thorough understanding of the techniques described in this chapter. Care should be taken to suction the airway gently, as vigorous suctioning and stimulation of the posterior pharynx may induce bradycardia and/or apnea. Providing tactile stimulation with methods other than those recommended may result in bruising or fractures. When using an overhead warmer in the servo mode, the skin probe should always remain in contact with the skin and in direct line with radiation from the warmer. Displacement of the probe can result in overheating and possible burning of the newborn. Rectal temperature should never be used to control skin temperature. Radiant warming also results in increased insensible water losses, and attention to the fluid balance is necessary. During PPV, chest excursions and pressure gauge readings should be closely monitored to avoid producing a pneumothorax.

▶ SUMMARY

The overall goals of neonatal resuscitation are to assist the newborn in making the transition to neonatal life and to avoid the dire consequences of asphyxia. Neonates are more often vulnerable to asphyxia and are far more likely to require resuscitation than children in any other age group. The effects of asphyxia can usually be avoided or minimized by (a) having skilled staff readily available who are able to function as a team, (b) having proper equipment available, and (c)

SUMMARY: FURTHER EVALUATION

1 Continuously monitor respirations, umbilical or brachial pulse, and color.

2 If newborn has spontaneous respirations and heart rate above 100, then evaluate color; provide oxygen if central cyanosis is present.

3 If newborn displays no spontaneous respirations or heart rate below 100, provide PPV with 100% oxygen.

4 If newborn's heart rate is between 60 and 100 and increasing, continue PPV until it is above 100 and spontaneous respirations develop.

5 If the heart rate is below 60 and not increasing despite adequate ventilation, begin chest compressions.

6 If heart rate remains below 60 after 30 seconds of PPV, initiate intubation and resuscitation medications.

promptly recognizing neonatal distress. The uncommon occurrence of ED deliveries mandates an organized and effective approach to the emergent resuscitation of newborns. More specific information and necessary skills, including management of meconium aspiration, techniques of intubation, and bag-mask ventilation, are discussed in great detail in other chapters. These should be reviewed to supplement the general approach delineated in this chapter.

▶ ACKNOWLEDGMENT

The authors would like to acknowledge the valuable contributions of Sigmund J. Kharasch to the version of this chapter that appeared in the previous edition.

▶ REFERENCES

1. Saugstad OD. Practical aspects of resuscitating asphyxiated newborn infants. *Eur J Pediatr*. 1998;157[Suppl 1]:S11–15.
2. Kattwinkel J. *Textbook of Neonatal Resuscitation*. 5th ed. Elk Grove Village, IL: American Heart Association, Academy of Pediatrics; 2006.
3. Fanaroff A, Martin R. *Neonatal-Perinatal Medicine: Diseases of the Fetus and Infant*. 7th ed. St. Louis: Mosby; 2002.
4. *World Health Report*. Geneva: World Health Organization; 1995.
5. Jain L, Ferre C, Vidyasagar D, et al. Cardiopulmonary resuscitation of apparently stillborn infants: survival and long-term outcome. *J Pediatr*. 1991;118:778–782.
6. Yeo CL, Tudehope DI. Outcome of resuscitated apparently stillborn infants: a ten year review. *J Paediatr Child Health*. 1994;30:129–133.
7. Gandy GM, Adamson SK, Cunningham N, et al. Thermal environment and acid-base homeostasis in human infants during the first few hours of life. *J Clin Invest*. 1964;43:751–758.
8. Lieberman E, Lang J, Richardson DK, et al. Intrapartum maternal fever and neonatal outcome. *Pediatrics*. 2000;105:8–13.
9. Allen MC, Donohue PK, Dusman AE. The limit of viability: neonatal outcome of infants born at 22 to 25 weeks gestation. *N Eng J Med*. 1993;329:1597–1600.
10. 2005 American Heart Association Guidelines for Cardiopulmonary Resuscitation and Emergency Cardiovascular Care. Pat 13: Neonatal Resuscitation Guidelines. *Circulation*. 2005;112:IV-188–195.
11. Funato M, Tamai J, Noma K, et al. Clinical events in association with timing of intraventricular hemorrhage in preterm infants. *J Pediatr*. 1992;121:614–619.
12. Cochrane Injuries Group Albumin Reviewers. Human albumin administration in critically ill patients: systematic review of randomized controlled trials. *BMJ*. 1998;317:235–240.
13. Lokesh L, Kumar P, Murkae S, et al. A randomized controlled trial of sodium bicarbonate in neonatal resuscitation: effect on immediate outcome. *Resuscitation*. 2004;60:219–223.
14. Hein HA. The use of sodium bicarbonate in neonatal resuscitation: help or harm? *Pediatrics*. 1993;91:496–497.
15. Recommendations for neonatal surfactant therapy. Fetus and Newborn Committee, Canadian Pediatric Society (CPS). *Paediatr Child Health*. 2005;10:109–116.

37

JORDAN D. LIPTON

Prevention and Management of Meconium Aspiration

▶ INTRODUCTION

Meconium staining of the amniotic fluid is thought to indicate fetal distress and is seen predominantly in infants who are postmature or small for their gestational age. It rarely occurs in newborns of less than 38 weeks gestation. Meconium is present in the amniotic fluid in 10% to 15% of deliveries (1–3) and is best managed quickly and aggressively when there is evidence of fetal distress or neonatal depression during a delivery room or emergency department (ED) delivery. Meconium aspiration syndrome is defined as the presence of meconium below the vocal cords associated with some degree of respiratory distress and hypoxia. With appropriate management, only 5% of neonates born through meconium-stained amniotic fluid develop the syndrome (4). Unfortunately, for those infants who do develop the syndrome, meconium can be responsible for severe pulmonary complications (5).

▶ ANATOMY AND PHYSIOLOGY

Meconium first appears in the fetal ileum between the 10th and 16th week of gestation. It is a viscous liquid composed of gastrointestinal secretions, cellular debris, bile, pancreatic secretions, mucus, blood, hair, and vernix. Passage of meconium before birth may be a normal physiologic event, and the maturation of peristaltic activity may account for the increased incidence of meconium-stained amniotic fluid seen with increased gestation. An increase in the passage of meconium is also associated with fetal asphyxia.

Respiratory movements are normal in utero. The general direction of amniotic flow is from the lungs and kidneys to the amniotic sac. Asphyxia of the fetus stimulates deep breaths and gasping, which results in aspiration of amniotic contents into the lungs (Fig. 37.1). As a result, meconium aspiration may occur both in utero and at the time of delivery and may indicate fetal distress or asphyxia.

Meconium aspiration syndrome is associated with a wide range of respiratory symptoms, from mild to severe. Meconium has been shown to produce mechanical obstruction, chemical pneumonitis, pulmonary vessel vasoconstriction, surfactant inactivation, and complement activation. In severe cases, meconium aspiration results in pulmonary hypertension and persistent fetal circulation with right-to-left shunting. Air leak also has been noted as a complication of significant meconium aspiration (1,5).

▶ INDICATIONS

Meconium is a dark brownish-green material. The distinction between thin and thick refers to its density, which varies from liquid to semisolid. This consistency is dictated by the quantity of meconium that is passed and the amount of amniotic fluid in which it is diluted. With increasing gestational age, the relative amount of amniotic fluid decreases, resulting in thicker meconium. Fetal stress also may be responsible for increased passage of meconium and therefore a thicker consistency.

Two approaches have been advocated to prevent meconium aspiration. The first alternative—selective intubation—involves visualizing the glottis using a laryngoscope, followed by intubation and suctioning of the infant, but only if the infant is depressed. This approach is taken by authorities who

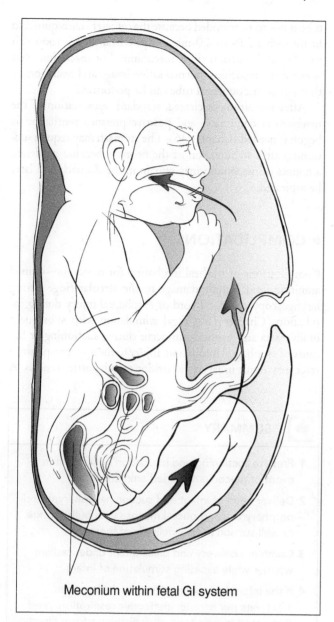

Meconium within fetal GI system

Figure 37.1 In utero flow of meconium predisposing to aspiration.

believe that when signs of distress are absent, an infant is unlikely to have a significant amount of meconium in the trachea. The second option—universal intubation—involves endotracheal intubation and suctioning whenever thick meconium is present in the amniotic fluid. The latter approach has fallen out of favor since it has been found that tracheal suctioning of the vigorous infant with meconium-stained fluid does not improve outcome and may cause iatrogenic complications (6,7). This is in spite of the fact that one study found 9% of meconium-stained infants had meconium suctioned from their tracheas when no meconium was visible in the mouth, in the pharynx, or at the vocal cords (3).

Thus, vigorous infants with meconium-stained amniotic fluid (whether thick or thin) rarely require special intervention.

However, meconium-stained amniotic fluid in association with a depressed neonate requires endotracheal suctioning. It is estimated that 95% of cases of meconium aspiration syndrome develop in the presence of thick meconium (2). A vigorous infant with a heart rate greater than 100 beats per minute, effective spontaneous respirations, and good muscle tone within the first several seconds after birth will likely not benefit from immediate tracheal suctioning, but continued assessment is mandatory (7).

▶ EQUIPMENT

Suction capable of generating up to 100 mm Hg negative pressure
Connective tubing (1/4 inch)
Suction trap or canister
Suction catheters (10 to 14 French)
DeLee suction trap apparatus
Bulb syringe
Endotracheal tubes, uncuffed (3.0, 3.5, and 4.0 mm)
Endotracheal tube stylettes
Laryngoscope and straight blades (Miller 0 and 1)
Meconium aspirator

▶ PROCEDURE

To prevent aspiration, the oropharynx and nasopharynx of infants born with meconium staining should be suctioned after the head is delivered but before delivery of the thorax (Fig. 37.2). A bulb syringe or wall suction apparatus with suction catheter is used for this process. Suctioning should occur along the buccal mucosa to avoid overstimulation of the posterior pharynx, which can result in a severe reflex vagal bradycardia.

Delivery is then completed, the umbilical cord is cut, the infant is placed under a radiant warmer, and residual meconium is suctioned from the hypopharynx under direct vision. Overstimulation, such as vigorous drying, should be avoided during the intubation procedure, as this may promote gasping or deep breathing. Cardiac and oxygen saturation monitoring can be performed by an assistant during the resuscitation but should not delay resuscitative efforts.

When indicated by an infant's distress or depression, direct laryngoscopy is performed while maintaining the infant's neck in a slightly extended position, and the infant is intubated (Chapter 16). Once placed, the endotracheal tube should be secured with a free hand resting on the infant's head while preparing for suctioning. The entire intubation procedure, excluding suctioning, should be limited to approximately 20 seconds to avoid significant hypoxia. Free flow blow-by oxygen should be provided over the infant's face to minimize hypoxia during suctioning.

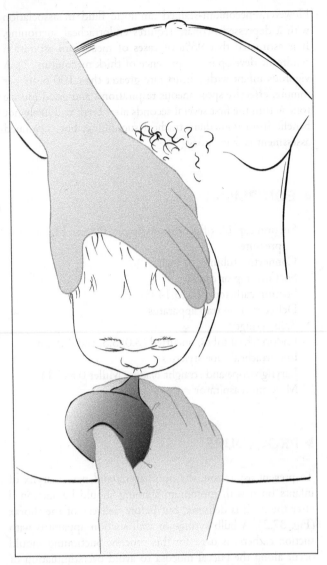

Figure 37.2 Suctioning of a meconium-stained infant at the perineum.

Tracheal suctioning should be limited to 10 seconds per pass. Wall suction devices should be set at 60 to 80 mm Hg negative pressure, with a maximum of 100 mm Hg. Suction tubing can be connected to a DeLee suction apparatus or directly to the endotracheal tube with a special adapter called a meconium aspirator. Suction is applied continuously as the endotracheal tube is slowly withdrawn from the trachea (Fig. 37.3). Oral suction through a face mask functioning as a filter with or without a DeLee suction apparatus is not recommended because of the infectious risks to the physician (chlamydia, *Neisseria gonorrhoeae, Trichomonas vaginalis,* group B streptococcus, cytomegalovirus, herpes simplex virus, hepatitis, and human immunodeficiency virus) (8).

Reintubation and repeat suctioning is necessary until no further meconium is collected in the trap. If the endotracheal tube becomes obstructed with thick meconium, a new one should be used for subsequent intubation. Using a small, disposable plastic catheter to suction through the endotracheal

tube is not recommended because the catheter size required to fit through a 3.0- to 4.0-mm endotracheal tube is too small to adequately suction thick meconium. For meconium that is especially tenacious, normal saline lavage and resuctioning through an endotracheal tube can be performed.

After the airway is cleared, standard resuscitation of the newborn is continued, and positive pressure ventilation is begun if needed (Chapter 36). The stomach may require suctioning after stabilization of the neonate, because moderate amounts of meconium may remain in the stomach and later be aspirated.

▶ COMPLICATIONS

Complications of tracheal intubation for meconium-stained amniotic fluid include damage to the alveolar ridge during laryngoscopy and vocal cord or esophageal injury during intubation (Chapter 16). Vagal stimulation with subsequent bradycardia and hypoxia can occur during suctioning or because of esophageal intubation. Injury to the upper respiratory tract may result in laryngeal stridor or subglottic stenosis. A

 SUMMARY

1 Prepare suctioning and intubation equipment in event of meconium-stained amniotic fluid.

2 Deliver head of infant and suction nasopharynx and oropharynx along buccal mucosa with bulb syringe or wall suction before delivery of thorax.

3 Complete delivery and place infant under radiant warmer while avoiding stimulation of infant.

4 If the infant is depressed (heart rate less than 100 beats per minute, ineffective respirations, and decreased muscle tone after birth), perform direct laryngoscopy and endotracheal intubation with 3.0-, 3.5-, or 4.0-mm endotracheal tube.

5 Apply continuous suction at 60 to 80 mm Hg negative pressure to endotracheal tube as it is withdrawn.

6 Repeat laryngoscopy, intubation, and tracheal suctioning until no further meconium is suctioned.

7 Begin positive pressure ventilation if needed, and resume standard newborn resuscitation.

8 Suction stomach for residual meconium.

9 For infants who develop meconium aspiration syndrome despite preventive measures, provide warmed nasal or endotracheal oxygen with ventilatory support and transfer to neonatal intensive care unit.

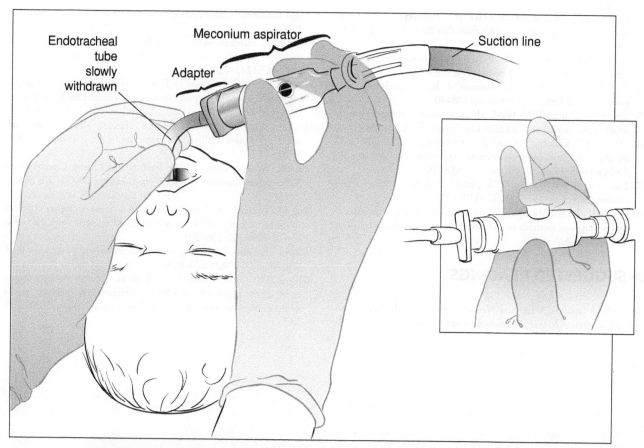

Figure 37.3 Using the meconium aspirator in suctioning meconium from the trachea of an intubated (depressed) newborn.

physician who performs oral suctioning also is at risk for infection. The performance of this procedure results in a delay in the usual resuscitative procedures for the newborn, especially the provision of adequate oxygenation and ventilation.

 CLINICAL TIPS

▶ After the head is delivered at the introitus, suction is applied along the buccal mucosa to avoid overstimulation of the posterior pharynx during suctioning.

▶ Stimulation before and during intubation should be avoided, as this may promote gasping or deep breathing.

▶ The stomach should be suctioned to clear any residual meconium following stabilization of the neonate.

▶ When multiple passes are necessary, the endotracheal tube should be replaced between each attempt.

▶ Intubation and suctioning should be repeated until no significant meconium is obtained.

▶ SUMMARY

Amniotic fluid stained with meconium during delivery generally requires removal and clearance from an infant's respiratory tract only if the infant is depressed or becomes depressed. First bulb syringe or wall suctioning is performed at the perineum after delivery of the infant's head. If the infant is depressed, the trachea is suctioned using direct laryngoscopy and repetitive endotracheal intubation following delivery of the body. Finally, the stomach is suctioned. Aggressive management is thought to reduce the incidence of meconium aspiration syndrome and its severe complications.

▶ ACKNOWLEDGMENT

The authors would like to acknowledge the valuable contributions of Robert W. Schafermeyer to the version of this chapter that appeared in the previous edition.

▶ REFERENCES

1. Cleary GM, Wiswell TE. Meconium-stained amniotic fluid and the meconium aspiration syndrome: an update. *Pediatr Clin North Am.* 1998;45:511–529.

2. Holtzman RB, Banzhaf WC, Silver RK, et al. Perinatal management of meconium staining of the amniotic fluid. *Clin Perinatol.* 1989;16:825–838.

3. Gregory GA, Gooding CA, Phibbs RH, et al. Meconium aspiration in infants: a prospective study. *J Pediatr.* 1974;85:848–852.

4. Wiswell TE. Advances in the treatment of the meconium aspiration syndrome. *Acta Paediatr.* 2001;90(suppl):28–30.

5. Gelfand SL, Fanaroff JM, Walsh MC. Controversies in the treatment of meconium aspiration syndrome. *Clin Perinatol.* 2004;31:445–452.

6. Halliday HL. Endotracheal intubation at birth for preventing morbidity and mortality in vigorous, meconium-stained infants born at term. *Cochrane Database Syst Rev.* 2001;No. 1:CD000500.

7. Niermeyer S, Van Reempts P, Kattwinkel J, et al. Resuscitation of the newborn. *Ann Emerg Med.* 2001;37:S110–125.

8. Ballard JL, Musial MJ, Myers MG. Hazards of delivery room resuscitation using oral methods of endotracheal suctioning. *Pediatr Infect Dis.* 1986;5:198–200.

▶ SUGGESTED READINGS

Bloom RS, Cropley C; AHA/AAP Neonatal Resuscitation Program Steering Committee. *Textbook of Neonatal Resuscitation.* Rev. ed. Elk Grove Village, IL: American Heart Association, American Academy of Pediatrics; 1996.

Falciglia HS, Henderschott C, Potter P, et al. Does DeLee suction at the perineum prevent meconium aspiration syndrome? *Am J Obstet Gynecol.* 1992;167:1243–1249.

Locus P, Yeomans E, Crosby U. Efficacy of bulb vs. DeLee suction at deliveries complicated by meconium-stained amniotic fluid. *Am J Perinatol.* 1990;7:87–91.

Newborn resuscitation. In: Chameides L, Hazinski MF, eds. *Pediatric Advanced Life Support.* Dallas, TX: American Heart Association; 1997: 9–10.

Pediatric Working Group of the International Liaison Committee on Resuscitation. Neonatal resuscitation. *Circulation.* 2000;102[8 Suppl]: 1343–1357.

Peng TC, Gutcher GR, Van Dorsten JP. A selective aggressive approach to the neonate exposed to meconium-stained amniotic fluid. *Am J Obstet Gynecol.* 1996;175:296–301.

Wiswell TE, Fuloria M. Management of meconium-stained amniotic fluid. *Clin Perinatol.* 1999;26:659–668.

Wiswell TE, Gannon CM, Jacob J, et al. Delivery room management of the apparently vigorous meconium-stained neonate: results of the multicenter international collaborative trial. *Pediatrics.* 2000;105: 1–7.

ARIS C. GARRO AND JAMES G. LINAKIS

38

Umbilical Vessel Catheterization

▶ INTRODUCTION

Umbilical vessel catheterization is used frequently in the newborn period for transfusion therapy, blood pressure monitoring, emergency delivery of medications and fluids, delivery of parenteral nutrition, and blood sampling. Although most likely to be performed in the neonatal ICU setting, arterial or venous catheterization also can be performed in the emergency department (ED) for the resuscitation of infants delivered in the prehospital or ED setting. Peripheral intravenous access should be attempted first; however, such access can at times be difficult to obtain. Umbilical vessel catheterization provides a reliable means of emergency vascular access in the newborn. In addition, the umbilical vein should be considered as an option for emergency access in the neonate up to 2 weeks of age. Although it is associated with a higher complication rate, this method has the advantage of providing central venous access and allowing direct visualization of the vessels to be catheterized.

▶ ANATOMY AND PHYSIOLOGY

The fetal cardiovascular system serves prenatal needs and allows for modifications after birth that lead to a postnatal circulatory pattern (Fig. 38.1) (1). In the fetal circulatory system, well-oxygenated blood (~80% saturated) returns from the placenta through the umbilical vein, which courses through the hepatic sinusoids and ductus venosus to the inferior vena cava. High pressure in the fetal pulmonary vascular system results in the majority of blood being shunted from the right atrium across the foramen ovale into the left atrium. One third of the blood that reaches the right ventricle is distributed to the lungs, while two thirds is shunted to the aorta by way of the ductus arteriosus. Umbilical arteries receive approxi-

mately 40% to 50% of the mixed blood in the descending aorta (~58% saturated with oxygen) and return it to the placenta, where O_2, CO_2, nutrients, and waste products are exchanged. The remainder of the blood from the descending aorta circulates through the gut, kidney, and lower extremities.

Numerous changes occur in the circulatory system following birth. With the first breath and the inflation of alveoli, pulmonary vascular resistance falls. Elevations in PaO_2 and pH contribute to pulmonary vasodilation and further reduction of pulmonary vascular resistance. In contrast, neonatal systemic resistance is immediately increased when the umbilical cord is clamped. These dramatic changes in pressure result in a reversal of the gradient across the atrial septum and closure of the foramen ovale.

The ductus arteriosus begins to constrict almost immediately following birth, stimulated by increased oxygen tension and decreased circulating prostaglandins. Functional closure generally occurs 1 to 2 days after birth. The ductus venosus also closes once the umbilical cord is clamped. The umbilical arteries begin to constrict within minutes of birth and close before the umbilical vein. The umbilical vein may retain some degree of patency for up to 2 weeks after the cord is clamped and cut.

The umbilical arteries and vein can be differentiated in a cross section of the umbilical cord based on a number of characteristics. The vein is generally located on the cephalad end of the umbilicus. It is thin walled, with a large lumen, and only a single vein is present within the cord. The umbilical artery possesses a thicker wall and a smaller lumen and may appear slightly protuberant above the cut umbilical surface. Two arteries generally are present in the umbilical cord; however, approximately 0.5% of newborns will have only one umbilical artery. A patent urachus is a persistent embryologic connection to the bladder that may rarely be present and can appear similar to the umbilical vein but without bleeding.

483

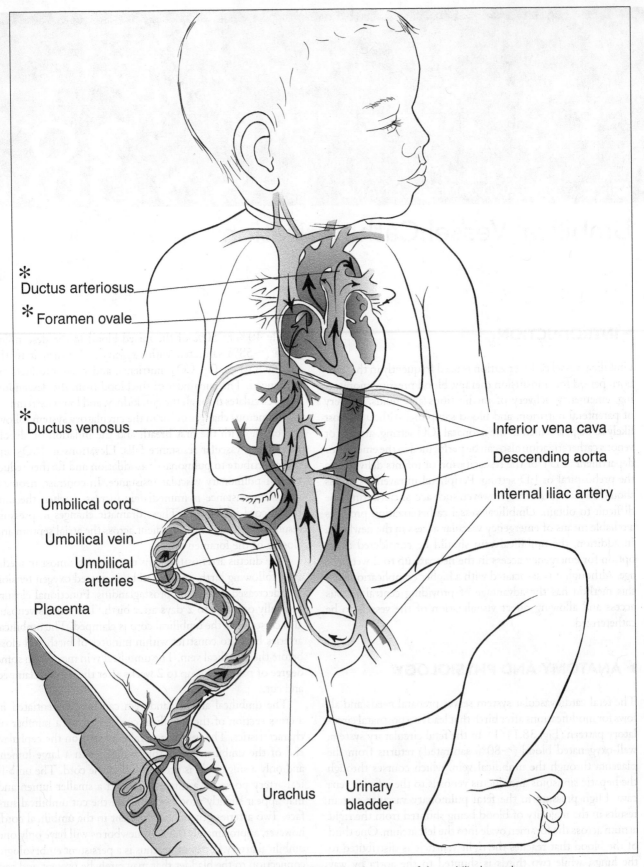

Figure 38.1 The fetal cardiovascular system illustrating the course of the umbilical vessels. Structures marked with an asterisk (*) close soon after birth.

▶ INDICATIONS

Umbilical artery catheterization is indicated for newborns with severe cardiopulmonary insufficiency requiring mechanically assisted ventilation. The umbilical artery catheter allows for frequent arterial blood gas determinations and can be used for administration of fluids, medications, and exchange transfusion. It is usually quite simple to catheterize the umbilical artery in a sick infant during the first hour of life, and most infants can be catheterized within the first 24 hours. Occasionally this route can be used up to 7 days of age.

Umbilical vein catheterization in the ED or delivery room is recommended for emergent situations in which delivery of resuscitative medications, volume expanders, or blood products is the desired goal. Catheterization of the umbilical vein is easiest in newborns but has been successful in infants up to 2 weeks of age.

An umbilical vessel catheter (arterial or venous) should never be inserted in the presence of omphalitis or impetiginous skin lesions. It is also generally contraindicated when a possibility of intestinal hypoperfusion or necrotizing enterocolitis exists, both of which are often suggested by abdominal distention. Finally, inserting an umbilical catheter for routine administration of parenteral fluids or medications or for routine blood sampling is inappropriate.

▶ EQUIPMENT

Radiant warmer with light source
Prep solution (povidone-iodine), sterile drape, gauze pads
Mask, cap, goggles, sterile gloves, gown
Scalpel (No. 11 or 15)
Curved, nontoothed iris forceps (4″) or pointed, solid metal dilator
Small, smooth curved hemostat(s)
Straight Crile forceps
Iris scissors
Needle holder
Nonthrombogenic, molded-tip umbilical catheters (3.5, 4, 5, and 8 French with end hole)
3.0 or 4.0 silk suture on curved or straight needle
Linen umbilical tape (~15″)
Adhesive tape
10-cc syringe filled with normal saline (NS) (with or without heparin 1 unit/mL)
D5W (5% dextrose in water), D10W (10% dextrose in water), or NS infusion setup (with heparin 1 unit/mL, unless medications incompatible with heparin)
Fluid chamber, i.v. tubing, infusion pump, 0.22-μm filter
Three-way stopcock, cardiac monitor, pulse oximeter

▶ PROCEDURE

Preparation

Treatment for cardiorespiratory disturbances should begin before commencing the procedure. The child is placed be-

neath a radiant warmer and the extremities are restrained in a supine frog-leg position (Fig. 38.2). The cardiac rate should be monitored, and adequate oxygenation should be made available throughout the procedure. The clinician performing the procedure should wear a surgical gown, gloves, cap, mask, and goggles (Chapter 7). The infant's abdomen and remaining umbilical cord is scrubbed with a bactericidal solution, such as povidone-iodine, from the xiphoid process to the symphysis pubis. Pooling of solution at the infant's side should be avoided because this may result in skin blistering. The umbilical area is draped in a sterile fashion, and the infant's head is left exposed for observation.

A purse-string suture or umbilical tape loosely tied with a surgeon's knot is placed at the base of the umbilical cord to provide hemostasis and an anchor after line placement.

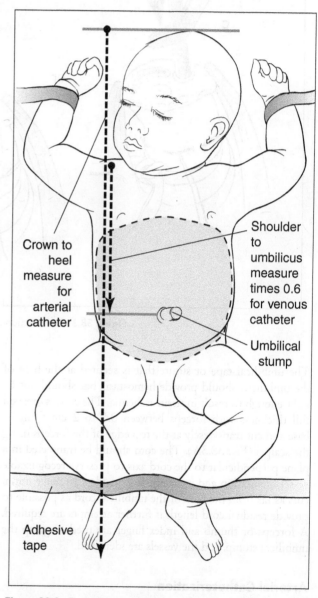

Crown to heel measure for arterial catheter

Shoulder to umbilicus measure times 0.6 for venous catheter

Umbilical stump

Adhesive tape

Figure 38.2 Positioning and restraint of the neonate for umbilical vessel catheterization. Note shoulder to umbilicus and crown to heel (total body length) measurements. Shading represents area to be cleansed with bactericidal solution.

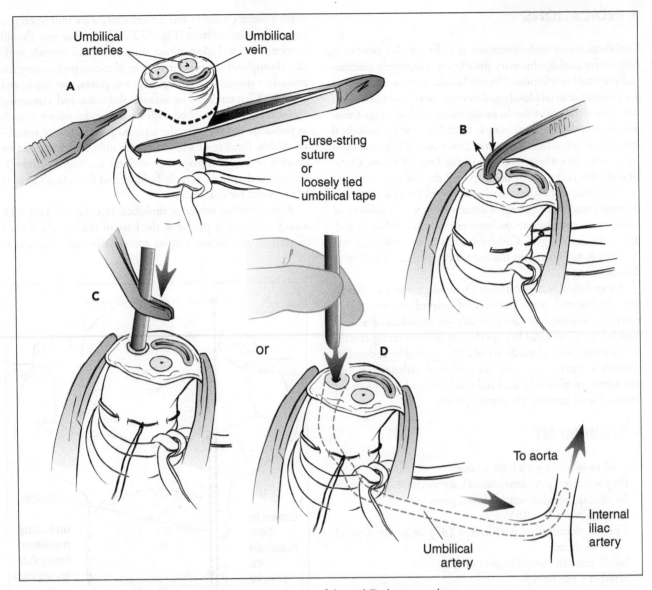

Figure 38.3 Introduction of the umbilical artery catheter.

The umbilical tape or suture that is secured at the base of the umbilicus should provide hemostasis but should not be tight enough to result in tissue ischemia. The cord is grasped full thickness with forceps between 0.5 to 2 cm from its base and cut transversely at the top edge of the forceps using the scalpel (Fig. 38.3A). The cord should be transected in a plane perpendicular to the cord axis to preserve recognizable vessel orientation and anatomy. It is prudent to make initial cuts as far from the base of the umbilical cord as possible to provide residual cord length if further attempts are required. A forceps or thumb and index finger are used to grasp the umbilical stump, and the vessels are identified.

Arterial Catheterization

A curved hemostat is used to grasp the cut edge of the cord near the artery selected for catheterization, or two hemostats are used to grasp opposite sides of the umbilicus. The edges are then everted (Fig. 38.3B). Using curved iris forceps without teeth, approximately 1 cm of arterial lumen is gently dilated by repetitively introducing and opening the tips of the forceps within the lumen. A pointed, solid metal dilator can be used in place of the iris forceps, with careful attention directed toward not tearing the arterial wall.

The catheter, previously flushed with heparinized solution, is grasped approximately 1 cm from its tip with thumb and index finger or with small forceps, and the tip is inserted into the arterial lumen (Figs. 38.3C–D). A 3.5 to 4 French catheter is used for infants weighing less than 2 kg, and a 5 French catheter for infants weighing more than 2 kg. During insertion, tension is placed cephalad on the cord so that the catheter can be advanced more directly toward the feet. The catheter is passed using gentle, constant pressure to overcome resistance, which is usually felt at two points. Slight resistance is first met at 1 to 2 cm, where the umbilical artery curves toward the feet; placing tension cephalad on the cord helps to reduce this resistance. The clinician will feel greater resistance at the junction of the internal iliac artery at 5 to 6 cm, where the artery turns upward (Fig. 38.1). A slight twisting motion of the catheter will help to overcome resistance. Resistance during arterial catheter insertion may occur as a result of vasospasm. This can sometimes be relieved by removing the catheter, filling its tip with 0.1 to 0.2 mL of 2% lidocaine, reinserting the catheter to the point of resistance, flushing the lidocaine into the vessel, and waiting 1 to 2 minutes before reattempting to advance the catheter.

Resistance at 4 to 5 cm generally indicates that a false tract has been created, with subintimal cannulation. If this occurs to both arteries, a vessel may still be cannulated by performing a subumbilical cutdown. This latter procedure does, however, carry the risk of hemorrhage and accidental entry into the peritoneum and should therefore only be performed by personnel experienced with the procedure.

Two insertion depths for the distal end of an umbilical artery catheter are generally accepted, and data supporting the advantage of one location over the other are equivocal. For positioning above the diaphragm, the tip is placed at the level of the thoracic aorta between the ductus arteriosus and the origin of the celiac axis (spinal level T6 through T9). For placement below the diaphragm, the tip is positioned between the inferior mesenteric artery and the bifurcation of the aorta (spinal level L3 through L5) (Fig. 38.4). A Cochrane database systematic review in 2000 concluded that more superiorly placed umbilical artery catheters (tip resides above the diaphragm)

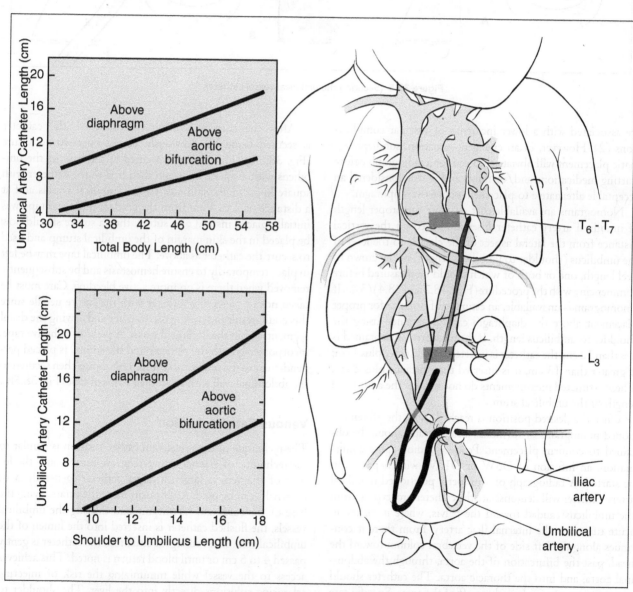

Figure 38.4 Nomograms for estimating umbilical artery catheter length based on total body or shoulder to umbilicus measurement. (Adapted from Dunn PM. Localization of the umbilical catheter by postmortem measurement. *Arch Dis Child.* 1966;41:69.)

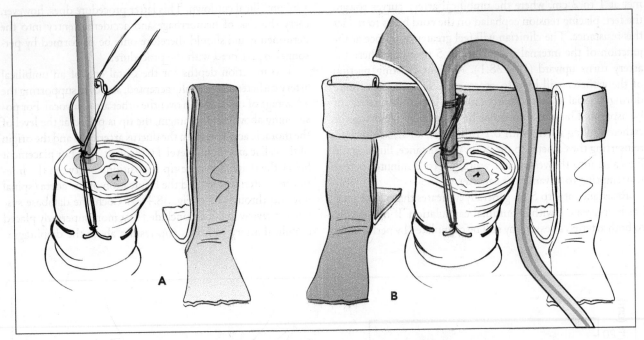

Figure 38.5 Securing the umbilical vessel catheter.

are associated with a lower incidence of vascular complications (2). However, in an emergent situation, subdiaphragmatic placement will obviate the need for a radiograph before starting medications and/or fluids and is still considered an acceptable alternative to placement above the diaphragm.

Nomograms are available that estimate the proper length of umbilical artery catheter insertion based on the vertical distance from the lateral aspect of the clavicle to the level of the umbilicus (shoulder to umbilicus length) or the crown to heel length, one or both of which should be measured before commencing with the procedure (Figs. 38.2 and 38.4)(3,4). If a nomogram is unavailable, an estimate of distance for proper placement above the diaphragm can be obtained using the shoulder to umbilicus length. If the measurement obtained is less than 13 cm, the catheter is inserted that distance plus 1 cm; if greater than 13 cm, it is inserted that distance plus 2 cm. These estimated measurements do not include the additional length of the umbilical stump.

Once the desired position is reached using the aforementioned nomograms or formulas, a radiograph should be obtained to confirm placement. Pending radiographic confirmation, an infusion of D5W or D10W with heparin can be started. A radiograph of a properly positioned umbilical artery catheter will demonstrate the catheter proceeding from the umbilicus caudad toward the pelvis, where it makes an acute turn into the internal iliac artery. From there it continues along the left side of the vertebral column toward the head, past the bifurcation of the aorta, through the abdominal aorta, and into the thoracic aorta. The catheter should not enter any arteries branching off of the aorta. Specific care should be taken to avoid cannulation of the renal or spinal arteries.

After the correct position is confirmed, the catheter is secured using the previously placed purse-string suture (Fig. 38.5A). This suture is secured at the base of the umbilicus with a square knot and then tied to the catheter with square knots at the entrance to the umbilical vessels and at a distance of 2 to 4 cm from the cord. If umbilical tape was initially placed instead of a suture, then a suture should now be placed in the skin margin of the umbilical stump and used to secure the catheter as above. The umbilical tape may be left in place temporarily to ensure hemostasis and be subsequently removed when there is no more active bleeding. Care must be taken not to pierce the catheter with the suture needle since this could result in severing the catheter and leaving the distal segment within the umbilical vessel. A piece of adhesive tape, incorporating both the catheter and the suture, is placed perpendicular to the umbilical stump. This tape is then secured to the abdominal wall with additional strips of tape (Fig. 38.5B).

Venous Catheterization

The technique of umbilical vein catheterization is similar to the technique of arterial catheterization, but because the lumen of the vein is larger, a larger catheter (generally 5 or 8 French) can be used. After positioning the infant, tying the base of the cord, and identifying and dilating the umbilical vessels, the flushed catheter is inserted into the lumen of the umbilical vein. In an emergent situation, the catheter is gently passed 4 to 5 cm or until blood return is noted. This achieves access to the vessel while minimizing the risk of injecting sclerosing solutions directly into the liver. The shoulder to umbilicus length multiplied by 0.6 approximates the length of the catheter that needs to be inserted in order to place

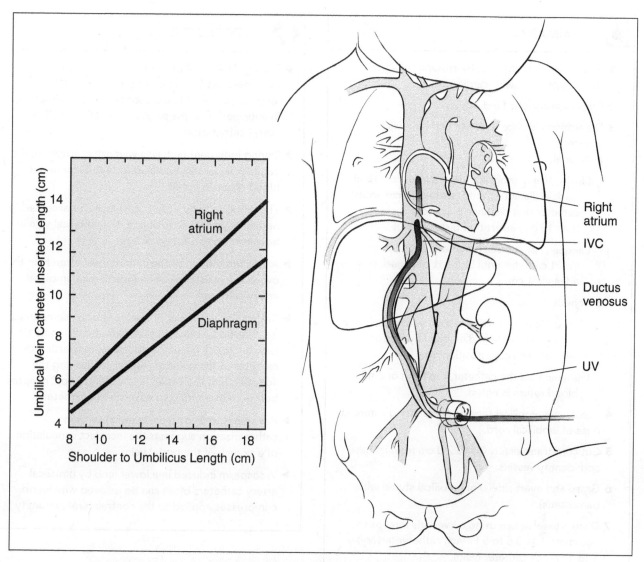

Figure 38.6 Nomogram for estimating umbilical vein catheter length based on shoulder to umbilicus measurement. (Adapted from Dunn PM. Localization of the umbilical catheter by postmortem measurement. *Arch Dis Child.* 1966;41:69.)

its tip above the diaphragm at the junction of the inferior vena cava and the right atrium (5). Alternatively, a nomogram is available to estimate the proper length of umbilical vein catheter insertion based on the shoulder to umbilicus length (Fig. 38.6) (3). This distance (10 to 12 cm) will allow for central venous pressure monitoring or infusion of medications or hyperalimentation solutions. However, if obstruction is encountered at 5 to 10 cm, the catheter has likely passed into a branch of the portal vein within the liver, into which the injection of high osmolar solutions can result in hepatic necrosis.

Common malpositions to be identified on radiograph (6) include catheterization of the right portal vein (catheter tip in the right upper quadrant directed to the right) and middle hepatic vein (tip turns in caudal direction before reaching the diaphragm). Also, the catheter tip should not be advanced past the foramen ovale into either the left atrium or pulmonary vein.

The venous catheter is secured in the same manner as the arterial catheter.

Removal of Catheters

As soon as an umbilical catheter is no longer indicated, it should be removed. In preparation for removal, the stopcock is turned off. Loosely tied umbilical tape is placed around the umbilical stump, and over 3 to 5 minutes the catheter is gradually withdrawn. If bleeding occurs, the umbilical tape can be tightened. If bleeding persists, the vessel can be grasped with a curved hemostat.

▶ COMPLICATIONS

The most life-threatening complication of umbilical vessel catheterization is pericardial tamponade from penetration of

SUMMARY

1 Place infant under radiant warmer in supine frog-leg position with cardiac monitor.

2 Prepare antiseptic field.

3 Determine distance to which catheter will be inserted:

 a Arterial:

  Elective: Use nomogram for umbilicus to lateral clavicle distance, or if less than 13 cm, insert catheter that distance plus 1 cm; if greater than 13 cm, insert that distance plus 2 cm.

  Emergent: For subdiaphragmatic positioning, insert catheter until blood is obtained, then advance 1 cm.

 b Venous:

  Elective: Measure vertical distance from umbilicus to lateral clavicle and multiply by 0.6 for inferior vena cava positioning.

  Emergent: Pass the catheter 4 to 5 cm or until blood return is noted.

4 Loosely tie umbilical tape or purse-string suture at base of umbilical cord.

5 Cut cord transversely 0.5 to 2.0 cm from its base and identify vessels.

6 Grasp and evert side(s) of umbilical stump with hemostat(s).

7 Dilate vessel lumen using curved iris forceps to accommodate 3.5 to 5 French catheter (artery) or 5 to 8 French catheter (vein).

8 Insert catheter tip into vessel lumen and pass catheter using gentle, constant pressure.

9 Techniques to overcome resistance during arterial catheterization:

 a Place tension cephalad on the cord.

 b Apply twisting motion to catheter.

 c Flush with 0.1 to 0.2 mL of 2% lidocaine.

10 Obtain radiograph of thorax and abdomen to confirm placement.

11 Secure catheter in place using purse-string suture and adhesive tape.

CLINICAL TIPS

▶ During delivery of preterm or potentially ill neonates, it is important to preserve a relatively large length of umbilical cord (several centimeters) in anticipation of the possible need for umbilical vessel catheterization.

▶ During emergent umbilical vein catheterization, the catheter is passed cephalad for 4 to 5 cm or until blood return is noted.

▶ The umbilical artery can occasionally be accessed in neonates up to 7 days of age, the umbilical vein in neonates up to 14 days of age.

▶ A twisting motion of the catheter will often help to overcome resistance when inserting an umbilical artery catheter.

▶ Resistance as a result of vasospasm can sometimes be relieved by removing the catheter, filling its tip with 0.1 to 0.2 mL of 2% lidocaine, reinserting the catheter to the point of resistance, flushing the lidocaine into the vessel, and waiting 1 to 2 minutes before reattempting to advance the catheter.

▶ Resistance at 5 to 10 cm in umbilical vein catheterization suggests the incorrect cannulation of a branch of the portal vein.

▶ Vasospasm induced in a lower limb by umbilical artery catheters often can be relieved with warm compresses applied to the contralateral extremity.

the atrial wall and infusion into the pericardial space (7). This may occur even in the setting of radiographic confirmation of correct catheter tip location. Another potential complication is lower extremity or buttock ischemia caused by umbilical artery catheter–induced vasospasm (8–10). This can often be treated with warm compresses applied to the contralateral

extremity, triggering a reflex vasodilation in the affected limb. The catheter should be removed if no improvement in limb color or pulse is seen within 15 minutes, which may indicate inadvertent cannulation of the left internal iliac artery. Similarly, ischemia of the bowel or kidneys can occur with improper positioning of the catheter at the origin of a renal or mesenteric artery (10,11). This may respond to repositioning of the catheter. Thrombus formation associated with umbilical artery catheters is common (5,8–12), but risks are minimized by using nonthrombogenic catheters and heparin-containing solutions.

Bacterial colonization of umbilical catheters has been reported with frequencies as high as 57%; however, bacteremia is unusual (5,10–12). Significant blood loss is most commonly the result of an accidentally dislodged arterial catheter or stopcock and is much less likely to occur when locking connectors are used and the catheter is sutured and taped securely in place (5,8,9,11,12). Pericardial perforation can occur when an umbilical venous catheter is placed into the right atrium. Systemic hypertension can result from renovascular stenosis or renal artery thrombosis as a result of umbilical vessel catheter placement. Other complications include vessel perforation (9,10), peritoneal perforation, organ perforation, hepatic necrosis, arrhythmias, aneurysm formation, and portal hypertension.

Air embolism, which is more common with umbilical vein catheters (5,9–12), can be avoided by flushing the catheter and intravenous tubing with intravenous fluid before insertion and by using a three-way stopcock.

▶ SUMMARY

Vascular access is frequently difficult to obtain in the newborn. Although associated with higher complication rates, umbilical vessel catheterization provides a useful alternative to peripheral lines in this age group. Once cannulated, these vessels can be used for transfusion of blood products, blood pressure monitoring, delivery of medications and fluids, and blood sampling.

▶ ACKNOWLEDGMENT

The authors would like to acknowledge the contributions of Joseph Bliss, MD, PhD, who provided valuable suggestions regarding the content of this chapter, and the authors would also like to acknowledge the valuable contributions of Jordan D. Lipton and Robert W. Schafermeyer to the version of this chapter that appeared in the previous edition.

▶ REFERENCES

1. Moore KL. *The Developing Human: Clinically Oriented Embryology.* 7th ed. Philadelphia: WB Saunders; 2003.

2. Barrington KJ. Umbilical artery catheters in the newborn: effects of position of the catheter tip. *Cochrane Database Syst Rev.* 2000;No. 2:CD000505.

3. Dunn PM. Localization of the umbilical catheter by postmortem measurement. *Arch Dis Child.* 1966;41:69–75.

4. Rosenfeld W, Biagtan J, Schaeffer H, et al. A new graph for insertion of umbilical artery catheters. *J Pediatr.* 1980;96:735–737.

5. Prinz SC, Cunningham MD. Umbilical vessel catheterization. *J Fam Pract.* 1980;10:885–890.

6. Burton EM, Brody AS. *Essentials of Pediatric Radiology.* New York: Thieme Medical Publishers; 1999.

7. Onal EE, Saygili A, Koc E, et al. Cardiac tamponade in a newborn because of umbilical venous catheterization: is correct position safe? *Paediatr Anaesth.* 2004;14:953–956.

8. Dorand RD, Cook LN, Andrews BF. Umbilical vessel catheterization: the low incidence of complications in a series of 200 newborn infants. *Clin Pediatr.* 1977;16:569–572.

9. Kitterman JA, Phibbs RH, Tooley WH. Catheterization of umbilical vessels in newborn infants. *Pediatr Clin North Am.* 1970;17:895–912.

10. Tooley WH, Myerberg DZ. Should we put catheters in the umbilical artery? *Pediatrics.* 1978;62:853–854.

11. Cowett RM, Peter G, Hakanson DO, et al. Prophylactic antibiotics in neonates with umbilical artery catheter placement: a prospective study of 137 patients. *Yale J Biol Med.* 1977;50:457–463.

12. Thomas DB. Umbilical vessel catheterization. *Med J Aust.* 1974;1: 404–407.

▶ SUGGESTED READINGS

Kattwinkel J, ed. *Neonatal Resuscitation Textbook.* 4th ed. Elk Grove Village, IL: American Heart Association, American Academy of Pediatrics; 2000.

Chameides L, ed. *Textbook of Pediatric Advanced Life Support.* Dallas, TX: American Heart Association; 1990.

Klaus MH, Fanaroff AA. *Care of the High-Risk Neonate.* Philadelphia: WB Saunders; 1986.

Paster S, Middleton P. Roentgenographic evaluation of umbilical artery and vein catheters. *JAMA.* 1975;231:742–746.

39

GAIL S. RUDNITSKY AND SONIA O. IMAIZUMI

Emergency Management of Selected Congenital Anomalies

▶ INTRODUCTION

Congenital anomalies requiring surgical intervention in the immediate postnatal period are not uncommon. Approximately 2% of all newborns will have a serious surgical or cosmetic anomaly (1). With improvements in monitoring capabilities and increased use of high-resolution ultrasonography, most babies with congenital anomalies are diagnosed in utero and delivered in a tertiary care center with the appropriate specialists standing by to care for these high-risk infants. However, unforeseen circumstances, such as lack of prenatal care or unexpected premature deliveries, may result in an infant being born in an emergency center or delivery room of a hospital not equipped to care for an infant with such an anomaly. Therefore, it is necessary for the treating physician to be able to stabilize an infant before transport to a hospital that is capable of caring for an infant born with a congenital malformation. Stabilization should include standard neonatal resuscitative measures (Chapter 36), including stabilizing the airway and cardiovascular system when necessary, keeping the infant warm, and preventing any exposed organs from injury or drying out. The accepting hospital should be a tertiary care center with the appropriate surgeons and subspecialists available to provide definitive care for these children. Discussion in this chapter will be limited to several of the more common and severe malformations that require immediate attention.

▶ ABDOMINAL WALL DEFECTS

Anatomy and Physiology

The more common abdominal wall defects include gastroschisis, omphalocele, bladder exstrophy, and cloacal exstrophy. All these defects require immediate intervention to prevent loss of heat and fluids and to minimize the chance of fatal infections.

Gastroschisis

Gastroschisis is a full-thickness defect of the abdominal wall, varying from a few centimeters in length to a large defect that extends from the xiphoid process to the pubic symphysis and with herniation of uncovered intestinal contents through the defect (2) (Fig. 39.). The origin of this disorder is still unknown, but gastroschisis may arise from incomplete closure of the lateral folds during the fourth week of gestation or from rupture of the lateral umbilical ring (3). This anomaly can be differentiated from an omphalocele by the generally smaller size of the defect, which is located lateral to the umbilicus. In gastroschisis, the umbilical cord is normally attached to the abdominal wall to the left of the defect (1). Because no amniotic or peritoneal sac covers the bowel, it is exposed to the chemical irritation of amniotic fluid in utero and is often edematous, matted together, and covered with a gelatinous exudate (4). All infants have nonrotation and abnormal fixation of the intestines. Of infants with gastroschisis, 16% will have gastrointestinal malformations consisting of atresias and stenoses. Other associated congenital anomalies are rare (5). The incidence of gastroschisis is approximately 1 per 10,000 live births (6).

Omphalocele

Omphalocele, by contrast, is a 2- to 15-cm defect of the umbilical ring resulting from failure of fusion of the four somatic folds that define the abdominal wall early in gestation (1), with herniation of varying amounts of abdominal viscera into a sac composed of amnion and peritoneum (Fig. 39.1B). This sac may be ruptured before or at the time of delivery,

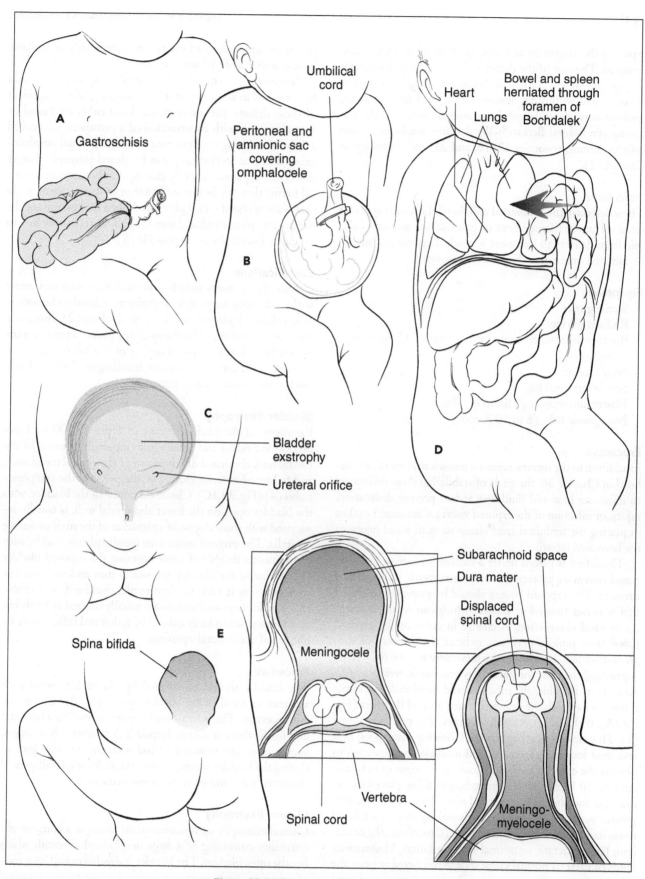

Figure 39.1 Selected congenital anomalies.
A. Gastroschisis.
B. Omphalocele.
C. Exstrophy of the bladder.
D. Diaphragmatic hernia.
E. Spina bifida.

exposing the viscera to amniotic fluid or the ambient environment. The size of the defect and covering sac determines the amount of viscera that is herniated. Omphalocele may be associated with other abnormalities (cardiac, neurologic, genitourinary, skeletal, and chromosomal) as well as the following syndromes: Beckwith-Wiedemann syndrome; prune belly syndrome; trisomies 13, 18, and 21; and pentalogy of Cantrell (2).

Indications

These defects in the abdominal wall should be readily apparent on observation. Management of gastroschisis and omphalocele from delivery to transport is nearly identical and should be initiated once either diagnosis is suspected.

Equipment

    Sterile gloves
    Radiant warmer
    Routine neonatal resuscitation equipment (Chapter 36)
    Sterile gauze
    Sterile saline
    Sterile intestinal bag
    Plastic film wrap (e.g., Saran or Glad)
    Nasogastric tube (8 to 10 French)

Procedure

In addition to the routine neonatal resuscitative measures outlined in Chapter 36, the goals of stabilizing these infants are to minimize heat and fluid loss and to prevent desiccation, injury, or infection of the exposed viscera. Care must be taken in placing the umbilical cord clamp so as to avoid injury to the herniated intestine.

The infant is placed under a radiant warmer, and the exposed viscera are protected with a warm, sterile, saline-soaked dressing. The exposed viscera should be inspected to ensure that it is not twisted or kinked, which can result in vascular or caval obstruction. A change in color of the exposed bowel from pink to gray may indicate the presence of such an obstruction. Tension on the mesentery may be reduced by supporting the bowel on packs of warm, sterile, wet gauze (2). As soon as possible, the infant should be placed in a sterile intestinal bag with the drawstring tied around the chest (Fig. 39.2A). If the infant is small, the arms also can be enclosed (1). This clear plastic bag has the following advantages: heat and fluid loss are minimized, and it allows the physician to observe the color of the bowel, looking for signs of ischemia. An 8 to 10 French nasogastric tube should be placed to free drainage and should be aspirated every 10 to 15 minutes to prevent vomiting and to keep the bowel decompressed. Fluid resuscitation should be initiated with 10 to 20 mL/kg of colloid, Ringer lactate, or normal saline solution. Maintenance fluids of D10 $^1/_4$ normal saline should be started at twice the calculated normal maintenance volume and continued until the urine output is 2 to 3 mL/kg/hour (4). Broad-spectrum antibiotics (ampicillin and gentamicin) should be started after a baseline blood culture is obtained. Transport should be promptly arranged to a tertiary care center with an available neonatologist and pediatric surgeon.

Gastroschisis is considered a surgical emergency and should be corrected as soon as possible. In the surgical management of these defects, the infant is stabilized either by fascial or skin closure or with construction of a prosthetic sac (called a "silo") enclosing the herniated viscera (5). Small omphaloceles (5 cm or less) usually can be closed primarily. Larger defects are repaired either by closing skin but leaving a vertical hernia that can be repaired later or by constructing a silo that is compressed on a daily basis. When the contents of the site are completely reduced into the abdomen (usually in 7 to 10 days), fascial closure is possible (5).

Complications

Despite the measures already described, the infant may arrive at the accepting hospital with problems related to hypothermia, volume depletion, acidosis, or all three (2). Insensible fluid loss is minimized by the overlying plastic wrap but must be watched closely to avoid drying of the viscera or hypovolemia in the patient. Excessive handling of the bowel may predispose to infection or injury.

Bladder Exstrophy

Exstrophy of the bladder occurs in 1 per 10,000 to 1 per 50,000 live births and results from incomplete fusion of the caudal fold, abnormal development of the cloacal membrane, and failure of anterior closure of the pelvis at the symphysis pubis (4) (Fig. 39.1C). Classic exstrophy of the bladder, with the bladder open on the lower abdominal wall, is usually associated with some degree of epispadias of the male or female genitalia. The ureteral orifices are usually plainly visible, with a continuous dribble of urine covering the exposed bladder (7). At birth, the bladder mucosa is thin and smooth, but with exposure it becomes hyperemic, thickened, and friable (2). The kidneys and ureters are usually normal at birth but may become secondarily dilated by reflux and infection or by fibrosis of the ureteral openings.

Procedure

The bladder should be covered by plastic film wrap such as Saran or Glad or by Vaseline gauze (4). Antibiotics are not necessary. The infant should be transferred to a neonatal unit for further evaluation. Repair is done electively in stages, beginning in the neonatal period with the ultimate goal of closing the bladder, reconstructing the abdominal wall, genital reconstruction, and eventual urinary continence.

Cloacal Exstrophy

Cloacal exstrophy or vesicointestinal fissure is a complex abnormality consisting of a large omphalocele beneath which lies the open bladder. The bladder is divided in half by a zone of intestine, with an upper orifice leading to the terminal ileum and a lower orifice leading to a short colon (5 cm) that ends blindly (2,7). Almost all infants with this defect have either a meningomyelocele or a tethered cord (2,7). Other

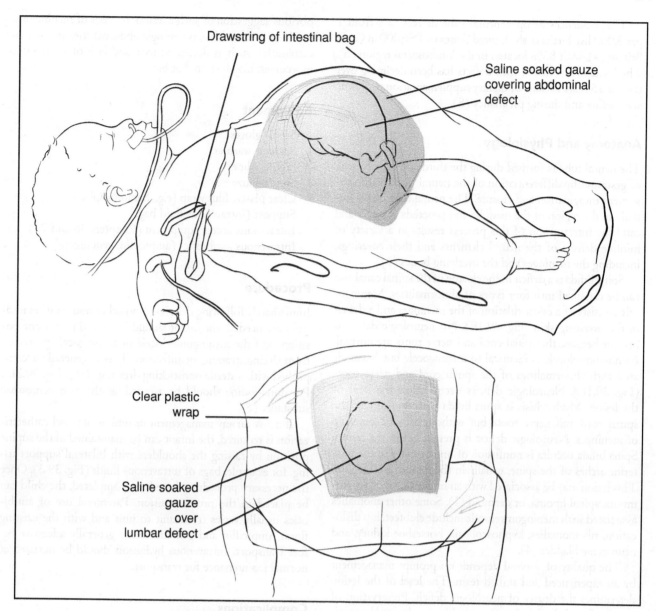

Figure 39.2 Initial management of selected congenital anomalies.
A. Gastroschisis and omphalocele.
B. Neural tube defects.

associated anomalies include undescended or absent testes, bicornate uterus, and absent or duplicated vagina and epispadias. In addition, 50% of infants have abnormalities of the kidneys or ureters (2). Cardiovascular, musculoskeletal, diaphragmatic, and other small intestinal abnormalities may occur (2).

Management

Complete functional repair is difficult or impossible (7). However, without surgical intervention, infants with cloacal exstrophy usually die shortly after birth (2). Because of the ethical and moral issues involved, these children should be treated as previously described in the section on omphalocele and should be transferred to a tertiary care center where

the staff is available to give the parents complete information concerning the infant's condition and long-term prognosis.

▶ NEURAL TUBE DEFECTS

Defects in enclosure of the neural tube are the most common of the major malformations of the central and peripheral nervous systems. They include meningocele, meningomyelocele, myeloschisis, and spina bifida occulta. The latter is not functionally or cosmetically obvious and, as a result, is not diagnosed until later in life (30% of cases are diagnosed in adults) (1).

The incidences of open neural tube defects vary from I per 3,000 live births in the United States to 1/1,000 in Great Britain (4), with 85% located in the lumbosacral region (6). The incidence of neural tube defects has been declining over the last 15 years because of dietary supplementation with folic acid before and during pregnancy (8).

Anatomy and Physiology

The neural tube is formed during the third and fourth week of gestation by differentiation of the neural plate, with subsequent invagination and closure. The neural tube closes initially in the region of the medulla and proceeds rostrally and caudally. Interruption of this process results in a variety of midline defects of the neural elements and their coverings, including the meninges and the overlying bones (I).

Spina bifida is a deficit in the closure of the spinal canal and can be classified into four types of abnormalities. Meningocele consists of a cystic dilation of the meninges and a deficit in the overlying skin (Fig. 39.IE). No neurologic deficit is present because the spinal cord and nerve roots are normal. Meningomyelocele is identical to meningocele but is associated with abnormalities of the spinal cord and nerve roots (Fig. 39.IE). Neurologic deficits occur below the level of the lesion. Myeloschisis is spina bifida with exposure of the spinal cord and nerve roots but without a cystic covering of meninges. Neurologic deficit is present below the lesion. Spina bifida occulta is nonfusion of one or more of the posterior arches of the spine, usually in the lumbosacral region. This lesion may be associated with an underlying diastematomyelia, spinal lipoma, or dermoid (I). Some other anomalies associated with meningomyelocele include clubfeet, hip dislocation, rib anomalies, kyphoscoliosis, horseshoe kidney, and neurogenic bladder (4).

The quality of survival depends on prompt management by an experienced and skilled team. The level of the lesion determines the degree of neurologic deficit. Preservation of existing function of the lower extremities is enhanced by surgical correction within the first 48 hours, although with higher lesions earlier surgery does little to improve the quality of survival (I). The decision to repair a high meningomyelocele or myeloschisis involves moral and ethical considerations beyond the scope of this chapter. With immediate closure, infants born with spina bifida have a 90% chance of survival (I). Without repair, many die from untreated hydrocephalus, infection, or renal failure secondary to their neurogenic bladder.

Indications

Initial management of neural tube lesions is conservative, noninvasive, and not associated with adverse effects and is therefore indicated in those instances in which the diagnosis is known or suspected. Early temporizing measures are important in avoiding infection, desiccation, and injury to the involved structures and in improving the eventual outcome. The physical finding of a midline defect along the back is the most obvious suggestion of such a lesion. In cases of meningomyelocele or myeloschisis, neurologic abnormalities in the lower extremities, such as decreased tone and lack of spontaneous movement, may be noted at birth.

Equipment

Sterile gloves
Radiant warmer
Sterile saline
Sterile gauze
Clear plastic film wrap (e.g., Saran or Glad)
Support (intravenous fluid bags)
Intravenous access equipment (Chapters 38 and 73)
Intravenous antibiotics (ampicillin, gentamicin)

Procedure

Immediately following delivery, if no other resuscitation measures are needed, the infant should be placed in a prone position, and the meningomyelocele or meningocele protected from drying, trauma, or infection. This is generally accomplished with a sterile nonsticking dressing (6,8) (Fig. 39.2B). Povidone-iodine should be avoided, as this is a neurotoxic substance (8).

If active airway management or umbilical vessel catheterization is required, the infant can be maintained in the supine position by raising the shoulders with bilateral support using, for example, bags of intravenous fluids (Fig. 39.3). Once the necessary procedures have been completed, the child can be placed in the prone position. Parenteral use of antibiotics usually varies from unit to unit and with the existing flora. Ampicillin and gentamicin are generally adequate before transport. Intravenous hydration should be initiated at normal maintenance for transport.

Complications

Excessive handling or force may result in perforation of the cystic lesion, introduction of infection, or further injury to involved neurologic structures.

▶ DIAPHRAGMATIC HERNIA

Anatomy and Physiology

When the fusion of the diaphragmatic leaflets fails to happen by 8 weeks' gestation, a defect occurs in the diaphragm that can vary from several centimeters to complete absence of the involved hemidiaphragm (I). Of these defects, 85% are left sided at the foramen of Bochdalek, and 1% are bilateral and uniformly fatal. They occur as an isolated defect in I to 2 per 1,000 live births (1,6). Improvements in prenatal ultrasonography have resulted in approximately 50% of these infants being diagnosed between weeks 16 and 24 of gestation (9).

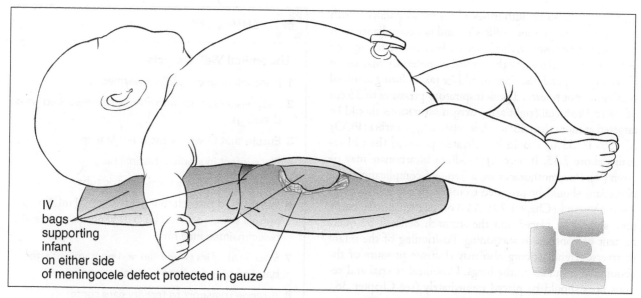

IV
bags
supporting
infant
on either side
of meningocele defect protected in gauze

Figure 39.3 Support for infant with a neural tube defect requiring supine positioning.

Major morbidity and high fatality rates for infants with diaphragmatic hernia occur because of the effects of the herniated abdominal viscera on the thoracic cavity and interference with the normal development of the lungs (Fig. 39.1D). The severity of the defect is related to the timing and degree of the prenatal visceral herniation (1). The subsequent lung hypoplasia is more severe on the side of the hernia, but the contralateral side also is affected. An infant with congenital diaphragmatic hernia suffers both hypoperfusion and hypoventilation of the lungs by the herniated bowel (4). The latter occurs as a result of the arrested development (hypoplasia) and compression of the lung (4). Hypoventilation leads primarily to hypoxia, hypercarbia, and acidosis, decreasing further the already compromised pulmonary blood flow by increasing the pulmonary vascular resistance.

Pulmonary hypoperfusion is a result of a decrease in the cross-sectional arterial surface area and of vascular smooth muscle cell hyperplasia. Both contribute to the exaggerated vasoconstriction caused by the hypoxia and acidosis. Cardiac dysfunction with a subsequent increase in pulmonary venous pressure and decrease in systemic pressure may occur as a consequence of the hypoxia or the associated left-sided cardiac hypoplasia (4).

Indications

A diaphragmatic hernia should be considered in infants who develop respiratory distress within the first day of life. These infants clinically may have a scaphoid abdomen and an asymmetric or distended chest (5). As the infant feeds or swallows air, the herniated bowel becomes distended and the infant's clinical condition deteriorates. Tachypnea and cyanosis may occur (cyanosis without dyspnea is more commonly associated with a congenital heart lesion) (2). On physical examination, the apex of the heart is frequently displaced to the patient's

right. Breath sounds may not be heard on the affected side, although this may be difficult to appreciate, as transmitted breath sounds from the opposite side are frequently heard. Retractions and grunting may be present. Bowel sounds in the chest are not a reliable finding (2).

Diagnosis of a diaphragmatic hernia is usually made by a plain radiograph of the chest and abdomen showing intestinal loops in the chest cavity on the affected side and the lung compressed into a small area at the apex. Placement of a nasogastric tube before the radiograph may aid in the diagnosis if the stomach is in the chest. If the examiner is in doubt, a small amount of contrast material can be given through the nasogastric tube.

The diagnosis can be confused with eventration of the diaphragm, pentalogy of Cantrell, an esophageal hiatus, Morgagni hernia, and congenital cystic disease of the lung (5). The stomach bubble in the chest may be misdiagnosed as a pneumothorax, which might prompt inappropriate chest tube insertion.

Equipment

Standard neonatal resuscitation equipment (Chapter 36)
Endotracheal intubation equipment (Chapter 16)
8 and 10 French nasogastric tubes
Umbilical vessel catheterization equipment (Chapter 38)
Sedative agent
Paralytic agent
Dopamine and dobutamine

Procedure

All infants should be intubated and ventilated with 100% O$_2$. If the diagnosis is suspected, bag-valve-mask (BVM) ventilation should be avoided to prevent filling the gastrointestinal tract with air. Some authorities recommend paralysis with pancuronium to prevent swallowing and noncompliance with ventilation (2); however, this has never been shown to improve outcome (9). Sedation with fentanyl as necessary may be an alternative to paralysis. Care should be taken during artificial ventilation not to exceed peak inspiratory pressures of 25 cm of water. Preductal (right arm) oxygen saturations should be targeted at more than 85%, while relative hypercarbia (PCO_2 of 45% to 55%) should be tolerated provided the pH remains above 7.35. If necessary, sodium bicarbonate may be given (9). Pneumothoraces are a frequent complication, and physicians should be prepared to insert thoracostomy tubes when necessary (Chapter 29). An 8 or 10 French nasogastric tube should be placed and the stomach deflated by intermittent or continuous suctioning. Positioning of the infant in reverse Trendelenburg also may decrease pressure of the abdominal contents on the lungs. Umbilical arterial and venous lines should be placed immediately (see Chapter 38). The venous line provides access for resuscitation. The arterial line minimizes repeated punctures for blood sampling, as these can cause the infant to desaturate. Oxygenation can be determined with arterial blood gases drawn either from the right radial artery (preductal) or a pulse oximeter probe placed on the right hand. This should be compared with postductal measurements from the umbilical arterial line. Dopamine and dobutamine are generally used for blood pressure support.

Arrangements should be made for transfer of the infant to a neonatal center with extracorporeal membrane oxygenation (ECMO) capabilities, because adequate oxygenation and ventilation of these infants is difficult, if not impossible. ECMO has improved the survival rates for infants diagnosed with a diaphragmatic hernia to 60% according to the Extracorporeal Life Support Organization Registry (9).

Complications

Infants with congenital diaphragmatic hernias require accurate diagnosis and aggressive management to survive. High inspiratory pressures necessary to adequately oxygenate and ventilate infants with diaphragmatic hernias place them at high risk for pneumothoraces.

▶ CHOANAL ATRESIA

Anatomy and Physiology

Choanal atresia is theorized to be the result of a failure of the invaginating nasal pits to rupture through the oronasal membrane separating the nasal pits from the oral cavity. This process normally occurs during the seventh week of gestation. Choanal atresia occurs in approximately 1 per 5,000 live births and can be unilateral or bilateral, although the unilateral form is more common. Obstruction generally occurs at a distance of approximately 3 cm from the opening of the nares (1). Ninety percent of the time the obstruction is bony, and it is

SUMMARY

Abdominal Wall Defects

1 Place infant under radiant warmer.

2 Keep viscera moist with sterile, saline-soaked gauze dressings.

3 Ensure that bowel or sac is not kinked.

4 Place infant in sterile intestinal bag.

5 Insert 8- or 10-French nasogastric tube.

6 Initiate fluid resuscitation with 10 to 20 mL/kg normal saline followed by D10 ¼ normal saline at twice maintenance rate.

7 Start antibiotics (ampicillin and gentamicin) after baseline blood culture is obtained.

8 Arrange transport to tertiary care center.

Neural Tube Defects

1 Place infant in prone position for initial resuscitation.

2 If intubation or umbilical vessel catheterization is required, place infant in supine position with bilateral support to prevent pressure against lesion.

3 Apply a sterile, non-sticking dressing to lesion.

4 Begin broad-spectrum antibiotics (ampicillin and gentamicin).

5 Initiate D10 ¼ normal saline maintenance intravenous hydration.

Diaphragmatic Hernia

1 Intubate and ventilate with 100% oxygen; avoid BVM ventilation.

2 Paralyze or sedate infant.

3 Place 8- or 10-French nasogastric tube and connect to continuous or intermittent suction.

4 Place infant in reverse Trendelenburg position.

5 Place umbilical artery and umbilical vein lines.

6 Obtain preductal arterial blood gas or pulse oximeter reading from right arm.

7 Maintain pH at or above 7.35 and preductal (right arm) oxygen saturations above 85%.

8 Maintain blood pressure with dopamine or dobutamine.

Choanal Atresia

1 Assess nasal airway with 6-French catheter or respiratory motion of cotton wisp.

2 Relieve respiratory distress with oral airway or endotracheal intubation as necessary.

CLINICAL TIPS

- ▶ In the presence of one congenital anomaly, be aware of additional associated abnormalities.

- ▶ Goals in the management of exposed organs include the prevention of heat loss, desiccation, injury, and infection.

- ▶ A dusky appearance of exposed intestines may be a sign of vascular insufficiency or mechanical obstruction.

- ▶ In gastroschisis the hernia occurs on the right of the umbilical cord.

- ▶ In gastroschisis, as opposed to an omphalocele, the umbilical cord remains attached to the abdomen.

- ▶ Diaphragmatic hernias occur almost exclusively on the left.

- ▶ Placement of a nasogastric tube before radiograph may be helpful in the diagnosis of a diaphragmatic hernia.

- ▶ Failure to pass a 6-French catheter through the nasopharynx, or failure of inspiration and expiration to move a wisp of cotton held in front of the nares is suggestive of choanal atresia.

membranous in the remainder (4). Associated anomalies are common. When the diagnosis is missed, infants with choanal atresia are at risk for developing respiratory insufficiency if they do not establish oral breathing (1).

Indications

Because newborn infants are obligate nasal breathers, if the obstruction is bilateral, infants with choanal atresia will present immediately after birth with a cyclic respiratory obstruction pattern that improves when the infant cries or when an oral airway is in place (4). Diagnosis is suspected by failure to pass a 6-French suction catheter down the infant's nostril. A wisp of cotton also can be placed in front of the infant's nostril while occluding the opposite nostril and mouth. If the nos-

tril is patent, the cotton should move toward the nose with inspiration and away with expiration (4). Confirmation is by computerized tomography.

Procedure

If the emergency physician suspects the diagnosis, an oral airway can be placed or endotracheal intubation may be performed as temporizing measures in the distressed infant until surgery. Unilateral choanal atresia may remain undetected for years.

▶ SUMMARY

Initial management of infants with congenital anomalies follows standard resuscitation procedures. In addition, certain exposed structures will require protection from desiccation, infection, and injury. Early temporizing measures are crucial in determining the eventual outcome for patients with congenital anomalies, independent of the definitive surgical procedures. Initial management can be performed with equipment available in the standard emergency department or delivery room. Infants diagnosed with congenital anomalies require timely transport to tertiary care centers equipped with experienced surgeons and subspecialists capable of providing definitive care.

▶ REFERENCES

1. Fanaroff AA, Martin RJ. *Neonatal-Perinatal Medicine: Diseases of the Fetus and Infant.* 7th ed. St. Louis: Mosby; 2002.
2. Lister J, Irving IM. *Neonatal Surgery.* London: Butterworth; 1990.
3. Lockridge T, Caldwell AD, Jason P. Neonatal surgical emergencies: stabilization and management. *J Obstet Neonatal Nurs.* 2002;31:328–339.
4. Donn SM, Faix, RG. *Neonatal Emergencies.* Mount Kisco, NY: Futura Publishing Co.; 1991.
5. Altman PR, Stylianos S. Pediatric surgery. *Pediatr Clin North Am.* 1993: 4016.
6. Seeds JW, Azizkhan RG. *Congenital Malformations, Antenatal Diagnosis, Perinatal Management and Counseling.* Rockville, MD: Aspen Publishers; 1990.
7. Raffensperger JG. Swenson's Pediatric Surgery. 5th ed. Norwalk, CT: Appleton & Lange; 1990.
8. Kaufman BA. Neural tube defects. *Pediatr Clin North Am.* 2004;51: 389–419.
9. Bohn D. Congenital diaphragmatic hernia. *Am J Respir Crit Care Med.* 2002;166:911–915.

40

SUSAN DUFFY AND DALE STEELE

Heel Sticks

▶ INTRODUCTION

Capillary blood sampling by means of a heel stick is used to obtain blood for hematologic, biochemical, and blood gas analysis in elective and emergent situations. It is most useful in young infants in whom venous access is difficult or limited. It is a relatively simple procedure that can be performed by physicians, nurses, emergency medical technicians, and other trained personnel.

▶ ANATOMY AND PHYSIOLOGY

The primary arterial and venous blood supply for the heel skin is located at the junction of the dermis and subcutaneous tissues. In infants, the distance from the surface of the heel to this junction is quite constant at 0.35 to 1.6 mm (1). The distance to the calcaneus from the heel surface increases with infant weight. The mean depth from the skin to the calcaneus is greater in the medial and lateral portions of the heel than in the posterior aspect. Calcaneal depth also increases with growth; however, after 1 year of age, callus formation in the heel precludes using this site (2,4).

The boundaries of the calcaneus can be located by extending a line posteriorly from between the fourth and fifth toes running parallel to the lateral aspect of the heel and a line extending posteriorly from the middle of the great toe running parallel to the medial portion of the heel. To avoid calcaneal puncture, heel sticks should be performed only in the areas delineated in Figure 40.1.

▶ INDICATIONS

Heel puncture samples are useful for most common laboratory studies that require frequent measurement, including hemoglobin, hematocrit, and electrolyte determination. It is most practical in the newborn and especially the premature infant but can be performed in children up to 1 year of age. If hemolysis, venous stasis, or bacterial contamination will interfere with interpretation, samples are better obtained by vascular puncture.

Heel puncture is not recommended when poor peripheral perfusion (e.g., shock) is present. It is not recommended in the setting of compromised blood flow to an extremity, local infection or edema, or significant polycythemia or if there is a need for an accurate measurement of PaO_2.

▶ EQUIPMENT

Gloves
Warm, wet towel or hot pack
Alcohol swab
Sterile petroleum jelly
Sterile gauze
Detachable capillary blood collector
Collection tubes
    Capillary blood gases: heparinized glass capillary tubes
    Chemistries: Microtainer tube with serum separator available
    Complete blood count: Microtainer tube with heparin or EDTA
    Hemoglobin/hematocrit (spun): heparinized glass capillary tube
Capillary cap adapters
Clay pad
Incision device (choose one)
    No. 11 surgical blade
    Heel lancet device (e.g., Microlance, Minilancet, Microtainer Safety Lance)
    Automated disposable incision device (e.g., Tenderfoot, Surgicutt, Nicky, Unistik, Autolet)

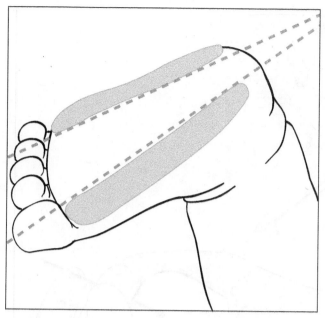

Figure 40.1 Acceptable sites for heel stick puncture illustrated by shaded area.

The blade and the lancet are subject to variability in operator technique and lack features to control puncture depth. The lancet compresses the dermis and does not allow for free flow of blood. Automated heel stick devices provide consistent penetration depths and standard incisions and allow the collection of increased volumes of blood more quickly and with reduced hemolysis (2).

▶ PROCEDURE

A warm, wet towel is applied to the heel for approximately 5 minutes before the procedure to increase blood flow to the skin surface. The heel is cleansed with alcohol and allowed to dry (alcohol on the skin may lead to erroneously high glucose values) (3). The leg is held in a dependent position while the patient is supine. The heel is held at an 80- to 90-degree angle to the leg. The incision device is then used to puncture the heel perpendicular to the skin on the most medial or lateral portion of the heel, as demonstrated in Figure 40.2A. The posterior curve of the heel should not be punctured, and any previous puncture sites that may be infected should be avoided. The puncture should not exceed 2.5 mm in depth. Milking the heel may activate clotting and cause hemolysis (4,5).

The first drop of blood is wiped away with gauze in order to reduce the chance of contaminants or tissue fluids impacting test results (4) (Fig. 40.2B), and subsequent drops are collected using the plastic lip on the capillary blood collector (Fig. 40.2C). Most heparinized collection tubes are marked with two lines. Tubes must be filled to the first line and not filled above the second line for adequate sampling. A thin

layer of sterile petroleum jelly promotes droplet formation on the skin surface and facilitates collection. Once collection is completed, the clinician applies pressure to the puncture site with a sterile gauze for 2 to 3 minutes. The detachable capillary blood collector is removed with a twisting motion, and the specimen is capped; some practitioners follow this with a brief rocking motion in an effort to prevent clotting, although documentation of the efficacy for this technique is sparse (Fig. 40.2C). For collection in a glass capillary tube, one end of the heparinized capillary tube is touched to the drop of blood. The tube is held at about a 20-degree angle from horizontal and fills by capillary action (Fig. 40.2C). Both ends of the tube should remain unoccluded during the collection. For blood gas sampling, the tube should be filled as completely as possible to minimize exposure to the external air. Once the tube is full, the free end is occluded with a gloved fingertip to prevent air entry when removing it from the site. The collection end of the tubes for chemistry or hematocrit samples is inserted into clay to form a plug. Both ends are plugged for blood gases. Plugging should be done gently to avoid inadvertent tube breakage. Alternatively, plastic capillary cap adapters may be used in place of clay but must be applied to both sides of the capillary tube (Fig. 40.2C).

▶ COMPLICATIONS

The most significant potential complication from heel puncture is infection subsequent to puncture of the calcaneus. This can result in necrotizing chondritis or osteomyelitis. Additional complications include (a) calcified nodules of the heel; (b) hemolysis of the blood sample, resulting in falsely elevated

---

 CLINICAL TIPS

▶ Warming the heel prior to the procedure will improve blood flow.

▶ Automated incision devices more consistently gauge depth and result in improved flow with less hemolysis.

▶ Punctures should only be performed within the relatively small "safe" area of the heel.

▶ "Milking" the heel activates clotting and causes hemolysis.

▶ The first drop of blood should be discarded.

▶ A thin layer of petroleum jelly will promote the beading of blood droplets.

▶ Capillary tubes for blood gas samples should be filled completely and capped at both ends.

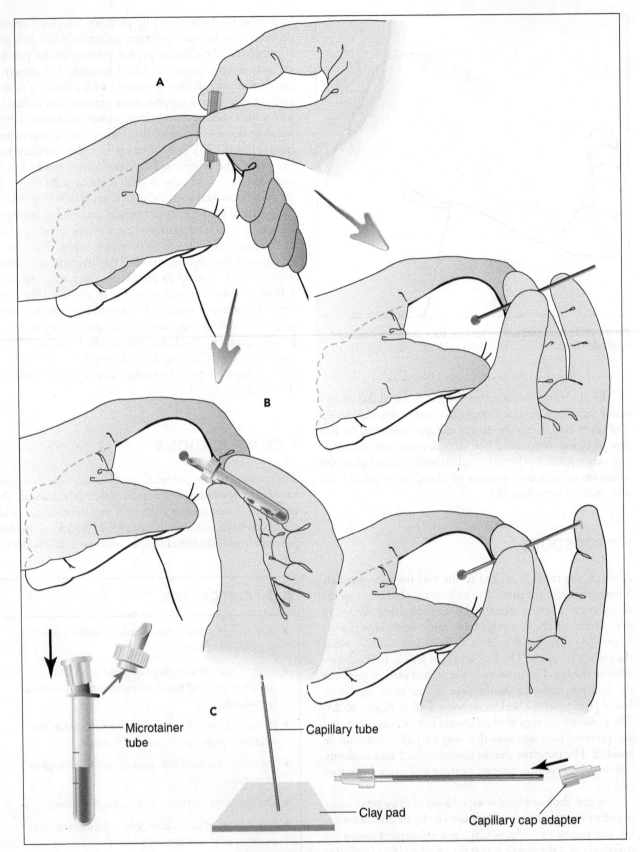

Figure 40.2
A. Heel puncture in safe area.
B. Collection of specimen.
C. Capping of specimen.

Microtainer
tube

Capillary tube

Clay pad

Capillary cap adapter

> ### SUMMARY
>
> **1** Warm heel with wet towel.
>
> **2** Wipe heel with alcohol and allow to dry.
>
> **3** Puncture heel perpendicular to skin on medial or lateral portion.
>
> **4** Wipe away first blood drop with gauze pad.
>
> **5** Collect specimen of blood.
>
> **6** Micro tube collection:
>   **a** Collect subsequent drops of blood against plastic lip of capillary blood collector.
>   **b** Remove capillary blood collector and cap specimen.
>
> **7** Capillary tube collection:
>   **a** Touch one end of glass capillary tube to subsequent drops of blood.
>   **b** Allow tube to fill by capillary action.
>   **c** Occlude free end of tube gently with fingertip once collection is complete.
>   **d** Cap ends of tube gently with clay or plastic capillary adapters.
>   **e** Use caution to avoid inadvertant tube breakage during handling.
>
> **8** Apply pressure to puncture site with sterile gauze.

bilirubin and potassium levels from mechanical trauma; (c) erroneously high glucose values secondary to alcohol from the swab; (d) inaccurate PCO_2 and PO_2 values from poor blood flow; (e) elevated hematocrit from hemoconcentration from inadequate blood flow to the region; and (f) pain from the procedure (6–12).

An inadequate volume of blood collected for a complete blood count in relation to the amount of anticoagulant may result in an inaccurately low hematocrit and hemoglobin. An excessive volume will frequently result in clotting of the specimen. Capillary tube breakage during plugging may result in injury and expose the physician to percutaneous blood.

▶ SUMMARY

Heel puncture is a quick and simple procedure that is particularly useful in young infants. If performed correctly, it is a safe method for obtaining interpretable laboratory samples when venipuncture is difficult (13).

▶ REFERENCES

1. Blumenfeld TA, Turi GK, Blanc WA. Recommended site and depth of newborn heelstick punctures based on anatomical measurements and histopathology. *Lancet.* 1979;1:230–233.
2. Meites S. Skin-puncture and blood-collecting technique for infants: update and problems. *Clin Chem.* 1988;34:1890–1894.
3. Meites S, Linn SS, Thompson C. Studies on the quality of specimens obtained by skin puncture of children: tendency to hemolysis, and hemoglobin and tissue fluids as contaminants. *Clin Chem.* 1981;27:875–878.
4. Paes B, Janes M, Vegh P, et al. A comparative study of heel stick devices for infant blood collection. *Am J Dis Child.* 1993;147:346–348.
5. Reiner CB, Meites S, Hayes JR. Optimal sites and depths for skin puncture of infants and children as assessed from anatomical measurements. *Clin Chem.* 1990;36:547–549.
6. Boris LC, Helleland H. Growth disturbance of the hind part of the foot following osteomyelitis of the calcaneus in the newborn. *J Bone Joint Surg.* 1986;68A:302–305.
7. McLain BI, Evans J, Dear PR. Comparison of capillary and arterial blood gas measurements in neonates. *Am J Dis Child.* 1988;63:743–747.
8. Lauer BA, Altenberger KM. Outbreak of staphylococcal infections following heel puncture for blood sampling. *Am J Dis Child.* 1981;135:277–278.
9. Sell EJ, Hansen RC, Struck-Pierce S. Calcified nodules on the heel: a complication of neonatal intensive care. *J Pediatr.* 1980;96:473–475.
10. Larsson BA, Tannfeldt G, Lagercrantz H, et al. Venipuncture is more effective and less painful than heel lancing for blood tests in neonates. *Pediatrics* 1998;101:882–886.
11. Vertanen H, Fellman V, Brommels M, et al. An automatic incision device for obtaining blood samples from the heels of preterm infants causes less damage than a conventional manual lancet. *Arch Dis Child Fetal Neonatal Ed.* 2001;84:F532.
12. Short BL, Avery GB. Capillary blood sampling. In: Fletcher MA, MacDonald MG, Avery G, eds. *Atlas of Procedures in Neonatology.* Philadelphia: JB Lippincott; 1983:68–74.
13. Shah V, Ohlsson A. Venepuncture versus heel lance in term neonates (Cochrane Review). *Cochrane Library.* 2001:No. 1.

SECTION 6 ▶ NEUROLOGIC AND NEUROSURGICAL PROCEDURES

SECTION EDITOR: JAMES F. WILEY, II

KATHLEEN M. CRONAN AND JAMES F. WILEY, II

41

Lumbar Puncture

▶ INTRODUCTION

Lumbar puncture (LP) is used to obtain cerebrospinal fluid (CSF) for diagnostic and therapeutic purposes. In most cases, it is a relatively simple procedure, although it can sometimes prove challenging even for the experienced practitioner. LP is most commonly performed in neonates and infants who, due to both anatomic characteristics and the types of illness they experience, are prone to respiratory compromise during the procedure (1,2). The potential for complications during and following LP therefore dictates that it be performed in an area equipped for resuscitation. Moreover, although not technically complex, LP is by no means a trivial procedure, and it should only be performed or supervised by a health professional with appropriate training who is knowledgeable about the indications and contraindications for the procedure. For some patients, LP can only be safely performed after brain imaging excludes a space-occupying central nervous system (CNS) lesion and/or elevated intracranial pressure. For patients with shock or respiratory compromise also suspected of having meningitis or encephalitis, stabilization of the patient and presumptive antibiotic therapy must precede LP. These considerations require careful patient evaluation and selection before performing LP.

▶ ANATOMY AND PHYSIOLOGY

CSF is found in the space between the pia mater and the arachnoid mater that surrounds the brain, spinal cord, ventricles, aqueduct, and central canal of the spinal cord. Most CSF is formed in the choroid plexuses of the lateral ventricles. After formation, CSF flows out the foramina of Luschka and Magendie into the subarachnoid space, around the spinal column, and over the cerebrum. The CSF is primarily absorbed by the arachnoid villi located adjacent to the sagittal sinus and then returned to the venous circulation (3).

The average total volume of CSF in children is approximately 90 mL. For full-term infants, the volume is about 40 mL. One quarter of the volume is located in the ventricles, and the remainder in the subarachnoid space. CSF provides physical cushioning between bony structures and the brain and spinal cord (4). It expands and contracts to offset changes in the size of the brain (e.g., cerebral edema) as well as changes in arterial and venous volumes (e.g., cortical atrophy, parenchymal injury) (5). CSF also has an important role in transferring chemical byproducts of metabolism from the brain to the venous circulation.

At birth, the inferior end of the spinal cord is opposite the body of the third lumbar vertebra (L3). As the child's

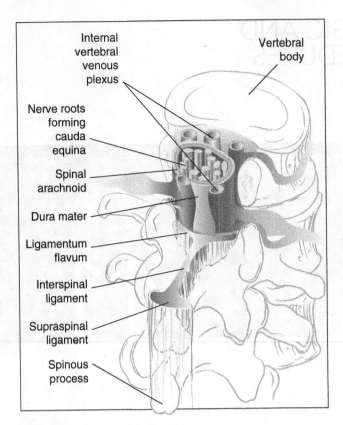

Figure 41.1 Anatomy of the lumbar spine.

spinal cord grows, the vertebral column grows more rapidly. In the adult, the caudal aspect of the cord lies opposite the inferior border of the first lumbar vertebra. Of note, the spinal cord rises slightly when the trunk of the body is bent forward (3,6).

Structures pierced during median LP are (in order) skin, subcutaneous fat, supraspinal ligament, interspinal ligament, ligamentum flavum, dura mater, and arachnoid mater (Fig. 41.1). In older patients, supraspinal and interspinal ligaments are sometimes calcified, which may require a lateral approach (Fig. 41.2). However, this is rare in children, and the median approach is therefore most commonly used (7).

▶ **INDICATIONS**

For the pediatric patient, the primary emergent reason for LP is suspicion of CNS infection (meningitis, encephalitis). Fever, paradoxic irritability (increased crying when held), and bulging anterior fontanel are classic findings associated with bacterial meningitis in the infant. Fever, headache, neck pain/stiffness, confusion, or meningismus manifested by Brudzinski sign (pain on flexion of the neck) or Kernig sign (pain on extension of the knee when the hips are flexed to 90 degrees) may be present in older children with bacterial meningitis. The hallmark of encephalitis is meningeal irritation accompanied by abrupt onset of mental status changes. Signs of meningitis may be subtle in neonates, young infants,

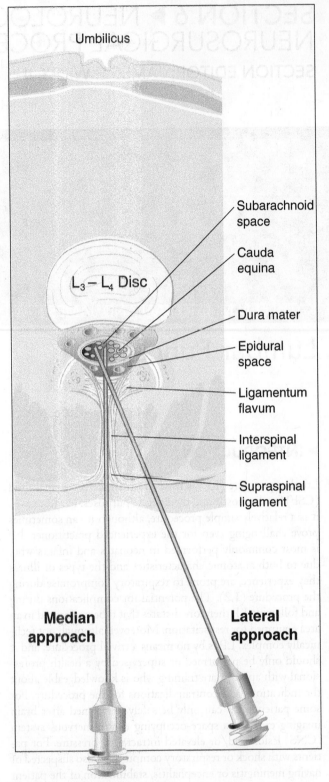

Figure 41.2 Spinal needle access into the subarachnoid space by the median or lateral approach.

and patients taking oral antibiotics (i.e., with so-called "partially treated" meningitis) (8). Furthermore, patients with viral or Lyme meningitis often have fewer clinical signs. Patients with a complex febrile seizure are also at increased risk for concurrent meningitis (9). It is important to remember that meningismus may not be detectable in patients with meningitis who are comatose or have neurologic impairment. Furthermore, meningismus may be present in children who have conditions other than meningitis, such as a posterior fossa brain tumor, retropharyngeal abscess, upper lobe pneumonia, cervical diskitis, and pyelonephritis (8).

Suspected spontaneous subarachnoid hemorrhage constitutes another urgent indication for LP. Patients with suspected intracranial bleeding should have a brain imaging study before LP in most instances. A small percentage of subarachnoid hemorrhages are not detectable on a CT scan of the head, and LP becomes the sole method of diagnosing this problem (9). LP also is performed in a variety of nonacute situations, such as the administration of chemotherapeutic agents, injection of radiopaque dye for spinal cord imaging, diagnosis of CNS metastases, treatment of pseudotumor cerebri, and measurement of opening pressure to rule out specific disease entities.

Contraindications to LP include the presence of infection in the tissues near the proposed puncture site, evidence of spinal cord trauma or spinal cord compression, an uncorrected severe coagulopathy, and signs of progressive cerebral herniation. LP may also be contraindicated based on the condition of the patient. If a patient has an unstable airway, a potentially dangerous breathing problem (e.g., apnea), and/or severe circulatory instability, the stress of being restrained in the correct position for LP may cause an abrupt (and often undetected) decompensation. As mentioned previously, this is especially true of young infants. In these situations, suspected infection should be treated presumptively, without performing the LP, using appropriate antimicrobial therapy (8).

Extreme caution should be exercised, and the procedure generally avoided, when a patient has elevated intracranial pressure resulting from a space-occupying intracranial lesion. Such conditions include brain tumor, cerebral hemorrhage, cavernous sinus thrombosis, brain abscess, and epidural or subdural collection. Focal neurologic findings in conjunction with one of these conditions should be interpreted as signs of impending herniation and serve as an absolute contraindication to LP. Although an unlikely outcome, dexamethasone or mannitol infusion may be helpful if increased intracranial pressure from an unsuspected mass lesion is encountered or signs of cerebral herniation occur during or after LP (10,11).

Patients with a known spinal column deformity should have the procedure performed under fluoroscopy. LP cannot access the subarachnoid space in patients who have undergone posterior spinal fusion in the lumbar region, because needle entry is blocked by bone. These patients require a cisternal tap for CSF collection, a procedure that is performed by a neurosurgeon. In all circumstances where LP might cause harm to the patient, risks and potential benefits must be evaluated thoroughly before performing the procedure.

TABLE 41.1	SPINAL NEEDLE SIZE BY AGE
Premature infant	22 gauge or smaller, 1.5 inch, plastic hub preferred
Neonate–2 y	22 gauge, 1.5 inch, plastic hub preferred
2–12 y*	22 gauge, 2.5 inch
Over 12 y	20 or 22 gauge, 3.5 inch

*May need larger needle depending on patient habitus.

An important point to remember is that for the great majority of patients managed in the ED, LP is merely a test, not a therapy. A patient will rarely have an adverse outcome simply because they did not undergo LP. A common mistake that must be avoided is delaying treatment that *will* affect outcome (e.g., administration of antibiotics) for the sake of obtaining a "clean" LP. If a patient is suspected of having a potentially life-threatening CNS infection, and LP cannot be performed on a timely basis (e.g., the patient is currently unstable, the clinician is uncomfortable with the procedure), then appropriate antimicrobial therapy must be administered as quickly as possible to protect the patient. The consequences of an imperfect test can be dealt with later.

▶ EQUIPMENT

Sterile gloves
Betadine solution
LP tray:
    Sterile drapes
    Betadine swabs or tray to pour Betadine
    Sterile sponges for preparing the puncture site
    Sterile 3-mL syringe with needle for lidocaine injection
    Sterile collecting tubes
    Sterile spinal needle (Table 41.1)
    Manometer (may be a separate sterile item to be added to tray)
Injectable lidocaine 1% without epinephrine
Eutectic mixture of lidocaine and prilocaine (EMLA) or lidocaine 4% cream (LMX-4)
Midazolam or other anxiolytic agent

▶ PROCEDURE

The indication for LP and potential complications should be explained fully to the patient (if appropriate) and the parents. Many institutions require written informed consent before the procedure. The consent form may be standardized within the hospital or tailored to the individual setting. The consent form should include a description of the procedure as well as the benefits and risks of the procedure. Monitoring of heart rate, respirations, and oxygen saturation should be strongly considered during the procedure, particularly in neonates, young infants, and children with any degree of cardiorespiratory compromise. Airway and resuscitation equipment should be immediately available. If the LP is being performed for elective reasons, 4% lidocaine cream (LMX-4) or eutectic mixture of lidocaine and prilocaine (EMLA) may be applied over the puncture site to anesthetize the area (see also Chapter 35). LMX-4 is effective after about 30 minutes, and EMLA is effective after about 45 to 60 minutes (12,13). Given the shorter time frame for onset of effect with LMX-4, it may be the preferred agent for this purpose.

Achieving and maintaining proper patient position is the most crucial and challenging aspect of LP in children. Having an experienced assistant to perform this task is invaluable. The patient is placed on the examining table, and the operator is typically seated next to the bed, although some clinicians choose to stand with the bed elevated. The goals of positioning are to stretch the ligamenta flava and increase the interlaminar spaces. The two positions most widely used in the pediatric population are the lateral recumbent position and the sitting position (Fig. 41.3).

For the lateral recumbent position, the patient lays on his or her side near the edge of the bed next to the operator. For the right-handed operator, the patient's head is usually facing left. The patient's neck is flexed and the knees are drawn upward by the assistant. This is done by placing one arm under the child's knees and the other arm around the posterior aspect of the neck. By grasping his or her own wrists (with smaller patients), the assistant can maintain a greater degree of control over the restraint of the child. The assistant also should ensure that the shoulders and hips are perpendicular to the bed, thus keeping the spinal column in line, with no rotation. To increase the size of the interlaminar spaces, the cooperative patient can be asked to fully bend his or her back toward the physician.

The sitting position can be used with older children who are cooperative and with very young infants who are unlikely to struggle and may have increased respiratory distress in the lateral recumbent position (2). An older child may sit with feet over the side of the bed and with neck and upper body flexed over a pillow or a pile of blankets held in the lap. With an infant, the assistant holds the patient in a sitting position with an arm and a leg in each hand while supporting the head to prevent excess flexion of the neck (Fig. 41.3).

Once the patient is positioned, the upper aspects of the posterior superior iliac crests are palpated, and an imaginary line between them is pictured. This line intersects the midline just above the fourth lumbar spine. The interspaces between L3-L4 and L4-L5 can then be located, and one site is chosen for puncture (Fig. 41.3). In children outside infancy, the interspace between L2-L3 also may be used for LP.

After the puncture site has been selected, it should be cleansed with Betadine-soaked, sterile gauze or sponge using enlarging circles that begin at the puncture site. The Betadine solution may then be removed with alcohol in the same manner. Sterile towels are draped around the procedure site in such a way as to allow for good exposure. The puncture site should be relocated as previously described, and the site can be marked with a fingernail depression in the skin.

If EMLA or LMX-4 has not been used, the skin and subcutaneous tissues are next anesthetized by local infiltration using 1% lidocaine. It may be necessary to use lidocaine infiltration in addition to topical anesthetic in some cases. The practice of withholding local anesthesia for this procedure is discouraged. Local anesthesia has been shown to decrease the pain response to LP without hampering its successful completion in neonates (14). Certainly, all older children should receive some form of local anesthesia. Additionally, administration of an anxiolytic (e.g., midazolam) may be appropriate to facilitate the procedure when a patient is especially upset or frightened. For the rare older child who is combative to the extent that adequate positioning will be impossible or the safety of the procedure cannot be ensured, formal procedural sedation may be necessary.

When inserting the spinal needle, two possible approaches can be used (Fig. 41.2). Using the median approach, the needle is inserted through the supraspinal ligament. Using the lateral approach, the needle is inserted just lateral to the ligament. With both approaches, the needle may be held in one hand or both hands. When the needle is held in one hand, the clinician can ensure good alignment of the needle by placing the tip of the thumb of the noninserting hand on the spinous process above the space being entered. When holding the needle with both hands, the thumbs are placed on either side of the needle hub, and the index fingers are used to support the needle (Fig. 41.4).

Using the median approach, the needle (with the stylet in place) is inserted exactly in the midline. The bevel of the spinal needle should be positioned horizontally if the lateral recumbent position is used or vertically if the sitting position is used so that the dura mater is pierced parallel to its fibers (which run longitudinally down the spinal cord). This precaution minimizes the amount of CSF leakage and thereby decreases the likelihood of post-LP headache (4). The needle is then advanced cephalad toward the umbilicus if the patient is in the lateral recumbent position or slightly caudad if the patient is in the sitting position. Using the lateral approach, the needle should be inserted lateral to the upper border of the spinous process of L3 or L4. It should then be directed slightly medial and slightly upward (cephalad) to avoid contact with the supraspinal ligament.

With either the median or lateral approach, a degree of resistance during insertion of the needle is normally appreciated. When the ligamentum flavum is penetrated, a loss of resistance may be felt, especially in older children. This change in resistance is again experienced when the dura is penetrated. This second loss of resistance is often referred to as a "pop." If a pop is felt, the stylet is removed from the needle and fluid is obtained. In neonates and infants, the pop may not be evident. Consequently, it is easy to "overshoot" by inserting the needle too far, which often results in a traumatic LP with peripheral blood contaminating the CSF specimen. The most effective way to avoid this problem is by inserting the needle slowly and methodically, in increments of a few millimeters at a time, and frequently checking for return of CSF. For infants

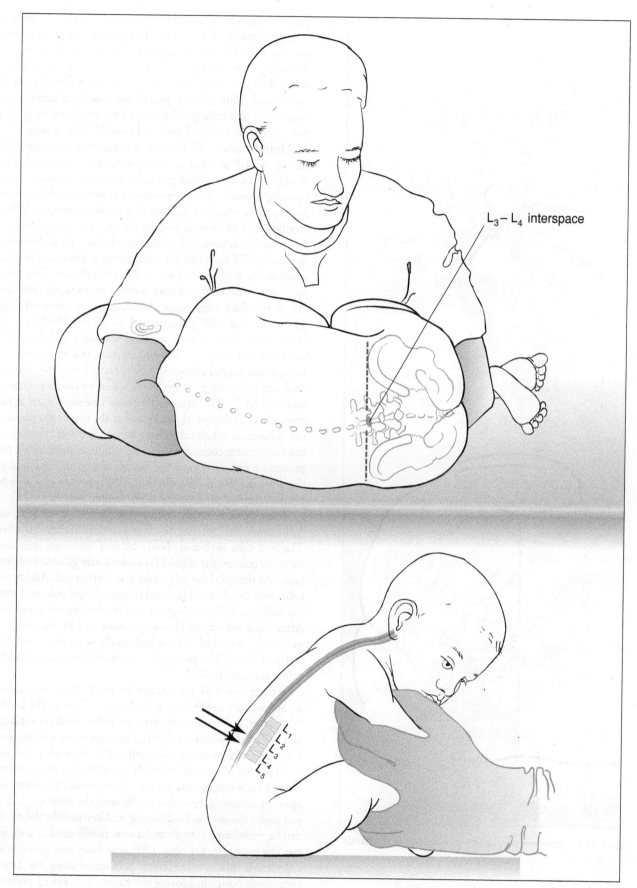

L₃–L₄ interspace

L₁
L₂
L₃
L₄
L₅

Figure 41.3 Lateral recumbent and sitting positions for lumbar puncture.

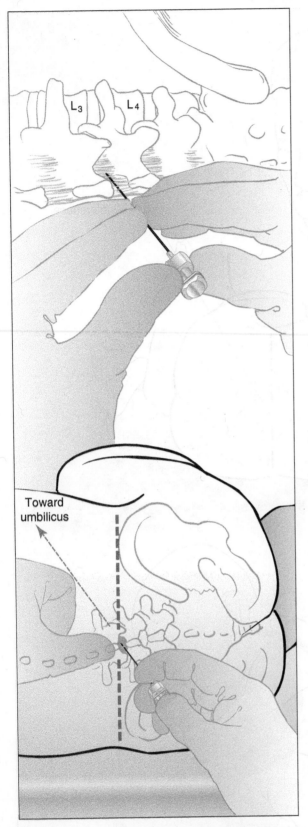

L₃ L₄

Toward
umbilicus

Figure 41.4 Spinal needle placement using one or two hands.

under 6 months of age, the appropriate depth of insertion is approximately 1 to 2 cm. The proper depth of needle insertion for LP can be calculated more exactly using the following formula: depth (in cm) = 0.77 + [2.56 × BSA], where BSA is the body surface area in square meters (15). The spinal needle should be supported with one hand during fluid collection (particularly in infants) to prevent dural tugging, a potential source of local pain and post-LP CSF leakage.

Measurement of CSF opening pressure is recommended during any LP in which it can be accurately performed. The struggling infant or child precludes accurate measurement of opening pressure. The measurement is most reliable in a relaxed patient who is in the lateral recumbent position. When free flow of CSF is obtained, the pressure manometer should be immediately attached to the needle hub via a three-way stopcock. CSF then fills the manometer column and is measured at the highest level reached in the column. This measurement should not end until respiratory variation (rise and fall of the fluid meniscus with breathing) is observed (Fig. 41.5). Normal CSF pressure is 5 to 20 cm H_2O in a relaxed child who has neck and legs extended and 10 to 28 cm H_2O in a relaxed child who has neck and legs flexed. Of note, a meaningful change in CSF pressure may not depend on lower extremity position, as indicated by recent studies in adults (16,17). The manometer should be supported at the connection to the spinal needle and at the top of the measuring column. It is helpful to have an assistant hold the top of the manometer column so that the clinician performing the procedure can determine the measurement and manipulate the stopcock for fluid collection. CSF pressure can also be estimated based on drops of CSF counted over time (18).

The CSF is normally collected in a series of sterile tubes. Approximately 1 mL per tube is required for standard studies. The first tube specimen should be sent for Gram stain and bacterial culture, the second for quantitative glucose and protein, and the third for cell count and differential. Additional tubes may be obtained for viral culture, fungal culture, bacterial antigens, cell pathology, or special chemistries, as needed. After fluid collection, closing pressure can be measured as previously described. The spinal needle is removed with the stylet in place. The puncture area should be cleansed and a sterile dressing applied.

If there is no CSF return after the needle has been inserted an appropriate depth, it may be helpful to rotate the needle 90 degrees. If this is not effective, the stylet should be replaced and the needle advanced slightly. In some cases, withdrawing the needle incrementally will result in CSF flow when the procedure is initially unsuccessful. If spinal fluid is not obtained despite such maneuvers, the procedure should be attempted again by removing the spinal needle with the stylet in place to just under the skin and redirecting it. Alternatively, the needle can be withdrawn entirely and a new needle used at a different insertion site. Of note, CSF may flow very slowly with dehydrated infants when LP is performed using the lateral recumbent position. Moving the patient to a sitting position may increase flow in this situation.

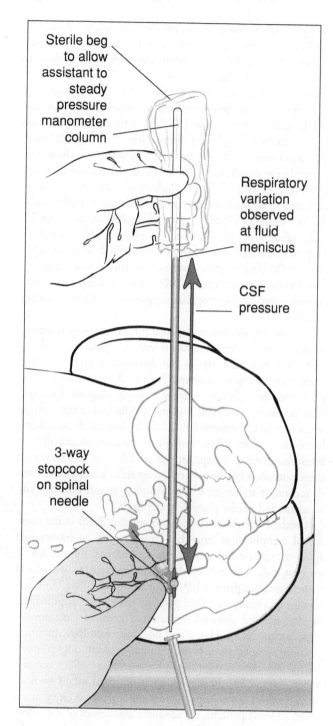

Sterile beg to allow assistant to steady pressure manometer column

Respiratory variation observed at fluid meniscus

CSF pressure

3-way stopcock on spinal needle

Figure 41.5 Manometer measurement of CSF pressure.

Occasionally, bony resistance is felt upon spinal needle placement. This situation may occur when the skin is punctured over the spine of the vertebral body instead of the vertebral interspace or when the patient's position does not achieve adequate spinal flexion to open the interlaminar space. If bony resistance is felt superficially, then puncture over the spinous process is likely, and the needle should be withdrawn to just below the skin and redirected through the interspace. If bony resistance is felt more deeply, then inadequate spinal flexion

is likely. Directing the needle more cephalad in conjunction with improved positioning usually overcomes this problem in the infant. In the older child, directing the needle more caudad (or straight in) may be necessary to find the interspace.

As mentioned previously, a traumatic LP may result from improper technique, limiting the usefulness of the CSF cell count. Causes include inserting the needle too far to one side into an epidural venous plexus or through the subarachnoid space into or adjacent to the vertebral body. If blood is seen during fluid collection but the spinal needle is in proper position, the CSF normally clears and the specimen does not clot. If the bloody fluid does not clear and clots form in the collection tube, then the spinal needle should be removed and LP attempted at a different interspace with an unused needle. Unfortunately, a traumatic LP can sometimes result even when the procedure is performed correctly.

Rarely, LP fails despite proper positioning and technique. In this instance, ultrasound may be useful to determine the reason for failure and the likelihood of success on continued attempts. In one study of infants and neonates who underwent ultrasound after failed LP, about two-thirds of the patients had intrathecal and/or epidural hematomas that obliterated the CSF space, and 12% had minimal CSF (19). Under ultrasound guidance, an adequate volume of CSF for culture was obtained for only 2 of 9 patients with no visible CSF, usable CSF samples were obtained for 4 of 6 patients with minimal CSF, and all 11 patients with clearly visualized CSF had LP performed successfully.

▶ COMPLICATIONS

LP is frequently associated with the minor complications of localized back pain without neurologic abnormalities, transient paresthesia during the procedure, and post-LP headache. Localized back pain typically resolves with symptomatic treatment such as acetaminophen and applied heat. Severe back pain associated with neurologic signs such as decreased sensation or incontinence may be indicative of a subdural or epidural spinal hematoma and requires emergent investigation and treatment. Extradural CSF collections have also been demonstrated in the setting of severe post-LP back pain (20). Paresthesias may occur as the spinal needle contacts nerves in the cauda equina and are ameliorated by repositioning the spinal needle. Permanent peripheral nerve damage is rare, because the spinal needle does not pierce the nerve, although it may move or stretch the nerve (4).

Post-LP headaches occur most commonly in children over 10 years of age and are more frequent among females (21,22). Post-LP headaches are caused by continued leakage of spinal fluid through the dural hole, which decreases the cushioning of intracranial contents (20). Associated symptoms include vertigo and tinnitus from decreased endolymph volume in the semicircular canals, as well as diplopia and blurry vision from stretching of cranial nerve VI as it passes over the petrous portion of the temporal bone. Headache is best prevented by using the smallest spinal needle possible and limiting the amount of cerebrospinal fluid removed. Headache occurs in as many as 80% of cases after LP with a 16-gauge needle but in only 1% of cases after puncture with a 25-gauge needle (23). The incidence of post-LP headache in adults may be further reduced by the use of atraumatic LP needles, such as the Sprotte, Whitacre, and Pajunk types, instead of the Quincke cutting needle. However, one study found that atraumatic needles were associated with a higher failure rate for LP than the standard needle (24). Another study failed to find a decrease in post-LP headache when an atraumatic needle was used in children (25). Placing the patient supine immediately following LP does not affect the occurrence of headache (26). Treatment of postspinal headache depends on its severity. Symptomatic treatment of pain and nausea suffice in most cases. Severe or prolonged symptoms (longer than 4 to 5 days) have been successfully treated with intravenous caffeine in adults and epidural blood patching in adults and children (23). Epidural blood patching requires the injection of 5 to 15 mL of autologous fresh blood into the epidural space at the same level as the previous LP. The epidural patch has efficacy approaching 90% in relieving post-LP headache in adults (27).

Major complications after LP include LP-induced meningitis, epidural or subdural hematoma, acquired epidermoid tumor, damage to adjacent structures (disk herniation, retroperitoneal abscess, spinal cord hematoma), and cerebral herniation. Fortunately, these complications are quite rare. As previously discussed, the lateral recumbent position for LP can cause respiratory obstruction, hypoxemia, and cardiovascular instability, particularly in the young infant (2). Consequently, LP is sometimes contraindicated simply because the patient is too ill to safely undergo the procedure.

LP through an area of cellulitis predictably causes meningitis. For this reason, cellulitis overlying the LP site is an absolute contraindication to this procedure. An association has also been made between performing LP in children with bacteremia and the occurrence of meningitis (28). However, an analysis of risk factors found that the development of bacterial meningitis in children with occult bacteremia was very strongly related to the infecting organism but not to whether LP was performed (29). Eng and Seligman reported the incidence of LP-induced meningitis to be no greater than 2.1%, which does not exceed the incidence of spontaneous meningitis in patients with bacteremia (30). They also found possible LP-induced meningitis to be most common in critically ill patients who underwent LP multiple times. Although LP may lead to meningitis in a small percentage of children with bacteremia, LP-induced meningitis is a rare event and should not deter the physician from performing the procedure if clinically indicated.

Subdural or epidural hematoma following LP has been reported with all forms of bleeding dyscrasias. Subdural spinal hematoma has been reported in thrombocytopenic children with leukemia, cancer, and ITP who had platelet counts from 1,000 to 73,000/mm³. Signs and symptoms of spinal cord

compression, including pain, sensory deficits, paralysis, and incontinence, developed 1 hour to 6 days after the procedure. In most cases, the LP was difficult and yielded bloody fluid. In these patients, platelet counts were low or falling, and platelet transfusion was not provided before LP (31). However, in one report of children with acute lymphoblastic leukemia (ALL) undergoing elective LP, there were no complications in 941 cases with platelet counts less than 50,000/mm³. These authors concluded that children with ALL do not require platelet transfusion prior to LP if platelet counts exceed 10,000/mm³ (32). Of note, epidural spinal hematomas have occurred spontaneously after anticoagulation in patients who did not undergo LP, after epidural anesthesia, and after LP in an infant with undiagnosed hemophilia A (33,34). LP can be performed safely in patients with thrombocytopenia less than 10,000/mm³ if they receive transfusion to a peripheral platelet count greater than 50,000/mm³ and in patients with coagulopathy after appropriate correction of factor deficiency (32,34).

Acquired epidermal spinal cord tumors can arise from implantation of epidermal material into the spinal canal during LP. The tumor manifests as gait disturbance, pain, and neurologic dysfunction occurring 1.5 to 23 years after LP. Experimental and clinical evidence strongly suggests that these tumors can be avoided if a spinal needle with a tight fitting stylet is used to perform LP (35,36). Osteomyelitis, diskitis, herniated vertebral disk, and spinal cord hematoma all have been described as complications of LP. The occurrence of these outcomes can be minimized by strict adherence to sterile technique and by careful attention to proper puncture site selection and needle placement depth (37).

Cerebral herniation leading to sudden death is the most feared complication from LP. Patients with an intracranial space-occupying lesion (abscess, hematoma, tumor) are at greatest risk. The risk of death among patients with focal neurologic signs prior to LP may be as high as 40% (38). Conversely, in a study of 1,053 patients with either papilledema or documented elevated intracranial pressure (manometry greater than 20 cm H₂O) and no focal neurologic findings, possible complications from LP were noted in only 5% and 1.2%, respectively, regardless of the etiology of intracranial hypertension (39). Risk of herniation in an infant with an open fontanel and no focal neurologic findings is likely much lower. In most patients, an adequate assessment of the safety of performing LP can be made based on clinical grounds. Patients who have a history of focal neurologic symptoms (e.g., focal seizures, unilateral motor paralysis), focal neurologic findings on physical examination, signs of impending herniation (posturing, Glasgow coma score less than 8, bilateral dilated pupils, respiratory abnormalities, abnormal tone, absent Doll eye reflex), or papilledema should not undergo LP until further imaging and treatment establish that the procedure can be safely performed (8). If meningitis or other CNS infection is strongly considered, the patient should receive appropriate antibiotic therapy prior to the imaging study.

SUMMARY

1 Determine the patient's ability to safely undergo lumbar puncture.

2 Explain procedure to the parents and patient (if applicable); obtain informed consent.

3 Correctly position the patient in a lateral recumbent or sitting position.

4 Consider the application of a topical anesthetic (LMX-4, EMLA) and the possible need for procedural sedation.

5 With the patient positioned, choose the puncture site by imagining a line across the superior margins of the posterior superior iliac crests and finding the L3-L4 or L4-L5 spinal interspace.

6 Cleanse the area with povidone-iodine solution, and drape and relocate the puncture site.

7 Anesthetize the skin and subcutaneous tissue by infiltration with 1% lidocaine if a topical anesthetic is not used.

8 For the median approach (preferred if there is no ligamentous calcification), identify the interspace with the thumb of one hand and direct the needle as follows:

   a Lateral recumbent position: parallel to the bed and cephalad (toward the umbilicus).
   b Sitting: perpendicular to the skin (slightly caudad).

9 For the lateral approach, puncture the skin just above transverse process of L3 or L4, and direct it medially and upward (cephalad).

10 Keeping the stylet in place, advance the spinal needle until a loss of resistance or a "pop" is felt; in infants, a pop may not be felt, and the spinal needle should be advanced approximately 1 to 2 cm.

11 If performing manometry, attach the manometer and stopcock to the spinal needle; extend the patient's neck and legs as much as possible and read the CSF pressure.

12 Remove the stylet or manometer and collect fluid in sterile tubes.

13 Once fluid is obtained, remeasure the CSF pressure (if indicated), replace the stylet, and remove the spinal needle.

14 Dress the lumbar puncture site with an adhesive bandage.

 CLINICAL TIPS

▶ Correct positioning of the patient, with adequate flexion of the spine and good vertebral alignment, is key to successfully performing a lumbar puncture.

▶ For nonemergent cases, transdermal topical anesthetic cream (LMX-4, EMLA) can be used to minimize overall pain experience by the child.

▶ Injected lidocaine anesthesia has not been shown to interfere with performing lumbar puncture and is recommended for all patients.

▶ If no CSF return is obtained after needle insertion to an appropriate depth, the spinal needle should be rotated 90 degrees.

▶ If rotation of the spinal needle does not produce fluid, then the needle should be advanced slightly.

▶ If CSF flow is slow in the lateral recumbent position, the patient may be moved to the sitting position.

▶ If bony resistance is felt immediately below the skin, then the puncture site is likely over the spinous process and not over the spinal interspace.

▶ If bony resistance is felt more deeply, the spinal needle should be withdrawn to the skin surface and redirected more cephalad while ensuring that the patient's back is properly flexed.

▶ If bloody fluid that does not clear or forms clots, then the spinal needle should be withdrawn and the procedure attempted at a different lumbar interspace.

▶ A slow, methodical approach that includes advancing the needle incrementally and frequently checking for CSF return is usually the best way of avoiding a traumatic ("bloody") lumbar puncture.

▶ Ultrasound may be a useful adjunct in situations where attempts at lumbar puncture have failed despite proper positioning and technique.

Infants in whom the fundus cannot be visualized can undergo LP if no other findings suggest cerebral herniation, increased intracranial pressure, or a focal neurological process.

▶ SUMMARY

LP is commonly performed in the care of sick infants and children. The potential for cardiorespiratory decompensation during the procedure, especially in neonates and young infants, requires that it be performed in an area equipped for resuscitation. Its successful completion depends on proper positioning, judicious analgesia, and a thorough knowledge of the anatomy of the lumbar spine. Complications may be avoided by careful clinical assessment of the patient before LP and strict adherence to proper technique.

▶ REFERENCES

1. Weisman LE, Merenstein GB, Steenbarger JR. The effect of lumbar puncture position in sick neonates. *Am J Dis Child.* 1983;137:1077–1079.
2. Gleason CA, Martin RJ, Anderson JV, et al. Optimal position for a spinal tap in preterm infants. *Pediatrics.* 1983;71:31–35.
3. Kiernan JA. *Barrs' The Human Nervous System.* 8th ed. Philadelphia: Lippincott Williams & Wilkins; 2004.
4. Swaiman KF. Spinal fluid examination. In: Ashwal S, Swaiman KF, eds. *Pediatric Neurology: Principles and Practice.* 3rd ed. St. Louis: Mosby; 1999.
5. Truex RC, Carpenter MB. Cerebrospinal fluid. In: Truex RC, Carpenter MB, eds. *Human Neuroanatomy.* Baltimore: Williams & Wilkins; 1971.
6. Boon JM, Abrahms PH, Meiring JH, et al. Lumbar puncture: anatomical review of a clinical skill. *Clin Anat.* 2004;17:544–553.
7. Lachman E. *Case Studies in Anatomy.* 2nd ed. New York: Oxford University Press; 1996:25–44.
8. Riordan FAI, Cant AJ. When to do a lumbar puncture. *Arch Dis Child.* 2002;87:235–237.
9. Earnest MP. Safe and effective use of lumbar puncture. In: Earnest MP, ed. *Neurologic Emergencies.* New York: Churchill Livingstone; 1983.
10. Clarke MA. Timing of lumbar puncture in severe childhood meningitis. *BMJ.* 1985;291:899.
11. Horwitz SJ, Boxerbaum B, O'Bell J. Cerebral herniation in bacterial meningitis in childhood. *Ann Neurol.* 1980;7:524–528.
12. Eichenfeld L, Funk A, Fallon-Friedlander S, et al. A clinical study to evaluate the efficacy of ELA-Max (4% liposomal lidocaine) as compared with eutectic mixture of local anesthetics cream for pain reduction of venipuncture in children. *Pediatrics.* 2002;109:1093–1099.
13. Kaur G, Gupta P, Kumar A. A randomized trial of eutectic mixture of local anesthetics during lumbar puncture in newborns. *Arch Pediatr Adoles Med.* 2003;157:1065–1070.
14. Pinheiro JMB, Furdon S, Ochoa LF. Role of local anesthesia during lumbar puncture in neonates. *Pediatrics.* 1993;91:379–382.
15. Bonadio WA, Smith DS, Metrou M, et al. Estimating lumbar puncture depth in children [Letter]. *N Eng J Med.* 1988;319:952–953.
16. Ellis RW III. Lumbar cerebrospinal fluid opening pressure measured in a flexed lateral decubitus position in children. *Pediatrics.* 1994;93:622–623.
17. Abbrescia KL, Brabson TA, Dalsey WC, et al. The effect of lower-extremity position on cerebrospinal fluid pressures. *Acad Emerg Med.* 2001;8:8–12.
18. Ellis RW III, Strauss LC, Wiley JM, et al. A simple method of estimating cerebrospinal fluid pressure during lumbar puncture. *Pediatrics.* 1992;89:895–897.

19. Coey BD, Shiels WE II, Hogan MJ. Diagnostic and interventional ultrasonography in neonatal and infant lumbar puncture. *Pediatr Radiol.* 2001;31:399–402.
20. Atabaki S, Ochsenschlager D, Vezina G. Post-lumbar puncture headache and backache in pediatrics: a case series and demonstration of magnetic resonance imaging findings. *Arch Pediatr Adolesc Med.* 1999;153:770–773.
21. Tobias JD. Postdural puncture headache in children: etiology and treatment. *Clin Pediatr.* 1994;33:110–113.
22. Ebinger F, Kosel C, Pietz J, et al. Headache and backache after lumbar puncture in children and adolescents: a prospective study. *Pediatrics.* 2004;113:1588–1592.
23. Choi JE, Chang JY, Sin JY, et al. CSF leakage after diagnostic lumbar puncture: case reports. *Clin Pediatr (Phila).* 2004;43:769–771.
24. Thomas SR, Jamieson DRS, Muir KW. Randomised controlled trial of atraumatic versus standard needles for diagnostic lumbar puncture. *BMJ.* 2000;321:986–990.
25. Kokki H, Salonvaara M, Herrgard E, et al. Postdural puncture headache is not an age-related symptom in children: a prospective, open-randomized, parallel group study comparing a 22-gauge Quincke with a 22-gauge Whitacre needle. *Paediatr Anaest.* 1999;9:429–434.
26. Ebinger F, Kosel C, Pietz J, et al. Strict bed rest following lumbar puncture in children and adolescents is of no benefit. *Neurology.* 2004;62:1003–1005.
27. Crawford JS. The prevention of headache consequent upon dural puncture. *Br J Anaesth.* 1972;44:598–600.
28. Teele DW, Dashefsdy B, Rakusan T, et al. Meningitis after lumbar puncture in children with bacteremia. *N Eng J Med.* 1981;305:1079–1081.
29. Shapiro ED, Aaron NH, Wald ER, et al. Risk factors for development of bacterial meningitis among children with occult bacteremia. *J Pediatr.* 1986;109:15–19.
30. Eng RHK, Seligman SJ. Lumbar puncture-induced meningitis. *JAMA.* 1981;245:1456–1459.
31. Edelson RN, Chernik NL, Posner JB. Spinal subdural hematomas complicating lumbar puncture: occurrence in thrombocytopenic patients. *Arch Neurol.* 1974;31:134–137.
32. Howard SC, Amar G, Ribeiro RC, et al. Safety of lumbar puncture for children with acute lymphoblastic leukemia and thrombocytopenia. *JAMA.* 2000;184:2222–2224.
33. Faillace WJ, Warrier I, Canady AI. Paraplegia after lumbar puncture in an infant with previously undiagnosed hemophilia A: treatment and perioperative considerations. *Clin Pediatr.* 1989;28:136–138.
34. Silverman R, Kwiatkowski T, Bernstein S, et al. Safety of lumbar puncture in patients with hemophilia. *Ann Emerg Med.* 1993;22:1739–1742.
35. Batnitzky S, Keucher TR, Mealey J, et al. Iatrogenic intraspinal epidermoid tumors. *JAMA.* 1977;237:148–150.
36. Gibson T, Norris W. Skin fragments removed by injection needles. *Lancet.* 1958;2:983–985.
37. Dripps RD, Vandam LD. Hazards of lumbar puncture. *JAMA.* 1952;247:1113–1122.
38. Duffy GP. Lumbar puncture in the presence of raised intracranial pressure. *BMJ.* 1969;1:407–409.
39. Korein J, Cravioto H, Leicach M. Reevaluation of lumbar puncture: a study of 129 patients with papilledema or intracranial hypertension. *Neurology.* 1959;9:290–297.

42

ANN-CHRISTINE DUHAIME AND JAMES F. WILEY, II

Ventricular Shunt and Burr Hole Puncture

▶ INTRODUCTION

Children with ventricular shunts can present to the emergency department (ED), office, or clinic with signs or symptoms of two major shunt complications—obstruction or infection. Shunt puncture, or "tapping" the shunt, refers to withdrawing cerebrospinal fluid (CSF) from the shunt apparatus percutaneously to aid in diagnosing a shunt malfunction or infection. In some cases, elevated intracranial pressure may be acutely relieved by removing some ventricular fluid. However, because shunt puncture carries an approximately 1% risk of introducing infection, and because improperly performed taps can damage certain types of shunt components, the physician should try to identify shunt problems without tapping the shunt when possible (1). Ideally, shunt punctures should be performed by a neurosurgeon who is familiar with the particular type of shunt in question and who has assessed the patient and can weigh the relative risks and benefits to be derived from a shunt tap. Because some shunt problems require immediate attention, however, the goal of this chapter is to review the basics of shunt anatomy and evaluation and to describe the indications and techniques for shunt puncture and burr hole puncture when a neurosurgeon is unavailable. Because of the potential for cardiorespiratory instability in the child with a shunt obstruction or infection, a physician should only perform this procedure in an area where monitoring, resuscitation equipment, and personnel are sufficient to handle sudden decompensation, such as in the ED, intensive care unit, or operating room.

▶ ANATOMY AND PHYSIOLOGY

The majority of shunts placed for hydrocephalus consist of the following four main components (Fig. 42.1):

1 A proximal catheter, usually in the lateral ventricle
2 A distal catheter, usually in the peritoneal cavity or, less commonly, in the right atrium, pleural cavity, or other site
3 A reservoir, which is usually a single or double bubble or button, often located on the head near the burr hole entry site of the proximal catheter
4 A valve to control flow, which most often is a device located within or adjacent to the reservoir but in some cases is integrated into or part of the distal catheter (in-line or slit valve)

There are many types of valves, ranging from simple designs to more complex programmable valves that can be adjusted to increase or decrease resistance to flow by the application of an external magnetic device (Fig. 42.2).

Shunts are described according to their proximal and distal drainage sites; therefore, a ventriculoperitoneal (VP) shunt drains from the ventricle to the peritoneal cavity, a ventriculojugular (VJ) or ventriculoatrial (VA) shunt drains the ventricle through the jugular vein into the right atrium, and a lumboperitoneal (LP) shunt drains the lumbar subarachnoid space into the peritoneum. In addition, shunts have "brand names," which often identify the manufacturer and the model of the shunt. As the number of valves available has increased, the terminology can be quite confusing. Clinicians can often sort out which valve is present in the patient by asking the family, by checking the operative report, or by looking at the plain films (shunt survey). Most major manufacturers have websites on which specific valve types are pictured; by searching these sources and comparing them to the appearance on plain films, most valves can be identified when this becomes necessary during shunt "troubleshooting."

Figure 42.1 Selected ventricular shunt components.

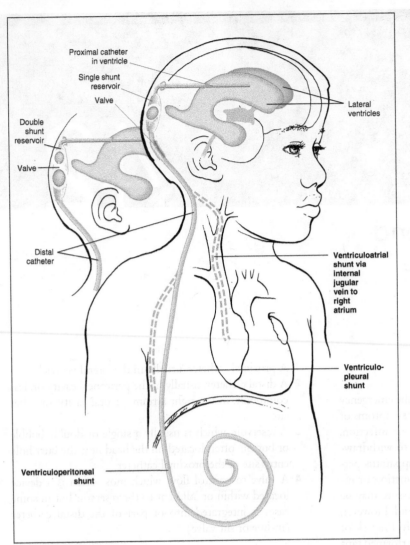

Proximal catheter in ventricle

Single shunt reservoir

Valve

Double shunt reservoir

Valve

Distal catheter

Lateral ventricles

Ventriculoatrial shunt via internal jugular vein to right atrium

Ventriculo-pleural shunt

Ventriculoperitoneal shunt

"Pumping" the shunt to assess its function involves pressing on the reservoir or valve and assessing how it refills; this requires experience with the specific shunt type and can be interpreted only in the context of the ventricular size or volume of fluid in the space being drained. Tapping the shunt requires identifying the reservoir, which is specifically designed for this purpose. A shunt survey (plain radiographs of the shunt along its course) will usually show its location. The part of the shunt that is "pumped" usually, but not always, is the part that is tapped. For example, with a Holter-type valve, a separate (Rickham) reservoir is usually placed in the burr hole itself (Fig. 42.3); tapping the pumping chamber of the cylindrical Holter valve may cause it to be damaged.

As always, there are exceptions and variations in shunt components. Proximal catheters are sometimes multiple and may drain other cavities such as cysts, a trapped fourth ventricle, or the subdural space. Some shunts do not have reservoirs or valves, and some components may be radiolucent on radiograph. The consulting neurosurgeon can usually help sort out these less common situations.

▶ INDICATIONS

Shunt Malfunction

Children with a ventricular shunt malfunction often present with signs and symptoms of increased intracranial pressure, such as headache, vomiting, irritability, and lethargy. Sunsetting (inability to look up) or crossed eyes may be seen, and in infants the fontanel may be full. Occasionally, less common symptoms will herald malfunction, such as seizures or other neurologic symptoms. In severe cases, coma, herniation, arrest, and death can occur (2). Families often recognize and diagnose shunt problems with a high degree of accuracy, especially because each shunt malfunction tends to present with the same signs in a given child. Their opinion is a valuable resource not to be overlooked.

Shunt malfunction may result from obstruction of the proximal catheter (usually with choroid plexus) or the distal system from one of the following: (a) malfunction of a valve; (b) improper setting of a programmable valve due to application of a strong magnetic field, as with magnetic resonance

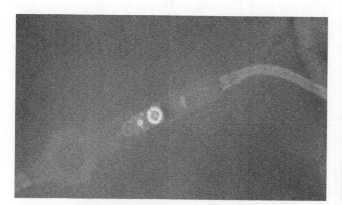
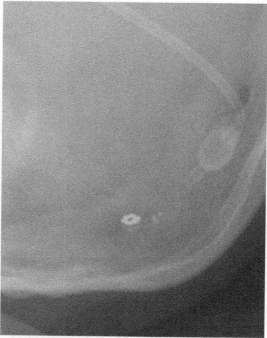

Figure 42.2 Lateral skull views from shunt surveys of children with two types of commonly used programmable valves. *Left:* Codman programmable valve with intrinsic antisiphon device (SiphonGuard). *Right:* Medtronic programmable valve (Strata). Because the Strata is similar to the Medtronic line of nonprogrammable valves (Delta), it is often referred to as the "Delta programmable." The pressure setting on these valves can be read with a "key" that is specific to the manufacturer, and the setting can be changed with a special "magnet" or "wand." Because new models of valves are developed continuously, terminology and radiologic appearance will be variable.

imaging (MRI); (c) a short shunt due to growth; (d) shunt fracture or disconnection, or (e) distal catheter occlusion. Proximal obstructions, which are the most common cause of shunt malfunction, are diagnosed by a slowly refilling shunt or minimal flow on shunt tap in the presence of ventricular enlargement on computed tomography (CT) scan or MRI. Shunt disconnections or insufficient distal length are diagnosed by shunt survey. Most other cases of shunt malfunction involve distal obstruction or valve malfunction (2).

In general, proximal obstructions cause the most acute neurologic symptoms—and may require urgent surgical correction—because a high-grade proximal obstruction precludes relief of pressure by a shunt puncture. If the problem is elsewhere in the shunt, or if the proximal obstruction is partial, tapping the shunt will usually allow withdrawal of sufficient CSF to relieve the more severe symptoms temporarily until definitive surgical repair can be performed. The CSF pressure and the ease with which fluid can be withdrawn also help evaluate shunt function. If symptoms are mild, and if the diagnosis of shunt malfunction is clear by noninvasive means, temporary medical management with diuretics such as acetazolamide can be helpful until surgical correction is accomplished, as the risks associated with shunt puncture can thus be avoided (Table 42.1). Consequently, not every child with a suspected shunt malfunction will need to undergo a shunt tap.

Shunt Infection

Shunt infections nearly always present with fever, which may be low grade, intermittent, or high grade. Abdominal pain or, uncommonly, frank peritonitis may be seen with infected VP shunts. Redness or tenderness over the shunt may also be apparent. With VA shunts, nephritis is a rare but serious complication of shunt infection. Although a severe shunt infection may lead to obstruction and shunt failure, the majority of infected shunts continue to function, so increased intracranial pressure is not part of the typical picture of early shunt infection (2).

VP shunt infections almost always result from bacteria that have been introduced into the shunt at the time of surgery. Therefore, infections generally manifest as fever during the first few months after an operation. If it has been more than 6 months since any invasive VP shunt procedure, fever is highly unlikely to be the result of a shunt infection (3). Exceptions include obvious contamination of the shunt by an intraperitoneal process, such as a ruptured appendix, or erosion of a shunt component through the skin. In contrast, shunts that terminate in the bloodstream (VJ/VA shunts) may become contaminated by any episode of bacteremia and thus are suspect as a source of fever regardless of time of last revision (4). The febrile child with a shunt who demonstrates an obvious source (e.g., otitis media, upper respiratory infection,

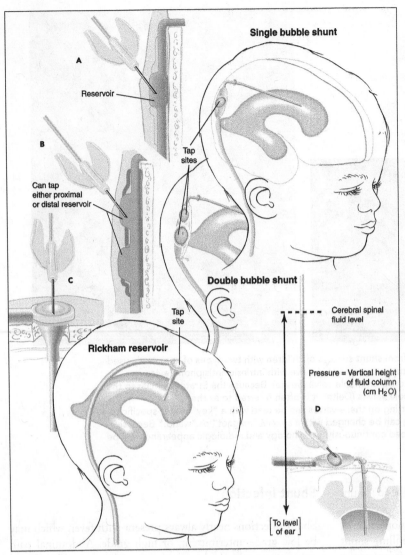

Single bubble shunt

Reservoir

Tap sites

Can tap either proximal or distal reservoir

Double bubble shunt

Tap site

Rickham reservoir

Cerebral spinal fluid level

Pressure = Vertical height of fluid column (cm H$_2$O)

[To level of ear]

Figure 42.3 Ventricular shunt tap and measurement of intraventricular pressure.
A. Single reservoir shunt.
B. Double reservoir shunt: either the proximal or distal reservoir may be tapped.
C. Rickham reservoir.
D. Measurement of CSF pressure during ventricular shunt tap.

TABLE 42.1	**INDICATIONS FOR VENTRICULOPERITONEAL SHUNT PUNCTURE**

Malfunction
1. Problem not clear by physical examination and radiograph evaluation
2. Severe symptoms of elevated intracranial pressure that cannot be managed medically until definitive repair

Infection
Ventriculoperitoneal shunt
1. Persistent fever without known source
2. Fever with recent (<6 months) shunt surgery or recent shunt tap
3. Suspected intra-abdominal soilage/contamination
4. Incisional CSF leakage or exposed shunt
Ventriculojugular/atrial shunt
1. Fever without known source
2. Sepsis
3. Suspected shunt nephritis

Note: Individual exceptions may occur and should be discussed with the patient's neurosurgeon.

---

gastroenteritis) can be treated for the presumed underlying infection. Tapping the shunt in this setting is usually unnecessary (Table 42.1).

As mentioned, infection can be introduced by a shunt puncture. A shunt should never be tapped through compromised or inflamed skin. Additionally, a partial shunt obstruction can be worsened by forceful suction on the choroid plexus. Withdrawal of a large volume of fluid before CT scan can also compromise the interpretation of ventricular size, and therefore a shunt tap should not be performed until after imaging unless symptoms are severe.

Cerebral Herniation Due to Proximal Shunt Obstruction

Burr hole puncture can be a life-saving procedure in the setting of a complete proximal shunt obstruction with severely elevated intracranial pressure. The goal is to relieve intracranial hypertension acutely by inserting a spinal needle directly into the ventricle using the burr hole through which the shunt enters the skull. A ventricular tap through the burr hole almost always damages the shunt and carries a significant risk of parenchymal brain injury, intracranial hemorrhage, and infection. It should therefore *only* be performed if cerebral herniation is occurring despite medical management of increased intracranial pressure and no alternative, such as immediate surgery, is available.

▶ VENTRICULAR SHUNT PUNCTURE

Equipment

> Isopropyl alcohol
> Betadine
> 23-gauge butterfly needle
> Sterile test tubes or syringe with cap
> Razor

Procedure

Although a shunt puncture is not very painful (for most children, it is less painful than venipuncture), reassurance should be provided. The child is placed in the lateral position for posterior shunts and supine for frontal shunts. With small children, this can be accomplished in the parent's lap, which aids in controlling crying and facilitates more effective pressure measurement. Contamination is prevented by keeping the child calm and stationary. The use of surgical drapes and towels is usually unnecessary. Although most neurosurgeons prefer that the tap site be shaved, some believe that shaving increases the risk of infection and prefer to simply cleanse the hair. In either case, the first step is to clean and degrease the scalp with alcohol in an area that includes the part of the shunt to be tapped and a surrounding margin of several centimeters. The hair is then clipped or shaved, if desired; a dime-sized area is all that is required. A thorough, repetitive, center-to-circumference Betadine cleansing is then performed for several minutes. Importantly, a shunt tap breaches a foreign

body; therefore, three brief wipes with the lumbar puncture tray sponges do not constitute adequate preparation for this procedure. Ideally, the Betadine should be allowed to dry on the skin while equipment is readied.

As mentioned, the reservoir is the component to puncture. For most dome-shaped pumping reservoirs, the needle should be inserted tangentially to a depth of a few millimeters (Fig. 42.3). The clinician should feel the needle pop through the reservoir dome. If the needle is advanced too far, it may embed in the back wall of the reservoir and become occluded. Firm, button-type reservoirs (usually Rickham reservoirs) are situated in the burr hole. These are most easily punctured by inserting the needle straight down, perpendicular to the scalp.

Once CSF flow is established and the child is reclining and quiet, the butterfly tubing is held perpendicular to the floor. Pressure measurements are not accurate if the child is not placed in the full reclining position. If fluid does not immediately flow, gentle syringe suction is applied. An assistant can measure the distance between the external ear canal and the top of the CSF column in the butterfly tubing with a metric rule or tape measure after the syringe is removed from the tubing. This is easier than using a manometer and provides an accurate opening pressure.

Rapid flow of CSF under pressure suggests a shunt obstruction distal to the reservoir with a patent proximal shunt catheter. Slow or absent flow in the presence of large ventricles (relative to the patient's baseline) indicates a proximal shunt obstruction, and pressure measurements are not accurate in this setting. Slow flow, with good respiratory variation and a normal pressure, is usually normal in the setting of small ventricles seen on brain imaging.

If the ventricles are large, the proximal catheter is unobstructed, and the pressure is high, at least 10 mL of fluid can be withdrawn through a syringe to acutely lower the pressure. Small ventricles or a partially occluded proximal catheter will result in slow flow, and fluid is best removed by gentle suction through a small (5 mL or less) syringe. Only a small amount of fluid can be obtained in this case. After fluid is withdrawn,

---

 SUMMARY: VENTRICULAR SHUNT PUNCTURE

1 Position child:
  a Supine for frontal shunt.
  b Lateral for posterior parietal shunt.

2 Clean shunt site and adjacent scalp with isopropyl alcohol.

3 Clip or shave a dime-sized area over reservoir (optional).

4 Carefully clean site for several minutes with Betadine and allow to dry.

5 For dome-shaped pumping reservoirs, insert needle tangentially approximately 2 to 5 mm; Rickham (firm

"button") reservoirs should be punctured perpendicular to scalp.

6 Measure opening pressure by holding butterfly tubing perpendicular to floor and measuring from ear to top of CSF column in tubing.

7 Remove CSF until ventricular pressure is at or below approximately 10 cm H_2O (10 to 20 mL); with proximal obstruction (slow flow), pressure measurement may be inaccurate.

8 Transfer CSF to sterile test tubes for further studies.

9 Remove butterfly needle and apply sterile dressing.

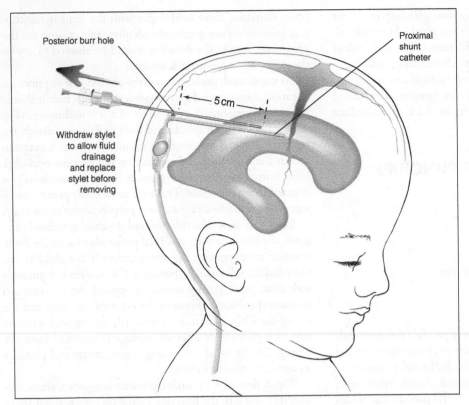

Figure 42.4 Ventricular puncture through the burr hole.

Posterior burr hole

Proximal shunt catheter

5 cm

Withdraw stylet to allow fluid drainage and replace stylet before removing

either specimens are transferred to sterile tubes or the syringe is tightly capped. Helpful laboratory tests include CSF cell count, Gram stain, and culture.

If the shunt tap is not successful, and if severe symptoms of increased intracranial pressure exist and are not amenable to medical management (hyperventilation and diuretic therapy), then a ventricular tap through the burr hole should be considered.

▶ BURR HOLE PUNCTURE

Equipment

> Isopropyl alcohol
> Betadine
> 3.5-inch, 21-gauge spinal needle
> Razor
> Sterile towels

Procedure

After shaving and cleansing the scalp thoroughly with isopropyl alcohol and Betadine, the burr hole is palpated, and a 3.5-inch, 22-gauge needle is slowly inserted straight in, perpendicular to the skull, through either a frontal or an occipital burr hole (Fig. 42.4). With some shunts, the burr hole will contain a reservoir, and this also is punctured by the spinal needle. The ventricle usually will be reached by a depth of 5 cm. The stylet is withdrawn after advancing the needle, and

fluid is allowed to drain spontaneously until it begins to slow down, indicating relief of pressure. The stylet is replaced and the needle is slowly withdrawn along its entry tract. Most patients will then proceed directly to the operating room for definitive shunt repair (5).

▶ COMPLICATIONS

Ventricular shunt puncture with large-volume fluid removal and burr hole puncture carry a significant risk for

---

 SUMMARY: BURR HOLE PUNCTURE

1 Locate burr hole.

2 Wash site with isopropyl alcohol.

3 Shave or clip hair in 3 cm circumference (optional).

4 Wash site thoroughly with Betadine.

5 Advance a 22-gauge, 3.5-inch spinal needle perpendicularly through burr hole; check every 0.5 cm for CSF flow (up to 5 cm).

6 Withdraw fluid.

7 When pressure is relieved, replace stylet and slowly remove.

CLINICAL TIPS

Ventricular Shunt Puncture

No Flow

▶ The physician should ensure that the reservoir is being tapped.

▶ The angle or depth of the needle should be adjusted slightly to see if flow improves.

▶ In young infants, the physician can push on the fontanel.

▶ If the bubble collapses when suction is applied, the proximal catheter is likely to be blocked, and the procedure should be abandoned.

▶ In a child with signs of herniation, a ventricular tap through the shunt burr hole should be considered.

Slow Flow

▶ Partial proximal obstruction may be present.

▶ Low ventricular pressure may be present.

Burr Hole Puncture

▶ The direction of the spinal needle should not be changed during the puncture to avoid shearing of brain parenchyma.

▶ Burr hole puncture inevitably damages the shunt, necessitating operative intervention soon after alleviation of ventricular pressure.

▶ Risk of intracranial injury following ventricular puncture through the burr hole necessitates close observation and possible brain imaging after the procedure.

complications. The abrupt change in relative pressure among brain compartments can cause upward, lateral, and subdural fluid shifts. Upward and lateral pressure gradients can cause rapid intraparenchymal brain expansion along with bleeding and edema. Rapid removal of ventricular fluid can lead to tearing of subdural bridging veins and subdural hematoma formation. These complications must be weighed against the risk of acute herniation in a patient who is unresponsive or deteriorating rapidly. With a diagnostic ventricular shunt puncture, limiting the amount of cerebrospinal fluid removed and

collecting the fluid slowly and without using excessive suction should avoid most of the dangers related to fluid shifts. A ventricular puncture through the burr hole carries a greater risk for intraparenchymal damage than a shunt puncture. For this reason, patients who undergo burr hole puncture must be closely monitored after the procedure and may require reassessment by CT or MRI. As mentioned, most of these patients will proceed directly to surgery.

Risk of shunt infection after a shunt tap approaches 1%. *Staphylococcus epidermidis* is the most common pathogen isolated when a shunt is infected (2,4,6,7). Infectious complications of these procedures underscore the need for strict adherence to sterile technique.

▶ SUMMARY

Ventricular shunt puncture allows the physician to diagnose a shunt malfunction or infection and to alleviate intracranial hypertension until definitive neurosurgical intervention can be arranged. Appropriate use of this procedure requires a thorough knowledge of the proper indications and an understanding of the shunt mechanism. Careful clinical assessment and, in most cases, radiographic evaluation must precede this procedure. Ventricular tap through the burr hole is indicated in a shunted patient with cerebral herniation who has a complete proximal shunt obstruction. When successful, this procedure may be life-saving, but it must be immediately followed by revision of the ventricular shunt. Both procedures carry significant risks, including infection and hemorrhage, and should be performed only when indicated.

▶ REFERENCES

1. Noetzel MJ, Baker RP. Shunt fluid examination: risks and benefits in the evaluation of shunt malfunction and infection. *J Neurosurg.* 1984;61:328–332.

2. Kanev PM, Park TS. The treatment of hydrocephalus. *Neurosurg Clin North Am.* 1993;4:611–619.

3. Michell JJ, Ward JD. Evaluation and treatment of increased intracranial pressure. In: Kelley VC, ed. *Practice of Pediatrics.* Vol. 9. Philadelphia: Harper & Row; 1987:28–29.

4. McLaurin RL. Ventricular shunts: complications and results. In: Schut L, Venes JL, Epstein F, eds. *Pediatric Neurosurgery.* 2nd ed. Philadelphia: WB Saunders; 1989:219–229.

5. Duncan CC. Management of proximal shunt obstruction. *J Neurosurg.* 1988;68:817–819.

6. Odio C, McCracken GH, Nelson JD. CSF shunt infections in pediatrics: a 7-year experience. *Am J Dis Child.* 1984;138:1103–1108.

7. Yogev R. Cerebrospinal fluid shunt infections: a personal view. *Pediatr Infect Dis.* 1985;4:113–118.

43

GEORGE A. WOODWARD AND CAROLYN M. CAREY

Subdural Puncture

▶ INTRODUCTION

A subdural puncture (commonly referred to as a subdural "tap") is used to evacuate subdural blood or fluid. This procedure can be performed in infants when an acute or chronic subdural fluid collection is causing the child to experience symptoms of increased intracranial pressure. The procedure also can be used for diagnostic purposes in a child with potentially infected cerebrospinal fluid (subdural empyema and meningitis with effusions). Neurosurgical consultation should be obtained before this procedure whenever possible. As for the recommended age group, subdural puncture is usually performed in infants, preferably those with an open fontanelle. The procedure can also be performed in patients with fibrous or split sutures (up to approximately 18 months of age). A similar procedure has been described in adults (1).

▶ ANATOMY AND PHYSIOLOGY

The subdural space lies beneath the skin, subcutaneous tissue, skull, and dura (Fig. 43.1). The major landmark for a subdural tap is the lateral margin of the anterior fontanelle, which is formed by the coronal suture. Subdural fluid collections can be acute, subacute, or chronic and can result from trauma or infection (2,3). Disruption of the bridging veins that traverse the dura is a major factor leading to formation of a subdural hematoma (4). Dural or sinus tears and repeated needle punctures of the fontanelle also are known causes. Transudates and exudates can occur and may be loculated. Identification of a subdural fluid collection as the etiology of increased intracranial pressure can allow rapid reversal of symptoms with the successful removal of fluid. These collections are best diagnosed by computed tomography (CT) or magnetic resonance imaging (MRI) of the brain.

▶ INDICATIONS

Physiologic parameters that suggest the therapeutic need for a subdural tap include those signs and symptoms associated with increased intracranial pressure. These include mental status changes, irritability, somnolence, pallor, lethargy, vomiting, full or bulging fontanelle, third or sixth nerve palsies, respiratory irregularity, unconsciousness, coma, posturing, seizures, hypotonia, hemiparesis, and spasticity (see also Chapters 42 and 44). The fluid can be an acute or subacute blood collection from trauma or a transudate or exudate that accompanies a central nervous system infection.

Subdural puncture can be used as a therapeutic and diagnostic tool to verify the presence of fluid, identify the type of fluid, and decrease the intracranial pressure (5,6). This invasive procedure should always be reviewed with a neurosurgical consultant before proceeding if time allows. Imaging of the brain using ultrasound (if the patient has an open fontanelle), CT, or MRI should also be performed before undertaking this procedure whenever possible. MRI of the head prior to the tap can be especially useful in cases of suspected intentional trauma to document the presence and age of the blood collection before evacuation. Repeated subdural taps to remove residual fluid are rarely indicated; reaccumulation of fluid generally warrants drain placement by a neurosurgeon. Contraindications to performing subdural puncture include bleeding abnormalities, overlying infected skin, and age outside the infant-toddler group.

▶ EQUIPMENT

Sterile gloves, drapes
Mask
Immobilizer (papoose board) (see Chapter 3)

522

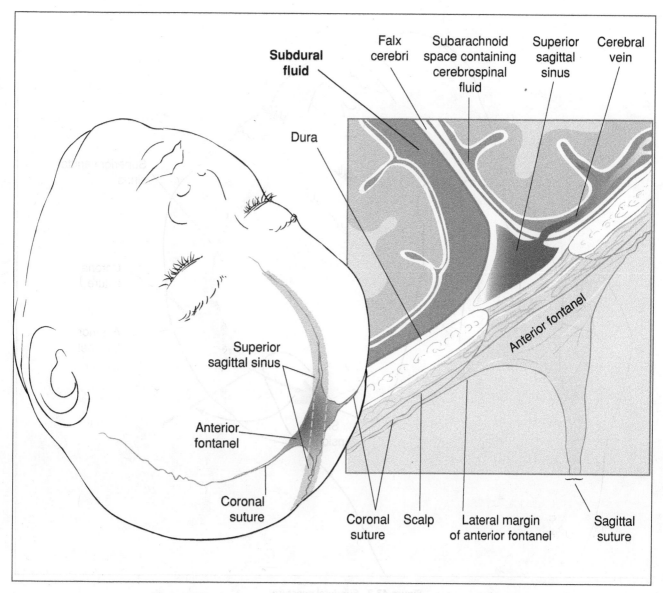

Figure 43.1 Anatomy of the subdural space adjacent to the anterior fontanelle.

Povidone-iodine solution

Alcohol

18- to 22-gauge, 1.5-inch subdural or spinal needle with stylet (can also use an 18- to 22-gauge over-the-needle intravenous catheter)

Local anesthetic if desired (lidocaine with epinephrine)

Sterile gauze, cotton

Dressing material

Cardiac monitor, pulse oximeter

Resuscitative equipment, personnel as needed

▶ PROCEDURE

The child should be in the supine position and secured in an immobilizer, with additional head stabilization provided by an experienced assistant. Sedation can be considered for the agitated patient. Resuscitative equipment should be identified and readily available for immediate use as needed. All appropriate resuscitative maneuvers should have been attended to before this point. The patient should be physically and mechanically monitored at all times during the procedure. A small area of hair should be clipped or shaved around the intended puncture site. The skin is then cleansed with povidone-iodine or another appropriate sterilizing solution. Local anesthetic can be infiltrated in the skin at the area of intended puncture. Strict aseptic technique should be observed, including sterile gloves, masks, instruments, and field.

Once the area has been prepared, a subdural needle (18- to 22-gauge, 1.5-inch spinal needle) or an 18- to 22-gauge over-the-needle intravenous catheter should be inserted at a 90-degree angle (to the transverse plane of the skull) through stretched skin at the lateral margin of the anterior fontanelle (Fig. 43.2). The site can be identified at the junction of the

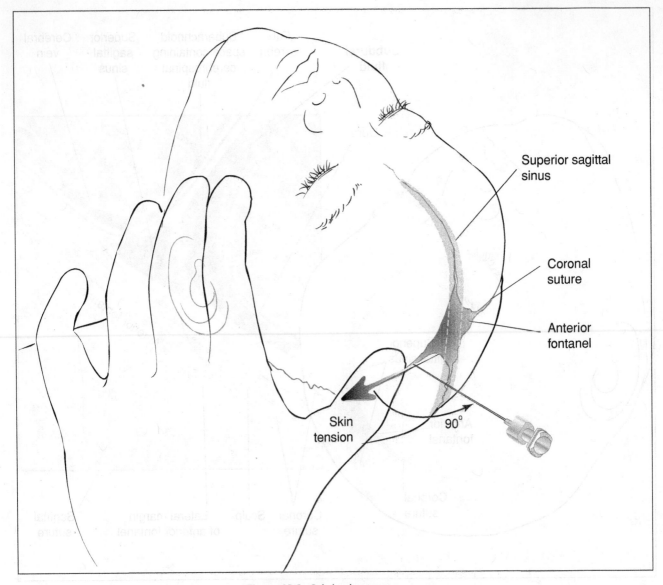

Superior sagittal
sinus

Coronal
suture

Anterior
fontanel

Skin
tension

90°

Figure 43.2 Subdural puncture.

coronal and parietal sutures, where the coronal suture forms the lateral margin of the anterior fontanelle. If the anterior fontanelle is small, the physician should make the puncture 5 to 10 mm laterally in the coronal suture (at least 2 cm from the midline) to avoid entering the sagittal sinus and associated vessels. As a rule of thumb, the site of needle insertion should be either the most lateral area of the fontanelle or the point where an imaginary line drawn from the ipsilateral pupil intersects the suture line, whichever is farther from the midline (7).

By stretching the skin before inserting the needle through the fontanelle, the physician can effectively establish a Z-track and help minimize the possibility of postprocedure fluid leak. The needle should be secured in the physician's hand and with the heel of the hand against the infant's scalp to prevent a deep puncture with inadvertent head or table motion. The needle should be advanced slowly through the skin and suture line until the subdural space is entered. The physician may feel decreased resistance as the needle enters the subdural space. This should be at a distance of approximately 5 to 10 mm. Once the space is entered, the stylet is removed from the subdural or spinal needle or the needle is removed from the intravenous catheter. Correct positioning of a subdural or spinal needle can be maintained by clamping the needle at the skin with a hemostat. This prevents inadvertent and potentially dangerous advancement of the needle.

The fluid should drain spontaneously. Extension tubing placed on a T-connector may assist drainage by the siphoning effect. Suction should not be applied to the needle (8). Cessation of fluid flow does not necessarily indicate that the subdural space has been completely emptied (and should not be an anticipated endpoint of the procedure) but rather that pressures are now equal between the intracranial and extracranial areas. Drainage of up to 80 mL can be tolerated (7). The procedure can also be terminated when the child becomes asymptomatic and the fontanelle becomes soft or scaphoid (3). After the needle or catheter is removed, a gentle pressure dressing should be applied to the puncture site (5,9).

The fluid should be collected for laboratory tests (e.g., hematocrit, bacterial or fungal culture, Gram stain, glucose, protein, cell count, differential) as indicated. The procedure can be performed on the opposite side, although most subdural cavities will communicate, and bilateral taps are therefore rarely needed. Repeated subdural punctures, if indicated, should be accomplished under the direct guidance of a pediatric neurosurgeon. External drain placement should be con-

 CLINICAL TIPS

▶ If possible, a cerebral imaging study should be performed before subdural puncture, especially when intentional head trauma (child abuse) is suspected.

▶ Bilateral or repeated subdural punctures are rarely needed.

▶ Consultation with a pediatric neurosurgeon is indicated whenever possible before a subdural puncture.

sidered if repeated subdural taps are necessary, and a shunt may be required if external drainage fails (6,10).

▶ COMPLICATIONS

Suction applied to the indwelling subdural needle or inadvertent vessel puncture can cause vascular tears or lacerations and increase the blood component of the already compromised subdural space. In addition, overly rapid decompression of the cerebral cortex may cause venous engorgement and/or cerebral edema (5). However, a pial vessel, if lacerated, will usually stop bleeding without intervention. A persistent leak can occur from the site of the subdural puncture. If this occurs, a gentle pressure dressing with cotton or collodion usually suffices to seal the leak.

Other complications include contusion or laceration of the underlying cerebral cortex and introduction of infection. It should be noted that a subdural tap in the recommended location may not identify localized or loculated occipital or basal subdural fluid collections.

▶ SUMMARY

A subdural puncture to remove fluid from the subdural space in infants can be a diagnostic, stabilizing, and/or life-saving procedure. The procedure should always be performed with careful attention to sterile technique and with an awareness of the complications that may be encountered. As with all invasive pediatric procedures, resuscitative personnel and equipment should be immediately available if needed.

 SUMMARY

1 Seek neurosurgical consultation prior to the procedure if time allows.

2 Immobilize the patient in a supine position and ensure that appropriate monitoring, ancillary personnel and resuscitation equipment are available.

3 Wear a surgical mask and sterile gloves.

4 Prepare the puncture site (lateral margin of the anterior fontanelle) by shaving a small area of hair.

5 Vigorously clean the site with povidone-iodine solution applied in a circular fashion from the puncture site outward.

6 Drape the area with sterile surgical towels.

7 Inject local anesthetic intradermally if desired; aspirate prior to injection to ensure that inadvertent subdural injection of anesthetic does not occur.

8 Stretch skin overlying the puncture site to form a Z-track.

9 Insert spinal needle or over-the-needle intravenous catheter and release skin.

10 Advance the needle slowly to a maximum depth of 1 cm at the lateral margin of the anterior fontanelle at a 90-degree angle to the transverse plane; if the fontanelle is closed but the suture is still fibrous (up to 18 months of age), insert the needle in a similar fashion at least 2 cm from the midline through the coronal suture, in line with the ipsilateral pupil.

11 Secure the needle in place with a hemostat applied at the base of spinal needle.

12 Allow fluid to drain without using suction.

13 Apply a gentle, sterile pressure dressing when the procedure is completed.

▶ REFERENCES

1. Aoki N. Percutaneous subdural tapping for the treatment of chronic subdural haematoma in adults. *Neurol Res.* 1987;9:19–23.
2. McLaurin RL, Towbin R. Posttraumatic hematomas. In: McLaurin RL, Schut L, Venes JL, et al., eds. *Pediatric Neurosurgery.* 2nd ed. Philadelphia: WB Saunders; 1989:277–289.

3. Aronyk KE. Subdural and epidural hematoma. In: McLone DG, ed. *Pediatric Neurosurgery: Surgery of the Developing Nervous System.* 4th ed. Philadelphia: WB Saunders; 2001:646–653.

4. Choux M, Lena G, Genitori L. Intracranial hematomas. In: Raimondi AJ, Choux M, Di Rocco C, eds. *Head Injuries in the Newborn and Infant.* New York: Springer-Verlag; 1986:203–216.

5. Ingraham FD, Matson DD. Subdural hematoma in infancy. *J Pediatr.* 1944;24:1–37.

6. Till K. Subdural hematoma and effusion in infancy. *Br Med J.* 1968;3:400–402.

7. Punt J. Congenital defects, vascular malformations, and other lesions.

In: Levene MI, Chervenek FA, Whittle MJ, eds. *Fetal and Neonatal Neurology and Neurosurgery.* London: Churchill Livingstone; 2001:775–787.

8. Sauter KL. Percutaneous subdural tapping and subdural peritoneal drainage for the treatment of subdural hematoma. *Neurosurg Clin North Am.* 2000;11:519–524.

9. McLaurin RL. Posttraumatic hematomas. In: Section of Pediatric Neurosurgery of the American Association of Neurologic Surgeons, ed. *Pediatric Neurosurgery: Surgery of the Developing Nervous System.* New York: Grune & Stratton; 1982:309–319.

10. Collins WF, Pucci GL. Peritoneal drainage of subdural hematomas in infants. *J Pediatr.* 1961;58:482–485.

44

JAMES F. WILEY, II AND ANN-CHRISTINE DUHAIME

Ventricular Puncture

▶ INTRODUCTION

Ventricular puncture refers to the removal of cerebrospinal fluid directly from the intracranial ventricular system by way of an open fontanel or suture. The procedure is appropriate for young patients with signs of impending brain herniation from acute untreated hydrocephalus. Once excess fluid is removed, definitive treatment with a ventriculoperitoneal (VP) shunt follows. A ventricular puncture requires a thorough knowledge of anatomy and an understanding of the risks and benefits of the procedure. Ideally, a neurosurgeon should perform a ventricular puncture. When a neurosurgeon is unavailable, only the most experienced physician should attempt this procedure. The need for a ventricular puncture implies that the patient is unstable from untreated intracranial hypertension. For this reason, the physician should perform the procedure in an area where acute decompensation can be quickly managed, such as an emergency department (ED), intensive care unit, or operating room.

▶ ANATOMY AND PHYSIOLOGY

The anterior horn of the lateral ventricle lies directly beneath the lateral border of the anterior fontanel, an area of nonossified tissue in the skull that allows for brain growth (Fig. 44.1). The anterior fontanelle remains "open" until it is gradually replaced by bony skull at around 12 to 18 months of age. This area corresponds to the coronal suture in an older child, which is approximately 2 cm from the midline. In a patient with hydrocephalus, dilation of the ventricles creates a large potential site for puncture. Most importantly, the physician must not puncture too close to the sagittal midline, where the venous sagittal sinus is located (Fig. 44.1).

Hydrocephalus occurs under two conditions: obstructive hydrocephalus, in which a physical blockage of the ventricular system is present, and communicating hydrocephalus, in which the capacity to absorb cerebrospinal fluid is exceeded by the production of cerebrospinal fluid. Common causes of chronic obstructive hydrocephalus include congenital aqueductal stenosis, posterior fossa tumors, and other congenital anomalies (e.g., Dandy-Walker malformation). Meningitis is the most common cause of communicating hydrocephalus. Acute decompensation with cerebral herniation is more likely to occur in a patient with acute obstructive hydrocephalus, which may complicate head trauma, intracranial hemorrhage, or space-occupying lesions (e.g., abscess, tumor) that impinge on the ventricular system (I).

▶ INDICATIONS

The primary indication for ventricular puncture is cerebral herniation due to hydrocephalus that is unresponsive to hyperventilation and diuretics in a patient with an open fontanel or coronal suture. Physical findings suggestive of this condition include unilateral or bilateral pupillary dilation, ocular cranial nerve abnormalities, focal neurologic findings, and decorticate or decerebrate posturing (see also Chapters 42 and 43). Before performing ventricular puncture, the physician must consider other potential causes of these findings for which this procedure would not be indicated, such as brain tumor without hydrocephalus, head trauma with cerebral edema, subdural hematoma, and epidural hematoma. Consultation and concurrent management with a neurosurgeon, as well an imaging study such as computed tomography (CT) or magnetic resonance imaging (MRI) of the head or cerebral ultrasound, should precede the procedure whenever possible. Ventricular puncture is not indicated for the patient with hydrocephalus who is asymptomatic. Furthermore, a patient with a closed fontanel and sutures requires a surgical approach to the ventricular system.

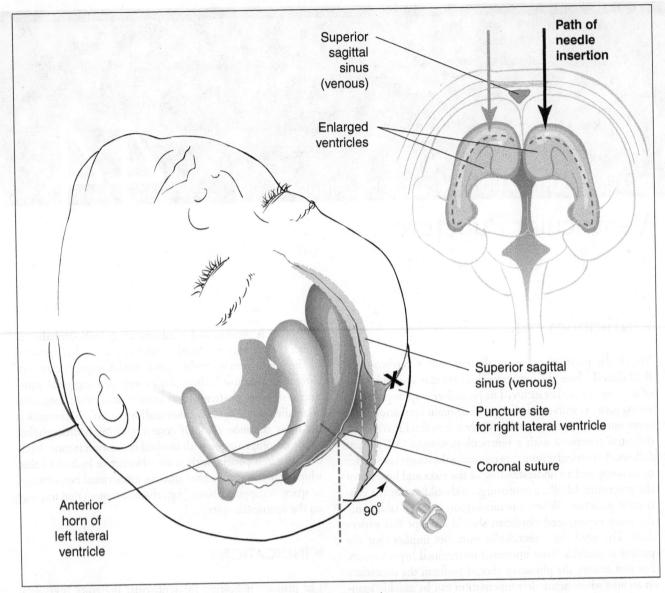

Figure 44.1 Ventricular puncture.

▶ EQUIPMENT

Isopropyl alcohol
Betadine
18-gauge, 2.5-inch spinal needle
Sterile 10 mL syringe
Sterile test tubes
Sterile towels

▶ PROCEDURE

Because performance of this procedure assumes ongoing herniation, the patient should be positioned with the head elevated at 30 degrees. The child must be restrained to prevent inadvertent movement (see Chapter 3). The puncture site is first cleansed with alcohol. The hair may be clipped or shaved to provide a 2 cm diameter area at the lateral border of the anterior fontanel or over the coronal suture approximately 2 cm from the midline. The site should then be thoroughly cleansed with Betadine using repetitive center-to-circumference motions (Images).

The needle enters the skin perpendicular to the skull at the lateral border of the anterior fontanel or through the coronal suture at least 2 cm from the sagittal midline (Fig. 44.1). The needle is advanced slowly, with a check for fluid return every centimeter. The direction of the spinal needle should not be changed while it is advanced. Alternatively, the stylet may be removed from the spinal needle after the skin is punctured, followed by attachment of a syringe that is advanced with gentle suction until cerebrospinal fluid is obtained. Enough fluid is removed to reverse signs and symptoms of herniation (2,3).

SUMMARY

1 Restrain the patient to prevent inadvertent motion.

2 Position the patient with the head elevated at 30 degrees.

3 Prepare the site (lateral border of anterior fontanel or coronal suture 2 cm from the midline) using alcohol.

4 Shave or clip hair to provide a 2 cm diameter area around the site.

5 Cleanse the puncture site vigorously with Betadine.

6 If possible, stretch skin over the puncture site to displace it slightly before the puncture; this will "zigzag" the puncture tract to help seal it after completion.

7 Puncture the skin at the lateral border of the anterior fontanel or through the coronal suture 2 cm from the midline with an 18-gauge, 2.5- or 3.5-inch spinal needle.

8 Release the skin, then direct and advance the needle perpendicular to skull (straight in).

9 Advance the needle slowly, checking for fluid return every centimeter *or* remove the stylet and attach a syringe and advance slowly with gentle suction.

10 Remove fluid until the signs and symptoms of herniation subside.

11 Withdraw the spinal needle slowly.

 CLINICAL TIPS

▶ Once symptoms are relieved, the needle should be removed slowly until CSF flow ceases. If repeated punctures are likely to be needed, it may be helpful to note the depth at which drainage is no longer obtained as an estimate of cortical width.

▶ The direction of the spinal needle should not be changed, nor should the needle be rotated in the skull. To change the direction of puncture, the spinal needle must be withdrawn to skin level.

▶ COMPLICATIONS

A ventricular puncture carries a high risk of potentially life-threatening complications, such as intracranial hemorrhage, parenchymal damage, and subdural hematoma. Ventriculitis or even cerebral abscess may occur following a ventricular puncture if a lapse in sterile technique occurs. Inadvertent puncture of the sagittal venous sinus results from a ventricular puncture performed too close to the midline. Subsequent bleeding may be difficult to control, potentially leading to severe brain injury or death. By necessity, a ventricular puncture causes damage to brain parenchyma. This damage is increased if the spinal needle is passed in multiple directions, with shearing of the brain matter. Finally, rapid removal of fluid may lead to a shrinkage in brain size that can cause transection of subdural bridging veins, with subdural hematoma formation. The serious nature of potential complications after a ventricular puncture dictates close assessment of the patient after the procedure, ideally with immediate imaging by CT or MRI once the patient is stabilized.

▶ SUMMARY

A ventricular puncture is indicated for a patient with hydrocephalus and an open anterior fontanel or coronal suture who shows advanced signs of cerebral herniation that are unresponsive to hyperventilation and diuretic therapy. This procedure may be life-saving in this setting but carries significant risks of infection, parenchymal brain damage, and intracranial bleeding. After a ventricular puncture, the patient requires close observation and immediate brain imaging.

▶ REFERENCES

1. Milhorat TH. Acute hydrocephalus. *N Engl J Med.* 1970;283:857–859.
2. Perret G, Meyers R. Neurosurgery in infants and children. *Pediatr Clin North Am.* 1960;7:543–582.
3. Mapstone TB, Ratcheson RA. Techniques of ventricular puncture In: Wilkins RH, Rengachary SS, eds. *Neurosurgery.* 2nd ed. New York: McGraw-Hill; 1996:180.

SECTION 7 ▶ OPHTHALMOLOGIC PROCEDURES

SECTION EDITOR: RICHARD M. RUDDY

45

ALEX V. LEVIN

General Pediatric Ophthalmologic Procedures

▶ INTRODUCTION

Physicians caring for children will be confronted with a number of ocular problems, including trauma, infection, inflammation, and ocular manifestations of systemic disease. Although management of some ocular conditions will require consultation by an ophthalmologist, initial diagnosis and management can be greatly facilitated by a familiarity with basic ocular procedures that lie within the skills of pediatricians and emergency physicians (1–4).

▶ OPENING THE LIDS

One of the most challenging procedures is to adequately visualize the external ocular structures when obscured by lid swelling or when a noncompliant, fearful child refuses to voluntarily allow the eyelids to be opened. Selection of the appropriate technique depends on circumstance and equipment availability. Once the eyeball is visualized, the examiner then can make the appropriate triage decision: ophthalmology consultation (hyphema, full thickness or lid margin laceration, corneal ulcer, corneal/scleral laceration), treatment (bacterial conjunctivitis, corneal abrasion), or observation (viral conjunctivitis). The eye can be evaluated in a logical, progressive anatomical fashion, with consideration given to each structure separately and in order—eye movements, visual acuity,

conjunctiva, cornea, anterior chamber, pupil, lens, optic nerve, and retina.

Anatomy and Physiology

The skin of the eyelids is quite loose and redundant, which allows for the marked accumulation of fluid. As the tissues become increasingly distended, the lids become tense and more difficult to open. The eyelashes are inserted in the lid margin at the edge of each lid. The lid margin acts as a focal point for the application of mechanical devices designed to separate the lids for visualization of the underlying eyeball (Fig. 45.1). Forced lid closure is largely accomplished by contraction of the orbicularis oculi muscle. If the examiner places pressure on the bony insertions of this muscle, its contractile force is greatly disadvantaged.

Manual Lid Opening

Indications

This technique is best used for the noncompliant child who is firmly squeezing the eyelids closed. It also can be used to facilitate the instillation of eye drops or ointments. This procedure also can be used in any type of lid swelling, including trauma, as it allows for the lids to be opened without putting undue pressure on the globe.

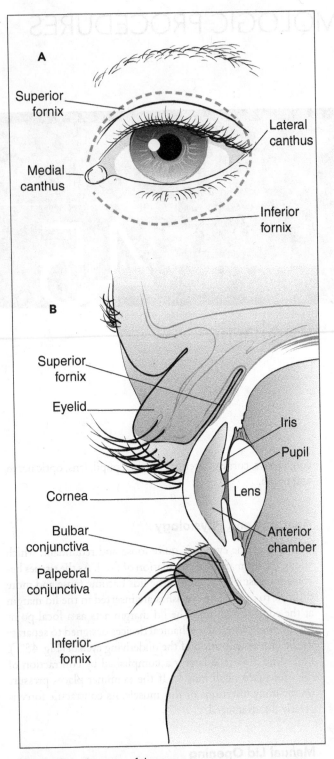

Figure 45.1 Anatomy of the eye.

Equipment
None.

Procedure
With the child's head gently restrained in the supine position (or in an examining chair with the head tilted back), the thumb of one hand is placed on the supraorbital rim (eyebrow), and

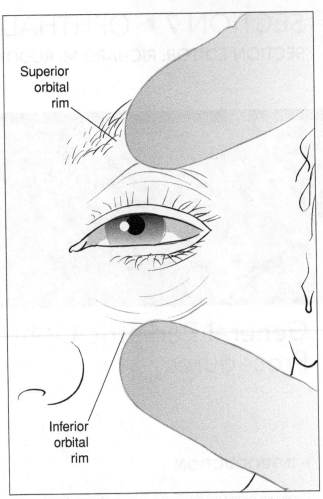

Figure 45.2 Manual eye opening. Pressure on the bone at the insertion of the orbicularis oculi disadvantages the muscle and prevents forced eyelid closure. Do not exert any pressure on the globe.

the fingers or thumb of the other hand on the infraorbital rim. Pressure is applied at these two locations compressing the underlying muscle firmly against the bone (Fig. 45.2). This is not a painful procedure. While pressure is being applied, the thumbs and underlying tissue are moved superiorly (upper hand) and inferiorly (lower hand), thus dragging the lids open. The thumbs or fingers should not be placed on the eyelids, as this may cause lid eversion or pressure on the eyeball.

Complications
The major complication of this technique is extrusion of intraocular contents if an underlying unrecognized laceration of the globe is present. This risk is reduced in the setting of trauma by selecting this procedure only for compliant children.

Summary
Manual lid opening is an excellent technique that requires no equipment and allows for the opening of virtually any lids.

Care must be taken in a trauma setting to avoid putting manual pressure on a potentially ruptured globe.

Lid Opening with Cotton-Tipped Swabs

Indications

Although this procedure can be very useful in opening swollen or forcibly closed lids, particularly in infants, it should *not* be used in the traumatized eye until the presence of a ruptured globe has been ruled out, as this procedure will put pressure on the globe.

Equipment

The examiner should use a cotton-tipped applicator of the usual bulk but with a short wooden or plastic stick handle. If only applicators with long sticks are available, then the examiner should either break the stick to within a few inches of the tip or be sure to grasp the stick close to the tip. This helps to avoid potentially harmful breakage of the stick during the procedure.

Procedure

While standing beside the supine patient's head, ipsilateral to the eye to be examined, and with the child's head gently restrained, one applicator tip is placed on the midbody of the upper lid, and the other in a similar position on the lower lid (Fig. 45.3A). With just enough pressure to engage the skin, the swabs are rotated (i.e., twirled) approximately one-quarter to one-half turn in the direction of the lashes (Fig. 45.3B). This will begin to draw the lid margins apart. The tips are then depressed with some firmness posteriorly (towards the underlying eyeball), engaging the entire thickness of the lid, and simultaneously the swabs are separated from each other in the direction of the orbital rims—the upper lid swab moving superiorly and the lower swab inferiorly (Fig. 45.3C).

Complications

If the swabs are not applied firmly to the lids or if the rotation is in the wrong direction, the lids will evert, thus making visualization even more difficult. If the swab sticks are too long, they may break during the procedure, possibly causing injury to the globe. Rolling the swabs too far toward the eyelid margin might allow the swabs to roll onto the corneal surface and can result in a corneal abrasion.

Summary

Using cotton-tipped swabs allows for wide, controlled separation of the lids. Swabs should not be used in the traumatized eye until rupture of the globe has been excluded.

▶ LID SPECULA

Indications

Virtually no contraindications to speculum insertion exist. Specula do not put pressure on the globe and can therefore be used to open lids swollen by trauma. They are also useful in noncompliant children with voluntary forced lid closure, provided the child is not old enough to generate more force than the speculum can apply. A speculum can be used to open eyelids that are swollen or otherwise involuntarily closed for virtually any reason.

Equipment

A variety of pediatric lid specula are commercially available. When purchasing a speculum, considerations should include tensile strength (to resist spontaneous extrusion with the child's voluntary forced lid closure), size (to allow easy insertion, particularly in infants), cost, and ease of handling. The Alfonso eye speculum is useful in the greatest number of

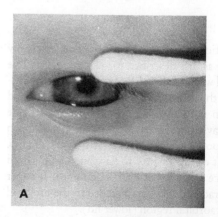 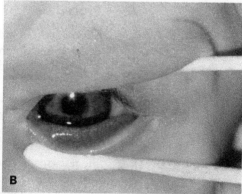 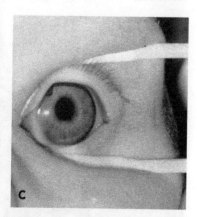

Figure 45.3 Opening eye with cotton-tipped swabs.
A. Swabs are placed against upper and lower lids.
B. Gentle pressure and a one-quarter rotation toward the lid margin have engaged the upper lid without eversion. However, the lower swab has been rotated away from the margin, resulting in lid eversion.
C. Lower lid swab now rotated correctly toward lid margin to avoid eversion. Swabs are separated to visualize the eyeball.

situations because it has good tensile strength, a small open blade that can be inserted into palpebral openings of virtually any size, reasonable cost, and a thumb rest to facilitate ease of handling. Specula that are bulky or that require screw mechanisms to keep them in place are usually not desirable in the emergency setting and require more skill to insert. Specula and retractors should be sterilized between patients.

Procedure

Before inserting the speculum, the child should be supine and gently restrained to prevent spontaneous movement of the head. A drop of topical anesthetic (proparacaine or tetracaine) must be instilled. Onset of action of these drugs is within 30 seconds. Arms of the speculum are grasped between the thumb and forefinger. The first blade can be inserted onto the margin of either the upper or lower lid. The examiner should gently retract the lid away from its fellow lid to expose the lid margin so that the corresponding speculum blade can be placed on the lid margin (Fig. 45.4). The speculum is then compressed closed while the engaged lid is pushed away so that the fellow lid can be engaged with the remaining speculum blade on its lid margin. The speculum is then slowly and gently released to allow the lids to separate with it.

Complications

Although specula are fashioned in such a way that, with the assistance of the normally present corneal tear film, they glide easily over the ocular surface, they may on rare occasion induce corneal abrasion. Despite the use of topical anesthetic, some patients object to the periocular "stretching" sensation, which might in turn increase agitation and combative behavior. Specula also may cause the extension of a pre-existing lid laceration.

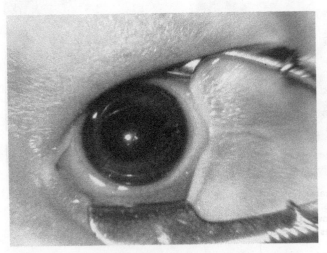

Figure 45.4 Lid speculum in use. Topical anesthetic should be instilled before lid speculum placement.

Summary

Specula can be expensive but provide an easy and effective way to achieve lid separation. They can be used in any situation to facilitate examination of the eyeball.

▶ LID RETRACTORS

Indications

Retractors can be used in virtually any situation where the lids need to be separated in an assisted fashion. They tend to be less disturbing to the agitated patient than specula, as they cause less stretching discomfort.

Equipment

Lid retractors operate on only one lid at a time, although two can be used simultaneously to retract both lids. The most commonly used commercial type is the Desmarres retractor, which is available in a number of sizes. A small (size I) Desmarres is perhaps most practical in the pediatric emergency setting because it can be used on any size patient. If this commercial retractor is too costly or not available, the examiner can easily construct a disposable retractor out of paper clips (Fig. 45.5A). The paper clip type chosen for this usage should be smooth metal and not coated. The coating on some clips may fragment when the clip is bent, creating particles that can disperse onto the conjunctiva or cornea. After bending, it would be prudent to double-check the bent clip to be certain no such particles have formed. Such paper clip retractors are intended for single usage and should be prepared by cleansing with an alcohol swab prior to use. Like specula, retractors do not put pressure on the globe.

Procedure

The patient is positioned and the eye anesthetized topically in the same fashion as just described for using specula. The retractor can be held with the thumb and forefinger, approaching one lid (usually the upper) at a 90-degree angle to the lid margin. The margin is then engaged by the retractor blade and pulled back away from the fellow lid while care is taken not to lift the lid too far off the surface of the eyeball (Fig. 45.5B). If needed, it can be helpful to have an assistant hold the retractor in place while the eyeball is examined. If paper clips are used as retractors, they can be taped to the forehead (upper lid) and infraorbital region (lower lid).

Complications

Like specula, retractors can result in corneal abrasion or extension of a pre-existing lid laceration. Paper clip retractors may

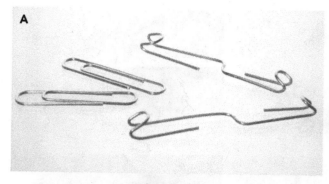

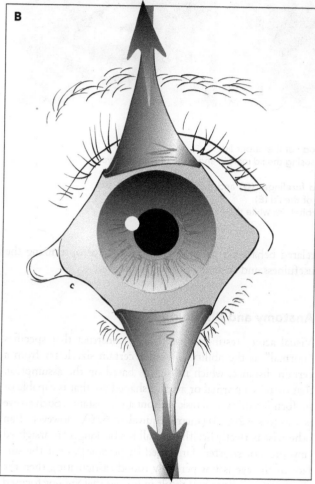

Figure 45.5
A. Lid retractors fashioned out of paper clips.
B. Desmarres lid retractors separate lids after topical anesthetic is instilled.

allow for the deposition of tiny particulate matter loosened from the clip surface when it is bent into position.

Summary

Retractors offer the examiner a handy, comfortable way to move the lids apart. When used properly, retractors are safe even in the setting of eye trauma.

▶ EVERTING THE UPPER EYELID

Introduction

This is a basic technique that should be mastered by all primary care physicians and emergency personnel. It allows for rapid inspection of the undersurface of the upper lid with minimal discomfort.

Anatomy and Physiology

The upper lid contains a band of dense collagenous tissue (tarsal plate) that spans the majority of the horizontal width of the lid and rises to occupy approximately 60% of the lid height from the lid margin upward. If pressure is applied to the lid just above the superior border of this plate, a fulcrum point is created whereby the lower section of the lid can be rotated upward, thus folding the lid back on itself so that its undersurface (the palpebral conjunctiva) comes into view.

Indications

Eversion of the eyelid is useful when the examiner wishes to view the palpebral conjunctiva of the upper lid. The lid is everted to search for foreign bodies, to facilitate complete lavage following chemical exposure, and to visualize changes diagnostic of various types of conjunctivitis.

Procedure

The key to success when performing upper lid eversion is to have the child keep the eyes in downward gaze (Fig. 45.6A). Repetitively reminding the child to keep looking down throughout the procedure is very helpful. The procedure is extremely difficult in the noncompliant child who is crying or refusing to open the eyes. Examination with sedation or ophthalmology consultation may be required. In the compliant patient, the lid can be everted with the patient supine, cradled in the arms of the parent, or sitting.

A cotton-tipped applicator (vide supra) is placed on the midbody of the upper lid with just enough pressure to engage the skin (Fig. 45.6B). The applicator is rotated toward the lid margin with just enough pressure against the eyelid skin to draw the skin up under the applicator, causing the lid margin and lashes to rotate away from the eyeball (Fig. 45.6C). The lashes or the full thickness lid margin are grasped between the thumb and forefinger and then simultaneously pulled upward (toward the forehead) while applicator tip is pushed into the body of the lid in a downward direction: the lid margin and the swab are moving in directly opposite but parallel directions (Fig. 45.6D,E). The lower half of the lid should abruptly "flip" over the swab. The examiner can then use the thumb of the hand holding the lashes to pin the lashes against the superior orbital rim or eyebrow while the examination is conducted (Fig. 45.6F). At this point, the swab is removed by

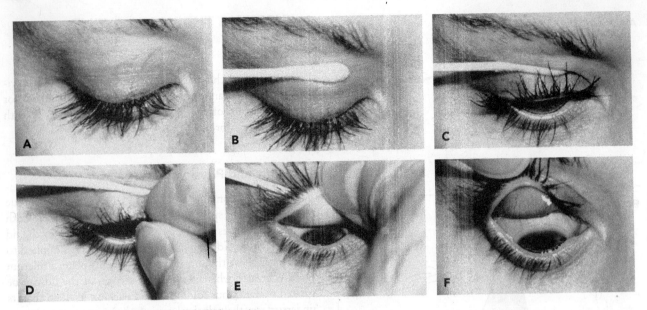

Figure 45.6 Upper eyelid eversion.
A. The child is asked to look downward.
B. A cotton-tipped applicator is placed on the midbody of the upper lid.
C. The applicator is rotated toward the lid margin, causing the lid margin and lashes to rotate away from the eyeball.
D,E. The lashes are grasped between the thumb and forefinger **(D)** and pulled upward while the applicator tip is pushed downward into the body of the lid **(E)**.
F. The thumb pins the lashes against the superior orbital rim while the examination is conducted.

pulling it straight out laterally away from the face. Removal of the swab may require a firm tug.

If a foreign body is seen, it can be removed gently with a cotton swab or, if embedded, plucked away with a nontoothed forceps. This type of manipulation usually requires topical anesthetic.

Complications

Lid eversion is a painless procedure when done properly, although it may be associated with an unfamiliar and uncomfortable sensation. Instillation of topical anesthetic may be helpful. Extension of a corneal laceration can occur if pressure is inadvertently put on the underlying eyeball following trauma. This procedure should be avoided if a ruptured globe is present or suspected.

Summary

Lid eversion is a technique used for inspection of the undersurface of the upper lid, particularly when searching for a foreign body or during ocular lavage. It is relatively easy to perform on most compliant children and very useful in the emergency care of children.

▶ VISUAL ACUITY TESTING

Introduction

Visual acuity testing is the foundation of the eye examination. A basic understanding of the pediatric visual system and age-

related behavioral patterns is important for optimizing the usefulness and accuracy of this procedure.

Anatomy and Physiology

Visual acuity testing is based on a construct that specifies "normal" as the ability to read a certain size letter from a certain distance, which in turn is based on the assumption that there is a normal or average shaped eye that is capable of performing this visual task without any assistance. Such an eye is said to see 20/20 (metric equivalent 6/6). However, if an otherwise perfectly healthy eyeball is a bit longer (nearsighted [myopic]) or shorter (farsighted [hyperopic]), or if the surface of the eye is not perfectly round (astigmatic), then the abnormal eye shape will result in images that are not focused on the desired spot on the retina. This results in a blurry image. For example, a person who sees 20/60 (metric 6/18) has to stand at 20 feet (6 meters) to see what the normal 20/20 (metric 6/6) individual can see standing at 60 feet (18 meters). Glasses can correct this problem by altering the pathway of light so that the image that is being viewed is redirected to fall crisply on the retina. It is this corrected visual acuity that is the true measure of ocular health. Only if an organic abnormality exists (e.g., retinal trauma, optic nerve problem, cataract, hyphema) will a reduction occur in the best corrected visual acuity.

Although the visual acuity of each eye is independent of the visual acuity of the other eye, another important consideration is the unconscious desire for the immature pediatric visual system to use the better eye. Not only will children demonstrate behavioral alterations when their better eye is covered, but they also may engage in somewhat unconscious behaviors in an attempt to use their better eye for testing, despite the efforts of the examiner to prevent this from occurring. As a result, the child will capitalize on any breech in technique to allow the better eye to become the seeing eye. The child will look around a handheld occluding device, look through the tiny gaps between the fingers of the hand that is covering the eye, or turn his or her face to look around an occluding device or hand while reading a chart straight ahead. The examiner must constantly be alert for these behaviors to avoid inaccuracy. It is this demanding preference for the better eye that results in amblyopia, a condition unique to the developing visual system in which the brain ignores the development of vision in an eye that is not preferred and instead solely uses the better eye without the child sensing that he or she is functioning with only one eye.

Indications

Virtually all patients who present with an ocular complaint, and many who present with neurologic complaints, should have their visual acuity measured. Even the preverbal patient and the supine patient, both of whom are unable to read the standard wall chart, should have some estimation made of their visual acuity.

Equipment

Occlusion of the eye that is not being tested is perhaps best achieved by covering this eye with a broad (2 inch), lightly adhesive, hypoallergenic tape. In the absence of tape, or when the child objects to the application of tape, the palm of an examiner's or caretaker's hand can be used. Never cover the eye with fingers, as this will always allow peeking through tiny cracks between fingers.

Selection of a testing chart is based on the child's developmental age and reading capabilities. The illiterate child can be tested with an Allen picture chart in black and white that uses standardized figures representing a cake, car, hand, telephone, and person on a horse. Color picture charts are available for use, but it is recommended that the yellow figures be ignored, as low-contrast differential between the yellow and background white, particularly in a brightly lit emergency department, can lead to errors not reflective of the true visual acuity. Other charts are available for the illiterate child, including the tumbling E chart (also known as the "illiterate E"), in which the child is asked to indicate the direction in which a capital letter E is pointing. However, this can often be quite confusing to younger children, who are not yet able to describe and point appropriately due to insufficient coordination and poorly developed handedness. Matching systems, such as the HOTV card or the Sheridan Gardiner testing cards, allow the child who is entering the age of literacy to use a rudimentary knowledge of letters to match projected or letters hand held at a distance with a card that is held in his or her own hand and contains identical letters. This is also particularly helpful in children between the ages of 3 and 6 years who are capable of performing visual recognition and identification but too frightened or developmentally immature to venture a spoken guess. For children who are fluently familiar with the letters of the alphabet, the readily available standard Snellen letter chart is recommended. Although the charts are available in different sizes, a standard chart designed to be read at 20 feet (6 m) can be used at virtually any distance. If the chart location only permits the patient to stand at 10 feet (3 m), then the value of each line is approximately doubled (the 20/20 line would have a 20/40 value).

Procedure

With visual acuity testing, the unaffected eye is tested first. This is particularly helpful in young children who may be fearful or shy. They can become familiar with the testing procedure and gain confidence in their performance using their better eye. The appropriate chart is selected and the desired eye occluded. When using occluding tape, the examiner must ensure that the child is not able to peek out medially or laterally around the edge of the tape, which should be pressed firmly against the bridge of the nose and the lateral orbital rim. The patient should be placed at the proper distance, while the examiner stands next to the wall chart. This allows the examiner to observe the child during testing to ensure that no cheating by the better eye occurs.

The examiner should have no need to go through every letter on the chart. To do so would certainly risk losing the child's attention. The examiner can start by testing the better eye with the 20/20 line and ask the child to identify the first one or two letters. If the child fails this line, then the examiner can go down a few lines to larger print and try from there. The child may then progress surprisingly to the 20/20 line that he or she could not read before. This is a common childhood behavior with no visual significance. Using cheerful, positive reinforcement encourages the child's best performance. Telling the child that he or she is wrong repeatedly may inhibit the child from volunteering responses on lines that he or she is able to see. Likewise, the examiner should indicate that all guesses the child makes, particularly if the child is young, are correct even when they are not. It is acceptable for the child to make minor mistakes, such as reading an F as a P or a D as an O. If a child correctly identifies two letters on a row, that can be used as the visual acuity.

Testing of both eyes allows for comparison. If, for example, both the injured eye and the uninjured eye have poor vision, the examiner might suspect that the poor vision is unrelated to the trauma (the child may simply need glasses). Likewise, children should always have their vision tested when wearing their glasses. This allows for measurement of the best corrected visual acuity. If the child does not have his or her glasses along, the examiner can try testing the child's vision while the child views the eye chart through pinholes. Any vision that gets better while viewing through a pinhole is indicative of a refractive error (need for glasses) rather than an ocular disorder. Although commercially available pinhole occluders can be purchased, the examiner can take any piece of paper, create a cluster of holes using an 18-gauge needle, and then hold this up to the tested eye. For example, if the traumatized eye initially reads 20/400 and the vision then improves to 20/25 or 20/30 (often the best testable using this crude pinhole method), the examiner knows that the child has no serious visually compromising injury: the child simply needs eyeglasses.

Although a numerical visual acuity cannot be generated for a preverbal child in the emergency department or pediatric office, the examiner can alternately cover each eye and look for an adverse change in behavior (irritability, pushing the examiner's hand away) when the better eye is covered, which forces the child to view with the weaker eye. These behaviors, or closing of the eye and going to sleep, can be seen starting in the first weeks of life.

If the injured or ill child is unable to stand while using a chart, a commercially available near card can be used to test the vision. If the child is able to see the 20/20 line at near, it is highly unlikely that any serious visually disturbing abnormality is present. If a near card is not available, the child can be asked to read or identify letters on any form of common use print (usually roughly equivalent to the 20/60 line or better).

If a child is unable to read print, the examiner should at least indicate the presence or absence of vision (light perception versus no light perception), a test which can be done even through a closed lid with the use of a bright light. The child who is able to see light can then be asked to identify a hand moving in front of the affected eye (record as "hand motion") and perhaps to count the fingers on that hand, noting the distance at which the child is still able to count fingers (record as "counting fingers at 2 feet").

A critical part of visual acuity testing is the recording of the results. The examiner should indicate the numerical value of the visual acuity and the type of method used for testing. When quantitative acuity is not possible, gross acuity is recorded as a preference for either eye (preverbal), fixing and following, counting fingers distance, hand motions, light perception, or no light perception.

Complications

Perhaps the greatest risk of visual acuity testing lies in obtaining an inaccurate measurement. This is most often the result of either the child's noncompliance or cheating. The examiner also must be careful that the occlusion of the injured eye does not lead to further discomfort or harm. In children with infectious conjunctivitis, tape used to cover the infected eye(s) should be discarded to prevent fomite transmission to the other eye.

Summary

Visual acuity testing is an essential part of any emergency examination of the eyes. Both eyes should be tested with the patient wearing his or her glasses. Proper attention to testing procedures will lead to optimal accuracy.

▶ DIRECT OPHTHALMOSCOPY

Introduction

Direct ophthalmoscopy is the procedure used to view the optic nerve and the posterior retina (Fig. 45.7). The direct ophthalmoscope is also useful to illuminate the eye for inspection or performing the Hirschberg and red reflex tests (see below).

Anatomy and Physiology

The optic nerve enters the sclera nasal to the center of vision (the fovea). The optic nerve carries with it the retinal blood vessels, which fan out onto the surface of the retina. The region temporal to the optic nerve between the major superior and inferior vessels (superior and inferior arcades) is the macula. The fovea appears as a small, dark area in the center of the macula and is used for straight-ahead fixation. The optic nerve usually appears to have a pink or salmon colored hue and contains a central white area called the cup, which contains the emerging retinal vessels. The size of the cup in children is quite variable. In papilledema, swelling of the optic nerve fibers causes the cup to be obliterated. The optic nerve margin should be sharply demarcated. Otherwise the examiner might suspect the presence of papilledema. Sometimes a normal variant collection of hyper- or hypopigmentation occurs around the nerve.

The basic principle of direct ophthalmoscopy relies on the illumination of the interior of the eye posterior to the iris.

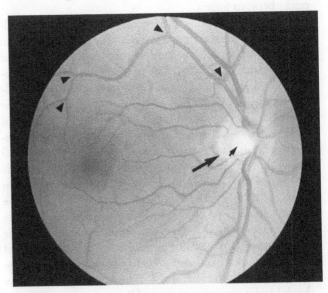

Figure 45.7 Normal posterior retina. *Large arrow:* Sharp optic disk margin. *Small arrow:* Optic cup. *Triangles:* Vessel branch points direct examiner toward the optic nerve.

Indications

Direct ophthalmoscopy is used to look for abnormalities of the optic nerve (e.g., papilledema), retinal hemorrhages (as in shaken baby syndrome), or other abnormalities of the retina.

Equipment

Several direct ophthalmoscopes are commercially available. It is beyond the scope of this chapter to discuss their relative merits. However, it is recommended that the chosen brand be full size, easily rechargeable, and equipped at least with a blue light (for the detection of fluorescein staining of a corneal abrasion) and at least two sizes of illuminated circular spot beams.

Occasionally, the child's pupil will be too small to allow for an acceptable view of the optic nerve with the direct ophthalmoscope. Under these circumstances, phenylephrine 2.5% and cyclopentolate 1% eye drops can be used to dilate the pupil provided that the child is post term.

Procedure

The examiner may use the direct ophthalmoscope with or without their own glasses on or contact lenses in. The patient's glasses should be removed. Contact lenses may be left in place (provided the examiner finds no other reason to remove them). The instrument is held in the hand that corresponds to the eye being examined (right hand for right eye, left hand for left eye). The examiner stands on the side of the patient ipsilateral to the eye being examined. The cooperative patient should be asked to sit on an examining table or chair and to fixate on a distant target. This method allows the child to keep the eyes still while the examiner looks in through the pupil. However, if the examiner's head blocks the view of the eye not being examined, then the child's eyes may wander. To avoid this complication, the examiner's face should approach the child's face with the direct ophthalmoscope in front of the same eye of the examiner as the eye being examined (i.e., the examiner's right eye is used to examine the patient's right eye) and the examiner's head should be parallel to the child's head. This method prevents obstruction of the other eye by the examiner's head. If the child is seated below the standing examiner, then the examiner can either sit in a chair facing the child or lean over from a standing position while tilting the child's head away so that his or her head is still parallel to that of the child.

In infants and younger children, the examiner cannot hope for continued fixation with the unexamined eye. It is usually easiest to place such children in the supine position. The examiner should be in a position as close to the examined eye as possible, shine the light in from an angle about 30 to 45 degrees temporal to the straight-ahead visual axis of the child, and patiently wait for the optic nerve to move briefly, albeit intermittently, into view. The examiner should not "chase" the optic nerve, as the movements of the eye will usually render these attempts futile and frustrating. Pharmacologic dilation of the pupil is helpful in examination of the optic nerves of infants and toddlers.

Some examiners find that they have difficulty using one of their eyes to perform direct ophthalmoscopy. Following the procedures outlined above, this would result in a difficulty using that eye to examine the same sided eye of the patient. By placing the patient in a supine position and standing at the head of the bed and leaning down over the patient, the examiner can use his or her good eye to examine the opposite eye of the patient without obstructing the vision of the nonexamined eye.

The examination is facilitated by darkening the room as much as possible to induce natural pupillary dilation. It is best to use the smallest circle of light provided by the direct ophthalmoscope to maximize the amount of light entering the pupil and to minimize the amount of light not entering the pupil, which reflects off the iris and causes glare for the examiner.

The direct ophthalmoscope focusing wheel is set on zero. Standing approximately 1 foot away from the patient, the examiner should look through the direct ophthalmoscope while shining the light in the eye to be examined to obtain a red reflex. As the examiner moves closer to the patient, a retinal blood vessel will be sighted within this red reflex. The examiner focuses on this vessel by spinning the focusing dial and follows the vessel toward the optic nerve. The apices of branches in the vessel always point in the direction of the optic nerve and therefore guide the examiner in the proper direction, like arrows pointing the way (Fig. 45.7). The examiner moves closer to the patient, ultimately arriving at a distance of less than 3 inches from the eye. The focusing wheel may be turned in either direction to keep the retinal blood vessel that is being tracked in focus.

Once the optic nerve is localized, its circumferential border is identified and assessed for clarity and sharpness. To aid in viewing the macula and fovea, compliant children can be asked to look directly into the direct ophthalmoscope light.

Complications

Occasionally, particularly in younger children, the direct ophthalmoscope may increase anxiety and induce photophobia (particularly in the presence of ocular surface disease). Although dilating drops may sting when administered, they have virtually no contraindications in children, with the exception of ectopia lentis, previously diagnosed narrow-angle glaucoma (dilation may occur in other forms of childhood glaucoma), and known allergy to the drops—all of which are rare. If the child has a neurologic disorder or injury, it may be wise to consult with a neurologist, neurosurgeon, and/or ophthalmologist before dilating the pupils so the dilation is not misinterpreted.

Summary

Direct ophthalmoscopy is a critical tool in the evaluation of many ocular disorders, brain injury, and neurologic conditions. Proper preparation will help to ensure an optimal view.

▶ THE DIRECT OPHTHALMOSCOPE AS A HANDHELD MAGNIFIER

Introduction

The direct ophthalmoscope can be used as a high-power magnifier to view the front surface of the eye.

Anatomy and Physiology

The cornea is a clear dome covering the anterior segment of the eye and has dimensions that appear to match that of the iris. The space between the iris and the inner corneal surface (endothelium) is filled with optically clear fluid (aqueous humor). The aqueous can become contaminated with red (hyphema) or white (iritis, hypopyon) blood cells. The pupil is a central hole in the iris that should appear round and reactive. Among normal individuals, 20% may have a slight difference in pupil size between the two eyes (anisocoria). It is also common to find that the pupil margin is lined with chocolate brown tissue regardless of the color of the rest of the pupil. When the cornea is lacerated, fluid from the anterior chamber will leak out through the hole. The rapid change in hydrostatic pressure will cause the iris to come forward to plug the leak. Therefore, any change in iris anatomy or pupillary roundness after trauma may be a sign of a ruptured globe, an indication to stop further examination and seek urgent ophthalmologic consultation. Foreign bodies may come to lie on the surface of the cornea or the tissue (conjunctiva) covering the white (sclera) of the eye. Both the cornea and conjunctiva may be abraded by mechanical forces.

Indications

As a magnifier, the direct ophthalmoscope is helpful in assessing the conjunctiva, cornea, and anterior chamber structures for the presence of abrasions, foreign bodies, lacerations, blood in the anterior chamber (hyphema), or cataract.

Equipment

    Direct ophthalmoscope
    Lid speculum or lid retractors (see above) if needed

Procedure

The examination should be conducted with the patient's glasses off, but contact lenses can be left in place if the examiner wishes. Once the lids are opened to allow a view of the eyeball, the examiner may approach the ocular surface from a close distance (within inches) by dialing in the green or black numbers on the focusing wheel (the color of the numbers depends on the brand of ophthalmoscope) while viewing through the direct ophthalmoscope. These "plus" lenses will convert the instrument into a handheld magnifier. When looking for a conjunctival or corneal abrasion that has been stained with fluorescein, the largest spot beam is used with a blue light. In the absence of a blue light, a white light is used rather than the green (red free), which may make it more difficult to see the characteristic yellow-green fluorescence. When looking for a small hyphema clot in the anterior chamber, the examiner concentrates on the peripheral iris, moving from the superior (12 o'clock) position in a clockwise pattern for 360 degrees. Following trauma, subtle irregularities in pupil shape may be a sign of more serious injury such as a subluxed lens or a ruptured globe.

The conjunctiva and corneal surface also can be scanned for foreign bodies with the direct ophthalmoscope. Lateral, inferior, and superior conjunctival recesses (fornices, Fig. 45.1) must be carefully inspected. This is facilitated by asking the patient to look in the direction opposite the fornix being examined and then pulling the surrounding lid or periocular tissue in the opposite direction (e.g., have patient look up to examine the inferior conjunctival fornix while pulling the lower lid down). The position of the lashes also can be inspected (e.g., for trichiasis) using the direct ophthalmoscope as a magnifier.

Complications

Provided that the ocular surface is not touched, no complications other than photophobia should occur.

Summary

The direct ophthalmoscope can be used as a high-power, handheld magnifier to assess the anterior structures of the eye.

▶ RED REFLEX TEST

Introduction

The red reflex test allows for rapid screening of the visual axis to ensure that light is passing clearly without obstruction by ocular abnormalities.

Anatomy and Physiology

The visual axis consists of the central cornea, anterior chamber, pupil, central lens, vitreous, and fovea. The pupil is usually black, as the inside of the eye is not being directly illuminated. The direct ophthalmoscope allows a focused beam of light to be projected into the eye, creating sufficient illumination to enable the examiner to see a reflection. This reflection usually has a red, orange, or yellowish glow due to the similar colors of the inside of the eye. An opacity can occur anywhere along the light's path. For example, a corneal scar, hyphema, vitreous hemorrhage, or retinal detachment can obstruct the visual axis. A cataract is an opacity in the normally clear lens that sits behind the pupil. When a cataract is present, the pupil may appear to the naked eye as white rather than the usual black.

Indication

The red reflex is a rapid screening test that should be part of virtually every examination for an ocular emergency. It is particularly helpful in the noncompliant child and following trauma.

Equipment

Direct ophthalmoscope
Lid speculum or lid retractors (see above) if needed

Procedure

The examiner should stand approximately 3 feet (1 m) away from the patient. While sighting through the direct ophthalmoscope, the entire face is illuminated with the largest white spot beam. The examination should be conducted with the patient's glasses off, but contact lenses can be left in place. To allow for comparison, the red reflex of both eyes should be assessed simultaneously while the patient is looking directly at the ophthalmoscope light. The red reflex is actually red, pink, orange, yellow, or some combination of these colors. The color is less important than the symmetry between the eyes. Any black area within the reflex is abnormal and should prompt closer inspection of the anterior segment, optic nerve, and retina, as discussed previously. The most common cause of a black reflex is small pupils or a patient who is not looking at the examiner. In the former case, the reflex can be rechecked after instillation of dilating drops. The reflex also is enhanced by turning off the room lights.

Any frankly white area also is abnormal, usually indicating the presence of a white abnormality inside the eye that would require urgent ophthalmologic consultation (cataract, retinal detachment, retinoblastoma).

Complications

Photophobia is the only complication that may occur. It is always better to err on the side of referral for ophthalmology consultation when there is a concern about a possibly abnormal red reflex test.

Summary

The red reflex test is an essential tool to rule out abnormalities in the visual axis.

▶ THE HIRSCHBERG TEST

Introduction

Children may present to the emergency department with misaligned eyes (strabismus), usually as the result of acute trauma or neurologic conditions. The Hirschberg test is designed to give the clinician a rapid assessment of whether or not the eyes are aligned properly.

Anatomy and Physiology

Normally, our eyes are aligned so that both eyes point in the same direction and view the world simultaneously in all directions that the eyes can move. Any misalignment of the two eyes is called "strabismus." Strabismus may be idiopathic or due to a need for glasses; poor vision; an injured or entrapped muscle (e.g., blowout fracture of the orbit); infiltration of the muscles (e.g., thyroid eye disease); a paresis or paralysis of cranial nerve III, IV, or VI; or an abnormality in the orbit behind the globe that is restricting movement (e.g., tumor, hemorrhage). It is beyond the scope of this chapter to discuss the differential diagnosis of strabismus or its full evaluation. The Hirschberg test is designed to determine if strabismus is present.

The orbits and globes point somewhat lateral to the sagittal plane, yet the eyes are focused straight ahead and parallel to the sagittal plane. As a result, if a light is shined at the eye, it will appear to fall slightly nasal to the middle of the pupil (Fig. 45.8A). Should the eyes be misaligned, the light reflex will not fall symmetrically on the two eyes. If one is crossed (esotropic), the light reflex in that eye will be more temporal relative to the center of the pupil (Fig. 45.8B). If one eye is turned out (exotropic), the light reflex will be more nasal (Fig. 45.8C). If one eye is too high or low, the reflex will be displaced vertically.

Indications

The Hirschberg test is performed when there is a concern about possible strabismus or unequal eye movements. For example, if there is a concern about high intracranial pressure resulting in a sixth cranial nerve palsy, one eye may be esotropic and have poor abduction. The Hirschberg test will show asymmetry of the light reflex on the cornea in the straight-ahead position that will be even more apparent when the child tries

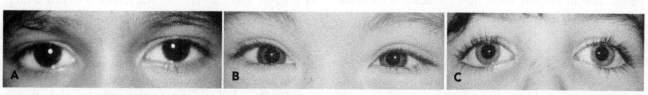

Figure 45.8
A. Normally aligned eyes (no strabismus). Hirschberg light reflex falls symmetrically in each eye.
B. Left esotropia. Light reflex in left eye falls laterally relative to pupil center.
C. Left exotropia. Light reflex in left eye falls medially relative to pupil center.

to look in the direction ipsilateral to the paretic lateral rectus muscle.

Equipment

Direct ophthalmoscope

Procedure

From straight ahead and virtually any distance close enough that the examiner can see the child's eyes clearly, one of the white circle beams of the direct ophthalmoscope is shined toward the open eyes of the patient. The examiner notes the reflection of this light on the surface of the eye relative to the center of the pupil in both eyes simultaneously and assesses the symmetry. The test can be repeated in different fields of gaze should there be a concern about unequal eye movements. The relative symmetry should be preserved regardless of the direction of gaze unless strabismus is present. For example, if the child has a right blowout fracture that prevents the right eye from looking upward fully, then the Hirschberg light reflex, which may be symmetrical in straight-ahead gaze, would become asymmetric in upgaze, with the reflex in the affected eye being closer to the center of the pupil than the reflex in the affected eye (which will be seen toward the lower border of the pupil).

Complications

Photophobia might be possible.

Summary

The Hirschberg test is designed to identify the presence of ocular misalignment.

▶ INSTILLATION OF OPHTHALMIC DROPS AND OINTMENTS

Introduction

Many children seem to fear the instillation of ophthalmic medications as much as needles. With refinement of technique, the examiner can accomplish this task quickly and efficiently, thus minimizing the child's discomfort and anxiety. Instilling ophthalmic medications also creates an opportunity to teach parents how to properly instill these medications for home use.

Indications

Topical medications are used to treat a wide variety of ophthalmic conditions. However, neither drops nor ointments should be instilled when the clinician suspects that the globe has been ruptured. This recommendation is made not because the medications are particularly injurious but rather because the clinician should try to avoid *all* manipulations of the eye until an ophthalmologist arrives.

Equipment

Ophthalmic drops or ointment

Anatomy and Physiology

The ocular surface, including the inner aspect of each eyelid, is lined with nonkeratinized epithelium, which helps to make it remarkably absorbent. However, only approximately 20% of each drop can be utilized by the eye. For these reasons, only one drop, if administered correctly, is necessary. The drop can be instilled onto the inner surface (palpebral conjunctiva) of the lower lid, where it will act just as effectively as if it was dropped directly on the cornea. Absorption is rapid. Contrary to common myth, rubbing or dabbing the eyes after drop instillation does not cause the drops to be rubbed out of the eye. Because the conjunctival recesses can only use a portion of each drop that is instilled, it is expected that some of the dose will drip down onto the patient's cheek. This is not a concern (although some dilating drops such as phenylephrine may cause skin blanching in the path of the excess drop as it courses over the skin).

Many drops sting the eye when instilled. Children may react with a reflex resistance to administration of eye medications with forceful, voluntary contraction of the orbicularis oculi muscle, making instillation difficult. Although technically it is preferable to have a 5-minute waiting period between ocular instillation of different medications, the minimal benefit is probably outweighed by the increased anxiety and discomfort for the child. Rapid instillation of two different medications, one right after the other, will usually create acceptably effective dosing in most clinical situations.

In many clinical situations, the treating physician may have the option of using ointments or drops. Usually this is a matter of convenience more than medical indication or efficacy. Drops require more frequent dosing than ointments. However, some patients find ointments more difficult to instill. The patient may also have a preference.

Procedure

The technique of manual opening of the eyelids (see above) is particularly useful when the child is forcibly closing his or her eyes. Once *any* conjunctival surface is viewed, a drop can be instilled. The procedure is made easier by using an assistant to instill the medication once the lids are separated. Alternatively, the clinician can hold the bottle between the forefinger and thumb in one hand while using the ulnar side of that hand to place pressure on the orbicularis either above or below the palpebral fissure (replacing the use of the thumb by that hand, as explained in "Manual Lid Opening" above). Even if the conjunctiva cannot be viewed, as long as the lid

SUMMARY

Opening the Eye

1 Manually compress orbicularis muscle against bones and separate lids.

2 Use cotton swabs with short sticks and roll skin toward lid margin to avoid eversion (Not for trauma).

3 Instill topical anesthetic before using lid specula or lid retractors.

Upper Lid Eversion

1 Recommended for lavage and identification of foreign body under lid.

2 Have child look downward.

3 Gently press cotton-tipped swab into body of upper lid and pull lashes to fold back upper lid.

Visual Acuity Testing

1 Assess in all patients with ocular complaints.

2 Test each eye with glasses on; use pinhole if glasses are not available.

3 Occlude eye not being tested with tape to prevent cheating.

4 Choose appropriate chart for child's developmental stage and degree of literacy.

5 Record results.

Direct Ophthalmoscope

1 Assess visual axis by checking red reflex with largest circle of light from 1 m away.

2 Examine optic nerve and retina in darkened room with smallest circle of light.

3 Use "plus" lenses (green or black numbers) as a magnifier to examine anterior structures.

4 Assess ocular alignment by examining symmetry of light reflex in each pupil.

Drop and Ointment Instillation

1 Do not instill any medications until rupture of globe is excluded.

2 Open eye and apply one drop to any conjunctival surface.

3 Apply 1 cm of ointment to the lower lid palpebral conjunctiva.

 CLINICAL TIPS

Opening the Eye

1 Manual—no equipment, no pressure on globe.

2 Cotton-tipped swabs—inexpensive but exerts pressure on globe.

3 Lid specula—specialized equipment, no pressure on globe.

4 Lid retractors—less discomfort than speculum, may fashion from paper clips.

Upper Lid Eversion

1 Keep reminding patient to look down during procedure.

Visual Acuity Testing

1 Positive reinforcement improves cooperation.

2 Assess light perception or finger counting if standard test cannot be administered.

Direct Ophthalmoscopy

1 Minimize ambient light to dilate pupils.

2 Smallest circle of light decreases glare on retinal examination.

3 For infants, do not chase the moving eye. Hold position and wait for optic nerve to move into view.

4 Stand 1 m away for red reflex test.

5 Check Hirschberg reflex in different gazes to rule out strabismus due to muscle weakness or restriction.

Drop Instillation

1 One drop is enough.

2 No need to see eyeball.

margins are separated, a significant portion of the drop will usually reach the ocular surface.

In the extremely noncompliant patient, when the examiner feels that achieving any eye opening using the manual technique is impossible and/or when specula or retractors are either not available or not desired, he or she can try an alternative method to get drops onto the ocular surface. The child is placed in the supine position with eyes closed. A single drop can then be placed into the sulcus between the medial corner of the palpebral fissure (medial canthus) and the ipsilateral side of the nose. Eventually, the child will open the eye and the drop will run onto the ocular surface, provided that the child is kept in the supine position.

Topical ophthalmic ointments are instilled by pulling down the lower lid and expressing an approximately 1- to 2-cm strip onto the lower lid palpebral conjunctiva. This procedure is made easier by having the compliant patient look upward. After the ointment has been instilled, many patients find it more comforting to close their eyes for a few minutes as the ointment begins to melt on the ocular surface. The child should be warned that when the eyelids open he or she may feel a sticky sensation and experience some temporary blurring of vision. Excess ointment on the lashes can be wiped away with a tissue.

One special situation deserves mention. Fluorescein is sometimes delivered in the form of an impregnated paper strip. This strip should be wetted (with water, saline, or topical anesthetic) before instillation. Dry, stiff paper in contact with the cornea can cause an abrasion.

Complications

Although each drop and ointment has its own associated side effects, instillation of drops should be atraumatic. Anxiety and fear are usually short lived. One must be careful not to scratch

the ocular surface with the tip of the bottle or tube. Likewise, the medication bottle or tube should not be contaminated by the lid, tears, or conjunctiva. Both ophthalmic drops and ointments should be stored with the caps on securely.

Summary

Instillation of topical ophthalmic medication is an essential process that can be done effectively while minimizing discomfort and anxiety for the child.

▶ REFERENCES

1. Levin AV. Eye-strabismus. In: Fleisher GR, Ludwig S, Henretig FM, eds. *Textbook of Pediatric Emergency Medicine.* 5th ed. Philadelphia: Lippincott Williams & Wilkins; 2005:273–280.
2. Levin AV. Ophthalmic emergencies. In: Fleisher GR, Ludwig S, Henretig FM, eds. *Textbook of Pediatric Emergency Medicine.* 5th ed. Philadelphia: Lippincott Williams & Wilkins; 2005:1653–1662.
3. Sit M, Levin AV. Direct ophthalmoscopy in pediatric emergency care. *Pediatr Emerg Care.* 2001;17:199–204.
4. McLaughlin C, Levin AV. The red reflex. *Pediatr Emerg Care.* 2006; 22:137–140.

ALEX V. LEVIN

46

Slit Lamp Examination

▶ INTRODUCTION

Slit lamp biomicroscopy is a diagnostic procedure that requires experience and specific skills. It is unlikely that the majority of pediatricians and emergency physicians will have the opportunity to repetitively use the slit lamp enough to acquire and refine the skills needed to use it well in many situations. Therefore, this chapter will address the basic theory and practice of slit lamp illumination, along with a few common applications that may fall into the scope of practice of nonophthalmologists treating children in the emergency setting. It would of course be appropriate to seek ophthalmology consultation whenever the physician does not feel comfortable using the slit lamp, the diagnosis remains in question, or the evaluation and treatment of the patient requires slit lamp techniques beyond the basics discussed herein.

Purchasing a slit lamp is an individual decision that should take into account cost, need, and frequency of use. If it is unlikely to be used often, then it is unlikely that the physicians will have the opportunity to acquire the skills necessary for proper use. In this setting, it may be more harmful than beneficial. The slit lamp is best placed in a dedicated area, with an adjustable patient chair and with ocular medications, forceps, and cotton swabs readily available. Purchasing a slit lamp on wheels is an alternative. Another consideration is the utility of having the slit lamp available on-site for the consulting ophthalmologist. In some situations, this may obviate the need for the patient to make a trip to the ophthalmologist's office and may allow the ophthalmologist to optimize the examination on-site.

▶ ANATOMY AND PHYSIOLOGY

Light can only be seen when it is reflected off an object. If a person were to hold a flashlight and shine it into an endless

vacuum, the beam of light emanating from the bulb would be invisible. Only if a person were to place a substance or object within the path of the light would the light become visible. For example, if smoke or dust were allowed to enter our theoretical vacuum, the beam of light would readily become apparent, as it would be reflected by the particles. This is called the Tyndall phenomenon. Likewise, if a person were to erect a piece of semitransparent plastic several centimeters thick in the vacuum and then several meters thereafter erect a cement slab, the beam of light would become visible as it strikes the plastic, as it moves through the plastic (being reflected by the continuous substance of the plastic), and again as it hits the opaque cement slab (Fig. 46.1A). Because the vacuum itself contains no reflective materials, the beam would remain invisible at all other places.

These principles are directly applicable to the eyeball. If a person shines a beam of light (in this case, the slit lamp beam) into the eyeball, it will only be visible where it is reflected. Between the bulb and the eyeball it is invisible, as, for the most part, air is relatively nonreflective from an optical standpoint. However, as the beam hits the surface of the cornea, it can be seen (Fig. 46.1B,C). As it passes through the corneal substance, it is continuously visible, just as the light passing through the plastic in the previous example would be continuously visible. The beam then becomes invisible as it leaves the back of the cornea and travels to the surface of the iris, where it is once again reflected and therefore becomes visible to the observer. The space between the back of the cornea and the iris (anterior chamber) is filled with optically clear fluid (aqueous humor), which prevents the beam from being visualized. The pupil is simply a hole in the iris through which the beam continues to pass, invisible to the observer until it strikes the front surface of the lens, which is just beyond the pupil. Again, the beam becomes visible as it hits the surface of the lens and passes through the substance of

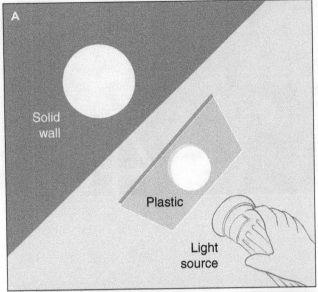

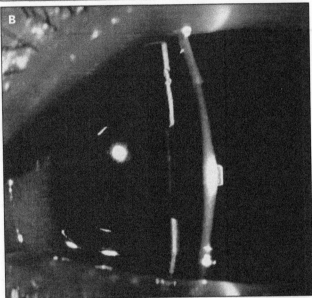

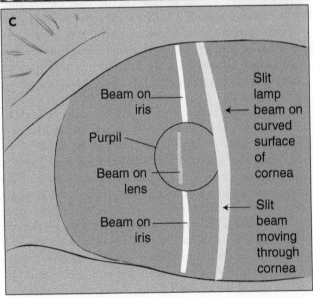

the lens. Visualization of the interior of the lens is difficult without pharmacologic dilation of the pupil, but the anterior surface is easily seen with the pupil in its usual state. After pupillary dilation, the skilled observer can also visualize strands of vitreous behind the lens. Using special lenses, the ophthalmologist also can direct the slit lamp beam to allow visualization of the posterior vitreous, optic nerve, and retina.

The slit lamp is given its name because of its ability to create a slit beam of light. Using a slit allows for a topographic appreciation of each surface because the light appears to bend along the curvature of that surface. The observer can appreciate the corneal curvature, the iris architecture, and the curved surface of the lens (Fig. 46.1). In disease states, the observer can assess the elevation and contour of ocular structures. For example, a foreign body on the cornea would cause an elevation of the beam as it bends to go over the material. The slit beam also allows for the delineation of the internal anatomy of translucent structures such as the cornea and lens. The skilled observer can visually distinguish the corneal layers and therefore recognize the depth of a lesion, such as foreign body or corneal laceration.

When the aqueous humor loses its optical clarity, the beam of light becomes visible as it passes from the cornea to the iris and lens. This occurs with iritis and hyphema. The white blood cells and protein that leak out of inflamed iris vessels in iritis and the red blood cells of a hyphema reflect the beam to the observer so that the particles can actually be seen floating in the aqueous, similar to the beam of an automobile headlight in the fog. The visualization of red or white blood cells is called "cells" and graded on a scale of 1+ to 4+ by an experienced examiner. The presence of protein is referred to as "flare" and graded on a similar scale.

▶ INDICATIONS

It is likely that the slit lamp will be most useful to the physician as a unique diagnostic magnification system to examine the ocular surfaces, in particular for the identification of corneal or conjunctival injury or foreign bodies on these surfaces. For the physician who is well versed in slit lamp techniques,

---

Figure 46.1

A. A person shines a flashlight through a thick piece of semitransparent plastic onto a cement slab. The beam is only visible as it contacts and passes through the plastic and contacts the solid, opaque slab. It is not visible between the flashlight and the plastic or between the plastic and the slab because air is optically clear.

B. Slit lamp beam is visible as an arc of light on the curved surface of the cornea and on the iris above and below the pupil. The beam passes invisibly through the optically clear aqueous humor. The lens located just behind the pupil is also visible.

C. Schematic drawing of B.

it also may be helpful for minor procedures such as foreign body removal (Chapter 47) and for the diagnosis of iritis and microscopic (no clot) hyphema.

▶ EQUIPMENT

Slit lamps are available in many models from several manufacturers. Although some have novel configurations, the basic principles are identical, and the discussion here should be applicable to all slit lamps. When purchasing a slit lamp, especially if one is not experienced in this area, it is advisable to examine at least two models and to request the sales representative to loan a sample for trial use. All potential examiners should become familiar with the purchased model and perhaps with the repeated assistance of volunteer adult subjects before using it on patients. An ophthalmologist consultant may be useful in providing "hands-on" instruction. Exercises that may be helpful include identification of the corneal layers, grasping eyelashes with a forceps, identifying a contact lens on the cornea, and especially manipulation of the slit lamp beam up, down, from side to side, and from cornea to iris while maintaining a well-focused view. Only after these skills are mastered should the examiner begin using the slit lamp on pediatric patients.

▶ PROCEDURE

For the most part, successful use of the slit lamp requires a compliant patient. This large machine is often quite imposing for the young child. Examination of infants and those toddlers who are unable to follow directions well and unable to easily get their chin to the chinrest should be deferred to the ophthalmologist. Very compliant toddlers, sometimes as young as 2 or 3 years old, will cooperate, particularly if they are allowed to sit on a parent's lap. This is often facilitated by telling the child that the slit lamp is a type of television in which the child can see his or her favorite character. Fortunately, the child's imagination will often allow him or her to see the imaginary figure promised! Another approach is to tell the child that slit lamp examination is like riding a bicycle or motorcycle. Most slit lamps have handles for the patient that extend out from either side. These can be likened to handlebars and, with the appropriate noises and encouragement from the examiner, can lead to some fun role-playing for the child while being examined.

All of these techniques are made easier by using an electric examination chair that can be raised or lowered by foot pedal or hand control to place the child at a comfortable height. Most slit lamps have an adjustable chinrest that is moved up or down so that the eyes of the patient are level with an indicator line next to the face to ensure optimal ease of focus and adjustment. Slit lamps have a forehead bar or band to prevent the child's face from moving too far forward toward the beam. The patient's forehead must be against this band even if it requires gentle pressure on the occiput by the parent.

Once in position, the slit lamp is turned on. Most models have a power switch for which several levels of voltage may be available. Using the lowest setting is adequate and adds to bulb longevity. Filter switches change the intensity of the illumination and also allow for other options (e.g., red-free light). A knob will be available to change the height of the beam (using a fully extended vertical height is usually easiest for the nonophthalmologist), and another knob for adjustment of beam width. A beam 2 to 3 mm wide is usually the best for the nonophthalmologist. For simple magnification of the eyeball without the need for assessing corneal layers or aqueous clarity, the beam can be opened fully in its horizontal direction until it becomes a large circle. Slit lamps also have variable magnification controlled by a knob or lever. The lowest power is usually adequate and easiest to use.

The part of the machine from which the beam emanates may be moved through a 180-degree arc between the patient and the examiner. In general, the patient's eye is examined with the beam swung to the side ipsilateral to that eye and projected onto the eye at approximately 30 to 45 degrees from the visual axis. This allows maximal illumination of the ocular structures while optimizing the observer's ability to sense depth in the cornea, anterior chamber, and lens. The slit beam becomes "a slice of light" imaging a section of each structure as it passes through. The observer's view is then somewhat oblique to the beam, allowing its full anterior-to-posterior course to be appreciated as it passes through a structure such as the cornea.

Focusing the beam onto a structure of interest is usually the most difficult task for the beginner. The slit lamp is equipped with a joy stick or adjusting knob(s) that allow the beam to be elevated, lowered, moved from side to side, or toward and away from the patient. Since the eye is curved, as the machine is moved, the relationship between the beam and the surface of the eye is changed, causing alterations in focus. Also, because the beam is projected onto the eye from an angle, as the machine is moved forward the beam will move to the side such that the object of regard is no longer illuminated in the same location. Coordination of focus and beam movement is not teachable in the text of a chapter. Rather, this is a skill that can be acquired only through practice.

Although the slit lamp offers the ophthalmologist the opportunity to perform a multitude of procedures under high magnification, only physicians with considerable experience should attempt the following procedures.

Special Uses

Iritis and Hyphema
Photophobia is often the first obstacle to recognizing iritis or hyphema. Using a lower power of illumination, a narrower beam, and/or a beam of reduced height may be helpful to

reduce the patient's reaction to direct light. Sometimes the cells and flare are best appreciated using a vertically short, moderately wide, nonfiltered, bright beam. The examiner should try to focus on the midaqueous, with the beam coming from an angle in such a way that the observer's line of sight would be extrapolated into the pupil. The black of the pupil then serves as a backdrop, which makes appreciation of the aqueous abnormalities easier.

When looking for hyphema, the physician should be sure to examine the entire iris surface, in particular its far peripheral edges, for tiny adherent clots. It is helpful to do this in a systematic fashion starting superiorly (at the 12 o'clock position) and working around the iris clockwise. The slit lamp provides a green light, which is a red-free beam. Red blood cells are only visible by virtue of the reflection of red wavelength light. By using a red-free beam, the red blood cells become invisible. Any remaining visible cells are either liberated pigment cells (as in trauma) or white blood cells (as in iritis). This technique, although reserved for the experienced and skilled observer, can be helpful in distinguishing iritis from a microhyphema (no clot). In both situations, management requires ophthalmology consultation.

Corneal Abrasion

The slit lamp provides the observer with a blue beam (cobalt blue), which can be used to examine the cornea after instillation of fluorescein. The blue light causes the fluorescein to fluoresce such that it will appear yellow-green. This technique is useful for viewing surface abnormalities such as corneal and conjunctival abrasion, foreign bodies, and lesions associated with corneal herpetic infection (dendritic keratitis).

Intraocular Pressure Measurement

All slit lamps are capable of measuring intraocular pressure by Goldmann applanation tonometry. This advanced technique is particularly difficult in children, noncompliant patients, and photophobic patients—the very patients that are most likely to be encountered in an emergency setting.

Epilation

An eyelash may be turned toward the cornea such that its tip rubs the corneal epithelium, causing microscopic abrasions that can be quite irritating and even painful. This is called trichiasis. The lash can be grabbed at its base with a fine, non-toothed forceps (epilation forceps are available) and quickly tugged along the line of origin away from the lid margin. The lash will come out with its root. Care must be taken not to twist the forceps or pull in a direction that is not parallel to the lash's origin as this may fracture the lash, leaving a stub that is more difficult to grasp and that is potentially even more injurious to the corneal surface. The procedure may be facilitated by the instillation of a topical anesthetic. The physician also must be sure to establish the cause of the trichiasis to prevent recurrence. The lash will grow back.

Removal of a Foreign Body

For a description of the removal of a foreign body, see Chapter 47.

▶ COMPLICATIONS

Slit lamp biomicroscopy is usually free from complications, with the exception of induced photophobia and anxiety. The procedure should be otherwise painless, although some children may need to be held in place. Care must be taken not to back the machine away while the child is still on the chin rest. This could result in the child falling forward. When not in use, the tonometer should be moved laterally to its resting position to avoid trauma to the cornea when moving the machine from one eye to the other. If the tonometer tip is used, appropriate cleaning techniques should be undertaken before the next patient.

Epilation can cause mild pain. Corneal or conjunctival abrasion or perforation can occur during attempted removal of a foreign body, particularly if the examiner is using a needle or pointed forceps, if he or she is not well versed in the procedure, or if the child moves unexpectedly forward should the forehead be allowed to drift away from the rest. Deeply embedded foreign bodies should not be removed because of the possibility of an unrecognized perforation of the globe. Ophthalmology consultation is recommended.

SUMMARY

1 The child may sit on a caretaker's lap for comfort; position the chin on the rest with the forehead fully forward.

2 Use the lowest magnification and illumination that is adequate for examination.

3 Examine structures systematically—conjunctiva, cornea, aqueous humor, iris, lens.

4 Use fluorescein plus blue light to identify abrasions, foreign bodies, or herpetic lesions on the corneal surface.

5 For epilation, grasp the lash at its base and pull sharply along the axis of the hair shaft.

6 Use green (red-free) light to differentiate red and white blood cells in the anterior chamber.

7 Consult ophthalmology in cases where there is diagnostic uncertainty, a foreign body not easily removed, a noncompliant patient, hyphema, iritis, herpetic keratitis, corneal laceration, an abnormal pupil or other anatomic structures or when the examiner is unfamiliar with slit lamp use.

CLINICAL TIPS

▶ Slit lamp use requires practice, understanding of the theory of operation, and experience.

▶ Consult ophthalmology for noncompliant patients.

▶ A smaller, less intense beam is better tolerated by photophobic patients.

▶ Look for small clots of hyphema carefully around 360 degrees of the iris. Red cells opacifying the aqueous humor represent hyphema without clot.

▶ The slit lamp green (red-free) light can help distinguish red blood cells from white blood cells and liberated pigment cells.

▶ SUMMARY

The slit lamp can be a valuable tool in the emergency setting for diagnosis of ocular disorders affecting the conjunctiva, cornea, or anterior segment. An understanding of the theory behind slit lamp use helps the physician utilize the considerable capacity of the machine. Proper use requires experience that this chapter cannot provide. Children are not usually compliant patients, making their ocular evaluation with a slit lamp more difficult. Ophthalmologic consultation will frequently be necessary for full evaluation of children with ocular complaints requiring slit lamp examination.

▶ REFERENCE

1. Stein HA, Stein RM, Freeman M. *The Ophthalmic Assistant*. 8th ed. New York: Elsevier; 2006.

47

WINNIE T. WHITAKER AND WENDY J. POMERANTZ

Ocular Foreign Body Removal

▶ INTRODUCTION

Foreign bodies commonly become lodged on the eye surface, whether blown in by wind or propelled at high velocity. Patients with ocular foreign bodies often present to the emergency department (ED) because of pain or, in the case of young children, irritability. Foreign bodies may be located superficially in the cornea or conjunctiva or may be embedded. It is important to distinguish a superficial foreign body from a penetrating eye injury. Objects embedded in the cornea are not always associated with pain and therefore may be difficult to identify.

A high index of suspicion for an ocular foreign body necessitates careful examination of the eye. The promptness of the exam and the technique used depends on the type of injury and the patient's ability to cooperate. Management of ocular foreign bodies may be challenging in children. While irrigation does not require full cooperation, a child must be completely still if an instrument is to be used for foreign body removal. For children in whom irrigation is not successful, sedation or general anesthesia is occasionally required.

▶ ANATOMY AND PHYSIOLOGY

The conjunctiva covers the sclera and lines the inner surfaces of the upper and lower eyelids (see Fig. 45.1). It secretes a mucous film that helps to capture particulate matter on the eye surface. The cornea is a tough covering over the iris a few millimeters thick and consists of three layers: the outer surface, the stroma, and the endothelium. The outer surface is composed of five layers of epithelial cells, which, unlike the skin epithelium, is not keratinized. Below this, the stroma gives the cornea structural integrity. It is this layer that glows yellow-green when a corneal abrasion is stained with fluorescein. A single-cell layer of endothelium below the stroma regulates fluid and nutrient supply.

The eye will respond to the presence of a foreign body with injection of the conjunctiva, tearing, and blinking. The patient usually has associated pain; however, not all foreign body injuries, even with globe perforation, are associated with pain. Visual acuity may be affected if the foreign body is in the visual axis or if associated corneal edema is present (1).

Intraocular foreign bodies of inert materials, such as some plastics or glass, may be well tolerated and may not necessitate immediate removal. Metallic foreign bodies precipitate inflammatory reactions that can further damage the eye, whereas organic materials increase the risk of infection (2).

▶ INDICATIONS

All foreign bodies in the eye must be removed; however, not all are removed immediately. In some circumstances, such as with the uncooperative child or when equipment is needed that is not available, removal may best be performed in an ophthalmologist's office or in an operating room. A corneal foreign body is best removed as soon as possible, because the cornea may epithelialize over the foreign body in several hours (1) and make removal more difficult.

Foreign bodies may be located on the inner surface of the eyelids, in the fornices, on bulbar conjunctiva and sclera, or on the cornea or may have penetrated the globe. Corneal foreign bodies are most commonly found on the lower two thirds of the cornea.

Examination to rule out foreign body is indicated when a child complains of foreign body sensation. Foreign body sensations are not uncommon, however, and may represent other conditions, such as conjunctivitis. A patient may complain of foreign body sensation when the foreign body is no longer in the eye but has resulted in a residual corneal abrasion.

Vertical, linear corneal abrasions often result when foreign bodies adherent to the inside of the upper lid injure the cornea during blinking. If noted on eye examination with fluorescein, a thorough search for an ocular foreign body on the upper lid is indicated.

The presence of a metallic foreign body in the eye, even for a few hours, may result in a brownish rust ring at the site of the injury. Removal of the foreign body and the rust ring is required, but the rust ring can be removed at follow-up by an ophthalmologist (see "Complications").

A ruptured globe should be considered in patients with a history of high-velocity wounds and in those with hyphema, irregular or sluggish pupil, and a decrease in visual acuity. Attempts at foreign body removal by the emergency physician are contraindicated if a ruptured globe is suspected, if lack of patient cooperation precludes safe removal, or if the foreign body appears to be embedded. In these circumstances, and when attempts at foreign body removal are unsuccessful or the foreign body is incompletely removed, immediate referral to an ophthalmologist is indicated. When the possibility of a ruptured globe exists, the eye should be protected with an eye shield. This keeps the patient from rubbing the eye and prevents any contact of the eye that can cause extrusion of orbital contents.

Indications for immediate ophthalmologic consultation include the presence of an embedded foreign body, the presence of multiple foreign bodies, unsuccessful foreign body removal attempts, a patient who is unable to cooperate with the procedure, any indication of possible ruptured globe such as hyphema or an irregular or sluggish pupil, and a decrease in visual acuity.

▶ EQUIPMENT

Visual acuity chart
Topical anesthetic drops (e.g., proparacaine HCl 0.5% or tetracaine HCl 0.5%)
Sterile water, syringe, and plastic catheter
Sterile cotton-tipped applicators
Fluorescein drops or strips
Wood's lamp or slit lamp
Eye spud or 25-gauge needle on 3-mL syringe
Topical dilating drops (e.g., homatropine 2% or 5%, cyclopentolate 0.5% or 1%, tropicamide 1%)
Antibiotic ointment or drops

▶ PROCEDURE

Evaluation for Ocular Foreign Body

Emergency personnel should ask the child or parent how the foreign body entered the eye. An object blowing or falling into the eye is unlikely to penetrate the globe, whereas an object entering the eye at high velocity, such as when hammering on metal or working with industrial tools, should alert the clinician to the possible rupture of the globe.

Before the eye is anesthetized, the physician may ask the older child where the foreign body sensation is located. Kaye-Wilson demonstrated that adult patients indicating a foreign body sensation in either the temporal, nasal, or central regions were generally correct in identifying the area of the cornea where a foreign body was located. Localization to the lower lid indicated a foreign body in the lower half of the cornea. Localization of the foreign body sensation to the upper lid was less reliable, and foreign bodies were located in any region of the cornea (3). This information may be particularly useful to the physician who does not have access to a slit lamp.

It is often difficult for children to cooperate with techniques involving direct removal of ocular foreign bodies. Minimal cooperation may be required for the irrigation technique. Pharmacologic sedation can be helpful in children who may not be able to remain still during foreign body removal (Chapter 33). Administering pharmacologic sedation requires a physician trained in its use and careful monitoring of the patient. If the patient is sedated and the attempt at foreign body removal is unsuccessful, immediate ophthalmologic referral is indicated.

A thorough examination of the eye is necessary for all children in whom a foreign body of the eye is suspected (Chapter 45). Any associated injuries, especially a ruptured globe, must be identified before attempts to remove an ocular foreign body are made. Intraocular foreign bodies (within the globe rather than superficial) may be subtle in up to 20% of patients (4) and should be suspected if the patient has a history of high-velocity injuries. Diffuse, chemotic subconjunctival hemorrhage raises the suspicion of corneal laceration and therefore a ruptured globe (4,5).

Careful observation of pupil size, shape, and reactivity is critical. Prolapse of the iris with distortion of pupillary shape indicating a ruptured globe may look deceptively like a foreign body. If a ruptured globe is clinically suspected, a metal shield is placed over the eye with no pressure applied to the eye; an eye patch is contraindicated. No drops or ointments are instilled in the eye. The patient is instructed to have nothing by mouth. Broad-spectrum intravenous antibiotics are administered, and tetanus immunization, if not current, is given. Urgent ophthalmologic consultation is obtained. Plain radiographs and computerized tomography may be helpful in ruling out an intraocular foreign body, but magnetic resonance imaging should be avoided if any possibility of intraocular metal foreign body exists (6).

A small but reactive pupil may indicate traumatic iritis. A pupil with abnormal reactivity may indicate intracranial injury or optic nerve injury from blunt or penetrating trauma (2).

Once the possibility of a ruptured globe is excluded, two drops of topical anesthetic, such as proparacaine 0.5% or tetracaine 0.5%, are instilled in the eye. Prompt relief of pain after topical anesthetic drops should be noted. In adults, Sklar et al. found that pain relief in response to topical anesthetic was more likely when the pain was the result of corneal injury (foreign body or abrasion) rather than conditions such as iritis or conjunctivitis (7).

The patient should not be sent home with topical anesthetics. Not only do they delay corneal re-epithelialization, but the anesthetized eye is prone to further injury (4). Recent literature has shown that ophthalmic nonsteroidal anti-inflammatory drugs (NSAIDs), such as ketorolac 0.5%, diclofenac 0.1% and indomethacin 0.1%, provide significant pain reduction in patients with traumatic corneal abrasions when compared to placebo (8). Systemic analgesics may be necessary when a significant corneal abrasion has resulted and topical medications have failed.

When possible, visual acuity should be assessed in each eye, before the injured eye is manipulated. If the child is unable to cooperate, the ability to follow objects or response to light perception is noted. Routine use of glasses or contact lenses should be documented.

The eye should then be examined after instillation of fluorescein. A corneal foreign body will often be surrounded by a circular area of fluorescein staining. Vertical abrasions on the cornea are typical of foreign bodies located on the undersurface of the upper lid that scrape the corneal surface during blinking. A positive Seidel test, with a stream of aqueous humor stained with fluorescein draining from the site of corneal injury, indicates globe perforation. In this situation, a shield is placed immediately over the eye using care not to put pressure on the globe, and immediate ophthalmologic consultation is obtained.

The eye is examined carefully for the location of one or more foreign bodies. Both eyelids are everted (Chapter 45) and the undersurface is examined. Tiny foreign bodies may not be visible in the upper fornix, but the object may be discovered and removed during gentle wiping across the fornix with a moistened cotton swab (9).

Localization of the foreign body is made easier by the use of a slit lamp, loupes (magnifying lenses worn by the physician), or other magnification, when available. Indirect lighting, by shining a light at an angle, may cast a shadow from the foreign body. The conjunctival cul-de-sacs and the undersurface of the lids (see Fig. 45.1) must be carefully inspected. The anterior chamber is examined for evidence of hyphema or a foreign body; if either is found, the eye is protected with an eye shield, and immediate ophthalmologic consultation is obtained.

Plain films of the orbit may be indicated if the patient has a history of high-velocity injuries (BB pellet, metallic splinter propelled during hammering, etc.). A history of high-velocity injuries, especially combined with an inability to locate the foreign body on physical examination, is an indication for radiography. Plain radiographs may reveal radiopaque foreign bodies such as metallic fragments. Computerized tomography is very useful for foreign body localization, and sonograms may be used in some institutions. The patient with a suspected metallic intraocular foreign body should not undergo magnetic resonance imaging. A history of blast injuries should alert the physician to the possibility of multiple foreign bodies.

Foreign Body Removal

Several techniques are used for foreign body removal. The choice of technique depends on the location and nature of the foreign body. Superficial foreign bodies are often most easily removed with irrigation, whereas embedded foreign bodies may require using a spud or needle for removal.

Superficial Foreign Bodies

Small foreign bodies on the surface of the eye can often be removed most easily by simple irrigation with sterile water or a commercially prepared eye solution (Chapter 48). Irrigation may be performed with an irrigation solution bag attached to intravenous tubing.

A cotton swab premoistened with sterile saline is best reserved for foreign bodies on the bulbar or palpebral conjunctiva. A cotton swab, especially if dry, may cause an abrasion if used on the cornea.

Embedded Foreign Bodies

Removal of an embedded foreign body in a child may be challenging and often is best left to an ophthalmologist. Embedded corneal foreign bodies generally require using either a 25- or 27-gauge needle on a small syringe or an eye spud device (Fig. 47.1). In a cooperative older child, the head should be secured against a slit lamp frame, and the child instructed to focus on an object in the distance. The needle or spud is held tangentially to the eye while the foreign object is gently scooped off the cornea (Fig. 47.2). The physician's hand may be braced against the child's face during foreign body removal.

If difficulty is encountered in removing the foreign body, penetrating ocular trauma should be suspected, and immediate referral to an ophthalmologist is indicated. Incomplete foreign body removal or multiple foreign bodies also necessitate referral to an ophthalmologist. An eye shield may be placed over the eye to prevent the child from rubbing it, thereby forcing a foreign body deeper into the eye or causing extrusion of ocular contents when the globe is ruptured.

After Foreign Body Removal

When the foreign body has been successfully removed, an examination with fluorescein is useful to determine if a corneal

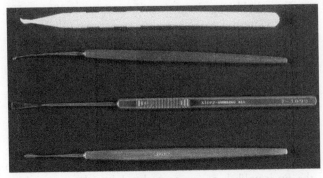

Figure 47.1 Spud devices used for removing embedded foreign bodies. A hypodermic needle on a syringe also can be used.

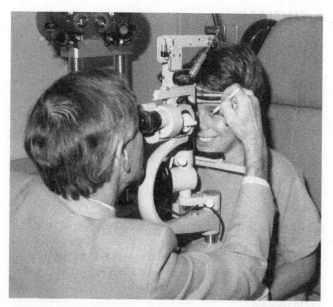

Figure 47.2 A physician with experience uses a spud device held tangential to the eye with the slit lamp to remove an embedded foreign body in a cooperative child.

abrasion has resulted. The presence of a corneal abrasion requires that the eye be examined again within 24 to 36 hours to ascertain the degree of healing. Patients with larger or deeper corneal abrasions should receive follow-up evaluation by an ophthalmologist.

Ciliary spasm or iritis may cause pain after foreign body removal. A drop of topical cycloplegic (e.g., homatropine 2% or 5%, cyclopentolate 0.5% or 1%, tropicamide 1%) can reduce this discomfort. For reasons stated previously, patients should not be discharged with a topical anesthetic agent. Ophthalmic NSAIDs may provide safe and effective analgesia while avoiding potential systemic side effects; these agents include ketorolac 0.5%, diclofenac 0.1%, and indomethacin 0.1% (8). If cycloplegics and non-narcotic analgesics prove ineffective, pain should be managed with oral narcotics. Instillation of antibiotic solution or ointment has not been shown to be of much value for superficial corneal abrasions after foreign body removal (9). In some instances in which risk of infection is increased, such as when the foreign body is of organic material or the patient is a contact lens wearer, an antibiotic ointment with antipseudomonal coverage may help prevent infection.

Routine patching of the eye for conjunctival or corneal abrasions is no longer recommended (see also Chapter 49). Although widely used in the past, recent data suggests that eye patching offers no advantage in the treatment of small, superficial corneal abrasions resulting from foreign bodies. Several studies, including one in children, have shown that eye patching is associated with no difference in the rate of corneal abrasion healing but may be associated with more discomfort after foreign body removal (10–12). There is also concern that eye infections may go undetected when covered by an eye patch (10).

▶ COMPLICATIONS

Complications may occur as a consequence of either the foreign body or the removal procedure. Infection may occur as simple conjunctivitis; however, infection resulting from a corneal abrasion may be more severe and should be referred to an ophthalmologist.

Metallic foreign bodies may leave rust rings that stain the cornea secondary to iron oxidation (see "Indications"). Physicians with experience in rust ring removal and with a highly cooperative child may attempt removal in the emergency setting at the time of foreign body removal. This is accomplished by picking away at the rust with a 25- or 27-gauge needle or spud device, with care not to cause further corneal damage. If this is unsuccessful, antibiotic ointment should be applied to the eye and a referral made to an ophthalmologist for follow-up in 24 hours. The rust ring will continue to oxidize and migrate to the corneal surface. As it does, the underlying cornea typically becomes softer, facilitating removal of the rust ring. Occasionally, the rust ring will fall out spontaneously. Young children may be uncooperative for rust ring removal and should be referred to an ophthalmologist without any removal attempt in the ED.

Retained foreign bodies may be surprisingly well tolerated (5). Foreign bodies may have penetrated into but not through the corneal stroma. In this case, some inert substances such as glass or sand are relatively noninflammatory, whereas organic materials such as plant or insect matter and ionizing metals precipitate a significant inflammatory reaction. Foreign bodies composed of organic material have an increased

 CLINICAL TIPS

▶ Check the pupils carefully. A deformed pupil or an area of prolapsed iris may indicate a ruptured globe.

▶ Beware of an intraocular foreign body if there is a history of high-velocity projectiles. Plain radiographs or computerized tomography can localize a foreign body. Magnetic resonance imaging is contraindicated with metallic foreign bodies.

▶ If a globe rupture is suspected, protect the eye with a shield and obtain an immediate ophthalmologic consultation.

▶ Moist cotton-tipped swabs may be useful for finding and removing conjunctival foreign bodies.

▶ Consider ophthalmologic referral for the child who has multiple foreign bodies or an embedded foreign body and is not able to cooperate with an examination.

risk of infection. Retained intraocular foreign bodies may be suspected when either a history of high-velocity injuries or an irregularly shaped pupil is found.

Although not common, vigorous attempts at foreign body removal with a needle or spud in uncooperative, poorly restrained children may cause corneal abrasion or penetrating trauma. This highlights the need for good judgment in deciding which children to refer and which to sedate for ocular foreign body removal. Consultation with an ophthalmologist should be readily employed. Recurrent abrasions may occur later in an area of corneal injury, particularly at night when lubrication from tears is decreased (5,13).

Allergic reactions to anesthetics and antibiotics may occur. Topical antibiotics containing neomycin may be particularly sensitizing. A history of medication allergies, if present, may prevent these reactions.

SUMMARY

1 Obtain a history. High-velocity injuries often result in penetration of the globe.

2 Assess for a ruptured globe. If at any point a penetrating injury is suspected, stop the examination, shield the eye, and immediately call an ophthalmologist.

3 Anesthetize the eye.

4 Perform a thorough physical examination of the eye, including visual acuity testing and fluorescein examination.

5 Locate the foreign body. Evert the eyelids and inspect with magnification. Tiny foreign bodies adherent to the conjunctiva may be found by wiping a moist cotton-tipped applicator across the superior fornix.

6 Remove superficial foreign bodies with irrigation.

7 Conjunctival foreign bodies may be removed with a moistened cotton-tipped applicator.

8 Embedded corneal foreign bodies in cooperative children may be removed with a 25-gauge needle on a syringe or with a spud device.

9 Perform a fluorescein examination after foreign body removal to look for corneal abrasion.

10 Relieve the pain of ciliary spasm or iritis with a drop of topical cycloplegic.

11 Consider instillation of antibiotic ointment or drops.

12 Arrange for re-evaluation of the patient in 24 hours.

▶ SUMMARY

Ocular foreign bodies must be removed, although not all are appropriate for removal in the emergency setting. Before foreign body removal, a careful eye examination must be performed to rule out associated injuries, in particular a ruptured globe and intraocular foreign body. Children with foreign body sensation in the eye need a thorough examination to locate material that may be in the recesses of the upper or lower fornices or embedded in the cornea. Some children with foreign body sensation may have corneal abrasions, conjunctivitis, or other eye injuries without foreign bodies being present.

Removal of ocular foreign bodies may be accomplished by irrigation or by using a moistened cotton swab for conjunctival foreign bodies or a needle or spud for corneal foreign bodies. Care must be exercised to avoid damage to the eye. Many children will require ophthalmologic consultation for foreign body removal.

▶ ACKNOWLEDGMENT

The authors would like to acknowledge the valuable contributions of Jennifer Pratt Cheney to the version of this chapter that appeared in the previous edition.

▶ REFERENCES

1. Santen SA, Scott JL. Ophthalmologic procedures. *Emerg Med Clin North Am.* 1995;13:681–701.
2. Linden JA, Renner GS. Trauma to the globe. *Emerg Med Clin North Am.* 1995;13:581–605.
3. Kaye-Wilson LG. Localization of corneal foreign bodies. *Br J Ophthalmol.* 1992;76:741–742.
4. Shingleton BJ. Eye injuries. *N Engl J Med.* 1991;325:408–413.
5. McMahon TT, Robin JB. Corneal trauma, I: classification and management. *J Am Optom Assoc.* 1991;62:170–178.
6. Janda AM. Ocular trauma: triage and treatment. *Postgrad Med.* 1991;90(7):51–60.
7. Sklar DP, Lauth JE, Johnson DR. Topical anesthesia of the eye as a diagnostic test. *Ann Emerg Med.* 1989;18:1209–1211.
8. Weaver C, Terrell K. Update: do ophthalmic nonsteroidal anti-inflammatory drugs reduce the pain associated with simple corneal abrasions without delaying healing? *Ann Emerg Med.* 2003;41:134–140.
9. Knoop KJ, Dennis WR, Hedges JR. Ocular foreign body removal. In: Roberts JR, Hedges JR, eds. *Clinical Procedures in Emergency Medicine.* 4th ed. Philadelphia: WB Saunders; 2004:1252–1258.
10. Hulbert MFG. Efficacy of eyepad in corneal healing after corneal foreign body removal. *Lancet.* 1991;337:643.
11. Michael JG, Hug D, Dowd MD. Management of corneal abrasion in children: a randomized clinical trial. *Ann Emerg Med.* 2002;40:67–72.
12. LeSage N, Verreault R, Rochette L. Efficacy of eye patching for traumatic corneal abrasions: a controlled clinical trial. *Ann Emerg Med.* 2001:38:129–134.
13. Elkington AR, Khaw PT. ABC of eyes: injuries to the eye. *Br Med J.* 1988;297(6641):122–125.

MANANDA S. BHENDE AND ERIC THAM

48

Ocular Irrigation and Decontamination of Conjunctiva

▶ INTRODUCTION

Eye irrigation is the crucial first step in the treatment of chemical injuries to the eye. Chemical burns are among the most urgent of ocular emergencies. The procedure dilutes the chemical (acid or base) and, if accomplished within seconds or minutes after the event, can decrease the damage caused by the chemical and improve the long-term prognosis.

Chemical burns are more common in adult patients and may occur as industrial accidents, in agricultural work, or in the household. In children, household accidents are the most common source of ocular chemical exposure. Ideally, irrigation of the eye begins immediately at the location where the incident occurred and is continued by emergency medical technicians (EMTs) and then completed in the hospital emergency department. The procedure can be performed by the parent, the patient, a bystander, EMTs, nurses, and physicians (1–6).

Chemical injuries to the eye can occur accidentally or unintentionally in all age groups and also may occur intentionally in adolescents. Because household agents are a major cause of chemical burns of the eye, active toddlers and preschoolers are at particular risk (Table 48.I).

▶ ANATOMY AND PHYSIOLOGY

The conjunctiva is a thin, transparent mucous membrane that covers the posterior surface of the lids (the palpebral conjunctiva) and the anterior surface of the sclera (the bulbar conjunctiva) (see Fig. 45.I). It is continuous with the skin at the lid margin and with the corneal epithelium at the limbus (sclerocorneal junction). The palpebral conjunctiva is firmly adherent to the tarsus. At the superior and inferior margins of the tarsus, the conjunctiva is reflected posteriorly at the superior and the inferior fornices and attaches to the sclera to become the bulbar conjunctiva, which is loosely attached to the orbital septum in the fornices and the sclera. The fornices and the medial and lateral canthi are locations where chemicals can pool or become trapped, especially if in the solid state. The eye, therefore, must be irrigated well in these difficult-to-reach areas (7).

The cornea is a transparent, avascular membrane that functions as a refracting and protective window through which light rays pass en route to the retina. The epithelium comprises the outer layer of the cornea, and the endothelium lines the anterior chamber of the eye. Chemical or physical damage to the endothelium of the cornea is far more serious than epithelial damage and can cause marked swelling, scarring, and loss of transparency, which can lead to loss of vision. Therefore it is vital to limit damage to the cornea during chemical exposure by prompt and thorough irrigation.

The irrigation process is more difficult in a child who is uncooperative. Such a child may need to be immobilized for the procedure; however, sedation is rarely indicated.

The severity of a chemical burn varies depending on the nature of the chemical, its volume, its concentration, the duration of contact, and the reaction with tissue components. Gases are less injurious than liquids or solid particles.

Alkaline substances are usually more damaging to the ocular structures than acids. Acids with pH of 2.5 or less coagulate and precipitate tissue proteins, which create a physical barrier against further penetration. Buffering by surrounding tissue proteins also helps localize damage to the initial area of contact. Exceptions include burns from hydrofluoric acid and from acids containing heavy metals, which rapidly penetrate

TABLE 48.1	COMMON HOUSEHOLD AGENTS CAPABLE OF CAUSING CHEMICAL BURNS TO THE EYE

Household ammonia (ammonium hydroxide 9%, pH 12.5)
Other ammonia-containing agents such as window cleaner and jewelry cleaner
Dishwasher detergent (sodium tripolyphosphate, pH 12)
Drain cleaner (sodium or potassium hydroxide, pH 14)
Oven cleaner (sodium hydroxide, pH 14)
Toilet bowl cleaner (sulfuric acid 80%, pH 1.0)
Battery fluid (sulfuric acid 30%, pH 1.0)
Pool cleaner (sodium or Ca hypochlorite 70%)
Bleaches (sodium hypochlorite)
Disinfectants
Deodorizing cleaners
Automotive cleaners and degreasers
Whitewall tire cleaners
Lime (calcium hydroxide) and plaster

the cornea. Organic solvents result in epithelial damage and do not penetrate into deeper structures.

An alkali burn is usually more severe because it thromboses blood vessels, denatures collagen, and damages cell membranes by saponification, a process by which the alkali reacts with fats to form soaps, thereby allowing further penetration of the alkali into the eye (1,3–6,8–9).

▶ INDICATIONS AND CONTRAINDICATIONS

Any suspected contact with the eyes by a caustic or irritant warrants irrigation. Children with acute onset of burning, pain, itch, or redness should have the affected eyes irrigated for possible chemical exposure.

Small foreign bodies of the conjunctiva that are not embedded often can be removed with irrigation. Children with foreign body sensation in the eye without a visible foreign body also may benefit.

For moderate or severe burns, irrigation should begin immediately on arrival to the ED. Consultation with ophthalmology should occur promptly while instituting treatment. Irrigation is indicated in children with suspected chemical exposure of the eye even if the parent or prehospital care providers have already irrigated.

Irrigation of the eye is not contraindicated when penetrating injury occurs to the eye, but extra care must be taken to avoid exerting any pressure on the globe (10).

▶ EQUIPMENT

Irrigation solution (normal saline solution or lactated Ringer 1-L bags or Balanced Salt Solution Plus at room temperature)
Intravenous tubing
Towels or linen saver pads
Emesis basin, pail, or bucket
Topical anesthetic (tetracaine 0.5% or proparacaine 0.5%)
pH paper
Papoose board, if needed
4″ × 4″ gauze
Eyelid retractor (rarely needed)
Moist cotton-tip swabs
Gloves
Fluorescein strips
Morgan therapeutic lenses (optional)

▶ PROCEDURE

Irrigation with water or saline is the first step in diluting the chemical in the eye so as to decrease the duration of exposure. At home or in the workplace, eye irrigation can be accomplished by placing the patient's face in a bowl of water with eyes open and by frequently changing the water. Alternatively, tap water can be run over the patient's open eyes. The water need not be sterile. In the ED setting, using isotonic normal saline or lactated Ringer solution is ideal. The ocular solution Balanced Salt Solution Plus (BSS Plus) is an alternative that may be better tolerated if available. There has not been shown to be a therapeutic difference between the different solutions (4–5).

Before the procedure, both the parents and the child should be given a brief explanation about what is going to be done. Although it is important to explain the details, prolonged description should not delay the procedure. Time is of the essence. Parents usually know that the chemical substance has to be washed off the eye. While preparing the child and the equipment for irrigation, parents can be informed about the procedure. Signed informed consent is usually not necessary. Parents should be offered the option of remaining with their child during the irrigation (see Chapter 1).

A quick history and brief physical examination is performed while the equipment is prepared. Gloves should be worn because of the potential contact with a caustic substance. Immobilization is appropriate if the child is uncooperative.

An older child can lie on the examining table with his or her head just beyond or over the end. This enables the irrigating fluid to be collected in a pail placed directly underneath the back of the child's head.

The pH should be measured if a strip is easily available. Measurement is accomplished by simply placing the strip into the pocket that is formed when the lower eyelid is retracted. This baseline value, although not crucial, will help to determine the effectiveness of the therapy. Instillation of a topical anesthetic (tetracaine 0.5% or proparacaine 0.5%) also is advisable, but the search for pH paper and topical anesthetic must not delay the irrigation. For this reason, it is advisable to keep these materials together in a single location.

Irrigation is begun by holding the end of the intravenous tubing just above the eyeball and allowing free flow of the irrigation fluid (Fig. 48.1). During irrigation, the eyelids must

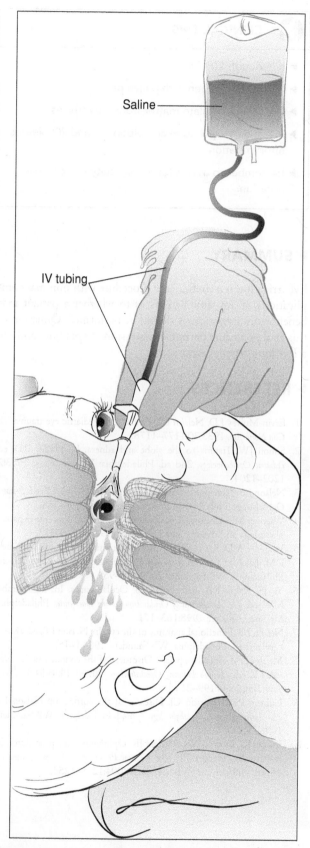

Saline

IV tubing

Figure 48.1 While an assistant retracts the eyelids with gauze pads or lid retractors, the eye is copiously irrigated with saline using a standard intravenous setup. It is important to expose and irrigate the upper and lower conjunctival sacs.

be held maintained open. This is best accomplished by an assistant rather than the physician performing the irrigation. Gauze pads enable the holder to better grip the wet, slippery eyelids. If retractors are necessary (see Chapter 45), the physician must ensure that the eye is well anesthetized.

Alternatively, a Morgan lens can be inserted into the anesthetized eye. This device is a large, soft contact lens with an irrigation nipple extending from its anterior aspect. The nipple is connected to a bag of saline, and the saline drains into the eye. The patient can close the lids around the lens without affecting the irrigation. Some concern exists, however, that this device may allow pooling of chemicals beneath the lens. Some authorities therefore recommend using the lens when prolonged irrigation is required after the more traditional technique (Fig. 48.1) has been performed. Additionally, maximum patient comfort during lens irrigation requires a well-anesthetized eye. The lens causes topical anesthetic to be rapidly washed out of the eye, and recurrent dosing (which is not without risk) may be necessary.

Towels or linen pads should be placed on either side of the head to catch the irrigating fluid, and an emesis basin also can be used. If the patient's head is extended beyond the end of the table, a pail can be placed on the floor to catch the drops of irrigating fluid.

Saline exiting from the intravenous tubing should be directed over the globe, into the upper and lower fornices, and over the canthi. The saline should flow from medial to lateral so that it can be easily collected. The child is instructed to look straight up and then to move his or her eyes in all directions—medial, lateral, up, and down—allowing all areas of the conjunctival sac to be well irrigated.

Care should be taken not to cause trauma to the cornea by touching it with the tubing, retracting the eyelids, or forcing the saline directly against the cornea.

Particulate matter is swept from the conjunctival fornices and the medial and lateral canthi with moistened cotton-tipped applicators. This may require eversion of the upper lid (see Chapter 45).

Irrigation with 1 to 2 L of saline over 20 minutes is usually more than adequate. Severe alkaline burns may benefit from prolonged irrigation with larger volumes. One cannot overirrigate the eye. As mentioned, a scleral contact lens for continuous irrigation may be used. The pH in the conjunctival fornices should be measured after irrigation. If still alkaline or acidic, irrigation should continue until pH normalizes (normal ocular pH is 7.4). The pH is measured again in 20 minutes to make sure it remains normal. Delayed pH changes are usually the result of incomplete irrigation or residual particulate matter in the fornices.

When adequate irrigation has been accomplished, the face is dried and the child is released from the securing device. The patient's eyes are checked for corneal abrasion with aseptic fluorescein liquid or fluorescein strips. It is extremely important to test for visual acuity and document the findings in the record. This is usually done after irrigation to avoid a delay and prolonged chemical contact with the eye.

SUMMARY

1 Obtain brief history and perform examination as the equipment is prepared.

2 If necessary, secure the child and separate the eyelids manually with gauze pads.

3 Check the pH of the conjunctivae.

4 Instill topical anesthetic.

5 Sweep away any particulate matter with moistened cotton-tipped swabs.

6 Irrigate with 1 to 2 L normal saline or lactated Ringer solution for about 20 minutes; direct irrigation fluid over globe, into upper and lower fornices, and over canthi.

7 Measure the pH of tears; if still alkaline or acidic, continue until the pH normalizes to 7.4.

8 Recheck the pH in 20 minutes.

9 Check for corneal abrasions with fluorescein.

10 Assess visual acuity.

11 Consult ophthalmology as needed and arrange for follow-up.

Ophthalmologic consultation should be sought immediately for all serious injuries. Follow-up for ophthalmologic evaluation should be recommended for all but the most minor injuries (1–6,8–10).

▶ COMPLICATIONS

Complications from irrigation of the eye are rare. Most injuries noted after irrigation are the result of the injury for which irrigation was performed. Irrigation may cause abrasion of the cornea or conjunctiva. A linear abrasion may occur from attempts to keep the eyelids open, or a fine punctate keratitis from the force of the irrigation fluid on the cornea. Superficial corneal abrasions are treated in the usual manner. Deep or penetrating injuries are likely to be the result of the chemical and require immediate ophthalmologic evaluation (1–6,8–10).

 CLINICAL TIPS

▶ If in doubt, IRRIGATE.

▶ Hold the lids open with gauze pads.

▶ Remove particulate matter from the fornices.

▶ Measure the pH upon completion of and 20 minutes after irrigation.

▶ Remember to assess for visual acuity and corneal abrasion.

▶ SUMMARY

Eye irrigation is a useful, easy procedure with minimal complications. If any doubt exists as to whether a patient may benefit from irrigation, it should be performed. Omission of this vital procedure permits progression of eye injury and can affect long-term prognosis.

▶ REFERENCES

1. Ervin-Mulvey LD, Nelson LB, Freeley DA. Pediatric eye trauma. *Ped Clin North Am.* 1983;30:1177–1178.

2. Simon JW. Trauma to the globe and adnexa. In: Harley RD, ed. *Pediatric Ophthalmology.* 2nd ed. Philadelphia: WB Saunders; 1983:2: 1202–1204.

3. Nelson LB. Management of ocular trauma. In: Nelson LB, ed. *Pediatric Ophthalmology.* Philadelphia: WB Saunders; 1984:227–228.

4. Wagoner MD. Chemical injuries of the eye: current concepts in pathophysiology and therapy. *Surv Ophthalmol.* 1997;41:275–313.

5. Wagoner MD, Kenyon KR. Chemical injuries of the eye. In: Albert DM, Jakobiec FA, eds. *Principles and Practice of Ophthalmology.* 2nd ed. Philadelphia: WB Saunders; 2000:943–959.

6. Yu JS, Ralph RA, Rubenstein JB. Ocular burns. In: MacCumber MW, ed. *The Management of Ocular Injuries and Emergencies.* Philadelphia: Lippincott-Raven; 1998:163–171.

7. Nelson LB. Functional anatomy of the eye. In: Nelson LB, ed. *Pediatric Ophthalmology.* Philadelphia: WB Saunders; 1984:1–18.

8. Meisler DM, Beauchamp GR. Disorders of the conjunctiva. In: Nelson LB, ed. *Harley's Pediatric Ophthalmology.* 4th ed. Philadelphia: WB Saunders; 1998:199–214.

9. Laibson PR, Rapuano CJ. Diseases of the cornea. In: Nelson LB, ed. *Harley's Pediatric Ophthalmology.* 4th ed. Philadelphia: WB Saunders; 1998:215–257.

10. Knopp KJ, Dennis WR, Hedges JR. Ophthalmologic procedures. In: Roberts JR, Hedges JR, eds. *Clinical Procedures in Emergency Medicine.* 4th ed. Philadelphia: WB Saunders; 2004:1248–1252.

49

MICHAEL SHANNON

Eye Patching and Eye Guards

▶ INTRODUCTION

Because of its prominence and delicateness, the eye is frequently injured. Eye injuries occur despite a large number of physiologic protective mechanisms and structures, including the eyelids and eyelashes, the tarsal plates, the orbicularis oculi muscles, the lacrimal apparatus, the corneal reflex, and the lid reflexes. Severe injury can lead to significant disability, especially if the injury is bilateral. Evaluating eye injuries in children is often challenging. The clinician's goal is to identify the type and severity of injury without causing further damage.

Eye patches, which are designed to maintain the eye in a closed position, are to be distinguished from eye guards or shields, which are fenestrated metal guards used to protect the eye. Eye patching may reduce discomfort and promote healing. In contrast, eye guards play an important role in preventing further injury. Proper use of these techniques and appropriate consultation with an ophthalmologist are important in optimizing visual outcome in children with eye injuries.

▶ ANATOMY AND PHYSIOLOGY

The most important ocular structures to identify are the conjunctivae (bulbar and palpebral), the cornea, the iris, the ciliary apparatus, and the anterior chamber (see Fig. 45.1). The epithelium of the cornea is directly continuous with the conjunctiva. The cornea is extensively innervated by the ciliary nerves. It is unique in being avascular, having no direct blood supply. Oxygen and nutrients are supplied to the cornea by tears and by their diffusion from the ciliary circulation. Nonetheless, after corneal injuries, healing and re-epithelialization occur rapidly.

Full-thickness lacerations of the cornea or sclera allow extrusion of aqueous or vitreous humor. The underlying iris or choroid often plugs the wound, preventing ongoing leakage. Further trauma or pressure on the globe or physical agitation can disrupt this delicate protective mechanism and cause further extrusion of intraocular contents. Helping the child to be as calm as possible and placing an eye guard protects the ruptured globe from additional injury. Eye patches should be avoided in possible globe injury, since they put pressure on the globe, which can worsen the eye injury.

▶ INDICATIONS AND CONTRAINDICATIONS

The goals of eye patching are to provide comfort and facilitate healing. Eye patching can reduce photophobia (light-induced ciliary spasm) and pain associated with blinking by keeping the eyelid closed. Patching may facilitate healing of corneal injuries by preventing the surface abrasion that may occur during eye blinking. Eye patches are contraindicated in (a) patients with possible penetrating eye injury or open globe, (b) patients with glaucoma, (c) patients in whom corticosteroid ophthalmic solutions have been instilled, (d) wearers of extended-wear contact lenses, and (e) patients with chemical eye injuries, whose eyes should remain open to allow residual chemical to drain until thorough irrigation has been completed. Patches also are relatively contraindicated in the treatment of abrasions secondary to contact lens wear (see "Complications").

Although eye patching is virtually always recommended in the treatment of corneal abrasion, almost no literature demonstrates that patching has advantages over treatment without patching in minor corneal abrasions. In fact, some studies indicate that patients who have not been patched have faster

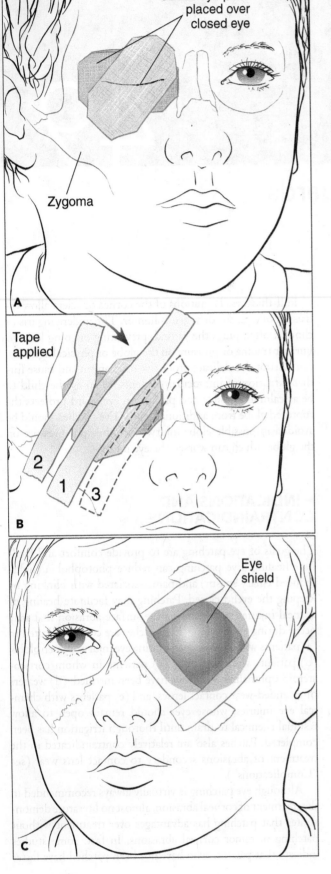

healing and are more comfortable (1,2). Furthermore, the possibility exists that patching may predispose the eye to infection by creating a warm, moist environment that favors bacterial growth. Placing antibiotic cream into the eye provides a false sense of security because effective antibiotic levels in the eye fall within 6 hours after cream instillation and within 2 hours after instilling antibiotic eye drops. In adolescents and young adults who drive, patching has the additional disadvantage of eliminating stereoscopic vision, which can increase the risk of an automobile crash. Reading is also difficult or impossible with a patch in place. If a child or adolescent who has a simple corneal abrasion will not keep a patch in place or finds a patch too inconvenient or uncomfortable, then he or she should be treated without one.

Eye guards are used for patients awaiting or being transported for ophthalmologic evaluation with a known or suspected rupture of the globe (1–3). They should be applied gently, with every effort made not to place pressure on the globe.

▶ EQUIPMENT

Eye pads
Gauze cut into ovals if eye pads are not available
Eye guard or shield
Tape

▶ PROCEDURE

Eye Patching

The only equipment necessary for eye patching consists of eye pads and tape. Gauze cut into an oval shape is an acceptable alternative to an eye pad. Before the eye is patched, a thorough ophthalmologic examination should be performed that includes an assessment of visual acuity, pupil shape, light response, and extraocular movements; an inspection for a retained foreign body; an examination of adjacent bony structures; and a presumably positive corneal fluorescein examination (see Chapter 45). An ophthalmologist should be

---

Figure 49.1 The purpose of an eye patch is to hold the eyelid tightly closed.
A. Two pads are placed over the eye with the lid closed.
B. Tape is applied from the center of the forehead to the zygomatic arch on the affected side and continued until the patch is securely taped. In contrast to patching, the purpose of the eye shield is to prevent the application of undue pressure on an injured eye.
C. The shield is placed over the eye, and tape is placed along the edges of the shield, securing it against the underlying bone. Pressure directly over the eye must be avoided. If an eye shield is unavailable, a plastic, paper, or Styrofoam cup may be used as a substitute.

SUMMARY

Eye Patching

1 Thoroughly examine the eye before patching.

2 Use at least two eye pads.

3 Place over the closed eyelid on an angle, with the narrow end toward nose.

4 Apply tape from the forehead to the zygoma, using benzoin if better adhesion is required.

Eye Shielding

1 Place the eye guard as soon as a ruptured globe is suspected.

2 Ensure that the eye guard does not contact the eyelid or globe.

3 Apply tape from the forehead to the zygoma.

CLINICAL TIPS

▶ Do not place an eye patch on a child who may have a ruptured globe.

▶ If the eye patch will not keep the eyelid completely closed, consider treatment without a patch.

▶ Secure tape on eye patches and eye guards firmly. Supply the parent with tape and patches in case the patch needs to be replaced.

▶ If a patient with a simple corneal abrasion cannot or will not wear a patch, then he or she should be managed without a patch.

Occasionally eye shielding is required in the absence of a plastic or metal eye shield. In these cases, a plastic, paper, or Styrofoam cup may be used as a temporary alternative, provided the cup is large enough to protect the eye without putting pressure on the globe itself (3,4).

consulted before eye patching in patients with chemical eye injuries, suspicion of penetrating globe injuries, or identified abnormalities of extraocular movement or pupillary action. If warranted, ophthalmic medications (cycloplegics, antibiotics) are applied before patching.

At least two eye pads should be placed against the closed eyelid. The pad is applied on a slant, with the narrow end toward the nose (Fig. 49.1A). Tape is applied from the center forehead to the cheek overlying the zygoma of the affected side (Fig. 49.1B); benzoin may be necessary to improve tape adhesion to the facial skin. In young children, instructions regarding patch reapplication and extra pads and tape should be provided to the parents in the event the patch falls off or is removed. An improperly placed patch may be worse than no patch at all. If the patch will not maintain the eyelid in the closed position, then treatment without a patch should be considered (3,4).

Eye Shielding

The eye guard is positioned over the injured eye, with avoidance of direct contact with the eyelid or globe. The edges are placed against the underlying bone of the nose, supraorbital ridge, and zygoma. Tape is applied from the forehead to the cheek of the affected side, and the guard is checked to ensure that it is firmly positioned without contact with the orbital structures (Fig. 49.1C).

▶ COMPLICATIONS

Eye patches are always to be removed 24 to 48 hours after initial application for re-examination of the eye. Complications from eye patching are rare but include corneal drying or abrasion secondary to forced partial opening, infection (particularly in extended-wear contact lens wearers), and intraocular hypertension. Eye patches also are relatively contraindicated in the treatment of corneal abrasion secondary to contact lens use. These injuries are predisposed to *Pseudomonas* infections, and patching appears to increase the risk of this very serious condition.

Improper placement of an eye guard can further injure the affected eye, particularly if the globe is ruptured.

▶ REFERENCES

1. Long J, Tann T. Orbital trauma. *Ophthalmol Clin North Am.* 2002;15:249–253.

2. Hamid RK, Newfield P. Pediatric eye emergencies. *Anesthesiol Clin North America.* 2001;19:257–264.

3. Ophthalmologic procedures. In: Roberts JR, Hedges JR, eds. *Clinical Procedures in Emergency Medicine.* 3rd ed. Philadelphia: WB Saunders; 2003:995–1019.

4. Michael JG, Hug D, Dowd MD. Management of corneal abrasion in children: a randomized clinical trial. *Ann Emerg Med.* 2002;40:67–72.

50

TIMOTHY G. GIVENS

Contact Lens Removal

▶ INTRODUCTION

As the number of persons wearing contact lenses steadily increases, so does the chance that a physician in the emergency department (ED) will encounter problems related to contact lens use. Familiarity with indications and techniques for contact lens removal is therefore essential. These skills also may prove valuable for the office-based practitioner.

Contact lens use requires a certain level of maturity, so children do not usually become contact lens wearers until approximately 10 years of age. At that age, children are less likely to be meticulous in regard to the proper wear, removal, and cleaning of their lenses. They are therefore at increased risk of complications such as eye trauma or infection. Children also are less likely to be cooperative with contact lens removal, which can make this procedure much more challenging.

▶ ANATOMY AND PHYSIOLOGY

The cornea is a transparent window at the most anterior portion of the eye (see Fig. 45.1). It is a dense layer of tissue that is uniformly about 1 mm thick. Because it has a greater curvature than the sclera, the cornea resembles a watch crystal. The cornea is avascular and receives nutrients from the capillaries associated with the anterior ciliary arteries at its margin. It is well supplied with sensory nerves from the ciliary nerves. Aside from the cornea, the remainder of the visible portion of the anterior eyeball is covered by the conjunctiva. The conjunctiva joins the corneal epithelium at the limbus, or corneal margin. The conjunctiva and cornea are lubricated by mucous-containing secretions from the lacrimal gland and from the conjunctiva itself (1,2).

A contact lens is designed to float on the tear film overlying the surface of the centrally located cornea and to modify its refractive power. When the lens slides out of position and is lost in the eye, it may commonly hide on the undersurface of either eyelid, especially in the fornices, which are the upper and lower recesses where the conjunctiva reflects onto the eyeball. Tinted lenses are usually easy to locate and remove, but localization and recovery of a clear lens may require topical anesthesia and slit lamp examination (1,3,4).

Lack of vascularity of the cornea makes it dependent on the movement of tears beneath the contact lens for oxygen delivery. Both hard and soft contact lenses may, with prolonged wear, cause mechanical irritation, hypotonic tear production, and resultant corneal edema. The subsequent reduction in oxygen-rich tear flow can produce ischemia of segments of the cornea. The symptoms of this overwear syndrome are similar to a foreign body sensation and include eye pain, redness, itching, and tearing. Symptoms may not appear until several hours after removal of the contact lens from the eye as a result of transient anesthesia of the eye caused by buildup of anoxic metabolites over the course of wear. Chemical irritants such as cigarette smoke and anything that decreases blinking and normal tear flow, such as the ingestion of sedatives (e.g., alcohol), also may produce a similar syndrome of corneal edema and ischemic injury.

The cornea is easily abraded by trauma to the eye, whether it is from a fingernail during contact lens insertion or removal, or from foreign material trapped beneath the improperly cleaned lens. Many abrasions and foreign bodies are visible to the naked eye with fluorescein staining and a Wood's (UV) lamp, although a complete examination should involve using a slit lamp. Mechanical trauma to the cornea may predispose to infection and ulceration if untreated. Few organisms are capable of penetrating an intact corneal epithelium without antecedent injury (1–5).

Soft contact lenses, made of a hydrophilic gel that may contain in excess of 60% water, carry added risk in terms of predisposition to infection. Soft lenses readily absorb water and, along with it, pathogenic organisms. Even minor trauma caused by simple lens insertion and wear may provide a portal of entry for organisms that then invade the cornea and lead to the development of a bacterial or fungal corneal ulcer. In the contact lens wearer who presents with eye pain, tearing, photophobia, and/or decreased vision in the affected eye, a suspicion of a corneal ulcer should be raised. The lens should be removed and a fluorescein slit lamp examination performed. Corneal opacity with shaggy debris and a flocculent stromal infiltrate indicate ulceration. Such a lesion represents an emergency and requires immediate ophthalmologic consultation for appropriate cultures and antimicrobial therapy (5).

Soft contact lenses also may be associated with other forms of nonemergent ocular injury, including corneal neovascularization, giant papillary conjunctivitis, and sensitivity reactions to contact lens solutions (2).

▶ INDICATIONS

The emergency physician may need to remove a contact lens from a patient's eye for several reasons. The first is to allow for a more detailed evaluation of the eye. This is especially true for the contact lens wearer who sustains trauma to the eye with a lens in place. The lens should be removed before a more thorough inspection of the patient's cornea, including instillation of fluorescein. Contact lenses, particularly the soft variety, absorb stains and chemicals and will become permanently stained if fluorescein is instilled before their removal from the eye (1,6).

Complaint of eye pain in a contact lens wearer is a second common indication for lens removal. Because of the cornea's rich nerve supply, pain is the classic presenting symptom of corneal injury. Photophobia also may be a significant component if the abrasion is large or is present for an extended period of time. As discussed previously, pain may represent traumatic injury to the eye, presence of a foreign body, infection, or "overwear" syndrome (1,6).

Inability of the patient to remove a contact lens is a third indication for removal by a physician. The patient with an altered sensorium who may not be able to express the need to have his or her lenses removed, the patient who needs assistance in locating a lost contact lens in the eye, and the patient who cannot physically remove a lens as a result of corneal edema from prolonged wear all fall into this category. All patients who are unconscious on presentation to the ED should undergo an examination of the eyes aimed at identifying eye injuries and locating and removing contact lenses (1,6).

The only relative contraindication to contact lens removal is the presence of a corneal perforation. Pressure on the globe must be avoided in this setting. Removal by an ophthalmologist using the suction cup technique is preferred.

▶ EQUIPMENT

Sterile gloves
Sterile saline or lubricating eye drops
Topical anesthetic solution
Several cotton-tipped applicators
A rubber-tipped suction cup device (DMV Corporation)
Pincer-type device for removal of soft contact lenses
Penlight
Slit lamp

▶ PROCEDURE

If possible, visual acuity should be assessed in each eye before contact lens removal. If perforation of the globe is suspected, an eye shield should immediately be placed and ophthalmologic consultation sought. Hands should be clean and/or sterile gloves worn when removing a lens. Because most pediatric patients wearing contact lenses will be 10 years of age or older, restraint or sedation is seldom necessary if the patient is approached calmly and all procedures are explained beforehand. However, patients with altered mental status or in severe pain as a result of eye trauma may require appropriate restraint devices. Slit lamp examination is impossible for the patient who must remain supine because of immobilization for trauma or other reasons. Unless contraindicated, topical ophthalmic anesthetic should be administered before attempts to remove the lens (1,6).

Hard Contact Lens

If the patient is alert and cooperative, his or her face should be held over a table surface or a clean cloth. The thumbs are placed on the upper and lower eyelids from the lateral palpebral margin and pulled to secure the lids tightly against the edges of the contact lens (Fig. 50.1). The patient is instructed to look toward the nose and then downward. This maneuver allows the lower eyelid to work itself under the lower lens edge and lift the lens off the eye (1).

If the patient is uncooperative or must remain supine, the physician can actively remove the contact lens with a modification of this technique. The location of the lens may be identified by shining a pen light across the surface of the eye from the lateral side. (This should be done in all unconscious adolescents once they are stable.) If the lens is in proper position, the thumbs are placed on the upper and lower eyelid near the margins. The eyelids are opened so that the lid margins pull away beyond the lens edges. Both eyelids are then pressed gently but firmly on the globe so that the lid margins just touch the contact lens edges. Firmer pressure on the lower

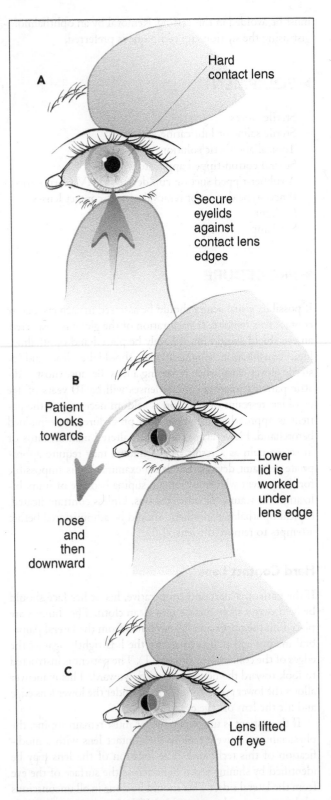

Figure 50.1 Removal of a hard contact lens.
A. Using the thumbs of both hands, pull the eyelids apart and then bring the lids down, trapping the lens between the lids.
B. If possible, have the patient look downward and medially as the lower lid is worked under the lower edge of the lens.
C. The lower edge of the lens will lift off the eye as the lid passes beneath it.

lid will manually work the lid margin under the bottom lens edge. As the lower lens edge tips away from the surface of the eye, the lids are moved together and the contact lens is slid out to where it may be grasped (1,6).

Alternatively, the lens can be removed from the cornea with a cotton-tipped applicator. After a drop of topical anesthetic solution is placed into the eye, the lens is moved laterally onto the sclera, and the tip of the applicator worked beneath a lens edge, lifting the lens off the eye. Applicator contact with the cornea may cause an abrasion.

If available, a moistened suction cup device applied directly to the contact lens allows for easy removal from the cornea. Suction cup devices appropriate for this purpose should be stocked in all EDs (1,6). A reasonable substitute that may be effective is a drop of honey on a gloved fingertip or cotton-tipped applicator. The honey can be later removed from the lens by simple washing (1).

If the lens is present but not in proper position, a drop of sterile saline or lubricating eye drops may be used to "float" it into a better location (6).

Soft Contact Lens

The lower eyelid is pulled down with the examiner's middle finger (Fig. 50.2). Placing the tip of the index finger on the lower edge of the contact lens, the examiner then slides the lens downward onto the sclera and is able to pinch the lens between the thumb and the index finger. The soft lens will fold, allowing easy removal from the eye. An alternative is to use a specially designed rubber tweezers made for this purpose. The tweezers serve the same purpose as the thumb and index finger, pinching the lens and causing it to fold. If the lens is dry and therefore relatively adherent to the eye, a drop of saline or an eye drop may be used to moisten and loosen it (1,6).

The Lost Contact Lens

Occasionally a patient presents with the complaint that he or she is unable to locate a contact lens and is uncertain whether it remains in the eye. As in all other eye examinations, evaluation must begin with an assessment of visual acuity in both eyes. The eye is then directly inspected for the contact lens. Though transparent, when appropriately located over the cornea, a lens is readily visible as a fine line on the sclera a few millimeters peripheral to the limbus. Shining a light from the lateral margin of the eye (sidelighting) may help to identify the location of a lens. If the lens is not apparent on initial inspection, topical anesthetic should be instilled and the eyelids everted (Chapters 45 and 47), as in a search for a foreign body, and an attempt to locate the lens beneath the lids is made. If the lens is not found, then, with the patient looking toward his or her chin, the examiner should sweep over the fornix with a moistened cotton-tipped applicator. If the lens remains elusive yet the patient insists that it is present in the eye, a fluorescein examination may be performed. The fluorescein will pool around the outside of the lens and its

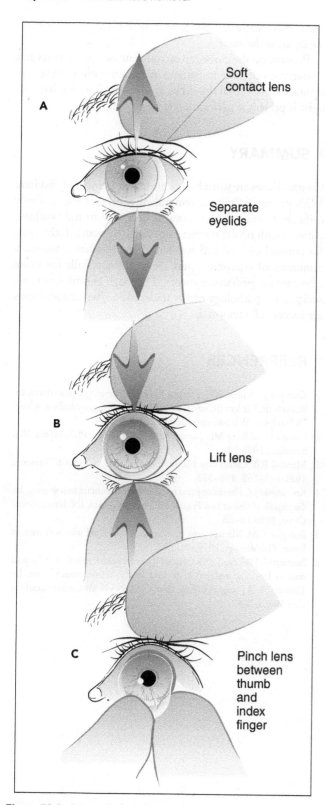

Figure 50.2 Removal of a soft contact lens.
A. Separate eyelids.
B. Use the index finger to work the lens onto the sclera. If the lens proves difficult to move, it may be moistened with a drop of saline.
C. Pinch the lens between the thumb and forefinger and remove it.

location will become apparent. It is important to inform the patient that the dye will permanently stain the soft contact lens if it is present.

If after an exhaustive search the contact lens is not found, the patient should be reassured that a thorough examination has not located the missing lens. It is useful to check that the patient has not inadvertently placed one contact lens over the top of the other in the same eye (1,6).

 SUMMARY

All Lenses and All Patients

1 Check the patient's visual acuity and perform a complete eye examination.

2 Appropriately restrain the patient, if necessary.

Hard Contact Lens and Cooperative Patient

1 Pull the eyelids from the lateral palpebral margin to secure the lids tightly against the edges of the contact lens.

2 Instruct the patient to look medially toward his or her nose, then downward.

3 Grasp the lens as it flips off the eye.

4 Alternatively, use a suction device to remove the lens.

Hard Contact Lens and Uncooperative Patient

1 Place thumbs on the upper and lower eyelids at the lid margins.

2 Open the eyelids beyond the margins of the contact lens.

3 Press both eyelids firmly on the globe so the lid margins touch the contact lens edges.

4 Press slightly more firmly on the lower lid to work the lower lid margin under the lens edge.

5 Move the lids together so the contact lens slides out and is able to be grasped.

6 Alternatively, use a suction device to remove the lens.

Soft Contact Lens

1 Pull down the lower eyelid with the middle finger.

2 Place the tip of the index finger on the lower edge of the contact lens.

3 Slide the lens downward onto the sclera and pinch it between the thumb and index finger or use a pincer-type removal device.

CLINICAL TIPS

▶ Assume that all unconscious adolescents are wearing contact lenses until an appropriate examination proves otherwise.

▶ If the patient feels a foreign body in his or her eye, determine the approximate location of the sensation before instilling a topical anesthetic.

▶ Do not hesitate to use fluorescein if a lens cannot be located. This will stain a soft contact lens, but finding the displaced lens is more important.

▶ Ensure that a proper eye examination is performed after the lens is removed. If the lens has been overworn, an underlying corneal infection is possible and requires careful assessment for diagnosis.

itself. Nevertheless, management of both types of corneal abrasions is the same.

Pressure on the globe can extrude intraocular contents and worsen the outcome in patients with perforation of the eye. Contact lens removal should be deferred until an ophthalmologist is present if perforation is suspected.

▶ SUMMARY

Contact lenses are worn by a considerable number of children. With proper technique, removal of a contact lens is rarely difficult. Contact lens removal is necessary to fully evaluate patients with ocular trauma or ocular symptoms. Techniques for removal of hard and soft lenses and lost lenses require a minimum of equipment and are important skills for those who care for pediatric patients. Thorough evaluation for associated eye pathology can be undertaken after contact lenses are successfully removed.

▶ COMPLICATIONS

Complications of contact lens removal include the production of a corneal abrasion and contamination of the eye with bacterial or viral organisms. Risk can be minimized by using aseptic technique and exercising care in gently removing lenses. A fluorescein examination of the eye is indicated in the evaluation of all suspected abrasions, foreign bodies, or eye infections. Thus any patient who is symptomatic either before or following contact lens removal should undergo a fluorescein examination. Typically, injury to the cornea from "overwear" results in a centrally located, brightly stippled staining pattern, referred to as "superficial punctate keratitis." This is in contrast to the usual sharp, linear staining pattern typical of mechanical trauma, such as might be caused by lens removal

▶ REFERENCES

1. Knoop KJ, Dennis WR, Hedges JR. Ophthalmologic procedures. In: Roberts JR, Hedges JR, eds. *Clinical Procedures in Emergency Medicine.* 4th ed. Philadelphia: WB Saunders, 2004:1261–1264.
2. Paton D, Goldberg MF. *Management of Ocular Injuries.* Philadelphia: WB Saunders; 1976:194.
3. Mandell RB. *Contact Lens Practice.* Springfield, IL: Charles C Thomas; 1981:142–168, 496–513.
4. Krezanoski JZ. Physiology and biochemistry of contact lens wearing. In: *Encyclopedia of Contact Lens Practice.* Vol. 4. South Bend, IN: International Optic; 1959:18–26.
5. Bohigian GM. Management of infections associated with soft contact lenses. *Ophthalmology.* 1979;86:1138.
6. Buttaravoli PM, Stair TO. Contact lens overwear, removal of dislocated contact lens, and removal of contact lens in unconscious patient. In: *Common, Simple Emergencies.* Englewood Cliffs, NJ: Brady Communications Co.; 1985:47–52.

SECTION 8 ▶ OTOLARYNGOLOGIC PROCEDURES

SECTION EDITOR: JOHN M. LOISELLE

51

MICHAEL P. POIRIER

Acute Upper Airway Foreign Body Removal: The Choking Child

▶ INTRODUCTION

Annually in the United States more than 300 deaths of children are due to choking secondary to upper airway obstruction (1). These incidents are usually due to foods, toys, or other small objects. More than 90% occur in infants and children younger than 5 years of age and 65% in infants younger than 2 years of age. Foods continue to be the most common objects involved in reported choking episodes in the infant and the child, with round or cylindrical foods most often cited (2) (Table 51.1).

In 1979, the U.S. Consumer Product Safety Commission passed regulations to control the marketing of non-food choking hazards (3). Small toys, rubber balloons, nails, tacks, and bolts are the main objects responsible for nonfood-related choking episodes in children (4–9). Rubber balloons are the leading cause of choking deaths from toys. Of these deaths, 75% are in children under 6 years of age (10).

Treating the child with an acutely obstructed airway is an emergent procedure. Although usually performed in the pre-hospital setting, it may be necessary to perform the procedure in the emergency department (ED). The first-aid approach is routinely taught to the lay public by emergency medicine and other health care providers. The laryngoscopic procedure may be performed by any qualified physician.

▶ ANATOMY AND PHYSIOLOGY

The nose, mouth, and pharynx comprise the upper airway. The upper airway has numerous functions, which include acting as a filter to prevent foreign material from entering the lower airway, humidifying and heating inspired gases, and acting as a system for conducting inspired gases to the lungs.

Ciliated and nonciliated mucous cells line the nose. The function of these cells is to help humidify inspired gases and to filter foreign material. Hair follicles and thick, sticky mucous secretions of the nose also help filter foreign material from the upper airway.

The laryngopharynx extends from the base of the tongue to the esophagus, which lies posterior to the trachea. Closure of the glottis protects the tracheobronchial tree from foreign material. This reflex mechanism is crucial in protecting the airway during the process of swallowing. Patients with neuromuscular illness, anatomically abnormal airways, or poorly protected airways are at the highest risk for foreign body aspirations and choking episodes.

The trachea begins at the level of the cricoid cartilage; it descends in the middle of the neck to the level of the fifth to sixth thoracic vertebra and then bifurcates into the right and left mainstem bronchi. Unlike in adults, the angle of takeoff at the carina is almost equal on both sides in young children. In the older child and young adult, the trachea at the bifurcation

TABLE 51.1	SPECIFIC FOODS CAUSING CHOKING EPISODES IN CHILDREN
Hot dog	17%
Candy	10%
Peanut/nut	9%
Grape	8%
Cookie/biscuit	7%
Meat	7%
Carrot	6%
Apple	5%
Popcorn	5%
Peanut butter	5%
Bean	4%
Bread	4%
Macaroni/noodle	3%
Chewing gum	3%
Others	7%

Source: Tinswarth DK. Analysis of chokingrelated hazards associated with children's products. Washington, DC: U.S. Consumer Product Safety Commission; 1989.

is slightly angled to the right, making the opening to the right bronchus a less acute angle.

The airway has protective mechanisms in place that continuously remove foreign debris. Tiny foreign bodies are continually swept up by cilia and mucus to the supraglottic region, where they can be swallowed down the esophagus. Coughing, which results from stimulation of receptors in the mucosa of the large respiratory passages, is an important means of expelling secretions and foreign matter from the airway. A cough begins with a deep inspiration followed by a forced expiration against a closed glottis. The glottis is then suddenly opened, producing a forceful outflow of air.

▶ INDICATIONS

Four assumptions form the rationale for the current recommended treatment of acute airway obstruction in infants and children (11). First, airway obstruction with secondary cardiac arrest is far more common in pediatric patients than the sudden cardiac arrest with secondary airway obstruction seen in adults. Second, a foreign body completely obstructing the upper airway is an immediate threat to life and must be removed. Third, if the child can speak, breathe, or cough, the foreign body is only partially obstructing the airway, yet it may be dislodged or moved to a position that totally obstructs the airway. This can make first-aid airway maneuvers potentially dangerous. Finally, partial airway obstruction with poor air exchange or complete airway obstruction with cyanosis requires immediate relief.

Importantly, any child who has choked on a foreign body but who is coughing, crying, or speaking should merely be observed, at least initially, since the normal airway reflexes will likely be sufficient to fully clear the obstruction. However, if acutely worsening or complete obstruction develops, if the child or infant is unable to make sounds, or if there is no evidence of respiratory air movement, immediate first aid

to establish a patent airway and deliver basic life support is required to avoid permanent disability or death (12).

The abdominal-thrust (Heimlich) maneuver is thought to be the most effective method of relieving complete airway obstruction in children over 1 year of age (13). This method is based on several physiologic factors: (a) 80% of respiratory effort is from diaphragmatic contraction; (b) abdominal inward pressure compresses the diaphragm upward, thereby raising intrathoracic pressure; (c) a sudden, rapid increase in intrathoracic pressure may expel the obstructing object; and (d) patients with airway obstruction who become unconscious from hypoxia lose muscle tone, which improves the effectiveness of the maneuver (13). If the abdominal-thrust maneuver is initially ineffective, continued attempts using this method should be made, as it may prove successful after the patient loses consciousness (12).

The American Academy of Pediatrics (AAP), the American Heart Association (AHA), and the Red Cross all recommend that the abdominal-thrust maneuver be used in children over 1 year of age for complete airway obstruction. Some controversy exists, however, about which maneuver—the abdominal thrust or the combination back blow and chest thrust—is best for the choking patient under 1 year of age. In infants, the stomach, liver, and spleen are relatively larger than they are in older children. Damage and even rupture of abdominal organs with the abdominal-thrust technique have been reported (14,15). Additionally, infants have greater chest wall compliance than older children. A compliant chest wall absorbs some of the energy from the abdominal-thrust maneuver by allowing increased chest wall expansion, which in turn decreases the extent of lung and airway compression. This can make the abdominal-thrust maneuver less effective in producing pressure changes adequate to expel a foreign object from the obstructed airway.

For infants under 1 year of age, the technique currently recommended by the AAP and AHA involves two steps: the head-down back-blow maneuver and the chest-thrust maneuver (12). The head-down back-blow maneuver is designed to compress the chest with a posteriorly applied force while the anterior chest is held. Ideally, this will generate a rapid increase in intrathoracic pressure that propels the foreign body out of the airway (16). Similarly, the chest-thrust maneuver uses sternal compression to increase intrathoracic pressure in an effort to expel the foreign object. This maneuver is much like performing chest compressions in the setting of cardiopulmonary arrest.

A concern has been raised that the sudden acceleration produced by the back-blow maneuver in an awake patient may actually worsen airway obstruction. Back blows in an awake patient might stimulate inhalation at the same time as the pressure is increased, possibly opening the airway and allowing the foreign body to advance in the wrong direction. Some evidence has indicated that the back-blow maneuver may in fact cause caudal movement of the object, in concordance with Newton's third law of motion: to every action there is an opposed equal reaction (17). Nevertheless, it appears that, in the case of an infant, when the maneuver is performed with the infant held head down and prone over the rescuer's leg (Fig. 51.1), further intrusion of the foreign body is unlikely (12).

▶ EQUIPMENT

No specific equipment is needed to manage a pediatric patient with an obstructed airway in the field. Prehospital in-

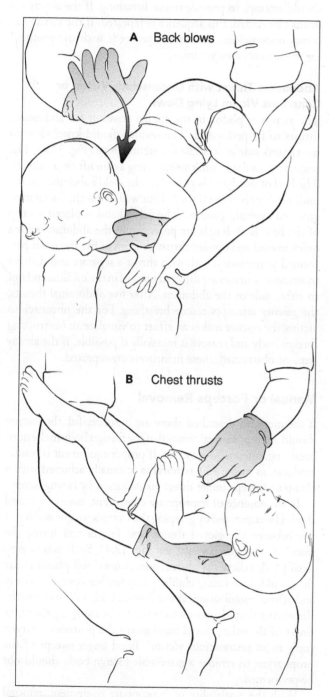

Figure 51.1
A. Back blows and
B. Chest thrusts are attempted to relieve foreign body airway obstruction in the infant.

terventions consist of abdominal thrusts, back blows, and chest compressions as well as other basic life support maneuvers (see Chapter 12). For this reason, any qualified medical professional or trained layperson can perform the necessary procedures without specialized devices. In the ED or other hospital setting, supplemental oxygen, a laryngoscope handle with an array of blade sizes, a forceps for removing the foreign body if visualized, a bag-valve-mask setup, suctioning equipment, and capabilities for ensuring an emergent airway must be readily available (see also Section 2 for details of equipment needs associated with these interventions).

▶ PROCEDURE

The following recommendations of the AAP and AHA for the acute treatment of the choking child are based on the current consensus regarding pediatric emergency care (12).

Infants 1 Year of Age and Younger

The following steps should be performed immediately in the field to relieve the airway obstruction. The infant is initially held prone, resting on the rescuer's forearm. The infant's head is supported by firmly holding the jaw. The rescuer's forearm should lie on his or her thigh to support the infant, with the patient's head lower than the trunk. Five back blows are delivered forcefully between the infant's shoulder blades using the heel of the hand (Fig. 51.1A). After delivering the back blows, the rescuer's free hand is placed on the infant's back, holding the infant's head. The patient is thus held between the two hands of the rescuer—one hand supporting the neck, jaw, and chest while the other supports the back. The infant is turned while the head and neck are carefully supported, and the infant is held in the supine position across the rescuer's thigh. The infant's head is turned to one side and held lower than the trunk. Five quick downward chest thrusts are performed in the lower half of the sternum, approximately one fingerbreadth below the nipple line (the same location used for external chest compressions). The rescuer should use two or three fingers to compress the sternum approximately one third to one half the depth of the chest, or 0.5 to 1.0 inch (Fig. 51.1B), at a rate of one per second. Attempts should then be made to provide rescue breathing. If the infant becomes unconscious, the rescuer may attempt a tongue-jaw lift, and if a foreign body is visible in the posterior pharynx, an effort can then be made to remove it with a finger sweep. If the airway remains obstructed, the maneuvers as described are repeated in sequence.

Children over 1 Year of Age

Abdominal Thrust with a Conscious Victim

These thrusts are performed with the rescuer standing behind the victim, who may be sitting or standing. The rescuer positions his or her arms directly under the victim's axilla and encircles the victim's chest (Fig. 51.2). The thumb side of one fist is placed against the victim's abdomen in the midline, slightly above the navel and well below the tip of the xyphoid process. The rescuer grasps this fist with the other hand and administers five quick inward and upward thrusts. The fist should not impact on the xyphoid process or the lower costal margins, because force applied to these structures may damage internal organs. Each thrust should be a separate, distinct movement. The thrusts are continued until the foreign body is expelled or five thrusts are completed. Again, the rescuer should attempt to provide rescue breathing. If the airway remains obstructed, this sequence is repeated. If the victim becomes unconscious, the rescuer proceeds with the protocol for the unconscious victim.

Abdominal Thrust with Unconscious Victim or Conscious Victim Lying Down

The victim is placed in the supine position for abdominal thrusts to be performed. The rescuer should kneel close to the victim's side or straddle the victim's hips (Fig. 51.3). The rescuer opens the victim's airway using a chin lift or jaw thrust. The heel of one hand is placed on the child's abdomen in the midline slightly above the navel but well below the costal margins and xyphoid process. The other hand is placed on top of the first. Both hands are pressed into the abdomen with a quick inward and upward thrust. A series of five thrusts is performed as necessary, with each thrust a separate and distinct movement. Thrusts are directed upward in the midline and not to either side of the abdomen. After five abdominal thrusts, the rescuer attempts rescue breathing. For the unconscious victim, the rescuer makes an effort to visualize an obstructing foreign body and remove it manually if possible. If the airway remains obstructed, these maneuvers are repeated.

Manual or Forceps Removal

If the methods described above are unsuccessful, the rescuer should attempt manual removal of the foreign body in the non-breathing, unconscious victim. If proper equipment is readily available, as in the ED, removal is optimally achieved with a clamp or forceps under direct visualization by laryngoscopy.

In the absence of appropriate equipment, manual removal should be attempted by grasping the victim's tongue and lower jaw between the gloved thumb and fingers and lifting the mandible (tongue-jaw lift; see Fig. 12.4). Such action may itself partly relieve the obstruction. A towel roll placed under the shoulders in young children may further open the airway and afford visualization. If the foreign body becomes visible, the rescuer should attempt to remove it by sweeping the index finger of the other gloved hand across the posterior pharynx (only in an unconscious victim). Blind finger sweeps of the oropharynx to remove a nonvisible foreign body should not be performed.

With the availability of appropriate equipment, removal under direct visualization should be attempted (18). Laryngoscopy should be performed during careful visualization of the oropharynx (see Chapter 16) so that the laryngoscope

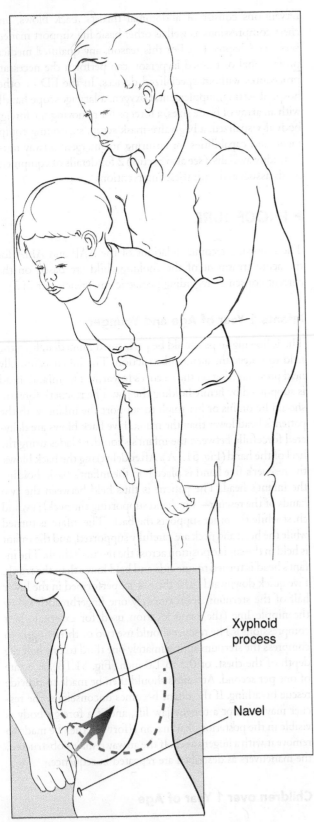

Figure 51.2 Abdominal thrusts with older conscious child standing or sitting.

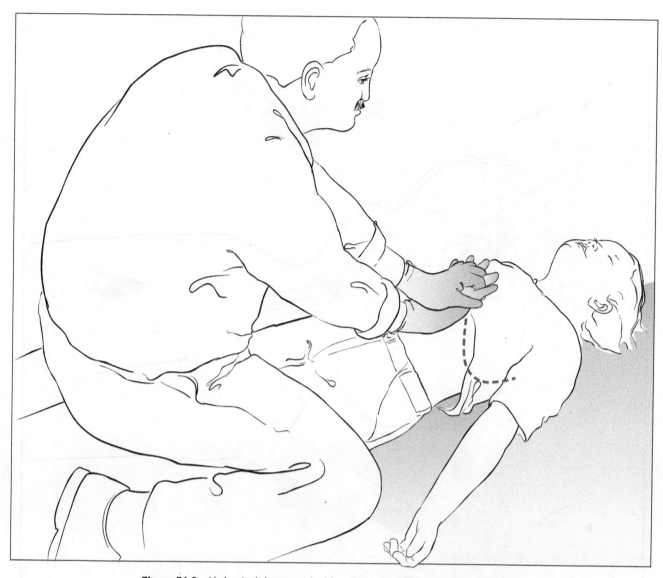

Figure 51.3 Abdominal thrusts with older child lying (conscious or unconscious).

 SUMMARY: FIRST AID FOR THE CHOKING CHILD 1 YEAR OF AGE AND YOUNGER

1 Hold the infant head downward, prone, resting on the rescuer's forearm, with the head supported.

2 Deliver five back blows between the infant's shoulder blades using the heel of the hand (Fig. 51.1A).

3 Place the free hand on the infant's back and turn the infant supine, with the head dependent across the rescuer's thigh.

4 Perform five quick downward chest thrusts in the same location as external chest compressions (lower half of sternum, approximately one finger breadth below the nipple line) but at a slower rate (Fig. 51.1B).

5 Attempt to provide rescue breathing.

6 If the airway remains obstructed and the infant becomes unconscious, attempt to visualize the foreign body and remove it manually.

7 Repeat the sequence as necessary.

Source: Adapted from Committee on Pediatric Emergency Medicine. Revise first aid for the choking child. *Pediatrics.* 1993;92:477–479.

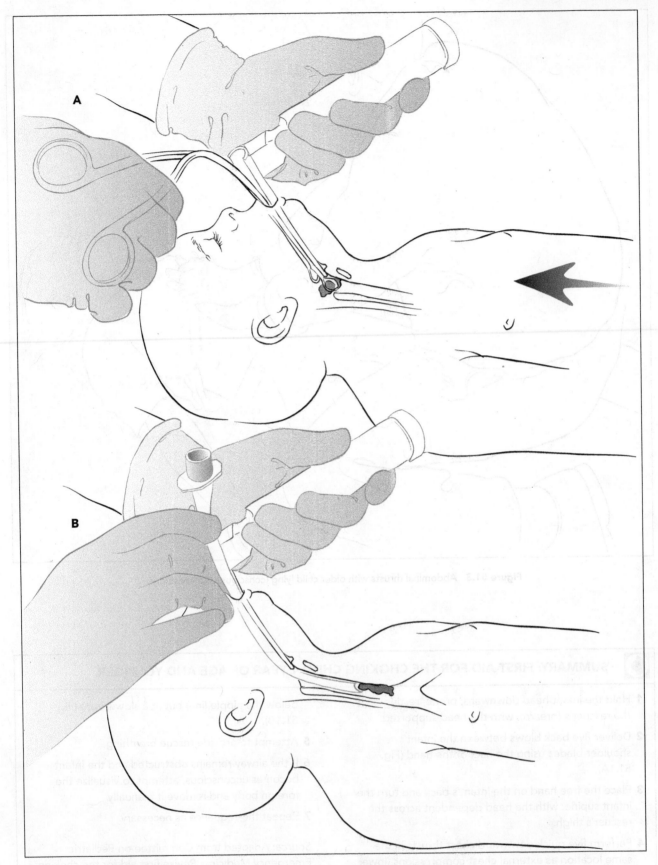

Figure 51.4
A. Magill forceps is used to extract a foreign body visualized by direct laryngoscopy.
B. Endotracheal intubation may force the foreign body distally into one mainstream bronchus. The patient can then be temporarily supported by ventilating the unobstructed lung.

SUMMARY: FIRST AID FOR THE CHOKING CHILD OVER 1 YEAR OF AGE

Abdominal Thrust with a Conscious Patient Sitting or Standing

1 Stand behind the child with arms directly under the child's axilla and encircling the chest (Fig. 51.2).

2 Place the thumb side of one fist against the patient's abdomen in midline, just above the navel but below the tip of the xiphoid process.

3 Grasp the fist with the other hand and exert five quick inward and upward thrusts.

4 Continue the thrusts until the foreign body is expelled or five thrusts are completed. If the airway remains obstructed, repeat the sequence. If the patient becomes unconscious, attempt to visualize the foreign body and remove it manually. If unsuccessful, modify the approach as described in the next section.

Abdominal Thrust with an Unconscious or Conscious Patient Lying Down

1 Place the patient supine, with the rescuer at the patient's side or straddling the patient's hips (Fig. 51.3).

2 Open the patient's airway using a chin lift or jaw thrust.

3 Place the heel of one hand on the child's abdomen in the midline just above the navel and below the costal margins and xiphoid. Place the other hand on top of the first hand.

4 Press both hands into the abdomen with a quick upward thrust in the midline. If necessary, perform a series of five thrusts, with each thrust a separate and distinct movement.

5 After the delivery of five abdominal thrusts, attempt rescue breathing. If the airway remains obstructed, attempt to visualize and remove the foreign body manually. If unsuccessful, repeat the sequence.

Source: Adapted from Committee on Pediatric Emergency Medicine. Revise first aid for the choking child. *Pediatrics.* 1993;92:477–479.

CLINICAL TIPS

▶ First-aid airway maneuvers should not be performed in children with partial airway obstruction as evidenced by cough, presence of breath sounds, and maintenance of consciousness.

▶ The abdominal-thrust (Heimlich) maneuver is the mainstay for airway foreign body obstruction in children over 1 year of age.

▶ Back blows and chest thrusts are the preferred maneuvers in children under 1 year of age.

▶ Each maneuver should be attempted five times in unconscious patients, and then ventilation reattempted. If possible, visualized foreign bodies may be removed by finger sweep in the unconscious patient.

▶ In the ED, prompt visualization of the airway by direct laryngoscopy followed by removal of the foreign body with Magill forceps and/or endotracheal intubation as necessary should be attempted in the unconscious patient while preparing for surgical airway interventions if unsuccessful (Chapters 17 and 26).

helpful to have an assistant perform abdominal or chest thrusts in an effort to move the object to a point where it can be visualized and grasped.

Inability to remove a foreign body from the mouth does not necessarily mean failure. By performing endotracheal intubation, it may be possible to force a subglottic foreign body into a mainstem bronchus and then support the patient temporarily by ventilating the unobstructed lung (Fig. 51.4B). The object can then be removed later using rigid bronchoscopy. In this situation, the pop-off valve of the bag-valve system should be occluded to deliver sufficient volume for effective oxygenation and ventilation. If these attempts fail to oxygenate the patient, the physician should proceed to create a surgical airway immediately (see Chapters 17 and 26).

▶ COMPLICATIONS

Although rib and cardiac damage are theoretical risks of the chest compression maneuver in infants and small children, a large review of infants who underwent chest compressions found no significant rib injuries or fractures (19). Severe complications have been reported when the Heimlich maneuver was performed incorrectly in the emergent treatment of airway obstruction (20). Reported complications include pneumomediastinum, ruptured stomach, and a thrombosed aorta. A possible explanation for these complications is that

blade does not push a foreign body partly obstructing the airway further down and cause complete obstruction. Most such foreign objects are located at the base of the tongue or around the tonsillar pillars. If the foreign body is visualized, a Magill forceps (or Kelly clamp) is used to grasp the foreign body and extract it (Fig. 51.4A). If the foreign body is not visualized at the time of initial laryngoscopy, it is sometimes

as many as 70% of maneuvers are done by untrained individuals, and 50% of the individuals learned the technique in lay magazines or newspapers. For example, one male infant is reported to have suffered a nonfatal pneumomediastinum as a result of a "bear hug" attempt at the Heimlich maneuver by his father (20). When performed properly, the complication rate of the abdominal thrusts appears to be quite low, particularly given the life-threatening potential of airway obstruction. Complications related to forceps removal of a foreign body under direct visualization should be largely related to those of instrumenting the airway and are detailed in Chapter 16.

▶ SUMMARY

Despite advances over the past decade, from changes in product regulation to increased awareness of first aid, choking deaths still remain a significant problem. Primary prevention and anticipatory guidance play a key role in addressing this problem. Secondary prevention by understanding and using the recommended emergent maneuvers for the obstructed airway can be life-saving. In the prehospital setting, when airway equipment is unavailable, the rescuer must rely on the first-aid measures for choking as delineated by the AHA and AAP. Recent studies have shown that the majority of airway foreign bodies are cleared by basic first-aid procedures prior to the arrival of emergency medical services (21). Techniques for abdominal-thrust, chest-thrust, back-blow, and finger-sweep maneuvers should be acquired through appropriate training courses. In the ED or in any setting with access to proper equipment, laryngoscopy and forceps extraction under direct visualization must be rapidly undertaken when indicated. If all such efforts are unsuccessful, a surgical airway should be performed.

▶ ACKNOWLEDGMENT

The authors would like to acknowledge the valuable contributions of Richard M. Ruddy to the version of this chapter that appeared in the previous edition.

▶ REFERENCES

1. National Safety Council. *Accident Facts*. Itasca, IL: National Safety Council; 1992:5.
2. Harris CS, Baker SP, Smith GA, et al. Childhood asphyxiation by food: a national analysis and overview. *JAMA*. 1984;251:2231–2235.
3. U.S. Consumer Product Safety Commission. *Method for Identifying Toys and Other Articles Intended for Use by Children under 3 Years of Age Which Present Choking, Aspiration, or Ingestion Hazards Because of Small Parts (16 CFR 1501)*. Washington, DC: General Services Administration; 1979.
4. Tinsworth DK. *Analysis of Choking-related Hazards Associated with Children's Products*. Washington, DC: U.S. Consumer Product Safety Commission; September 1989.
5. Becker PG, Turow J. Earring aspiration and other jewelry hazards. *Pediatrics*. 1986;78:494–496.
6. Press S, Liberman JG. Aspiration through a "sip-up" straw. *Am J Dis Child*. 1986;140:1090–1091.
7. Ross MN, Janik JS. "Foil tab" aspiration and retropharyngeal abscess in a toddler. *JAMA*. 1988;260:3130.
8. Arnold RW, Hoffman AD, Brutinel WM, et al. Barbie doll curler aspiration into the upper trachea. *Am J Dis Child*. 1987;141:1325–1326.
9. Myer CM. Foreign body aspiration. *Am J Dis Child*. 1988;142:485–486.
10. Ryan CA, Yacoub W, Paton T, et al. Childhood deaths from toy balloons. *Am J Dis Child*. 1990;144:1221–1224.
11. Committee on Accident and Poison Prevention. Revised first aid for the choking child. *Pediatrics*. 1986;78:177–178.
12. Basic life support for the PALS healthcare provider. In: Hazinski MF, Zaritsky AL, Nadkarni VN, et al., eds. *PALS Provider Manual*. Dallas, TX: American Heart Association; 2002:43–80.
13. Heimlich HF. A life-saving maneuver to prevent food choking. *JAMA*. 1975;234:398–401.
14. Visintine RE, Baick CH. Ruptured stomach after Heimlich maneuver. *JAMA*. 1975;234:415.
15. Croom DW. Ruptured stomach after attempted Heimlich maneuver. *JAMA*. 1975;234:415.
16. Gordon AS, Belton MK, Ridolpho PF. Emergency management of foreign body airway obstruction. In: Safar PJ, Elam JO, eds. *Advances in Cardiopulmonary Resuscitation*. New York: Springer-Verlag; 1977:39–50.
17. Day RL, Crelin ES, Dubois AB. Choking: the Heimlich abdominal thrust vs. back blows: an approach to measurement of inertial aerodynamic forces. *Pediatrics*. 1982;70:113–119.
18. Young GP, Pace SA. Esophageal foreign bodies. In: Roberts JR, Hedges JR, eds. *Clinical Procedures in Emergency Medicine*. Philadelphia: WB Saunders; 1985:638.
19. Spevak MR, Kleinman PK, Belanger PL, et al. Cardiopulmonary resuscitation and rib fractures in infants. *JAMA*. 1994;272:617–618.
20. Fink JA, Klein RL. Complications of the Heimlich maneuver. *J Pediatr Surg*. 1989;24:486–487.
21. Andazola JJ, Sapien RE. The choking child: what happens before the ambulance arrives? *Prehosp Emerg Care*. 1999;3:7–10.

HOLLY W. DAVIS AND KALA PARKER

52

Otoscopic Examination

▶ INTRODUCTION

Symptoms referable to the ears account for over one third of all pediatric visits to a medical facility (1,2). Patients can present with localized symptoms, such as otalgia and otorrhea, or with nonspecific complaints, such as fever, irritability, and decreased appetite. A small number may be asymptomatic. For this reason, the pediatric physical examination is not complete without an otoscopic examination. Pediatricians, emergency physicians, and family practitioners must therefore be skilled in the techniques of assessment. Otoscopic examination not only is used as a diagnostic procedure for external auditory canal problems and middle ear disease but also can serve as an indirect evaluation of intracranial injury in children with a history of trauma. Otoscopy also provides a means to directly visualize procedures that occur within the ear canal (see Chapters 53, 54, and 56).

▶ ANATOMY AND PHYSIOLOGY

The external ear includes the pinna, auricle, the outer cartilaginous canal, the inner bony canal, and the outer surface of the tympanic membrane (Fig. 52.1). The middle ear includes the inner portion of the tympanic membrane, the three ossicles, and the mastoid air cells (Fig. 52.2). The inner ear is composed of the semicircular canals, the cochlea, and the seventh and eighth cranial nerves. The eustachian tube connects the middle ear with the nasopharynx. When functioning normally, the eustachian tube vents the middle ear, serves as a conduit for drainage of middle ear secretions, and protects the middle ear from nasopharyngeal sound pressure and secretions (1,3). The tympanic membrane is perpendicular to the external auditory canal in children over 1 year of age, while in infancy it is tilted at a more horizontal angle, making

visualization of landmarks more difficult (1,2). Additionally, the external auditory canal itself is often slightly angulated in infancy and early childhood. This necessitates applying gentle lateral traction on the auricle to help visualize the tympanic membrane (1,2,4). During the first 4 to 6 months of life, the canal mucosa is somewhat loosely attached to supporting structures and moves readily on insufflation. If care is not taken to inspect the canal as the speculum is inserted, thereby ensuring that the transition between the canal wall and tympanic membrane is visualized, movement of the canal wall during insufflation may be mistaken for a normally mobile drum (1,2).

The wall of the external auditory canal is protected by a waxy layer of cerumen, formed by a combination of viscous secretions from sebaceous glands, watery secretions of apocrine glands, and exfoliated epithelial cells. While the canal is colonized by normal skin flora, the acidic pH of the secretions acts as a chemical barrier against infection (5). Infection of the external canal (otitis externa) can result from a variety of factors. Repeated wetting of the canal wall from swimming, bathing, or high humidity alters the protective coating of wax and renders the surface more susceptible to infection. Conditions causing excessive dryness, underlying skin disorders (e.g., eczema or psoriasis), and trauma to the external canal (from fingernails, cotton swabs, or the presence of a foreign body) predispose this area to infection. Finally, perforation of the tympanic membrane in a patient with acute otitis media, by releasing purulent material into the external auditory canal (1,3,5), can also cause external canal infection.

The major predisposing factor for development of acute middle ear infection (otitis media) is eustachian tube dysfunction. The high incidence of otitis media in young children who are otherwise healthy partly reflects the immaturity of the eustachian tube of the young child. It is shorter, less rigid, and more horizontally oriented in younger children, thus allowing organisms from the nasopharynx to reach the middle ear

575

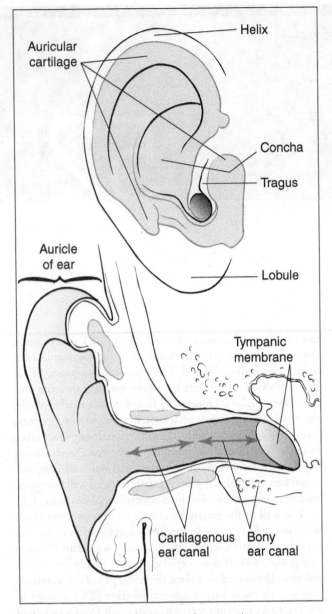

Figure 52.1 Anatomy of the external ear.

region more easily (1–3,6). These features of the eustachian tube also can result in impairment of pressure regulation and clearance of fluid from the middle ear. Furthermore, infants and young children are prone to functional obstruction of the eustachian tube. Lack of stiffness in the cartilaginous supporting structures predisposes to collapse of the tube, which impairs venting of the middle ear (4). As oxygen is absorbed by mucosal cells, negative pressure develops within the middle ear. When venting of air eventually does occur, the vacuum created facilitates aspiration of nasopharyngeal secretions into the middle ear (4).

The anatomic and physiologic abnormalities associated with cleft palate and other craniofacial anomalies produce similar functional impairment and obstruction (1–3,6). Tonsillar enlargement can also cause mechanical obstruction of the eustachian tube, predisposing to infection. The tonsils and

adenoids normally enlarge over the first 8 to 10 years of life and then gradually decrease in size. Less commonly, nasopharyngeal tumors may be the source of mechanical obstruction (1–3,6). In addition, organisms can enter the middle ear space from the external canal through a tympanic membrane perforation or via hematogenous spread (1,6).

Acute otitis media consists of inflammation of the mucoperiosteal lining of the middle ear. Respiratory viruses set the stage for a substantial proportion of cases of bacterial otitis by inducing respiratory epithelial injury and by causing congestion of the respiratory mucosa of the nose, nasopharynx, and eustachian tube. The resulting eustachian tube inflammation and edema impair middle ear drainage and make it easier for pathogenic bacteria that have colonized the nasopharynx to gain access to the middle ear. With infection, the mucosal lining becomes inflamed and weeps, resulting in accumulation of mucopurulent material in the middle ear space (1,2,6). As pressure in the middle ear increases, the membrane tends to bulge. Rupture may occur if pressure becomes great enough to cause ischemic necrosis. When the middle ear is filled with fluid, tympanic membrane mobility is markedly reduced on both positive and negative pressure. If, however, some venting of the eustachian tube occurs, air and fluid may be present with a milder decrease in mobility, and an air fluid level or bubbles can be seen (2,6).

Otitis media with effusion refers to the presence of clear, uninfected fluid within the middle ear. The membrane is neither opacified nor inflamed and does not tend to bulge out. Typically, it is seen in children with eustachian tube dysfunction, often following resolution of an acute infection. On pneumatic otoscopy, there is decreased tympanic membrane mobility with both positive and negative pressure (1,2,6). If negative pressure has developed within the middle ear, the drum may move primarily when negative pressure is applied (2). This condition may persist for weeks to months. Some affected children experience a decrease in hearing, but most patients are asymptomatic (1,2,6).

▶ INDICATIONS

Because otitis media is so common in early childhood and presenting symptoms are often nonspecific, otoscopic examination is indicated as a routine part of the evaluation of every infant or young child, especially those with fever, irritability, upper respiratory symptoms, or sore throat (1,2,6). Symptoms specific to the ear, such as otalgia, otorrhea, auricular swelling and/or erythema, hearing loss, tinnitus, vertigo, nystagmus, sensation of a foreign body, and ear injury are also obvious indications. Chronic cough in children has been associated with a foreign body in contact with the tympanic membrane. Any patient being evaluated for head and/or facial trauma must undergo otoscopy to check for canal wall laceration, hemotympanum, and cerebrospinal fluid (CSF) leak, which all may be seen with a basilar skull fracture. Patients exposed to the severe concussive force of an explosion also

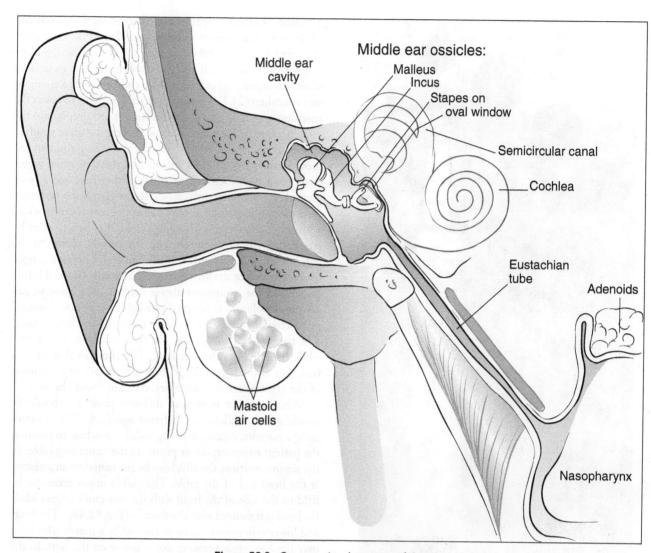

Figure 52.2 Cross-sectional anatomy of the ear.

must be assessed for possible traumatic perforation of the tympanic membrane and hearing loss (1,2,5,6).

Indications for consultation and/or referral to an otolaryngologist include (a) frequent recurrences of acute otitis media (more than three in a 6-month period), (b) persistence of otitis media with effusion for over 3 months, (c) persistent tympanic membrane perforation following an episode of otitis media, (d) otologic trauma other than canal wall abrasions, and (e) the presence of suppurative complications of otitis media (mastoiditis, intracranial abscess, seventh cranial nerve involvement) or otitis externa (auricular or periauricular cellulitis).

▶ EQUIPMENT

Items and materials that may be useful in performing pneumatic otoscopy are listed in Table 52.1. The minimum necessary equipment consists of the following:

Pneumatic otoscope with 3.5-V halogen illumination and an airtight head (Fig. 52.3)

Bulb insufflator and rubber tubing
Specula (sizes 2 through 5)

▶ PROCEDURE

Before otoscopic examination, the equipment should be tested to ensure an adequate air seal, which is essential for accurate pneumatic otoscopy. To do this, the speculum is attached to

TABLE 52.1	EQUIPMENT

Pneumatic otoscope
Insufflator bulb
Specula (sizes 2, 3, 4, 5)
Surgical otoscope head (optional)
Rubber tubing
Blunt cerumen curette
3% hydrogen peroxide solution
20-mL syringe, 23-gauge butterfly without the needle
Suction

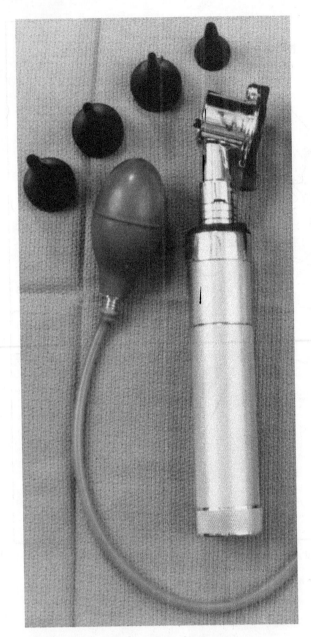

Figure 52.3 Equipment for pneumatic otoscopy.

speculum is usually appropriate, whereas older children and adolescents may require a 5-mm speculum. Putting a piece of rubber tourniquet tubing around the end of the speculum may give a better seal if the clinician encounters an air leak while attempting to examine older children with a 4- or 5-mm speculum (2). Extra caution should be taken to insert the speculum gently and to avoid inserting it too deeply into the bony portion of the canal, because this can be quite painful.

Otoscopic examination of infants and young children can prove challenging, as older infants and toddlers often vigorously resist the procedure, especially if they have had a prior painful experience. In such cases, effective restraint is necessary to prevent injury and another bad experience. Nevertheless, with the toddler or preschool-age child, it is best to start by attempting the examination with the patient sitting in the parent's lap, using a puppet, stuffed animal, or even a tongue blade with a face drawn on it as a distractor. Gradual introduction of the equipment also is helpful. The clinician can ask preschoolers to try to catch the light as it is moved around or to blow it out as the clinician turns off the light source. The parent or physician also can serve briefly as a "patient" while the child is offered a look. The clinician then takes a turn (see also Chapter 2). If these efforts fail, or if cleaning of the external canal is necessary, restraint should be used.

When restraint is needed, different positions should be considered for children of different ages (2,4). When examining a neonate, infant, or young toddler, it is best to position the patient either supine or prone on the examining table. In the supine position, the child can be restrained by an assistant at the head end of the table. The child's upper arms can be held to the side of the head with the assistant's fingers while the head is stabilized with the thumbs (Fig. 52.4A). The body and lower extremities can be restrained by a parent who leans over the legs while pressing down firmly on the hips. In the prone position, the assistant can hold the arms and body from the caudal end while leaning firmly over the child's buttocks. The clinician then stabilizes the head using the hand that holds the pinna of the ear. Toddlers and preschoolers sometimes can be restrained in a sitting position on the parent's lap. The child's legs are secured between the parent's legs, and the arms and body are held tightly against the parent's chest with one arm while the other arm stabilizes the child's head against the parent's chest (Fig. 52.4B). Although this may work for an examination, the degree of restraint afforded often is not adequate for cleaning the external auditory canal.

The examination begins with inspection of the auricle and periauricular tissues. The external auditory canal is then viewed as the speculum is gradually inserted. Adequate visualization often necessitates removal of cerumen using a curette and/or irrigation of the canal (see Chapter 53). To examine the right ear, the otoscope is held in the right hand like a pencil, with thumb and forefinger around the handle near the junction of the barrel and otoscope head (Fig. 52.5). The ulnar aspect of the clinician's right hand rests on the child's cheek to prevent deep insertion of the speculum with sudden movement of the child's head. With the left hand, the pinna is

the head of the otoscope, the tip is occluded with the thumb or finger, and positive pressure is applied by pressing on the bulb. No air leak should occur. The clinician should also test the light source on the otoscope, as a good high-intensity light source is essential. With a wall-mounted unit, absence of light when the device is turned on usually means that the bulb has burned out and needs to be replaced. With a battery-operated unit, a dim yellow light indicates that the batteries must be replaced or recharged.

The largest speculum that can be inserted to about one third the distance into the ear canal should be used. Neonates and young infants may require a 2-mm aural speculum. The ear canal of an older infant or toddler will normally accommodate a 3-mm speculum. For children 2 to 7 years of age, a 4-mm

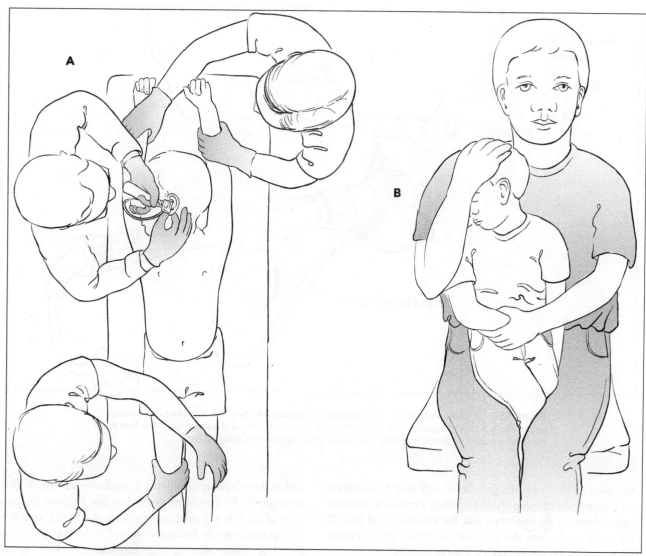

Figure 52.4
A. Restraint in the supine position for otoscopic examination. This method is often most effective for an infant or younger child. A similar approach with the child in the prone position also can be used.
B. Restraint by a parent in the seated position for otoscopic examination.

pulled outward and backward to straighten the canal for better visualization. To examine the left side, the clinician changes hands to hold the otoscope with the left hand and the pinna with the right. The clinician should look through the otoscope lens as the speculum is inserted, taking care to ensure that the transition between the canal wall and the tympanic membrane is seen clearly. Once the membrane is visualized, the color, position, degree of translucency, and visibility of the bony landmarks should be assessed, and evidence of scarring and/or the presence of air-fluid or air-pus levels should be noted. The light reflex is of limited value, as it does not reliably indicate middle ear pathology (1,2,4,6,7).

The next task is to check the mobility of the tympanic membrane (2,4,6,7). Use of the insufflator bulb while at the same time holding the otoscope and the ear is the most dif-

ficult step to master in this procedure. The bulb of the insufflator can be held between the fingers or in the palm of the same hand that holds the otoscope (Fig. 52.5). While maintaining a view of the tympanic membrane, the clinician should press the bulb gently to create positive pressure in the canal. In a normal ear, this causes the tympanic membrane to move briskly backward. When the bulb is released, negative pressure is automatically applied, and the drum moves forward toward the clinician. A normal membrane moves about 1 to 2 mm in each direction. Movement is decreased or absent when middle ear effusion is present. A retracted or scarred membrane also may have decreased mobility on insufflation, whereas a thinned or dimeric area, often formed when a perforation reseals, may have exaggerated movement (1,2,4,6,7). It should be remembered that a true assessment of the

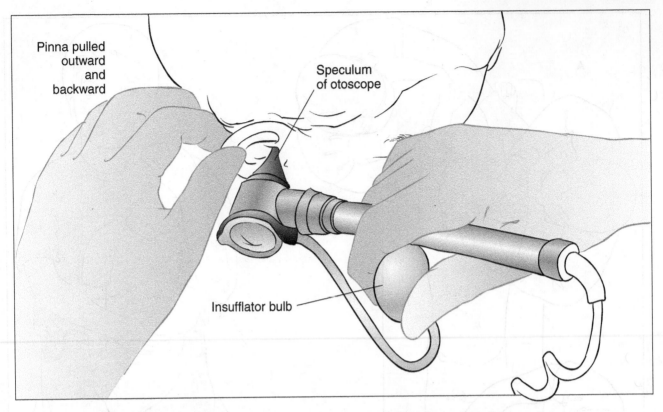

Figure 52.5 Proper hand position for pneumatic otoscopy. Holding the otoscope like a pencil allows the clinician to squeeze the insufflator bulb with the thumb and index finger. The free hand can then be used to gently pull back the auricle to straighten the external canal.

mobility of the tympanic membrane will only be obtained with an airtight otoscope head and when a good seal is maintained between the speculum and the external canal wall. If the seal is inadequate, the tympanic membrane will not move with insufflation even though it may be healthy.

▶ INTERPRETATION

Acute Otitis Media

The normal tympanic membrane is thin and translucent, and its landmarks are easily visualized. In contrast, classic findings during an episode of acute otitis media include opacification and thickening of the tympanic membrane, often with erythema. Landmarks are obscured, and the membrane bulges outward. Mobility is absent or markedly decreased on pneumatic otoscopy when performed with a good air seal (1,2,6).

In some cases, the drum appears highly injected and hyperemic, with dilated vessels, and may be frankly hemorrhagic, whereas in other patients erythema can be minimal or even absent. Fluid is generally somewhat cloudy, and often frank yellow or white pus can be visualized behind the membrane (1,2,6,7). When bubbles or an air-fluid level are seen, reflecting some venting of the eustachian tube, mobility may be less severely decreased. Occasionally, painful bullae may form

within the tympanic membrane, a condition termed "bullous myringitis" (8). Erythema alone does not confirm the presence of middle ear infection, because the blood vessels of the eardrum rapidly become engorged with crying, repeated sneezing, or nose blowing or at times with fever. Likewise, evidence of middle ear effusion with constitutional symptoms but without opacification or frank pus and without bulging or poor mobility does not meet diagnostic criteria for acute otitis media (1,2,7,9).

Otitis Media with Effusion

Otitis media with effusion is not infrequently mistaken for acute otitis media. It is important for practitioners to learn to differentiate between the two conditions, as otitis media with an effusion does not require antibiotic therapy and is not treated unless it becomes chronic (i.e., persistent for more than 3 months). Affected patients often have no symptoms, or they may complain of hearing loss or, less commonly, tinnitus or vertigo. On otoscopic exam, the membrane may appear full (but not bulging), retracted, or normal, depending on the chronicity of the process. The color of the fluid may be yellow, amber, or gray, but it is clear, and the membrane is not opacified. The mobility of the tympanic membrane is reduced on pneumatic otoscopy and is often greater with negative pressure (1,2,6).

Acute Otitis Externa

The pain from acute otitis externa is exacerbated by movement of the pinna, which is a distinguishing feature, as well as by insertion of the speculum to perform otoscopy. The canal typically appears quite inflamed and friable and may be filled with exudate. With severe cases, attendant mucosal edema may produce marked narrowing, and even complete closure, of the canal. The discharge is usually white or yellow but may become bloody with particularly severe inflammation and/or if associated with tympanic membrane perforation.

Hemotympanum

Direct trauma to the middle ear or a basilar skull fracture can result in hemotympanum. The appearance may vary depending on the time elapsed since injury, with the color of the membrane ranging from blue to purple (2). Patients with basilar fracture may also have bruising behind the external ear

 SUMMARY

1 Select a speculum of the proper size for the patient:
   ▶ 2 mm for neonate or young infant
   ▶ 3 mm for older infant or toddler
   ▶ 4 mm for child aged 2 to 7 years
   ▶ 5 mm for older child or adolescent

2 Test equipment
   ▶ Occlude the tip of the speculum with one finger, and apply positive pressure with the insufflator bulb to ensure that no air leak occurs.
   ▶ Ensure that the otoscope provides a high-intensity light source.

3 Restrain the patient appropriately if necessary.

4 Inspect the auricle and periauricular tissues.

5 Examine the right ear by holding the otoscope in the right hand, and examine the left ear by holding the otoscope in the left hand.

6 Pull the pinna outward and posteriorly to straighten the canal if necessary.

7 Examine the external auditory canal while inserting the speculum.

8 Remove cerumen if necessary to visualize the tympanic membrane.

9 Assess the color, position, and condition of the tympanic membrane as well as the bony landmarks.

10 Assess the movement of the tympanic membrane by pressing and releasing the insufflator bulb.

 CLINICAL TIPS

▶ The external auditory canal should be carefully examined as the otoscope is inserted to ensure that the transition between the canal wall and tympanic membrane is visualized. Otherwise, movement of the canal wall during insufflation may be mistaken for a normally mobile drum.

▶ Any patient being evaluated for head and/or facial trauma must undergo otoscopy to check for canal laceration, hemotympanum, or cerebrospinal fluid leak, which are all signs of a basilar skull fracture. Traumatic rupture of the tympanic membrane may also result from a blow to the side of the head or the concussive force of an explosion.

▶ In the presence of serous otitis or otitis media with effusion, the mobility of the tympanic membrane is reduced and often is greater when applying negative pressure on pneumatic otoscopy.

▶ The largest speculum that can be inserted to about one third the distance into the ear canal should be used. Extra caution should be taken to avoid inserting the speculum too deeply into the bony part of the canal because this causes pain.

▶ Putting a piece of rubber tourniquet tubing around the end of the speculum may provide a better seal if a significant air leak is encountered while attempting to examine an older child or adolescent with a 4- or 5-mm speculum.

▶ A normal tympanic membrane moves approximately 1 to 2 mm in each direction. Movement is decreased or absent when a middle ear effusion is present. When a child cries, both tympanic membranes may appear erythematous. Asymmetric dullness, bulging, or movement between the two sides often indicates the presence of an effusion in this situation.

(Battle sign) or persistent leakage of clear fluid (CSF) from the external canal.

▶ COMPLICATIONS

The most common complication of otoscopy is nicking the canal wall as a result of overly forceful insertion of the speculum, sudden movement by the patient, or overly vigorous curettage of cerumen. This can result in both pain and bleeding. The likelihood of this complication is minimized with proper preparation, positioning, and restraint as well as careful visualization and avoidance of abrupt movements. If bleeding should occur, instillation of hydrogen peroxide (which is left in for a few minutes and then wicked out with cotton) followed by instillation of Cortisporin otic suspension can minimize discomfort and prevent secondary infection. Using Cortisporin for a few days after extensive cleaning, even if bleeding does not occur, is also advisable.

▶ SUMMARY

"Earache" is one of the more common chief complaints of children seen in an emergency department, clinic, or office practice. However, otitis media may present with a number of other more subtle and nonspecific symptoms, such as fussiness or crying, fever, and anorexia. This is particularly true in younger children. For this reason, the pediatric physical examination is generally not complete without an otoscopic evaluation. In addition, findings such as hemotympanum and tympanic membrane perforation due to trauma also must be recognized. Otoscopic skills are also essential for visualization during procedures such as removal of cerumen or a foreign body. For older children, making the examination a game will often enhance the child's cooperation. With toddlers, it may be necessary to enlist the aid of a parent or other assistant to restrain the child appropriately to perform an adequate otoscopic examination. Taking extra care to avoid causing any true pain (as opposed to the psychological pain of being restrained and having one's ears "invaded") may help reduce the child's fear of subsequent examinations.

▶ ACKNOWLEDGMENT

The authors gratefully acknowledge the work of Dr. Hnin Khine on this chapter in the first edition of this text.

▶ REFERENCES

1. Bluestone CD, Klein JO, eds. *Otitis Media in Infants and Children*. 3rd ed. Philadelphia: WB Saunders; 2001.
2. Yellon RF, McBride TP, Davis HW. Otolaryngology. In: Zitelli BJ, Davis HW, eds. *Atlas of Pediatric Physical Diagnosis*. 4th ed. Philadelphia: Mosby; 2002:65–84.
3. Durrant JD. Embryology and developmental anatomy of the ear. In: Bluestone CD, Stool SE, Scheetz MD, eds. *Pediatric Otolaryngology*. 3rd ed. Philadelphia: WB Saunders; 2003:51–63.
4. Bluestone CD, Klein JO. Methods of examination in clinical exam. In: Bluestone CD, Stool SE, Scheetz MD, eds. *Pediatric Otolaryngology*. 3rd ed. Philadelphia: WB Saunders; 2003:82–101.
5. Bergstrom L. Diseases of the external ear. In: Bluestone CD, Stool SE, Scheetz MD, eds. *Pediatric Otolaryngology*. 3rd ed. Philadelphia: WB Saunders; 2003:102–122.
6. Bluestone CD, Klein JO. Otitis media and eustachian tube dysfunction. In: Bluestone CD, Stool SE, Scheetz MD, eds. *Pediatric Otolaryngology*. 3rd ed. Philadelphia: WB Saunders; 2003:64–81.
7. Kaleida PH, Hoberman A. *Otoendoscopic Examination* [Videotape]. Test videotape 3. Pittsburgh: University of Pittsburgh; 1995.
8. Rosenfeld RM, Bluestone CD. *Evidence-based Otitis Media*. 2nd ed. London: BC Decker; 2003.
9. Wald ER. To treat or not to treat. *Pediatrics*. 2005;115:1087–1089.

53

Removal of Cerumen Impaction

▶ INTRODUCTION

Removing cerumen from the external auditory canal of pediatric patients is a procedure that is performed daily in the emergency department (ED) and a variety of other medical settings. Authorities estimate that cerumen removal by syringing occurs 150,000 times per week. Visualization of the tympanic membrane is critical for completing a physical examination in pediatric patients presenting with symptoms where the underlying cause may involve the middle ear or tympanic membrane (see also Chapter 52).

The two basic methods for cerumen removal are syringing and débridement. Syringing (irrigation) uses an emulsifying agent to soften and break up cerumen, followed by irrigation. Débridement (curettage) is performed using either a blind technique or by direct visualization with a light source.

▶ ANATOMY AND PHYSIOLOGY

As shown in Chapter 52, the ear is divided into internal, middle, and external portions (see Figs. 52.1 and 52.2). The internal ear is composed of a system of tubes and spaces called the "membranous labyrinth," and these are contained within the bony labyrinth. The middle ear is composed of three ossicles. From lateral to medial, they are the malleus, incus, and stapes. All three are contained within the tympanic space, but only the malleus contacts the tympanic membrane. The border separating the middle ear and the external ear is the tympanic membrane. The external auditory canal and the auricle comprise the external ear. The external canal is divided into two parts: the superficial segment, which is supported by cartilage, and the deep segment, which is supported by bone. The deeper bony segment has significantly greater sensitivity to pain.

Cerumen is a mixture of desquamated keratin, dust and debris, hair, and secretions from ceruminous and sebaceous glands in the ear canal (1–5). Long-chain fatty acids, alcohols, squalene, and cholesterol form the major organic components of cerumen (2). Cerumen type is an inherited trait. Wet cerumen is autosomal dominant and is found in most African Americans and Caucasians. It is soft, sticky, and yellow-gold in color. Dry cerumen is common among Asians. It crumbles easily and is light gray. The lysosomes, immunoglobulins, and proteins contained in cerumen, as well as its acidic pH, are believed to have bacteriostatic or bacteriocidal activity (1,4,5).

Indications

Visualization of the tympanic membrane is indicated for any complaint that may stem from middle ear pathology. In children, this would most commonly be otitis media or tympanic membrane perforation. Symptoms may include ear pain or fullness, hearing difficulty, drainage from the ear canal, and headache. Fever, vomiting, diarrhea, poor appetite, ear pulling, cough, and irritability are nonspecific symptoms that may be seen in infants and toddlers with middle ear infections. Symptoms of cerumen impaction alone include vertigo, hearing loss, cough, tinnitus, ear pain, and fullness (1,4–7).

Syringing and débridement with direct visualization work best in older, cooperative pediatric patients. Blind débridement, although sometimes necessary in the older patient, is normally best used for infants and toddlers. Syringing is a less painful procedure than blind débridement and has fewer iatrogenic risks but is frequently unsuccessful. Débridement by direct visualization can often be accomplished without pain. The advantages of débridement are that it is less time consuming and has a higher success rate.

A suspected perforated tympanic membrane, tympanostomy tubes, and an uncooperative patient are contraindications to cerumenolytics and syringing. A history of otitis

TABLE 53.1	CERUMENOLYTICS

Glycerine
Vegetable oils
Spirit of turpentine
Formaldehyde 10%
Alcohol 95%
Mineral oil
Propylene glycol
Water
Sodium bicarbonate 5%, 10%, 15%
Hydrogen peroxide 3%
Sialic acid 2.5%
Buro-sol (0.5% aluminum acetate, 0.03% benzothoniun chloride)
Cerumenex (triethanolamine polypeptide oleate-condensate 10%, chlorbutanol 0.5% in propylene glycol)
Cerumol (paradichlorobenzene 2%, chlorbutal 5%, terebinth 5%)
Auralgan (benzocaine 14 mg and antipyrine 54 mg in glycerine made up to 1 mL)
Waxsol (docusate sodium 0.5% in a water miscible base)
Exterol (urea hydrogen peroxide 5% in glycerin)

externa, a single hearing ear, and previous ear surgery are relative contraindications to syringing (8). Bleeding disorders are a relative contraindication to blind débridement. Syringing is the preferred method for patients with a bleeding disorder because trauma to the ear canal is avoided.

▶ EQUIPMENT

Items and materials that may be useful for removal of a cerumen impaction are listed in Tables 53.1 to 53.3.

    Otoscope
    Emulsifying agents. Several compounds can be used to emulsify and lubricate cerumen and thereby facilitate its removal from the ear canal. Sodium bicarbonate 10% and saline are popular noncommercial products. The most popular commercial products are paradichlorobenzene 2%, chlorbutol 5%, oil of terebinth 5% (Cerumol), triethanolamine polypeptide oleate-condensate 10%, docusate sodium, and chlorbutanol 0.5% in propylene glycol (Cerumenex).
    Irrigant: room temperature saline or tap water. A recent study found commercial products had no advantage over

TABLE 53.2	SYRINGING EQUIPMENT

Warm water or saline
Emulsifying agent
Syringe
Intravenous catheter
Otoscope
Cotton
Emesis basin or bowel
Towel
Gauze

TABLE 53.3	DÉBRIDEMENT EQUIPMENT	
Direct visualization		**Blind technique**
Light source		Otoscope
Alligator forceps		Cerumen curette
Cerumen curette		Gauze or towel
Gauze or towel		Auralgan

normal saline in visualizing the tympanic membrane when syringing was used for disimpaction (9).
    Irrigation device:
        16- or 18-gauge intravenous catheter or short section of tubing cut from a butterfly needle
        Luer-Lok syringe (20 cc)
    There are also many commercial jet-type irrigation devices available for use in the patient with a normal, healthy tympanic membrane (8,10,11).
    Emesis basin or towels
    Gauze
    Alligator forceps
    Cerumen curette. The choice of curette material and shape is largely a personal one (Fig. 53.1). The metal curette may be best for the novice due to its heavier weight, which allows the clinician to gently guide the instrument into the auditory canal, as opposed to the lightweight plastic curette, which frequently must be pushed into the canal with the attendant risk of perforation. The softer tip of a plastic curette has less potential to cause bleeding from abrading the lining of the auditory canal during cerumen removal. Other advantages of plastic curettes are that they are made in a variety of tip shapes and styles, they are disposable, and they are now available with lighted tips for use with direct visualization.

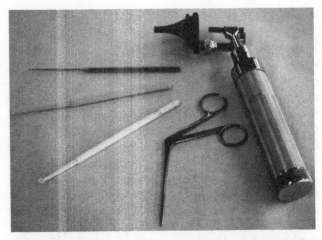

Figure 53.1 An operating otoscope with (clockwise) an alligator forceps, two flexible plastic cerumen spoons, and a metal cerumen spoon.

▶ PROCEDURE

Syringing

Patients should wear a hospital gown and be placed in the lateral decubitus position with the affected side up. The emulsifying agent of choice is gently placed in the ear canal until the ear canal is full. A compacted piece of cotton is placed in the canal to prevent the solution from dripping out. The other ear canal also may be treated in a similar fashion, and the emulsifying solution is given a minimum of 20 minutes to work. The best results are obtained when a patient has an emulsifying agent repeatedly instilled in the ear for 2 to 7 days before syringing, but this obviously is not possible for ED patients.

Next, the ear canal is irrigated. Commonly used agents include saline, water, or a 1:1 mixture of saline or water with hydrogen peroxide. All solutions should be warmed to body temperature to minimize discomfort. Some clinicians prefer to use a Frazier suction catheter to remove the emulsifying agent at this point; however, noise from the suction catheter frequently frightens children and may make them less cooperative with the procedure. The patient should be placed in the supine position so that the irrigating solution will easily spill out of the ear. It is important that the irrigating fluid easily exit the ear canal and not be blocked by the irrigating equipment, because excessive pressure can lead to perforation of the tympanic membrane. An emesis basin or several towels may be held next to the patient's mastoid region to catch the irrigating solution. A syringe with an attached 16- or 18-gauge intravenous catheter (or a short section of tubing with attached hub cut from a butterfly needle) is used with mild to moderate force to irrigate the canal. The volume of the syringe should be at least 20 mL to generate adequate pressure. The catheter tip is inserted approximately 1.0 to 1.5 cm into the ear canal and directed toward the posterosuperior wall of the canal (Fig. 53.2). The stream of fluid should not impact the tympanic membrane directly. Often the clinician will observe pieces of cerumen being flushed out of the ear. However, even if this is not the case, the ear should be frequently examined with the otoscope during the procedure because the cerumen may partially dislodge to the extent that the clinician can visualize a section of the tympanic membrane. In many cases, this will allow an adequate examination. It is important to always visualize the tympanic membrane when syringing is completed to check for iatrogenic tympanic membrane rupture.

Débridement

Débridement may be accomplished by either direct visualization or the blind method. Direct visualization requires a light source, preferably a head mirror, or an operating otoscope (Fig. 53.1). The patient is positioned either in the lateral decubitus position or sitting upright against a headrest. Parents (and patients) should be forewarned that a minimal amount of unavoidable discomfort may occur and that some bleeding

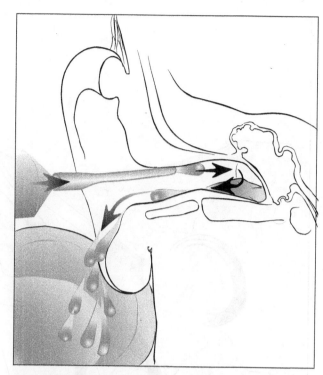

Figure 53.2 Syringing cerumen or a foreign body from the auditory canal with an intravenous catheter attached to a 20-mL syringe. The irrigating stream is directed at the posterosuperior wall of the canal.

postdébridement is not uncommon but is rarely serious. The clinician applies traction to the auricle by grasping the helix to straighten the external auditory canal and allow visualization. Cerumen that is visible may now be removed with alligator forceps or a curette (Fig. 53.3). This technique requires a high degree of patient cooperation and thus is not the method of choice in the very young child.

The blind method is the quickest and most commonly used means of cerumen removal in infants and small children. It is imperative that the child be well restrained and with the head rotated so that the opposite ear is held against the stretcher. Some clinicians recommend a drop of an emulsifying agent and then a drop of antipyrine-benzocaine solution (e.g., Auralgan) as a topical anesthetic a few minutes before the procedure. When ready to proceed, the clinician gently retracts the helix of the auricle to straighten the auditory canal and briefly visualize the location of the impacted cerumen. This may help identify where the curette can most easily pass beyond the impaction. The cerumen spoon is then grasped with the tips of the thumb and index and middle fingers, and the ulnar side of the hand is braced against the child's head. This position will prevent the curette from plunging deeper into the ear if an unexpected movement occurs. The curette is then gently introduced into the external auditory canal (Fig. 53.4). A plastic cerumen spoon will usually require some gentle downward pressure before scooping out the cerumen, and therefore this technique requires patience and practice to

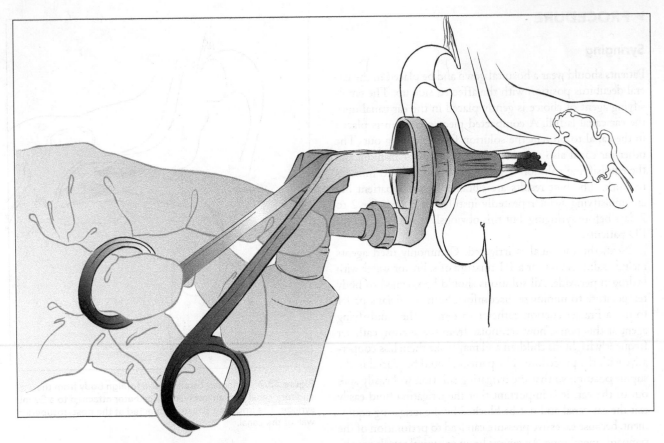

Figure 53.3 Cerumen (or a foreign body) can be removed from the auditory canal under direct visualization with an alligator forceps and an operating head otoscope.

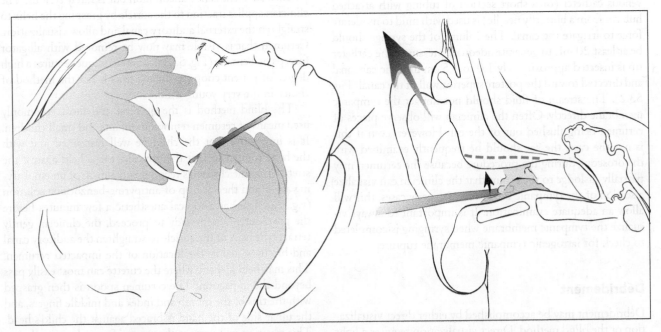

Figure 53.4
A. Blind débridement of cerumen is accomplished with the child well restrained and the clinician's hand braced against the child's head.
B. The cerumen spoon is passed into (and ideally beyond) the impaction and then withdrawn while scooping out the cerumen.

be done safely. A metal cerumen spoon will normally pass through the canal by gravity alone due to its heavier weight.

If the clinician is successful in retrieving a piece of cerumen, the spoon is wiped off on a towel or piece of gauze. The clinician should frequently attempt to visualize the tympanic membrane due to the pain associated with this procedure. Visualization should be attempted even when no cerumen is found on the end of the spoon, because often a partial dislodgment of cerumen will enable the clinician to see enough of the tympanic membrane to make a diagnosis.

 SUMMARY

Syringing

1 Position or restrain the child as needed with the affected ear facing up.

2 Instill emulsifying agent followed by a cotton plug and allow 20 minutes to work.

3 Reposition the child in supine position with an emesis basin or towels below the affected ear.

4 Fill a 20-mL syringe with saline or tap water at body temperature (may be mixed 1:1 with hydrogen peroxide).

5 Attach a 16- or 18-gauge intravenous catheter (or a short section of butterfly needle tubing with attached hub) to a 20-mL syringe.

6 Insert the catheter 1.0 to 1.5 cm into the auditory canal.

7 Direct the stream posteriorly and superiorly in the canal (not directly at the tympanic membrane).

8 Repeat until the tympanic membrane can be visualized.

Débridement

1 Warn parents (and patient) that a certain minimal amount of unavoidable discomfort will occur and that bleeding postprocedure is common but generally not serious.

2 For blind débridement, brace the hand holding the curette against the child's head, with the child securely restrained and the head held firmly against the stretcher.

3 Gently lower the curette into the canal to the estimated level of cerumen impaction, then withdraw with scooping motion.

4 Frequently examine the canal to ascertain if the tympanic membrane is visible, even in absence of overt cerumen removal.

▶ COMPLICATIONS

Complications of cerumen removal include pain, bleeding, infection, tympanic membrane perforation, contact dermatitis, ossicle disruption, vertigo, vomiting, and even cardiac arrest (10,12–17). It is estimated that the complication rate of ear syringing is 1 in 1,000 (18). Iatrogenic perforation of the tympanic membrane during syringing or syringing an ear with a pre-existing tympanic membrane perforation can cause a middle ear infection, disruption of the ossicles, or both. Overzealous use of the cerumen spoon may cause tympanic membrane perforation, significant pain, and bleeding. Accidental

---

 CLINICAL TIPS

▶ Instilling an emulsifying agent into the ear before débridement will soften the cerumen, making it easier to remove.

▶ Instilling Auralgan before débridement may decrease pain.

▶ Proper positioning of the patient and bracing the ulnar side of the hand against the child's head before débridement prevents injury from sudden movements.

▶ Straightening the auditory canal by applying traction to the auricle will aid direct visualization and/or passing a cerumen curette.

▶ The irrigating stream should be directed posteriorly and superiorly against the wall of the external canal to prevent iatrogenic tympanic membrane injury.

▶ Allowing gravity alone to guide the metal cerumen spoon in and down the auditory canal decreases the likelihood of injury to the external canal and tympanic membrane.

▶ If one tympanic membrane is visualized and the diagnosis of otitis media is made, it may not be necessary to débride the other side. Emulsifying drops can often be prescribed along with antibiotics, and the ears can be re-examined subsequently to assess for resolution of infection and clearing of the cerumen impaction.

▶ Permitting the child to see and touch the equipment, such as the irrigating setup and the cerumen curette, may aid in gaining cooperation.

▶ Débridement under direct visualization requires full patient cooperation and thus is rarely chosen for infants or toddlers. With visualization, cerumen may be removed using a curette or alligator forceps.

perforation of the tympanic membrane during débridement of cerumen is treated like any other perforation, that is, with otic antibiotic drops and a follow-up examination to ensure that proper healing has occurred. Bleeding and pain are not uncommon complications and are usually caused by abrasion of the external auditory canal. Bleeding can become serious in the patient with a bleeding disorder. Extra care, or syringing alone, should be considered for these patients. Blind débridement almost always causes some discomfort. Pain and bleeding episodes will diminish as the clinician gains experience. If the ear canal is abraded, some clinicians advocate the prophylactic use of otic antibiotic drops.

▶ SUMMARY

Cerumen removal is a common procedure in the ED and other outpatient settings. Removal may be performed by direct or indirect débridement, by syringing, or by using a commercial jet-irrigation apparatus. Blind débridement is the method most commonly used in infants and small children in the ED because it is the quickest and most reliable method. Care should be taken to prevent iatrogenic injury and minimize discomfort.

▶ REFERENCES

1. Hanger HC, Mulley GP. Cerumen: its fascination and clinical importance: a review. *J R Soc Med*. 1992;85:346–349.
2. Okuda I, Bingham B, Stoney P, et al. The organic composition of earwax. *J Otolaryngol*. 1991;20:212–215.
3. Naiberg JB, Robinson A, Kwok P, et al. Swirls, wrinkles and the whole ball of wax (the source of keratin in cerumen). *J Otolaryngol*. 1992;21:142–148.
4. Pray WS, Pray JJ. Earwax: should it be removed? *US Pharm*. 2005;5:21–27.
5. Guest JF, Greener MJ, Robinson AC, et al. Impacted cerumen: composition, production, epidemiology and management. *QJM*. 2004;97:477–488.
6. Harkess CK. Clearing the occluded auditory canal. *Pediatr Nurs*. 1982;8:23–25.
7. Raman R. Impacted ear wax: a cause for unexplained cough? [Letter]. *Arch Otolaryngol Head Neck Surg*. 1986;112:679.
8. Marcuse EK. Removal of cerumen [Letter]. *JAMA*. 1984;251:1681.
9. Whatley VN, Dodds CL, Paul RI. Randomized clinical trial of docusate, triethanolamine polypeptide and irrigation in cerumen removal in children. *Arch Pediatr Adolesc Med*. 2003;157:1177–1180.
10. Dinsdale RC, Roland PS, Manning SC, et al. Catastrophic otologic injury from oral jet irrigation of the external auditory canal. *Laryngoscope*. 1991;101[1 Pt. 1]:75–78.
11. Watkins S, Moore TH, Phillips J. Clearing impacted ears. *Am J Nurs*. 1984;84:1107.
12. Lindsey D. It's time to stop washing out ears! [Letter]. *Am J Emerg Med*. 1991;9:297.
13. Drysdale AJ. Earwax removal [Letter]. *Br Med J*. 1991;302(6769):182.
14. Robinson AC, Hawke M. The efficacy of cerumenolytics: everything old is new again. *J Otolaryngol*. 1989;18:263–267.
15. Andaz C, Whittet HB. An in vitro study to determine efficacy of different wax-dispersing agents. *J Otorhinolaryngol Relat Spec*. 1993;55:97–99.
16. Mehta AK. An in vitro comparison of the disintegration of human earwax by five cerumenolytics commonly used in general practice. *Br J Clin Pract*. 1985;39:200–203.
17. Shreeve C. Ear wax solvents. *Nurs Mirror*. 1984;159(5):33.
18. Sharp JF, Wilson JA, Ross L, et al. Ear wax removal: a survey of current practice. *Br Med J*. 1990;301(6763):1251–1253.

54

Foreign Body Removal from the External Auditory Canal

▶ INTRODUCTION

Foreign bodies in the external auditory canal (EAC) are a frequent problem in children. The objects found in children's ears are diverse and include beads, pebbles, popcorn kernels, paper, toy parts, earring parts, and eraser tips (1,2). Pain from pre-existing otitis media may occasionally prompt children to place foreign bodies in the ear. Although the presence of a foreign object in a body orifice is usually a presentation of inquisitive younger children, older children and adolescents will sometimes present after a cockroach has crawled into the EAC during sleep. The majority of superficially located soft or irregularly shaped objects with graspable parts can be successfully removed without otolaryngologic consultation, while firm, rounded, and/or deeply imbedded objects can be much more challenging and may warrant referral (2–5).

▶ ANATOMY AND PHYSIOLOGY

Objects frequently lodge at the narrow junction between the cartilaginous and bony portions of the EAC (see also Chapter 52). In children, pulling the pinna superiorly and laterally will straighten the external auditory canal for adequate visualization (see Fig. 52.5). Skin over the bony canal lacks subcutaneous tissue and is tightly adherent to the periosteum. The canal is exquisitely sensitive to touch, with sensory innervation supplied by branches of the vagus and trigeminal nerves. Nerve blocks of the external ear canal require painful, four-quadrant injections that are impossible to perform without significant emotional distress in an awake child and are not recommended. Topical anesthesia is minimally effective due to the impermeable keratinized epithelial surface of the

EAC. Procedural sedation or analgesia should be considered when instruments are used or patient immobility is essential (see Chapter 33) (6).

▶ INDICATIONS

Objects may be found on routine examination, or asymptomatic patients may have been observed putting something in the ear. Symptoms consistent with a foreign body in the EAC include ear pain, decreased hearing, cough, and otorrhea. Live insects such as roaches in the EAC often cause extreme discomfort. Triage protocols should facilitate early instillation of mineral oil to kill live insects and to prioritize care for patients suspected of having a button battery in the ear. While urgent removal may be indicated (e.g., in the case of a button battery), most objects are safe to leave in place if necessary until removal can be performed by an otolaryngologist.

▶ EQUIPMENT

Most equipment for foreign body removal is readily available in the office or emergency department (ED) (Table 54.1). The diagnostic-type otoscope head commonly available is not ideal for direct visualization during instrument removal. The operating-type head (see Fig. 53.1) facilitates introduction of an instrument under continuous direct visualization.

▶ PROCEDURE

Preparation

For the frantic child with a live insect in the ear, it is reasonable to instruct parents and triage nurses to immediately instill

TABLE 54.1	EQUIPMENT FOR FOREIGN BODY REMOVAL FROM THE EXTERNAL AUDITORY CANAL

Operating otoscope
Alligator forceps
Cerumen curette
Irrigation setup:
    20-mL Luer-Lok syringe
    14- or 16-gauge plastic catheter or butterfly needle tubing
    Sterile water
Suction device:
    Soft-tip catheter
    Frazier suction catheter
Mineral oil
Right-angle ball hook
Bayonet forceps
Cyanoacrylate glue
Wood or plastic swab stick
Paper clip
Papoose board

mineral oil (e.g., baby oil) to kill the insect. Mineral oil is superior to lidocaine in its ability to kill insects rapidly (7).

Patient cooperation is the critical factor for success. An important point is that the first attempt should be the best attempt. Stimulation of the exquisitely sensitive ear canal will quickly reduce the level of cooperation in even the most tractable patient. If the clinician is not confident that an object can be removed on the first attempt, then referral is advisable when possible. A younger child should be restrained by first wrapping the patient in a sheet and then applying the papoose board. An assistant then immobilizes the patient's head against the bed with the involved ear upwards. Parents should be warned that minor bleeding may occur with any method of removal.

The removal technique used must be tailored to the location and type of foreign body. As mentioned previously, procedural sedation (Chapter 33) should be considered before attempts at removal using instruments if the object is not easily grasped or amenable to irrigation. Foreign body removal by irrigation and by instrumentation under direct visualization are closely analogous to these same methods of removing a cerumen impaction, which are discussed and illustrated in Chapter 53.

Irrigation

Irrigation is the technique of choice for small, nonvegetable foreign bodies and dead insects. Irrigation is better tolerated than instrumentation and does not require direct visualization. However, pneumatic otoscopy should first be performed to document an intact tympanic membrane. Water at body temperature will minimize vestibular stimulation. Irrigation is performed using a 20-mL syringe attached to either a 1- to 2-inch section of butterfly needle tubing that has been cut to remove the needle or a 14- or 16-gauge intravenous catheter. This apparatus is used to produce a pulsatile stream directed

against the posterosuperior canal wall (see Fig. 53.2). The stream should not be directed directly at the tympanic membrane, as this risks injury. Presence of a hygroscopic foreign body (e.g., a bean) is a relative contraindication to irrigation because the object may swell, making subsequent attempts more difficult. Electronic ear syringes and special irrigation tips designed for ear irrigation may also be used. Irrigation should not be attempted in an ear with a myringotomy tube. Devices designed for oral (dental) irrigation generate excessive pressures and should not be used for irrigation of the ear (8). Disc batteries should never be irrigated, as wetting the battery leads to leakage of electrolyte solution and may exacerbate tissue damage (2). After removal of a disc battery, the EAC should be irrigated to remove any chemical residue.

Instrument Removal

An alligator forceps can be introduced under direct vision via an operating otoscope head to remove irregular objects such as insects or paper (see Fig. 53.3). Bayonet forceps are useful for superficial irregular objects. The hand holding the instrument should be stabilized against the patient's head to avoid excessive penetration if the child moves. For smooth, round objects such as beads, a right-angle ball hook or plastic or metal ear curette often can be passed beyond the object, which, if superficial, may not require otoscopic visualization (see Figs. 53.4 and 59.3A). Hair beads can be rotated until the central hole is lined up with the ear canal, allowing removal by threading the hole with a straightened paper clip.

Blind attempts or attempts to remove deeply placed firm, round objects with forceps are rarely successful, increase the pain and risk of injury to the tympanic membrane and middle ear structures, and complicate subsequent removal. Frequently, impacted, nongraspable objects, sharp objects, and objects adjacent to the tympanic membrane are best referred to an otolaryngologist, with no attempt at removal (2–5).

Miscellaneous Techniques

Suction can be used for removal of foreign bodies for which irrigation is inappropriate or has failed. Continuous wall suction is attached to a handheld suction catheter with a soft tip. Frazier suction catheters can be modified by attaching a segment of intravenous tubing or a tympanostomy tube to the end (9). A disposable commercial soft-tipped catheter is also available (Schuknecht Foreign Body Remover, Memphis, TN). Metallic foreign bodies may sometimes be removed using a magnet of the type used to remove ocular foreign bodies (10).

Cyanoacrylate glue (Super Glue) has been successfully used to remove smooth dry, nongraspable objects (11–13). A small amount of glue is applied to the blunt end of a wood or plastic swab stick that is then introduced into the EAC and held to the foreign body surface for 25 to 60 seconds. This technique requires patient immobility and operator patience so that a firm bond is formed, allowing subsequent withdrawal of the stick with the foreign body attached.

Postprocedure Care and Referral

Regardless of the technique used, it is essential to set reasonable limits for time and number of attempts and to recognize defeat. After failed removal, children should be referred to an otolaryngologist, who may choose to perform the procedure with the aid of an otomicroscope, sometimes under general anesthesia. Button batteries in the EAC have potentially corrosive effects and should be removed as soon as possible. Follow-up evaluation should include postprocedure pneumatic otoscopy of both ears to ensure the object has not fragmented, to exclude multiple foreign bodies, and to document that the tympanic membrane remains intact (see Chapter 52).

▶ COMPLICATIONS

A small amount of excoriation and minimal bleeding from the EAC are common after foreign body removal. If this

---

 SUMMARY

Syringing (see Fig. 53.2)

1 Use irrigation for nonvegetable foreign bodies.

2 Fill a 20-mL syringe with saline or tap water at body temperature.

3 Connect the syringe to a 14- or 16-gauge intravenous catheter or a 1- to 2-inch section of butterfly needle tubing that has been cut to remove the needle.

4 Insert the catheter 1.0 to 1.5 cm into the auditory canal.

5 Direct the stream posteriorly and superiorly.

Instrument Removal (see Figs. 53.3, 53.4 and 59.3A)

1 Perform under direct visualization for foreign body removal, when possible.

2 Using right angle, gently insert the instrument into the canal and attempt to pass the hooked end beyond the foreign body, rotate the end behind the object. and use the hooked end to pull out the object.

3 Use alligator forceps for irregular, graspable objects.

4 Consider suction and cyanoacrylate techniques for removal of some smooth objects.

 CLINICAL TIPS

▶ The first attempt should always be the best attempt, especially with younger children. As a corollary, lack of confidence that a foreign body can be removed on the first attempt should be taken as a sign that, when possible, referral is likely the best option.

▶ The technique used should be tailored to the location and type of foreign body.

▶ Reasonable limits must be set on time and number of attempts.

▶ Live insects should first be killed with mineral oil, as this will greatly reduce patient discomfort and anxiety.

▶ Button battery impaction is an emergency and requires immediate otolaryngologic consultation if ED removal is unsuccessful, as does any evidence of middle ear pathology.

▶ Initial attention to proper patient preparation and restraint will ultimately result in a quicker, less traumatic procedure with a greater likelihood of success.

▶ Procedural sedation may be appropriate to facilitate foreign body removal in selected cases.

---

occurs, a topical antibiotic such as Floxin otic suspension should usually be prescribed. Hematoma formation and iatrogenic perforation of the tympanic membrane can occur. Prior attempts at removal by the patient, parents, or referring physician decrease the chances of success and increase the risk of complications. Patients who present with or develop middle ear symptoms (e.g., severe bleeding, marked hearing loss, vertigo, facial paralysis) require immediate otolaryngologic consultation, as do patients with button batteries that cannot be removed or have already had corrosive effect.

▶ SUMMARY

Foreign bodies in the EAC are a common problem in children. Many can be removed in the ambulatory setting without consultation. To avoid complications and enhance success, the first attempt should be tailored to the type and location of the foreign body. Reasonable limits on time and number of attempts should be set. Direct visualization with adequate restraint and/or sedation is essential if instruments are used.

▶ REFERENCES

1. Baker MD. Foreign bodies of the ears and nose in childhood. *Pediatr Emerg Care*. 1987;3:67–70.

2. Ansley JF, Cunningham MJ. Treatment of aural foreign bodies in children. *Pediatrics*. 1998;101:638–641.

3. Thompson SK, Wein RO, Dutcher PO. External auditory canal foreign body removal: management practices and outcomes. *Laryngoscope*. 2003;113:1912–1915.

4. DiMuzio J, Deschler DG. Emergency department management of foreign bodies of the external auditory canal in children. *Otol Neurotol*. 2002;23:473–475.

5. Schulze SL, Kerschner J, Beste D. Pediatric external auditory canal foreign bodies: a review of 698 cases. *Otolaryngol Head Neck Surg*. 2002;127:73–78.

6. Brown L, Denmark TK, Wittlake WA, et al. Procedural sedation use in the ED: management of pediatric ear and nose foreign bodies. *Am J Emerg Med*. 2004;22:310–314.

7. Leffler S, Cheney P, Tandberg D. Chemical immobilization and killing and intraaural roaches: an in vitro comparative study. *Ann Emerg Med*. 1993;22:1795–1798.

8. Dinsdale RC, Roland PS, Manning SC, et al. Catastrophic otologic injury from oral jet irrigation of the external auditory canal. *Laryngoscope*. 1991;101:75–78.

9. Fritz S, Kelen GD, Sivertson KT. Foreign bodies of the external auditory canal. *Emerg Med Clin North Am*. 1987;5:183–193.

10. Davies PH, Benger JR. Foreign bodies in the nose and ear: a review of techniques for removal in the emergency department. *J Accid Emerg Med*. 2000;17:91–94.

11. Pride H, Schwab R. A new technique for removing foreign bodies of the external auditory canal. *Pediatr Emerg Care*. 1989;5:135–136.

12. Benger JR, Davies PH. A useful form of glue ear. *J Accid Emerg Med*. 2000;17:149–150.

13. McLaughlin R, Ullah R, Heylings D. Comparative prospective study of foreign body removal from external auditory canals of cadavers with right angle hook or cyanoacrylate glue. *Emerg Med J*. 2002:43–45.

55

NESTOR J. MARTINEZ AND MARLA J. FRIEDMAN

External Ear Procedures

▶ INTRODUCTION

The external ear is vulnerable to injury because of its exposed position. Injuries to the external ear occur in all age groups and are common among those engaged in sports activities (e.g., wrestling, cycling, martial arts) (1). Lacerations of the external ear are the most frequent form of accidental ear trauma (2). Auricular hematomas usually result from shearing injury and are often seen in boxers and wrestlers (3). Other types of external ear injury include abrasions, burns, and avulsions. Additionally, earring studs or backs may become embedded as a result of infection or excessive pressure. This usually involves the earlobe but can occur in other parts of the ear where a piercing has been done (4). The goal of treatment of these conditions is to restore the normal appearance of the ear while preventing complications such as infection or abnormal cartilage formation.

▶ ANATOMY AND PHYSIOLOGY

The external ear consists of the auricle and the external auditory canal. The auricle is composed of cartilage covered by tightly attached perichondrium and skin on the external surface. The lobule is without cartilage and is composed of soft tissue and skin only. Anteriorly, the skin of the helix and antihelix region is firmly adherent to the cartilage. The perichondrium and skin behind the auricle are separated from the cartilage by a thin layer of subcutaneous tissue and are more loosely attached. The vascular supply to the skin and perichondrium is provided by the superficial temporal artery and the posterior and deep auricular branches of the external carotid artery. Four nerve branches provide sensory innervation to the outer ear. The outer portion of the auricle receives its innervation from the greater and lesser auricular nerves, while the more medial portion receives innervation from the

auriculotemporal nerve (Fig. 55.1). The auricular branch of the vagus nerve innervates the external auditory meatus and much of the concha (5,6).

The cartilaginous tissue of the auricle lacks its own blood supply. Instead, the cartilage of the ear is nourished by the surrounding perichondrium. Blunt trauma can disrupt the normal relationship between these two structures. If the cartilage becomes denuded or separated from the perichondrium by an auricular hematoma, ischemia may occur without proper treatment, potentially resulting in infection or necrosis of the cartilage. As the cartilage dies, it is replaced by fibrocartilaginous scar tissue, resulting in the cosmetic deformity known as "cauliflower ear" (7). Hematoma or seroma can occur after closure of a laceration to the external ear, but this is less likely when a proper dressing is applied.

▶ INDICATIONS

More than half of all ear lacerations occur in the pinna, and the extent of injury is usually immediately obvious (2). However, in some cases blood from ear or other facial lacerations may conceal exposed perichondrium, cartilage, or additional lacerations, especially behind the ear. Small, simple lacerations of the ear should undergo primary skin closure. It is important not to leave any exposed cartilage after closure, as this increases the risk of infection and chondritis. If the cartilage is minimally injured, closing the skin over the cartilage should result in an adequate repair. However, if the cartilage requires suturing to maintain its stability, or if there is exposed cartilage that may require skin grafting, a surgical consultation should be obtained. Consultation is also advisable in cases of complex cartilage injury that may require débridement. When the laceration involves the external ear canal, surgical consultation is recommended, because stenosis of the canal is possible without the appropriate management and follow-up (3,8).

A mastoid dressing or a customized pressure dressing should be applied to the ear following the repair of most complicated ear lacerations and following drainage of auricular hematomas. This dressing serves to prevent further bleeding and hematoma or seroma formation (8). It also helps to maintain the normal contour of the external ear.

Embedded earring backs must be removed to prevent foreign body impaction, scarring, disfigurement, and infection. Removal of an earring back is a simple procedure once adequate anesthesia is performed. Proper wound care following extraction should be provided.

▶ EQUIPMENT

Auricular Block
Antiseptic solution
Syringe, 10 mL
Needle, 25 to 27 gauge, 1½ inch
Lidocaine 1% without epinephrine, 10 to 15 mL

External Ear Laceration Repair
Antiseptic solution
Syringe, 20 mL, with protective shield for irrigation
Sterile water or saline for irrigation
Syringe, 10 mL
Needle, 25 to 27 gauge, 1½ inch
Lidocaine 1% without epinephrine
Skin sutures, 6.0 nonabsorbable monofilament
Cartilage sutures, 6.0 absorbable Vicryl

Auricular Hematoma Aspiration
Antiseptic solution
Lidocaine 1% without epinephrine, if needed
Syringe, 10 mL
Needle, 18 gauge
Scalpel with No. 15 blade
Curved hemostat

Mastoid or Pressure Dressing
Cotton balls soaked in saline or mineral oil or petroleum gauze
Gauze pads (4) 4″ × 4″ with partial cut in center
Gauze pads (4) 4″ × 4″ without center cut
Gauze wrap-around bandage, 4 inch

Removal of Embedded Earring Backs
Antiseptic solution
Syringe, 1 mL
Needle, 25 to 27 gauge, ½ inch
Lidocaine 1% without epinephrine
Small forceps or hemostatic clamp
Scalpel with No. 15 blade
Skin sutures, 6.0 nonabsorbable monofilament

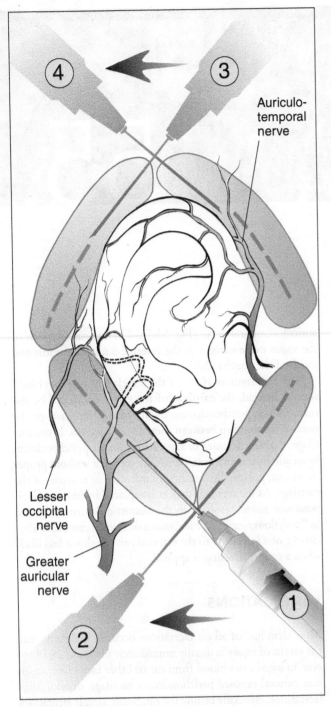

Figure 55.1 Regional auricular block.

Auriculo-temporal nerve

Lesser occipital nerve

Greater auricular nerve

Auricular hematomas require prompt, meticulous drainage in order to prevent ensuing complications. Drainage must be complete, and the appropriate dressing should be applied. Timely follow-up within 24 hours is of paramount importance in the management of these injuries, since blood frequently accumulates again after the initial drainage (3,9).

▶ PROCEDURE

Regional Auricular Block

Many external ear procedures require anesthetizing the ear. This may be accomplished by either local infiltration of anesthetic or by the use of a regional auricular block. The regional block is used in extensive lacerations and when the intent is to avoid distortion of the wound edges from the injection of local anesthetic. Lesions that involve the meatus and the concha may require a combination of both local and regional anesthesia, since vagus nerve innervation of these areas will not be blocked by regional anesthesia (8).

Local infiltration or a regional block is used to achieve anesthesia during laceration repairs or hematoma drainage of the ear. Anesthesia can be attempted via local infiltration if the laceration is small and distortion of the wound edges can be avoided. Hematoma drainage may not require any anesthetic.

When performing an auricular block, the ear and the surrounding skin area are first cleaned with an antiseptic solution. A 10-mL syringe with a 1.5-inch, 25- to 27-gauge needle is filled with 1% lidocaine without epinephrine and is used to inject a track of lidocaine around the entire ear (Fig. 55.1). This is achieved by first entering a point just above the ear and fully inserting the needle along the back of the ear. Lidocaine (3 to 5 mL) is injected as the needle is withdrawn. Without withdrawal of the needle from the skin, a second track is made in the same fashion, this time extending along the front of the ear, thus forming an inverted V. Similar anterior and posterior tracks are made at the bottom of the ear (i.e., an upright V) by entering the skin just below the lobe in the sulcus, so that a complete circumference around the ear is anesthetized. Maximum anesthetic effect is achieved approximately 10 minutes after injection (8).

Auricular Laceration Repair

Prior to beginning laceration repairs, the skin of the ear should be cleaned with antiseptic solution, and the ear should be anesthetized using the techniques previously described. The wound should then be irrigated using copious amounts of saline solution. Thorough wound irrigation is the most effective way to remove debris and reduce bacterial contamination of the wound (8). If the cartilage is not involved or is only minimally involved, adequate repair can be accomplished by simple skin closure using 6.0 nonabsorbable monofilament sutures (3,8). If necessary, a few absorbable 6.0 Vicryl sutures can be placed in the cartilage to add support (7). Cartilage should not be débrided, as débridement may result in notching of the ear contours. Finally, any exposed cartilage must be covered with skin. Failure to do so may result in chondritis and subsequent ear deformities. Suture removal may take place as soon as 5 days following repair, although a wound check should be scheduled within 24 hours of repair to check for

infection and possible formation of a hematoma or seroma. Surgical consultation is indicated for complex cartilage lacerations, wounds that may need graft placement, and lacerations involving the ear canal (3,8).

Auricular Hematoma Drainage

To evacuate an auricular hematoma (Fig. 55.2), the area to be drained should first be cleaned with antiseptic solution. An anesthetic may not be necessary for a single needle aspiration of the hematoma. An 18-gauge needle attached to a

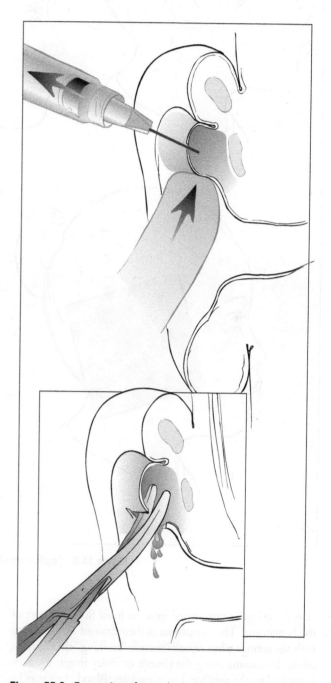

Figure 55.2 Evacuation of auricular hematoma.

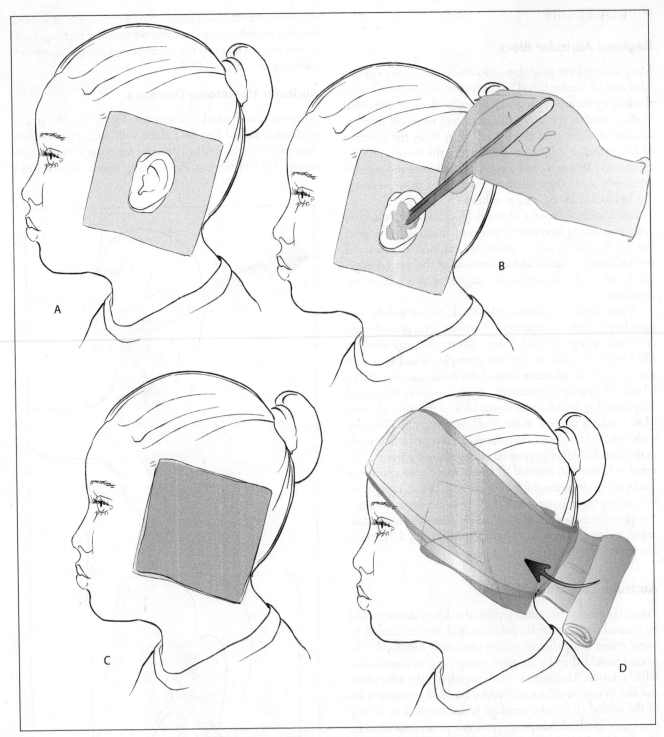

Figure 55.3 Application of mastoid pressure dressing.

10-mL syringe is introduced into the most fluctuant part of the hematoma. The hematoma is then drained by aspirating with the syringe while simultaneously "milking" the contents of the hematoma using the thumb or index finger. Pressure is applied to the area for 3 to 5 minutes. Blood clots may be difficult to remove by needle aspiration alone. In this case, a small incision is made into the hematoma using a No. 15 scalpel blade. A curved hemostat is then inserted into this incision and used to break up the clot. The hematoma must be completely evacuated in order to prevent possible cartilage necrosis. After the auricular hematoma has been drained, a pressure dressing is applied to prevent reaccumulation of fluid and to provide support and protection to the ear. A repeat examination is required within 24 hours to check for

SUMMARY

Regional Auricular Block

1 Restrain the child appropriately and prepare the involved area using aseptic technique.

2 Insert the needle into the subcutaneous tissue layer just above the ear.

3 Direct the needle posteriorly and then anteriorly to form an inverted V track of anesthetic.

4 Insert the needle into the subcutaneous tissue layer just below the earlobe.

5 Direct the needle posteriorly and then anteriorly to form an upright V track of anesthetic.

6 Maximum anesthetic effect is attained in approximately 10 minutes.

Auricular Laceration Repair

1 Restrain the child appropriately.

2 Anesthetize the wound as indicated.

3 Prepare the area using aseptic technique and create a sterile field.

4 Clean and thoroughly irrigate the wound with saline.

5 For simple lacerations involving only skin, carefully align and close the wound edges using 6.0 nonabsorbable sutures.

6 For cartilage lacerations that require suturing, use the least possible number of 6.0 Vicryl sutures, and employ large needle bites to prevent cartilage tearing.

7 Avoid cartilage débridement or exposure of cartilage after wound closure.

8 Apply a mastoid pressure dressing.

9 Arrange for follow-up within 24 hours to check for early signs of infection or fluid accumulation.

Auricular Hematoma Drainage

1 Restrain the child appropriately.

2 Prepare the area using aseptic technique and create a sterile field.

3 If needed, anesthetize the area to be drained.

4 Puncture the hematoma using an 18-gauge needle or a No. 15 scalpel blade.

5 Drain the hematoma completely by milking the fluid.

6 Maintain manual pressure for 3 minutes and then place a mastoid pressure dressing.

7 Follow-up within 24 hours to check for reaccumulation of serous fluid or blood.

Application of Pressure Dressing

1 Place two to four 4″ × 4″ gauze pads with central cutouts completely around the ear.

2 Mold petroleum gauze or cotton balls soaked in saline or mineral oil into the contours of the outer ear.

3 Cover the entire ear with two to four intact gauze pads.

4 Wrap the ear and the head with a 4-inch gauze bandage.

Removal of Imbedded Earring Backs

1 Restrain the child appropriately.

2 Prepare the area using aseptic technique.

3 Infiltrate the earlobe with 0.5 mL of lidocaine without epinephrine.

4 Apply pressure to the anterior aspect of the lobe with the nondominant hand to position the earring back.

5 Insert a small, closed forceps or hemostatic clamp into the rear earring opening of the earlobe.

6 Firmly grasp the earring back and gently pull it out of the earlobe through the rear opening.

7 If necessary, separate and remove the stud of the earring from the back by spreading the "rings" of the back with a forceps.

8 Apply antibiotic ointment and a sterile dressing.

---

fluid reaccumulation and, if necessary, to perform additional drainage (10).

Pressure Dressing Application

A pressure dressing should be placed on the ear following complicated laceration repairs and hematoma drainage. The goal is to provide constant pressure to the ear without producing ischemia (8). Two to four gauze pads (4″ × 4″) with the centers cut out are placed around the entire ear (Fig. 55.3). These pads provide support posteriorly and help to prevent distortion and excessive pressure on the ear. Next, petroleum gauze or cotton balls soaked in saline or mineral oil are positioned and molded to conform to the contours of the external ear.

Four intact gauze pads are then placed over the entire ear, and a 4-inch gauze bandage is wrapped around the head and over the ear several times. Patients should be advised to return to the emergency department within 24 hours for reassessment. In addition, they should be instructed to return immediately if they experience signs of chondritis or perichondritis, such as increasing pain, swelling, redness, warmth, and tenderness at the site.

Removal of Embedded Earring Backs

Local infiltration of lidocaine into the earlobe is usually sufficient anesthesia for the removal of an embedded earring back. The area is cleaned with povidone-iodine, and a small amount (usually less than 0.5 mL) of 1% lidocaine without epinephrine is injected into the lobe through the existing rear earring opening. Aseptic technique should be used, as difficulty in removal can necessitate making an incision into the ear that may require suturing. Using the fingers of the non-dominant hand, the operator applies pressure to the anterior portion of the patient's earlobe to push the earring back either through or near the earring opening on the posterior of the earlobe. Sometimes the earring stud will still be attached, with the back imbedded in the earlobe. In such cases, the stud may be used to direct the back out of the earlobe by applying pressure on the stud with the thumbs while simultaneously spreading the skin on the rear of the earlobe with the fingers. The technique is analogous to reducing a paraphimosis as shown in Figure 98.1. If the earring back is not immediately visualized, a small forceps or a pair of hemostatic clamps is then inserted into the rear opening and gently opened in order to grasp the earring back. Once the earring back is firmly gripped, it can simply be pulled through the rear opening of the earlobe if the stud has previously been removed. Most earring backs consist of a central flange with two metal strips that have been bent inward to form rings. The sides of these "rings" hold the earring stud in place. If the stud is still in place, it can be removed by spreading these rings outward with a forceps once the earring back has been externalized. The tissue of the earlobe normally has sufficient elasticity to allow extraction of the earring back through the pre-existing opening without an incision. If an incision is required for exposure and removal, simple closure may be needed using 6.0 nonabsorbable monofilament sutures. Although the patient may wish differently, the stud should not be left in place after the earring back is removed. The wound site is covered with antibiotic ointment and a bandage. Parenteral antibiotic therapy may be required if there are signs of infection (4).

▶ COMPLICATIONS

Complications of ear laceration repair include poor skin or cartilage alignment, loss of cartilage from improper débridement, damage due to suture placement into the cartilage, and infection. Notching of the ear contour may re-

CLINICAL TIPS

▶ Complete drainage of an auricular hematoma is essential for a good outcome. Follow-up should occur within 24 hours to check for reaccumulation of fluid.

▶ Application of a mastoid pressure dressing is advisable for any external ear injury that may subsequently result in a significant accumulation of serous fluid or blood.

▶ Placement of sutures into cartilage should avoided if possible.

▶ Surgical consultation is indicated for complex cartilage lacerations, wounds that may need graft placement, and lacerations involving the ear canal.

▶ Cartilage débridement is best left to the consultant.

▶ Most earring backs have metal strips bent into "rings" that hold the stud in place. Once the earring back is exposed, the stud can be removed by spreading these rings with a forceps.

▶ When performing a regional auricular block, it is important to ensure that a track of anesthetic is deposited around the entire circumference of the ear.

sult from any of the above complications. The most effective means of avoiding these complications is to thoroughly clean and irrigate wounds, avoid débridement of cartilage, carefully align wound edges, cover any exposed cartilage, and avoid placing sutures into the cartilage. Surgical consultation should be obtained for complicated ear injuries. Incomplete drainage of an auricular hematoma or failure to drain reaccumulated fluid following initial drainage may lead to infection, with possible perichondritis, cartilage destruction, and disfigurement of the external ear (3).

▶ SUMMARY

The external ear is subject to trauma causing laceration and/or auricular hematoma. Local infiltration or regional auricular block can be used to provide anesthesia for external ear procedures. Repair of simple lacerations and drainage of an auricular hematoma are within the scope of primary care providers, emergency physicians, and other health care providers familiar with the management of simple wounds. Complex lacerations involving the cartilage and those requiring graft placements require surgical consultation. An auricular hematoma must be completely drained and a pressure dressing applied. If additional fluid reaccumulates following initial treatment, drainage may again be indicated. All but the most trivial wounds of the external ear should be rechecked within 24 hours of treatment. Failure to properly manage ear injuries may result in damage to the ear cartilage, with possible cosmetic deformity or abnormal appearance of the auricle. Complications can be avoided by ensuring a combination of proper technique and judicious follow-up.

▶ ACKNOWLEDGMENT

The authors would like to acknowledge the valuable contributions of Mary Clyde Pierce to the version of this chapter that appeared in the previous edition.

▶ REFERENCES

1. Lane SE, Rhame GL, Wroble RL. A silicone splint for auricular hematoma. *Phys Sports Med.* 1998;26:77–78.

2. Steele BD, Brennan PO. A prospective survey of patients with presumed accidental ear injury presenting to a paediatric accident and emergency department. *Emerg Med J.* 2002;19:226–228.

3. Templer J, Renner GJ. Injuries of the external ear. *Otolaryngol Clin North Am.* 1990;23:1003–1018.

4. Turhan-Haktanir N, Demir Y. Embedded earrings as a result of misuse: case report. *Indian J Plast Surg.* 2004;37:134–135.

5. Kenna MA. Embryology and developmental anatomy of the ear. In: Bluestone CD, Stool SE, eds. *Pediatric Otolaryngology.* 2nd. ed. Philadelphia: WB Saunders; 1990:77–79.

6. Hollinshead WH, Tosse C. *Textbook of Anatomy.* 4th ed. Philadelphia: Harper & Row; 1985:944–946.

7. Serafin D, Georgiade NG. *Pediatric Plastic Surgery.* Vol. 2. St. Louis: Mosby; 1984:648–651.

8. Trott A. *Wounds and Lacerations: Emergency Care and Closure.* St. Louis: Mosby; 1991:41–42, 55–63, 163–168.

9. Rahman WM, O'Connor TJ. Facial trauma. In: Barkin RM, Caputo GL, Jaffe DM, et al., eds. *Pediatric Emergency Medicine Concepts and Clinical Practice.* 2nd ed. St. Louis: Mosby; 1997:274–276.

10. Ruddy RM. Procedures. In: Fleisher GR, Ludwig S, eds. *Textbook of Pediatric Emergency Medicine.* 4th ed. Philadelphia: Lippincott Williams & Wilkins; 2000:1821.

56

MARLA J. FRIEDMAN

Tympanocentesis

that appeared in the previous edition.

REFERENCES

▶ INTRODUCTION

Tympanocentesis involves needle aspiration of middle ear contents to obtain fluid for culture or to provide symptomatic relief in cases of especially painful otitis media. It can be safely performed by pediatricians, emergency physicians, and other qualified clinicians in the outpatient setting (1–5).

Otitis media is one of the most common childhood infections, with a peak incidence during the first 2 years of life. The incidence of otitis media is on the rise, with approximately 70% of children having at least one episode in the first year of life (6,7). The growing number of cases may be due to the increased use of day-care facilities in this country (7–9). Otitis media is a general term used to describe acute or chronic inflammation of the middle ear. Acute otitis media is defined as the presence of middle ear effusion with symptoms (pain, fever, irritability) and signs (redness, fullness, bulging of the tympanic membrane) of acute suppurative inflammation. Otitis media with effusion describes the presence of fluid in the middle ear without the signs or symptoms of acute suppurative inflammation (8,10,11). Otitis media with effusion frequently follows an episode of acute otitis media and usually resolves within about 3 months (12).

Middle ear infections must be effectively treated to prevent complications and minimize the morbidity that can be associated with otitis media. Conductive hearing loss due to middle ear fluid is the most common complication of otitis media. Even a mild unilateral hearing impairment can lead to speech and language problems and affect both the school performance and the social interactions of a young child. Other less common complications include chronic suppurative otitis media, tympanic membrane perforation and scarring, cholesteatoma, facial paralysis, and extension of the infection into the mastoids or intracranial structures (7,9).

Antibiotic therapy is generally effective in treating acute otitis media, and it remains the initial recommended approach. Tympanocentesis is recommended for patients who fail antimicrobial therapy (13,14). With the increasing prevalence of antimicrobial resistance, tympanocentesis is likely to have an increasingly important role in the management of otitis media.

▶ ANATOMY AND PHYSIOLOGY

The anatomy of the ear is illustrated in Figure 52.2. The tympanic membrane separates the external auditory canal from the middle ear. The middle ear, or tympanic cavity, consists of the auditory ossicles (malleus, incus, and stapes), muscles, nerves, blood vessels, and the eustachian tube. The eustachian tube, which opens and closes during swallowing, connects the nasopharynx with the middle ear cavity and functions to equalize the pressure in the middle ear with atmospheric pressure. It protects the middle ear from reflux of nasopharynx secretions and drains secretions from the middle ear into the nasopharynx. Most cases of otitis media occur as a result of an abnormally functioning eustachian tube (15,16).

The structure of the middle ear is illustrated in Figure 56.1A. Landmarks that must be clearly identified before performing tympanocentesis include (a) the lateral (short) process of the malleus, a protrusion at the superior aspect of the malleus that points toward the anterior quadrant; (b) the handle (long) process of the malleus, the thin structure that divides the membrane into anterior and posterior segments; and (c) the umbo, which is the inferior tip of the malleus that separates the superior and inferior quadrants of the tympanic membrane. The four quadrants of the tympanic membrane are roughly delineated by drawing one line through the long handle of the malleus and a second perpendicular line through the umbo (16,17). The umbo is perhaps the most important

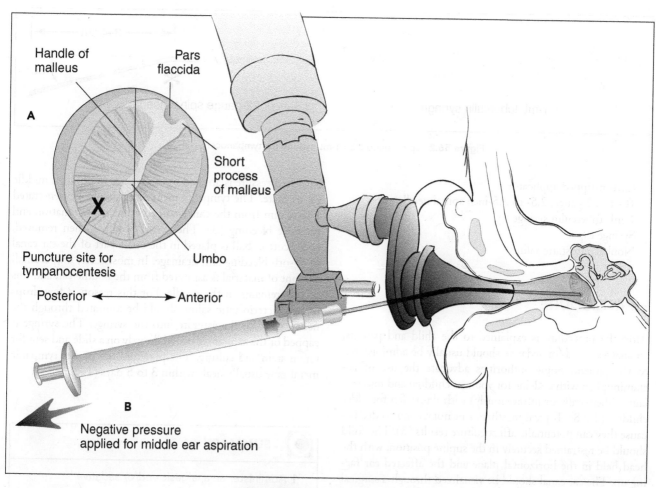

Handle of
malleus

Pars
flaccida

A

Short
process
of malleus

X

Puncture site for
tympanocentesis

Umbo

Posterior ◀──────▶ Anterior

B

Negative pressure
applied for middle ear aspiration

Figure 56.1
A. Landmarks of the middle ear.
B. Technique for tympanocentesis.

bony landmark to identify. It points toward the posteroinferior quadrant of the tympanic membrane, which is where tympanocentesis should be performed. The ossicles and nerves, including a branch of the facial nerve, lie within the superior quadrants of the tympanic membrane. Consequently, this area should be avoided during tympanocentesis.

▶ INDICATIONS

Uncomplicated cases of otitis media do not require aspiration, because cultures are likely to yield common pathogens that will be effectively treated by a first-line antibiotic regimen. However, with the dramatic rise in cases of refractory otitis media due to drug-resistant pathogens, tympanocentesis is becoming an increasingly useful procedure in the management of acute otitis media. Aspiration of middle ear fluid is indicated to determine the causative organisms in patients who fail to respond to conventional antimicrobial therapy (1,3,8,13,14). It may also be appropriate when acute otitis media is identified in a septic-appearing child or a neonate suspected of having serious bacterial illness. Needle aspiration should be

performed in patients with suppurative complications (e.g., mastoiditis, brain abscess) and should be considered in patients with isolated facial paralysis associated with otitis media (1,2,5,15,18,19). Occasionally, a child will present with an extremely painful case of otitis media, and tympanocentesis may be warranted to provide immediate pain relief (1).

Tympanocentesis should not be performed when the clinician is unable to adequately visualize the landmarks of the tympanic membrane, as this increases the likelihood of damaging middle ear structures (19). The procedure is contraindicated in patients with a bleeding diathesis and is not recommended for those with severe bone marrow suppression, because manipulation from the procedure could lead to septicemia.

▶ EQUIPMENT

Analgesic or sedative medications
Body restraint system (e.g., papoose board)
Otoscope with surgical operative head
70% isopropyl alcohol
Ear curette

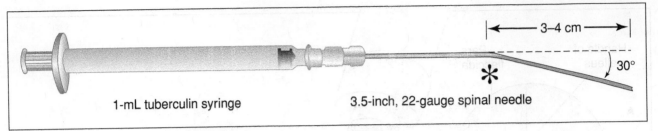

Figure 56.2 Spinal needle on 1-mL syringe for tympanocentesis.

Cotton-tipped applicator
18- to 22-gauge, 2.5- to 3.5-inch spinal needle
1-mL tuberculin syringe
Syringe cap
Nonbacteriostatic saline

▶ PROCEDURE

After the procedure is explained to the child and parents, an analgesic and/or sedative should usually be administered to the patient. Some authorities advocate the use of acetaminophen with codeine for younger children and midazolam (either orally or intravenously) with ibuprofen for older children (1,3,8). Topical anesthetics are not recommended because they can potentially affect culture results (3). The child should be restrained securely in the supine position, with the head held in the horizontal plane and the affected ear facing up. The ear canal should be visualized through a surgical otoscope head and carefully cleared of cerumen and debris. A culture of material from the ear canal can help differentiate between contaminants from the external meatus and true pathogens from the middle ear (2,19). The external ear canal should then be cleansed by filling the canal with 70% alcohol for 60 seconds and drained by turning the ear down toward the table. Alternatively, an alcohol-soaked cotton-tipped applicator can be used to sterilize the canal (3). With either method, the alcohol must dry completely before the procedure is performed.

The otoscope is reinserted to ensure a clear view of the entire tympanic membrane. All landmarks must be identified before proceeding. A spinal needle (18 to 22 gauge, 2.5 to 3.5 inch) is bent approximately 30 degrees 3 to 4 cm from the distal end, as shown in Figure 56.2. Bending the needle in this way allows a better view of the tympanic membrane during the procedure and facilitates puncture of the membrane in the posteroinferior quadrant. A 1-mL tuberculin syringe is attached to the spinal needle, and the clinician uses the dominant hand to insert the spinal needle through the otoscope speculum (Fig. 56.1B). With the bevel facing up, the needle is advanced into the canal toward the posterior aspect of the tympanic membrane. The ulnar aspect of the clinician's dominant hand should rest on the child's cheek or head to prevent deep penetration if the child moves suddenly. The membrane is punctured in the posteroinferior quadrant, and

negative pressure is applied to the syringe to obtain a middle ear aspirate. The tympanic membrane should be penetrated 1 to 2 mm from the canal wall to avoid contamination and excessive bleeding (3). The spinal needle is then removed, and a cotton ball is placed in the outer part of the ear canal to absorb bleeding and drainage. In most cases, only a small amount of material is aspirated from the middle ear, and this usually remains in the needle. For this reason, a few drops of nonbacteriostatic saline should be aspirated through the needle to flush the aspirate into the syringe. The syringe is capped or the aspirate is plated directly on a slide and sent for Gram stain and culture. The puncture site on the tympanic membrane usually heals within 3 to 5 days (1–3,18,19).

⬤ **SUMMARY**

1 Administer an analgesic and/or sedative medications as needed.

2 Restrain the child securely in the supine position with the affected ear facing up.

3 Clear the ear canal of cerumen and debris.

4 Sterilize the canal with 70% alcohol and allow to dry.

5 Visualize the tympanic membrane and identify landmarks using a surgical otoscope head.

6 Attach a spinal needle (18 to 22 gauge, 2.5 to 3.5 inch) to a 1-mL (tuberculin) syringe.

7 Bend the needle approximately 30 degrees 3 to 4 cm from the tip.

8 Advance the needle through the otoscope into the ear canal with the bevel facing upward.

9 Puncture the membrane in the posteroinferior quadrant, and apply negative pressure on syringe.

10 Remove the needle and place a cotton ball in the ear canal.

11 Flush the needle by aspirating a small amount of saline.

12 Send the aspirate for Gram stain and culture.

CLINICAL TIPS

▶ Secure restraint of the child is critical to a successful procedure.

▶ It is important to fully visualize the tympanic membrane and identify landmarks prior to initiating the procedure.

▶ The proper site for tympanocentesis is the posteroinferior quadrant of the tympanic membrane. The superior quadrants must be carefully avoided to minimize the risk of complications.

▶ COMPLICATIONS

Proper restraint of the child is the key to avoiding complications from tympanocentesis. Unexpected movement could cause a tear in the tympanic membrane, leading to persistent perforation, otorrhea, and continued contamination of the middle ear with bacteria from the external canal. Puncture in the superior half of the tympanic membrane could result in injury to the bones, nerves, and blood vessels that lie just behind this quadrant. Dislocation of a bony ossicle may lead to significant hearing loss. Injury to a branch of the seventh cranial nerve could result in either a transient facial paralysis or an impairment of taste on the corresponding side of the tongue. Bleeding into the middle ear from a laceration to the internal carotid artery is another potentially serious complication of superior quadrant tympanocentesis. Despite these risks, experience has shown that when tympanocentesis is performed appropriately and in the correct location, complications associated with this procedure are rare (1,18,19).

▶ SUMMARY

Otitis media is one of the most common childhood infections. In an era of refractory otitis media due to drug-resistant pathogens, middle ear aspiration can definitively identify the etiology of the infection. Other possible indications include the presence of acute otitis media in a septic-appearing child or a neonate with suspected serious bacterial illness. Tympanocentesis can also provide immediate pain relief in the unusually severe earache caused by acute otitis media. It is likely to become an increasingly valuable skill for both primary care providers and emergency physicians to master.

▶ ACKNOWLEDGMENT

The authors would like to acknowledge the valuable contributions of Mary Clyde Pierce to the version of this chapter that appeared in the previous edition.

▶ REFERENCES

1. Block SL. Tympanocentesis: why, when, how. *Contemp Pediatr.* 1999;16:103–127.
2. Guarisco JL, Grundfast KM. A simple device for tympanocentesis in infants and children. *Laryngoscope.* 1988;98:244–246.
3. Hoberman A, Paradise JL, Wald ER. Tympanocentesis technique revisited. *Pediatr Infect Dis J.* 1997;16:S25–26.
4. Hoberman A, Paradise JL. Acute otitis media: diagnosis and management in the year 2000. *Pediatr Ann.* 2000;29:609–620.
5. Pichichero ME. Acute otitis media, I: improving diagnostic accuracy. *Am Fam Phys.* 2000;61:2051–2056.
6. Lanphear BP, Byrd RS, Auinger P, et al. Increasing prevalence of recurrent otitis media among children in the United States. *Pediatrics.* 1997;99:EI.
7. Kenna MA. Otitis media: the otolaryngologist's perspective. *Pediatr Ann.* 2000;29:630–636.
8. Hoberman A, Marchant CD, Kaplan SL, et al. Treatment of acute otitis media consensus recommendations. *Clin Pediatr.* 2002;41:373–390.
9. Klein JO. The burden of otitis media. *Vaccine.* 2001;19:S2–8.
10. Rovers MM, Schilder AG, Zielhuis GA, et al. Otitis media. *Lancet.* 2004;363:465–473.
11. Perkins JA. Medical and surgical management of otitis media in children. *Otolaryngol Clin North Am.* 2002;35:811–825.
12. Roddey OF, Hoover HA. Otitis media with effusion in children: a pediatric office perspective. *Pediatr Ann.* 2000;29:623–629.
13. Dowell SF, Butler JC, Giebink GS, et al. Acute otitis media: management and surveillance in an era of pneumococcal resistance: a report from the Drug-resistant *Streptococcus pneumoniae* Therapeutic Working Group. *Pediatr Infect Dis J.* 1999;18:1–9.
14. AAP, AAFP Subcommittee on Management of Acute Otitis Media. Clinical practice guideline: diagnosis and management of acute otitis media. *Pediatrics.* 2004;113:1451–1465.
15. Cotton RT. The ear, nose, pharynx, and larynx. In: Rudolph CD, Rudolph AM, Hostetter MK, et al., eds. *Rudolph's Pediatrics.* 21st ed. New York: McGraw Hill, 2003:1239–1283.
16. Kenna MA. Embryology and developmental anatomy of the ear. In: Bluestone CD, Stool SE, eds. *Pediatric Otolaryngology.* 2nd ed. Philadelphia: WB Saunders; 1990:77–79.
17. Rosse C, Gaddum-Rosse P, Hollinshead WH. *Hollinshead's Textbook of Anatomy.* 5th ed. Philadelphia: Lippincott Williams & Wilkins; 1997:801–837.
18. Ruddy RM. Procedures. In: Fleisher GR, Ludwig S, eds. *Textbook of Pediatric Emergency Medicine.* 4th ed. Philadelphia: Lippincott Williams & Wilkins; 2000:1819.
19. Hickerson SL, Cross JT, Schutze GE, et al. Diagnostic procedures. In: Dieckmann RA, Fiser DH, Selbst SM, eds. *Pediatric Emergency and Critical Care Procedures.* St. Louis: Mosby; 1997:522–524.

57

PARUL B. PATEL AND SUSANNE I. KOST

Management of Epistaxis

▶ INTRODUCTION

Epistaxis is a common complaint in the pediatric population, especially among toddlers and school-aged children. Most episodes of bleeding from the nose will resolve before the child arrives at a medical care facility, but persistent or recurrent bleeding requires intervention (1,2). Because specialized equipment is needed for visualization and treatment of epistaxis, a definitive procedure should not be attempted in the prehospital setting. Prehospital management of a nosebleed should consist of applying pressure to the external nares and providing supportive care as necessary. The child who is still bleeding upon arrival at a medical care facility can usually be managed by cautery or anterior packing. An emergency physician or an experienced pediatrician or family practitioner should be capable of performing both of these procedures. In the unusual situation when posterior packing is required for a pediatric patient or when epistaxis is severe or recurrent, consultation with an otolaryngologist should be obtained whenever possible (3).

▶ ANATOMY AND PHYSIOLOGY

The relatively high incidence of epistaxis in otherwise healthy children can be explained by a combination of physiologic and behavioral factors. The nasal mucosa is lined with a rich vascular network that facilitates warming of inspired air. In children, this mucosa is thinner and more likely to bleed than in adults. Children also are prone to manipulate the septal mucosa (nose picking) and are therefore predisposed to anterior bleeding. The most common source of epistaxis is the Kiesselbach plexus in the Little area of the anterior septum (Fig. 57.I). Attempts to localize and treat the typical nose-

bleed in a child should focus on this area (1,2,4). Because blood supply to the Kiesselbach plexus comes in part from the superior labial artery, application of pressure to the upper lip may aid in the initial management.

In addition to minor trauma from nose picking, environmental, local, and systemic factors may influence the incidence of epistaxis. Environmental factors, including cold air or dry heat in the winter, may irritate the mucosa, a condition known as "rhinitis sicca." It has been shown that hospital admissions for epistaxis increase during the winter months (5). A local factor that commonly causes epistaxis in children is injury due to accidental trauma (6). Other local factors—for example, inflammation from viral or bacterial infection, foreign body reaction (see Chapter 59), allergic rhinitis, and chemical irritants (such as cigarette smoke)—may increase the friability of the anterior nasal mucosa (7,8). In adolescents, chronic inhalation of recreational drugs may lead to epistaxis. Although much less common, nasal septal deviation and lesions such as polyps, vascular malformations, and tumors may act as focal points for anterior or posterior bleeding in children (1,2,4).

Systemic conditions that may produce or exacerbate epistaxis include hypertension, hematologic disease, renal disease, menstruation, and the use of anticoagulant medication. Extensive testing for systemic illness should not be undertaken unless current or past medical history, family history, or physical examination leads to suspicion of a systemic disorder. Although hypertension is unusual in children, blood pressure should be measured routinely in a child presenting with epistaxis. Anxiety over the nosebleed and the hospital environment may cause transient hypertension; consequently, a finding of elevated systemic pressure should be confirmed with a repeat reading and then evaluated appropriately on an acute and/or outpatient basis. Hematologic disease may include congenital coagulation defects or acquired conditions such as idiopathic

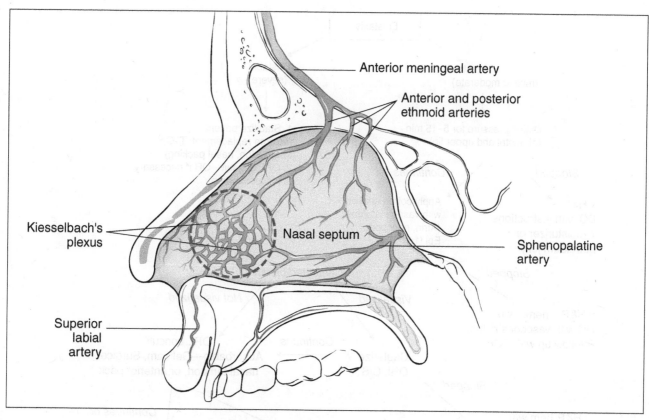

Anterior meningeal artery

Anterior and posterior ethmoid arteries

Kiesselbach's plexus

Nasal septum

Sphenopalatine artery

Superior labial artery

Figure 57.1 Anatomy of nasal septum.

thrombocytopenic purpura and malignancy (7,9). Assessing the child for bruising, petechiae, and lymphadenopathy should therefore be routinely included as part of the physical examination. An adolescent female who has episodes of epistaxis that always coincide with menstruation may have vicarious menstruation, a rare condition thought to be caused by increased capillary permeability resulting from hormonal changes. Ingestion of drugs that affect coagulation (e.g., Coumadin or aspirin) should be suspected in a setting where these drugs are available, especially in the toddler age group (1,2,10). Patients with chronic renal failure undergoing hemodialysis may present with persistent epistaxis due to coagulopathy from underlying disease or prolonged use of low-molecular-weight heparin (6).

▶ INDICATIONS

Any child who continues to bleed after properly applied nasal pressure, or a child with recurrent episodes of bleeding over a period of hours or days, deserves a more definitive procedure. An adequate trial of digital nasal pressure consists of at least 5 minutes of squeezing the cartilaginous segment of the nares together between a thumb and finger. Using a rolled gauze pad to compress the upper lip (and thus the labial artery)

also may be performed if the child is cooperative. If bleeding persists despite an adequate trial of pressure, vasoconstrictive medication (Afrin, Neosynephrine) may be applied to the affected area on a cotton pledget and the pressure regimen repeated. If vasoconstriction with pressure fails to control bleeding or if a presumptive source of bleeding is identified, chemical cautery should be considered. Continued epistaxis from an anterior site despite cautery requires placement of an anterior nasal pack. The persistent appearance of blood in the hypopharynx with no identifiable anterior source or after placement of an anterior nasal pack indicates a posterior site of epistaxis and necessitates placement of a posterior nasal pack (Fig. 57.2).

When the patient has a known history of an intranasal lesion (e.g., a polyp or hemangioma) or a known bleeding disorder, consultation with an otolaryngologist should be sought before attempting to cauterize or pack the affected area (7). Attempts at cauterization in a patient with a bleeding diathesis may exacerbate the bleeding. These patients may require treatment with packing and replacement of the appropriate blood product (factor or platelets). Consultation is also recommended if a posterior site of bleeding or a facial fracture is suspected. In addition, immediate consultation should be obtained in the rare instance of a severe nasal bleed resulting in unstable vital signs or signs of hemorrhagic shock (3,4,10).

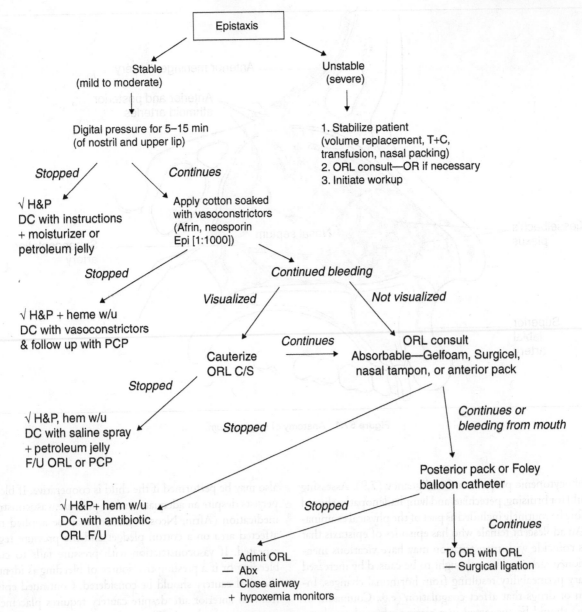

Figure 57.2 Management approach to Epistaxis.

▶ EQUIPMENT

General
Adequate light source (preferably a headlight)
Suction with Frazier tip (5 to 9 French)
Nasal speculum (small, medium, large)
Cotton pledgets or swabs
Bayonet forceps
Alligator forceps

Cautery
Topical vasoconstrictors and anesthetics:
   Phenylephrine 0.25% (Neosynephrine)
   Oxymetazoline 0.05% (Afrin)
   Lidocaine 2% to 4% (maximum dose 3 to 5 mg/kg)
   Epinephrine 1:1000

Commercially premixed 2% lidocaine with epinephrine
   (maximum dose 5 to 7 mg/kg)
Silver nitrate sticks
Trichloroacetic acid
Petroleum or KY jelly

Anterior Packing
Vaseline gauze, 1/4- and 1/2-inch strips
Topical antibiotic ointment
Nasal tampon (Merocel, Rapid Rhino, Rhino Rocket)
Topical absorbable hemostatic agents such as Gelfoam and
   Surgicel

Posterior Packing
Small red rubber or flexible latex-free catheters
Hemostat

Silk ties or umbilical tapes
Foley catheters (10 to 16 gauge)
Syringe, 30 mL
Gauze, 2″ ×2″, 4″ × 4″
Plastic cuff (2-inch length of suction tubing)
Hoffman clamp
Topical thrombin

Combined Anterior-Posterior Packing
Gottschalk Nasostat or Xomed Epistat

▶ PROCEDURE

Examination and Preparation

The most important task in the treatment of epistaxis is locating the site of bleeding. In an ideal situation, the patient sits upright, leaning slightly forward, and looking directly at the clinician, although with many pediatric patients, this will not be possible. An adequate light source is essential for good visualization of the nasal mucosa. A headlight provides direct illumination of the nose and frees both hands for treatment. Young or uncooperative patients may require procedural sedation before the procedures described in this section can be performed successfully (see Chapter 33). Certain patients, such as those with severe bleeding or complicated medical histories, may merit evaluation under general anesthesia in the operating room. Uncooperative or sedated patients must be positioned supine on a stretcher using appropriate restraint (e.g., a papoose), with an assistant stabilizing the head. It may be helpful to apply a topical decongestant and anesthetic to the patient's nasal mucosa prior to the examination (see below). This can be done using sterile long cotton swabs or a spray device, depending on the formulation available.

Once the patient is calm and positioned properly, the clinician can use a nasal speculum to visualize the anterior septum. The speculum blades should be opened vertically rather than horizontally so that the septum is better visualized without being directly instrumented, thus avoiding additional pain and mucosal trauma that may result from applying pressure against the septum. Keeping the speculum blades slightly open on insertion and removal will prevent plucking nasal hairs. Clots are carefully suctioned from the nose with a Frazier tip suction catheter until the source of bleeding can be identified. If active bleeding obscures the septal mucosa, cotton pledgets soaked in a topical vasoconstrictor such as phenylephrine (Neosynephrine) or oxymetazoline (Afrin) may be inserted with bayonet forceps (Fig. 57.3). Oxymetazoline is preferred when available because it has no effect on systemic blood pressure. A success rate of 65% in the treatment of epistaxis has been reported with the use of oxymetazoline alone (6). If cautery or packing is anticipated, an anesthetic such as 4% lidocaine may be mixed with the vasoconstrictor and applied simultaneously. Phenylephrine or oxymetazoline provides vasoconstriction but not anesthesia. Either a commercially premixed preparation of lidocaine with epinephrine or

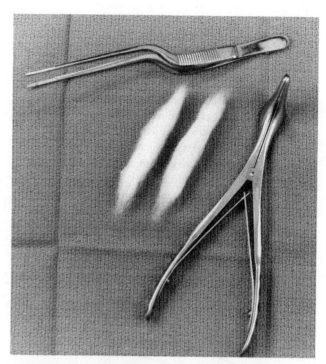

Figure 57.3 Bayonet forceps, nasal speculum, and cotton pledgets.

a mixture prepared at the time of the procedure (0.25 mL of epinephrine 1:1000 in 20 mL of 4% lidocaine) also has been recommended. The maximum allowable dose of lidocaine alone is 3 to 5 mg/kg, and the maximum allowable dose of lidocaine with epinephrine is 5 to 7 mg/kg (11). Although total systemic absorption of lidocaine does not occur after topical administration, the maximum recommended dosages should not be exceeded. While still used by pediatric otolaryngologists, liquid cocaine, an agent that provides both vasoconstriction and anesthesia, is rarely used now for children in the emergency department because of its expense and potential for serious complications. After a topical vasoconstrictor has been properly applied for about 5 to 10 minutes, a persistent anterior source of bleeding will often be visible (3,12).

Cauterization

Cautery is recommended for persistent or recurrent epistaxis. After adequate anesthesia and hemostasis are obtained and the source of bleeding is visualized, the excoriated area may be chemically cauterized with silver nitrate or trichloroacetic acid. Chemical cautery is preferred over electrocautery in a pediatric outpatient setting because the latter is more painful and requires proper grounding of equipment. The silver nitrate stick should be applied to the affected area in concentric circles, starting at the outer limits of the area and working inward. If the affected area is small, the end of the stick may simply be rolled over the excoriation or vessel. Petroleum jelly, a water-based jelly (e.g., KY), or antibiotic ointment smeared on the unaffected areas of mucosa will prevent unwanted exposure to the chemical (4). Areas in contact with the silver nitrate will turn gray or black. If the nostril is too small to allow adequate passage of the silver nitrate stick, a small cotton-tipped applicator or a wisp of cotton wrapped around a metal applicator may be soaked in trichloroacetic acid and applied in the same concentric manner.

Cauterization alone will not always stop active bleeding; adequate hemostasis with a topical vasoconstrictor before cautery is usually an essential step. Following cautery, twice daily application of petroleum jelly and antibiotic cream or ointment to the nose and frequent applications of saline nasal spray should be initiated to prevent drying or crusting (with possible rebleeding) and infection (6). Children must be encouraged to refrain from manipulating the area while it is healing; aspirin and ibuprofen should also be avoided. If the site of bleeding cannot be visualized, topical thrombin provides a useful alternative to cautery. Thrombin is applied directly on the bleeding septal mucosa in powdered form or as a spray to achieve hemostasis.

Anterior Packing

If epistaxis recurs after local measures and cautery or if the site of bleeding cannot be located, then anterior nasal packing is indicated. Whenever possible, the site of bleeding should be located and cauterized before the pack is placed. A pack placed blindly is less likely to control bleeding; in fact, it may actually exacerbate bleeding by creating friction against the septal mucosa.

The traditional method of anterior nasal packing consists of layering Vaseline gauze ($1/4$ or $1/2$ inch), as shown in Fig. 57.4. The patient is positioned and the mucosa is

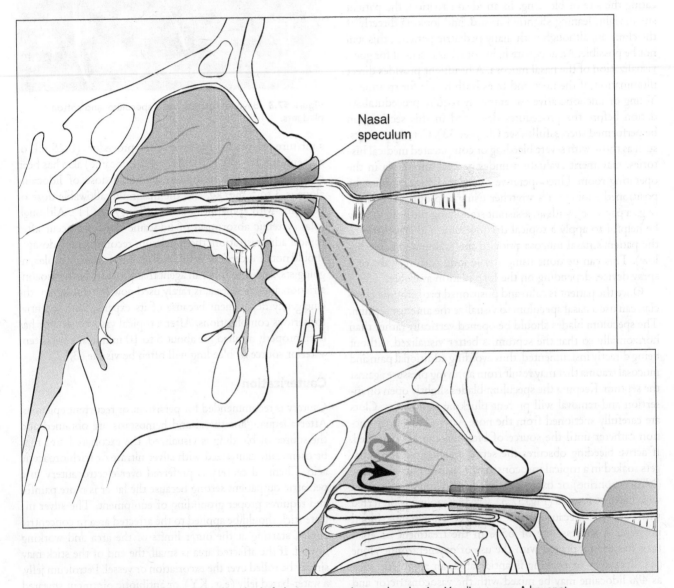

Figure 57.4 Traditional method of placing an anterior nasal pack using Vaseline gauze. A bayonet forceps is used to insert the gauze straight back along the floor of the nasal cavity. The speculum is removed after each layer is applied and then reinserted to gently pack the gauze down. The gauze is layered in accordion fashion until the nasal cavity is filled.

prepared as described previously. A length of Vaseline gauze is first coated with antibiotic ointment. It is then grasped with bayonet forceps 5 to 7 cm from the end and inserted through a nasal speculum straight back along the floor of the nose. Approximately 2 to 3 cm of gauze should protrude from the nostril to keep the pack from sliding posteriorly into the pharynx. After the first layer is placed, the bayonet forceps should be withdrawn and reinserted to place another layer of gauze in accordion fashion. Each time the bayonet forceps is inserted, it is used to gently pack down the gauze. Alligator forceps may be used instead of bayonet forceps in patients with a small nasal opening. Layering the gauze in this manner should continue until the nasal cavity is filled. The goal is to place the packing from the back and bottom of the nose forward. The most common error with this procedure is failure to adequately pack the posterior portion of the anterior nasal cavity (6). Taping the protruding gauze end to the face will help stabilize the pack (3,4,12).

With the development of improved commercial sponge products for anterior nasal packing which are both effective and convenient to use, the traditional method of layered gauze packing is now rarely performed (13). Examples include the Merocel nasal tampon and oxycellulose (Surgicel). The nasal tampon, which is available in pediatric and adult sizes, consists of dehydrated material that expands when exposed to moisture, filling the surrounding cavity. It is inserted with bayonet forceps along the floor of the nose. Insertion must be rapid, as the material expands almost immediately on contact with fluid. Coating the tampon with antibiotic ointment will facilitate both insertion and later removal (3,10,12). Oxycellulose is supplied as knitted fabric strips in a variety of sizes that can be cut for a custom fit. This material differs from mechanical packs in that it requires contact with blood to form a clot, it provides intrinsic bacteriostatic action, and it is spontaneously absorbed. Of note, both prior mucosal cautery and application of antibiotic ointment to oxycellulose will interfere with the action and absorption of this product. A small amount of the material is applied directly to the site of bleeding until hemostasis is obtained. Oxycellulose should not be confused with the absorbable gelatin sponge (Gelfoam), which has similar properties but potentiates bacterial growth and has been associated with toxic shock syndrome (14). Other commercially available products for anterior nasal packing include Rapid Rhino (ArthroCare, Sunnyvale, CA) and Rhino Rocket (Shippert Medical Technologies, Centennial, CO).

Because anterior nasal packs are foreign bodies that lead to stasis of nasal secretions, patients with a pack in place for more than a few hours should be put on oral antibiotics to prevent sinus infection and possible toxic shock syndrome. Nonabsorbable packing material is usually removed within 3 to 5 days. Ideally, the child should be re-evaluated on an outpatient basis within 24 hours. Absorbable packing material residue should be left in place, as attempts to remove it may cause rebleeding (3,10,12). Saline sprays can be used to facilitate dissolution. The previously described regime of twice

SUMMARY: ANTERIOR NASAL PACKING

1 Position the patient sitting upright facing the clinician whenever possible (younger patients who are unable to cooperate may be positioned supine with appropriate restraint); administer sedation as needed.

2 Apply a topical vasoconstrictor and topical anesthetic to the nasal mucosa.

3 Insert a nasal speculum into the nostril and open vertically to expose the septum and locate the site of bleeding.

4 Attempt cautery with silver nitrate or trichloroacetic acid (continue with anterior packing if ineffective).

5 Coat Vaseline gauze ($1/4$ inch or $1/2$ inch) with an antibiotic ointment.

6 Grasp the gauze with a bayonet forceps 5 to 7 cm from the end and insert it straight back along the floor of the nose (allow 2 to 3 cm of gauze to protrude from the nose).

7 After the first layer is placed, remove the speculum and replace it on top of the gauze to gently pack it down as the next layer is placed in accordion fashion.

8 Continue applying layers of gauze until the nasal cavity is filled.

9 Place a piece of tape on the gauze protruding from the nose to stabilize the pack.

10 Initiate a course of prophylactic oral antibiotics.

daily applications of petroleum jelly or antibiotic ointment, along with frequent use of saline nasal spray, will generally prevent crusting and rebleeding after removal of the pack.

Posterior Packing

If packing of both anterior chambers fails to stop an episode of epistaxis or if bleeding persists in the posterior pharynx, a posterior pack may be required. Consultation with an otolaryngologist is always advisable in this situation. Either the rolled gauze or the inflatable balloon method may be used. The balloon method has become more popular because it is technically easier and is somewhat more comfortable for the patient. Because both methods are painful, appropriate analgesia should be administered as required before placing a posterior pack. Additionally, application of topical anesthetic to the posterior pharynx (e.g., Cetacaine spray) will reduce discomfort and gagging during the procedure.

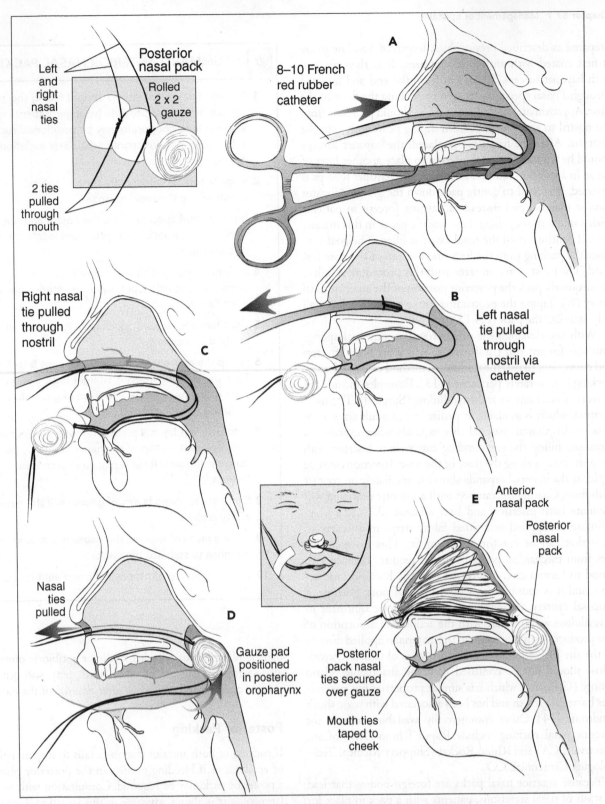

Figure 57.5 Traditional method of placing a posterior nasal pack using gauze pads.
  A. A small catheter is inserted into one nostril, advanced to the posterior pharynx, and withdrawn through the mouth.
  B. One end of a tie is then fastened to the end of the catheter, and the catheter is removed to pull the tie out through the nose.
  C. This is repeated on the opposite side with the other tie.
  D. The pack is drawn into the posterior pharynx by pulling both nasal ties and positioned manually against the vomer. An anterior nasal pack is then applied.
  E. The ends of the ties protruding from the mouth are taped to the cheek. The ends protruding through the nostrils are tied around a gauze pad under the septum of the nose.

Labels within figure:

Left and right nasal ties

Posterior nasal pack

Rolled 2 x 2 gauze

2 ties pulled through mouth

A 8–10 French red rubber catheter

B Left nasal tie pulled through nostril via catheter

Right nasal tie pulled through nostril **C**

Nasal ties pulled

D Gauze pad positioned in posterior oropharynx

E Anterior nasal pack

Posterior nasal pack

Posterior pack nasal ties secured over gauze

Mouth ties taped to cheek

The traditional posterior gauze pack is made from cylindrically rolled $2'' \times 2''$ gauze pads or an open gauze pad wrapped around cotton filling (Fig. 57.5). Two silk ties sutures (No. 0) or umbilical tapes are tied around the gauze roll, leaving a long (8- to 12-inch) length of tie on each end. A small (8 or 10 French) red rubber or flexible catheter is inserted into one nostril, advanced to the posterior pharynx, and withdrawn through the mouth with a hemostat. One end of a tie is fastened to the end of the catheter that protrudes from the mouth. The nasal end of the catheter is then withdrawn from the nose, pulling out the tie with it. This is repeated on the other side so that one end of each tie protrudes through the nares. The pack is drawn into the posterior pharynx by pulling both nasal ties and quickly positioned manually against the vomer. Care must be taken to not entrap the uvula. The opposite ends of the ties (protruding from the mouth) are taped to the cheek so that they can be used later in removing the pack. The anterior nose is then packed as previously described, and the nasal ties from the posterior pack are tied over a second rolled gauze pad under the nostrils to hold the pack in place. This second pad should be snug against the nose but not tight enough to cause ischemia and potential necrosis of the nasal cartilage. An alternative method of placing the pack is to insert a red rubber catheter in each nostril, fasten each tie separately to a catheter, and withdraw both catheters simultaneously (3).

A Foley catheter also may serve as a posterior pack (Fig. 57.6). The catheter size should approximate the diameter of the external nares (10 to 16 gauge). Before using the catheter, the balloon should be inflated to ensure that no air leak is present, and the end of the catheter distal to the balloon should be cut off to prevent irritation of the posterior pharynx. The catheter is lubricated with antibiotic ointment and inserted into the anesthetized bleeding nostril until the balloon is visible in the posterior pharynx. The balloon is then inflated with 10 to 15 mL of water or saline, and the proximal end of the catheter is withdrawn until the balloon is snug against the vomer. If the pressure exerted by the balloon causes any significant pain, the balloon should be deflated slightly. The catheter may be secured by placing a length of plastic suction tubing, split lengthwise, around the catheter just under the nostril. A Hoffman clamp, umbilical clamp or hemostat fastened under the plastic cuff will hold the catheter in place. An anterior pack should then be placed around the Foley catheter (4,10,12).

An alternative to placing both anterior and posterior packs separately is to place a double-balloon tamponade device, such as the Gottschalk Nasostat (Sparta Surgical, Pleasanton, CA; available in multiple sizes) or the Xomed Epistat (Medtronic ENT, Jacksonville, FL; available in one size) (Fig. 57.7). Such systems, which consist of both an anterior and a posterior balloon, are inserted in a manner similar to using a Foley catheter as a posterior pack. After the posterior balloon is inflated with water, the device is withdrawn to secure the posterior balloon against the vomer, and then the anterior balloon is gradually inflated. As with a Foley balloon, pain associated with inflation of either segment of the tam-

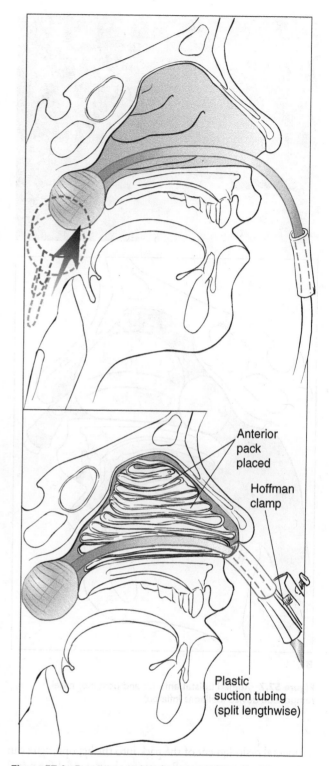

Anterior pack placed

Hoffman clamp

Plastic suction tubing (split lengthwise)

Figure 57.6 Posterior nasal pack using a Foley catheter.

ponade device requires that the balloon be deflated slightly (4,10).

Patients with posterior packs have complete nasal obstruction and should be monitored in the hospital. Posterior packs are known to cause hypoxia and hypoventilation and may cause significant pain, dysphagia, and infection. In addition,

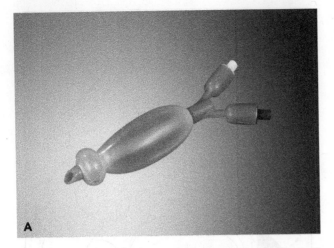

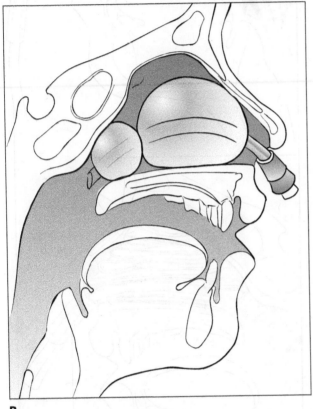

Figure 57.7 Xomed Epistat anterior and posterior nasal tamponade device (balloons inflated).

SUMMARY: POSTERIOR NASAL PACKING

1 Position the patient sitting upright facing the clinician whenever possible (younger patients who are unable to cooperate may be positioned supine with appropriate restraint); administer sedation as needed.

2 Apply a topical anesthetic to the nasal mucosa and posterior pharynx.

3 Tie two silk sutures or umbilical tapes around cylindrically rolled 2″ × 2″ gauze pads or an open gauze pad wrapped around cotton filling, leaving a long (8- to 12-inch) length of tie on each end.

4 Insert a small (8 or 10 French) red rubber catheter through anesthetized bleeding nostril until it can be retrieved from the posterior pharynx through the mouth.

5 Fasten one end of a tie to the catheter and withdraw the catheter so the tie protrudes from the nostril.

6 Repeat the same procedure on the opposite side with the other tie.

7 When one end of each tie protrudes through each nostril, draw pack into the posterior pharynx and quickly position it manually against the vomer.

8 Tape the opposite ends of ties (protruding from mouth) to the cheek so that they can be used later in removing pack.

9 Pack the anterior nose.

10 Secure the nasal ties of the posterior pack over a rolled gauze pad placed under the nostrils.

Note: A more simplified method of placing a posterior nasal pack using a Foley catheter is described in the text (see also Fig. 57.6).

accidental dislodgment of the pack into the hypopharynx can cause airway compromise. Because of the potential for respiratory complications, patients with posterior packs should be sedated with caution.

▶ COMPLICATIONS

Complications of the procedures described in this chapter are chiefly related to ischemia, scarring, infection, and air-

way control. Overzealous cauterization (especially bilateral cauterization of the septum) or packing under pressure can lead to septal ischemia and possible necrosis. Circumferential cautery of a nostril can cause subsequent scarring and stenosis (4,12). Both anterior and posterior packs lead to stasis of nasal secretions and potentiate bacterial growth. Using topical and systemic antibiotics is recommended in patients with nasal packs to reduce the likelihood of this complication. The risk of developing toxic shock syndrome may be minimized with antistaphylococcal antibiotics and timely removal of the packing material (generally within 3 days).

Improperly secured nasal packs, especially posterior packs, create a risk of aspiration of the packing material. If a patient

CLINICAL TIPS

▶ When the patient has a known history of an intranasal lesion (e.g., a polyp or hemangioma) or a known bleeding disorder, consultation with an otolaryngologist should be sought before attempting to cauterize or pack the affected area.

▶ When using a speculum to examine the nose, the blades should be opened vertically rather than horizontally so that the septum is better visualized without being directly instrumented.

▶ When using silver nitrate to perform chemical cautery, it should be applied to the affected area in concentric circles, starting at the outer limits of the area and working inward. Cautery of both sides of the septum can lead to necrosis. Circumferential cautery around the entire margin of one nostril can lead to scarring and stenosis.

▶ Patients with packs in place for more than a few hours should be placed on oral antibiotics to prevent sinus infection and toxic shock syndrome.

▶ Posterior nasal packs can cause hypoxia and hypoventilation, significant pain, and dysphagia. In addition, accidental dislodgment of the pack into the hypopharynx can cause airway compromise. Patients with a posterior pack should therefore be monitored in the hospital.

▶ The risk of rebleeding after treatment may be minimized by having the parents humidify the child's home environment, by preventing the child from picking or manipulating the nose, and by lubricating the anterior septum with petroleum or water-based jelly as well as saline nasal spray or drops.

▶ With younger patients who are unable to cooperate, it may be necessary to administer procedural sedation to successfully perform the procedures used for managing epistaxis.

▶ Although complete systemic absorption of lidocaine does not occur after topical administration, the maximum allowable doses of this agent (3 to 5 mg/kg for lidocaine alone; 5 to 7 mg/kg for lidocaine with epinephrine) should not be exceeded.

may interfere with the obligatory nasal breathing pattern in young infants.

Although sedation may be necessary to place a nasal pack, it should be used with caution in the setting of potential airway and breathing disturbances. In addition, patients with epistaxis are prone to nausea and vomiting as a result of swallowed blood, thus increasing the risk of aspiration (2,3,4,10,12).

▶ SUMMARY

The vast majority of episodes of epistaxis in the pediatric population stem from an anterior source of bleeding, and most episodes can be managed with external nasal pressure and reassurance. In children with persistent or recurrent bleeding, application of a topical vasoconstrictor helps locate the site of bleeding and permits treatment with cauterization. If cautery fails to control the bleeding, placement of an anterior nasal pack is indicated. Posterior packing may be required as a last resort if the source of bleeding is not visible and/or bleeding persists after appropriate placement of an anterior pack. Consultation with an otolaryngologist is recommended if posterior packing is performed. Any patient with persistent bleeding that results in hemodynamic compromise requires emergent intervention by an otolaryngologist.

The risk of rebleeding after treatment may be minimized by (a) having the parents humidify the child's home environment, (b) lubricating the anterior septum with petroleum or water-based jelly or antibiotic ointment as well as frequent use of saline nasal spray or drops, and (c) preventing the child from picking or otherwise manipulating the nose. Referral to an otolaryngologist and laboratory evaluation for a bleeding disorder are not necessary unless the bleeding is severe and prolonged or the history and/or physical examination are abnormal.

▶ ACKNOWLEDGMENT

The authors would like to acknowledge the valuable contributions of Christopher Post to the version of this chapter that appeared in the previous edition.

▶ REFERENCES

1. Nadel F, Henretig FM. Epistaxis. In: Fleisher GR, Ludwig S, eds. *Textbook of Pediatric Emergency Medicine*. 4th ed. Philadelphia: Williams & Wilkins; 2000:227–230.
2. Mulberry PE. Recurrent epistaxis. *Pediatr Rev.* 1991;12:213–216.
3. Potsic WP, Handler SD. Otolaryngology emergencies. In: Fleisher GR, Ludwig S, eds. *Textbook of Pediatric Emergency Medicine*. 4th ed. Philadelphia: Williams & Wilkins; 2000:1575–1576.
4. Culbertson MC, Manning SC. Epistaxis. In: Bluestone CD, Stool SE, Scheetz MD, eds. *Pediatric Otolaryngology*. 2nd ed. Philadelphia: WB Saunders; 1990:672–679.

with a traditional gauze posterior pack develops any signs of airway obstruction, the personnel caring for the patient should be instructed to remove the pack immediately using the mouth tie after first cutting the nasal tie. All patients with bilateral anterior packs or posterior packs in place should be monitored for respiratory complications. Nasal packing also

5. Tomkinson A, Bremmer-Smith A, Creaven C, et al. Hospital epistaxis admission rate and ambient temperature. *Clin Otolaryngol.* 1995;20:239–240.

6. Tan LK, Calhoun KH. Otolaryngology for the internist. *Med Clin North Am.* 1999;83:43–56.

7. Guarisco JL, Graham HD III. Epistaxis in children: causes, diagnosis, and treatment. *Ear Nose Throat J.* 1989;68:522, 528–530, 532.

8. Kucik CJ, Clenney T. Management of epistaxis. *Am Fam Physician.* 2005;71:305–311.

9. Bennett JD, Giangrande PL. Nosebleeds: the importance of taking a history. *J R Army Med Corps.* 1990;136:167–169.

10. Josephson GD, Godley FA, Stierna P. Practical management of epistaxis. *Med Clin North Am.* 1991;75:1311–1320.

11. Bauman B, McManus JG. Pediatric pain management in the emergency department. *Emerg Med Clin North Am.* 2005;23:393–414.

12. Abelson TI, Witt WJ. Otolaryngologic procedures. In: Roberts JR, Hedges JR, eds. *Clinical Procedures in Emergency Medicine.* 2nd ed. Philadelphia: WB Saunders; 1991:1029–1037.

13. Wilson W, Nadal J Jr, Randolph G. *Clinical Handbook of Ear, Nose, and Throat Disorders.* Lancaster, England: Parthenon Publishing Group; 2002:211–220.

14. *Physicians' Desk Reference.* 59th ed. Singapore: Thomson Medical; 2005.

COLETTE C. MULL AND MARK A. GINSBURG

58

Drainage and Packing of a Nasal Septal Hematoma

▶ INTRODUCTION

A nasal septal hematoma forms when blood collects in the potential space between the cartilage of the nasal septum and its overlying mucoperichondrium. The presence of a hematoma impairs blood flow into the septal cartilage and can thereby lead to cartilage necrosis. Blunt trauma is by far the most common cause of a septal hematoma (1–4). Septal hematoma may also present as a complication of septoplasty or recurrent rhinitis or sinusitis (5). In children, the most common causes of nasal trauma are unintentional household injuries and sports injuries (4). Other etiologies in older children and adolescents include motor vehicle crashes and fights (1,6). Published case reports have described the occurrence of nasal septal hematoma in infant victims of nonaccidental injury (4,6–8). Provided no reaccumulation of blood occurs, drainage and packing of a septal hematoma is a curative procedure.

Drainage and packing of a septal hematoma is moderately complex and requires good technical skill. It fulfills the criteria for minor surgery and therefore should be performed by physicians only. The difficulty of treating a septal hematoma in a pediatric patient is usually inversely proportional to the age of the child. For a very young or extremely fearful child, this procedure is often most easily done in the operating room. However, if timely treatment by an otolaryngologist is unavailable, drainage and packing of a septal hematoma in such patients can be performed in an emergency department (ED) setting with procedural sedation (Chapter 33). For a cooperative older child or adolescent, the procedure normally can be successfully accomplished using local anesthesia alone.

▶ ANATOMY AND PHYSIOLOGY

The nasal septum is formed by the perpendicular plate of the ethmoid bone, the vomer bone, and the quadrangular cartilage (9). The thin septal cartilaginous plate supports the nasal tip and is lined by a closely adherent perichondrium and its overlying mucosa (Fig. 58.1) (9). The rich vascular network within the mucoperichondrium constitutes the blood supply to the nasal septal cartilage. Because of a relative lack of bony support, the nasal septum is often damaged as it bends and buckles under pressure. Forces generated by nasal trauma cause a separation of the mucoperichondrium from the cartilage; a septal hematoma is formed as torn submucosal blood vessels fill the potential space with blood (7). Without timely incision and drainage, the hematoma exerts increasing pressure on septal vasculature. With no alternative blood supply to the area, this pressure can impede perfusion of the nasal cartilage, potentially resulting in cartilage necrosis, cartilage resorption, septal abscess, saddle-nose deformity of the nose, and/or varying degrees of nasal obstruction (2,3,5,7,10). An untreated septal abscess can progress by direct extension and/or by hematogenous spread to involve intracranial structures (5). With or without disruption of the integrity of the septum (e.g., septal fracture), the patient may present with bilateral hematomas, an entity that carries a greater risk for permanent complications (3,5,7). Drainage of a nasal septal hematoma improves blood flow to the area but may not reverse antecedent cartilage destruction.

▶ INDICATIONS

Any child who sustains trauma to the midface should be carefully examined to exclude the presence of a septal hematoma

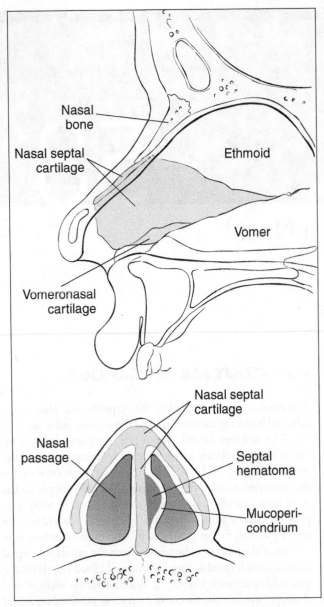

Figure 58.1 Anatomy of the nose with location of nasal septal hematoma.

or other injuries to the nose. Because of the potential for adverse long-term sequelae with such injuries, this aspect of the overall physical examination must not be overlooked. A septal hematoma will appear as a discolored (usually red, dark blue, or purple), fluctuant bulge. It has a doughy consistency and is tender to palpation. As mentioned, a septal hematoma may occur on one or both sides of the nasal septum (5,10–12). A septal hematoma should be drained as soon as is possible but certainly within 48 hours of its onset to avert the potential complication of irreversible septal necrosis that occurs by day 3 to 4 (13).

Because a septal hematoma in a young or extremely fearful child is most easily treated under general anesthesia, these cases are usually managed in the operating room. If drainage is attempted in the ED using procedural sedation, great care

must be taken to prevent any movement of the patient during the procedure so that inadvertent perforation of the septum does not occur. Although deviation of the nasal bone and/or nasal septum is not necessarily a contraindication for drainage, it does increase the complexity of the procedure and merits otolaryngology consultation (14–16).

▶ EQUIPMENT

Topical anesthesia: 4% liquid cocaine (maximum dose 3 mg/kg) or 4% liquid lidocaine (maximum dose 7 mg/kg)
Topical vasoconstrictor: 0.25% phenylephrine nasal solution (Neosynephrine)
Scalpel, No. 15 blade
Wall suction, tubing, and Frazier tip suction catheter
Sterile rubber band
Sterile gauze
Anterior nasal pack (see also Chapter 57)
Light source (a head lamp is ideal)
Nasal speculum
Monitoring and resuscitation equipment for procedural sedation, as needed (see Chapter 33)
Gloves
Eye protection

▶ PROCEDURE

Draining a septal hematoma in an awake patient should be done with the patient in a seated position, which minimizes the patient's discomfort and potential for swallowing or aspirating blood during the procedure. A young or fearful child who requires procedural sedation should have the procedure performed in the supine position using appropriate restraint techniques (see Chapter 3). For these patients, standard monitoring equipment for procedural sedation should be used, and necessary resuscitation equipment must be readily available. Reversal agents, when applicable, should be drawn up in labeled syringes (see Chapter 33). An older, cooperative child should not generally require sedation or any extensive monitoring.

Adequate anesthesia of the nasal mucosa is crucial for all patients. Sudden movement by the patient can result in iatrogenic perforation of the nasal septum, and it is therefore essential that painful or noxious stimuli be minimized. Local anesthesia is achieved with topical application of 4% liquid cocaine or 4% liquid lidocaine. A cotton pledget is soaked in the liquid anesthetic chosen and then wrung out prior to insertion into the nose (see also Fig. 57.3). The pledget is removed from the nose after approximately 10 minutes. If lidocaine is used, a topical vasoconstrictor such as 0.25% phenylephrine nasal solution (Neosynephrine) (2 to 3 drops per application every 3 to 4 hours) can be added to the pledget prior to its insertion or dripped directly onto the nasal mucosa immediately after pledget removal. The local anesthetic with or without the topical vasoconstrictor should be applied at least 10 minutes before performing any instrumentation of the nasal mucosa so that peak effect of the selected agent(s) is achieved. Although unlikely with topical application, the clinician should ensure that the toxic doses for these agents (3 mg/kg for cocaine and 7 mg/kg for lidocaine) are not exceeded. For all patients, oxygen and suction should be readily available.

To ensure good visualization of the hematoma, use of a high-intensity, easily directed light is essential. A head lamp with an attached light source is generally most effective. A nasal speculum should be used to open the naris and provide exposure of the area involved. The speculum blades should be opened vertically rather than horizontally so that the septum is better visualized without being directly instrumented. Leaving the speculum blades slightly open on insertion and removal will avoid plucking nasal hairs. When available, an assistant should be enlisted to hold the speculum in place, so that both hands of the clinician are free to perform the incision and drainage procedure.

At this point, a vertical incision is made into the hematoma using a No. 15 scalpel. At its base, the incision is then extended posteriorly to make an L shape (Fig. 58.2). Extreme care must be taken not to make the incision too deep, as this increases the risk of septal perforation. Cotton pledgets, 4″ × 4″ gauze pads, and suction should be available to drain the blood from the incised hematoma. If pus is visualized at the time of drainage, the diagnosis of concurrent septal abscess can made, and a culture should be obtained (7). It is important to keep the incision open for as long as possible, which is best accomplished by placing a small sterile rubber band (or a small segment trimmed from a Penrose drain) into the evacuated hematoma. The rubber band is simply held with a forceps and inserted deep into the incision. It can then be secured in place with an anterior nasal pack or Merocel sponge (see Chapter 57). To ensure that the drain stays in place, the clinician must apply the nasal pack securely against the overlying nasal mucosa. It is preferable to insert a nasal pack into both nostrils to avoid creating a deviation of the nasal septum. Because abscess formation is a complication of this procedure and because placement of an anterior nasal pack has been associated with sinusitis and toxic shock syndrome, all patients should be started on oral antimicrobial therapy with coverage to include *Staphylococcus aureus*, *Haemophilus influenzae*, group A β-hemolytic streptococci, and *Streptococcus pneumoniae* (2–4,8,10,12,17–20). An intravenous dose of an appropriate antibiotic is often given at the time of the procedure (4,5,18). Local antimicrobial resistance patterns and culture results, when available, should guide antibiotic selection (7). Duration of antibiotic prophylaxis or treatment of an abscess has not been firmly established. Nonabsorbable packing material should be left in place for no longer than 3 to 5 days. Ideally the child should be re-evaluated on an outpatient basis by an otolaryngologist in 24 hours.

If the patient is found to have bilateral septal hematomas, drainage involves greater potential risk. Consultation with an

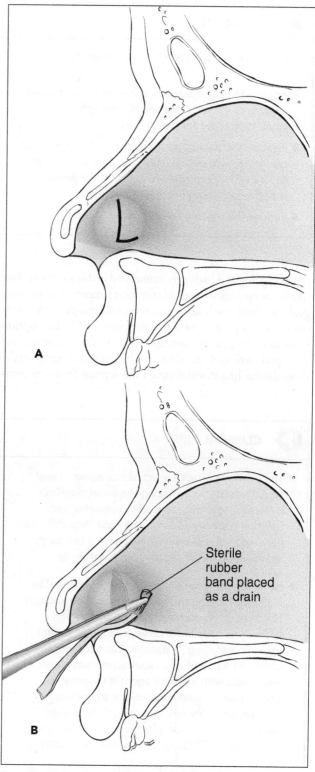

Figure 58.2 Incision and drainage of a septal hematoma.
A. An L-shaped incision is made through the hematoma, and the blood is suctioned from the nasal cavity.
B. A sterile rubber band (or a small segment trimmed from a Penrose drain) is inserted through the incision to prevent closure of the wound. The anterior nose is then packed as described in Chapter 57.

SUMMARY

1 Perform procedural sedation as necessary (see Chapter 33).

2 Apply a topical anesthetic and vasoconstrictor (4% cocaine or 4% lidocaine and Neosynephrine) and allow 10 minutes for peak effect.

3 Position the patient upright if the procedure is performed without sedation; position the patient supine with appropriate restraints if the procedure is performed using procedural sedation.

4 Expose the septum using a nasal speculum.

5 Make a vertical incision through the hematoma with a No. 15 scalpel.

6 Extend the incision at its base in a posterior direction to create an L-shape.

7 Place a sterile rubber band through the incision to serve as a drain.

8 Apply an anterior nasal pack to the affected side (preferably to both sides) (see Chapter 57).

---

otolaryngologist is highly recommended in this situation. Two treatment options are available for these patients. The primary goal with both methods is to achieve bilateral drainage without causing a permanent septal perforation. The first option involves making an incision through both the hematoma and the septal cartilage from one side. This permits drainage of the contralateral hematoma through the septum from one incision site. When this method is used, it is extremely important not to penetrate the overlying mucosa of the opposite side. The second option is to create L-shaped incisions on both mucosal surfaces, leaving the septal cartilage intact. The incisions must be staggered (offset) somewhat, because placing them directly opposite one another increases the chances for the development of a permanent septal perforation.

 CLINICAL TIPS

▶ The most important aspect of managing a nasal septal hematoma is making the initial diagnosis. Delayed treatment can lead to cosmetic and functional abnormalities of the nose. Any child with nasal or midfacial trauma must have a thorough examination of the septum and nasal cavity.

▶ Minimizing any patient movement is essential to avoid perforating the nasal septum. With younger children, this is accomplished by performing procedural sedation and restraining the patient appropriately (e.g., a papoose board). Even with older children and adolescents, adequate local anesthesia with a topical agent is essential to prevent sudden movements due to noxious stimulation of the nasal mucosa. If the patient continues to move despite these measures, the procedure should be performed in the operating room.

▶ Enlisting the aid of an assistant to hold the nasal speculum frees both hands of the clinician to perform the procedure and apply the necessary hemostasis. With younger children, a second assistant should hold the patient's head completely still even when procedural sedation is performed.

▶ Adequate lighting is essential. A head lamp with a high-intensity light source is usually most effective.

▶ Any continued bleeding after drainage of the hematoma can normally be controlled by simply pinching the nose for 5 to 10 minutes. Persistent bleeding after an adequate trial of nasal pressure necessitates evaluation by an otolaryngologist.

▶ To ensure that the drain stays in place, the anterior nasal pack must be placed securely against the overlying nasal mucosa. Applying an anterior pack to both nares prevents creating a deviation of the septum.

▶ Because placement of an anterior nasal pack has been associated with toxic shock syndrome, all patients should be started on an oral antibiotic with antistaphylococcal coverage. Nonabsorbable packing material should remain in place no longer than 3 to 5 days. All patients should be re-evaluated within 24 hours, preferably by an otolaryngologist.

▶ Although total systemic absorption of cocaine and lidocaine does not occur after topical administration, the maximum allowable doses of these agents (3 mg/kg for cocaine and 7 mg/kg for lidocaine) should not be exceeded.

▶ COMPLICATIONS

Nasal deformity may occur despite early and complete drainage of the hematoma (21). This can result from reaccumulation of blood or pre-existing necrosis of the cartilage at the time of treatment (1,5,10). Consequently, close follow-up of these patients is mandatory.

A serious but avoidable complication is the development of a permanent septal perforation, potentially leading to cosmetic deformity and chronic nasal whistling (1,5,21). This can generally be prevented by using great caution to incise only the overlying perichondrium without extending the incision into the septal cartilage. Even if a small incision is inadvertently made in the septal cartilage, a permanent septal perforation is unlikely as long as the mucosa on the opposite side remains intact. However, the septum should be avoided to the extent possible. Clearly, the technical precision required to prevent this complication underscores the importance of having a motionless patient during the procedure. It is in part for this reason that treatment of very young or fearful patients in the operating room is recommended. Otherwise, restraint techniques and procedural sedation should be used as indicated.

Infection introduced during the procedure can remain localized (septal abscess) or can extend to adjacent cartilage (perichondritis) (5). If left unchecked, infection can progress, leading to such complications as cavernous sinus thrombosis or meningitis (5). Re-evaluation of the incision and drainage site within 24 to 48 hours will generally allow the clinician to identify these problems and initiate early treatment as needed.

As with any invasive procedure involving the airway, the potential exists for aspiration of blood into the lungs during drainage and packing of a septal hematoma. Bleeding associated with this procedure is normally minimal, with only the small amount of blood in the hematoma being evacuated. Careful suctioning will generally be adequate to avoid any complications. With more extensive bleeding, pinching the nose, as with any other anterior epistaxis, will usually provide adequate hemostasis. In those rare cases when bleeding persists despite an adequate trial of nasal pressure (e.g., an unrecognized coagulopathy), evaluation of the patient by an otolaryngologist will be necessary (8).

▶ SUMMARY

Drainage of a septal hematoma involves making an L-shaped incision into the involved area, inserting a small drain to keep the incision open and placing an anterior nasal pack to tamponade the bleeding and secure the drain. Caution must be used to avoid incising the cartilaginous nasal septum, as this can lead to a permanent septal perforation. This procedure requires good technical skill and optimal patient cooperation. With younger and/or uncooperative patients, the procedure is often best done in the operating room under general anesthesia. Careful technique, antibiotic prophylaxis/treatment, and close follow-up are the most effective means of avoiding potential complications.

▶ ACKNOWLEDGMENTS

We would like to take this opportunity to acknowledge the work of Daniel J. Isaacman and J. Christopher Post the authors of this chapter in the first edition of this text. We thank them for providing us with the foundation for this chapter.

▶ REFERENCES

1. Kryger H, Dommerby H. Hematoma and abscess of the nasal septum. *Clin Otolaryngol.* 1987;12:125–129.
2. Olsen KD, Carpenter RJ III, Kern EB. Nasal septal injury in children: diagnosis and management. *Arch Otolaryngol.* 1980;106:317–320.
3. Ginsburg CM, Leach JL. Infected nasal septal hematoma. *Pediatr Infect Dis J.* 1995;14:1012–1013.
4. Canty PA, Berkowitz RG. Hematoma and abscess of the nasal septum in children. *Arch Otolaryngol Head Neck Surg.* 1996;122:1373–1376.
5. Hengerer AS, Klotz DA. Complications of nasal and sinus infections. In: Bluestone CD, Stool SE, Alper CM, et al., eds. *Pediatric Otolaryngology.* Philadelphia: WB Saunders; 2003:1021–1031.
6. East CA, O'Donaghue G. Acute nasal trauma in children. *J Pediatr Surg.* 1987;22:308–310.
7. Toback S. Nasal septal hematoma in an 11-month-old infant: a case report and review of the literature. *Pediatr Emerg Care.* 2003;19: 265–267.
8. Feinberg AN, Gushurst CA, Purdy WK, et al. Picture of the month: bilateral nasal septal hematomas. *Arch Pediatr Adolesc Med.* 1998;152: 601–602.
9. Cressman WR, Naclerio RM. Nasal physiology. In: Bluestone CD, Stool SE, Alper CM, et al., eds. *Pediatric Otolaryngology.* Philadelphia: WB Saunders; 2003:876–885.
10. Olsen KD, Carpenter RJ III, Kern EB. Nasal septal trauma in children. *Pediatrics.* 1979;64:32–35.
11. Wilson SW, Milward TM. Delayed diagnosis of septal hematoma and consequent nasal deformity. *Injury.* 1994;25:685–686.
12. Lopez MA, Liu JH, Hartley BE, et al. Septal hematoma and abscess after nasal trauma. *Clin Pediatr.* 2000;30:609–610.
13. Wilson SW, Milward TM. Delayed diagnosis of septal haematoma and consequent nasal deformity. *Injury.* 1994;25:685–686.
14. Altreuter RW. Nasal trauma. *Emerg Med Clin North Am.* 1987;5: 293–300.
15. Votey S, Dudly JP. Emergency ear, nose and throat procedures. *Emerg Med Clin North Am.* 1989;7:130–154.
16. White MJ, Johnson PC, Heckler FR. Management of maxillofacial and neck soft-tissue injuries. *Clin Sports Med.* 1989;8:11–23.
17. Eavey RD, Malekzackch MM, Wright HT. Bacterial meningitis secondary to abscess of nasal septum. *Pediatrics.* 1977;60: 102–104.
18. McCaskey CH. Rhinogenic brain abscess. *Laryngoscope.* 1951;18: 460–467.
19. Ambruss PS, Eavey RD, Baker AS, et al. Management of nasal septal abscess. *Laryngoscope.* 1981;91:575–582.
20. Chundu KR, Naqvi SH. Nasal septal abscess caused by *Haemophilus influenzae* type B. *Pediatr Infect Dis.* 1986;5:276.
21. Alvarez H, Osorio J, De Diego JI, et al. Sequelae after nasal septum injuries in children. *Auris Nasus Larynx.* 2000;27:339–342.

59

JONATHAN E. BENNETT

Nasal Foreign Body Removal

► INTRODUCTION

Nasal foreign bodies are a common problem among pediatric patients. Children have a sincere curiosity about placing objects in body orifices, and the nose seems to be a favorite choice for this behavior. At times, the diagnosis will be obvious, as the parent's presenting complaint will be "He stuck something in his nose." The task at that point is to find and remove the offending object. Diagnosis of an intranasal foreign body in a child, however, can be subtle when the parent has not witnessed the object being inserted. The classic presentation in this situation is an unexplained, foul-smelling nasal discharge that is unilateral and persistent. Other less specific complaints include chronic sinusitis, recurrent epistaxis, and halitosis (1–4). Body odor in a child also has been reported as a presenting complaint for intranasal foreign body (5,6). In addition, objects may be found incidentally, often during routine radiographic procedures (7,8). It is not unusual for the patient to be evaluated on multiple occasions with the same symptoms before the correct diagnosis is made. The physician must therefore maintain a high index of suspicion to detect this problem.

A veritable encyclopedia of small objects have been removed from the noses of children (9,10). Common items include toy parts, beads, tissue paper, and foam rubber (2). More recently, button batteries (i.e., those used in watches, calculators, and electronic toys and games) have increasingly been found as intranasal foreign bodies (11,12). These small alkaline batteries are a special concern, as they can cause liquefaction necrosis, leading to severe local tissue destruction (11). Objects that are hygroscopic, such as seeds or beans, may enlarge substantially as they absorb moisture from the nasal cavity, making extrication more difficult. Less commonly, animate objects (insects) may become lodged in the nose (13).

Goals for the physician suspecting this diagnosis are three-fold: to conduct a thorough inspection of the nasal cavity, to maximally visualize the object (assuming one is found), and to remove the object while causing as little trauma (both physical and emotional) as possible. The difficulty of achieving these goals depends on several factors, including the size, shape, and location of the object; the level of cooperation from the child; and the skill of the physician. In cases of pediatric nasal foreign bodies, 90% occur in children under 4 years of age (2). Achieving adequate cooperation with these younger patients often is the primary factor determining the success or failure of the procedure.

Several techniques have been advocated for removing nasal foreign bodies. Most are similar to methods used for retrieving foreign bodies from the external auditory canal (see Chapter 54). In general, removal should be performed only by a physician, because a failed attempt can result in advancing the object further into the nasal cavity, making subsequent attempts far more difficult. In addition, younger children become much more fearful and uncooperative after an initial attempt is unsuccessful. The procedure should be performed in a setting that has proper lighting, suction, and a variety of specialty instruments, including a right angle, an alligator forceps, and a curette. Airway equipment should be readily available in the unlikely event that an object is aspirated into the proximal airway.

► ANATOMY AND PHYSIOLOGY

There are a few points about the anatomy of the nasal cavity that are important to keep in mind when attempting foreign body removal (Fig. 59.1). One is that the turbinates are essentially perpendicular to the face rather than parallel to the nasal bone. Instruments inserted into the nose should therefore be oriented in an anteroposterior (i.e., straight in) direction,

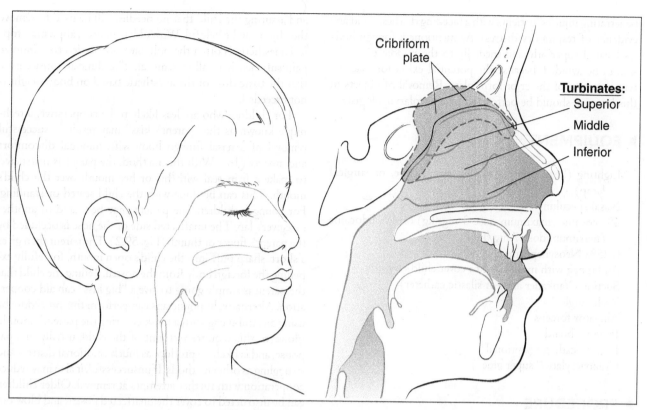

Figure 59.1 Anatomy of the nasal cavity.

perpendicular to the plane of the face. Additionally, objects lodged superiorly and medially to the middle turbinate are precariously close to the cribriform plate. The clinician should not attempt removal from this area without involving an otolaryngologist. Inferior and medial to the middle turbinates are the nasal ostia, which drain the maxillary and anterior ethmoid sinuses. Foreign bodies may occlude these and lead to sinusitis (3). Persistent nasal discharge after the clinician is certain that the foreign body has been completely removed may be due to this cause. The patient should be started on an appropriate oral antibiotic regimen after the possibility of a retained foreign body has been excluded. Finally, the nasal septum consists of a thin cartilaginous plate with a closely adherent perichondrium and mucosa (see Fig. 57.1). This mucosa, which is lined with a rich vascular network, is thinner and more likely to bleed in children than adults. Bleeding is especially common at the Kiesselbach plexus in the Little area of the anterior nasal septum. Special care should be taken to prevent any significant injury to the septal mucosa, as this may result in bleeding to an extent that visualization and removal of a foreign body become impossible. Parents should be warned that minor bleeding after this procedure is common and generally benign.

▶ INDICATIONS

A thorough inspection of the nasal cavity is obviously indicated whenever a child has reportedly placed a foreign body

in the nose. This information may come from a parent or other caretaker, a sibling, or the child. As described previously, other complaints that should prompt suspicion of an intranasal foreign body include a persistent nasal discharge (particularly when unilateral), recurrent epistaxis, and halitosis (1–4). Diagnosis of clinical sinusitis, a common finding in the outpatient setting, is often based on a history of purulent nasal discharge for longer than 7 to 10 days. These children also should be routinely evaluated for a nasal foreign body (3). A more exotic presentation, such as body odor in a young child, which would be unusual before the development of apocrine glands during adolescence, should cause the physician to at least consider the diagnosis of a nasal foreign body as one possibility (5,6).

In a review of 212 cases of ear and nose foreign bodies in children presenting to an urban emergency department (ED), Baker found that approximately 90% of the objects could be removed by ED personnel with readily available equipment (2). If necessary, procedural sedation may be performed in the ED to facilitate the procedure with a young or fearful child (see Chapter 33). Consultation with an otolaryngologist, however, is indicated for any case in which the clinician is not confident of successful removal. In the combative young child who may be difficult to sedate adequately, a few minutes of general anesthesia often is preferable to a prolonged and potentially unsuccessful struggle. In addition, cases that are appropriate for immediate consultation include embedded foreign bodies, a button battery that cannot be removed, penetrating injuries, patients with a bleeding diathesis, and any evidence of respiratory distress. As mentioned, foreign bodies located superiorly and medially to the middle turbinate should be avoided, because the potential exists for inadvertent puncture of the cribriform plate. Removal of objects in this location should be performed by an otolaryngologist.

▶ EQUIPMENT

Lighting (head light, operating microscope, or surgical lamp)
Nasal speculum
4% cocaine (maximum dose 3 mg/kg) or 4% lidocaine (maximum dose 7 mg/kg)
0.25% Neosynephrine
Ambu bag with mask sized to cover child's mouth
Suction (Yankauer and/or silastic catheter)
Right angle
Alligator forceps
Papoose board
Fogarty catheter (optional)
Cyanoacrylate ("super glue")

▶ PROCEDURE

The clinician should first explain to the parents the planned approach and outline the risks of the procedure. As with any procedure, parental concerns should be completely discussed before proceeding. For this procedure to be successful, it is particularly important that the child remain still, and therefore every attempt should be made to calm the patient. Atraumatic removal is rarely accomplished with a struggling child. If the child is verbal, honestly explaining what should be expected

and assuring the child that no needles will be used to remove the object can be helpful. With older children, applying a topical anesthetic is often the only measure needed to minimize pain sufficiently to allow removal. The clinician must ensure that the toxic dose of the anesthetic based on body weight is not exceeded.

For children who are less likely to be cooperative, a technique known as the "parent's kiss" may result in successful removal of a nasal foreign body with minimal discomfort and anxiety (14). With this method, the parent is instructed to make a firm seal with his or her mouth over the child's mouth. This can be done with the child seated or standing. For younger children, the patient may be seated in another caregiver's lap. The unaffected side of the nose is occluded by the parent's finger or thumb (Fig. 59.2). The parent then gives a short, sharp puff into the child's open mouth, forcefully expelling the foreign body from the nostril. Telling the child that the parent is simply going to give a "big kiss" can aid cooperation. Alternatively, physicians can perform this procedure by using an Ambu bag with a mask covering the patient's mouth. However, this requires restraint of the child, usually in a papoose, and is likely to produce as much emotional distress and struggling as other methods. If unsuccessful, it also may reduce cooperation with further attempts at removal. Older children can be instructed to cover the unaffected nostril and blow out of the nose, which may be enough to dislodge the object.

For more invasive methods of extraction, younger or fearful children may require administration of rectal midazolam to facilitate the procedure, and in some cases standard intravenous procedural sedation techniques will be necessary (see Chapter 33). Patients should be positioned supine with appropriate restraint. Restraining an older child may only require gently holding the arms down to avoid having the patient grab the clinician's hands as the foreign body is manipulated.

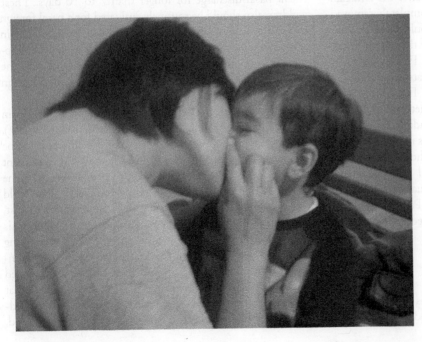

Figure 59.2 Positive-pressure method for removal of intranasal foreign body (parent's kiss).

Younger children should generally be placed in a papoose or other comparable restraint device (see Chapter 3). Above all, the clinician must ensure that the head will be completely immobilized during the procedure. Assigning one assistant to concentrate solely on stabilizing the head will greatly enhance the likelihood of successful removal on the first attempt.

A key step in removing the nasal foreign body is to gain as much visualization as possible. A good view of the nasal cavity should always be obtained before any instrumentation. Blind passage of removal devices is rarely successful and increases the risk of injury. If significant edema or blood is present, the clinician should administer a vasoconstrictor such as Neosynephrine and allow 10 minutes for maximal clinical effect. Applying a local anesthetic such as lidocaine will often enhance patient cooperation so that a better view of the nasal cavity can be obtained. Although still used by pediatric otolaryngologists, liquid cocaine is now rarely used for children in the ED because of its expense and potential for serious complications. A fiberoptic headlight provides excellent lighting and allows two-hand manipulation, which is a distinct advantage. A nasal speculum should be placed in the nose to open the nostril and maximize visualization. The speculum is held between the palm of the hand and the third, fourth, and fifth fingers. The thumb and index fingers are used to stabilize the instrument against the nose (Fig. 59.3). It is important that the blade of the speculum open in a cephalad-caudad (superoinferior) orientation so as not to put pressure on the nasal septum. Gentle upward pressure on the tip of the nose may aid visualization. Suctioning with a narrow-width suction tip, such as a tonsil suction tip, may also be helpful. Once the object is adequately visualized, the clinician should assess its size and orientation.

Several techniques have been described for direct removal of an intranasal foreign body (15–18). In many cases, the nature of the foreign body will determine the optimal method. For example, a firm or rounded foreign body can generally be extracted by placing a right angle or curette behind the object and gently pulling it out (Fig. 59.3A). The right angle or curette should be advanced through the largest gap between the object and the nasal wall, parallel to the palate. Leverage can by used to roll the object along the nasal floor but not the septum. Alternatively, cyanoacrylate ("super glue") can be used with this type of foreign body. The glue is first applied to the tip of a wooden stick that is then pressed directly to a surface of the foreign body. Great care must be taken to avoid touching the interior of the nasal cavity, as the glue also will bond to the mucosal surfaces. The stick should be kept in place against the foreign body for 15 to 30 seconds to allow a strong bond to form. The object can then be retrieved by slowly withdrawing the stick (19). Another option with firm or rounded foreign bodies is to insert a Fogarty biliary catheter beyond the object, inflate the balloon with air, and then gently remove the catheter. For metallic objects, rod magnets may be used to try to dislodge the foreign body from the nostril (20). Foreign bodies made of softer materials (e.g., rubber or paper) can generally be grasped with a bayonet or alligator forceps and removed (Fig. 59.3B,C).

Occasionally, an irregularly shaped foreign body will have to be manipulated to ensure that the long axis is parallel to the direction of removal. It is important to emphasize that objects should never be pushed deeper into the nose to move them into the oropharynx, as the risk of aspiration is significant. The procedure should be terminated if the object is being inadvertently pushed deeper into the nose, if adequate visualization of the object is lost, or if significant bleeding occurs. After removal of the object, the nares should be reinspected to confirm complete patency because the object may have broken into pieces or more than one foreign body may have been inserted. Generally, no specific follow-up is required for the asymptomatic patient. Parents should be instructed to return for any signs or symptoms of a retained foreign body, primarily a persistent purulent nasal discharge or recurrent epistaxis.

Once the approach and instrument have been chosen, the clinician should proceed with removal as quickly and efficiently as possible. It is important to give the patient positive feedback for cooperating and to let the patient know when the procedure is drawing to a close. As described, removing the object on the first pass is highly desirable, as cooperation will quickly diminish after an initial failed attempt, particularly with younger patients.

▶ COMPLICATIONS

A few important complications are associated with this procedure. One is local trauma to the nasal mucosa. It is quite common to induce minor epistaxis during removal of an intranasal foreign body, particularly one that has been present over a longer period of time. The formation of granulation tissue in the area can result in transient bleeding when the object is extricated. Abrasion or laceration of the mucosa also can occur if the child moves suddenly during instrumentation. When using instruments to grasp the foreign body, one should be careful not to inadvertently grasp the turbinates. If cyanoacrylate is used, inadvertent application of glue to the interior of the nasal cavity can cause mucosal injury. Although bleeding from any of these causes is usually self-limited, the clinician should carefully avoid traumatizing the richly vascularized nasal septum, as this can sometimes lead to more extensive epistaxis. Applying a topical vasoconstrictor before the procedure will often limit any bleeding. If a local anesthetic is used, the clinician must ensure that the maximum allowable dose based on the child's body weight is not exceeded. Toxicity due to either cocaine or lidocaine can produce seizures and circulatory compromise. Unless the child has a congenital or acquired coagulopathy, bleeding can normally be stopped without difficulty by pinching the cartilaginous portion of the nose for 5 to 10 minutes. If necessary, an anterior nasal pack can be applied (see Chapter 57).

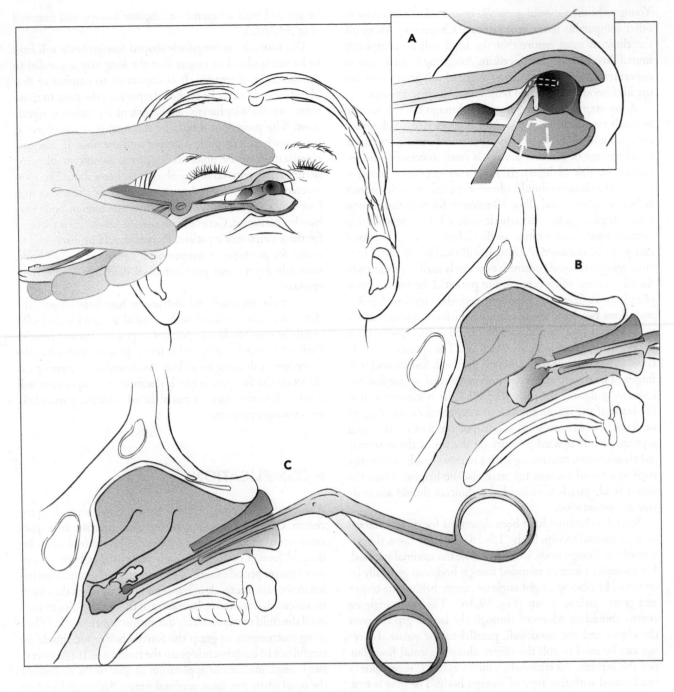

Figure 59.3 Removal of an intranasal foreign body.
A. A right-angle curette can be used to remove firm or rounded objects.
B, C. A forceps (bayonet or alligator) can be used to remove softer materials (e.g., rubber or paper).

As mentioned previously, the clinician should be cognizant of the proximity of the superior aspect of the nasal cavity to the intracranial cavity. Overzealous instrumentation with a metal probe can result in fracture of the thin cribriform plate, producing a cerebrospinal fluid leak and allowing entry of bacteria into the cranium. The area superior and medial to the middle turbinate is immediately adjacent to the cribriform plate and thus represents a danger zone. A foreign body lodged in this position should only be removed by an otolaryngologist.

One significant but avoidable complication is aspiration of the foreign body into the proximal airway. This normally results when the object is pushed backward into the nasal cavity during attempts at removal or realignment. Sudden deep inspiration by the patient (e.g., crying) also may contribute to this complication. If the clinician finds that the foreign body is progressively moving posteriorly as it is manipulated, the procedure should be terminated and appropriate consultation sought. In the unlikely event that aspiration of the foreign body

SUMMARY

1 Ascertain the nature of the foreign body (if possible).

2 Explain the procedure to the parent and child.

3 Assemble the necessary equipment.

4 Attempt noninvasive positive-pressure removal ("parent's kiss"): (a) the parent occludes the unaffected nostril with a finger; (b) the parent administers a forceful mouth-to-mouth breath to the child; (c) if unsuccessful after two attempts, proceed with the following steps.

5 Restrain the child appropriately; assign one assistant to stabilize the child's head.

6 Perform sedation as necessary.

7 Insert a nasal speculum and visualize the object to determine its size, location, and orientation.

8 Apply a topical anesthesia (e.g., 4% lidocaine) as needed.

9 Apply a topical vasoconstrictor (e.g., 0.25% Neosynephrine) as needed.

10 Remove the foreign body:
   a For a hard, smooth foreign body, insert the removal instrument parallel to the nasal turbinates (straight in) until the tip is behind the object and pull outward.
   b Grasp a soft object with forceps and remove.

11 Reinspect the nasal cavity after removal to ensure that the object (or objects) is completely removed and that the mucosa has not been injured.

 CLINICAL TIPS

▶ A nasal foreign body should never be intentionally pushed back into the hypopharynx in an attempt to remove it, as this may result in aspiration of the object into the proximal airway.

▶ If it is apparent that a foreign body is only being pushed further into the nasal cavity during attempted removal, the procedure should not be continued. In such cases, removal by an otolaryngologist in the operating room will likely be necessary.

▶ Visualization of the object can generally be improved by (a) applying a topical vasoconstrictor to the nasal mucosa, (b) using a high-intensity light source (a head lamp is ideal), (c) pressing the tip of the nose up and back, and (d) using suction to remove any blood or secretions.

▶ The noninvasive, nontraumatic "parent's kiss" method of positive-pressure removal may be tried as a first attempt. While typically performed by a parent, this technique can also be performed by the physician using an Ambu bag with a mask that covers the child's mouth.

▶ The child must be very still during this procedure to prevent injury to the nasal cavity, and the clinician should take appropriate measures to accomplish this goal (restraint and/or procedural sedation). If the clinician is not confident that the child will remain motionless, the procedure should likely be performed in the operating room.

▶ With a verbal child, explaining each step of the procedure in a friendly, calming voice is often the most effective means of avoiding any sudden movements by the patient.

▶ A firm, smooth foreign body that cannot be readily removed using a curette or right angle can often be retrieved by applying cyanoacrylate ("super glue") to the tip of a wooden stick, pressing the tip against the object for 15 to 30 seconds to form a secure bond, and then slowly withdrawing the stick.

▶ Although total systemic absorption of cocaine and lidocaine does not occur after topical administration, the maximum allowable doses of these agents (3 mg/kg for cocaine, 5 mg/kg for lidocaine, 7 mg/kg for lidocaine with epinephrine) should not be exceeded.

does occur, standard methods of addressing this problem must be performed (see Chapter 51).

A final complication concerns the emotional trauma caused by an injudicious use of force to remove the foreign body. Unlike many procedures performed in the acute care setting, time is not a factor when removing an intranasal foreign body. Therefore, the clinician should try to minimize the discomfort experienced by the child as much as possible. Attempts at simply overpowering a struggling child often are met with failure and subject the patient to needless anxiety and fear. In addition, should the procedure prove unsuccessful, subsequent efforts to remove the foreign body will be complicated by the distrust and apprehension of the patient. For this reason, some authorities recommend sedation to facilitate this procedure for young or extremely fearful children, unless the object is in a shallow position and easily retrievable with one quick pass. If adequate sedation is not feasible in this situation, then removal should be performed in the operating room by an otolaryngologist. In most cases, time spent preparing the child by explaining what can be expected in a calm and nonthreatening manner will be rewarded with a successful procedure that causes a minimum of emotional distress to both patient and family.

▶ SUMMARY

Removing a foreign body from a child's nose is a task frequently performed in the outpatient setting. Success primarily depends on the size and location of the object, the duration of time it has been in the nose, and the ability to adequately immobilize the child during the procedure. As with most procedures, proper lighting and the appropriate instruments are essential. Above all, the physician should make a judgment about the difficulty of the procedure before undertaking removal and proceed only when confident of success on the first attempt.

▶ ACKNOWLEDGMENTS

The authors would like to acknowledge the valuable contributions of Daniel J. Isaacman and J. Christopher Post to the version of this chapter that appeared in the previous edition.

▶ REFERENCES

1. Brownstein DR, Hodge D. Foreign bodies of the eye, ear, and nose. *Pediatr Emerg Care.* 1988;4:215–218.
2. Baker MD. Foreign bodies of the ears and nose in childhood. *Pediatr Emerg Care.* 1987;3:67–70.
3. Fireman P. Diagnosis of sinusitis in children: emphasis on the history and physical examination. *J Allergy Clin Immunol.* 1992;90:433–436.
4. Bennett JD. An unexpected cause of halitosis. *J R Army Med Corps.* 1988;134:151–152.
5. Eun HC, Kim KH, Lee YS. Unusual body odor due to a nasal foreign body in a child. *J Dermatol.* 1984;11:501–503.
6. Wesley RE, Arterberry JF. Soft tissue intranasal foreign bodies. *Ann Emerg Med.* 1980;9:215–217.
7. Kittle PE, Aaron GR, Jones HL, et al. Incidental finding of an intranasal foreign body discovered on routine dental examination: case report. *Pediatr Dent.* 1991;13:49–51.
8. Jones DC, O'Bree WD, Macintyre DR. Intranasal foreign body: an incidental radiographic finding. *Dent Update.* 1987;14:408.
9. Harun S, Montgomery P, Ajulo SO. An unusual oronasal foreign body. *J Laryngol Otol.* 1991; 105: 1118–1119.
10. Fosarelli P, Feigelman S, Pearson E, et al. An unusual intranasal foreign body. *Pediatr Emerg Care.* 1988;4:117–118.
11. Gomes CC, Sakano E, Lucchezi MC, et al. Button battery as a foreign body in the nasal cavities: special aspects. *Rhinology.* 1994;32:98–100.
12. Palmer O, Natarajan B, Johnstone A, et al. Button battery in the nose: an unusual foreign body. *J Laryngol Otol.* 1994;108:871–872.
13. Werman HA. Removal of foreign bodies of the nose. *Emerg Med Clin North Am.* 1987;5:253–263.
14. Botma M, Bader T, Kubba H. "A parent's kiss": evaluating an unusual method for removing nasal foreign bodies in children. *J Laryngol Otol.* 2000;114:598–600.
15. Backlin SA. Positive-pressure technique for nasal foreign body removal in children. *Ann Emerg Med.* 1995;25:554–555.
16. Nandapalan V, McIlwain JC. Removal of nasal foreign bodies with a Fogarty biliary balloon catheter. *J Laryngol Otol.* 1994;108:758–760.
17. Cohen HA, Goldberg E, Horev Z. Removal of nasal foreign bodies in children [Letter]. *Clin Pediatr.* 1993;32:192.
18. Wavde V. Removal of foreign body from nose or ear. *Aust Fam Physician.* 1988;17:904.
19. Hanson RM, Stephens M. Cyanoacrylate-assisted foreign body removal from the ear and nose in children. *J Paediatr Child Health.* 1994;30:77–78.
20. Douglas SA, Mizra S, Stafford F. Magnetic removal of a nasal foreign body. *Int J Pediatr Otorhinolaryngol.* 2002;62:165–167.

60

Pharyngeal Procedures

▶ INTRODUCTION

Three pharyngeal problems in children that may be treated in the emergency department (ED)—pharyngitis, tonsillar foreign body, and peritonsillar abscess—require careful and complete historical investigation and physical examination before any diagnostic or ameliorative procedure is initiated.

Pharyngitis is one of the more common reasons for which children and adolescents seek emergency care. Pharyngitis may manifest in several different clinical ways, including nasopharyngitis, tonsillopharyngitis, and tonsillitis. It is essential that diagnostic procedures are used that may enable the clinician to distinguish between viral and bacterial causes of pharyngitis. Treatment of viral pharyngitis with antibiotics is unnecessary and may result in an allergic response to the antibiotic and development of antibiotic resistance in the community. Failure to identify and treat group A streptococcal pharyngitis may lead to complications such as peritonsillar and retropharyngeal abscess and rheumatic fever (1,2).

Foreign body ingestion is not an uncommon problem in both the pediatric and adult age groups. However, tonsillar foreign body is an infrequent finding, although in older children and adolescents it is no less common than in the adult population. Jones et al. described 388 patients aged 0 to 90 years in whom 60 of 121 foreign bodies retained in the throat were located in the tonsil and 67 of 71 fishbones were found in the tonsil or posterior third of the tongue (3). Management of a tonsillar foreign body depends on the particular foreign body and its location, but it is often a straightforward procedure performed by the emergency physician.

Peritonsillar abscess (quinsy), one of the most common abscesses of the head and neck, is thought to be rare in children younger than 8 years but has been reported in children only 4 months (4) and 15 months (5) of age. In fact, in one study of children with peritonsillar abscess, 31% of patients were younger than 10 years of age (6), whereas in another, the mean age was 10 years (range, 3 to 16 years) (7). Management of peritonsillar abscess has undergone considerable and controversial change over the last century. Management options include medical (antibiotic) treatment, transmucosal needle aspiration, incision and drainage, acute tonsillectomy, and delayed tonsillectomy (8–11). The emergency physician is involved in medical treatment and, in selected cases, may perform needle aspiration or incision and drainage prior to or instead of admission to the hospital. When available, consultation with an otolaryngologist should be sought in such cases.

▶ ANATOMY AND PHYSIOLOGY

The palatine tonsils—the lateral component of the Waldeyer ring of lymphatic tissue (composed of the palatine, lingual, and pharyngeal tonsils)—lie in the tonsillar fossa (Fig. 60.1) (12). The deep or lateral surface of the palatine tonsil is a fibrous connective tissue capsule that opposes the superior constrictor muscle; the palatopharyngeal muscle lies posteriorly and the palatoglossal muscle lies rostral (13,14). Importantly, the tonsillar and ascending palatine branches of the facial artery are just lateral to the constrictor muscle, whereas the internal carotid artery is no more than 2 cm dorsal and lateral.

Pharyngitis

Primary bacterial pathogens account for approximately 30% of cases of pharyngitis in children, the most common being *Streptococcus pyogenes* and group A β-hemolytic streptococci. Less common causes include group G streptococci and *Neisseria gonorrhoea* (cultured from sexually active adolescents and

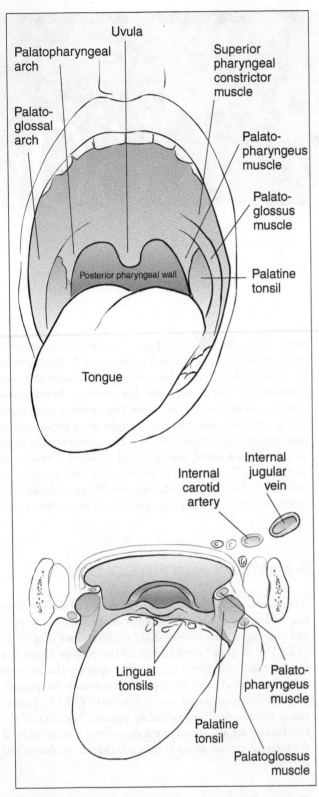

Figure 60.1 Anatomy of the palatine tonsils and associated structures.

as a coincident infection in some young victims of sexual abuse). Fortunately, widespread childhood immunization has made *Corynebacterium diphtheriae* very uncommon. Most bacterial pharyngitis requires antibiotic treatment. Common viral causes include adenovirus, influenza virus, rhinovirus, and parainfluenza virus. Coxsackievirus and herpes simplex virus may cause pharyngitis marked by the presence of vesicles. Ebstein-Barr virus (infectious mononucleosis) causes pharyngitis primarily in older children and adolescents. The atypical organisms *Chlamydia trachomatis* and *Mycoplasma pneumoniae* are less common causes of childhood pharyngitis.

Tonsillar Foreign Body

Up to 12% of foreign bodies found in the aerodigestive tract of children are fish or chicken bones (13). Although the majority of objects that children swallow are not retained in the throat, foreign bodies with a spicular shape may be become lodged in the tonsil. These include fish bones, meat bones, and hard seed husks as well as man-made objects such as glass, plastic toothbrush bristles, straight and safety pins, ballpoint pen caps, and countless other spicate household items that arouse the curiosity of children (14–17).

Tonsilloliths, most commonly seen in young adults with chronic or recurrent tonsillitis, are composed of retained caseous secretions in exaggerated tonsillar crypts that may contain vegetable matter and calcium salts. Tonsilloliths are therefore often rocklike and radiopaque (18–20).

Peritonsillar Abscess

Peritonsillar abscess is the most common complication of tonsillitis (6,21) and is a result of suppurative infection of the tonsil. This infection penetrates the tonsillar capsule and extends into the connective tissue space between the fibrous wall of the capsule and the posterior wall of the tonsillar fossa overlying the superior constrictor muscle. Localized purulent material (pus) extends superiorly into the soft palate. Although 85% to 90% of abscesses occur in the superior pole of the tonsillar space, pus can accumulate in the midaspect or lower pole (9,21,22). Peritonsillar abscesses are almost always unilateral (22,23). Further dissection of the infected space may result in the extension of organisms through the constrictor muscle and in deep neck infection if a peritonsillar abscess remains untreated.

The microbiology of peritonsillar abscess cultures is polymicrobial in 30% to 75% of aspirates, with *S. pyogenes* being one of the primary pathogens (7,24). In several recent series of pediatric patients, *S. pyogenes* was isolated in 25% to 30% of aspirate cultures, other *Streptococcus* species in 20% to 40%, and anaerobic pathogens in 12% to 33% (6,7,9). In two of these studies, 30% of aspirate cultures yielded both aerobic and anaerobic bacteria such as *Streptococcus* and *Bacteroides* species (6,9). Interestingly, 20% to 35% of abscess cultures will not grow bacterial pathogens (6,7,9,25).

▶ INDICATIONS

Pharyngitis

Except for patients with a classical scarlatiniform rash, streptococcal pharyngitis cannot be reliably diagnosed based on clinical grounds. The presence of sore throat, enlarged tonsils, palatal petechiae, and anterior cervical adenopathy in the absence of symptoms of a viral upper respiratory infection warrant obtaining a diagnostic test for group A β-hemolytic streptococci. In children under 2 years of age, these typical symptoms may be absent, and therefore testing for group A β-hemolytic streptococci may be indicated in this population despite a paucity of findings when there is an exposure history.

Tonsillar Foreign Body

Older patients with tonsillar foreign bodies will report swallowing a foreign body or choking on food with spicular bones or fragments. Most will have sudden onset of discomfort, and as many as 68% of patients who localize their pain to the tonsil have been found to have foreign bodies (3). Otalgia is not uncommon, and odynophagia can progressively worsen. However, it should be noted that foreign body sensation is not reliably reported (13). Younger (especially preverbal) children may have subtle presentations, such as an unwitnessed or unexplained choking episode during a meal or while playing with small objects. Children with developmental delay are at higher risk for foreign body ingestion, with late presentation not uncommon (3,13).

Careful inspection of the tonsillar fossae and palate will detect most tonsillar foreign bodies. Using an indirect mirror or fiberoptic nasopharyngoscopy will lead to a more effective examination when the foreign body cannot be adequately or fully visualized (see Chapter 61). Radiographs will corroborate clinical findings of radiopaque foreign bodies such as meat and poultry bones, pins, and most glass. Of note, not all fish species bones are radiographically visible. Ell and Sprigg assessed the radiopacity of the bones of 14 species of fish in a swine head and neck preparation. On plain radiograph, bones of the cod, gurnard, haddock, cole fish, lemon sole, monk fish, and red snapper were moderately or clearly visible in the tonsil, larynx, vallecula, and esophagus (Fig. 60.2). In contrast, bones of the salmon, trout, pike, mackerel, herring, and plaice were not radiopaque (26).

The uncooperative patient or young child with a tonsillar foreign body should be examined carefully by both the emergency physician and a consulting otolaryngologist. Removing a foreign body in such a patient may require general anesthesia in the operating room. For the older and cooperative patient, removal is usually straightforward if the site and depth of the foreign body is established. A lateral radiograph of the soft tissues of the neck can be helpful before removal.

Contraindications for removal of a tonsillar foreign body in the ED include an uncooperative or young child, difficulty visualizing the appropriate anatomy or the foreign body, and anticipation of a difficult removal or difficult management of the airway.

Peritonsillar Abscess

The child with a peritonsillar abscess will typically present with a sore throat and fever of a few to several days duration. Dysphagia and odynophagia can worsen acutely, and changes in phonation can progress to a so-called "hot potato" voice, when the patient speaks with limited movement of the tongue and pharynx (10,23). Pyrexia increases and trismus can develop due to spasm of the internal pterygoid muscle (23). Tender cervical adenopathy accompanies the tonsillopharyngitis, and inflammatory torticollis is occasionally seen (27).

Physical examination of a patient with a peritonsillar abscess reveals a mildly to moderately ill-appearing febrile child. Swallowing may be difficult or painful, and the patient may drool as a result (10,23). Trismus often limits

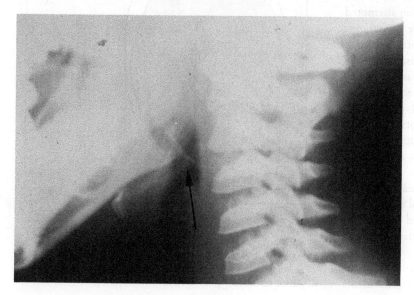

Figure 60.2 Radiograph of a fish bone lodged in the palatine tonsil and hanging into the hypopharynx of a 3-year-old boy.

examination, but an exudative tonsillopharyngitis is usually present on inspection of the pharynx. The abscess usually displaces the affected tonsil forward and inferomedially, and the uvula is consequently deviated toward the unaffected tonsil (23) (Fig. 60.3). Other characteristic findings include a red, swollen soft palate, halitosis, and tender ipsilateral cervical adenopathy.

These findings do not always differentiate peritonsillar cellulitis from abscess (28), although the pharyngotonsillar bulge is usually of greater magnitude with abscess (10). Gentle palpation with the examiner's gloved finger inserted into the patient's mouth will normally reveal fluctuance when a true abscess is present. Imaging studies such as ultrasound (29,30) and computerized tomography (31,32) may be helpful in confirming the presence of an abscess. Consultation with an otolaryngologist is mandatory if the clinician is unsure of the diagnosis. Other diagnoses that should be considered include severe tonsillopharyngitis, retropharyngeal abscess, lymphoma, deep neck tumor, and carotid artery aneurysm. Most of the pediatric literature supports hospitalizing patients with potential peritonsillar abscess for intravenous antibiotic therapy. Those patients who do not respond within 24 to 48 hours undergo acute tonsillectomy (8,10). The management strategy used should be individualized, and postprocedure care plans should be made in consultation with an otolaryngologist.

Transmucosal needle aspiration or incision and drainage in the ED is a safe option for acute management of the nontoxic, cooperative patient with peritonsillar abscess. Ill-appearing or uncooperative patients and very young children should be admitted to the hospital, with consideration given to operative or closely supervised sedation for the procedure.

The cure rates for incision and drainage versus needle aspiration of peritonsillar abscess have been compared in several studies. Stringer et al. found similar cure rates for needle aspiration and incision and drainage of peritonsillar abscess (22 of 24 vs. 26 of 28 patients) (33), as did Spires et al. (39 of 41 vs. 21 of 21) (23). Likewise, Ophir et al. studied 104 patients with abscesses who had needle aspiration attempted (25). Seventy-five of 104 patients had positive aspirations; of these, 64 (85%) resolved with oral antibiotic treatment and only 9 required hospitalization. Transmucosal needle aspiration for peritonsillar abscess in children was studied by Weinberg et al. (9). Of 41 patients with a suspected abscess, 31 had pus obtained on aspiration. Of the 31 patients, 27 (87%) had resolution of the abscess after aspiration and parenteral antibiotics. Of the 10 children with negative aspirates, 7 resolved with parenteral antibiotics. Recently, an evidence-based review of the treatment of peritonsillar abscess was performed by Johnson et al. (34). A Medline search resulted in the return of 42 articles. Five level I clinical studies were identified and analyzed. These studies showed that needle aspiration, incision and drainage, and tonsillectomy were all effective for initial management.

Current management strategies for children with peritonsillar abscess differ among institutions. In general, the

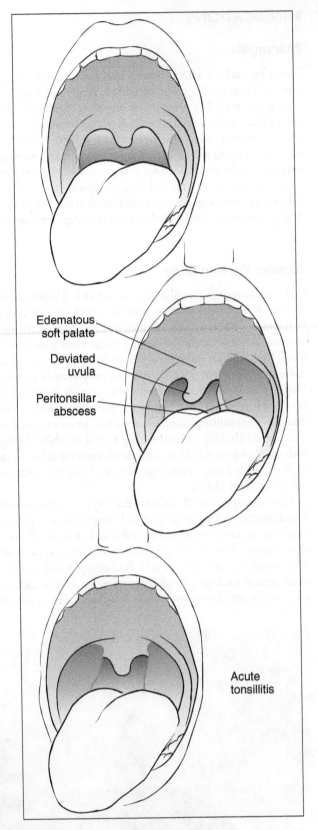

Figure 60.3
A. Normal tonsil.
B. Peritonsillar abscess. The tonsil is displaced forward and inferomedially, the uvula is deviated toward the unaffected tonsil, and the soft palate is edematous and ruborous.
C. Acute tonsillitis.

TABLE 60.1	EQUIPMENT FOR TONSILLAR FOREIGN BODY REMOVAL AND MANAGEMENT OF PERITONSILLAR ABSCESS	
	Equipment	**Comments**
Airway management	Oxygen	Place at bedside
	Bag-valve-mask apparatus	
	Oral, nasal airways	
	Endotracheal tubes	
	Suction apparatus	Large tonsil (Yankauer) suction tube
Anesthesia	Topical: anesthetic spray, viscous lidocaine 4%, cocaine 4%	
	Injectable: lidocaine 1%, 2%	Luer-Lok syringe
		3-inch dental needle
Removal of tonsillar foreign body	Fine-tipped biopsy (alligator) forceps	
	Straight hemostat; curved hemostat	
Transmucosal needle aspiration of a peritonsillar abscess	3.5-inch, 20-gauge or 22-gauge needle	Use a needle guard
Incision and drainage of a peritonsillar abscess	No. 11 or 12 surgical blade	Use a blade guard
	Curved hemostat	

management approach includes parenteral antibiotic therapy and either transmucosal needle aspiration or incision and drainage of the abscess. Some otolaryngologists will, however, recommend incision and drainage if purulent fluid is obtained by needle aspiration.

Contraindications for performing needle aspiration or incision and drainage of a peritonsillar abscess in the ED include uncertainty of the diagnosis, an uncooperative or very young child, and anticipation of a difficult airway. Any patient with a potential coagulopathy should have correction before the drainage procedure. Such cases are generally best managed in the operating room.

▶ EQUIPMENT

Obtaining a Throat Culture

Whether a single or double swab should be used in swabbing the oropharynx to identify the presence of group A β-hemolytic streptococci depends on the availability of rapid antigen testing. The advantages of early diagnosis using a rapid antigen test include decreased transmission and earlier return to school of the older child. Delayed treatment (waiting for the results of a traditional throat culture) is urged by some authors based on limited data suggesting that recurrences of streptococcal pharyngitis are less common if the patient is permitted to mount an immune response (35,36). Moreover, treatment within 9 days of onset is believed to be sufficient to prevent rheumatic fever (1,2). A single swab transported on specialized media (Thayer-Martin) is used for diagnosis of pharyngitis due to *N. gonorrhoea*.

When a rapid antigen test is used, it is reasonable to initiate antibiotic treatment based on a positive result, since these tests have a specificity of up to 99% (37). However, the sensitivity is only about 70% (i.e., a 30% false-negative rate). It is therefore essential to perform a traditional throat culture if the rapid antigen test is negative (37).

Tonsillar Foreign Body Removal

Equipment used for removing a tonsillar foreign body is listed in Table 60.1. The optimal instrument for this procedure depends on the type of foreign body. Most are managed with fine-tipped biopsy (alligator) forceps or a straight or curved hemostat. Mishandling a tonsillar foreign body or tonsillolith may result in airway compromise. Consequently, equipment required for management of the airway should always be readily available. A topical or local anesthesia is sometimes a helpful adjunct in the removal of a foreign body.

Management of Peritonsillar Abscess

Equipment used for transmucosal needle aspiration or incision and drainage of a peritonsillar abscess is listed in Table 60.1. Topical or local anesthesia is generally recommended for these procedures. As with the removal of a tonsillar foreign body, appropriate airway equipment should be readily available. Needle and surgical blade guards should be prepared before beginning the procedure.

▶ PROCEDURE

A thorough inspection of the neck, cervical lymph chain, ears, nose, paranasal sinuses, dentition, and the nasopharynx, oropharynx, and hypopharynx is mandatory when a pharyngeal procedure is being considered. Chronic or acute examination findings and associated disease may influence the management strategy.

The examination of the oropharynx is especially threatening to the young child. Time spent establishing rapport and trust with the patient is imperative for cooperation during the examination and subsequent procedures. An external examination (neck, ears, nose, paranasal sinuses) should precede oropharyngeal manipulation. An explanation of the different phases of the examination and instruments used will allay some children's fears and will also enhance parental acceptance of the examination and procedure. Inspection of the oral cavity and pharynx is aided by using a wooden tongue blade and should include an assessment of the floor of the mouth and the gingiva, palate, dentition, and retropharynx.

Obtaining a Throat Culture

Obtaining a specimen by throat swab can be difficult with a struggling child (who might gag, cough, or vomit), but it is important to obtain an adequate specimen. Assistance from another person may be required to accomplish this goal. Younger children should generally be positioned sitting in a parent's lap or supine on the examination table. Older children and adolescents will usually tolerate the procedure sitting upright with the head firmly back against a headrest. A tongue depressor is inserted to provide better exposure, and the area is illuminated. The swab is inserted into the posterior pharynx, with avoidance of the tongue and uvula. Phonation with the traditional "ah" in older children and crying in younger children decrease the gag reflex, which, if unanticipated, can interfere with obtaining a specimen. The swab is rubbed against the posterior pharynx and both tonsils (especially if exudates are present). Although suboptimal, intentionally inducing the gag reflex using the tongue blade may be the only way to obtain an adequate throat culture in a young or uncooperative child who is forcefully resisting mouth opening. This obviously causes greater discomfort to the patient and increases the likelihood of vomiting, and it should therefore be reserved as a method of last resort. The specimen must be obtained quickly in such cases, as the "window of opportunity" is brief.

Tonsillar Foreign Body Removal

The patient should be sitting upright with the head firmly back against a headrest. An alternative position is used if the foreign body is located posteriorly in the tonsil and the operator is concerned that the foreign body may endanger

CLINICAL TIPS: OBTAINING A THROAT CULTURE

▶ Having on older child say the traditional "ah" decreases gagging, which, if unanticipated, can interfere with obtaining an adequate specimen. Crying sometimes serves the same purpose in younger children.

▶ Intentionally making a younger or uncooperative child gag is sometimes the only means of obtaining an adequate throat culture. Intentionally caused gagging results in great discomfort to the child and increases the likelihood of vomiting, and it should there be reserved as a method of last resort.

the airway if not secured during the procedure. In such cases, the patient is positioned in a lateral decubitus position, the tonsil with the foreign body oriented in the "down" position. Younger or less cooperative children may require gentle but firm restraint. Using topical anesthesia such as Cetacaine spray or viscous lidocaine will often aid removal of a tonsillar foreign body. A tongue blade should be used to fully depress the tongue and expose the foreign body.

Fishbones, meat bones, pins, and plastic spicular matter should be grasped firmly with a straight or curved hemostat or fine biopsy forceps and gently removed. Nonregular man-made and vegetable matter foreign bodies and tonsilloliths can be loosened with a probe and then grasped with a hemostat or forceps. Care should always be taken to protect the airway during the entire procedure. Removal of a tonsillolith by a surgeon is sometimes necessary to establish a diagnosis. The differential diagnosis of tonsillolith includes granulomatous disease (tuberculosis, syphilis, actinomycosis) and infection.

SUMMARY: OBTAINING A THROAT CULTURE

1 Seat the child on parent's lap or supine on the examination table.

2 Depress the tongue with a tongue blade; illuminate the oropharynx.

3 Insert the swab into the oropharynx and rub against the posterior oropharynx and both tonsils.

SUMMARY: TONSILLAR FOREIGN BODY REMOVAL

1 Place the required equipment at the bedside.

2 Have the patient seated with his or her head firmly against the headrest; consider a lateral decubitus position (affected tonsil facing "down") if the foreign body is overlying the posterior oropharynx in close proximity to the glottic opening.

3 Firmly grasp spicular foreign bodies with a fine-tipped biopsy (alligator) forceps or with a straight or curved hemostat.

4 Carefully loosen nonregular foreign bodies and tonsilloliths with a probe and grasp with a hemostat or forceps and gently remove.

CLINICAL TIPS: TONSILLAR FOREIGN BODY REMOVAL

▶ A high degree of suspicion should be maintained during the investigation of a possible retained foreign body, especially in young, preverbal children or those with developmental delay.

▶ Acute onset of pain and progressively worsening discomfort and odynophagia are common presenting symptoms.

▶ Most foreign bodies in the tonsil are spicular; most, but not all, are radiopaque. A lateral radiograph of the soft tissues of the neck should be obtained to identify the shape, size, and location of a foreign body. Of note, not all fish species bones are radiographically visible.

▶ The differential diagnosis for tonsilloliths includes infection and granulomatous disease.

▶ Suction equipment and equipment for advanced airway management should be readily available whenever a tonsillar foreign body is removed.

Management of Peritonsillar Abscess

Evaluation and management of a peritonsillar abscess requires careful examination of the oropharynx and should take place in an examining chair with a headrest or in the lap of the parent, who can stabilize the child's head. Optimal visualization requires good light; direct lighting is provided by a handheld source or headlight, and indirect lighting by a head mirror. Careful inspection of the tonsils and peritonsillar region should note size, symmetry and displacement, surface appearance and the presence of rubor, pus, and site of an abscess point or a foreign body. The uvula also should be inspected and deviation from the midline noted.

Before transmucosal needle drainage or surgical incision and drainage, application of a topical or local anesthesia will reduce the risk of the child moving during the procedure. Topical anesthesia is preferred over injection to avoid contamination of uninvolved tissues; application of viscous lidocaine with a cotton-tipped swab or spraying of an anesthetic liquid such as Cetacaine reduces both the pain of incision and the gag reflex. The glossopharyngeal nerve can be anesthetized by an injection of lidocaine through the mucosa and into the tonsillar fossa (38). A Luer-Lok syringe attached to a 3-inch dental needle (22 gauge) is used to inject 1% lidocaine, although anesthesia can be incomplete due to the low pH in the abscess. Adequate local anesthesia often is not attainable in young children or uncooperative patients, and procedural sedation with appropriate monitoring may be necessary (see Chapter 33)(39). In such cases, it may be advisable to consult

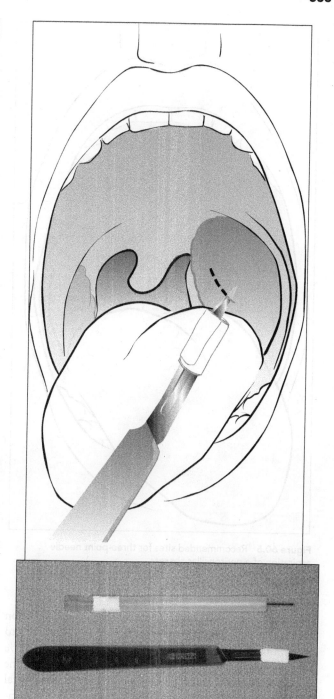

Figure 60.4 The depth of the needle and blade is controlled using a needle guard or an adhesive tape blade guard.

an otolaryngologist for possible incision and drainage in the operating room.

Transmucosal needle aspiration is a straightforward procedure but requires a cooperative patient. The patient is positioned sitting up with the head firmly against a headrest. A 3.5-inch, 20- or 22-gauge needle (a spinal needle will suffice) with a needle guard taped in place is attached to a Luer-Lok 3- or 5-mL syringe. A needle guard is used to limit the depth

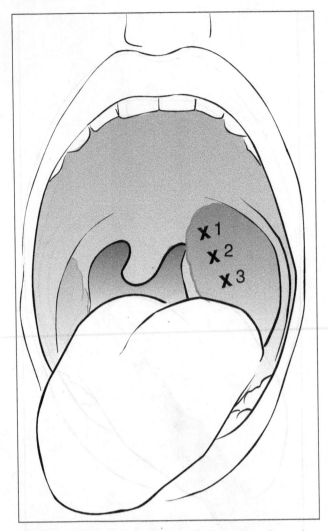

Figure 60.5 Recommended sites for three-point needle aspiration of a peritonsillar abscess.

SUMMARY: MANAGEMENT OF PERITONSILLAR ABSCESS

1 Place the required equipment at the bedside.

2 Have the patient seated with his or her head firmly against the headrest.

3 Use a needle guard or tape a No. 11 or 12 blade to control the depth of needle insertion or incision.

4 For transmucosal needle aspiration, use a three-point technique until pus is obtained:

   a Insert the needle 0.5 to 1 cm and aspirate first at the superior pole; aspirate as much pus as possible.

   b If unsuccessful, insert the needle 0.5 to 1.0 cm inferior to the initial site.

   c If again unsuccessful, aspirate at the inferior pole (yield is lower at this relatively inaccessible location).

5 For incision and drainage:

   a Make a 1- to 2-cm vertical incision through the mucosa overlying the area of greatest pharyngotonsillar bulge or fluctuance.

   b Insert a curved hemostat through the incision and gently spread to break loculations of pus.

   c Suction with rigid suction as necessary.

6 Send aerobic and anaerobic cultures of pus for analysis.

of needle insertion during aspiration—the terminal portion of the plastic needle cover is trimmed beyond which 0.5 to 1.0 cm of the needle will protrude (Fig. 60.4). Up to 90% of abscess collections are located in the superior pole of the peritonsillar space (9,22). The first attempt in the typical three-point needle aspiration is therefore made at the supratonsillar area of the greatest pharyngotonsillar bulge (23). This is superior and medial to the tonsil, at the junction of the anterior tonsillar pillar and the soft palate (Fig. 60.5). A second aspiration is made 0.5 to 1.0 cm below the first if pus is not obtained. A third aspiration may be attempted 0.5 to 1.0 cm lower, near the inferior pole. As much purulent fluid as possible should be drained, and the aspirated fluid sent for aerobic and anaerobic culture.

The site for incision and drainage is similar to that used for aspiration. A No. 11 or 12 surgical scalpel blade is typically used for incision and drainage of a peritonsillar abscess. Adhesive tape is wrapped 0.5 cm from the point of the blade to control the depth of incision (Fig. 60.4). The tip of the

scalpel blade is used to incise 1 to 2 cm of mucosa overlying the area of greatest pharyngotonsillar bulge or fluctuance. A curved hemostat is then placed through the incision and gently spread to extend the incision and break loculated abscess pockets. The abscess cavity should be swabbed for cultures. Large amounts of drainage should be suctioned using a rigid Yankauer suction device.

During either needle aspiration or incision and drainage, great care should be taken to avoid the arterial vessels just lateral to the constrictor muscles. This is accomplished by accurately controlling the direction and depth of the needle or incision with both hands and maintaining complete control of the patient's head at all times.

▶ COMPLICATIONS

Obtaining a Throat Culture

Although uncommon, obtaining a throat culture can result in vomiting. Biting of the swab with ingestion may also occur, although this is rare and the swab is nontoxic. A more likely and significant "complication" is the failure to obtain an adequate

CLINICAL TIPS: MANAGEMENT OF PERITONSILLAR ABSCESS

▶ Signs and symptoms characteristic of a peritonsillar abscess include trismus, dysphagia, odynophagia, drooling, fever, "hot potato" voice, deviation of the uvula away from the abscess, and bulging of the posterolateral soft palate.

▶ It may be difficult to differentiate peritonsillar abscess from cellulitis. In such cases, management usually involves parenteral antibiotic therapy and hospitalization. The decision to perform needle aspiration or incision and drainage should be made in consultation with an otolaryngologist.

▶ Up to 90% of peritonsillar abscesses are localized in the superior pole; this is the optimum site for aspiration or incision.

▶ Laterally directed aspiration or incision should be avoided. Branches of the facial artery are just lateral to the constrictor muscles, and the carotid vessels are located no more than 2 cm lateral to the tonsillar fossae.

▶ Suction equipment and equipment for advanced airway management should be readily available whenever aspiration or incision and drainage of a peritonsillar abscess is performed.

specimen so that the diagnosis of streptococcal pharyngitis is missed, increasing the risk of rheumatic fever and suppurative complications.

Tonsillar Foreign Body Removal

Although unlikely, aspiration of the foreign body by the patient is the most significant risk. The clinician must carefully grasp the object with whatever instrument is used and ensure that the child remains motionless. A rare complication is puncture of or erosion into peritonsillar vessels by the foreign body, resulting in significant hemorrhage upon removal. This is a much greater risk for chronic foreign bodies. Prompt direct pressure should be applied to any bleeding that occurs. If bleeding cannot be controlled in this fashion, exploration of the bleeding site is performed by an otolaryngologist in the operating room.

Management of Peritonsillar Abscess

Local bleeding usually occurs at the site of aspiration or incision and drainage of a peritonsillar abscess, but this is generally brief and self-limited. Hemorrhage from the carotid or jugular vessels may result from direct surgical injury or from erosion of the vessel wall due to the abscess itself, although this is rare (40). Direct pressure should be applied to any bleeding site. Surgical exploration is indicated if bleeding cannot be controlled easily in 5 to 10 minutes or if bleeding is severe. The patient may aspirate blood or purulent material, and this should be anticipated by arranging ready access to suction equipment.

▶ SUMMARY

Procedures involving the pharynx that are most commonly performed on an outpatient basis by physicians who care for children and adolescents include obtaining a throat culture, removal of a tonsillar foreign body, and needle aspiration or incision and drainage of a peritonsillar abscess. In most cases, the techniques involved are straightforward, particularly when the patient is cooperative. The physician can usually enhance patient cooperation with potentially painful procedures by liberally anesthetizing the oropharyngeal mucosa with a topical agent and by carefully explaining each step in a calm and reassuring manner. Light sedation may also be used for a more anxious child. Because the patient must remain motionless for foreign body removal and for aspiration or incision and drainage of a peritonsillar abscess, younger children who clearly cannot cooperate are usually best managed by an otolaryngologist in the operating room. In the outpatient setting, airway equipment and suction should be readily available when any invasive procedure involving the oropharynx is performed.

▶ REFERENCES

1. Denny FW, Wannamaker LW, Brink WR, et al. Prevention of rheumatic fever: treatment of preceding streptococcal infection. *JAMA.* 1950;143:151–153.
2. Denny FW, Wannamaker LW, Brink WR, et al. Landmark article, May 13, 1950. *JAMA.* 1985;254:534–537.
3. Jones NS, Lannigan FJ, Salama NY. Foreign bodies in the throat: a prospective study of 388 cases. *J Laryngol Otol.* 1991;105:104–108.
4. Lapetus VF. Peritonsillar abscess in a 4-month-old child. *J Laryngol Otol.* 1987;101:617–618.
5. Shenoy P, David VC. A case of quinsy in a 15-month-old child. *J Laryngol Otol.* 1993;107:354–355.
6. Dodds B, Maniglia AJ. Peritonsillar and neck abscesses in the pediatric age group. *Laryngoscope.* 1988;98:956–959.
7. Holt GR, Tinslet PP. Peritonsillar abscesses in children. *Laryngoscope.* 1981;91:1226–1230.
8. Parker GS, Tami TA. The management of peritonsillar abscess in the 90s: an update. *Am J Otolaryngol.* 1992;13:284–288.
9. Weinberg E, Brodsky L, Stanievich J, et al. Needle aspiration of peritonsillar abscess in children. *Arch Otolaryngol Head Neck Surg.* 1993;119:169–172.
10. Brodsky L, Sobie SR, Korwin D, et al. A clinical prospective study of peritonsillar abscess in children. *Laryngoscope.* 1988;98:780–783.
11. Sexton DG, Babin RW. Peritonsillar abscess: a comparison of a conservative and a more aggressive management protocol. *Int J Pediatr Otolaryngol.* 1987;14:129–132.

12. Clemente CD, ed. *Gray's Anatomy*. 30th ed. Philadelphia: Lea & Febiger; 1985.

13. Binder L, Anderson WA. Pediatric gastrointestinal foreign body ingestions. *Ann Emerg Med*. 1984;13:112–117.

14. Gracia C, Frey CF, Bodai BI. Diagnosis and management of ingested foreign bodies: a 10-year experience. *Ann Emerg Med*. 1984;13:30–34.

15. Norris CM. Foreign bodies in the air and food passages: a series of 250 cases. *Ann Otol Rhinol Laryngol*. 1948;57:1049–1071.

16. Osborne EA. Unusual foreign body in tonsil: case report. *J Laryngol Otol*. 1966;80:962–963.

17. Pruett CW, Duplan DA. Tonsil concretions and tonsilloliths. *Otolaryngol Clin North Am*. 1987;20:305–309.

18. Dale JW, Wing G. Clinical and technical examination of a tonsillolith: a case report. *Aust Dent J*. 1974;19:84–87.

19. Shrimali R, Bhatia PL. A giant radiopaque tonsillolith. *J Indian Med Assoc*. 1972;58:174–175.

20. Marshall WG, Irwin ND. Tonsilloliths. *Oral Surg Oral Med Oral Pathol*. 1981;51:113.

21. Maisel RH. Peritonsillar abscess: tonsil antibiotic levels in patients treated by acute abscess surgery. *Laryngoscope*. 1982;92:80–87.

22. Zalzal GH, Cotton RT. Pharyngitis and adenotonsillar disease. In: Cummings CW, Fredrickson JM, Hanker CA, et al., eds. *Otorhinolaryngology: Head and Neck Surgery*. 2nd ed. St. Louis: Mosby; 1993:1180–1198.

23. Spires JR, Owens JJ, Woodson GE, et al. Treatment of peritonsillar abscess: a prospective study of aspiration versus incision and drainage. *Arch Otolaryngol Head Neck Surg*. 1987;113:984–986.

24. Brook I, Frazier EH, Thompson DHL. Aerobic and anaerobic microbiology of peritonsillar abscess. *Laryngoscope*. 1991;101:289–292.

25. Ophir D, Bawnik J, Poria Y, et al. Peritonsillar abscess: a prospective evaluation of outpatient management by needle aspiration. *Arch Otolaryngol Head Neck Surg*. 1988;114:661–663.

26. Ell SR, Sprigg A. The radiopacity of fishbones-species variation. *Clin Radiol*. 1991;44:104–107.

27. Bredenkamp JK, Maceri DR. Inflammatory torticollis in children. *Arch Otolaryngol Head Neck Surg*. 1990;116:310–313.

28. Shoemaker M, Lampe RM, Weir MR. Peritonsillitis: abscess or cellulitis? *Pediatr Infect Dis J*. 1986;5:435–439.

29. Ahmed K, Jones AS, Shah K, et al. The role of ultrasound in the management of peritonsillar abscess. *J Laryngol Otol*. 1994;108:610–612.

30. Strong EB, Woodward PJ, Johnson LP. Intraoral ultrasound evaluation of peritonsillar abscess. *Laryngoscope*. 1995;105:779–781.

31. Suskind DL, Park J, Piccirillo JF. Conscious sedation: a new approach for peritonsillar abscess drainage in the pediatric population. *Arch Otolaryngol Head Neck Surg*. 1999;125:1197–1200.

32. Scott PM, Loftus WK, Kew J. Diagnosis of peritonsillar infections: a prospective study of ultrasound, computerized tomography and clinical diagnosis. *J Laryngol Otol*. 1999;113:229–233.

33. Stringer SP, Schaefer SD, Close LG. A randomized trial for outpatient management of peritonsillar abscess. *Arch Otolaryngol*. 1988;114:278–298.

34. Johnson RF, Stewart MG, Wright CC. An evidence-based review of the treatment of peritonsillar abscess. *Otolaryngol Head Neck Surgery*. 2003;128:332–343.

35. Pinchichero ME, Disney FA, Talpey WB, et al. Adverse and beneficial effects of immediate treatment of Group A beta-hemolytic streptococcal pharyngitis with penicillin. *Pediatr Infect Dis J*. 1987;6:635–643.

36. Gerber MA. Effect of early antibiotic therapy on recurrence rates of streptococcal pharyngitis. *Pediatr Infect Dis J*. 1991;10(suppl):56–60.

37. Roosevelt GE, Kulkarni MS, Shulman ST. Critical evaluation of a CLIA-waived streptococcal antigen test in the emergency department. *Ann Emerg Med*. 2001;37:377–381.

38. Scott BA, Stiernberg CM. Deep neck space infections. In: Bailey BJ, ed. *Head and Neck Surgery-Otolaryngology*. Philadelphia: JB Lippincott; 1993.

39. Suskind DL, Park J, Piccirillo JF. Conscious sedation: a new approach for peritonsillar abscess drainage in the pediatric population. *Arch Otolaryngol Head Neck Surg*. 1999;125:1197–2000.

40. Blum DJ, McCaffrey TV. Septic necrosis of the internal carotid artery: a complication of peritonsillar abscess. *Otolaryngol Head Neck Surg*. 1983;91:114–118.

ERIN D. PHRAMPUS AND ROBERT F. YELLON

61

Diagnostic Laryngoscopic Procedures

▶ INTRODUCTION

The larynx, hypopharynx, and posterior nasopharynx cannot be adequately visualized by simple examination, and results obtained on plain radiograph may be incomplete or misleading. Special equipment and techniques are therefore necessary to gain accurate information regarding the anatomy and function of these structures. Children who present with complaints such as recurrent or persistent stridor, chronic hoarseness, or a suspected airway foreign body (without respiratory distress) may be candidates for these procedures. A preliminary examination in the emergency department (ED), office, or other outpatient setting can aid the physician in determining the appropriate management, disposition, and follow-up studies for the patient. Thus diagnostic laryngoscopy is a valuable skill for emergency physicians, pediatricians, and family physicians.

The upper airway can be divided anatomically into the extrathoracic and intrathoracic regions. The extrathoracic region can further be divided into the supraglottic area (nasopharynx, epiglottis, larynx, aryepiglottic folds, and false vocal cords) and the glottic/subglottic area (extending from the vocal cords to the extrathoracic segment of the trachea). With indirect laryngoscopy, the glottis, vocal cords, and supraglottic structures are visualized using an angled mirror placed above the patient's larynx. Direct laryngoscopy involves visualization of the larynx through an eyepiece using an angled telescope or flexible fiberoptic laryngoscope. Advances in fiberoptic technology have led to the development of progressively smaller devices that are appropriate for pediatric use and have excellent image resolution. The flexible fiberoptic laryngoscope can also be used to examine the nasal cavity.

These techniques can be used for most stable pediatric patients. Infants and younger children are not developmentally capable of cooperating with indirect laryngoscopic procedures. Older children and adolescents may be able to tolerate an indirect laryngoscopic examination if the procedure is thoroughly explained and carefully performed. The procedures described in this chapter are intended for the outpatient examination of pediatric patients who are generally well. If there are signs of respiratory distress, an otolaryngologist should perform the procedure, preferably in the operating room. Even with the well child, airway equipment should be readily available when these procedures are performed, as inadvertent contact with the larynx in rare instances can precipitate laryngospasm.

▶ ANATOMY AND PHYSIOLOGY

A detailed discussion of distinguishing features of pediatric airway anatomy can be found in Chapter 16. The upper airway starts with the nasal cavity and continues with the nasopharynx and oropharynx to the larynx and the extrathoracic segment of the trachea. The structures of greatest interest during diagnostic laryngoscopy are the posterior nasopharynx and adenoids, the hypopharynx, and the vocal cords and supraglottic region (Fig. 61.1).

The upper airways are protected from infection by a system of lymphatic tissue known as the Waldeyer ring, which comprises the lymphoid tissue in the nasopharynx (adenoid tissue), the lymphatic tissue at the base of the tongue (lingual tonsils), and the two palatine tonsils. However, this lymphatic system can also become a site of acute or chronic infection. Adenoidal hypertrophy can occur with or without infection, and extensive hypertrophy can result in blockage of the nasal passages. Enlarged adenoids can obstruct the eustachian tube orifice, leading to otitis media. Chronic upper airway obstruction often presents with evidence of obstructive sleep apnea syndrome. In severe cases, these children may present with pulmonary hypertension and cor pulmonale (1).

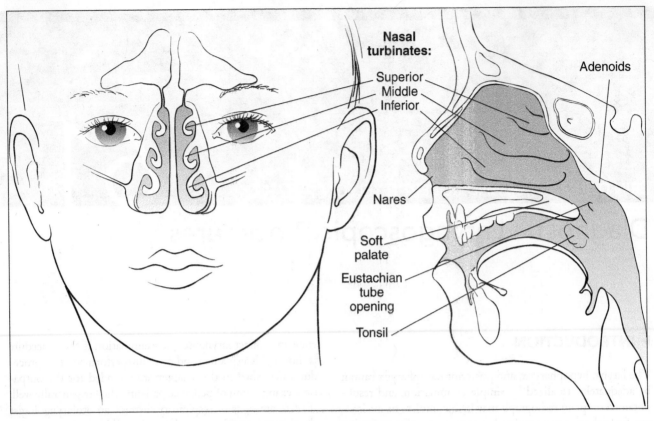

Figure 61.1 Anatomy of the nasal cavity.

Foreign bodies can become embedded in the hypopharynx and supraglottic areas, and these may be undetectable on routine physical examination of the oropharynx. In addition, plain radiographs may not identify certain types of items, including tiny fish bones, wooden splinters, and organic materials such as sunflower seeds and nuts. Indirect or direct laryngoscopy may be the only means of detecting such a foreign body (2).

The larynx is part of the anterior hypopharynx (Fig. 61.2). In newborns, the larynx is at the level of C3–C4 and gradually descends to the level of C6–C7 around adolescence. The hyoid bone forms the upper limit of the larynx, which is divided into the supraglottic, glottic, and subglottic regions. The supraglottic region encompasses the area above the vocal cords and includes the epiglottis, arytenoids, aryepiglottic folds, and the false vocal cords. The glottic region includes the vocal cords and the subglottic structures extending 1 cm below the vocal folds in the upper cervical trachea. The true vocal cords are paired, V-shaped structures with the point facing anteriorly. The vocal cords vibrate to produce the sound of the voice. Abnormalities may result in hoarseness or stridor.

Phonation results from a series of minute changes in the muscular tension exerted on the vocal cords as air is forced out through the glottic opening. The vocal cords vibrate to produce the sound of the voice. In pediatric patients, common causes of hoarseness or stridor include laryngomalacia, vocal cord paralysis or paresis, vocal cord nodules, subglottic hemangioma, and juvenile laryngeal papillomatosis (3–5).

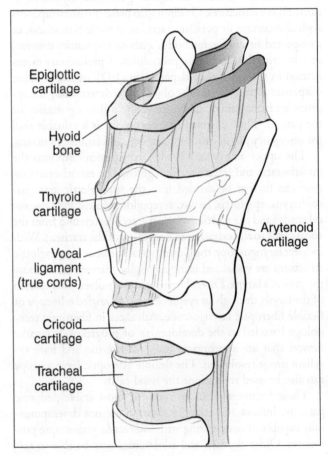

Figure 61.2 Anatomy of the larynx.

Infants with a low-pitched cry who have findings suggestive of a neuromuscular disorder, a congenital anomaly of the mediastinum (e.g., tracheoesophageal fistula, vascular ring), or Arnold Chiari malformation should be suspected of having unilateral or bilateral vocal cord paralysis. The large, floppy epiglottis of an infant often will fall back and forth over the glottis during respiration, giving the clinician an intermittent view of the vocal cords on laryngoscopy.

▶ INDICATIONS

A variety of presenting complaints may serve as indications for performing indirect or direct laryngoscopic procedures (Table 61.1). In general, any child with persistent symptoms believed to involve the nasopharynx, supraglottic region, or vocal cords that cannot be explained based on findings from a routine physical examination may be a candidate for a diagnostic laryngoscopic procedure. The safety of these techniques when performed properly has been demonstrated in both the inpatient and outpatient settings (6–16).

Complaints such as voice changes, chronic stridor or hoarseness, an unusual cry, and persistent odynophagia should generally prompt the physician to examine the vocal cords and supraglottic region using indirect or direct laryngoscopy. Abnormalities of vocal cord function or the presence of a penetrating foreign body warrant evaluation by an otolaryngologist. One relatively common cause of stridor in infancy is laryngomalacia. It accounts for 65% to 75% of all cases of stridor and is caused by the collapse of the supraglottic structures during respiration. It is a self-limited condition that typically resolves without therapy by 12 to 18 months of age. However, in about 5% of affected children the upper airway obstruction is severe enough to cause apnea or failure to thrive. The etiology of laryngomalacia is unknown, and some investigators believe it represents a form of laryngeal "hypotonia," while others believe that increased flexibility of the cartilage is the cause. Infants with laryngomalacia typically have inspiratory stridor that is more pronounced when supine and decreases when prone. Abnormalities of swallowing may occur in up to 50% of patients (17). Laryngoscopy will reveal the epiglottis and the arytenoids collapsing into the glottis with inspiration during spontaneous ventilation (18). No-

tably, children exposed to hot fumes or a house fire may have no stridor or voice change initially, despite thermal injury. In such children, a laryngoscopic examination that shows edema or carbonaceous deposits requires that the patients be subject to close observation and often early endotracheal intubation.

Children with chronic mouth breathing, snoring respirations, or persistent nasal drainage often require an examination of the nasopharynx with a fiberoptic laryngoscope (19–22). Obstruction of the nasal cavity in children is commonly caused by adenoidal hypertrophy. The finding of significantly enlarged adenoid tissue, particularly when the orifice of the eustachian tube is occluded, is an indication for referral to an otolaryngologist. Other conditions causing chronic nasal obstruction include nasal polyps, the presence of a foreign body, and encephalocele, which can communicate directly with cerebrospinal fluid (23). Polyps appear as gray, grapelike masses in the nasal cavity and are highly associated with cystic fibrosis. A foreign body not seen on a more limited examination may be visible during an examination of the posterior nasal cavity with a fiberoptic laryngoscope. Care should be taken not to push the object posteriorly, which may result in aspiration.

Indirect laryngoscopy offers the advantage of providing a wide, panoramic view that direct techniques cannot achieve. Success with this procedure requires cooperation from the patient and a clinician who has had ongoing experience. Indirect laryngoscopy is unsuitable for neonates, infants, and young children, as a high degree of cooperation is required. This technique will usually be successful in older children and adolescents if the clinician thoroughly explains what is expected and is careful not to stimulate the patient's gag reflex. The flexible fiberoptic laryngoscope is better tolerated by children of all ages and can be used even in crying infants and children. With proper training and repeated experience, an emergency physician can become adept at performing the preliminary examination. Patients should be advised to follow up with an otolaryngologist if there are concerning findings on the examination, an inadequate examination has been performed, or there are continued symptoms.

Diagnostic evaluation in the ED or office using laryngoscopic techniques is contraindicated for the patient with respiratory distress. The child with a high-grade obstruction of the extrathoracic airway due to a foreign body is not a candidate for diagnostic laryngoscopy outside the operating room. The patient's marginal respiratory status may be further compromised during the procedure, and total obstruction may result if the object is inadvertently advanced into the proximal airway. In such situations, the stable patient should be immediately transferred to the operating room, where rigid bronchoscopy or emergent tracheotomy can be performed by an otolaryngologist. An unstable patient should undergo direct laryngoscopy using a standard laryngoscope blade and handle to allow removal of the foreign body (see Chapter 51). Direct diagnostic laryngoscopy also is contraindicated in situations when advanced airway management techniques would not be possible. Although a rare complication, laryngospasm can result when a fiberoptic laryngoscope is inadvertently introduced below the level of the vocal cords. For this reason,

TABLE 61.1	INDICATIONS FOR DIAGNOSTIC LARYNGOSCOPY

Acute change in voice
Unusual cry (low pitched or breathy)
Chronic hoarseness
Persistent stridor
Chronic mouth breathing
Snoring respirations while sleeping
Chronic nasal discharge
Persistent odynophagia
Chronic cough
Suspected exposure to hot fumes or gases (e.g., a house fire)

the clinician must be fully prepared to secure the airway by emergent intubation or a surgical technique if necessary.

▶ EQUIPMENT

Indirect Laryngoscopy
Examination chair
Light source (two options):
   Head mirror with high-intensity lighting behind patient
   Electric headlamp
Angled mirror
Laryngeal mirror warmer or other defogging method
Gauze to hold patient's tongue
Cetacaine spray (2% tetracaine hydrochloride, 14% benzocaine)
Personal protection gear (minimum of gloves and eye protection)

Flexible Direct Laryngoscopy
Suction machine and catheters (tonsil tip, 8 French)
Topical vasoconstrictor:
   For infants, 0.25% phenylephrine
   For children, one of the following:
      0.5% phenylephrine (Neosynephrine) spray
      1% ephedrine sulfate spray
      0.05% oxymetazoline (Afrin) spray
Topical anesthetic (one of the following):
      2% tetracaine hydrochloride solution (maximum dose 0.75 mg/kg)
      4% lidocaine solution (maximum dose 5 mg/kg)
Cotton pledgets or spray device
Forceps (bayonet or alligator)
Nasal speculum
Pulse oximeter
Flexible fiberoptic laryngoscope
Rigid direct laryngoscopy angled telescope
Personal protection gear (minimum of gloves and eye protection)

Diagnostic laryngoscopy can be performed using almost any type of chair (or stretcher); however, the procedure is greatly facilitated by an examination chair that can swivel, has a headrest for the patient, and has a foot pedal that allows the clinician to automatically adjust the height.

As mentioned previously, advances in fiberoptic technology have led to the development of smaller laryngoscopic devices suitable for use with any pediatric age group (24). Manufacturers of pediatric units include Machida, Olympus, and Welch-Allen. The basic elements of a fiberoptic laryngoscope are the eyepiece, through which the image is visualized, and the insertion tube containing the fiberoptic bundles (Fig. 61.3). The insertion tube must hold at least two fiberoptic bundles—one that transmits light to illuminate the structures being viewed and another that transmits the desired image back to the eyepiece. The number of glass strands in each bundle largely determines the image quality (and cost)

of the laryngoscope. If available, a portable light source permits the clinician to use a fiberoptic laryngoscope in any room of the ED. Some units also have a capability for video monitoring and recording, which can be useful for teaching purposes and documenting the examination. Currently, fiberoptic laryngoscopes with an outer diameter of 2.2 mm are available, a size that can easily be passed through the nasal cavity of even an infant. The primary limitation of these smaller devices is the lack of a suction port to allow removal of secretions, which can make visualization of the airway anatomy more difficult.

After each use, the fiberoptic laryngoscope should be immediately cleansed with a detergent solution to prevent drying of secretions on the insertion tube. The laryngoscope is then sterilized according to the manufacturer's instructions. Not surprisingly, inadequate cleaning and sterilization have been demonstrated to cause transmission of a variety of infectious agents among patients (25,26).

Special care must be taken when wiping the insertion tube. Grasping the laryngoscope with gauze and pulling vigorously causes the material covering the fiberoptic bundles to bunch up at the tip, making subsequent passage difficult. In addition, bending the insertion tube excessively can cause breakage of the glass bundles. Disposable sheaths for single use are available from commercial suppliers for fiberoptic laryngoscopes.

▶ PROCEDURE

Indirect Laryngoscopy

The patient should be seated and leaning forward in the "sniffing" position—that is, with the head slightly extended

---

SUMMARY: INDIRECT LARYNGOSCOPY

1 Position the patient seated and leaning forward in the "sniffing" position.

2 Spray a topical anesthetic in the posterior oropharynx to reduce the patient's gag reflex.

3 Warm the laryngeal mirror to prevent fogging.

4 Grasp the tongue with gauze and gently pull forward.

5 Illuminate the oropharynx with a direct light source or a head mirror.

6 Insert the mirror into the patient's mouth, and position it over the back of the tongue with the mirror angled downward.

7 Visualize the larynx and surrounding structures by tilting the mirror as necessary.

8 Assess vocal cord function by having the patient say "EEEEE" and hum a tune.

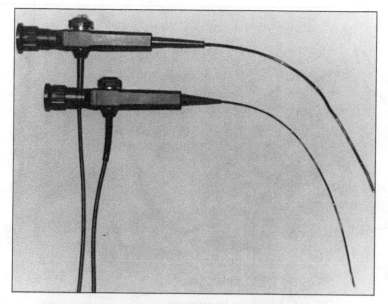

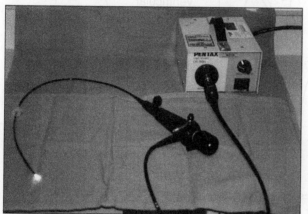

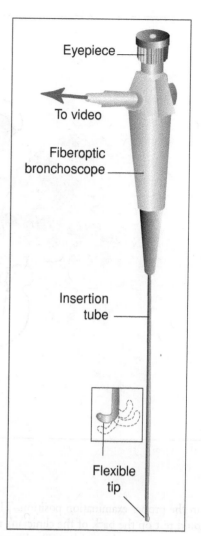

Figure 61.3 Flexible fiberoptic laryngoscopes for pediatric use.

(rotated) and the neck flexed. Spraying Cetacaine or another topical anesthetic may be helpful in controlling the patient's gag reflex. If a head mirror is used to illuminate the airway, a strong light source should be positioned over the patient's shoulder so that the light can be reflected from the mirror into the patient's mouth. Adequate lighting is essential to successfully complete the procedure. For the physician who performs this technique less frequently, an electric headlight provides excellent illumination and is usually much easier to use. The laryngeal mirror should be warmed to prevent fogging. If a laryngeal mirror warmer is not available, the angled mirror can be placed under warm running water and then dried before use to prevent fogging. The temperature of the mirror is tested against the back of the clinician's hand before use to avoid burning the patient.

The patient is first instructed to breath in and out through the mouth during the entire procedure. This may be better understood if the child is periodically reminded to pant "just like a dog." Next the tongue is grasped with gauze and gently pulled forward. The clinician inserts the mirror into the patient's mouth and positions it over the back of the tongue and

angled downward (Fig. 61.4). Care must be taken to avoid contacting the tongue or posterior pharyngeal wall with the mirror, as this usually will induce gagging. The light source is directed onto the mirror and down the airway. The larynx and surrounding structures then can be visualized by tilting the mirror back and forth as necessary. Vocal cord function is initially assessed by observing as the patient says "EEEEE," which should cause the cords to adduct. The clinician then can ask the patient to hum a tune, which results in adduction and abduction of the cords throughout their full range of motion.

Direct Laryngoscopy with an Angled Telescope

The patient is positioned in the same manner as with the indirect technique. The angled telescope is passed into the patient's mouth until the tip is over the base of the tongue. As with the use of an angled mirror, the best way to prevent gagging and emesis is to avoid inadvertent contact with the tongue and posterior pharynx. For this reason, the clinician should not look through the eyepiece until the instrument

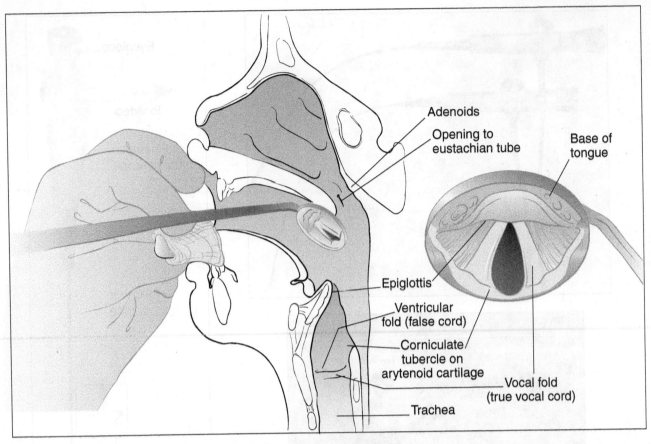

Figure 61.4 Indirect laryngoscopy.

is in the proper examination position. The angled telescope should rest on the back of the clinician's nondominant hand to maintain a steady position. The larynx and hypopharynx can then be viewed. Vocal cord function is assessed as with indirect laryngoscopy.

  SUMMARY: DIRECT LARYNGOSCOPY WITH AN ANGLED TELESCOPE

1 Position the patient seated and leaning forward in the "sniffing" position.

2 Spray a topical anesthetic in the posterior oropharynx to reduce the patient's gag reflex.

3 Insert an angled telescope into the patient's mouth until the tip is positioned over the back of the tongue.

4 Steady the telescope by resting it on the operator's nondominant hand.

5 View the larynx and hypopharynx.

6 Assess vocal cord function by having the patient say "EEEEE" and hum a tune.

Direct Laryngoscopy with a Flexible Fiberoptic Laryngoscope

The clinician first should examine the patient's nose with a nasal speculum to determine the more patent side and to identify any obstruction to airflow. The laryngoscope should be passed on the more patent side. If the nasal cavity is a primary area of interest, the clinician will insert the laryngoscope into both nares during the examination.

The topical vasoconstrictor and anesthetic are applied to one or both nares using cotton pledgets with a nasal speculum and forceps or by spraying. As mentioned previously, 1% ephedrine sulfate and 2% tetracaine hydrochloride are effective for this purpose. In order to achieve the full effects of these agents, the clinician should wait 5 to 10 minutes after application. Most local anesthetics are bitter, and the patient often will complain of the taste. The clinician should explain that it is not harmful to swallow any medicine that accumulates in the back of the patient's throat. It also is advisable to warn the patient that the resulting sensation of numbness may make swallowing or even breathing seem more difficult. Reassurance is all that is necessary for these complaints. The patient should not be fed for 1 hour following administration of a topical anesthetic to avoid aspiration.

A cooperative patient can be positioned sitting upright with the neck flexed and the head slightly extended (rotated),

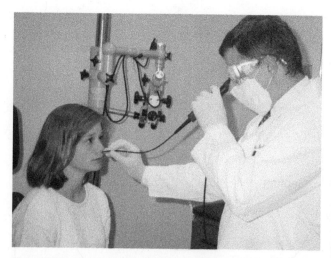

Figure 61.5 Positioning for flexible fiberoptic laryngoscopy.

similar to the positioning for indirect laryngoscopy (Fig. 61.5). Infants and younger children should be placed in the supine position and appropriately restrained. Before inserting the fiberoptic laryngoscope, the clinician should view an object through the eyepiece to ensure that the tip is clean and the focal length correct. The tip also should be manipulated to determine how much force is needed to move it a given amount. Great care must be taken to not bend the laryngoscope excessively, as this can cause the fiberoptic bundles to break. The lens may be rinsed with a minute amount of soap to prevent fogging of the scope.

The tip of a flexible fiberoptic laryngoscope is directed by the clinician using a combination of two motions. Rotating the eyepiece along its axis translates to rotation of the entire insertion tube. The flexible tip of the insertion tube also can be directed back and forth along a single plane using a control

lever on the eyepiece. By systematically deflecting the tip and rotating the insertion tube, the clinician can obtain a complete view of the airway.

While viewing through the eyepiece, the clinician inserts the fiberoptic laryngoscope along the floor of the nasal cavity parallel to the septum and medial to the inferior turbinate (Fig. 61.6). Importantly, the laryngoscope should never be advanced blindly, because this increases the likelihood of causing injury to the nasal or pharyngeal mucosa. Gentle suctioning may be required to remove secretions. If the landmarks are lost during insertion, the clinician should withdraw the laryngoscope until recognizable structures are again seen. Likewise, if the tip of the laryngoscope fogs, the patient should be instructed to breathe in and out through the mouth until the image reappears. The laryngoscope then can be advanced once again under direct visualization. As appropriate, the clinician should carefully examine the posterior nasal cavity to identify adenoid hypertrophy (Fig. 61.7), the orifice of the eustachian tube, nasal polyps, and/or the presence of an intranasal foreign body.

As the posterior nasal cavity is approached, the tip of the laryngoscope should be deflected inferiorly so that it can be passed atraumatically over the posterior aspect of the soft palate. Injury to the posterior pharyngeal wall can be avoided by maintaining direct visualization at all times and never using excessive force to advance the laryngoscope. Once this turn is negotiated, the base of the tongue will come into view. By rotating the laryngoscope from side to side, the clinician also can identify the medial aspect of each tonsil. The laryngoscope is then further advanced until the larynx can be fully visualized (Fig. 61.8).

As mentioned previously, the clinician must be careful to avoid contacting supraglottic structures and the vocal cords with the tip of the laryngoscope, as this can precipitate

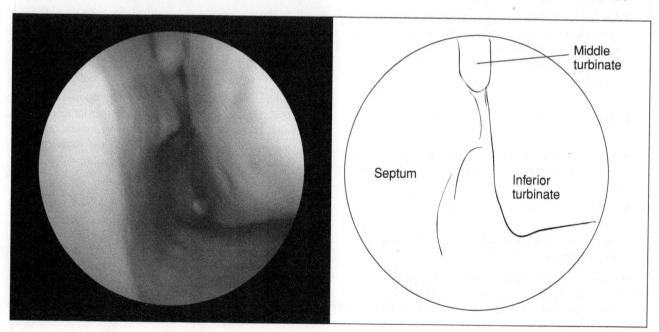

Figure 61.6 View of the left nasal cavity with fiberoptic laryngoscopy.

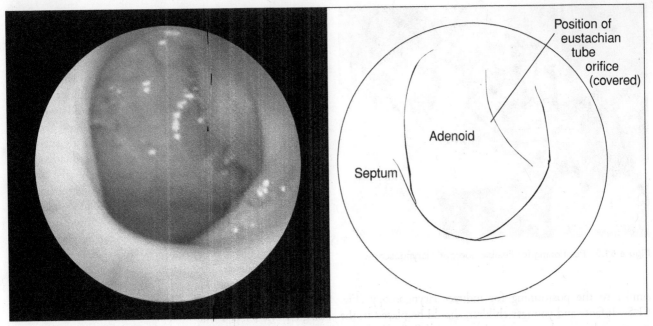

Figure 61.7 Adenoid hypertrophy.

laryngospasm. Vocal cord function is assessed by having the patient say "EEEEE" or humming a tune, as with indirect laryngoscopy. With younger children who are unable to co-operate, the cords are observed for any abnormal movement as the patient phonates or cries. Polyps or other lesions of the vocal cords should be noted. In addition, the clinician should carefully examine the epiglottis and arytenoid cartilages. Because a complete view of the entire supraglottic region is not obtainable in one field of vision, the clinician must system-atically rotate the laryngoscope while deflecting the tip to

---

 SUMMARY: DIAGNOSTIC LARYNGOSCOPY USING A FLEXIBLE FIBEROPTIC LARYNGOSCOPE

1 Identify the more patent nostril using a nasal speculum and use that side for insertion (unless both nasal cavities are to be examined).

2 Apply a topical vasoconstrictor and an anesthetic to one or both nares using cotton pledgets or a spray device (1% ephedrine sulfate and 2% tetracaine hydrochloride is a good combination); allow 5 to 10 minutes for these agents to achieve their full effect.

3 Position the patient seated and leaning forward in the "sniffing" position.

4 Before inserting the fiberoptic laryngoscope, view an object through the eyepiece to ensure that the tip is clean and the focal length is correct.

5 Deflect the tip back and forth using the control lever on the head of the laryngoscope to determine the force necessary to move the tip a given amount.

6 While viewing through the eyepiece, insert the fiberoptic laryngoscope along the floor of the nasal cavity parallel to the septum and medial to the inferior turbinate.

7 Examine the entire nasal cavity and nasopharynx, noting adenoid size, patency of eustachian tube orifice, nasal polyps, etc.

8 At the posterior nasal cavity, deflect the tip of the fiberoptic laryngoscope inferiorly and advance the tip around the posterior aspect of the soft palate; identify the landmarks of the base of the tongue and the medial aspect of each tonsil.

9 Advance the laryngoscope into supraglottic region and carefully examine all important structures; deflect the tip and rotate the laryngoscope in a systematic fashion to obtain a complete view of the area; note abnormal lesions, injuries, the presence of a foreign body, etc.

10 Assess vocal cord function:

   a With an infant or younger child, observe the movement of the cords with phonation or crying.

   b With an older child or adolescent, have the patient say "EEEEE" and hum a tune.

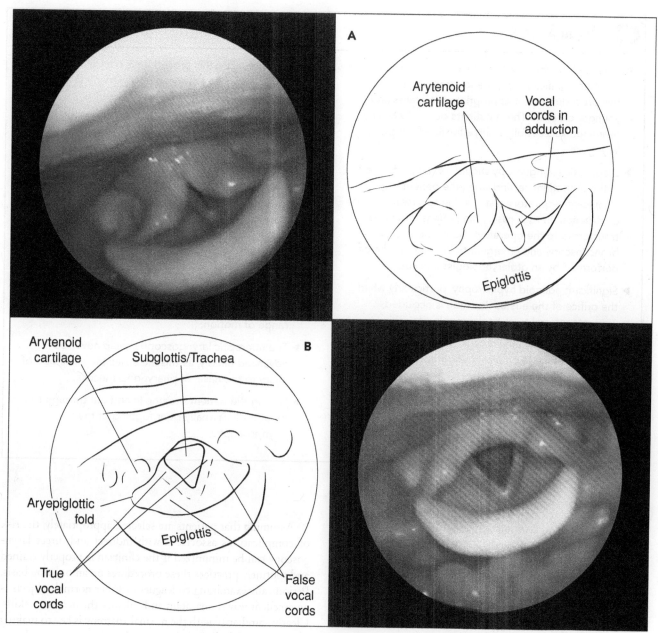

Figure 61.8 View of the larynx with fiberoptic laryngoscopy.
A. Adduction of vocal cords.
B. Abduction of vocal cords.

visualize all the important structures. Any edema, erythema, bleeding, or disruption of the mucosa should be noted. The base of the tongue and piriform sinuses lateral to the larynx must be examined to exclude the presence of a foreign body.

▶ COMPLICATIONS

Although both indirect laryngoscopy and direct laryngoscopy have proven to be safe when used appropriately, certain hazards must be avoided. Proper patient selection is one of the most important factors in reducing the risk of complications.

It cannot be overemphasized that any child with severe respiratory distress is not a suitable candidate for diagnostic laryngoscopy outside the operating room. Conditions such as an expanding hematoma in the supraglottic region or high-grade airway obstruction due to a foreign body can cause a tenuous respiratory status. Agitating a child in this situation may lead to full respiratory arrest. Diagnostic laryngoscopy in the outpatient setting should only be performed on patients who are well appearing and are not experiencing airway compromise.

Complications that are less severe but more frequently encountered relate to problems with technique. Mucosal injuries of the airway can result when a fiberoptic laryngoscope is

CLINICAL TIPS

▶ Because indirect laryngoscopy with an angled mirror requires significant cooperation from the patient, this procedure is not appropriate for infants and younger children. These patients generally can be examined successfully using a flexible fiberoptic laryngoscope.

▶ Diagnostic laryngoscopy should not be performed in the outpatient setting when the patient is in significant respiratory distress due to airway obstruction. In such cases, the patient should be transferred to the operating room where rigid bronchoscopy and emergent tracheostomy can be performed by an otolaryngologist if necessary.

▶ Significant adenoid hypertrophy, particularly when the orifice of the eustachian tube is occluded, warrants referral to an otolaryngologist.

▶ Foreign bodies of the supraglottic region that may not be identifiable on plain radiographs (e.g., wooden splinter, certain types of fish bone) are commonly found using diagnostic laryngoscopy.

▶ Inadvertently introducing a fiberoptic laryngoscope that contacts the supraglottic structures or the vocal cords can in rare cases precipitate laryngospasm.

Consequently, this procedure is contraindicated in situations when advanced airway management techniques would not be possible.

▶ If a laryngeal mirror warmer is not available, the angled mirror can be placed under warm running water and then dried before use to prevent fogging.

▶ Special care must be taken when cleaning the insertion tube of a fiberoptic laryngoscope. Grasping it with gauze and pulling vigorously causes the material covering the fiberoptic bundles to bunch up at the tip, making subsequent passage difficult. In addition, bending the insertion tube excessively can cause breakage of the glass bundles.

▶ Having the patient hum a tune produces adduction and abduction of the vocal cords throughout the full range of motion.

▶ The fiberoptic laryngoscope should never be advanced blindly, as this increases the likelihood of injury to the nasal or pharyngeal mucosa.

▶ Having the patient breathe in and out through the mouth will normally clear fogging of the laryngoscope.

passed blindly (i.e., without maintaining direct visualization through the eyepiece). As with blind nasal passage of an endotracheal tube, abrasions and lacerations of the soft tissues can occur at multiple sites, typically the nasal turbinates, adenoids, and posterior pharynx. Bleeding induced by this type of injury often makes further examination impossible. If airway anesthesia is inadequate or the clinician inadvertently contacts the posterior hypopharynx with an instrument, the patient may cough, gag, or vomit. Although this does not generally lead to any serious consequences because the patient's normal airway reflexes are preserved, subsequent examinations of a previously cooperative child who has undergone serious gagging are likely to be difficult or impossible.

One significant complication related to poor technique is laryngospasm due to accidental passage of a fiberoptic laryngoscope to the point where it touches the supraglottic or glottic structures. Care must therefore be taken to advance the laryngoscope only as far as necessary to fully visualize the larynx and supraglottic region. Although it is a rare occurrence, the risk of laryngospasm requires that all equipment necessary for advanced airway interventions must be available whenever this procedure is performed, and the clinician and the staff should be prepared to initiate such interventions if they are needed.

Assuming that patients are selected appropriately, the risk of complications associated with indirect and direct laryngoscopy can be minimized if the clinician is properly trained and routinely practices these procedures on an ongoing basis. Periodically examining colleagues or other normal subjects is an excellent way to maintain and enhance the necessary skills. Clearly, familiarity with the normal anatomy is key to making any meaningful clinical decisions. In addition, honestly explaining what should be expected to older children and adolescents in a calm and unhurried manner often will reduce the likelihood of complications. Because diagnostic laryngoscopy requires significant cooperation, gaining the trust and compliance of a pediatric patient is usually the most important factor in completing an examination successfully and atraumatically.

▶ SUMMARY

Diagnostic laryngoscopy for pediatric patients of all ages may be performed in the outpatient setting by emergency physicians, pediatricians, and family physicians with proper training and experience. These techniques are performed to obtain a preliminary evaluation of patients with hoarseness, chronic nasal discharge, a suspected foreign body, and other common complaints. Referral to an otolaryngologist for a more definitive examination should be arranged when necessary. Indirect laryngoscopy gives a panoramic view of the larynx but requires practice and is not suitable for infants and younger children. Direct laryngoscopy with a flexible fiberoptic laryngoscope can be used to examine the nasal cavity, supraglottic region, and vocal cords in any age group. Although complications with these procedures are unlikely, good technique and proper patient selection are essential. Children with respiratory distress are not appropriate candidates for outpatient diagnostic laryngoscopy. A thorough knowledge of the anatomy, a gentle technique, and practice will allow the physician to successfully complete this examination.

▶ ACKNOWLEDGMENTS

The authors would like to acknowledge the valuable contributions of J. Christopher Post and Clark A. Rosen to the version of this chapter that appeared in the previous edition.

▶ REFERENCES

1. Pohunek P. Development, structure and function of the upper airways. *Paediatr Respir Rev.* 2004;5:2–8.
2. Karakoc F, Karadag B, Akbenlioglu C, et al. Foreign body aspiration: what is the outcome? *Pediatr Pulmonol.* 2002;34:30–36.
3. Swift AC, Rogers J. Vocal cord paralysis in children. *J Laryngol Otol.* 1987;101:169–171.
4. Grundfast KM, Harley E. Vocal cord paralysis. *Otolaryngol Clin North Am.* 1989;22:569–597.
5. McBride JT. Stridor in childhood. *J Fam Pract.* 1984;19:782–790.
6. Riley RH, Dally FG, Fisher PH. Fiberoptic techniques in the emergency department [Letter]. *N Z Med J.* 1991;104:296.
7. Schafermeyer RW. Fiberoptic laryngoscopy in the emergency department. *Am J Emerg Med.* 1984;2:160–163.
8. Handler SD. Direct laryngoscopy in children: rigid and flexible fiberoptic. *Ear Nose Throat J.* 1995;74:100–104, 106.
9. Hocutt JE Jr, Corey GA, Rodney WM. Nasolaryngoscopy for family physicians. *Am Fam Phys.* 1990;42:1257–1268.
10. Lancer JM, Jones AS. Flexible fiberoptic rhinolaryngoscopy: results of 338 consecutive examinations. *J Laryngol Otol.* 1985;99:771–773.
11. Selkin SG. Clinical use of the pediatric flexible fiberscope. *Int J Pediatr Otorhinolaryngol.* 1985;10:75–80.
12. Hawkins DB, Clark RW. Flexible laryngoscopy in neonates, infants, and young children. *Ann Otol Rhinol Laryngol.* 1987;96:81–85.
13. Wood RE, Postma D. Endoscopy of the airway in infants and children. *J Pediatr.* 1988;112:1–6.
14. Selner JC. Concepts and clinical application of fiberoptic examination of the upper airway. *Clin Rev Allergy.* 1988;6:303–320.
15. Holinger LD. Diagnostic endoscopy of the pediatric airway. *Laryngoscope.* 1989;99:346–348.
16. McDonald RJ. Flexible fiberoptic bronchoscopy in children. *West J Med.* 1990;153:646–647.
17. Yellon RF, Goldberg H. Update on gastroesophageal reflux disease in pediatric airway disorders. *Am J Med.* 2001;11[Suppl 8A]:78S–84S.
18. Olney DR, Greinwald JH, Smith RJ, et al. *Laryngoscope.* 1999;109:1770–1775.
19. Ransom JH, Kavel KK. Diagnostic fiberoptic rhinolaryngoscopy. *Kans Med.* 1989;90:105–108, 115.
20. Chait DH, Lotz WK. Successful pediatric examinations using nasoendoscopy. *Laryngoscope.* 1990;101:1016–1018.
21. Wang DY, Clement P, Kaufman L, et al. Fiberoptic examination of the nasal cavity and nasopharynx in children. *Acta Otorhinolaryngol Belg.* 1991;45:323–329.
22. Weir N, Bassett I. Outpatient fiberoptic nasolaryngoscopy and videostroboscopy. *J R Soc Med.* 1987;80:299–300.
23. Dinwiddie R. Congenital upper airway obstruction. *Paediatr Respir Rev.* 2004;5:17–24.
24. Bailey BJ, Strunk CL, Jones JK. Methods of examination. In: Bluestone CD, Stool SEW, eds. *Pediatric Otolaryngology.* 2nd ed. Philadelphia: WB Saunders; 1990.
25. Wheeler PW, Lancaster D, Kaiser AB. Bronchopulmonary cross colonization and infection related to mycobacterial contamination of suction valves of bronchoscopes. *J Infect Dis.* 1989;159:954–958.
26. Hanson PJV, Jeffries DF, Batten JC, et al. Infection control revisited: dilemma facing today's bronchoscopists. *Br Med J.* 1988;297:185–187.

complaints. Referred to an otolaryngologist for a more definitive examination should be arranged when necessary. Indirect laryngoscopy gives a panoramic view of the larynx but requires practice and is not suitable for infants and younger children. Direct laryngoscopy with a flexible fiberoptic laryngoscope can be used to examine the nasal cavity, supraglottic region, and vocal cords in any age group. Although complications with these procedures are unlikely, good technique and proper patient selection are essential. Children with respiratory distress are not appropriate candidates for outpatient diagnostic laryngoscopy. A thorough knowledge of the anatomy, a gentle technique, and practice will allow the physician to successfully complete this examination.

◀ ACKNOWLEDGMENTS

The authors would like to acknowledge the valuable contributions of L. Christopher Post and Clark A. Rosen to the version of this chapter that appeared in the previous edition.

◀ REFERENCES

1. Polnara B. Developmental structure and function of the upper airways. Pediatr Respir Rev 2004;5:2–8.

2. Foltran F, Ballali S, Akbarshadeh C, et al. Foreign body aspiration: what is the outcome? Pediatr Pulmonol 2002;34:30–36.

3. Swift AC, Rogers J. Vocal cord paralysis in children. J Laryngol Otol 1987;101:166–171.

4. Chandhok KM, Holite E. Vocal cord paralysis. Otolaryngol Clin North Am 1989;22:589–597.

5. Michaels L. Stridor in childhood. Med Pract 1981;19:782–790.

6. Richards BW, Dajani FG, Faber PH. Fiberoptic techniques in the emergency department. Pediatr Clin North Am 1991;104:304–306.

7. Seidenstein RW. Fiberoptic laryngoscopy in the emergency department. Ann Emerg Med 1984;21:450–454.

8. Handler SD. Direct laryngoscopy in children: rigid and flexible approaches. Pediatr Rev Rep 1993;74:100–109.

9. Hoeve JJ, de Core GA, Ruben WM. Nasolaryngoscopy for infant physician. Int J Pediatr Otorhinolaryngol 1990;9:1247–1248.

10. Lancer JM, Jones AS. Flexible fiberoptic rhinolaryngoscopy: results of 228 consecutive examinations. J Laryngol Otol 1985;99:771–773.

11. Selkin SG. Clinical use of the pediatric flexible fiberoptic rhinolaryngoscope. Otolaryngology 1983;10:3–580.

12. Hawkins DB, Clark RW. Flexible laryngoscopy in neonates, infants, and young children. Ann Otol Rhinol Laryngol 1987;96:81–85.

13. Wood RE, Postma D. Endoscopy of the airway in infants and children. J Pediatr 1988;112:1–6.

14. Selner JC. Concept and clinical application of fiberoptic examination of the upper airway. Clin Rev Allergy 1988;6:303–320.

15. Hollinger LD. Endoscopic radiography of the pediatric airway. Laryngoscope 1989;99:319–345.

16. McDonald RE, Ludwig E. Topic bronchoscopy in children. Pediatrics 1990;73:645–647.

17. Yellon RF, Goldberg H. Update on gastroesophageal reflux disease in pediatric airway disorders. Am J Med 2001;111 Suppl 8A:78S–84S.

18. Olney DR, Greinwald JH, Smith RJ, et al. Laryngomalacia. 1999;109:1770–1775.

19. Ramon JH, Koltai PJ. Diagnostic fiberoptic rhinolaryngoscopy. Am J Otolaryngol 1990;10:105–112.

20. Chait DH, Lotz WK. Successful pediatric examinations using nasoendoscopy. Laryngoscope 1990;101:1018–1018.

21. Wang DY, Clement P, Kaufman L, et al. Fiberoptic examination of the nasal cavity and nasopharynx in children. Acta Otolaryngol 1991;11:323–326.

22. Wea A, Braren L. Outpatient fiberoptic tracheobronchoscopy and endobronchoscopy. J Clin Anesth 1995;80:296–300.

23. Linwelker R. Conventional upper airway obstruction. Pediatr Resp Rev 2004;5:17–24.

24. Bailey BJ, Spirak CL, Jones JG. Atlas of otolaryngologic examination. Scott SEW, eds. Pediatric Otolaryngology. 2nd ed. Philadelphia, WB Saunders, 1990.

25. Wheeler PW, Lancaster D, Kirca AR. Bronchopulmonary cross colonization and infection related to mycobacterial contamination of suction valves of bronchoscopes. J Infect Dis 1989;159:954–958.

26. Hanson PJV, Jeffries DL, Bateman DL, et al. Infection control revisited: dilemma facing today's bronchoscopist. Thorax 1988;207:185–187.

SECTION 9 ▶ DENTAL PROCEDURES

SECTION EDITOR: JOHN LOISELLE

ZACH KASSUTTO

Orofacial Anesthesia Techniques

62

▶ INTRODUCTION

Orofacial nerve blocks and infiltrations can be used for regional anesthesia in the event of orofacial pathologies such as dental caries, tooth and alveolar fractures, and soft-tissue trauma to the lower half of the face. These procedures are most commonly performed by dentists and oral surgeons in the outpatient setting. Patients requiring these types of procedures also are seen regularly in the emergency department (ED). Given the numerous approaches and types of procedures available, this chapter will review only those procedures that have the greatest utility and success rate and the lowest rate of complications.

When used for the relief of pre-existing pain, these procedures are temporizing only. Using a longer-acting anesthetic agent can extend their effect. These procedures can be performed successfully in children of any age. In younger and uncooperative children, the procedures are more difficult to carry out. Adjuncts to the procedure include emotional preparation and support (Chapter 2), procedural sedation (Chapter 33), appropriate restraint (Chapter 3), and mucosal topical anesthetics. Honesty and sincerity also must be used, as they are perhaps the most important preparation for any procedure with pediatric patients.

▶ ANATOMY AND PHYSIOLOGY

Orofacial anesthesia blocks transmission of painful stimuli via one or several afferent branches of the fifth cranial (trigeminal) nerve. Three primary divisions of the fifth cranial nerve on each side of the face are designated V_1, V_2, and V_3 (Fig. 62.1).

V_1, the ophthalmic division, innervates structures above the mouth. V_2, or the maxillary division, supplies sensory fibers to the various structures in and around the maxilla. These include all the maxillary teeth and their associated gingivae; the entire palate and tissues posterior to this, including the tonsillar region; the lower eyelid; the side of the nose; the upper lip; and the mucous membranes of most of the nasal cavity. The palatine branches (greater, lesser, and nasopalatine nerves) branch off before the nerve enters the infraorbital canal. These nerves innervate the soft-tissue structures of the posterior mouth and the throat.

The posterior superior, middle superior, and anterior superior alveolar nerves are the next branches of V_2. The posterior superior alveolar nerve branches off before entering the infraorbital canal and innervates the maxillary sinus and the maxillary molars and their gingivae. The middle superior and anterior superior alveolar nerves separate from the maxillary nerve trunk as it traverses the infraorbital canal (where it is called the "infraorbital nerve"). Together, these nerves supply the anterior maxillary teeth and their associated structures as far posterior as the maxillary premolars or primary molars. The infraorbital nerve exits the skull via the infraorbital foramen and its terminal branches innervate the lower eyelid, the alae of the nose, and the upper lip. Anesthetic applied at the infraorbital foramen allows repair of ala or upper lip injuries without the swelling associated with direct infiltration.

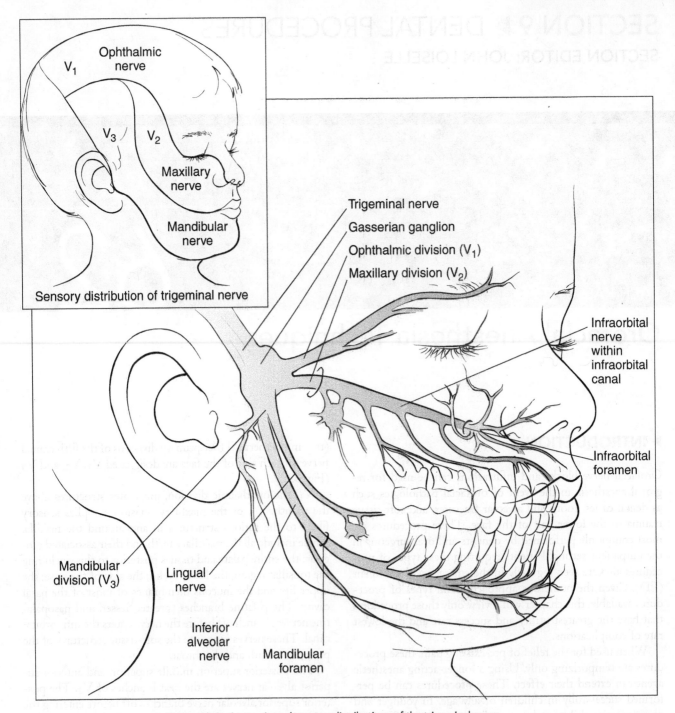

Figure 62.1 Anatomic and sensory distributions of the trigeminal nerve.

The mandibular division, or V_3, supplies motor innervation to the muscles of mastication and sensory fibers to the mandible. The inferior alveolar nerve is the largest branch of the mandibular nerve. It enters the mandible via the mandibular foramen, which is located on the internal surface of the ramus. It then traverses the mandible through the mandibular canal, where the nerve and its branches innervate all the teeth of the mandible on each respective side. The lingual nerve is an early branch of the mandibular division. This branch travels with the inferior alveolar nerve until it enters the mandibular canal. Then the lingual nerve enters the base of the tongue. There it supplies sensory fibers to the anterior two thirds of the tongue, the floor of the mouth, and the lingual aspect of the mandibular gingivae. Anesthetic applied near the mandibular foramen will usually anesthetize both the lingual and inferior alveolar nerves.

The alveolar bone of the pediatric patient is usually less dense than that of the adult. This advantage allows for more rapid and complete dissemination of the anesthetic solution when infiltration anesthesia is used (1,2).

▶ INDICATIONS

Orofacial anesthesia can be used for pain relief (e.g., dental abscess, caries) or for the prevention of pain (e.g., tooth extraction, facial and/or oral laceration repair, facial and/or dental abscess drainage). Procedures are classified as nerve blocks or direct infiltration.

Nerve blocks allow the use of small amounts of anesthetic applied to a small area for anesthesia of larger areas. In this way, manipulation of infected tissues can be avoided and anatomical landmarks are not distorted. An example is using an infraorbital nerve block for repair of the vermilion border in upper lip lacerations. Nerve blocks also decrease the risks of using larger amounts of anesthetic and avoid the need for injection of anesthetic in areas that are more susceptible to pain. Infiltration anesthesia is used when smaller areas of anesthesia are needed. Examples include tooth pain from caries or isolated tooth injury from trauma. Nerve blocks and infiltration anesthesia for other parts of the body are described in Chapters 35 and 55.

The need for consultation depends on the patient's exact injury and the practice at a given institution. Possible consultants include dentists, oral surgeons, otorhinolaryngologists, and plastic surgeons. Consultation should be considered for cases involving mandibular fractures, nerve injury from trauma, difficulty achieving anesthesia, or any contraindications to the procedure.

Absolute contraindications to the procedures in this chapter include known allergy to the anesthetic agent and grossly distorted anatomical landmarks. Injecting through infected tissue (e.g., tooth abscess) is a relative contraindication (2). Local anesthetics are less effective when applied in regions of inflammation (3). Manipulating a needle through infected tissues also increases the risk of spreading the infection to other adjacent areas or into the blood stream. Whenever possible, a nerve block (as opposed to direct infiltration) should be used in this type of situation.

▶ EQUIPMENT

See also Table 62.1.

1″ × 1″ sterile gauze pads
Cotton-tipped applicators

TABLE 62.1	EQUIPMENT FOR OROFACIAL ANESTHESIA

1″ × 1″ sterile gauze pads
Cotton-tipped applicators
Suction
Supplies for universal precautions (latex gloves, protective eyewear, surgical mask, and moisture-repellent gown)
Anesthetic agents
Sterile syringe and needle
Resuscitation equipment

Yankauer suction (a large-bore suction device such as a Yankauer device is preferred for removing any secretions, blood, or emesis; see Chapter 13)
Syringe
27-gauge, 1- or 1.25-inch straight needle or aspirating dental syringe

Orofacial anesthesia can be performed using medical syringes and needles commonly available in the ED but is more easily accomplished using dental equipment specifically designed for this task, such as an aspirating dental syringe that uses cartridges (carpules) of anesthetic solution and disposable needles (4). This type of syringe affords the physician a better grasp of the instrument and the ability to aspirate with the same hand that is holding the syringe. This frees the other hand to hold, stabilize, and retract the involved tissues.

Various suggestions have been made as to the best size needle to use for the procedure. Large bore needles make the procedure unduly painful and could compromise exact placement of the needle tip. Narrower needles make aspiration more difficult and increase the risk of needle breakage. Some authorities believe that a needle smaller than 25 gauge may increase the risk of inadvertent intravascular injection (i.e., no blood on aspiration despite the needle being inside a vessel). Others believe that this risk is small and that slow injection after aspirating further minimizes this risk. Most sources recommend a 27-gauge "short needle" (1 inch) for most infiltrations and blocks and a 27-gauge "long needle" (1.25 inch) for older adolescents.

Orofacial anesthesia techniques in children differ from adults because of the smaller size of the skull and the characteristics of the bone. In general, the depth of needle insertion needs to be adjusted for the size of the child's anatomy. Relevant variations in size will be discussed under each procedure.

Topical anesthetic
- 20% benzocaine
- 5% to 10% lidocaine

Commercial topical dental anesthetics are available in liquids, gels, ointments, and sprays. The most commonly used preparations contain benzocaine (e.g., Hurricane, a flavored preparation of 20% benzocaine). If a specific dental preparation is unavailable, 5% to 10% lidocaine or 20% benzocaine can be used. Less concentrated anesthetics usually prove to be ineffective (4).

The oral mucosa is supplied by a rich vascular network. Anesthetics applied topically may be absorbed into the systemic circulation. The dose of topical anesthetic, although often difficult to quantify, must be considered when calculating the overall dose of anesthetic that a patient receives. Benzocaine is the preferred agent because it has little systemic absorption when applied topically (5) (although methemoglobin has been reported rarely after its topical use). Anesthetic sprays are discouraged because they tend to cover larger areas than required for the procedure.

Injectable anesthetic
- 2% lidocaine with epinephrine 1:100,000
- 3% mepivacaine
- 0.5% Bupivacaine

Many dental anesthetics are commercially available for injection in dental anesthetic carpules. These carpules each contain 1.8 mL of anesthetic and insert into standard dental aspirating syringes. They cannot be directly adapted for use with other injecting devices commonly available in EDs. The contents, however, can be drawn into a standard disposable syringe through the carpule's rubber stopper. Care must be taken to use sterile technique when doing this. The standard solution used by dentists is 2% lidocaine with epinephrine 1:100,000. In cases where a prolonged effect is desired, longer-acting agents such as bupivacaine also are available. Long-acting agents are usually avoided for intraoral anesthesia when the oral mucosa or tongue may be involved (e.g., inferior alveolar block). This is especially important in preadolescent or developmentally delayed children who may self-inflict injury by biting their numbed oral tissues. Less commonly used agents include Novocain, prilocaine, and etidocaine.

Anesthetics are available with or without vasoconstrictors. Most practitioners prefer using a vasoconstrictor (such as epinephrine 1:100,000 or 1:50,000), as it slows anesthetic absorption into the surrounding tissues. This allows injection of smaller doses of anesthetic, prolongs the anesthetic effect, and provides for hemostasis. For patients in whom vasoconstrictors are contraindicated (as with certain cardiac anomalies or conduction abnormalities), 3% mepivacaine without epinephrine is the agent of choice. Some dentists advocate warming anesthetic solutions to body temperature before injection to make the injection less painful and anesthesia onset more rapid.

Universal precaution supplies
- Latex-free examination gloves
- Protective eye wear
- Surgical mask
- Moisture-repellent gown

Standard cardiopulmonary resuscitation equipment should be readily available in the unlikely event of an adverse reaction to the medications or procedure.

▶ PROCEDURE

Topical anesthesia of mucous membranes can reduce the pain associated with orofacial anesthesia and should be considered before any intraoral injection. In the apprehensive patient, the physician must weigh the extra time involved in undertaking this procedure versus the transient pain of passing a thin needle through the oral mucosa. Most topical anesthetics are pleasant tasting, but if unpleasant, can increase the patient's apprehension (5).

First, the area to be injected must be dried with gauze. The anesthetic is applied to a cotton-tipped swab or a small piece of cotton or gauze. The dose of topical anesthetic should be included in calculating the total anesthetic dose that the patient receives. Application of the anesthetic to the mucosa is limited to the site where the needle is expected to pass. According to the manufacturer, topical anesthesia should occur within 15 to 30 seconds of using 20% benzocaine. Others have suggested that it takes at least 2 minutes for this drug to exert its effect (2). Application of the anesthetic to the tongue should be avoided, as this may result in excessive salivation. Before injection, any residual topical anesthetic should be removed with gauze.

Infraorbital Nerve Block

An effective infraorbital nerve block places local anesthetic at the infraorbital foramen. This nerve block should effectively anesthetize the anterior and middle superior alveolar nerves, which innervate the anterior maxillary teeth. Also anesthetized are the terminal branches of the infraorbital nerve, which innervate the upper lip, the nasal alae, and the lower eyelid (see Fig. 62.1). This block is especially useful for repair of facial lacerations. It avoids the distortion of anatomy usually associated with direct infiltration of the soft facial tissues. This block can be performed by either an extraoral or an intraoral approach. For the sake of clarity, only the latter technique will be described here.

The physician and the patient must be seated comfortably, with bright overhead lighting that can be directed into the oral cavity. Ideally the patient sits semi-reclined in a dental chair that supports the head and can tilt the maxillary occlusal plane to about 45 degrees relative to the floor. This position allows for control of the head to reduce movement and is advantageous should the patient have a vasovagal reaction (2). The physician is seated so as to be above the patient's mouth and to have easy access to the equipment. Whenever possible, the help of an assistant who is familiar with the equipment and the procedure should be obtained. If a dental chair is unavailable, the above positioning can be attained with a cooperative patient using an adjustable reclining stretcher. In younger or uncooperative children, the patient should be restrained with a papoose board or bed sheet (Chapter 3). The procedure can then be carried out with the patient supine on a stretcher. Ideally, the clinician should be positioned on the side of the patient that will be anesthetized.

The patient's supraorbital and infraorbital notches are palpated. An imaginary line between these two landmarks should cross the patient's pupil (6) (Fig. 62.2A). Further inferiorly, this line will cross the bicuspid teeth and the mental foramen. About 0.5 cm inferior to the infraorbital notch, a shallow depression can be palpated. The infraorbital foramen lies within this depression. One finger is used to mark the site of the foramen while the other fingers of the same hand retract the lip. The exact position of the physician's hand will depend on his or her handedness and the side of the patient on which

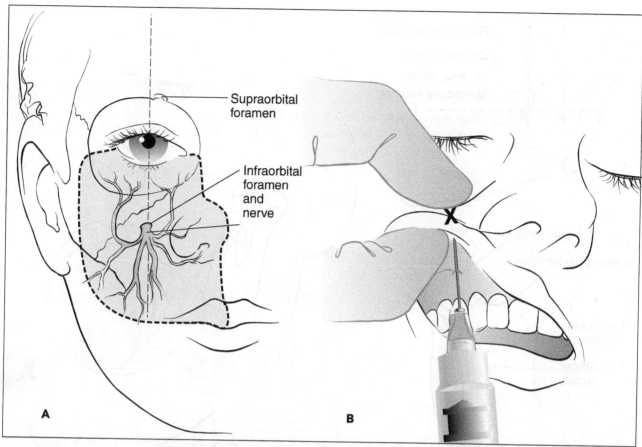

Figure 62.2
A. Anatomic landmarks and needle position for infraorbital nerve block.
B. Localization of infraorbital nerve.

the physician is standing. The foramen can be marked with either the thumb or middle finger. In either case the lip is retracted with the index finger. Topical mucosal anesthesia can be applied as previously described. The syringe is best held in the dominant hand. The needle is inserted in the mucolabial fold (where the mucosal aspect of the upper lip meets the maxillary bone) just anterior to the apex of the first premolar tooth. The needle tip should be advanced along the axis of the tooth toward the infraorbital foramen. The digit over the foramen helps direct the needle tip into contact with the bone at the opening of the foramen (Fig. 62.2B). Advancing the needle into the foramen should be avoided, as this may damage the nerve (3). If the patient complains of paresthesias before the injection of anesthetic, the needle has entered the nerve and must be withdrawn slightly. After aspirating to exclude intravascular needle placement, about 1 to 2 mL of anesthetic is slowly deposited. The needle should be advanced no more than 0.5 to 0.75 inches (1 to 2 cm) from the insertion point. It is important to limit the depth of needle insertion and to mark the infraorbital foramen with a digit, as these precautions prevent accidental entrance of the needle into the orbital cavity. If the location of the needle tip is uncertain, the needle should be withdrawn and insertion reattempted.

If the needle is angled excessively toward the skull, the malar eminence will prevent the advancement of the needle to the foramen. If this occurs, a less acute angle of needle insertion should be used.

The anesthetic requires about 5 minutes to take effect. Effective anesthesia is confirmed by a subjective feeling of numbness or tingling and an absence of pain with manipulation of the targeted tissues.

Inferior Alveolar Nerve Block

The inferior alveolar nerve block is difficult to perform successfully without practice. Even in the most experienced hands, the failure rate is approximately 15%. Failures are mostly the result of improper technique. Anatomical variation and accessory innervation play less of a role. It is recommended that this technique be practiced initially under experienced supervision.

A well-placed inferior alveolar nerve block eliminates pain sensation from all the mandibular teeth as well as the skin of the chin and lower lip on the side of the block. Because of its proximity, the lingual nerve is almost always anesthetized when attempting a block of the inferior alveolar nerve. This results in anesthesia to the tongue on the side of the block.

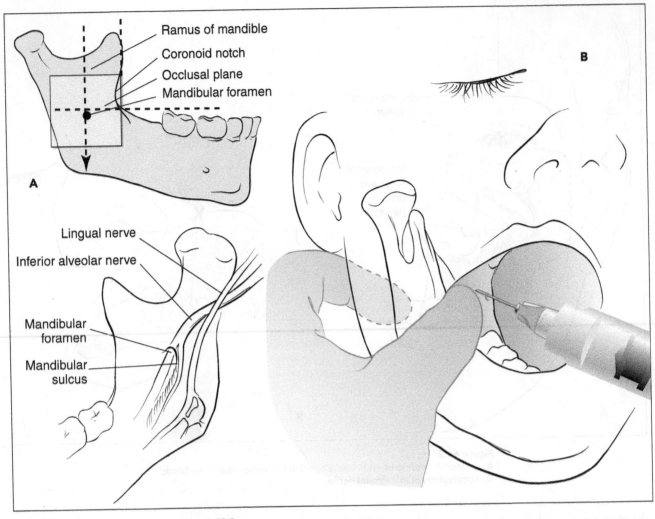

Figure 62.3
A. Localization of inferior alveolar nerve.
B. Hand and needle positions for inferior alveolar nerve block.

The buccal mucosa also may be anesthetized by blocking the long buccal nerve, which lies just lateral to the lingual nerve.

The goal of this block is to place the anesthetic in the mandibular sulcus, the notch that funnels into the mandibular foramen. This is where the inferior alveolar nerve enters the mandible. The location of these structures is best approximated by conceptualizing the inner surface of the mandibular ramus roughly as a rectangle (Fig. 62.3A). The target site for injection is the intersection of two imaginary lines. The horizontal line is identified relative to the occlusal plane of the teeth or relative to the deepest portion of the anterior aspect of the ramus of the mandible. This depression is sometimes called the coronoid notch. The vertical line is at the midpoint of the rectangle and is approximated by the midpoint between two fingers grasping the ramus from either side. To identify the coronoid notch, the ramus of the mandible is clasped between the thumb and index fingers. One finger grasps the extraoral posterior ramus while the other palpates the intraoral anterior ramus. The intraoral digit slides up and down

the anterior border of the ramus of the mandible. The deepest area is the coronoid notch. A horizontal line through the middle of the coronoid notch should transect the mandibular sulcus. The same digit that marks the coronoid notch is used to retract the soft tissues of the cheek outwardly, thus exposing the injection site. The tip of the intraoral digit should remain in contact with the coronoid notch. To confirm the horizontal position of the mandibular foramen, the clinician should note its location relative to the occlusal plane. In children, the mandibular foramen is located below the occlusal plane of the primary teeth. Toward adulthood, its location rises to several millimeters above the occlusal plane (1,3,5). No age-related difference is found in the anteroposterior location of the foramen.

The patient is positioned and restrained as previously described. Topical anesthesia is applied and maximal exposure is gained by having the patient open his or her mouth as wide as possible. The syringe is held with the dominant hand, and the injection site is approached from the opposite side of the patient's mouth (Fig. 62.3B). The barrel of the syringe should

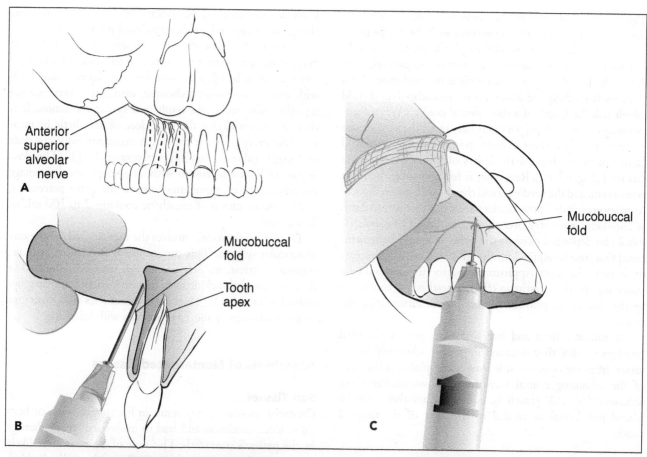

Figure 62.4 Supraperiosteal infiltration.
A. Nerve supply of the maxillary teeth.
B. Needle insertion at the mucobuccal fold allows deposition of anesthesia close to the tooth apex.
C. Minimal depth of needle insertion (about 2 mm) is required for the anterior primary maxillary teeth.

lie over the primary molars of the opposite side of the mouth. The needle should be directed slightly below the occlusal plane of the mandibular teeth in children and at the occlusal plane in older adolescents and adults. The needle is inserted at a point that bisects the coronoid notch and is midway between the intraoral and extraoral digits that are grasping the mandible. The needle is advanced gently until it contacts the bony surface of the inner aspect of the mandible. The penetration depth should be about 15 mm, although this may vary from patient to patient. This site should closely approximate the mandibular sulcus, where the inferior alveolar nerve enters the mandible (Fig. 62.3A). The needle is withdrawn slightly (about 1 mm). Intravascular needle placement is excluded by aspirating, and then up to 1.8 mL of anesthetic (or the maximum dose based on the patient's weight) is injected over 30 to 60 seconds. Injecting more rapidly may cause unnecessary pain. If the patient complains of paresthesias before the injection of anesthetic, the needle has entered the nerve and must be withdrawn slightly.

Approximately 5 minutes is necessary for complete anesthetic effect. Effective anesthesia is confirmed by a subjective feeling of numbness or tingling and an absence of pain with manipulation of the lower lip on the side of the injection.

Infiltration Anesthesia (Supraperiosteal Infiltration)

Using infiltration technique, anesthetic is deposited near the periosteum of the bone that supports a given tooth. Solution then diffuses through the periosteum and underlying bone and contacts the nerve supplying that tooth (Fig. 62.4A). The maxillary bone remains relatively porous throughout life, allowing easy permeability of anesthetic. The mandibular bone is more dense and less permeable to anesthetic. As a result of these characteristics, this procedure is limited in adults to anesthesia of the maxillary teeth. In children, the mandible is less dense and therefore allows for the additional use of this technique for anesthesia of the anterior primary teeth or their surrounding gingivae.

The patient is positioned and topical anesthesia is applied as described previously. The lip in front of the involved tooth is grasped with a dry gauze to prevent slippage. The lip is retracted from the mouth to best expose the mucobuccal fold

(Fig. 62.4B). The bevel of the needle is oriented toward the bone to avoid scraping the periosteum with the needle point (2). The needle is introduced through the mucobuccal fold and advanced slowly along the anterior or buccal surface of the tooth toward its apex. The needle is inserted about 1 cm in a preschool child and about 1.5 cm in a school-aged child (about half the length of a short dental needle). When anesthetizing the anterior primary maxillary teeth, the needle must be inserted only a short distance past the mucobuccal fold (2 mm at most), because the apices of primary teeth are at this level (Fig. 62.4C). Resistance is felt on contact with the periosteum, and the needle should then be withdrawn slightly. Aspiration excludes intravascular needle placement; 1 to 2 mL of anesthetic is injected over about 1 minute. The anesthetic should be deposited close to the bone. It should be remembered that time is required for the anesthetic to diffuse across the bone to the nerve. Approximately 5 to 10 minutes is necessary for the full anesthetic effect. Anesthesia is confirmed by the absence of pain in the soft tissues surrounding the tooth.

Permanent central and lateral incisors pose a potential problem, in that they occasionally receive additional innervation from the opposite side. Anesthetic placed at the apex of the adjoining central incisor should anesthetize these accessory fibers. Alternatively, additional anesthetic can be placed just lateral or medial to the apex of the targeted tooth.

▶ COMPLICATIONS

Anesthetic Reactions

A larger percentage of dental anesthesia morbidity and mortality occurs in children than in adults. This is probably related to overdosing of local anesthetic. Since the introduction of the amide local anesthetics (e.g., lidocaine, mepivacaine) (Table 62.2) (7), allergic reactions have been less frequent.

Ester anesthetics (e.g., Novocain) are more likely to cause allergic reactions and are therefore used infrequently.

As with other uses of local anesthetics, the total dose of drug administered must be monitored to avoid systemic toxicity. Care must be taken to avoid intravascular injection. Even with careful aspiration technique, inadvertent intravascular injection may occur and result in a systemic reaction. It is therefore essential that the total dose of anesthetic be measured for every pediatric patient. A maximum lidocaine dose of 2 mg/lb (about 4 mg/kg) is recommended (1). This dose applies to lidocaine with or without epinephrine. Percentage concentrations of anesthetics refer to the gram percentage. A 2% concentration of anesthetic contains 2 g/100 mL or 20 mg/mL.

Dose-related toxicity involves the nervous and/or the cardiovascular systems. This can include hypotension, asystole, respiratory arrest, and seizure. Allergic reactions unrelated to dose are rare and include rash, urticaria, edema, and anaphylactoid reactions (3). Most local anesthetics have toxicities qualitatively comparable to those seen with lidocaine.

Anesthesia of Nontargeted Tissues

Soft Tissues

Orofacial anesthesia may result in lip, tongue, face, or buccal mucosa numbness and lead to inadvertent tissue damage by the patient's own teeth. This type of injury is more likely to occur in the young or the mentally or physically disabled. These injuries can be minimized by selecting shorter-acting anesthetic agents or anesthetics without vasoconstrictors. The patient and the family should be carefully instructed to avoid solid foods and hot substances by mouth for as long as anesthesia persists (5).

Other Nerves

Nontargeted nerves may inadvertently be anesthetized. Examples of this include inadvertent anesthesia of the facial nerve

TABLE 62.2	CHARACTERISTICS OF DENTAL ANESTHETICS			
Anesthetic agent	Relative toxicity*	Maximum dose (mg/kg)	Maximum total dose (mg)	Class
Lidocaine 2%	2	4.0	300	Amide
Lidocaine 2% with epinephrine	2	4.0	500	Amide
Mepivacaine 3%	1.5	6.6	400	Amide
Mepivacaine 2% with epinephrine	1.5	6.6	400	Amide
Bupivacaine 0.5%	3+	2	175	Amide
Bupivacaine 0.5% with epinephrine	3+	2	225	Amide
Novocain 4%	1	20	1000	Ester†

*Refers to cardiac and neurologic toxicities.
†The esters have a much greater allergic potential than the amides.
Adapted from Bennett CR. Monheim's local anesthesia and pain control in dental practice. 7th ed. St. Louis: CV Mosby; 1984.

with attempted infraorbital nerve block (3) or anesthesia of the lingual nerve with inferior alveolar nerve block.

Bleeding/Hematoma

Puncture or laceration of blood vessels by the needle tip is uncommon with proper technique. Clinically significant bleeding from application of dental anesthesia is rare (2). In the rare event that a blood vessel is entered, direct pressure should be applied to the site for 2 to 5 minutes. The patient and family should be instructed to watch for signs of soft tissue swelling as a result of extravasation of blood.

Infection

Like bleeding, infection is a theoretical concern that rarely occurs. Injecting through infected tissues, however, should be avoided. This may serve to spread the infection, and anesthesia may be less effective because of the low pH in infected areas.

Neuronal Damage

If the patient experiences paresthesia over the distribution of the targeted nerve before the injection of anesthetic, the needle tip is in the nerve. Anesthetic should not be injected at this point, as permanent nerve damage may result. The needle

---

 SUMMARY

Infraorbital Nerve Block

1 Position the patient with the maxillary occlusal plane 45 degrees relative to the floor.

2 Restrain or sedate the patient as necessary.

3 Locate the site of the infraorbital foramen by palpation and mark the spot with the thumb or middle finger.

4 Apply topical anesthesia to the mucous membrane.

5 Insert the needle at the mucolabial fold just anterior to the first premolar. The needle axis should follow the axis of the tooth. pointing toward the finger marking the infraorbital foramen. Do not insert the needle more than 2 cm, as this increases the risk of entering the orbit.

6 When the needle tip has contacted bone at the foramen, aspirate, then slowly inject 1 to 2 mL of anesthetic.

7 Withdraw the needle, wait 5 minutes, then test for anesthesia.

Inferior Alveolar Nerve Block

1 Position the patient with the maxillary occlusal plane 45 degrees relative to the floor.

2 Restrain or sedate the patient as necessary.

3 Grasp the mandibular ramus between the thumb and index finger. Approximate the location of the mandibular sulcus on the interior surface of the ramus midway between the thumb and index finger and just above or below the level of the occlusal plane of the teeth, depending on the child's age.

4 Apply topical anesthesia to the mucous membrane.

5 Hold the barrel of the syringe over the contralateral molars of the patient, with the needle tip just over the mucosa that overlies the mandibular sulcus.

6 Advance the needle through the mucosa until bone is contacted (about 15 mm); withdraw the needle about 1 mm, aspirate, and then inject 1 to 1.8 mL of anesthetic over about 1 minute.

7 To guarantee anesthesia of the lingual nerve, withdraw the needle to half the insertion depth and instill additional anesthetic.

8 Withdraw the needle, wait about 5 minutes, then test for anesthesia by absence of sensation on ipsilateral lower lip.

Infiltration Dental Anesthesia

1 Position the patient with the maxillary occlusal plane 45 degrees relative to the floor.

2 Restrain or the sedate patient as necessary.

3 Apply topical anesthesia to the mucous membrane.

4 Grasp the lip with a piece of gauze and retract it to expose the mucobuccal fold.

5 Insert the needle through the mucobuccal fold with the bevel oriented toward bone.

6 Advance the needle to the level of the apex of the tooth (2 mm for primary anterior maxillary teeth, 1 cm for permanent teeth in preschool children, 1.5 cm for permanent teeth in school-aged children).

7 Aspirate, then inject 1 to 2 mL of anesthetic over 1 minute.

8 Withdraw the needle, then wait 5 to 10 minutes for anesthesia to take effect; confirm anesthesia by the absence of pain with manipulation.

CLINICAL TIPS

▶ Younger or uncooperative patients may require sedation using nitrous oxide or intravenous procedural sedation.

▶ It may be helpful to suggest that the child close his or her eyes just before the injection. The child should be warned of the pinch or pain that is about to occur. The needle should be concealed as long as possible to reduce anxiety.

▶ Distraction techniques can be very effective. Singing or talking to the child by the physician or parent may make the patient more comfortable. Another technique involves pressing the lip firmly at some site away from the injection site. While inserting the needle and injecting the anesthetic, the lip is gently shaken.

▶ Having an uncooperative patient keep the mouth open may be difficult. This can be facilitated using a mouth prop. This device is commonly used by dentists. It is available in various sizes. Alternatively, several tongue blades covered with layers of gauze and held together by tape may serve the same purpose.

▶ Younger and uncooperative children should be restrained appropriately to avoid unexpected movements. Both the injecting and supporting hands should be anchored against the patient's face or teeth when anesthetic is injected.

▶ Treatment should begin immediately after the onset of anesthesia. A delay from the time of anesthesia to the start of treatment is a common cause of anesthesia failure. This is especially true in children, as both diffusion and absorption of anesthetic may be rapid.

should be withdrawn 0.5 to 1.0 mm, and then the anesthetic is injected.

Needle Breakage

As with any procedure involving hypodermic needles, the needle has the potential to break while still in the patient. Although this is a rare occurrence, care must be taken to properly restrain the patient to avoid sudden unexpected movements.

▶ SUMMARY

Orofacial nerve blocks and anesthetic infiltrations are not commonly used in the pediatric emergency setting. When indicated, however, these nerve blocks allow for the temporary relief of pain, greater patient comfort, and improved outcomes with several orofacial procedures.

▶ ACKNOWLEDGMENTS

The author would like to acknowledge the valuable contributions of Mark Helpin, MD, who provided valuable suggestions regarding the content of this chapter.

▶ REFERENCES

1. Malamed SF. *Handbook of Local Anesthesia*. 4th ed. St. Louis: Mosby; 1996.
2. Evers H, Haegerstam G. *Introduction to Dental Local Anaesthesia*. Fribourg, Switzerland: Mediglobe; 1990.
3. Haglund J, Evers H. *Local Anaesthesia in Dentistry*. 9th ed. Sodertalje, Sweden: Astra Lakemedel; 1988.
4. Roberts JR, Hedges JR. *Clinical Procedures in Emergency Medicine*. 4th ed. Philadelphia: WB Saunders; 2004.
5. McDonald RE, Avery DR. *Dentistry for the Child and Adolescent*. 5th ed. St. Louis: Mosby; 1988.
6. Brammer-Graham K. *Local Anesthesia and Pain Control: A Modular Approach* [video handbook]. Kansas City: Kansas City School of Dentistry; 1979.
7. Bennett CR. *Monheim's Local Anesthesia and Pain Control in Dental Practice*. 7th ed. St Louis: Mosby; 1984.

ELLIOTT M. HARRIS

63

Incision and Drainage of a Dental Abscess

▶ INTRODUCTION

A dental abscess is an area of localized infection involving the structures surrounding the teeth. Often this becomes a fluctuant swelling that requires drainage to promote healing. Usually dental abscesses are seen in older children and are more likely to involve the permanent dentition. However, abscesses may be seen in younger patients with poor oral hygiene and carious teeth (1). Although the vast majority of cases are managed by a dentist or an oral surgeon, the emergency physician is occasionally called upon to perform incision and drainage for patients with simple abscesses when referral is delayed. Emergency care will help speed the recovery process and provide some relief from pain. Further dental care will normally be needed once the infectious process subsides.

The most common types of dental abscesses include periapical and periodontal abscesses. The periapical abscess is by far the most common dental abscess in children and results from spread of infection or inflammation from the pulp to the periapical tissues via the apical foramen of the tooth (1). Periodontal abscesses, which involve the periodontal structures (such as the gingivae or periodontal ligament), are more common in adults and are usually a complication of periodontal disease. When seen in children, periodontal abscesses are most often the result of a foreign body introduced into previously healthy periodontal tissue (1).

▶ ANATOMY AND PHYSIOLOGY

The most common predisposing factor to formation of a dental abscess in children is the presence of caries. Once the carious process has extended through the hard structures of the tooth (the enamel and the dentin) and into the pulp cav-ity (Fig. 63.1), pulpal infection and/or inflammation occur. This process usually results in pulp necrosis. The inflammatory process then extends to the periapical tissues via the apical foramen, leading to the formation of a periapical abscess. Although caries are the most common predisposing factor, any process that causes or predisposes to pulp necrosis (e.g., trauma, recent dental procedures) may lead to abscess formation (2–4).

Primary teeth have thinner enamel than permanent teeth, and therefore the pulp of the primary dentition has relatively less protection. In addition, because of a more abundant blood supply, the pulp of primary teeth tends to have a greater inflammatory response to injury. One advantage primary teeth have is that they are better at forming dentin beneath carious lesions. This provides some extra protection for the pulp in the face of the poor oral hygiene practiced by many children.

As mentioned previously, periodontal abscesses in children, unlike in adults, are not associated with periodontal disease. Often a cause cannot be elucidated, but frequently they are due to impaction of a foreign body in the periodontal tissues. In contrast to periapical abscesses, periodontal abscesses are associated with vital teeth (1).

Dental abscesses may be found on either side of the gingiva, but lesions are found more frequently on the buccal aspect than on the lingual side. The vast majority (more than 80%) of abscesses are found in the maxillary arch (2). Such infections can be complicated by the spread of infection through the soft-tissue planes of the head and neck via paths of least resistance. Infection of the orbit, maxillary sinuses, infratemporal fossa, and sublingual and submandibular regions may result from untreated dental abscesses. Chronically draining fistulas also may occur. The buccinator muscle often serves as a barrier to the spread of infection to other areas of the head and neck. In children (who have a shorter facial height), the apices of

659

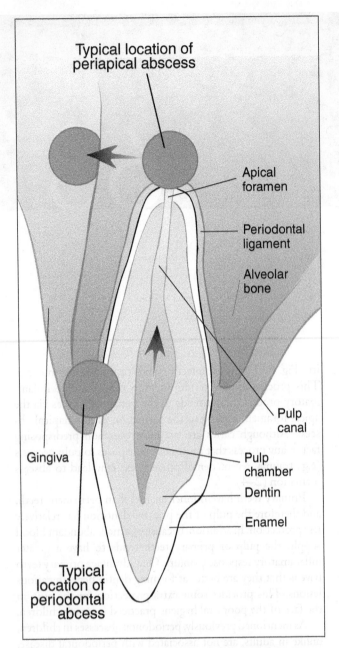

Figure 63.1 Location of periodontal and periapical abscess.

the teeth—especially the permanent first molars, incisors, and canines—lie outside the muscle attachments. This leads to an increased risk of extraoral spread in younger patients (1).

Bacteria in dental abscesses tend to correspond to normal oral flora. Gram-positive cocci and anaerobes are the usual pathologic bacteria. Although *Streptococcus viridans* tends to predominate in caries, once the pulp chamber is entered, anaerobes become the more frequently cultured offending organisms (3,4). Penicillin is still considered by most to be the drug of choice when antibiotics are required (2–4); however, longer standing infections tend to have a higher incidence of penicillin-resistant organisms (4). Clindamycin has become the recommended empiric therapy for those with more chronic

presentations or allergy to penicillin (2,4). Erythromycin has fallen out of favor as a second-line agent (2,4). Amoxicillin, although broader in spectrum than penicillin, has not been shown to have any significant advantage except in dosing interval and palatability (4).

▶ INDICATIONS

All dental abscesses will require drainage at some point. The question is, when does this need to occur? The vast majority should be handled by expedient referral to a dentist or an oral surgeon. However, abscesses that have become fluctuant but are not yet draining in a stable patient for whom referral might be delayed may be treated in the emergency department (ED). Reasons the procedure would be desirable include relief of pain and prevention of spontaneous drainage, with resulting formation of a chronic sinus tract (5). Even if incision and drainage is performed by an emergency physician, referral will still be required for definitive treatment and/or follow-up in virtually all patients.

With periapical abscesses, the pulp is almost always nonvital. This necessitates either tooth extraction or endodontic treatment. If the initial procedure permits sufficient drainage, definitive therapy may wait until the infection is under control (6). For periodontal abscesses, initial treatment may be definitive, but a retained foreign body may still need to be removed to prevent recurrence.

The only absolute contraindication to performance of incision and drainage in the ED is a patient who cannot be sedated and/or restrained sufficiently to enable the procedure to be performed safely. Such patients may require general anesthesia to perform the operation and thus are not amenable to treatment in the emergency setting. Relative contraindications to the procedure are patient toxicity and nonfluctuant lesions. The emergency physician needs to determine the risks versus the benefits of proceeding in these situations.

▶ EQUIPMENT

Topical benzocaine
1% lidocaine
3- or 5-mL syringe for anesthetic administration
25-gauge needle
20-gauge Angiocath and 10-mL syringe (wound irrigation)
Saline for irrigation
Scalpel with No. 11 blade (may substitute No. 15 blade if preferred)
Small, curved hemostat
10 2″ × 2″ gauze sponges
Forceps (without teeth)
Suction tip connected to suction
Culture swab
Bite block or mouth prop for uncooperative patients

Monitoring equipment (if sedation is to be used)

Plain gauze or petroleum gauze

Optional equipment (if drain is to be placed):

- T-drain (T-shaped latex drain) or small Penrose drain
- Suture kit
- 3.0 nonabsorbable (silk) suture

▶ PROCEDURE

Anesthesia is difficult to achieve in an area of infection due to the acidic nature of pus. Liberal application of a topical anesthetic such as benzocaine may help. In many cases, a regional block (Chapter 62) may be more effective, but usually the procedure can be accomplished with local infiltration. A topical disinfectant such as chlorhexidine may be used, but this practice is rare (7). Infiltration into the buccogingival fold or circumferential to the lesion should be accomplished with lidocaine (see Fig. 62.4). This should be done slowly to minimize patient discomfort. The anesthetic requires several minutes to work. The level of anesthesia should be tested before proceeding.

For uncooperative patients, it may be necessary to use either a bite block (a rubber block that is placed between the molars) or a mouth prop (an adjustable metal prop). As this is usually a relatively short procedure, these items are needed infrequently once anesthesia is established. The physician needs only to visualize the lesion. Lip retraction is usually of little added benefit.

With the scalpel blade perpendicular to the bone, a horizontal incision is made through the area of fluctuance. The incision should extend down to the level of the alveolar bone if dealing with a periapical abscess (Fig. 63.2B,C) and should be long enough to allow proper drainage without premature closure. Entry into the abscess cavity is sufficient for periodontal lesions. Gauze sponges or suction should be readily available to remove the pus and avoid the possibility of aspiration. The incision should be widely opened by dissection using the hemostat along the abscess tract. For periapical infections, the dissection should proceed through the bone to the periapical area to allow drainage of the source of infection (Fig. 63.2D). A culture should be obtained and the wound thoroughly irrigated with saline through a 20-gauge Angiocath. Lidocaine may be added to the irrigation solution to decrease sensitivity if desired.

Although most dental texts recommend using a drain (8), many dentists feel this may not be necessary in all cases. Use of a drain tends to be reserved for very extensive abscesses or those with extraoral spread (e.g., those with periorbital or malar swelling). The wound can be packed with either iodoform or petroleum gauze, which should be changed within 24 to 48 hours after the procedure. If a latex drain is to be used, it will need to be sutured in place to prevent dislodgment. A single stitch to the gingival surface is generally sufficient. The drain should remain in place for 24 to 48 hours (7).

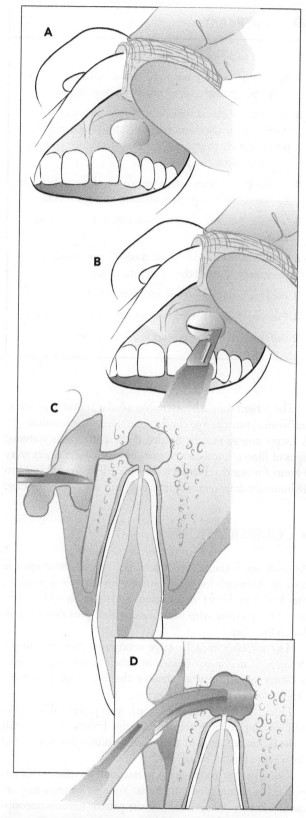

Figure 63.2 Incision and drainage of a periapical abscess.
A. External appearance of a periapical abscess.
B,C. Incision of a periapical abscess.
D. Dissection along abscess tract.

SUMMARY

1 Provide sedation when necessary.

2 Apply topical anesthesia, followed by local infiltrative anesthesia or regional nerve block.

3 Make a horizontal incision through the area of fluctuance and extend the incision to the bone for a periapical abscess; have suction or a gauze sponge ready to catch any pus.

4 Widen the incision with a hemostat; dissect through the bone for a periapical abscess when possible.

5 Irrigate the wound with saline through a 20-gauge Angiocath.

6 Place a drain or packing (if desired, but usually not necessary); suture the drain into place.

7 Begin a 5-day course of oral antibiotics.

8 Encourage warm water rinses for the first 24 hours.

9 Refer for dental follow-up at 24 to 48 hours.

The patient should be started on a 5-day course of systemic antibiotics (penicillin or clindamycin) after the procedure (6). A longer course may be needed if the patient has systemic signs of illness. Local care consists of warm water rinses every 4 hours for one day. Dental follow-up will be needed in 24 to 48 hours for drain removal (if placed) and more definitive care.

▶ COMPLICATIONS

As with any intraoral procedure, the risk of bacteremia is present. Although for most patients this is rarely a problem, the American Heart Association guidelines should be followed for patients with heart disease that puts them at risk for endocarditis.

The incision must be large enough to promote proper drainage. If drainage is inadequate, the infection may worsen and may spread to other areas of the face, leading to more serious soft-tissue infections.

Despite optimal care, most teeth with periapical abscesses will die due to necrosis of the pulp. Follow-up care with a dentist is required to more fully evaluate the tooth and determine if it can be salvaged.

Good patient cooperation is essential; therefore, it is important to attain good anesthesia. Younger patients may require sedation (Chapter 33). If the patient remains uncooperative, dental referral would be appropriate.

CLINICAL TIPS

▶ Acute drainage in the ED is indicated only in stable patients for whom dental referral will be delayed or when pain relief is necessary and a dentist is unavailable.

▶ Carious teeth are suggestive of a periapical rather than a periodontal abscess.

▶ Good anesthesia is crucial. Treatment is rarely successful if a child feels any significant pain.

▶ All patients will require dental follow-up for more definitive treatment.

▶ SUMMARY

Dental abscesses are not uncommon in the pediatric population. In children, periapical abscesses are more common and are usually the result of pulpal inflammation secondary to caries. Although incision and drainage is usually left to the dentist or oral surgeon, this procedure can be performed by the emergency physician on stable patients for whom referral might be delayed. The procedure is done to relieve pain and to prevent the spread of infection to other areas of the head and neck. Close follow-up and dental referral for definitive treatment are imperative.

▶ REFERENCES

1. Winter GB, Hill FJ. Local oral pathology in children and adolescents. In: Braham RL, Morris ME, eds. *Textbook of Pediatric Dentistry*. 2nd ed. Baltimore: Williams & Wilkins; 1985:322–349.

2. Judd PL, Sandor GK. Management of odontogenic orofacial infection in the young child. *Ont Dent.* 1997;74(8):39–45.

3. Brook I. Microbiology and management of endodontic infections in children. *J Clin Pediatr Dent.* 2003;28:13–18.

4. Wynn RL, Bergman SA, Meiller TF, et al. Antibiotics in treating oralfacial infections of odontogenic origin: an update. *Gen Dent.* 2001; 49:238–244.

5. Hutton CE. Oral surgery for the child patient. In: McDonald RE, Avery DR, eds. *Dentistry for the Child and Adolescent*. 5th ed. St. Louis: Mosby; 1987:652–659.

6. Cummings RR, Ingle JI, Frand AL, et al. Endodontic surgery. In: Ingle JI, Taintor JF, eds. *Endodontics*. 3rd ed. Philadelphia: Lea & Febiger; 1985:618–707.

7. Kilgore TB. Minor oral surgery in pediatric dentistry. In: Braham RL, Morris ME, eds. *Textbook of Pediatric Dentistry*. 2nd ed. Baltimore: Williams & Wilkins; 1985:407–430.

8. Thoma KH. *Oral Surgery*. 5th ed. St. Louis: Mosby; 1969.

JOHN M. LOISELLE AND MELANIE PITONE

Management of Dental Fractures

64

▶ INTRODUCTION

Certain tooth fractures are considered dental emergencies. Fractures can occur as the result of isolated mouth trauma or as part of multisystem injury. The severity of fractures ranges from minor cracks to complex transections of the tooth. The primary goal in the acute management of tooth fractures is to maintain the vitality of the pulp, which is the neurovascular tissue within the tooth. Viability of the tooth in many cases is time dependent, and prognosis is best when treatment is initiated shortly after the injury (1,2). Predictions of the future health of an injured tooth must be made cautiously. The extent of injury to the dental pulp is difficult to determine, and response of the pulp to injury is varied. One child may have multiple dental injuries from one incident, and each tooth may have a different outcome (3).

Three peak ages predict when pediatric dental trauma is most likely to occur. The first peak is between 1 and 3 years of age, when the child is learning to walk. Bicycle and playground injuries predominate in the 7- to 10-year-old age group. The onset of athletic endeavors and aggressive or violent activities bring the third peak, at ages 16 to 18 (4).

Patients commonly seek treatment for dental injuries in the emergency department (ED), although it is not unusual to see these injuries in the office or outpatient clinic setting. Optimal management of a tooth fracture is immediate evaluation by a dentist capable of performing a definitive restoration of the tooth. This approach should be taken when it is available. However, in considering time constraints involved with tooth viability and potential inability to obtain timely dental consultation during off hours, emergency physicians should be familiar with early management options for these injuries. Application of a protective covering (described in this chapter) and splinting (described in Chapter 66) are temporizing procedures performed before eventual aesthetic restoration of the tooth in an outpatient setting.

▶ ANATOMY AND PHYSIOLOGY

The primary (deciduous) teeth and the secondary (permanent) teeth share a common anatomy, as illustrated in Figure 64.1. The external anatomy of the tooth is divided into two segments, with the gingival margin serving as the dividing line. The clinical crown is the part of the tooth exposed above the margin, whereas the remainder of the tooth below the margin comprises the root. Each tooth is composed of several layers. The external coating of the crown is the enamel, which is the hardest substance in the body. The underlying calcified layer is the dentin. The neurovascular supply, or pulp, is located in the center of the tooth and runs the length of the root. The cementum is an outer layer of calcified material on the root of the tooth. Each tooth is supported in the alveolar bone by fibrous connective tissue known as the periodontal ligament.

Several characteristics, including size, shape, and color, help to distinguish primary from secondary teeth (Table 64.1). This differentiation can frequently be an issue with anterior teeth in the presence of mixed dentition. The age of the child also is a helpful indicator of tooth type. Eruption of the permanent central incisors and first molars generally does not occur until the child has reached 6 to 8 years of age (Table 64.2). Permanent teeth are larger than primary teeth, and their color ranges from white to a yellowish gray. Primary teeth are a milky, opalescent white and have therefore acquired the name "milk teeth." Primary incisors tend to have a smooth incisal edge, in contrast to the permanent incisors, which are often ridged, especially on the incisal surface. In questionable cases, a radiograph may be useful in demonstrating the presence or absence of a developing permanent tooth.

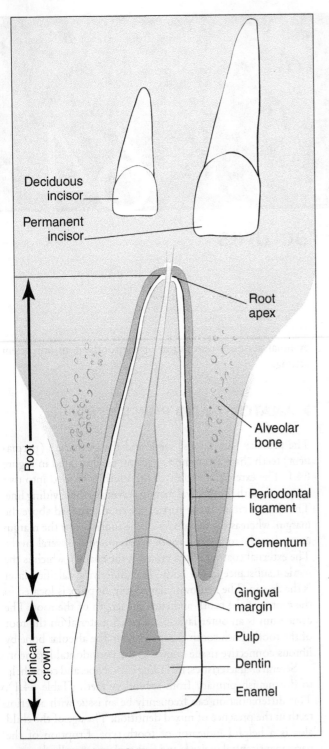

Figure 64.1 Basic tooth anatomy.

TABLE 64.1	DIFFERENTIATING CHARACTERISTICS OF PRIMARY AND SECONDARY TEETH	
Characteristics	**Primary teeth**	**Secondary teeth**
Age	<6 y	>5 y
Color	Milky white, opalescent	White to yellowish gray
Size	Smaller	Larger
Clinical crown length	Shorter	Wider
Shape	Smooth	Ridged
Radiographic appearance	Developing permanent tooth visible	No apical structures visible

tures are those involving only the enamel. The enamel may also sustain an internal fracture or crack that is not evident on visual inspection. An internal fracture line may be seen on transillumination of the tooth. Internal fractures are important to identify because they cause a weakness in the tooth, which can fracture at a later time. These fractures can be easily diagnosed upon dental referral with radiographs. Fractures that involve the dentin can be identified by the presence of a yellow area within the fracture site and an associated sensitivity of the tooth. Because dentin consists of microtubules that communicate with the pulp, exposure of dentin allows insult to the pulp, which can result in inflammation, infection, and eventual necrosis. Fractures resulting in pulp exposure are identified by the presence of a pink area or an actual bleeding spot located in the center of the tooth. Early treatment of dentin and pulpal exposure is crucial in preserving the viability of these teeth (12–14).

Fractures limited to the visible portion of the tooth above the gingiva are crown fractures and involve the enamel, dentin, and occasionally the pulp. Those that are visible above the gingiva but extend into the root of the tooth are crown-root fractures. They involve the enamel, dentin, cementum, and frequently the pulp. These complicated fractures are best handled through dental referral. Isolated root fractures are not visible on the exposed portion of the tooth. The diagnosis is suggested by mobility of the tooth and is confirmed with

TABLE 64.2	ERUPTION SCHEDULE FOR SECONDARY DENTITION	
	Age (y)	
	Lower	**Upper**
Central Incisors	6–7	7–8
Lateral Incisors	7–8	8–9
Cuspids	9–10	11–12
First bicuspids	10–12	10–11
Second bicuspids	11–12	10–12
First molars	6–7	6–7
Second molars	11–13	12–13
Third molars	17–21	17–21

Adapted from Lunt RC, Law DB. A review of the chronology of eruption of deciduous teeth. *J Am Dent Assoc.* 1974;89:872–879.

The maxillary central incisors are prominent and consequently are the most commonly fractured primary and permanent teeth (3,5–10). Children with excessive protrusion of the maxillary incisors are especially susceptible to injury. Teeth can fracture in a number of ways (Fig. 64.2). Fractures are classified as complicated or uncomplicated depending on whether the pulp is exposed or not (11). The simplest frac-

cally distinguishable from luxation injuries; thus suspicion of either should lead to referral to the dentist (3).

Despite timely management of tooth injuries, death of the pulp may be unavoidable. The initial traumatic event can result in a disruption of blood flow to the pulp, which is not detectable at the time of presentation. Fractures that expose the dentin or pulp are associated with a risk of inflammation and infection, which can progress to pulp necrosis and eventual loss of the tooth. Infection and death of the pulp when left untreated can lead to a local abscess or cellulitis.

Tooth discoloration can occur following fractures as breakdown products of hemoglobin become deposited in the microtubules of the dentin. In some cases, this staining resolves over time. Pulp damage can result in permanent discoloration of the tooth due to tissue necrosis (13).

▶ INDICATIONS

Treatment of tooth fractures with the goal of improving tooth survival is generally limited to the secondary dentition (Table 64.3). Primary teeth are more commonly cracked than fractured. Exposure of the pulp is rare. If pulpal exposure occurs in primary dentition, treatment is determined by the amount of pulp exposed and the involvement of the root. These teeth may be observed by the dentist for possible maintained vitality; others will be extracted to protect the patient from infection or damage to the underlying permanent teeth (13). Survival of a primary tooth once a significant fracture has occurred is not significantly improved by immediate active interventions. Normal exfoliation of these teeth results in an altered cosmetic appearance that is only a temporary condition.

Fractures that are limited to the enamel require minimal intervention in the acute care setting, and patients can generally be referred for aesthetic repair by a dentist.

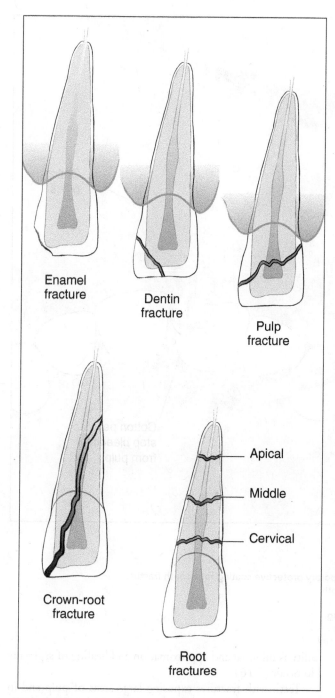

Figure 64.2 Fractures through various layers of the tooth and location of root fractures.

radiographs. Root fractures are classified according to their location along the length of the root. They may be classified as cervical, middle, or apical based on their location in relation to the crown of the tooth (Fig. 64.2). The cervical third is adjacent to the clinical crown, and the apical third is located at the root apex. Root fractures usually result in an extruded tooth, with bleeding at the gingiva. The site of the fracture determines the degree of mobility of the tooth, as apical fractures are less mobile. Root fractures are not clini-

TABLE 64.3	EMERGENCY DEPARTMENT MANAGEMENT OF DENTAL FRACTURES	
Injury type	**Clinical findings**	**Treatment options**
Primary teeth	See Table 64.1	Extraction
		Dental referral
Secondary teeth		
Enamel	Chip of top layer	Dental referral
Dentin	Exposed yellow area below enamel	Dental referral
	Tooth sensitivity	Temporary Ca(OH)₂ or glass ionomer coating
Pulp	Exposed pink area	Temporary Ca(OH)₂ or glass ionomer coating
	Frank bleeding dot	
	Tooth sensitivity	
Crown-root fracture	Fracture line visible above gingiva and extending into root	Dental referral
Root fracture	Tooth mobility	Splinting for cervical and middle third root fractures
	Bleeding at gingiva	
	Fracture on radiograph	

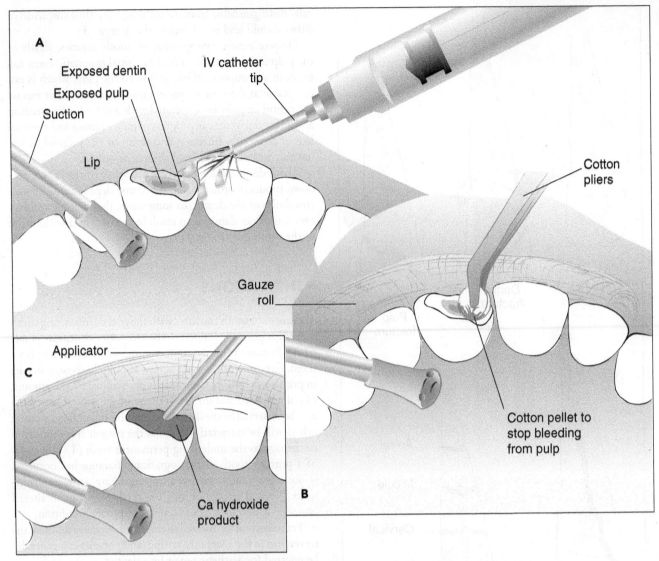

Figure 64.3 Application of a temporary protective coating for a tooth fracture.
A. Saline irrigation of fractured tooth.
B. Drying and hemostasis.
C. Application of protective coating.

Fractures through dentin (identified by its yellowish tint) that do not involve the pulp also can be referred to a dentist for definitive treatment. Damage involving deep or large areas of exposed dentin may be reversible if care is obtained within 24 to 48 hours of the injury.

Tooth fractures that result in frank pulpal exposure or occur adjacent to the pulp, as suggested by the presence of a pink area or frank bleeding dot, require emergent dental treatment. Pulp exposure to the oral environment and surrounding bacteria should be minimized by applying a temporary protective coating. Crown-root fractures are best handled through dental referral. Acute management of cervical and middle third root fractures of the permanent dentition consists of stabilization through splinting (Chapter 66), a process that is generally not practical in the primary dentition (6,9,15). Fractures in the apical third of the root often do not require splinting, as mo-

bility is minimal and approximation and healing of segments do occur (7,16).

Teeth with fractures exposing large areas of pulp and in which treatment is delayed for several hours or in which the pulp appears grossly contaminated have a low rate of survival and do not benefit from applying a protective coating in the ED (1,2). Treatment of dental injuries may be deferred to the inpatient setting when associated with more urgent medical priorities (16).

▶ EQUIPMENT

Mouth mirror
Gloves
Protective eyewear

Dental explorer
Cotton rolls
Calcium hydroxide or glass ionomer product
Calcium hydroxide applicator
Mixing pad
Gauze rolls
Cotton pliers
Cotton pellets
Suction catheter
Aspirating syringe
27-gauge, 1-inch needles
Local anesthetic (2% lidocaine with epinephrine
  1:100,000)
McKesson or Molt mouth prop
Monitoring as needed for procedural sedation

▶ PROCEDURE

All tooth fragments must be accounted for, because they may become lodged in lacerations, aspirated, or swallowed. A chest radiograph is indicated in the event of a missing tooth fragment. Radiographs that include the lip or tongue are necessary to rule out the presence of tooth fragments within lacerations of these structures. Original tooth fragments have a chance for reattachment at a later time if they can be stored in physiologic saline until definitive treatment by the dentist (17).

Young children and the occasional older child may require some combination of restraint and/or procedural sedation for this procedure. For those patients in whom cooperation is hard to obtain, a mouth prop should be inserted to allow adequate visualization and working space. In the most common scenario, a maxillary central incisor injury, the patient is placed in a supine position with the physician seated at the head or side of the bed where control and access are greatest. Both the dentin and the pulp can be extremely sensitive, and regional anesthesia may be required before initiation of the procedure (Chapter 62). The area around the fractured tooth is irrigated with normal saline through a syringe and intravenous catheter or splash shield while simultaneously oral suction is used to remove any loose material or blood (Fig. 64.3A). Once the area has been cleaned, it is dried but not desiccated, using a combination of a suction catheter and gauze pads. Gauze rolls are placed between the lip and tooth, and generous oral suction is used to prevent obstruction or contamination of the field by oral secretions. Any bleeding from the pulp can usually be controlled with pressure from cotton pellets on the end of the cotton pliers (Fig. 64.3B). Calcium hydroxide base and catalyst or glass ionomer product is mixed on a mixing pad, and a thin layer is applied directly to the pulp and the surrounding 2 mm of dentin using the applicator instrument or the wooden end of a cotton-tipped swab (Fig. 64.3C). This is *only* a temporizing measure, and follow-up with a dentist should occur within 24 hours. A soft diet is recommended until that time. Prophylactic antibiotics are of unproven bene-

fit in acutely traumatized teeth and should not be given unless other indications for antibiotics are present (11,12,14).

▶ COMPLICATIONS

A poor outcome is more likely to result from failure to provide timely treatment or from irreversible damage occurring at the time of the injury than from poor technique in applying the protective coating.

Excessive stimulation or drying of the pulp during the procedure may adversely affect its viability. Inadequate coverage of the pulp results in continued exposure to infection and irritation, which seriously harms the tooth's chance for survival. The need for early dental referral to minimize these complications cannot be overemphasized.

SUMMARY

1 Account for any missing tooth fragments.

2 Use restraint, procedural sedation, and a bite block as needed.

3 Inject regional or local anesthesia.

4 Irrigate the fractured tooth and surrounding area with normal saline.

5 Dry the fractured tooth and surrounding area with suction and gauze pads.

6 Apply calcium hydroxide or glass ionomer product to the fracture with an applicator stick or the wooden end of a cotton-tipped swab.

CLINICAL TIPS

▶ Follow-up care with a dentist is essential for optimal outcome.

▶ Extreme sensitivity is common following a tooth fracture involving dentin or pulp.

▶ Prognosis for teeth with pulpal exposure or deeper dentin involvement is time dependent.

▶ Calcium hydroxide or glass ionomer application is not indicated if delay in treatment is greater than several hours or if the tooth is grossly contaminated, because more extensive pulp treatment will be required.

▶ Visualization of a central pink area or bleeding from the tooth is diagnostic for pulp involvement.

▶ SUMMARY

Children experience a wide variety of tooth fractures. A fracture of a permanent tooth in which the pulp is exposed is considered a true dental emergency, and survival is time dependent. When a dentist is not immediately available, application of a protective covering of a calcium hydroxide or glass ionomer product may temporarily preserve the viability of the tooth. Follow-up by a dentist is necessary for definitive repair.

▶ ACKNOWLEDGMENT

The authors would like to acknowledge the valuable contributions of Mark L. Helpix to the version of this chapter that appeared in the previous edition.

▶ REFERENCES

1. Basrani E. *Fractures of the Teeth*. Philadelphia: Lea & Febiger; 1985.
2. Klokkevold P. Common dental emergencies, evaluation and management for emergency physicians. *Emerg Med Clin North Am*. 1989;7:29–63.
3. Garcia-Godoy F. Treatment of trauma to the primary and young permanent dentitions. *Dent Clin North Am*. 2000;44:597–632.
4. Berkowitz R, Ludwig S, Johnson R. Dental trauma in children and adolescents. *Clin Pediatr*. 1980;19:166–171.
5. Lombardi SM, Sheller B, Williams BJ. Diagnosis and treatment of dental trauma in a children's hospital. *Pediatr Dent*. 1998;20:112–120.
6. Andreasen JD, Andreasen FM. *Essentials of Traumatic Injuries to the Teeth*. Copenhagen: Munksgaard; 1990.
7. Comer RW, Fitchie JG, Caughman WF, et al. Oral trauma. *Postgrad Med*. 1989;85(2):34–41.
8. Josell SD, Abrams RG. Managing common dental problems and emergencies. *Pediatr Clin North Am*. 1991;38:1325–1342.
9. Josell SD, Abrams RG. Traumatic injuries to the dentition and its supporting structures. *Pediatr Clin North Am*. 1982;29:717–741.
10. McDonald RE, Avery DR. *Dentistry for the Child and Adolescent*. 6th ed. St. Louis: Mosby; 1986.
11. Andreasen JD. *Traumatic Injuries of the Teeth*. 2nd ed. Copenhagen: Munksgaard; 1981.
12. McTigue DJ. Management of orofacial trauma in children. *Pediatr Ann*. 1985;14:125–129.
13. Nelson LP, Shusterman S. Emergency management of oral trauma in children. *Curr Opin Pediatr*. 1997;9:242–245.
14. McTigue DJ. Diagnosis and management of dental injuries in children. *Pediatr Clin North Am*. 2000;47:1067–1084.
15. American Academy of Pediatric Dentistry. Clinical guideline on management of acute dental trauma. *Pediatr Dent*. 2004;26(7):120–127.
16. Dierks EJ. Management of associated dental injuries in maxillofacial trauma. *Otolaryngol Clin North Am*. 1991;24:165–179.
17. Dewhurst SN, Mason C, Roberts GJ. Emergency treatment of orodental injuries: a review. *Br J Oral Maxillofac Surg*. 1998;36:165–175.

BRUCE L. KLEIN AND BERNARD J. LARSON

65

Reimplanting an Avulsed Permanent Tooth

▶ INTRODUCTION

An avulsed tooth is a tooth that has been totally displaced from its socket. Children and adolescents sustaining this type of injury commonly present to the emergency department (ED). If the tooth is part of the permanent (secondary) dentition, the physician may be able to salvage it. It is emphasized that avulsion of a permanent tooth is a true dental emergency. An early study found that when avulsed teeth were reimplanted within 30 minutes, there was a 90% success rate; when they remained out for several hours, less than 5% exhibited long-term "survival" (1). More recent studies report an even shorter extraoral time period is required to achieve a good prognosis (2–6).

▶ ANATOMY AND PHYSIOLOGY

Maxillary central incisors are avulsed most frequently, followed by maxillary lateral incisors (7). Children with prognathism (buck teeth) are particularly prone to incur such injuries (8). Mandibular incisors and canines are avulsed less often, and posterior teeth only rarely (7).

The emergency physician must distinguish an avulsed deciduous (primary) tooth from a permanent one because their management differs greatly. Deciduous incisors are smaller and have less pronounced serrations along the edges. In addition, a deciduous maxillary central incisor is approximately the same size as its lateral counterpart, whereas a permanent maxillary central incisor is noticeably larger than the corresponding lateral incisor (see Table 64.1). Another clue is that deciduous incisors are most often exfoliated between 6 and 9 years of age. Mandibular central incisors are shed first (6 to

7 years of age), followed by maxillary central and mandibular lateral incisors (7 to 8 years of age), and maxillary lateral incisors (8 to 9 years of age) (see Table 64.2) (9).

Avulsions of permanent teeth occur most often in 7- to 10-year-old boys (8,10). Bicycle and skateboard accidents and sports injuries are the typical causes (11,12). Several factors predispose to exarticulations at this age. Between 7 and 10 years of age, the roots of the permanent teeth are immaturely formed, the periodontal ligaments are loosely structured and weakly connect the roots to the alveolar bone, and the alveolar bone is relatively soft (11,13). In contrast, older individuals with mature roots, strong periodontal ligaments, and hard alveolar bone are more likely to sustain a dental fracture rather than an avulsion.

The key to successful reimplantation is maintaining the viability of the periodontal ligament fibers. These surround the root and secure it to the adjacent alveolar bone. Following a traumatic avulsion, some fibers remain attached to the root whereas others remain on the surrounding alveolus. To avoid traumatizing the periodontal ligament fibers, one should only handle the tooth by its crown. In addition, the fibers are quite sensitive and do not tolerate drying or prolonged lack of nutrition. Therefore, if for some reason the tooth cannot be reimplanted immediately, it must be stored in a suitable liquid medium. Although a commercially prepared medium such as ViaSpan (which is used for transplant organ storage) or Hank's balanced salt solution is best, this type of solution is rarely available, even in the ED (14–16). Cool milk, which is readily available in the home, is a good next choice, followed by intraoral saliva and physiologic saline solution (8,10,11,17,18). Storing the tooth in water is least preferable but is better than letting it dry (16,19).

▶ **INDICATIONS**

The sole indication for reimplantation is avulsion of a permanent tooth that is not severely fractured. In general, a tooth with a root fracture or a vertical fracture more than half its length should not be reimplanted.

Because the long-term success rate of reimplantation is inversely related to the time the tooth remains out of its socket, the tooth must be reimplanted as rapidly as possible. A tooth that has sustained a prolonged extraoral dry time has an especially poor prognosis. Recent recommendations caution against reimplanting an avulsed permanent tooth with an incompletely developed root that has suffered a prolonged extraoral dry time (e.g., greater than 60 minutes) because of concerns regarding replacement root resorption (20–22). However, we advise the emergency physician to consult a dentist before making this decision.

An avulsed deciduous tooth should not be reimplanted because its root may damage the developing permanent tooth bud during reimplantation (8,10–13,17). Potential sequelae to the immature permanent tooth include enamel dysplasia, root deformation, and discontinuance of tooth development (23). We suggest that the child place it under a pillow for the tooth fairy instead.

▶ **EQUIPMENT**

> Hank's balanced salt solution, milk, or ViaSpan
> Light source
> Monojet syringe (5 or 10 cc)
> Mouth prop (commercial version or taped stack of tongue depressors)
> Physiologic saline solution
> Sterile gauze
> Sterile gloves
> Suction (wall or portable)
> Suction catheter (Yankauer)
> Tongue depressor

▶ **PROCEDURE**

What follows is a general but reasonable approach that is intended for emergency physicians in the ED until a dentist arrives (16,18,20–22,24). If a dentist is immediately available or the patient presents directly to a dental office, management may differ or be expanded upon, based on factors such as the extraoral dry time, whether or not the root is immature or completely developed, and the availability of special equipment and materials like doxycycline, fluoride and EDTA solutions, and Emdogain.

The avulsed tooth must be located first. This seems obvious, but sometimes a frantic parent forgets to search for the tooth, rushing the child to the ED without it. If the tooth cannot be found at the scene, it may be embedded in the child's lip or the child may have aspirated or swallowed it.

Whenever possible, the parent should be instructed to reimplant the tooth before leaving for the ED. However, this is not always feasible. Often the parent does not call the ED before leaving or is simply too upset or otherwise unable to reinsert the tooth at home. Similarly, if the physician thinks the child may aspirate or swallow the tooth en route, it is safest to defer this procedure. In such cases, the tooth should be transported to the ED in cool milk. An alternative is for the child or parent to hold it under the tongue or in the buccal pouch. Although acceptable, this is less optimal, both because saliva is contaminated by bacteria and because the carrier might aspirate or swallow the tooth.

To minimize damage to the periodontal ligament, the tooth must always be handled by its crown, never by its root. After identifying it as a permanent tooth, it should be inspected for fractures. Reimplantation is contraindicated if a root fracture or a vertical fracture more than half its length is discovered. The best way to cleanse visible debris off the tooth is to hold it by the crown and gently swirl it in ViaSpan, Hank's balanced salt solution, milk, or physiologic saline solution (Fig. 65.1A) or rinse it gently with a stream of saline. If necessary, the tooth can be rinsed under slowly running water, although obviously this should never be done over an open drain. Importantly, the tooth must never be scrubbed, because this will injure the periodontal ligament fibers.

Before reimplanting the tooth, the empty socket from which it was avulsed must be located. When multiple teeth have been avulsed, this may not be a trivial task. A hematoma or ecchymosis of the gingival mucosa near the socket suggests the possibility of an alveolar bone fracture. To help visualize the socket better, the surrounding area can be lightly swabbed with a wet gauze pad or cleared with low suction (Fig. 65.1B). The socket should be flushed gently with saline to remove any clot. There is some evidence to suggest that the presence of a clot in the socket at the time of reimplantation predisposes to ankylosis. When the patient has delayed seeking care, suction may be necessary to disrupt and dislodge a hardening clot.

Reimplanting the avulsed tooth is actually a relatively simple procedure. First, the tooth is positioned and aligned correctly at the socket opening. Then, with firm but gentle pressure, it is reinserted into the depth of the socket (Fig. 65.1C). Administering a sedative or local anesthetic is usually not necessary. If there is resistance to reinsertion, the alveolus should be inspected for fractures. When present, the displaced alveolar bone can be repositioned using a flat instrument placed inside the socket. Often the reimplanted tooth protrudes a little more than its nonavulsed equal. The tooth must be stabilized manually until the dentist arrives; the child can bite on a gauze pad or tongue depressor, or a responsible adult can hold the tooth in place with finger pressure (Fig. 65.1D).

Emergency dental consultation is mandatory. Even when the tooth has been reinserted, it remains unstable. To secure

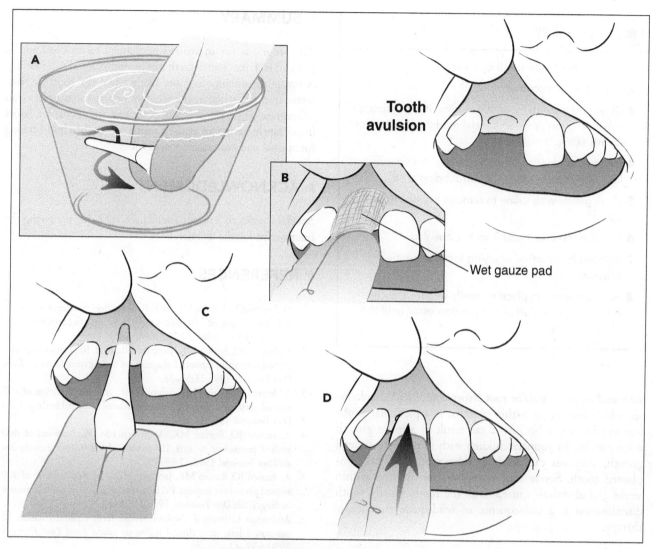

Figure 65.1 Reinserting an avulsed tooth.
A. Cleansing the avulsed tooth.
B. Clearing blood and secretions from the surrounding area.
C. Reimplanting the tooth.
D. Stabilizing the reimplanted tooth.

it better, the tooth must be splinted to the adjacent teeth; a slightly flexible splint, such as an acid etch splint, is ideal for this purpose (see Chapter 66). Generally, a dental radiograph is taken to confirm proper tooth positioning and to diagnose any associated alveolar bone fractures.

In one study, inflammatory root resorption was greatly reduced when systemic antibiotics were administered following reimplantation (25). Therefore, we recommend prescribing a 7-day regimen of prophylactic penicillin, which is started before discharge. The patient should also be started on a soft diet, be instructed to brush regularly with a soft toothbrush, and be given prescriptions for chlorhexidine mouth rinse and an analgesic. A tetanus booster should be administered if required. A follow-up appointment with the dentist should be scheduled for 7 to 10 days. At this visit, the splint is removed

and endodontic therapy is usually begun. In an older child or adolescent, root canal treatment is essential because the neurovascular structures of the pulp are virtually always destroyed and will not regenerate. Root canal therapy removes necrotic tissue and, hopefully, arrests inflammatory root resorption. In contrast, a 6- to 8-year-old child may not need endodontic therapy; the root of an immature permanent tooth still retains an open apex, so revascularization is possible (2,4).

▶ COMPLICATIONS

Local infection, especially abscess formation, is the principal short-term concern. The most important long-term complications are ankylosis of the reimplanted tooth to the

SUMMARY

1 Always handle the tooth by its crown.

2 Inspect it for fractures.

3 Cleanse the tooth by gently swirling it in physiologic saline solution or a commercial medium or irrigating it with saline.

4 Locate the empty socket; for better visualization, lightly suction or swab the surrounding area.

5 Flush gently with saline to remove any clot from the socket.

6 Position the tooth at the socket opening.

7 Reinsert it smoothly, applying firm but gentle pressure.

8 Hold the tooth in place manually or have the child bite on a gauze pad or tongue depressor until the dentist arrives.

surrounding bone and/or root resorption (24,25). Ankylosis, which may occur within months, is a particular problem in adolescents because it can result in alveolar growth discrepancies. In younger children with incomplete skeletal growth, ankylosis can result in submergence of the reimplanted tooth. Severe root resorption can develop within weeks and ultimately cause loss of the tooth. Finally, tooth discoloration is a consequence of inadequate endodontic therapy.

CLINICAL TIPS

▶ Reimplantation is only indicated for an avulsed permanent tooth, not for a deciduous (primary) tooth.

▶ The tooth must be reimplanted immediately. Delay greatly reduces the chance of success.

▶ If the parent or physician cannot reimplant the tooth, it should be stored in ViaSpan, Hank's balanced salt solution, cool milk, or physiologic saline. Do not allow it to dry.

▶ Always handle the tooth by its crown. Never touch the root.

▶ The dentist should be consulted as soon as the physician is notified about the case.

▶ SUMMARY

The prognosis for an avulsed permanent tooth need not be grim; in fact, many such teeth can be reimplanted successfully. A favorable outcome is more likely when the tooth is reinserted immediately after the accident occurs and the physician adheres strictly to the protocol described in this chapter. Most importantly, saving an avulsed tooth spares the child lifelong functional and cosmetic consequences.

▶ ACKNOWLEDGMENT

Special thanks to Jennifer Pacella, D.M.D., for reviewing the manuscript for the chapter.

▶ REFERENCES

1. Andreasen JO, Hjorting Hansen E. Replantation of teeth: radiographic and clinical study of 110 human teeth replanted after accidental loss. *Acta Odontol Scand.* 1966;24:263–286.
2. Andreasen JO, Borum MK, Jacobsen HL, et al. Replantation of 400 avulsed permanent incisors, I: diagnosis of healing complications. *Endod Dent Traumatol.* 1995;11:51–58.
3. Andreasen JO, Borum MK, Jacobsen HL, et al. Replantation of 400 avulsed permanent incisors, II: factors related to pulpal healing. *Endod Dent Traumatol.* 1995;11:59–68.
4. Andreasen JO, Borum MK, Andreasen FM. Replantation of 400 avulsed permanent incisors, III: factors related to root growth. *Endod Dent Traumatol.* 1995;11:69–75.
5. Andreasen JO, Borum MK, Jacobsen HL, et al. Replantation of 400 avulsed permanent incisors, IV: factors related to periodontal ligament healing. *Endod Dent Traumatol.* 1995;11:76–89.
6. Andersson L, Bodin I. Avulsed human teeth replanted within 15 minutes: a long-term clinical follow-up study. *Endod Dent Traumatol.* 1990;6:37–42.
7. Coccia CT. A clinical investigation of root resorption rates in reimplanted young permanent incisors: a 5-year study. *J Endod.* 1980;6:413–420.
8. Henry RJ. Pediatric dental emergencies. *Pediatr Nurs.* 1991;17:162–167.
9. Barone MA, ed. *The Harriet Lane Handbook.* St. Louis: Mosby; 1996:274.
10. Mueller WA. Emergency dental care. *Pediatrician.* 1989;16:147–152.
11. McIlveen LP. Orofacial trauma in children. *Pediatr Basics.* 1990;54:7–16.
12. Josell SD, Abrams RG. Managing common dental problems and emergencies. *Pediatr Clin North Am.* 1991;38:1325–1342.
13. Dierks EJ. Management of associated dental injuries in maxillofacial trauma. *Otolaryngol Clin North Am.* 1991;24:165–179.
14. Hiltz J, Trope M. Vitality of human lip fibroblasts in milk, Hanks balanced salt solution and ViaSpan storage media. *Endod Dent Traumatol.* 1991;7:69–72.
15. Krasner P, Person P. Preserving avulsed teeth for replantation. *J Am Dent Assoc.* 1992;123:80–88.
16. American Academy of Pediatric Dentistry, Council on Clinical Affairs. Clinical guideline on management of acute dental trauma. *Pediatr Dent.* 2004-2005;26(reference manual):120–125.
17. Nelson LP. Pediatric emergencies in the office setting: oral trauma. *Pediatr Emerg Care.* 1990;6:62–64.

18. Barrett EJ, Kenny DJ. Avulsed permanent teeth: a review of the literature and treatment guidelines. *Endod Dent Traumatol.* 1997;13:153–163.

19. Lindskog S, Blomlof L. Influence of osmolarity and composition of some storage media on human periodontal ligament cells. *Acta Odontol Scand.* 1982;40:435–441.

20. American Association of Endodontists. Treatment of the avulsed permanent tooth. *Dent Clin North Am.* 1995;39:221–225.

21. Flores MT, Andreasen JO, Bakland LK, et al. Guidelines for the evaluation and management of traumatic dental injuries. *Dent Traumatol.* 2001;17:193–196.

22. Ram D, Cohenca N. Therapeutic protocols for avulsed permanent teeth: review and clinical update. *Pediatr Dent.* 2004;26:251–255.

23. Holan G, Topf J, Fuks AB. Effect of root canal infection and treatment of traumatized primary incisors on their permanent successors. *Endod Dent Traumatol.* 1992;8:12–15.

24. Andreasen JO, Andreasen FM. *Essentials of Traumatic Injuries to the Teeth.* 2nd ed. Copenhagen: Munksgaard; St. Louis: Mosby; 2000.

25. Hammarstrom L, Blomlof L, Feiglin B, et al. Replantation of teeth and antibiotic treatment. *Endod Dent Traumatol.* 1986;2:51–57.

66

MARIA CARMEN G. DIAZ

Splinting Teeth

▶ INTRODUCTION

Children often present to the emergency department with traumatic dental injuries. Most of these injuries affect the maxillary central incisors. In primary dentition, these injuries are most frequently caused by falls, whereas in permanent dentition, these injuries often occur in motor vehicle accidents or during sporting events. Emergency physicians should be aware of the management of these common injuries.

The emergent care of traumatized teeth should first and foremost optimize healing of the injured area and the supporting structures. Splinting teeth is an easy technique that allows the traumatized region to gain stability and support from neighboring unaffected teeth while the injured area is undergoing the healing process. It is vital that physicians be aware of proper splinting methods in order to enhance and ensure proper healing. Splinting is best done in the emergency department so that the regeneration process is initiated in a timely manner.

▶ ANATOMY AND PHYSIOLOGY

Teeth are composed of enamel, dentin, and cementum. They contain a neurovascular supply within the root canal and pulp chamber and are suspended in the supporting alveolar bone by fibrous periodontal ligaments. By providing stability and preventing further damage, splints permit and promote the regeneration of the periodontal ligaments (1). It is these ligaments that maintain the integrity of the root and form the attachment between the root and the bone. Absence of these periodontal ligaments results in ankylosis, a bony union between the tooth and the alveolar bone. Persistence of this bony union may eventually result in facial deformities. Splints also enhance the regeneration of cementum, which is most critical

for the development of root resorption and ultimately tooth vascularity and viability.

Clinical healing of the periodontium takes place within the first 7 days after a traumatic injury. It is crucial that the recovery period enhance the regeneration of these junctional fibers. The alveolar socket is continuously remodeling in response to functional stimuli. The splint applied should not impair but rather augment this remodeling process (2).

▶ INDICATIONS

Types of injuries that require dental splints include reimplanted avulsed permanent teeth, luxated or extruded permanent teeth that have been repositioned, crown-root fractures in permanent dentition, and alveolar fractures (3–6). It is best not to splint injured teeth that have minimal mobility. Also, care should be taken in attempting to splint teeth when there are surrounding artificial crowns or large fillings, as these synthetic structures do not provide adequate support for the splint. Injured primary teeth should not be splinted, as immobilization in these types of teeth increases the risk for ankylosis. Attempting to apply a splint in a very uncooperative patient may be difficult and may require the assistance and expertise of a dental consultant. The duration of the splint varies depending on the type of injury but ranges between 1 and 3 weeks (7).

▶ PRINCIPLES OF SPLINTING TEETH

The ideal splint should create an environment in which tooth movement can be contained within physiologic limits while restoring function and patient comfort. An acceptable splint should be simple to apply directly on the teeth and not cause

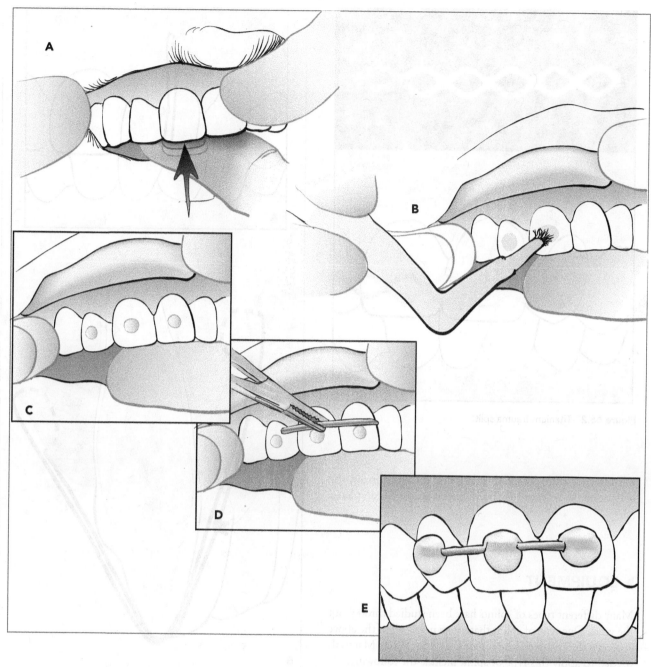

Figure 66.1
A. The traumatized teeth are repositioned.
B. Etchant is placed on the labial surface of the tooth while the tooth is held in place with a gloved finger.
C. After washing off the etchant, bonding material and then composite has been applied to the tooth.
D. Wire is placed on top of the composite.
E. A second layer of composite has been placed on top of the wire. The composite is then smoothed and the wire ends are covered.

any trauma during its application. It should immobilize the injured tooth in a normal position while allowing physiologic mobility in order to promote regeneration of periodontal fibers but discourage ankylosis and external root resorption. The fixation provided by the splint should last during the entire period of immobilization and not permanently alter the tooth structure. Additionally, the patient needs to feel com-

fortable while wearing the splint. The splint should therefore not interfere with occlusion or articulation and should not impinge on the gingiva. Any damage to the surrounding soft tissues may disrupt the healing process and may lead to bacterial infection. It is imperative that the patient be able to maintain good oral hygiene while the splint is in place. The splint should not predispose the teeth to caries and should

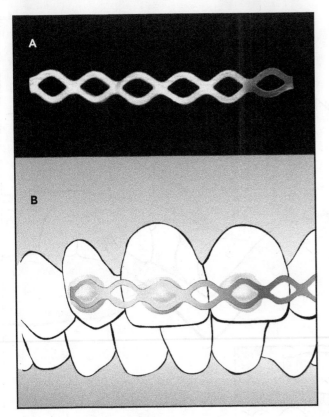

Figure 66.2 Titanium trauma split.

not interfere with potential endodontic therapy. Finally, the splint should be easy to remove once therapy is completed (8,9).

▶ EQUIPMENT

Many different types of splints have been studied throughout the years. One type of splint that meets nearly all of the above criteria is the acid-etch wire composite splint (9,10). Materials needed to apply this type of splint include the following:

> Light-cured composite material
> Etchant
> Bonding material
> Flat plastic applicator
> 0.6- to 0.7-mm stainless steel orthodontic wire
> Wire cutters and pliers
> Cotton wool rolls
> Gauze
> Gloves
> Irrigation
> Suction
> Light-curing machine

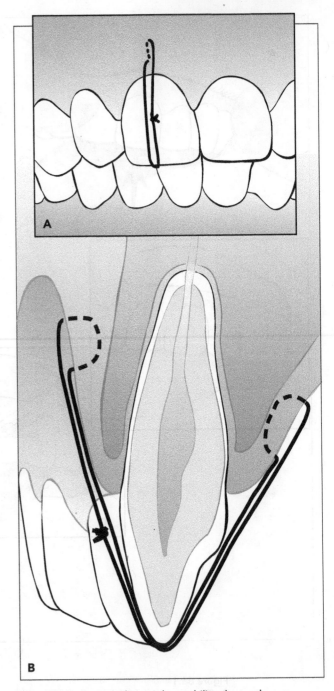

Figure 66.3 Suture splint used to stabilize the tooth.

▶ PROCEDURE

The patient should not require local or general anesthesia in order to for the splint to be placed. It is ideal to do this procedure with the patient in the supine position so that excess blood and saliva may be easily suctioned and cleared away from the teeth.

After the appropriate materials are gathered, the orthodontic wire should be measured and cut to a distance that would include the injured tooth and one stable tooth on either side.

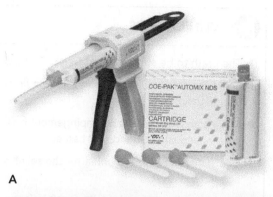

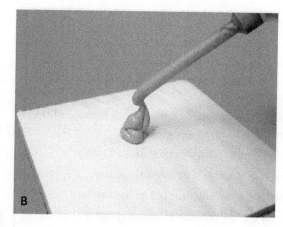

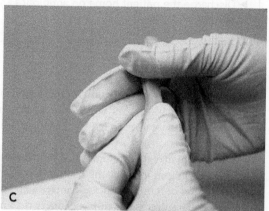

Figure 66.4 Application of Coe-Pak. The base and catalyst may be mixed using a tongue depressor. The paste is rolled and then applied to dry enamel and gingiva.

The wire is then bent to follow the normal contour of the dental arch. The injured tooth should now be reimplanted or repositioned (Chapter 65) and the teeth isolated using cotton wool rolls (Fig. 66.1A). Using gauze, all blood, debris, and saliva should be removed from the injured tooth and the surrounding teeth. The center of the labial surface of each tooth to be splinted should be spot etched in the position where the wire is to be placed (Fig. 66.1B). Etching time varies depending on the composite system used but usually takes 30 to 60 seconds. After the appropriate time period, the etchant should then be washed and removed and the teeth dried. A small amount of bonding material is next placed on top of the etched areas. Once the bonding material has been placed, a small amount of composite is applied, and the wire is then placed on top of the composite (Fig. 66.1C,D). With the wire in place, a second layer of composite is applied on top of the wire at the site of the initial layer of composite. This top layer of composite may then be compressed and smoothed using a gloved finger (Fig. 66.1E). Finally, the composite is light cured. The light source is held directly in front of the composite compound for a certain period of time so that the material is polymerized. Curing times vary depending on the type of system used, but usually 30 seconds is required for polymerization. Occlusion must be evaluated before and after curing. Thus, the stable surrounding teeth should be cured first and the injured tooth last in case repositioning is needed. Composite should not bond teeth together. If there

is excess composite, this needs to be removed (9,11,12). Self-curing systems are available. However, they allow minimal manipulation time, and care must be taken to avoid malocclusion (11).

If available, a titanium trauma splint may be used in place of the orthodontic wire. This splint is made of pure titanium and is only 0.2 mm thick. It is easily bent without pliers. The unique shape allows physiologic mobility while withstanding shearing forces (Fig. 66.2) (13,14).

Alternatives to the Acid-Etch Wire Splint

Many institutions do not have dental consultants nor light-curing or self-curing systems available. If these are lacking, a temporary splint may be placed and removed in 1 to 2 days in the dentist's office. This alternative may also be used in uncooperative patients or in cases where there are no adjacent teeth or not enough exposed tooth to attach the acid-etch resin. The alternatives that will be discussed are the suture splint and Coe-Pak.

Suture Splint

After anesthetizing the surrounding affected gingiva and reimplanting the injured tooth, the tooth may be sutured into place. This is done by passing the suture through the labial surface of the gingiva and carrying it over the incisal edge of the tooth into the lingual gingival tissue. The suture is then

SUMMARY

1 Measure and cut the orthodontic wire to include the injured tooth and one stable tooth on each side.

2 Bend the wire to follow the normal contour of the dental arch.

3 Reimplant or reposition the injured tooth.

4 Remove blood and debris with gauze.

5 Spot etch the labial surface of the teeth.

6 Apply a small amount of bonding material on top of the etched areas.

7 Apply a small amount of composite on top of the bonding material.

8 Place wire on top of the composite.

9 Apply a second layer of composite on top of the wire at the site of the initial composite layer.

10 Compress and smooth the top layer of the composite with a gloved finger.

11 Confirm accurate occlusion.

12 Light cure the composite.

CLINICAL TIPS

▶ The teeth to be splinted must be clean and dry.

▶ Splint the surrounding supporting teeth first and the traumatized teeth last.

▶ Make sure that there is no impingement on the gingiva and surrounding soft tissue.

▶ Check occlusion before and after the splint is applied.

▶ Discharge the patient home on antibiotics and ensure close dental follow-up.

by dentists. It is therefore vital that occlusion be assessed before and after curing. Antibiotics should be administered after tooth reimplantation to reduce the risk of inflammatory resorption.

Wire splints may cause gingivitis. Gingivitis is usually reversible and disappears after the fixation has been removed. The likelihood of more significant damage and destruction is increased if the splint is left in place longer than needed (2).

passed through the lingual surface of the gingiva. It is once again passed over the incisal edge and into the labial gingival tissue, where it is tightened and tied (Fig. 66.3) (15,16).

Coe-Pak

Coe-Pak is a periodontal paste composed of a base and catalyst. These two components are mixed and form a sticky dressing that becomes firm once applied. This composite is placed over the affected enamel and gingiva as well as the adjacent teeth. Once again, it is best applied when the affected surfaces are clean and dry. The patient is then advised to follow up with a visit to the dentist in 24 hours (Fig. 66.4) (17).

▶ COMPLICATIONS

The major complications associated with splinting teeth are infection and ankylosis. These complications may be avoided by adhering to the aforementioned principles and procedures. If splinting results in malocclusion, the splint has been improperly applied and needs to be removed, as malocclusion increases the risk of ankylosis. Suture splints are easily cut, removed, and replaced. Coe-Pak paste may be peeled off and reapplied. Acid-etch wire splints require a diamond bur and abrasive discs for removal, tools that are usually used only

▶ SUMMARY

The presence of an intact, viable periodontal ligament is the most important factor in ensuring proper healing of a traumatized tooth. The use of splints in traumatized teeth has been shown to enhance the healing process (18). Splints are easy to apply and should be used in the ED setting. The type of injury dictates the duration of the splint. However, regardless of the type of injury or the type of splint applied, immediate outpatient follow-up with the dentist is recommended.

▶ REFERENCES

1. Kehoe JC. Splinting and replantation after traumatic avulsion. *J Am Dent Assoc.* 1986;112:224–230.

2. Oikarinen K. Tooth splinting: a review of literature and consideration of the versatility of a wire-composite splint. *Dent Traumatol.* 1990;6:237–250.

3. Flores MT, Andreasen JO, Bakland LK, et al. Guidelines for the evaluation and management of traumatic dental injuries (part 1 of series). *Dent Traumatol.* 2001;17:1–4.

4. Flores MT, Andreasen JO, Bakland LK, et al. Guidelines for the evaluation and management of traumatic dental injuries (part 3 of series). *Dent Traumatol.* 2001;17:97–102.

5. Flores MT, Andreasen JO, Bakland LK, et al. Guidelines for the evaluation and management of traumatic dental injuries (part 4 of series). *Dent Traumatol.* 2001;17:145–148.

6. Flores MT, Andreasen JO, Bakland LK, et al. Guidelines for the evaluation and management of traumatic dental injuries (part 5 of series). *Dent Traumatol.* 2001;17:193–198.

7. Andreasen JO, Andreasen FM, Mejare I, et al. Healing of 400 intra-alveolar root fractures, II: effect of treatment factors such as treatment delay, repositioning, splinting type and period and antibiotics. *Dent Traumatol.* 2004;20:203–211.

8. Neaverth EJ, Goerig AC. Technique and rationale for splinting. *J Am Dent Assoc.* 1980;100:56–63.

9. Brown CL, Mackie IC. Splinting of traumatized teeth in children. *Dent Update.* 2003;30:78–82.

10. Camp J. Management of trauma in the child and adolescent. *Pediatr Dent.* 1995;17:379–383.

11. Klokkevold P. Common dental emergencies: evaluation and management for emergency physicians. *Emerg Med Clin North Am.* 1989;7:29–63.

12. McDonald N, Strassler HE. Evaluation for tooth stabilization and treatment of traumatized teeth. *Dent Clin North Am.* 1999;43:135–149.

13. von Arx T, Filippi A, Buser D. Splinting of traumatized teeth with a new device: TTS (titanium trauma splint). *Dent Traumatol.* 2001;17:180–184.

14. von Arx T, Filippi A, Lussi A. Comparison of a new dental trauma splint device (TTS) with three commonly used splinting techniques. *Dent Traumatol.* 2001;17:266–274.

15. Gupta S, Sharma A, Dang N. Suture splint: an alternative for luxation injuries of teeth in pediatric patients: a case report. *J Clin Pediatr Dent.* 1997;22:19–21.

16. Herrmann HJ. Dental and facial emergencies. In: Auerbach PS, ed. *Wilderness Medicine.* 4th ed. St. Louis: Mosby; 2001:563–564.

17. Benko K. Emergency dental procedures. In: Roberts JR, ed. *Clinical Procedures in Emergency Medicine.* 4th ed. St. Louis: Elsevier; 2004:1323–1325.

18. Qin M, Ge LH. Use of a removable splint in the treatment of subluxated, luxated, and root fractured anterior permanent teeth in children. *Dent Traumatol.* 2002;18:81–85.

67

MAGDY W. ATTIA AND JOHN LOISELLE

Management of Soft-Tissue Injuries of the Mouth

▶ INTRODUCTION

The physician who deals with the pediatric age group is frequently called on to evaluate oral trauma (1,2). Children often present to the emergency department (ED) after apparently minor trauma with fractured teeth or lacerations to the oral soft tissues.

Blunt trauma is the most common source of orofacial injuries in children and is usually the result of striking the mouth on a piece of furniture or from a fall. In the younger age groups, the possibility of child abuse should always be considered (3). Animal bites are another frequent cause. Children are at greater risk than adults for being the victim of an animal bite. Three fourths of all bites involve the extremities; however, because of their small size, children are more likely to suffer bites to the face. Bites to the lips are particularly common, sustained while "kissing" an animal (4).

Electrical burns of the lips and tongue are not an uncommon injury among young children, who are predisposed to mouthing electrical outlets and cords. It is important to elicit an adequate history relative to the nature of the trauma, because these scenarios will differ in pattern and extent of injury (5).

Closure of oral mucosal lacerations will result in decreased healing time, decreased propensity for infection, and adequate hemostasis and cosmesis (5–7). The issue of cosmesis is one of utmost importance for the parent and patient, particularly if there is an injury involving the lips.

The complexity of injuries varies greatly. The majority heal well without intervention. Those that require repair can, in most cases, be handled by any experienced physician. A small number require surgical expertise. It is imperative to rule out associated injuries, but most facial lacerations are simple and are easily managed by ED personnel. Occasionally, other medical priorities necessitate deferring treatment to the inpatient setting. Extensive facial lacerations are preferably closed by a specialist in the operating room. Consultants may include a general, plastic, or oral surgeon; a dentist; or an otorhinolaryngologist.

▶ ANATOMY AND PHYSIOLOGY

The generous blood flow to the face and mouth contributes to its excellent healing potential (Fig. 67.1). The upper lip is supplied by the superior labial arteries, which branch from the facial arteries. The lower lip also is supplied by branches of the facial artery known as the "inferior labial arteries." The labial arteries join to form a ring about the mouth. The inferior labial arteries have anastomoses with the mental and submental arteries, which are branches of the maxillary and facial arteries, respectively.

The tongue receives its main blood supply from the lingual arteries (Fig. 67.1). Branches of the lingual artery and the inferior alveolar artery provide blood supply to the mucosa of the floor of the mouth. The maxillary and palatal mucosa are supplied by branches of the maxillary arteries. The buccal mucosa is supplied by branches of both the facial and maxillary arteries (8).

The nerve supply to the area is equally complex and is mostly derived from the trigeminal and glossopharyngeal nerves (see Fig. 62.1).

The structure of a lip is multilayered, as shown in Figure 67.2. The skin comprises the external layer and the mucosa the internal layer. The middle layer is composed of muscle (the orbicularis oris), which encircles the mouth. A fibrofatty

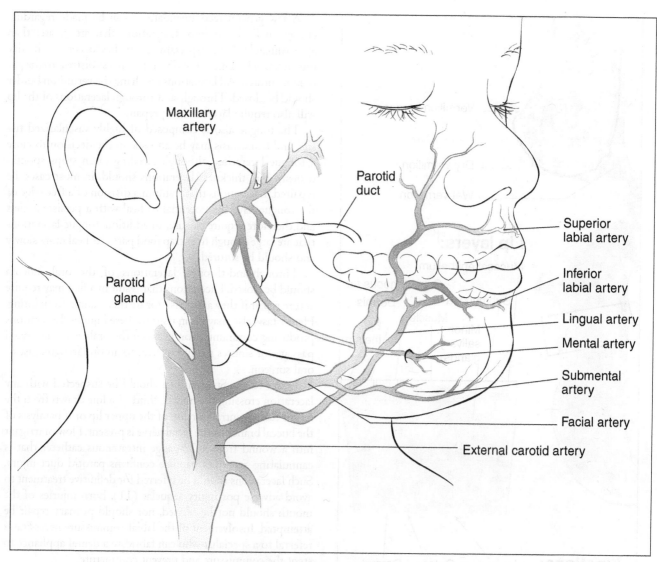

Maxillary artery

Parotid duct

Parotid gland

Superior labial artery

Inferior labial artery

Lingual artery

Mental artery

Submental artery

Facial artery

External carotid artery

Figure 67.1 Blood supply to the face and mouth.

junction borders both the inside and the outside surfaces of the muscle. Between the inner fibrofatty junction and the mucosa, a layer of submucosal or minor salivary glands is present.

The vermilion border is the mucocutaneous junction of the lips where the mucosa meets the skin. A common lip injury treated in the ED is a through-and-through laceration. These lacerations often involve the vermilion border, which is a fixed and obvious landmark.

The tongue is composed almost entirely of eight separate muscle groups, which confer a wide variation of movement. It is covered on the dorsal and inferior surfaces by mucous membrane. The anterior two thirds of the dorsal surface contains the numerous papillae or taste buds.

When a child mouths an electrical outlet or two bared wires, saliva will complete the arc. A spark burn will result. Fortunately, the immediate reaction of the victim is to jerk away. When a child bites into a cord, current courses through the soft tissue and produces a muscle contraction. The victim

is unable to release the cord because of the ongoing perioral muscle contraction, and the burn progresses (5).

Spark burns produce a limited white blister and will not result in much deep tissue necrosis. Current burns are more diffuse. Necrosis of deep tissues will occur, and the eschar will break down approximately 5 to 10 days postinjury. Without vital connective tissue support, damaged circumoral vessels also will necrose, tear, and bleed (5,9). Although this is a rare scenario, parents should be alerted to the possibility of delayed bleeding and the need to seek medical attention at the first indication of bleeding (10). Pain and edema may prevent adequate oral hydration or, in more severe cases, result in airway compromise.

The parotid duct is an additional structure within the mouth that may be injured. It originates at the anterior parotid gland and courses anteriorly. The duct turns medially at the anterior border of the masseter muscle and penetrates the buccinator muscle. It then courses obliquely forward to exit

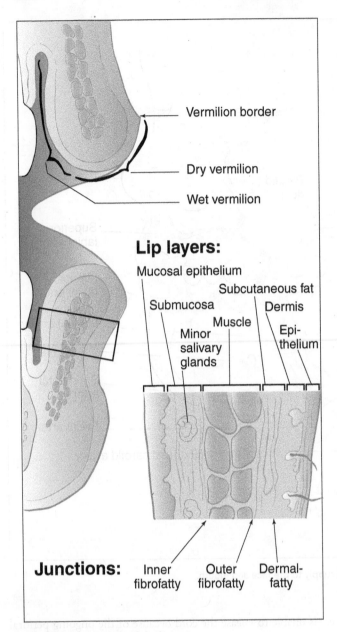

Lip layers:

Mucosal epithelium

Subcutaneous fat

Submucosa   Dermis

Minor   Muscle   Epi-
salivary   thelium
glands

Junctions: Inner   Outer   Dermal-
                  fibrofatty   fibrofatty   fatty

Vermilion border

Dry vermilion

Wet vermilion

Figure 67.2 Anatomy of the lip.

the mucosa at Stensen's papillae opposite the maxillary second molar (8).

▶ INDICATIONS

The generous blood supply of the face and mouth allows the vast majority of intraoral lacerations to heal well on their own. This benefit is counterbalanced by the fact that even the smallest lacerations in the facial area can leave cosmetically disfiguring scars. The elapsed time from wound occurrence and the degree of contamination of wound are additional concerns for infection. These issues must be considered when deciding on the need for primary closure.

A few general recommendations can be made regarding closure of lip lacerations. Lacerations that are greater than approximately 2 cm, especially when they occur on the dry mucosa, will heal more rapidly and with less distress to the patient if sutured. All lacerations involving the vermilion border should be closed. Through-and-through lacerations of the lip will also require layered suture repair.

The tongue also is composed of highly vascularized tissue, and hemostasis may be an issue in the decision to close a tongue laceration, although bleeding often stops spontaneously. Full thickness lacerations should, in most cases, be repaired. Lacerations that result in a division of a free edge of the tongue have the potential to heal with a persistent cleft and therefore require closure. In addition, tongue lacerations that are large enough to entrap food particles heal more slowly and should be sutured.

Through-and-through lacerations of the oral mucosa should be closed. Lacerations that result in a flap may require suture repair if they are at risk for further trauma from biting. Hemostasis also may be an issue in these injuries. Lacerations producing communication between the oral cavity and nasal passages or sinuses require referral to an otolaryngologist or oral surgeon.

Injury to the Stensen duct should be suspected with any laceration crossing the middle third of a line drawn from the tragus to the central portion of the upper lip or if paralysis of the buccal branch of the facial nerve is present. Flow of irrigant into a wound from a 22-gauge intravenous catheter that is cannulating Stenson's papillae confirms parotid duct injury. Such lacerations should be referred for definitive treatment to avoid adverse postinjury sequelae (11). Burn injuries of the mouth should not be excised, nor should primary repair be attempted. Involvement of the labial commissure necessitates referral to a specialist who can fabricate a dental appliance to stent the commissure and prevent contracture.

Tear wounds from animal bites about the face and mouth, like any other laceration, can be closed following thorough wound cleansing, irrigation, and débridement of devitalized tissue (12). True puncture wounds should not be closed but be allowed to granulate. Because of the rich vascular supply to the face and mouth, human bite wounds to this region treated within 24 hours of injury may be closed primarily. This is unlike human bites to other regions of the body, which are not closed and allowed to granulate. If more than 24 hours has elapsed since the injury, delayed primary closure of facial bite wounds is performed after resolution of infection.

▶ EQUIPMENT

Dental anesthetic syringe or 5-mL Luer-Lok syringe
25-gauge or smaller, 1.5-inch needle
Yankauer and Frazier suction catheters
1% or 2% lidocaine with or without 1:100,000 epinephrine
Gauze sponges

Bite block
Suture tray (fine scissors, needle holder, nontraumatic forceps)
Saline for irrigation
20-mL irrigation syringe
Splash shield or 18-gauge intravenous catheter tip
Resorbable sutures 3.0, 4.0, and 5.0 chromic gut, Vicryl, Dexon
Nonresorbable sutures 5.0 and 6.0 nylon, Ethilon, Prolene

▶ PROCEDURE

The approach to these injuries, as with all trauma, is to initially assess for concurrent life-threatening injuries to the airway, cervical spine, or brain. Once any such injuries have been stabilized, a regional head and neck examination should evaluate for signs and symptoms of facial bone or skull fracture, such as hemotympanum, paresthesia of the divisions of the trigeminal nerve, diplopia, cerebrospinal fluid rhinorrhea, cerebrospinal fluid otorrhea, trismus, malocclusion, temporomandibular joint pain, and deviation of the mandible on opening (11). Injuries to the temporomandibular joints or mandibular condyles should be suspected in patients who have sustained blows to the mental symphysis region.

Intraoral examination should evaluate for the integrity of the oral and pharyngeal mucosa, the stability of dental occlusion, and the presence of luxated, mobile, fractured, or avulsed teeth. Ecchymosis of the floor of the mouth or near the ramus of the mandible may indicate an underlying mandibular fracture. Similarly, palatal ecchymosis or ecchymosis near the zygomatic buttress suggests a maxillary fracture. Once the presence of occult facial bone fractures has been excluded, treatment can turn to facial and mucosal lacerations (11).

Oral mucosal lacerations may contain tooth fragments and other foreign bodies such as glass and gravel. These must be identified either through direct or radiographic examination and removed before proceeding with the repair. Oral mucosal lacerations can also be quite painful, and administration of regional anesthetic blocks before examination may be helpful. Sensory and motor examinations of the cranial nerves should be documented before the administration of anesthetics. Placement of a bite block or a taped stack of tongue depressors may improve exposure for intraoral procedures.

Anesthesia

Clinical evaluation of the child's interaction with the physician may be helpful in determining the need for restraint. Thorough evaluation and treatment of oral injuries is difficult with an uncooperative child. If necessary, restraint should be used, physically by a papoose board and/or pharmacologically through procedural sedation (Chapters 3 and 33). Topical anesthesia with combination lidocaine-epinephrine-tetracaine gel ("LET") is not recommended in the management of soft-tissue injuries of the mouth due to the potential

systemic effects. Likewise, there is no role for tissue glue in the repair of these injuries. Procedural sedation should be considered if extensive repair is anticipated; however, all precautions should be taken to avoid upper airway compromise.

Upper Lip

The infraorbital nerve block is the preferred method for obtaining anesthesia in this region (see also Chapter 62). A regional block will cause minimal distortion of the vermilion border and will result in anesthesia of the lower eyelid, the skin overlying the malar prominence, and the skin and mucosa of the upper lip from the commissure to the midline on the injected side.

Supraperiosteal infiltration in the mucobuccal fold over the laceration also will provide anesthesia of the skin and mucosa of the lip directly distal to the injection site (Chapter 62). This method results in greater distortion of the vermilion border and soft-tissue landmarks than an infraorbital block. Several injections will be needed. Injections should be made above the apex of each tooth to which the laceration is adjacent.

Direct infiltration of the laceration margins (Chapter 35) will provide adequate anesthesia and hemostasis but also will result in the greatest distortion of the vermilion border. If epinephrine is contained in an anesthetic solution used for direct infiltration, blanching of the mucosa will occur, which may result in obliteration of the vermilion border (13).

Lower Lip

A regional nerve block is again the preferred method for anesthesia of the lower lip region. As with the upper lip, a regional nerve block will produce less distortion of soft-tissue landmarks and requires less total anesthetic injection than the techniques of supraperiosteal injection and direct infiltration.

A mental nerve block will result in anesthesia of the buccal gingiva anterior to the mental foramen as well as the mucosa and skin of the lower lip from the midline to the labial commissure on the side of the injection. The mental nerve is located near the apex of the second primary molar of a young child or near the apex of the second premolar of an adolescent (Fig. 67.3). The lip and buccal tissues are tautly retracted with fingers of the clinician's nondominant hand. A 25-gauge or smaller needle penetrates the mucosa directly over or slightly anterior to the mental foramen. The needle is advanced approximately 5 mm. If no blood is aspirated, 0.5 to 1.0 mL of 1% lidocaine is injected.

An inferior alveolar or mandibular block will result in a distribution of anesthesia that encompasses the region anesthetized by a mental block. In addition, the remainder of the buccal mucosa, the lingual gingiva, the anterior two thirds of the tongue, and the dentition on the side of the injection will be anesthetized. The target area for this block is the mandibular foramen, where the inferior alveolar nerve enters the mandibular canal (Chapter 62, Fig. 62.3).

Supraperiosteal injections and direct infiltration techniques also may be used in anesthesia of the lower lip, although

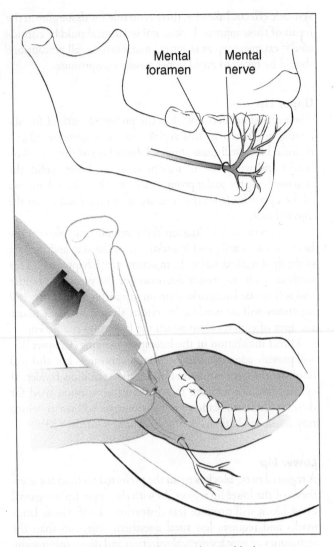

Figure 67.3 Administration of a mental nerve block.

described, a mandibular block also will result in block of the lingual nerve.

Direct infiltration of laceration margins with an anesthetic solution containing a vasoconstrictor will provide both anesthesia and hemostasis. Tongue lacerations can bleed quite briskly. The added hemostatic effect of a vasoconstrictor, although temporary, can aid visualization when suturing (12).

Direct infiltration of the buccal and palatal mucosal soft tissues will provide anesthesia and hemostasis (if vasoconstrictors are used) and will not distort any vital landmarks. Although techniques of regional anesthetic blocks exist, their use in the ED will be rare, and therefore these methods are not described.

Repair

The basic principles of suturing are described in Chapter 108. The following discussion is limited to specific techniques for closure of oral soft-tissue wounds.

Lip

Repair of a lip laceration should be performed layer by layer from the inside out and from the wound apex to the free margin (5,6). It is of paramount importance to identify the vermilion border before initiating infiltration anesthesia or wound débridement. Regional block anesthesia can be administered without distortion of the vermilion border. Some clinicians advocate approximation of the vermilion border with a tacking stitch (5.0 or 6.0 nonabsorbable suture) at the outset. Others recommend simply marking the junction with a pen or a scratch from a needle tip or the back of a scalpel blade (5,6).

Once the vermilion border is marked, the wound is débrided, and any obviously traumatized minor salivary glands are removed. If these remain in a wound, delayed formation of a mucocele is likely to occur. Any obviously necrotic tissue should be excised. The face has a rich vascular supply and a tremendous healing potential. Tissue with a minimal blood supply can survive and become revascularized. Care should be taken not to excise tissue that contains the vermilion cutaneous junction. The wound should be thoroughly inspected for foreign bodies, particularly tooth fragments, and all foreign material should be removed. Once débridement is complete, the wound is irrigated with a copious amount of saline, and the surrounding skin is prepped with povidone-iodine solution.

Closure of a through-and-through lip laceration occurs in at least three layers (Fig. 67.4). As described previously, a stitch that aligns the vermilion border may be placed at the beginning of the closure. The inner fibrofatty junction at the wound apex is then reapproximated using a resorbable 4.0 or 5.0 suture. Interrupted, inverted sutures will provide adequate reapproximation without protrusion of the suture material through the wound. The outer fibrofatty junction is approximated next, and the two fibrofatty junctions are united at the free edge. If the muscle is not approximated

they have the same caveats as those described for the upper lip (12).

Tongue

A lingual nerve block will provide anesthesia to the anterior two thirds of the tongue, lingual gingiva, and mucosa of the floor of the mouth on the side injected. Although this technique will provide excellent anesthesia in the region described, vasoconstrictors contained in the anesthetic solution will have minimal hemostatic effect on the mucosa and muscles of the tongue.

A 25-gauge or smaller needle is inserted through the mandibular mucosa immediately posterior and medial to the most posterior tooth in the arch (see also Chapter 62; the lingual nerve location in relation to the inferior alveolar nerve is illustrated in Fig. 62.3). The needle should penetrate to a depth of approximately 5 mm. If aspiration is negative for blood, 0.5 to 1.0 mL of anesthetic is injected. As previously

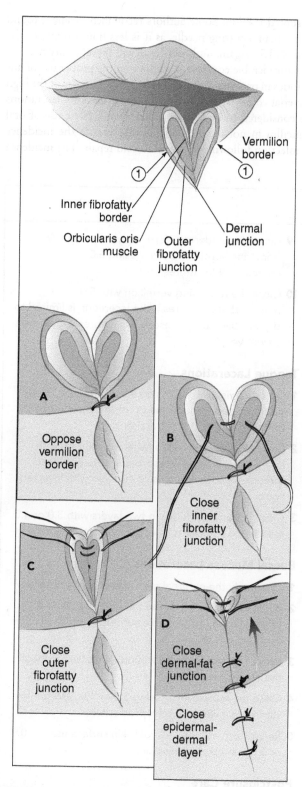

Figure 67.4 Three-layer repair of a through-and-through lip laceration.
A. Opposition of vermilion border.
B. Closure of the inner dermal-fat junction.
C. Closure of the outer dermal-fat junction.
D. Closure of the epidermal layer, with joining of the dermal-fat junction at the free wound edge.
Note: Closure of muscle layer (orbicularis oris) not shown in diagram.

both anteriorly and posteriorly, it will contract away from the wound edge. This will produce an unobtrusive scar with the lip at rest, but when the lip is in function, a contraction will produce an obvious ridging or depression of the scar. If suturing of the inner and outer fibrofatty junctions is not joined at the free edge, a notch in the scar over this region will develop (5).

If the laceration extends well beyond the vermilion border, one has to suspect involvement of the orbicularis oris muscle. If this is identified, it should be repaired as a separate layer. This can be accomplished by using 5.0 absorbable material.

The dermal-fat junction is then closed with an inverted interrupted stitch using resorbable 4.0 suture. Alignment of the vermilion border must remain perfect before and after this layer is sutured. The presence of any malalignment necessitates removal of the sutures and reapproximation of the tissue until alignment is achieved.

The final epidermal-dermal layer is approximated by placing the sutures adjacent to the vermilion-cutaneous junction and working toward the wound apex in the skin using a 6.0 nonresorbable material such as nylon.

If the laceration is limited to the dry vermilion (see Fig. 67.2), nonresorbable suture material may be used. If the laceration extends onto the wet vermilion, 5.0 chromic gut is used in an interrupted or continuous stitch.

Some clinicians prefer an alternative or simple three-layered closure (14). Using this technique, the outer fibrofatty junction is approximated as previously described. Next, the mucosa and the inner fibrofatty layer are closed as a unit. A 3.0 chromic gut suture is used to penetrate the mucosa, engage the fibrofatty layer on both sides of the laceration, and then exit the mucosa on the other side of the wound. The skin is approximated as previously described.

A two-layer closure, in which the skin and outer fibrofatty layer are closed as a unit and the mucosa and posterior fibrofatty layer are closed as a unit, is not recommended, as it can result in great variability in the approximation of tissue layers. Nonresorbable sutures should be removed in 3 to 5 days.

Tongue

Most tongue lacerations do not require repair. When repair is indicated, all layers can be closed with interrupted sutures penetrating through mucosa and muscle. Sutures should be inverted to avoid untying. A 4.0 or 3.0 resorbable suture material such as Vicryl or chromic gut should be used. Because the tongue is slippery and difficult to grasp, it may be helpful to place one 3.0 silk suture through the anesthetized tip of the tongue and pull the ends gently through the open mouth to obtain better control and exposure of the wound.

Gingiva

Gingival lacerations are rare, and those requiring closure are even more rare. When indicated, they should be closed using interrupted simple sutures with multiple knots to avoid untying. A 3.0 or 4.0 chromic gut is an ideal choice.

Buccal Mucosa

Through-and-through lacerations should be closed in layers, as described for lip lacerations. When possible, only the external surface is closed. When both surfaces must be sutured, the inner surface is closed first. The wound is irrigated thoroughly through the external open wound. The muscle layer and then the skin should be closed sequentially. Lacerations involving only the oral mucosa should be closed with 3.0 or 4.0 chromic gut or 4.0 coated Vicryl in a continuous or in-

terrupted fashion. Some authors recommend using a round rather than a cutting needle, as it is less traumatizing to the tissues (15). Again, multiple knots will prevent untying.

Considerable controversy exists over the proper use of antibiotics in patients with facial lacerations. Because of the high bacterial count within the mouth, most intraoral lacerations are considered to be contaminated. Prophylactic use of oral penicillin in nonallergic patients may reduce the incidence of infection following intraoral wound repair. The incidence

---

 SUMMARY

1 Assess and stabilize life-threatening injuries.

2 Examine for associated injuries such as underlying fractures or foreign bodies.

3 Document sensory and motor examinations of cranial nerves, preferably before local anesthesia.

4 Administer procedural sedation as needed.

5 Physically restrain the patient with a papoose board if necessary.

6 Place a bite block or stent mouth open with taped tongue depressors.

7 Administer regional nerve block or local infiltrative anesthetic as indicated.

8 Carry out any necessary débridement or excision.

9 Irrigate wound with saline.

10 Alert the parents to the possibility of the child chewing the sutures and advise distracting the child until the local anesthesia is worn off.

Lip Lacerations

1 Identify and mark the vermilion border before initiating anesthesia or débridement.

2 Prepare the wound borders with povidone-iodine solution.

3 Reapproximate the vermilion border.

4 Reapproximate the inner fibrofatty junction with resorbable 4.0 or 5.0 suture using interrupted stitches with inverted knots.

5 Close the outer fibrofatty junction in the same manner.

6 Unite the fibrofatty junction at the free edge.

7 Close the dermal-fat junction with inverted interrupted resorbable 4.0 sutures.

8 Ensure the vermilion border is reapproximated exactly.

9 Close the epidermal-dermal layer sewing "away from" the vermilion border using 6.0 nonresorbable sutures.

10 Close the remaining vermilion with 5.0 nonresorbable sutures if the laceration is limited to dry vermilion or 5.0 resorbable sutures if it extends to wet vermilion.

Tongue Lacerations

1 Optimize visualization using a bite block or 3.0 silk suture placed through the tip of the anesthetized tongue and used for retraction.

2 Close smaller lacerations, when warranted, with interrupted 3.0 or 4.0 resorbable sutures placed through mucosa and muscle and tied with inverted knots.

3 Close larger lacerations in two layers with 3.0 or 4.0 resorbable sutures in inverted interrupted stitches.

Buccal Mucosa Lacerations

1 Close only the external skin surface when possible.

2 When necessary, close the internal mucosa first, using 3.0 or 4.0 resorbable sutures in interrupted or continuous fashion.

3 Repeat irrigation of the wound with saline through the external surface.

4 Close the muscle layer using 3.0 or 4.0 resorbable sutures in inverted interrupted stitch.

5 Reapproximate the external skin surface using 5.0 or 6.0 nonresorbable sutures.

Postclosure Care

1 Consider using prophylactic antibiotics.

2 Recommend liquids until the anesthetic effect has resolved and then soft diet for 1 to 2 days.

3 Administer a tetanus booster if necessary.

CLINICAL TIPS

▶ The vermilion border should be marked or approximated before infiltration anesthesia or débridement.

▶ Using epinephrine in infiltration anesthesia will blanch and obscure the vermilion border.

▶ Using a regional anesthetic block will avoid distortion of soft-tissue landmarks.

▶ Inverted sutures and multiple knots are less likely to become untied.

▶ The orbicularis oris must be approximated or it will result in a depressed scar when in motion.

of infection is relatively low in lacerations involving only the mucosa. The infection rate is higher in through-and-through lacerations, and patients with these wounds may benefit more from prophylaxis (16). It is recommended that antibiotics be given before or during ED procedures. No evidence indicates the superiority of a cephalosporin over penicillin or clindamycin as long as the proper dose is prescribed (5).

Patients should be advised to adhere to a soft diet for 24 to 48 hours following repair. In addition, only liquids should be taken until the anesthetic has completely worn off. All patients should have a tetanus booster administered if needed.

COMPLICATIONS

Obliteration of landmarks secondary to infiltration anesthetics resulting in volume distortion and blanching of the vermilion mucosa can result in poor approximation of this sensitive area. Knots are more likely to become untied when they are placed in the mouth. The occurrence of untying can be lessened with the inversion of knots and the tying of multiple knots.

Repeat injury to anesthetized tissues following the repair can occur secondary to cheek and lip biting. This is especially problematic in the young child, who may not comprehend the consequences of this action. Extensive manipulation of tissues or anesthetic infiltration may result in airway compromise secondary to edema or excessive hemorrhage. Mucocele formation may result from damage to minor salivary glands and ducts in the lips.

SUMMARY

Oral mucosal and lip injuries are common in the pediatric age group. While some of these injuries are of great cosmetic importance, many will require no repair, and most heal well because the area is highly vascularized. The majority of injuries requiring surgical repair can be closed by an experienced physician. Success is largely dependent on the ability to accurately visualize and assess the injury. Administration of local or regional anesthesia, with the use of procedural sedation when necessary, will greatly facilitate this task in young children. A layered closure of deep wounds with accurate approximation of key landmarks like the vermilion border is essential for a good functional and cosmetic outcome. Although antibiotic prophylaxis is controversial, penicillin is commonly prescribed following intraoral repairs.

ACKNOWLEDGMENT

The authors would like to acknowledge the valuable contributions of Peter D. Quinn to the version of this chapter that appeared in the previous edition.

REFERENCES

1. Nelson LP. Pediatric emergencies in the office setting: oral trauma. *Pediatr Emerg Care.* 1990;16:147–152.
2. Berkowitz R, Ludwig S, Johnson R. Dental trauma in children and adolescents. *Clin Pediatr.* 1980;3:166–171.
3. Maniglia AJ, Kline SN. Maxillofacial trauma in the pediatric age group. *Otolaryngol Clin North Am.* 1983;16:717–730.
4. Newton E. Mammalian bites. In: Schwartz CR, Cayten CG, Mangelsen MA, et al., eds. *Principles and Practice of Emergency Medicine.* 3rd ed. Philadelphia: Lea & Febiger; 1992:2750–2761.
5. Dushoff IM. About face. *Emerg Med.* 1974;25–77.
6. Dushoff IM. A stitch in time. *Emerg Med.* 1973;21–43.
7. Potsic WP, Handler SD. *Primary Care Pediatric Otolaryngology.* New York: Macmillan; 1986:116–119.
8. Goss CM, ed. *Gray's Anatomy.* 29th ed. Philadelphia: Lea & Febiger; 1973.
9. Hammond JS, Ward GG. Burns of the head and neck. *Otolaryngol Clin North Am.* 1983;16:679–695.
10. McDonald RE, Avery DR, Hennon DK. Management of trauma to the teeth and supporting tissues. In: McDonald RE, Avery DR, eds. *Dentistry for the Child and Adolescent.* 6th ed. St. Louis: Mosby; 1993.
11. American Association of Oral and Maxillofacial Surgery. *Oral and Maxillofacial Surgery Services in the Emergency Department.* Rosemont, IL: American Association of Oral and Maxillofacial Surgery; 1992:4–5.
12. American Academy of Pediatrics. Bite wounds. In: Pickering L, ed. *2003 Red Book: Report of the Committee on Infectious Diseases.* 26th ed. Elk Grove Village, IL: American Academy of Pediatrics; 2003: 182–186.
13. Malamed SF. *Handbook of Local Anesthesia.* St. Louis: Mosby; 1980.
14. Peterson LJ. *Contemporary Oral and Maxillofacial Surgery.* St. Louis: Mosby; 1988:554–555.
15. Selbst SM, Attia M. Minor trauma: lacerations. In: Fleisher GR, Ludwig S, Henretig FM, eds. *Textbook of Pediatric Emergency Medicine.* 5th ed. Philadelphia: Lippincott Williams & Wilkins; 2006:1571–1586.
16. Steele MT, Riedel C, Robinson WA, et al. Prophylactic penicillin for intraoral wounds. *Ann Emerg Med.* 1989;18:847–852.

68

AMANDA PRATT AND JOHN M. LOISELLE

Reduction of Temporomandibular Joint Dislocation

▶ INTRODUCTION

Temporomandibular joint dislocation is the displacement of the mandibular condyle from the mandibular fossa, rendering the patient unable to achieve reduction without assistance. It is an uncommon condition in children but may occur in adolescents. Due to the associated pain and anxiety, patients in the acute period typically present to the emergency department (ED) or to a dental or primary care office.

The procedure for reducing a temporomandibular joint dislocation has changed little since Hippocrates, who is generally credited with the earliest description of the technique.

The goal in treatment is to reduce the dislocation, restore function, and alleviate pain. The earlier the reduction is attempted, the greater the likelihood of success (1,2). Reduction is most frequently performed in the office or ED setting by a physician, dentist, or oral surgeon and is relatively uncomplicated, assuming that proper technique is followed.

▶ ANATOMY AND PHYSIOLOGY

The temporomandibular joint consists of the head of the mandibular condyle sitting within the mandibular fossa of the temporal bone (Fig. 68.1A). The articular surfaces are lined by a synovial membrane and separated by a disk or meniscus composed of fibrous connective tissue. The structure of the joint allows for hinge, gliding, and side-to-side motions. The capsular ligament attaches to both the mandibular fossa and the neck of the condyle. Its laxity allows for the flexible movement of the joint. The joint is also supported by two ligaments on the medial surface, the sphenomandibular and stylomandibular ligaments, and one on the lateral surface, the temporomandibular ligament. Recurrent dislocation may be associated with excessive laxity in these ligaments, as occurs in Ehlers-Danlos or Marfan syndrome.

The lateral pterygoid muscle and several neck muscles are responsible for opening the jaw. Closure is controlled by the masseter, medial pterygoid, and temporalis muscles.

Acute dislocation of the temporomandibular joint occurs most frequently in an anterior direction, causing the mandibular condyle to become locked in front of the articular eminence (Fig. 68.1B). Dislocation can occur bilaterally or unilaterally. Spasms of the lateral pterygoid and temporalis muscles maintain the dislocation and often make reduction difficult. Conditions that predispose to dislocation include prior stretching of the joint capsule, a low articular eminence, increased tonicity of the muscles of mastication, and excessive ligamentous laxity.

A number of mechanisms are associated with anterior dislocation, including extreme mouth opening, as occurs during episodes of laughing, yawning, or vomiting, and prolonged mouth opening, as occurs with tonsillectomy or dental therapy (1,3). Dislocation also can occur as a result of convulsions, dystonic reactions, or trauma.

Although unusual, posterior and superior dislocations may be seen. Posterior dislocation is generally the result of trauma and often is associated with damage to the nearby auditory system. Disruption of the external auditory canal or fracture of the temporal plate is common (4). Superior dislocation occurs with severe trauma and is associated with fractures of the mandibular fossa. Lateral dislocations occur only with concomitant fractures of the mandibular body (5).

▶ INDICATIONS

Patients with an acute anterior dislocation of the temporomandibular joint complain of severe pain in the preauricular

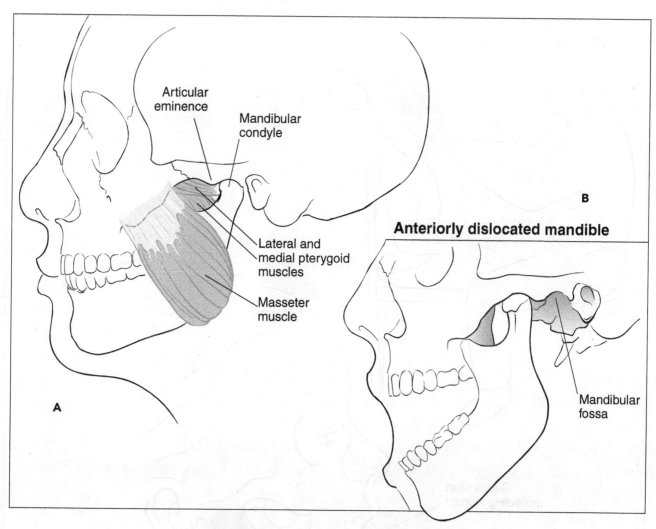

Figure 68.1
A. Anatomy of the temporomandibular joint.
B. Anterior dislocation of the temporomandibular joint.

area. They present with an open mouth, a protruding mandible, and an inability to occlude the anterior teeth. A visible depression is evident in the preauricular area. In the case of a unilateral dislocation, the jaw will be displaced toward the unaffected side.

Before reduction is attempted, radiographs should be obtained to confirm the dislocation and exclude any associated fractures. A panoramic view is considered best for this purpose, although transcranial, transpharyngeal, or transorbital temporomandibular joint views are generally adequate. A dislocation associated with a fracture of the mandibular condyle often requires open reduction and internal fixation. Referral to an oral surgeon is recommended in this situation.

Damage to the cartilage within the temporomandibular joint can produce a hemarthrosis and a subsequent subluxation but not a true dislocation of the mandible. Attempts at manual reduction will fail for obvious reasons and are contraindicated if this condition is recognized.

▶ EQUIPMENT

Gauze, preferably with an attached string or trailing appendage to avoid aspiration
Gloves
2% lidocaine with 1:100,000 epinephrine
3-mL syringe
21- or 25-gauge, 1.5-inch needle
Yankauer suction
McGill forceps

▶ PROCEDURE

The patient is positioned in a chair facing the physician performing the reduction (1). Stimulation of the gag reflex has been described in adults as a successful alternative to manual reduction, and this approach might be

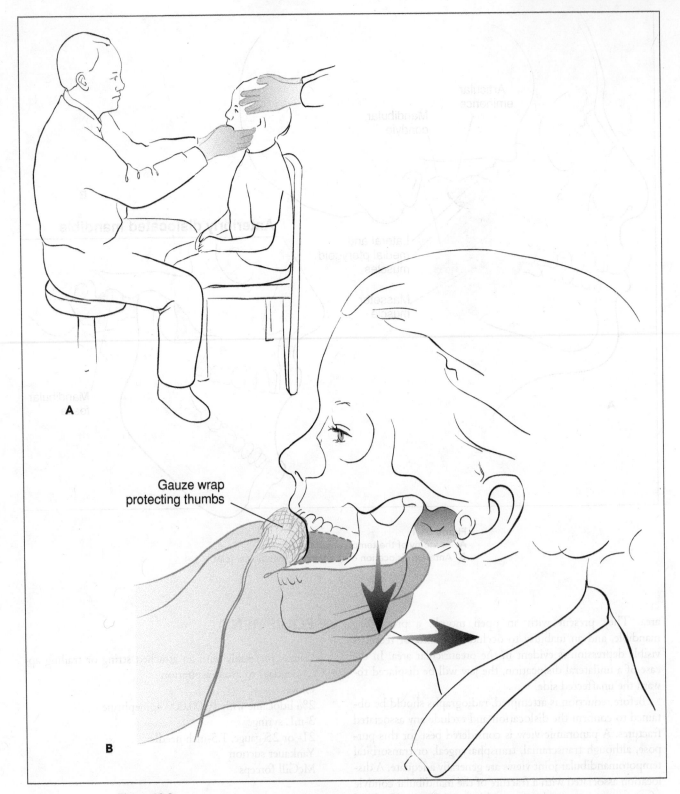

Figure 68.2
A. Position of the patient, assistant, and physician in preparation for reduction.
B. Application and direction of forces in the reduction of an anteriorly dislocated temporomandibular joint.

Gauze wrap
protecting thumbs

considered as an initial effort in an older adolescent patient (6). For manual reduction, the head is held firmly by an assistant or stabilized posteriorly against a wall or headrest. Alternatively, the patient may be placed in a supine position with the physician located at the head of the bed. In the seated patient, further control is gained by straddling the patient's lap (Fig. 68.2A).

Both thumbs are swathed in gauze to avoid injury when the mandible snaps back into place. The thumbs are placed against the surface of the lower molars as far posteriorly as possible. The fingers of each hand are wrapped under the angle and body of the mandible with the elbows flexed at a 90-degree angle. Pressure is applied first in a downward motion to release the condyle from the articular eminence and then posteriorly to move the condyle back into the fossa (Fig. 68.2B). A less common but also effective method is performed by seating the patient upright in a chair and standing behind the patient. The physician presses downward with his or her thumbs over the posterior lower molars. The physician's fingers are used to provide counteraction by pulling upward along the inferior aspect of the patient's anterior mandible. In this way, the patient's head can be braced against the physician's abdomen, thereby minimizing any movement. Care must be taken to avoid a crushing injury to the fingers or teeth once reduction is achieved. Placing the thumbs in the buccal aspect of the mandibular ridge rather than on the surface of the molars may avoid this risk but provides less leverage for the reduction. When severe muscle spasm is present, reduction may be facilitated by gently rocking the mandible back and forth until the muscles fatigue. With a bilateral dislocation, reducing one side at a time may prove easier and more successful (3,7).

Because significant pain and anxiety inevitably accompany this condition, using procedural sedation is recommended for reducing both the level of anxiety and the degree of muscle spasm (Chapter 33). Frequently, reduction may not be possible without the concomitant use of anesthetic agents to facilitate patient cooperation and muscle relaxation. In some cases, intra-articular or intramuscular administration of lidocaine may aid reduction by relaxing the lateral pterygoid and temporalis muscles, which tend to force the mandible forward (7,8).

Displacement of the meniscus may simulate temporomandibular joint dislocation and is an additional cause for reduction failure. Patients with temporomandibular joint dislocation that fails to reduce should be referred to an oral surgeon for closed or open reduction under general anesthesia.

Patients who have undergone a successful reduction should be warned against opening the mouth widely for approximately 3 weeks to allow the involved ligaments and muscles to resume their normal tone and strength. The mandible should be supported when yawning. The patient should be started on a mild analgesic and advised to eat a soft diet (9).

 SUMMARY

1 Administer procedural sedation as needed.

2 Position patient upright in chair and straddle patient's lap.

3 Protect thumbs by generously wrapping them in gauze.

4 Place thumbs against lower posterior molars and wrap fingers around angle and body of mandible.

5 Apply slow, steady pressure, first downward and then posteriorly.

▶ COMPLICATIONS

Complications associated with the reduction of a temporomandibular joint dislocation are mainly related to the muscular spasm that accompanies the dislocation. Muscles controlling the mandible are capable of generating forces in excess of 300 lb/in^2 (10). If reduction does not occur in a controlled fashion, these forces are capable of producing crush injuries of the physician's thumbs and fractures of the patient's teeth.

Aspiration of gauze used as protection for the physician's thumbs has been described (11). The reflex withdrawal of the thumbs on reduction may result in gauze that is not tightly bound to the thumbs remaining in the posterior pharynx. The sedated patient is at additional risk for this problem. Suction and airway equipment, including McGill forceps, should therefore always be available. Using gauze with trailing appendages may decrease the risk of this complication (12).

 CLINICAL TIPS

▶ Using sedation is highly recommended to alleviate anxiety and decrease the degree of muscle spasm.

▶ Stimulation of the gag reflex has been described in adults as a successful alternative to manual reduction.

▶ Gentle rocking of the mandible or digital massage may fatigue muscles that are in spasm and ease reduction.

▶ With a bilateral dislocation, reduction of one condyle at a time may be useful when spasm is severe.

▶ Dislocations associated with fractures should be referred to an oral surgeon for reduction.

▶ SUMMARY

Temporomandibular joint dislocation is a painful and anxiety-provoking condition that occurs only rarely in children. Those afflicted generally seek immediate care in the office or ED. Unilateral and bilateral anterior dislocations of the mandible are the most common presentations, and most can be manually reduced. Other dislocations have a higher incidence of associated fractures and complications and require the expertise of an oral surgeon.

▶ ACKNOWLEDGMENT

The authors would like to acknowledge the valuable contributions of William Ahrens to the version of this chapter that appeared in the previous edition.

▶ REFERENCES

1. Kruger GO. The temporomandibular joint. In: Kruger GO, ed. *Textbook of Oral and Maxillofacial Surgery*. St. Louis: Mosby; 1979.
2. Upton LG. Management of injuries to the temporomandibular joint. In: Fonseca RF, Walker RV, eds. *Oral and Maxillofacial Trauma*. Philadelphia: WB Saunders; 1991.
3. Wessberg GA. Mandibular condylar dislocation. *Hawaii Dent J.* 1987;18:9–11.
4. Bradley PF. Injuries of the condylar and coronoid process. In: Rowe NL, Williams JL, eds. *Maxillofacial Injuries*. Edinburgh: Churchill Livingstone; 1985.
5. Lentrodt G. Treatment of dislocation of the TMJ. In: Kruger E, Schili W, Worthington P, eds. *Oral and Maxillofacial Traumatology*. Chicago: Quintessence Publishing Co.; 1986.
6. Awang MN. A new approach to the reduction of acute dislocation of the temporomandibular joint: a report of three cases. *Br J Oral Maxillofac Surg.* 1987;25:244–249.
7. Luyk NH, Larsen PE. The diagnosis and treatment of the dislocated mandible. *Am J Emerg Med.* 1989;7:329–335.
8. Littler BO. The role of local anesthesia in the reduction of longstanding dislocation of the temporomandibular joint. *Br J Oral Surg.* 1980;18:81–85.
9. Dolwick MF. Management of temporomandibular joint disorders. In: Peterson LJ, Ellis E, Hupp JR, et al., eds. *Contemporary Oral and Maxillofacial Surgery*. St. Louis: Mosby; 1993.
10. Awang MN. A new approach to the reduction of acute dislocation of the temporomandibular joint: a report of three cases. *Br J Oral Maxillofac Surg.* 1987;25:244–249.
11. Wagner DK, ed. *1985 Year Book of Emergency Medicine*. Chicago: Year Book; 1985.
12. Mariani PJ. Avoiding "death in the dental chair" [letter]. *Am J Emerg Med.* 1989;8:85.

69

SRIKANT B. IYER

The Electrocardiogram in Infants and Children

▶ INTRODUCTION

The surface electrocardiogram (ECG) remains an efficient and inexpensive aid in the initial and emergent evaluation of dysrhythmias, conduction disturbances, myocardial damage and chamber hypertrophy and dilatation. Important differences exist between children of various ages and adults in ECG procedure and interpretation. This chapter provides an overview of the indications for obtaining a pediatric ECG, details of the ECG procedure and a suggested stepwise approach for the interpretation of pediatric ECGs.

▶ ANATOMY AND PHYSIOLOGY

Figure 69.1A shows a diagrammatic representation and ECG tracing of a cardiac cycle (see also Chapters 22 and 70). The heart beats in response to an electrical signal that is generated by the heart's "pacemaker," normally the sinoatrial (SA) node located in the right atrium. This electrical signal is conducted through the atria and ventricles, creating an electrical impulse that may be recorded from electrodes applied to the skin. The recording of this impulse comprises the ECG. The appearance of an impulse will vary depending on which electrodes are used to make the recording.

The SA node impulse depolarizes the right and left atria, producing a P wave on the ECG. The impulse then arrives at the atrioventricular (AV) node, which conducts at a much slower velocity than other parts of the heart. This "delay" in the AV node is represented by the PR interval. The impulse then travels rapidly through the bundle of His, the left and right bundle branches, the Purkinje fibers, and finally the ventricular muscle. This rapid conduction is represented by the QRS complex. If the QRS complex begins with a negative deflection, this negative deflection is called the Q wave. If the complex begins with a positive deflection, this positive deflection is called the R wave. The first negative deflection after the R wave is called the S wave. A second positive or negative deflection is called R′ or S′, respectively. Finally, repolarization of the ventricles produces the T wave.

The anatomy of the chest wall and the heart of the pediatric patient differs from that of an adult in a number of ways that directly affect the recording of the ECG. The heart of an infant or child is larger relative to the size of the thoracic cavity. The normal adult heart occupies about half the transverse diameter of the thorax, whereas the normal pediatric heart occupies up to two thirds of this space, depending on the age of the child. In general, the younger the patient, the larger the area that the heart occupies. As described below, this proportionally wider anterior chest surface area in infants and younger children is addressed when recording an electrocardiogram by adding one or two extra right-sided chest leads and, if necessary, an extra left-sided lead. Many of the other age-related differences in pediatric ECGs are related to changes in ventricular dominance. The normal right ventricular (RV) dominance of the newborn period is gradually replaced by left ventricular

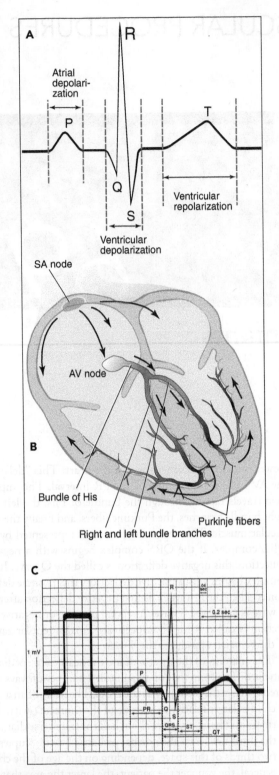

Figure 69.1 Cardiac conduction.
A. Cardiac cycle as represented on a rhythm strip tracing.
B. Diagrammatic representation of the conduction system of the heart.
C. Waves and intervals in a P-QRS-T complex (PR, PR interval; QRS, QRS interval; ST, ST segment; QT, QT interval). Standard calibration is 1 mV = 10 mm; paper speed is 25 mm/sec. (B is redrawn from Park MK, Guntheroth WG. *How to Read Pediatric ECGs.* 4th ed. New York: Mosby; 2006. C is reprinted with permission from Gessner IH, Victorica BE. *Pediatric Cardiology: A Problem Oriented Approach.* Philadelphia: WB Saunders; 1993:51.)

(LV) dominance in adulthood. Because the ECG reflects these changes in heart size and ventricular dominance, there is great variation in the normal values for various ECG measurements. The following changes occur with increasing age:

- The PR interval, QRS duration, and QT interval increase.
- The QRS axis changes from a right anterior direction in infants to a left posterior direction in adults.
- The R/S ratio in the right precordial leads decreases.
- The R/S ratio in the left precordial leads increases.

The T vector also changes significantly depending on patient age. During the first 3 days of life (and up to 8 to 10 days of age), the T vector is directed anteriorly, resulting in upright T waves in the anterior precordial leads. Immediately after this period and throughout early adolescence, the T vector is directed posteriorly, resulting in inverted T waves in the anterior precordial leads. During adolescence, the T vector gradually shifts to an anterior direction again, resulting in upright T waves in the anterior precordial leads. Therefore, correct interpretation of the T vector requires knowing these expected age-based normal conduction patterns.

An exhaustive explanation of the physiologic and electromechanical principles of electrocardiography and vectorcardiography is beyond the scope of this chapter. The references listed at the end of this chapter provide more detailed explanations of these principles.

▶ INDICATIONS

The most common indications for obtaining an ECG in the pediatric patient are listed in Table 69.1. History of palpitations, heart racing, and fluttering of the heart should lead the clinician to consider an underlying electrocardiac abnormality or a structural lesion. Tachycardias, bradycardias, or irregular rates and/or rhythms should be detectable on examination of the patient, and the ECG can be used as a confirmatory and diagnostic tool.

Signs of cardiac failure may be subtle in infants and young children (e.g., poor feeding, sweating during feeds), and the differentiation from primary pulmonary disease can be difficult. Pediatric patients with heart failure may manifest nonspecific electrocardiographic changes or changes associated with

TABLE 69.1	INDICATIONS FOR ECG TRACING IN PEDIATRIC ACUTE CARE

▶ Extreme tachycardia
▶ Extreme bradycardia
▶ Irregularity of rhythm, palpitations, sensation of fluttering of heart
▶ Clinical suggestion of cardiac failure
▶ Clinical suggestion of myocarditis or pericarditis
▶ Significant murmur not readily explainable
▶ Cyanosis not ameliorated by oxygen
▶ Chest pain and/or syncope
▶ Suspected calcium or potassium abnormalities
▶ Ingestion of cardiac toxic drug and any symptomatic overdose

a specific underlying cardiac lesion. An electrocardiogram can be helpful in determining previously undiagnosed congenital heart disease or onset of acquired heart disease such as pericarditis or myocarditis.

The presence of a heart murmur sometimes constitutes an indication for performing an ECG with a pediatric patient. The significance of the murmur—that is, whether it may represent underlying cardiac disease—is determined by the intensity, radiation, and point of maximum loudness. Children in a high output state, such as hyperpyrexia, may present with a loud murmur that is not significant. However, if the patient has no known prior history of murmur and the clinical picture cannot be defined, an ECG may be helpful.

Cyanosis related to pulmonary disease usually improves significantly with oxygen. Cyanosis not ameliorated by oxygen may be related to a hemoglobinopathy but may also be related to previously undiagnosed cyanotic congenital heart disease. An electrocardiogram can be useful in screening for the cardiac causes of cyanosis.

While the differential diagnosis of chest pain in children is extensive, this complaint does not often relate to cardiac disease. The most common causes are respiratory and musculoskeletal etiologies as well as gastroesophageal reflux, costochondritis, and functional problems. However, the occasional pediatric patient with chest pain will show ECG findings consistent with cardiac strain, pericarditis, or myocarditis. In rare instances, there may be signs of ischemia. Additionally, chest pain without overt palpitations will sometimes be found in children with an aberrant atrial pathway such as Wolff-Parkinson-White syndrome.

TABLE 69.2	EQUIPMENT FOR RECORDING AN ELECTROCARDIOGRAM

Electrocardiograph
  Fully automated and computerized (Fig. 69.2)
Electrode wires, appropriately labeled
Electrodes
  Prepackaged, imbued with adherent conducting substance, possibly with conducting button or clip holder
Recording paper

Syncope in children is usually related to noncardiac causes, such as vasovagal episodes, orthostatic syncope, and breath-holding spells. However, an electrocardiogram should be considered for all pediatric patients presenting with syncope to screen for arrhythmia as the cause. Syncope may be the only manifestation of prolonged QT syndrome, a condition that puts the patient at risk for subsequent sudden death.

▶ EQUIPMENT

An electrocardiograph and its associated equipment are used to obtain an ECG (Table 69.2). These machines have evolved dramatically over the years from Einthoven's galvanometer to today's electronically sophisticated computerized devices. The keyboard, monitor, and simultaneous three-channel paper recording of an automated modern electrocardiograph are shown in Figure 69.2. These machines must be preprogrammed but after preprogramming are relatively simple to operate.

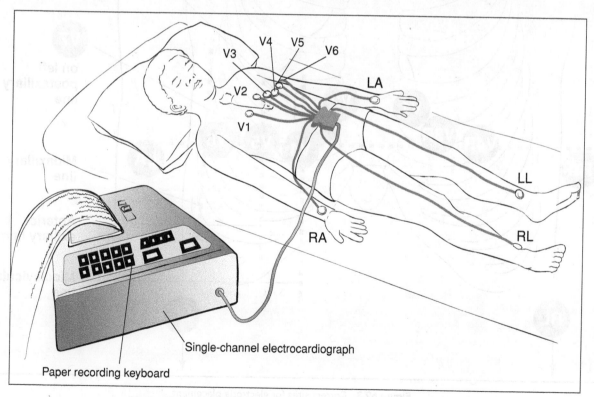

Figure 69.2 Keyboard and monitor of fully automated electrocardiograph.

Electrodes are usually conveniently prepackaged. They are coated on one side with an adherent conducting material that holds the electrode in place on the patient's skin. On the other side, they have a conducting button or clip holder that attaches to the electrode wires. The appropriate electrode wires, recording paper, and plugs are supplied with the machine.

▶ PROCEDURE

The patient should be lying supine on an examining table or crib that is free of vibration, electrical interference, and human contact. The usual array of distractors and tricks may calm the crying infant or frightened child. If these are not successful, sedation may be required, depending on the urgency with which the tracing is required and the general clinical status of the patient.

The proper sites for placement of the electrodes are listed in Table 69.3 and are shown in Figure 69.3. Proper place-

TABLE 69.3	ELECTRODE LOCATION

Extremity Leads

RA and LA*—anywhere on the right and left arms. In infants less than 1 year of age, place midway between elbow and shoulder.

RL and LL*—anywhere on the right and left legs. In infants place above knee and close to hip.

Chest Leads

V_4R—Midclavicular line (MCL) in right 5th intercostal space (ICS)

V_3R—Halfway between V_4R and V_1

V_1—4th ICS at right border of sternum

V_2—4th ICS at left border of sternum

V_3—Halfway between V_2 and V_4

V_4—MCL in 5th left ICS

V_5—Left anterior axillary line (AAL) on same horizontal level as V_4

V_6—Left midaxillary line (MAL) on same horizontal level as V_4

V_7—Left posterior axillary line (PAL) on same horizontal level as V_4

*RA, LA, RL, LL—right and left arms and legs.

ment is essential, particularly when sequential ECG tracings will be required over time for a given patient. For effective

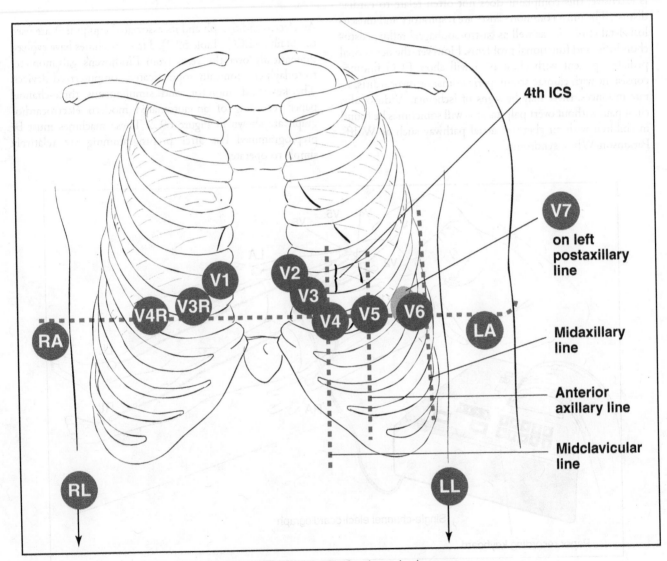

Figure 69.3 Correct sites for electrode placement.

lead attachment, it may be necessary to clean the skin with isopropyl alcohol to remove oils before placement of the electrodes. Some adolescents will have enough body hair that the electrode sites may need to be abraded slightly by rubbing with dry gauze or, rarely, to be shaved.

The number and sites of electrode placement for the chest leads depend on the age of the patient. For infants and children up to approximately 1 year of age, the electrodes shown in Figure 69.3 will normally be required. Children between 1 and 12 years of age should have leads V_4R through V_6 recorded. For patients older than 12 years of age, only leads V_1 through V_6 are necessary.

Depending on the design of the machine, the electrode lead wires must be attached to the electrode by the appropriate clip, button, or probe. The wires are marked near their distal ends with symbols corresponding to those in Figure 69.3 and Table 69.3. Modern machines that are designed primarily for adult use have chest lead wires that are only dedicated for leads V_1 through V_6, and an additional "nondedicated" wire is available for V_4R, V_3R, and V_7.

The connector located at the proximal end of the lead wires should be inserted into the designated socket on the electrocardiograph. The power switch should then be turned on, and the operator should check the machine for sufficient recording paper. The patient's name and other pertinent data are then entered. Paper speed is normally set to the standard rate of 25 mm/sec. The standard electrical calibration is 1 mV equivalent to a 10-mm deflection.

On modern machines (Fig. 69.2), pressing a single button labeled "Record" will print the entire ECG. Such machines are usually preprogrammed for automatic recording. They are usually set to record one to three leads simultaneously for a specific time period (usually 2.5 to 3 seconds), and they will automatically identify the leads on the recording paper. These machines often store readings that can be sent by modem to the ECG laboratory as a permanent electronic record.

▶ STEPWISE APPROACH FOR PEDIATRIC ECG INTERPRETATION

Once an ECG has been obtained, the next task is to interpret the tracing. Interpretation of pediatric ECGs is made more challenging by age-based variations in "normal" values for various measurements, as mentioned previously. The following is intended as a useful quick reference for interpreting pediatric ECGs in the acute care setting. It is not meant to replace the more comprehensive explanations provided in reference texts such as those listed at the end of this chapter.

Step 1: Assess the Rhythm

The normal rhythm for any person regardless of age is sinus rhythm. The following two criteria must be met in order to prove that the ECG shows sinus rhythm:

1 There must be one P wave (and only one) prior to each QRS complex.
2 The P axis must be between 0 and +90 degrees.

In order to determine the P axis, one must be familiar with the hexaxial reference system (Fig. 69.4). If the P waves are upright (deflections are positive) in leads I and aVF, the P axis must be between 0 and +90 degrees. The rhythm strips shown in Figures 69.5 through 69.8 are examples of various types of sinus rhythm. An example of nonsinus rhythm is shown in Figure 69.9, as there are no P waves seen on the tracing.

Step 2: Calculate the Rate

Table 69.4 shows five methods for calculating the heart rate from the ECG. All are valid, but one may be preferred over the others depending on the ease of use for a given tracing. For example, Figure 69.7 shows the tracing of a child with sinus tachycardia. To measure the actual heart rate using Method 1, approximately 3.75 R-R intervals can be counted in six large divisions on the ECG graph paper (1.2 seconds at a standard paper speed of 25 mm/sec), so the patient's rate is 188 ($3.75 \times 50 = 188$). As another example, Figure 69.6 shows the tracing of a child with sinus bradycardia. Using Method 2, 6.7 large divisions are in one R-R interval. Thus, the heart rate is 44 ($300/6.7 = 44$). The calculated heart rate should be compared to expected age-based normal values (listed in Table 69.5).

In the two previous examples, only one rate was calculated for each tracing because the patient had an underlying sinus rhythm. If, however, a nonsinus rhythm was present, individual rate calculations for both the atria and ventricles might be necessary. For example, Figure 69.10 shows a tracing of complete atrioventricular block. Using Method 2 from Table 69.4, five large divisions are in one R-R interval, giving a ventricular rate of 60 ($300/5 = 60$). Two large divisions are in one P-P interval, giving an atrial rate of 150 ($300/2 = 150$).

Step 3: Determine the QRS Axis

Similar to the determination of the P axis, the hexaxial reference system (Fig. 69.4) may be used to determine the QRS axis. Directionality of the R-wave deflections in leads I and aVF may be used to localize the QRS axis to a particular quadrant, as shown in Figure 69.11. After the quadrant is determined, the tracing should be examined to find the most isoelectric lead (i.e., the lead in which the R and S waves are nearly equal in length). The QRS axis is perpendicular to the isoelectric lead in the previously localized quadrant. An example is shown in Figure 69.12. Net positive deflections in leads I and aVF localize the QRS axis somewhere between 0 and +90 degrees. The most isoelectric lead is aVL. The QRS axis is calculated to be +60 degrees, since this is perpendicular to aVL *and* in the previously localized quadrant. The calculated QRS axis should be compared to expected age-based normal values (Table 69.4).

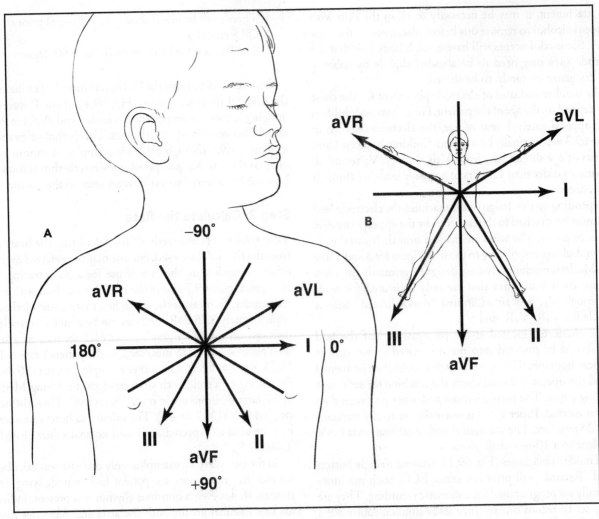

Figure 69.4

A. Hexaxial reference system (viewed from the patient's front). The positive pole of each lead is indicated by a + sign. The angle between two adjacent limb leads in 30 degrees.

B. Easy method for memorizing the hexaxial reference system. (Redrawn from Park MK, Guntheroth WG. *How to Read ECGs.* 4th ed. New York: Mosby; 2006.)

TABLE 69.4	METHODS FOR DETERMINING HEART RATE

1. Count R-R intervals in six large divisions (equivalent to 1.2 seconds) and multiply by 50 (best method for fast rates).

OR

2. Count number of large divisions in one R-R interval and divide into 300 (best method for slow rates).

OR

3. Count R-R intervals in 15 large divisions (3 seconds) and multiply by 20 (best for irregular rhythms).

OR

4. Heart rates of 300, 150, 100, 75, 60, and 50 have approximate R-R intervals of 5, 10, 15, 20, 25, and 30 small spaces, respectively.

OR

5. Use calibrated ECG "ruler" for direct reading.

Step 4: Measure Intervals

Figure 69.1 shows a diagram representing the various intervals on an ECG. Calculations for these intervals should be compared with age-based normal values for interpretation.

The PR interval is calculated by measuring the distance from the beginning of the P wave to the beginning of the QRS complex. Figure 69.13 shows an example of a tracing with a short PR interval.

The QRS duration is calculated by measuring the distance from the beginning of the Q wave to the end of the S wave. Figure 69.14 shows an example of a tracing with prolonged QRS complexes. Figure 69.15 shows an example of a tracing with QRS complexes that occur irregularly and in rapid sequence.

The QT interval corrected for rate (QTc) is calculated by first measuring the distance from the beginning of the

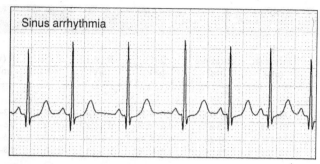

Figure 69.5 Tracing from a 5-year-old child.

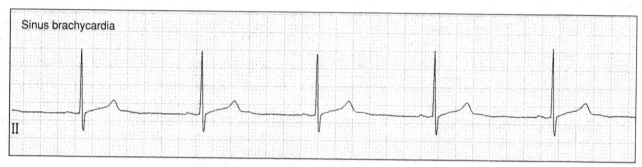

Figure 69.6 Sinus bradycardia in a 14-year-old child.

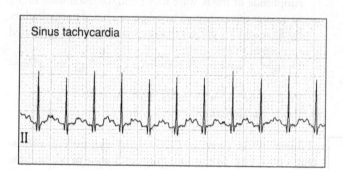

Figure 69.7 Sinus tachycardia in a 2-month-old child.

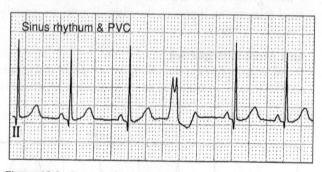

Figure 69.8 Sinus rhythm with a premature ventricular contraction seen in a 2-year-old child.

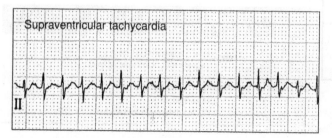

Figure 69.9 Supraventricular tachycardia in a 7-month-old child.

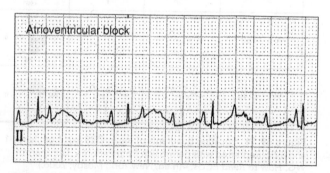

Figure 69.10 Complete atrioventricular block in a 3-month-old child.

			PR	QRS							S
Age	Heart rate (beats/min)	QRS axis (degrees)	interval (ms)	duration (ms)	Q (III) (mV)	R (V₁) (mV)	S(V₁) (mV)	R (V₄) (mV)	S (V₄) (mV)	R (V₄) (mV)	(V₄) (mV)
Days											
0–1	93–155	59–193	79–161	21–76	0.01–0.51	0.5–2.6	0.1–2.3	0.3–3.0	0.3–2.8	0–1.2	0–1.0
1–3	91–158	64–196	81–139	22–67	0.01–0.51	0.5–2.7	0.1–2.1	0.6–3.0	0.2–2.7	0–1.2	0–1.0
3–7	90–166	77–193	73–136	21–68	0.01–0.48	0.3–2.4	0.1–1.7	0.6–2.9	0.3–2.6	0–1.2	0–1.0
7–30	106–182	65–161	72–138	22–79	0.01–0.56	0.3–2.1	0.1–1.1	0.8–2.9	0.3–2.3	0.2–1.7	0–1.0
Months											
1–3	120–179	31–113	72–130	23–75	0.01–0.54	0.3–1.8	0.1–1.3	1.3–3.8	0.5–2.2	0.5–2.2	0–0.7
3–6	106–186	7–104	73–146	22–79	0–0.66	0.3–2.0	0.1–1.7	1.1–4.3	0.3–2.3	0.6–2.2	0–1.0
6–12	108–169	6–99	72–157	23–76	0–0.63	0.2–2.0	0.1–1.8	1.2–3.6	0.2–2.3	0.6–2.3	0–0.7
Years											
1–3	90–151	7–101	81–148	27–75	0–0.53	0.3–1.8	0.1–2.1	1.1–3.5	0.3–2.0	0.6–2.3	0–0.7
3–5	72–138	6–104	83–161	30–72	0–0.42	0.2–1.8	0.2–2.2	1.3–4.5	0.2–1.8	0.8–2.4	0–0.5
5–8	64–132	11–143	90–163	32–79	0–0.32	0.1–1.4	0.3–2.3	1.1–4.2	0.2–1.9	0.8–2.7	0–0.4
8–12	62–130	9–114	88–171	32–85	0–0.27	0.1–1.2	0.3–2.5	1.1–4.2	0.2–1.9	0.9–2.6	0–0.4
12–16	61–120	11–130	92–176	34–88	0–0.30	0.1–1.0	0.3–2.2	0.7–3.9	0.1–1.8	0.7–2.3	0–0.4

TABLE 69.5 | NORMAL VALUES FOR PEDIATRIC ECG

Source: Adapted from Davignon A, Rautaharju P, Boisselle E, et al. Normal ECG standards for infants and children. *Pediatr Cardiol.* 1979;1:123.

QRS complex to the end of the T wave. This number is then divided by the square root of the distance of the prior R-R interval (Table 69.6).

Step 5: Assess Chamber Size

Right Atrial Enlargement

P waves greater than 3 mm in height are an indication of right atrial enlargement. If present, these large P waves are typically best seen in leads I, 2, V₁, and V₂.

Left Atrial Enlargement

Broad P waves (greater than 80 msec in infants and greater than 100 msec in children) are an indication of left atrial enlargement. These are usually seen in leads I and 2. Another sign of left atrial enlargement is the presence of a biphasic P wave in lead V₁.

Right Ventricular Hypertrophy

The following are some of the common criteria for right ventricular hypertrophy (RVH):

Amplitude of the R wave in V₁ and/or the S wave in V₆ greater than expected based on age-based normal values

R/S ratio in V₁ greater than expected based on age-based normal values

Upright T wave in V₁ between 5 days of age and adolescence

Presence of a Q wave in V₁, V₃R, or V₄R

Right axis deviation

Figure 69.16 shows an ECG tracing with findings consistent with RVH. In this example, the S wave in V₆ and the R/S ratio in V₁ are greater than the upper limits of normal for age, there is right axis deviation, and Q waves are present in V₁.

Figure 69.11 Locating quadrants of mean QRS axis from leads 1 and aVF. (Reprinted with permission from Park MK, Guntheroth WG. *How to Read ECGs.* 4th ed. New York: Mosby; 2006.)

TABLE 69.6 | CORRECTED QT INTERVAL (QTc)

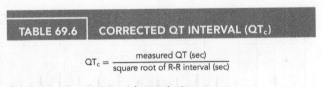

$$QT_c = \frac{\text{measured QT (sec)}}{\text{square root of R-R interval (sec)}}$$

QTc should not exceed: 0.45 in infants under 6 mo
0.44 in children
0.425 in adolescents and adults

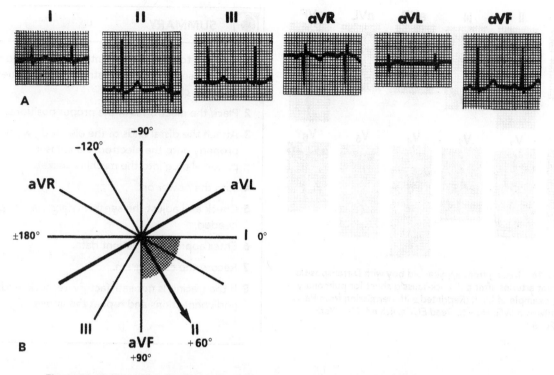

Figure 69.12 Example of QRS axis determination. (Reprinted with permission from Park MK, Guntheroth WG. *How to Read ECGs.* 4th ed. New York: Mosby; 2006.)

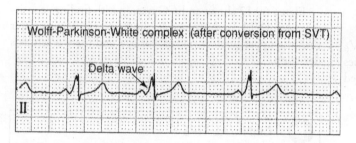

Figure 69.13 Wolff-Parkinson-White syndrome after conversion from SVT in 14-year-old child.

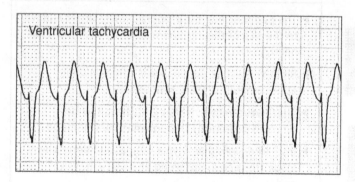

Figure 69.14 Ventricular tachycardia in a 2-year-old child.

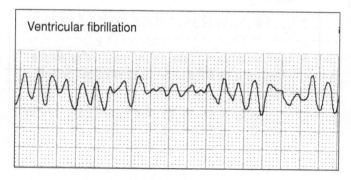

Figure 69.15 Ventricular fibrillation in a 10-month-old child.

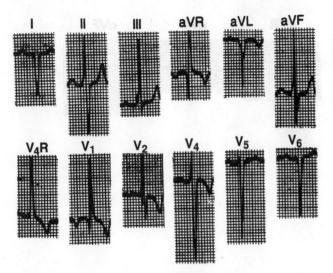

Figure 69.16 Tracing from a 9-year-old boy with D-transposition of the great arteries after a Blalock-Taussig shunt for pulmonary stenosis; example of RVH. (Reprinted with permission from Park MK, Guntheroth WG. *How to Read ECGs.* 4th ed. New York: Mosby; 2006.)

Left Ventricular Hypertrophy

The following are some of the common criteria for left ventricular hypertrophy (LVH):

Amplitude of the S wave in V_1 and/or the R wave in V_6 greater than expected based on age-based normal values

R/S ratio in V_1 less than expected based on age-based normal values

Left axis deviation

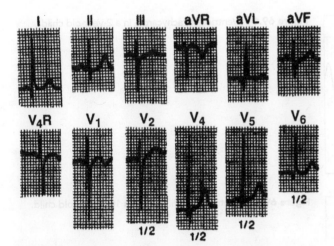

Figure 69.17 Tracing from a 4-year-old boy with moderate ventricular septal defect; example of LVH. (Reprinted with permission from Park MK, Guntheroth WG. *How to Read ECGs.* 4th ed. New York: Mosby; 2006.)

SUMMARY

1 Attempt to calm the patient before proceeding and/or use appropriate distraction techniques to have the child lie still.

2 Place the electrodes in the proper positions.

3 Attach the distal ends of the electrode wires properly onto the electrodes and insert the proximal plug into the machine socket.

4 Turn the power on.

5 Check and adjust the sensitivity and paper speed as needed.

6 Enter appropriate patient data.

7 Record the cardiogram.

8 If the tracing is not satisfactory, recheck leads and connections and repeat the above steps.

Figure 69.17 shows an ECG tracing with findings consistent with LVH. In this example, the R wave in V_6 is greater than the upper limit of normal for age, and there is left axis deviation.

CLINICAL TIPS

▶ The pediatric heart is proportionately larger relative to the size of the intrathoracic cavity than the adult heart.

▶ Right ventricular dominance is common until approximately 3 years of age.

▶ The T-wave vector of the right chest may be directed posteriorly through much of childhood.

▶ In children less than 1 year of age, additional chest leads are used in obtaining an ECG: V_3R, V_4R, and V_7.

▶ In children 1 to 12 years of age, leads V_4R through V_6 are used.

▶ Age-based normal values from standard reference tables must be used to properly interpret pediatric ECGs.

▶ **SUMMARY**

Although used less frequently for children than adults, the ECG is an important tool in the management of pediatric patients who present with complains such as chest pain, syncope, and cyanosis. The ECG of a child differs from that of an adult in several important respects, and characteristics of the ECG change from infancy to adolescence. An understanding of these changes is necessary for correct pediatric ECG interpretation. The procedure for obtaining an ECG is essentially the same for children and adults, except that different leads may be needed depending on the age of the child. By using a stepwise, systematic approach as well as appropriate information regarding age-based normal values, clinicians can learn to interpret pediatric ECGs reliably and use the information obtained to guide the management of children in the ED and other acute care settings.

▶ **ACKNOWLEDGMENTS**

The authors would like to acknowledge the valuable contributions of Michele R. Wadsworth and Benjamin K. Silverman to the version of this chapter that appeared in the previous edition.

▶ **REFERENCES**

1. Garson A. The electrocardiogram in infants and children: a systematic approach. Philadelphia: Lea & Febiger; 1983:19–35.
2. Gessner IH, Victorica BE. *Pediatric Cardiology: A Problem Oriented Approach.* Philadelphia: WB Saunders; 1993.
3. Park MK. *Pediatric Cardiology for Practitioners.* 3rd ed. St. Louis: Mosby-Year Book; 1996.
4. Park MK, Guntheroth WG. *How to Read Pediatric ECGs.* 3rd ed. St. Louis: Mosby-Year Book; 1992.
5. Surawicz B, Knilans TK. *Chou's Electrocardiography in Clinical Practice.* 5th ed. Philadelphia: WB Saunders; 2001.

70

KATHY N. SHAW

Converting Stable Supraventricular Tachycardia Using Vagal Maneuvers

▶ INTRODUCTION

Many different vagal maneuvers have been used to convert stable supraventricular tachycardia (SVT). The procedures are relatively simple and can be performed by a variety of medical personnel, including physicians, physicians-in-training, nurses, and paramedics. However, because these techniques may in rare instances result in profound bradycardia or asystole, supervision by individuals experienced in pediatric resuscitation is recommended when the procedures are performed in medical settings. Vagal maneuvers are usually temporary measures to re-establish normal sinus rhythm, because medication is often required to maintain the child in this rhythm.

SVT is an abnormal tachycardia, usually due to a re-entrant mechanism, which is narrow complex (of the QRS) in about 90% of cases. In older children and adolescents, SVT is often present at rates above 150 beats per minute (bpm). In infants, the heart rate is usually at or above 240 bpm but may be as high as 300 bpm. SVT must be distinguished from sinus tachycardia (ST), which is usually less than 200 bpm but can occasionally produce heart rates of up to 265 bpm in infancy. However, signs of fever, hypovolemia, or sepsis usually are coexistent (1,2). It is important to distinguish SVT from ventricular tachycardia (VT). In general, the patient with wide complex tachycardia in the range of 150 to 240 bpm must have an assessment to determine whether there is a risk factor for VT, such as cardiac disease, an electrolyte abnormality, or a poisoning from overdose. If a past history of recurrent SVT is indicated, it is usually safe to assume the patient is again in SVT.

SVT is the most common significant dysrhythmia in children. Its incidence ranges from 1:1,000 to as high as 1:250. The majority of children presenting with SVT will be under 1 year of age, and close to half of the cases will occur in infants less than 4 months of age. These young babies usually have a normal underlying heart, although there will occasionally be a predisposing factor such as myocarditis, congenital heart disease, thyrotoxicosis, or infection/sepsis (2). Of note, many infants will present with SVT after receiving an over-the-counter cold preparation or other medication with sympathomimetic properties.

▶ ANATOMY AND PHYSIOLOGY

Most pediatric patients with SVT that is not associated with a specific cause (medication overuse, etc.) have an accessory atrioventricular (AV) pathway. This developmental abnormality may change the heart's electrophysiologic characteristics during the child's growth (1). At birth, autonomic cardiovascular control is not fully developed and may be under hormonal control. This concept of autonomic imbalance or immaturity is one hypothesis of why SVT is more common in young infants (3). SVT from AV node re-entry or primary atrial tachycardia is more common after infancy or postcardiac surgery (1).

Parasympathetic stimulus via the vagus nerve to the sinus and AV nodes slows heart rate. At birth, the infant has a predominance of vagal tone due to an immature sympathetic system. However, despite this parasympathetic predominance, few vagal maneuvers are usually successful in converting SVT in young children, with the exception of the diving reflex (bradycardia following submersion or ice water to the forehead) (3). The diving reflex, which occurs in many aquatic mammals and also in young children, is a very potent stimulus to the afferent limb of this vagally mediated reflex (4).

▶ INDICATIONS

Vagal maneuvers should be used only in children with SVT who do not exhibit signs of hemodynamic compromise. Patients with severe congestive heart failure or shock should have immediate cardioversion (see Chapter 23) (5). With stable SVT, vagal maneuvers often are tried first. If unsuccessful, IV adenosine is then used (Fig. 70.1) (5).

Consultation with a pediatric cardiologist is warranted for all children with SVT, even after an uncomplicated return

TABLE 70.1	EQUIPMENT

Monitor
  Electrocardiographic machine
  Cardiac monitor
  Oximetry
  Bag-valve-mask for age, airway equipment, suction
Intravenous access
  Intravenous catheter
  Alcohol swab
  Normal saline
Resuscitation medications
  Epinephrine 1:10,000
  Atropine
  Amiodarone or lidocaine
Defibrillator/cardioversion machine
  Pediatric paddles
  Electrode gel
Ice bag
  Plastic bag
  Water
  Ice
Gagging or rectal stimulation
  Sterile tongue depressor
  Gloves
  Lubricating jelly

to sinus rhythm. Vagal maneuvers may only be effective temporarily. Furthermore, additional diagnostic workup may be needed, including electrophysiologic studies, and long-term medical treatment is often indicated.

▶ EQUIPMENT

Table 70.1 lists the equipment used for conversion of stable supraventricular tachycardia. All children should have an intravenous line placed, and resuscitation drugs and emergency airway equipment should be readily available.

▶ PROCEDURE

Vagal maneuvers include facial immersion in cold water or saline, placing an ice bag on the face, carotid sinus massage, Valsalva maneuvers, rectal stimulation, stimulation of a gag reflex with a tongue depressor, breath holding, and coughing. Ocular pressure also has been used but is not recommended due to the risk of serious eye injury such as retinal detachment.

The only vagal maneuver that is likely to be successful for a child under 4 years of age is stimulating the diving reflex by applying an ice bag to the face (2). Breath holding, facial immersion in iced saline, coughing, and Valsalva maneuvers are impractical for an infant or uncooperative young child. An attempt at gentle rectal stimulation with a gloved, lubricated finger, induction of the gag reflex with a tongue blade, or brief carotid massage also may be attempted before using

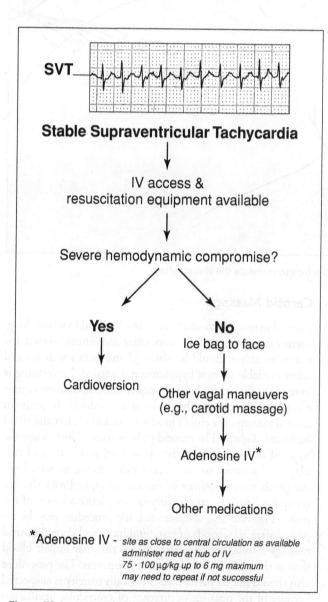

Figure 70.1 Approach to stable supraventricular tachycardia.

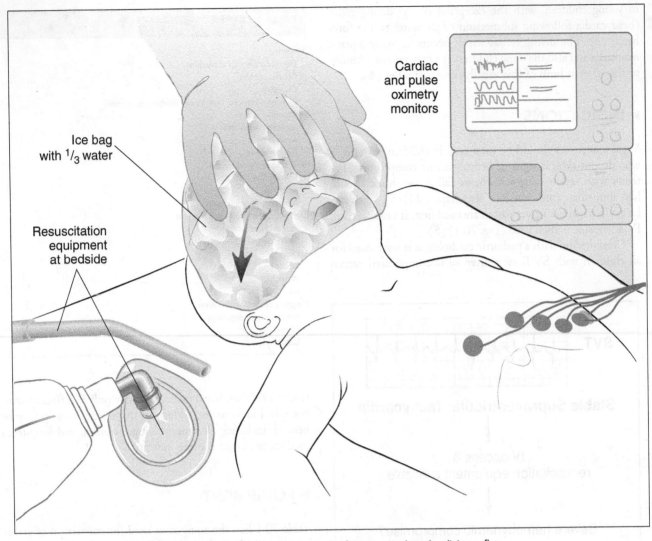

Figure 70.2 Ice bag application to the face to stimulate the diving reflex.

adenosine, but these are less effective. If vagal maneuvers fail, administration of intravenous adenosine is recommended to convert stable SVT in pediatric patients (9,10).

Ice Bag Technique

The infant or child should have intravenous access established, continuous ECG monitoring, and pulse oximetry. Resuscitation equipment and medications should be available at the bedside. A plastic bag is filled one third with water and an equal volume of ice. The bag should be large enough to completely cover the child's face with overlap to the preauricular area (Fig. 70.2). When the procedure is explained to older children, they are asked to hold their breath at the end of a deep inspiration. Young children are immobilized. The bag is applied so that it covers the areas of the nose and mouth and prevents breathing for up to 15 seconds. If conversion to sinus rhythm is noted earlier, the bag is immediately removed (2,4).

Carotid Massage

Carotid massage is most effective in older children with long, narrow necks who will be cooperative and remain relaxed. Intravenous access should be obtained and intravenous normal saline available to treat hypotension if needed. Monitoring is initiated as for the ice bag technique, and resuscitation equipment and medications should be at the bedside. To perform carotid massage, the child's head is turned to the left and tilted backward slightly. The carotid pulse is located just below the angle of the mandible at the upper level of the thyroid cartilage and anterior to the sternocleidomastoid muscle. Firm but gentle rotary pressure or massage is applied with the fingertip for 5 to 10 seconds without complete occlusion of the pulse (Fig. 70.3). If unsuccessful, the procedure may be repeated after 30 seconds of rest. Simultaneous bilateral carotid massage should not be performed, as this may impair blood flow to the brain and induce unconsciousness. The procedure also should not be performed if digitalis toxicity is suspected because of the possible occurrence of ventricular fibrillation in such situations (5,7).

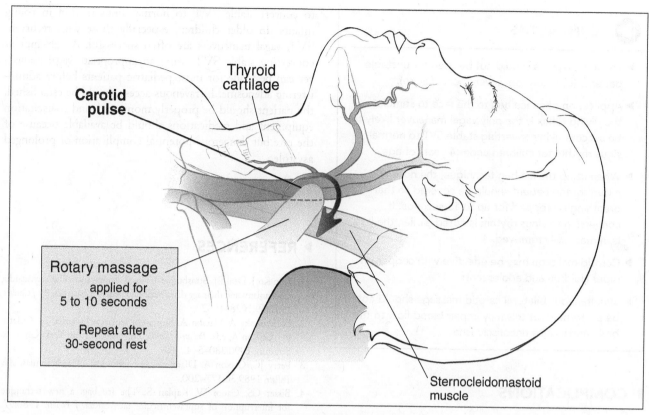

Figure 70.3 Carotid massage technique.

TABLE 70.2	VAGAL MANEUVERS: COMPLICATIONS	
Vagal maneuver	**Advantage**	**Possible disadvantage**
All	Noninvasive	▶ Transient effect ▶ Asystole ▶ Dysrhythmias
Ice bag to face	Most successful	▶ Apnea ▶ Unpleasant
Immersion of face in iced saline with breathing holding	Older children can perform themselves	▶ Unpleasant ▶ Aspiration
Carotid massage	Easy to perform on older children	▶ Transient ischemic attack/CVA ▶ Not with digoxin toxicity
Rectal stimulation	Can be used in noncooperative or young child	▶ Tissue trauma ▶ Unpleasant
Valsalva	Older, cooperative child	▶ Subconjunctival hermorrhages ▶ Rupture of tympanic membrane ▶ Syncope
Coughing	Older, cooperative child	▶ Aspiration ▶ Subconjunctival hemorrhage ▶ Ruptured tympanic membrane ▶ Syncope
Gag reflex	Easy to perform on all ages	▶ Tissue trauma ▶ Emesis/aspiration ▶ Unpleasant

CLINICAL TIPS

▶ Vagal maneuvers should not be used for unstable patients (hypotension, severe heart failure).

▶ Application of an ice bag to the face to stimulate the diving reflex is the only vagal maneuver likely to be successful in converting stable SVT to normal sinus rhythm for children under 4 years of age.

▶ When using the ice bag technique, the nose and mouth of the patient should be covered so that breathing is stopped for up to 15 seconds. If conversion to sinus rhythm is noted earlier, the bag is immediately removed.

▶ Carotid massage may be effective with cooperative older children and adolescents.

▶ Simultaneous bilateral carotid massage should not be performed, as this may impair blood flow to the brain and induce unconsciousness.

COMPLICATIONS

Vagal maneuvers should not be attempted without first obtaining intravenous access, initiating ongoing continuous cardiac and pulse oximetry monitoring, and ensuring that resuscitation medications and equipment are available. Prolonged asystole and other dysrhythmias are rare but potentially unavoidable side effects from vagal maneuvers. A brief period of asystole, lasting a few seconds with no hemodynamic effects, commonly precedes spontaneous conversion to sinus rhythm (6). Potential complications associated with each of the vagal maneuvers are listed in Table 70.2.

SUMMARY

With the exception of stimulating the diving reflex by applying an ice bag to the face, vagal maneuvers are unlikely to convert stable SVT to normal sinus rhythm in young infants. In older children, especially those with recurrent SVT, vagal maneuvers are often successful. An attempt at converting stable SVT using an appropriate vagal maneuver can be made for most pediatric patients before administering adenosine. Intravenous access should be established, the patient should be properly monitored, and resuscitation equipment and medications should be available because of the rare but dangerous potential complication of prolonged asystole.

REFERENCES

1. Kon Ko J, Deal BJ, Strasburger JF, et al. Supraventricular tachycardia mechanisms and their age distribution in pediatric patients. *Am J Cardiol.* 1992;69:1028–1032.
2. Ludomirsky A, Garson A. Supraventricular tachycardia. In: Gillette PC, Garson A, eds. *Pediatric Cardiac Dysrhythmias.* New York: Grune & Stratton; 1990:380–514.
3. Perry JC, Garson A. Diagnosis and treatment of arrhythmias. *Adv Pediatr.* 1989;36:177–200.
4. Bisset GS, Gaum W, Kaplan S. The ice bag: a new technique for interruption of supraventricular tachycardia. *J Pediatr.* 1980;97:593–595.
5. *PALS Provider Manual.* Elk Grove Village, IL: American Academy of Pediatrics, American Heart Association, 2006.
6. Waxman MB, Wald RW, Sharma AD, et al. Vagal techniques for termination of paroxysmal supraventricular tachycardia. *Am J Cardiol.* 1980;46:655–664.
7. Burdick W. Carotid sinus massage. In: Roberts JR, Hedges JR, eds. *Clinical Procedures in Emergency Medicine.* 4th ed. Philadelphia: WB Saunders; 2004.
8. Roberge R, Anderson E, MacMath T, et al. Termination of paroxysmal supraventricular tachycardia by digital rectal massage. *Ann Emerg Med.* 1987;16:1291–1293.
9. Till J, Shinebourne EA, Rigby ML, et al. Efficacy and safety of adenosine in the treatment of supraventricular tachycardia in infants and children. *Br Heart J.* 1989;62:204–211.
10. Overholt ED, Rheuban KS, Gutgesell HP, et al. Usefulness of adenosine for arrhythmias in infants and children. *Am J Cardiol.* 1988;61:336–340.

71

SCOTT D. REEVES

Pericardiocentesis

▶ INTRODUCTION

Pericardiocentesis is the use of a needle-syringe system to aspirate fluid from the pericardial space. Although not often required in the emergency department (ED), the prompt and efficient removal of pericardial fluid can be life-saving in cases of cardiac tamponade. Pericardiocentesis also may be performed electively as a diagnostic procedure in cases of pericardial effusion and as a means of improving cardiac output with chronic pericardial accumulations. The technique for pericardiocentesis is relatively straightforward, but studies in both children and adults report variable success rates in the emergency setting. In addition, a number of severe complications have been reported, and the overall complication rate is fairly high. For these reasons, emergent pericardiocentesis should be performed only by physicians who are comfortable managing critically ill children and when the procedure is necessary to improve cardiac output in the face of life-threatening cardiac tamponade.

▶ ANATOMY AND PHYSIOLOGY

The pericardial sac is a thin, transparent fibrous membrane that surrounds the heart and the trunk of the great vessels. The sac comprises two layers—the visceral pericardium and the parietal pericardium. The interface of these two layers is a potential space that, when filled with fluid, becomes the pericardial space. The normal pericardium may contain 20 to 30 mL of free fluid if it is accessed by a surgical procedure.

Animal studies have shown that large volumes of fluid may occupy the pericardial space with relatively little impairment of cardiac function. This is especially true for subacute accumulations, when the pericardial space can be greatly expanded in the face of increasing fluid volume. Eventually, however, additional relatively small increases in pericardial fluid volume

lead to marked increases in pressure, with a resultant decrease in cardiac filling and cardiac output. The end result of this chain of events is cardiac tamponade with sudden hemodynamic compromise and shock. The point at which this decompensation occurs depends primarily on three factors: the absolute volume of pericardial fluid, the rate of accumulation of pericardial fluid, and the compliance of the pericardium. For trauma patients, rapid accumulation of pericardial blood, even in a relatively compliant space, may lead to precipitous deterioration. Conversely, for patients with collagen vascular disease or chronic infection, the slower accumulation may allow the compliant pericardium to expand to much larger volumes of fluid with fewer clinical symptoms.

In addition, the pressure-volume relationship of the pericardium demonstrates hysteresis; that is, removal of a given amount of fluid diminishes intrapericardial pressure more than its addition raised the pressure. The therapeutic effect of pericardiocentesis largely depends on this characteristic. Prompt removal of even small amounts of fluid may dramatically lessen intrapericardial pressure and restore cardiac output to an acceptable range.

Accumulation of pericardial fluid will alter the clinician's findings on physical examination and detailed cardiac evaluation. On auscultation, changes may be as subtle as minimal reduction of the amplitude and tone of the heart sounds (muffling). With a subacute effusion, auscultation may reveal a pericardial friction rub resulting from movement of the heart within the inflamed fluid and sac, which can also translate to reduced voltages on the cardiac monitor and electrocardiogram (ECG) leads. As the fluid volume increases, findings begin to reflect the impact of reduced cardiac filling with reduced stroke volume and compensatory tachycardia, narrowing of the pulse pressure, pulsus paradoxus, and ultimately decreased cardiac output and poor perfusion. With trauma patients, these physiologic changes may occur in minutes to hours. In less acute scenarios, they may occur over hours to days. Beck's triad (distant heart sounds, distended neck veins, and hypotension) is the classic sign of cardiac tamponade; however, these findings are both late and inconsistent indicators of tamponade. Although 90% of patients with tamponade will display at least one characteristic of the triad, fewer than one third of patients exhibit the full triad on diagnosis.

▶ INDICATIONS

The only emergent indication for pericardiocentesis is the development of cardiac tamponade that is endangering the patient's life. A less urgent indication is to obtain pericardial fluid for diagnostic testing (especially culture) in patients who have effusion but are not in tamponade.

Pericardial effusions leading to cardiac tamponade are commonly divided into two categories: traumatic and atraumatic. This classification scheme emphasizes the importance of traumatic tamponade as a rapidly developing condition that often poses an immediate threat to the patient's life. Traumatic tamponade commonly is the result of direct penetration of the pericardium, such as by a knife blade. This results in the rapid accumulation of blood in the pericardial space and the sudden onset of cardiac decompensation. Less commonly, traumatic tamponade may develop as the result of blunt trauma, such as that produced by a vehicular crash. The patient suffers injuries caused by rapid acceleration/deceleration when the chest impacts against a hard surface (e.g., steering wheel, handle bars, solid ground). Whatever the cause, prompt attention to the characteristic signs and symptoms of traumatic tamponade is imperative for successful management.

Causes of atraumatic pericardial effusions are numerous and varied, and a complete discussion is beyond the scope of this chapter. Neoplasm, infection, connective tissue disease, drugs, and metabolic disorders are the most common causes. Of particular interest in the pediatric population is purulent pericarditis, an inflammation of the pericardium secondary to pyogenic bacteria (most commonly *Staphylococcus aureus*). Purulent pericarditis primarily affects younger children, with about one third of patients being under 6 years of age.

Atraumatic tamponade occurs less frequently than traumatic tamponade and tends to be less acute. This is primarily the result of the slower rate of accumulation of atraumatic effusions, which allows the pericardium to compensate for the increased volume with a less dramatic increase in pressure. This slower rate of accumulation has clinical implications for the emergency physician. Most patients with atraumatic effusions who are not rapidly deteriorating can be managed without emergent ED drainage or at least can undergo pericardiocentesis in a more controlled fashion than those with traumatic tamponade.

It must be emphasized, however, that any patient with evidence of hemodynamic instability secondary to tamponade, whatever the etiology, should undergo prompt drainage of the pericardial space. Contraindications to pericardiocentesis in the unstable patient are few. Perhaps the most reasonable contraindication is the availability of a better form of therapy (e.g., immediate pericardial window or thoracotomy for the unstable trauma patient). If immediate therapeutic alternatives are lacking, however, no absolute contraindications to pericardiocentesis exist. An important consideration in patients with pericardial effusion or tamponade is whether they have problems with coagulation, which could make hemorrhage more likely with pericardiocentesis if the hemostatic disorder is not corrected.

Although the diagnosis of life-threatening pericardial tamponade must often be made presumptively in the emergency setting, the rapid availability of bedside ultrasonography in the ED greatly enhances the physician's ability to accurately identify this process in a timely manner (see Chapter 133). When time and circumstances permit, use of this modality can clarify potentially uncertain presentations with an almost immediate and virtually definitive diagnosis. Absence of a pericardial effusion, even in the face of signs and symptoms that may be suggestive of possible pericardial tamponade, require the physician to search for a different underlying process that explains the patient's condition.

▶ EQUIPMENT

The necessary equipment for this procedure is listed in Table 71.1. The needle system can be a standard over-the-needle catheter, although with more chronic effusions, it may

TABLE 71.1	EQUIPMENT	
All children	**Infants/young children**	**Older children**
Sterile drapes	20-gauge spinal needle	1.5-inch 16- to 18-gauge over-the-needle catheter
Betadine solution	1.5-inch, 18- to 20-gauge over-the-needle catheter	50-mL syringe
Local anesthetic	1.5-inch 16- to 18-gauge over-the-needle catheter	
3 syringes (10, 20, 50 mL)		
3-way stopcock		
Alligator clip		
Flexible guidewire		
Scalpel blade		
22-gauge needle		
ECG monitor		

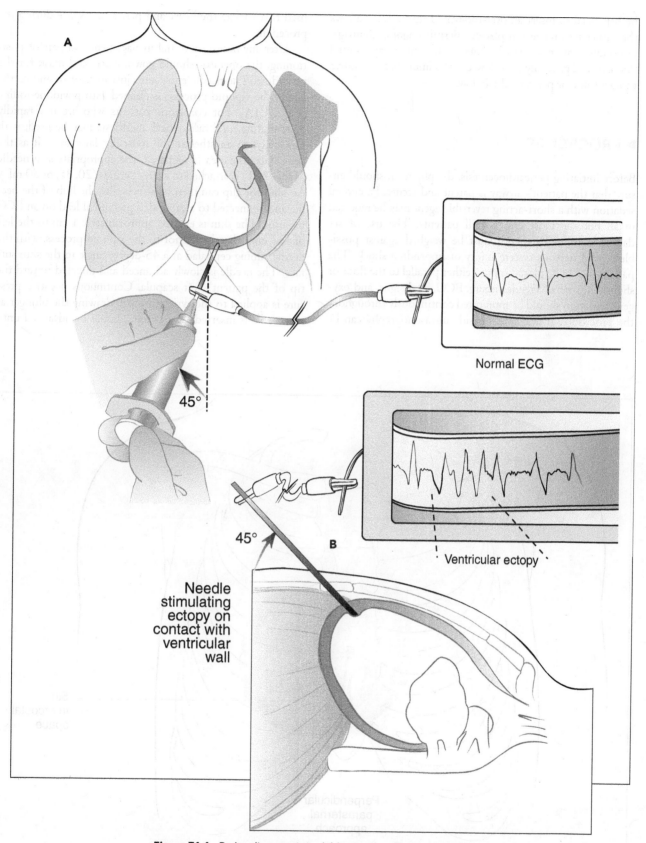

A

45°

Normal ECG

Ventricular ectopy

45°

B

Needle
stimulating
ectopy on
contact with
ventricular
wall

Figure 71.1 Pericardiocentesis in child using the substernal approach.

be beneficial to insert an over-the-wire catheter. This allows the catheter to remain in place to permit ongoing drainage. For trauma patients, a needle alone is sufficient, because initial drainage will generally be followed by an immediate operative thoracotomy or pericardial window.

▶ PROCEDURE

Before initiating pericardiocentesis, the physician should ensure that the patient's airway is patent and secure. Parenteral sedation with a short-acting reversible agent may be required in all but the most critically ill patients. The use of sedation in injured patients must be weighed against possible central nervous system injury or impending shock. The patient should be placed supine, either parallel to the floor or slightly in reverse Trendelenburg. ECG, vital signs, and oxygen saturation should be monitored continuously throughout the procedure. If available, bedside ultrasonography can be used to visualize the heart and pericardial space during the procedure.

After any necessary initial management and patient positioning, the operator should gown, glove, and mask for the procedure. The needle entry site (just inferior to and to the left of the xiphoid process) is cleaned with povidone-iodine (Fig. 71.1A). For conscious patients who are not rapidly deteriorating, infiltrative local anesthesia may be used, with care taken to anesthetize the muscular layer as well as the skin. After the area is prepared, the appropriate size needle (Table 71.1) is attached to a large syringe (20, 35, or 50 mL). An alligator clip can then be attached to the hub of the needle and connected to a grounded precordial lead on an ECG monitor. The skin is entered approximately 1 cm to the left of and immediately inferior to the xiphoid process, with the needle aiming cephalad at a 45-degree angle to the skin surface. The needle is slowly advanced and directed toward the tip of the patient's left scapula. Continuous negative pressure is applied to the syringe by withdrawing the plunger as the needle is inserted. The needle should be advanced until

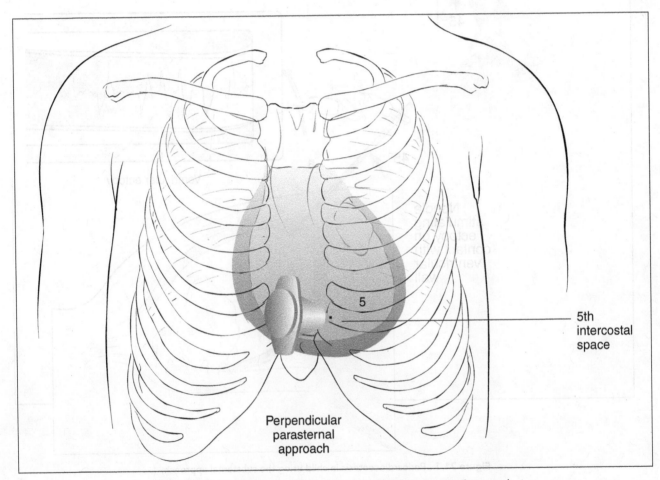

5

5th intercostal space

Perpendicular parasternal approach

Figure 71.2 Pericardiocentesis in adolescent using the parasternal approach.

pericardial fluid is obtained or ECG changes are observed. If fluid is obtained, the clinician should drain as much as possible, although, as mentioned previously, removal of even a relatively small amount of fluid will often reduce or eliminate the deleterious effects of cardiac tamponade. With atraumatic tamponade, the fluid obtained is typically clear or, in cases of bacterial infection, cloudy/purulent. With traumatic tamponade, blood obtained from the pericardial space is usually nonclotting and has a lower hematocrit than venous (ventricular) blood. In patients who will be managed nonoperatively, a catheter can be inserted into the pericardial space using a guidewire by the Seldinger technique (see Chapter 19). The catheter is then attached to a stopcock, which may be opened and aspirated if symptoms of tamponade recur.

Acute ECG abnormalities during attempted aspiration indicate contact with the ventricular wall, which should be avoided (Fig. 71.1B). These usually appear as ST-T wave changes, QRS widening, or premature ventricular beats with wide complexes. If ECG changes are encountered, the needle should be withdrawn until the original electrical pattern returns; then if no fluid has been obtained, the needle should be redirected slightly and reinserted. If ECG changes do not disappear, the needle should be completely withdrawn.

In some cases, the patient's clinical condition may preclude both ECG monitoring via the needle and the use of ultrasound guidance during the procedure. In these instances, pericardiocentesis is performed blindly using the landmarks outlined previously. An assistant should continuously observe the cardiac monitor so that any rhythm disturbance can be immediately identified. The best indicator of successful pericardiocentesis is rapid improvement in the patient's hemodynamic status after withdrawal of fluid or blood.

Adult studies using ultrasound guidance have advocated the parasternal approach as having a higher success rate and a lower complication rate. Using this approach, the needle is inserted perpendicular to the skin surface into the left fifth intercostal space (Fig. 71.2). Insertion should occur at a point just lateral to the sternum. This approach has not been validated in children, but its use can be considered for the older adolescent.

Following the procedure, the patient should be carefully monitored. An upright chest radiograph should be obtained to rule out a pneumothorax and to assess heart size. Finally, arrangements should be made for transfer to a unit or facility that is appropriately equipped to provide ongoing intensive care.

▶ COMPLICATIONS

Pericardiocentesis is associated with significant risks, and complication rates as high as 15% have been reported. Known complications include dysrhythmias, puncture of the ventricle, hemopericardium, and pneumothorax. Almost any vascular structure in the thorax (including coronary arteries and the inferior vena cava) may be punctured or lacerated. In addition, the esophagus, diaphragm, and peritoneal cavity may be penetrated. Delayed complications include pericardial leak, cutaneous fistula formation, and local infection. Use of bedside ultrasonography to visualize the heart and pericardial space is likely the most effective means of reducing the incidence of such complications when pericardiocentesis is performed in the ED (see Chapter 133). When an ultrasound device is available and the patient's condition permits, routine use of this modality is strongly encouraged.

 SUMMARY

1 Assess the patient—airway, breathing, circulation.

2 Recognize the presence of cardiac tamponade:

   a Check for Beck's triad: distant heart sounds, increased jugular venous distention, hypotension.

   b Suspect in an appropriate clinical setting in the absence of Beck's triad.

3 Position the patient in reverse Trendelenburg to maximize the chance of success.

4 Select the appropriate sizes of equipment for the patient's age; consider using a catheter-over-wire system if chronic effusion is present in order to allow continued drainage.

5 Attach the needle to a grounded ECG lead (if time allows) using the chest lead.

6 Insert the needle at 45-degree angle 1 cm to left of the xiphoid process; consider using a parasternal approach in adolescents.

7 Advance the needle (with constant traction on the plunger) until fluid is obtained or ECG abnormalities (e.g., ST-T wave changes, QRS widening) are seen; if ECG changes occur, withdraw the needle until normal electrical activity resumes, and if no fluid has been obtained, redirect the needle and reinsert.

8 Assess patient response:

   a Pulses, blood pressure

   b Heart sounds

   c Jugular venous distention

9 After the procedure, transfer the patient to an appropriate unit or facility for appropriate intensive care monitoring or, in the case of a trauma patient, to an operating room for possible surgical intervention.

CLINICAL TIPS

▶ The only indication for emergent pericardiocentesis is cardiac tamponade, which is characterized by distant heart sounds, increased jugular venous distension, and hypotension.

▶ Airway control should be ensured before this procedure is performed.

▶ The optimal patient position is slight reverse Trendelenburg.

▶ Bedside cardiac ultrasound can be used to confirm the diagnosis of cardiac tamponade. Using ultrasound during the procedure will increase the likelihood of success and minimize complications.

▶ The needle should be aimed 45 degrees from perpendicular 1 cm left of the xiphoid process and advanced toward the left scapula.

▶ As the needle is advanced, the ECG should be observed for premature ventricular beats, ST-T wave changes, or QRS widening. Such changes indicate contact with the ventricular wall, which should be avoided.

▶ SUMMARY

Pericardiocentesis is an infrequently performed but potentially life-saving procedure. Although not technically difficult, its high complication rate dictates that it be performed by skilled personnel and only when clearly indicated. When available, bedside ultrasonography can be highly useful for both making the diagnosis of pericardial tamponade and facilitating pericardiocentesis.

▶ SUGGESTED READINGS

American College of Surgeons. *Advanced Trauma Life Support Course for Physicians: Student Manual.* Chicago: American College of Surgeons; 1993: 139–140.

Callaham ML. Pericardiocentesis. In: Roberts JR, Hedges JR, eds. *Clinical Procedures in Emergency Medicine.* 2nd ed. Philadelphia: WB Saunders; 1991:210–228.

Krikorian JG, Hancock EW. Pericardiocentesis. *Am J Med.* 1978;65:808–814.

Lindenberger M, Kjellberg M, Karlsson E, et al. Pericardiocentesis guided by 2-D echocardiography: the method of choice for treatment of pericardial effusion. *J Intern Med.* 2003;253:411–417.

Morgan CD, Marshall SA, Ross JR. Catheter drainage of the pericardium: its safety and efficacy. *Can J Surg.* 1989;32:331–334.

Noren GR, Staley NA, Kaplan EL. Nonrheumatic inflammatory diseases. In: Adams FH, Emmanoulides GC, Riemenschneider TA, eds. *Heart Disease in Infants, Children and Adolescents.* 4th ed. Baltimore: Williams & Wilkins; 1989:740–746.

Pories W, Goudiani A. Cardiac tamponade. *Surg Clin North Am.* 1975;55: 573.

Ruddy R, ed. Pericardiocentesis. In: Fleisher GR, Ludwig S, Henretig FM, eds. *Textbook of Pediatric Emergency Medicine.* 5th ed. Baltimore: Lippincott Williams & Wilkins; 2005:1908–1909.

Shoemaker W, Carey S, Yao S. Hemodynamic monitoring for physiologic evaluation, diagnosis and therapy of acute hemopericardial tamponade from penetrating wounds. *J Trauma.* 1973;13:36.

Spodick DH. Acute cardiac tamponade. *N Engl J Med.* 2003;349:684–690.

Wong B, Murphy J, Chang CJ, et al. The risk of pericardiocentesis. *Am J Cardiol.* 1979;44:1110–1114.

72

SUSAN B. TORREY AND RICHARD A. SALADINO

Arterial Puncture and Catheterization

▶ INTRODUCTION

Arterial blood sampling is necessary in the evaluation and management of many seriously ill or injured children (1,2). Precise measurements of pH, Po_2, and Pco_2 are important adjuncts in assessing respiratory and acid-base status. Although advances in noninvasive technology have reduced the need for arterial sampling, arterial blood may be required to clarify an abnormal pulse oximetry reading, and arterial access may be the most reliable source of blood in patients with difficult venous access. Arterial puncture is used for limited sampling and is a routine part of emergency medical care for pediatric patients.

Repeated access to arterial blood is best accomplished by catheterization of an artery. Indwelling catheters have long been used for hemodynamic monitoring in critically ill patients in the intensive care unit (ICU) (2–4). Arterial catheter placement is also important for monitoring the unstable ill or injured child in the emergency department (ED) (1). The most common indications for arterial catheterization are continuous blood pressure monitoring and repeated sampling of blood. Although noninvasive techniques for the continuous monitoring of arterial blood pressure are being developed, none are yet routinely available for use in infants and children (5). Data from both the pediatric ICU and ED show that arterial catheterization is a useful and appropriate procedure for children and that complications are few (1–4).

Arterial puncture is of moderate technical complexity. Nurses and respiratory therapists have been trained to perform this procedure in many institutions; however, it is more difficult to perform in infants and smaller children. Arterial catheterization in children is technically complex and should be performed by health care providers specifically trained in the technique, usually physicians. Both arterial puncture and catheterization can be performed in children of all ages as indicated by their clinical condition.

▶ ANATOMY

Radial Artery

The radial artery is the most frequently used artery for both puncture and cannulation. Collateral circulation in the wrist and hand is provided by the superficial and deep palmar arches (6). The superficial palmar arch is formed by the superficial branch of the radial artery, which communicates with the terminal aspect of the ulnar artery. The deep palmar arch is likewise a communication of the deep branches of the radial and ulnar arteries.

The strongest radial artery impulse is felt at its most superficial course on the volar aspect of the wrist (Fig. 72.1), that is, lateral to the flexor carpi radialis tendon and median nerve and medial to the superficial radial nerve and lateral radius, just before the artery descends under the extensor pollicis brevis and abductor pollicis longus tendons to the anatomical snuffbox area. This usually corresponds to a site just lateral to the flexor carpi radialis tendon at the second skin crease proximal to the hand.

Femoral Artery

The femoral artery is a common site for arterial access in children. The femoral artery courses though the anterior thigh as a continuation of the iliac artery into the inguinal region after passing under the inguinal ligament (6). In particular, its most superficial and easily palpated course lies in the femoral triangle, bounded above by the inguinal ligament, laterally by the sartorius muscle, and medially by the adductor longus muscle. This site is most easily located as the midpoint

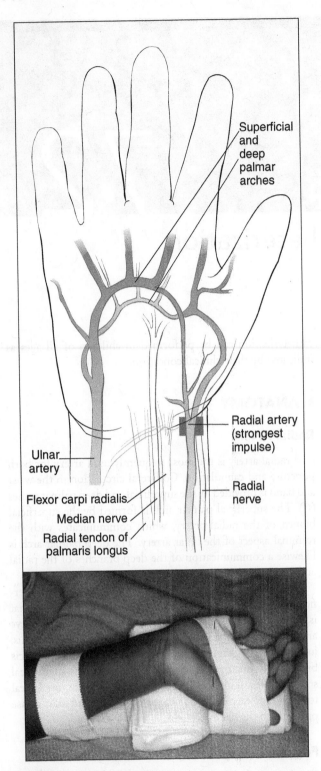

Figure 72.1 Radial artery anatomy.

(labels in figure)
Superficial and deep palmar arches

Ulnar artery

Flexor carpi radialis

Median nerve

Radial tendon of palmaris longus

Radial artery (strongest impulse)

Radial nerve

Posterior Tibial and Dorsalis Pedis Arteries

The posterior tibial artery courses the posterior aspect of the leg as the posterior branch of the popliteal artery, terminating in the plantar arteries and arch (6). Its most superficial and accessible site is a point between the medial malleolus and the calcanean (Achilles) tendon (Fig. 72.3).

The dorsalis pedis artery is a direct continuation of the anterior tibial artery, which passes down the dorsum of the foot to the proximal end of the first intermetatarsal space (6). Cannulation of the dorsalis pedis artery should be done at the dorsal midfoot, where the artery is most easily palpated; this is medial to the extensor hallucis longus and the extensor digitorum longus of the second toe (Fig. 72.4).

Axillary Artery

The subclavian artery becomes the axillary artery at the lateral border of the first rib, which in turn becomes the brachial artery at the tendon of the teres major muscle (6). It is important to locate the most superficial course of the axillary artery so as to avoid trauma to the terminal branch nerves of the brachial plexus. With the patient supine, the arm is positioned in 90-degrees abduction with the dorsum of the hand on the examination table, preferably near the ipsilateral ear or under the occiput. The axillary arterial pulse is palpated high in the axilla medial to the pectoralis major muscle insertion.

More data are available in the medical literature regarding cannulation of the axillary vein (7–9) than the axillary artery. The safety of axillary arterial catheterization has been documented in neonates and children (10–12); however, catheterization at this site is rarely indicated.

Brachial Artery

The brachial artery can be easily palpated in the antecubital fossa, where it lies atop the brachialis muscle (6). The median nerve is located along the medial side of the artery. Because there is little collateral circulation in this area, the brachial artery should not be routinely used for puncture or cannulation.

Umbilical Artery

Catheterization of the umbilical vessels in the neonate is useful and possible for hours to days after delivery. A detailed discussion of this procedure is provided in Chapter 38.

Temporal Artery

The superficial temporal artery, a terminal branch of the external carotid artery, ascends through the parotid gland, crosses the zygomatic arch, and terminates in the frontal and parietal branches (6). The course of either branch is easily palpated. The temporal artery may be a useful site for cannulation in

between the anterior superior iliac spine and the symphysis pubis (Fig. 72.2). Importantly, the operator should keep in mind the close proximity of the femoral nerve (lateral to the artery) and the femoral vein (medial to the artery). In addition, the femoral head lies posterior to the femoral triangle and can be potentially traumatized during femoral artery puncture.

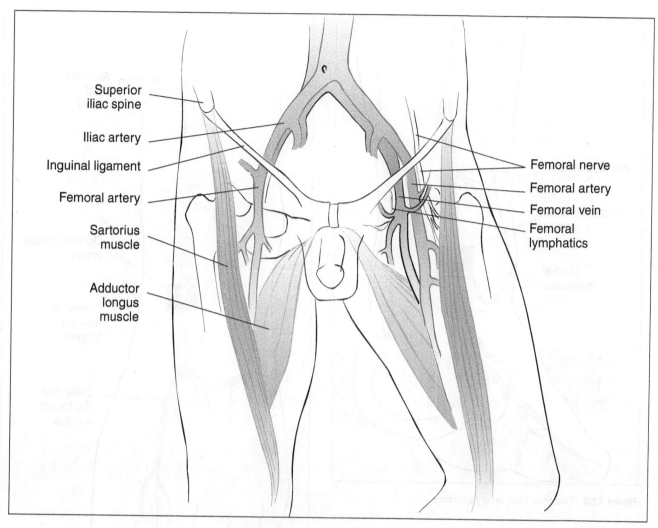

Figure 72.2 Femoral artery anatomy.

neonates once an umbilical artery catheter has been discontinued (3,13).

▶ INDICATIONS

Analysis of pH, PO_2, and PCO_2 is often needed for patients with severe respiratory compromise. Although pulse oximetry (SaO_2) and capnography have become important tools in the assessment of oxygenation and ventilation, arterial samples are often necessary to clarify abnormal readings or when the noninvasive technology is not available. Finally, many conditions require an accurate assessment of acid-base status for optimal management, including diabetic ketoacidosis, shock, dehydration, metabolic diseases, and certain drug and poison ingestions.

The most common indications for arterial catheterization are continuous blood pressure monitoring and serial blood sampling (1–3,14). Repeated arterial puncture may injure a vessel, resulting in thrombosis, infection, or an arteriovenous fistula. Serial blood pH and gas tension analysis are easily performed after arterial cannulation. Repeated blood samples can also be obtained for other indications from an indwelling arterial catheter.

Puncture or cannulation of an artery is contraindicated if compromise of arterial circulation will result. These situations are unusual but must be considered. Examples include anatomic variants and patients with artificial arteriovenous shunts. Care must be taken when performing these procedures on anticoagulated patients or those with a bleeding diathesis.

▶ EQUIPMENT

Arterial puncture can be performed with a minimum of equipment, although prepackaged kits are available that include a needle and heparinized syringe. A 25-gauge needle should be used in the newborn, whereas a 23-gauge needle is appropriate for older infants and small children. The procedure is most easily performed with a 1-inch butterfly needle. A heparinized syringe must then be prepared by aspirating 1 mL heparinized saline (1,000 units/mL) into a syringe, coating

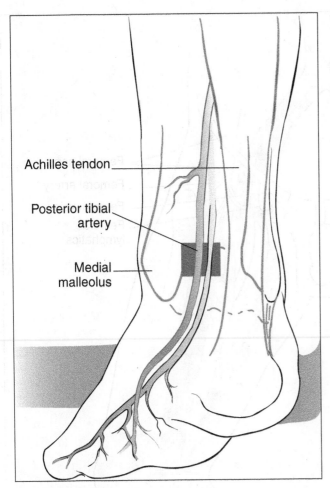

Figure 72.3 Posterior tibial artery anatomy.

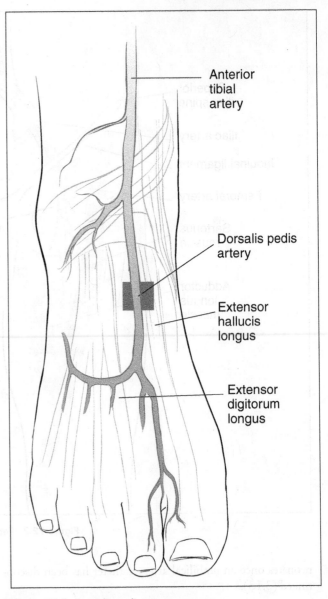

Figure 72.4 Dorsalis pedis artery anatomy.

the barrel with the solution, and then expelling it. If too much heparin remains, the measured P_{CO_2} may be falsely low (15).

The equipment required for percutaneous arterial cannulation includes supplies to ensure aseptic technique and catheters of appropriate size and length for the age and size of the patient (Table 72.1). Equipment also is required for maintenance of the indwelling catheter and for measurement

TABLE 72.1	ARTERIAL CATHETER SIZES BY SITE AND BODYWEIGHT					
	Infants <10 kg		10–40 kg		>40 kg	
Site*	Catheter size	French size†	Catheter size	French size	Catheter size	French size
RA, PTA, DPA, TA	Angiocath 24/22g		Angiocath 22g		Angiocath 22/20g	
Femoral artery, axillary artery	Angiocath 20/18g	3.0/4.0	Angiocath 18/16g	4.0/5.0	Angiocath 18/16/14g	5.0/5.5/6.0
Umbilical artery		Umbilical catheter 3.5/5.0				

*RA, radial artery; PTA, posterior tibial artery; DPA, dorsalis pedis artery; TA, temporal artery.
†Single-lumen central catheters are manufactured in standard French sizes, and lengths: 3.0 French (5 or 8 cm); 4.0 French (12 cm); 5.0 French (15, 20, or 25 cm); 5.5 French (5 cm with introducer); 6.0 French (15, 20, or 25 cm). The diameter of wires used for over-a-wire catheter technique correspond to the inner diameter of the catheter used: 3.0 French: 0.018 inches; 4.0 French: 0.021 inches; 5.0 French: 0.035 inches; 6.0 French: 0.035 inches.

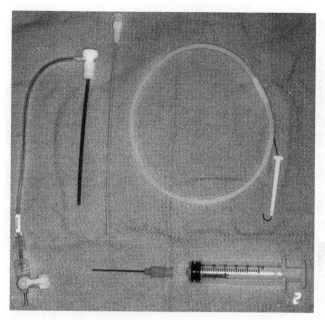

Figure 72.5 Catheterization tray equipment for arterial line placement by the Seldinger technique.

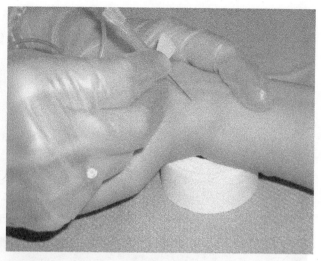

Figure 72.6 Technique and positioning for arterial puncture with a butterfly needle.

of blood pressure. Prepackaged kits are available that include the equipment necessary for performing arterial catheterization by the catheter-over-a-wire technique (e.g., Cook Critical Care, Bloomington, IN; Arrow International, Reading, PA) (Fig. 72.5).

▶ PROCEDURE

Site Selection and Preparation

Radial Artery

The radial artery is the most frequently used artery for both arterial puncture and cannulation (1–3). It is convenient both for performing the procedure and for maintaining an indwelling line. In children, it is often helpful to stabilize the hand and wrist on an arm board, placing the wrist in approximately 30 to 45 degrees extension over several gauze pads (Fig. 72.6).

Importantly, if the radial artery is selected for puncture or catheterization, adequacy of the palmar arterial arch should be assessed. Collateral flow has been shown to be adequate in approximately 93% to 98% of patients tested (16,17). In 1929, Allen described a method for diagnosis of occlusion of the radial or ulnar artery distal to the wrist (18) that can, with slight modification, be performed even in young or uncooperative patients. The Allen test is used to assess collateral flow in the hand; in particular, the Allen test will indicate adequacy of ulnar collateral flow such that the radial artery can safely be punctured or cannulated (Fig. 72.7). First, the patient clenches the fist to exsanguinate the hand. Firm digital pressure (17) is then used to occlude both the radial and

ulnar arteries at the pulse over the wrist. Of note, failure to accurately and completely occlude arterial flow at each artery leads to unreliable results with the Allen test (19). The hand is opened without hyperextending the fingers (20), and the occlusion of the ulnar artery is released. The open hand is observed for return of perfusion (rubor) (Fig. 72.6B). The Allen test is normal if pallor resolves and rubor returns within 5 seconds, indicating adequate collateral flow. The Allen test is considered abnormal if pallor persists beyond 5 seconds, indicating inadequate palmar arch collateral circulation, and radial arterial puncture should not be performed at that site. Finally, the test should be repeated, this time with release of digital pressure over the radial artery to assess radial arterial flow and thereby ensure that the radial artery pulsation is not due solely to ulnar flow (21). In the young, uncooperative, or unconscious patient, occlusion of the arteries is preceded by manual exsanguination, either by having an assistant "milk" a manually clenched hand or by using an elastic bandage wrapped around the hand. Distal arterial flow may also be assessed using a pulse oximeter on the thumb or finger, although this modification may not be reliable (22–26). The Allen test, or a modification thereof, should be performed and documented in the medical record before radial arterial puncture or catheterization is attempted.

Femoral Artery

Cannulation of the femoral artery is technically straightforward and is frequently chosen in unstable patients (1,2). The routine use of this artery is discouraged because of the possibility of traumatizing the head of the femur. The catheter-over-a-wire technique is primarily used owing to the relatively deeper location of the femoral vascular bundle.

In children, optimal positioning is achieved by externally rotating the leg at the hip and comfortably flexing the leg at the knee before femoral site preparation (Fig. 72.8). With appropriate sterile preparation and placement technique, along

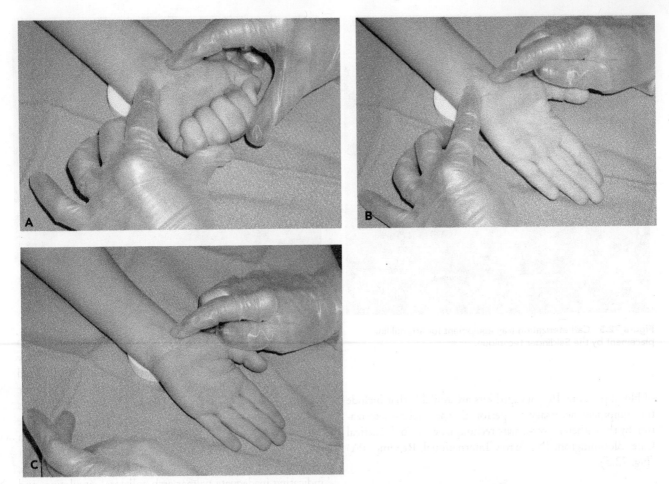

Figure 72.7 Demonstration of the Allen test for ulnar arterial collateral flow.

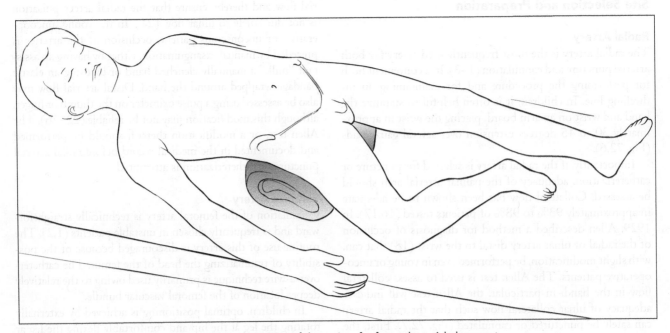

Figure 72.8 Positioning of the patient for femoral arterial placement.

with proper nursing care, the potential duration in situ and complication rates of femoral vessel cannulation are no different than those for cannulation at any other site.

Posterior Tibial and Dorsalis Pedis Arteries

The dorsalis pedis and posterior tibial arteries are suitable for cannulation, but they are easier to use for puncture. Cannulation of the posterior tibial artery is facilitated by holding the foot in comfortable dorsiflexion. Cannulation of the dorsalis pedis artery is best performed with the foot in mild plantar flexion.

Axillary Artery

Axillary artery cannulation is rarely indicated for pediatric patients. This site is technically difficult to access and should only be attempted in the ED when all other options prove unsuccessful. The catheter-over-a-wire technique is the preferred method for cannulation of the axillary vessels.

Brachial Artery

The brachial artery should only be used for puncture when other sites are unavailable and should not be used for cannulation.

Temporal Artery

Temporal artery cannulation is indicated in the young infant only when attempts at sites that are technically less difficult and easier to secure have failed.

Arterial Puncture

This procedure begins with identifying the optimal site for puncturing the artery, which can be accomplished by palpating the pulse of the artery at two points along its most superficial course. The depth and orientation of the vessel will determine

the best angle and direction for puncture. Transillumination of the extremity may also help to define the course of the artery (27,28). In addition, bedside ultrasound has been used to locate the femoral artery and to facilitate puncture or cannulation (29,30).

Once a site is chosen, the most superficial course of the artery is identified by palpation using the operator's nondominant hand. The patient's skin is cleansed with alcohol or other antiseptic solution. A small amount of 1% lidocaine without epinephrine can be injected to provide local anesthesia using a 27- or 30-gauge needle. A small intradermal wheal is created at the puncture site, with care taken not to obscure the pulse proximally. The arterial pulse is palpated continuously just proximal to the puncture site. Using an uncapped butterfly needle or a prepackaged syringe, the needle is inserted at an angle 30 to 45 degrees from the horizontal and aimed toward the pulse (Fig. 72.7). The needle is advanced slowly until arterial blood flows into the butterfly tubing. At this point, the heparinized syringe is attached to the tubing, and the appropriate volume of blood is aspirated. If a prepackaged syringe is used, blood will passively flow into the syringe once the needle has punctured the artery. The needle is withdrawn once the desired amount of blood is obtained. After the needle is withdrawn, manual pressure must be applied to the puncture site for a full 5 minutes to prevent leakage from the puncture site and subsequent hematoma formation.

Peripheral Arterial Catheterization

Once the site for arterial catheterization has been selected, the skin should be thoroughly cleansed with an iodophor solution, a sterile field should be established, and meticulous aseptic technique should be maintained throughout the procedure. The over-a-needle catheter is inserted at a 30- to 45-degree angle relative to the skin (Fig. 72.9A), entering the artery as described for puncture. Bright red blood should appear in

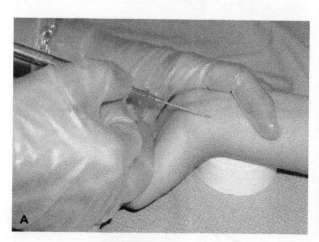
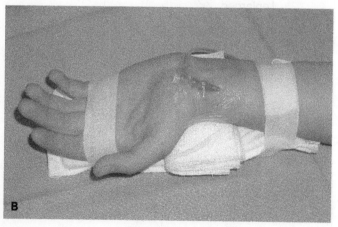

Figure 72.9
A. Catheter-over-a-needle arterial line placement.
B. The catheter is secured by silk sutures. A transparent sterile dressing should then be applied over the site.

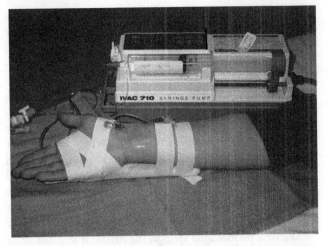

Figure 72.10 Flushing of the arterial catheter with a pump system.

the transparent flash chamber of the catheter. It is helpful to lower the angle of the catheter somewhat and advance it slightly to ensure that the catheter itself enters the lumen of the vessel. The catheter is then advanced over the stabilized needle. Pulsatile blood will appear through the hub of the catheter as the needle is withdrawn. If blood does not appear, it may be that puncture of the back wall of the vessel has occurred. In this case, the catheter should be withdrawn slowly until pulsatile flow is noted, and the catheter is then advanced into the lumen. This is in fact an alternate method of catheterization: the operator may puncture both walls of the artery, withdraw the needle, slowly withdraw the catheter, and then advance it into the lumen when pulsatile flow is detected in the hub of the catheter.

The catheter is secured using nylon or silk (4.0 or 5.0) suture material. Sutures are placed in the skin, tied, and then

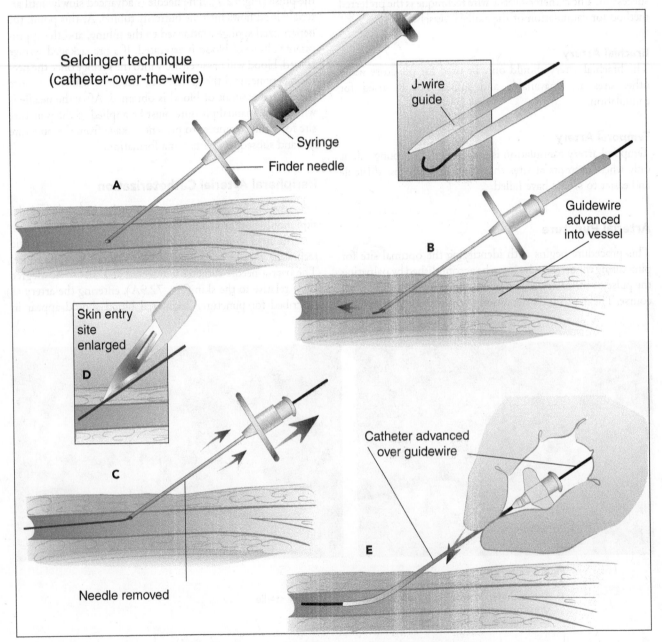

Figure 72.11 Arterial line placement using the Seldinger technique.

looped around the suture ring of the hub of the catheter or through the fenestrations in the wing clips of the catheter (Fig. 72.9B). Antibiotic ointment may be applied to the catheter entry site, over which a transparent sterile dressing (e.g., OpSite, Smith and Nephew; Tegaderm, 3M Health Care) is placed. The catheter hub and extension tubing are further secured with tape.

The catheter is attached to tubing appropriate for pressure transduction if arterial access is to be used for continuous blood pressure monitoring. A three-way stopcock is attached to the tubing proximal to the patient whereas the pressure transducer is located distally. Blood sampling is possible from this stopcock system. Care must be taken to draw adequate waste blood before the sample and to avoid air embolism

(31). Continuous flushing (2 to 4 mL/hr) of the arterial catheter with heparinized saline (2 units/mL) to prevent clotting is accomplished via a pump system distal to the transducer (Fig. 72.10).

Catheter-over-a-Wire Technique

An alternative method of arterial catheterization uses the Seldinger technique of introducing a catheter over a guidewire (Fig. 72.11) (32). This procedure is discussed in detail

CLINICAL TIPS

Arterial Puncture

▶ Site selection is a key aspect of this procedure. Knowledge of the anatomy is therefore crucial. The most commonly used sites in the child include the radial, femoral, and posterior tibial arteries.

▶ Failure to detect a pulse may be due to low blood pressure, occlusion of an artery from excessive pressure by the assistant, or ill-timed inflation of a blood pressure cuff.

▶ An Allen test for ulnar collateral flow should be performed and documented if the radial artery is to be used for puncture or catheterization.

▶ Local infiltration of lidocaine may enhance patient cooperation and increase the likelihood of success with arterial puncture or catheterization.

▶ After arterial puncture, direct pressure should be applied over the site for a full 5 minutes.

Arterial Catheterization

▶ Once a flash of blood appears in the transparent chamber, the angle of the needle/catheter to the skin should be lowered, and the needle/catheter should be advanced 1 to 2 mm to ensure that the catheter is in the lumen of the artery.

▶ As the catheter is advanced into the artery, the needle should not be withdrawn. The needle should remain stationery until the catheter hub reaches the skin.

▶ Failure to observe pulsatile blood flow from the catheter may indicate that the back wall of the artery has been punctured. When this occurs, the catheter should be slowly withdrawn and, if a flash of blood is seen, advanced again into the artery.

▶ The catheter should be secured with a transparent dressing so that a "window" is available to observe any blanching of the skin around the site of the catheter.

SUMMARY

1 Assess the indications and contraindications for arterial puncture or catheterization.

2 Identify the optimal site for arterial access.

3 Establish a sterile field and maintain aseptic technique throughout the procedure.

4 Use a finger of nondominant hand to locate the most superficial (easily palpable) course of the artery.

5 Insert the needle at an angle 30 to 45 degrees from the horizontal; for catheterization, lower the angle slightly once flashback is observed, and advance the catheter into the lumen of the artery.

6 Advance the catheter over the needle; do not withdraw the needle until the hub of the catheter is at the skin.

7 For the catheter-over-a-wire technique:

  a Insert the needle until flashback is seen.

  b Insert the wire through the needle into the artery.

  c Remove the needle, controlling the wire at all times.

  d Thread the catheter over the wire into the artery.

  e Remove the wire.

8 Secure the catheter to the skin with nylon or silk suture material (4.0 or 5.0) and a sterile transparent dressing.

9 Connect the catheter to an appropriate extension or pressure tubing.

10 Use heparinized (2 units/mL) saline to prevent clotting of the catheter.

in Chapter 19. Briefly, an introducer needle attached to a non-Luer-Lok syringe is placed into the lumen of the selected artery, it is stabilized after aspiration of arterial blood into the syringe, and the syringe is then disconnected. A guidewire is inserted through the introducer needle into the lumen of the artery. The needle is then withdrawn over the guidewire, with care taken to control both the proximal and the distal ends of the wire. A catheter is then threaded over the guidewire into the artery (note that the distal end of the guidewire must be kept beyond the hub of the catheter). The guidewire is removed and the catheter is connected to the appropriate tubing.

▶ COMPLICATIONS

The most serious complication of arterial puncture is permanent damage to the artery, interrupting the arterial supply to the distal extremity. With selection of an appropriate puncture site and proper technique, this is an exceedingly rare occurrence. Arterial spasm may temporarily impede distal circulation, but this is generally self-limited and benign. Injury to the adjacent nerve or underlying bony structures may cause transient pain. As mentioned previously, injury to the developing femoral head can occur in children during cannulation or puncture of the femoral artery. Hematoma formation at the site also may be uncomfortable.

Complications during or after arterial catheterization include entry into a false lumen in the intima surrounding the vessel, puncture of the artery by the guidewire during its use, kinking or shearing of the catheter and air embolism, as well as arterial spasm, hematoma, or thrombus formation (1–4,32–34). Bedford demonstrated that thrombosis is inversely related to catheter diameter (35), so care must be taken in selecting the appropriate catheter size for the patient. Local skin necrosis or infection also may occur secondary to poor technique or arterial occlusion (3,4,35–37).

▶ SUMMARY

Arterial puncture and catheterization are important procedures in the care of critically ill or injured children. When performed properly, these procedures are safe, and the blood sampling and monitoring provided may be valuable adjuncts in the management of pediatric patients with respiratory and/or cardiovascular compromise.

▶ REFERENCES

1. Saladino R, Bachman D, Fleisher G. Arterial access in the pediatric emergency department. *Ann Emerg Med*. 1990;19:382–385.
2. Sellden H, Nilsson K, Larsson L, et al. Radial arterial catheters in children and neonates: a prospective study. *Crit Care Med*. 1987;15:1106–1109.
3. Randel SN, Tsang BHL, Wung JT, et al. Experience with percutaneous indwelling arterial catheterization in neonates. *Am J Dis Child*. 1987;141:848–851.
4. Smith-Wright DL, Green TP, Lock JE, et al. Complications of vascular catheterization in critically ill children. *Crit Care Med*. 1984;12:1015–1017.
5. Cua SL, Thomas K, Zurakowski D, et al. Comparison of the Vasotrac with invasive arterial blood pressure monitoring in children after pediatric cardiac surgery. *Anesth Analg*. 2005;100:1289–1294.
6. Clemente CD, ed. *Gray's Anatomy*. 30th ed. Philadelphia: Lippincott Williams & Wilkins; 1985.
7. Metz RI, Lucking SE, Chaten FC, et al. Percutaneous catheterization of the axillary vein in infants and children. *Pediatrics*. 1990;84:531–533.
8. Oriot D, Defawe G. Percutaneous catheterization of the axillary vein in neonates. *Crit Care Med*. 1988;16:285–286.
9. Martin C, Eon B, Auffray JP, et al. Axillary or internal jugular central venous catheterization. *Crit Care Med*. 1990;18:400–402.
10. Cantwell GP, Holzman BH, Caceres MJ. Percutaneous catheterization of the axillary artery in the pediatric patient. *Crit Care Med*. 1991;18:880–881.
11. Lawless S, Orr R. Axillary arterial monitoring of pediatric patients. *Pediatrics*. 1989;84:273–275.
12. Piotrowski A, Kawczynski P. Cannulation of the axillary artery in critically ill newborn infants. *Eur J Pediatr*. 1995;154:57–59.
13. Gauderer M, Holgerson LO. Peripheral arterial line insertion in neonates and infants: a simplified method of temporal artery cannulation. *J Pediatr Surg*. 1974;9:875–877.
14. Filston HC, Johnson DG. Percutaneous venous cannulation in neonates and infants: a method for catheter insertion without "cutdown." *Pediatrics*. 1971;48:896–901.
15. Roberts JR, Hedges JR, eds. *Clinical Procedures in Emergency Medicine*. 2nd ed. Philadelphia: WB Saunders; 1991:255–287.
16. Hosokawa K, Hata Y, Yano K, et al. Results of the Allen test on 2940 arms. *Ann Plast Surg*. 1990;24:149–151.
17. Gelberman RH, Blasingame JP. The timed Allen test. *J Trauma*. 1981;21:477–479.
18. Allen EV. Thromboangiitis obliterans: methods of diagnosis of chronic occlusive arterial lesions distal to the wrist with illustrative cases. *Am J Med Sci*. 1929;178:237–244.
19. Hirai M, Kawai S. False positive and negative results in Allen test. *J Cardiovasc Surg*. 1980;21:353–360.
20. Greenhow DE. Incorrect performance of Allen's test: ulnar artery flow erroneously presumed inadequate. *Anesthesiology*. 1972;37:356–357.
21. Meyer RM, Katele GV. The case for a complete Allen's test. *Anesth Analg*. 1983;62:947–948.
22. Rozenberg B, Rosenberg M, Birkhan J. Allen's test performed by pulse oximeter [letter]. *Anaesthesia*. 1988;43:515–516.
23. Duncan PW. An alternative to Allen's test [letter]. *Anaesthesia*. 1986;41:88.
24. Spittell JA Jr, Juergens JL, Fairbairn JF II. Radial artery puncture and the Allen test [letter]. *Ann Intern Med*. 1987;106:771–772.
25. Levinsohn DG, Gordon L, Sessler DI. The Allen test: analysis of four methods. *J Hand Surg*. 1991;16:279–292.
26. Fuhrman TM, Reilley TE, Pippin WD. Comparison of digital blood pressure, plethysmography, and the modified Allen's test as means of evaluating the collateral circulation to the hand. *Anaesthesia*. 1992;47:959–961.
27. Cole FS, Todres ID, Shannon DC. Percutaneous catheterization of the radial artery in the newborn infant. *J Pediatr*. 1978;92:105–107.
28. Kastogridakis YL, Seshadri R, Sullivan C, et al. Veinlite transillumination in the pediatric emergency department: a therapeutic interventional trial. Paper presented at the meeting of the Pediatric Academic Societies; May 15, 2005; Washington, D.C.

29. Kanter RK, Gorton JM, Palmieri K, et al. Anatomy of femoral vessels in infants and guidelines for venous catheterization. *Pediatrics.* 1989;83:1020–1022.

30. Yeow KM, Toh CH, Wu CH. et al. Sonographically guided antegrade common femoral artery access. *J Ultrasound Med.* 2002;21:1413–1416.

31. Chang C, Dughi J, Shitabata P, et al. Air embolism and the radial arterial line. *Crit Care Med.* 1988;16:141–143.

32. Seldinger SI. Catheter replacement of the needle in percutaneous angiography: a new technique. *Acta Radiol.* 1953;39:368.

33. Brown MM. Another complication of arterial cannulation. *Anaesthesia.* 1991;46:326.

34. Pettenazzo A, Gamba P, Salmistraro G, et al. Peripheral arterial occlusion in infants: a report of two cases treated conservatively. *J Vasc Surg.* 1991;14:220–224.

35. Bedford RF. Radial artery function following percutaneous cannulation with 18- and 20-gauge catheters. *Anesthesiology.* 1977;47:37–39.

36. Furfaro S, Gauthier M, Lacroix J, et al. Arterial catheter-related infections in children: a 1-year cohort analysis. *Am J Dis Child.* 1991;145:1037–1043.

37. Ducharme FM, Gauthier M, Lacroix J, et al. Incidence of infection related to arterial catheterization in children: a prospective study. *Crit Care Med.* 1988;16:272–276.

73

MANANDA S. BHENDE AND MIOARA D. MANOLE

Venipuncture and Peripheral Venous Access

▶ INTRODUCTION

Venipuncture and peripheral venous access remain two of the most common yet most challenging procedures in pediatric medical care. Many providers who do not treat infants and children on a regular basis are uncomfortable performing these procedures. Consequently, children, parents, and health care professionals alike may be anxious when obtaining blood or inserting an intravenous catheter becomes necessary.

Venipuncture, as the name implies, consists of puncturing a vein, and it continues to be the primary method of obtaining blood samples in children, usually preferred to finger stick, heel stick, and arterial puncture. Peripheral venous access provides a means of maintaining or replacing body stores of fluids or blood volume, restoring acid-base balance, and administering medications. These two procedures can be used for all pediatric age groups. They are commonly performed by many health care professionals in hospital and prehospital settings, offices, outpatient facilities, and, through the efforts of trained visiting nurses, in the patient's own home. If peripheral venous access is not easily obtained in emergent settings, alternative routes include central venous access (Chapter 19), intraosseous access (Chapter 21), and venous cutdown catheterization (Chapter 20). Peripheral venous access is a short-term, definitive procedure that can be used for 48 to 72 hours. After that time, access should be changed because of increased incidence of thrombophlebitis and infection. If long-term access is needed or hyperosmolar solutions must be administered, the patient will generally require central venous access.

▶ ANATOMY AND PHYSIOLOGY

Sites available for peripheral venous cannulation and venipuncture include multiple locations in the upper and lower extremities, the scalp, and the external jugular vein. The veins are larger and generally easier to locate in adults than in children. In states of intravenous depletion or shock or in the well-nourished toddler with chubby hands and feet, intravenous access can be difficult for even the most experienced personnel.

Upper Extremity

On the dorsum of the hand, the most commonly used veins are the tributaries of the cephalic and basilic veins and the dorsal venous arch (Fig. 73.1). The cephalic vein, which is located on the radial border of the forearm just proximal to the thumb, is predictable in its location. It is a large vein that is well secured to the fascia, making it unlikely to move or "roll" during venipuncture or venous cannulation. In the forearm, the cephalic, basilic, and median cubital veins may be difficult to locate in a younger child because of subcutaneous fat. Veins on the volar side of the wrist, if visible, can also be cannulated. It is important to avoid puncturing the radial or ulnar arteries or nerves that lie in close proximity to these vessels. The axillary vein is a continuation of the basilic vein and should be used with caution for peripheral venous cannulation.

Lower Extremity

The saphenous vein, which is situated about 1 cm above and in front of the medial malleolus, is a good choice for cannulation (Fig. 73.2). It is large and well secured by fascia, which prevents it from rolling when cannulation is attempted. Because of its reliably predictable location, it is one of the few veins appropriate for attempting access by location alone (i.e., a "blind stick"). The median marginal veins and the veins of the dorsal arch of the foot also may be accessed. The anterior and posterior tibial veins form the popliteal vein, which continues

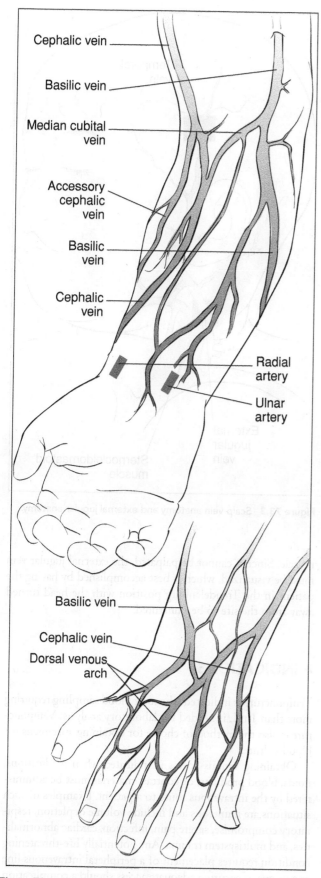

Figure 73.1 Veins of the upper extremity.

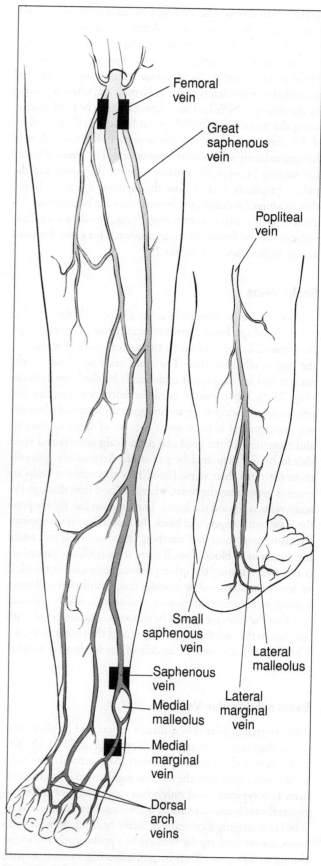

Figure 73.2 Veins of the lower extremity.

as the femoral vein. The long saphenous vein drains into the femoral vein. When the patient is critically ill and peripheral venipuncture proves impossible, the femoral vein, which is a site for central catheterization, may be used for venipuncture. In the femoral triangle, the anatomic relationship from lateral to medial is nerve, artery, vein, and lymphatic, often expressed by the acronym NAVL. This relationship can be remembered using the mnemonic "NAVL towards the navel." Therefore, if the clinician can palpate the arterial pulsations, the vein lies immediately medial to the pulsations. The femoral artery lies midway between the anterior superior iliac spine and the pubic symphysis 1 cm below the inguinal ligament. Using this anatomic landmark, the femoral vein can be punctured in cases when the artery is not palpable (e.g., hypotension). Cannulation of the femoral vein, an approach for central venous access, is described in Chapter 19.

Scalp Veins

Scalp veins are prominent in infants, especially those under 3 months of age. From a practical standpoint, scalp veins may be accessed in patients up to the age of about 9 months if the hair is relatively thin. The scalp veins are closer to the surface and are supported underneath by the bony cranium (Fig. 73.3). They can be used for both venipuncture and venous access. Scalp veins are not generally accessed when airway management is in progress because of space limitations and movement of the head and neck. Scalp arteries and veins should be differentiated by palpation. Arteries are generally more tortuous than veins. Blood flow through the scalp arteries is away from the heart, whereas blood flow through the scalp veins is toward the heart. The clinician can lightly press the vessel with fingers and block the blood flow at two points. Releasing one point and watching the vessel refill will reveal the direction of blood flow. If there is no refill, the procedure is repeated releasing the other pressure point on the vessel. If an artery is cannulated by mistake, fluid instillation will cause immediate blanching in the surrounding area, which will indicate that the catheter should be removed. The temporal veins anterior to the earlobe are the largest and the easiest to locate. The frontal vein down the middle of the forehead is another good choice.

External Jugular Vein

The external jugular vein is usually cannulated by physicians rather than nurses because of its location (Fig. 73.3). Despite its location in the neck and proximity to the central circulation via the subclavian vein, the external jugular vein is a peripheral vein. It is typically used only when cannulation of other peripheral sites is unsuccessful or when considerable time may be saved in managing a critically ill infant or child. As with scalp veins, the external jugular vein can be a problematic site to use during resuscitative efforts because accessing it interferes with airway management. It extends from the lower lobe of the ear to the medial clavicular head across the sternocleidomastoid

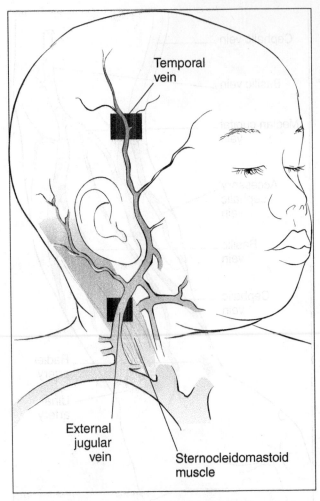

Figure 73.3 Scalp vein anatomy and external jugular anatomy.

muscle. Since it cannot be palpated, the external jugular vein must be visualized, which is best accomplished by having the patient in the Trendelenburg position with the head turned away from the site to be punctured.

▶ INDICATIONS

Venipuncture is indicated whenever blood sampling requiring more than 1 mL is needed for laboratory analysis. Venipuncture is also the method of choice for obtaining specimens for blood culture.

Obtaining venous access is indicated when medications, fluids, blood products, or contrast material must be administered by the intravenous route to a patient. Examples of such situations are numerous and include volume depletion, respiratory compromise, severe pain, infection, cardiac abnormalities, and multisystem trauma. Any potentially life-threatening condition requires placement of a peripheral intravenous line as a means of ensuring adequate access should a complication develop.

For pediatric resuscitations, peripheral venous access is the accepted mode to treat the patient. With adult resuscitations, central venous drug administration may provide more rapid onset of action and higher peak concentrations than peripheral venous administration (1). However, this has not been demonstrated in pediatric arrest models. In pediatric animal and human resuscitation, peripheral administration, central administration, and intraosseous administration result in comparable onset of drug action and peak drug levels, particularly if the drug is followed by a bolus of normal saline (2).

Absolute contraindications to venous cannulation are cutaneous infection overlying the vein chosen for cannulation, presence of phlebitis or thrombosis of the vein, poor perfusion, and marked edema of the extremity. Relative contraindications include burns overlying the venipuncture site and trauma of the extremity. In a patient with neck or upper chest trauma, the ipsilateral arm should not be used to place an intravenous line because the integrity of the proximal veins cannot be ensured. With a gunshot wound or massive trauma to the abdomen, intravenous lines should preferably be started in the upper extremities rather than the lower extremities for the same reason. Care must be also taken when starting intravenous lines in patients with coagulation defects or abnormal blood vessels.

▶ EQUIPMENT

It is important to have all the equipment ready and organized so that the clinician does not have to look for necessary items in the midst of the procedure. Mobile intravenous carts that have all the equipment stored in one place are a good solution (Table 73.1). These carts should be stocked at least daily.

TABLE 73.1	INTRAVENOUS CART EQUIPMENT LIST

Tourniquet or rubber bands (for scalp veins)
Povidone-iodine (Betadine) wipes or sticks
Alcohol wipes (70% alcohol)
Butterfly needles—different sizes 21, 23, 25 (large to small)
Over-the-needle catheters (intracaths, Angiocaths)—various sizes 14, 16, 18, 20, 22, 24, 26 (large to small)
Normal saline (nonbacteriostatic)
3- and 5-mL syringes
T-connectors
Tape—½-, 1-, and 2-inch (tapes cut and kept ready on the side)
2″ × 2″ sterile gauze packets
4″ × 4″ unsterile gauze
Transparent dressing (Tegaderm)
Padded arm boards (infant, pediatric, and adult size)
Razors
Betadine ointment
Gloves—sterile and nonsterile
Intravenous infusion microtubing setup
Vacutainers for blood samples for different studies
Plastic medicine cups cut lengthwise in half and sharp edges protected by tape to act as transparent covering for i.v. sites in infants and children in order to protect i.v.
Intravenous infusion pumps on stands

The top of the cart can be used as the area where equipment needed for the patient is placed. The cart should also have its own sharps disposal unit.

Tourniquets can be round or flat rubber tubing. They are applied proximal to the desired vein to produce temporary venostasis by occlusion. For scalp veins, a rubber band is used. A piece of tape is placed at some point on the rubber band with the two sticky sides together so that the rubber band can be removed using the tape as a "handle." This prevents the rubber band from snapping against the infant's head. Ten percent povidone-iodine (Betadine) prep pads or sticks, which are antiseptic and microbicidal, are first used to prepare the area. Then 70% alcohol pads can be used to clean off the Betadine, allowing visualization of the veins. Povidone-iodine is superior to alcohol as an antiseptic agent (3). In fact, using alcohol pads alone has been shown to be no better than using no antiseptic agent in terms of infectious complications.

Butterfly needles are fine metal cannulas also known as scalp needles. Needles and catheters are sized by their diameter using an inverse measurement known as "gauge"—the smaller the diameter, the larger the gauge. Butterfly needles were once synonymous with pediatric vascular access but now range in size from 25 gauge (smallest) to 19 gauge (largest). Butterflies are used for venipuncture, arterial puncture, and, very rarely, short-term vascular access. In children they are preferred over a needle attached to a syringe for venipuncture because it is easier to manipulate a butterfly into tiny veins and it offers better control while drawing the blood. Butterfly needles are not optimal for providing vascular access, as any movement can lead to vessel perforation by the sharp needle tip even after securing it in place.

Intravenous over-the-needle catheters are used most commonly for venous access. They are composed of thin-walled, semiflexible plastic tubing over a hollow needle. Once inside the vein, the plastic covering is threaded in the vein, and the needle is withdrawn and discarded. Over-the-needle catheters range in size from 26 to 14 gauge. Appropriate catheter sizes for pediatric patients are as follows: 22 and 24 gauge for infants; 20, 22, and 24 gauge for young children; 16 and 18 gauge for adolescents. For adolescents with multisystem trauma and/or severe shock, a 14-gauge catheter may be needed. Over-the-needle infusion catheters cause minimal endothelial irritation and therefore are the most popular choice for peripheral venous access. As mentioned previously, however, they are not indicated for long-term use. Attention to blood and body fluid precautions has led to the development of closed systems where blood stays within the capped tubing (4) as well as intravenous catheters that are retractable inside a plastic shield, plastic shields that slide over the needle, and self-sheathing angiocatheter needles (see also Chapter 8).

Padded armboards of different sizes should be available to immobilize an extremity as needed. Sterile gauze pads (2″ × 2″) are placed near the intravenous site, but around the taping area 4″ × 4″ clean (nonsterile) gauzes may be used. Sterile, transparent occlusive dressings (e.g., OpSite, Smith and

Nephew; Tegaderm, 3M Health Care), which allow visualization of the puncture site, can also be used to secure the catheter.

▶ PROCEDURE

Preparing the Patient

Verbal consent is usually sufficient before venipuncture or placement of a peripheral intravenous catheter. It is essential to prepare the patient and the parent for the procedure, which they may view as an ordeal. In an emergent situation (e.g., cardiac arrest or a seizing child), the clinician should not take time to explain all details of the procedure. A quick explanation that an intravenous line needs to be started to give medications is adequate. This can be explained by a staff member helping with the care of the patient (5).

When obtaining venous access is not emergent, it is important to discuss the reason for the procedure with the parents and patient in terms they understand. The clinician should explain that there will be a "pinch" when the needle and plastic catheter go into the vein but that the needle will be removed, leaving only the catheter in the vein to give fluids and medications. The child may understand better if told that it is like a straw through which "water and medicine" that will make the child better can be given. Because the pinch hurts, the child should be told that it is okay to cry but that it is important to remain as still as possible. If time allows, explaining with dolls or stuffed animals may also help. This is usually possible for elective procedures done outside the ED and occasionally in the urgent setting. While such measures do not lessen the pain of the procedure, taking time to allay fears will decrease the amount of emotional trauma experienced by the child.

Parents should be encouraged to remain in the room for the procedure if they so desire. They should be told that it is helpful for them to remain calm and supportive. Anxiety and agitation can be conveyed by the parents to the child, who may become even more apprehensive and fearful. The child should remain in a parent's arms for as long as possible while the clinician prepares for the procedure (see Chapters 1 and 3).

It is important to look carefully for potential intravenous access sites. While looking, the clinician should describe to the child what is happening and explain that the tourniquet will be used to choose the best site. Whenever possible, each aspect of the procedure should be explained as it takes place. Speaking in a calm and soothing manner at all times greatly assists in relaxing the child. Offering a choice about where the needle puncture will be performed (e.g., in the nondominant arm) increases a child's sense of control, but if offered, it should be honestly explained that fulfilling such a request cannot be guaranteed. The child should not be given food or a bottle to drink during the procedure to reduce the risk of choking. Parents should be informed that while the procedure will ideally require only one needlestick, success may require more than one attempt. Finally, praise and compliments should be

TABLE 73.2	PAIN RELIEF METHODS AND TIME OF ONSET
Method	**Onset**
EMLA	1 hr
ELA-Max	30 min
Lidocaine iontophoresis	10 min
Nitrous oxide	Immediate
Amethocaine	30–45 min

given after the procedure regardless of the child's behavior. Obviously, an extremely critical situation allows no time for such psychological preparation, but even in these cases, a kind manner and genuine expressions of concern will lessen the fear and anxiety of the children and their parents.

Methods of Pain Relief during Venous Cannulation

The pain of a needle is significant for a child. Adjuncts for decreasing this pain include eutectic mixture of local anesthetics cream (EMLA), lidocaine 4% cream (ELA-Max), amethocaine 4% gel (Ametop), nitrous oxide, and low-dose lidocaine iontophoresis (Table 73.2) (see also Chapters 34 and 35). Local anesthetic creams or gels are the most commonly used in the ED for children. It should be remembered, however, that if attempts at access are unsuccessful in the anesthetized area, another area that is not anesthetized may have to be used.

EMLA cream is absorbed through intact dermis and induces local anesthesia (6). The disadvantage in the ED setting is that it takes approximately 45 to 60 minutes for the skin to become anesthetized. It is primarily useful for elective procedures. In children with chronic conditions requiring frequent venipuncture or intravenous access (e.g., hemophilia, sickle cell disease), parents can administer it at home before coming to the office or ED. ELA-Max is as effective as EMLA in achieving pain reduction, with an onset of 30 minutes and potentially less local vasoconstriction (7). Ametop gel, most often used in Europe, provides adequate analgesia with an onset of 30 to 45 minutes (8). Lidocaine iontophoresis (transfer of lidocaine into the skin using low-level electrical current) provides effective topical anesthesia for venous cannulation in about 10 minutes (9). Local injection of bacteriostatic saline 0.5 mL can also cause a temporary local anesthetic effect. Before large-bore catheter placement, lidocaine injected intradermally with a small-bore needle (27 to 30 gauge) can be used to decrease the pain. Buffering lidocaine with sodium bicarbonate (9:1 solution) and injecting slowly minimize the pain caused by the medication itself. Nitrous oxide inhaled with oxygen has been shown to decrease pain and anxiety associated with venipuncture and venous cannulation and is as effective as EMLA in pain reduction. Additionally, the combination of EMLA and nitrous oxide provides superior analgesia to EMLA alone (10). Biofeedback, music therapy, and hypnotherapy have been studied in other settings as measures for decreasing pain from venous cannulation in patients with chronic illness.

Choosing the Vein

During cardiopulmonary resuscitation, the largest vein that does not interfere with resuscitation should be accessed (2). For stable patients, obtaining venous access should be attempted first in more distal veins, such as on the dorsum of the hand and feet, so that proximal veins can be saved for later use, especially in chronically ill children. The clinician should try not to use the child's dominant hand because this will limit subsequent activities. For obvious reasons, it may be wise to avoid the feet of active toddlers. However, the clinician may not have this luxury, as only a few veins may be accessible. Except in critical emergencies, it is important to evaluate multiple intravenous sites before the first attempt to maximize the chances of success. Inserting intravenous lines over joints should be avoided, because movement may dislodge the line and make stabilization more difficult. When veins cannot be visualized, it is advisable to attempt obtaining access at sites where the vein has a fixed anatomic location, such as the saphenous vein at the ankle, the median cubital vein, and the cephalic vein just proximal to the thumb.

Methods for Making Veins Prominent

Applying a tourniquet around the extremity just proximal to the vein makes it more prominent by blocking venous return. The tourniquet should not be kept on longer than 3 to 5 minutes because prolonged pressure can make the vein tortuous and fragile. The tourniquet should not be so tight as to impede arterial flow. After choosing the vein, it is important to remove the tourniquet and then reapply it just before venipuncture or catheter placement.

Other techniques may also enhance visualization of the vein (Table 73.3). Tapping the vein gently often makes it more prominent by increasing vasodilation. Keeping the extremity in a dependent position also helps to fill the vein. Using warm compresses for a few minutes helps dilate the vein. In patients with darker pigmented skin, wiping with Betadine swabs reportedly helps the clinician see veins more easily.

In children with chubby hands, it is useful to press the skin with alcohol swabs and release it to allow brief visualization

TABLE 73.3	METHODS FOR MAKING VEINS MORE VISIBLE

Tourniquet
Tapping on the vein (vasodilatation)
Milking the vein from proximal to distal
Keep extremity in dependent position
Fist clenching
Betadine swab (dark skin)
Alcohol swab press-release
Landry light
Nitroglycerin

of the vein as it fills. To keep the location of the vein in mind, a superficial thumbnail impression can be made or the alcohol gauze can be held at the specific point. In the antecubital fossa, it is often easy to palpate a cordlike structure. Rotating the arm back and forth can help distinguish a vein from a tendon because a tendon will roll as the arm is rotated.

Another method is to turn the lights off and place a flashlight under the hand or wrist to help illuminate small veins. This is also helpful when the skin is darkened by a hematoma from prior sticks because the linear vein will still look darker than the hematoma. The Landry light is also useful for visualizing veins (11–13). In infants, 4% nitroglycerin ointment applied on the area for 2 minutes has been shown to cause local venodilation and to facilitate venous cannulation (14).

Immobilization

Usually two health care staff members will be involved in performing venipuncture or venous access with a child—one person to hold the child and one to perform the procedure. If the child is uncooperative and strong, more assistants may be needed. It is best but not always possible to have an adult other than the parent assist in restraint of the child. Parents should ideally be providing support to calm their child. It should be emphasized that proper immobilization is a crucial aspect of venipuncture and obtaining venous access. While immobilization does not guarantee success, failure is very likely with an inadequately immobilized child.

If the dorsum of the hand is used, the wrist and fingers should generally be slightly flexed when restrained. Small infant hands can be held between the thumb and fingers of the nondominant hand of the person performing the procedure. In older children, the restraining person can hold the forearm and the fingers (Fig. 73.4A). To make the antecubital veins more prominent, a towel can be placed beneath the elbow. For the foot, the ankle should be extended so that the veins can be easily visualized (Fig. 73.4B). If the long saphenous vein is to be cannulated, the foot also should be turned laterally. For scalp veins, an assistant must immobilized the infant's head. The veins are distended by using a rubber band, and the head is turned to the opposite side so it lies flat against the bed.

As mentioned previously, the external jugular vein may be cannulated in a child when other peripheral veins are not accessible. The child should lie in Trendelenburg position with the head turned away from the side where cannulation will be performed. Alternatively, a towel can be placed under the child's shoulders or an assistant can support the child's head tilted down slightly beyond the end of the bed. Because the external jugular vein cannot be palpated, it must be visualized crossing the sternocleidomastoid muscle from the angle of the jaw to the lower one third of the muscle. Valsalva maneuver and hepatic compression augments venous return to the right atrium and results in external jugular vein distention (15). For femoral puncture in the critically ill patient, the thigh is held with the hip flexed and abducted.

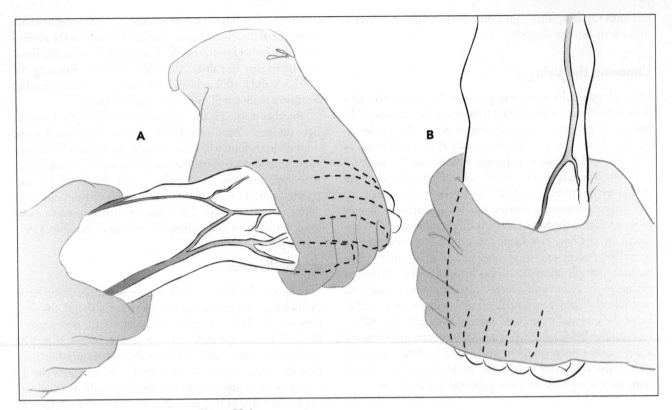

Figure 73.4
A. Immobilization of the hand for intravenous line placement.
B. Immobilization of the foot for intravenous line placement.

Preparing the Site

Both the clinician and the assistant(s) providing restraint should wear clean gloves, and universal precautions should always be followed. A tourniquet is applied proximal to the selected vein. As mentioned, it should not be applied so tightly that it obstructs the arterial supply. To prevent the tourniquet from pinching the skin or pulling hair, a 4″ × 4″ gauze pad can be placed under the area where the tourniquet is applied.

Next the puncture site should be cleaned. When blood is drawn that will not be used for blood cultures, this is often done with an alcohol swab. Otherwise, the area should be wiped with povidone-iodine swabs starting from the central area where the skin will be pierced and working out in a circular fashion to a radius of 3 to 4 cm. To ensure bactericidal effect, this should be allowed to dry before cleansing with alcohol swabs.

Butterfly Needles

The butterfly needle is often the preferred method of venipuncture for obtaining blood samples (Fig. 73.5). Usually a 23- or 25-gauge needle is used, but the clinician may opt to use a 21-gauge needle for the larger veins of school-aged children. Tension is applied to the skin and vein distal to the puncture site so that the vein is straightened. This affords easier penetration, decreases the chance of puncturing the posterior vessel wall, and enhances visualization of the vein. At this point, the child should be reminded of the upcoming "little pinch."

The tip of the needle is placed about 0.5 to 1 cm distal to the site selected for entering the vein. With the needle held at a 30- to 45-degree angle above the skin surface, the skin and underlying tissue are firmly pierced (Fig. 73.5A). The angle of the needle is then made closer to parallel to the skin surface, and the vein is entered slowly. Penetration of the vein is verified by a flashback of blood into the clear plastic tubing of the butterfly set. For intravenous placement, the needle is advanced carefully, with the butterfly lifted upward by the wings to avoid piercing the posterior vessel wall. For venipuncture, the needle is advanced only if required to improve blood flow, and then the syringe is attached. If this is awkward for the clinician performing the procedure, an assistant can attach the syringe and withdraw the blood by slowly applying suction. Aspirating the syringe with excessive negative pressure should be avoided, as the vein may collapse. The clinician may place a piece of clear tape over the needle or butterfly wings when drawing the sample to help stabilize the needle (Fig. 73.5B).

Sometimes blood will drip from the tubing but cannot be aspirated with the syringe. In such cases, the blood may be allowed to drip directly into the specimen tubes. This cannot be done for a blood culture, because the blood must be injected into vacuum-sealed blood culture containers using a syringe.

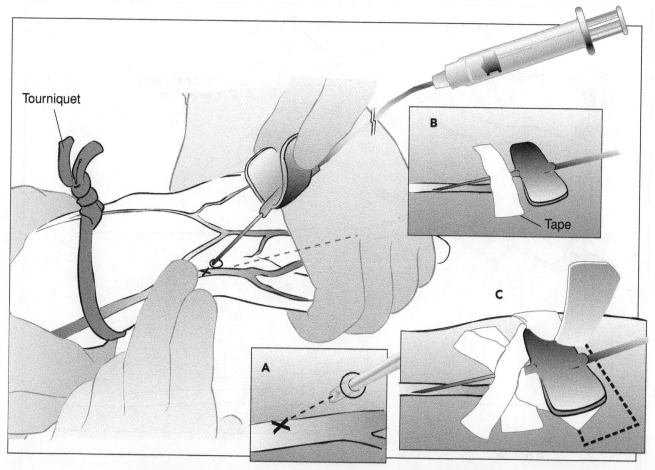

Figure 73.5 Using a butterfly needle for intravenous access or blood sampling.

However, blood can be allowed to drip into a syringe and then transferred to a blood culture container.

When blood drawing is complete, the tourniquet is removed. The butterfly needle is withdrawn from the skin, and pressure is applied to the venipuncture site with a 4″ × 4″ gauze pad. If blood is aspirated from the antecubital veins, holding pressure on the site with the elbow extended is believed to cause a smaller hematoma and less bruising than holding gauze or cotton with the elbow flexed.

When a butterfly needle is used for intravenous access, a syringe of normal saline is attached to the tubing. If the saline flushes easily and there is no infiltration of fluid indicated by swelling or induration around the needle tip, correct intravenous placement is confirmed. The butterfly is then secured with tape (Fig. 73.5C). Unfortunately, it is difficult to maintain butterfly needles as indwelling intravenous lines for prolonged periods. The only site for which this method of access is used with any frequency for pediatric patients is a scalp vein.

Over-the-Needle Catheters

Insertion of an over-the-needle catheter is preferred for intravenous access in most instances. The sizes most commonly used in infants and children are 22- and 24-gauge catheters,

although a 20-gauge catheter may be used if a higher rate of infusion is needed. For the older child or adolescent who requires rapid administration of large fluid volumes (e.g., trauma, septic shock), large-bore catheters (e.g., 14, 16, and 18 gauge) are used.

The limb is positioned optimally and the skin stretched taut (Fig. 73.6A). The needle cover is removed and the needle enters the skin about 0.5 to 1 cm below the intended site of entry into the vein at an angle of about 30 to 45 degrees. The bevel should generally be kept facing up to allow smooth entry through the skin. For small veins, some experts advise inserting the needle with the bevel facing down so that once the vein is entered, the chance of puncturing the opposite wall is reduced (16). This usually works best when the catheter appears larger than the vein.

Next, the operator should lower the angle of entry so that the needle-catheter is almost parallel to the skin surface and then advance slowly to puncture the vein (Fig. 73.6B). The operator should verify entry into the vein by visualizing a flashback of the blood inside the clear hub. The needle-catheter is advanced an additional 1 to 2 mm to ensure that the catheter also has entered the vein and not the needle tip only.

The operator should feed the catheter over the needle while holding the needle steady so that only the catheter advances

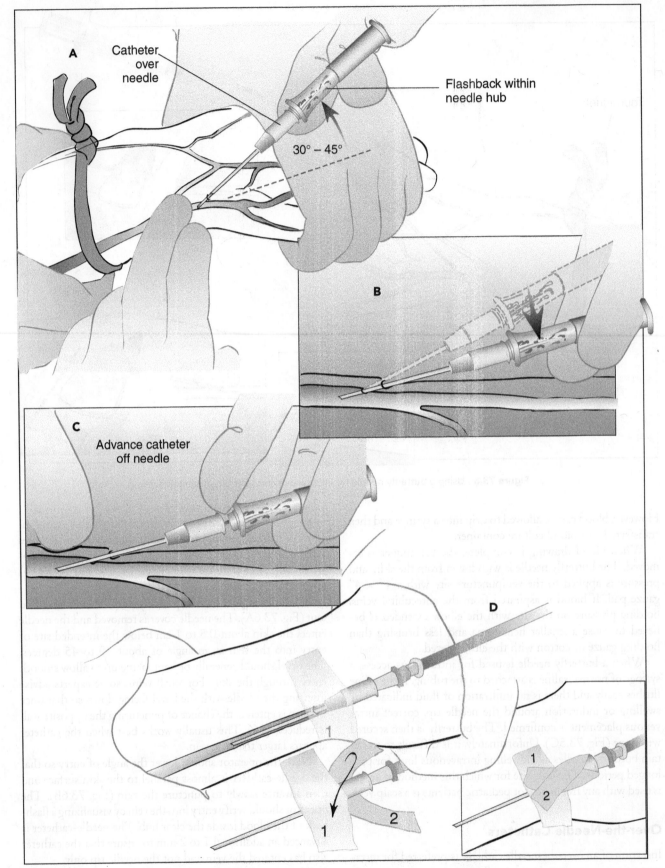

Figure 73.6 Intravenous line placement in a young child.

into the vein. The thumbnail of the nondominant hand may fit between the needle and the catheter to advance the catheter (Fig. 73.6C). Once the catheter is inserted, a T-connector is attached and the line is flushed with saline to ensure that the catheter is in the vein. Sometimes when the catheter tip is against a valve or wall of the vein, feeding it into the vein may be difficult. In such cases, it may be helpful to remove the needle and rotate the catheter while flushing with saline as the catheter is advanced.

Blood can be aspirated into the syringe for specimens with slow negative pressure. In small hand veins, some authorities prefer to have the specimen drip directly from the intravenous hub into the sample tubes or into a syringe for blood culture. Care must be taken to avoid having blood clot in the intravenous catheter or tubing, with resulting loss of the line. If not enough blood returns, the tourniquet is removed, and the extremity is "milked" by applying and releasing pressure alternately to obtain blood, followed by reapplication of the tourniquet. If too much suction is used, the vein may collapse, which will preclude specimen collection. Before flushing with intravenous fluids, the tourniquet or rubber band is removed. Otherwise, distending the fragile vein against pressure may infiltrate the tissue.

After the catheter has been inserted and the needle removed, most safety needles cannot be placed back into the catheter to help thread it. This practice is not recommended with standard nonsafety intravenous catheters, as it can cause shearing of the catheter tip, along with possible catheter embolism or intravenous infiltration. The thumb of the nondominant hand of the clinician placing the intravenous line can be used to physically secure the line until it can be taped in place. Sharps should be discarded immediately in an approved sharps container to avoid accidental needle puncture. It is usually advisable to limit intravenous attempts to 2 or 3 tries per clinician, especially if a more experienced individual is available to make additional attempts. For children with difficult veins, such as those with chronic illness, the more experienced clinician should consider trying first.

Securing the Intravenous Catheter

After an intravenous catheter has been successfully inserted, antibiotic ointment should be applied to the puncture site. The catheter is then secured with tape. This is done by first placing a piece of tape across the catheter, making sure that the hub is not covered so that intravenous tubing can be removed and replaced if necessary. A second piece of tape is placed under the hub of the catheter with the adhesive side away from the skin, and both sides of the tape are then crossed over the front of the catheter onto the skin (Fig. 73.6D). This may be repeated, but it is important to ensure that the area of skin over the tip of the catheter can be visualized so that infiltration or phlebitis can be detected early. It is helpful to tear off appropriately sized pieces of tape and to have them close by (e.g., on the side of the intravenous cart) prior to performing cannulation. After the catheter has been taped in

SUMMARY

1 Prepare the patient and organize all equipment at the bedside; ensure good lighting and obtain appropriate assistance for immobilizing the patient.

2 Observe universal precautions.

3 Carefully search for the best vein before starting.

4 Immobilize and then apply a tourniquet or rubber band to best visualize the vein.

5 Cleanse the area with povidone-iodine and allow to dry, then cleanse with alcohol (when time permits).

6 Pull the skin taut and insert the needle 0.5 to 1 cm distal to the actual point of entry and with the bevel facing up; when the vein is collapsed or small, entry with the bevel facing down may be preferred.

7 Puncture the vein and, after flashback, aspirate blood (venipuncture) or insert the needle-catheter into the vein 1 to 2 mm more to ensure that the catheter tip enters the vein (venous access).

8 Thread the catheter in the vein by feeding the catheter over the needle using the thumbnail of nondominant hand while stabilizing the needle; withdraw the needle when the catheter hub reaches the skin.

9 Attach the hub to a T-connector and syringe; flush the catheter to make sure it is still in the vein.

10 To collect a blood specimen, aspirate the syringe using slow negative suction without purging the T-connector beforehand; alternatively, collect blood by allowing it to drip into a specimen tube or syringe.

11 Secure the intravenous site with adhesive tape alone or tape and a clear dressing; tape the T-connector tubing away from the intravenous site.

12 Tape the extremity to a padded board if necessary.

13 Consider protecting the site with a plastic cover, especially if it is on the scalp.

14 Attach the catheter to an intravenous fluid line or convert to a heparin lock.

place, a transparent sterile dressing (e.g., OpSite, Tegaderm) can be applied to further secure the catheter, again making sure that the catheter hub is accessible. If used, T-connector tubing should be taped at least 2 cm away from the intravenous site.

The extremity is then placed on a soft board, usually covered with gauze for comfort and taped above and below the

CLINICAL TIPS

▶ Taking time to prepare the patient and parents reduces anxiety and increases the likelihood of success.

▶ Having an experienced assistant to properly immobilize a fearful or uncooperative child is crucial.

▶ Several techniques can be used to enhance visualization of a vein, including (a) using a tourniquet for extremities and a rubber band for the scalp, (b) tapping the vein gently to enhance filling, (c) keeping the extremity in a dependent position, (d) applying a warm compress to increase vasodilation, (e) using a flashlight under an extremity in a darkened room, and (f) applying topical 4% nitroglycerine to increase vasodilation.

▶ If veins are not visualized at all, veins with relatively fixed locations can be used for attempts (saphenous vein at the ankle, median cubital or cephalic vein proximal to the thumb).

▶ When inserting an intravenous catheter, the needle should be advanced an additional 1 to 2 mm after flashback of blood is seen to ensure that the catheter has also entered the vein.

▶ When the clinician has difficulty advancing the catheter over the needle, rotating the catheter or flushing with saline may be helpful.

intravenous site. To prevent the tape from irritating the skin, gauze can be placed below the tape that circles the extremity. When securing the hand, the fingers are allowed to curl up under the board and are taped over the distal metacarpals. It is best to allow the thumb to remain unrestrained. To the extent possible, an extremity should be secured in a position of function in order to minimize discomfort.

One final measure of security that can be used is a plastic "house" fashioned by cutting a clear medicine cup in half and taping it over the intravenous catheter (Table 73.1). This method is often used for scalp veins but is effective for any area that may be bumped (e.g., the hand or forearm). It is also useful in preventing a child from picking off the tape or dressing securing the catheter.

Parents should be instructed how to assist in caring for and preserving the intravenous line. Similar instructions can be given to the child, if appropriate. This may help the intravenous site stay protected and avoid undue pulling at the site.

▶ COMPLICATIONS

Complications of venipuncture include hematoma formation, injury to adjacent structures such as nerves or tendons,

local infection, phlebitis, cellulitis, and thrombosis. All except hematoma formation are uncommon. Poor technique in performing a puncture of the external jugular vein can result in injury to vital structures of the neck. Related problems include those associated with inadvertent infiltration of medications or other agents with local toxic effects, possibly resulting in necrosis or sloughing of the skin (e.g., phenytoin). Rarely, air embolism can occur with a peripheral intravenous line. Catheter embolism is now unlikely with the widespread use of safety devices that prevent reinsertion of the needle into an intravenous catheter.

▶ SUMMARY

Venipuncture and peripheral intravenous access are commonly performed in all pediatric age groups and are vital in the management of critically ill children. These procedures allow collection of blood samples for laboratory analysis and provide access for administration of parenteral fluids and medications. They are performed by a variety of health professionals in the ED, hospital wards, operating room, and outpatient settings. Using a calm, methodical approach, taking time to prepare the patient and parents, and organizing all the necessary equipment prior to the procedure are the best measures for ensuring success.

▶ REFERENCES

1. Hedges JR, Barsan WB, Doan LA, et al. Central versus peripheral intravenous routes in cardiopulmonary resuscitation. *Am J Emerg Med.* 1984;2:385–390.
2. *PALS Provider Manual.* Elk Grove Village, IL: American Academy of Pediatrics, American Heart Association; 2002.
3. Jacobsen C-JB, Grabe N, Damm MD. A trial of povidone-iodine for prevention of contamination of intravenous cannulae. *Acta Anaesthesiol Scand.* 1986;30:447–449.
4. Friedland LR, Brown R. Introduction of a "safety" intravenous catheter for use in an emergency department: a pediatric hospital's experience. *Infect Control Hosp Epidemiol.* 1992;13:114–115.
5. Frederick V. Pediatric i.v. therapy: soothing the patient. *RN.* 1991;54: 40–42.
6. Cooper CM, Gerrish SP, Hardwick M, et al. EMLA cream reduces the pain of venipuncture in children. *Eur J Anaesthesiol.* 1987;4:441–448.
7. Eichenfield FL, Funnk A, Fallon-Friedlander S, et al. A clinical study to evaluate the efficacy of ELA-Max (4% liposomal lidocaine) as compared with eutectic mixture of local anesthetics cream for pain reduction of venipuncture in children. *Pediatrics.* 2002;109:1093–1099.
8. Arowsmith J, Campbell C. A comparison of local anesthetics for venipuncture. *Arch Dis Child.* 2000;82:309–310.
9. Zempsky WT, Sullivan J, Paulson DM, et al. Evaluation of a low-dose lidocaine iontophoresis system for topical anesthesia in adults and children. *Clin Ther.* 2004;26:1110–1119.
10. Hee HI, Goy RW, Ng ASB. Effective reduction of anxiety and pain during venous cannulation in children: a comparison of analgesic efficacy conferred by nitrous oxide, EMLA and combination. *Paediatr Anaesth.* 2003;13:210–216.

11. Zimerman E. The Landry vein light: increasing venipuncture success rates. *J Pediatr Nurs.* 1991;6:64–66.

12. Nager AL, Karasic RB. Use of transillumination to assist placement of intravenous catheters in the pediatric emergency department [abstract]. *Pediatr Emerg Care.* 1992;8:307.

13. Sieh A, Brentin L. A little light makes venipuncture easier. *RN.* 1993;56: 40–43.

14. Vaksmann G, Rey C, Breviere G-M, et al. Nitroglycerine ointment as aid to venous cannulation in children. *J Pediatr.* 1987;111:89–91.

15. Verghese ST, Nath A, Zenger D, et al. The effects of the simulated Valsalva maneuver, liver compression, and/or Trendelenburg position on the cross-sectional area of the internal jugular vein in infants and young children. *Anesth Analg.* 2002;94:250–254.

16. Filston HC, Johnson DG. Percutaneous venous cannulation in neonates and infants: a method for catheter insertion without "cutdown." *Pediatrics.* 1971;48:896–901.

▶ SUGGESTED READINGS

Campbell LS, Jackson K. Pediatric update: starting intravenous lines in children: tips for success. *J Emerg Nurs.* 1991;17:177–178.

Hutchinson DB. Pediatric i.v. therapy: starting the line. *RN.* 1991;54: 43–48.

Lin SW, Zane Z. Peripheral intravenous access. In: Roberts JR, Hedges JR, eds. *Clinical Procedures in Emergency Medicine.* Philadelphia: WB Saunders; 1998:401–412.

Lozon MM. Pediatric vascular access and blood sampling techniques. In: Roberts JR, Custalow C, Hedges JR, eds. *Clinical Procedures in Emergency Medicine.* Philadelphia: WB Saunders; 1998:355–382.

Millam DA. How to insert an i.v. *Am J Nurs.* 1979;79:1268–1271.

O'Brien R. Starting intravenous lines in children. *J Emerg Nurs.* 1991;17: 225–231.

74

SUSAN M. FUCHS

Accessing Indwelling Central Lines

▶ INTRODUCTION

In children, numerous illnesses exist that require long-term parenteral pharmacologic or nutritional therapy and repetitive blood drawing. Several long-term central venous access devices (indwelling lines) have been developed that allow the administration of antibiotics, chemotherapy, blood, hyperalimentation, and fluids, often on an outpatient basis. When a child with one of these indwelling lines is evaluated in the emergency department (ED), the ability to properly access the device can be an important skill for providing optimal management. Because these devices directly access the central circulation, it is always necessary to follow sterile procedures to reduce the risk of infection. Air embolism and central vein thrombosis are additional risks.

▶ TYPES OF EQUIPMENT

Several indwelling lines are currently available, and clinicians should become familiar with the ones used most commonly in their own medical center. Differences among the devices include access, flushing, and aftercare.

The first partially implanted catheter was developed in 1973 by Broviac and consisted of a Silastic catheter that was used to administer total parenteral nutrition (TPN). The Broviac catheter was 18 gauge (1.0 mm internal diameter) and was inserted into the external jugular, subclavian, or cephalic vein, with the distal tip positioned in the right atrium. The proximal end was tunneled under the skin to exit on the chest (1). The same procedure for placement is used today. A Dacron cuff located on the catheter is positioned in the subcutaneous tunnel and serves two purposes: (a) a fibrin

sheath develops around it within about 2 weeks that anchors the line in the tunnel, and (b) it acts as a mechanical barrier to infection (1,2). In 1979, Hickman enlarged this catheter (16 gauge, 1.6 mm) to administer chemotherapy and to facilitate blood drawing (1,2). More recently, single-, double-, and triple-lumen catheters with a wider range of sizes (0.5 to 2.6 mm internal diameter) have been developed. In addition to the Broviac (Evermed) and Hickman (Fig. 74.1), other commonly used catheters include the Leonard, Raaf, Hemed, and Corcath (2). Another recent advance is the development of the Groshong catheter, which has an antireflux slit valve near the distal (implanted) tip (Fig. 74.2). The slit opens outward for administrating fluid and inward for aspirating blood, but it otherwise remains closed. The advantage of this type of catheter is that blood does not remain in the lumen of the catheter after it is flushed, so only saline flushes (no heparin) are used (2).

In 1982, the totally implantable central venous access device was introduced. It consists of a silastic catheter attached to a subcutaneous injection port or reservoir (Fig. 74.3). The catheter is placed in a central vein until the distal tip is at the junction of the superior vena cava and right atrium. The proximal portion is tunneled under the skin, but rather than exiting the skin, it is attached to a reservoir that is sutured into a subcutaneous pocket on the chest (1,2). The reservoir, which can be single or double lumen, is covered with a silicone septum that is self-sealing for up to 2,000 punctures (1). A special needle (Huber), which is noncoring and has a solid tip and a side hole opening, is used for access (Fig. 74.4). Most have a 90-degree bend, although some are straight (1,3). The reservoirs are made of plastic, stainless steel, or titanium. The plastic and titanium ports are light and do not interfere with magnetic resonance imaging studies (4). The Port-A-Cath (Pharmacia) comes in two sizes—an infant size

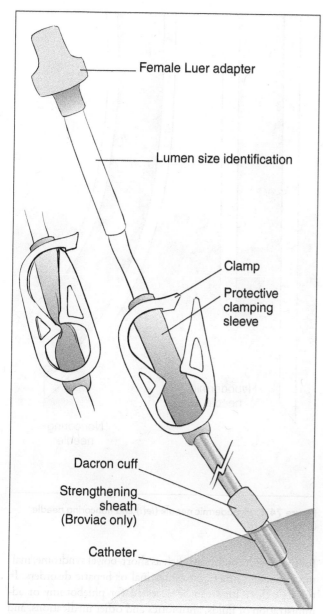

Figure 74.1 Schematic of Hickman and Broviac single-lumen catheters.

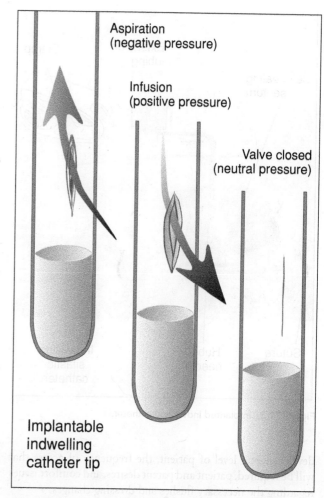

Figure 74.2 The Groshong three-position valve.

(outer diameter 2 mm, internal diameter 0.5 mm) and a child size (outer diameter 2.8 mm, internal diameter 1 mm) (1,3). Other available devices include the Infuse-A-Port, Mediport, and Babyport (1,2,4).

Two additional types of central line that have seen increased use in the neonatal and pediatric populations include the peripherally inserted central catheter (PICC) (see also Chapter 19) and the percutaneous central venous catheter (PCVC). The PICC is made of either silicone (Intrasil) or polyurethane (Intracath). These catheters may be single or double lumen and are generally 2 to 7 Fr in size (1,3). A Hohn PICC has a Dacron cuff, similar to the Broviac and Hickman catheters, which is placed in the subcutaneous tissue and is used to help hold the PICC in place (3). The PCVC is used in neonatal

patients, with sizes 1.1, 1.9, and 2.8 Fr. Because of their small size and risk of clot formation, use of the 1.1 and 1.9 Fr PCVC lines for blood sampling or blood transfusions is not recommended (3). Also because of their small size, PCVC lines require a heparin flush every 12 hours (3). Use of the PCVC is limited to the neonatal intensive care unit and therefore will not be discussed here; however, the 2.8 Fr PCVC can be treated in the same way as a small PICC, described below.

▶ ANATOMY AND PHYSIOLOGY

The basic purpose of using these catheter systems is to have a long-term intravenous line positioned within a central vein with a port that can be readily accessed. The benefits of accessing the central circulation over a peripheral vein include the ability to administer certain antibiotics and chemotherapeutic agents that may cause sclerosis of peripheral veins and the ability to infuse solutions containing higher concentrations of dextrose or potassium than can safely be administered through a peripheral vein. The decision about which type of catheter to use is based on several factors, including the age and

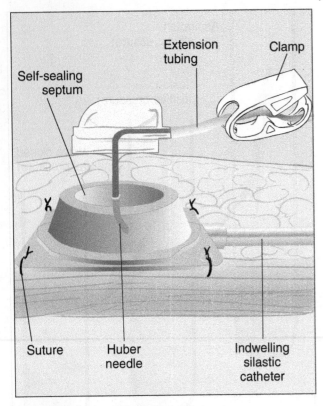

Figure 74.3 Implanted indwelling catheter.

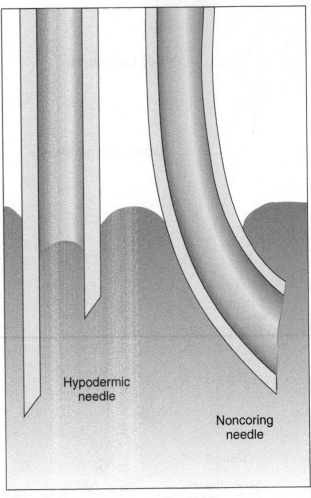

Figure 74.4 Hypodermic needle (*left*) and noncoring needle (*right*).

developmental level of patient, the frequency of access that will be required, patient and parent desires, and comfort issues regarding the necessary flushes and dressing changes.

For the partially implanted external catheters, the most common sites include the external jugular, subclavian, and cephalic veins. For the implantable device, the catheter is usually placed in the subclavian vein, although the internal jugular vein also can be used. With both of these types of catheter, the distal tip is positioned at the junction of the superior vena cava and right atrium or within the right atrium (1,2). The PICC and PCVC are inserted in the upper arm through the basilic, brachial, or cephalic vein and passed to the superior vena cava until the tip of the catheter lies at the junction of superior vena cava and right atrium. Another option for these catheters is insertion in the lower leg through the saphenous vein to the inferior vena cava, with the tip positioned at the junction of the inferior vena cava and right atrium (3,5).

▶ **INDICATIONS**

Children undergo placement of an indwelling line for a variety of reasons, including chronic illnesses requiring long-term intravenous antibiotic therapy (e.g., osteomyelitis, pulmonary infection associated with cystic fibrosis); administration of chemotherapy treatments for childhood cancers; difficult intravenous access in a child who frequently requires blood draws or intravenous medications; and parenteral nutrition for those with conditions such as short-bowel syndrome, malnutrition, and other gastrointestinal or hepatic disorders. In the ED, these lines can be accessed for phlebotomy or administration of fluids, antibiotics and other medications, and blood products. Catheter-related problems that may result in ED visits include catheter occlusion or breakage, unintentional displacement, and skin irritation and/or infection at the site of insertion. Contraindications to access for therapy would include a dislodged catheter, an inability to confirm that a catheter has been placed properly, and a suspicion of significant clot or infection within the catheter that may be dislodged with use.

▶ **EQUIPMENT**

Partially Implantable Catheters (Broviac, Hickman), PICC, and 2.8 Fr PCVC

Sterile gloves (two pairs), mask, gown and eyewear
10% povidone-iodine solution and alcohol *or* 2% chlorhexidine (for those older than 2 months and not sensitive to this product)

Sterile drapes

10-mL syringe filled with normal saline

Heparin flush

- For patients up to 6 months of age, 3 mL heparin (10 U/mL)
- For patients over 6 months of age, 5 mL heparin (100 U/mL)
- For 2.8 Fr PCVC, 2 mL heparin (10 U/mL)
- Note: for the Groshong catheter, 5 mL saline is used to flush the catheter, not heparin

Catheter clamp or hemostat *without teeth*

Fluids and medications to be administered

Dressing and tape for procedure completion (gauze or transparent dressing such as Opsite or Tegaderm), povidone-iodine ointment

10-mL syringes (2 to 3 empty) if blood drawing is desired

Heparin lock, normal saline flush, and cap

Totally Implanted Devices (Port-A-Cath)

Sterile gloves (two pairs), mask, gown, and eyewear

10% povidone-iodine solution and alcohol *or* 2% chlorhexidine (for those older than 2 months and not sensitive to this product)

Sterile drapes

10-mL syringe filled with normal saline

Heparin flush

- For patients up to 6 months of age, 3 mL heparin (10 U/mL)
- For patients over 6 months of age, 5 mL heparin (100 U/mL)

Two noncoring (Huber) needles with a 90-degree bend, using (preferably) the following sizes:

- 20-gauge for drawing blood
- 22-gauge for administration of intravenous fluids or medications or 19-gauge for administration of blood
- Note: in an emergency, a standard 19-gauge needle can be used

T-extension tubing with side clamp

Several sterile gauze squares (2″ × 2″) to stabilize needle

Tape

Gauze dressing for procedure completion

10-mL syringes (2 to 3 empty) if blood drawing is desired

Additional Equipment Needed for Special Procedures

Dissolving a Clot in the Catheter

Recombinant tissue plasminogen activator (CathFlo, Alteplase), 2 mg

Broken Catheter Repair

Catheter repair kit (Evermed) containing plastic clamps, silicone adhesive, injection caps, and 12 Fr catheter re-placement segment (three sizes of catheter repair kits are available, based on the internal diameter of the patient catheter– 0.8, 1.0, and 1.3 mm)

▶ PROCEDURE

Several key points should be made about accessing an indwelling line: (a) a sterile field and sterile technique should be maintained during the entire procedure; (b) acetone or tincture of iodine should not be used on the external catheter, as this can lead to drying or cracking of the catheter (povidone-iodine is acceptable); (c) forceps with teeth should not be used on the external catheter, as these can damage the catheter and cause breakage or make holes; (d) a catheter clamp should always be readily available to access partially implantable devices; (e) only 10-mL syringes should be used to draw fluid or flush the catheter, as smaller syringes generate higher pressure, which can rupture the catheter; (f) heparin flush and parenteral fluids should be ready to administer; (g) fluids should not be administered if no blood return is obtained after the catheter is flushed; and (h) the clinician should infuse 10 mL of saline flush between any medications to flush the catheter, except PCVC lines, for which a 2-mL flush is adequate (1–3,5).

Accessing a Partially Implantable Catheter (Broviac, Hickman), PICC, or 2.8 Fr PCVC

The clinician should prepare all the necessary equipment, wash his or her hands, and don sterile gloves. The catheter is clamped at least 3 inches from the cap. Most patients will have their own clamp, but hemostats without teeth also can be used. (If only hemostats with teeth are available, the teeth should be wrapped in gauze to reduce the risk of damaging the catheter.) A sterile towel is positioned under the catheter, and the cap is removed. The catheter is wiped with alcohol and allowed to dry for 5 to 10 seconds. A 10-mL syringe filled with normal saline is then attached. The catheter is unclamped, and 3 to 5 mL of saline is slowly injected into the catheter. Fluid is aspirated back into the catheter to check for blood return.

If there is resistance to the instillation of saline or no blood is aspirated, the catheter is likely occluded, and the clinician should reclamp the catheter and attempt maneuvers described below (see "Establishing Patency"). Importantly, fluids or medications should not be injected if resistance is met or no blood is aspirated. If there is no resistance and a good blood return, the clinician should inject the remaining 5 to 7 mL of fluid into the catheter (or 0.5 mL of fluid for a PCVC line), reclamp the catheter, and remove the syringe. The intravenous fluid tubing is purged of any air bubbles and attached to the catheter. The catheter is then unclamped and fluids are administered.

After completion of the procedure, the clinician should inject heparin into the catheter (or saline for a Groshong catheter) using the guidelines listed above (see "Equipment"). The cap is replaced, and a gauze or transparent dressing is applied according to preference (gauze must be changed daily, whereas a transparent dressing can be changed weekly). The catheter should be flushed with heparin on a daily basis, except for a Groshong catheter, which is flushed with 5 mL of saline weekly (3).

Accessing a Totally Implanted Device (Port-A-Cath)

If access of a totally implantable device is not needed emergently, a topical anesthetic (LMX$_4$ or EMLA) should be applied over the site, because this procedure involves a skin puncture. The reservoir should be palpated to identify the site. The topical anesthetic is applied to the skin overlying the reservoir, and the area is covered with an occlusive dressing for 20 minutes (LMX$_4$) or 40 minutes (EMLA) prior to performing the skin puncture.

Necessary equipment should be organized beforehand. If an anesthetic cream is used, the dressing should be removed and the cream wiped away with a gauze pad. The clinician should wash his or her hands and don sterile gloves. The skin overlying the reservoir is prepared by washing in a circular motion from the center of the device outward with povidone-iodine. The skin is allowed to dry, and the same procedure is repeated with an alcohol swab. Another option for cleaning is 2% chlorhexidine, although it should not be used for infants under 2 months or those who are sensitive to it. A 10-mL syringe filled with saline should be attached to T-connector tubing and flushed through the tubing. The extension tubing is attached to the Huber needle, and the needle is flushed with saline to remove air. The extension tubing is clamped and placed on a sterile field.

The clinician should then don a new pair of gloves and other sterile apparel and locate the center of the septum (reservoir membrane). While stabilizing the reservoir with the thumb and index finger, the clinician inserts the needle with slow but firm pressure through the septum to the posterior wall of the reservoir, taking care not to penetrate the posterior wall (Fig. 74.5). The extension tubing is unclamped and 2 mL of saline slowly instilled. If there is resistance to flow, the catheter is likely occluded, and the clinician should reclamp it and attempt maneuvers described below (see "Establishing Patency"). Force should not be used in such situations to inject the saline. If there is no resistance to flow, another 3 mL of saline should be infused into the port. At this point, blood should be aspirated. If blood appears, the remaining 5 mL of saline should be injected into the reservoir. If no blood return is seen, the catheter is likely occluded, and the clinician should reclamp it and attempt maneuvers described below (see "Establishing Patency"). Importantly, the clinician should not administer fluids or medications through the catheter if there is no blood return with aspiration. Once catheter patency is ensured, the needle is taped in place so as

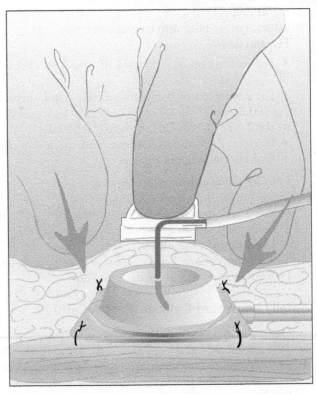

Figure 74.5 Stabilizing a reservoir with the thumb and index finger while accessing an implanted device.

to maintain it at a right angle to the septum. This is best done by placing gauze pads around the needle and then applying tape. A sterile dressing should be placed over the needle when in use. The extension tubing should be reclamped and the syringe removed. Intravenous fluid tubing is carefully purged of any air bubbles and attached to the catheter. The catheter is unclamped and fluids are administered.

After completion of the procedure, the clinician should inject heparin through the extension tubing through the Huber needle into the catheter using the guidelines listed above (see "Equipment"). The extension tubing is then clamped and the needle removed. A dressing (gauze or adhesive strip) is applied over the puncture site and left in place for 24 hours. Heparin flushes are required every 3 to 4 weeks (1,3).

Establishing Patency

Catheter occlusion can be classified as complete or partial (withdrawal occlusion). Complete occlusion is when no solution can be infused and no blood withdrawn. This is usually due to a blood or fibrin clot, drug precipitate, catheter malposition (against a vein wall), or a kinked catheter. Partial occlusion is when there is resistance to flush and sluggish or absent blood withdrawal; it is usually due to a fibrin sheath around the distal catheter tip (3,6). Noninvasive methods to evaluate for this include altering the patient's position, raising the patient's hands above his or her head, having the patient cough or perform a Valsalva maneuver, and placing the bed in reverse Trendelenburg. All these actions may change the venous pressure gradient along the catheter and improve patency (2,3). It must be emphasized that the clinician should never use excessive force to infuse saline or withdraw blood, as this may damage the catheter, necessitating repair or replacement.

If noninvasive methods are ineffective in clearing a catheter occlusion, this may be due to either a blood clot within the catheter or a fibrin clot at the tip. If the patient is not actively bleeding and does not have cerebrovascular disease, declotting the catheter using a fibrinolytic such as recombinant tissue plasminogen activator (r-tPA) (CathFlo, Alteplase) should be attempted. (It is the practice in some hospitals to require a physician to perform this procedure.) Although the use of r-tPA has not been approved by the U.S. Food and Drug Administration for those under 2 years of age, studies on its use in this population have yielded good results (6,7). The dose is based on the child's weight and the catheter type (ideally 100% of the internal lumen volume of the catheter), with a concentration not exceeding 1 mg/mL. For children weighing 10 kg or less, 0.5 mg r-tPA is diluted in normal saline to the volume required to fill a partially implantable device (each lumen if needed), or 0.5 mg r-tPA is diluted with normal saline to 2 mL for a totally implanted device. For children weighing more than 10 kg, a concentration of 1 mg/mL of t-PA (maximum 2 mg) is used to fill a partially implanted device (each lumen if needed), or 2 mg r-tPA is diluted with normal saline to 3 mL for a totally implanted device (7). This should be left in the line for a minimum of 2 hours and then withdrawn. The line is then tested for patency. If patency is not restored, this can be repeated in 2 hours (3), or another agent can be used. Occlusion due to mineral precipitates on the catheter can often be cleared with 0.1 N hydrochloric acid (1.0 mL), which is slowly injected and allowed to remain in the catheter for 20 minutes, after which time aspiration is attempted (3). If the occlusion is believed to be due to waxy clots associated with hyperalimentation and intralipids, 70% ethanol can be used. The catheter is filled with 70% ethanol for 1 hour and aspiration is reattempted (3). If this is not successful, 0.1 N hydrochloric acid can then be used. In general, using hydrochloric acid or ethanol to improve patency should be done after consultation with the physician responsible for catheter placement and ongoing care.

Drawing Blood from a Partially Implantable Catheter (Broviac, Hickman), PICC, or 2.8 Fr PCVC

The clinician should prepare any necessary supplies and arrange them on a sterile field. The catheter is then clamped, and the cap of the catheter is removed and discarded. The catheter is wiped with alcohol and allowed to dry for 5 to 10 seconds. An empty 10-mL syringe is attached and the catheter unclamped. Approximately 2 to 5 mL of blood is withdrawn, the catheter is reclamped, and the syringe is discarded. An second empty syringe is attached, and the catheter is unclamped. The desired amount of blood is withdrawn, and the catheter is reclamped. It is best to reclamp the catheter each time before a syringe is removed. A 10-mL syringe filled with saline is then attached, the catheter is unclamped, and saline is injected slowly into the catheter (for a 2.8 Fr PCVC, only 0.5 mL of flush is required). The catheter is clamped once again, the syringe is removed, and a new heparin cap is attached. Then the cap is swabbed and injected with 1 to 2 mL of 100 U/mL heparin (or 10 U/mL heparin for infants under 6 months of age).

Drawing Blood from a Totally Implanted Device (Port-A-Cath)

The clinician should prepare all the supplies and follow the steps previously outlined for access [see "Accessing a Totally Implanted Device (Port-A-Cath)"]. An empty 10-mL syringe is attached to the extension tubing, and the tubing is unclamped. Approximately 2 to 5 mL of blood is withdrawn, the tubing is reclamped, and the syringe is removed and discarded. The clinician should attach another empty syringe and withdraw the desired amount of blood, remembering that the extension tubing should be reclamped every time before a syringe is removed. After the blood is drawn, a 10-mL syringe filled with normal saline is attached, the extension tubing is unclamped, the saline is slowly injected into the reservoir, and the tubing is reclamped. The clinician should mix 1 mL of 100 U/mL heparin (10 U/mL heparin for infants under 6 months of age) with 4 mL of saline in a 10-mL syringe and attach the syringe to the extension tube. The tubing is unclamped and the heparin flush instilled into the reservoir. The tubing is then clamped and the Huber needle is pulled straight out. If no bleeding occurs, a gauze dressing or adhesive strip can be applied and left in place for 24 hours.

Catheter Breakage

Catheter breakage can result inadvertently from (a) cutting the catheter with a scissors while trying to remove the dressing, (b) piercing the catheter with a needle, (c) a child pulling away during access, (d) a child playing with the implantable port site, and (e) injury from contact sports. The catheter can separate from the port of the implanted device. For partially implantable devices, it is important to clamp the catheter proximal to the point of breakage and to cover the torn region with a sterile gauze if available. If no external catheter is present, pressure should be applied at the catheter entrance site into the vein (not at the exit site) (2,3,5). Repair kits are available for partially implantable catheters. For totally implanted devices, a radiograph should be obtained to determine the integrity of the system. Both the physician managing the catheter-related treatment and the surgeon need to be contacted.

SUMMARY

Accessing a Partially Implantable Catheter (Broviac, Hickman), PICC, or 2.8 Fr PCVC

1 Prepare the equipment.

2 Wash hands and don sterile gloves.

3 Clamp the catheter at least 3 inches from the cap; most patients will have their own clamp, but hemostats without teeth also can be used (if only hemostats with teeth are available, wrap the teeth in gauze).

4 Position a sterile towel under the catheter.

5 Remove the cap from the catheter, wipe the catheter hub with alcohol, and it allow to dry for 5 to 10 seconds; attach a 10-mL syringe filled with normal saline.

6 Unclamp the catheter and slowly inject 3 to 5 mL of saline.

7 Aspirate fluid back into the syringe to check for blood return.

8 If resistance is met to the instillation of saline or no blood is aspirated, reclamp the catheter and perform maneuvers for establishing patency (see text); do not inject fluids or medications if resistance is met or no blood is aspirated.

9 If blood return is obtained, inject the remaining 5 to 7 mL of fluid into the catheter, reclamp the catheter, and remove syringe (use only 0.5 mL of saline to flush a PCVC).

10 Attach intravenous fluid tubing to the catheter after purging the tubing of any air bubbles, unclamp the catheter, and administer fluids.

11 After completion of the procedure, inject 3 to 5 mL of heparin into the catheter (2 mL of 10 U/mL for 2.8 Fr PCVC, 3 mL of 10 U/mL heparin for patients under 6 months, 5 mL of 100 U/mL heparin for patients 6 months or older), replace the cap, and apply the preferred dressing; for the Groshong catheter, use 5 mL of saline (not heparin) to flush the catheter.

Accessing a Totally Implanted Device (Port-A-Cath)

1 Prepare the equipment.

2 If LMX₄ or EMLA cream and dressing was applied, remove the dressing and swab the cream away with gauze.

3 Wash hands and don sterile gloves.

4 Palpate the reservoir and prepare the overlying skin by washing in a circular motion from the center of the device outward with povidone-iodine, then alcohol; alternatively, use 2% chlorhexidine (for those over 2 months and not sensitive to this product).

5 Attach a 10-mL syringe filled with saline to T-connector tubing and flush saline through the tubing; set on a sterile field.

6 Attach extension tubing to a Huber needle and flush the needle with saline to remove air; clamp the extension tubing closed and set on a sterile field.

7 Don a new pair of gloves and other sterile apparel.

8 Locate the center of the septum and stabilize the reservoir with the thumb and index finger.

9 Slowly but firmly insert the needle through the septum to the back of the reservoir.

10 Unclamp the extension tubing and slowly instill 2 mL of saline.

11 If resistance is met, do not force fluid into the reservoir; reclamp the extension tubing and perform procedures for establishing patency (see text).

12 If no resistance is met injecting saline, infuse another 3 mL into the port.

13 Aspirate fluid back into the syringe and check for blood return.

14 If blood is seen, inject the remaining 5 mL of saline into reservoir and tape the needle in place, maintaining it at a right angle to the septum; apply a sterile dressing over the needle while in use; if no blood return is obtained, reclamp the extension tubing and perform procedures for establishing patency (see text).

15 Reclamp the extension tubing and remove the syringe.

16 Attach intravenous fluid tubing to the catheter after purging the tubing of any air bubbles, unclamp the catheter, and administer fluids.

17 After completion of the procedure, inject 3 to 5 mL of heparin (3 mL of heparin 10 U/mL for patients under 6 months, 5 mL of 100 U/mL for patients 6 months or older) into the catheter through the extension tubing and the Huber needle, clamp the extension tubing and remove the needle, and apply a dressing.

SUMMARY (CONTINUED)

Drawing Blood from a Partially Implantable Catheter (Broviac, Hickman), PICC, or 2.8 Fr PCVC

1 Prepare supplies and arrange on a sterile field.

2 Clamp the catheter.

3 Remove the cap and discard.

4 Wipe the catheter hub with alcohol and allow to dry for 5 to 10 seconds.

5 Attach an empty 10-mL syringe and unclamp the catheter.

6 Withdraw 2 to 5 mL of blood, reclamp the catheter, and discard the syringe.

7 Attach another empty syringe, unclamp the catheter, and withdraw the desired amount of blood; clamp the catheter.

8 Attach a 10-mL syringe filled with saline and unclamp the catheter; slowly inject saline into the catheter (only 0.5 mL of saline is needed to flush a PCVC).

9 Reclamp the catheter, remove the syringe, and attach a new heparin cap; swab the cap and inject with 1 to 2 mL of heparin (100 U/mL heparin for patients 6 months or older, 10 U/mL heparin for patients under 6 months); apply a dressing.

Drawing Blood from a Totally Implanted Device (Port-A-Cath)

1 Prepare supplies and arrange on a sterile field.

2 Follow Steps 2–9 from "Accessing Totally Implanted Devices."

3 Attach an empty 10-mL syringe to the extension tubing and the unclamp tubing.

4 Withdraw 2 to 5 mL of blood, reclamp the tubing, and remove the syringe and discard.

5 Attach another empty syringe and withdraw the desired amount of blood.

6 Attach a 10-mL syringe filled with normal saline, unclamp the tubing, slowly inject the saline into the reservoir, and reclamp the extension tubing.

7 Mix 1 mL of 100 U/mL heparin (10 U/mL heparin for patients under 6 months) with 4 mL of saline in a 10-mL syringe.

8 Attach the syringe to the extension tubing, unclamp the tubing, and instill the heparin flush into the reservoir.

9 Clamp the tubing and pull the Huber needle straight out.

10 Apply a dressing.

Aftercare Instructions for Partially Implantable Catheters (Broviac, Hickman) and PICC and PCVC Lines

Patient instructions should include the following:

Always keep the site covered and dry.

Change the dressing every other day (gauze), weekly (transparent), and as necessary to reduce the risk of contamination.

Flush the line daily with heparin solution. If this cannot be done, notify the physician most responsible for the catheter.

Look for bruising, bleeding, and signs of infection (redness, pain, purulent drainage, fever) each day. If present, call your physician immediately.

For PICC lines, the extension tubing should be looped on top of the dressing. The arm is secured with an elastic bandage (Ace wrap) placed loosely to cover the dressing. The extension tubing is looped over the first layer of elastic bandage, but the line should be covered with elastic bandage (3). For PCVC lines, the catheter should be anchored with tape across the silicone "heart," and then a transparent dressing is placed over the insertion site (although not over the heart). A strip of tape should be placed with the adhesive side up under the catheter extension next to the heart and then crossed over the heart so that it adheres to the transparent dressing rather than the skin. A third piece of tape can be placed over the crossed tape (3).

Aftercare Instructions for Totally Implanted Devices (Port-A-Cath)

Patient instructions should include the following:

Avoid direct pressure over device (includes seatbelts with shoulder harness).

Flush line at least weekly. If this cannot be accomplished, then notify your physician.

Look for bruising, bleeding, and signs of infection (redness, pain, purulent drainage, fever) every day. If present, call your physician immediately.

Patients do not have to wear a dressing over the device, and swimming and bathing are allowed.

Medication Incompatibility

Two medications that possibly should not be administered by central access lines are diazepam and phenytoin. It is thought that these medications interact with the silicone lining of the catheter and could crystallize with it. Such crystallization cannot be reversed by fibrinolytic agents. Because debate exists around this issue, it is probably advisable to find another method of administration if these medications are required. It is also important to avoid administering agents that are not compatible with each other or may react when given in succession (e.g., calcium and bicarbonate) without an adequate saline flush between them.

▶ COMPLICATIONS

Infection

One of the main risks of a central line is line infection. The likelihood of this complication is increased if sterile technique is not maintained during procedures. Although accessing a line or withdrawing blood can introduce organisms into the line, infection from the line also may be the presenting problem. Organisms cultured from infected lines include coagulase-negative staphylococci (usually *S. epidermidis*), *Staphylococcus aureus*, streptococcal species, gram-negative organisms (e.g., *Pseudomonas aeruginosa*, *Klebsiella pneumoniae*, *Escherichia coli*), and fungi (especially *Candida albicans*) (2,4,8,9). Even when proper sterile technique is practiced, there is a risk of introducing infection any time an indwelling line is accessed.

Possible catheter infections include bacteremia, fungemia, and sepsis as well as soft-tissue infections at the exit site, subcutaneous tunnel, and subcutaneous pocket ("pocket infection"). The rate of infection for partially implantable catheters is higher than for totally implanted devices (2,9). The risk of a soft-tissue infection, especially a "pocket infection," is greatest in the first 100 days after insertion (4,9). *S. aureus* and *S. epidermidis* are the most common pathogenic organisms (2). Management of potential line infections requires obtaining a blood culture from both the indwelling line and a peripheral site. Appropriate intravenous antibiotic therapy is then initiated, typically consisting of vancomycin and a third- or fourth-generation cephalosporin (until cultures results are known) based on regional resistance patterns (2,8). For skin exit site infections of partially implantable catheters, aggressive local care and topical antibiotics may suffice (2). For tunnel and pocket infections, catheter removal is recommended, combined with intravenous antibiotic therapy (8).

Air Embolism

Because these catheter systems end in blood vessels near the heart, there is a risk of air embolism. To minimize this risk, it is vital to keep the system clamped whenever instillation of fluid or withdrawal of blood is not taking place. Signs and symptoms of air embolism include the sudden onset of tachypnea,

hypotension, and loss of consciousness (2,3). Treatment includes clamping the system immediately, placing the patient on his or her left side in the Trendelenburg position, administering oxygen, and obtaining alternate intravenous access (2).

Catheter-Related Thrombosis and Embolization

The tip of an indwelling line can be a site of thrombus formation or the formation of fibrin sheaths, which may result in occlusion of the catheter or possible embolization. Although the thrombi at a catheter tip are generally small fragments, a large one can result in a clinically significant pulmonary embolism if dislodged during flushing. Signs and symptoms include tachycardia, palpitations, dyspnea, hypoxia, and chest pain (2).

Another complication is central venous thrombosis. This can occur when a catheter rubs chronically against the wall of a vein, causing thrombus development. If the thrombus becomes large enough, it can obstruct venous flow and result in superior vena cava syndrome. Symptoms include a fullness in the head or neck, vertigo, and blurred vision. Signs include edema of the periorbital area, neck, chest, or arms as well as dyspnea and tachycardia. Treatment requires catheter removal and anticoagulation (6).

 CLINICAL TIPS

▶ A sterile field should be established and sterile procedures followed.

▶ Acetone or tincture of iodine should not be used on an external catheter. Povidine-iodine is acceptable.

▶ Forceps with teeth should not be used on an external catheter.

▶ A clamp should always be readily available when a partially implantable device is accessed.

▶ Only 10-mL syringes should be used to reduce the risk of high-pressure line damage.

▶ Fluids should not be administered if there is no blood return seen. Maneuvers to clear a catheter occlusion should be tried, followed by r-tPA and, as warranted, 70% ethanol and/or 0.1 N hydrochloric acid.

▶ A 10-mL saline flush (or a 2-mL saline flush for a 2.8 Fr PCVC) should be administered between any medications.

▶ When access of a totally implantable device is not needed emergently, a topical anesthetic should be applied over the site before skin puncture. Applying LMX₄ or EMLA cream to the skin overlying the reservoir and covering with an occlusive dressing for 20 or 40 minutes, respectively, significantly reduces discomfort.

Catheter Displacement

Catheter displacement can occur accidentally due to patient movement or during catheter care, especially if the cuff (if present) has not had time to develop a fibrin sheath. In such cases, a chest radiograph should be obtained to determine the position of the catheter tip prior to attempting access (9). Occasionally a catheter can migrate from its original location. In rare cases, this can result in arrhythmias, cardiac tamponade, or pneumothorax (2,3).

▶ SUMMARY

Many central venous access devices are currently used by children on an outpatient basis. When problems develop due to the device or to underlying illness, these patients will present for emergency evaluation. Clinicians who provide acute and emergency care for children should be familiar with the specific devices currently being used in the region and be knowledgeable about potential complications. Necessary equipment for access should be available. Strict aseptic technique is mandatory whenever these devices are accessed.

▶ REFERENCES

1. Wesley JR. Permanent central venous access devices. *Semin Pediatric Surg.* 1992;1:188–201.
2. Krywko DM, Colone PD. Indwelling vascular devices: emergency access and management. In: Roberts JR, Hedges JR, eds. *Clinical Procedures in Emergency Medicine.* 4th ed. Philadelphia: WB Saunders; 2004:462–474.
3. Owen K, Rae-Zahradnik ML. *Care and Maintenance of a Central Venous Access Catheter Procedure.* Chicago: Children's Memorial Medical Center, Department of Nursing; 2004.
4. Hengartner H, Berger C, Nadal D, et al. Port-A-Cath infection in children with cancer. *Eur J Cancer.* 2004;40:2452–2458.
5. Dyer BJ, Gardner Weiman M, Ludwig S. Central venous catheters in the emergency department: access, utilization, and problem solving. *Pediatr Emerg Care.* 1995;11:112–117.
6. McCloskey DJ. Catheter-related thrombosis in pediatrics. *Pediatr Nurs.* 2002;28:97–106.
7. Choi M, Massicotte P, Marzinotto V, et al. The use of alteplase to restore patency of central venous lines in pediatric patients: a cohort study. *J Pediatr.* 2001;139:152–156.
8. Mermel LA, Farr BM, Sherertz RJ, et al. Guidelines for the management of intravascular catheter-related infections. *Clin Infect Dis.* 2001;32:1249–1272.
9. Wiener ES, Albanese CT. Venous access in pediatric patients. *J Intraven Nurs.* 1998;21(5S):S122–133.

SECTION 11 ▶ PULMONARY PROCEDURES
SECTION EDITOR: RICHARD M. RUDDY

RONNIE S. FUERST

75

Use of Pulse Oximetry

▶ INTRODUCTION

The pulse oximeter, an electronic monitor used to noninvasively measure arterial oxygen saturation, is standard equipment in the emergency department (ED) and other places, such as the operating room, the intensive care unit, and outpatient settings, where the information would be valuable for patient care. An understanding of its applicability, interpretation, and limitations is essential in the modern practice of emergency medicine.

The origin of this technology lies in the 1930s, when the first in vivo device to measure oxygen saturation by transillumination was developed. The 1970s heralded two important developments. The first was the discovery of arterial pulsations in the microvasculature, and the second was the use of light-emitting diodes (LEDs) as a light source and photodiodes as light detectors. These latter findings assisted greatly in overcoming the size and weight problems associated with previous devices. In the early 1980s, microprocessors were added for self-calibration and improved accuracy through the use of algorithms (1).

The pulse oximeter has distinct advantages over other measures of oxygenation. First, it is at most an uncomfortable attachment to an extremity but can measure both absolute SaO_2 and trends in patients requiring monitoring for acute medical and traumatic illness in an emergency setting. Second, it can be a stand-alone monitor or be integrated into more complex monitoring of a patient's vital functions. Its

only disadvantage is that it is unable to distinguish other molecules attached to the hemoglobin moiety, such as carboxyhemoglobin and methemoglobin. It may read a normal value in their presence. Improvements in microprocessor performance in the past 10 years have vastly improved the performance of pulse oximeters overall and, in particular, when there is patient movement, when oxygen saturation drops below 80%, in low-perfusion states, and when monitoring sites are vasoconstricted (2). Pulse oximeter readings under these conditions should still be viewed with a cautious eye and correlated with other clinical information.

▶ ANATOMY AND PHYSIOLOGY

Pulse oximetry is a measure of the percent saturation of hemoglobin by the oxygen molecule. This is only one part of the oxygen transport system (Fig. 75.1), and other methods of observation and monitoring are required to evaluate other aspects of oxygen delivery (2). The remainder of this section presents a review of the physiology of hemoglobin saturation and the oxyhemoglobin dissociation curve, followed by a review of the mechanism of the equipment.

The hemoglobin molecule is almost entirely responsible for oxygen transport when oxygen is within the cardiovascular system. Only 1.5% of oxygen is dissolved in plasma. Hemoglobin saturation (SaO_2) is the amount of oxygenated hemoglobin (O_2Hb) compared with the total amount of hemoglobin

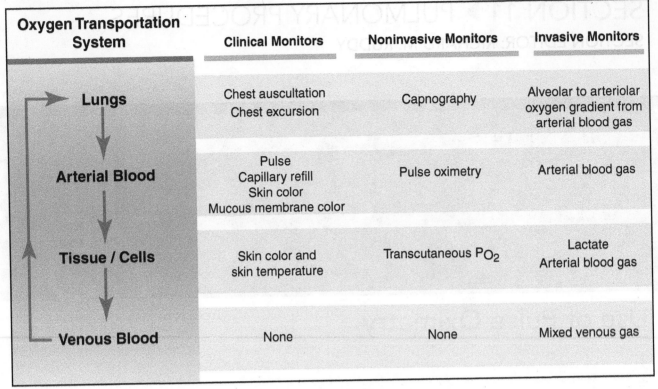

Figure 75.1 Oxygen transport system.

available for oxygenation, expressed as a percentage (3):

$$SaO_2 = \frac{\text{Oxygenated hemoglobin}}{(\text{Oxygenated hemoglobin} + \text{Reduced hemoglobin})} \times 100$$

The oxyhemoglobin dissociation curve (Fig. 75.2) demonstrates the nonlinear relationship between hemoglobin satu-

ration and the partial pressure of oxygen in plasma (PO_2). Normal SaO_2 is between 95% to 100%, and hypoxemia is defined as PO_2 less than 70 mm Hg (SaO_2 below 90%). Small changes in the SaO_2 in the upper, flat part of the oxyhemoglobin dissociation curve result in larger changes in PO_2. In the steep part (lower and middle part of the curve), large changes in the SaO_2 result in small changes in PO_2. Under normal physiologic conditions, the body operates at the upper portion of the curve, as depicted in Figure 75.2. Changes in the oxyhemoglobin dissociation curve either to the left or to the right change the relationship of SaO_2 to PO_2. The factors that shift the oxyhemoglobin curve to the left and increase the affinity of oxygen to hemoglobin at lower PO_2 are increased pH, decreased temperature, decreased PCO_2, and decreased 2,3-DPG. The 2,3-DPG levels are altered by a number of physiologic effects, and increases of 2,3-DPG are seen when anemia, chronic hypoxemia, high-altitude adaptation, chronic alkalosis, and hyperthyroidism are present.

Pulse oximetry uses the principles of spectrophotometry and the Beer-Lambert law together with complex signal-processing algorithms and calibrations to calculate the percentage of oxyhemoglobin concentration. Four types of hemoglobin are clinically significant to pulse oximetry: oxygenated hemoglobin (O_2Hb), reduced hemoglobin (Hb), carboxyhemoglobin (COHb), and methemoglobin (MetHb). For the purposes of pulse oximetry, both fetal hemoglobin and sickle hemoglobin are assumed to have the characteristics of adult hemoglobin. The oximeter emits two wavelengths of light—one in the red region (660 nm) and one in the infrared region (920 nm)—to differentiate the absorption of light by

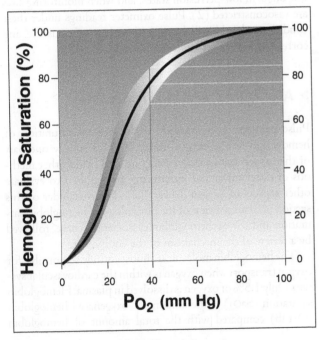

Figure 75.2 Oxyhemoglobin dissociation curve.

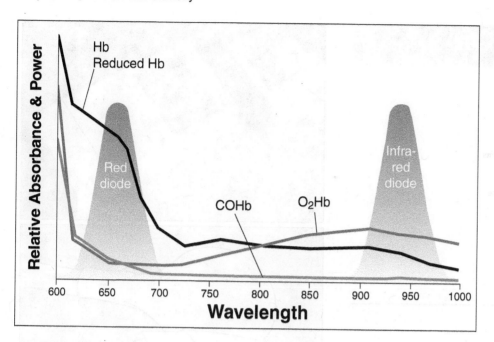

Figure 75.3 Absorbance spectrum curves for O_2Hb and $COHb$.

the oxygenated and deoxygenated hemoglobin species in the microcirculation. Figure 75.3 shows the wavelength absorption of different hemoglobin moieties as they relate to this phenomenon.

Carboxyhemoglobin (COHb) behaves as O_2Hb in regard to its absorption spectra, and so the oximeter misinterprets the CoHb and reads a falsely high SpO_2. Methemoglobin (MetHb) absorbs light at both wavelengths emitted by the LED. Therefore, MetHb will always cause a falsely high SpO_2, but as MetHb levels rise, the SpO_2 level measured will be less because of the effects on both wavelengths where it causes interference. When the MetHb reaches 30%, the SpO_2 will not be above 85% and will remain at that level regardless of increasing MetHb concentrations. Other dyshemoglobinemias may not reliably quantitate the actual oxyhemoglobin percentage. In patients suspected of MetHb or COHb, an arterial or venous blood gas should be sent with co-oximetry to assess their measured concentration in blood. The pulse oximeter also must measure absorption differences between the maximal and minimal arterial pulsations to enable it to separate the signals from arterial blood and exclude the background (i.e., venous blood and tissues). After obtaining the separate signals for bound and unbound hemoglobin, the formula above can be used to calculate the percentage saturation of hemoglobin in the circulation measured.

Pulse oximeters commonly used in the ED have been found to correlate with arterial blood gas oxygen saturation (SaO_2) in patients with systolic blood pressures between 80 and 206 mm Hg, heart rates between 40 and 180 beats per minute, and hematocrits between 20% and 56% (4). The accuracy of pulse oximeters, as reported by manufacturers, is ±4% (with a 95% confidence interval) when the SpO_2 is above 70%. There is much statistical variability when the SpO_2 is below 70%. Thus, the trend of readings may be more accurate and useful than the individual SpO_2 readout.

There are other important technical issues worthwhile to consider (5–10). Motion near the sensor site may mimic the pulsations of small arteries and affect the reading. In this instance, the pulse on the oximeter will not produce a normal curve and will not trace the patient's actual heart rate. In low-flow states, the lack of blood flow in the vessels may not transmit sufficient change in light emittance for the monitor to read the saturation adequately. This may be demonstrated by the monitor indicating "pulse search." During high venous pressure, the venous pulsation may transmit falsely low SpO_2 to the monitor. In children, this rarely occurs in heart failure but may be present in traumatic venous obstruction or when a manometer cuff is inflated or a tourniquet is applied. Lastly, other ambient light sources, such as sunlight, warming lights, phototherapy, and bright fluorescent bulbs, may interfere with the reading by increasing the light to the photodetector. The patient ought to have the sensor shielded with a more light-resistant covering. Manufacturers have improved pulse oximeter performance by dealing with many of these confounding factors (2,11–14).

▶ INDICATIONS

Common uses of pulse oximetry in the emergency setting are as an adjunct in triage to determine level of acuity, monitoring during a procedure, monitoring for a decline or improvement in a patient's cardiopulmonary state, and ascertainment of the effectiveness of therapy affecting oxygen delivery. Table 75.1 lists the most common indications for pulse oximetry. As regards the monitoring of procedures, pulse oximetry is cited in the American Academy of Pediatrics guidelines for the sedation of pediatric patients (15). It is particularly useful to monitor SaO_2 closely during procedural sedation, such as that used for fracture reduction and complex laceration

TABLE 75.1	INDICATIONS FOR USE OF PULSE OXIMETRY

Monitoring during procedures
  Sedation
  Airway procedures
  Lumbar punctures in infants
Monitoring clinical status
  Apnea monitoring
  Confirmation of periodic breathing in infants
  Monitoring during mechanical ventilation
  Sedation
  Detection of misplaced or blocked ET tube
  Monitoring during analgesia
  Monitoring during transport
  Maximizing ventilator settings
Response to therapy
  Asthma/reactive airway disease
  Bronchiolitis
  Pneumonia
  Congestive heart failure

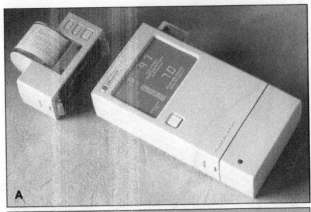

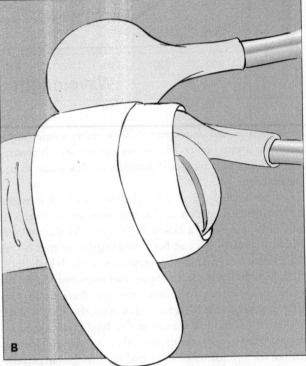

Figure 75.4
A. Pulse oximeter.
B. Pulse oximetry probe attached to the finger of a child.

repair. Young infants, potentially septic, should have continuous SaO_2 monitoring during all procedures but particularly during lumbar puncture, when observation for apnea may be difficult. Patients requiring an airway intervention, such as bag-valve-mask, endotracheal intubation, nasopharyngeal, and oropharyngeal airways, should have continuous SaO_2 monitoring. As listed in Table 75.1, several additional categories of emergency patients should have continuous SaO_2 monitoring.

Lastly, a number of illnesses are better managed when the SaO_2 is monitored either continuously or intermittently. Illnesses at risk of leading to hypoxemia in childhood include clinically significant upper airway obstruction, pneumonia, bronchiolitis, and asthma. The list also includes the baby with apnea, and congenital heart disease, including both congestive heart failure and cyanotic heart disease. In illnesses for which acute therapy may reverse the process, such as asthma, SaO_2 is best continuously monitored to evaluate improvement or decline. It is vital to remember that *SaO_2 measures the oxygenation and not the ventilation*. Therefore, children with upper airway obstruction, large airway–lower airway disease, or central hypoventilation (e.g., an overdose of a respiratory depressant drug) may have normal SaO_2 until late in deterioration. Pulse oximeters should be used for transferring high-risk pediatric patients between medical units, such as from the ED to the operating room or intensive care unit, and for interhospital transfer. Emergency medical services carry pulse oximeters that enable the paramedics to assess for hypoxia, which may have been difficult to recognize clinically (16).

▶ EQUIPMENT

Pulse oximeters found in EDs are usually freestanding portable devices or integrated into remote patient monitors. The typical unit will display heart rate and arterial oxygen saturation (Fig. 75.4A). Some units display the wave form or plethysmograph. Typical controls include a power on/off switch, an alarm on/off switch, and a high/low alarm limit control for both pulse rate and saturation level. Many freestanding units have internal battery power for transport. The externally attached component is the probe that is placed on the patient and connected to the oximeter with a standard adapter. Most manufacturers make only probes that are compatible with their own instrument. The probe is made of an LED and a sensor (photodiode). Probes can be reusable in that they are usually clipped on to a toe or finger. The disposable probes are typically held to the extremity with a mild adhesive and are malleable. Disposable probes have distinct advantages; in particular, they often conform to different children's fingers or toes better and lead to less false alarms from loss of signal transduction.

SUMMARY

1 Choose a sensor of the appropriate type and size.

2 Affix the sensor to the forehead or a finger, toe, or earlobe (rarely, to the nose or penis or a lip, hand, or foot in a small child).

3 Observe for capture of the pulsation signal; be sure the LED is aligned opposite the detector.

4 Set alarm limits for SpO₂ and heart rate 5% from the baseline.

5 Remember that oxygenation, not ventilation, is monitored.

 CLINICAL TIPS

▶ Be sure the pulse signal matches patient's heart rate; check the alignment of the LED and detector.

▶ Consider a replacement sensor if there is poor signal recognition.

▶ If in doubt, obtain an arterial blood gas for correlation.

▶ Carboxyhemoglobin and methemoglobin will cause falsely high SpO₂ readings; methylene blue causes falsely low SpO₂ readings.

▶ Observe chest rise and respiratory rate in addition to SpO₂.

▶ Supplemental oxygen may delay recognition of hypoventilation when there is sole reliance on oximetry.

▶ PROCEDURE

Orientation to the operation of the pulse oximeter can be accomplished in just a few minutes. The operator must first decide on a location for the sensor placement. The sensor must be placed on a part of the body that will allow light to pass through from one side to the other. Fingers, toes, and the earlobe are the most common sites for children and adults. The hand, foot, nose, or penis also may be used. There is now a forehead sensor available. Most operators initially attempt placement on a finger or toe. Once the site has been chosen, the appropriate size sensor must be selected. The available sizes include infant, child, and adult sizes depending on the model. Nondisposable clip-on sensors are self-aligning but at times more difficult to use in young children. Disposable sensors are placed in a circular or longitudinal fashion, with care taken to ensure that the LED is aligned directly across the digit from the light detector (Fig. 75.4B).

After the sensor has been placed, the unit is turned on and observed for capture of the signal. If the oximeter is able to detect pulsations, it will display the rate of pulsations (equivalent to the heart rate) and an SpO₂ value. If no signal is captured, the oximeter may print a message such as "pulse search" or display a heart rate that will not correlate with the true heart rate or not display the SpO₂. If a disposable sensor has been reused, it is often of value to reattempt monitoring with a new sensor.

After the signal is picked up, alarm limits for the rate and the SpO₂ need to be set. Alarm limits are a subject of varied opinion. Alarm limits should be set to the patient's age and clinical condition in order to warn health care providers of changes in heart rate and SpO₂. Most clinicians would set the lower-limit SpO₂ to at least 90% and as high as 94%. As a general guideline, a SpO₂ of 95% is close to a PO₂ of 75, a SpO₂ of less than 90% correlates with a PO₂ of approximately 60, indicating moderate hypoxemia. At 90%, in most circumstances, the level is at the top of the steep portion of the oxyhemoglobin desaturation curve where hypoxemia is defined. Some clinicians set low limits 5% below baseline. It is important to verify that the alarm switch is in the desired position should the clinician walk away from the bedside of the child.

If any doubt exists about the accuracy of the pulse oximeter, or if no correlation is found between the clinical situation and the oximeter reading, then an arterial blood gas should be obtained. It must be remembered that the pulse oximeter yields information regarding oxygenation without reflection of ventilation.

▶ COMPLICATIONS

Modern pulse oximeters are extremely safe devices with few reported complications. Thermal burns have been reported from connecting a sensor made by one manufacturer to an instrument made by a different manufacturer (17). Theoretically, ischemia could be induced by applying disposable sensors too tightly. Reusable sensors need to be cleaned with bactericidal and viricidal agents between uses for infection control.

Common complications result from over-reliance on the device in place of clinical judgment or from misinterpretation of the data obtained. Both over-reliance and misinterpretation are due to lack of training and/or experience (18,19). This is especially true in clinical states where hypoxemia may be masked by falsely elevated oximeter readings of SpO₂ (e.g., carbon monoxide poisoning) or in states of methemoglobinemia. Also, misinterpretation is possible in patients with edema, anemia, intravascular dyes (e.g., methylene blue therapy for methemoglobinemia, which transiently causes falsely low SpO₂), venous pulsations from restrictive taping, and elevated venous pressure.

▶ REFERENCES

1. Tremper KK, Barker SJ. Pulse oximetry. *Anesthesiology.* 1989;70:98–108.

2. Giuliano KK. New generation pulse oximetry in the care of critically ill patients. *Am J Crit Care.* 2005;14:26–39.

3. Ehrenwerth J, Eisenkraft JB. *Anesthesia Equipment: Principals and Applications.* St. Louis: Mosby; 1993:249.

4. Jones J, Heiselman D, Cannon L, et al. Continuous emergency department monitoring of arterial saturation in adult patients with respiratory distress. *Ann Emerg Med.* 1988;17:463–468.

5. Barker SJ, Tremper KK, Hyatt J. Effects of methemoglobin on pulse oximetry and mixed venous oximetry. *Anesthesiology.* 1989;70:112–117.

6. Barker SJ, Tremper KK, Hyatt J. The effect of carbon monoxide inhalation on pulse oximetry and transcutaneous Po_2. *Anesthesiology.* 1987;66:677–679.

7. Tremper KK, Hustedler SM, Barker SJ, et al. Accuracy of a pulse oximeter in the critically ill adult: effect of temperature and hemodynamics. *Anesthesiology.* 1985;63:3A.

8. Scheller MS, Unger RJ, Kelner MJ. Effects of intravenously administered dyes on pulse oximetry readings. *Anesthesiology.* 1986;65:550–552.

9. Veychemans F, Baele P, Guillaume JE, et al. Hyperbilirubinemia does not interfere with hemoglobin saturation measured by pulse oximetry. *Anesthesiology.* 1989;70:118–122.

10. Lawson D, Norley I, Korbon G, et al. Blood flow limits and pulse oximetry signal detection. *Anesthesiology.* 1987;67:599–603.

11. Bonhurst B, Peter CS, Poets, CF. Pulse oximeters' reliability in detecting hypoxemia and bradycardia: comparison between conventional and two new generation oximeters. *Crit Care Med.* 2000;28:1565–1568.

12. Gehring H, Hornberger C, Matz H, et al. The effects of motion artifact and low perfusion on the performance of new generation pulse oximeters in volunteers undergoing hypoxemia. *Respir Care.* 2002;47:48–60.

13. Hay WW, Rodden DJ, Collins SM, et al. Reliability of conventional and new generation pulse oximetry in neonatal patients. *J Perinatol.* 2002;22:360–366.

14. Jopling MW, Mannheimer PD, Bebout DE. Issues in the laboratory evaluation of pulse oximeter performance. *Anesth Analg.* 2002;94 (1 suppl):S62–68.

15. Committee on Drugs, American Academy of Pediatrics. *Guidelines for Monitoring and Management of Pediatric Patients during and after Sedation for Diagnostic and Therapeutic Procedures.* American Academy of Pediatrics; 1992;89:1110–1113.

16. McGuire TJ, Pointer JE. Evaluation of a pulse oximeter in the prehospital setting. *Ann Emerg Med.* 1988;17:1058–1062.

17. Murphy K, Secunda JA, Rockoff MA. Severe burns from a pulse oximeter. *Anesthesiology.* 1990;73:350–352.

18. Alshehri M. Pulse oximetry: are health personnel aware of its clinical applications and limitations? *Ann Saudi Med.* 2000;20:75–77.

19. Salyer JW. Neonatal and pediatric pulse oximetry. *Respir Care.* 2003;48:386–396.

JAVIER A. GONZALEZ DEL REY

76

End-Tidal Carbon Dioxide Monitoring

▶ INTRODUCTION

Measurement of variations in the respiratory cycle of expired carbon dioxide (CO_2) by displayed waveform and by absolute numerical values is defined as capnography and capnometry, respectively. Measurement of exhaled CO_2 at the level of the upper airway at the end of the expiration (when CO_2 is at its maximum) is referred to as end-tidal CO_2 ($EtCO_2$) (1–4). This noninvasive measurement of blood gases has been used since the 1950s. Initially described by Luft in 1943 (5), it was not until this past decade that its clinical applications made this technique popular in the intensive care unit (ICU) and the operating room (OR). Primitive attempts at crude CO_2 measurement were made in the anesthesia suite by the barium hydroxide agglutination reaction and the Einstein CO_2 detector, which was capable of sensing 4 to 6 volume percentage (volume %) CO_2 (6). Modern technology designed monitors that use infrared absorption spectroscopy to measure the amount of CO_2 in an exhaled breath. These sensors may be located in the patient's artificial breathing circuit (mainstream) or away from the patient as part of the CO_2 monitoring circuit system (sidestream).

In the late 1980s, another practical method that documents concentrations of CO_2 usually present in the trachea was introduced. It is based on a device that demonstrates colorimetric changes that reflect levels of carbon dioxide above 2%. This technique has been particularly useful for the documentation of endotracheal tube placement in emergency situations and for the assessment of a patient's respiratory status. Recent studies in urban emergency medical services found that up to 25% of medical and trauma pediatric and adult patients had esophageal intubations on presentation to the emergency department (ED) (7,8). These devices have had a tremendous impact in the rapid detection of unrecognized esophageal intubations in prehospital and hospital settings.

Although unrecognized esophageal placement may be rapidly fatal, it is not harmful if it is recognized quickly, especially in prehospital settings (9,10).

Transcutaneous CO_2 monitoring, a technique developed in the 1970s primarily for the neonatal intensive care patient, has not proven useful in the ED setting. This is because transcutaneous CO_2 measurements take time to calibrate, and skin thickness in older children and adults makes the test inaccurate.

With the development of emergency and transport medicine, $EtCO_2$ measurement has become a very popular and useful tool for monitoring ventilated patients and for confirming endotracheal tube placement. Portable and disposable units have been designed, making the technology user-friendly and less costly.

All critically ill or injured children requiring ventilatory support, in particular where the outcome may be affected by the adequacy of ventilation or special techniques (e.g., cases of acute head trauma and status epilepticus and in the transport of ventilated patients), should ideally be monitored by pulse oximetry and capnography. Thus, physicians, nurses, and respiratory therapists managing these patients in the ED should be familiar with capnography. The American Academy of Pediatrics recommends this type of device to ensure correct placement of the endotracheal tube because other physical findings, such as breath sounds or condensation mist in the endotracheal tube, are more subjective to the clinician (11).

▶ ANATOMY AND PHYSIOLOGY

Carbon dioxide (CO_2), one of the waste products of cellular metabolism, is transported in blood predominantly in the form of bicarbonate ion (60%). One third of CO_2 is bound to blood proteins, and the rest is carried as dissolved gas in plasma (pCO_2). The dissolved CO_2 concentration in the arterial end of the skin capillaries approximates the pCO_2 of an arterial sample. Carbon dioxide then diffuses in lung capillaries to the alveolar unit and enters the gaseous phase. During exhalation, the pCO_2 concentration at the end of each breath will be nearly equal to the $PaCO_2$, when the ventilation and perfusion (V/Q) are well matched. $EtCO_2$ represents the approximation of pCO_2 from all ventilated alveoli whether or not they are perfused. $PaCO_2$ represents the pCO_2 of perfused alveoli. In normal conditions, $EtCO_2$ is 2 to 6 mm Hg less than arterial pCO_2 (12).

To further understand the $EtCO_2$ concept, it is important to understand the physiology of lung ventilation and perfusion. In normal lungs, the apical segments have a tendency to be more aerated relative to perfusion (Fig. 76.1). At the base, secondary to the opposite phenomenon, the lung is more perfused and not as well aerated. The V/Q constant in most individuals is 0.8 (4 parts ventilation to 5 parts perfusion). The normal respiratory cycle has nonused (or wasted) ventilation. Some of this is alveolar gas that does not get exchanged (alveolar dead space). Other gas travels only within the large or conducting airways and also is not part of the CO_2 exchange (large airway dead space). The sum of the alveolar dead space and the large airway dead space is the physiologic dead space. The $EtCO_2$ concentration is related to the arterial carbon dioxide tension ($PaCO_2$), the segmental perfusion of lung units, and the percentage of dead space ventilation.

For example, in cases when pulmonary capillary bed perfusion is less than normal but ventilation is normal, the $EtCO_2$ may significantly underestimate $PaCO_2$. In airways with no perfusion, CO_2 will approach zero if ventilation is adequate, whereas perfused airways will diffuse CO_2. The net effect is that the $EtCO_2$ will represent the combination of normal and close to zero CO_2 diffusion and thereby underestimate $PaCO_2$. Conditions that affect a V/Q mismatch include shock, heart failure, pulmonary emboli or thrombi, cardiac arrest, pneumothorax or hydrothorax, and persistence in a lateral decubitus position. This V/Q mismatch develops because inadequate perfusion to well-ventilated areas results in a widened difference between the arterial pCO_2 ($PaCO_2$) and alveolar CO_2. In these cases $EtCO_2$ underestimates $PaCO_2$ because of the effect of abnormal perfusion.

A different scenario occurs when the lung has adequate perfusion but inadequate ventilation (shunt perfusion). Conditions that reduce alveolar ventilation or increase the production of carbon dioxide will elevate the arterial CO_2, decreasing the V/Q ratio. Although the $EtCO_2$ rises as $PaCO_2$ does from this state, $EtCO_2$ may underestimate $PaCO_2$ because the contribution of dead space ventilation makes it difficult to have a real-time steady-state $EtCO_2$. This is frequently observed in patients with asthma, atelectasis, mucous plugging, right main stem bronchial intubation, emphysema, pneumonia, pleural effusion, and pneumothorax.

During normal respiration, some dead space ventilation travels through the esophagus instead of down the airway. In the proximal esophagus, the measured CO_2 closely corre-

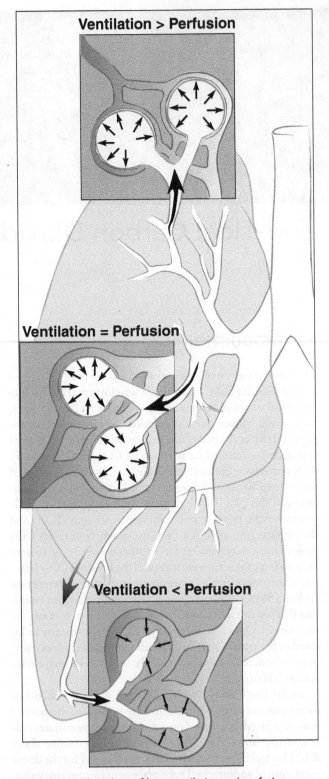

Figure 76.1 Physiology of lung ventilation and perfusion.

lates with the concentration in inhaled air. In patients with tracheal trauma or tracheoesophageal fistulas measured CO_2 at esophagus may show concentration closer to that in main airway.

Endotracheal intubation is associated with a complication rate reported to be as high as 26% (13). Unrecognized esophageal intubation is probably the most serious complications. Utting et al. in 1979 reported that 15% of anesthesia-related accidents resulting in brain injury or death were the result of unrecognized esophageal intubation (14). In the prehospital setting, Stewart et al. and Shea et al. noted a 1.8% and 2% incidence of recognized esophageal intubation, respectively (15,16). In recent years, the colorimetric $EtCO_2$ detector has become available, which indicates the presence of CO_2 by a color change. The premise is that with intact pulmonary circulation, CO_2 is present in the trachea but not in the esophageal gas reflux. Studies have revealed that the gastric CO_2 expired is lower and usually less than 0.7 volume % (mL/100 mL) (17,18). Initially the waveform during esophageal intubations may appear normal, but with successive ventilations (three to six) it dissipates. This occurs even under the influence of carbonated beverage consumption or the presence of antacids in the stomach. Several studies have demonstrated the accuracy and convenient ease of use in animal models, children, and adults in the ED, ICU, and OR and in transport and prehospital settings (19–23).

▶ INDICATIONS

Indications and uses of capnography are multiple and based on the determination of $EtCO_2$. In the OR, it is used primarily to monitor intubated patients during anesthesia, alerting physicians to inadequate ventilation, ventilatory circuit disconnection, or airway leaks. Most importantly, it can detect inadvertent placement of the endotracheal tube in the esophagus. In the ED, it is used to confirm the proper placement of the endotracheal tube, assess the effectiveness of cardiopulmonary resuscitation, and monitor patients ventilated due to trauma, respiratory failure, or status epilepticus (24). It is important during the delivery of special ventilatory therapy, such as controlled hyperventilation in head trauma. Most recently, esophageal $EtCO_2$ monitoring has been used in the monitoring of patients under conscious sedation for a procedure or diagnostic study and in the evaluation of patients in impending respiratory failure from pneumonia, asthma, and neurologic illness.

▶ EQUIPMENT

$EtCO_2$ partial pressure can be measured either by mass or by infrared spectroscopy. Mass spectroscopy separates and counts ionized molecules of the gas to determine its concentration. Most commonly used is infrared spectroscopy, which compares the amount of infrared light absorbed by the sample with that absorbed by a non-carbon-dioxide-containing chamber. Carbon dioxide strongly absorbs infrared light at a wave length of 4.28 nm. In the sample chamber, CO_2 absorbs the light energy emitted by the infrared source corresponding to its wave length. At the end of the chamber, a detector converts the light energy into an electrical signal proportional

to the intensity of the incidental radiation, reflecting in this way the $EtCO_2$ of the sample. Most capnometers will usually report concentrations of end-tidal expired CO_2 in mm Hg or volume % CO_2 by dividing the CO_2 partial pressure by the atmospheric pressure. The normal concentration is approximately 38 mm Hg or 5 volume % at an atmospheric pressure of 760 mm Hg.

The gas sample may be obtained from the patient's airway using either a mainstream or a sidestream method (Fig. 76.2). Mainstream sampling places a chamber in the airway between

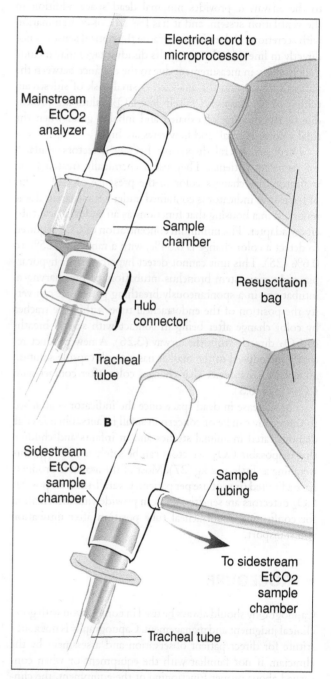

Figure 76.2 Gas sampling methods.
A. Mainstream.
B. Sidestream.

the patient and the ventilatory unit. The sidestream aspirates gas from the ventilatory system and draws the gas sample to the analyzer via the side sample tubing. The advantages of using the mainstream system are mostly related to the location of the infrared source. Because it is placed in the airway in series, no mixing of gases occurs, nor is there aspiration of secretions into the side circuit. Continuous reading of the CO_2 concentration also occurs, avoiding lag time to measurement.

The sidestream method collects a sample of gas from the patient's airway and withdraws it down the side tubing to the analyzer. Its advantages are that it does not add weight to the airway, it provides minimal dead space addition in the ventilation system, and it has less risk of contamination with secretions and moisture because the optical sensor is not directly in line with the airway. Its disadvantages may include a slight delay in measurement due to the distance between the patient's airway and the analyzer. A small risk of sidestream tubing obstruction and falsely low CO_2 values are present due to the mixture of exhaled and inhaled gases when the tidal volume is small and flow rates are high.

There are several disposable $EtCO_2$ detectors available for pediatric patients. They use a chemically treated foam indicator that changes color in the presence of CO_2. This pH-sensitive indicator is contained under a transparent dome mounted in a housing that functions as an endotracheal tube elbow adapter. The minimum concentration of CO_2 required to detect a color change is 0.54%, with a range of 0.25% to 0.6% (25). This unit cannot detect hypercarbia or hypocarbia, right main stem bronchus intubation, or oropharyngeal intubations in a spontaneously breathing patient. It can verify the position of the endotracheal tube within the trachea by color change after being in contact with several breaths of CO_2 directly from the airway (3,26). A new product recently introduced in the market has a crush capsule solution attached to the device that changes color after contact with CO_2 (Fig. 76.3).

The increase in dead space once the indicator is attached to the airway can be of concern in small infants. Bhende et al. demonstrated in animal studies and in infants and children that disposable CO_2 detectors can be safely used in patients weighing as little as 2 kg (27). Most of the available products have a limited time of use per patient. Overall, these disposable CO_2 detectors are sensitive and can provide vital information for confirming endotracheal tube position after intubation and transport.

▶ PROCEDURE

Capnography should always be used in conjunction with good clinical judgment and management. Capnography is not a substitute for direct patient observation and assessment by the clinician. If not familiar with the equipment or when concerned about proper functioning of the equipment, the clinician may often be better off to not use it at all. Providers should always follow the manufacture's recommendations

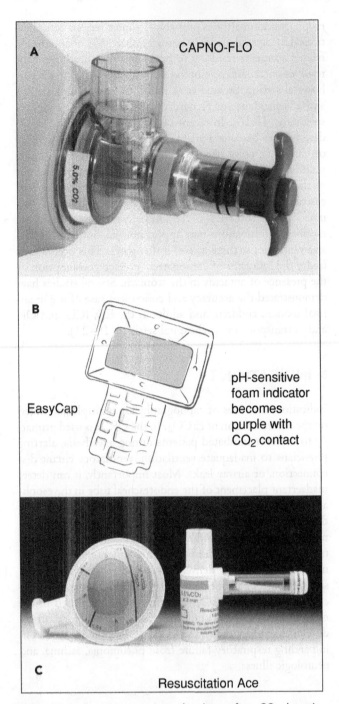

Figure 76.3 Capnometer using color change from CO_2 detection to verify endotracheal intubation.

regarding equipment setup, calibration, and maintenance and remember to place the sensor or sampling probe as close as possible to the patient-ventilator (bag) interface.

Appropriate and repeated clinical evaluation of the ABCs is indicated even when $EtCO_2$ monitoring is in place. In the prehospital care setting, the colorimetric capnometers are very practical. Once a patient is intubated, the clinician should ensure that the endotracheal tube is in the correct place clinically, which is accomplished by assessing the patient's

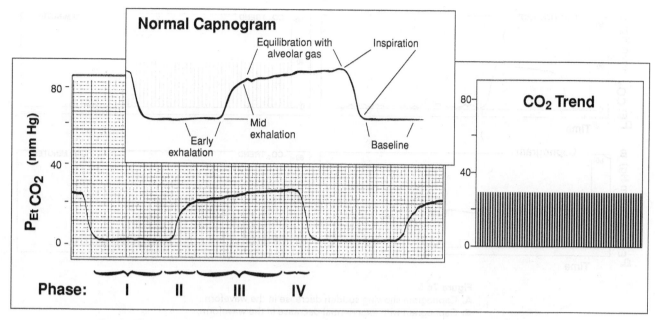

Figure 76.4 Normal capnogram: Phase I, baseline during inspiration; Phase II, CO_2 ascent during exhalation; Phase III, plateau of CO_2 measurement; Phase IV, CO_2 descent during early inspiration.

responsiveness, chest movements, breath sounds, and condensation of air in the endotracheal tube. If a disposable detector is available, the clinician should attach it to the endotracheal tube and then connect the Ambu bag to it. If CO_2 is present in concentrations indicating exhaled air from the trachea, the color will change after several breaths, confirming the position of the endotracheal tube within the trachea. These disposable units have some limitations. Because they may be affected adversely by humidity, they should not be used continuously for more than 2 hours. If used in conjunction with humidified oxygen, the disposable units may not remain reliable after 15 minutes of continuous use (28).

If a portable unit with mainstream or sidestream sampling is available, the unit is turned on and the analyzer (mainstream) or sampler (sidestream) is inserted in series with the endotracheal tube. After several breaths, the analyzer should be equilibrating EtCO2. In this case, the reading is presented to the operators on liquid display bar graphs in either mm Hg or volume % CO_2. Waveforms will be discussed in the following section on clinical applications.

In the hospital setting, EtCO2 modes have been incorporated into the ICU, OR, and ED monitors. Different EtCO2 manufactures have different ways of initiating or activating the EtCO2 probe. The operator should be familiar with the monitors used in his or her institution. These monitors usually have the capability to provide numerical and trend information on monitored ventilatory status. The process is the same. Once the airway has been established and clinically checked for position, the adaptor is attached to the end of the endotracheal tube and then connected to the Ambu bag or ventilator. In nonintubated patients, sidestream technology is more convenient. A nasal probe is placed in the patient's nostrils to collect gases for monitoring.

▶ CLINICAL APPLICATIONS

Capnogram: Normal Waveform

A normal capnogram is shown in Figure 76.4. It includes a zero baseline (or Phase I), which represents most of the early exhalation. This is followed by a sharp ascent (Phase II), which indicates the presence of CO_2 as the result of combined alveolar and dead space gas during midexhalation. Phase III represents the plateau; during this period, alveolar gas is measured. The end of this steady state represents the maximum CO_2 concentration exhaled. After this point, inspiration will bring fresh gas and the removal of CO_2 from the analyzer, causing a sharp downstroke and return to baseline (Phase IV). The continuous recording of these changes generates a CO_2 trend. In monitoring ventilated patients, the trend may be more critical for assessing the patient's ventilation than the absolute value of expired CO_2 at a given time, and for identifying specific events that may not be clinically apparent.

Abnormal Capnograms

Abnormal EtCO2 wave patterns have been associated with specific clinical situations. Elevations in the baseline from zero are unusual but generally not a risk for the patient; they indicate that CO_2 is being reinspired. They could represent a malfunction in the artificial ventilating system, a slow flow rate in the circuit, or extremely shallow respiration, causing the rebreathing of exhaled CO_2.

Decrease in the EtCO2 waveform (Phases II, III, and IV) may be sudden or exponential (Fig. 76.5). Both cases indicate an immediate danger or potential high-risk event. An EtCO2

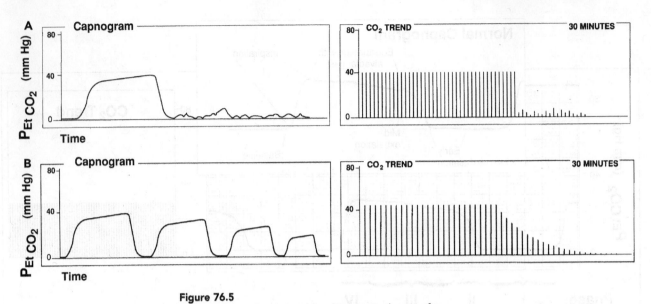

Figure 76.5
A. Capnogram showing sudden decrease in the waveform.
B. Capnogram with exponential decrease in the waveform.

wave that maintains near zero values could be the result of ventilator malfunction, patient extubation (esophageal intubation), or an obstructed endotracheal tube (Fig. 76.5A). In cases when pulmonary perfusion is compromised (i.e., shock, pulmonary embolism, cardiac arrest), an exponential decrease occurs (Fig. 76.5B) in the $EtCO_2$ waveform as the result of a functional increase in dead space ventilation from lung units not being perfused.

Steady rises in the CO_2 trend may be associated with hypoventilation, partial airway obstruction, or an increase in CO_2 production associated with a rising body temperature or increased metabolism (Table 76.1). If the trend shows a rapid rise in $EtCO_2$, malignant hyperthermia should be considered as a possibility (Fig. 76.6A). Conversely, a low $EtCO_2$ trend

may indicate hyperventilation or an increase in dead space ventilation resulting, for example, from asthma, pneumonia, or pulmonary embolism (Fig. 76.6B).

▶ COMPLICATIONS

As with other monitoring equipment, most of the problems or complications associated with $EtCO_2$ monitoring are directly related to a mechanical malfunction or misinterpretation of data by the operator. Most of these situations, such as esophageal intubation, ventilator malfunction, complete or partial obstruction of the endotracheal tube, and rebreathing of CO_2, have been discussed previously. Misinterpretation occurs when the operator does not understand changes in the baseline or waveforms based on the physiology of gas exchange, which can lead to an inappropriate reaction.

The initial capnometers were impractical for pediatric patients. Those using mainstream sampling had a bulky airway adaptor positioned on the endotracheal tube that added significant weight to the tube, increasing the risk of unplanned extubation or changes in endotracheal tube location. The adaptor required to accommodate the sensor housing also created a problem by increasing the dead space in the ventilator circuit when it was attached in series on the circuit. This was of concern especially in small children. New designs have made available disposable and portable equipment that has minimized or solved these problems.

All capnography readings should be correlated with the clinical presentation, and the clinical evaluation should be used to intervene when in doubt. Capnometers using sidestream sampling have a main disadvantage: if water and mucus obstruct the flow of gas to the analyzer, occasionally falsely low

TABLE 76.1	CONDITIONS THAT AFFECT THE ASSESSMENT OF END-TIDAL CO_2

Conditions that may lead to an underassessment of end-tidal CO_2
   Esophageal intubation
   Shock
   Cardiopulmonary arrest
   Asthma
   Pneumonia
   Pulmonary embolism
   Hyperventilation
   Hypothermia
   Accidental extubation or endotracheal tube obstruction
Conditions that increase end-tidal CO_2
   Hypoventilation
   Hyperthermia
   Administration of bicarbonate

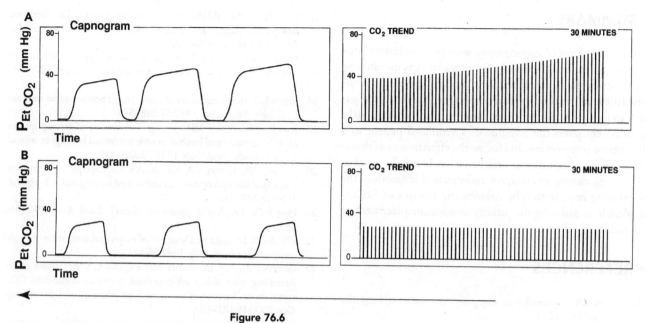

Figure 76.6
A. Capnogram with rise in CO₂ trend.
B. Capnogram with low CO₂ trend.

EtCO₂ readings are obtained. It is also important to note that if ventilator flow rates are high and the tidal volume is small, some of the inhaled gases will be aspirated with the exhaled gas and may give a falsely low CO₂ reading. In general, patients with severely diminished pulmonary flow (e.g., during CPR) may present with falsely low EtCO₂ results (29–32).

Problems associated with the disposable colorimetric units are related to duration of use. Although they are not affected by temperature, they are affected by humidity. For this reason, if used for too long, they will not give accurate results. In cases when humidified O₂ is used, they may not be accurate after even 15 minutes. Contamination of the indicator with secretions, gastric contents, or endotracheal drugs used during resuscitation can produce permanent yellow discoloration of the detector. In this case, a new detector should be used (30,33–35).

 SUMMARY

1 Once the patient's airway has been secured and the position of the endotracheal tube has been clinically confirmed, the clinician should use an EtCO₂ monitor to reconfirm the position and monitor ventilation.

2 If a disposable colorimetric EtCO₂ monitor is used, it must be attached to the endotracheal tube. It takes approximately six breaths to change the color of the membrane in the presence of CO₂. If no changes in color are noted, the patient's airway should be evaluated immediately, and if doubt exists, removal of the endotracheal tube and bag-mask ventilation should be initiated.

3 If an infrared capnometer is used, the operator should evaluate the quality of the curve and the numeric values in relation to the clinical presentation before making any changes in the patient's management.

 CLINICAL TIPS

▶ Become familiar with the equipment available before using.

▶ Always assess the adequacy of endotracheal tube placement clinically. Follow the ABCs and then use the CO₂ indicator to confirm endotracheal tube position.

▶ Esophageal intubation, if near the airway, may closely mimic the EtCO₂ pattern of tracheal intubation.

▶ When using a disposable unit, use the pediatric size for patients weighing 1 to 15 kg; avoid its use in patients less than 1 kg.

▶ Avoid prolonged use of the colorimetric indicators and be aware of their limited life when used in conjunction with humidified oxygen.

▶ SUMMARY

The combination of capnography with pulse oximetry provides complete and continuous (noninvasive) gas monitoring for the critically ill or injured ventilated patient in the pediatric ED. It can be used to great advantage in the intubated patient to follow the patient's ventilatory function continuously, immediately assess the response of a ventilated patient to a therapeutic intervention, and follow the effectiveness of therapies during cardiopulmonary resuscitation. In a prehospital or ED setting during an emergent endotracheal intubation, the monitoring or detection by colorimetric changes of $EtCO_2$ is valuable in assessing the patency or adequate placement of the endotracheal tube.

▶ REFERENCES

1. Sanders AB. Capnometry in emergency medicine. *Ann Emerg Med.* 1989;18:1287–1290.
2. Nobel JJ. Carbon dioxide monitors: exhaled gas (capnographs, capnometry, end tidal CO_2 monitors). *Pediatr Emerg Care.* 1993;9:244–246.
3. Gravenstein JS, Paulus DA, Hayes TJ. Clinical indications. In: Gravenstein JS, Paulus DA, Hayes TJ, eds. *Capnography in Clinical Practice.* Stoneham, MA: Butterworth Publishers; 1989:43–49.
4. Bhende MS. End-tidal carbon dioxide monitoring in pediatrics: clinical applications. *J Postgrad Med.* 2001;47:215–218.
5. Kalenda Z. Capnography during anesthesia and intensive care. *Acta Anaesthesiol Belg.* 1978;29:3.
6. Berman JA, Fuirgiure JJ, Marx GF. The Einstein CO_2 detector. *Anesthesiology.* 1984;60:613–614.
7. Katz SH, Falk JL. Misplaced endotracheal tubes by paramedics in an urban emergency medical services system. *Ann Emerg Med.* 2001;37:32–37.
8. Falk JL, Sayre MR. Confirmation of airway placement. *Prehosp Emerg Care.* 1999;3:273–278.
9. O'Connor R, Levine B. Airway management in the trauma setting. In: Ferrara PC, Colucciello SA, Marx J, et al. *Trauma Management: An Emergency Medicine Approach.* St. Louis: Mosby; 2001:39–51.
10. DeBoer S, Seaver M, Arndt K. Verification of endotracheal tube placement: a comparison of confirmation techniques and devices. *J Emerg Nurs.* 2003;29:444–450.
11. American Academy of Pediatrics. *NRP Instructor Update.* April 2004; 12(1):1, 4, 8. http://www.aap.org/nrp/pdf/nrp_sprsum03.pdf.
12. Burton GW. The value of CO_2 monitoring during anesthesia. *Anaesthesia.* 1966;21:173–183.
13. Craig I, Wilson ME. A survey of anesthetic misadventures. *Anaesthesia.* 1981;36:933–936.
14. Utting IE, Gray TC, Shelley FC. Human misadventure in anesthesia. *Can Anaesth Soc J.* 1979;26:472–478.
15. Stewart RD, Paris PM, Winter PM, et al. Field endotracheal intubation by paramedical personnel: success rates and complications. *Chest.* 1984;85:341–343.
16. Shea SR, MacDonald IR, Gruzinski G. Prehospital endotracheal tube airway or esophageal gastric tube airway: a critical comparison. *Ann Emerg Med.* 1985;14:102–112.
17. Linko K, Paloheim M, Tammisto T. Capnography for detection of accidental esophageal intubation. *Acta Anaesthiol Scand.* 1983;27:199–202.
18. Triner L. A simple maneuver to verify proper position of an endotracheal tube. *Anesthesiology.* 1982;57:548–549.
19. Sum Ping ST, Mehta MP, Symreng T. Reliability of capnography in identifying esophageal intubation with carbonated beverage or antacid in the stomach. *Anesth Analg.* 1991;73:333–337.
20. Garnett AR, Gervin CA, Gervin AS. Capnograph waveforms in esophageal intubation: effect of carbonated beverages. *Ann Emerg Med.* 1989;18:387–390.
21. Ping STS. Esophageal intubation [letter]. *Anesth Analg.* 1987;66:483.
22. Zbinden S, Schupfer G. Detection of esophageal intubation: the cola complication. *Anesth Analg.* 1987;66:483.
23. Gonzalez del Rey JA, Poirier MP, Digiulio GA. Evaluation of an Ambu-bag valve with a self-contained, colorimetric end-tidal CO_2 system in the detection of airway mishaps: an animal trial. *Pediatr Emerg Care.* 2000;16:121–123.
24. Soubani AO. Noninvasive monitoring of oxygen and carbon dioxide. *Am J Emerg Med.* 2001;19:141–146.
25. Jones BR, Dorsey MJ. Disposable end tidal CO_2 detector: minimal CO_2 requirements. *Anesthesiology.* 1989;71:A358.
26. Bhende MS, Thompson AE, Orr RA. Utility of an end tidal CO_2 detector during stabilization and transport of critically ill children. *Pediatrics.* 1992;89:1042–1044.
27. Bhende MS, Thompson AE, Howland DF. Validity of a disposable end tidal CO_2 detector in verifying endotracheal tube position in piglets. *Crit Care Med.* 1991;19:566–568.
28. Ponitz AL, Gravenstein N, Banner MJ. Humidity affecting a chemically based monitor of exhaled carbon dioxide [abstract]. *Anesthesiology.* 1990;73:A515.
29. MacLeod BA, Heller MB, Gerard J, et al. Verification of endotracheal tube placement with colorimetric end tidal CO_2 detection. *Ann Emerg Med.* 1991;20:267–270.
30. Ornato J, Shipley J, Racth EM, et al. Multicentre study of a portable, hand-size, colorimetric end tidal carbon dioxide detection device. *Ann Emerg Med.* 1992;21:518–523.
31. Varon AJ, Morrina J, Civetta JM. Clinical utility of a colorimetric end tidal CO_2 detector in cardiopulmonary resuscitation and emergency intubation. *J Clin Monit.* 1991;7:289–293.
32. Bhende MS, Gavula DP, Menegazzi JJ. Comparison of an end tidal CO_2 detector with a capnometer during CPR in a pediatric asphyxial arrest model [abstract]. *Pediatr Emerg Care.* 1991;7:383.
33. Bhende MS, Thompson AD. Gastric juice, drugs and end tidal carbon dioxide detectors [letter]. *Pediatrics.* 1992;90:1005.
34. Muir JD, Randalls PB, Smith GB. End tidal carbon dioxide detector for monitoring cardiopulmonary resuscitation [letter]. *BMJ.* 1990;301:41–42.
35. Hayes M, Higgins D, Yau EHS, et al. End tidal carbon dioxide detector for monitoring cardiopulmonary resuscitation [letter]. *BMJ.* 1990;301:42.

NIRANJAN KISSOON

77

Peak Flow Rate Measurement

▶ INTRODUCTION

Peak expiratory flow is the greatest flow that can be obtained during a forced expiration starting from full inflation of the lung (i.e., total lung capacity) (I). It is the most convenient of all indirect tests of ventilatory capacity. Peak expiratory flow rate (PEFR) assessment is an excellent tool for monitoring the severity of respiratory insufficiency from airway obstruction and for following the progress of children with lower airway obstruction such as asthma. PEFR assessment offers an objective and accurate measurement of lung function in asthma. The procedure is relatively simple to perform using a handheld spirometer. Recently, portable, handheld spirometers have become available for clinical use, and pager-sized monitoring systems are available for patient home recordings. PEFR assessment can be performed by the physician, nurse, or respiratory therapist in the emergency department (ED) or office setting or by a properly trained individual at home or at school. To obtain reliable results, full cooperation of the patient is required, making the test generally useful only for children older than about 5 years of age. The ability to successfully complete the procedure varies widely in the 5- to 7-year age group. Results may not reflect the severity of airway obstruction in patients who are not fully cooperative and delivering a full effort. Therefore, PEFR assessment should not be attempted in severely symptomatic patients before emergency bronchodilator therapy.

PEFR measurement has been endorsed by the National Asthma Education Program (2) for assessing the degree of airflow obstruction and severity, monitoring response to therapy, diagnosing exercise-induced asthma, and detecting asymptomatic deterioration. To help an asthma patient use home PEFR monitoring, a system of PEFR zones can be established based on the patient's personal best PEFR or the predicted value for the patient's height (3,4). When the zone system is

adapted to a traffic light pattern for the zones, it may be easier to use and remember. The following are the common guidelines used: green (80% to 100% of personal best) signals all is clear (i.e., no asthma symptoms are present), yellow (50% to 80% of personal best) signals caution (i.e., an acute exacerbation may be present), and red (below 50% of personal best) signals a medical alert. A medical alert indicates that a bronchodilator should be administered immediately and a clinician should be notified (2).

In the ED, PEFR assessment in a cooperative, trained patient is obtained with the help of a respiratory therapist, emergency physician, or nurse. Periodic assessments may be required at baseline and post β-agonist therapy to demonstrate reversibility (minimum of 15% improvement) and reassure patients and families that the drug is effective and pulmonary function has improved. PEFR assessment is an effort-dependent procedure, which means that the best result requires a fully cooperative patient. A supervisor needs to closely monitor, coach, and give cues to the patient in order to ensure optimal performance.

▶ ANATOMY AND PHYSIOLOGY

The airway and lung anatomy of children differs from that of adults. The chest wall in young children is more compliant than in adults. This tends to enhance ventilation by requiring small efforts for tidal breathing in the healthy child. As children grow, the chest wall becomes more stiff (less compliant), and recoil of the lung on expiration is more effortless. The pressure necessary to expand the lungs is increased in pathophysiologic states that reduce the lung compliance or increase the "stiffness" of the lungs. Airflow resistance is an important determinant of respiration and is greatest in the upper and nasal airway during inspiration and greatest on

763

expiration in the intrathoracic airways. In addition, the airways of young children are relatively narrow compared with those of adults. Because flow is related to the radius of the airway to the fourth power, small reductions in the airway caliber in children due to inflammatory processes greatly reduce the flow of air per given amount of generated work. In the healthy state, these differences lead to minimal effort in chest expansion and airway ventilation. The growth of the distal airways lags behind that of the proximal airway in the first 5 years of life. These narrow distal airways account for high peripheral airway pressures necessary to optimize air flow.

In lower airway disease such as asthma, airway narrowing is caused by bronchial smooth muscle constriction, airway inflammation, and increased mucous production. This inflammation affects more distal small airways not measurable by the PEFR. Small airway measurements such as the mid-expiratory flow rate (FEF_{25-75}) more accurately relate to the small airways. Air trapping associated with airway obstruction of the small airways places the end of inspiration and the initiation of expiration higher on the flow-volume curve, where more effort is used for a given tidal volume change. Even with the patient's best effort, the exhalation of a breath from maximal inspiration (from total lung capacity) through the narrowed airways cannot produce the same maximal flow that occurs without this obstruction. The point of maximal flow in expiration (PEFR) is almost at the onset of expiration. It is expressed in liters per second, is effort dependent, and is a measure of large airway flow rates.

▶ INDICATIONS

Although it is not a sophisticated method of assessing pulmonary function, PEFR assessment provides objective evidence of the severity of airway obstruction and assists in judging the response to bronchodilator therapy. It can also provide warning signs of increasing severity of asthma or resistance to bronchodilator therapy.

Children will present to the ED because of increasing severity of symptoms or more commonly in status asthmaticus that has not responded to home therapy. Cough, dyspnea, and wheezing are the major clinical features, but presentation may vary with age. In some cases, children may present with persistent cough at night or during exercise, while in others, shortness of breath may be the predominant symptom. The degree of wheezing does not correlate well with the severity of the attacks, but the relative absence of wheezing in the presence of respiratory distress, poor air entry, or hypoxia signifies severe obstruction. The use of accessory muscles of respiration and the presence of pulsus paradoxus are other indicators of marked severity. However, these signs and symptoms are subjective, and hence objective measures of the severity of airway compromise can be useful adjuncts.

Peak flow monitoring in the ED is a useful objective tool to assist in the evaluation and treatment of children. Several indications for ED use are listed in Table 77.1. PEFR

TABLE 77.1	INDICATIONS FOR PEAK FLOW TESTING IN THE ED (AGE GREATER THAN 5 TO 7 YEARS)

Acute asthma in the cooperative patient to grade severity of airway obstruction
Monitoring the response to therapy of the patient with acute asthma
Confirming the findings of home asthma program in acute asthma patients in the ED
Acute respiratory symptoms or signs suggestive of lower airway obstruction before and after bronchodilator response

measurements should be done in all patients with asthma in the ED who are able to perform this maneuver. In the ED, PEFR assessment will be useful as an adjunct in determining the need for bronchodilator therapy or admission. It is also useful when referring these patients to specialists and when discussing these patients via telephone. The importance of documenting and quantitating airway obstruction cannot be overemphasized, because patients' reports of their symptoms and physicians' physical findings may not correlate with the variability and severity of airflow obstruction (5,6). However, peak flow assessment should not be attempted in the severely compromised patient who is very dyspneic or in impending respiratory failure. Under these circumstances, therapy should be determined by clinical findings and other ancillary data such as transcutaneous oxygen saturation monitoring. Measurement of PEFR can then be used to follow clinical response to therapy.

▶ EQUIPMENT

A standard office peak flow meter is the simplest and easiest meter to use (7). Several peak flow meters are commercially available (Table 77.2). Specific instructions, including a step-by-step chart to assist in performing the maneuver, are contained in the literature accompanying each meter. Because different peak flow meter brands and models often yield different values when used by the same person, children should be encouraged to use the same model in the home, in the clinician's office, and, when possible, in the ED. Although meters may have different configurations, they all usually have a disposable mouthpiece and gauge (upright, horizontal, balls, arrows, etc.) and function on the same principles.

▶ PROCEDURE

PEFR measurement is one of a series of measurements that can be obtained from a full and maximal expiration starting from full inspiration. Patients must breathe in fully, seal lips completely around the mouthpiece, and blow out as fast and hard as possible for at least six seconds. The moment of most rapid expiratory flow, the peak flow, is brief and occurs early in the maximal expiratory effort (Fig. 77.1). As shown in the graph, peak flow occurs early and close to maximal lung

Name	Clinical range of flow	Manufacturer
AsmaPLAN+ peak flow meter	Standard range: 50–800 L/min	Vitalograph Lenexa, KS
Assess	Standard range 100–890 L/min Low range: 50–390 L/min	Respironics Health Scan Products Cedar Grove, NJ
Asthma Check	Standard: 60–810 L/min Low range: 50–390 L/min	Respironics Health Scan Products Cedar Grove, NJ
DeVilbiss peak flow meter	Standard range 50–720 L/min	Sunrise Medical Longmont, CO
Model 4200 peak flow meter	Standard range: 100–600 L/min Low range: 30–200 L/min	Boehringer Laboratories Norristown, PA
Peak Flow Meter	Standard range 50–750 L/min	Sammons Preston (Rolyan) Cedarburg, WI
Personal Best peak flow meter	Full range: 90–810 L/min Low range: 50–390 L/min	Respironics Health Scan Products Cedar Grove, NJ
Pocket Peak	Standard range: 50–720 L/min	Hudson RCI Temecula, CA
Truzone	Standard range: 60–800 L/min	Monaghan Medical Corp. Plattsburg, NY

Wright	Standard range: (2 scales)
	  Wright-McKerrow scale: 60–800 L/min
	  American Thoracic Society scale: 60–880 L/min
	Low range: (2 scales)
	  Wright-McKerrow scale: 30–370 L/min
	  American Thoracic Society scale: 30–400 L/min
		Clement Clark Inc.
		Columbus, OH

TABLE 77.2 COMMERCIALLY AVAILABLE SPIROMETERS FOR PEFR ASSESSMENT

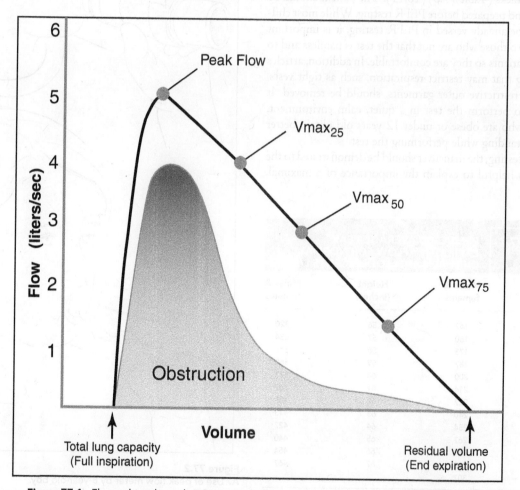

Figure 77.1 Flow-volume loop showing normal effort and loop showing reduced flow from lower airway obstruction.

volume, where variability and dependency on patient effort and muscular strength affect the reliability of the measurement. In addition, chest wall restriction from pain or tight clothing also may result in a suboptimal effort. These factors may result in a 10% to 15% variance of PEFR in a given subject on consecutive repeated best efforts with no change in clinical status. Clinicians should expect a minimum increase of 15% after bronchodilator treatment to substantiate clinically significant improvement. PEFR may be underestimated if the patient does not generate an adequate effort, if air leaks occur from the corners of the mouth (inadequate seal), or if the mouthpiece is blocked by the tongue. Conversely, a tremendous effort by a patient with lower airway obstruction may produce a close to normal peak flow by expulsion of air from compressible airways and may give the impression of better ventilation than is the case. Despite these limitations, PEFR can correlate well with other measures of lower airway obstruction, such as forced expiration volume (FEV) in 1 second (8,9).

The patient's demographic data (age, sex, height, weight) need to be obtained. Measured PEFRs are compared with the standard values for the same height and sex or with baseline values established by the patient during a healthy period between attacks (Table 77.3) (10,11). The patient should be educated and prepared before PEFR testing. While most children may be already versed in PEFR testing, it is important to explain to those who are not that the test is painless and to position patients so they are comfortable. In addition, articles of clothing that may restrict respiration, such as tight vests, belts, and restrictive outer garments, should be removed. It is better to perform the test in a quiet, calm environment. Children who are obese or under 12 years old obtain better results if standing while performing the test.

Before testing, the maneuver should be demonstrated to the child. It is helpful to explain the importance of a maximal,

prolonged effort to squeeze as much air out of the lungs as possible. It is a good idea to demonstrate by blowing into a similar mouthpiece reserved for that purpose. The child should then be instructed to take a few slow breaths and then breathe in as much as possible. The child should then hold his or her breath and concentrate on proper placement of the mouthpiece (Fig. 77.2). The mouthpiece should be placed in the mouth and the lips closed around it to prevent air

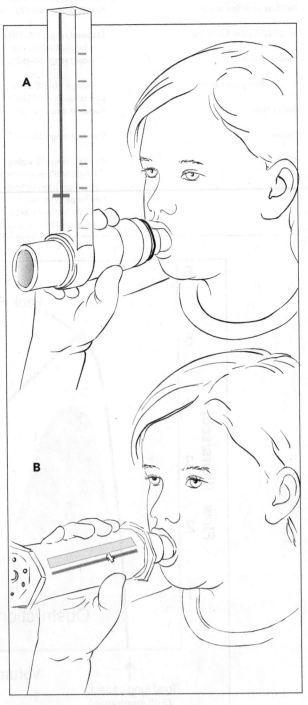

Figure 77.2
A. Use of peak flow meter by 8-year-old boy.
B. Peak flow meter with targeted green and red zone for a normal and reduced PEFR.

TABLE 77.3	PREDICTED AVERAGE PEAK EXPIRATORY FLOW FOR NORMAL CHILDREN AND ADOLESCENTS L/MIN		
Height (inches)	**Males & females**	**Height (inches)**	**Males & females**
43	147	56	320
44	160	57	334
45	173	58	347
46	187	59	360
47	200	60	373
48	214	61	387
49	227	62	400
50	240	63	413
51	254	64	427
52	267	65	440
53	280	66	454
54	293	67	467
55	307		

Adapted from Polger G, Promedhar V. Pulmonary function testing in children techniques and standards. Philadelphia: WB Saunders; 1971.

from escaping between the lips and the meter. It also should be placed on the top of the tongue so that the tongue will not obstruct the meter. The hole at the back of the meter from which the breath exits should not be obstructed by the patient's hands when the meter is held properly. The child then should blow out as hard as possible.

During the procedure verbal prompting and cheerleading such as "start now, blast off, hard and fast" usually results in a greater effort during exhalation. The operator should maintain close attention to the patient to discourage distractions during the procedure. A useful trick to maximize effort is to ask the child to take a deep breath in and "blow out the candles on a birthday cake" a few feet away.

The goal of testing is to obtain at least two test results that appear acceptable and reproducible. Because it is common for PEFR variation in testing of up to 10%, results that are closer to each other for several attempts are of the greatest value. The highest PEFR obtained is considered to be the most representative. Problems that may produce unacceptable results include a slow start of exhalation, coughing during the procedure, and premature termination of the effort. Recognition of these are important for successful testing. These faults

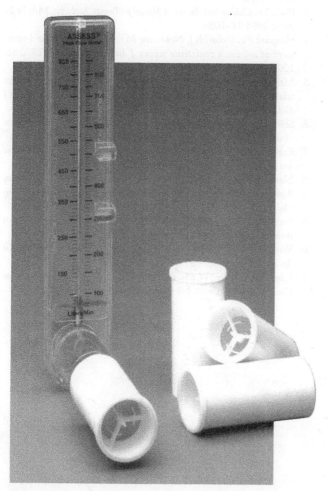

Figure 77.3 Peak flow meter attached to side measure with zone clips to assist in setting levels of management.

SUMMARY

1 Perform clinical evaluation, including assessment of degree of airway obstruction. If moderately severe obstruction is present, administer β-agonist aerosol with supplemental oxygen to the patient.

2 Determine if the patient is capable of performing the maneuver. Has the patient done the maneuver before? Exclude all children younger than 5 years of age except where the procedure is elective.

3 Obtain demographic data (age, sex, height, weight) to enable a review of the standard for the particular patient. Obtain the history of personal best PEFRs when available.

4 Review the procedure with patient, including a demonstration on how to hold the meter, how to purse the lips around the meter, and how to perform the maximal inspiratory effort and expiratory maneuver. Demonstrating the procedure yourself may be most helpful.

5 Have the patient take a few normal breaths.

6 Have the patient make a maximal inspiratory effort and hold the breath at full inspiration.

7 Have the patient place the meter in the mouth and over the tongue.

8 Have the patient *maximally exhale* to full end expiration; coach the patient to best effort.

9 Have the patient breathe normally for a minimum of 30 to 60 seconds.

10 Have the patient repeat the PEFR test two to three times to obtain the best result.

11 Assume the "best" PEFR obtained is the patient's current PEFR.

12 Establish the percentage predicted from the chart.

should be identified and explained to the patient in an effort to eliminate them on the next try.

PEFR testing is sometimes useful in determining the efficacy of bronchodilator therapy (Fig. 77.3). In these instances, the best of three measurements, as previously outlined, should be accepted as the PEFR. The testing should be done a minimum of 10 minutes after inhaled bronchodilators or at the end of the time of observation before another intervention or before discharge.

▶ COMPLICATIONS

Spirometry may provoke an increase in airways obstruction in a few patients with asthma. If this occurs, it should be

CLINICAL TIPS

▶ Avoid the maneuver in patients with severe airway obstruction, as it may worsen bronchospasm acutely.

▶ Do not attempt in a child less than 5 to 7 years of age unless the child has previous experience before the present ED visit.

▶ Review the procedure before the patient performs it.

▶ Be sure the patient has a tight seal on the mouthpiece, the exhalation hole on the meter is not blocked, and the meter measuring gauge is unimpeded by the patient.

▶ Coach the patient with encouraging words during the maneuver.

▶ Take the best of three measures for the current peak flow.

▶ If done after use of a bronchodilator, wait 10 to 15 minutes to obtain an adequate response. A clinically relevant bronchodilator response is an improvement in PEFR of greater than 15%.

▶ Check the result against the standard for this child or against the standard nomograms for the patient's size.

▶ Observe the technique for:
  ▶ Poor maximal inspiration
  ▶ Less than maximal effort
  ▶ Occlusion of the exhalation hole or gauge
  ▶ Premature cessation of the exhalation

immediately brought to the attention of a physician. An inhaled bronchodilator may be necessary to relieve this obstruction. Performing spirometry can delay administration of bronchodilators or supplemental oxygen, which can be harmful in severe status asthmaticus. Improper techniques will yield incorrect results, which may lead to over- or undertreatment with bronchodilators.

▶ SUMMARY

Peak flow measurement is a relatively simple and useful objective measurement of large airway obstruction in the lower airways. It is useful for titration of therapy and early identification of worsening of symptoms. Proper performance relies on the cooperation of the patient and is generally not possible in children less than 5 years of age.

▶ REFERENCES

1. National Heart, Lungs and Blood Institute. *Guidelines for the Diagnosis and Management of Asthma.* Expert Panel Report 2. Washington, DC: U.S. Government Printing Office; 1997. Pub No. 97-4051.
2. American Thoracic Society, Committee on Proficiency Standards for Clinical Pulmonary Function Laboratories. Standardization of spirometry: 1994 update. *Am J Respir Crit Care Med.* 1994;152:1007–1036.
3. Plaut TF. *Children with Asthma: A Manual for Parents.* Amherst, MA: Pedipress; 1988:94–108.
4. Hargeave FE, Dolovich J, Newhouse MT. The assessment and treatment of asthma: a conference report. *J Allergy Clin Immunol.* 1990;85:1098–1111.
5. McFadden ER Jr, Kiser R, DeGroot WJ. Acute bronchial asthma: relationships between clinical and physiologic manifestations. *N Engl J Med.* 1973;288:221–225.
6. Shim CS, Williams H. Relationship of wheezing to the severity of obstruction in asthma. *Arch Intern Med.* 1983;143:890–892.
7. Enright PL, Hyatt RE. *Office Spirometer: A Practical Guide to the Selection and Use of Spirometers.* Philadelphia: Lea & Febiger; 1987.
8. Nowak RM, Pensler MI, Parker DD. Comparison of peak expiratory flow and FEV: admission criteria for acute bronchial asthma. *Ann Emerg Med.* 1982;11:64–69.
9. Eichenhorn MS, Beauchamp RK, Harper PA, et al. An assessment of three portable peak flow meters. *Chest.* 1982;82:306–309.
10. Weng T, Levison H. Standards of pulmonary function in children. *Am Rev Respir Dis.* 1969;99:879–894.
11. Rarey KP, Youtsey JW, eds. *Pulmonary Function Testing in Respiratory Patient Care.* Englewood Cliffs, NJ: Prentice Hall; 1981:328–330.

MORTON E. SALOMON AND FRANK A. ILLUZZI

78

Use of Metered Dose Inhalers, Spacers, Dry Powder Inhalers, and Nebulizers

▶ INTRODUCTION

Respiratory diseases such as asthma, croup, and bronchopulmonary dysplasia (BPD) are among the most common childhood diseases and account for 10% to 15% of visits to the emergency department (ED) each year. Medications delivered by inhalation are being used with increasing frequency to treat respiratory disease, both acutely and on a maintenance basis. Aerosol therapy permits the delivery of small quantities of medication directly to the site of action (1–3).

Studies comparing the effectiveness of medications delivered via inhalation with that of oral or parenteral delivery have demonstrated that the inhalation route provides more rapid onset, equal duration of activity, and comparable improvement in pulmonary function testing, with fewer side effects (2–5). Because inhalation therapy can be administered without painful or invasive procedures, it also has the added benefit of eliciting less fear and resistance when a child visits the ED. Inhalation treatment should be viewed as a significant therapeutic advance and is now the mainstay of our treatment for many respiratory illnesses, particularly asthma.

▶ ANATOMY AND PHYSIOLOGY

Lung Receptor Pathophysiology

The human respiratory system is under the control of the nervous system through autonomic nerve fibers originating in cranial nerve X. It is also controlled by multiple receptor sites with or without accompanying nerve fibers.

Autonomic influences on the lung are contributed by parasympathetic (cholinergic) forces and by sympathetic (adrenergic) receptors. The adrenergic system contains both α- and β-receptors.

Parasympathetic innervation is provided by fibers of the vagus nerve. Stimulation of the parasympathetic efferent fibers causes bronchoconstriction of the large and midsize airways, increased mucous gland secretion, and vascular dilatation. Postganglionic parasympathetic fibers terminate in bronchial smooth muscle, mucus-secreting goblet cells, and mast cells. These parasympathetic nerve fibers are present from the trachea to the bronchioles but are found in greatest density in midsize airways 3 to 8 mm in diameter. These same parasympathetic effects also can be induced by direct administration of cholinergic agents such as acetylcholine and methacholine (6).

The parasympathetic nervous system plays a role in airway response to irritants through what is referred to as the vagally mediated "cholinergic reflex." When specific irritants activate receptors in the airways, these receptors initiate impulses via afferent fibers of the vagal system. The afferent vagal stimuli trigger reflexive responses via efferent fibers that release acetylcholine at multiple neuroeffector sites, leading to bronchoconstriction, mucus secretion, and mediator release from mast cells and cell membranes. This cholinergic reflex can be triggered by immunologic or nonimmunologic stimuli. The role of this parasympathetic reflex in chronic hyperreactive airway diseases, such as bronchitis and asthma, is not well defined and is likely to vary from one patient to another. Moreover, the cholinergic reflex is not the only mechanism by which irritants exert influence on the airways (6).

Sympathetic nerve fibers have not been found in the tracheobronchial tree of the human lung. Adrenergic influences on the lung are exerted at α- and β-receptor sites that receive no neuronal innervation. These adrenergic receptors are found in bronchial smooth muscle, blood vessels, and goblet cells and can be stimulated by either sympathomimetic endogenous agents (e.g., epinephrine) or exogenous agonists (e.g., terbutaline).

In contrast to parasympathetic receptors, adrenergic receptors are mostly concentrated in the smaller peripheral airways. Stimulation of β-receptors produces smooth muscle relaxation and subsequent bronchodilatation. β-agonists also are potent inhibitors of mast cell release and thus exert a strong anti-inflammatory effect. This anti-inflammatory control is most effective in the earliest phases of inflammation. Prolonged inflammation, with late phase reaction, is not as responsive to β-agonist stimulation. Glucocorticoids, in fact, exert some of their anti-inflammatory effect by restoring the availability and binding affinity of β-receptors (6).

At the intracellular level, cholinergic and adrenergic receptor stimulation is mediated by alterations in cyclic AMP and cyclic GMP. Increases in cyclic AMP (c-AMP) relax bronchial smooth muscle and inhibit mast cell degranulation. Increases in cyclic GMP (c-GMP) exert the opposite effect, contracting smooth muscle and stimulating mast cell release. Stimulation of parasympathetic effectors produces increases in intracellular c-GMP. Conversely, β-adrenergic stimulation increases c-AMP, whereas α-receptor stimulation decreases c-AMP (6). Thus, β-sympathomimetic activity produces bronchial relaxation, and both parasympathetic activity and α-sympathetic activity produce bronchoconstriction. Excessive parasympathetic tone, excessive α-sympathetic stimulation, or β-sympathetic blockade may be the predominant cause of hyper-reactive airways in different patients.

Two common categories of medication available by aerosol and used to treat common pulmonary illnesses are β-adrenergic agonists and parasympathetic antagonists. β_2-agonists relax bronchial smooth muscle, producing bronchodilatation; inhibit inflammatory mediator release from mast cells; and stimulate mucociliary clearance. These effects are produced by activating adenyl cyclase with subsequent increased intracellular c-AMP.

Parasympatholytic agents include atropine and its derivatives. They are competitive inhibitors of acetylcholine at the neuroeffector junction and block the cholinergic reflex and parasympathetic receptor stimulation, thereby preventing a rise in intracellular c-GMP. The net effect, therefore, is to inhibit bronchoconstriction. Anticholinergic agents currently available for aerosolized treatment include atropine sulfate, which may lead to significant side effects when used in therapeutic respiratory doses, and ipratropium, a quaternary derivative of atropine that has a much wider therapeutic margin. Theoretically, α-adrenergic blocking agents should have a beneficial effect in the treatment of bronchoconstrictive respiratory diseases. By blocking α-stimulation and thereby inhibiting decreases in c-AMP, α-blockers should enhance bronchodilation. To date, however, α-receptor blockers have not been shown to have a convincing role in treating asthma or bronchitis. Their application is usually reserved for the patient with severe disease who is already being treated maximally with other agents (6).

Inflammation, not bronchospasm, is the basic pathologic condition encountered in chronic asthma. Airway inflammation results from injury to the lung possibly caused by trauma, inhalation of noxious or toxic or allergenic substances, respiratory infection, or even systemic infection. The most common chronic inflammatory disease of the lung is asthma.

Once triggered by injurious stimuli, the inflammatory process starts with the release of several chemical mediators from mast cells, leukocytes, and endothelial cell phospholipids. Chemical mediators in turn activate specific receptor sites on the cell wall surface of the lung. These receptors then decrease c-AMP concentration or increase calcium ion concentration inside the cell. The net result includes smooth muscle contraction, chemotaxis of inflammatory cells, microvascular leaks, increased mucus secretion, and parasympathetic neuronal reflex stimulation. The immediate response to fast-acting inflammatory mediators, such as histamine, is primarily bronchoconstriction. This reaction often responds to bronchodilators. If the inflammatory response continues and the slower-acting metabolites of arachidonic acid accumulate, mucosal swelling, mucus secretion, and desquamation of cells occur. This produces a late-phase inflammatory response that is less sensitive to bronchodilator therapy (6).

Corticosteroids exert an anti-inflammatory response principally by stabilizing mast cells. They also restore the availability and sensitivity of β-agonist receptors. The glucocorticoids currently used for aerosol therapy are synthetic analogs of hydrocortisone. When compared with cortisol or dexamethasone, they have the distinct advantage of having less systemic absorption, rapid inactivation when reaching the central circulation, high local potency in the lung, and less systemic potency. The aerosolized glucocorticoids currently in use in the United States via metered dose inhalers (MDIs) include beclomethasone, triamcinolone, and flunisolide. The glucocorticoids commonly available via dry powder inhalers (DPIs) include fluticasone and budesonide.

Aerosols

An aerosol is a suspension of either solid particles or liquid droplets in a stream of air. By incorporating medication in these droplets, aerosols can deliver therapy directly to the lung. Large droplets are often trapped and filtered by the upper airway. To be effective in treating respiratory illnesses, the droplets must reach their receptor sites in the smaller airways. Drug delivery to the peripheral lung depends on three factors: aerosol droplet size, inspiratory flow, and disease state in the lung (1,2).

Droplets created by jet nebulizers and MDIs vary in size. Droplets greater than 8 μm are always deposited in the mouth and nasopharynx by inertial impaction. β-Agonists are not well absorbed by this mucosa and therefore will not exert any demonstrable effects (1).

To reach the distal airways, droplets must be less than 5 μm in size. Once they reach the bronchiole, they settle out by gravitational sedimentation. However, very small droplets (less than 1 μm) generally remain suspended in the airstream and are exhaled without deposition on the tissue surface (1).

Regardless of droplet size, particles are unlikely to get beyond the oropharynx if significant turbulence occurs in the airstream. Turbulence can be created by rapid inspiratory flow rates, partial mechanical obstructions, or sudden changes in airstream direction. Inspiratory flow rates through the patient's airways greater than 1.0 L/sec will create turbulent airflow. Under these conditions, inertial forces keep droplets from remaining suspended in the mainstream, and droplets of any size will deposit on the nasal and oropharyngeal airways. At slower inspiratory rates—generally less than 0.5 L/sec—laminar airflow is evident, and the droplets may reach the peripheral lung. Slow flow rates of less than 0.5 L/sec are best achieved by inhalations of 6-second duration. The airstream slows even further on reaching the smaller airways, allowing the droplets to deposit by gravitational sedimentation. Sedimentation at peripheral sites can be further enhanced by breath holding at the end of inspiration, which postpones the reversal of airflow (1,2).

Airflow through diseased airways, narrowed by spasm, edema, or mucus, is much more turbulent than through healthy airways. More drug is deposited before reaching the targeted airways. This may lead to the patient with acute respiratory illness requiring larger doses of aerosolized medication to obtain the same therapeutic effect.

▶ INDICATIONS

Aerosol therapy is most commonly applied in pediatric emergency settings to the treatment of asthma, bronchiolitis, bronchopulmonary dysplasia (BPD), and laryngotracheobronchitis (LTB).

Asthma is the most common chronic disease of childhood, affecting up to 15% of the pediatric population in the United States. It is characterized by hyper-responsive airways that are prone to develop edema, mucus hypersecretion, and muscular constriction in response to offending stimuli. Triggers most commonly associated with airway inflammation in asthmatics include inhaled irritants such as cigarette smoke, changes in weather, exposure to cold air, exercise, environmental allergens, and minor respiratory illnesses such as sinusitis and otitis. Patients with asthma generally manifest their airway hyperactivity with symptoms such as cough and wheezing. In more severe cases, patients also will have shortness of breath, tachypnea, retractions, diminished peak expiratory flow rates, and hypoxia. Aerosolized medications are currently the mainstay of bronchodilator therapy for asthma. Corticosteroids and sodium cromolyn are anti-inflammatory agents commonly used in children to reduce the inflammatory aspects of exacerbations. Inhaled β-agonists, such as albuterol, are used as both prophylactic therapy and acute therapy. The role of inhaled anticholinergic agents in the treatment of acute childhood asthma is not as well substantiated, although these agents are known to have measurable bronchodilator effect. Atropine sulfate is available only as a nebulizer solution. Ipra-

tropium bromide, an anticholinergic agent with much fewer side effects than atropine, is available in the United States in a metered dose inhaler and as a nebulizer solution (7). Inhaled ipratropium added to albuterol demonstrates added benefit in children with acute severe asthma and leads to fewer admissions (8).

Bronchiolitis is a pulmonary infection generally occurring in late fall and winter that mostly affects young infants. Its peak incidence occurs between the age of 2 and 8 months. Bronchiolitis is characterized by coryza and cough progressing to wheezing, prolonged expiration, and respiratory distress. Most cases of bronchiolitis are caused by respiratory syncytial virus (RSV), but other viruses such as parainfluenza and influenza can be isolated from patients with this illness. Mild bronchiolitis has been treated with nebulized bronchodilators, such as albuterol, and improved symptoms and signs are found in subgroups of patients. Corticosteroids are not clearly beneficial but are under investigation. In some children, however, it is difficult to differentiate acute asthma from bronchiolitis, because the symptoms are so similar. Aerosolized ribavirin can be effective in ameliorating the course of severe bronchiolitis caused by RSV when administered continuously over a 3- to 5-day period in high-risk patients (9,10). This antiviral agent is not commonly useful and is generally reserved for patients with severe respiratory compromise or an underlying illness such as congenital heart disease or BPD (7,10).

Bronchopulmonary dysplasia (BPD) is a chronic pulmonary disorder of infancy that results from treatment by mechanical ventilation of hyaline membrane disease or other congenital lung disorders. It generally occurs in newborns undergoing prolonged ventilation during the first several weeks of life. Approximately 15% of premature infants develop BPD. Its etiology has been ascribed to many factors, including high concentrations of oxygen and barotrauma from positive pressure ventilation. Infants with BPD often have chronic tachypnea, wheezing, and asymmetric breath sounds. In more severe cases, arterial blood gases show chronic hypercarbia and hypoxia. Chest radiographs of BPD patients usually demonstrate hyperinflation and interstitial nodularity or multiple cystic areas. Home management of patients with BPD and treatment of acute exacerbations of respiratory difficulties can be similar to the treatment of asthma. These patients are frequently improved with daily nebulized β-agonists and occasionally by aerosolized corticosteroids. Acute exacerbations are treated by intensified β-agonist treatment, systemic steroids, and other therapies as necessary (7).

Laryngotracheobronchitis (LTB), or croup, is a viral infection of the upper airways affecting the larynx, trachea, and bronchi. Sixty percent of cases appear to be caused by parainfluenza virus, mostly in early fall. Influenza virus, adenovirus, and RSV also have been recovered from croup patients. LTB is characterized by mild to moderate fever, barking cough, and inspiratory stridor. Croup is the most common cause of stridor in childhood. Milder cases can be treated simply with normal saline mist. Moderate to severe bouts of LTB receive treatment with either racemic or L-epinephrine in a nebulized

TABLE 78.1	AVAILABLE FORMATS		
	MDIs	**DPI**	**Nebulizer**
β-Agonists	✓	✓	✓
Corticosteroids	✓	✓	X
Sodium cromolyn	✓	✓	✓
N-acetylcysteine	X	X	✓
Ipratropium	✓	✓	✓
Atropine	X	X	✓
Nystatin suspension	X	X	✓
Pentamadine	X	X	✓
Racemic and L-epinephrine	X	X	✓

format. Studies have demonstrated a role for nebulized or systemic corticosteroids as well (11).

In patients with cystic fibrosis, aminoglycosides can be aerosolized to suppress *Pseudomonas aeruginosa* and other organisms. Aerosolized pentamidine is indicated for prophylaxis against pneumocystis carinii in patients over the age of 5 years who have AIDS and are unable to tolerate trimethoprim-sulfa (7).

Table 78.1 summarizes the medications available in the MDI format, in nebulized solution, or in both. A large variety of adrenergic medications are available by MDI, including nonselective β_1- and β_2-agonists such as epinephrine, isoproterenol, and metaproterenol and β_2-selective agents such as terbutaline, pirbuterol, and albuterol. Corticosteroids are currently only available in MDIs or DPIs for inhalation therapy. These preparations have been difficult to aerosolize when incorporated into nebulizer solutions.

All adrenergic drugs available in MDIs are also available for nebulization. Ipratropium and sodium cromolyn are similarly available in both MDI and nebulizer formats. Drugs only available in nebulizer format include atropine, ribavirin (which requires a special particle generator), pentamidine, racemic (L- and R-) epinephrine or L-epinephrine, and nystatin suspension (for laryngeal candidiasis) (1–3). Cromolyn powder also can be delivered using a spinhaler.

Spacers are small canisters that attach to MDIs to allow patients who cannot easily hold their breath to inhale their medication more effectively. Spacers are indicated for use with MDIs in patients who are likely to have difficulty correctly coordinating the MDI inhalation, such as younger patients (generally less than 10 years of age), neurologically impaired patients, patients with arthritis of the hands, and adults who are unable to master the MDI technique. Spacers also are helpful for patients of all ages with significant acute distress, who are more likely to have difficulty taking slow deep breaths and holding it at the end of inspiration. This may include anyone with acute respiratory distress. Indications for nebulizer use are similar to those for spacer need. Nebulizers are indicated for younger patients, patients with coordination problems, and patients with moderate to severe asthma or distress. Patients who are maintained chronically on β-agonist therapy by MDI or nebulizer at home often require higher and more

frequent doses during acute exacerbations of bronchospasm. Home use should not exceed a frequency of less than every 3 hours without physician contact. Failure to seek emergent care in a timely manner in patients on bronchodilators without anti-inflammatory therapy is an important contributor to asthma mortality. In the monitored setting, such as the hospital, MDIs can be used with significantly more intensity. One hospital regimen that has been suggested is four puffs over 2 minutes followed by one puff every minute until dyspnea is relieved or the patient develops a significant tremor (1). It is key to augment β-agonists with anti-inflammatory therapy early in the treatment course. Continuous nebulization therapy (CNT) should be applied only to patients with severe asthma, and its use restricted to the ED or a monitored inpatient setting. Indications for CNT might include patients whose chests are too tight to perform peak flow testing, patients with $PaCO_2$ greater than 40, and patients with asthma scores in the severe range. CNT is also indicated for hospitalized patients who repeatedly deteriorate clinically between β-agonist treatments performed every 1 to 2 hours (12).

▶ EQUIPMENT: TECHNICAL CONSIDERATIONS

Metered Dose Inhalers

A **metered dose inhaler** is an inhalation device that contains medication dissolved or suspended in a pressurized propellant solution. The MDI has two components—the drug canister and the inhalation device (Fig. 78.1). Within the canister, the therapeutic medication is mixed with the propellant at high pressure to maintain a liquid phase. The inhalation device consists of a hollow canister holder, an actuator, a valve, and a mouthpiece with cover. The actuator, when depressed, opens the valve. The valve is designed to release a precise, premeasured amount of aerosol with each actuation.

Sudden decompression of the liquid in the canister produces an aerosol of propellant plus medication. As the liquid exits the mouthpiece, heterodisperse (various size) particles average 35 μm in diameter. These large droplets travel away from the mouthpiece at a high velocity, and the propellant evaporates within a few centimeters, leaving smaller droplets consisting primarily of medication.

When the drug is released from the MDI, approximately 5% to 10% is deposited on the inhaler device or escapes into the air, and another 80% is deposited in the oropharynx and eventually swallowed. This means that only 10% to 15% of the drug released actually reaches the lung, even under ideal conditions. It is likely that only 3% of the total dose reaches the bronchioles and alveoli. The proportion of drug reaching the lung is greatly influenced by the patient's technique. Factors such as the position of the inhaler at the mouth, slow inspiratory flow rate, adequacy of breath holding, adequate interval between puffs of at least 1 minute, and volume of air inhaled can all influence the delivery of medication to the peripheral lung sites (2).

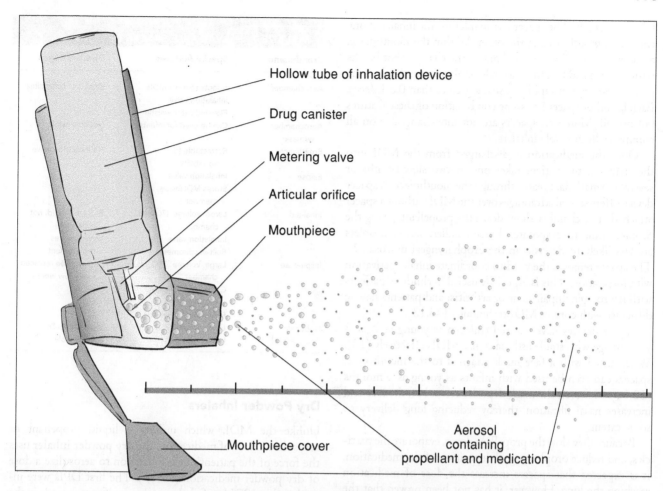

Hollow tube of inhalation device

Drug canister

Metering valve

Articular orifice

Mouthpiece

Mouthpiece cover

Aerosol containing propellant and medication

Figure 78.1 Metered dose inhaler with aerosol cloud.

Most package inserts instruct the patient to close the lips around the mouthpiece of the inhaler. However, the open mouth technique can deliver up to twice as much medication to the lower lung. By holding the inhaler 1 to 2 inches (two adult fingerbreadths) away from the mouth, less medication is deposited on the oropharynx. Studies have demonstrated that the open mouth technique produces less oropharyngeal deposition, more peripheral lung delivery, and better pulmonary function response (2). A variation on the open mouth technique has the patient hold the MDI between opened lips, which reduces the problems of improper aiming and provides the same pharmacologic benefits (2).

As mentioned, slow inspiratory flow rates create more laminar flow and deliver more drug to the distal airways. Ideally the patient should inhale the released medication for a minimum of 6 seconds (2). Breath holding at the end of inhalation allows more time for the inhaled medication to sediment on the lung surface. Breath holding for up to 10 seconds has been shown to incrementally increase drug absorption. Beyond 10 seconds, breath holding does not add benefit (2). If patients are unable to hold their breath for 10 seconds, they should do so as long as is comfortably possible. Larger, deeper breaths bring a larger tidal volume into the lung and more medication with it. Optimal dosing can be achieved by beginning with a

full exhalation to functional residual capacity, then inhaling. Such maneuvers are unnecessary, however, are likely to cause additional turbulence or coughing, and are difficult for acutely ill patients (1).

Theoretically, waiting several minutes between puffs of bronchodilator aerosol should enhance delivery of drug. The minimum time recommended is 1 minute. Allowing time for the first puff to exert some therapeutic effect should open the airway to deeper penetration by subsequent bursts. Moreover, if the patient is to receive both bronchodilator therapy and anti-inflammatory therapy, it would be logical to suppose that bronchodilator therapy should precede anti-inflammatory therapy. This would allow the anti-inflammatory to penetrate deeper after the bronchodilator exerts its benefit.

Although the mechanisms for optimizing drug delivery in MDIs are understood in some detail, studies have estimated that only 11% to 40% of adult patients use MDIs correctly (2,3).

Spacer Devices

Spacer devices are holding systems or reservoirs that collect the aerosol from an MDI, momentarily, before inhalation. The spacer holding chamber varies in volume but can be as large as 750 mL. The spacer has an inlet for the inhaler at one end and a mouthpiece at the other. Within the mouthpiece, a one-way valve allows aerosol out of the chamber but blocks return of exhaled breath. A whistle or alarm sounds when the patient inhales too rapidly (usually greater than 0.3 L/sec). Each brand of spacer has some combination of these features but not all. Moreover, spacers are not interchangeable on all commercially available inhalers.

Once the medication is discharged from the MDI into the chamber, the patient takes one or two slow breaths or several normal tidal breaths through the mouthpiece. A spacer device offers several advantages over the MDI without a spacer attached. The chamber slows down the propellant, giving the droplets time to evaporate. These smaller, slower droplets are less likely to deposit on the oropharyngeal mucosa (2). The spacer removes the need to coordinate inhaler activation with inspiration. This is especially useful in children, patients with neurologic impairment or arthritis, and patients having difficulty with correct MDI technique (1–3,13).

Spacer devices have allowed children as young as 2 or 3 years of age with stable asthma to use MDIs effectively (13). When fitted with a face mask attached to the mouthpiece, spacers can even be used with infants as young as 4 months (12,14). However, the mask deposits aerosol on the face and increases nasal filtration, thereby reducing lung delivery to some extent.

Because they slow the propellant down, evaporate the particles, and reduce oropharyngeal deposition of the medication, it is expected that spacers increase the dose of medication reaching the lung. However, it has not been proven that the amount of medication reaching the alveoli is increased. In terms of clinical benefits, studies have produced mixed results when comparing the bronchodilating effects of MDIs with spacers against MDIs used alone. Currently, it appears that spacer devices do not add any measurable clinical benefit when the MDI without spacer is used properly (1). Even results in children are inconclusive. However, it is safe to say that in both children and adults there is no drawback to the use of spacers, and they are likely to produce equivalent or better lung function with generally greater convenience (13).

By decreasing the oropharyngeal deposition of the medication, the spacer provides two particularly significant advantages when used with inhaled corticosteroid. It reduces the incidence of oropharyngeal candidiasis. In one study, the incidence decreased from 22% without spacer use to 0% with spacer use (2). Moreover, spacers also seem to decrease the systemic absorption of the steroid, indicated by reduced hypothalamic-pituitary-adrenal suppression (15,16).

Table 78.2 lists commonly available spacer devices and the particular advantages and disadvantages of each device. Of the currently available spacers, the Aerochamber is one of the best devices available for use with children. It adapts to the widest variety of MDIs, and it contains a flow indicator whistle that warns the child if he or she is inhaling too rapidly. The Aerochamber is also available with a face mask for use in children under 3 years of age.

TABLE 78.2	AVAILABLE SPACER DEVICES	
Brand name	**Special features**	**Disadvantages**
Aerochamber	Adapts to most MDIs Inhalation valve Flow indicator whistle	Rigid, not collapsible
Aerochamber w/mask	Can be used for infants	Not collapsible
Breathancer	Retractable for portability	No inhalation valve
Ellipse	Inhalation valve Stores MDI inside chamber	
Inhal-aid	Large volume (700 mL) chamber Inhalation valve Built-in spirometer	Bulky and rigid, not collapsible Valve requires replacement
Inspir-ease	Large volume (700 mL) chamber Collapsible for easy carrying Flow indicator whistle	Bag must be replaced every few weeks
Nebuhaler	Large volume (750 mL) Inhalation valve	Rigid and bulky, not collapsible

Dry Powder Inhalers

Unlike the MDI, which utilizes a liquid propellant to aerosolize a dose of medication, the **dry powder inhaler** uses the force of the patient's own inhalation to aerosolize a dose of dry powder medication (17,18). The first DPIs were introduced in 1971 but failed to make significant inroads in the United States until the 1987 Montreal Protocol promoted a phase out of CFCs as a propellant in MDIs (19,20). A list of their advantages and disadvantages is presented in Table 78.3.

While there are several types of DPIs on the market today, the basic configuration consists of a drug depository

TABLE 78.3	PROS AND CONS OF DRY POWDER INHALERS
Advantages	**Disadvantages**
Portable, convenient, and easy to use	More expensive to produce than MDIs
No spacer required	Multiple device types available; patients need specific instructions and training for each
At least as effective as MDIs with spacer at pulmonary drug delivery	
Higher resistance devices may be more effective at pulmonary drug delivery in patients able to use them	No single device available to deliver all classes of respiratory drugs
CFC-free; no effect on environment	Higher PIFRs required; may be unsuitable for patients with severe illness unable to generate the necessary inspiratory forces
Breath activated; aerosolization is coordinated with inhalation; major cause of MDI misuse avoided	Not suitable for patients younger than 6 years
Able to deliver β-agonists, corticosteroids, anticholinergics, and cromolyn sodium preparations	Efficacy reduced by exposure to humidity or extremes in temperature

(e.g., a multidose reservoir of powdered medication, a disk of individually wrapped foil blisters of powdered medication) and a hollow breathing chamber with a mouthpiece through which the patient inhales and aerosolizes the drug. The device needs to be "primed" or "activated" by releasing a single measured dose of the powder from the drug depository into the breathing chamber. A deep and forceful inhalation—at a flow rate that is intrinsic to each device—causes a valve to open and initiates turbulent airflow through the powder, resulting in aerosolization of the powder (21). Since aerosolization is coordinated with the patient's inhalation, a major cause of improper technique of MDI use (discoordination error) is avoided (22). Ensuring that the powdered drug becomes aerosolized, inhaled, and deposited into the lung requires precise engineering of both the drug particles and the geometry of the breathing chamber.

A particle size of 2 to 5 μm in diameter is ideal for deposition in the tracheobronchial tree (17,23–25). However, particles micronized to this size tend to become densely packed and generate significant electrostatic forces on their surface. This results in increased cohesion and poor flow, increasing the airflow requirements (i.e., the force of patient inspiration) for aerosolizing the drug (26).

Most dry powder devices add larger and coarser "carrier" particles to the micronized drug to facilitate aerosolization. These carriers increase the spaces between particles (thus reducing the forces of attraction between them) in addition to providing bulk to the unit dose of active drug (17,27). Although bound aggregates of the actual drug are sometimes mixed with the micronized particles to fulfill this purpose, the two most commonly used carrier particles are lactose and glucose. Due to their irregular shape and larger size (30 to 100 μm), they greatly reduce the cohesive forces between the micronized drug particles. In addition, due to their weaker cohesive forces, the carrier particles only loosely bind to the micronized drug and readily release the drug particles at flow rates generated by patient inspiration (approximately 30 to 90 L/min) (17,27,28). It should be noted that at these significant flow rates, the larger and heavier carrier particles are deposited on the tongue and impact the back of the oropharynx. This is especially important when delivering inhaled corticosteroids. The lactose and sugar particles are inert and will not cause oral thrush (unlike larger particles of active drug used as carriers). In addition, they leave a sweet taste, giving the patient a positive feedback that the dose has been correctly delivered (17).

The internal geometry of the breathing chamber contributes to the success of aerosolization of the drug by controlling the resistance to inspiration through the device. Each drug preparation requires a unique airflow rate to overcome the cohesive forces between the drug particles. Each DPI device has a unique resistance to airflow that must be overcome by the patient's inhalation in order for the drug to be properly administered. As the resistance of the device increases, the minimum inspiratory flow rate required from the patient's inhalation also increases.

Some DPI devices are designed to deliver drug doses with a relatively low peak inspiratory flow rate (e.g., Diskus inhaler, 28 L/min), whereas other inhalers require higher flow rates to deliver drug doses (e.g., Turbuhaler inhaler, 60 L/min) (29–32). At optimal flow rates (peak inspiratory flow rate [PIFR] greater than 60 L/min), higher resistance DPIs appear to improve drug delivery to the lower respiratory tract (30,31,33,34). At suboptimal flow rates (PIFR 28 to 60 L/min), lower-resistance devices appear to deliver more consistent drug doses to the lower respiratory tract, comparable to those of MDIs with a spacer (24,30–32,35). The clinician should consider these factors when prescribing a DPI. A high-resistance device may be preferred for maintenance medications given to otherwise healthy patients to prevent asthma exacerbations but may not be appropriate for rescue medications in the acutely ill or in chronically decompensated patients who cannot generate the necessary inspiratory flow rates. In addition, children under the age of 6 years have a limited PIFR and may not be appropriate candidates for all DPI devices (36). When compared with MDIs, DPIs appear to be at least as effective at delivering medication into the lung.

When the drug is first aerosolized, approximately 15% to 25% is deposited on the DPI apparatus, and 12% to 40% is deposited in the lung (17,37–41). Decreased drug delivery to the lung is attributed to inefficient aerosolization of the micronized drug particles from the carrier particles (42). Factors that contribute to this are improper technique (low inspiratory flow rate), high humidity (high ambient humidity or improper storage of the device without a securely fitting cap), and rapid temperature changes (travel between two climates can create condensation on the inside of the device) (43,44). It is important to be aware of these factors and instruct patients accordingly when teaching them to use these devices. Patients who have previously been taught to use an MDI have been told to inhale slowly and deeply to create laminar flow and thereby enhance pulmonary drug delivery. When teaching patients proper DPI use, it is necessary to emphasize that it is best to seal the lips over the mouthpiece and inhale deeply, quickly, and forcefully in order to create enough turbulence to aerosolize the powdered drug and maximize pulmonary delivery. In addition, it must also be emphasized that exposure to humidity and temperature extremes reduces the efficacy of all DPI devices. All caps and covers must be replaced when the device is not in use, and the device should not be stored where it will be exposed to extremes in temperature.

Nebulizers

Technically, a **nebulizer** is any device that produces aerosols. In common parlance, the term "nebulizers" usually refers to jet nebulizers. These devices create aerosols by passing a gas stream (either air or oxygen) through a fluid. When the fluid is released into the jet of gas, it is shattered into small particles, and an aerosol of various size particles is created (1,45). To produce droplets small enough to reach the distal lung,

TABLE 78.4	DOSE DEPOSITION PERCENTAGES			
	Percentage of total dose exhaled	Percentage of total dose adherent to apparatus[1]	Percentage deposited in the oropharynx	Percentage of dose deposited in lung[2]
Dry powder inhaler	1%	18%	54%	27%
Metered dose inhaler	1%	5–10%	80%	9%
MDI used with a spacer	1%	78%	1%	20%
Jet nebulizer	20%	66%	2%	12%

[1] and/or lost to atmosphere.
[2] A smaller percentage of medication reaches the small airways.

nebulizers commonly use a high gas flow rate and baffling devices. Slow gas jets will produce only large particles. To obtain particle sizes in the 1 to 5 μm range, a gas jet must generally exceed 12 L/min. A baffle—any object placed within a container that obstructs the path of the aerosol particles—will generate smaller particles at lower flow rates. Large particles "rain out," and the smaller particles continue on in the gas stream (1,45).

Jet nebulizers are considerably easier to use than MDIs. They deliver significant amounts of medication to the lung without any special respiratory maneuvers. Moreover, they can be used with normal tidal breaths and no coordination between activation and inhalation. They are probably even more effective if the patient takes slow inhalations and breath-holds at the end of inspiration. With a face mask attached, nebulizers also can deliver medication to less cooperative patients such as infants.

Even nebulizers are relatively inefficient, with more than 90% of the drug not reaching the desired site of delivery (Table 78.4). About one third of the nebulized medication is deposited on the apparatus, and another third is lost to the atmosphere. Attaching a face mask reduces this environmental loss but deposits more drug on the face and the nasopharynx. Less than 10% of the drug reaches the lower airways, and a much smaller proportion reaches the distal airways (1). To minimize this dissipation, medication being aerosolized in a jet nebulizer is usually diluted to a total of 3 to 5 mL with normal saline. Ready-made diluted unit dose medication is available for most bronchodilators.

Continuous Nebulization

Continuous nebulization therapy (CNT) uses large-volume aerosol generators (up to 240 mL) to deliver β-agonists continuously for as long as 24 hours to asthmatic patients in severe distress. Because they do not require repeated filling, CNT nebulizers are more convenient and can be more cost-effective

than intermittent nebulizer therapy (INT). They require significantly less respiratory therapist time with the equipment, but patients generally need closer observation because they are sicker.

CNT provides a mechanism for maximizing the dose-response curve without exceeding tolerable side effects. When used with patients in impending respiratory failure, CNT may avoid more toxic treatments such as intravenous β-agonist therapy or mechanical ventilation (46).

When CNT is compared with INT for the treatment of acute asthma, the clinical outcomes are generally similar. Intermittent therapy is more likely to cause more acute elevations in heart rate (46). Moreover, when used in the ED, CNT appears to reduce ICU admission (46) and, in adults, may increase the likelihood of discharge home (47).

Devices most widely used for continuous nebulization are the high-output extended aerosol respiratory therapy (HEART) nebulizers. These nebulizers, which come in large and mini sizes, produce a high-density aerosol of small particles using a sonic spray and baffle. The MiniNEB (also called the "MiniHEART") is especially suitable for use in children (Fig. 78.2). These nebulizers contain a 20-mL reservoir, operate at a flow rate of 8 L/min, generate especially small particles (1.0 to 2.5 μm), have a Luer-Lok intravenous adapter port that permits medication refill without interruption of therapy, and can be connected via an adapter to a mechanical ventilator.

Intermittent Positive Pressure Breathing

Intermittent positive pressure breathing (IPPB) devices automatically coordinate a jet nebulizer aerosol burst with the patient's inspiration. As a result, the patient does not have to learn special techniques to use the device, and the medication is not wasted by continuous gas flow.

However, both short- and long-term studies have failed to demonstrate any clinical advantage of IPPB therapy over ordinary jet nebulization in the treatment of asthma or chronic obstructive pulmonary disease (COPD). Moreover, IPPB therapy is more expensive than nebulization and has a greater risk of causing barotrauma and infection (1). Consequently, IPPB devices are no longer routinely used for the treatment of common respiratory illnesses.

Aerosol Therapy for Intubated Patients

Children with respiratory diseases frequently require intubation and mechanical ventilation. Aerosol medication can be delivered to the intubated patient, but only with some technical difficulty. Sidestream actuators have been designed that use jet nebulization to produce aerosol near the origin of the endotracheal tube. However, studies of these actuators demonstrate that only 11% to 66% of the particles produced are in the 1 to 5 μm range. The larger particles created impact on the adaptor and endotracheal tube without entering the patient's lower airways (48). Moreover, the high inspiratory

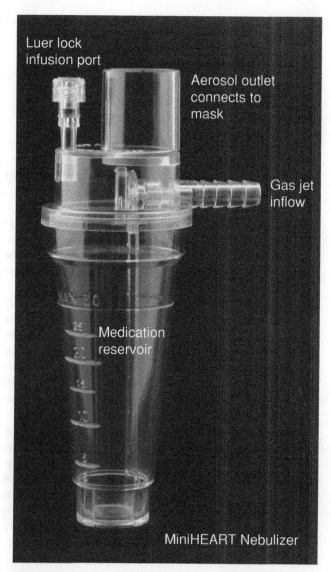

Luer lock
infusion port

Aerosol outlet
connects to
mask

Gas jet
inflow

Medication
reservoir

MiniHEART Nebulizer

Figure 78.2 Continuous nebulizer canister (MiniHEART or MiniNEB).

flow rates of the mainstream airflow delivered by the ventilators lead to significant upper airway deposition of medication due to turbulence and inertial forces. Therefore, less than 3% of the dose arrives in the lung even if the nebulizer adaptor is placed immediately adjacent to the endotracheal tube. Thus, larger doses of medication are needed to achieve the same efficacy (1).

In-line MDIs appear to be more efficient than jet nebulizers in treating the intubated patient. If the MDI is activated during the inspiratory flow stream of the ventilator, drug delivery is enhanced. To maximize therapy, the ventilator should be set at a slower than normal flow rate, with large inspiratory volume and an inspiratory pause (3,49). Even though aerosol treatment by means of MDIs in the intubated patient is probably more effective than jet nebulizer treatment, the efficiency of drug delivery is still less than that obtained from normal MDI use in the nonintubated patient (49).

Nebulizers versus MDIs versus DPIs for Acute Attacks

MDIs have many obvious advantages over nebulizers (see Table 78.3). They are less expensive, require less time to deliver a therapeutic dose, are more portable and more convenient to use, and are less likely to become contaminated. Moreover, at the present time, MDIs are available with a wider variety of respiratory medications than can be administered using nebulizers (3,13).

Conventional wisdom holds that MDIs are better for the provision of maintenance therapy in the stable patient, but nebulizers may be required for the treatment of acute exacerbations. This belief, however, is not supported by the literature. Whether studied in adults or in children, in the ED or in inpatient wards, there seems to be no difference in the treatment of mild to moderate asthma in terms of clinical outcome or adverse effects between nebulizer therapy and the use of an MDI with a spacer (13,50).

The argument has been made that tachypneic and dyspneic patients might do better with nebulizers because they are unable to use an MDI with the correct technique. However, a spacer can overcome the impediments to proper technique. If jet nebulizers are perceived by some patients to be more effective, this is probably because a much larger dose of medication is used in nebulizers, especially for acute attacks. The standard nebulizer dose of β-agonist is 10 times that in an MDI.

Although clinical studies comparing DPIs to MDIs and jet nebulizers in the acute setting of moderate to severe asthma need to be performed, the DPI is probably not the delivery system of choice because seriously ill patients may not be able to generate the necessary PIFR.

It should also be pointed out that studies comparing the financial cost of MDIs plus spacers to the cost of nebulizers in the treatment of hospitalized patients have estimated that patients treated with MDIs required 80% less respiratory therapist time and have their respiratory supply charges reduced by 75% (1,3). Nebulizers may have the additional disadvantage of carrying a greater risk of infection to the patient, especially if they are not adequately cleaned between usage, when colonization rises. Also, in-hospital use of MDIs with spacers—either in the ED or inpatient ward—provides an excellent opportunity to train patients in proper technique for outpatient use. In conclusion, it seems likely that MDIs with spacer devices provide comparable efficacy in the treatment of acute bronchospasm and have several secondary advantages over nebulizers (1,51).

Cleaning the Equipment

MDIs should be cleaned once a day by removing the canister and rinsing the inhaler, mouthpiece, and cap in warm water and then air drying before using again. Twice a week, the mouthpiece should be cleaned with a dishwashing soap and then rinsed.

The spacer mouthpiece should be rinsed in warm running water once a day, with care taken not to damage the one-way inhalation valve. The reservoir should be rinsed with warm water at least once a week to remove medication buildup. Both components should be shaken and air dried after cleaning. Never clean a spacer device in a dishwasher.

The face mask or T-piece used with a nebulizer is rinsed under running warm water and then air dried after each use. Once a day, along with the medication dropper or syringe, it is washed with dishwashing soap and water. Once a week, these components should be soaked in white vinegar and water (1:2 solution) for 30 minutes. Air compressors should be covered after each use to prevent dust accumulation.

MDIs, spacers, and nebulizer masks are designed for single patient use and should not be shared.

Determining How Much Medication Is Left in a Metered Dose Inhaler

The number of aerosol puffs in an MDI canister varies with the type of medication. Most β-agonist canisters contain 200 puffs. Figure 78.3 illustrates how to approximate the amount of medication left in a canister by floating it in water. This

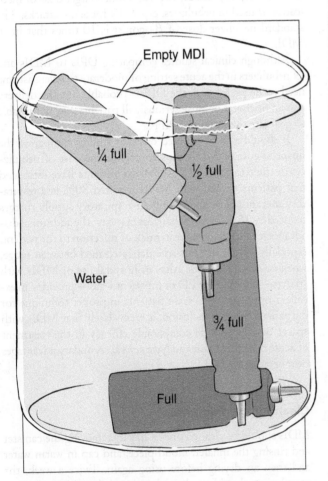

Figure 78.3 MDI canisters floating in tap water to demonstrate the amount of medication remaining.

method does not apply to all canisters, so the patient should consult the package insert.

▶ PROCEDURE

Metered Dose Inhaler Use

Before starting, the patient should ensure that the canister is inserted properly into the inhaler mechanism. The patient should remove the cap from the mouthpiece of the inhaler and inspect for foreign materials. The canister-inhaler assembly is shaken immediately before each puff.

Holding the inhaler upright (mouthpiece is below canister), the patient breathes out fully without forcing exhalation. The head is tilted back slightly, and the mouthpiece of the inhaler is placed 1 to 2 inches away from the mouth or, alternatively, between open lips (Fig. 78.4A,B).

The patient or assistant presses down on the canister fully with his or her index finger while the patient starts to breathe in slowly at the same time. The patient should inhale the medication as slowly as possible, taking up to 6 seconds for inspiration. Once the medication is inhaled, the patient holds his or her breath as long as is comfortable and up to 10 seconds. Having completed the breath holding, the patient then exhales.

If additional puffs are required, the patient should wait at least 1 minute between puffs and then repeat the procedure, starting with shaking the canister and ending with exhaling. Once the medication is completely administered, the patient replaces the cap over the mouthpiece and stores the inhaler in a clean, dry place. If corticosteroid inhalers are used, the patient should rinse the mouth with water after treatment to avoid oral candida infection.

Spacer Use

The patient using a spacer device with the MDI should prepare for medication administration by first removing the dust cap from the spacer mouthpiece and inspecting the spacer for foreign material. The patient should then remove the cap from the mouthpiece of the MDI and look for foreign material there as well. Some MDIs adapt to spacers by attaching the canister directly to the spacer device without using the MDI mouthpiece. If this is the case, the canister should be removed from the MDI and inspected for foreign materials. The entire MDI (or just the canister) is then inserted into the spacer in an upright position.

The patient starts the treatment by breathing out fully without forcing exhalation, then places the spacer mouthpiece in the mouth and closes the lips snuggly around it (Fig. 78.4C). One puff of medication is released into the spacer reservoir by pressing down fully on the inhaler canister with the index finger. The patient then breathes the medication in slowly from the reservoir for up to 6 seconds. A whistle sound indicates that the patient is breathing too rapidly and should

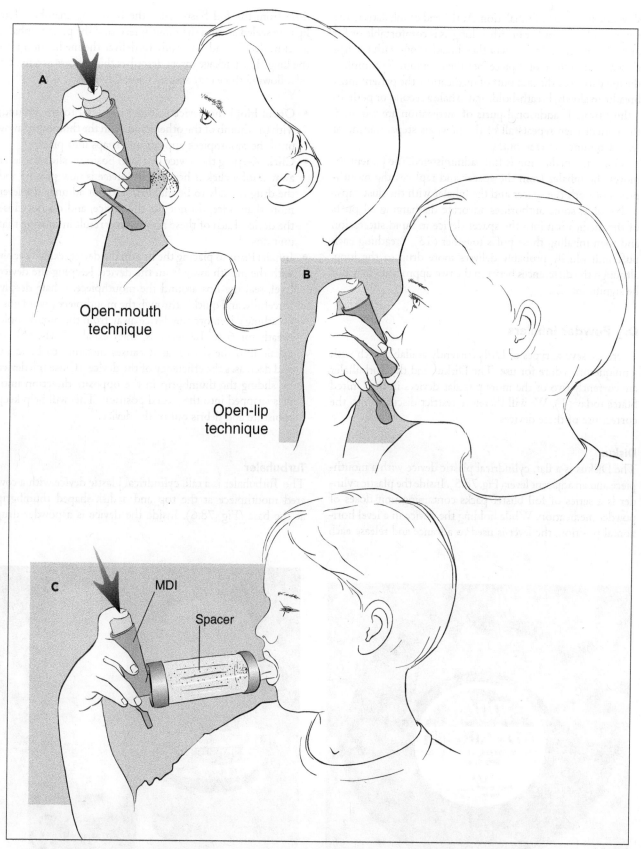

Open-mouth technique

Open-lip technique

MDI

Spacer

Figure 78.4
A. MDI usage with open mouth technique (1 to 2 inches from mouth).
B. MDI usage with canister mouthpiece surrounded by lips.
C. MDI usage with a spacer attached.

slow down the rate of inhalation. At the end of inhalation, the patient holds his or her breath as long as is comfortable or for up to 10 seconds. The patient then breathes out with the lips closed around the mouthpiece into the reservoir. To complete the inhalation of the first puff of medication, the patient must breathe in slowly, breath-hold, and exhale a second or perhaps a third time. If additional puffs of medication are required, the patient then repeats all of the previous steps, waiting at least 1 minute between puffs.

Once the medication is fully administered, the patient removes the inhaler from the spacer and replaces the mouthpieces of both the spacer and the inhaler with the dust caps.

Notably, some authorities advocate discharging all puffs of the medication into the spacer device in rapid succession and then inhaling these puffs together (13). Breathing each puff individually probably delivers more drug to the lung, although the differences between the two approaches may not be significant (2).

Dry Powder Inhalers

There are several types of DPIs currently available, each with a unique procedure for use. The Diskus and the Turbuhaler are currently two of the more popular devices in the United States today (1). We will therefore restrict discussion to the correct use of these devices.

Diskus

The Diskus is a flat, cylindrical plastic device with a mouthpiece and an adjacent lever (Fig. 78.5). Inside the plastic cylinder is a series of foil blister packs containing unit doses of powder medication. While holding the device in a level horizontal position, the lever is used to advance and release each

dose from the foil blister into the breathing chamber. The lips are sealed around the mouthpiece, and the patient inhales quickly, deeply, and forcefully to deliver the medication into the lung. The package insert describes this process as a matter of following three easy steps: "*Open, Click, Inhale.*" (52).

- **Open:** Hold the device in one hand level to the ground; with the thumb of the other hand push the thumbgrip away until the mouthpiece appears and snaps into place.
- **Click:** Keeping the device in a level position, slide the lever away until a click is heard. The device is now primed and the drug is ready to be inhaled. (Do not advance the lever more than once, do not tilt the device, and do not close the device. Each of these actions may result in wasting that unit dose.)
- **Inhale:** Prior to placing the lips on the device, exhale deeply with the mouth away from the device. Keeping the device level, seal the lips around the mouthpiece. Inhale deeply, forcefully, and quickly through the mouthpiece (avoid nose breathing). Remove the device away from the mouth, hold breath for 6 to 10 seconds, then exhale slowly. (Never exhale into the device, as it causes moisture to build up and decreases the efficiency of the device.) Close the device by sliding the thumbgrip in the opposite direction until it is snapped into the closed position. This will help keep moisture and debris out of the device.

Turbuhaler

The Turbuhaler is a tall, cylindrical plastic device with a covered mouthpiece at the top and a disk-shaped thumbgrip at the base (Fig. 78.6). Inside the device is a powder drug

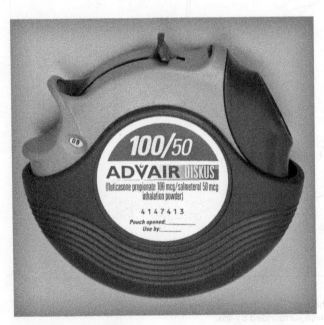

Figure 78.5 Advair Diskus.

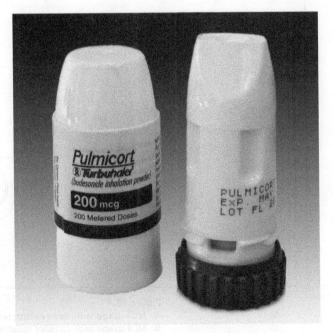

Figure 78.6 Pulmicort Turbuhaler.

reservoir from which each unit dose is measured and deposited into the breathing chamber when the device is primed. The device is primed in the upright position (mouthpiece up) by twisting the thumbgrip base as far right as it will go, then as far left to produce a click. The device is now primed and the dose of medication ready to be inhaled. The lips are sealed around the mouthpiece (with the device in either an upright or horizontal position), and the patient inhales quickly, deeply, and forcefully to deliver the medication into the lungs. Again using *Open, Click, Inhale* as the three main steps, the procedure as described in the package insert is as follows (53):

- **Open:** Hold the device in the upright position. Remove the protective cover, exposing the mouthpiece.
- **Click:** Keeping the device in the upright position, twist the thumbgrip at the base all the way to the right, then all the way to the left until it clicks. (Do not twist the thumbgrip more than once, and do not tilt the device. Each of these actions may result in wasting the unit dose.)
- **Inhale:** Prior to placing the lips on the device, exhale deeply with the mouth away from the device. Keeping the device upright or turning it to the horizontal position, seal the lips around the mouthpiece. Inhale deeply, forcefully, and quickly through the mouthpiece (avoid nose breathing). Remove the device away from the mouth, hold breath for 6 to 10 seconds, then exhale slowly. (Never exhale into the device, as it causes moisture to build up and decreases the efficiency of the device.) Close the device by securely placing the protective cover over the mouthpiece. This will help keep moisture and debris out of the device.

Nebulizer Use

Starting with a clean medication reservoir, the clinician measures the correct amount of normal saline (usually 3 mL) and places it in the reservoir, then adds the measured amount of medication to the saline. Once the medication is in the reservoir, the reservoir can be attached to its jet source (air compressor or oxygen line) using gas tubing. The T-connector mouthpiece or the face mask is attached to the other end of the medication cup. It is better to use a T-connector and mouthpiece than a face mask if the patient is able to cooperate with the breathing in of the medication. Face masks deposit a large portion of the aerosol on the face and in the nasopharynx. T-connectors with a mouthpiece waste less medication than face masks and are the device of choice in cooperative patients.

Once the mask is placed around the face or the T-connector mouthpiece set is placed in the mouth, the clinician turns on the jet source at 8 L/min flow. Taking deep breaths, the patient inhales slowly (over 6 seconds if possible) and then holds each breath as long as is comfortable (up to 10 seconds). The patient continues inhaling in this manner until all fluid is gone from the reservoir. After the treatment is completed, the compressed air or oxygen is turned off.

Continuous Nebulization Therapy: Operating the MiniHEART Nebulizer

To prepare for continuous nebulization treatment with a mininebulizer, the clinician connects a low-flow oxygen meter (0 to 15 L/min) to the oxygen source. Because continuous nebulization therapy is reserved for severely ill patients, oxygen should always be used as the jet source. The oxygen is connected to the medication reservoir using gas tubing. The reservoir is filled with a mixture of β-agonist and normal saline through the aerosol outlet at the top (up to a maximum of 20 mL of solution). The aerosol outlet port is then connected to a face mask, and the face mask is placed on the patient. It should be noted that T-connectors are usually not used in continuous nebulization therapy if treatment is expected to continue more than 1 hour because it would be impractical for the patient to hold the T-connector in the mouth for prolonged periods of time.

The oxygen jet should be run at 8 L/min to produce an aerosol output from the miniHEART of approximately 20 mL/hr. If the clinician wishes to provide continuous nebulization beyond the capacity of the miniHEART reservoir, he or she can mix β-agonist with respiratory normal saline in the medication bag and place this mixture in an infusion pump. The infusion pump is then connected with intravenous tubing to a Luer-Lok inlet on the miniHEART. The fluid infusion rate is adjusted to match the aerosol output rate, thus keeping the reservoir fluid level at a steady 10 to 20 mL. As an infection control precaution, the miniHEART reservoir, tubing, and mask should be changed every 24 hours.

Notably, the optimal dose of continuous nebulization medication for children and adults has not been determined. The dosage delivered should be titrated to the individual patient's tolerance of the β-agonist. As a rule of thumb, however, the clinician can start the patient on an hourly dose of β-agonist that is three times the usual single intermittent dose. For example, if using 0.15 mg/kg (.03 mL/kg) of 5% albuterol and 3 mL of normal saline as a single dose, start the patient on 0.45 mg/kg (.09 mL/kg) of albuterol in enough normal saline to make a total of 20 mL.

For the adult size patient, the clinician can use the full-size HEART nebulizer instead of the miniHEART. The HEART nebulizer has a larger reservoir, and when driven at an oxygen flow rate of 9 to 10 L/min, it produces 20 mL of aerosol per hour.

Teaching Patients to Use Equipment Correctly

A survey from a general medical practice in 1989 indicated that only 25% of adult MDI users had perfect technique and more than a third had poor technique (54). Therefore, every medical visit, including every visit to the ED, should be viewed as an opportunity to demonstrate correct technique. It is preferable to use a placebo inhaler and observe the patient's use of it (2). The teaching should emphasize using the open mouth technique, the coordination of inhalation with activation, slow inspiration, and breath holding.

SUMMARY

MDI Use

1 Shake the canister immediately before each aerosol release.

2 Breathe out fully without forcing exhalation.

3 Hold the MDI with the mouthpiece down and the canister above.

4 Place the mouthpiece of the inhaler 1 to 2 inches away from open mouth or between open lips.

5 Pressing the canister down with the index finger to release a measured medication burst, start inhaling slowly over 6 seconds.

6 Hold breath up to 10 seconds.

7 Wait at least 1 minute before the next puff.

8 If using a corticosteroid inhaler, rinse mouth after each treatment.

Spacer Use with MDI

1 Close lips snugly around the spacer mouthpiece.

2 Place one puff of medication in the reservoir at a time.

3 Breathe in the medication slowly over 6 seconds.

4 If the whistle sounds, slow down the rate of inhalation.

5 Hold breath as long as possible up to 10 seconds.

6 Repeat Steps 3 to 5 for each aerosol puff taken (one or two more times).

7 Wait at least 1 minute before inhaling an additional burst of medication.

DPI Use

1 Position the device in the proper orientation.

2 Remove the cover and expose the mouthpiece.

3 Prime the device (load the medication dose).

4 Away from the mouthpiece, exhale completely.

5 Maintain proper orientation of the device, and seal lips over the mouthpiece.

6 Inhale deeply and forcefully.

7 Remove the device from mouth.

8 Hold breath for 6 to 10 seconds.

9 Exhale slowly.

10 Close the device securely.

Nebulizer Use

1 Add medication to respiratory saline in the reservoir, being sure to measure both liquids accurately.

2 It is better to use a T-connector than a mask if the child is old enough to cooperate.

3 Turn on the air compressor or oxygen after placing the T-connector in the patient's mouth.

4 Take deep, slow breaths (each breath up to 6 seconds long).

5 Hold each breath up to 10 seconds.

For the patient using a spacer device, teaching should emphasize placing the lips tightly around the mouthpiece, inhaling slowly, and breath holding at the end of inhalation. These same points, as well as the correct measurement of medication, should be emphasized for the patient using a home nebulizer.

▶ COMPLICATIONS

The complications of inhalation therapy are limited and are mostly related to use of the medications. For example, the principal complications of β-agonist inhalation are tremor, hypokalemia, tachycardia, and dysrhythmias. Abuse of β-agonist MDIs has been associated with a higher incidence of asthma deaths, but the higher incidence is probably also partly caused by delays in seeking hospital care and lack of early treatment with anti-inflammatory therapy (55). Similarly, principal complications of corticosteroid inhalation are oral thrush and hypothalamic-pituitary-adrenal suppression.

However, a few complications have been associated with the actual inhalation devices and not just the medications they are delivering. One of the principal concerns raised regarding MDIs is their use of chlorofluorocarbons (CFCs) and the environmental effects. Although CFCs from MDIs make up only a small percentage of the total CFC burden in the environment, this environmental impact is undesirable. Fortunately, many MDIs have replaced the CFC propellant with hydrofluoroalkanes (HFAs), which are not known to be harmful to the environment. CFCs, HFAs, and other halogenated hydrocarbons can sensitize the myocardium to the effects of catecholamines. It has been estimated that a patient must use an inhaler 20 times over 2 minutes before the CFC concentration in the blood becomes great enough to make the myocardium irritable (3). It also should be noted that inhalation of the dust cap of a MDI, with subsequent airway obstruction, has been reported. Use of an MDI with the open mouth technique provides an opportunity for the patient to misdirect the burst of aerosol. Spraying into the eyes can be a problem, especially with ipratropium, which has been reported to cause blurry vision when squirted in the eye (2). To avoid this complication, it is recommended that only the closed mouth technique be used for ipratropium MDIs.

A theoretical complication of all aerosol therapies is infection. The small aerosol particles can carry micro-organisms far down the airways. In practice, this seems to be principally a complication of nebulizers and to a lesser extent spacers. The problem here is probably related to poor cleaning of the reservoirs and mouthpieces. With regard to spacers, those made with one-way inhalation valves can cause difficulty for patients with severe airway obstruction. These patients cannot mount enough expiratory pressure to close the valve (1). A similar problem applies to DPIs as well.

Continuous nebulizer therapy carries the most risk of medication toxicity because of the high doses of β-agonist that are used. In addition to tremor, muscle cramps with elevation in creatine phosphokinase (CPK) (MM fraction) and lactate dehydrogenase (LDH) have been reported. Moreover, one patient was reported to develop unifocal premature ventricular contractions (PVCs) on high-dose therapy. Mild hyperglycemia with blood glucose in the 200 to 250 mg/dL range and hypokalemia have also been reported (46). Conversely, continuous nebulizer therapy has not been found more toxic than frequent intermittent treatments.

▶ SUMMARY

The advent of inhalation therapy has made it possible to treat a variety of respiratory illnesses with fewer side effects by delivering small doses of medication directly to their site of action. MDIs are capable of delivering a wide variety of medications to the lungs in a convenient and cost-effective manner. However, their effectiveness is dependent on their being used with correct technique. For those patients unable to use MDIs with ideal technique, spacer devices offer an effective adjunct. MDIs with spacers seem to be at least as effective as nebulizers, even in the treatment of acute asthma, and these devices have even been successfully used in very young children. For the treatment of severe bronchospasm, continuous nebulization therapy might prevent the need for intubation with mechanical ventilation and even intensive care admission.

▶ REFERENCES

1. Lee DKP, Ingbar DH. Aerosol delivery: what's best for your patient? *J Respir Dis.* 1989;10:97–116.
2. Whelan AM, Hahn NW. Optimizing drug delivery from metered dose inhalers. *DICP.* 1991;25:638–645.
3. Hofford JM. Metered dose inhaler therapy for asthma, bronchitis and emphysema. *J Fam Pract.* 1992;34:485–492.
4. Kemp JP, Meltzer EO. β_2 adrenergic agonists: oral or aerosol for the treatment of asthma. *J Asthma.* 1990;27:149–157.
5. Kelly HW, Murphy S. β-adrenergic agonists for acute, severe asthma. *Ann Pharmacother.* 1992;26:81–91.
6. Rau JL. *Respiratory Care Pharmacology.* 4th ed. St. Louis: Mosby; 1994.
7. Baker MD, Ruddy RM. Pulmonary emergencies. In: Fleisher GR, Ludwig S, Henretig FM, eds. *Textbook of Pediatric Emergency Medicine.* 5th ed. Philadelphia: Lippincott Williams & Wilkins; 2005:1137–1150.
8. Schuh S, Johnson DW, Callahan S, et al. Efficacy of frequent nebulized ipratropium bromide added to frequent high-dose albuterol therapy in severe childhood asthma. *J Pediatr.* 1995;126:639–645.
9. Hall CB, McBride JT, Walsh EE, et al. Aerosolized ribavirin treatment of infants with respiratory syncytial viral infection. *N Eng J Med.* 1983;308:1443–1447.
10. Feldstein TJ, Swegarden JL, Atwood GF, et al. Ribavirin therapy: implementation of hospital guidelines and effect on usage and cost of therapy. *Pediatrics.* 1995;96:14–17.
11. Klassen TP, Feldman ME, Watters LK, et al. Nebulized budesonide with mild to moderate croup. *N Eng J Med.* 1994;331:285–289.
12. Karem D, Levinson H, Schuh S, et al. Efficacy of albuterol administered by nebulizer versus spacer device in children with acute asthma. *J Pediatr.* 1993;123:313–317.
13. Noble V, Ruggins NR, Everard ML, et al. Inhaled budesonide for chronic wheezing under 18 months of age. *Arch Dis Child.* 1992;67:285–288.
14. Conner WT, Dolovich MB, Frame RA, et al. Reliable salbutamol administration in 6- to 36-month-old children by means of a metered dose inhaler and Aerochamber with mask. *Pediatr Pulmonol.* 1989;6:263–267.
15. Selroos O, Halme M. Effect of volumatic spacer and mouth rinsing on systemic absorption of inhaled corticosteroids from a metered dose inhaler and dry powder inhaler. *Thorax.* 1991;46:891–894.
16. Farrer M, Francis AJ, Pearce SJ. Morning serum cortisol concentrations after 2 mg inhaled beclomethasone diproprionate in normal subjects: effect of a 750 mL spacing device. *Thorax.* 1990;45:740–742.
17. Fink JB. Metered doses inhalers, dry powder inhalers, and transitions. *Respir Care.* 2000;45:623–635.
18. Dhand R, Fink J. *Respir Care.* 1999;44:940–951.
19. Bell JH, Hartley PS, Cox JS. Dry powder aerosols. *J Pharm Sci.* 1971;60:1559–1564.
20. *Montreal Protocol.* Washington, DC: U.S. Government Printing Office; 1987:26 ILM 1541.
21. Richards R, Saunders M. Need for a comparative performance standard for dry powder inhalers. *Thorax.* 1993;48:1186–1187.
22. Crompton GK. Problems patients have using pressurized aerosol inhalers. *Eur J Respir Dis.* 1982;199(suppl):101–104.
23. Byron PR. Prediction of drug residence times in regions of the respiratory tract following aerosol inhalation [published correction appears in *J Pharm Sci.* 1986;75:1207–1208]. *J Pharm Sci.* 1986;75:433–438, 1207–1208.
24. Byron P. Drug delivery devices: issues in drug development. *Proc Am Thorac Soc.* 2004;1:321–328.
25. Celga UH. Pressure and inspiratory flow characteristics of dry powder inhalers. *Respir Med.* 2004:(suppl A):S22–28.
26. Staniforth JN. Order out of chaos. British Pharmaceutical Conference Science Aware Lecture 1986. *J Pharm Pharmacol.* 1987;39:329–334.
27. Dalby RN, Byron P, Farr SY, eds. *Respiratory Drug Delivery.* Vol. 5. Buffalo Grove, IL: Interpharm Press; 1996:332–335.
28. Engel T, Heinig JH, Madsen F, et al. Peak inspiratory flow and inspiratory vital capacity of patients with asthma measured with and without a new dry powder inhaler device (Turboinhaler). *Eur Respir J.* 1990;3:1037–1041.
29. Prime D, Grant AC, Slater AL, et al. A critical comparison of the dose delivery characteristics of four alternative inhalation devices delivering salbutamol: pressured metered dose inhaler, Diskus inhaler, Diskhaler inhaler, and Turbohaler inhaler. *J Aerosol Med.* 1999;12:75–84.

30. O'Riordan T. Optimizing delivery of inhaled corticosteroids: matching drugs with devices. *J Aerosol Med.* 2002;15:245–250.

31. Bisgaard H, Klug B, Sumby BS, et al. Fine particle mass from the Diskus inhaler and Turbohaler inhaler in children with asthma. *Eur Respir J.* 1998;11:1111–1115.

32. Hill LS, Slater AL. A comparison of the performance of two modern multidose dry powder asthma inhalers. *Respir Med.* 1998;92:105–110.

33. Pedersen S, Hansen OR, Fuglsang G. Influence of inspiratory flow rate upon the effect of a Turbohaler. *Arch Dis Child.* 1990;65:308–310.

34. Thorsson L, Edsbacker S, Conradson TB. Lung deposition of budesonide from Turbohaler is twice that from a pressurized metered dos inhaler P-MDI. *Eur Respir J.* 1994;7:1839–1844.

35. Fuller R. The Diskus: a new multi-dose powder device: efficacy and comparison with Turbohaler. *J Aerosol Med.* 1995;8:S11–17.

36. Pedersen S. Delivery options for inhaled therapy in children over the age of 6 years. *J Aerosol Med.* 1997;10(suppl 1):S37–40.

37. Dolovich M. New propellant-free technologies under investigation. *J Aerosol Med.* 1999;12 (suppl 1):S9–17.

38. Pedersen S. Inhalers and nebulizers: which to choose and why. *Respir Med.* 1996;90:69–77.

39. Fink JB, Tomin MJ, Dhand R. Bronchodilator therapy in mechanically ventilated patients. *Respir Care.* 1999;44:53–69.

40. Newman SP, Moren F, Trofast E, et al. Deposition and clinical efficacy of terbutaline sulphate from Turbohaler, a new multi-dose powder inhaler. *Eur Respir J.* 1989;2:247–252.

41. Newman SP. Aerosol generators and delivery systems. *Respir Care.* 1991;36:939–951.

42. Labris NR, Dolovich M. Pulmonary drug delivery, II: the role of inhalant delivery devices and drug formulations in therapeutic effectiveness of aerosolized medications. *Br J Clin Pharmacol.* 2003;56:600–612.

43. Newhouse MT, Kennedy A. Condensation due to rapid, large temperature (t) changes impairs aerosol dispersion from Turbuhaler (T). *Am J Respir Cell Mol Biol.* 2000;161:A35.

44. Newhouse MT, Kennedy A. Inspiryl Turbuhaler (ITH) DPI vs. Ventolin MDI + Aerochamber (AC): aerosol dispersion at high and low flow and relative humidity/temperature (RH/T) in vitro. *Am J Respir Crit Care Med.* 2000;161:A35.

45. McPherson SP. *Respiratory Therapy Equipment.* 4th ed. St. Louis: Mosby; 1990:93–107.

46. Portnoy J, Nadel G, Amado M, et al. Continuous nebulization for status asthmaticus. *Ann Allergy.* 1992;69:71–79.

47. Rudnitsky G, Eberlein RS, Schoffstall JM, et al. Comparison of intermittent and continuously nebulized albuterol for treatment of asthma in an urban emergency department. *Ann Emerg Med.* 1993;22:1842–1846.

48. Bishop MJ, Larson RP, Buschman DL. Metered dose inhaler aerosol characteristics are affected by the endotracheal tube actuator-adapter used. *Anesthesiology.* 1990;73:1263–1265.

49. Crogan SJ, Bishop MJ. Delivery efficiency of metered dose aerosols given via endotracheal tubes. *Anesthesiology.* 1989;70:1008–1010.

50. Kisch GL, Paloucek FP. Metered dose inhalers and nebulizers in the acute setting. *Ann Pharmacother.* 1992;26:92–95.

51. Zainudin BM, Biddiscombe M, Tolfree SE, et al. Comparison of bronchodilator responses and deposition patterns of salbutamol inhaled from a metered dose inhaler as a dry powder and as a nebulizer solution. *Thorax.* 1990;45:469–473.

52. GlaxoSmithKline. Research Triangle Park, NC. Package insert. Advair Diskus.

53. AstraZeneca Pharmaceuticals. Pulmicort Turbuhaler. Södertälje, Sweden. Package insert.

54. Buckley D. Assessment of inhale technique in general practice. *Irish J Med Sci.* 1989;158:297–299.

55. Spitzer WO, Suissa S, Ernest P, et al. The use of β-agonists and the risk of death and near death from asthma. *New Eng J Med.* 1992;326:501–506.

MARY E. LACHER

79

Suctioning the Trachea

▶ INTRODUCTION

Suctioning is a technique used to maintain airway patency by removing pulmonary secretions, blood, vomitus, saliva, or other foreign material. Removal of these materials allows for the maintenance of gas exchange to provide adequate oxygenation and ventilation. In addition, suctioning removes potentially infective material from the upper airway and trachea. Suctioning may be nasal, oral, nasopharyngeal, or tracheal, depending on the patient's particular problem. Tracheal suctioning began to be performed in the 1950s, concurrent with the development of positive pressure ventilation (1–5).

Even though suctioning is a common, basic procedure, it may be associated with complications and risks if not done properly. It is frequently performed in pediatric patients of all age groups and may be performed by health care providers with different training backgrounds (emergency medical technicians, nurses, physicians, respiratory therapists, etc.). Suctioning the upper airway is detailed in Chapter 13.

▶ ANATOMY AND PHYSIOLOGY

The upper airway includes the nose, mouth, and pharynx (Fig. 79.1). The upper airway has several functions, including (a) conducting inspired gases to the lungs, (b) acting as a filter to prevent foreign material from entering the lower airway, and (c) humidifying and heating inspired gases.

The nose is lined with ciliated and nonciliated mucous cells. These cells help humidify inspired gases and filter foreign material. The filtering of foreign material is aided by the hair follicles and the thick, sticky mucous secretions of the nose. When an artificial airway (i.e., endotracheal tube or tracheotomy) is in place, the protective mucociliary clearance system is bypassed, leading to a reduction in airway humidity and thus drying and thickening of the secretions. The generous blood supply to the nares helps to warm and humidify inspired gases. As much as 1,000 mL of water per day humidifies the inspired air by mucous and serous secretions (1). These glands also are stimulated to produce more secretions from inflammatory processes such as respiratory infections, allergies, and inhalation of toxic substances (e.g., smoke, chemicals).

From the base of the tongue, the laryngopharynx extends to the esophagus, which lies posterior to the trachea (Fig. 79.1). The proximity and function of these structures around the larynx serve to protect the airway from microbial organisms. Closure of the glottis during swallowing prevents food or other substances from contaminating the tracheobronchial tree. Patients with neuromuscular illness, anatomically abnormal airways, or poorly protected airways are at the greatest risk for aspiration of gastrointestinal contents.

Within the neck, the trachea begins at the level of the cricoid cartilage. The trachea descends in the middle of the neck to the vertebral level of T5-6 and bifurcates into the right and left bronchi. This bifurcation is positioned slightly angled to the right, making the opening to the right bronchi a less acute angle. This allows an endotracheal tube or suction catheter to enter the right mainstem bronchus if passed beyond the carina.

Gas flow during respiration in normal healthy airways occurs by laminar flow, with the molecules traveling parallel to the walls of the airway. Laminar flow is governed by the law of Poiseuille, which states that at a constant driving pressure, the resistance to flow of a gas will vary with the fourth power of the radius of the tube it transverses. For example, if the internal diameter of the tube is halved, resistance to flow will be increased 16-fold. Therefore, small changes in airway caliber, even in local parts of the tracheobronchial tree (e.g., secretions or debris causing obstruction, insertion of a suction catheter), can greatly increase resistance to gas exchange.

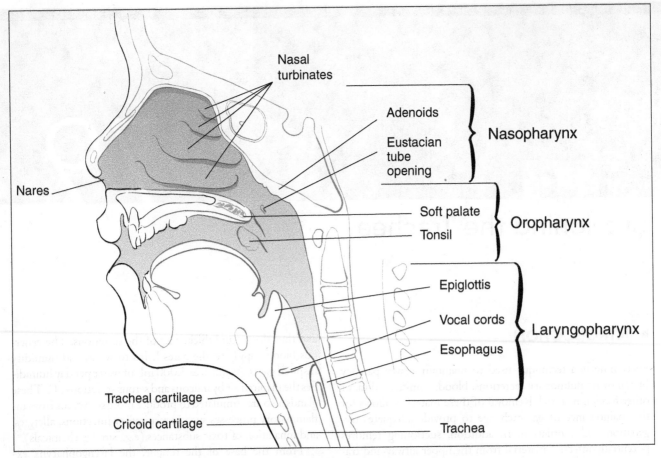

Figure 79.1 Anatomy of the upper (pharyngeal) airway.

Airway secretions can affect respiratory function in several ways (Fig. 79.2). Initially, these secretions may provoke a local inflammatory response that leads to increased resistance to airflow by the narrowing secondary to hyperemia and edema. This increases the work of breathing necessary to move gases past the secretions and inflamed airways. Ventilation-perfusion mismatch occurs because plugging, inflammation, and retained secretions lead to uneven distribution of oxygen reaching the distal pulmonary bed. Perfused lung segments may not receive fresh air, which leads to hypoxemia and triggers increased ventilatory effort in an attempt to compensate. If retained secretions cause total plugging of the bronchioles, atelectasis will develop, leading to a reduction in lung compliance, thereby worsening the ventilation-perfusion mismatch. Atelectatic or inflamed lung segments also continue to produce secretions that further act as a culture media for bacteria.

Defense mechanisms exist to remove foreign debris and excess secretions from the airway that are caused by artificial airways or primary disease. Small amounts of foreign material are continually swept up by cilia and mucus to the supraglottic region, where they can be swallowed down the esophagus. Coughing also is a means by which the secretions

and foreign material can be expelled from the airway. Receptors in the mucosa of the large respiratory passages are stimulated by irritation from secretions or foreign material, producing cough. Coughing begins with a deep inspiration, followed by a forced expiration against a closed glottis. The glottis is then suddenly opened, producing a forceful outflow of air.

Endotracheal or tracheotomy tubes tend to reduce effective cough and ciliary clearance, potentially leading to further inspissation of secretions. This is in part due to the need for a closed glottis for truly effective cough to be maintained. This is not possible with an endotracheal tube in place. Because the normal upper airway humidification systems are bypassed, secretions may be drier and thicker with artificial airways. The endotracheal tube impedes ciliary function. A foreign body can stimulate increased secretions.

▶ INDICATIONS

Tracheal suctioning may be necessary any time foreign material is interfering with adequate ventilation or oxygenation of a patient with natural or artificial airways. A number of medical

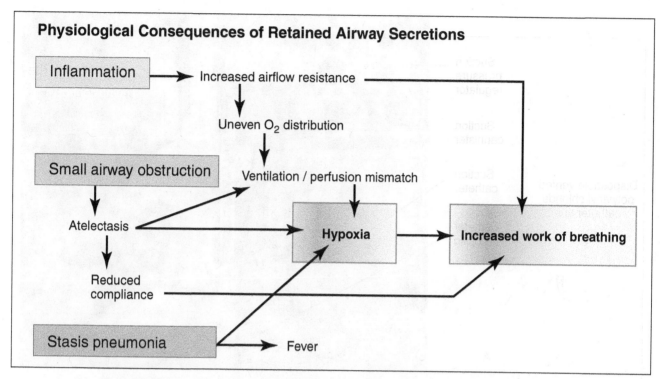

Figure 79.2 Physiologic consequences of retained secretions. (Adapted from Shapiro BA, Kacmarek RM, Cane RD, et al. *Clinical Applications of Respiratory Care.* St. Louis: Mosby; 1991.)

conditions affect the production and clearance of secretions to the degree that tracheal suctioning is indicated. Children with pneumonia or cystic fibrosis often have increased thick secretions that are difficult to clear. Victims of smoke inhalation or other inhalation injury may have edema and increased secretion production. Head injury or intoxicated patients may have reduced or absent protective reflex mechanisms that assist in the maintenance of clear airway. Patients with poor pulmonary mechanics (due to thoracic-abdominal surgery, rib fracture or chest trauma, or neuromuscular disorders such as muscular dystrophy) may not be able to clear their secretions. In addition to suctioning to clear the airway, suctioning may be used to obtain sputum for a culture to aid diagnosis.

Patients with artificial airways (tracheotomy cannula or endotracheal tube) have a routine need for suctioning. It is common for children with small artificial airways (endotracheal tube size 2.5 to 4.0) to require more frequent suctioning than older children or adults with larger airways just to ensure continued patency of the smaller tube.

Suctioning is performed frequently in the emergency department in patients with increased secretions or foreign material in the airway. The most common form is oral and nasopharyngeal suctioning (Chapter 13). Suctioning is routinely performed when a patient is being intubated to improve the visualization of landmarks and after the artificial airway is in place to maintain its patency and provide adequate oxygenation and ventilation.

▶ EQUIPMENT

The necessary equipment for suctioning is listed in Table 79.1. Various types of catheters are available, depending on the type of suctioning to be performed (Fig. 79.3). One major type is a disposable, vented polyvinyl chloride plastic catheter (Fig. 79.3A); another is a Yankauer-type tube (Fig. 79.3B). When suctioning the upper airway, the catheter should be soft and pliable but not collapsible when suction is applied. The distal end should be open and have at least two holes and smooth edges. The catheter should allow for intermittent suction with a thumb control valve (Fig. 79.3C). With this valve, no suction occurs when the valve port is open. To create suction, the clinician places a thumb over the valve opening. The Yankauer catheter is frequently used to suction the pharynx before endotracheal intubation or when initially

TABLE 79.1	EQUIPMENT

1. Pair of sterile gloves, protective eyewear and mask
2. Appropriate size suction catheter (Table 79.2)
3. Suction set at appropriate pressure (Table 79.3)
4. Resuscitation bag (Ambu) attached to high-flow oxygen
5. Sterile water or saline to flush catheter (minimum 100 mL)
6. Saline vial (3–5mL) for instillation into airway for very thick secretions
7. Pulse oximeter and cardiac monitor

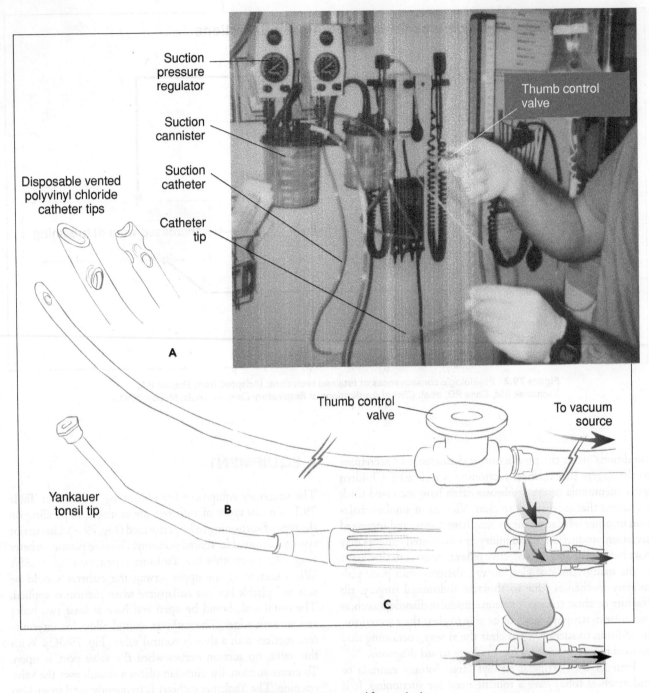

Figure 79.3 Equipment used for suctioning.

clearing the oropharynx in children who are at risk for aspiration. In these instances, after intubation of the airway, the soft, vented polyvinyl catheter is used.

Catheter size plays a role in the effectiveness of this procedure. A catheter that is too small may not clear sections. Too large a catheter can induce mucosal trauma and contribute to hypoxia. For endotracheal or tracheotomy tube suctioning, the catheter should be one half the size of the inner diameter of the tube into which the clinician is suctioning. For intraoral suctioning, the larger the catheter, the better, especially if clearing vomitus. A Yankauer-type catheter is recommended

for vomitus or large amounts of blood or other material in the oropharynx (Table 79.2).

▶ PROCEDURE

Tracheal Suctioning (via Endotracheal Tube or Tracheotomy Site)

Ideally, two people should be available to assist in the tracheal suctioning. One assistant monitors oxygenation and

TABLE 79.2	SUGGESTED AGE/WEIGHT APPROPRIATE SIZES OF SUCTION CATHETER AND ENDOTRACHEAL TUBES	
Age/weight	Endotracheal tube Internal diameter (mm)	Suction catheter
<1000 g	2.5	5 Fr
1000–2000 g	3.0	6 Fr
2000–3000 g	3.0–3.5	6–8 Fr
Term newborn	3.0–3.5	6–8 Fr
6 mo	3.5	8 Fr
12–18 mo	4.0	8 Fr
3 y	4.5	8 Fr
5 y	5.0	10 Fr
6 y	5.5	10 Fr
8 y	6.0	10 Fr
12 y	6.5	10 Fr
16 y	7.0	12 Fr
Adult (F)	7.5–8.0	12 Fr
Adult (M)	8.0–8.5	14 Fr

SUMMARY

1 Explain the procedure.

2 Wash hands and wear protective equipment.

3 Set up equipment.

4 Assess the patient's cardiorespiratory status.

5 Hyperoxygenate with 100% oxygen (minimum of six breaths).

6 Insert the catheter without suction applied to just past the distal end of the artificial airway or just above the carina.

7 Withdraw the catheter with intermittent suction up to 5 seconds (catheter should be in airway less than 10 seconds total).

8 Repeat hyperoxygenation with 100% oxygen.

9 Repeat Steps 4–8 as necessary and reassess the patient.

ventilation and helps to position the child while the other assistant performs the procedure. Because the area below the pharynx is sterile, it is important to use aseptic technique to reduce the risk of airway colonization or nosocomial infection.

Whenever possible, the clinician should explain the procedure to the patient and family beforehand. Sedation may need to be considered in the head injury patient for whom increases in intracranial pressure are a concern. After washing his or her hands, the clinician must don protective equipment (gloves, eyewear, and mask). The clinician should then set up the necessary equipment using aseptic technique. This includes determining the correct catheter size for the endotracheal tube (see Table 79.2) and setting the suction to the appropriate pressures (Table 79.3). The clinician should then assess the patient's cardiorespiratory status, noting color, auscultatory findings, oxygen saturation, respiratory rate, heart rate, and blood pressure. At the start, the clinician should hyperoxygenate the patient with 100% oxygen by bag-valve ventilation for a minimum of six breaths. The amount of hyperoxygenation should be lengthened in the extremely ill patient. After removing the bag, the clinician should gently insert the catheter without suction, advancing it a short distance past the distal end of the artificial airway (Fig. 79.4). When the clinician meets resistance (typically at the carina), he or she should pull back the catheter slightly (0.5 cm). While

occluding the suction, the clinician should gently and slowly withdraw the catheter. Most authorities suggest using a rotating motion between the thumb and forefinger as the catheter is withdrawn. No more than 5 consecutive seconds of suction should be applied, and the catheter should not be allowed to be in the airway more than 10 seconds total. After the catheter is removed, hyperoxygenation should be repeated with 100% oxygen and manual bag ventilation. The procedure should be repeated until the secretions or foreign materials are sufficiently cleared. It was previously thought that the use of sterile water or saline may help with particularly thick secretions. If secretions are particularly thick, sterile saline may be placed down the endotracheal tube, followed by a few spontaneous or assisted breaths (saline volumes: neonate, 0.25–0.5 mL; infant, 0.5–1.0 mL; older child, 1–3 mL; adolescent or adult, 5–10 mL). There has been a recent debate in the literature regarding this practice, as there is an association between suctioning with normal saline and more significant drops in oxygen saturation (6,7). If necessary, the clinician can selectively suction the airway past the carina by varying the patient's head position from side to side. Entry into the left mainstem bronchus is facilitated by turning the patient's head to the right, and, conversely, entry into the right mainstem bronchus is facilitated by turning the patient's head to the left (1).

▶ COMPLICATIONS

Some potential complications can be minimized or prevented with monitoring and proper and sterile technique. The most common potential complication is hypoxemia. Risk is increased by a failure to adequately hyperoxygenate and/or by

TABLE 79.3	SETTINGS FOR SUCTIONING PRESSURE
Neonates	60–80 mm Hg
Infants	80–100 mm Hg
Children	100–120 mm Hg
Adults	100–150 mm Hg

Source: Adapted from AARC clinical practice guideline: nasotracheal suctioning: revisions and updates. *Respir Care.* 2004;49:1080–1084.

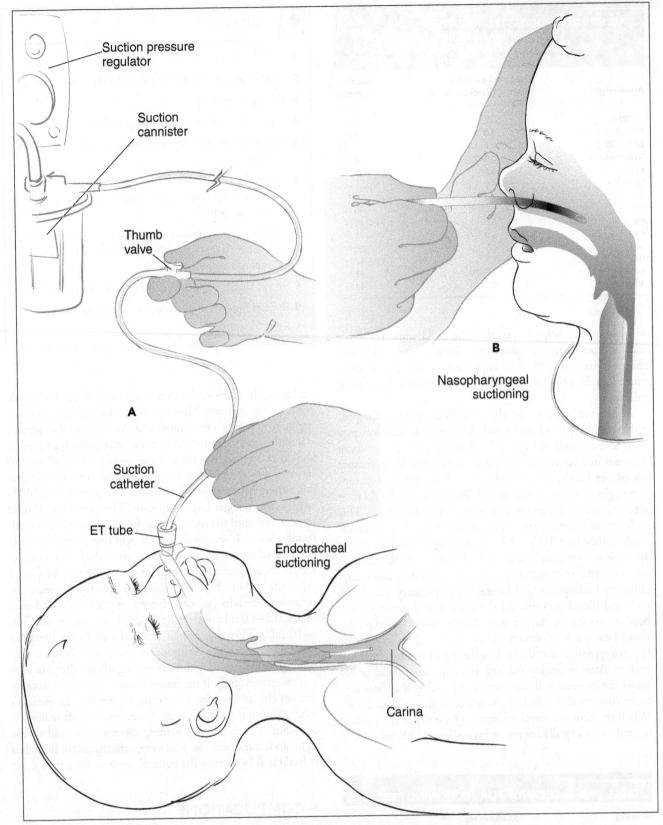

Suction pressure regulator

Suction cannister

Thumb valve

Suction catheter

ET tube

Endotracheal suctioning

Carina

A

Nasopharyngeal suctioning

B

Figure 79.4 Proper techniques for endotracheal and nasopharyngeal suctioning.

prolonged duration of the suctioning (8–11). Hypoxia may manifest itself as a significant reduction in oxygen saturation (less than 85%), cyanotic color, altered mental status, and/or cardiac dysrhythmia. Initially, tachycardia may be present, but many young infants develop bradycardia (especially neonates).

Bradycardia secondary to vagal stimulation may be the result of overstimulation of the gag reflex or secondary to hypoxemia. Hemodynamic changes (hypertension or hypotension) and dysrhythmia have been noted secondary to hypoxia or vagal stimulation (12). If bradycardia occurs, the clinician should immediately hyperoxygenate the child. If the patient does not respond and continues to have symptomatic bradycardia after adequate oxygenation, the clinician needs to consider administering atropine intravenously at 0.02 mg/kg (minimum dose 0.1 mg; maximum single dose 1 mg) because the bradycardia may also be secondary to vagal stimulation. It is important to consider hypoxemia as the primary cause before giving atropine. Cardiac output may decrease secondary to a decrease in venous return if the patient is hyperventilated.

Although this complication is less common, improper technique by overzealous suctioning can lead to airway collapse or atelectasis. This can be avoided by choosing the correct catheter size and limiting the amount of time suction is applied.

Tissue injury, including hemoptysis, may on occasion be caused by excessive pressure, local trauma, a catheter of too large a caliber, or prolonged duration of suctioning. Using too much pressure can damage mucosal tissue and denude airways of cilia. Acute bronchoconstriction may result from the irritative stimulation of bronchial smooth muscle but may be present as the primary problem and not be a consequence of suctioning. A risk of introducing infectious material and causing a nosocomial infection is also present. Transient increases in intracranial pressure from tracheal suctioning have been noted, but these can be minimized in patients requiring suctioning by utilizing careful techniques, avoiding hypoxia, and possibly using presedation (13,14). Increases in intracranial pressure may be of significance in a head injury patient, and sedation may be of great benefit if the patient is hemodynamically stable.

CLINICAL TIPS

▶ Perform procedure with an assistant if possible.

▶ Always have a resuscitation bag (Ambu) readily available and attached to high-flow oxygen.

▶ If bradycardia occurs, try oxygen first, then atropine.

▶ Limit time (less than 10 seconds) and use appropriate pressures (Table 79.3).

▶ SUMMARY

Suctioning is an important procedure for maintaining a patent airway and for oxygenating and ventilating patients with impaired pulmonary function, excessive secretions, and/or artificial airways. It carries the potential serious risk of hypoxemia or local airway injury. The procedure should be performed only by a trained individual with strict adherence to proper sterile technique.

▶ REFERENCES

1. Shapiro B, Kacmarek R, Cane R, et al. *Clinical Applications of Respiratory Care.* St. Louis: Mosby; 1991.
2. Standards for CPR and ECC. *JAMA.* 1986;255:2962.
3. American Heart Association. *Textbook of Pediatric Advanced Life Support.* Dallas, TX: American Heart Association; 2002:92.
4. Koff P, Eitzman D, Neu J. *Neonatal and Pediatric Respiratory Care.* St. Louis: Mosby; 1988:252–254.
5. Burton G, Hodgkin JE, Ward JJ, et al. *Respiratory Care: A Guide to Clinical Practice.* Philadelphia: Lippincott-Raven; 1991:498–502.
6. Ridling DA, Martin LD, Bratton SL. Endotracheal suctioning with or without instillation of isotonic sodium chloride in critically ill children. *Am J Crit Care.* 2003;12:212–219.
7. Kinlock, D. Instillation of normal saline during endotracheal suctioning: effects on mixed venous oxygen saturation. *Am J Crit Care.* 1999;8:231–240.
8. Langrehr EA, Washburn SC, Guthrie MP. Oxygen insufflation during endotracheal suctioning. *Heart Lung.* 1981;10:1029.
9. Skelley BF, Deeren SM, Powaser MM. The effectiveness of preoxygenation methods to prevent endotracheal suction induced hypoxemia. *Heart Lung.* 1980;9:316.
10. Naigow D, Powaser MM. The effects of different endotracheal procedures on arterial blood gases in a controlled experiment model. *Heart Lung.* 1977;6:808.
11. Barnes CA, Kirchhoff KT. Minimizing hypoxemia due to endotracheal suctioning: a review of the literature. *Heart Lung.* 1986;15:164.
12. Shim C, Fine N, Fernandez R, et al. Cardiac arrhythmias resulting from tracheal suctioning. *Ann Intern Med.* 1969;71:1140.
13. Rudy EB, Baun M, Stone K, et al. The relationship between endotracheal suctioning and changes in intracranial pressure: a review of the literature. *Heart Lung.* 1986;15:488.
14. Gemma M, Tommasino C, Cerri M, et al. Intracranial effects on endotracheal suctioning in the acute phase of head injury. *J Neurosurg Anesthesiol.* 2002;14:50–54.

▶ SUGGESTED READINGS

AARC clinical practice guideline: nasotracheal suctioning: revisions and updates. *Respir Care.* 2004;49:1080–1084.
Dantzer DR, et al. *Comprehensive Respiratory Care.* St. Louis: WB Saunders; 1995.
West JB. *Respiratory Physiology: The Essentials.* 7th ed. Baltimore: Lippincott Williams & Wilkins; 2005.

80

JEAN MARIE KALLIS

Replacement of a Tracheostomy Cannula

▶ INTRODUCTION

Replacing a tracheostomy cannula is typically a routine and simple procedure. Parents of children with tracheostomies perform this task on a regular basis without the assistance of a health care professional (1).

Although the actual skills involved are generally no more complicated than those used by parents at home, the degree of anxiety present in an emergent situation can make this task more challenging. In addition, with those children who present acutely in the emergency department (ED) for cannula replacement, other factors may be present that increase the complexity of the procedure. These include such things as recannulation in the very young infant, a tracheostomy performed in the previous week or two, the absence of an alternative upper airway, and certain underlying airway conditions. A calm, methodical approach is usually the key to success.

▶ ANATOMY AND PHYSIOLOGY

A tracheostomy is designed to bypass the upper airway and to provide a direct opening to the trachea. Tracheostomies are performed after endotracheal intubation or for an immediate airway because of three broad and often overlapping clinical problems: acute or chronic airway obstruction, prolonged assisted ventilation, and problems requiring improved pulmonary toilet. More recent data demonstrate a trend toward a larger number of pediatric tracheotomies being performed for prolonged ventilation, congenital anomalies, and severe neurologic disorders, whereas inflammatory upper airway diseases

have become less and less of an indication (2–6). Following a tracheostomy, a tract of healing tissue forms between the cervical epithelium and the tracheal endothelium. Until this is well granulated, recannulation may be difficult. Patients are usually hospitalized for a number of days, often in an intensive care setting, to reduce the risk of accidental decannulation, allow sufficient healing, and ensure the primary process is better controlled. Except in unusual circumstances, ED physicians tend to deal with the more mature tracheostomies, which makes reinsertion less challenging (1,2,7–9).

The younger the patient, the more likely the occurrence of accidental decannulation or obstruction. Infants have short, thick necks that make them prone to dislodgment of the tracheostomy tube (9,10). Tracheostomy ties may not be snug enough to prevent decannulation. The smaller tracheostomy tubes of young infants also have a narrower internal lumen, making the tubes more susceptible to acute obstruction. Mucous plugging occurs when viscous upper airway secretions occlude the lumen of the cannula, which may already be narrowed by secretions that have previously accumulated and dried. Because infants have less fully developed intercostal and diaphragmatic musculature, they are more likely to be unable to adequately clear a mucous plug from the cannula when it occurs.

▶ INDICATIONS

The need to replace a tracheostomy cannula in the ED typically occurs after accidental decannulation or obstruction of the tracheostomy tube (secretions, mucous plug, foreign body) (6,9,11,12). The most life-threatening complications for a child with an artificial airway are cannula obstruction or

TABLE 80.1	EQUIPMENT FOR TRACHEOSTOMY CHANGE

Suction—source, catheters
Oxygen—high-flow source of 100% O_2 (preferably humidified)
Bag-valve-mask—appropriate sizes to cover mouth and nose
Tracheostomy cannulas—appropriate sizes
Endotracheal tubes—appropriate sizes
Laryngoscope—blade, handle, bulb, battery
Tape—tracheostomy twill tape, "cloth tape"
Bandage scissors
Sterile saline

dislodgement (2,10). The pediatric patient who decannulates or obstructs a tracheostomy tube while in the ED for another problem can often be managed routinely. However, the child who is brought to the ED for the specific purpose of replacing a tracheostomy cannula may be in significant respiratory distress. Such a patient may arrive via an emergency services ambulance or be carried into the ED by a worried parent. As mentioned previously, the physician who is calm, unhurried, and armed with an awareness that the skills required to manage this situation are relatively straightforward will generally be most effective.

▶ EQUIPMENT

The equipment required for tracheostomy replacement is listed in Table 80.1, and the sizes for different ages are listed in Table 80.2. There are numerous tracheotomy tubes on the market, and the more commonly used tubes are noted in the latter table. Special features are also available (e.g., cuffs, swivel devices, fenestrated tubes) (6,10,11,13), but these should not distract from establishing a patent airway in the emergency setting.

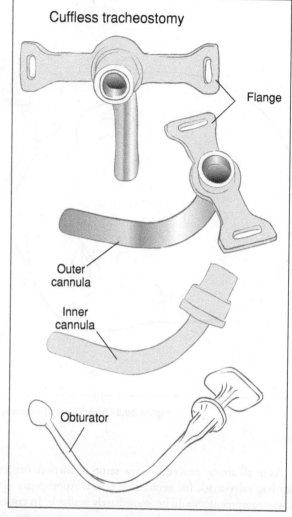

Figure 80.1 Tracheostomy tubes with tube, inner cannula, and obturator. (If the tracheostomy tube is rigid at the distal end, an obturator is necessary to pass the cannula, to reduce the risk of tissue damage. Softer cannulas may not require the use of an internal obturator.)

TABLE 80.2	APPROXIMATE SIZE OF TRACHEOSTOMY CANNULAS, ENDOTRACHEAL TUBES, AND SUCTION CATHETERS

Bivona				Shiley				ETT			Suction catheter
Size	I.D. (mm)	O.D. (mm)	Length (mm)	Size	I.D. (mm)	O.D. (mm)	Length (mm)	Size/I.D. (mm)	Length (mm)		Size (Fr)
2.5 neo	2.5	4.0	30					2.5	12		6
3.0 neo	3.0	4.7	32	3.0 neo	3.0	4.5	30	3.0	14		6–8
3.5 neo	3.5	5.3	34	3.5 neo	3.5	5.2	32	3.5	16		6–8
4.0 neo	4.0	6.0	36	4.0 neo	4.0	5.9	34	4.0	18		6–8
				4.5 neo	4.5	6.5	36	4.5	20		6–8
2.5 ped	2.5	4.0	38								6
3.0 ped	3.0	4.7	39	3.0 ped	3.0	4.5	39				6
3.5 ped	3.5	5.3	40	3.5 ped	3.5	5.2	40				6–8
4.0 ped	4.0	6.0	41	4.0 ped	4.0	5.9	41				6–8
4.5 ped	4.5	6.7	42	4.5 ped	4.5	6.5	42				6–8
5.0 ped	5.0	7.3	44	5.0 ped	5.0	7.1	44	5.0	22		8–10
5.5 ped	5.5	8.0	46	5.5 ped	5.5	7.7	46	5.5	25		10–12

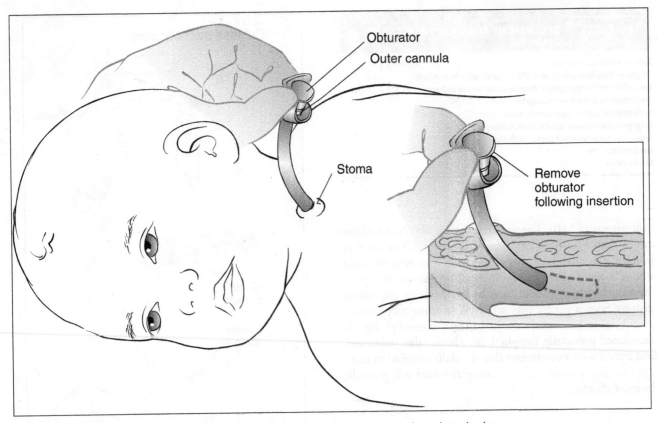

Figure 80.2 Inserting tracheostomy cannula into airway through tracheal stoma.

As in all airway procedures, the setup of suction, oxygen, and bag-valve-mask for ventilation is key. Appropriate size airway equipment should be immediately available. In critical emergencies, the physician should have endotracheal tubes the same size and one size smaller available (see Table 80.2 for exchange sizes). Lastly, the equipment necessary to secure the new airway must be readied.

▶ PROCEDURE

Initial assessment of the patency or placement of the tracheostomy tube requires proper positioning. The patient should be positioned with the head and neck hyperextended to expose the tracheostomy site and improve the accessibility of the tracheocutaneous fistula (8–11). In the nondistressed, alert, cooperative patient, it is wise to have the parent assist in finding the best position for the child. This may reduce the child's anxiety when the physician accesses the airway. Oxygen should be delivered by face mask over the nares and mouth or tracheostomy stoma. The physician needs to evaluate the patient for signs of tracheostomy cannula dislodgment or obstruction, including pallor, cyanosis, agitation, labored breathing, and inability to ventilate. If the child is unstable, assistance should be obtained to provide immediate advanced life support.

Replacing Cannula after Accidental Dislodgment

Accidental decannulation is obvious—the cannula is no longer in the stoma (a partial dislodgment should not be overlooked and may present more insidiously with respiratory distress or failure). Ideally, a new tracheostomy cannula of the same size and model should be reinserted, but if one is not immediately available, the dislodged tube can be used if it is patent. The obturator should be placed within the outer cannula before insertion, after first removing the inner cannula, if present (Fig. 80.1). The obturator helps maintain the appropriate curvature for insertion and also provides a rounded end for the tracheostomy tube, decreasing the risk of tissue damage during insertion (8). If time allows, lightly lubricating or wetting the tip of the cannula with a water-soluble gel or sterile saline may help ease passage (8,12). The cannula is most easily manipulated by holding it with the dominant hand either by the flange or like a pencil. It is then gently inserted in a posterior then caudal direction in a single sweeping motion (Fig. 80.2) (6,8–12). Once the tracheostomy tube is in place, the obturator is removed and the inner cannula (if needed) is reinserted. A bag should then be attached with high-flow oxygen, and manual breaths provided to check patency and to hyperoxygenate the child.

If resistance is met when reinserting, care must be taken not to force the tube in place, creating a false passage in the subcutaneous tissues of the neck. This may have potentially

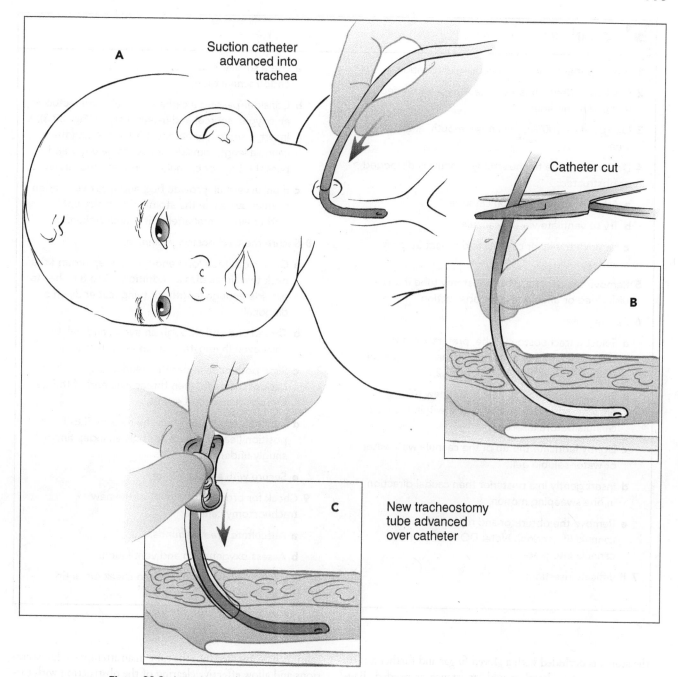

A Suction catheter advanced into trachea

Catheter cut

B

C New tracheostomy tube advanced over catheter

Figure 80.3 Inserting tracheostomy over red rubber catheter into the airway through the stoma.

devastating consequences (i.e., subcutaneous air, pneumomediastinum, pneumothorax, or obstruction) (6,9,12). Notably, the stoma may close after decannulation, even if the tube has been out for only a few hours. A smaller size tracheostomy cannula or an endotracheal tube may be used if the physician is unable to pass the original size cannula (8–10,12). When using an endotracheal tube, it is advisable to compare it with the tracheostomy tube length and note the markings to assist in determining the depth of insertion. A more appropriate cannula can be placed at a later time, after dilation of the tract.

Another aid for reinsertion in a difficult recannulation involves the passage of a small suction catheter attached to

an oxygen source (approximately 0.5 to 1.0 L/min) a short distance into the trachea (9,10,12). After oxygenation via the catheter on high-flow oxygen, it is necessary to cut the catheter proximally, leaving a length of it outside the stoma to thread under a tracheostomy or endotracheal tube. Care should be taken not to let go of the catheter. This is then used as a stylet for the advancement of the new tracheostomy or endotracheal tube over it, which avoids creation of a false passage (Fig. 80.3). Once the tube is in place, the patient must be re-evaluated to ensure the adequacy of the airway. If all attempts at recannulation fail, the patient usually can be ventilated via the nose and mouth with a bag and mask while

SUMMARY

1 Assess patient—airway, breathing, circulation.

2 Position patient—head and neck hyperextended (roll under shoulder).

3 Oxygenate—100% O_2 via nose, mouth, and/or stoma.

4 Determine if the tracheostomy cannula is dislodged or obstructed:

   a Attempt to pass suction catheter.

   b Try to ventilate via the cannula.

   c Remove the inner cannula and repeat Steps a and b.

5 Remove the complete tracheostomy tube if it is dislodged or unable to clear obstruction.

6 Recannulate:

   a Select a tracheostomy tube, preferably of the same size and model as the original tube (parents often carry a spare one) (Table 80.2).

   b Remove the inner cannula of the new tube, if present, and place the obturator within the outer cannula before insertion.

   c Lightly lubricate the tip of the cannula with water or water-soluble gel.

   d Insert gently in a posterior then caudal direction in one sweeping motion.

   e Remove the obturator and replace the inner cannula (if needed). Note: DO NOT FORCE cannula into place.

7 If difficult insertion:

   a Use a smaller size tracheostomy tube or endotracheal tube.

   b Consider passing a catheter (ideally connected to an oxygen source) and use as a stylet (Fig. 80.3). Insert it and oxygenate; cut it longer than the cannula length outside of the stoma entry and pass the tube or cannula over it into the airway.

   c If unsuccessful, provide bag-and-mask ventilation from above while the stoma is covered, until further airway management is undertaken.

8 Secure the tracheostomy cannula:

   a Cut a cloth tape long enough to wrap around the neck two times plus an additional 6 to 8 inches to provide enough length for tying (cut ends on a diagonal).

   b Thread one end through an eyelet and pull the ends even (hemostats can assist in threading).

   c Slide both ends under the head and around the back of the neck, then thread one end of the tie through the second eyelet.

   d Pull the ends snugly with the neck in FLEXED position (leaving space for only an index finger snugly under tie).

   e Secure with a square knot.

9 Check for proper placement of the new tracheostomy cannula:

   a Auscultate breath sounds.

   b Assess oxygenation and ventilation.

   c Perform chest radiograph to check distal tip placement.

---

the stoma is occluded with a gloved finger and further airway management is undertaken with assistance as needed. Bag-and-mask ventilation may fail, however, in rare cases when the upper airway is obstructed due to a prior medical condition or surgery.

Replacing an Obstructed Tracheostomy Cannula

A child who presents to the ED with a tracheostomy tube in place and is experiencing respiratory distress, inadequate oxygenation, or ventilation should be assumed to have a mechanical obstruction of the cannula until proven otherwise (2,8,10). The patient should be properly positioned and oxygen delivered as previously described. An immediate effort to carefully pass a suction catheter and clear the offending obstruction is made. If this is unsuccessful, 1 to 4 mL of sterile saline can be instilled into the tube in an attempt to thin secretions and allow effective clearing of the obstruction with further suctioning. Attention to suction pressure, duration, and depth is important, especially if frequent passes are necessary. Ideally, suction pressure should not exceed 80 to 100 mm Hg, duration not last for more than 10 seconds, and depth not exceed more than 0.5 cm beyond the tracheotomy tube distally. These measures will help avoid such complications as hypoxemia, hypotension, hypertension, bronchospasm, increased intracranial pressure, vasovagal responses, and trauma to the airway (8,10,11). The patient should be ventilated with 100% oxygen between suctioning attempts. The inner tracheal cannula can be removed, if present, to aid in relieving the obstruction. The clinician should not hesitate to remove the entire tracheostomy tube if the above-mentioned measures are unsuccessful—or immediately if the patient is

CLINICAL TIPS

▶ Have equipment set up before an elective procedure.

▶ If initial attempts fail, most children can be oxygenated by bag-valve-mask from the natural airway.

▶ To maximally open the tracheostomy stoma, hyperextend the child's neck by placing towel rolls under the shoulders.

▶ Choose appropriate size equipment. When an appropriate size tracheostomy tube is unavailable in the ED, remember that parents may have a spare tube.

▶ If a tracheostomy tube is unavailable, use an endotracheal tube of the same or a smaller diameter through the stoma (Table 82.2).

that both nurses and physicians recognize a patient with a compromised airway and intervene immediately. In a patient with a tracheostomy, this should include attempting to clear the obstruction, replacing the cannula, and/or providing bag-and-mask ventilation until further airway management is undertaken.

Life-threatening pneumomediastinum and pneumothorax can potentially result from formation of a "false track" in the subcutaneous tissues of the neck (6,9,12). This is more likely to occur in the operative or immediate postoperative period, with interruption of a tissue plane outside the tracheal lumen. In the ED, disruption can be avoided by never attempting to force the cannula into place.

Occasionally granuloma or stricture formation at the stoma or where the tip of the tube meets the tracheal wall can lead to localized bleeding from manipulation of the cannula (6,8,11,13). This small amount of bleeding is typically not a problem. Erosion into the innominate artery is a rare occurrence (11,14), usually related to a inferiorly located tracheostomy stoma and not a consequence of replacement of a tracheostomy cannula.

decompensating. Most patients will breathe easier through just the stoma than through a significantly obstructed cannula.

A new tracheostomy cannula is inserted as described earlier. Often the parents have a spare tube if one of the same size and type is not readily available in the ED. Once the cannula is in place, the patient should be reassessed to check for correct positioning (breath sounds, oxygenation, ventilation).

Securing the Airway

An appropriate method for securing the tube is essential to prevent extubation. Tracheostomy twill tape is used and should be cut at a length long enough to wrap around the patient's neck twice and an additional 6 to 8 inches for tying. Cutting the ends diagonally will aid insertion through the eyelets of the flange. One end of the tie is threaded through the eyelet and then the ends are pulled even. Both ends of the tape are then slid behind the head and around the neck and one tie is threaded through the second eyelet. With the neck in a flexed position, the ends are pulled snugly and secured to the flange with a square knot, allowing space for only one finger under the tape once it is tied (8,9,11,12). After the tube is secured and the patient stabilized, a chest radiograph can be obtained to check placement of the distal tip and assess for any pulmonary parenchymal changes.

▶ COMPLICATIONS

Complications are rare if decannulation or obstruction is promptly identified and properly managed. Certainly if adequate oxygenation and ventilation are not provided in a timely fashion, hypoxia and hypercarbia can ensue. It is imperative

▶ SUMMARY

In the ED, replacing a tracheostomy cannula is frequently performed in anxiety-provoking circumstances. When the physician remains calm, this task is often no more difficult than a routine tracheostomy tube change. Certain factors may contribute to making recannulation more challenging. The goal in any case is to allow for optimal oxygenation and ventilation, whether by clearing the obstruction, replacing the cannula, or providing bag-and-mask ventilation until further airway management is undertaken.

If the clinician elects to replace the cannula, he or she needs to remember to properly position the patient and use correct technique to increase the ease and success of insertion. Care must be taken not to force the cannula into place, potentially leading to further complications. Once the cannula is successfully replaced, it must be adequately secured. The patient should be repeatedly assessed to ensure proper positioning of the cannula and optimal oxygenation and ventilation.

▶ REFERENCES

1. Duncan BW, Howell LJ, DeLarimier AA, et al. Tracheostomy in children with emphasis on home care. *J Pediatr Surg.* 1992;27:432–435.
2. Kremer B, Botos-Kremer AI, Eckel HE, et al. Indications, complications, and surgical techniques for pediatric tracheostomies: an update. *J Pediatr Surg.* 2002;37:1556–1562.
3. Wetmore RF, Thompson ME, Marsh RR, et al. Pediatric tracheostomy: a changing procedure? *Ann Otol Rhinol Laryngol.* 1999;108: 695–699.
4. Ward RF. Current trends in pediatric tracheotomy. *Pediatric Pulmonol Suppl.* 1997;16:290–291.

5. Carron JD, Derkay CS, Strope GL, et al. Pediatric tracheostomies: changing indications and outcomes. *Laryngoscope.* 2000;110:1099–1104.

6. Wetmore RF. Tracheotomy. In: Bluestone CD, Stool SE, Cuneyt AM, et al., eds. *Pediatric Otolaryngology,* 4th ed. Philadelphia: WB Saunders; 2004:1583–1598.

7. Carr MM, Poje CP, Kingston L, et al. Complications in pediatric tracheostomies. *Laryngoscope.* 2001;111:1925–1928.

8. Fiske E. Effective strategies to prepare infants and families for home tracheostomy care. *Adv Neonatal Care.* 2004;4:42–53.

9. Mirza S, Cameron DS. The tracheostomy tube change: a review of techniques. *Hosp Med.* 2001;62:158–163.

10. Posner JC. Acute care of the child with a tracheostomy. *Pediatr Emerg Care.* 1999;15:49–54.

11. American Thoracic Society. Care of the child with a chronic tracheostomy. *Am J Respir Crit Care Med.* 2000;161:297–308.

12. Handler SD. Replacement of a tracheostomy cannula. In: Fleisher GR, Ludwig S, Henretig FM, eds. *Textbook of Pediatric Emergency Medicine.* 5th ed. Philadelphia: Lippincott Williams & Wilkins; 2006:1901–1904.

13. Raouf SA, Fittan CM. Tracheostomy and home ventilation in children. *Semin Neonatol.* 2003;8:127–135.

14. Neacy KA. Tracheostomy care and tracheal suctioning. In: Roberts JR, Hedges JR, eds. *Clinical Procedures in Emergency Medicine.* 4th ed. Philadelphia: WB Saunders; 2004:133–145.

▶ SUGGESTED READINGS

Aaron's Tracheostomy Page. www.tracheostomy.com.

American Thoracic Society. Care of the child with a chronic tracheotomy. *Am J Respir Crit Care Med.* 2000;161:297–308.

Wetmore RF. Tracheotomy. In: Bluestone CD, Stool SE, Cuneyt AM, et al., eds. *Pediatric Otolaryngology.* 4th ed. Philadelphia: WB Saunders; 2003:1583–1598.

Thoracentesis

81

▶ INTRODUCTION

A pleural effusion is a collection of fluid in the potential space that exists between the visceral and parietal pleurae of the lung. The causes of an effusion are varied. In the pediatric patient, acute pulmonary infection is the most common etiology, whereas some other less common etiologies include collagen-vascular disease, congestive heart failure, hypoalbuminemic states, trauma, and neoplasm (1,2). Table 81.1 lists some of the various etiologies of pleural effusions. Children with an effusion are usually older than 2 years of age but may be younger when the cause is a parapneumonic effusion (1,3).

A thoracentesis is a method to remove fluid or air from the pleural space (4). In this chapter, the discussion is limited to removal of fluid from the pleural space. A discussion relevant to the appropriate management and approach to the treatment of a pneumothorax is contained in Chapter 29.

Thoracentesis is indicated to remove pleural fluid that has caused respiratory embarrassment or to determine the etiology of the effusion (5). Depending on the volume and the characteristics of the pleural fluid, the procedure itself may be either definitive or temporizing. A tube thoracostomy is considered definitive therapy when an empyema is present or when continuous drainage is required, as in a traumatic hemothorax (4,5). The thoracentesis is most frequently performed on a semi-elective basis in a monitored setting. If the effusion is causing significant respiratory distress, however, a more urgent procedure is required.

▶ ANATOMY AND PHYSIOLOGY

The pleural space is a potential space that exists between the visceral and parietal pleura. Normally this space contains less than 15 mL of pleural fluid (6). The formation of pleural fluid is controlled in part by the effect of Starling forces. The forces affecting net fluid movement across the pleura depend on the capillary and intrapleural hydrostatic pressures, the plasma and intrapleural oncotic pressures, and the capillary filtration coefficient. These forces are summarized in Figure 81.1. In a healthy person, the forces are such that protein-free extracellular fluid enters the pleural space from the parietal pleura and is absorbed at the visceral pleura (6–8). A small amount of protein in the pleural space leaks into the space from the pleural capillaries. The protein and approximately 10% of the pleural fluid leave the space through the rich lymphatic supply (7).

In the healthy state, no net accumulation of fluid is evident because of a balance between the Starling forces. A pleural effusion develops when various disease processes alter these forces and lead to net fluid accumulation (7,8). For example, in the hypoproteinemic state, a decrease in the serum oncotic pressure leads to a gradient favoring fluid transport to the pleural space. Pleural fluid collects in inflammatory diseases, such as pneumonia and serositis caused by a collagen-vascular disease, through an alteration in the capillary filtration coefficient. A pleural effusion also may develop if obstruction of the lymphatic drainage would occur, as with traumatic rupture of the thoracic duct.

The consequence of fluid collecting in the pleural cavity is an affect on normal respiratory physiology that may interfere with normal respiratory function. A large or rapidly expanding effusion may clinically cause respiratory embarrassment (9). The pleural fluid initially reduces the lung volume and consequently diminishes the vital capacity. If sufficient fluid accumulates, the vital capacity and the functional residual capacity decrease to the point where distal lung units collapse (i.e., atelectasis). The enlarging effusion also impedes diaphragmatic function and reduces chest wall compliance, which increases the work of breathing and makes deep sigh breaths more difficult. The ultimate effect is an impairment of alveolar gas exchange.

TABLE 81.1	CAUSES OF PLEURAL EFFUSIONS

Transudates
Congestive heart failure
Cirrhosis
Nephrotic syndrome
Hypothyroidism
Hypoalbuminemia
Atelectasis
Superior vena cava obstruction
Exudates
Pneumonia (parapneumonic effusions)
Empyema
Collagen vascular disease
Pancreatitis
Esophogeal perforation
Subphrenic abscess
Chylothorax
Urinary tract obstruction (urinothorax)
Hemothorax
Drug hypersensitivity
Malignancy
Pulmonary infarction

▶ INDICATIONS

When the etiology of the pleural effusion is unknown or when respiratory embarrassment occurs because of the effusion, a thoracentesis should be performed. In certain circumstances,

it may be reasonable to defer thoracentesis and institute therapy when the cause of the effusion is readily apparent. This would be the case in nephrotic syndrome with effusion or from left ventricular heart failure (10).

Clinical suspicion of a pleural effusion arises when a child presents with pain on inspiration, shortness of breath, dyspnea, decreased breath sounds, and dullness to percussion over the affected area. Occasionally, a pleural friction rub is heard.

An upright posteroanterior and lateral chest radiograph will confirm the clinical impression. When the effusion is small, the only radiographic abnormality may be a meniscus or "blunting" at the costophrenic angle on upright chest radiograph (11). This meniscus occurs with small or larger amounts of fluid (175 to 525 cc) (12). As the effusion enlarges, there is extension of the fluid up the lateral chest wall on the upright view (11). Large effusions may appear to be consolidation or "whiteout" of the entire lung and may include mediastinal shift away form the affected side (11). Ultrasound can be helpful in differentiating an effusion draping the lungs from a complete consolidation of the lung (11). Computerized tomography (CT) is also an excellent way to visualize pleural disease, distinguish and localize loculations, and aid in the differentiation of other causes of pleural effusions (13,14).

The appearance of a pleural effusion is somewhat different in recumbent films. If the fluid collection is less than

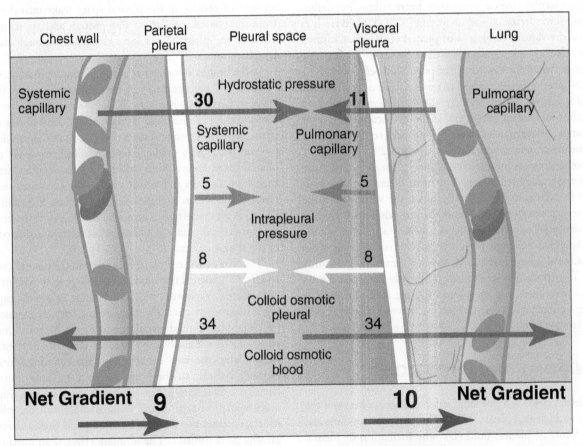

Figure 81.1 Schematic of Starling forces on the formation of pleural fluid.

125 mL, a recumbent film may appear normal despite the presence of an effusion (15). Moderate size effusions appear as a homogeneous density in the lower lung fields, and as the collection enlarges, the entire lung field takes on a ground glass appearance (15). For all suspected pleural effusions, a lateral decubitus radiograph is valuable, as it helps identify questionable effusions and also aids in determining whether an effusion is free flowing or loculated (10). Loculated pleural fluid does not shift with position changes. When the fluid appears loculated, consideration should be given to a radiologically guided thoracentesis to ensure proper drainage and decrease the incidence of complications.

The most frequent indication for performing a thoracentesis is as a diagnostic aid. In adults, results of a thoracentesis give diagnostic or clinically useful information in over 90% of examinations when taken in the context of the clinical presentation (16). Before attempting the procedure, it may be helpful to consult a specialist in pediatric pulmonary medicine or infectious disease to review issues and determine which laboratory studies should be performed on the fluid.

Once fluid is obtained, the most useful information to be determined is whether the fluid is a transudate or an exudate. An exudate implies a breakdown of vascular integrity, as seen in infection, neoplasms, and other inflammatory processes. In contrast, a transudate is an ultrafiltrate of plasma. Table 81.1 categorizes the etiologies of pleural effusions as to whether they are associated with an exudative or a transudative process.

Although the laboratory diagnosis of an exudate is not absolute, the criteria established by Light and his colleagues are generally accepted to define an exudative process (10). Light et al. (17) defined an exudate as having any one of the three following characteristics:

1 A pleural/serum protein ratio greater than 0.5
2 A pleural/serum LDH ratio greater than 0.6
3 A pleural fluid LDH of more than two thirds the upper limits of normal for the serum LDH

A transudate will have none of these characteristics. In the initial study by Light et al., the sensitivity and specificity of the criteria approached 100%. Later studies on unselected populations have confirmed the high sensitivity of these criteria (18,19).

If initial studies indicate that the effusion is a transudate, some authorities have suggested that further laboratory evaluation of the fluid is costly and does not increase the diagnostic yield (19,20). These authorities suggest a two-step approach in which the initial laboratory studies are sent to determine whether an exudate or a transudate exists. During the initial collection of fluid, samples should be "held" so that they can be used at a later time. If the laboratory evaluation suggests an exudative process, the history and physical examination should guide further laboratory and diagnostic evaluation.

For a transudate, the physician should treat the underlying disease process (5).

▶ PLEURAL FLUID LABORATORY STUDIES

This section reviews the potential laboratory studies that can be performed in the evaluation of pleural fluid. This is not meant to imply that all studies need to be sent for every patient. Clinical circumstances should guide the subsequent laboratory evaluation.

The gross appearance of the pleural fluid can be helpful. Transudates are often pale yellow. Milky white fluid suggests a chylothorax. Bloody fluid has been associated with neoplasms, pulmonary infarction, and trauma. This finding is tempered by the fact that 2 mL of blood into 1,000 mL of fluid can give a bloody appearance (21). A thick, purulent fluid is diagnostic of an empyema.

Pleural fluid is frequently sent for cytologic examination. Some authorities question the utility of cytologic examination for red and white blood cells (10,21,22). Light et al., in a prospective study of 182 patients, concluded that a red cell count of above $100,000/mm^3$ suggested neoplasm, pulmonary infarct, or trauma, but red cell counts between 10,000 and $100,000/mm^3$ were not specific for any disease process (21). They also concluded that the absolute white blood cell count is of limited utility due to a lack in both sensitivity and specificity. The differential count, however, may be helpful. A predominance of polymorphonuclear cells usually results from an acute inflammatory process such as pneumonia, pulmonary infarction, or a sympathetic effusion from pancreatitis. The presence of more than 50% lymphocytes strongly correlates with the presence of a malignancy or tuberculosis in patients with exudative effusions. The study did confirm the utility of cytologic examination for malignant cells, with a sensitivity of 77% when performed on one sample and of 90% when performed on three samples (21).

Although serosanguineous fluid has no predictive value (10,21), truly bloody fluid may indicate a traumatic hemothorax. If the hematocrit of the bloody fluid approaches that of serum, a traumatic hemothorax should be suspected and tube thoracostomy considered (5).

The pH, glucose, and Gram stain of the pleural fluid aid in discriminating between complicated parapneumonic effusions (effusions behaving like empyemas and requiring chest tube drainage for resolution) and uncomplicated parapneumonic effusions (which can be managed expectantly with antibiotic therapy). Unfortunately, clinical and radiologic indicators are not sufficiently distinct to separate children with uncomplicated effusions from those with empyema (2). A pleural fluid pH of less than 7.0 to 7.2, a glucose less than 40 mg/dL, or a positive Gram stain suggests a complicated parapneumonic effusion requiring tube thoracostomy (23,24). Pleural fluid glucose levels also are decreased in tuberculosis, malignancy, and rheumatoid diseases (5,25). Caution should be used when interpreting the pH value from a single measurement from a patient with multiloculated effusions. The pH can vary significantly between loculations and may give a false sense of security that one is dealing with an uncomplicated effusion if only one sample is obtained (26).

When differential diagnosis of the pleural effusion includes parapneumonic effusion or an empyema, a Gram stain and an aerobic culture, with consideration of an anaerobic culture, should be obtained (10). *Staphylococcus aureus* and *Streptococcus pneumoniae* cause the majority of empyemas in children and adolescents (1–3,27,28). *Streptococcus pyogenes*, Gram-negative bacteria, and now *Haemophilus influenzae* are found less frequently (1,28). In adult patients, anaerobic bacteria frequently are found alone or in a mixed infection (29). Their role in childhood empyemas is less clear, although some authorities suggest that anaerobes may play a significant role when aspiration pneumonia, lung abscess, subdiaphragmatic abscess, or abscesses of dental origin are the underlying cause of the empyema (28).

If tuberculosis is suspected, mycobacterial culture and acid-fast staining of the fluid should be performed. A culture of the pleural fluid for mycobacteria is of low yield, and the diagnosis is best confirmed by acid-fast staining of a needle biopsy of the pleura, sputum culture, or skin test conversion (10,30). Newer markers such as adenosine deaminase and gamma interferon are highly diagnostic for tuberculosis (31,32).

Several other tests may be helpful in certain clinical circumstances. The amylase will be elevated in effusions caused by acute pancreatitis or esophageal rupture (7,8). In patients with a malignant effusion, the amylase is elevated 10% of the time (7). A creatinine level of the fluid may be elevated in urinothorax from genitourinary injury to the ureter or bladder (5). In patients with a pleural effusion due to systemic lupus erythematosus, an antinuclear antibody titer is frequently greater than 1:160, and the lupus erythematosus (LE) cell prep may be positive. Complement levels may be decreased in lupus or other rheumatoid diseases. An elevated rheumatoid factor suggests an effusion due to rheumatoid arthritis (33). In the case of a true chylothorax, the triglyceride levels will be greater than 110% of the serum triglyceride level, and a Sudan III stain of fluid will be positive for chylomicrons (17).

Relative contraindications to performing a thoracentesis include an uncooperative patient, a skin infection at the insertion site, bleeding diathesis, and an insufficient volume of pleural fluid (5,10). The presence of pleural adhesions increases the risk of a pneumothorax, and therefore a thoracentesis should be performed cautiously in these patients (4).

▶ EQUIPMENT

Assemble the necessary equipment (Table 81.2). Use the thoracentesis needle on the tray or the largest over-the-needle

TABLE 81.2	EQUIPMENT AND SUPPLIES

For procedure:
  Pillow
  Sterile gloves
  Povidone-iodine solution
  Sterile gauze sponges
  Sterile basin for skin preparation
  Sterile towels or drape
  5-mL syringe
  27- and 22-gauge needles
  1% lidocaine
  Hemostat or metal spring
  15-mL or 30-mL syringe
  One 14- to 22-gauge Angiocath or a thoracentesis needle
  Three-way stopcock
  Intravenous tubing (optional)
  Vacuum bottle (optional)
  Sterile dressing
  Tape to secure bandage
For specimen collection:
  Aerobic and anaerobic culture bottles
  Sterile tubes for mycobacterial or fungal cultures
  Sterile tube for cytology
  Blood gas syringe
  Specimen tube for hematology
  Specimen tube for chemistry
  Other specimen tubes as needed

catheter possible for the thoracentesis, which is usually an 18- to 22-gauge catheter, depending on the size of the child. Commercial kits are available that contain a similar list of supplies.

▶ PROCEDURE

The following method is recommended when an effusion is felt to be free flowing. If the effusion is loculated, one should strongly consider performing the procedure with ultrasound or fluoroscopic guidance to more successfully obtain fluid and decrease the risk of complications (11,34,35).

The physician and nurse should explain the procedure to the child in an age-appropriate manner, with the family included in the discussion. The time spent preparing the child is well compensated for in terms of the cooperation that the physician will gain. A peripheral intravenous catheter is started in the event that a complication arises, for i.v. therapy, or for parenteral sedation as indicated. A venous blood sample is drawn to determine the serum LDH and protein levels and other studies as indicated. Monitoring includes continuous pulse oximetry and heart rate, with frequent vital signs. Supplemental oxygen is supplied for patients with respiratory distress or hypoxemia and should be available as needed afterwards (see "Complications"). For the younger or anxious child, mild, short-acting sedation may be considered. If parenteral sedation is used, follow the appropriate monitoring guidelines established by the American Academy of Pediatrics (36) (see Chapter 33 for sedation guidelines).

A thoracentesis is usually performed with the child in a sitting position (Fig. 81.2). This is best accomplished by having the child lean forward over a pillow that is placed over the back of a chair or table. If the child is unable to sit, the procedure is performed in the lateral decubitus position. The level of dullness percussed and the findings on the chest radiograph are used to identify the best location to perform the thoracentesis. The midscapular line is frequently used, although the posterior axillary line also is acceptable (4). When choosing which intercostal space to use, it is important to recall the level of the diaphragm throughout the respiratory cycle. The height of the diaphragm is most superior during expiration. The right arch is higher than the left because of the size of the liver. During maximal expiration, the level of the right dome is at the fourth costal cartilage anteriorly, at the sixth rib laterally, and at the eighth rib posteriorly. The dome of the left diaphragmatic arch is one to two ribs below that of the right (37). This makes the seventh intercostal space posteriorly a reasonable place to attempt a thoracentesis most of the time, and it will help prevent accidental puncture of the liver or spleen. When a child raises his or her arm, the tip of the scapula lies at the level of the seventh intercostal space in the posterior axillary line (6).

The area is widely prepared in a sterile manner with an antiseptic. Sterile towels are used to drape the area. With a 27-gauge needle attached to 5-mL syringe filled with local anesthetic, such as 1% or 2% lidocaine with epinephrine, a wheal is raised over the insertion site, identified by the rib below the desired intercostal space. The needle is removed and replaced by a 22-gauge needle. Entering directly over and perpendicular to the rib and through the previously raised wheal and by slowly advancing and injecting, the clinician should anesthetize to the periosteum. Then, the clinician should "walk" the needle over the superior margin of the rib, infiltrate, and proceed to aspirate while advancing the needle. The clinician needs to remember to keep the needle perpendicular to the skin surface to minimize the risk of accidental laceration of one of the intercostal arteries that lie along the inferior border of the rib superior to the entry site. Once fluid is aspirated, the clinician should stop infiltrating and mark the depth of the needle at the skin surface by cross-clamping the needle with a hemostat or a metal spring. The needle, hemostat, and syringe together are then removed from the entry site.

If no fluid is aspirated on entering the pleural space, it is sometimes necessary to enter one intercostal space inferior to the previously selected one. Again the clinician needs to recall the levels of the diaphragm during the respiratory cycle to minimize the risk of injury to the abdominal contents.

A 15- or 30-mL syringe and an over-the-needle catheter are now attached to a three-way stopcock. The previously identified depth of insertion is transferred to this needle by

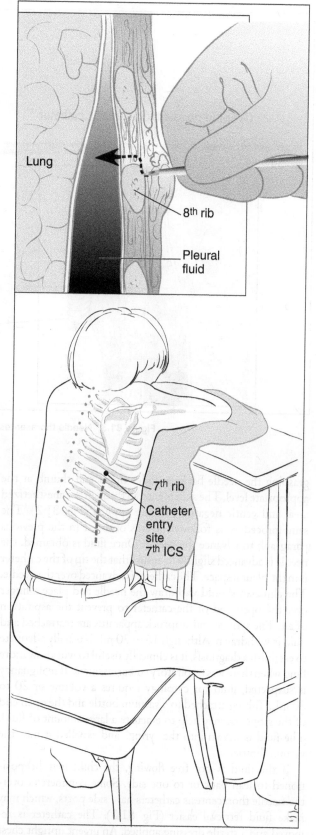

Figure 81.2 Thoracentesis. Placement of intravenous catheter into pleural fluid.

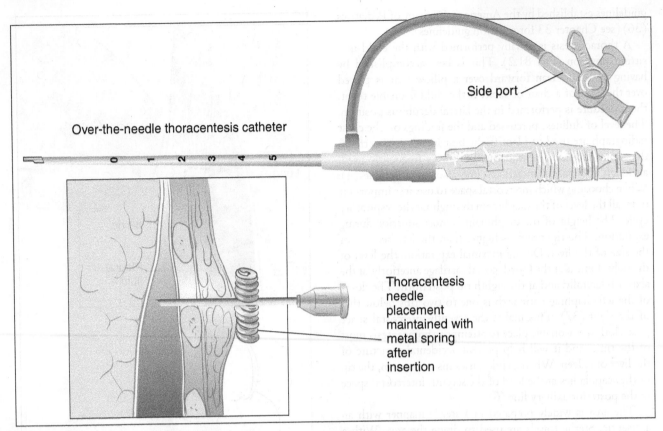

Figure 81.3 Needle thoracentesis with spring and thoracentesis catheter.

grasping the needle between index finger and thumb at the appropriate level. The skin is entered through the anesthetized area, and gentle negative pressure applied (Fig. 81.2). The same procedure is followed as was outlined in the previous paragraph to advance the needle. Once fluid is obtained, the needle is advanced slightly to ensure that the tip of the catheter is in the pleural space. The catheter is advanced over the needle. The clinician should withdraw the needle and place a finger over the open end of the catheter to prevent the aspiration of air. The syringe and stopcock apparatus are reattached and fluid is withdrawn. Although 15 to 30 mL is usually adequate to establish a diagnosis, it is clinically useful to withdraw more fluid when there was respiratory embarrassment. If malignancy is suspected, fluid for cytology requires a volume of 20 to 30 mL. Tubing attached to a vacuum bottle and the open end of the stopcock may help to evacuate a large amount of fluid. The fluid is drawn into the syringe and expelled it into the vacuum bottle.

If the fluid is not free flowing, the child may be positioned to lean back or to one side. Some commercial over-the-needle thoracentesis catheters have side ports, which may make fluid retrieval easier (Fig. 81.3). The catheter is removed and a sterile dressing applied. An urgent upright chest radiograph is obtained in order to check for an iatrogenic pneumothorax.

Needle Thoracentesis

The above mentioned procedure also may be done with a needle rather than an over-the-needle catheter. The procedure is performed as previously described, except that after the depth of the needle is identified during anesthetic infiltration, this depth should be transferred to the thoracentesis needle by placing a hemostat or metal spring across the thoracentesis needle (Fig. 81.3). This will help prevent accidental advancement of the needle into the lung and a subsequent pneumothorax. The level of the hemostat sometimes needs to be adjusted slightly.

Other Techniques

Other techniques include using pigtail catheters (34,38) and semiflexible catheters (39,40) for the thoracentesis. Procedures with these catheters can be performed under ultrasound or fluoroscopic guidance (34) or directly if the fluid is free flowing (38). The catheters are introduced into the thoracic cavity via the Seldinger technique (catheter over a wire). An advantage of this technique is that the catheters, once in place, can be attached to water seal suction drainage and provide continuous drainage (34,38,41). The patient can be moved with minimal risk of puncture or injury to the underlying lung. Patient preparation and follow-up is as described previously.

SUMMARY

1 Identify effusion and whether it is free flowing with posteroanterior and lateral decubitus chest radiograph.

2 Monitor with pulse oximetry and frequent vital signs.

3 Consider pharmacologic sedation as necessary.

4 Position the child in sitting position leaning forward over the chair.

5 Identify the insertion site—frequently the seventh intercostal space in the posterior or posterior axillary line.

6 Prepare the sterile field and anesthetize the skin and tissue to pleura.

7 Attach the needle or a catheter over the needle to a three-way stopcock and syringe and walk the needle over the top of the rib while applying negative pressure to the syringe.

8 Once fluid is obtained, thread the catheter over the needle into the pleural space.

9 Reattach the syringe and stopcock to the catheter and remove pleural fluid.

10 Remove the catheter and cover with a dressing.

11 Obtain a chest radiograph to check for an iatrogenic pneumothorax.

12 Send pleural fluid for protein and LDH. Send the patient's serum for protein and LDH. "Hold" other samples in appropriate sterile containers.

13 If a transudate is identified, treat the underlying cause.

14 If an exudate is identified, consider further laboratory analysis relative to the presenting history and physical examination.

▶ COMPLICATIONS

A diagnostic thoracentesis does carry the risk of significant complications. The most frequent major complication is a pneumothorax, which occurs in up to 11% to 30% of

 CLINICAL TIPS

▶ A lateral decubitus chest radiograph identifies free-flowing pleural fluid.

▶ A loculated effusion is best approached with an ultrasound-guided thoracentesis.

▶ The neurovascular bundle lies along the inferior border of the rib.

▶ The seventh intercostal space posteriorly is a safe landmark for attempting a thoracentesis and is located at the tip of the scapula when the arm is completely abducted.

▶ If the pleural fluid does not flow freely, try having the child lean back or to the side. If using the needle approach, care must be taken to prevent accidental puncture of the underlying lung. Commercial thoracentesis needles with side ports may ease fluid retrieval.

▶ Empyemas and hemothorax require tube thoracostomy.

procedures (16,35,42). Risk is reduced when the procedure is performed by a clinician well trained in the technique and in a monitored setting with a cooperative patient (43). Ultrasound guidance of the procedure appears to significantly decrease the rate of pneumothorax (35). Using mild sedation and measures to suppress the child's cough may lessen the risk of a pneumothorax. Other less common complications include laceration of the intercostal vessels and subsequent hemothorax, laceration of the liver or spleen, cough, vasovagal reactions, and persistent local pain (5,16,43).

In an adult, no more than 1,000 to 1,500 mL of fluid should be removed at a time. Re-expansion pulmonary edema or severe hypotension has been described if larger volumes are rapidly removed (5,10,44). Larger volumes can be safely removed if intrapleural pressure is monitored during the procedure and kept above −20 cm H_2O (44). No comparable data are available for children.

Hypoxemia predictably occurs after thoracentesis and correlates directly with the volume of fluid removed (45). Hypoxemia resolves after 24 hours, and supplying oxygen during and after the procedure prevents this complication.

▶ SUMMARY

When used to remove pleural fluid causing respiratory embarrassment, a thoracentesis is considered therapeutic. When used to assist in identifying the underlying cause of the effusion, it is considered diagnostic. Important information to obtain is whether the effusion is an exudate or a transudate.

The causes of a pleural effusion are diverse, and the evaluation of pleural fluid is particularly useful when taken in the context of the clinical presentation. The procedure itself is straightforward, and either a needle or a flexible catheter can be used. No matter which method is used, care must be taken so that the risk of a pneumothorax is minimized.

▶ REFERENCES

1. Wolfe WG, Spock A, Bradford WD. Pleural fluid in infants and children. *Am Rev Respir Dis.* 1968;98:1027–1032.
2. Chonmaitree T, Powell KR. Parapneumonia pleural effusion and empyema in children. *Clin Pediatr.* 1983;22:414–419.
3. Freij BJ, Kusmiesz H, Nelson JD, et al. Parapneumonia effusions and empyema in hospitalized children: a retrospective review of 227 cases. *Pediatr Inf Dis.* 1984;3:578–591.
4. Blok B, Ibrado A. Thoracentesis. In: Roberts JR, Hedges JR, eds. *Clinical Procedures in Emergency Medicine.* 4th ed. Philadelphia: WB Saunders; 2004:171–186.
5. Jay SJ. Diagnostic procedures for pleural disease. *Clin Chest Med.* 1985;6:33–48.
6. Zeitlin PL. Pleural effusions and empyema. In: Laughlin GM, Eigen H, eds. *Respiratory Disease in Children.* Baltimore: Williams & Wilkins; 1994:453–463.
7. Light RW. Pleural effusions. *Med Clin North Am.* 1977;61:1339–1352.
8. Sahn SA. The pathophysiology of pleural effusions. *Ann Rev Med.* 1990;41:7–13.
9. Pagtakhan RD, Chernick V. Liquid and air in the pleural space. In: Chernick V, ed. *Kendig's Disorders of the Respiratory Tract in Children.* 5th ed. Philadelphia: WB Saunders; 1990:545–557.
10. American College of Physicians, Health and Public Policy Committee. Diagnostic thoracentesis and pleural biopsy in pleural effusions. *Ann Intern Med.* 1985;103:799–802.
11. Swischuk LE. *Emergency Radiology of the Acutely Ill or Injured Child.* 3rd ed. Baltimore: Williams & Wilkins; 1994.
12. Collins JD, Burwell D, Furmanski S, et al. Minimum detectable pleural effusions: a roentgen pathology model. *Radiology.* 1972;105:51–53.
13. Davies CL, Gleeson FV. Diagnostic radiology. In: Light RW, Lee GYC, eds. *Textbook of Pleural Diseases.* London: Arnold; 2003:210–237.
14. McLoud TC. CT and MR in pleural disease. *Clin Chest Med.* 1998;19:261–276.
15. Woodring JH. Recognition of pleural effusion on supine radiographs: how much fluid is required? *AJR Am J Roentgenol.* 1984;142:59–64.
16. Collins TR, Sahn SA. Thoracentesis: clinical value, complications and experience. *Chest.* 1987;91:817–822.
17. Light RW, MacGregor I, Ruchsinger PC, et al. The diagnostic separation of transudates from exudates. *Ann Intern Med.* 1973;132:854.
18. Romero S, Candela A, Martin C, et al. Evaluation of different criteria for the separation of pleural transudates from exudates. *Chest.* 1993;104:339–404.
19. Peterman TA, Speicher CE. Evaluating pleural effusions: a two-stage laboratory approach. *JAMA.* 1984;252:1051–1053.
20. Sahn SA. The differential diagnosis of pleural effusions. *West J Med.* 1982;137:99–108.
21. Light RW, Erozan YS, Ball WC. Cells in pleural fluid: their value in differential diagnosis. *Arch Intern Med.* 1973;132:854–860.
22. Dine DZ, Pierce AV, Franzen SS. The value of cells in the pleural fluid in the differential diagnosis. *Mayo Clin Proc.* 1975;50:571–572.
23. Houston MC. Pleural fluid pH: therapeutic and prognostic value. *Am J Surg.* 1987;154:333–337.
24. Light RW, Giraud WM, Jenkinson SG, et al. Parapneumonia effusions. *Am J Med.* 1980;69:507–512.
25. Lillington GA, Carr DT, Mayne JG. Rheumatoid pleurisy with effusion. *Arch Intern Med.* 1971;128:764–768.
26. Maskell NA, Gleeson FV, Darby M, et al. Diagnostically significant variations in pleural fluid pH in loculated parapneumonic effusions. *Chest.* 2004;126:2022–2024.
27. Fajardo JE, Chang MJ. Pleural empyema in children: a nationwide retrospective study. *South Med J.* 1987;80:593–596.
28. Brook I. Microbiology of empyema in children and adolescents. *Pediatrics.* 1990;85:722–726.
29. Bartlett JG, Gorbach SL, Thadepalli H, et al. Bacteriology of empyema. *Lancet.* 1974;1:338–339.
30. Van Hoff DD, LiVolsi V. Diagnostic reliability of needle biopsy of the parietal pleura. *Am J Clin Pathol.* 1975;64:200–203.
31. Valdes L, Alvarez D, San Jose E, et al. Tuberculous pleurisy: a study of 254 patients. *Arch Intern Med.* 1998;158:2017–2021.
32. Villegas MV, Labrada LA, Saravia NF. Evaluation of polymerase chain reaction, adenosine deaminase, and interferon-gamma in pleural fluid for the differential diagnosis of pleural tuberculosis. *Chest.* 2000;118:1355–1364.
33. Halla JT, Schrohenloher RE, Volanakis JE. Immune complexes and other laboratory features of pleural effusions. *Ann Intern Med.* 1980;92:748–752.
34. Westcott JL. Percutaneous catheter drainage of pleural effusion and empyema. *AJR Am J Roentgenol.* 1985;144:1189–1193.
35. Grogan DR, Irwin RS, Channick R, et al. Complications associated with thoracentesis: a prospective randomized study comparing three different methods. *Arch Intern Med.* 1990;150:873–877.
36. Committee on Drugs. Guidelines for monitoring and management of pediatric patients during and after sedation for diagnostic and therapeutic procedures. *Pediatrics.* 1992;89:1110–1115.
37. Pick TP, Howden R, eds. *Gray's Anatomy.* Philadelphia: Running Press; 1974.
38. Fuhrman BP, Landrum BG, Ferrara TB, et al. Pleural drainage using modified pigtail catheters. *Crit Care Med.* 1986;14:575–576.
39. Cooper CM. Pleural aspiration with a central venous catheter. *Anaesthesia.* 1987;42:217.
40. Clarke JM. A new instrument for thoracentesis. *Surg Gyne Obstet.* 1984;159:587–588.
41. Crouch JD, Keagy BA, Delany DJ. "Pigtail" catheter drainage in thoracic surgery. *Am Rev Respir Dis.* 1987;136:174–175.
42. Seneff MG, Corwin W, Gold LH, et al. Complications associated with thoracentesis. *Chest.* 1986;89:97–100.
43. Bartter T, Mayo PD, Pratter MR, et al. Lower risk and higher yield for thoracentesis when performed by experienced operators. *Chest.* 1993;103:1873–1876.
44. Light RW, Jenkinson SG, Minh V, et al. Observations on pleural fluid pressures as fluid is withdrawn during thoracentesis. *Am Rev Resp Dis.* 1980;121:799–804.
45. Brandstetter RD, Cohen RP. Hypoxemia after thoracentesis. *JAMA.* 1979;242:1060–1061.

JOSEPH W. LURIA

82

Introduction to Conventional Mechanical Ventilation

▶ INTRODUCTION

The appropriate use of mechanical ventilation is a requisite skill for all physicians caring for children who are critically ill. The first widespread use of ventilators in a nonoperative setting occurred during the polio epidemic of the 1950s. Since that time, ventilators and ventilation strategies have become more sophisticated and, for some, more challenging. Although ventilators may seem to be complex machines, a few basic principles govern their function. Once these principles are understood and applied correctly, ventilator management can proceed in an effective manner (1–14).

▶ ANATOMY AND PHYSIOLOGY

The respiratory cycle consists of inspiration and exhalation. Inspiration is an active process initiated by contraction of the intercostal musculature and diaphragm. The actions of these muscles cause an expansion of the chest cavity, which generates a negative transpleural pressure. Air flows along the resultant pressure gradient (between the atmosphere and pleural space), through the airways, and into the lungs. Exhalation, which eliminates air after alveolar gas exchange, is largely a passive process due to the elastic recoil of the lung.

The two forces that affect airflow through the respiratory tree are compliance and resistance. Compliance represents the elasticity of the respiratory system and is defined as the unit change in lung volume per unit change in pressure. When respiratory compliance decreases, the lung is often described as being "stiff." The lung and chest wall have separate compliances, and each contributes to the total compliance of the respiratory system. Adult respiratory distress

syndrome (ARDS), neonatal RDS, and the presence of pulmonary edema are examples of clinical scenarios in which respiratory compliance is decreased.

Resistance is the impedance of airflow due to friction. It is defined as the unit change in pressure per unit change in gas flow. Respiratory resistance is greatest in the airways. Processes that cause a narrowing of the airways, such as asthma, will increase respiratory resistance.

Work of breathing is the amount of effort required to overcome both the respiratory compliance and resistance. Processes that decrease compliance or increase resistance will increase the total work of breathing. In these settings, patients will compensate by adopting a respiratory pattern that minimizes their work of breathing. Generally, acute lung processes that decrease compliance are associated with rapid, shallow breathing. In contrast, processes that increase respiratory resistance are associated with slow, deep breathing. These breathing patterns can be useful clinical clues when determining a patient's underlying pathophysiology.

The volume of air that is moved into the lungs during a normal inspiration is termed the tidal volume. Normal tidal volume at all ages is 6 to 8 mL/kg. Functional residual capacity (FRC), or resting volume, is the amount of air remaining in the lungs at the end of a normal, quiet exhalation. FRC is determined by two opposing forces that are equal at the end of exhalation. These are the elastic properties of the lung and chest wall. At FRC, the elasticity of the lung exerts a force that favors a reduction in lung volume. The elastic force of the chest wall favors expansion. Processes that alter the relationship between these two forces will alter the FRC. Closing capacity is the volume of air in the lung below which small airways begin to collapse. Any disease state that increases the closing capacity or decreases the FRC can result in airway collapse and atelectasis. One objective of mechanical ventilation

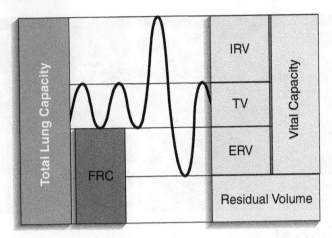

Figure 82.1 Spirogram illustrating lung volumes. ERV, expiratory reserve volume; FRC, functional residual capacity; IRV, inspiratory reserve volume; TV, tidal volume. (Adapted from Rogers MC, ed. *Textbook of Pediatric Intensive Care*. Baltimore: Williams & Wilkins; 1987:115.)

is to optimize the relationship between closing capacity and FRC. For example, closing capacity occurs at greater lung volumes in premature infants with surfactant deficiency (RDS). The goal of positive pressure ventilation in this setting is to increase the FRC above closing capacity by using positive end-expiratory pressure (PEEP). This will prevent further atelectasis and assist in the re-expansion of collapsed segments of the lung. These lung volumes are illustrated in the spirogram in Figure 82.1.

The central nervous system (CNS) coordinates the actions of the respiratory muscles. The respiratory muscles are responsible for the bellows-like action that brings oxygen into the lungs and expels carbon dioxide. The lungs provide the interface for the transfer of oxygen into the blood and the removal of carbon dioxide. The circulatory system is responsible for delivering oxygen to the tissues and bringing carbon dioxide back to the lung for removal. In a simplistic manner, this describes the big picture of normal respiration. Processes that depress the CNS (e.g., traumatic brain injury, narcotic intoxication), weaken the respiratory musculature (e.g., Guillain-Barré syndrome, poliomyelitis, myopathies), or damage the lung or heart can lead to respiratory failure.

A large number of pulmonary and cardiac processes can result in respiratory failure. The end result of these processes is impaired pulmonary gas exchange with or without increased work of breathing. Impaired gas exchange results in the inability of the circulation to deliver adequate amounts of oxygen to peripheral tissues. To meet the oxygen demands of the body, minute ventilation and/or cardiac output must be increased. To accomplish this, the respiratory musculature and cardiac musculature are forced to work harder. This additional work of breathing increases the oxygen consumption of the cardiopulmonary system. To meet the higher oxygen demand, minute ventilation and/or cardiac output must be further increased. If the underlying insult is severe or is not corrected, this cycle will continue until demand cannot be met. Then it

will not be possible to meet the oxygen requirements of the body, the respiratory musculature will fatigue, and respiratory failure will ensue. This concept as it pertains to specific pathophysiologic processes is discussed in the "Procedure" section later in this chapter.

▶ INDICATIONS

Respiratory failure is the primary indication for initiating mechanical ventilation. Respiratory failure is characterized as the inability to maintain adequate oxygenation and/or ventilation despite using more conservative respiratory therapies. Traditionally, hypoxemic respiratory failure is defined as a PaO_2 of less than 55 to 60 torr in the face of inspired oxygen concentrations of greater than 60%. Inadequate ventilation is defined as the presence of respiratory acidosis, an elevated PaO_2, and an arterial pH of less than 7.2 to 7.25. These numbers are guidelines and should not be used as absolute values. The clinician, in deciding whether to begin mechanical ventilation, should consider the disease process present and its anticipated progression, the patient's clinical assessment and response to other therapies, and the risks associated with mechanical ventilation.

Impending respiratory failure with or without increased work of breathing constitutes a relative indication for mechanical ventilation. It is always preferable to initiate mechanical ventilation under controlled conditions rather than to wait for worsening acidosis, exhaustion, or cardiorespiratory failure.

In some medical and surgical conditions, it may be best for a patient to assume a specific respiratory pattern. When this occurs, mechanical ventilation can be used to achieve this goal. The most common example of this is the need for hyperventilation in a patient with intracranial hypertension and lateralizing signs or impending herniation. Table 82.1 reviews these indications for initiating mechanical ventilation.

Mechanical ventilation may be an indicated treatment in a number of clinical diseases. Specific details of ventilator management are highly dependent on the disease state present

TABLE 82.1	INDICATIONS FOR INITIATING MECHANICAL VENTILATION

Absolute Indications
Apnea
Inadequate oxygenation (despite F_IO_2 >60%)
  1. PaO_2 <55–60 torr
  2. O_2 saturation <90%
Inadequate ventilation—respiratory acidosis (hypercapnia, Pco_2 >50) with pH <7.2–7.25
Relative Indications
Increased work of breathing
  1. Circulatory insufficiency
  2. Prolonged respiratory distress
Need to control respiratory pattern—intracranial hypertension and lateralizing signs or impending herniation.

Source: Adapted from Rogers MC, ed. *Textbook of Pediatric Intensive Care*. Baltimore: Williams & Wilkins; 1987.

and its severity; therefore, specific pathophysiologic processes and how they relate to ventilator management are discussed in the "Procedure" section later in this chapter.

▶ EQUIPMENT

To use a ventilator effectively, it is important to have a basic understanding of how it works and a common vocabulary for describing its function. Similar to spontaneous respiration, mechanical breaths may be divided into four phases: transition from exhalation to inspiration, inspiration, transition from inspiration to exhalation, and exhalation. The goal of the operator is to select ventilator settings to perform these phases of respiration in a manner that is optimal for the patient.

Transition from exhalation to inhalation refers to the way in which a ventilator initiates a mechanical breath. For practical purposes, initiation of a mechanical breath can be controlled by either time or pressure. When a breath is initiated because a preset time has elapsed, the ventilation is said to be time triggered. A pressure-triggered breath is initiated in response to a spontaneous respiratory effort. Contraction of the respiratory musculature from a spontaneous breath results in a negative transpleural pressure. This negative pressure is transmitted through the respiratory tree to the endotracheal tube and into the ventilator circuit. The ventilator will sense this decrease in the circuit pressure, and a positive pressure breath will be delivered.

Once a mechanical breath has been initiated, the ventilator must deliver an effective tidal volume, which is accomplished by preselecting limits for the inspiration. For instance, if the inspiratory pressure reaches a constant value before inspiration ends, it is a pressure-limited breath. If a constant volume or flow rate is reached before the end of inspiration, the breath is volume or flow limited, respectively. Some ventilators also have the capability to select an inspiratory flow pattern (constant, sinusoidal, accelerating, or decelerating). Despite a number of studies, the data fail to demonstrate any advantage of one gas flow pattern over the others in all circumstances.

Cycling refers to the manner by which a ventilator transitions from inspiration to exhalation. If inspiration ceases after a preset time, the breath is said to be time cycled. Likewise, if inspiration ceases after a preset volume or inspiratory pressure is reached, the breath is volume or pressure cycled, respectively.

Exhalation proceeds after a valve is opened within the exhalatory limb of the ventilator circuit. As with normal respiration, exhalation is a passive process. During mechanical ventilation, the patient will remain in the exhalation phase until another breath is triggered.

Ventilators are described by the manner in which they operate during the first three phases of respiration. For example, an infant ventilator may be described as providing time-triggered, pressure-limited, and time-cycled breaths. Most clinicians, however, do not routinely refer to ventilator function in this manner. Rather, they refer to a particular mode of ventilation.

Referring to a mode of ventilation is a shorthand method for describing how a ventilator performs the phases of the respiration. Modes of ventilation are selected based on the clinical situation.

Control Mode Ventilation

Control mode ventilation (CMV) is time triggered. Each breath is initiated at a preset time interval. By definition, the ventilator will not respond to the patient's spontaneous respiratory efforts. CMV should be reserved for patients who are apneic. A patient who is breathing spontaneously would be uncomfortable on this mode of ventilation. CMV is not responsive to patient respiratory effort and gives breaths to the alert patient asynchronously with his or her spontaneous respiration.

Assist Mode Ventilation

In assist mode ventilation, mechanical breaths are initiated by the patient's spontaneous respiratory effort. The ventilator accomplishes this by sensing a change in circuit pressure or gas flow (pressure or flow triggered). This mode allows the patient to "interact" with the ventilator. That is, the ventilator is responsive to the patient's needs in a synchronous fashion. It may be used for fully awake intubated patients. The assist mode should not be used with apneic patients because no respiratory support would be afforded.

Assist/Control Mode Ventilation

Assist/control mode breaths are initiated in response to the patient's spontaneous respiratory efforts. The ventilator will deliver a controlled breath at a preset time interval or when it detects a patient-initiated breath. This combination of assisted and controlled breaths offers the advantages of both modes. It allows the patient to interact with the ventilator, thereby serving the patient's respiratory needs. Should the patient become apneic or too weak to initiate a mechanical breath, the ventilator would continue to provide support in the form of controlled breaths triggered by a period of apnea.

Intermittent Mandatory Ventilation

Intermittent mandatory ventilation (IMV) was initially developed as a means of weaning patients from CMV back to total independent spontaneous respiration. During IMV, mechanical breaths are delivered at a preset frequency (time triggered). In between mechanical breaths, the patient is allowed to breathe spontaneously. Spontaneous breaths are permitted by one of two mechanisms. The ventilator will either have a continuous flow of gas in the circuit or an intermittent flow of fresh gas accessed by the patient's spontaneous effort, which opens a demand valve. The ventilator does not deliver a controlled breath during spontaneous breathing.

IMV is thought to have a number of benefits. First, it decreases the amount of positive pressure to which the lung is subjected. It has been suggested that this will decrease the impedance of venous return to the right heart associated with positive pressure ventilation. Spontaneous respiration also is associated with improved ventilation to the dependent areas of the lung, which theoretically should result in less ventilation-perfusion ($\dot{V}/\dot{Q}$) mismatching. In addition, allowing spontaneous breathing will assist in preserving the patient's respiratory muscular tone.

Synchronized Intermittent Mandatory Ventilation

Synchronized intermittent mandatory ventilation (SIMV) is similar to IMV except that mechanical breaths are triggered by the patient's respiratory effort instead of being time triggered. If no effort is detected during a preset time interval, a controlled breath is delivered. Like IMV, the patient breathes spontaneously between ventilator breaths. The advantage of SIMV is that it allows the patient to interact with the ventilator to a greater degree and thus allows the patient to be more comfortable while on the ventilator. If a high enough rate is selected, this mode is similar to the assist/control mode.

Pressure Support Ventilation

Pressure support ventilation (PSV) is pressure triggered, pressure limited, and flow cycled. This means that mechanical breaths are initiated by the patient's spontaneous effort. The ventilator then delivers a preset pressure into the circuit. This pressure can be set to provide any fraction of the total respiratory support needed by the patient. The ventilator cycles to exhalation when the flow in the circuit decreases below some preset level. This allows the patient to determine the length and volume of the delivered breath. Pressure support can be used solely or to assist spontaneous respiration between mandatory breaths as a method of weaning.

Continuous Positive Airway Pressure/Positive End-Expiratory Pressure

The application of a continuous airway distending pressure in the absence of mechanical breaths is referred to as "continuous positive airway pressure" (CPAP). When mechanical breaths are present, this baseline airway pressure is termed "positive end-expiratory pressure" (PEEP). The advantage of CPAP/PEEP is that it increases FRC by maintaining open airways and re-expanding atelectatic areas of the lung, which improves respiratory compliance and ultimately decreases the patient's work of breathing. The recruitment of atelectatic areas of the lung also decreases $\dot{V}/\dot{Q}$ mismatch, improving oxygenation. A lower, less toxic concentration of oxygen can be used.

CPAP/PEEP must be used with caution. It should be used sparingly or not at all in respiratory diseases associated with overinflation, such as asthma. When used in these settings, CPAP/PEEP is associated with a number of complications related to increased alveolar distention. Overdistention can result in decreased venous return to the right heart and thus will decrease cardiac output and impair oxygen delivery to the tissues. Intravascular volume expansion may minimize this effect. Increased distention also increases the likelihood of complications from pulmonary overinflation "volutrauma." Additionally, overdistention of alveoli can cause increased $\dot{V}/\dot{Q}$ mismatching, resulting in decreased oxygen delivery to peripheral tissues.

CPAP/PEEP also is associated with an increase in intracranial pressure. Consequently, elevated levels of CPAP/PEEP should be avoided in patients with intracranial hypertension.

▶ PROCEDURE

Initiation of mechanical ventilation begins with selecting an appropriate ventilator. In most situations, choices are limited to either a volume controller or a pressure controller. Volume controllers are used most commonly in children weighing more than 10 kg. They offer the advantage of being able to track changing respiratory compliance. When a patient's compliance decreases, pulmonary pressures increase, as the delivered tidal volume remains constant. Ventilators of this type are equipped with an alarm to indicate increasing airway pressures, which assists clinicians in delivering effective ventilator management.

Pressure controllers are most commonly used in smaller children and neonates. In contrast to volume controllers, delivered tidal volumes depend on the patient's respiratory compliance and resistance. A decrease in compliance will result in a smaller tidal volume, as peak inspiratory pressure is constant. Adequacy of ventilation should be assessed clinically (i.e., chest excursion and auscultation of breath sounds), by blood gas determination, and by the measured tidal volume displayed on the ventilator (if available).

As with most procedures, the use of a systematic approach helps to avoid errors and omissions. The following information provides a starting point for initiating mechanical ventilation. It is not meant to imply that a "cookbook approach" to mechanical ventilation is available that will work in all situations. The method by which a patient is ventilated is largely determined by the underlying disease process.

Volume-Controlled Ventilation

The first step in initiating volume-controlled ventilation is selecting a mode (Table 82.2). The most commonly used modes are SIMV and assist/control. They allow the most patient-ventilator interaction and will ensure adequate ventilation should the patient become apneic or too weak to initiate a breath. SIMV offers a number of advantages over the assist/control mode and is often the first choice. When initiating mechanical ventilation, a higher ventilator respiratory rate

TABLE 82.2	INITIAL VENTILATOR SETUP	
	Volume controller	**Pressure controller**
1. Select a ventilatory mode	Usually SIMV, but assist/control may be used	Infant ventilators usually have only one mode (time triggered, pressure limited, time cycled)

2. Provide adequate inspiration	Children: 8–10 mL/kg
	Adolescent: 6–8 mL/kg
		PIP to cause adequate inspiration to rise and fall of chest with good breath sounds
		Newborn
		  Well 15 cm H_2O
		  RDS 25 cm H_2O
		1 year 20–30 cm H_2O

3. Set the ventilator frequency	Physiologic norm for age (Table 82.3)	Physiologic norm for age (Table 84.3)
4. Set the inspiratory time (I time)	Calculated to keep I:E ratio of 1:2 unless clinically contraindicated	Calculated to keep I:E ratio of 1:2 unless clinically contraindicated
5. Set the F_iO_2	100% initially, then wean to maintain adequate O_2 saturation	100% initially, then wean to maintain adequate O_2 saturation
6. Set the PEEP	5 cm H_2O pressure unless clinically contraindicated	3–5 cm H_2O pressure unless clinically contraindicated
7. Assess the patient	Clinically and by blood gas determination to ensure adequate oxygenation and ventilation	Clinically and by blood gas determination to ensure adequate oxygenation and ventilation

can be selected, and the ventilator will perform in a manner similar to the assist/control mode. As the patient's respiratory status improves, the ventilator rate can be decreased, allowing the patient to take a larger number of unassisted breaths, which will provide a means for weaning the patient from the ventilator. In the assist/control mode, both spontaneous and time-triggered breaths are assisted. This exposes the patient to more positive airway pressure and its associated risks.

Regardless of the type of mode selected, it is important to ensure adequate alveolar ventilation and tissue oxygenation. Alveolar ventilation is determined by tidal volume and frequency of ventilation (rate). As previously stated, tidal volume of a normal patient is approximately 6 to 8 mL/kg. The tidal volume set on the ventilator, however, should range from 8 to 10 mL/kg in an infant or child and 6 to 8 mL/kg in an adolescent or adult. One reason for the difference is that uncuffed endotracheal tubes are utilized in prepubertal patients. Some of the delivered tidal volume may leak around the tube and escape into the atmosphere. Another reason is that the ventilator circuit is compressible, and some of the delivered tidal volume will remain within it. Ventilator rate is usually set at the age-specific norm (Table 82.3).

Next, the operator must select an inspiratory time. Inspiratory time is calculated after determining the desired respiratory rate. Under normal circumstances, one third of a normal respiratory cycle is spent in inspiration (I:E ratio of I:2). If a respiratory rate of 20 is desired, for example, each breath will take 3 seconds. The inspiratory time should be set at one third this value, or I second.

Oxygenation is determined by F_iO_2 and mean airway pressure. Initially the ventilator should be set to deliver 100% oxygen. This setting should be weaned provided oxygenation is adequate (SaO_2 greater than 93%). Mean airway pressure is most commonly augmented by the application of PEEP, which is usually set at 5 cm H_2O, unless clinically contraindicated. If the F_iO_2 can be weaned to less than 60%, this level of PEEP should be maintained. Under certain clinical situations, it will be necessary to further increase the PEEP so that the F_iO_2 can be weaned to less toxic levels.

Assessment of Settings

After selecting these parameters, it is important for the clinician to assess the adequacy of mechanical ventilation, which is accomplished by observing the rise and fall of the chest and auscultating breath sounds. If ventilation appears to be inadequate, the tidal volume should be increased. In contrast, the tidal volume should be decreased if the observed chest movement is hyperdynamic. Alveolar overdistention is the primary determinant of ventilator-induced lung injury, so excessive tidal volumes should be avoided. Adequate oxygenation should be assessed both clinically (i.e., color, heart rate) and by measurement of the oxygen saturation. After the patient has been stabilized, these observations should be verified by blood gas determination.

TABLE 82.3	SUGGESTED VENTILATOR RATES BASED ON AGE
Age	**Rate (per min)**
<2 mo	40
2–6 mo	35
6–12 mo	30
12 mo–6 y	25
>6 y	20

If concerns exist regarding the patient's oxygenation or ventilation, use of the ventilator should be discontinued and the patient ventilated with a bag-valve device with 100% oxygen. If the patient can be adequately ventilated with a bag-valve device but deteriorates when placed on the ventilator, either a mechanical problem exists or inadequate ventilation parameters were selected. The ventilator should be checked to ensure proper setup. Respiratory therapy staff can be an excellent resource for this problem. If the patient's clinical condition does not improve with manual ventilation, a problem with the patient may exist. The position and patency of the endotracheal tube should be assessed. The patient also should be evaluated for any possible complications of positive pressure ventilation, such as a pneumothorax. When the specific problem is identified and corrected, the patient can then be reconnected to the ventilator and another assessment performed. Afterward a blood gas determination should be done to ensure adequate CO_2 elimination and oxygenation. Adjustments in the ventilation parameters are made on the basis of these observations. Table 82.2 summarizes the steps for initiating volume-controlled ventilation.

Most conscious patients who are being mechanically ventilated will have some degree of pain and/or anxiety. Clinically, the patient will appear to be fighting the ventilator, which can result in difficulties with oxygenation and ventilation. When this occurs, it is important for the clinician to exclude any problems with patient condition or ventilator function. Sedatives and/or analgesics can then be used to make the patient more comfortable and thus enhance patient-ventilator interaction.

Pressure-Controlled Ventilation

The major difference between pressure-controlled and volume-controlled ventilation is that a peak inspiratory pressure (PIP) is selected instead of a tidal volume. An easy method for determining the initial PIP is to use a manometer attached to the endotracheal tube through a bag-valve device. While manually ventilating, the clinician notes the peak pressure required to demonstrate an adequate rise of the chest. This pressure should then serve as the PIP when initiating mechanical ventilation. As with volume-controlled ventilation, the clinician should not select a PIP that causes hyperdynamic rise and fall of the chest. If a manometer is not available, clinical experience will help dictate the initial PIP setting. In general, a neonate with no lung disease will require a PIP of about 15 cm H_2O, whereas a neonate with RDS will need about 25 cm H_2O. In children weighing closer to 10 kg, a PIP of 20 to 25 is commonly needed to provide an adequate tidal volume. An even higher PIP may be necessary depending on the severity of the lung disease. Ventilatory frequency and inspiratory time should be set at the age-appropriate physiologic norm. As with volume-controlled ventilation, the F_iO_2 should be initially set at 100% and the PEEP at 5 cm H_2O pressure.

Once the patient is connected to the ventilator, a clinical assessment of the adequacy of ventilation should be performed after the setup of volume ventilation. Blood gas determination is often necessary to assist in gauging the patient's clinical condition. Noninvasive monitoring with pulse oximetry (Chapter 75) and end-tidal capnometry (Chapter 76) can also be helpful. As described earlier, sedatives and/or analgesics (Chapter 33) should be used to maintain patient comfort while on the ventilator. Table 82.2 summarizes the steps for initiating pressure-controlled ventilation.

When determining the best strategy for ventilating a patient, the pathophysiology of the underlying disease process must be considered. This is important not only for providing effective ventilation but for avoiding complications. Ventilator management as it pertains to specific pathophysiologic processes is discussed next.

Parenchymal Lung Disease

The hallmark of most parenchymal lung diseases is the formation of pulmonary edema. The decrease in FRC and the increase in closing capacity may lead to subsegmental atelectasis. Ultimately, difficulties in maintaining adequate oxygenation ensue because of ventilation-perfusion mismatch. Therapy should be directed at increasing FRC above closing capacity, which can be accomplished through the application of increased levels of PEEP. The amount of PEEP needed will directly correlate with the severity of the pulmonary insult. PEEP should be further increased in a stepwise fashion by 2 to 3 cm H_2O pressure until adequate oxygenation is achieved with nontoxic levels of oxygen (F_iO_2 of less than 60%). As discussed, increased PEEP can have adverse effects on venous return to the right heart and cardiac output. These adverse effects can be lessened by intravascular volume loading. Care must be taken to select the amount of PEEP that will optimize oxygenation and cardiac output.

Worsening parenchymal lung disease is associated with a decrease in respiratory compliance. If the tidal volume is held constant, peak inflating pressures will increase. High inflating pressures are associated with ventilator-induced lung injuries. One ventilation strategy used to avoid these complications is pressure-controlled ventilation with permissive hypercapnia. The goals of this strategy are to maintain adequate oxygenation while limiting maximal lung inflation pressures. This goal is accomplished by restricting the PIP to less than 35 to 40 cm H_2O pressure, PEEP to less than 15 cm H_2O pressure, and F_iO_2 to less than 60%. If oxygenation is still marginal (below 85% SaO_2), further increases in mean airway pressure are achieved by increasing the relative inspiratory time. In addition, careful attention to fever control and appropriate use of sedation will help decrease the end organ oxygen demands.

This combination of decreased peak inspiratory pressure, increased PEEP, and longer inspiratory time will reduce minute ventilation. The resultant increase in PcO_2 is termed permissive hypercapnia because this is the desired effect.

Under these conditions, attempts to normalize the P_{CO_2} would require an increase in the ventilatory frequency. Unfortunately, using a longer inspiratory time and increased ventilatory rate will result in the delivery of a mechanical breath before the preceding exhalation is complete. This "stacking of breaths" will lead to alveolar overdistention and higher airway pressures. The patient should, therefore, be managed in a hypercapnic state. Hypercapnia should be limited to a degree that allows an arterial pH of 7.2 or greater. Hypercarbia is well tolerated when developed chronically, due to a compensatory metabolic alkalosis. Permissive hypercapnia is contraindicated in patients with increased intracranial pressure, because carbon dioxide is a potent cerebral vasodilator, and under these conditions intracranial pressure may worsen.

Lower Airway Obstruction

Diseases such as asthma and bronchiolitis produce varying degrees of lower airway obstruction. Lower airway obstruction causes pulmonary hyperinflation due to mucous plugging and smooth muscle constriction. When positive pressure is applied, further hyperinflation occurs, which may produce a profound decrease in venous return and, therefore, cardiac output. The end result will be a decrease in peripheral tissue oxygenation. A strategy exists, however, to minimize this effect. First, mean airway pressure should be kept to a minimum. In general, this means providing no PEEP or limiting it to a maximum of 2 to 3 cm of H_2O pressure. Another method of decreasing pulmonary hyperinflation is by avoiding "inadvertent PEEP" or "auto-PEEP." When lower airway obstruction is present, more time is required to fully empty the lung. If the exhalatory time allowed by the ventilator is too short, another breath will be initiated before the lung has emptied back to the baseline FRC. Again, this stacking of breaths results in worsening hyperinflation and increased mean airway pressure (inadvertent PEEP or auto-PEEP). The amount of time required for exhalation should directly correlate with disease severity. In these situations the I:E ratio should be at least 1:2. It may be necessary to alter the I:E ratio to 1:3 or more in children requiring ventilation with asthma.

Lower airway obstruction also results in increased work of breathing by increasing respiratory resistance. As discussed earlier, this can contribute to respiratory failure. Providing mechanical ventilation will decrease the oxygen demands of the respiratory musculature and prevent further respiratory muscle fatigue, which should improve oxygen delivery to other peripheral tissues.

Cardiac Disease

Declining cardiac function places a number of stresses on the pulmonary system. The resultant pulmonary vascular congestion leads to the formation of interstitial edema. Interstitial edema can lead to alveolar collapse and to further $\dot{V}/\dot{Q}$ mismatch.

In addition, cardiac output falls as cardiac function worsens, impairing oxygen delivery to the peripheral tissues. Oxygen delivery is determined by cardiac output and the partial pressure of oxygen in the blood. When cardiac output falls, the body must increase the P_{O_2} in the blood to maintain oxygen delivery. The body accomplishes this by increasing respiratory rate and effort. The increased work of breathing required to accomplish this, however, places increased oxygen demands on the body. As discussed, this may ultimately result in respiratory failure.

The goal of mechanical ventilation in patients with cardiac dysfunction is therefore to re-expand areas of atelectasis and decrease the work of breathing. Areas of collapse are re-expanded by the application of PEEP. It is important to be cautious in using PEEP. Excessive PEEP will cause hyperinflation of the alveoli, which may result in increased pulmonary vascular resistance. Increased pulmonary vascular resistance has a negative effect on cardiac output due to a decrease in left ventricular filling. In the setting of heart disease, cardiac output is highly dependent on left ventricular filling. Therefore, higher mean airway pressures can significantly affect cardiac output. It is reasonable to start with a PEEP of 3 to 5 cm H_2O. The amount of PEEP can then be titrated to improve oxygenation while maintaining venous return.

Mechanical ventilation in patients with cardiac disease also will decrease the total work of breathing. When the work of breathing is decreased, the oxygen demanded by the respiratory musculature also is decreased. Oxygen that would have been used by the respiratory musculature can be used by other peripheral tissues. In this way, the total oxygen demand placed on the cardiopulmonary circulation is reduced.

▶ COMPLICATIONS

A number of complications are associated with using mechanical ventilation. In general, these complications are the result of endotracheal tube placement, alveolar overdistention, positive airway pressure, or ventilator failure. Careful attention to the specific details of ventilator management will assist in avoiding these complications.

Injuries resulting from the presence of an endotracheal tube are primarily the result of pressure placed on the airway mucosa. These injuries may range from mild swelling to severe ulceration and may occur at any point the airway is in contact with an endotracheal tube. A more comprehensive discussion of these complications appears in Chapter 16. To avoid endotracheal tube–related injuries, a proper size tube should be used. It is best if the air leak occurs around the tube beginning at no more than 20 cm H_2O pressure. To check for an air leak, the endotracheal tube should be connected to an anesthesia bag attached to a manometer. The airway pressure is slowly increased by carefully closing the pop-off valve. While watching the airway pressure rise on the manometer, the clinician should listen for an air leak. An air leak can be heard by listening at the patient's mouth or by placing a stethoscope over the cricothyroid membrane. Cuffed endotracheal tubes should not be used in prepubertal patients. If a cuffed tube is used, it should be inflated with air to less than 20 cm H_2O pressure.

Using excessive positive airway pressure can result in alveolar overdistension and possibly rupture. Overdistension of alveoli may decrease cardiac output by reducing venous return, as described in the "Procedure" section. Alveolar rupture results in the accumulation of air into sites outside the pulmonary tree. The clinical significance of these extrapulmonary air accumulations depends on their location and size. Pneumothorax, pulmonary interstitial emphysema, pneumomediastinum, pneumopericardium, pneumoperitoneum, and subcutaneous emphysema are possible complications that may result from alveolar rupture. The incidence of these complications can be reduced by using the smallest lung volumes and lowest airway pressures that will maintain adequate oxygenation and ventilation.

When a patient's clinical status deteriorates, it is important to assess whether a ventilator malfunction has occurred. As discussed, this is most easily accomplished by hand ventilating the patient with a bag and 100% oxygen. If the patient's condition improves, a problem most likely exists with the ventilator. Once the malfunction is identified and corrected, the patient can then be placed back on the ventilator. The patient should then be reassessed to ensure the malfunction has been remedied. Ventilator malfunctions can be kept to a minimum by frequently evaluating the patient's condition

CLINICAL TIPS

- ▶ Pressure-controlled ventilators should be used for patients weighing less than 10 kg.
- ▶ Volume-controlled ventilators should be used generally for patients weighing more than 10 kg.
- ▶ When mechanical ventilation is initiated, a systematic approach should be used that includes continuous reassessment of patient condition and ventilator function.
- ▶ Inspired oxygenation concentrations of less than 60% will generally avoid complications associated with oxygen toxicity.
- ▶ In patients with a reduction in function, a reduction in residual capacity, and a propensity toward atelectasis (e.g., pulmonary edema, ARDS), increased amounts of PEEP are often necessary to provide adequate oxygenation with acceptable inspired oxygen concentrations.
- ▶ In patients with severe parenchymal lung disease, pressure-controlled ventilation to maintain permissive hypercapnia may help reduce pulmonary barotrauma.
- ▶ In patients with severe lower airway obstruction (e.g., asthma), PEEP is contraindicated. Generally, these patients are best managed with lower ventilation rate and I:E ratio altered to allow longer exhalation time and a more complete exhalation.
- ▶ Use of sedatives and analgesics is an important adjunct to ventilator management.

SUMMARY

1 Select a ventilator—volume or pressure controlled.

2 Select a mode of ventilation.

3 Provide adequate ventilation:

  a Set tidal volume or peak inspiratory pressure (PIP).
  b Set the rate (Table 82.3).

4 Provide adequate oxygenation:

  a Set F_iO_2.
  b Set positive end-expiratory pressure (PEEP).

5 Set inspiratory time.

6 Assess patient for adequate ventilation:

  a Adequate rise and fall of chest
  b Adequate breath sounds
  c Arterial blood gas determination (adequate P_{CO_2})

7 Assess patient for adequate oxygenation:

  a Adequate heart rate and color
  b Adequate oxygen saturation (S_{aO_2})
  c Arterial blood gas determination (adequate P_{aO_2})

8 Make changes as necessary and reassess.

and the operation of the ventilator. All health care providers involved in the care of mechanically ventilated patients should have a thorough understanding of the ventilators used at their institution.

▶ SUMMARY

Mechanical ventilation can be a life-saving procedure in many clinical settings. Decisions regarding ventilator setup and management are based on the patient's physiology and underlying pathophysiology. Carefully repeated clinical assessments of patient condition and ventilator function will aid in the effective use of this treatment and help to avoid complications. The importance of this cannot be overstated, as the success of mechanical ventilation largely depends on the knowledge and expertise of the operator.

▶ REFERENCES

1. Chatburn RL. Assisted ventilation. In: Blummer J, ed. *A Practical Guide to Pediatric Intensive Care.* 2nd ed. St. Louis: Mosby; 1990:943–955.

2. Feihl F, Perret C. Permissive hypercapnia: how permissive should we be? *Am J Respir Crit Care Med.* 1994;150:1722–1737.

3. Hubmayr RD, Abel MD, Rehder K. Physiologic approach to mechanical ventilation. *Crit Care Med.* 1990;18:103–113.

4. Martin LD, Rafferty JF, Walker K, et al. Principles of respiratory support and mechanical ventilation. In: Rogers M, ed. *Textbook of Pediatric Intensive Care.* 2nd ed. Baltimore: Williams & Wilkins; 1992: 134–193.

5. Pfaff JK, Morgan WJ. Pulmonary function in infants and children. *Pediatr Clin North Am.* 1994;41:401–423.

6. Reynolds AM, Ryan DP, Doody DP. Permissive hypercapnia and pressure-controlled ventilation as treatment of severe adult respiratory distress syndrome in a pediatric burn patient. *Crit Care Med.* 1993; 21:468–471.

7. Ring JC, Stidham GL. Novel therapies for acute respiratory failure. *Pediatr Clin North Am.* 1994;41:1325–1362.

8. Rusconi F, Castagneto M, Gagliardi L, et al. Reference values for respiratory rate in the first 3 years of life. *Pediatrics.* 1994;94:350–355.

9. Schuster DP. A physiologic approach to initiating, maintaining, and withdrawing mechanical ventilatory support during acute respiratory failure. *Am J Med.* 1990;88:268–278.

10. Shapiro BA. A historical perspective on ventilator management. *New Horiz.* 1994;2:8–18.

11. Tobin MJ. Mechanical ventilation. *N Engl J Med.* 1994;330:1056–1061.

12. Venkataraman ST, Orr RA. Mechanical ventilation and respiratory care. In: Furhman B, ed. *Pediatric Critical Care.* St. Louis: Mosby; 1992: 519–543.

13. Rogers MC, ed. *Textbook of Pediatric Intensive Care.* Baltimore: Williams & Wilkins; 1987:115.

14. Marraro GA. Innovative practices of ventilatory support with pediatric patients. *Pediatr Crit Care Med.* 2003;4:8–20.

JEFF E. SCHUNK AND NANETTE C. DUDLEY

83

Management of Esophageal Foreign Bodies

▶ INTRODUCTION

Young children often swallow foreign bodies because of their inquisitive nature and propensity for pica (1). Esophageal impaction of these objects occurs frequently, and removal is often necessary to avoid serious complications (2–9). Most esophageal foreign bodies are blunt or smooth, and coins are the most common (1,10,11). Other esophageal foreign bodies include bones, meat, toys, and, less commonly, sharp objects. Esophageal foreign bodies may occur at any age, although they are found more commonly in children aged 6 months to 6 years.

A variety of techniques and settings may be used for esophageal foreign body removal, depending on the type of physician specialist who performs the procedure. Local referral patterns, the nature of the foreign body, the duration and extent of symptoms, and the physician's familiarity with various techniques will determine the method of choice. Removal methods include endoscopy (10–12) or the use of Magill forceps (13,14) in the operating room, flexible endoscopy in the outpatient setting (15), the Foley catheter technique (16–18), advancement with a Bougie dilator (19,20), and a newer method called the "penny pincher" (21).

▶ ANATOMY AND PHYSIOLOGY

Esophageal foreign bodies occur at predictable sites of normal anatomic narrowing (10,11). These sites include the thoracic inlet (cricopharyngeus), the level of the right mainstem bronchus-aortic arch, and the gastroesophageal junction (lower esophageal sphincter) (Fig. 83.1): (10,11,22,23). Children with underlying esophageal pathology are predisposed to foreign body impaction at sites of pathologic narrowing that may not correspond to the typical sites.

It is generally recommended that all esophageal foreign bodies should be removed. Local reaction, both inflammatory and muscular, may adversely affect esophageal motility and can lead to adjacent airway narrowing. Although esophageal perforation is most likely to occur from an impacted sharp object (24), complications also have been reported from impacted blunt objects. These include esophageal perforation (4), tracheoesophageal fistula (5), esophageal-aortic fistula (8), vocal cord paralysis (9), brain abscess (7), and upper airway compromise from local reaction (25). With the exception of disc ("button") batteries (26–28), no serious complications have been reported from blunt esophageal foreign bodies impacted for less than a few days. Removal of an esophageal foreign body

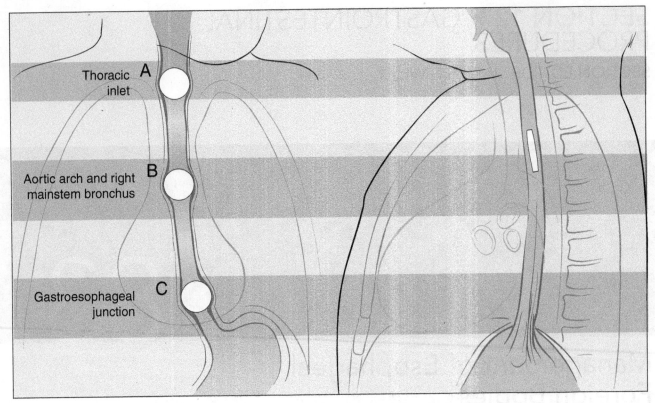

Figure 83.1 Common sites of esophageal impaction of smooth foreign bodies.

Labels in figure:
- Thoracic inlet — A
- Aortic arch and right mainstem bronchus — B
- Gastroesophageal junction — C

typically results in rapid return to normal esophageal function and relief of associated symptoms.

▶ INDICATIONS

Patients with esophageal foreign bodies often present with a foreign body sensation, pain, or symptoms of impaired esophageal function such as vomiting, drooling, and dysphagia. Airway compromise with stridor or wheezing also may occur. However, many children with esophageal foreign bodies have no symptoms. In two emergency department (ED) studies, 30% (22) and 44% (29) of children with a coin in the esophagus were asymptomatic. Patients with asymptomatic esophageal coins of less than 24 hours duration can be observed for spontaneous passage, as this will occur about 25% of the time (30–32).

Symptomatic patients and those with longer duration impaction should undergo emergent removal. Likewise, disc batteries should be removed emergently regardless of the duration of impaction because of the potential for rapid esophageal injury (26–28). Operative endoscopic removal is the traditional method of choice in such cases. It requires operating room personnel, an anesthesiologist and/or anesthetist, and an experienced surgeon. It is safe and efficacious in nearly all cases, and it allows for airway control and visualization of the esophagus (10,12,23). This method can be used for all esophageal foreign bodies. Rarely, thoracic surgery is required

due to mediastinal complications resulting from esophageal foreign bodies (perforation, mediastinitis, mediastinal mass). For coins in the upper esophagus, operative use of a Magill forceps has also been effective (13,14).

Flexible, nonoperative endoscopy is generally performed by a gastroenterologist. It is appropriate in selected cases (typically a blunt object impacted less than 1 week) but does require the use of pediatric equipment (15). In addition, procedural sedation may be necessary. This method affords advantages similar to those of operative endoscopy, except that airway control is not guaranteed. For this reason, some gastroenterologists will refer all children with an esophageal foreign body impacted above the clavicles (on plain radiograph) to an otolaryngologist.

The Foley catheter technique is typically performed by a radiologist under fluoroscopic guidance and has a success rate of 67% to 98% (16,18,33). It should only be used for uncomplicated blunt esophageal foreign bodies or foodstuffs with impaction duration less than 3 days. It can be used in patients with underlying esophageal conditions (17). This technique offers the main advantages of reduced cost, no risk of general anesthesia, and no need for hospitalization.

Advancement of an esophageal foreign body into the stomach with a Bougie dilator is typically performed by the pediatric surgeon in the ED or under fluoroscopy. This technique is reserved for patients who have no respiratory symptoms or underlying esophageal conditions and who have esophageal impaction with blunt objects (coins) of short duration (usually less than 24 hours) (6,19,20). This method offers the advantages of avoiding the cost and risk of general anesthesia and hospitalization and can be performed without fluoroscopy.

In general, patients with respiratory symptoms, recent esophageal procedures, sharp foreign objects, or objects impacted for a long duration should only be considered for operative endoscopic removal. Patients with blunt foreign bodies of shorter duration can be considered for flexible endoscopy or the Foley catheter technique. Bougie advancement is generally reserved for single coins impacted less than 24 hours in children without esophageal disease. The "penny pincher" technique has been successful for removing impacted esophageal coins of short duration (21).

▶ EQUIPMENT

Any esophageal foreign body removal attempt should be done with resuscitation equipment readily available, along with personnel experienced in its use. Specific techniques previously discussed require special equipment appropriately sized for the pediatric patient.

▶ PROCEDURE

The emergency physician is most often concerned with proper diagnostic evaluation to identify the location and nature of an ingested foreign object. This is followed by appropriate preparation for the expected procedure. Diagnosis is usually straightforward, as the typical radiopaque esophageal foreign body (coin) is visible on plain radiograph. Less frequently a barium swallow is needed to outline a nonopaque esophageal foreign body. Recently, some authorities have reported success with using a handheld metal detector for localization of ingested coins (34–37).

In preparation for operative endoscopy, the patient should have nothing orally, have intravenous access obtained, and undergo a preoperative lab evaluation. The same preparation is needed if the patient is to undergo flexible endoscopy, although preparation for outpatient conscious sedation and monitoring also is required.

The Foley catheter technique is usually done without sedation. The patient is placed in the prone oblique or prone Trendelenburg position. Under fluoroscopic guidance, a Foley catheter (8 to 12 Fr) is passed distal to the foreign body, and the balloon is inflated with 3 to 5 cc of barium. Gentle traction is applied to pull the esophageal foreign body out to the mouth, where it can then be grasped or expectorated. Alternatively, the esophageal foreign body may be pushed into the stomach (16–18,38).

Appropriately selected patients eligible for Bougie advancement are placed in the upright or prone position. An appropriately sized (based on the expected esophageal lumen diameter), well-lubricated dilator is gently advanced through the mouth and into the stomach. This technique has been used with and without fluoroscopy (19,20).

The "penny pincher" technique is performed without sedation or anesthesia. An endoscopic grasping forceps within a soft rubber catheter is advanced under fluoroscopic guidance, and the grasping forceps is used to retrieve the coin (21).

▶ NONINVASIVE TECHNIQUES

Several authors have noted that esophageal foreign bodies will commonly pass spontaneously (11,22,29). This was thought to occur more frequently with esophageal foreign bodies impacted at the gastroesophageal junction (11), but more recent studies have demonstrated spontaneous passage from all typical impaction locations (30,32). For this reason, expectant observation of short duration (24 hours) in asymptomatic children with a blunt foreign body impacted for less than 1 day is an acceptable alternative to active removal or advancement (30,32,39).

Anecdotal reports have supported the use of pharmacologic agents to promote passage of an esophageal foreign body (diazepam, glucagon, etc.). However, one study found no benefit (40), and these agents have not been compared to expectant observation for spontaneous passage. Consequently, routine use of such agents for pediatric patients cannot be recommended.

 SUMMARY

1 Identify the location of the foreign body by plain radiography, barium swallow, or metal detector.

2 Determine the duration of the esophageal impaction (if possible) and any patient history of esophageal abnormality or surgery.

3 If the object is sharp, causes respiratory distress or other significant symptoms, has a long duration of impaction, has failed to be removed by other methods or if the patient has an underlying esophageal abnormality, then prepare the patient for removal by operative endoscopy; impacted disc batteries should be removed emergently.

4 If the object is blunt, has been impacted for less than 1 day, and is not potentially harmful to the patient, observe for 24 hours to allow for possible spontaneous passage.

5 If the object is blunt, is not causing respiratory distress, and has been impacted for a short period of time, consider Foley catheter removal, advancement with a Bougie dilator, the "penny pincher" method, or nonoperative endoscopy.

CLINICAL TIPS

▶ Esophageal foreign bodies frequently cause no obvious symptoms in children.

▶ Pharmacologic methods to enhance foreign body passage have not been shown to be effective and are not recommended.

▶ Disc ("button") batteries impacted in the esophagus should be removed emergently.

▶ Each procedure for management of an esophageal foreign body is highly successful, with a low rate of complications, if performed by an experienced operator in carefully selected patients.

▶ COMPLICATIONS

Potential complications vary depending on the method of removal. Reported complications of operative esophagoscopy include dislodgment of the endotracheal tube; coughing at extubation; arrhythmia, vomiting, and laryngospasm during endoscopy; and stridor and laryngospasm after endoscopy (10,12). Complications from the Foley catheter technique include vomiting, epistaxis, transient respiratory distress, and, rarely, esophageal injury (16,18). Foreign body aspiration into the airway has not been reported with the Foley catheter technique. Significant complications from Bougie advancement in selected cases have not been reported (19,20). Any technique that involves manipulating the esophagus carries a risk of esophageal injury, perforation, and mediastinitis.

▶ SUMMARY

Esophageal foreign bodies are common in children. They are usually blunt and lodge at sites of anatomic narrowing. The nature of the foreign body, duration of impaction, clinical condition, past medical history, hospital practice, and local referral patterns influence the method of removal chosen. All techniques should only be attempted by those clinicians familiar with their use and capable of managing any potential complications.

▶ REFERENCES

1. Binder L, Anderson WA. Pediatric gastrointestinal foreign body ingestions. *Ann Emerg Med.* 1984:13:112–117.

2. Byard RW, Moore L, Bourne AJ. Sudden and unexpected death: a late effect of occult intraesophageal foreign body. *Pediatr Path.* 1990;10:837–841.

3. Katz KR, Emmens RW, Wood BP. Esophageal obstruction and abscess formation secondary to impacted, eroding tiddlywink. *Am J Dis Child.* 1989;143:961–962.

4. Nahmah BJ, Mueller CF. Asymptomatic esophageal perforation by a coin in a child. *Ann Emerg Med.* 1984;13:627–629.

5. Obiako MN. Tracheoesophageal fistula: a complication of foreign body. *Ann Otol Rhinol Laryngol.* 1982;91:325–327.

6. Jona JZ, Glicklich M, Cohen RD. The contraindications for blind esophageal bougienage for coin ingestion in children. *J Pediatr Surg.* 1988;23:328–330.

7. Louie JP, Osterhoudt KC, Christian CW. Brain abscess following delayed endoscopic removal of an initially asymptomatic esophageal coin. *Pediatr Emerg Care.* 2000;16:102–105.

8. Stuth EA, Stucke AG, Cohen RD, et al. Successful resuscitation of a child after exsanguination due to aortoesophageal fistula from undiagnosed foreign body. *Anesthesiology.* 2001;95:1025–1026.

9. Virgilis D, Weinberg JM, Fisher D, et al. Vocal cord paralysis secondary to impacted esophageal foreign bodies in young children. *Pediatrics.* 2001;107(6):E101.

10. Crysdale WS, Sendi KS, Yoo J. Esophageal foreign bodies in children: 15 year review of 484 cases. *Ann Otol Rhinol Laryngol.* 1991;100:320–324.

11. Spitz L. Management of ingested foreign bodies in childhood. *Br Med J.* 1971;20:469–472.

12. Hawkins DB. Removal of blunt foreign bodies from the esophagus. *Ann Otol Rhinol Laryngol.* 1990;99:935–939.

13. Janik JE, Janik JS. Magill forceps extraction of upper esophageal coins. *J Pediatr Surg.* 2003;38:227–229.

14. Mahafza TM. Extracting coins from the upper end of the esophagus using a Magill forceps technique. *Int J Pediatr Otorhinolaryngol.* 2002;62:37–39.

15. Bendig DW. Removal of blunt esophageal foreign bodies by flexible endoscopy without general anesthesia. *Am J Dis Child.* 1986;140:789–790.

16. Campbell JB, Condon VR. Catheter removal of blunt esophageal foreign bodies in children. *Pediatr Radiol.* 1989;19:361–365.

17. Nixon GW. Foley catheter method of esophageal foreign body removal: extension of applications. *Am J Radiol.* 1979;132:441–442.

18. Schunk JE, Harrison AM, Corneli HM, et al. Fluoroscopic Foley catheter removal of esophageal foreign bodies in children: experience with 415 episodes. *Pediatrics.* 1994;94:709–714.

19. Kelley JE, Leech MH, Carr MG. A safe and cost-effective protocol for the management of esophageal coins in children. *J Pediatr Surg.* 1993;28:898–900.

20. Bonadio WA, Jona JZ, Glicklich M, et al. Esophageal Bougienage technique for coin ingestion in children. *J Pediatr Surg.* 1988;23:917–918.

21. Gauderer MW, DeCou JM, Abrams RS, et al. The "penny pincher": a new technique for fast and safe removal of esophageal coins. *J Pediatr Surg.* 2000;35:276–278.

22. Schunk JE, Corneli H, Bolte R. Pediatric coin ingestions: a prospective study of coin location and symptoms. *Am J Dis Child.* 1989;143:546–548.

23. Chaikhouni AJ, Kratz JM, Crawford F. Foreign bodies of the esophagus. *Am Surgeon.* 1985;51:173–179.

24. Nandi P, Ong GB. Foreign body in the oesophagus: review of 2394 cases. *Br J Surg.* 1978;65:5–9.

25. Pasquariello PS, Kean H. Cyanosis from a foreign body in the esophagus. *Clin Pediatr.* 1975;14:223–225.

26. Maves MD, Carithers JS, Birck HG. Esophageal burns secondary to disc battery ingestion. *Ann Otol Rhinol Laryngol.* 1984;93(4 pt I):364–369.

27. Sigalet D, Lees G. Tracheoesophageal injury secondary to disc battery ingestion. *J Pediatr Surg.* 1988;23:996–998.

28. Samad L, Ali M, Ramzi H. Button battery ingestion: hazards of esophageal impaction. *J Pediatr Surg.* 1999;34:1527–1531.

29. Hodge D, Tecklenburg F, Fleisher G. Coin ingestion: does every child need a radiograph? *Ann Emerg Med.* 1985;14:443–446.

30. Soprano JV, Fleisher GR, Mandl KD. The spontaneous passage of esophageal coins in children. *Arch Pediatr Adolesc Med.* 1999;153:1073–1076.

31. Sharieff GQ, Brouseau TJ, Bradshaw JA, et al. Acute esophageal coin ingestions: is immediate removal necessary? *Pediatr Radiol.* 2003;33:859–863.

32. Conners GP, Cobaugh DJ, Feinberg R, et al. Home observation for asymptomatic coin ingestion: acceptance and outcomes. The New York State Poison Control Center Coin Ingestion Study Group. *Acad Emerg Med.* 1999;6:213–217.

33. Kirks DR. Fluoroscopic catheter removal of blunt esophageal foreign bodies, a pediatric radiologist's perspective. *Pediatr Radiol.* 1992;22:64–65.

34. Ros SP, Cetta F. Metal detectors: an alternative approach to the evaluation of coin ingestions in children? *Pediatr Emerg Care.* 1992;8:134–136.

35. Ros SP, Cetta F. Successful use of a metal detector in locating coins ingested by children. *J Pediatr.* 1992;120:752–753.

36. Bassett KE, Schunk JE, Logan L. Localizing ingested coins with a metal detector. *Am J Emerg Med.* 1999;17:338–341.

37. Biehler JL, Tuggle D, Stacey T. Use of a transmitter-receiver metal detector in the evaluation of pediatric coin ingestions. *Pediatr Emerg Care.* 1993;9:208–210.

38. Towbin R, Lederman HM, Dunbar JS, et al. Esophageal edema as a predictor of unsuccessful balloon extraction of esophageal foreign body. *Pediatr Radiol.* 1989;19:359–360.

39. Schunk JE. Foreign body ingestion/aspiration. In: Fleisher GR, Ludwig S, eds. *Textbook of Pediatric Emergency Medicine.* 3rd ed. Philadelphia: Lippincott Williams & Wilkins; 2000:267–273.

40. Mehta D, Attia M, Quintana E, et al. Glucagon use for esophageal coin dislodgment in children: a prospective, double-blind, placebo-controlled trial. *Acad Emerg Med.* 2001:8:200–203.

84

HAROLD K. SIMON, MAIA S. RUTMAN, AND
WILLIAM LEWANDER

Gastric Intubation

▶ INTRODUCTION

Gastric intubation for medical purposes dates back to Hermann Boerhaave (1668–1738), who first suggested inserting gastric tubes, and John Hunter, who reported conveying food and medicine in 1790 for a case of "paralysis of the muscles of deglutition" (1). Occasional case reports followed, but it was not until 1921, when Levin introduced the smooth catheter-tipped tube, that gastric intubation became a routine medical procedure (2,3).

Abdominal obstruction, severe trauma, drug overdose, and upper gastrointestinal bleeding, among other processes, commonly require emergent gastric intubation. Gastric tubes are also utilized in patients following tracheal intubation in order to facilitate gastric decompression. The procedure is commonly performed by physicians and nurses in both the emergency department (ED) and intensive care settings. The placement of a gastric tube is straightforward but requires close attention to technique in order to avoid serious complications.

▶ ANATOMY AND PHYSIOLOGY

The approach to gastric intubation for children is similar to that for adult patients. Major anatomic obstacles to gastric tube placement are the nares, choanae, adenoids, tonsils, tongue, and epiglottis (Fig. 84.1). Unlike adults, however, children have increased tonsillar and adenoidal tissue size that may predispose them to traumatic bleeding during gastric intubation, especially if excessive force is used. In addition, the relative macroglossia in young children and the smaller nostril diameter may impede nasogastric intubation. Also, children are more likely than adults to have undiagnosed congenital anomalies that may act as an impediment to gastric intubation, such as choanal atresia, esophageal atresia, esophageal strictures, and tracheoesophageal fistula. Orogastric intubation may be necessary for some pediatric patients if it becomes evident that nasogastric intubation will result in excessive trauma.

The cribriform plate, an anatomic site deserving special emphasis, is a thin bone located in the superior aspect of the nasal cavity. It separates the intracranial cavity from the nasal cavity. This bone may be fractured following severe facial or head trauma, creating a point of potential access into the intracranial cavity. Placement of a nasogastric tube in the presence of such an injury has resulted in introduction of the tube into the cranial vault, an obviously catastrophic result (4). Care must therefore be taken before nasogastric intubation to ensure that a cribriform plate disruption is not present; if this cannot be assured, then orogastric intubation should be performed.

The gag reflex impedes gastric tube placement by closing the nasopharynx via the levator veli palatini and tensor veli palatini muscles (cranial nerve X) and constricting the pharyngeal musculature (cranial nerves IX and X). Impairment of the gag reflex often occurs in patients with a depressed level of consciousness. In such patients, passage of the tube may actually be easier because the patient does not struggle. However, the risk of aspiration of gastric contents into the lungs increases greatly because the tracheal protection afforded by an intact gag reflex is diminished or absent. Additionally, the gastric tube may be inadvertently passed into the trachea because the warning signs of cough or lack of phonation would not be present.

▶ INDICATIONS

Gastric intubation is widespread in the daily practice of pediatric emergency medicine. Emergent indications include

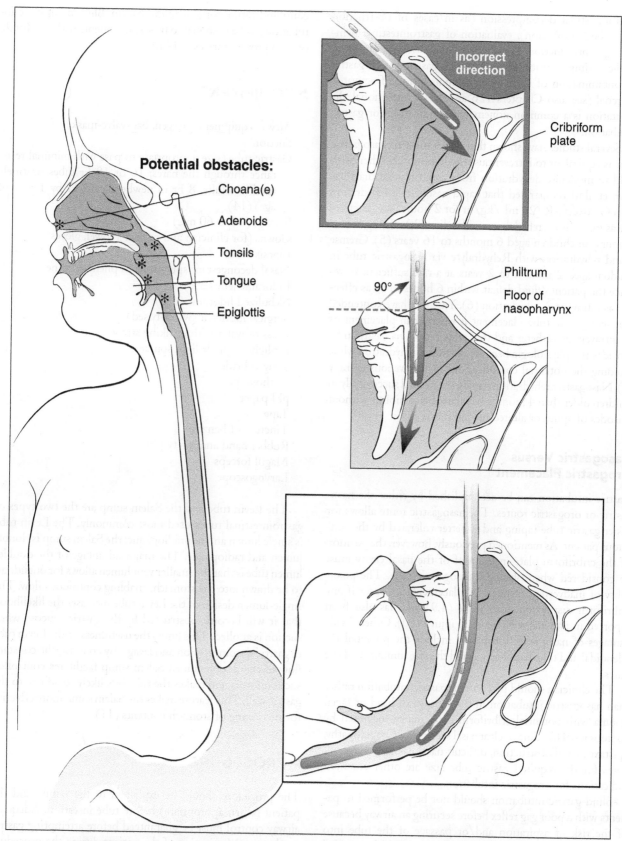

Figure 84.1 Anatomy of the oropharynx with potential sites of impedance during nasogastric intubation. Note the correct path for nasogastric tube insertion and the proximity to the cribriform plate.

gastrointestinal decompression (as in cases of obstruction or tracheal intubation), evaluation of gastrointestinal hemorrhage, introduction of radiographic contrast for imaging studies, administration of medications, gastric lavage, gastric decontamination of toxins, and administration of activated charcoal (see also Chapters 126 and 127). Nutritional alimentation is a common nonemergent indication for gastric intubation.

Several studies have shown that rehydration via nasogastric tube is equivalent to intravenous rehydration in children with mild to moderate dehydration from vomiting and diarrhea. Phin et al. demonstrated that rapid nasogastric rehydration with Gastrolyte-R (20 mL/kg/hr for 2 hours) was as effective as intravenous rehydration with saline (20 mL/kg/hr for 2 hours) in children aged 6 months to 16 years (5). Gremse found rehydration with Rehydralyte via nasogastric tube in children aged 2 months to 2 years at a rate sufficient to replace the patient's fluid deficit within 6 hours to be as effective as intravenous rehydration (6). Yiu et al. have contended that nasogastric tube placement is easier than placement of an intravenous catheter and that rehydration via gastric tube provides the physiologic benefits of enteral rehydration while avoiding the potential complications of intravenous therapy (7). Nasogastric rehydration has also been used successfully in children older than 4 months who have bronchiolitis without episodes of apnea or altered mental status (8).

Nasogastric Versus Orogastric Placement

Gastric intubation can be accomplished by either the nasogastric or orogastric routes. The nasogastric route allows for easier gastric tube taping and is better tolerated by the conscious patient. As mentioned previously, however, the position of the cribriform plate in the roof of the nasal cavity must be considered when placing a nasogastric tube. The possibility of inadvertent intracranial placement can occur if any cribriform disruption takes place (4,9) and has also been reported in patients with no skull injury (10). Other disadvantages of nasogastric intubation include the potential for adenoidal and tonsillar bleeding and the size limitation of the nares.

The clinician should perform orogastric intubation rather than nasogastric intubation in the settings of head or facial trauma with potential cribriform plate injury suggested by copious nasal bleeding or clear nasal secretions. Coagulopathy, epistaxis, nasal obstruction, difficult nasal passage, and small nares for the required gastric tube size are other common indications for orogastric intubation.

Blind gastric intubation should not be performed in patients with a poor gag reflex before securing an airway because of the risk of aspiration and/or passage of the tube into the trachea. Blind gastric intubation also should be avoided in patients with high-lying esophageal foreign bodies or in cases of caustic ingestions because of the risk of esophageal perforation. Of note, esophageal varices are not an absolute contraindication for gastric intubation. Blind nasogastric intubation has been shown to be safe in patients with suspected, or even proven, varices (11–13).

▶ EQUIPMENT

Airway equipment (oxygen, bag-valve-mask)
Suction
Gastric tube (size appropriate to pass with minimal resistance through the nares; 16 or 18 Fr tubes routinely used in adults, 8 Fr in newborns, 12 Fr by 1 year of age) (14)
Syringe (30 to 60 mL)
Gowns (for clinician and patient), towel, gloves
Emesis basin
Nasal decongestant spray such as phenylephrine
Lidocaine jelly (2%)
Nebulized lidocaine (4%)
Surgical lubricant (water-based)
Glass of water with drinking straw
Penlight or other light source
Tongue blade
Stethoscope
pH paper
Tape
Tincture of benzoin
Rubber band and safety pin
Magill forceps
Laryngoscope

The Levin tube and the Salem sump are the two types of gastrointestinal tubes used most commonly. The Levin tube is single lumen and nonradiopaque; the Salem sump is double lumen and radiopaque. The major advantage of the double-lumen tube is that the smaller vent lumen allows for outside air to be drawn into the stomach, enabling continuous flow. The single-lumen design of the Levin tube increases the likelihood that it will become obstructed by the gastric mucosa when suction is applied. This limits the usefulness of the Levin tube in gastric decompression and lavage. By contrast, the constant flow of the double-lumen Salem sump facilitates controlled suction forces and makes the tube less likely to adhere to the gastric wall. This feature makes the Salem sump more effective for suctioning of stomach contents (11).

▶ PROCEDURE

The procedure should be explained to the family and the patient (when appropriate) before tube insertion. Adequate airway control must be guaranteed before attempting gastric intubation. Monitoring of the patient during the procedure should include heart rate, respiratory rate, and pulse oximetry. If the patient is awake, the head of the bed should be raised so that the patient is sitting upright. If cervical spine injury is suspected, the neck must be stabilized. The comatose patient with an intact gag reflex should be placed in a decubitus position with the head down (when cervical spine injury is not suspected) to minimize the risk of aspiration. The comatose patient with a poor or absent gag reflex should undergo endotracheal intubation before proceeding with gastric intubation (see Chapter 16). All necessary equipment should be organized, and the help of one or more assistants should be enlisted. Suction equipment and oxygen must be immediately available and operating properly. A towel should be placed over the patient's chest, and an emesis basin in the patient's lap.

Next, the oropharynx is suctioned clear of secretions. For nasogastric intubation, the appropriate length tube for insertion can be estimated by combining the distance from the tip of the nose to the earlobe with the distance from the nose to the xiphoid (Fig. 84.2A) (15,16). Alternatively, the length of the tube can be measured by externally placing it from the tip of the nose (nasogastric) or the lip (orogastric) back to the ear and down to the left upper quadrant just below the costal margin. The tubing length can then be marked with a piece of tape. The patient's nose is examined to determine the larger naris and is cleared of secretions. An assistant should help secure the child's head in place.

A nasal decongestant such as phenylephrine may be sprayed into the nares to shrink the nasal mucosa at least 3 to 5 minutes before nasogastric intubation if the tube is not needed on a more emergent basis. Nebulized lidocaine (4%) delivered by face mask may be used to help anesthetize the pharynx, as this reduces gagging and vomiting and increases the chance of successful passage (17,18). A small amount of 2% lidocaine jelly can be placed in the naris with a syringe while the patient is supine 5 minutes before introducing the tube to limit the discomfort of the procedure (19). Placement of the tube is facilitated by coiling the tip around the finger prior to insertion and tilting the patient's head back against the pillow (20).

The tube should be well lubricated with lidocaine jelly (21) and gently passed through the naris perpendicular to the philtrum (*not* angled superiorly). Insertion is directed caudally and posteriorly toward the hypopharynx to avoid the cribriform plate and the nasal mucosa. If difficulty with passage is encountered, an attempt can be made on the contralateral side and/or a smaller tube can be tried. Difficult passage caused by curling of the tube may be lessened by stiffening the tube in ice, but excessive force should never be used. In cases when cervical injury is not suspected, flexion of the neck also may facilitate passage. If the relative macroglossia in young children and infants proves to be an impediment to placement, the tongue can be gently depressed with a tongue blade. Alternately, a soft, well-lubricated nasopharyngeal airway can be passed nasally and the lubricated gastric tube passed through it, both to facilitate placement and to protect the nasal mucosa if multiple placement attempts are necessary (22).

Palpating the neck to identify the site of impedance can be useful in guiding further efforts. When placing a gastric tube in a patient who has undergone endotracheal intubation,

the most common sites of resistance to placement are the arytenoid cartilages and piriform sinuses. It may be possible to palpate the tip of the tube impinging on these structures. In such cases, the operator can facilitate tube passage by using the fingers to apply medially directed pressure to the lateral aspect of the (ipsilateral) neck at the level of the thyrohyoid membrane (23).

As a last resort, direct visualization with a laryngoscope (see Chapter 16) is performed using appropriate sedation. The esophagus is visualized posterior to the larynx. The gastric tube is then passed directly into the esophagus. Guidance using McGill forceps may be necessary when passing a nasogastric tube in this manner (11).

Once the tube reaches the hypopharynx, insertion should be rapid and continuous as the patient swallows. The clinician can overcome esophageal resistance by having the older, cooperative patient sip water through a straw, which improves esophageal peristalsis. Flexing the neck at this point helps to direct the tube into the esophagus rather than the trachea. If coughing, choking, or changes in phonation occur (indicating tracheal insertion) or if significant gagging occurs (indicating coiling in the esophagus), the clinician should remove the tube and reattempt insertion. If the patient is crying or talking during the procedure, this is a good indication that the gastric tube has not been inadvertently placed in the trachea.

Tube placement is checked by aspirating stomach contents, which should have a pH less than 4 if the tube tip is in the stomach (24). Three to 10 mL of air (depending on the size of the child) is then introduced via a catheter-tipped syringe placed at the end of the tube (Fig. 84.2B). Auscultation over the epigastric region should reveal a rush of air (rumbling sound) as evidence of proper placement. If correct placement is questioned, the tube should be repositioned or removed. Placement should be confirmed with a radiograph in unconscious patients or whenever uncertainty about positioning exists.

Although several methods of securing the tube have been described (25), the basic approach involves securing a small piece of tape with tincture of benzoin to the nasal bridge or cheek (Fig. 84.2C). The distal end of the horizontally cut tape is wrapped around the segment of tube extending from the nostril. Orogastric tubes can be secured to the lateral cheek in a similar manner. Fastening the tube to the patient's gown by looping a rubber band around the tube and attaching it with a safety pin to the gown also helps to prevent inadvertent tube removal (19). The tube should then be clamped, allowed to drain by gravity, or be hooked up to wall suction, as appropriate for the specific circumstance.

▶ COMPLICATIONS

While gastric tube placement is generally well tolerated, several complications can occur. The primary method for avoiding most significant complications of gastric intubation is never to use excessive force during the procedure. This point

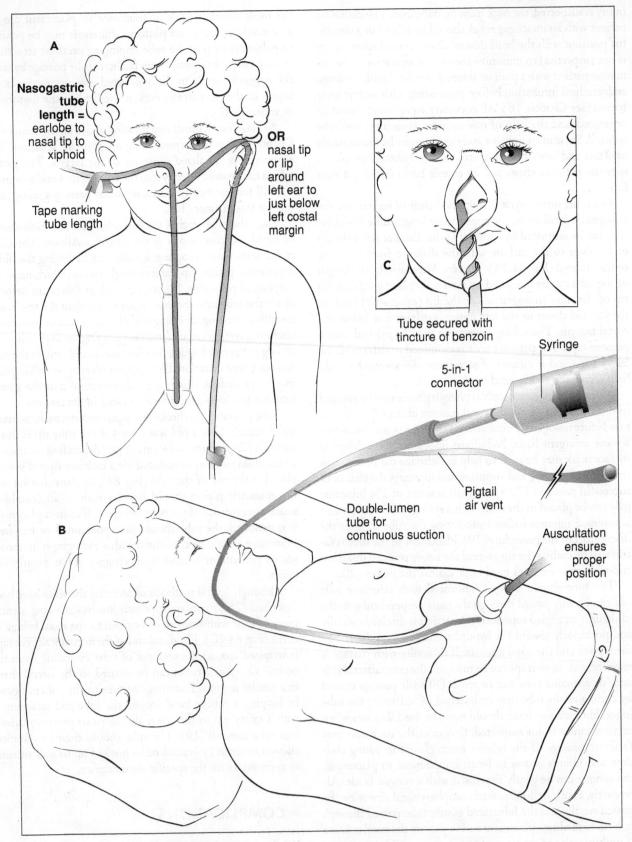

Figure 84.2
A. External landmarks for determining proper gastric tube length.
B. Confirmation of nasogastric placement.
C. Securing a nasogastric tube by applying tincture of benzoin and tape.

cannot be overemphasized. If the tube does not pass relatively easily, then another route should be used, or the tube should be passed under direct visualization using a laryngoscope. Creation of a false passage may occur when the tube is inserted into a natural cul-de-sac (such as a pyriform sinus) and persistent and inappropriate force is applied. Nasopharyngeal, laryngeal, esophageal, stomach, and duodenal perforations from gastric tube placement have all been reported (15,26–30). Forced passage of a gastric tube also may result in avulsion of tonsillar and adenoidal tissue, which may cause significant bleeding or airway obstruction if the dislodged segment of tissue is large enough to occlude the trachea (31–33).

Accidental intracranial passage of a gastric tube may be prevented by avoiding the nasogastric approach in patients

 SUMMARY

General Considerations

1 Fully discuss the procedure with the patient and family to limit anxiety.

2 Have the necessary equipment and assistants available.

3 Position the patient and protect the airway when indicated.

4 Stabilize the neck if there is any question of cervical spine injury.

5 Suction the nose and mouth clear of secretions.

6 Use a well-lubricated tube of the appropriate size.

7 Apply topical anesthetic for nasogastric placement; consider nebulized lidocaine for anesthesia of the pharynx.

8 Estimate the desired length of tube for insertion—the distance from the tip of the nose to the earlobe *plus* the distance from the nose to the xiphoid, or the distance from the nose back around the ear and down just below the left costal margin.

9 Gently pass the tube into the desired position in a caudally directed manner, going straight into the nostril (not "up" toward the cribriform plate).

10 Check placement with an injection of air; confirm placement with a radiograph as needed.

Specific Considerations in the Unconscious Patient

1 Consider head down, decubitus positioning and endotracheal intubation before gastric intubation in comatose patients to reduce the risk of aspiration.

2 Confirm the position of the tube with a radiograph in all unconscious patients.

 CLINICAL TIPS

▶ Topical anesthetic jelly (nasogastric tube) or topical anesthetic spray or nebulized lidocaine (orogastric tube) limits the discomfort of the procedure.

▶ If excessive choking or gagging occurs, the tube should be removed.

▶ Talking or crying during the procedure is a good indication that the gastric tube has not been inadvertently placed in the trachea.

▶ If difficulty is encountered, palpating the neck may allow the clinician to identify the site of impedance (e.g., piriform sinus, arytenoid cartilage).

▶ Gentle downward displacement of the tongue with a tongue blade may facilitate passage of a nasogastric tube in the young child or infant.

▶ If tube passage proves impossible, anatomic impediments due to congenital malformations (e.g., choanal atresia, esophageal atresia, esophageal strictures) should be considered.

▶ Excess force must never be used in passing a nasogastric tube.

with facial or head trauma who have possible cribriform plate disruption. However, it is possible to pass through the cribriform plate even in patients with no head injury (10). Passage of a gastric tube in an awake patient with a penetrating neck wound can worsen hemorrhage if gagging or coughing occur. Additionally, cervical spine injuries can be exacerbated by excessive neck motion during gastric tube placement.

It is possible to inadvertently place a gastric tube into the trachea or bronchial tree. Other possible pulmonary complications of gastric intubation include intrapleural placement leading to pulmonary hemorrhage or pneumothorax (34–37), pneumomediastinum from perforation of the posterior nasopharynx (38), and aspiration pneumonitis (39). Finally, prevention of endotracheal tube dislodgment when passing a gastric tube requires careful securing of the endotracheal tube (see Chapter 16) prior to gastric tube insertion.

▶ SUMMARY

Gastric intubation is a commonly used procedure in the ED and in the inpatient setting. Physicians and nurses should be knowledgeable regarding the use, placement, and potential complications of gastric intubation. If done with care and proper technique, this procedure can be performed successfully with minimal difficulty in most cases.

▶ REFERENCES

1. Paine JR. The history of the invention and development of the stomach and duodenal tubes. *Ann Intern Med.* 1934;8:752–763.

2. Levin AL. A new gastroduodenal catheter. *JAMA.* 1921;76:1007.

3. Hafner CD, Wylie JH, Brush BE. Complications of gastrointestinal intubation. *Arch Surg.* 1961;83:147–160.

4. Young RF. Cerebrospinal fluid rhinorrhea following nasogastric intubation. *J Trauma.* 1979;19:789–791.

5. Phin SJ, McCaskill ME, Browne GJ, et al. Clinical pathway using rapid rehydration for children with gastroenteritis. *J Paediatr Child Health.* 2003;39:343–348.

6. Gremse DA. Effectiveness of nasogastric rehydration in hospitalized children with acute diarrhea. *J Pediatr Gastroenterol Nutr.* 1995;21:145–148.

7. Yiu WL, Smith AL, Catoo-Smith AG. Nasogastric rehydration in acute gastroenteritis. *J Paediatr Child Health.* 2003;39:159–161.

8. Samartino L, James D, Gourtzamanis J, et al. Nasogastric rehydration does have a role in acute paediatric bronchiolitis. *J Paediatr Child Health.* 2003;38:321–323.

9. Wyler AR, Reynolds AF. An intracranial complication of nasogastric intubation. *J Neurosurg.* 1977;47:297–298.

10. Frejj RM, Mullett ST. Inadvertent intracranial insertion of a nasogastric tube in a non-trauma patient. *J Accid Emerg Med.* 1997;14:45–47.

11. Glauser JM. Nasogastric intubation. In: Roberts JR, Hedges JR, eds. *Clinical Procedures in Emergency Medicine.* 2nd ed. Philadelphia: WB Saunders; 1991:640–648.

12. Lopez-Torres A, Waye JD. The safety of intubation in patients with esophageal varices. *Am J Dig Dis.* 1973;18:1032.

13. Ritter DM, Rettke SR, Hughes RW, et al. Placement of nasogastric tubes and esophageal stethoscopes in patients with documented esophageal varices. *Anesth Analg.* 1988;67:283–285.

14. Carlson DW, Digiulio GA, Gewitz MH, et al. Illustrated techniques of pediatric emergency procedures, 10.1 nasogastric tube placement. In: Fleisher GR, Ludwig S, eds. *Textbook of Pediatric Emergency Medicine.* 4th ed. Philadelphia: Lippincott Williams & Wilkins; 2000:1847.

15. Simon RR, Brenner BE. Abdominal procedures. In: Simon RR, Brenner BE, eds. *Emergency Procedures and Techniques.* Philadelphia: Lippincott Williams & Wilkins; 2002:1–6.

16. Van Way CW, Nuerk C. Gastointestinal intubation. In: *The Pocket Manual of Basic Surgical Skills.* St. Louis: Mosby; 1986:179–185.

17. Wolfe TR, Fosnocht DE, Linscott MS. Atomized lidocaine as topical anesthesia for nasogastric tube placement: a randomized, double-blind, placebo-controlled trial. *Ann Emerg Med.* 2000;35:421–425.

18. Spektor M, Kaplan J, Kelley J, et al. Nebulized or sprayed lidocaine as anesthesia for nasogastric intubations. *Acad Emerg Med.* 2000;7:406–408.

19. Samuels LE. Nasogastric and feeding tube placement. In: Roberts JR, Hedges JR, eds. *Clinical Procedures in Emergency Medicine.* 3rd ed. Philadelphia: WB Saunders; 2004:794–816.

20. Volden C, Grinde J, Carl D. Taking the trauma out of nasogastric intubation. *Nursing.* 1980;10(9):64–67.

21. Singer AJ, Konia J. Comparison of topical anesthetics and vasoconstrictors vs. lubricants prior to nasogastric intubation: a randomized, controlled trial. *Acad Emerg Med.* 1999;6:184.

22. Lewis JD. Facilitation of nasogastric and nasotracheal intubation with a nasopharyngeal airway. *Am J Emerg Med.* 1986;4:426.

23. Ozer S, Benumof J. Oro- and Naso-gastric tube passage in intubated patients: fiberoptic description of where they go at the laryngeal level and how to make them enter the esophagus. *Anesthesiology.* 1999;91:137–143.

24. Metheny N, Reed L, Wiersema L, et al. Effectiveness of pH measurements in predicting feeding tube placement: an update. *Nurs Res.* 1993;42:324.

25. Sader AA. New way to stabilize nasogastric tubes. *Am J Surg.* 1975;130:102.

26. Reussner LA, Blebea J, Peterson P, et al. Nasopharyngeal perforation as a complication of nasogastric intubation. *Ear Nose Throat J.* 1993;72:755–757.

27. Friedman M, Baim H, Shelton V, et al. Laryngeal injuries secondary to nasogastric tubes. *Ann Otol Rhinol Laryngol.* 1981;90(5 pt. 1):469–474.

28. Jackson RH, Payne DK, Bacon BR. Esophageal perforation due to nasogastric intubation. *Am J Gastroenterol.* 1990;85:439–442.

29. Norman EA, Sosis M. Iatrogenic oesophageal perforation due to tracheal or nasogastric intubation. *Can Anaesth Soc J.* 1985;33:222–226.

30. Islam S, Counihan TC, Marik PE. Duodenal perforation caused by nasogastric intubation. *Am J Gastroenterol.* 1996;91:2439–2440.

31. Wald P, Stern J, Weiner B, et al. Esophageal tear following forceful removal of an impacted orogastric lavage tube. *Ann Emerg Med.* 1986;15:80–82.

32. Lind LJ, Wallace DH. Submucosal passage of a nasogastric tube complicating attempted intubation during anesthesia. *Anesthesiology.* 1978;49:145–147.

33. Weiner BC. Management of oral gastric lavage tube impaction of the esophagus. *Am J Gastroenterol.* 1986;81:1202–1204.

34. Fisman DN, Ward ME. Intrapleural placement of a nasogastric tube: an unusual complication of nasotracheal intubation. *Can J Anaesth.* 1996;43:1252–1256.

35. Gough D, Rust D. Nasogastric intubation: morbidity in an asymptomatic patient. *Am J Emerg Med.* 1986;4:511–513.

36. Eldar S, Meguid MM. Pneumothorax following attempted nasogastric intubation for nutritional support. *JPEN J Parenter Enteral Nutr.* 1984;8:450–452.

37. McDanal JT, Wheeler M, Ebert J. A complication of nasogastric intubation: pulmonary hemorrhage. *Anesthesiology.* 1983;59:356–358.

38. Siemers PT, Reinke RT. Perforation of the nasopharynx by nasogastric intubation: a rare cause of left pleural effusion and pneumomediastinum. *AJR Am J Roentgenol.* 1976;127:341–343.

39. Alessi DM, Berci G. Aspiration and nasogastric intubation. *Otolaryngol Head Neck Surg.* 1986;94:486–489.

JOHN W. GRANETO

85

Gastrostomy Tube Replacement

▶ INTRODUCTION

Percutaneous endoscopic gastrostomy (PEG) tube placement was introduced in 1980 in Cleveland, Ohio, as a procedure for children who required long-term nutritional support (1,2). The endoscopically placed PEG tube was found to be simpler and safer than surgical gastrostomy tube placement (3). It quickly became popular as a method of providing enteral access for children suffering from chronic illnesses that lead to impaired and insufficient oral intake, the most common being anoxic brain injury (3). Nutritional support and medication administration—either long term or for brief periods postoperatively—are easily achieved in these patients with a PEG tube. The increasing frequency with which these tubes are being used in pediatric patients, combined with the tendency of the tubes to dislodge or malfunction, make replacement of gastrostomy tubes a common procedure for the emergency physician.

▶ ANATOMY AND PHYSIOLOGY

Children can have impaired swallowing function for a variety of reasons, including anoxic brain injury, gastroesophageal reflux, esophageal injury from lye ingestion, congenital esophageal anomalies (e.g., stenosis, stricture, duplication, tracheoesophageal fistula), achalasia, familial dysautonomia, and any disease that interferes with oropharyngeal muscle tone and coordination (e.g., muscular dystrophy, Werdnig-Hoffmann disease, myasthenia gravis). These children may be unable to achieve sufficient oral intake to prevent eventual dehydration, or they may have such uncoordinated swallowing reflexes that they are highly prone to aspirate orally ingested substances into the lungs. Using a PEG tube avoids these problems by allowing direct access to the stomach, obviating the need for oral administration of medications and feedings.

The anterior or anterolateral surface of the stomach wall is the usual site of insertion of a PEG tube. The PEG site stoma traverses the stomach wall beginning at the internal mucosa and extending outward to the visceral lining, fixes these layers to the parietal peritoneal lining of the abdominal wall, and finally emerges through the skin surface externally. After several weeks, a fistulous tract forms, and adherence of these layers to each other becomes permanent.

▶ INDICATIONS

PEG tubes require replacement for several reasons. Tubes can deteriorate over time and become dysfunctional during the natural course of their use (4). PEG tubes also can become blocked, usually because of formula accumulations that dry and solidify. Certain formulas (Ensure, Pulmocare, and Osmolite) are more prone to clogging than others when exposed to acidic stomach contents (5). Tubes also can become blocked because of mechanical twisting, kinking, and undissolved medications. In general, attempts to unstop these types of blockages should not be made with stylets or other probing devices, as these efforts can potentially rupture the feeding tube below the skin surface, leading to intra-abdominal leakage. A blocked tube that cannot be made functional should be removed and replaced. Attempts to remove a well-positioned yet malfunctioning tube should be made only after assurance that the replacement equipment and personnel to perform the replacement are readily available.

Active children may cause their PEG tubes to become accidentally dislodged from the stomach. Although the specific incidence of this event is not known, it is likely a relatively frequent occurrence. Inadvertent dislodgement of a PEG tube requires timely tube replacement, because the stoma site will begin to close over in a short time (usually within hours). Furthermore, delays in tube replacement will increase the difficulty of passing a temporizing device such as a Foley catheter (6). If a Foley catheter is placed promptly, replacement of the PEG tube can usually be accomplished in the emergency department (ED) or office setting without requiring anesthesia or intervention by a subspecialist.

Immediate Postoperative Period

Although PEG tube replacement is usually a simple procedure, spontaneous expulsion of a tube that was recently placed (within 1 to 2 weeks of the initial operative procedure) is a special case. In such situations, the stomach wall may not have had time to adhere to the peritoneal lining and overlying skin. Attempts at re-establishing a PEG tube or temporizing with a Foley catheter can disrupt the fistula tract, resulting in the formation of a false lumen into the peritoneum. Instillation of formula through the improperly positioned tube can cause a chemical and bacterial peritonitis, with potentially life-threatening consequences. Therefore, patients requiring PEG tube replacement in the immediate postoperative period should have consultation from the ED with the surgeon, gastroenterologist, or interventional radiologist who originally placed the tube.

▶ EQUIPMENT

> Replacement tube
> Lubricant (e.g., K-Y Jelly, viscous lidocaine)
> 10-mL syringe
> 30- to 60-mL syringe
> Stethoscope
> Tape
> Benzoin
> Absorbent dressing

Replacing a gastrostomy tube in the ED does not necessarily mean that the dislodged tube must be replaced with the same type of tube. If the original type of tube is available, however, this is preferred. Additionally, a replacement tube that is the same size as the original should be used when possible. Usual catheter sizes range from 18 to 28 Fr.

A variety of PEG tubes are currently available on the market, most of which are made of silicone, rubber, or polyurethane. Many tubes are similar, with only minor differences in their design, connectors, and lengths (Fig. 85.1). The more common types are (a) balloon-ended, such as the MIC-KEY (Kimberly Clark, Roswell, GA); (b) mushroom-shaped (dePezzer), such as the Button (BARD Peripheral Vascular, Tempe, AZ); and (c) with collapsible wings, such as the Malecot.

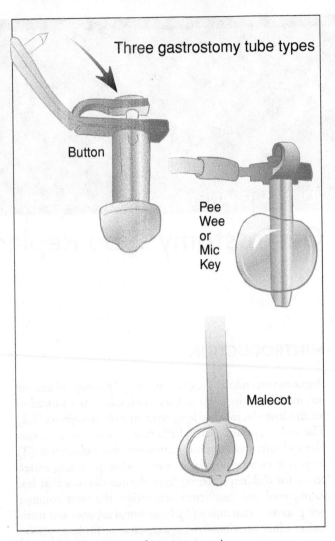

Figure 85.1 Three types of gastrostomy tubes.

The Button was first developed in 1984 (7). Its advantages over conventional gastrostomy tubes include less skin irritation, fewer problems with migration and dislodgment, and no awkward lengthy tube exposed externally. The Button tube does not have to be changed as frequently as other devices (8–10). The Button has gained popularity and is favored by both patients and families.

▶ PROCEDURE

When dealing with PEG tube problems, one goal of the clinician is to ensure that the patient does not have intra-abdominal pathology. Additionally, prior to removing or reinserting the tube, the use of procedural sedation and/or analgesia should be considered to diminish the degree of discomfort experienced by the child (see Chapter 33). The three clinical situations commonly encountered are (a) a malfunctioning tube, (b) a dislodged tube with an open stoma, and (c) a dislodged tube with a closed stoma.

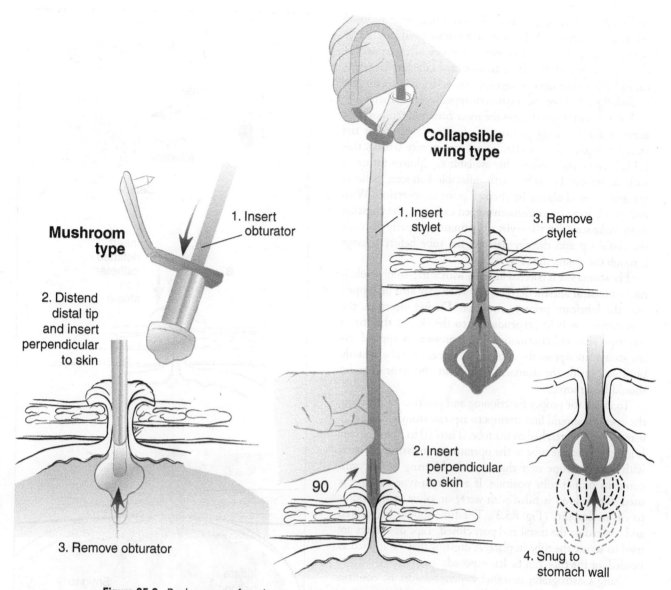

Figure 85.2 Replacement of mushroom-type and collapsible wing–type gastrostomy tubes.

Malfunctioning Tube

If a blockage has occurred, the clinician should gently instill warm water into the tube and allow it to flow back out repeatedly until patency is established. The effectiveness of carbonated soda, reputedly the best irrigant in such situations, has been studied, although with inconclusive results (11). Parents should be advised that the best way to avoid these occurrences is with proper flushing of the tube before and after each use. If the tube cannot be unclogged, the balloon should be deflated and the tube removed.

Before removing the malfunctioning tube, the clinician should detach any clamps or external sources of stabilization. If the dysfunctional catheter is balloon tipped, a Luer-Lok syringe or other adaptable syringe is connected to the balloon port of the old gastrostomy tube, and the balloon contents (water or saline) are withdrawn. If the tube requires a stylet or obturator for removal, it is inserted to extend the distal tip within the stomach wall.

If the child can follow commands, the clinician should instruct him or her to take a deep breath and hold it while the old tube is gently pulled out. If removal of the malfunctioning gastric tube is not possible by gentle traction, the tube may be cut at the abdominal wall surface. The distal portion will normally pass spontaneously through the gastrointestinal tract, or it may be removed later endoscopically (12).

Dislodged Tube with an Open Stoma

Balloon-type catheters such as the MIC-KEY tend to become dislodged after the balloon has been worn down by erosion. In one study, the average time for this to occur was about 5 months (13). The stoma of a recently dislodged tube may be bleeding or leaking gastric juices and may appear closed on first inspection. A lubricated cotton-tipped applicator (Q-tip) can be inserted to confirm patency of the stoma. If the stoma is patent, the clinician should obtain a replacement tube ideally of the same design and size as the malfunctioning or dislodged tube or use a balloon-tipped Foley catheter.

Foley catheter insertion is the most common temporizing measure for replacing gastrostomy feeding devices. For the emergency physician practicing in a community setting, this is likely to be the most readily available equipment to use in such situations. For tubes with inflatable balloons, balloon integrity should always be checked prior to insertion. With collapsible wing or mushroom-tipped catheters, the clinician must make sure that the stylet or obturator properly distends the distal tip and thereby narrows the tube before passage through the stoma site (Fig. 85.2).

The stoma site is covered liberally with water-soluble lubricant or topical anesthetic. The new tube may also be dipped into the lubricant prior to insertion. During insertion, the new catheter is held perpendicular to the skin at the stoma insertion site, and continuous gentle pressure is applied. As the stoma site opens, the clinician advances the tube steadily until well inside the stomach. If used, an obturator or stylet should be removed.

To check for proper functioning and position of the tube, the operator should first attempt to aspirate stomach contents using a syringe attached to the tube. Then 10 to 15 mL of air is injected into the tube as the operator or an assistant listens with a stethoscope over the stomach. Hearing borborygmi confirms proper tube position. If a balloon-type catheter is used, the balloon is filled with water or saline at this point to ensure stability (Fig. 85.3). The tube should be secured and covered or the distal end port closed. Tape or sutures are used to secure the tube in place. A dressing may be applied as needed, or the tube can be left exposed.

Using Gastrografin or other contrast media to confirm proper position radiographically is not generally necessary provided the two methods of placement confirmation described above are properly performed. If any question arises about the actual site of placement, radiographic studies are indicated. Likewise, if the clinician is suspicious of a perforated viscous, a noncontrast upright abdominal-chest radiograph is indicated to rule out free air in the peritoneum.

Dislodged Tube with a Closed Stoma

If a dislodged tube stays out for an extended period before the patient is seen, the stoma may become so tight that standard methods of inserting a new tube prove unsuccessful. Using a guidewire or stylet in a Malecot tube replacement for a recently closed stoma is an option that should be reserved for the surgeon, gastroenterologist, or interventional radiologist. For most patients, intravenous access can be established to administer maintenance hydration should the appropriate consultant not be immediately available. Improper technique in such situations can result in the creation of a "false lumen,"

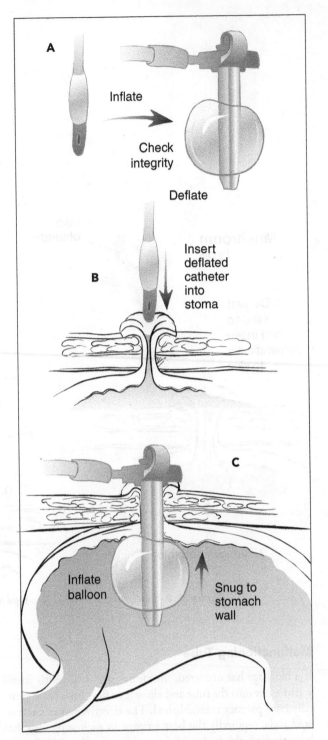

Figure 85.3 Replacement of balloon-type gastrostomy tube.

along with the potential serious complications of a ruptured viscous or separation of the gastric wall from the stoma site.

▶ COMPLICATIONS

Excessive force combined with using a tube that is too large may lead to accidental insertion into the peritoneal cavity

SUMMARY

1 Assess the child's condition and examine the stoma site.

2 Consider sedation and/or analgesia.

3 Obtain a replacement tube and check for proper function.

4 For a malfunctioning tube that must be removed:

   a Withdraw the balloon contents using a syringe OR

   b Insert a stylet or obturator.

5 Have the child take a deep breath and gently pull out the old tube.

6 To insert a replacement tube, lubricate the tube and stoma site generously.

7 Insert the tube into the stoma site perpendicular to the abdominal wall.

8 Advance with continuous steady pressure several centimeters into stomach.

9 Fill the balloon with saline/water OR

Remove the obturator/stylet.

10 Aspirate the stomach contents with a syringe and listen over the stomach for borborygmi while injecting air through the tube.

11 Secure the tube and cover the distal end.

 CLINICAL TIPS

▶ Tap water or saline is used for inflating catheter balloons.

▶ Prompt reinsertion with any tube into the opening of a fistulous tract of a recently dislodged tube is the most effective way to ensure continued patency.

▶ When inserting the tube, using continuous and steady pressure rather than intermittent "poking" or "jabbing" increases the likelihood of successful passage.

▶ Proper tube position is confirmed by aspirating gastric contents and auscultating over the stomach for borborygmi as air is injected through the tube. If these methods are inconclusive, radiopaque contrast material should be injected through the tube, and a plain radiograph of the abdomen should be obtained to confirm placement.

through a false lumen; separation of the stomach wall from the peritoneal wall, resulting in peritoneal insertion of the distal tube; or lysis of adhesions of the stomach wall away from the abdominal wall, causing pneumoperitoneum. If a false lumen is formed and is not recognized, formula may be instilled into the peritoneum, resulting in a potentially severe chemical peritonitis (14). These complications can be avoided by appropriately sizing the replacement tube and avoiding the use of excessive pressure when replacing the gastrostomy tube. Additionally, a gastrostomy tube should not be used unless correct positioning is confirmed, as previously described.

Insufficient advancement of the replacement tube, which leaves the distal tip in the fistula rather than in the stomach, can also lead to disruption of the fistula and pain when the stylet is withdrawn or the balloon is filled. Continued patient discomfort after tube placement is an indication of this problem. In most instances, the tube should be advanced several centimeters through the stoma to ensure intragastric placement.

As mentioned, delay in replacement may result in closure of the gastrostomy fistula before replacement of the tube. Other complications include wound infections at the skin site and bleeding at the site of insertion caused by trauma to the area. Adequate use of lubrication and avoidance of excessive force can minimize the potential for bleeding and infection. Finally, a replacement Foley catheter tube that is not secured adequately may migrate distally into the gastrointestinal tract and cause intestinal obstruction (15,16). The tube can also migrate into the esophagus, potentially causing perforation (17,18). This problem is easily avoided by pulling the Foley tube back against the stomach wall after the balloon has been inflated and ensuring that the excess tubing extending from the gastrostomy site is properly secured.

▶ **SUMMARY**

Various treatment options can be performed when a child presents with a gastrostomy tube that has been dislodged or is not functioning. When possible, a replacement tube of the same size and design as the original tube should be used. Otherwise, an appropriately sized Foley catheter can be inserted as a temporizing measure to allow continued feedings or administration of medications and to prevent closure of the stoma. To avoid complications, proper position of the tube should always be confirmed after insertion.

▶ **REFERENCES**

1. Gauderer MWL, Ponsky JL, Izant RJ. Gastrostomy without laparotomy: a percutaneous endoscopic technique. *J Pediatr Surg.* 1980;15:872–875.
2. Ponsky JL, Gauderer MW. Percutaneous endoscopic gastrostomy: a nonoperative technique for feeding gastrostomy. *Gastrointest Endosc.* 1981;27:9–11.

3. Gauderer MW. Percutaneous endoscopic gastrostomy: a 10-year experience with 220 children. *J Pediatr Surg.* 1991;26:288–294.

4. Kadakia SC, Cassaday M, Shaffer RT. Prospective evaluation of Foley catheter as a replacement gastrostomy tube. *Am J Gastroenterol.* 1992;87:1594–1597.

5. Marcuard SP, Perkins AM. Clogging of feeding tubes. *JPEN J Parenter Enteral Nutr.* 1988;12:403–405.

6. Ruddy RM. Illustrated techniques of pediatric emergency procedures. In: Fleisher GR, Ludwig S, eds. *Textbook of Pediatric Emergency Medicine.* Baltimore: Williams & Wilkins; 1993:1638–1639.

7. Gauderer MW, Picha GJ, Izant RJ Jr. The gastrostomy "button": a simple, skin-level, nonrefluxing device for long-term enteral feedings. *J Pediatr Surg.* 1984;19:803–805.

8. Steele NF. The Button: replacement gastrostomy device. *J Pediatr Nurs.* 1991;6:421–424.

9. Townsend LC. Practical considerations of the gastrostomy button. *Gastroenterol Nurs.* 1991;14:18–26.

10. Borge MA, Vesely TM, Picus D. Gastrostomy button placement through percutaneous gastrostomy tracts created with fluoroscopic guidance: experience in 27 children. *J Vasc Interv Radiol.* 1995;6:179–183.

11. Metheny N, Eisenberg P, McSweeney M. Effect of feeding tube properties and three irrigants on clogging rates. *Nurs Res.* 1988;37:165–169.

12. Korula J, Harma C. A simple and inexpensive method of removal or replacement of gastrostomy tubes. *JAMA.* 1991;265:1426–1428.

13. Michaud L, Guimber D, Blain-Stregloff AS, et al. Longevity of balloon-stabilized skin-level gastrostomy device. *J Pediatr Gastroenterol Nutr.* 2004;38:426–429.

14. Marshall JB, Bodnarchuk G, Barthel JS. Early accidental dislodgment of PEG tubes. *J Clin Gastroenterol.* 1994;18:210–212.

15. Cassaday M, Kadakia SC, Yamamoto K, et al. Foley feeding catheter migration into the small bowel. *J Clin Gastroenterol.* 1992;15:242–244.

16. Browne BJ, Kaufman B, Brown C. Internal displacement of a gastrostomy button: an unusual case of gastric outlet obstruction. *J Pediatr Surg.* 1993;28:1575–1576.

17. Whiteley S, Liu PH, Tellez DW, et al. Esophageal rupture in an infant secondary to esophageal placement of a Foley catheter gastrostomy tube. *Pediatr Emerg Care.* 1989;5:113–116.

18. Konigsberg K, Levenbrown J. Esophageal perforation secondary to gastrostomy tube replacement. *J Pediatr Surg.* 1986;21:946–947.

NATALIE E. LANE AND RONALD I. PAUL

86

Paracentesis

▶ INTRODUCTION

Paracentesis, or peritoneal tap, involves inserting a needle through the abdominal wall into the peritoneal cavity and aspirating fluid. The peritoneum is bathed in a small amount of fluid normally. Ascites, derived from the Greek word "askites," meaning bag or bladder, is a collection of fluid in the peritoneal cavity whose volume is in excess of the normal amount. Paracentesis may be used as a diagnostic tool in the evaluation of ascites and/or as a therapeutic procedure for the relief of respiratory distress secondary to large accumulations of ascites. An understanding of the patient's anatomy and the pathophysiology of ascites is essential to the correct performance of this procedure. Treatment rooms in the hospital, office, or clinic are appropriate settings for a diagnostic peritoneal tap. For the relief of respiratory distress, paracentesis should be performed in a facility equipped with monitoring and resuscitative equipment, such as an emergency department (ED) or intensive care unit, because the patient has the potential to rapidly deteriorate.

▶ ANATOMY AND PHYSIOLOGY

No one pediatric age group is predisposed to the development of ascites. Unlike adults, who often develop ascites secondary to acquired diseases, ascites in children is more often the result of congenital defects. Obstructive urinary tract anomalies are the most common cause of neonatal ascites (1). Other forms of ascites can be seen with a diverse group of conditions, including hydrops fetalis, occult perforations of the gastrointestinal tract, lymphatic obstruction, cardiac abnormalities with associated congestive heart failure, portal hypertension, peritonitis, metabolic diseases, malnutrition, neoplasias, and ventriculoperitoneal shunt obstruction. The basic pathologic

mechanisms resulting in ascites include (a) high venous hydrostatic pressure (congestive heart failure, portal hypertension), (b) decreased plasma colloid oncotic pressure (hypoproteinemia), (c) lymphatic obstruction, (d) genitourinary obstruction, (e) inflammation (peritonitis), and (f) ruptured viscus (2,3).

Marked ascites is clinically noted by a protuberant abdomen and bulging flanks in the supine position. Shifting areas of dullness may be noted by percussion of the abdomen as the patient moves from a supine to a decubitus position. The clinician can appreciate fluid waves by placing the hands on a supine patient's opposing flanks, gently thumping with one hand, and palpating the resulting wave on the opposite flank. (4). Regardless of the etiology of ascites, infants and small children may develop clinical symptoms by both direct and indirect effects on respiratory function. With marked ascitic fluid collections, restriction of diaphragmatic movement and compression of lower lung fields occur, resulting in decreased functional residual capacity, increased ventilation-perfusion mismatch, and resulting respiratory compromise.

In adult patients with cirrhosis and ascites, rapid removal of peritoneal fluid (8 L, or approximately 120 mL/kg, over 1 hour) has been associated with increased cardiac output 1 hour after paracentesis (5). However, prerenal azotemia, hyponatremia, decreased central venous pressure, decreased pulmonary capillary wedge pressure, and decreased cardiac output subsequently developed 24 hours later. Albumin replacement (8 g albumin for every 1 L of peritoneal fluid removed) prevented these effects.

▶ INDICATIONS

Paracentesis for therapeutic purposes is often temporizing until the etiology is determined and treated. In some situations,

835

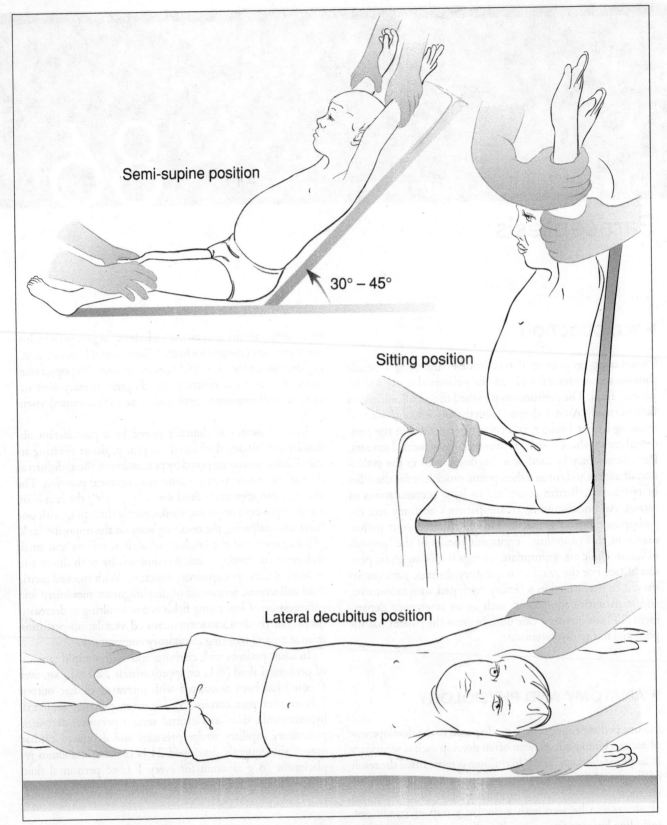

Figure 86.1 Patient positions for paracentesis.

ascitic fluid is difficult to locate, and a radiologist should be consulted. Ultrasound may detect as little as 10 mL in an optimal setting and can discern loculated areas of fluid (6,7). Radiographic films of the abdomen reflect indirect findings and only are helpful if a large amount of fluid is present.

Paracentesis should never be performed through an area of cellulitis. In addition, relative contraindications include a history of prior abdominal surgeries due to the possibility of perforating a bowel loop that is adherent to the abdominal wall. In these patients, paracentesis should be performed in consultation with a pediatric surgeon. Patients with abnormal coagulation studies are at risk of developing an expanding abdominal wall hematoma, and the clinician should be cognizant of this possibility (8). Coagulopathy, however, is not a contraindication to performing paracentesis. Pregnant patients also can undergo paracentesis with proper selection of the puncture site (see "Procedure").

▸ EQUIPMENT

Antiseptic solution
Intravenous catheter, 16 to 22 gauge
20-mL syringe
1% buffered lidocaine with or without epinephrine
5- to 10-mL syringe with 25- to 30-gauge needle
Sterile specimen vials
Sterile gauze dressings

Monitoring equipment should be used and intravenous access should be obtained in cases of large volume removal and for patients with respiratory distress. Monitoring in such situations should include heart rate, respirations, blood pressure, and oxygen saturation.

▸ PROCEDURE

Once ascites is identified either by physical examination or radiography, the child should be placed in one of three positions: sitting, semi-supine, or lateral decubitus (Fig. 86.1). The patient is secured by assistants or restraints. Consideration should be given to the use of procedural sedation in selected patients (see Chapter 33). The bladder should be emptied by catheterization (see Chapter 95). Gastric distension should be alleviated by gastric intubation and suction (see Chapter 84). The site of aspiration is prepped with an antiseptic solution, and sterile drapes are applied.

Needle insertion can be performed in various sites. In neonates, an area lateral to the rectus abdominis muscle and below the umbilicus is chosen to avoid the liver and spleen (Fig. 86.2) (9). The most common site in children is the midline at the avascular linea alba, 2 cm below the umbilicus (Fig. 86.2) (1). Needle insertion in pregnant patients should be above the umbilicus and lateral to the midline. Care should be taken

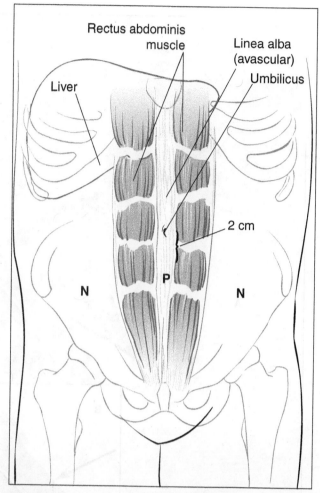

Figure 86.2 Neonatal insertion site (N) below the umbilicus and lateral to the rectus abdominis muscle. Pediatric insertion site (P) along the midline at the avascular linea alba and 2 cm below the umbilicus.

not to pierce the rectus abdominis muscle, as this increases the risk of puncturing the superior or inferior epigastric arteries.

Once the site is chosen, several milliliters of 1% buffered lidocaine, with or without epinephrine (maximum infiltration: 4 mg/kg lidocaine without epinephrine, 7 mg/kg lidocaine with epinephrine), are infiltrated subcutaneously down to the peritoneum using a small-gauge needle. The clinician then inserts an intravenous catheter at a 30 to 45-degree angle through the wheal of anesthesia while one hand pulls the skin caudally (Fig. 86.3). The clinician advances the needle and syringe with negative pressure applied until a "pop" is felt as the catheter passes through the peritoneum and fluid returns in the syringe. While holding the needle, the clinician advances the plastic sheath into the peritoneal cavity. The needle is removed and the syringe reapplied to the catheter to perform fluid collection and removal. Overly rapid removal of fluid can cause adverse effects (as described) if intravenous albumin replacement is not provided (see "Anatomy and Physiology"). On removing the catheter and syringe, the oblique angle and

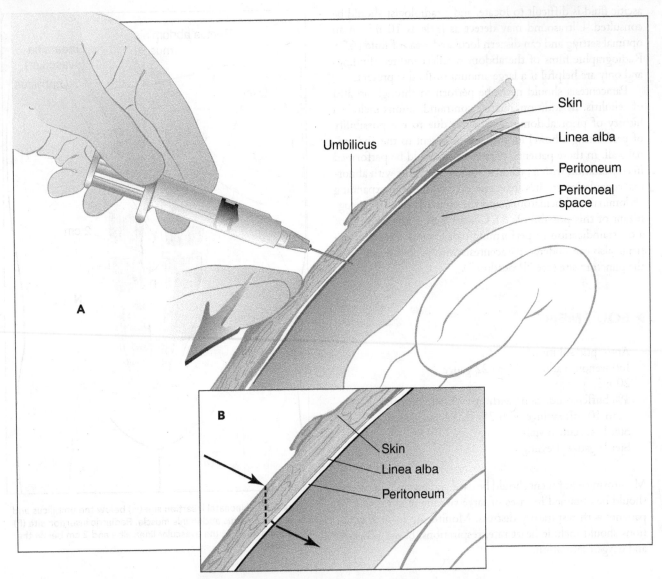

Figure 86.3 Z-track formation and controlled removal of ascitic fluid.
A. Needle insertion with caudal traction on the overlying skin.
B. Z-track formation after release of the skin and removal of the needle.

formation of a Z-track promote sealing and prevention of a leak (Fig. 86.3) (8).

Fluid (20 to 50 mL) is typically sent for diagnostic evaluation. Available tests include cell count and differential, Gram stain, cultures (bacterial, viral, fungal), acid-fast bacillus smear, cytology, total protein, albumin, glucose, lactic dehydrogenase, amylase, blood urea nitrogen, creatinine, potassium, ammonia, and specific gravity. The interpretation of peritoneal fluid studies is well described elsewhere (2).

▶ COMPLICATIONS

Complications occur in 1% to 3% of patients following paracentesis (10). Persistent peritoneal leak, abdominal wall

hematoma, and scrotal swelling are most common. Persistent fluid leaks can be minimized by creating a Z-track during the initial puncture, as described above. If a leak occurs, it can be stopped by a pressure dressing or suturing of the puncture site. Abdominal wall hematomas are usually self-limiting. Rarely, patients with pre-existing clotting abnormalities may develop expanding hematomas and hemorrhage. Correction of the underlying clotting disorder and blood transfusion are generally effective in treating this complication. Scrotal swelling results from dissection of ascites fluid through tissue layers and does not require specific treatment in most cases.

More serious complications include intraperitoneal hemorrhage, bowel or bladder puncture, and bacterial peritonitis. Appropriate patient selection, nasogastric tube placement, bladder catheterization, and careful attention to proper

SUMMARY

1 Insert a bladder catheter and consider nasogastric intubation to relieve gastric distension.

2 Position the patient (with restraint as needed) in sitting, semi-supine, or lateral decubitus position.

3 Prepare the puncture site using aseptic technique and establish a sterile field.

4 Anesthetize the puncture site with 1% buffered lidocaine.

5 Insert an intravenous catheter with a syringe attached while retracting the skin overlying the site caudally (to form a Z-track).

6 Advance the intravenous catheter with negative pressure applied to the syringe until a "pop" is felt and fluid fills the syringe.

7 Advance the catheter, remove the needle, and reattach the syringe.

8 Remove enough fluid for therapeutic results and/or diagnostic tests.

9 Remove the catheter when finished, and apply a clean gauze dressing.

CLINICAL TIPS

▶ The sitting or semi-supine position is more comfortable for patients in respiratory distress.

▶ Formation of the Z-track by applying caudal traction of overlying skin when placing the needle will seal the defect in the peritoneum and prevent leakage when the catheter is removed.

▶ Repositioning the patient may improve the flow of ascitic fluid through the catheter.

▶ Controlled flow of ascitic fluid may be accomplished by a three-way stopcock or intravenous tubing with a flow gauge.

▶ Large amounts of ascitic fluid may be safely removed if albumin replacement is given intravenously (8 g of albumin for 1 L of peritoneal fluid removed).

technique decrease the risk of viscous perforation and the potential sequelae of hemorrhage and bowel or bladder perforation. Bacteria can be introduced into the peritoneal cavity, causing peritonitis, if sterile precautions are not followed. Strict adherence to sterile technique during the procedure and avoidance of areas of skin infection decrease the likelihood of this complication.

▶ SUMMARY

Ascites occurs uncommonly in neonates and children. When present and causing respiratory distress or when fluid is needed for diagnostic purposes, paracentesis is indicated. The procedure is safe when performed in an appropriate setting by a physician familiar with the procedure and its potential complications.

▶ REFERENCES

1. Rice TB, Pontus SP. Abdominal paracentesis. In: Fuhrman BP, Bradley JJ, eds. *Pediatric Critical Care*. St. Louis: Mosby; 1992:147–151.
2. Cochran WJ. Ascites. In: McMillan JA, Feigin FD, DeAngelis CD, et al., eds. *Oski's Pediatrics: Principles and Practice*. 4th ed. Philadelphia: Lippincott Williams & Wilkins; 2006:2002–2009.
3. Dudley FJ. Pathophysiology of ascites formation. *Gastroenterol Clin North Am*. 1992;21:215–235.
4. Williams JW, Simel DL. Does this patient have ascites? How to divine fluid in the abdomen. *JAMA*. 1992;267:2645–2648.
5. Arroyo V, Gines P, Planas R. Treatment of ascites in cirrhosis: diuretics, peritoneovenous shunt, and large volume paracentesis. *Gastroenterol Clin North Am*. 1992;21:237–255.
6. Dinkel E, Lehnart R, Troger J, et al. Sonographic evidence of intraperitoneal fluid: an experimental study and its clinical implications. *Pediatr Radiol*. 1984;14:299–303.
7. Wyllie R, Fitzgerald D, Arasu T, et al. Ascites: pathophysiology and management. *J Pediatr*. 1980;97:167–176.
8. Runyon BA. Paracentesis of ascitic fluid: a safe procedure. *Arch Int Med*. 1986;146:2259–2261.
9. Valaes T. Neonatal ascites. In: Gellis S, Kagan B, eds. *Current Pediatric Therapy*. Philadelphia: WB Saunders; 1990:701–703.
10. Mallory A, Schaefer JW. Complications of diagnostic paracentesis in patients with liver disease. *JAMA*. 1978;239:628–630.

SHARON R. SMITH

87

SHARON R. SMITH

Inguinal Hernia Reduction

▶ INTRODUCTION

Two common causes of scrotal swelling in children are inguinal hernia and hydrocele. Inguinal hernias, which are classified as direct or indirect, occur when abdominal contents are present within a patent processus vaginalis. With an indirect inguinal hernia, the most common type in children, abdominal contents pass through the internal inguinal ring, whereas with a direct inguinal hernia, abdominal contents pass through the external inguinal ring. Direct inguinal hernias are rare in children and often occur after an indirect inguinal hernia repair (1).

The incidence of inguinal hernias in children ranges from 0.8% to 4.4% (1) and is highest in premature infants (16% to 25%). About one third of inguinal hernias occur in children under 6 months of age (1,2), with a peak incidence during the first 3 months of life. Inguinal hernias are six times more common in boys than girls and are more common on the right side (60% right, 30% left, 10% bilateral) (3).

A hydrocele develops if peritoneal fluid fills the processus vaginalis. It may occur along the spermatic cord or within the scrotal sac itself. Hydroceles are usually present at birth and often are bilateral; however, noticeable scrotal swelling may not develop until later in childhood. The hydrocele may decrease in size during sleep or when the child is relaxed. A hydrocele generally requires no acute treatment but can pose a clinical challenge when it must be distinguished from an inguinal hernia.

An incarcerated inguinal hernia occurs when the abdominal contents cannot be easily reduced into the abdominal cavity. Incarcerations occur more frequently in girls, in premature infants, and during the first year of life. In girls, the hernia sac may contain the fallopian tube, ovary, or uterus (1,4–9). A strangulated hernia compresses structures passing through the inguinal canal, such as viscera and blood vessels. Vascular compromise can lead to necrosis of the viscera and perforation of herniated intestine (1). Unlike adults, most children with irreducible incarcerated hernias rapidly progress to strangulation. Injury can occur to the testes, spermatic cord, or ovaries. Prompt reduction of the inguinal hernia before ischemia develops is the main goal of management.

▶ ANATOMY AND PHYSIOLOGY

The processus vaginalis is an outpouching of the peritoneum that develops approximately 3 months before birth. It descends through the inguinal canal into the scrotum or the labia. In boys, the testes descend with the processus and enter the scrotal sac between the seventh and ninth months of gestation (10). In girls, the processus ends in the labia majora. Normally, the processus vaginalis obliterates spontaneously after birth. When it does not obliterate, a patent processus vaginalis is created. Patency may remain in as many as 20% of normal adults (11). It is estimated that 80% to 94% of infants have patency of the processus at birth (1).

The partial or complete failure of the obliteration of the processus vaginalis predisposes to the formation of indirect inguinal hernias and hydroceles (Fig. 87.1). The processus vaginalis may remain widely patent, resulting in a scrotal hernia (complete inguinal hernia). A communicating hydrocele may develop when the proximal processus vaginalis remains patent but the neck of the communication is quite narrow. This allows peritoneal fluid to enter and exit the scrotal sac, although the patent neck is not large enough to allow entry of abdominal viscera. The processus may obliterate distally, leaving a patent proximal sac and the potential for an inguinal hernia. A commonly observed type of isolated hydrocele (noncommunicating hydrocele) occurs when fluid collects within the tunica vaginalis, and the inguinal processus obliterates

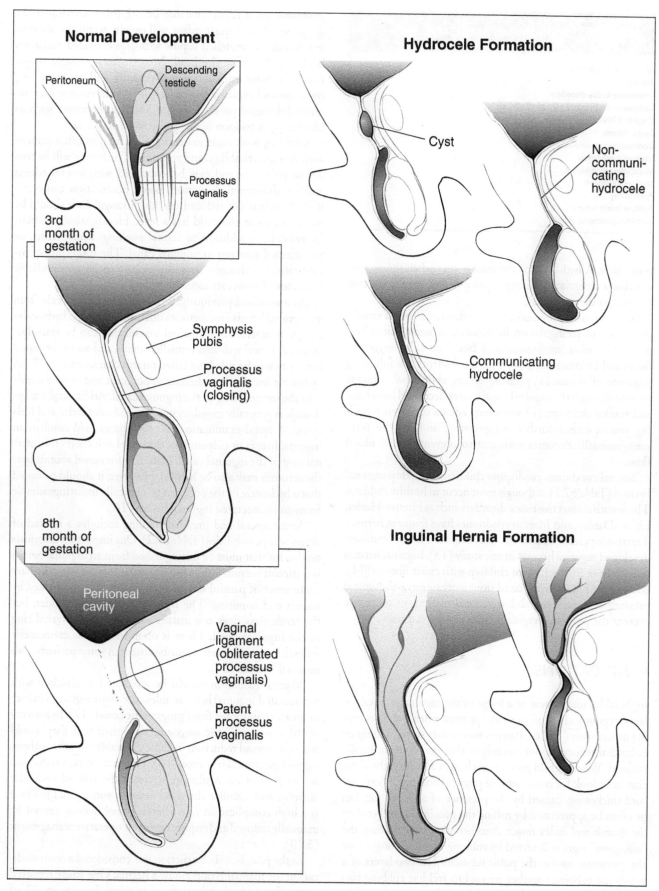

Figure 87.1 Common anomalies of the inguinal canal.

TABLE 87.1	CONDITIONS ASSOCIATED WITH INGUINAL HERNIA

Abdominal wall defects
Ascites
Connective tissue disorders
Continuous ambulatory peritoneal dialysis
Cryptorchidism
Cystic fibrosis
Genitourinary anomalies
Intersex syndromes
Mucopolysaccharidoses
Myelomeningocele
Prematurity
Positive family history
Ventriculoperitoneal shunt

proximally. A hydrocele of the cord occurs when the processus closes irregularly, leaving a patency and fluid collection isolated to the cord (12).

As mentioned previously, incarceration of a hernia rapidly progresses to strangulation in children. A strangulated hernia occurs when an incarcerated bowel or solid organ infarcts and becomes necrotic. This results from the following sequence of events: (a) pressure on the abdominal contents passing through the inguinal canal causes decreased lymphatic and venous drainage, (b) worsening edema of the surrounding tissues causes further compression, and (c) the pressure eventually becomes sufficient to prevent arterial blood flow.

Several conditions predispose children to develop inguinal hernias (Table 87.1), although most occur in healthy children. Those with connective tissue disorders such as Hunter-Hurler, Ehlers-Danlos, and Marfan syndromes have frequent hernias. Thirty-six percent of patients with Hunter-Hurler syndrome developed inguinal hernias in one study (13). Inguinal hernias also occur in 6% to 15% of children with cystic fibrosis (14). Most of the predisposing conditions increase intra-abdominal pressure or fluid, cause abdominal wall defects, or otherwise prevent the processus vaginalis from closing normally.

▶ INDICATIONS

Inguinal hernias appear as a bulge in the inguinal, scrotal, or labial region and are often more apparent when a child is crying or straining (15,16). Parents may report seeing a lump or bulge that reduced spontaneously or that the parent manually reduced. When a child presents with such a history, the clinician must look for corroborative physical findings. Spermatic cord thickening, caused by the presence of a hernia sac, can be often be appreciated by rolling the proximal cord between the thumb and index finger. Another suggestive finding, the "silk glove" sign, is detected by rubbing the index finger over the spermatic cord at the pubic tubercle. The two layers of a hernia sac rubbing together are said to feel like rubbing two layers of silk cloth together. Neither of these signs is patho-

gnomonic for a hernia but may be helpful in arriving at the diagnosis (17). A quiet infant will usually strain the abdominal muscles if stretched supine with legs extended and arms held straight above the head. Most infants struggle to get free, increasing intra-abdominal pressure and often causing the inguinal hernia to protrude. Older children may increase intra-abdominal pressure with a Valsalva maneuver such as blowing up a balloon or coughing while standing.

Children with incarcerated inguinal hernias often present with crying, irritability, and vomiting. The hernia will be tender to palpation and may be associated with scrotal edema and/or abdominal distention. Bowel obstruction can occur if the hernia is not reduced quickly. Strangulation should be suspected when the child has a fever, bloody stools, testicular swelling in addition to scrotal swelling, leukocytosis, or an inflamed scrotum or inguinal canal. The total time of incarceration is thought by most experts to be an unreliable predictor of bowel strangulation (18).

As mentioned previously, differentiating a hydrocele from an inguinal hernia is sometimes difficult. Although hydroceles are often described as inguinal masses that can be transilluminated, bowel will also transilluminate, and an incarcerated hernia cannot be ruled out based on this characteristic (19). A hydrocele usually has a definite upper limit and never extends into the internal ring of the inguinal canal. Additionally, a hydrocele is generally movable, smooth, and nontender and feels cystic. A rectal examination can sometimes help confirm an inguinal hernia by palpation of the bowel as it enters the internal ring of the inguinal canal. Listening for bowel sounds over the scrotum may also be helpful. However, it should be noted that a hydrocele of the cord can be clinically indistinguishable from an incarcerated inguinal hernia (10).

Acute scrotal and inguinal swelling includes a myriad of diagnostic possibilities (Table 87.2). One important diagnosis on this list that must be distinguished from an inguinal hernia is testicular torsion. Boys with testicular torsion typically have acute onset of painful scrotal swelling, often accompanied by nausea and vomiting. The testicle is exquisitely tender, but the tenderness does not usually extend to the external ring of the inguinal canal. There is often loss of the cremasteric reflex; however, this reflex may be absent in some patients with inguinal hernias (20).

Manual reduction should be attempted in children with incarcerated inguinal hernias unless they have signs of toxicity or an acute abdomen from gangrenous bowel (12). In a survey of 40 senior pediatric surgeons, all replied that they would attempt manual reduction in clinically stable patients without signs of peritoneal irritation (18). The goals of early reduction are to prevent strangulation, decrease the risk of testicular atrophy, and stabilize the child prior to surgery (21). There is a high complication rate when inguinal hernias cannot be manually reduced and require emergent operative management (5,19).

In the past, bowel obstruction was considered a contraindication for manual reduction of a hernia. One study reported successful manual reduction of inguinal hernias in 12 of

TABLE 87.2	DIFFERENTIAL DIAGNOSIS OF INGUINAL AND SCROTAL SWELLING

Testicular swelling
  Testicular torsion
  Testicular tumor
  Epididymitis
  Epididymoorchitis
  Testicular trauma
  Torsion of the appendage of epididymis or testicle
  Hydrocele of the tunica vaginalis
  Communicating hydrocele
  Varicocele
Inguinal swelling
  Retractable testicle
  Undescended testicle
  Hydrocele of the cord
  Incarcerated ovary
  Incarcerated dermoid cyst
  Appendicial abscess
  Groin abscess
  Inguinal lymphadenitis
Scrotal swelling
  Idiopathic scrotal edema
  Allergic scrotal edema
  Henoch-Schönlein purpura
  Kawasaki disease
  Insect bite

14 patients 2 years old and younger with radiographic evidence of bowel obstruction (6). A survey of pediatric surgeons revealed that 75% would attempt manual reduction for incarcerated inguinal hernias even if the child had abdominal distention and radiographic evidence of intestinal obstruction (18). For these reasons, abdominal radiographs are not routinely obtained, although radiographs should be considered for children with possible strangulation.

Manual reduction should not be attempted by the emergency physician in a child with (a) toxic appearance, (b) fever, (c) bloody diarrhea, (d) entrapped viscera that appear blue or black under the skin, (e) signs of peritonitis, or (f) leukocytosis greater than 15,000/mm^3 (12,18). Although the likelihood of reducing a necrotic segment of bowel is low, this undesirable outcome has been reported (22).

▶ EQUIPMENT

Gloves
Ice pack
Equipment for analgesia and/or mild sedation (see Chapter 33)

▶ PROCEDURE

Success rates for manual reduction of inguinal hernias have improved over time. Early studies reported successful reductions in 70% to 80% of patients (3,6). Two more recent

studies reported 95.5% (151 of 158) and 100% (30 of 30) success rates in the reduction of incarcerated inguinal hernia in children less than 2 years old, the age group in which incarceration occurs most commonly (23,24).

No prospective study has examined the success rate using different techniques of manual reduction. Instead, most authorities report using some combination of sedation, ice packs, elevation, and gentle taxis (manual reduction). Pediatric surgeons have reported the following frequencies for use of reduction techniques: gentle manipulation, 95%; sedation, 75%; elevation, 55%; and ice packs, 18% (18). There are two primary methods for manually reducing an inguinal hernia. One is to apply bimanual pressure along the inguinal canal using the distal hand to "milk out" the gas or contents of the incarcerated bowel (Fig. 87.2). After reducing the contents of the incarcerated bowel, pressure is slightly increased over the distal portion of the hernia as compared with the proximal portion to reduce the bowel. Up to 5 minutes of continual gentle pressure may be needed for successful reduction (25).

An alternate two-handed technique for manual reduction is shown in Figure 87.3 (10). The fingers of one hand (the left hand as depicted in the figure) are first used to sweep along the inguinal canal from the anterior iliac crest to the distal scrotum. The same hand is then used to grasp the testicle, hernia mass, or scrotal skin and apply gentle pressure (Fig. 87.3B). Next, the index finger and thumb of the opposite hand are used to apply "upward" and lateral traction over the hernia "neck" to help in keeping the internal and external inguinal rings open (Fig. 87.3C). The fingers of the hand on the scrotum are then used to "walk" the bottom of the hernia sac progressively up toward the inguinal rings until the hernia is reduced (Fig. 87.3D).

Placing the infant or child in Trendelenburg position and providing mild sedation may increase the success rate with either of these methods. A covered ice pack or cold pack to the groin has also been suggested, but there is little evidence to support its efficacy. Intravenous morphine sulfate or oral oxycodone can be used for both sedation and pain relief. Such medications can be used initially or administered after attempted reduction without medication proves unsuccessful. Deep sedation should not be used because of the risk of injuring the intestine or reducing gangrenous bowel.

▶ COMPLICATIONS

Reduction of necrotic or strangulated bowel is a rare but serious complication. Between 1960 and 1965, the intestinal resection rate among 351 patients with incarcerated inguinal hernias was 1.4%. A review of three series published since 1978 indicate no resection of bowel in 221 patients with incarcerated inguinal hernias (19). Although no cases have been reported of necrotic bowel being reduced, careful examination before reduction will help to avoid this problem (22).

After reducing an inguinal hernia, the physician should ensure that the inguinal canal is empty, especially the internal

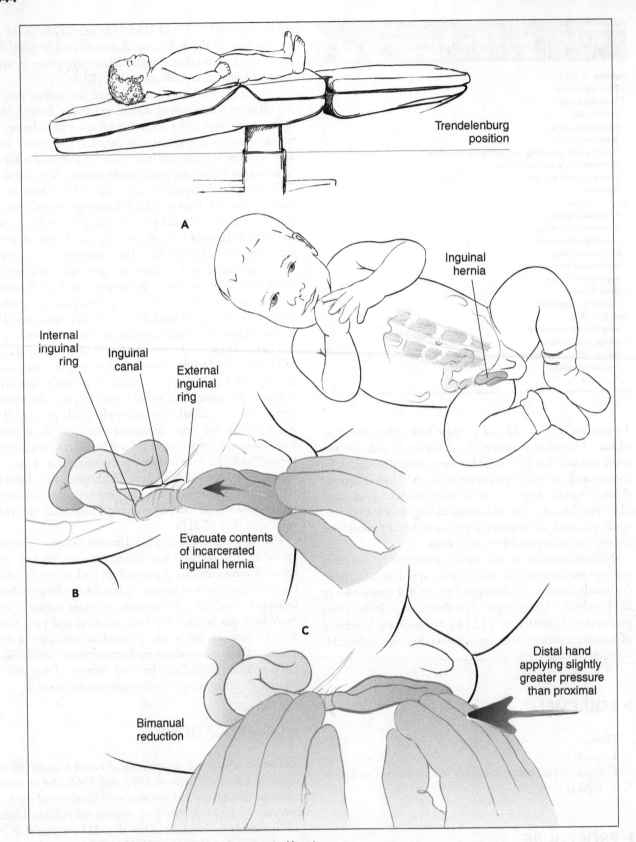

Figure 87.2 Reducing an indirect inguinal hernia.
A. Anatomy of an indirect inguinal hernia.
B. Gas and stool are first "milked out" of the bowel to reduce its size.
C. Constant pressure is applied for up to 5 minutes (distal to proximal) to reduce the hernia.

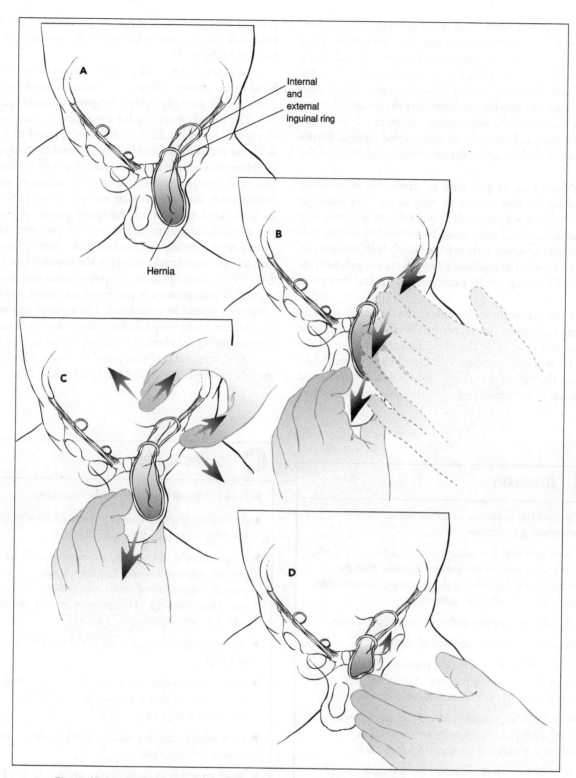

Figure 87.3 Alternate method for bimanual reduction of an inguinal hernia.
A. Anatomy of an indirect inguinal hernia. Note the position in the groin of the hernia "neck" extending through the internal and external inguinal rings.
B. The fingers of one hand are first used to sweep along the inguinal canal from the anterior iliac crest to the distal scrotum. The same hand is then used to grasp the testicle, hernia mass, or scrotal skin and apply gentle pressure.
C. The index finger and thumb of the opposite hand are used to apply "upward" and lateral traction over the hernia neck to help in keeping the internal and external inguinal rings open.
D. The fingers of the hand on the scrotum are then used to "walk" the bottom of the hernia sac progressively up toward the inguinal rings until the hernia is reduced.

ring. Emergent surgical referral is recommended if the reduction was difficult or there is concern about the completeness of reduction. Cases of incomplete reduction (one wall of the bowel still incarcerated) leading to bowel necrosis (Richter hernia) have been reported (1). Furthermore, incarceration often recurs and may happen soon after the initial reduction (8,26). Consequently, most experts recommend that children requiring reduction of an incarcerated inguinal hernia be admitted to the hospital for observation and repair of the hernia.

The hernia sac in girls with an irreducible incarcerated inguinal hernias may contain an ovary or other reproductive structures (6). It was previously thought that an asymptomatic irreducible herniated ovary could be managed by elective surgical reduction; however, there is a relatively high incidence of future torsion and strangulation. For this reason, girls with incarcerated ovaries generally require urgent surgical correction (6,7).

The vascular supply to the testis can be compromised by an incarcerated inguinal hernia, potentially resulting in ischemic necrosis and atrophy of the testis. Ischemic changes in the testes are relatively common with incarcerated inguinal hernias, but the rate of actual infarction is low. Patients most at risk for this complication are premature infants, infants younger than 6 months of age, and patients whose manual reduction was unsuccessful and who require emergency herniorrhaphy (6,9).

Two factors are most responsible for increasing the likelihood that a patient will have an irreducible incarcerated inguinal hernia: young age and prolonged duration of symptoms (6). The complication rate for irreducible hernias requiring emergency surgery is 22% to 33%, as opposed to 1.7% to 4.5% for manually reduced hernias repaired electively (3,27). Children with irreducible incarcerated inguinal hernias therefore need emergent pediatric surgery consultation, and their management should be similar to that of any patient with an acute surgical abdomen. Adequate parenteral pain control should be administered. Patients with persistent vomiting should receive intravenous fluids and may benefit from insertion of a nasogastric tube to empty the stomach (see Chapter 84) (19). Obtaining serum electrolyte values may also be indicated. If strangulation is present or suspected, intravenous antibiotics should be considered. The primary reason to admit children to the hospital after reduction of an incarcerated inguinal hernia for planned early surgical repair is to prevent recurrent incarceration (with possible irreducibility) and the attendant complications (3,4,6,8,15,18,23,26,27).

 SUMMARY

1 Confirm the presence of a true hernia before attempting reduction.

2 Make sure that the patient does not have signs of peritonitis and, to the extent possible, that the bowel is not ischemic; if there is any question, seek immediate surgical consultation.

3 Provide pain control and consider mild sedation.

4 Wear gloves before contacting patient.

5 Apply gentle, firm bimanual pressure along entire inguinal canal, using hand most distal to "milk out" contents or gas within incarcerated bowel.

6 After reducing contents of incarcerated bowel, apply increased pressure over the distal as compared with the proximal inguinal canal.

7 If the bowel is not reduced after 5 minutes of continuous pressure, try sedation (if not used on first attempt), Trendelenburg positioning, and/or ice pack to the groin, then repeat procedure (or use alternative method shown in Fig. 87.3).

8 For all incarcerated hernias, contact a surgeon to arrange for hospital admission and surgical correction.

 CLINICAL TIPS

▶ Direct inguinal hernias are rare in children.

▶ An indirect inguinal hernia presents with a mass at the internal ring of the inguinal canal.

▶ A hydrocele is usually smooth, nontender, and mobile. Although bowel can sometimes transilluminate, a hydrocele has brilliant transillumination, and it does not extend into the internal ring of the inguinal canal.

▶ A communicating hydrocele will often shrink during the night.

▶ When parents give a reliable history for an inguinal hernia, provocative maneuvers (e.g., Valsalva) may cause the hernia to protrude.

▶ Even with irreducible incarcerated inguinal hernias, strangulation is rare.

▶ Most attempts at reduction of an incarcerated inguinal hernia are successful.

▶ Irreducible inguinal hernias in girls are likely to include the ovary.

▶ Evidence of bowel obstruction is not a contraindication to manual reduction of an inguinal hernia.

▶ SUMMARY

Initial management of an incarcerated inguinal hernia involves recognition of the problem, proper technique in performing a manual reduction, and appropriate observation after hernia reduction. In most cases, the emergency physician can successfully perform reduction. Patients who have an irreducible hernia or signs of peritonitis require emergent surgical consultation.

▶ ACKNOWLEDGMENT

The authors would like to acknowledge the valuable contributions of Mark C. Clark to the version of this chapter that appeared in the previous edition.

▶ REFERENCES

1. Bronsther B, Abrams MW, Elboim C. Inguinal hernias in children: a study of 1,000 cases and a review of the literature. *JAMA*. 1972;27: 522–584.
2. Rajput A, Gauderer MWL, Hack M. Inguinal hernias in very low birth weight infants: incidence and timing of repair. *J Pediatric Surg*. 1992;27:1322.
3. Rowe MI, Clatworthy HW. The other side of the pediatric inguinal hernia. *Surg Clin North Am*. 1971;51:1371–1374.
4. Moss RL, Hatch EI. Inguinal hernia repair in early infancy. *Am J Surg*. 1991;161:596–599.
5. Rowe MI, Clatworthy HW. Incarcerated and strangulated hernias in children. *Arch Surg*. 1970;101:136–137.
6. Davies N, Najmaldin A, Burge DM. Irreducible inguinal hernia in children below 2 years of age. *Br J Surg*. 1990;77:1291–1292.
7. Boley SJ, Cahn D, Lauer T, et al. The irreducible ovary: a true emergency. *J Pediatr Surg*. 1991;26:1035–1038.
8. Stylianos S, Jacir NN, Harris BH. Incarceration of inguinal hernia in infants prior to elective repair. *J Pediatr*. 1993;28:582–583.
9. Friedman D, Schwartzbard A, Velcek FT, et al. The government and the inguinal hernia. *J Pediatr Surg*. 1979;14:356–359.
10. Kapur P, Caty MG, Glick PL. Pediatric hernias and hydroceles. *Pediatr Clin North Am*. 1998;45:773–789.
11. Tam P. Inguinal hernia. In: Lister J, Irving I, eds. *Neonatal Surgery*. 3rd ed. London: Butterworth; 1990:367–375.
12. Grosfeld JL. Current concepts in inguinal hernia in infants and children. *World J Surg*. 1989;13:506–515.
13. Curan AG, Erakis AJ. Inguinal hernia in the Hurler-Hunter syndrome. *Surgery*. 1967;61:302.
14. Maisonet L. Inguinal hernia. *Pediatr Rev*. 2003;24:34–35.
15. Skinner MA, Grosfeld JL. Inguinal and umbilical hernia repair in infants and children. *Surg Clin North Am*. 1993;73:439–449.
16. Dennis C, Enquist IF. Strangulating external hernia. In: Nyhus LM, Condon RE, eds. *Hernia*. Philadelphia: JB Lippincott Co.; 1978: 279–299.
17. Gilbert M, Clatworthy HW. Bilateral operations for inguinal hernia and hydrocele in infancy and childhood. *Am J Surg*. 1959;97: 255–259.
18. Rowe MI, Marchildon MB. Inguinal hernia and hydrocele in infants and children. *Surg Clin North Am*. 1981;61:1137–1145.
19. Rowe MI, Lloyd DA. Inguinal hernia. In: Welch KJ, Randolph JG, Ravitch MM, et al., eds. *Pediatric Surgery*. 4th ed. Chicago: Year Book Medical Publishers; 1986:779–793.
20. Rabinowitz R. The importance of the cremasteric reflex in acute scrotal swelling in children. *J Urol*. 1984;132:89–90.
21. Weber TR, Tracy TF. Groin hernias and hydroceles. In: Ashcraft KW, Holder TM, eds. *Pediatric Surgery*. 2nd ed. Philadelphia: WB Saunders; 1993:562–570.
22. Klein BL, Ochsenschlager DW. Scrotal masses in children and adolescents: a review for the emergency physician. *Pediatr Emerg Care*. 1993;9:351–361.
23. Puri P, Guiney EJ, O'Donnell L. Inguinal hernia in infants: the fate of the testis following incarceration. *J Pediatr Surg*. 1984;19: 44–46.
24. Stringer MD, Higgins M, Capps ANJ, et al. Irreducible inguinal hernia. *Br J Surg*. 1991;78:504–505.
25. Schnaufer L, Mahboubi S. Abdominal emergencies. In: Fleisher GR, Ludwig S, eds. *Textbook of Pediatric Emergency Medicine*. 3rd ed. Baltimore: Williams & Wilkins; 1993:1307–1335.
26. Sparnon AL, Kiely EM, Spitz L. Incarcerated inguinal hernia in infants. *Br Med J*. 1986;293:376–377.
27. Rescorla FJ, Grosfeld JL. Inguinal hernia repair in the perinatal period and early infancy: clinical considerations. *J Pediatr Surg*. 1984;19: 832–837.

88

ANGELA C. ANDERSON AND SEEMA SACHDEVA

Treatment of Umbilical Granuloma

▶ INTRODUCTION

An umbilical granuloma results from excessive growth of normal granulation tissue on the umbilical stump. Prevention of umbilical granuloma formation is usually accomplished by keeping the umbilical cord clean and dry and by applying a topical antimicrobial agent daily (e.g., isopropyl alcohol or bacitracin) (1). Removal of an umbilical granuloma is a simple procedure, usually performed in the office setting or a low-acuity area of the emergency department.

▶ ANATOMY AND PHYSIOLOGY

The umbilical cord normally comprises the umbilical vein and two umbilical arteries embedded in a gelatinous substance called Wharton's jelly. Umbilical cord separation usually occurs 1 to 2 weeks after birth; delayed cord separation beyond 7 to 8 weeks of age may be associated with defects in cellular immunity or chemotaxis (2–4). The remaining umbilical stump is covered by a thin layer of skin. This epithelialization typically occurs within 12 to 15 days following separation. Over time, the umbilical arteries become the lateral umbilical ligaments, and the umbilical vein becomes the ligamentum teres.

Although the blood vessels in the stump are functionally closed following cord separation, they remain anatomically patent. While patent, the blood vessels are potential portals of entry for invasive pathogens such as *Staphylococcus aureus*, group B streptococci, and *Clostridium tetani*.

An umbilical granuloma is formed when epithelialization of the umbilicus is incomplete and normal granulation tissue grows excessively. The resulting granuloma is soft and vascular, with pink or cherry-red coloration. It typically measures 3 to 10 mm in diameter and may be associated with small amounts of bleeding or drainage. It is unclear if low-grade infection or bacterial colonization plays a role in umbilical granuloma formation (4).

▶ INDICATIONS

Small umbilical granulomas often regress with continued application of isopropyl alcohol (5). However, large or pedunculated umbilical granulomas frequently bleed and may lead to umbilical disfigurement. In general, large or bleeding granulomas deserve removal.

Several umbilical abnormalities must be differentiated from an umbilical granuloma before any attempt is made at removal (Table 88.1 and Fig. 88.1). Omphalitis, characterized by periumbilical erythema and cord drainage, is caused by bacterial infection of the umbilical stump. Pathogens include group A streptococci, group B streptococci, and *S. aureus*. This condition represents a true cellulitis of the abdominal wall that may extend internally via the still patent umbilical vessels to cause liver abscess, portal vein thrombosis, and umbilical arteritis. Abscess formation within the cord may cause a red umbilical mass that might be mistaken for an umbilical granuloma. However, the presence of fever and periumbilical erythema should lead to the correct diagnosis.

An omphalomesenteric or vitelline duct results from the persistence of the embryologic connection between the umbilicus and the ileum. It presents as a pale pink orifice that releases flatus or feculent discharge and is often adjacent to an umbilical polyp. Umbilical polyps are remnants of the omphalomesenteric duct. An umbilical polyp appears bright red and nodular. It may be associated with mucoid discharge and is comprised of intestinal mucosa.

TABLE 88.1	DIFFERENTIATING FEATURES OF UMBILICAL ABNORMALITIES					
	Umbilical granuloma	**Patient omphalomesenteric duct**	**Patient urachus**	**Omphalitis**	**Umbilical polyp**	**Omphalocele**
Appearance	Reddish to pink mass	Pale pink orifice	Like the surrounding navel skin	Periumbilical erythema, discharge may be present	Red nodule	Protruding sac with glistening surface
Palpation	Dry, velvety feel	Moist velvety feel	Wet due to presence of urine	Indurated feel	Moist with some excoriation of surrounding skin	Usually soft, may feel firm if liver is a part of herniated contents
Presentation	Serous-serosanguinous foul smelling discharge or mass after cord separates off	Dischage (mucus, gas, meconium and fecal matter) present at birth or delayed until second week of life	Urinelike discharge at birth or soon after, sometimes delayed for several months	Mild local erythema, sometimes frank purulent discharge with extensive periumbilical involvement may be present	Mucous discharge and mass visible after cord separates	Protruding sac through umbilical area at birth
Orifice and tract	Absent	Present	Present	Absent	Absent	Absent
Diagnosis	Probe test is negative	Probe test is positive Injection of contrast material into the orifice demonstrates the tract and its communication with the gastrointestinal tract	Cystography and injection of contrast material into the orifice outlines the tract	Gram stain and culture	Biopsy confirms the presence of mucous membrane of small intestine	Physical examination
Treatment	Silver nitrate cauterization; if persistent, electrodesiccation, cryotherapy, or surgical treatment may be used	Surgical repair	Surgical repair	Oral or parental antibiotics	Cauterize if sure no tract present	Immediate surgical repair

A patent urachus (allantois) represents a continued connection between the umbilicus and the bladder and occurs when the allantoic duct fails to close. It is associated with obstruction of the bladder outlet or urethra. It appears as an opening at the base of the umbilicus and is occasionally associated with reddened surrounding mucosa. The diagnosis is made by careful observation for intermittent urine flow from the umbilicus.

An omphalocele is a protrusion of abdominal contents into the base of the umbilical cord. The abdominal organs within the omphalocele are visible through the transparent peritoneum. Although large omphaloceles will not be confused with an umbilical granuloma, small omphaloceles may appear as yellow-white protrusions within the cord.

▶ EQUIPMENT

75% silver nitrate on a wooden applicator stick
Clean gauze or cotton
Sterile 3.0 silk suture
Sterile scissors

Silver nitrate is an antiseptic cauterizing agent. Effective cautery requires aqueous activation of the silver nitrate.

The depth of silver nitrate cautery is limited by coagulation necrosis.

▶ PROCEDURE

The desired site for silver nitrate application is carefully inspected for evidence of infection, a sinus or fistula, fecal or urine discharge, or another anomaly, as described previously. Application of a partial skin barrier, such as petroleum jelly or bacitracin, to the surrounding normal skin may help prevent inadvertent spillage of silver nitrate. The tip of the silver nitrate stick is applied for 2 to 3 seconds to the umbilical granuloma, avoiding surrounding tissue (Fig. 88.2A). Cautery is signaled by a change in color from red to gray or black. If the surface of the lesion is dry, the tip of the applicator should be moistened with tap water before the procedure. Multiple applications with a single stick may be necessary with some large granulomas. Caution must be exercised to prevent contact of the silver nitrate with adjacent skin. Any excess silver nitrate or umbilical drainage should be wiped with gauze or cotton at the end of the procedure. Applications may be repeated every 3 to 5 days until the umbilical granuloma has resolved. Most granulomas resolve within

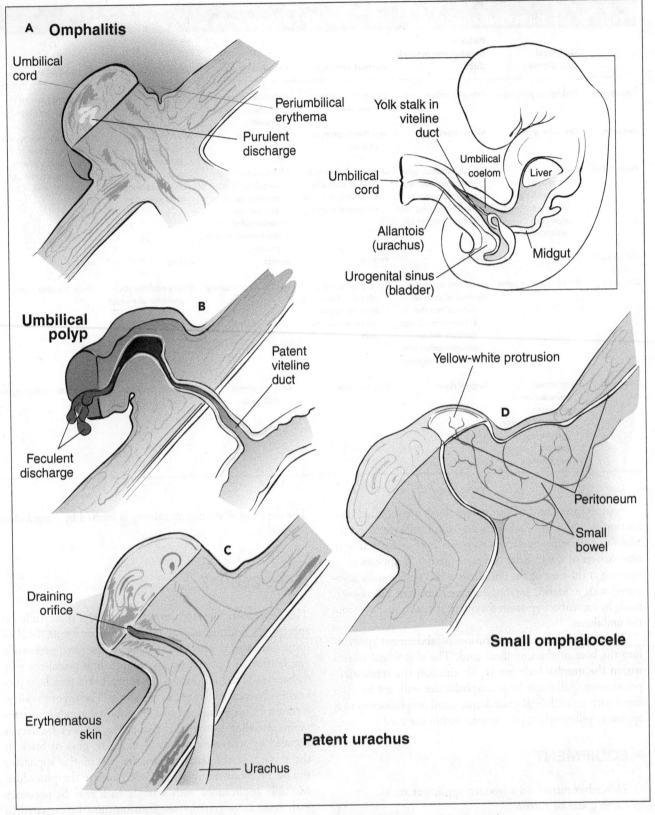

Figure 88.1 Anomalies of the umbilical cord to differentiate from an umbilical granuloma.
A. Omphalitis.
B. Umbilical polyp.
C. Patent urachus.
D. Small omphalocele.

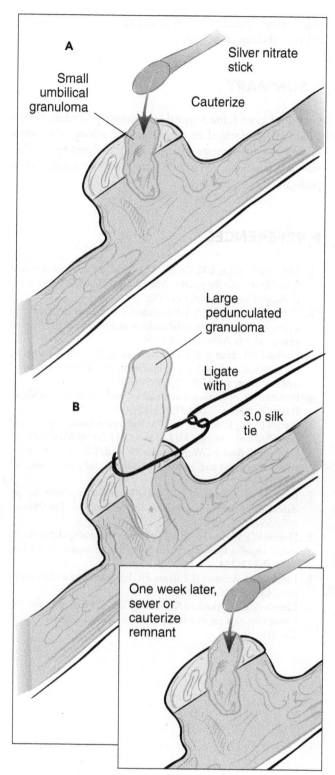

Figure 88.2 Umbilical granuloma removal.
A. Cautery with silver nitrate stick.
B. Ligation using thick silk or nylon tie.

SUMMARY

Large Nonpedunculated Granuloma

1 Apply a partial skin barrier such as petroleum jelly or bacitracin to the surrounding normal skin.

2 If the granuloma appears dry, wet the silver nitrate applicator with water.

3 Apply the silver nitrate to the granuloma for 2 to 3 seconds until the mucosa turns gray or black.

4 Apply repeatedly with a single stick, taking care to avoid inadvertent cautery of healthy skin or spillage of silver nitrate.

5 Blot excess silver nitrate off the granuloma and surrounding skin.

6 Repeat application in 3 to 5 days as needed.

Small Pedunculated Granuloma

1 Clean the area with an antiseptic solution.

2 Place a 3.0 silk tie on a superficial or distal area of the granuloma and have an assistant apply gentle traction.

3 Place a second 3.0 silk tie proximal to the first tie at the base of the granuloma; the granuloma should become necrotic and fall off in 7 to 14 days.

Large Pedunculated Granuloma

1 Tie off base of the granuloma using thick (1.0 to 3.0) silk or nylon surgical tie.

2 In 1 week, remove the remnant of the granuloma (if it does not fall off spontaneously) and cauterize the base of the granuloma with silver nitrate as described above.

3 weeks of the initiation of treatment. Persistence beyond that period may indicate the presence of one of the anomalies previously described, and surgical consultation is warranted (6).

Small pedunculated granulomas can be managed using the double-ligature technique (7). This technique is particularly helpful if the granuloma is situated deep within the umbilicus. The area is first cleaned with an antiseptic solution such as povidone-iodine or chlorhexidine. A 3.0 silk suture tie is then placed on a superficial or distal area of the granuloma. An assistant or parent uses this tie to provide gentle traction on the granuloma, and a second, more proximal 3.0 silk tie is placed at the base of the granuloma. The granuloma will become necrotic and fall off in 7 to 14 days.

> ## CLINICAL TIPS
>
> ▶ If the umbilical mass is bright red, flesh-colored, or excessively moist, cautery should not be performed until further evaluation for an orifice by probe test is performed.
>
> ▶ Fever and periumbilical redness suggest omphalitis and should preclude any attempts at umbilical cautery.
>
> ▶ No more than one applicator stick should be used when performing umbilical granuloma cautery.

Large pedunculated granulomas with a wide base can be managed by tightly ligating the granuloma at its base (Fig. 88.2B). The granuloma will subsequently fall off or can be cut off approximately 1 week after ligation. The base is then cauterized with silver nitrate, as previously described.

▶ COMPLICATIONS

Silver nitrate can cause chemical burns if applied to the skin, mucous membranes, or cornea (8,9). Careless application with spillage of silver nitrate-containing fluid onto the abdomen has caused significant burns. This problem can be avoided by limiting cautery to one silver nitrate stick per procedure, placing petrolatum on the surrounding skin, and carefully drying the treated area with gauze or cotton at the end of the procedure (10).

Cautery of vitelline duct remnants, a patent urachus, or omphalocele makes subsequent diagnosis and surgical treatment difficult. In the case of an omphalocele, cautery may risk peritonitis and underlying organ injury. Cautery of an omphalitis risks further spread of infection and creates a poorly healing, infected abdominal wound.

▶ SUMMARY

Umbilical granuloma removal is a simple procedure that is commonly performed in the outpatient setting. Care must be taken to differentiate an umbilical granuloma from other umbilical anomalies and to avoid damage to normal skin when performing this procedure.

▶ REFERENCES

1. McConnell TP, Lee CW, Couillard M. Trends in umbilical cord care: Scientific evidence for practice. *NBIN* 2004;4:211–222. http://www.medscape.com/viewarticle/497030.
2. Davies E, Levinsky R. A lethal syndrome of delayed umbilical cord separation, defective neutrophil mobility and absent natural killer cell activity. *Abstr Br Pediatr Assoc.* 1982;46.
3. Hayward AR, Harvey BA, Leonard J, et al. Delayed separation of the umbilical cord, widespread infections, and defective neutrophil mobility. *Lancet.* 1979;1(8126):1099–1101.
4. Pomeranz A. Anomalies, abnormalities, and care of the umbilicus. *Pediatr Clin North Am.* 2004;51:819–827.
5. Daniels J, Craig F, Wajed R, et al. Umbilical granulomas: a randomized controlled trial. *Arch Dis Child Fetal Neonatal Ed.* 2003;88(3):F257.
6. Campbell J, Beasley SW, McMullin N, et al. Clinical diagnosis of umbilical swellings and discharges in children. *Med J Aust.* 1986;145:450–453.
7. Lotan G, Klin B, Efrati Y. Double-ligature: a treatment for pedunculated umbilical granulomas in children. *Am Fam Physician.* 2002;65:2067–2068.
8. Fletcher PD, Wyman BS, Scopp IW. Acute necrotizing ulcerative gingivitis: sequelae following treatment with silver nitrate. *N Y J Dent.* 1976;46:122–124.
9. Laughrea PA, Arentsen JJ, Laibson PR. Iatrogenic ocular silver nitrate burn. *Cornea.* 1985;4:47–50.
10. Chamberlain JM, Gorman RL, Young GM. Silver nitrate burns following treatment for umbilical granuloma. *Pediatr Emerg Care.* 1992;8:29–30.

PHILIP R. SPANDORFER AND BRYAN D. UPHAM

89

Oral Rehydration

▶ INTRODUCTION

Children with acute gastroenteritis and dehydration are commonly treated in the emergency department (ED). Almost all children will have had rotavirus gastroenteritis, the most common etiology of acute gastroenteritis, by the age of 5 years. Morbidity and mortality are related to the acute loss of circulating fluid volume, ultimately resulting in diminished tissue perfusion, metabolic acidosis, and, in extreme cases, shock. The goals of therapy are the rapid restoration of circulating intravascular volume (water and electrolytes), the correction of acid-base disturbances, and the reduction of stool output and vomiting (1).

Oral rehydration therapy (ORT) is the administration of small volumes of an appropriate oral rehydration solution on a regular schedule (Fig. 89.1). For children with mild to moderate dehydration, ORT is recommended as the initial therapy of choice by the American Academy of Pediatrics, the World Health Organization, and the Centers for Disease Control (2–4). ORT can also be used for severely dehydrated children. Although ORT has been shown to be effective for treating moderately dehydrated children in an ED setting, its use in the United States has been limited (5). The most frequent obstacles to successful oral rehydration in the ED are false perceptions that oral rehydration is too slow or is not a definitive procedure. Physicians and nurses hold these beliefs as frequently as parents. Generally, 5 minutes spent preparing for and describing ORT to the family will reduce or eliminate these obstacles. ORT spares the child the pain of an intravenous line, promotes more direct parental involvement in the management of the child's dehydration, and teaches the parents a skill that can be used the next time the child becomes dehydrated.

▶ ANATOMY AND PHYSIOLOGY

Acute gastroenteritis is caused by a variety of viral and bacterial pathogens. Fluid losses from gastroenteritis often have an electrolyte composition similar to that of plasma. Most of the fluid deficit during the early stages of dehydration is from the extracellular space, but with time the fluid losses equilibrate and fluid leaves the intracellular space. During the recovery phase, fluid administered to the patient enters the extracellular space initially and then gradually re-equilibrates with the intracellular space.

Vomiting is controlled by the emetic center in the central nervous system in the area postrema. Of note, this center contains 85% of the body's 5HT-3 receptors. Diarrhea results when gastrointestinal fluid secretion exceeds fluid absorption. Regardless of the etiology, once fluid losses begin, a specific sequence of physiologic processes follow. Metabolic acidosis from decreased tissue perfusion causes further decline in end-organ function, such as decreased myocardial contractility, which may exacerbate the effects of shock. Reduced renal perfusion triggers the renin-angiotensin-aldosterone system, resulting in sodium and water retention at the expense of increased urinary potassium losses. Ultimately, hypokalemia results in decreased bowel motility, with the potential for further third-space fluid losses (6).

ORT can safely and rapidly restore circulating volume. Oral rehydration solutions consist of balanced mixtures of simple or complex carbohydrates and sodium. Small carbohydrate molecules promote absorption of sodium by "facilitated cotransport" (7), which in turn promotes water absorption. In the intestinal lining, this is most commonly glucose sodium cotransport, with an ideal stoichiometric ratio of one molecule of glucose to one molecule of sodium. Of note, when juice

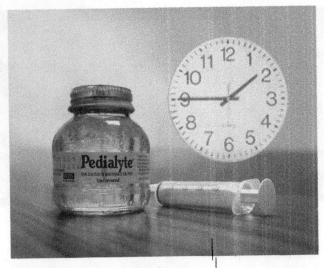

Figure 89.1 Oral rehydration therapy.

is added to oral rehydration solutions to make it "taste better," it alters the glucose-sodium ratio and disturbs the facilitated cotransport mechanism. ORT has been demonstrated to provide rehydration as rapidly as intravenous solutions and with equally good correction of electrolyte and acid-base disturbances.

▶ INDICATIONS

ORT may be used in any conscious infant, child, or adolescent with acute gastroenteritis. It should be considered the initial therapy for children with mild to moderate dehydration and can be used as a temporizing measure for children with severe dehydration. Patients with signs of shock should receive aggressive intravascular fluid replacement in the early stages. The fluid deficit should be replaced in the ED over the first 4 hours. The maintenance phase consists of the remaining time the child is symptomatic from acute gastroenteritis and is being managed with feeding and fluids at home.

Vomiting is not a contraindication to ORT but requires modification of the technique (e.g., decreasing the volume with each syringe feed). Ondansetron, a 5HT-3 receptor antagonist, is an effective antiemetic for children and can be used to facilitate ORT. In fact, one dose of oral ondansetron in the ED is often sufficient to stop the emesis caused by gastroenteritis and allow for successful treatment with ORT. Alternatively, vomiting children or those refusing to drink may receive fluid via a nasogastric tube (see Chapter 84), provided they have intact airway protective reflexes. Absolute contraindications to ORT include the suspicion of an acute surgical abdomen, obtundation, and loss of airway protective reflexes. Relative contraindications include severe dehydration, mental status changes that preclude tolerating oral feeds, and parents unwilling to assist in the process.

▶ EQUIPMENT

Specific equipment used depends on the child's age.

5-mL syringe
10-mL syringe
Clock
Oral rehydration solution: Pedialyte, Rehydralyte, Ricelyte, World Health Organization (WHO) oral rehydration solution (Jianas Brothers Packing Co., Kansas City, MO; Cera Products, Columbia, MD)
Optional: Flexible 5- or 8-Fr Silastic feeding tube and kangaroo pump

Fluids with high concentrations of sugars such as soft drinks, fruit juices, and fruit punch will actually exacerbate diarrhea by an osmotic effect. For purposes of discussion, the terms "physiologically appropriate solution" and "oral rehydration solution" refer to solutions containing no more than 3% glucose, 50 to 90 mEq/L of sodium, and potassium and base to correct losses. Although Pedialyte and Ricelyte are generally referred to as "oral maintenance" solutions, some authorities do not commonly differentiate between the oral maintenance and oral rehydration solutions. For practical purposes in the industrialized world, solutions containing 50 to 90 mEq/L of sodium provide adequate restoration of circulating volume in children with mild to moderate dehydration. Children with severe dehydration (more than 10%) or cholera should be given a true rehydration solution containing a sodium concentration of 70 to 90 mEq/L (Rehydralyte or WHO solution).

The compositions of various solutions commonly used in children with acute gastroenteritis are listed in Table 89.1. Of note, the high osmolality and low sodium content of cola, apple juice, and sports drinks make these products inappropriate for ORT. WHO has recently formulated a second oral rehydration solution that can be used for dehydration due to etiologies other than cholera.

▶ PROCEDURE

An algorithm for management of children with dehydration caused by gastroenteritis is shown in Figure 89.2. ORT works best when the clinician incorporates the child's parents into the process. The specific procedure undertaken will depend on parental and clinician preferences. The overriding principle is that continuous small quantities of oral rehydration solution must be provided. Giving an 8-kg infant 8 oz of fluid ad lib usually results in a messy and discouraging episode of vomiting. Most parents will not be able to restrict a thirsty infant to an ounce every few minutes unless they are given careful and explicit procedural instructions. The goal of ORT is to replace the entire deficit in 4 hours or less.

	Sodium (mEq/L)	Potassium (mEq/L)	Chloride (mEq/L)	Base (mEq/L)	Carbohydrate % (mmol/L)	Osmolarity (mmol/L)	Carb:Na
TABLE 89.1 COMPOSITION OF APPROPRIATE ORAL REHYDRATION SOLUTIONS AND INAPPROPRIATE LIQUIDS							
Appropriate Solutions							
WHO solution (1)	90	20	80	10	2% (111)	311	1:1
WHO solution (2)	75	20	65	10	1.4% (75)	245	1:1
Rehydralyte	75	20	65	30	2.5% (139)	329	2:1
Pedialyte	45	20	35	30	2.5% (139)	269	3:1
Inappropriate Liquids							
Gatorade	20	3	17	3	4.6% (58)	330	12:1
Coca-Cola	2	<1		13	12% (112)	>600	—
Apple juice	3	32	2	0	12.4% (120)	730	230:1
Chicken broth	250	8	250	0	0	500	—

The child's fluid deficit should be calculated from his or her present weight and degree of dehydration (Fig. 89.3) (8). This volume of fluid should be replaced during the ED visit. The total volume of fluid should be divided into 5-minute aliquots. As a general rule, a mildly dehydrated child will require 1 mL/kg and a moderately dehydrated child 2 mL/kg every 5 minutes. Table 89.2 has specific instructions for medical personnel to perform ORT. The child and parent should be placed in a relatively quiet place (although where they can still be observed), and the parent should be instructed to feed the child one aliquot of oral rehydration solution every 5 minutes (Table 89.3). A clock with a second hand should be provided. Ondansetron provided prior to the initiation of ORT will increase the likelihood of success. If the child vomits, the emesis should be collected in a basin for quantification. Physicians, nurses, and parents are equally inaccurate in estimating the volume of emesis after a child vomits. Importantly, the amount of emesis is almost always less than the amount of oral rehydration solution administered. It should be emphasized to all that children almost never really "throw up everything." The child who vomits can be given a 5- to 10-minute rest period, followed by the resumption of

ORT. The volume and timing of the aliquot administration should be adjusted to meet the specific needs of the child and family.

After 15 minutes, the physician should check that an appropriate volume of oral rehydration solution has been consumed. Parents may need frequent encouragement in the first 15 to 30 minutes. Periodically, emesis should be measured and compared with fluid intake. As the patient tolerates, the volume administered in the aliquot can be adjusted. If intake is going well, the volume can be increased. If it is difficult to administer the entire aliquot all at once, it can be administered in a smaller volume more frequently, with a goal of administering the same aliquot volume over a 5-minute period. Most infants and young children will readily absorb the oral rehydration solutions by this mechanism and will meet or exceed the calculated replacement volume in 2 to 4 hours.

The difference between an inability to tolerate ORT and ORT failure should be noted. Inability to tolerate ORT often revolves around compliance issues, either with the parents or the child. For example, the child refuses to drink the solution, the child falls asleep, the parent falls asleep, etc. ORT failure occurs when the ongoing losses exceed the fluid administered. ORT failure is rare, occurring in less than 4% of patients. However, the inability to tolerate ORT is more common, occurring in approximately 20% of patients. General guidelines for an inability to tolerate ORT include administration of only 50% of the hourly requirement, six consecutive oral refusals, or severe emesis.

Toddlers present a special challenge. Generally, their degree of dehydration is less severe than that experienced by infants. An active toddler with diarrhea and vomiting who vigorously refuses to drink oral rehydration solution can be sent home without formal rehydration in the ED in most instances. Such children may be given saltine crackers and half-strength apple juice. Consumption of 10 saltines along with 8 oz (240 mL) of half-strength juice provides approximately 70 mEq/L of sodium and 88 g/L of complex carbohydrates, comparable to oral rehydration solutions. The dilution of the juice is important to reduce the osmotic load presented to the gut. Half-strength sports drinks are another alternative for the child who refuses the preferred oral rehydration solutions.

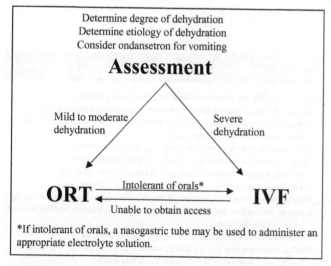

Figure 89.2 Rehydration therapy treatment algorithm.

Step 1. Calculate dehydration score by determining how many of the following clinical features are present (choose A or B).
A. 10-point dehydration score

Ill appearance	Tachycardia (HR >150)
Dry mucous membranes	Sunken eyes
Absent tears	Decreased skin elasticity
Capillary refill >2 sec	Abnormal radial pulse
Decreased urine output (parental report)	Abnormal respirations

B. 4-point dehydration score

Ill appearance
Dry mucous membranes
Absent tears
Capillary refill >2 sec

Step 2. Interpret the dehydration score.

Number of features present		Degree of dehydration	Approximate fluid deficit	Approximate fluid requirement
10-point scale	4-point scale			
0 out of 10	0 out of 4	Not dehydrated		
1–2 out of 10	1 out of 4	Mild dehydration	<5%	<50 mL/kg
3–6 out of 10	2 out of 4	Moderate dehydration	5–10%	50–100 mL/kg
7–10 out of 10	3–4 out of 4	Severe dehydration	>10%	>100 mL/kg

Note: The 4-point Dehydration score is derived from the full 10-point dehydration score and has the same diagnostic accuracy.

Step 3. Calculate the fluid replacement volume (to be administered over a 4-hour time frame).
50 mL/kg for mild dehydration
100 mL/kg for moderate dehydration
Note: Due to the density of water, 1,000 g approximately equals 1,000 mL. Hence, 5% dehydration equals 50 mL/kg.

Step 4. Calculate the amount to be administered every 5 minutes.
The fluid replacement volume divided by 4 divided by 12 determines the 5-minute requirement. The parents should be instructed to administer the volume over a 5-minute period.
Note: A mildly dehydrated child will need about 1 mL/kg every 5 minutes, and a moderately dehydrated child will need about 2 mL/kg every 5 minutes.

Step 5. Reassess patient.
The patient should be reassessed frequently to ensure that he or she is receiving the fluid and showing signs of improvement.

Figure 89.3 Rehydration protocol.

TABLE 89.2	ORT INSTRUCTIONS FOR MEDICAL PERSONNEL

ORT works via the sodium glucose cotransport mechanism.
Utilizing the correct electrolyte solution is critical for its success.
1. Chose appropriate solution:
   ▶ Use maintenance electrolyte solution (e.g., Pedialyte) as first line.
   ▶ May use half-strength sports beverage (e.g., Gatorade) with saltine crackers in older patients.
   Caution: Do not add juice to the oral rehydration solution, as it alters the sodium-to-glucose concentration, which is important for fluid absorption across the gastrointestinal tract.
2. Calculate the total volume to be administered over a 4-hour rehydration phase:
   ▶ Mild dehydration: 50 mL/kg
   ▶ Moderate dehydration: 100 mL/kg
3. Calculate the 5-minute aliquot volume:
   ▶ Total volume ÷ 4 ÷ 12 (4-hour rehydration period and 12 5-minute blocks per hour).
4. Administer each aliquot over the 5-minute period.
5. Increase the volume as tolerated.

TABLE 89.3	ORT INSTRUCTIONS FOR FAMILIES

ORT is a specific treatment technique for dehydrated patients.
A small amount of liquid is administered every few minutes with a syringe.
Although the child may want more, the stomach needs a chance to digest the liquid before the next syringe feed.
If the child has been vomiting, he or she may continue to vomit.
Please try to collect the vomit in a bucket so we can measure it.
If it is only a small amount of vomit, we will continue with ORT.
If it is a large amount of vomit, we may need to stop and place an i.v.
You should watch the clock and every 5 minutes administer liquid using the syringe.
It may be hard at first, but with a few feeds, it gets much easier, and the child will begin to take the feeds.
If your child refuses the feeds, then we may need to place an i.v.
This is a treatment that you are able to continue at home to treat this illness as well as any future cases of dehydration that may occur.

Complex carbohydrates are well tolerated with diarrhea because of their low osmotic contribution (9). As mentioned previously, adding undiluted juice to an oral rehydration solution such as Pedialyte significantly alters the glucose-to-sodium ratio, resulting in too much glucose and a high osmotic load.

Nasogastric feeding is appropriate for the truly dehydrated infant or toddler who refuses ORT, who has painful oral lesions, or who is simply too tired to drink. A soft, flexible feeding tube should be inserted and properly secured (see Chapter 84). A Kangaroo pump can be used to infuse oral rehydration solution at 20 to 30 mL/kg/hr. This technique can also be used as an initial measure for severely dehydrated children while intravenous access is being sought, especially when intraosseous access is felt to be unnecessary or inappropriate. A nasogastric tube should not be used for a child who lacks a gag reflex.

Laboratory evaluation is performed at the discretion of the clinician. ORT is effective for correcting electrolyte abnormalities such as hyponatremia and hypernatremia. In addition, at least a third of moderately dehydrated children under the age of 5 years are also hypoglycemic. With traditional intravenous rehydration, serum glucose must be checked and glucose added to the intravenous fluid if the patient is hypoglycemic. By contrast, ORT provides glucose to the patient as soon as this method of treatment is initiated. Although successful rehydration using ORT is generally based on the disappearance of clinical signs of dehydration, use of laboratory testing in making this determination may be indicated in some instances.

It is important to provide specific home care instructions for children who do not require inpatient hospital admission. Parents must understand that oral rehydration solution alone replaces fluid but does not reduce diarrheal symptoms. Symptomatic improvement will depend in large part on proper feeding practices (2). Appropriate feedings (selected from the entire range of foods normally taken by the child, including large proportions of complex carbohydrates and small quantities of simple sugars) should begin immediately following rehydration. Continuing clear liquids or dilute formulas is not necessary. Avoidance of dairy products and greasy foods will help keep the diarrhea under control, since children may develop a relative lactose deficiency during episodes of gastroenteritis. However, yogurt may be helpful, as it contains lactobacillus acidophilus, a normal bacterial component of the intestine. It is a probiotic, which helps restore the intestinal microbial milieu.

▶ COMPLICATIONS

Complications rarely occur with ORT. Overhydration (2% to 3%) may occur but is of no clinical significance. However, the clinician must be certain that the diagnosis of acute gastroenteritis is correct and that appropriate efforts are made to identify more serious processes that may cause vomiting and diarrhea (e.g., appendicitis). In well-nourished infants, hyper- or hyponatremia is not a risk, provided that appropriate and properly mixed solutions are used. Pre-existing electrolyte disturbances are usually corrected by proper oral therapy (2). A small proportion (approximately 1%) of infants may have acute glucose intolerance, resulting in explosive watery stools within hours of taking oral rehydration solution. These infants must receive intravenous hydration with nothing by mouth until improved. Prevention of complications

---

 SUMMARY

1 Calculate the fluid deficit based on the physical examination.

2 Begin fluid replacement with a physiologically appropriate solution.

3 Use a cup and spoon or a cup and syringe to provide the appropriate replacement volume in 5-minute intervals.

4 Replace the calculated deficit plus ongoing losses over 4 hours.

5 When the child is clinically rehydrated, discharge to home on alternating oral rehydration solution and regular feedings from a variety of high complex carbohydrate, low simple sugar feedings.

6 Be certain to remind parents that:

  a Oral rehydration therapy alone does not reduce stool output.

  b Full feedings will reduce both output and the duration of symptoms.

  c In general, an episode of acute gastroenteritis lasts 5 to 7 days.

  d As long as good hydration is maintained, diarrheal stools alone are not harmful.

7 If the child refuses oral rehydration solutions:

  a Give saltine crackers and half-strength apple juice.

  b Discharge the patient when he or she eats 10 crackers and drinks 8 oz (240 mL) of half-strength juice with instructions as indicated.

  c Consider insertion of a nasogastric feeding tube to administer rehydration.

CLINICAL TIPS

▶ Oral rehydration therapy is less invasive and takes no more time than intravenous rehydration.

▶ Parents should receive specific instructions to give 1 mL/kg of an appropriate oral rehydration solution every 5 minutes for a mildly dehydrated children and 2 mL/kg for moderately dehydrated children.

▶ The child should be checked approximately every 15 to 30 minutes and the volume of fluid consumed compared with the amount of emesis. In most cases, the amount of fluid consumed will greatly exceed the amount of fluid vomited.

related to technique depends on recognition of diminished airway protective reflexes and proper placement of nasogastric tubes if used.

Frequent observation and re-evaluation of patients undergoing ORT will permit prevention or detection of complications. Ongoing intake and output calculations allow the clinician to identify the occasional child who cannot keep up with losses and who requires parenteral therapy.

▶ SUMMARY

ORT is a simple and effective technique for rapid restoration of circulating volume when losses are due to acute gastroenteritis. ORT should be used for mild and moderate dehydration, even in vomiting children, and can be used as a temporizing measure in severely dehydrated children. Careful attention to teaching parents and staff increases the likeli-

hood of success. After rehydration, appropriate feeding should commence.

▶ ACKNOWLEDGMENT

The authors would like to acknowledge the valuable contributions of Julius G. Goepp to the version of this chapter that appeared in the previous edition.

▶ REFERENCES

1. Glass RI, Lew JF, Gangarosa RE, et al. Estimates of morbidity and mortality rates for diarrheal diseases in American children. *J Pediatr.* 1991;118:S27–33.
2. American Academy of Pediatrics, Provisional Committee on Quality Improvement, Subcommittee on Acute Gastroenteritis. Practice Parameter. The management of acute gastroenteritis in young children. *Pediatrics.* 1996;97:424.
3. World Health Organization. *The Treatment of Diarrhoea: A Manual for Physicians and Other Senior Health Workers.* 3rd ed. Geneva: World Health Organization, Division of Diarrhoeal and Acute Respiratory Disease Control; 1995. WHO/CDD/SER/80.2.
4. Centers for Disease Control and Prevention. Managing acute gastroenteritis among children: oral rehydration, maintenance, and nutritional therapy. *MMWR Recomm Rep.* 2003;52 (No. RR-16):1–20.
5. Spandorfer PR, Alessandrini EA, Joffe M, et al. Oral vs. intravenous rehydration of moderately dehydrated children: a randomized controlled trial. *Pediatrics.* 2005;115:295–301.
6. Hirschhorn N. The treatment of acute diarrhea in children: an historical and physiological perspective. *Am J Clin Nutr.* 1980;33:637–663.
7. Hirschhorn N, Greenough WB. Progress in oral rehydration therapy. *Sci Am.* 1991;264(5):50–56.
8. Gorelick MH, Shaw KN, Murphy KO. Validity and reliability of clinical signs in the diagnosis of dehydration in children. *Pediatrics.* 1997;99:1. Available at: http://www.pediatrics.org/cgi/content/full99/5/e6.
9. Khin-Maung-U, Greenough WB III. Cereal-based oral rehydration therapy, I: clinical studies. *J Pediatr.* 1991;118:S72–79.

Reducing a Rectal Prolapse

▶ INTRODUCTION

Rectal prolapse, a relatively uncommon clinical entity, is the prolapse of the rectal mucosa through the anus. In some instances, the rectal mucosa must be manually reduced if spontaneous reduction does not occur. Reduction can be easily performed by the pediatrician, emergency physician, or parent after adequate instruction. Although the procedure itself is not difficult, the presence of rectal prolapse in a young child should prompt the clinician to consider underlying causes for the condition.

▶ ANATOMY AND PHYSIOLOGY

Rectal prolapse begins with an internal prolapse of the upper rectum into the lower rectum. Further extension of the upper rectal mucosa through the anus creates a partial prolapse, the most common form seen in children. Continuation of this process results in a complete rectal prolapse (Fig. 90.1). Anatomic predisposing factors that may explain the predilection for rectal prolapse in certain children include vertical course of the rectum, flat sacrum and coccyx, and a lack of levator ani support (1).

Conditions that cause increased intra-abdominal pressure, hardening of the stool, or muscle weakness are also commonly associated with rectal prolapse (Table 90.1). Children under 3 years of age seem most susceptible to rectal prolapse, with the highest incidence found in children less than 1 year of age. The elderly comprise another high-risk group predisposed to rectal prolapse (2–4). Malnutrition most commonly causes rectal prolapse in underdeveloped countries, whereas in the United States most patients with rectal prolapse have stool abnormalities such as chronic constipation or diarrhea (1,2). Cystic fibrosis is the most serious of the potential etiologies

for rectal prolapse in an otherwise well patient. Patients with cystic fibrosis have an 18% overall incidence of rectal prolapse (5). For this reason, children with noninfectious diarrhea and no other etiology for rectal prolapse or with recurrent idiopathic prolapse should be considered for a sweat chloride determination or other diagnostic tests for cystic fibrosis.

▶ INDICATIONS

Children with rectal prolapse appear well. Rectal prolapse may even come to attention as an incidental finding by a clinician who notices a mass protruding from the anus. Often spontaneous reduction will occur before the patient is examined by medical personnel, and the clinician's examination may only reveal laxity of rectal tone. In such cases, a presumptive diagnosis of rectal prolapse is made based on the description of the finding by the parents.

Any patient with a visible rectal prolapse should have it reduced. Before reduction, other conditions that can mimic rectal prolapse, such as rectal hemorrhoids, a prolapsed rectal polyp, and an ileocecal intussusception protruding through the anus, should be considered. Of these, intussusception requires emergent diagnosis and treatment. Differentiating features of intussusception include (a) a history of intermittent episodes of abdominal pain and crying, (b) ill appearance and in some cases obtundation (a later finding), and (c) the ability to pass a finger between the prolapsed bowel and the anal sphincter. Hemorrhoids and rectal polyps should be easily identified because they do not involve the entire rectal mucosa.

Before reduction, sedation may be given, depending on the size of the rectal prolapse and the discomfort of the patient (see Chapter 33). Many small prolapses can be reduced with local comfort measures only. Patients who have undergone

859

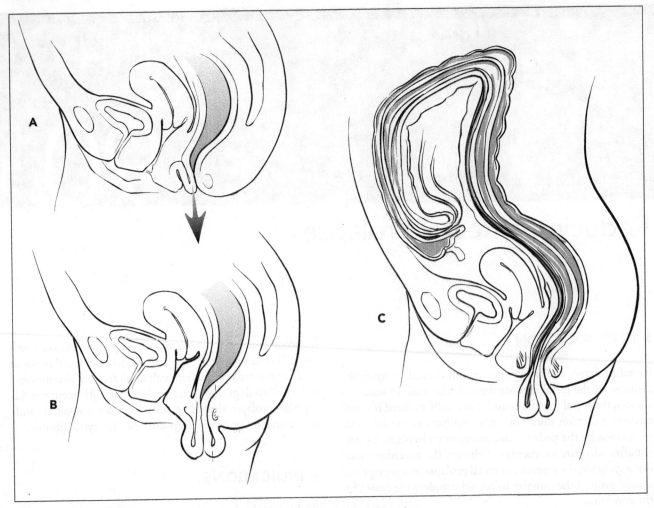

Figure 90.1 Anatomy of a rectal prolapse.
A. Partial prolapse.
B. Complete prolapse.
C. Prolapsed intussusception.

an unsuccessful attempt at reduction should receive sedation before renewed efforts.

▶ EQUIPMENT

Gloves
Lubricant
Gauze
Tape
Sedation (as needed)

TABLE 90.1	CAUSES OF RECTAL PROLAPSE

Constipation
Diarrhea
Cystic fibrosis
Malnutrition
Excessive straining
Meningomyelocele
Idiopathic causes

▶ PROCEDURE

As mentioned, this procedure may require sedation for the child who is crying or fighting, as this will increase intra-abdominal pressure and make reduction more difficult. The child is placed prone in the knee-chest position on the parent's lap or on the examination table. With gloved hands, the clinician should place gentle but firm pressure on the prolapsed mucosa (Fig. 90.2). A finger may be placed in the rectum to guide reversal of the prolapse. If the prolapsed mucosa has been out for a prolonged period of time, swelling may require manual compression of the prolapse before successful reduction. After reduction, a pressure dressing may be used between bowel movements. Parents must be warned that this reduction may be temporary and that rectal prolapse may recur for several months. As the child grows, the condition should resolve. Unlike inguinal hernias, rectal prolapses rarely become incarcerated in children. However, emergent surgical consultation is indicated if the prolapse cannot be reduced.

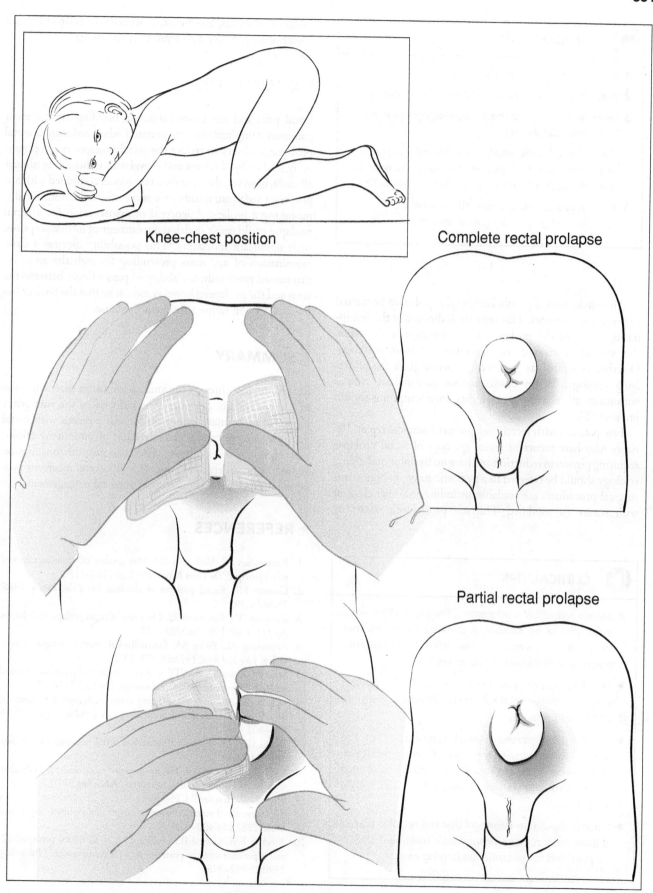

Knee-chest position

Complete rectal prolapse

Partial rectal prolapse

Figure 90.2 Rectal prolapse reduction.

SUMMARY

1 Sedate the child as needed.

2 Position the child prone in the knee-chest position.

3 Generously lubricate the prolapsed mucosa with water-soluble lubricant.

4 With gloved hands, apply circumferential pressure on the prolapsed mucosa while guiding the rectum internally with a finger placed in the central orifice.

5 Apply a pressure dressing with Vaseline-impregnated gauze, dry gauze, and tape.

After reduction, a prophylactic regimen should be started to prevent recurrences. This regimen is directed at the precipitating cause of the prolapse. If constipation is the cause, this should be treated with laxatives and stool softeners. Diarrhea is treated as indicated, depending on the underlying etiology. When cystic fibrosis patients are treated with pancreatic enzyme supplements, their symptoms should improve (5).

Few patients with rectal prolapse need surgical repair. Patients who have recurrent severe episodes of rectal prolapse requiring physician reduction and have no treatable underlying etiology should be referred to a pediatric surgeon. Numerous surgical procedures are available, including anal encirclement with suture (a modified Thiersch procedure), sclerosing

CLINICAL TIPS

▶ Before reduction is attempted, the protruding rectal mass should be carefully examined to ensure that the patient does not have hemorrhoids, a prolapsed polyp, or a prolapsed intussusception.

▶ The diagnosis of cystic fibrosis should be considered in an otherwise well child with noninfectious diarrhea and rectal prolapse.

▶ Sedation and careful manual compression of the mucosa to decrease edema may help when reduction of the rectal prolapse is difficult. Inability to reduce a rectal prolapse warrants emergent evaluation by a surgeon.

▶ Parents should be informed that the rectal prolapse is likely to recur, and prophylactic treatment should be provided for potential underlying causes.

solution injections, linear cauterization of the anorectum, and posterior suspension with levator repair (6–10).

▶ COMPLICATIONS

Local pain and self-limited mucosal bleeding are the most common complications encountered when reducing a rectal prolapse. Inability to reduce the rectal prolapse could potentially lead to local edema and bowel wall ischemia. In almost all cases, however, the described technique, combined with appropriate sedation, results in a successful reduction. Finally, mistaking a prolapsed ileocecal intussusception for a rectal prolapse could result in delayed treatment of intussusception, with significant morbidity. This possibility dictates a close examination of any mass protruding through the anus. As mentioned previously, the ability to pass a finger between the anus and the prolapsed bowel is indicative that the patient has intussusception rather than rectal prolapse.

▶ SUMMARY

Rectal prolapse through the anus, a condition most common in young children, can usually be reduced by the emergency physician or primary care provider. All patients with rectal prolapse deserve careful consideration of underlying etiologies, especially cystic fibrosis. Pediatric surgical consultation should be considered for patients with severe, recurrent prolapse unresponsive to conservative medical management.

▶ REFERENCES

1. Ramanujam PS, Venkatesh KS. Management of acute incarcerated rectal prolapse. *Dis Colon Rectum.* 1992;35:1154–1156.
2. Corman ML. Rectal prolapse in children. *Dis Colon Rectum.* 1985;28:535–539.
3. Zempsky WT, Rosenstein BJ. The cause of rectal prolapse in children. *Am J Dis Child.* 1988:142:338–339.
4. Armstrong AL, Bivins BA, Sachatello CR. Rectal prolapse: a brief review. *J Ky Med Assoc.* 1978;76:329–332.
5. Stern RC, Izant RJ, Boat TF, et al. Treatment and prognosis of rectal prolapse in cystic fibrosis. *Gastroenterology.* 1982;82:707–710.
6. Krasna IR. A simple purse string suture technique for treatment of colostomy prolapse and intussusception. *J Pediatr Surg.* 1979;14:801–802.
7. Wyllie GG. The injection treatment of rectal prolapse. *J Pediatr Surg.* 1979;14:62–64.
8. Kay NRM, Zachary RB. The treatment of rectal prolapse in children with injections of 30% saline solutions. *J Pediatr Surg.* 1970;5:334–337.
9. Hight DW, Hertzler JH, Philippart AI, et al. Linear cauterization for the treatment of rectal prolapse in infants and children. *Surg Gynecol Obstet.* 1982;154:400–402.
10. Ashcraft KW, Garred JL, Holder TM, et al. Rectal prolapse: 17-year experience with the posterior repair and suspension. *J Pediatr Surg.* 1990;25:992–995.

CINDY W. CHRISTIAN AND JOANNE M. DECKER

91

Prepubertal Genital Examination

▶ INTRODUCTION

Examination of the prepubertal genitalia should be part of a complete physical examination during well-child care visits. Although the performance of this examination is not routine in an acute care setting, under certain circumstances it is essential. The purpose is either to ensure normal anatomy during routine checkups or to evaluate for pathology in children who present with complaints specific to the genital area. The examination is generally done by physicians or specially trained nurses in a variety of outpatient and inpatient settings. Until recently, the physician has paid little attention to normal and abnormal prepubertal genital anatomy, particularly in girls. Although the technique of examining young patients is relatively simple, the interpretation of findings can be difficult. This chapter discusses the approach to performing a proper genital examination in the prepubertal child, basic genital anatomy, and common abnormalities and problems encountered. Specific indications for performing the examination also are discussed. If, by history or examination, sexual abuse is suspected, Chapter 94 may be used as a reference for the proper method of collecting forensic evidence. Examination of the genitalia in the adolescent patient is reviewed in Chapter 93.

Dr. Joanne M. Decker passed away in 2007 after a long battle with cancer.

▶ ANATOMY AND PHYSIOLOGY

Genital anatomy and physiology are largely influenced by hormonal changes throughout childhood, so individual patients have significant variation in the appearance of the genitalia, depending on age.

The normal full-term infant male should have a clearly identifiable penis with an average length of 3 to 4 cm. Any newborn boy with a penis measuring less than 2.5 cm should be referred to an endocrinologist (I). The examining physician should note if the urethral opening is in the normal position at the apex of the glans or displaced ventrally (hypospadias) or dorsally (epispadias). Infants with either of these abnormalities require urologic evaluation. In the uncircumcised newborn boy, the foreskin is rarely retractable and should not be forced. The scrotum should be fused. A bifid (partitioned) scrotum is abnormal and requires evaluation for ambiguous genitalia. Hydroceles are common in the newborn period and, in isolation, require only follow-up examinations. The testicles should be palpable in the scrotum or easily located in the distal inguinal canal. The child with a true undescended testicle should be referred to a surgeon.

Occasionally, a prepubertal boy can present with a painful, swollen penis. In the absence of a known trauma, this swelling may be due to inflammation of the glans (balanitis) or the foreskin and the glans (balanoposthitis). The inflammation will usually resolve if treated with warm soaks and an oral antibiotic such as cephalexin. In uncircumcised boys, a painful swollen penis could be caused by an unretractable foreskin (phimosis) or a foreskin that is retracted over the glans and now cannot be reduced to the normal position (paraphimosis). Procedures for paraphimosis reduction are described in Chapter 98. The clinician should remember, however, that it is normal to be unable to retract the foreskin back from the normal position in an uncircumcised boy until he is about 3 years of age. Essentially no other changes are apparent in the male external genitalia until the onset of puberty. The first genital change to occur is the enlargement of testicular diameter to greater than 2.5 cm. The average age of onset of testicular enlargement is 11.6 years, with a standard deviation of approximately 1 year (2). A boy younger than age 9 with testicular enlargement should be referred to an endocrinologist for evaluation of precocious puberty.

In a newborn girl, it is important to identify all normal genital structures (Fig. 91.1). In term infants, maternal estrogen causes the labia majora to appear well developed and plump. The labia generally cover the rest of the genitalia and must be separated to visualize the other structures. In preterm

infants, the labia majora are thinner and separated, and may actually make the clitoral prepuce appear unusually prominent. The labia majora should never be fused posteriorly nor demonstrate rugae. Either finding would indicate ambiguous genitalia. The clitoris is located ventrally at the anterior fusion of the labia minora. If any prepubertal girl is found to have a clitoris that measures greater than 3 mm in length and 2 mm in width, she should be referred to an endocrinologist for clitoromegaly. In the supine position, the urethral meatus should be located just inferior to the clitoris, between the labia minora. The vaginal orifice is located inferior to and separate from the urethra. The hymenal membrane should be seen surrounding the entrance to the vagina, partially obscuring visualization of the vagina. It is present in all girls with otherwise normally formed genitalia. Effects of maternal estrogen on the newborn hymen cause it to appear thickened and opaque. The newborn girl may have some white or blood-tinged vaginal discharge (also secondary to maternal hormone effect), which should resolve by 2 weeks of age. Finally, the inguinal areas should contain no palpable gonads or hernias.

In the prepubertal girl, the physician should pay more attention to the anatomy of the vulva. The appearance of the

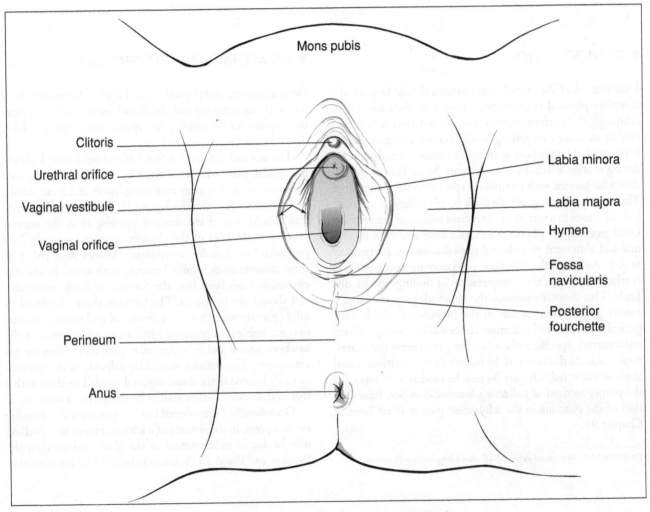

Figure 91.1 Anatomy of the female external genitalia.

vulva changes dramatically in the first years of life, as maternal estrogen effects wane. In the prepubertal girl, the vulvar mucosa may appear quite erythematous due to the normal appearance of the vasculature in the relatively thin tissue. The labia majora are less prominent than in an adolescent or an adult, exposing the vulvar structures to some extent, which leaves these structures more vulnerable to injury from straddle-type falls. Likewise, the labia minora in the prepubertal child are thin. They meet posteriorly to form the posterior fourchette, which may exhibit some friability in young girls. This friability does not necessarily indicate pathology. Occasionally the epithelium of the labia minora is fused as a result of nonspecific irritation. Fused labia minora may impede visualization of the hymen and vagina. In most cases, this is functionally insignificant and will eventually lyse with estrogen at puberty. Some children are symptomatic, however, with urinary dribbling and secondary vulvovaginitis. These children require a short course (no more than 2 weeks) of topical estrogen, followed by a nightly application of petrolatum. Manual lysis of the adhesions is not recommended as an initial therapy.

Some experts have devoted much attention in recent years to the hymenal anatomy in prepubertal children. Great variation exists in the appearance of the hymenal tissue and configuration of the hymenal orifice in young girls. Generally, the hymen is thin and may be translucent, with a lacy vascular pattern. In other children, a normal hymen may appear redundant and more opaque. Hymenal types are generally classified by both shape of the tissue and appearance of the opening (Fig. 91.2). Findings are described based on their location in relation to a clock face, with 12 o'clock at the ventral position. A crescentic hymen is probably the most common. The tissue is U shaped and appears slung between the 11 o'clock and 1 o'clock positions. Annular hymens are ring shaped, with a central orifice. A septate hymen is identified by a midline septum of tissue that creates two hymenal openings. The examiner should ensure that the septum is isolated to the hymen and does not continue internally. This can be done visually and/or with a small curved probe placed to encircle the septum if possible. A cribriform hymen contains multiple small openings and is an unusual variation. Microperforate hymens contain one small opening, which can be found anywhere on the hymenal surface. Unlike any of the discussed configurations, an imperforate hymen is abnormal and requires surgical correction.

The genitalia of prepubertal girls are susceptible to vulvovaginal irritation for several reasons. The prepubertal vagina lacks labial fat pads and pubic hair, which in the adolescent and adult serve to protect the vulva and vagina. The pH of the prepubertal vagina is neutral, providing a favorable milieu for bacterial overgrowth. Finally, prepubertal girls may not be meticulous about their hygiene, predisposing to fecal contamination of the vulvar and urethral areas. Unlike adolescent or adult patients, in whom a specific microbiologic cause of vulvovaginitis is usually identified, the majority of symptomatic prepubertal girls have nonspecific vulvovaginitis.

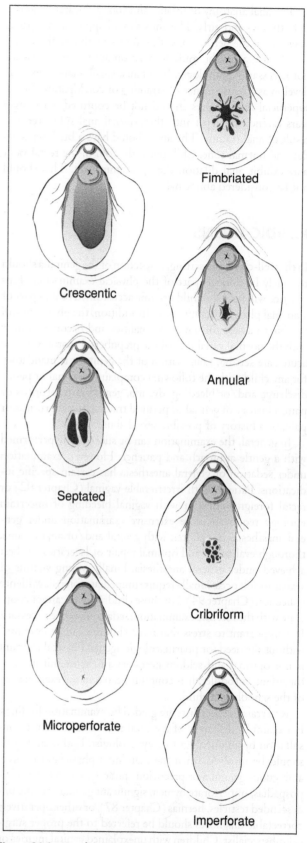

Crescentic

Fimbriated

Annular

Septated

Cribriform

Microperforate

Imperforate

Figure 91.2 Normal variants in hymenal structure.

The anal anatomy of infants and young children is similar in both boys and girls. The anus should appear as a separate opening on the perineum, with symmetric, thin radiating rugae. Anal tags in the midline position are common and are not necessarily pathologic. In infants, small anal fissures can develop as a consequence of straining or constipation. Small, superficial anal fissures should not be confused with larger tears extending deeper into the external anal sphincter as a result of anal trauma. The anus should have a brisk wink reflex and normal tone. Children with stool in the rectal vault may exhibit anal dilation during examination. This should not be considered abnormal.

▶ INDICATIONS

In the well-child care setting, inspection of the genitalia should routinely be done as part of the physical examination. This practice will help the child become accustomed to it as part of a normal physical examination. In addition, the physician will be able to assess for any abnormalities and become familiar with the normal variability of the prepubertal anatomy. In the acute care setting, examination of the genitalia is mandatory for any child with the following complaints: vaginal or penile discharge and/or bleeding, dysuria, genital rash, pruritus or pain, a history of genital or perineal trauma, rectal pruritus or pain, or a history of possible sexual abuse.

In general, the examination can be successfully performed with a gentle approach and patience. However, examination under sedation or general anesthesia has certain specific indications. Patients with irretrievable vaginal (Chapter 92) or rectal foreign bodies or with vaginal bleeding of uncertain etiology require a more extensive examination under general anesthesia. In children with genital and/or anal trauma, thorough evaluation and optimal repair of lacerations is best achieved under general anesthesia. Finally, young victims of sexual assault occasionally require immediate forensic evidence collection (Chapter 94). For those children who cannot cooperate with the forensic examination, sedation may be necessary. It is important to stress that most children can be examined without the need for pharmacologic agents. Physical restraint is not optimal and seldom necessary in the examination of the infant or toddler. It is contraindicated in the examination of the school-aged child.

Referrals to specialists are guided by examination findings. For example, discovery of a genital mass would require consultation by an oncologist or gynecologist. Endocrinologists should be involved when the examining physician discovers ambiguous genitalia or precocious puberty. Patients with hypospadias, imperforate hymen, significant genital trauma, undescended testicles, hernias (Chapter 87), or other operatively correctable diagnoses should be referred to the proper surgical subspecialist. Children with unexplained genital injuries or sexually transmitted diseases should be referred not only to a child protective service and the police but also, if possible, to a physician with expertise in the evaluation and follow-up of sexually abused children.

▶ EQUIPMENT

Examining gloves
Patient gown
Light source (e.g., goose-neck lamp)
Colposcope or otoscope
Several calcium alginate swabs (Calgiswabs) if cultures are indicated
Standard size culture swab
Sterile nonbacteriostatic saline
Microscopic slides
Culture and/or transport media for gonorrhea and chlamydia
Viscous lidocaine (optional)

▶ PROCEDURE

The patient should be informed before starting that a full physical examination, including an evaluation of the genitalia, will be done. To ensure that the child understands the precise nature of the examination, it is wise to use terms for anatomic parts with which the child is familiar. Parents of young children can relate the names for genitalia used in their household. The child may be given the choice of having the parent present during the examination. Most young children want a parent in the examining room during the evaluation, whereas older children often opt to be alone. If a parent is not going to be in the room, another member of the health care team should be present to chaperone during the procedure. After the examination is explained, the child should disrobe without the physician present. Examining gowns are typically used, except for very young patients, who either do not know the difference or want to be able to see everything that is happening. Before starting the examination, the physician should be sure all necessary equipment is easily accessible.

Genital examination of the young child should be preceded by a general physical examination to evaluate for evidence of systemic illness, which also allows the child to become familiar with the examiner and places the genital examination in a medical context. For children who are uncooperative, examination can be limited to the heart, lungs, and abdomen. The abdomen is auscultated and palpated for organomegaly, masses, and tenderness. The clinician should feel for inguinal adenopathy, which may indicate infection. Genital examination begins with assessment of Tanner staging of pubic hair for all patients, the breasts in girls, and penile and testicular size in boys.

Boys

Examination of the penis and scrotum is straightforward. With the patient in the supine position, the clinician should lift the penis off the scrotum. The penis should be evaluated for any abnormalities, including skin lesions such as warts, vesicles, and chancres. In an uncircumcised boy, the foreskin area should be examined for inflammation (balanoposthitis) or other abnormalities. In a boy under age 3 years, the

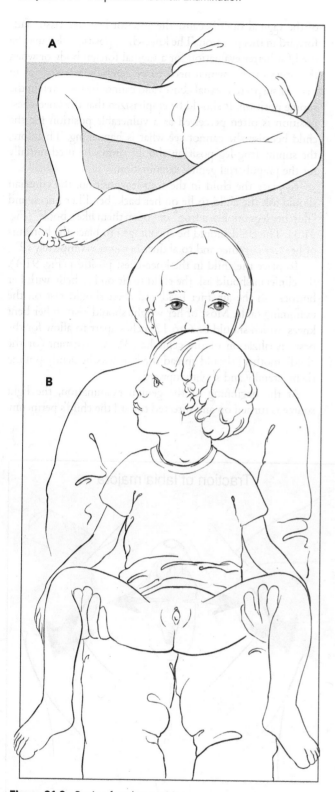

Figure 91.3 Supine frog-leg position.

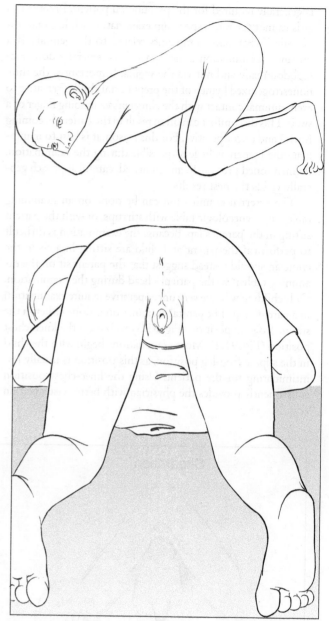

Figure 91.4 Knee-chest position.

foreskin may not yet be retractable and should not be forcibly retracted. An erection of the penis during the examination is not uncommon. If it occurs, it may be ignored or explained as a normal body response during a genital examination.

The scrotum is evaluated for any swelling, skin lesions, or bruising. Testicles should be palpable in the scrotum or in the inguinal canal. If a testicle is not obviously apparent, the clinician should press the index finger of one hand over the center of the ipsilateral inguinal canal, which should prevent the testicle from retracting proximally into the canal. The thumb and index finger of the opposite hand should palpate for the testicle beginning at the inguinal area and working gently down the canal to the scrotum. If the testicle is still not found, the patient should be examined in a standing position or sitting with his legs crossed. This technique uses gravity to assist in bringing down a retractile testicle. Inability to locate a testicle using any of these methods should prompt a referral to a urologist for presumed undescended testicle.

Girls

In contrast to the three stages of the adolescent pelvic examination (Chapter 93), a careful external examination is all that is generally required for the prepubertal patient. Prepubertal girls cannot tolerate a speculum examination while awake, especially if they have complaints related to the genitals. If a bimanual examination is necessary, it is generally done rectoabdominally and not via the vagina. Importantly, the thin, nonestrogenized hymen of the prepubertal child is sensitive to even minimal contact with the clinician's examining finger or a swab. This discomfort can often result in the patient becoming fearful and uncooperative. For this reason, it is best to manipulate the hymen as little as possible during the examination. As mentioned previously, an unhurried, careful approach generally yields the best results.

The external examination can be done on an examining table, on a gynecologic table with stirrups, or with the patient sitting in the parent's lap. Because the examination is difficult to perform if the parent and child are sitting in a chair, the clinician should instead suggest that the parent sit on the examining table near the patient's head during the examination. Only children who are very uncooperative require examination in a parent's lap. The genital examination is done either in the supine frog-leg position (Fig. 91.3) and/or in the knee-chest position (Fig. 91.4). Most examinations begin with the child in the supine frog-leg position, as this position is usually less intimidating for the patient. Using the knee-chest position subsequently provides the physician with better visualization

of the vaginal vault because the anterior hymenal tissue falls forward in this position. The knee-chest position also may be used for better evaluation for a vaginal foreign body or when the edges of the hymen need to be carefully assessed (as in cases of suspected sexual abuse) and cannot be seen well in the supine position. It should be emphasized that the knee-chest position is often perceived as a vulnerable position for the child because she cannot see what is happening. Therefore, the supine frog-leg position should always be used initially for the prepubertal genital examination.

To place the child in the frog-leg position, the clinician should ask the child to lie on her back, bend her knees, and "flop her legs out like a frog" or "open them like a book" (Fig. 91.3). The child should be encouraged to place the bottoms of her feet together and to abduct her knees completely (2).

To place the child in the knee-chest position (Fig. 91.4), the clinician should ask the child to lie on her belly with her buttocks in the air. Her head and chest should rest on the examining table. Most of her weight should rest on her bent knees, which should be 6 to 12 inches apart to allow for the best visualization of the genitalia (3). An assistant (or the child's mother) should spread the buttocks by gently pulling them laterally and slightly upward.

At the beginning of the genital examination, the light source is turned on and directed toward the child's perineum.

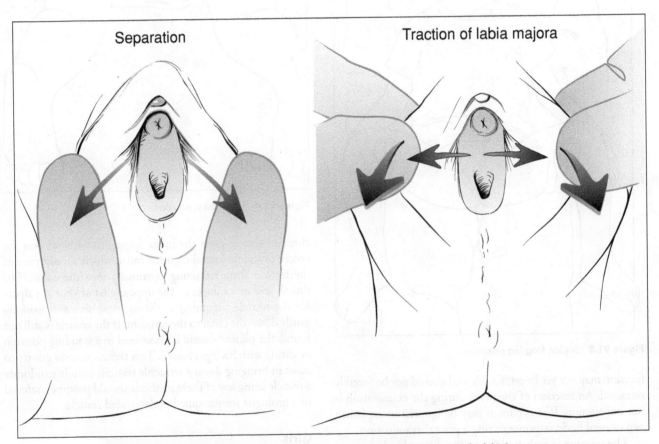

Figure 91.5 Techniques for inspection of the vulva. *Left:* labial separation. *Right:* labial traction—the labia majora are grasped between the thumbs and index fingers and gently pulled laterally, downward, and outward.

Talking casually to her throughout the examination often relaxes the patient and facilitates the evaluation. The child should be told when she will feel the gloved hand of the clinician on her thighs or genital areas. The labia majora, perineum, and buttocks should be inspected for discharge, rashes, warts, vesicles, and other abnormalities. The vulva is visualized using either the separation or the traction method (Fig. 91.5). The labial traction method is generally preferred. The separation method involves placing the thumbs or index fingers on the labia majora and displacing them laterally. In the labial traction method, the lower portions of the labia majora are held between the clinician's thumbs and index fingers, and the labia are pulled laterally, downward, and outward. This procedure should not hurt the patient and generally allows for better visualization of the vulvar structures than simply separating the labia.

The vulvar structures are examined for clitoromegaly, warts, vesicles, discharge, or signs of trauma. The clinician should identify the labia minora, the urethral meatus, and the hymen. The hymen should be assessed for patency and the configuration noted (Fig. 91.2). Some young girls have redundant hymenal tissue, which makes visualization of the vaginal orifice difficult. For these children, the knee-chest position may be preferable. Alternatively, a small moistened Calgiswab can be used to carefully manipulate the hymen and locate the opening. The Calgiswab may be bent to encircle a septate hymen and ensure that the septum does not extend internally. The clinician must remember, however, that the hymen is sensitive and that manipulation usually causes discomfort. If the hymenal tissue must be manipulated, the clinician can apply a small amount of viscous lidocaine. The posterior fourchette and perineum are then examined for any abnormalities.

Patients with a history of sexual abuse or with vaginal discharge identified during the examination may require laboratory or forensic evaluation (Chapter 94). Most sexually transmitted diseases in prepubertal girls cause vaginitis and not upper tract disease. Specimens for culture, therefore, can be obtained from the vaginal vault rather than the cervix. For children with copious discharge, a swab of the discharge handled correctly will usually lead to identification of the pathogen. For children with minimal discharge, intravaginal swabs are necessary. Calgiswabs are the appropriate swabs for obtaining vaginal cultures in a young girl. The swab should be premoistened with nonbacteriostatic saline. Labial traction should be performed with the nondominant, gloved hand. The clinician should pause for a few seconds to allow the child to relax. As the child relaxes, the hymenal orifice will enlarge, allowing for painless insertion of the swab past the hymenal tissue. The swab is inserted approximately 2 to 3 cm and kept there for 10 to 15 seconds (or less if the patient cannot tolerate the procedure) to absorb secretions. Gonorrhea, chlamydia, and general vaginal cultures are prepared in accordance with laboratory protocol. Rapid immunofluorescent tests for chlamydia are contraindicated in the evaluation of the prepubertal child with vaginitis due to high false-positive rates. Wet mounted and potassium hydroxide (KOH) preparations are prepared in the standard manner. Any vesicles noted should

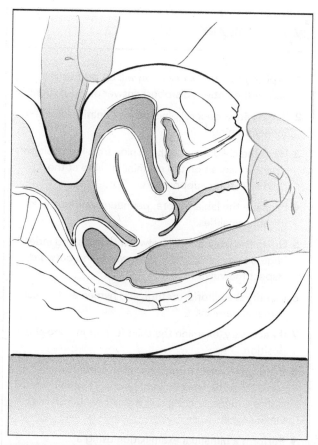

Figure 91.6 Rectoabdominal bimanual examination allows palpation of the uterus and adnexal areas in the prepubertal child.

be unroofed and swabbed for herpes culture using a swab premoistened with special transport medium (see Chapter 122). Nucleic acid amplification tests are not yet approved for use in prepubertal children and cannot replace culture at this time.

 CLINICAL TIPS

▶ An unhurried and sensitive approach will save time and make the examination more pleasant for both the clinician and the patient.

▶ Talking to the child during the examination helps the patient relax.

▶ Having a third person in the room can provide support to the patient and can protect the clinician from allegations of impropriety.

▶ Labial traction, accomplished by gently pulling the labia majora laterally, downward, and outward (Fig. 94.5), allows for better visualization.

▶ Pausing before inserting a swab lets the hymenal orifice enlarge to allow passage of the swab without touching the hymen.

SUMMARY

1 Explain how the examination will be performed before the patient disrobes; answer any questions.

2 Begin with a general physical examination and Tanner staging.

3 Have the child assume the supine frog-leg position; a parent may sit on the examining table at the child's head for support.

4 Examine the labia majora, perineum, and buttocks for abnormalities.

5 Grasp the labia majora between thumbs and index fingers and pull laterally, downward, and outward; inspect the vulva.

6 Identify the clitoris, urethra, and hymen and assess hymenal patency.

7 If necessary, examine the child further in knee-chest position.

8 If indicated, obtain specimens for culture by separating the labia majora, pausing so the hymenal orifice widens, and passing a small swab into the vaginal vault.

9 Perform a bimanual examination using a rectoabdominal approach to locate the uterus and assess for any abnormal masses, if indicated.

10 Allow the patient to dress privately and then discuss the findings of the examination and any necessary follow-up.

The bimanual examination of the prepubertal child is done with a finger in the rectum as opposed to the vagina (Fig. 91.6). Lubrication of the gloved finger is essential. The smallest finger possible should be used for the rectal examination in an infant. Gentle pressure on the abdomen and palpation with the finger that is inserted in the rectum is usually sufficient to locate the uterus. The adnexa are generally not palpable in the prepubertal child, and the detection of any mass in these areas should be further investigated.

Once the examination is complete, the patient should be allowed to dress in privacy. After the patient is clothed, examination findings are reviewed with the patient (as appropriate) and the parent, and any necessary follow-up is discussed.

▶ COMPLICATIONS

The most significant complication that can occur is psychological trauma to a child who is forcibly restrained during the examination. As previously discussed, most children will cooperate with the examination if the clinician provides a careful explanation and uses a calm, unhurried approach. If the clinician is still unable to gain cooperation, the examination should be stopped. At this point, either sedation should be considered or the examination should be deferred.

▶ SUMMARY

Genital examination of the prepubertal child should be part of routine well-child care. For girls, this allows the physician to appreciate the range of normal hymenal variation and assess for abnormalities. Indications for performing a genitoanal examination in other settings are based on complaints or symptoms related to the genitalia. The examining physician must be familiar with prepubertal anatomy. The examination should be brief and painless, allowing the child the opportunity to watch (if desired) and ask questions. Specimens for culture or forensic evaluation can be obtained in a painless manner to preserve the cooperation of the child. Any abnormalities or uncertain findings should be referred to the proper subspecialist.

▶ REFERENCES

1. Hoekelman R. The physical examination of infants and children. In: Bickley LS, Hockelman RA, Bates B, ed. *A Guide to Physical Examination and History Taking.* Philadelphia: JB Lippincott Co.; 1999:621–704.

2. Giardino AP, Finkel MA, Giardino ER, et al. *A Practical Guide to the Evaluation of Sexual Abuse in the Prepubertal Child.* Newbury Park, CA: Sage Publications; 1992.

3. Emans SJ, Laufer MR, Goldstein DP. *Pediatric and Adolescent Gynecology.* 5th ed. Philadelphia: Lippincott Williams & Wilkins; 2005.

ANGELO P. GIARDINO AND CINDY W. CHRISTIAN

92

Vaginal Foreign Body Removal

▶ INTRODUCTION

Vaginal foreign bodies in the prepubertal child frequently lead to vaginitis, vulvovaginitis, nonspecific genitourinary symptoms, and friability of the vaginal tissues with or without frank vaginal bleeding (1–3). Patients with vaginal foreign bodies commonly are symptomatic and present with either bright red vaginal bleeding or purulent, foul-smelling, sometimes bloody vaginal discharge (4,5). Asymptomatic foreign bodies have also been described. Once diagnosed, the object must be removed from the vagina to avoid a progression of genitourinary symptoms and superinfection of the vaginal area. Serious complications may occur as sequelae of long-standing vaginal foreign bodies, including traumatic lesions to the vagina, bladder, rectum, and urethra as well as fistula formation (6–8).

Early reports described a "veritable museum of curiosities" removed from the vagina, including batteries, beads, bits of toys, folded paper, cherries, cotton, corks, crayons, hairpins, insects, marbles, marker tips, nuts, paper clips, pencil erasers, pins, plum pits, safety pins, sand, shells, splinters of wood, stones, tampons, toilet tissue, and twigs (1,2,4,9,10). The most common material recovered is toilet tissue, which may be fecally contaminated (2,5,9). Owing to natural curiosity, body exploration, and hygienic habits, toddlers and school-age girls are the most likely to present with vaginal foreign bodies.

In the prepubertal child, irrigation of the vagina with normal saline or sterile water may be sufficient to dislodge the foreign body. If unsuccessful, removal under general anesthesia may be required. For use in the adult patient, forceps, vacuum suction, and other gynecologic and/or obstetrical instruments have been advocated (6,10–12). These are unlikely to be tolerated in the prepubertal child and are generally not appropriate for this age group. Occasionally, a moistened cotton swab can be used to retrieve toilet tissue visible in the vaginal vault. Examination for a foreign body should be done in accordance with the techniques described in Chapter 91. The knee-chest position allows for good visualization into the vaginal vault and may be helpful for cases of a possible foreign body. If a foreign body is suspected, saline irrigation should be performed by the examining physician or nurse practitioner. This procedure can be easily accomplished with equipment generally available in the ambulatory setting, including clinics, emergency departments, and primary care offices. It is a simple procedure whose success depends primarily on the cooperation of the child and the patience of the provider.

▶ ANATOMY AND PHYSIOLOGY

A full discussion of the anatomy and physiology of the prepubertal genitalia is included in Chapter 91. The foreign body, frequently fecally contaminated toilet tissue, causes an inflammatory reaction that leads to vaginitis with vaginal wall irritation, friability, vaginal bleeding, and/or discharge. Symptoms generally resolve promptly after removal.

Just as the hymen is not an obstacle to inserting foreign material, it also is not an obstacle to removing soft or solid foreign bodies in the vagina. The clinician frequently may encounter variations in hymenal configuration but should not change the basic approach to foreign body removal. It must be remembered, however, that the periurethral and hymenal tissues are highly innervated and sensitive to touch.

▶ INDICATIONS

The differential diagnosis in a prepubertal female who presents with vaginal bleeding with or without discharge should include vaginal foreign body. Additionally, nonspecific genitourinary symptoms with or without abdominal pain should raise the suspicion of a vaginal foreign body. Classically, the vaginal foreign body is associated with a purulent, foul-smelling, bloody vaginal discharge. Although vaginal bleeding is probably the most common presentation, routine vaginal inspection during a well-child examination may lead to visualization of a foreign body (4). Irrigation of the vagina is indicated if a foreign body is seen or strongly suspected based on the signs and symptoms.

If a foreign body is strongly suspected but is not visualized and irrigation fails to dislodge the object, or if symptoms persist, a surgical and/or gynecologic consult is necessary. Frank, uncontrolled bleeding requires more aggressive action than irrigation but rarely occurs with foreign bodies in young children. In cases of significant bleeding, a search for the source of the bleeding is warranted, with the goal of repairing a possible laceration or identifying a mass and/or oncologic process.

Foreign body removal from the vagina cannot be accomplished without some degree of cooperation by the patient. Rarely, a child may benefit from mild sedation. Forced removal in the uncooperative child is contraindicated.

▶ EQUIPMENT

Examination table
8 French feeding tube
60-mL syringe

Normal saline or sterile water (warmed and tested for temperature or at room temperature)
Viscous lidocaine
Cotton or Dacron swabs
Emesis basin (optional)
Absorbent underpads
Light source

▶ PROCEDURE

Early reports advocated instrumentation of the sedated or anesthetized child to visualize and remove the object (1,9). Recent experience suggests that irrigating the vagina is the initial procedure of choice for the prepubertal child (2–5). If there is a question as to the source of the bleeding, a small cotton or Dacron swab can be inserted into the vagina and removed and then inspected for evidence of blood. This swab can be sent for culture if the irrigation is unsuccessful. If the object is visualized and accessible, a premoistened cotton or Dacron swab can be used to "roll" the object out. Vigorous manipulation of the vagina with rigid instruments is contraindicated. Irrigation is less likely to cause discomfort than manipulation with rigid instruments.

Vaginal Irrigation of the Prepubertal Vagina

As mentioned previously, the child with a suspected vaginal foreign body should first be examined using the techniques

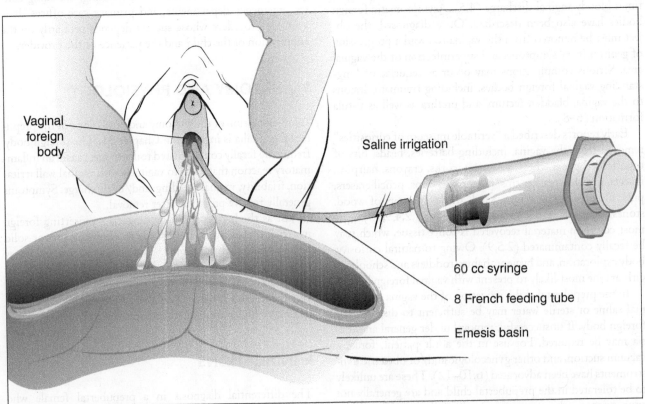

Vaginal foreign body

Saline irrigation

60 cc syringe

8 French feeding tube

Emesis basin

Figure 92.1 Vaginal irrigation with a feeding tube can remove some foreign bodies from the vagina.

described in Chapter 91. Examination in the knee-chest position may allow visualization of the foreign body in the vagina. Before irrigating the vagina, the procedure should be explained to the child. It is helpful to show the patient that the tubing used is flexible, soft, and thin in diameter.

The equipment is prepared by attaching a 60-mL syringe filled with saline (warmed and tested following standard protocol for warming crystalloid [13,14] or at room temperature) to an 8 French feeding tube (Fig. 92.1). Saline is run through the feeding tube.

The child is placed in the supine position on absorbent underpads to collect the fluid during irrigation. Alternatively, an emesis basin may be pressed against the buttocks to collect saline that runs out of the vagina during irrigation. The labia majora are separated with "down and out" traction. A small amount of viscous lidocaine may be applied with a cotton swab to the hymenal tissue to decrease discomfort. Because the feeding tube is flexible and thin, many children can cooperate without receiving a topical anesthetic. After separating the labia, the child is given time to relax so the hymenal orifice will open. The clinician gently inserts the distal end of the feeding tube past the hymenal orifice into the vagina until he or she encounters some resistance. The child is then informed that she will feel cool water "at her bottom." The tube is held in place and irrigation is begun. Asking the child to cough during the irrigation may help to expel small pieces of toilet tissue. Also, holding the labia downward toward the buttocks allows foreign bodies to easily exit the vagina.

CLINICAL TIPS

▶ An unhurried approach will ultimately save time.

▶ Examination in the knee-chest position improves vision into the vagina.

▶ Allowing the child to relax after separating the labia will enlarge the hymenal orifice. Avoiding contact with the hymenal tissue will decrease discomfort.

▶ Application of viscous lidocaine to the hymen may improve cooperation.

▶ Warmed saline is more comfortable for the child.

If irrigation results in recovering small bits of toilet paper, it should continue until the effluent is clear. It is unlikely that continued irrigation will successfully remove a foreign body after two or three unsuccessful attempts. After irrigating the vagina, the child is given a towel to dry herself and is allowed to dress. It is important to discuss the findings and further plans after the patient is dressed.

▶ COMPLICATIONS

Few complications are associated with this procedure if performed in an unhurried, careful manner. Inserting the feeding tube should not injure the tissues in any way. The pressure generated from the setup described is not great and should not cause injury to the vagina. Forceful restraint and irrigation of the vagina in an uncooperative child poses a risk of traumatic injury and should not be done. In such situations, examination under anesthesia is the safer option. The most common problem is failure to successfully remove a foreign body that is lodged in the proximal vagina.

▶ SUMMARY

Vaginal foreign body should be in the differential diagnosis of prepubertal girls who present with vaginal bleeding or malodorous discharge. Toilet paper is the most common foreign body found in the prepubertal vagina. Foreign bodies can occasionally be removed with a moistened cotton swab or with vaginal irrigation. Vaginal irrigation is a simple procedure that should be attempted before referring the child to a specialist. Some children, however, will ultimately require an examination under anesthesia.

▶ REFERENCES

1. Ambuel JP. Foreign bodies in the vagina of children. *J Pediatr.* 1959;54:113–114.

SUMMARY

1 Explain the procedure to the child.

2 Set up the equipment—fill a 60-cc syringe with saline and firmly attach to an 8 French feeding tube; prime the feeding tube with saline.

3 Visualize the hymenal orifice using labial traction; allow the child to relax before inserting the feeding tube.

4 Apply viscous lidocaine to the hymen with a cotton swab if necessary.

5 Gently pass the distal end of the catheter through the hymenal orifice into the vagina until slight resistance is felt.

6 Tell the child she may feel cold water "at her bottom."

7 Irrigate the vagina until the effluent is clear.

8 Ask the child to cough during the irrigation to help expel small pieces of toilet tissue.

9 Hold the labia downward toward the buttocks to help the foreign body exit.

2. Emans SJH, Laufer MR, Goldstein DP. *Pediatric and Adolescent Gynecology.* 5th ed. Philadelphia: Lippincott Williams & Wilkins; 2004.

3. Paradise JE, Willis ED. Probability of vaginal foreign body in girls with genital complaints. *Am J Dis Child.* 1985;139:472–476.

4. Wittich AC, Murray JE. Intravaginal foreign body of long duration: a case report. *Am J Obstet Gynecol.* 1983;169:211–212.

5. Henderson PA, Scott RB. Foreign body vaginitis caused by toilet tissue. *Am J Dis Child.* 1966;111:529–532.

6. Emge KR. Vaginal foreign body extraction by forceps: a case report. *Am J Obstet Gynecol.* 1992;167:514–515.

7. Pelosi MA, Giblin S, Pelosi MA. Vaginal foreign body extraction by obstetric soft vacuum cup: an alternative to forceps. *Am J Obstet Gynecol.* 1993;168:1891–1892.

8. Escamilla JO. Vaginal foreign body extraction by forceps: case report. *Am J Obstet Gynecol.* 1993;169:233–234.

9. Werwath DL, Schwab CW, Scholten JR, et al. Microwave ovens: a safe new method of warming crystalloids. *Am Surg.* 1984;50:656–659.

10. Leaman PL, Martyak GG. Microwave warming of resuscitation fluids. *Ann Emerg Med.* 1985;14:876–879.

11. Stricker T, Navratil F, Sennhauser FH. Vaginal foreign bodies. *J Paediatr Child Health.* 2004;40(4):205-207.

12. Smith YR, Berman DR, Quint EH. Premenarchal vaginal discharge: findings of procedures to rule out foreign bodies. *J Pediatr Adolesc Gynecol.* 2002;15:227–230.

13. Dahiya P, Agarwal U, Sangwan K, et al. Long retained intravaginal foreign body: a case report. *Arch Gynecol Obstet.* 2003;268:323–324.

14. Simon DA, Berry S, Brannian J, et al. Recurrent, purulent vaginal discharge associated with longstanding presence of a foreign body and vaginal stenosis. *J Pediatr Adolesc Gynecol.* 2003;16:361–363.

ANGELO P. GIARDINO AND CINDY W. CHRISTIAN

93

Adolescent Pelvic Examination

▶ INTRODUCTION

The adolescent pelvic examination allows thorough examination of the female external and internal genital structures and anus. A pelvic examination in the emergency setting is indicated for an adolescent female presenting with vaginal discharge, abnormal uterine or vaginal bleeding, amenorrhea, lower abdominal pain, severe dysmenorrhea, exposure to a sexually transmitted disease (STD), suspected pregnancy, genital or anal pruritus, suspected foreign body, pelvic inflammatory disease, or suspected sexual assault (1–4). Pelvic examinations have been traditionally indicated in the ambulatory setting for all sexually active teens, for patients seeking birth control, for STD surveillance, and for routine health assessment in all women over approximately 17 years of age (1,5,6). With the advent of nucleic acid amplification tests (NAATs), which offer the ability to screen for *Chlamydia trachomatis* and *Neisseria gonorrhoeae* noninvasively using urine samples, the need for pelvic examinations for STD surveillance has decreased, although obtaining pap smears and looking for other STDs such as herpetic lesions and human papillomavirus lesions still makes pelvic examinations necessary (7–9).

Properly trained pediatricians, emergency physicians, and other health care providers can perform pelvic examinations with skill and accuracy. Consultation with specialists is sometimes required. Patients with possible oncologic problems or those who are pregnant should be referred to an obstetrician and/or gynecologist (OB/GYN). Consultation with an endocrinologist may be necessary for hormonal aberrations such as virilization or delayed puberty.

Despite its value, the pelvic examination is often associated with dread by both patient and physician (10). Patient anxiety is especially great at the time of the first pelvic examination and may reach an anxiety level similar to that seen in patients before surgery (11). The most common patient concern is of pain from the procedure, and this fear is directly related to the information peers have passed on to the patient (11). Additional sources of anxiety include embarrassment over having breasts and genitals exposed and examined, feelings of vulnerability during the examination, perception of losing control of one's body, concern that a gynecologic disorder will be discovered, and concerns about personal cleanliness and hygiene (11,12). Positioning, presence of a support person, and gender of the clinician have all been associated with adolescents' perception of the discomfort and the level of anxiety associated with the procedure (12–14).

Reproductive and sexual functions are obviously sensitive subjects, and examinations of the genital and anal area require a thoughtful approach. Using force or restraint is always contraindicated. Sedation or anesthesia is acceptable only in the most extreme cases when examination cannot be deferred, such as patients with severe, uncontrollable vaginal bleeding. Patient requests regarding gender of clinician should be accommodated whenever possible (10,15).

Pelvic examination of the adolescent differs from the genital examination in the prepubertal child (Chapter 91) in its inclusion of an internal speculum and bimanual examination. Pelvic examinations are typically performed on adolescent patients with Tanner stages of 3 or above. Tanner stages are analogous to sexual maturity ratings and reflect the presence of secondary sexual characteristics (16).

Although few would argue that a pelvic examination is an important part of a comprehensive physical examination in the adolescent patient, it remains a procedure viewed as technically difficult. With adequate training, the correct equipment, an unhurried approach, and a sensitive demeanor, the procedure can be completed with a minimum of discomfort to the patient.

▶ ANATOMY AND PHYSIOLOGY

The external and internal structures of the adolescent female genital and anal anatomy are similar to those described in the prepubertal child. They differ, however, in terms of size and estrogen effect. The length of the vagina grows from approximately 3 to 4 cm in the infant to approximately 10 to 12 cm in the sexually mature adolescent female (17). The translucent hymenal membrane in the prepubertal child changes under the influence of estrogen and appears pink, thickened, and opaque on examination. With puberty, the labia majora, mons pubis, and perineal area increase in pigmentation and develop pubic hair. The vaginal pH becomes acidic, normal vaginal flora changes, and a physiologic leukorrhea composed of desquamated epithelial cells and cervical mucus develops (18).

▶ EQUIPMENT

Pelvic examination table with stirrups
Light source
Running water
Water-soluble lubricant
Culture materials—gonorrhea, chlamydia (in the adolescent patient, noninvasive NAATs may be appropriate, depending on the clinical situation [7,8])
Microscopic slides
Fixative and Ayre wooden spatulas for Pap smears (if performed)
Normal saline
KOH and Gram stain materials
Plastic test tubes
Sample swabs
Specula of different sizes
Hand mirror for patient use
Examining gloves, gowns, and sheets

Different specula exist and are recommended for different ages and sizes of patients: Huffman ($1/2'' \times 41/4''$) is used for nonsexually active adolescents; Pederson ($7/8'' \times 41/2''$) for sexually active, nulliparous adolescents; and Graves ($1\,3/8'' \times 3''$) for the parous female (19). Infant specula are not recommended.

▶ PROCEDURE

Before the procedure, the clinician should discuss the pelvic examination with the patient, specifically addressing issues related to discomfort during the examination and the presence of a support person in the room during the examination. A chaperone should be in the room regardless of the gender of the clinician.

During the examination, the clinician should inform the patient about what is happening and what sensations to ex-

pect. After the pelvic examination, the patient should be given the opportunity to dress in private, and, finally, the clinician should discuss findings and explain follow-up procedures.

Written consent for the pelvic examination is not necessary. Verbal consent should be obtained from the patient. Parental consent is not necessary in most situations, although institutional protocols should be consulted.

Pelvic examination of the adolescent patient contains the following basic steps, generally done in this order: (a) the external examination, (b) the speculum examination, and (c) the bimanual examination. The patient should empty her bladder before beginning the examination. She should be asked to take her clothes off, including her underwear, and cover herself with a sheet provided while the clinician waits outside the room.

The external examination begins by having the patient lie on the examining table. Placing a pillow under the patient's head makes the examination more comfortable and demonstrates concern for the patient's comfort. The abdomen is examined by first inspecting its shape and contour. Auscultation for bowel and/or fetal heart sounds and percussion for liver size and tenderness should follow. Tenderness of the liver may be present with Fitz-Hugh and Curtis syndrome. The remainder of the abdomen is palpated for masses, tenderness, guarding, or rebound. The inguinal area is palpated for adenopathy, which may indicate pelvic infection.

The patient is instructed in how to assume the lithotomy position, at which time the stirrups are adjusted for comfort. The patient should abduct her knees and relax her thighs into a frog-leg position. Phrases such as "separate your knees" are preferable to "spread your legs." This position will relax the pelvic musculature. First, a visual inspection of the external genitalia should note the Tanner stage as evidenced by pubic hair (and breasts). Before touching the patient, the clinician should inspect for lesions, bleeding, and discharge. If the patient complains of pruritus, the pubic hair is inspected for signs of pubic lice (pediculosis pubis). The clinician then places a gloved hand on the patient's thigh and, while maintaining a running dialogue with the patient, palpates the labia and mons pubis.

The labia majora are separated (Fig. 93.1), and the vulva is inspected for signs of infection or injury. Warts, vesicles, or signs of inflammation are identified. The perianal area is checked for condyloma. Palpation of the periurethral, Skene, and Bartholin glands for masses or discharge follows. Clitoromegaly, estrogen status of the mucosa, and the configuration of the hymen are noted. Assessing for hymenal patency is necessary to determine if a speculum examination should proceed. The majority of adolescents with normal anatomy can tolerate a speculum examination if appropriate equipment and technique are used. A Huffman speculum is narrow but long enough to allow for viewing the cervix. Sexually active adolescents are comfortably examined with a Pederson speculum. Obese or parous patients are best examined with the larger Graves speculum.

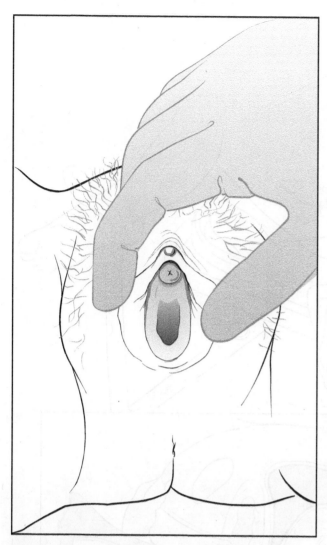

Figure 93.1 Labia majora are separated with thumb and index finger for inspection of the vulva.

The speculum examination begins by first running the speculum under warm water, which both warms and lubricates the speculum, allowing for a more comfortable examination. Lubricant gel is not necessary and may interfere with some specimen collections. The clinician inserts a gloved index finger of the dominant hand into the vagina, applying gentle pressure posteriorly, which will help relax the pubococcygeal muscle. In addition, identifying the location of the cervix at this time will help guide the speculum into proper position. The speculum is introduced into the vagina at a 45-degree angle in a downward direction, with the blades oriented vertically and inserted along the posterior vaginal wall (Fig. 93.2). This can be done before removing the finger from the vagina. After the speculum is inserted and rotated to the horizontal position, the blades are opened slowly to expose the cervix. Initially inserting the speculum with the blades oriented vertically minimizes patient discomfort caused when the blade edges impinge on the lateral vaginal walls. It should also be remembered that pressure applied anteriorly will compress the

urethra between the speculum blade and the pubic symphysis and cause pain. If the cervix is not visualized, the blades should be closed, repositioned, and reopened.

The surface of the cervix generally is smooth and pink. Many adolescents have columnar epithelium from the internal os extending onto the external cervix. This eversion of the mucosa is known as "ectropion" and may be normal or indicate infection.

If indicated, a Pap smear should be obtained first, before the cervical cells are disturbed. Cells from the endocervix and the cervical os are sampled (Fig. 93.3). A cotton-tipped swab or Cytobrush is rotated in the endocervical os in one direction. The swab is removed and rotated in the opposite direction on one half of a glass slide. Next, an Ayre wooden spatula is used to scrape the cervix. The spatula is rotated 360 degrees to sample the entire surface of the cervix and is smeared on the second half of the glass slide. Fixative is immediately applied to preserve the sample. Air drying of the sample will render the Pap smear unreliable.

Cultures for gonorrhea may be obtained by inserting a swab 1 to 2 cm into the cervical canal for 10 to 15 seconds (to allow the swab to absorb secretions). The specimen is applied to a culture plate with medium specific for identification of *N. gonorrhoeae*. Plates just taken from a refrigerator are too cold and can result in falsely negative culture results. The sample is transported to the laboratory in a sealed container with a carbon dioxide tablet. A sample obtained in the same manner can be placed on a slide for Gram stain.

Chlamydia cultures may be obtained by inserting a swab with either a plastic or metal stick (wood inhibits chlamydia growth) into the cervical canal and rotating the swab vigorously to pick up endocervical cells. The swab is removed and placed in culture medium. The swab is rotated onto a test slide if a rapid test is being used.

The introduction of noninvasive NAATs has decreased the need for chlamydia and gonorrhea cultures because the technology permits the detection of infections using urine samples (7). The clinical situation and consideration of the differential diagnosis will determine if NAATs or cultures are most appropriate.

Sampling of the vaginal secretions is necessary to diagnose trichomonas, bacterial vaginosis, and candida. A wet prep or potassium hydroxide (KOH) prep is performed by collecting a sample of vaginal secretions from the posterior fornix using a swab. The swab is then mixed with a few drops of normal saline, or slides are prepared directly.

Once all specimens are obtained, the speculum is slowly removed while the vaginal walls are inspected. After the cervix is released, the blades of the speculum are closed and the instrument withdrawn from the vagina while gentle pressure is maintained posteriorly.

The last part of the pelvic examination is the bimanual palpation (Fig. 93.4). This allows for assessment of the size, position, and configuration of the internal pelvic organs. The index and middle fingers of the clinician's gloved, dominant hand are lubricated with a water-soluble lubricant gel. One

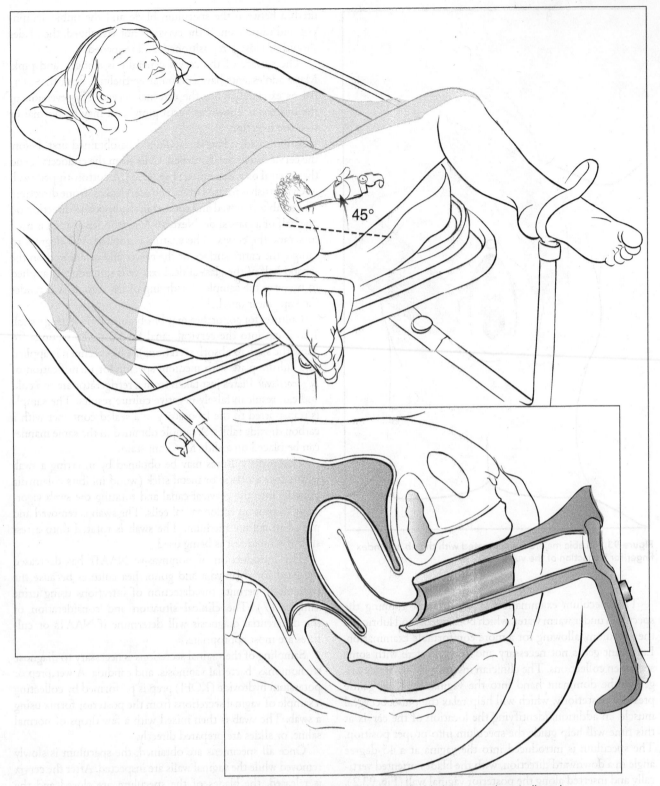

Figure 93.2 The speculum is inserted at a 45-degree angle with the blades oriented vertically and rotated into a horizontal position. Pressure on the sensitive periurethral tissues anteriorly is avoided.

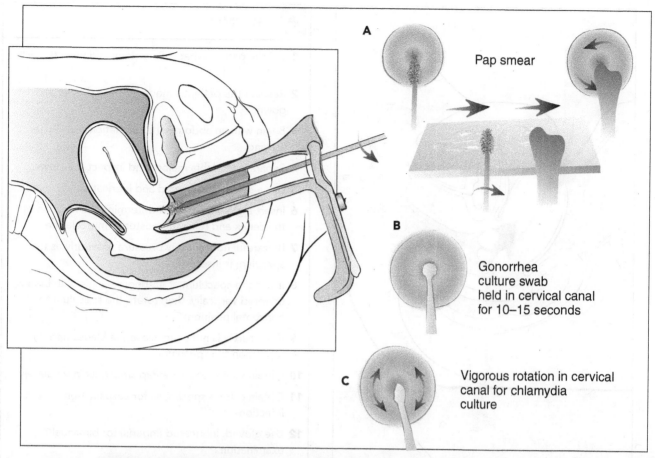

Figure 93.3 Specimen collection.
A. Sample for Pap smear is obtained with Cytobrush or swab and rotated onto slide. Spatula is rotated 360 degrees on cervix and smeared on glass slide.
B. Swab of cervical discharge is inoculated onto medium for gonorrhea culture.
C. Cervical cells are obtained for chlamydia culture or rapid test.

or two fingers are gently inserted into the vagina. When the patient is relaxed, external pressure to the abdomen is applied with the other hand. As the internal hand lifts and supports the uterus, the external hand palpates for size and position. Cervical motion or uterine tenderness is noted. The adnexa are palpated by placing the internal fingers laterally to one side of the fornix and pressing deeply on the ipsilateral lower abdominal wall. Finding the pulsations of the ovarian artery in the lateral vaginal recess and then sliding the fingers medially to locate the adnexa is sometimes helpful (2). The adnexa are smooth, walnut-size masses (normal ovary size is approximately 3 cm in diameter). Palpation of the adnexa can be uncomfortable for the patient. Any extreme tenderness, mass, enlargement, or asymmetry of the adnexa is abnormal. Both sides must be examined.

The rectoabdominal examination is especially helpful when the vaginal bimanual examination cannot be tolerated, when the uterus is retroverted and/or retroflexed, or when the patient has complaints specific to the rectum or anus (20). It is not mandatory in the adolescent patient. The rectal examination should follow the vaginal bimanual examination and is performed with one lubricated gloved finger.

After the examination is complete, the patient is offered tissues to wipe away lubricant and is left alone to dress. When the patient is clothed, the clinician then discusses the findings and arranges any necessary follow-up.

▶ COMPLICATIONS

Even with the most sensitive approach some discomfort from the pelvic examination is unavoidable. Complications due to technique include pain and anxiety, which may lead to avoidance of future health care interactions. Patient discomfort can be minimized by discussing the expected sensations associated with the examination before its performance and listening to the patient's concerns. Paying attention to techniques such as warming the speculum, avoiding pressure on the urethra, having patient void before the examination, using the appropriate speculum, using water to lubricate the speculum before insertion, and using drapes and gowns to ensure modesty can further reduce discomfort from a pelvic examination (21). Allowing the patient to assume a semirecumbent position and to use a handheld mirror to permit viewing of the examination

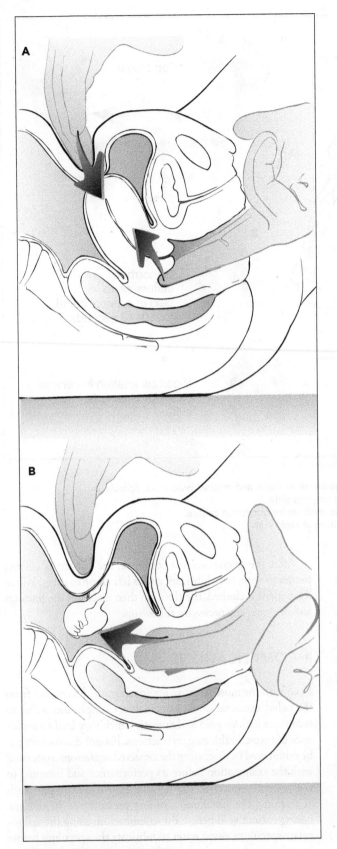

Figure 93.4 Bimanual examination.
A. The uterus is squeezed between the fingers on the cervix and the hand on the lower abdomen.
B. The adnexa on both sides are palpated.

  SUMMARY

1 Tell the patient what will be done and what she will feel.

2 Respect the patient's modesty—use drapes and gown.

3 Begin with an abdominal examination and Tanner staging.

4 Separate the labia majora and inspect the vulva.

5 Use a speculum warmed and lubricated with water.

6 Insert a gloved finger to determine the location of the cervix and relax the posterior musculature.

7 Be careful not to apply pressure anteriorly as the speculum is inserted.

8 Insert the speculum at 45-degree angle with blades oriented vertically, then rotate the speculum to a horizontal position.

9 If the cervix is not seen, close the blades and reposition the speculum.

10 Obtain specimens for a Pap smear; fix immediately.

11 Obtain culture specimens for sexually transmitted infections.

12 Use gloved, lubricated finger(s) for bimanual examination.

13 A rectoabdominal examination may be useful if a bimanual examination is not tolerated.

14 Discuss findings and arrange for follow-up.

  CLINICAL TIPS

▶ An unhurried and sensitive approach and talking the patient through the procedure will save time and make the examination more pleasant for both the clinician and the patient.

▶ In addition to the patient's support person, a chaperone should always be present during a pelvic exam (regardless of the sex of the clinician) to protect the clinician from allegations of impropriety.

▶ A speculum appropriate for the age and size of the patient should be selected.

▶ When inserting and removing the speculum, the clinician should be careful to avoid putting pressure anteriorly (against the urethra) and also to avoid trapping pubic hairs.

also may decrease anxiety and discomfort (14). A pelvic examination should never cause physical injury.

▶ SUMMARY

The pelvic examination is part of routine care for all sexually active adolescents and all adolescents older than 17 or 18 years. Pelvic examinations should be done on all female patients with complaints specific to the genital or rectal area and for those with unexplained abdominal pain. Proper training in the technical and interpersonal aspects of a pelvic examination can improve the diagnostic accuracy and reduce patient discomfort.

▶ REFERENCES

1. Beach RK. The adolescent pelvic examination: an office guide. *Adolesc Health Update.* 1991;4:3–7.
2. Wilson MD, Joffe A. Step-by-step through the pelvic exam. *Contemp Pediatr.* 1988;5:92–104.
3. Kreutner AK. Examination of the adolescent female. In: Kreutner AKK, Hollingsworth DR, eds. *Adolescent Obstetrics and Gynecology.* Chicago: Year Book Medical Publishers; 1978:47–65.
4. Nyirjesy P. Vaginitis in the adolescent patient. *Pediatr Clin North Am.* 1999;46:733–745.
5. Thibaud E. Gynecologic clinical examination of the child and adolescent. *Endocr Dev.* 2004;7:1–8.
6. Hubbard HS. Gynecologic examination of adolescents. *Am J Nurs.* 2001;101(3):24AAA–DDD.
7. Centers for Disease Control and Prevention. Screening tests to detect *Chlamydia trachomatis* and *Neisseria gonorrhoeae* infections—2002. *MMWR Recomm Rep.* 2002;51(No. RR-15):1–38.
8. Corneli HM. Nuclei acid amplification tests (polymerase chain reaction, ligase chain reaction) for the diagnosis of *Chlamydia trachomatis* and *Neisseria gonorrhoeae* in pediatric emergency medicine. *Pediatr Emerg Care.* 2005;21:264–270.
9. Centers for Disease Control and Prevention. Sexually transmitted diseases treatment guidelines 2002. *MMWR Recomm Rep.* 2002; 51(No. RR-6):1–79.
10. Braverman PK, Stasburger VC. Why adolescent gynecology? Pediatricians and pelvic examinations. *Pediatr Clin North Am.* 1989;36:471–487.
11. Millstein SG, Adler NE, Irwin CE. Sources of anxiety about pelvic examinations among adolescent females. *J Adolesc Health Care.* 1984;5:105–111.
12. Seymore C, DuRant RH, Jay MS, et al. Influence of position during examination, and sex of examiner on patient anxiety during pelvic examination. *J Pediatr.* 1986;108:312–317.
13. Phillips S, Friedman SB, Seidenberg M, et al. Teenagers' preferences regarding the presence of family members, peers, and chaperones during examination of genitalia. *Pediatrics.* 1981;68:665–669.
14. Swartz WH. The semisitting position for pelvic examination. *JAMA.* 1984;251:1163.
15. Pokorny S. Pediatric and adolescent gynecology. *Compr Ther.* 1997;23:337–344.
16. Christie D, Viner R. Adolescent development. *BMJ.* 2005;330:301–304.
17. Muram D. Anatomy: anatomic and physiologic changes. In: Heger A, Emans SJ, eds. *Evaluation of the Sexually Abused Child.* New York: Oxford University Press; 1992:71–73.
18. Wheeler MD. Physical changes of puberty. *Endocrinol Metab Clin North Am.* 1991;20:1–14.
19. Emans SJH, Laufer MR, Goldstein DP. *Pediatric and Adolescent Gynecology.* 5th ed. Philadelphia: Lippincott Williams & Wilkins; 2004.
20. Greydanus DE, Shearin RB. *Adolescent Sexuality and Gynecology.* Philadelphia: Lea & Febiger; 1990:17–42.
21. Primose RB. Taking the tension out of pelvic exams. *Am J Nurs.* 1984;84:72–74.

94

ROBERT A. SHAPIRO AND CHARLES J. SCHUBERT

Forensic Examination of the Sexual Assault Victim

▶ INTRODUCTION

Physicians are often called on to evaluate children who may have been victims of sexual abuse. It is estimated that 20% of American women and 5% to 10% of American men will experience some form of sexual abuse as children (I). Evaluation for sexual abuse includes a history from the alleged victim and/or guardian and a physical examination. When indicated, laboratory tests for sexually transmitted diseases and forensic specimens for the police are obtained. In this chapter, the term "forensic specimens" refers to samples collected for a police investigation, not for medical treatment. The procedure must be performed with precision and documentation must be complete because the evaluation may later be scrutinized in a court of law. Procedures presented in this chapter will satisfy legal requirements when performed properly.

Many communities have a multidisciplinary facility designated as a child advocacy center (CAC) that is equipped to evaluate allegations of sexual abuse. The medical evaluation of nonacute alleged sexual abuse, and in some communities acute assault, can often be provided by the CAC, and such an evaluation would be preferred to an evaluation in the emergency department. Protocols with the local CAC should be written so that guidelines for triage of alleged sexual abuse/assault patients are created.

Sexual assault nurse examiners (SANEs) are available to assist in the evaluation of forensic evidence in many communities. Because the evaluation of the child abuse victim is different from that of the adult victim, SANE nurses who evaluate children for suspected child sexual abuse/assault should complete appropriate training and demonstrate competency in child sexual abuse evaluations. Pediatric SANEs can collect laboratory specimens, forensic specimens, and diagnostic-quality photo documentation. If trained in forensic inter-view methods, the Pediatric SANE can also obtain a history from the child. Pediatric SANEs should document their involvement in the medical record using standard nursing methods and vocabulary. The interpretation and diagnosis should be made by an experienced physician or clinical nurse practitioner.

▶ ANATOMY AND PHYSIOLOGY

Before conducting an evaluation, the anatomy of the genitalia and the examination techniques presented in Chapters 91 and 93 should be reviewed. The appearance of the normal genitalia changes dramatically from infancy to childhood to adolescence. Many "normal" variants of the prepubertal and adolescent hymen are encountered, as well as great variation in the normal color and skin appearance of the anus. Errors in clinical judgment may occur if the physician is unfamiliar with the normal range of anatomic findings and the changes that occur with age.

The physical examination of most victims of sexual abuse will be normal (see Fig. 91.2) (2,3). Abuse by fondling and oral contact, for example, usually causes no identifying physical signs. Penetration of a young child's vagina may result in injury and recognizable findings on examination. Penetration of the vulva without introitus penetration in the young child, or introitus penetration in the pubertal female, most often causes no injury. Rectal and penile injuries are unusual. The amount of force used, the frequency of abuse, the use of lubricants, the size of the object penetrating the child, and the child's age are factors that will determine the likelihood of injury and an abnormal examination. Furthermore, when injuries heal, findings of trauma are often absent.

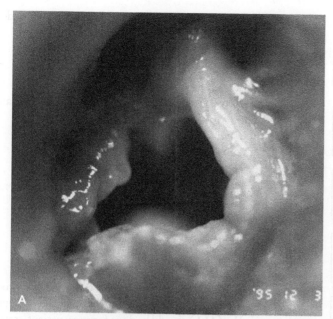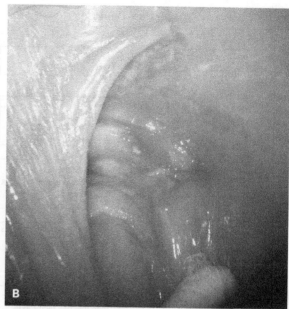

Figure 94.1 Traumatic vaginal injuries from sexual abuse.
A. Laceration of the hymen results in a deep tear at 8 o'clock.
B. A swab is used to lift the hymen, revealing a fresh laceration at 4 o'clock.

The most specific indicators of vaginal penetration are injuries to the hymeneal ring. Acute trauma is indicated by bleeding, fresh tears, abrasions, or bruising to the hymen or to one of the structures immediately adjacent to the hymen (Fig. 94.1). Healed trauma from vaginal penetration is difficult to recognize and should be diagnosed by a physician or clinical nurse practitioner skilled in this field. Small notches, bumps, minor irregularities, absence of hymen between 10 and 2 o'clock, redundant hymeneal tissue, labial adhesions, and erythema are examples of nonspecific findings (4). Speculum examinations in the prepubertal patient are indicated only when internal injury is suspected. An internal vaginal exam in the prepubertal patient will require anesthesia.

Penetration of the rectum in sexual abuse may cause lacerations or perianal bruising. Normal exams are common. Rectal tone should be assessed by observation of the anal diameter as the buttocks are spread apart. Stool in the rectal vault may cause decreased rectal tone and should be ruled out by re-examining the child after voluntary defecation. A digital rectal examination and anoscopy are necessary only when serious internal trauma is suspected.

Straddle injuries to the genitalia are a common cause of genital trauma and result in asymmetric bruising of and lacerations to (a) the skin overlying the pubic symphysis or (b) the labia majora. Because these injuries generally only involve the surface structures, sexual abuse should be suspected if the trauma involves the hymen.

▶ INDICATIONS

Evaluation for sexual abuse or assault is needed whenever illegal sexual activity has been alleged, disclosed, or discovered.

The definition of illegal sexual activity varies from state to state. When in doubt about whether a crime has been committed, police or social services from that jurisdiction should be consulted. In most states, any sexual activity with a child under 13 years of age is illegal and requires an evaluation. Teenagers between the ages of 13 and 15 who have sexual activity with a partner 4 or more years older may be engaging in illegal activity. Incest and any sexual activity that is forced on a minor against his or her will must be evaluated and reported.

Children who are victims of sexual abuse frequently report fondling of their genitalia or rectum, oral sex, attempted intercourse, sodomy, or demands to masturbate the perpetrator. Most often the perpetrator is a male who has access to the child, such as a member of the child's family, a close family friend, or one of the child's caretakers. Sexual abuse occurs in children of all ages. Of the victims, 85% are female. The child may disclose the abuse, or it may be discovered by others. The last incident of abuse before evaluation may have been years ago or within hours of presentation.

Experts differ on the indications for sexually transmitted infection (STI) testing in cases of sexual abuse. A suggested approach is presented in Figure 94.2. Testing all adolescent victims is warranted given the high incidence of STIs in this population. If the victim is an asymptomatic prepubertal child, testing is recommended if the prevalence of STIs is high in the community in which the child lives or if the history suggests an increased risk of infection. Symptomatic prepubertal children should have infections documented by culture or another gold standard test. Children diagnosed with one STI should be tested for others.

In most locations, forensic specimens must be collected if the last abuse or assault occurred within 72 to 96 hours of

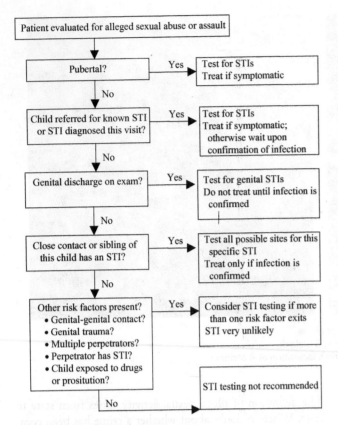

Figure 94.2 Indications for STI testing.

the evaluation and if the history suggests that semen, saliva, blood, or hair of the alleged perpetrator may be found on the victim's body or clothing (5,6).

Moderate sedation or examination under general anesthesia may be indicated for the uncooperative or combative patient whose examination cannot be deferred. This includes victims with acute genital or rectal trauma and victims for whom police evidence must be collected. Patients older than 2 or 3 years should not be restrained against their will because forced rectal and genital examinations may be psychologically harmful to them. Most patients, however, will cooperate if their fears are addressed by the physician and they are reassured that the evaluation will not be painful. Young children will cooperate more often with the evaluation if they are allowed to sit on a parent's lap.

▶ EQUIPMENT

If culturing for STIs:
Thayer-Martin plates or nucleic acid amplification kit (one for each culture site)
Chlamydia culture media or nucleic acid amplification kit (one for each culture site)
Calgiswabs (smaller swabs are most appropriate for young children; avoid swabs with wooden shafts for chlamydia culture)

Approximately 5 mL of sterile saline to moisten swabs (do not use bacteriostatic saline)
Pelvic examination tray (for adolescent patients)
Wet prep materials supplies

If collecting forensic specimens:
State-approved sexual assault evidence box (Note: not all evidence boxes are approved for pediatric use)
Woods lamp, BlueMax lamp, or equivalent
Pelvic examination tray (for the adolescent patient)

Photo documentation equipment:
Colposcope equipped with recording device or a camera (digital or film) with macro capability

▶ PROCEDURE

A series of procedures are described in this section. These procedures should typically be performed in the order listed. Steps accompanied by **(ALL)** should be done for every patient, steps accompanied by **(STI)** should be done for patients requiring STI cultures, and steps accompanied by **(FORENSIC)** should be done only for patients requiring forensic specimen collection. Patients receiving a forensic examination should also undergo the standard steps of STI testing if indicated.

A history of the abuse and/or assault is obtained **(ALL)**. If a skilled forensic interviewer is available, this interviewer should obtain the history of the alleged abuse from the patient. Those physicians and nurses untrained in forensic methods should limit their history to essential questions needed to provide medical care, determine the need for forensic evidence collection, and assist the child protection worker with discharge (safety) planning. This limited history would include a description of the sexual abuse and/or assault; any physical complaints or symptoms; the identity of the alleged perpetrator; the time, date, and place of last episode; the last menstrual period (if applicable); the date and time of last consensual intercourse (if any); and the method of birth control (if any). This information should reveal any indications for STI testing and forensic evidence collection and will be helpful in deciding the disposition of the patient. In many cases, a complete forensic interview can be done after discharge from the emergency department. Protocols for interviewing an alleged victim should include the local child protection agency, law enforcement, and/or the local CAC.

The patient is prepared for the examination **(ALL)**. The procedure is explained to the victim and family. If possible, the patient should not bathe, void, or defecate before forensic specimen collection. The patient is allowed to choose who he or she would like to be present during the examination. (The alleged perpetrator should not be allowed to stay with the patient.) The patient is reassured that the examination will not be painful. Young children should be allowed to sit on a parent's lap. A general examination is performed, with documentation of any signs of injury **(ALL)**. All injuries are photographed. Photographs should be clearly labeled, and photographs with injuries should include a measuring standard in the photographic frame.

Specific steps and procedures for forensic evidence collection will be included in the evidence kit. The following procedure is generic, and the procedure used with most approved kits will be similar.

Clothing of the patient that is or may be stained with blood, semen, or saliva is placed into a large paper bag (**FORENSIC**). The bag is sealed with tape and labeled with the date, the patient's name, and a description of the bag's contents. The patient's underwear is placed into a small paper bag, and the bag is sealed with tape. Underwear is collected even if the patient has changed underwear since the assault. The bag is sealed and labeled as described.

Oral specimens for semen are collected (**FORENSIC**). Using four cotton-tipped swabs, saliva from the victim's upper and lower gum lines is collected. These four swabs are placed into an envelope, sealed with tape, and labeled as described.

A pharyngeal culture for gonorrhea is collected if indicated (**STI**). A pharyngeal specimen is collected using a fresh cotton-tipped swab; culture media is inoculated and labeled as described.

The skin is examined for seminal stains and bite marks, particularly around the genitalia, thighs, and buttocks (**FORENSIC**). Stains are swabbed with four cotton-tipped swabs that have been lightly moistened with sterile saline. The center of bite marks are swabbed for saliva. The room is then darkened, and the victim's body is scanned with a Woods or BlueMax lamp. Fluorescence indicates other possible seminal stains. The swabs are placed into an envelope, sealed, and labeled as described. If more than one stain is found, each stain is collected separately and placed into separate envelopes.

The genitalia and rectum are inspected for signs of injury and infection (**ALL**). A detailed description of all findings should be documented.

A rectal specimen for semen is collected (**FORENSIC**). Four cotton-tipped swabs are lightly moistened with sterile saline and inserted into the victim's rectum. After 5 to 10 seconds, the swabs are withdrawn and placed into an envelope. The envelope is sealed and labeled as described.

Rectal and vaginal cultures for gonorrhea and chlamydia are obtained if indicated (**STI**). In prepubertal females, the vaginal mucosa is cultured just proximal or distal to the hymen using a small calcium alginate swab lightly moistened with nonbacteriostatic sterile saline. Avoid contact with the hymen because most prepubertal girls experience pain when the hymen is touched. In adolescent females, cervical specimens are obtained. Urethral cultures may be obtained in males. Swabs with plastic or aluminum shafts should be used for chlamydia culture, as wood is toxic to the organisms. "Gold standard" STI tests are preferable to other tests to minimize false-positive results, but nucleic acid amplification tests can be useful screening tests if followed up with culture.

Any loose pubic hairs are collected (**FORENSIC**). If the victim has pubic hair, a paper towel is placed under his or her buttocks, and the pubic hair is combed. Any loose hair that falls onto the towel is wrapped, along with the comb, in the paper towel and placed into an envelope. The envelope is sealed and labeled as described.

If the victim is a preadolescent and has no pubic hair, the skin near the child's genitalia and rectum is inspected carefully for stray hairs. If hairs are found, they are collected and wrapped in a paper towel. The folded towel is placed into an envelope, sealed, and labeled as described. If the victim has pubic hair, 5 to 10 pubic hairs are plucked or cut with the scissors as close to the skin as possible. The hairs are wrapped in a clean paper towel and placed into an envelope. The envelope is sealed and labeled as described. The scissors can be discarded.

A genital specimen for semen is collected (**FORENSIC**). If the patient is an adolescent female, four cotton-tipped swabs are used to collect vaginal secretions. If the patient is a male or a prepubertal female, four swabs lightly moistened with sterile saline are used to swab the external genitalia. The swabs are placed into an envelope, and the envelope is sealed and labeled as described.

Diagnostic quality photographs should be obtained of all genital and anal findings. Photographs should be properly labeled and stored for later diagnosis by skilled physicians or clinical nurse practitioners. Local protocol may require or encourage photo documentation of all exams.

Wet mount preparations for sperm and *Trichomonas* may be obtained from the mouth, genitalia, and rectum if requested in the kit or included in local protocol (**FORENSIC**). If they are to be examined in the hospital laboratory, they must be taken by the physician or nurse to maintain the chain of custody. If sperm are found, motility should be documented. The microscopic appearance of sperm is shown in Figure 94.3. Any slides prepared from the wet mount preparations are placed into cardboard slide holders, labeled, and placed into a large evidence envelope.

Blood is collected as indicated in the evidence box for DNA analysis. If a drug-facilitated sexual assault is suspected, blood and/or urine are also collected at this time. Drug testing is typically done by the forensic, not the hospital, laboratory. Specimens must remain refrigerated until tested.

Each envelope is examined to make certain that the outside surface contains a clear description of the specimen, the victim's name, and the current date (**FORENSIC**). Envelopes are sealed with tape. All forensic specimens are placed into a large envelope, and the envelope is labeled as described. The chain of custody—a legal term referring to the need to identify at all times the person possessing the evidence and to whom and at what time it was passed to another—is thus secured. Until the evidence is locked in a secure location or is given to the police, it must remain in the hands of the physician or nurse to secure the chain of custody. If the chain of custody includes periods of time when the evidence was not accounted for, such as a time when it was left on a counter unattended, an opportunity would have existed for tampering. This break in the chain might compromise the validity of the evidence

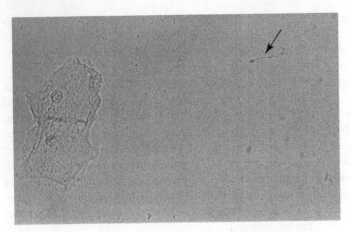

Figure 94.3 Microscopic view of sperm.

during a legal proceeding. The chain of custody should be thoroughly documented.

The completed evidence box is then sealed with tape and placed into a locked and secure closet or drawer until it is given to the investigating police officer **(FORENSIC)**. Written documentation is completed **(ALL)**.

Prophylaxis against STIs and pregnancy should be considered for the adolescent **(STI)**. The prevalence of STIs in sexually abused prepubertal children is low, and STI prophylaxis is generally not needed. Serum for HIV, hepatitis, and syphilis testing is obtained if indicated **(STI)**. Transmission

of HIV after sexual assault is low but must be considered whenever there is mucosal injury and perpetrator infection is possible. Current guidelines should be followed. HIV prophylaxis should be offered when indicated and follow-up arranged for clinical care and repeat testing at 3 and 6 months. Emergency contraception should be offered when clinically indicated.

The county children's protective service (CPS) and police should be called to report suspected child sexual abuse **(ALL)**. Discharge planning must be discussed with the CPS social worker in cases of abuse. In most instances, the child

---

⦿ SUMMARY

Procedure	ALL	STI	FORENSIC	Procedure	ALL	STI	FORENSIC
1 History and examination	✓			**11** Loose pubic hair specimen			✓
2 Outer clothing specimen			✓	**12** Cut or plucked pubic hair specimen			✓
3 Underwear specimen			✓	**13** Genital semen specimen			✓
4 Oral semen specimen			✓	**14** Wet prep collection			✓
5 Pharyngeal culture		✓		**15** Wet prep examination			✓
6 Skin stains specimen			✓	**16** Chain of custody			✓
7 Genital-rectal examination	✓			**17** HIV and syphilis testing		✓	
8 Photo documentation of genital and anal findings	✓			**18** Documentation	✓		
9 Rectal semen specimen			✓	**19** Reporting	✓		
10 Genital-rectal cultures		✓		**20** Discharge	✓		

Note: **ALL** denotes procedures that should be performed for all potential victims of sexual abuse or assault. **STI** denotes procedures that should be performed for patients requiring testing for sexually transmitted infections. **FORENSIC** denotes procedures that should only be performed for patients requiring collection of forensic specimens. Patients receiving a forensic examination should undergo routine STI testing as indicated.

can be safely discharged to home if he or she will not be in contact with the alleged perpetrator. Situations will arise when emergency placement into foster care or admission to the hospital will be required to ensure the child's safety. CPS has the legal authority to make this decision.

The victim and/or family should be told that the examination is complete and reassured that tests for any physical complications or problems resulting from the abuse have been done (ALL). The family's questions should be answered, and examination findings and the reporting process should be explained. Follow-up with the local CAC or the child's physician should be arranged.

▶ COMPLICATIONS

The alleged victim, whether in fact abused or not, has gone through an emotional ordeal and is asked to tolerate a sometimes uncomfortable and embarrassing evaluation. The physician can help the victim deal with the evaluation and begin the psychological healing by remaining sensitive and unhurried throughout the evaluation. Forcing an uncooperative victim to undergo an examination adds to the emotional trauma. Referral to a multidisciplinary center, such as a CAC, is indicated for the nonacute uncooperative patient.

Forensic evidence should not be left unattended, and the chain of custody must be documented and maintained to prevent legal invalidation of the collected evidence. All forensic specimens must be stored in paper envelopes. Specimens stored in plastic bags will not dry properly and may be rendered useless.

▶ SUMMARY

Physicians are required to evaluate and report all cases of suspected sexual abuse and/or assault. A report by telephone should be followed by a written report. Clear documentation and attention to details are required. Evaluation will vary depending on the details of the specific case. A sensitive and unhurried approach can minimize any additional distress caused by evaluation procedures. The physician is an important advocate for the victim of sexual abuse and should be available and willing to testify in court if necessary.

▶ REFERENCES

1. Finkelhor D, Hotaling G, Lewis IA, et al. Sexual abuse in a national survey of adult men and women: prevalence, characteristics, and risk factors. *Child Abuse Negl.* 1990;14:19–28.
2. Adams JA, Harper K, Knudson S, et al. Examination findings in legally confirmed child sexual abuse: it's normal to be normal. *Pediatrics.* 1994;94:310–317.
3. Berenson AB. The prepubertal genital exam: what is normal and abnormal. *Curr Opin Obstet Gynecol.* 1994;6:526–530.
4. Giardino AP, Finkel MA, Giardino ER, et al. *A Practical Guide to the Evaluation of Sexual Abuse in the Prepubertal Child.* Newbury Park, CA: Sage; 1992:75–79.
5. Jenny C. Forensic examination: the role of the physician as "medical detective." In: Heger A, Emans SJ, eds. *Evaluation of the Sexually Abused Child: A Medical Textbook and Photographic Atlas.* New York: Oxford University Press; 1992:51–61.
6. Kanda MB, Orr LA. Specimen collection in sexual abuse. In: Ludwig S, Kornbert AE, eds. *Child Abuse: A Medical Reference.* 2nd ed. New York: Churchill Livingstone; 1992:265–279.

CLINICAL TIPS

▶ Commercial rape kits will save time and increase the precision of forensic evidence collection.

▶ Examination and collection of specimens should not be rushed. Careful attention to details, labeling of specimens, and documentation are critical.

▶ Swabs moistened with sterile saline will be less painful.

▶ The number of persons handling specimens should be limited, and the chain of custody must be maintained.

▶ Diagnostic quality photographs should be obtained of genital and rectal exams.

▶ If the patient is uncooperative, the need for an emergency evaluation should be reassessed. If forensic specimens and emergency examination are not needed, the examination may be less stressful if completed at a later date in a facility geared for the multidisciplinary assessment (CAC) of alleged child abuse.

95

SUZANNE BENO AND SANDRA SCHWAB

Bladder Catheterization

▶ INTRODUCTION

Bladder catheterization is performed to obtain urine in a sterile manner for culture and urinalysis (1). The procedure allows for relatively easy and timely access to urine, particularly in the young child who cannot void on command. A bladder catheter also may be placed for monitoring urine output and relieving obstruction. Some obvious psychosocial issues impact on children of all age groups (and parents) regarding exposed genitalia and perceived violation of this sensitive area. Some cultural groups may even fear that a daughter's virginity will be compromised by urinary catheterization (2). All patients and/or parents thus deserve a brief but careful explanation of the relevant anatomy and details of the procedure. Respect for modesty and privacy is critical and will be highly appreciated by the older child and all parents.

▶ ANATOMY AND PHYSIOLOGY

The relevant anatomy of the prepubertal child is generally similar to that of the adult, except for the obvious differences in size and lack of secondary sexual characteristics. In boys, the urethral meatus is usually easy to locate, but the long course of the urethra and its relative fixation at the level of the symphysis pubis can make passage of the catheter difficult (3). Holding the penis straight with slight traction at 90 degrees vertical to the abdominal wall straightens the urethral course and facilitates catheter passage (Fig. 95.1).

In the uncircumcised neonate or infant boy, a tight foreskin can make the task of locating the urethral meatus challenging. Usually gentle retraction of the foreskin will expose enough of the glans to visualize the meatus. Infant males with hypospadias may require more exploration on the ventral surface of the shaft to identify the urethral meatus. Some infant boys with chronic ammoniacal diaper dermatitis may acquire meatal stenosis and thus require a smaller catheter than might otherwise be typical for their age. Whereas difficult catheterization in the adult male may result from prostatic hypertrophy, urethral obstruction in a young boy may indicate the presence of post-traumatic urethral stricture or congenital anomalies.

In the young female child, the urethra is short and generally easy to catheterize once the orifice is visualized. However, the opening is in close proximity to the vaginal introitus, and the mucosa of the introitus may cover the urethral meatus, making it difficult to locate (Fig. 95.2) (4). It may be noted that gentle lateral traction of the labia and gentle downward pressure on the cephalad aspect of the vaginal introital fold with a sterile cotton-tipped applicator allows visualization of the infantile female urethral meatus more readily (Fig. 95.3) (4). Alternatively, gently grasping the labia between thumb and forefinger and applying gentle lateral and outward traction (toward the clinician) may expose the urethral meatus (Fig. 95.4). Two additional considerations may complicate urethral visualization in girls. Female hypospadias results when the meatus opens into the distal anterior wall of the vagina. A catheter with a curved tip (coudé) may allow catheterization, usually just inside the introitus on the roof of the vagina. Additionally, labial adhesions may be present in infant girls. In this context, another technique, such as suprapubic aspiration, is generally preferred for simple collection of urine.

▶ INDICATIONS

The most common indication for catheterizing a young child in the ED or ambulatory setting is the need to obtain a sterile urine specimen for laboratory analysis with culture and sensitivity (1). In infants and small children with suspected urinary tract infection, no localizing signs of fever, or possible sepsis,

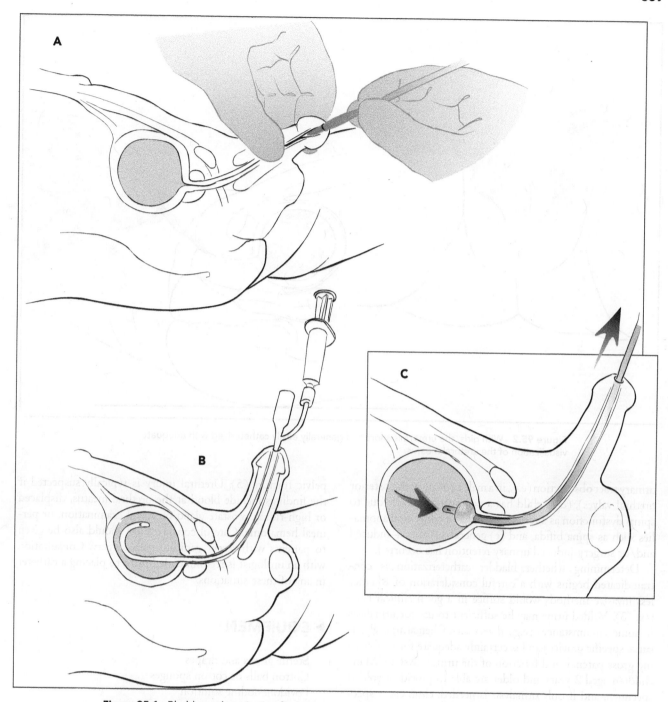

Figure 95.1 Bladder catheterization for boys.
A. The catheter is advanced gently with the penis held perpendicular to the suprapubic abdominal wall.
B. The catheter is fully advanced before an attempt is made to inflate the balloon.
C. The catheter is withdrawn slowly after balloon inflation until it sits against the trigone.

a sterile urine specimen is paramount to reaching a diagnosis. Commonly, either bladder catheterization or suprapubic aspiration is used. The latter procedure is considered by many authorities to be the gold standard for obtaining bacteriologically uncontaminated specimens; however, it is frequently unsuccessful with small bladder volumes of urine, which are common in ill or dehydrated infants (1). Other common indications for catheterization include preventing or relieving

urinary retention and close monitoring of urine output for fluid balance with an indwelling urinary catheter in the critically ill or injured child. Catheterization is also indicated on occasion in situations in which (a) urgent cystourethrography needs to be performed, (b) a child is suffering from contusions or burns (scald, flame, or chemical) to the perineum and thus at risk for meatal swelling and obstruction to urine outflow, (c) a temporizing measure is required to relieve lower

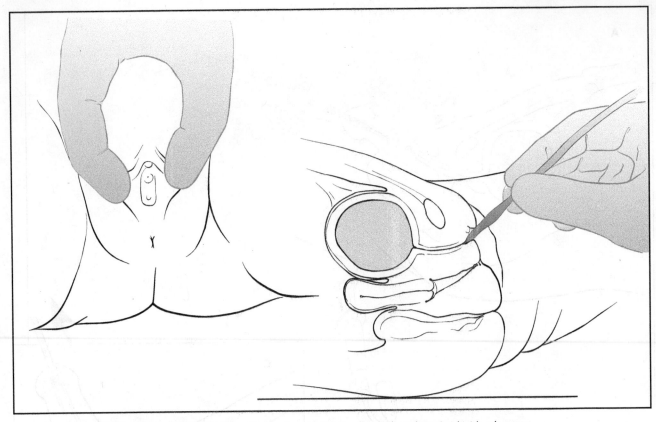

Figure 95.2 With girls, the urethra is short and generally easily catheterized with adequate visualization of the urethral meatus.

urinary tract obstruction (e.g., in a male neonate with posterior urethral valves), (d) a child has a neurogenic bladder due to spinal dysfunction as a result of trauma or congenital anomalies such as spina bifida, and (e) general anesthesia–induced and/or surgery-induced urinary retention has occurred.

Determining whether bladder catheterization is contraindicated begins with a careful consideration of whether less invasive methods would suffice in a given clinical context (3). Voided urine may be sufficient to use for urinalysis in some circumstances (e.g., detection of hematuria, glycosuria, specific gravity) and is certainly adequate for establishing gross patency and function of the urinary system. Many children aged 2 years and older are able to provide a voided specimen, and if only urinalysis is needed, clean catch specimens are usually adequate. Documentation of physiologic urine production (e.g., after intravenous hydration) can be accomplished in many patients by simply placing an adherent plastic urine bag on the child after adequately prepping the perineum. In the dehydrated child, invasive methods of obtaining urine should be postponed for 60 to 90 minutes after initiating intravenous hydration to allow for some bladder filling. Otherwise, a highly concentrated few milliliters of "sludge" will be obtained, rendering a urinalysis difficult to interpret and often necessitating a subsequent attempt at catheterization.

The primary absolute contraindication to placement of a catheter is trauma with possible urethral injury, such as a pelvic fracture (5). Urethral injury is typically suspected if the findings include blood at the urethral meatus, displaced or high-riding prostate gland on rectal examination, or perineal hematoma. Careful consideration should also be given to patients with recent genitourinary surgery. Consultation with an urologist is recommended prior to placing a catheter in any of these situations.

▶ EQUIPMENT

Sterile gloves and drapes
Cotton balls or cotton sponges
Povidone-iodine solution
Forceps
Lubricant
Catheter
Specimen collection cup
Connectible drainage bag and tubing (if desired)
Local anesthetic (if desired)

Most hospitals today use preassembled catheterization equipment trays (Fig. 95.5). Appropriate urinary catheter sizes are age and size dependent (see Table 6.2). The neonate can usually be catheterized with a 5 French feeding tube, while 8 French catheters are typically used in infants and 10 to 12 French catheters in older children. An extra specimen cup

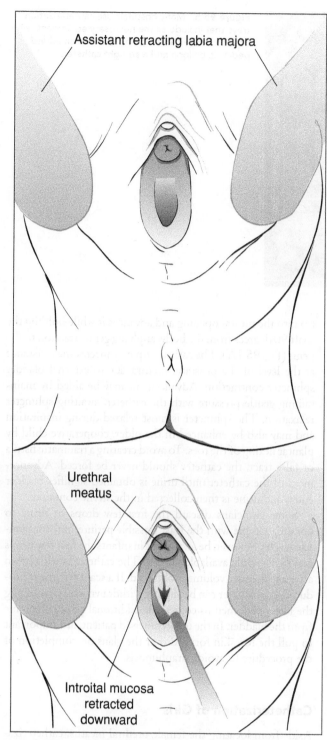

Figure 95.3 Applying gentle lateral traction to the labia with simultaneous downward traction applied to the introital mucosa may better expose the female urethral meatus.

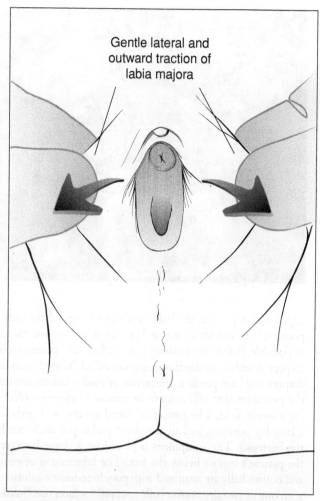

Figure 95.4 The female urethral meatus also may be exposed in some girls by gentle simultaneous lateral, outward, and upward traction on the labia majora.

Latex allergy is common in spina bifida patients, and thus latex-free equipment should be available particularly for this population.

▶ PROCEDURE

Verbal consent should be obtained and the procedure explained carefully to the caretaker and child, in age-appropriate language, avoiding medical jargon and anatomic terms (Chapter 9). Intermittent catheterization should be a quick procedure, with rare complications given adequate assistance, proper equipment, and appropriate restraint of and/or cooperation from the patient. A history of any previous difficulties with catheterization suggesting aberrant anatomy as well as a history of latex or iodine allergy should be sought.

Sterile technique is used throughout (Chapter 7). The catheterization tray is opened and inspected for appropriate contents, and any necessary equipment and assistance are gathered. The catheter should be examined for defects or sharp

may allow the discarding of the first few drops of collected urine, if sufficient quantity is present, so as to get the most uncontaminated specimen possible for microbiologic testing (6). An assistant is usually necessary with female infants and young children of either gender.

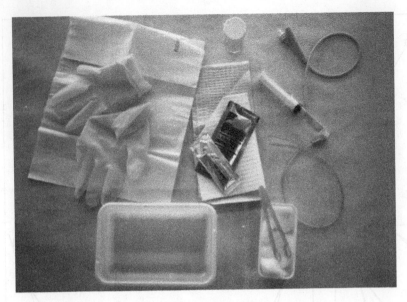

Figure 95.5 Many hospitals use catheterization trays that include all the necessary equipment, with or without the catheter. Photo shows an added pediatric balloon and a straight catheter.

edges, and if present, the balloon should be tested for competency. Curtains are drawn and privacy maintained as much as possible. Before establishing a sterile field, the perineum is inspected and the urethral opening identified. Many babies in diapers will have powder, ointments, or medicated creams on the perineum that will need to be removed before establishing a sterile field. The patient is placed supine, with girls in a frog-leg position, and an absorbent pad is put underneath the buttocks. The equipment is placed on a drape between the patient's legs or below the feet. The lubricant is opened and cotton balls are saturated with povidone-iodine solution, with one or two dry cotton balls reserved for later use. Sterile anesthetic (2% lidocaine hydrochloride jelly) can be used to locally anesthetize the area. Typically a soaked cotton ball is held over the urethral opening for 2 minutes, after which 0.5 to 2.0 cc of anesthetic is injected into the urethra, with 2 minutes allowed for it to take effect. This may be repeated two additional times for maximum anesthesia (7). Sterile drapes are placed on the perineum, with exposure of the genitalia. Direct over-the-shoulder lighting is a helpful adjunct for identifying the urethra in girls.

Catheterization of Boys

Intermittent catheterization is performed with a single-lumen (straight) catheter. Insertion of an indwelling catheter is described later in this section. For circumcised patients, the clinician holds the penis using the nondominant hand and swabs the glans and urethral meatus with povidone-iodine–saturated cotton held in tweezers or forceps. The dominant hand is maintained in sterile condition. In the uncircumcised patient, the foreskin is gently retracted, if possible, for cleaning and visualization of the meatus. Holding the catheter in the form of a loop will help to minimize contamination of the proximal part of the catheter via inadvertent contact with nonsterile areas. The clinician inserts the lubricated catheter

tip into the meatal opening and advances it while holding the shaft 90 degrees from the body, applying gentle traction to the penis (Fig. 95.1A). The catheter tip may meet some resistance at the level of the prostatic urethra due to external bladder sphincter contraction. Advancement may be aided by maintaining gentle pressure with the catheter, awaiting sphincter relaxation. The sphincter is most relaxed during inspiration and may also be enhanced in the older, cooperative child by plantar flexing of the toes. To avoid creating a traumatic fistula or false tract, the catheter should never be forced. Advancement of the catheter until urine is obtained signifies bladder entry, and urine is then collected in the sterile container.

Some clinicians discard the first few drops of urine to obtain a sample with the least possible periurethral contamination (6); however, be aware that in infants the first few drops may be the only available sample. The catheter is withdrawn after an adequate volume is obtained. If a scant volume is produced, the catheter can be slightly withdrawn while massaging the lower abdomen to coax some additional residual volume from the bladder. In the uncircumcised patient, it is important to pull the foreskin forward over the glans on completion of the procedure to avoid paraphimosis.

Catheterization of Girls

Aside from locating the female urethral meatus, catheterization of the female patient is often easier than that of the male patient. If the vagina is unintentionally catheterized, leaving the catheter in place might serve as a useful landmark during further attempts at locating the urethra. The female patient is positioned supine, with privacy maintained, while the necessary equipment and assistance are arranged. The perineum is prepared with sequential swabbing using a cotton ball and antiseptic from anterior to posterior. If an assistant is not available, the clinician uses the nondominant hand to keep the labia separated while inserting the lubricated catheter tip until urine is obtained (Fig. 95.2).

Indwelling Catheters

Indwelling bladder catheters have an expandable balloon near the distal tip to help secure them in the bladder. General preparation for catheterization is the same as for the intermittent procedure. The catheter balloon should be tested for competence before insertion by sequential filling with the recommended volume of sterile saline, observing for leakage, and then withdrawing saline to ensure complete emptying of the balloon. When inserting the catheter into the bladder, the balloon should be expanded only when urine flow is established and the catheter has been further advanced its full length to the Y-connector. The clinician thereby avoids inadvertent injury to the proximal urethra by an improperly positioned balloon (Fig. 95.1B). After balloon expansion, the catheter should be withdrawn until gentle resistance indicates that the balloon is positioned at the bladder neck (Fig. 95.1C). The catheter is then taped securely to the patient's leg and connected to a closed collecting system. In the combative child or adolescent, manual restraints and/or temporary sedation may be required to prevent urethral trauma.

▶ COMPLICATIONS

Unfavorable outcomes are generally rare and avoidable. These include inflicting urethral or bladder injury (8,9) or exacerbating existing injury by forceful passage of the catheter or failure to deflate the balloon. Failure to restore a retracted foreskin to its normal position may lead to paraphimosis, and infection may be introduced by failure to adhere to sterile procedure (3,10). Each of these complications may be anticipated and can be largely avoided by adherence to the methods described in this chapter. For most intermittent diagnostic catheterizations, the catheter is inserted for such a short time that infection is a rarely seen complication. Retained indwelling catheters may be due to intravesical knotting or balloon failure (3,11,12). A knotted catheter, often the result of coiling within the bladder, may be removed by passing a guidewire through the main lumen. Consultation with urology may be necessary if this technique is unsuccessful. Failure of a balloon to deflate is usually due to a flap valve defect in the inflating lumen or to syringe adaptor malfunction (3). A reasonable first course of action is to remove the adaptor plug, which may allow the saline from the balloon to flow out. If that is unsuccessful, a fine vascular access guidewire is gently passed, with rotation, through the inflating channel in an effort to disrupt the presumed flap valve defect. If this fails, the next step would be to cut the catheter off a few centimeters from the urethra in hope that the defect was external (distal) to the cut. If the balloon does not immediately deflate, it is then necessary to carefully attach a new, sterile, closed collecting system and to consult a urologist.

 SUMMARY

1 Provide a careful explanation of the relevant anatomy and procedural technique to the patient and family and seek a history of latex or iodine allergy.

2 Maintain strict adherence to sterile technique.

3 Inspect and test the catheter tip (and balloon) before insertion.

4 In boys, gently retract the foreskin as necessary and pull it back over the glans after completing the procedure.

5 In boys, hold the penis with gentle traction away from and perpendicular to the lower abdomen while advancing the catheter.

6 In girls, achieve visualization of the urethral meatus with gentle traction on the labia and/or downward displacement of the cephalad aspect of the vaginal introital fold with a cotton-tipped applicator.

7 With an indwelling catheter, it is important to advance the catheter well into the bladder before balloon inflation to avoid the urethral injury that would occur if the balloon were inadvertently placed in the proximal urethra.

 CLINICAL TIPS

▶ The physician should anticipate some patient and family anxiety related to urinary catheterization.

▶ It is often convenient to have an extra pair of gloves and catheter available before beginning the procedure in the event of inadvertent contamination.

▶ Latex allergy is common in patients with spina bifida and should be anticipated.

▶ An assistant usually should be available to help position female infants and young children of either gender.

▶ If resistance is met in attempting to pass the catheter in a boy, slow, gentle pressure with accentuation during inhalation and plantar flexion of the toes may help.

▶ If the vagina is inadvertently entered when attempting catheterization of a female infant, leaving the vaginal catheter transiently in place may facilitate visualization of the anteriorly located urethral meatus.

▶ SUMMARY

Diagnostic bladder catheterization is an important technique for obtaining a sterile urine sample for microscopic analysis and culture in the non-toilet-trained young child. The same procedural principles apply for initiating continuous monitoring of urine flow in critically ill or injured children. Pediatric patients and families need a careful explanation of the relevant anatomy and procedural methods. Anatomic considerations in children include tight foreskin in uncircumcised male infants, difficult visualization of the urethral meatus, hypospadias, and labial adhesions in girls. Appropriate size catheters are age and size dependent. Several simple guidelines exist to ease visualization of the urethral meatus. A urinary catheter should never be forced because forcing it may lead to complications related to urethral trauma. Indwelling catheters pose additional concerns, including increased risk of infection and a retained catheter. Nevertheless, both intermittent urinary catheterizations and indwelling urinary catheterizations of children have proven to be safe procedures and should be integral components of every emergency department's routine pediatric protocols.

▶ ACKNOWLEDGMENTS

We would like to thank Drs. Douglas A. Boenning and Fred M. Henretig for their work on the version of this chapter that appeared in the previous edition.

▶ REFERENCES

1. Pollack CV, Pollack ES, Andrew ME. Suprapubic bladder aspiration versus urethral catheterization in ill infants: success, efficiency, and complication rates. *Ann Emerg Med.* 1994;23:225–230.
2. Wong DL. The child who is hospitalized. In: *Nursing Care of Infants and Children.* 5th ed. St. Louis: Mosby; 1995:1176–1177.
3. Zbaraschuk I, Berger RE, Hedges JR. Emergency urologic procedures. In: Roberts JR, Hedges JR, eds. *Clinical Procedures in Emergency Medicine.* Philadelphia: WB Saunders; 1991:867–874.
4. Redman JF, Bissada NK. Direct bladder catheterization in infant females and young girls. *Clin Pediatr.* 1976;15:1060–1061.
5. Feeman S, Chapman J. Urologic procedures. *Emerg Med Clin North Am.* 1986;4:543–560.
6. Peniakov M, Antonelli J, Naor O, et al. Reduction in contamination of urine samples obtained by in-out catheterization by culturing the later urine stream. *Pediatr Emerg Care.* 2004;20:418–419.
7. Gerard LL, Cooper CS, Duethman KS, et al. Effectiveness of lidocaine lubricant for discomfort during pediatric urethral catheterization. *J Urol.* 2003;170:564–567.
8. Campbell JB, Moore KN, Voaklander DC, et al. Complications associated with clean intermittent catheterization in children with spina bifida. *J Urol.* 2004;171:2420–2422.
9. Lindehall B, Abrahamsson K, Hjalmas K, et al. Complications of clean intermittent catheterization in boys and young males with neurogenic bladder dysfunction. *J Urol.* 2004;172:1686–1688.
10. Matlow AG, Wray RD, Cox PN. Nosocomial urinary tract infections in children in a pediatric intensive care unit: a follow-up after 10 years. *Pediatr Crit Care Med.* 2003;4:74–77.
11. Kanengiser S, Juster F, Kogan S, et al. Knotting of a bladder catheter. *Pediatr Emerg Care.* 1989;5:37–39.
12. Turner TWS. Intravesical catheter knotting: an uncommon complication of urinary catheterization. *Pediatr Emerg Care.* 2004;20:115–117.

KATHLEEN M. CRONAN AND STEPHEN A. ZDERIC

96

Manual Detorsion of the Testes

▶ INTRODUCTION

Testicular torsion occurs when a testis rotates on the vascular pedicle, producing sharp pain secondary to ischemia. A final diagnosis of testicular torsion will be made in 20% to 25% of children presenting with acute scrotal pain. The differential diagnosis includes torsion of the testicular appendage, epididymitis, incarcerated inguinal hernia, and trauma. Clinicians should not be misled by a history of testicular trauma, which is often obtained in children with testicular torsion.

Time is of the essence, because many patients present after enduring ischemic pain for 12 or more hours. Studies suggest that the gonadal salvage rate is lower in the adolescent patient, which is felt to be secondary to patient delay in seeking medical attention (1). It is for this reason that manual detorsion of the testis can be quite useful as a temporizing therapeutic maneuver until surgeon and operating room availability is confirmed. Surgery should follow for definitive open surgical reduction and orchiopexy.

▶ ANATOMY AND PHYSIOLOGY

Testicular torsion occurs in children with testes that are not adequately fixed by the tunica vaginalis to the posterior scrotal wall. This "bell-clapper" deformity enables the testicle and spermatic cord to twist, causing either partial or complete obstruction of venous outflow and/or arterial inflow via the spermatic vessels. It is thought that after 8 hours of warm ischemia, there is an increased likelihood of testicular atrophy. However, gonadal salvage may still be possible after a period of prolonged symptoms if the obstruction is incomplete or intermittent.

Testicular torsion results in the triad of acute diffuse scrotal pain, a high-riding testicle, and an absent cremasteric reflex.

This triad occurs because twisting of the spermatic cord results in a retraction of the testis back toward the pubic tubercle. The twisting rotation shortens the cremasteric muscle fibers, leaving them unable to exert their normal pulling action, which forms the basis for the valuable cremasteric reflex test. Stroking the inner thigh causes stimulation that results in the cremasteric reflex, which is a sudden brisk upward deflection of the testicle (Fig. 96.1). This sign, if present, almost always excludes spermatic cord torsion in the acute setting (2). However, a case report does describe the presence of a cremasteric reflex in a patient with surgically confirmed testicular torsion, cites two other such cases, and thus serves as a reminder that this diagnosis should not be excluded entirely on one criterion alone (3). It must be stressed, however, that many normal male patients will not have a positive cremasteric reflex; hence this sign is helpful only if it is present. The deflection must be upward, and it must be significant (1 to 2 cm) to have the optimal reliability. Stroking the thigh may produce a wrinkling of the scrotal skin as the underlying dartos muscle contracts, and the inexperienced observer may mistake this for a cremasteric reflex. When testicular torsion is present, examination of the testis will reveal a tense and extremely tender gonad, with no ability to discriminate between the epididymis and the testis. On occasion, if the patient has been symptomatic for longer than 1 day, the pain may lessen over time as the infarction proceeds.

Testicular torsion is a clinical diagnosis, and the patient should be seen as quickly as possible by a urologist. For the patient with classic torsion who is seen and evaluated in the emergency department (ED) setting, no further testing is needed, and operative reduction and orchiopexy must occur. In many instances, with experienced ED and urology staff, the child is directed immediately to the operating room (OR), with no further testing. If the OR team is not assembled or OR time is not immediately available, manual detorsion can be performed to "buy time" until the OR and personnel

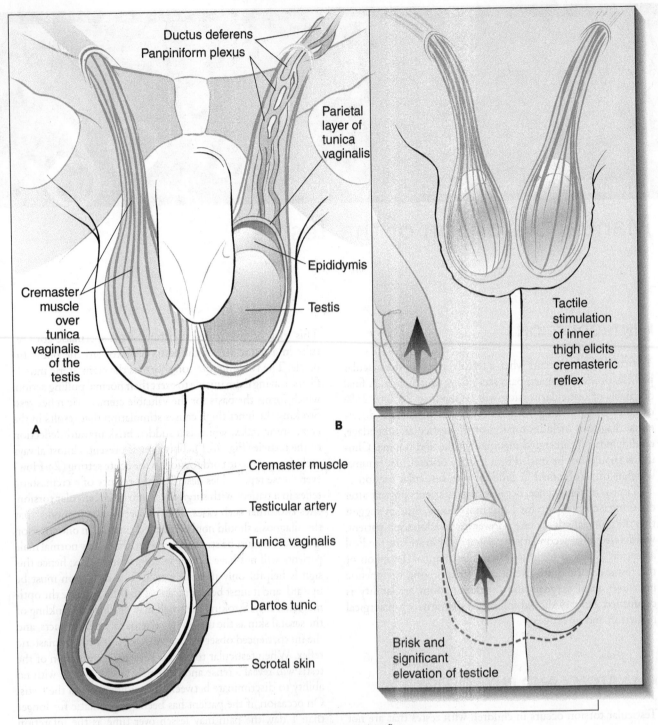

Figure 96.1 Normal scrotal anatomy and the cremasteric reflex.
A. The testes and epididymis are enveloped within the tunica vaginalis. Attached to the testes and epididymis are the gonadal artery and vein within the cremaster muscle fibers.
B. Stroking the inner thigh produces shortening of the cremaster muscle, with upward excursion of the gonad. This shortening should be significant (1 to 2 cm) so as to not be confused with simple wrinkling of the dartos muscle.

become available. Often the child presents with an equivocal history or the pain has lasted more than 12 hours, making the physical examination less reliable (4). In this setting the physicians, after a careful history and physical examination, often opt to obtain a Doppler flow ultrasound study to confirm that there is blood flow to the testis (5). With the improved spatial resolution and accuracy of Doppler sonography, this is a reasonable option. It is essential, however, that the sonographers be experienced in the use of such imaging technology, that the flow be clearly demonstrated within the testis itself, and that

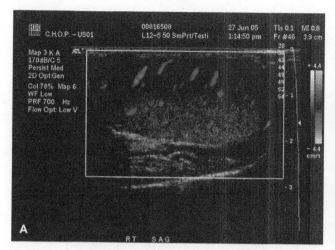

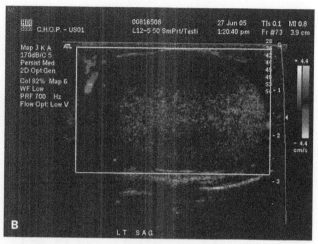

Figure 96.2

A. This Doppler ultrasound shows high flow to the testes with a normal arterial wave form pattern, thus excluding torsion as a cause of the patient's scrotal pain.

B. This ultrasound shows blood flow to the scrotal wall but none to the testes. The quality of the waveform is poor, indicating that this may represent venous flow to the scrotal wall. This patient was shown to have torsion at the time of exploration.

a clear and unequivocal arterial waveform be demonstrated (Fig. 96.2A). False-positive tests for blood flow to the testes have been reported that upon closer inspection are shown to represent flow to the inflamed scrotal wall (Fig. 96.2B).

▶ INDICATIONS

Manual detorsion of the testis may be used to acutely relieve the ischemic pain in patients with testicular torsion. It is highly effective if used early in the course (before 8 hours of symptoms). Manual detorsion is almost never successful after prolonged ischemia because the swelling and edema become so marked. If urologic consultation is unavailable or will be significantly delayed, the emergency physician, pediatrician, or family physician may attempt this maneuver. If the urologist will be arriving within a short period, he or she should be allowed to examine the patient before manual detorsion occurs.

A urologist should be consulted regarding any case of acute scrotal pain in a child. Detorsion is indicated only if the etiology of the acute scrotum is thought to be torsion of the spermatic cord. Although attempting this maneuver in the presence of epididymitis or torsion of the appendix testis will probably not produce any harm, it will be extremely painful and yield no benefit to the patient.

▶ EQUIPMENT (OPTIONAL)

Intravenous catheter
Opiate analgesic medications (e.g., morphine, fentanyl)
Anxiolytic medication (midazolam)

▶ PROCEDURE

Testes twist with inward rotation in 70% of all cases of testicular ttorsion, and the average number of twists in the cord is two (720 degrees) (6). Thus, a successful detorsion must involve gently grasping and rotating the testicle within the scrotum in an *outward* direction in a series of 360-degree twists (Fig. 96.3). A dose of intravenous analgesic and/or short-acting anxiolytic to blunt the discomfort of detorsion may help the child cooperate and minimize the pain from the procedure. This practice is unlikely to confuse the clinical presentation in cases when the pain is severe. Manual detorsion often produces brief discomfort, followed by relief of pain that is almost instantaneous. Often, after initiating the detorsion maneuver, the testicle flips over into the normal configuration.

Following successful detorsion, orchiopexy should not be delayed despite relief of symptoms. Often, even after a clinically successful detorsion, exploratory surgery reveals a 180-degree twist, with persistent venous congestion. Some have advocated that manual detorsion, when successful, should be the primary treatment for testicular torsion and that orchiopexy may then be scheduled "electively" (7). When considering the possibility that a patient who suddenly improves may not return for follow-up and the potential consequences of not returning, we believe the urologist should proceed with scrotal exploration as soon as an operating room is available. Admission to the hospital for observation while waiting 2 to 4 hours for OR time is certainly preferable to gonadal loss.

▶ COMPLICATIONS

Other than discomfort, there are no notable complications of manual detorsion. Failure of manual detorsion does not worsen the ischemia of the gonad. It is imperative, however,

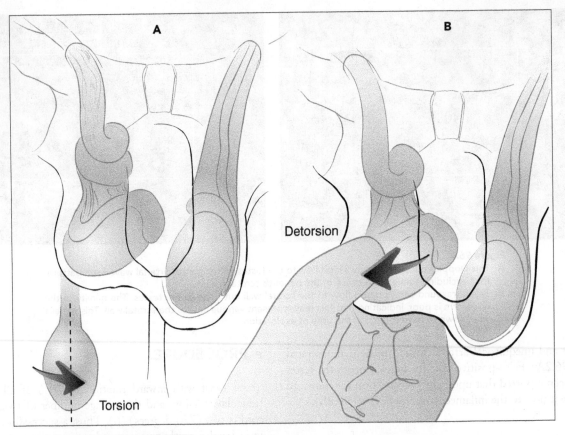

Figure 96.3 Manual detorsion.
A. Torsion of the testis with two inward twists has resulted in a new high-lying position.
B. The testis is grasped with the fingers and rotated outwardly with two full 360-degree twists.

 SUMMARY

1 The triad of acute scrotal pain, a high-riding testis, and an absent cremasteric reflex suggest testicular torsion.

2 Always seek urologic consultation for initial assessment and follow-up.

3 Manual detorsion may be successful and of value in the first 8 to 12 hours of symptoms.

4 Administer intravenous analgesia and/or anxiolytic.

5 Torsion almost always occurs with inward or internal rotation: rotate the testis within the scrotum in an outward direction one or two 360-degree turns.

6 Prompt relief of pain and return to normal position in the scrotum suggest successful detorsion.

7 Following successful detorsion, surgical exploration and orchiopexy should proceed as soon as possible.

 CLINICAL TIPS

▶ Torsion involves an average of two 360-degree inward twists.

▶ A positive cremasteric reflex usually excludes testicular torsion, but rare exceptions are reported. An absent cremasteric reflex does not confirm this diagnosis.

▶ Detorsion results in relief of pain and a normal configuration of the scrotum.

▶ Urologic consultation is vital and urgent for patients with suspected testicular torsion. Scrotal exploration is always indicated after manual detorsion.

that manual detorsion be viewed as a temporizing measure before surgical intervention. If the physician or patient does not fully understand this, the patient may be lost to follow-up and suffer a subsequent torsion of the testicle.

▶ SUMMARY

In most large metropolitan areas, prompt urologic consultation is available to assess children with acute scrotal pain. In other areas, transfer of the child to another facility may be necessary. Testicular torsion is an emergency in which duration of symptoms before treatment is inversely related to success in gonadal salvage. Manual detorsion can temporarily re-establish perfusion to the testis and may be safely used in the emergency setting when rapid consultation is unavailable. Definitive surgical therapy is always indicated in children with testicular torsion.

▶ REFERENCES

1. Barada JH, Weingarten JL, Cromie WJ. Testicular salvage and age-related delay in the presentation of testicular torsion. *J Urol.* 1989;142: 746–748.
2. Kadish HA, Bolte RG. A retrospective review of pediatric patients with epididymitis, testicular torsion, and torsion of testicular appendages. *Pediatrics.* 1998;102:73–76.
3. Nelson CP, Williams JF, Bloom DA. The cremasteric reflex: a useful but imperfect sign in testicular torsion. *J Ped Surg.* 2003;38: 1248–1249.
4. Kass EJ, Lundak B. The acute scrotum. *Pediatr Clin North Am.* 1997;44: 1251–1266.
5. Galejs LE, Kass EJ. Color Doppler ultrasound evaluation of the acute scrotum. *Tech Urol.* 1998;4:182–184.
6. Sessions AE, Rabinowitz R, Hulbert WC, et al. Testicular torsion: direction, degree, duration and disinformation. *J Urol.* 2003;169: 663–635.
7. Cornel EB, Karthaus HF. Manual derotation of the twisted spermatic cord. *BJU Int.* 1999;83:672–674.

97

JAMES F. PARKER

Management of Priapism

▶ INTRODUCTION

Priapism is defined as a sustained, unwanted, painful erection that continues hours beyond or is unrelated to sexual stimulation. It is characterized by a soft glans penis and spongy urethra in the presence of two erect corpora cavernosa.

Priapism is a relatively uncommon complaint presenting to the emergency department (ED). While the incidence of priapism in the general male population is reported as 1.5 episodes per 100,000 person years, children with sickle cell disease have an incidence in the range of 6% to 27% (1).

Priapism is a true urologic emergency that requires urgent intervention to avoid irreversible ischemic penile injury, scarring, and impotence. Numerous modes of therapy have been utilized in the treatment of priapism, with variable success. However, these therapies are not predictably effective at relieving priapism and may delay procedures that allow reperfusion of the corpora cavernosa.

▶ ANATOMY AND PHYSIOLOGY

The anatomy of the penis is shown in Figure 97.1. The penis consists of the two lateral corpora cavernosa, each with a centrally located deep artery and surrounded by the tunica albuginea. Located within the ventral aspect of the penis is the urethra, which is surrounded by the corpus spongiosum. These structures are enclosed within the Buck fascia, a septum of which also separates the corpus spongiosum from the corpora cavernosa. Of particular importance in the discussion of the treatment of priapism are the structures located in the dorsal aspect of the penis. The subcutaneous dorsal vein and the deep dorsal vein course along the midline of the penis. Immediately lateral to the deep dorsal vein are the dorsal artery and the dorsal nerve, structures that must be avoided when attempting aspiration of the penis during priapism. Finally, one must be aware of the lateral superficial veins of the penis, which are depicted in the illustration in approximately the 11 o'clock and 1 o'clock positions.

Physiologically, priapism is engorgement of the corpora cavernosa, resulting in dorsal penile erection with a relatively flaccid ventral penis and glans (Fig. 97.2). This engorgement may be the result of many factors, depending on the etiology of the priapism. Perhaps the most common etiology in the pediatric population is sickle cell disease, which accounts for 28% of all cases. Up to 64% of male patients with sickle cell disease will develop priapism at some point in their lives (2). Additional hematologic causes of priapism include anemia, leukemia, and multiple myeloma.

Other sources of priapism include pharmacologic agents (antihypertensives, psychotropic medications, hormones, etc.), illicit drug use (cocaine, marijuana), trauma, infectious agents (rabies, malaria), neurologic causes (cerebrovascular accidents, spinal stenosis), bladder tumors, black widow spider envenomation, and carbon monoxide poisoning (3).

Priapism can be classified into two types: low flow and high flow. The distinguishing characteristic between these two types is whether there is too much inflow of blood to the corpora or not enough outflow of blood from the corpora. Low-flow priapism (also referred to as "ischemic priapism" and "veno-occlusive priapism") is caused by little or no cavernous blood flow, resulting in the accumulation of hypoxic, hypercarbic blood. In this form of priapism, the corpora are rigid and tender to palpation. High-flow priapism is usually the result of trauma that causes unregulated inflow of arterial blood into the corpora. This results in corpora that are not fully rigid and are usually not painful (4). The best ways to distinguish between these two types are to use color duplex ultrasound and to measure blood gases from the corpora (2).

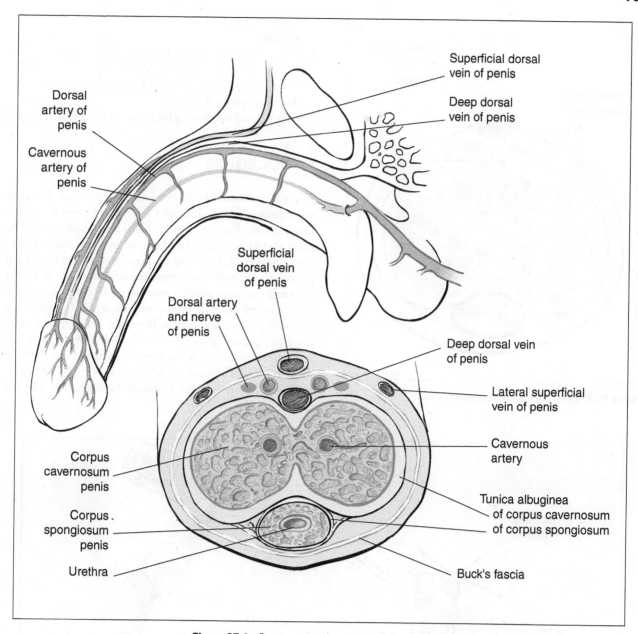

Figure 97.1 Cross-sectional anatomy of the penis.

▶ INDICATIONS

Not all cases of priapism require aspiration and irrigation. The goals of therapy should be to abort the erection, treat pain, and prevent long-term damage to the corpora. Often, treatment of the underlying cause of priapism will resolve the problem. However, it is important to remember that delaying definitive therapy may result in increased risk of long-term sequelae (including impotence). This risk increases dramatically if the erection is not resolved within 12 hours of onset.

Aspiration and irrigation may be indicated in cases of ischemic priapism, particularly if the erection has persisted for more than 6 hours. Aspiration should be performed in any case of ischemic priapism that has not responded to less invasive measures (3).

While the procedure should ideally be performed by a urologist, treatment should not be significantly delayed. An experienced emergency medicine physician is also capable of performing aspiration and irrigation.

▶ EQUIPMENT

Lidocaine for penile block (without epinephrine)
Appropriate needle for penile block
21 G or 19 G butterfly needle
10-cc syringes
Three-way stopcock
Sterile saline
Sterile gloves

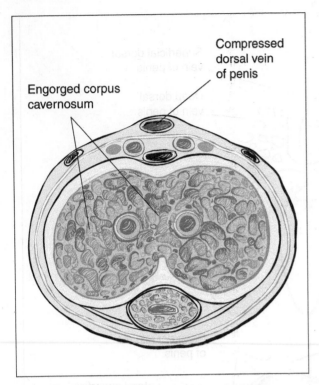

Figure 97.2 Pathophysiology of priapism.

Sterile towels

Betadine

Dilute solution of epinephrine or phenylephrine:
  Phenylephrine, 10 mg in 500 mL normal saline (1,3)
  Epinephrine, 1 mg in 1,000 mL normal saline (3,5)
Restraint system if needed
Supplies and monitoring for procedural sedation if needed

▶ PROCEDURE

The patient should be placed in supine position. Procedural sedation, if needed, should be initiated prior to further manipulation. Perform a penile block (see Chapter 35). The penis should be prepped and draped in sterile fashion. The physician should then grasp the penis in one gloved hand and palpate the engorged corpora cavernosa laterally. A 19- or 21-gauge butterfly needle (attached to a 10-mL syringe) is then inserted into one of the corpora at the 10 o'clock or 2 o'clock position approximately midway between the base of the penis and the glans (Fig. 97.3). Only one corpus needs to be punctured, as there are numerous anastomoses between the two sides. The needle is advanced slowly at a 45-degree angle while aspirating with the attached syringe. Once blood is

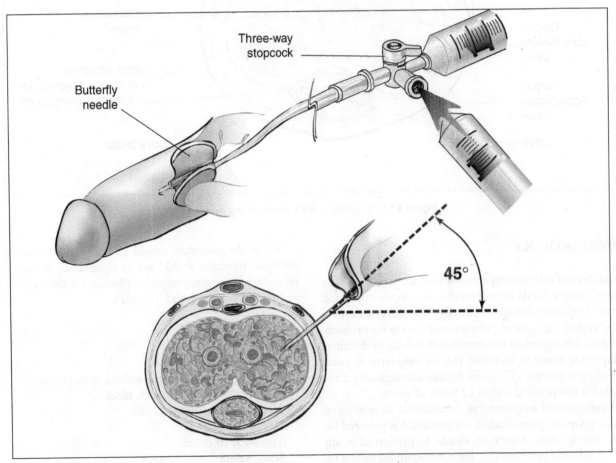

Figure 97.3 Aspiration (and irrigation, as needed) of the corpus cavernosum.

obtained, the needle is no longer advanced. The stopcock is then attached to the butterfly needle, and blood is aspirated from the corpora into dry 10-mL syringes with one hand while the corpus is milked with the other hand (1,3). Blood may be sent for blood gas analysis at this time to confirm the ischemic etiology of the priapism. If there is complete resolution of the erection, no further treatment may be necessary.

If, however, the erection persists or there is concern for retained blood, irrigation should be performed. To perform irrigation, a 10-mL syringe filled with the dilute solution of phenylephrine or epinephrine should be attached to the stopcock. The irrigation solution may then be introduced into the penis in 10-mL aliquots and then aspirated into dry 10-mL syringes (5). If the erection persists beyond this intervention, further surgical procedures may be necessary.

Once the erection has resolved, the needle may be withdrawn. Direct pressure should then be applied for a minimum of 5 minutes to prevent the formation of a hematoma. The patient should be observed for at least 1 hour following the procedure to assess for recurrence of priapism.

▶ COMPLICATIONS

The most common complication of aspiration of the corpus cavernosum is the development of an intrapenile hematoma. This risk can be minimized by providing direct pressure to the puncture site for at least 5 minutes after completion of the procedure. Some patients, particularly those with underlying medical conditions, may develop prolonged or excessive bleeding. Direct pressure should be continued in these patients until bleeding has stopped.

SUMMARY

1 Obtain a 19- or 21-gauge butterfly needle, 10-mL syringes, three-way stopcock, sterile saline, and phenylephrine or epinephrine.

2 Perform a penile block; use sedation if needed.

3 Prepare the penis in sterile fashion.

4 Palpate the engorged corpora cavernosa, insert a needle into the midshaft at the 2 o'clock or 10 o'clock position. Aspirate as the needle is advanced.

5 Aspirate 20 to 30 mL of blood into dry syringes. Consider blood gas analysis of the aspirated sample.

6 If not fully resolved, irrigate with 10-mL aliquots of dilute phenylephrine or epinephrine solution.

7 Apply direct pressure to the puncture site for at least 5 minutes after withdrawing the needle.

8 Monitor the patient for at least 1 hour for recurrence.

CLINICAL TIPS

▶ Strongly consider procedural sedation.

▶ The procedure is usually done by a urologist but may be initiated by an ED physician if specialist consultation is not available or is delayed.

▶ Avoid the dorsal aspect of the penis (veins, arteries, nerves).

▶ Aspirate as the needle is advanced to avoid damage to deeper structures.

Special care must be used to avoid damage to the nerves, arteries, and veins that traverse the dorsum of the penis. Puncture of these structures may result in future erectile difficulties as well as loss of sensation. One should also be careful to avoid puncture of the urethra, which could result in the development of a fistula.

As with any invasive procedure, there is a risk of introducing infection into the tissues. Care must be taken to maintain sterile conditions.

If irrigation is performed, the phenylephrine or epinephrine being used is essentially being infused intravascularly, and patients should be monitored closely for toxic effects of these medications. At the concentrations and volumes recommended, adverse reactions are rare.

▶ SUMMARY

Priapism is a relatively infrequent complaint presenting to the ED. It is, however, a surgical emergency comparable to compartment syndrome and therefore should be managed accordingly. Proper management of these patients in the ED can minimize long-term complications of priapism. Aspiration and irrigation is a useful clinical skill for the emergency medicine physician.

▶ REFERENCES

1. Vilke GM, Harrigan RA, Ufberg JW, et al. Emergency evaluation and treatment of priapism. *J Emerg Med.* 2004;26:325–329.
2. Walsh PC, Retik AB, Vaughn ED Jr, et al., eds. *Campbell's Urology.* 8th ed. Philadelphia: WB Saunders; 2002:1611–1613, 1661–1663.
3. Roberts JR, Hedges JR, Chanmugam AS, eds. *Clinical Procedures in Emergency Medicine.* 4th ed. Philadelphia: WB Saunders; 2004:1079–1084.
4. Monatgue DK, Jarow J, Broderick GA, et al. American Urological Association guideline on the management of priapism. *J Urol.* 2003;170:1318–1324.
5. Mantadakis E, Ewalt DH, Cavender JD, et al. Outpatient penile aspiration and epinephrine irrigation for young patients with sickle cell anemia and prolonged priapism. *Blood.* 2000;95:78–82.

98

PATRICIA CHAMBERS

Paraphimosis Reduction

▶ INTRODUCTION

Paraphimosis describes the condition when the foreskin of an uncircumcised male is retracted behind the glans penis, with resultant edema. As swelling of the glans increases, the prepuce can no longer return to its anatomic position. This condition is considered a urologic emergency, as prompt reduction is necessary to alleviate further swelling and tissue compromise (1).

Historically, paraphimosis reduction involved either manual reduction or surgical intervention via the dorsal slit technique. While these two modalities continue to be mainstays of definitive treatment, other methods of reduction have gained acceptance. Regardless of the method chosen, prompt recognition and treatment is crucial in preventing further swelling and long-term sequelae.

▶ ANATOMY AND PHYSIOLOGY

Paraphimosis occurs exclusively in the partially circumcised or the uncircumcised male. The uncircumcised penis is composed of the penile shaft, the coronal sulcus, the glans penis, and the foreskin. In a prepubertal population, the foreskin becomes increasingly mobile. In the mature penis, the foreskin can normally be retracted to expose the glans. Paraphimosis occurs when the foreskin is retracted proximal to the glans penis behind the coronal sulcus (2). This often occurs in a health care setting with preparation of the penis for catheterization. It can also occur with daily cleaning. Less often, paraphimosis has been reported with body piercing or sexual activity (1,2).

After the foreskin is trapped behind the coronal sulcus, swelling ensues. This swelling results in a tightening ring around the glans. Further edema, with impairment of ve-

nous and lymphatic drainage from the glans, leads to increased swelling (3,4). The resultant pressure can cause tissue ischemia and, if unrecognized, can ultimately result in infection or autoamputation (3). Young children can experience acute urinary obstruction (1). Once recognized, it is imperative that the foreskin be reduced to restore blood flow to the glans and prepuce. The edema then rapidly resolves following reduction (5,6).

▶ INDICATIONS

Paraphimosis reduction is indicated when the foreskin cannot be restored to its anatomic position. The penis should first be inspected and a history obtained to confirm the child is uncircumcised or partially circumcised. The genitals should be inspected for other causes of swelling, including circumferential foreign bodies such as hair or other objects (2). If a diagnosis of paraphimosis is confirmed, reduction techniques should be employed. In general, the least invasive method is first employed, with escalation of interventions as less aggressive measures fail.

▶ EQUIPMENT

Sterile gloves
Ice or compression dressing
Lubricant
Needles, syringes
Local anesthetic agent, lidocaine for injection or gel form
Babcock clamps
Gauze
Scalpel
Suture material

▶ PROCEDURE

Anxiety and pain are two key elements to consider in approaching paraphimosis reduction. Young children often require distraction or sedation to allow further interventions to successfully take place. Enlisting the help of the parents or a child-life specialist, if available, can greatly help in easing anxiety. If the child is still unable to cooperate, the use of sedative agents or restraints are then indicated (see Chapter 33).

Anesthesia for paraphimosis reduction can be achieved via several options. A dorsal penile nerve block (see Chapter 35) may be performed to allow manipulation. Another option is topical anesthesia using lidocaine gel. This must be applied in advance and covered in an occlusive dressing.

Manual reduction is the least invasive method. This method is best performed after reduction of swelling by a number of techniques. No prospective trials have been done to ascertain the best method of edema reduction. Therefore, local practice guidelines should dictate the method chosen (7). The easiest method is simply to apply circumferential pressure on the swollen glans and foreskin with the clinician's hand (Fig. 98.1). Constant gentle constriction alone can sometimes reduce the inflammation. If this fails, the use of ice packs to reduce swelling has been advocated. Granulated sugar applied to the edematous glans with an occlusive dressing can also be employed to reduce swelling. Sugar works by osmotic principles, drawing fluid out of the glans. Also advocated is the use of a compressive dressing. The penis is wrapped in rolled gauze or an ace wrap and frequently monitored (1).

After the tissue swelling has been minimized, manual reduction can be performed. The penis is held with the clinician's thumbs on the glans and the fingers behind the retracted prepuce. Slow, steady pressure is exerted to push the glans through the ring while the prepuce is gently pulled forward (Fig. 98.1). Adequate pain relief and anxiolysis is essential for achieving success by this method. Another approach to manual reduction involves the use of noncrushing Babcock clamps (Fig. 98.2). The clamps are applied to each quadrant of the foreskin and are used to pull the foreskin forward over the glans. This method allows for symmetrical traction of the foreskin (2).

Other methods to reduce paraphimosis include the puncture technique and the use of hyaluronidase. The puncture technique involves using a fine-gauge needle (21 gauge) to punch holes in the edematous foreskin to allow fluid to escape. This is done by first prepping the penis with antiseptic, then inserting the needle into the foreskin. Sources vary on the number of holes recommended. In general, the least number of punctures necessary to achieve decompression is suggested. After manually expressing the edema, the clinician then proceeds to replace the foreskin distally (2,8,9). The use of hyaluronidase causes the breakdown of hyaluronic acid, thus reducing tissue resistance and allowing substances to diffuse across tissue planes. It allows edematous fluid to be mobilized and expressed from the foreskin. Again, the penis is sterilely prepped. The hyaluronidase is injected into the prepuce using a tuberculin syringe. A volume of 1 cc is recommended. The fluid is then expressed out of the prepuce by manual reduction (10).

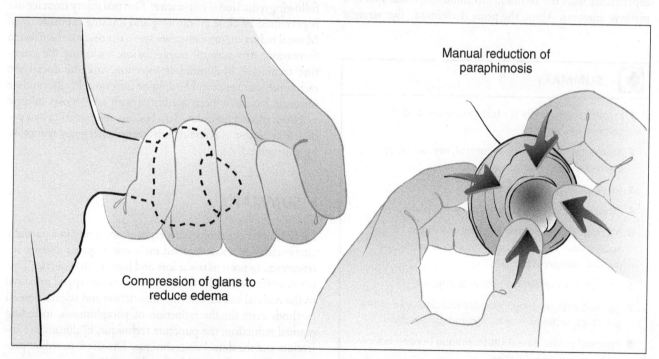

Compression of glans to reduce edema

Manual reduction of paraphimosis

Figure 98.1 With the thumbs on the glans penis and fingertips on the tight band of foreskin, the glans is pushed as the foreskin is pulled over the glans.

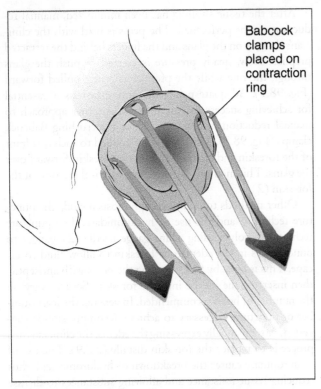

Babcock clamps placed on contraction ring

Figure 98.2 Noncrushing (Babcock) clamps are placed on the constricting portion of the foreskin in each quadrant. Gentle, continuous, equal traction is applied until reduction is achieved.

If less invasive methods fail, the dorsal slit procedure is employed. This procedure should be performed by a physician experienced with the technique to minimize tissue loss and preserve anatomy. Again, the penis is cleansed. Two straight

 SUMMARY

1 Inspect the genitals for foreign bodies and to confirm anatomy.

2 Assess the need for pain control, restraints, or distraction techniques.

3 Attempt manual reduction.

4 Proceed with the sedation/analgesia plan.

5 Attempt to reduce the swelling via sugar application, ice pack, compression dressing, or manual compression.

6 Repeat the manual reduction technique.

7 Consult with urology; consider judicious use of the puncture technique or hyaluronidase injection.

8 Proceed to the dorsal slit technique in conjunction with urology consultation.

9 Ensure follow-up with a urology specialist.

 CLINICAL TIPS

▶ Paraphimosis is a urologic emergency requiring prompt reduction to avoid tissue loss or infection.

▶ Adequate cooperation of the child is essential, and may necessitate distraction techniques, sedation, or restraints.

▶ Referral to a urology professional is required to monitor for the development of phimosis and to assess for the need for circumcision to prevent recurrence.

▶ Health care professionals and parents should be educated on the care of the uncircumcised penis and the importance of prompt recognition of paraphimosis.

hemostats are used to crush the foreskin at the dorsum of the penis. The foreskin is then incised between the hemostats to release the area of constriction. The two edges are then closed with absorbable suture material (1,3).

▶ COMPLICATIONS

Complications to consider depend on the method used to achieve reduction. Careful inspection of the glans and foreskin following reduction is imperative. Thermal injury from ice use is prevented by close monitoring and limiting exposure time. Manual reduction can cause damage to the tissue or hematoma formation. Any surgical manipulation, including the puncture technique, hyaluronidase injection, and the dorsal slit technique, can result in bleeding or infection. Hyaluronidase injection has rarely been associated with ecchymosis, allergic reaction, and hypotension (10). Follow-up evaluation by a pediatric urologist is recommended after emergency reduction by any method.

▶ SUMMARY

Paraphimosis is a urologic emergency occurring in a partially circumcised or uncircumcised male that requires decisive intervention to prevent tissue loss and long-term sequelae. This entity occurs when the foreskin becomes entrapped proximal to the coronal sulcus, causing constriction and edema. Several methods exist for the reduction of paraphimosis, including manual reduction, the puncture technique, hyaluronidase injection, and the dorsal slit technique. The aim is to reduce prepuce swelling and restore the foreskin to its anatomic position. Prompt therapy, in conjunction with referral to a pediatric urologist, is indicated in the management of paraphimosis.

▶ ACKNOWLEDGMENT

The authors would like to acknowledge the valuable contributions of Michael Green and Gary R. Strange to the version of this chapter that appeared in the previous edition.

▶ REFERENCES

1. Choe JM. Paraphimosis: current treatment options. *Am Fam Physician.* 2000;62:2623–2626.
2. Cantu S. Phimosis and paraphimosis. *eMedicine.* 2004. www.emedicine.com/EMERG/topic423.htm.
3. Choe JM. Paraphimosis. *eMedicine.* 2004. www.emedicine.com/med/topic2874.htm.
4. Gausche M. Genitourinary surgical emergencies. *Pediatr Ann.* 1996;25:458–464.
5. Cartwright PC, Snow BW. Office pediatric urology. In: Belman AB, King LR, Kramer SA, eds. *Guide to Clinical Pediatric Urology.* London: Martin Dunitz Ltd.; 2002:1–4.
6. Peppas DS. Pediatric urologic emergencies. In: Gearhart JP, ed. *Pediatric Urology.* Totowa, NJ: Humana Press; 2003:31–32.
7. Mackway-Jones K, Teece S. Ice, pins or sugar to reduce paraphimosis. *Emerg Med J.* 2004;21:77–78.
8. Barone JG, Fleisher MH. Treatment of paraphimosis using the puncture technique. *Pediatr Emerg Care.* 1993;9:298–299.
9. Reynard JM, Barua JM. Reduction of paraphimosis the simple way—the Dundee technique. *BJU Int.* 1999;83:859–860.
10. DeVries CR, Miller AK, Packer MG. Reduction of paraphimosis with hyaluronidase. *Urology.* 1996;48:464–465.

99

JOEL A. FEIN AND STEPHEN A. ZDERIC

Management of Zipper Injuries

▶ INTRODUCTION

Injury to the skin and soft tissues of the penis and scrotum commonly results from entrapment inside a zipper mechanism. Most of these injuries occur in school-age boys during opening or closing of the zipper, when tissue may be caught in the tracks or become entangled within the fastener mechanism (1). The goal of therapy is to provide a relatively painless and rapid extrication of the involved area without inflicting further injury. The techniques are straightforward and may be performed by physicians at any level of training. If local or regional anesthesia is not required, nonphysician health care providers also may perform the procedures outlined in this chapter.

▶ ANATOMY AND PHYSIOLOGY

The school-age boy who is dressing himself without using protective undergarments is at highest risk for zipper injuries. For this reason, parents should be wary of pajamas that contain such mechanisms. Although any loose tissue can become caught inside a zipper, the majority of zipper injuries involve uncircumcised penile foreskin. The redundant tissue located on the ventral aspect of the circumcised penis also is at risk for this type of injury. Once the tissue is caught inside the zipper, swelling may occur and may complicate the extrication procedure.

A zipper is composed of two opposing rows of teeth that interlock inside a sliding zipper fastener mechanism. The sliding portion consists of two face plates that are bridged by a "diamond" or median bar. As the fastener mechanism draws the two rows of teeth together on either side of the median bar, it aligns them such that the teeth interlock. Unless this alignment is maintained in a two-dimensional plane, the teeth

edges fall apart. This relationship is the basis for the following techniques, which work equally well for both metal and plastic zippers.

▶ INDICATIONS

Whenever tissue is entangled inside a zipper fastener or between the teeth of a zipper, the clinician should attempt to extricate the tissue. Using excessive force is not warranted and may cause further damage to the tissue. No absolute contraindications exist to these techniques, but if the extraction proves difficult, urologic referral is most appropriate. A urologist should be consulted for cases that involve the urethra or fail to respond to the following procedures. Any blood at the meatus or hematuria should alert the clinician to the possibility of an underlying urethral injury.

▶ EQUIPMENT

Betadine solution or alcohol pad
Mineral oil
Bone cutter or wire cutter
Bandage scissors

▶ PROCEDURE

The clinician can approach the extraction of tissue from a zipper mechanism using one of the following techniques: (a) mineral oil extraction, (b) cutting the zipper cloth, or (c) cutting the median bar.

Procedural sedation and analgesia (Chapter 33) should be considered before starting the procedure. Ice should be applied through a moist cloth to minimize swelling while setting

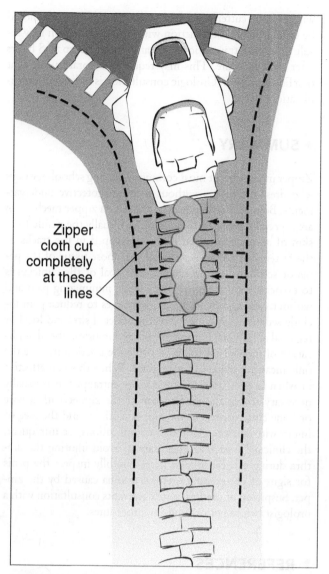

Figure 99.1 Cutting completely through the zipper cloth on both sides will enable the zipper teeth to be separated.

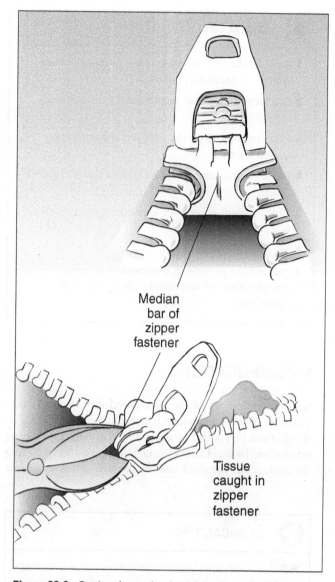

Figure 99.2 Cutting the median bar of the zipper fastener with a wire or bone cutter will allow the side plates to separate and the tissue to be freed.

up the sedation and anesthesia. Most children will require local or regional anesthesia after a superficial disinfectant is applied. A direct injection to the affected site may increase edema and complicate the extraction, so regional anesthesia techniques, such as dorsal penile block (Chapter 35) or circumferential penile block, should be considered.

The first attempt at extrication of the penile tissue does not involve much equipment. Mineral oil is applied liberally to the surface of the involved tissue and allowed to soak the area for several minutes. Then gentle traction is applied to the zipper (2). At this point, the tissue may be pulled free of the zipper without further injury. If penile tissue is entrapped in the zipper but does not involve the fastener mechanism, then isolate the zipper teeth from the surrounding clothing. Use a bandage scissors to make several cuts completely through the cloth on both sides of the zipper, above and below the entrapped skin (Fig. 99.1). Gentle traction on either side of

the zipper will easily separate the teeth, freeing the tissues that had been trapped.

If the tissue is entrapped in the zipper fastener mechanism, then the median bar of the zipper fastener should be cut with the wire cutters or bone cutter (3,4) (Fig. 99.2). A small hacksaw may be used if the penile tissue can be safely separated from the median bar area (5). With the median bar cut, the side plates of the zipper fastener separate and the zipper teeth fall apart.

After the tissue is freed from the zipper mechanism, any open wounds should be cleaned and dressed with sterile, dry gauze. Discharge instructions should address the possible complications of skin infections and urethral obstruction. Attempts to prevent recurrent injury should include a discussion of the protection afforded by undergarments and avoiding pajamas with zippers.

SUMMARY

1 Restrain the child and prepare entrapped tissues with an antiseptic solution.

2 Use local or regional anesthesia if extrication is difficult.

3 Place mineral oil on the involved area and apply gentle traction.

4 Separate the rows of teeth and free the entrapped tissue.

5 Cut the median bar with a wire or bone cutter if traction fails.

6 Provide local wound care.

7 Instruct the parents to observe at home for complications of wound infection or urethral obstruction.

▶ COMPLICATIONS

Some complications of the recommended procedures occur as a result of the initial injury; however, subsequent damage to the skin can be avoided by using only gentle traction during extrication. To avoid lacerating underlying skin when cutting the median bar, the child must be properly restrained, and a

CLINICAL TIPS

▶ Procedural sedation and analgesia may be necessary with an anxious patient.

▶ Ice may reduce the swelling and facilitate the extrication of the entrapped skin.

▶ Cutting the zipper out of the pants or pajamas makes it easier to cut the median bar.

▶ If the above-described techniques are unsuccessful, a urologist may need to perform a circumcision under general anesthesia.

wire or bone cutter with the smallest possible mouth should be used. Urethral obstruction with urinary retention may result from post-traumatic edema and can occur up to 8 hours after the procedure. This may require temporary placement of a Foley catheter. Urologic consultation is indicated if complications occur.

▶ SUMMARY

Zipper injuries occur most commonly among school-age boys who dress themselves without wearing protective undergarments. Boys who wear pajamas that have a zipper mechanism are especially prone to these injuries. Usually the penile foreskin of an uncircumcised boy is entrapped in the tracks or the fastener of a zipper, although any loose tissue of the penis or scrotum may be caught. The goal of the clinician is to extricate the entrapped tissue while minimizing pain and without causing further injury. Measures to reduce pain include sedation, applying ice to the affected site, and local or regional anesthesia. For uncomplicated injuries, liberal application of mineral oil followed by gentle traction may be the only measures required for removal. When this is ineffective or when larger segments of tissue are entrapped, it is usually necessary to cut the median bar of the zipper with a wire or bone cutter or to cut the zipper cloth around the area of injury with scissors. Although complications are infrequent, the clinician must take great care to avoid injuring the urethra during extrication and must carefully inspect the penis for signs of pre-existing urethral trauma caused by the zipper. Suspicion of urethral injury warrants consultation with a urologist before performing any procedures.

▶ REFERENCES

1. Saraf PS, Rabinowitz R. Zipper injury of the foreskin. *Am J Dis Child.* 1982;136:557–558.

2. Kanegaye JT, Schonfeld N. Penile zipper entrapment: a simple and less threatening approach using mineral oil. *Pediatr Emerg Care.* 1993;9: 90–91.

3. Nolan JF, Stillwell TJ, Sands JP. Acute management of zipper-entrapped penis. *J Emerg Med.* 1990;8:305–307.

4. Oosterlinck W. Unbloody management of penile zipper injury. *Eur Urol.* 1981;7:365–366.

5. Strait RT. A novel method for removal of penile zipper entrapment. *Pediatr Emerg Care.* 1999;15:412–413.

100

VIDYA T. CHANDE

Obstetrical Procedures for Adolescents

▶ INTRODUCTION

Emergency physicians and prehospital care providers must be familiar with the procedure for delivering a newborn, because transfer to a labor suite before delivery is not always possible. Even physicians who work solely in a pediatric emergency department (ED) and have ready access to inpatient obstetric services need a working knowledge of the steps involved. This chapter focuses on normal spontaneous vaginal delivery and the needs of the adolescent mother. A more extensive discussion of newborn delivery can be found in other textbooks (1,2).

The majority of women delivering babies today do so under the guidance of a health care professional who has special training in obstetrics. Women are encouraged to seek prenatal care and to contact their health care provider at the first signs of labor. Occasionally, however, young women unexpectedly present to the ED or clinic in active labor. It is the physician's job to decide if the pregnant adolescent can be transferred to a labor and delivery suite or if preparation on site for an imminent delivery is necessary.

The birth rate for teenage mothers has been dropping in the United States over the past decade (3). However, pregnant adolescents are still less likely to seek prenatal care and may be at greater risk for delivering in the ED because of their complex social situations. In fact, the pregnant adolescent may deny being pregnant even as the baby is about to be born. Therefore, providers of emergency care must assess the pregnant adolescent carefully, because her first medical contact for pregnancy may be at the time of delivery.

An adolescent patient presenting in labor is likely to be extremely anxious and complaining of severe abdominal pain. The patient may be screaming hysterically and may be unable to answer medical questions. The physician may have to rely solely on physical examination findings, such as the size of the uterus and observed uterine contractions, to determine that the patient is pregnant and about to deliver.

▶ ANATOMY AND PHYSIOLOGY

Labor is defined as progressive dilatation of the uterine cervix in association with repetitive uterine contractions. Normal labor is a continuous process that leads to delivery of the products of conception, including the baby and the placenta. The progress and outcome of labor are influenced by four factors: the bony and soft tissues of the maternal pelvis, the contractions of the uterus, the fetus, and the placenta (4). Just before the beginning of labor, a small amount of blood-tinged mucus is discharged from the vagina. This "bloody show" is a plug of cervical mucus mixed with blood and is evidence of cervical dilatation. Rupture of the fetal membranes occurs before onset of labor in approximately 10% of women. The majority of women whose membranes rupture first go into labor within 24 hours. If labor does not begin within 24 hours, the pregnancy is considered to be complicated by prolonged rupture of the membranes, a risk factor for neonatal sepsis. The diagnosis of true labor can be made when the following features exist: (a) contractions occur at regular intervals, (b) the intervals between contractions gradually shorten, (c) the intensity of contractions gradually increases, (d) discomfort localizes in the back and abdomen, (e) the cervix dilates, and (f) discomfort does not stop with sedation.

Labor is usually divided into three stages. The first stage begins with the onset of labor and ends when dilatation of the cervix is complete. The average duration of the first stage of labor is 8 to 12 hours in the primiparous patient and 6 to 8 hours in the multiparous patient. The progress of the first

911

stage of labor can be monitored by assessing the cervix for effacement and dilatation and determining the fetal station. Effacement of the cervix is a process in which thinning of the cervix occurs. Effacement is expressed in terms of the length of the cervical canal compared with an uneffaced cervix. For example, 0% indicates no effacement whereas 100% indicates that the cervix is very thin (less than 0.25 cm thick).

Dilatation of the cervical os is expressed by estimating the diameter of the cervical opening by direct palpation with the sterile gloved fingers. Complete dilatation occurs at 10 cm.

Fetal station is determined by the position of the presenting part in relation to the level of the ischial spines. If the presenting part is at the spines, it is at "zero station." If the presenting part is above the spines, the distance is reported in minus figures (e.g., −1 to −3 cm, or "floating"); if below the spines, the distance is reported in plus figures (e.g., +1 to +3 cm, or "on the perineum").

The second stage of labor extends from full dilatation of the cervix to complete birth of the infant. This stage varies from a few minutes to 1 to 2 hours. Many adolescents presenting in labor will be primiparous and therefore should be expected to labor for 8 to 12 hours before delivering the infant. The second stage of labor also may be longer in the primiparous patient. The third stage of labor is the period from the birth of the infant until completion of the delivery of the placenta. Separation and delivery of the placenta usually occurs within 10 minutes of the end of the second stage of labor.

The vertex (head) is the presenting part in 95% of deliveries. As shown in Figure 100.1, the sequence of events in vertex presentations is as follows:

1 *Engagement.* "Engagement" refers to the passage of the head through the pelvic inlet (Fig. 100.1A). This usually occurs in the last 2 weeks of pregnancy in the primiparous patient and at the onset of labor in the multiparous patient.
2 *Flexion and descent.* Flexion is necessary for passage of the smallest diameter of the head through the smallest diameter of the bony pelvis (Fig. 100.1B). Descent is gradual and is affected by the previously mentioned forces that influence labor.
3 *Internal rotation.* Internal rotation occurs with descent of the head and is necessary for the presenting part to traverse the ischial spines (Fig. 100.1C).
4 *Extension of head.* Extension occurs after the head has begun to pass through the introitus (Fig. 100.1D).
5 *External rotation of head.* External rotation occurs after delivery of the head as it rotates to the position it occupied at engagement (Fig. 100.1E). The shoulders then descend along the same pathway as the head, and the remainder of the fetus is delivered.

Vertex vaginal delivery usually occurs spontaneously. The primary role of the clinician is to help control the process to avoid sudden expulsion of the fetus, which could lead to injuries to the mother and infant.

▶ INDICATIONS

When a patient presents in labor, the clinician must assess the fetus and mother rapidly. If delivery is imminent, the infant should be delivered before transfer; if not, the mother should be transferred to a delivery suite, where personnel are more accustomed to obstetrical procedures.

If complete cervical effacement and dilatation are evident, immediate delivery may be necessary. Delivery is imminent when the contractions last 1 to 2 minutes and occur at intervals of 2 to 3 minutes, and the infant's head is at the perineum. An obstetrician should be contacted immediately while the physician prepares for the delivery. A box with equipment for emergency delivery should always be ready in the ED.

Every effort should be made for complicated deliveries to occur in a delivery suite. Heavy maternal bleeding and fetal distress are obstetrical emergencies requiring immediate involvement of an obstetrician and should not be managed by ED or clinic staff alone. Breech presentations also are more difficult to manage and have a higher risk of morbidity and mortality for the mother and fetus.

▶ EQUIPMENT

Mask, cap, gown
Goggles
Sterile gloves
Large basin (for placenta)
Scissors
2 Kelly clamps or umbilical tape
Bulb syringe
Cord clamp
Povidone-iodine solution
Sterile towels
Sterile drapes
Warm blankets
Heated isolette or overhead warming lights
Infant resuscitation tray
Name bands
Gauze sponges

▶ PROCEDURE

At least two clinicians should be present at the delivery. One person should attend to the mother while the other attends to the newborn. A support person for the mother, either a family member or another health care provider, also should be present. A social worker may be included as part of the team if the mother is particularly upset and difficult to manage.

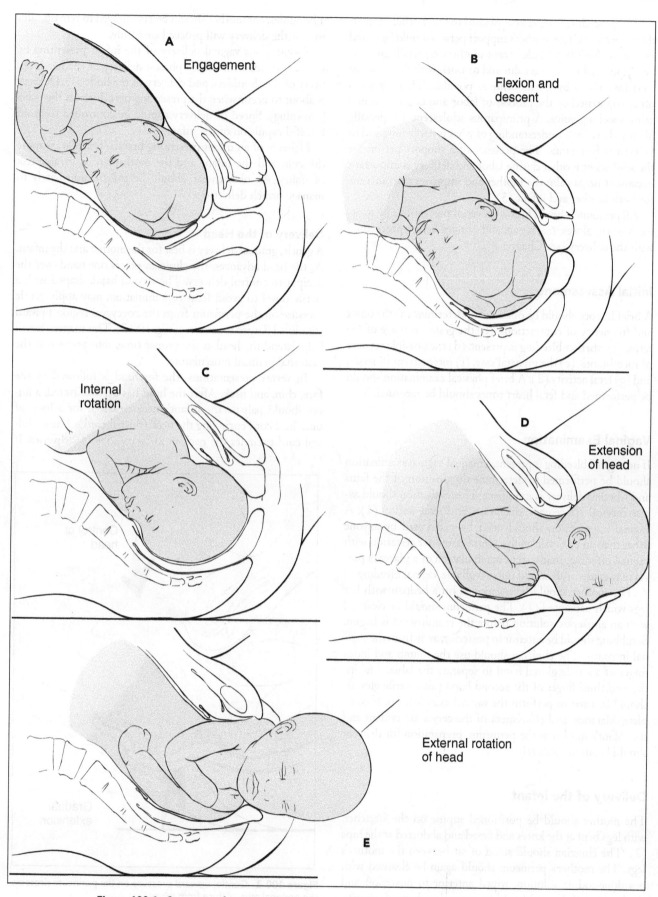

Figure 100.1 Sequence of events in vertex presentations (see text for description).

The procedure should be explained to the mother (and father, if present). The mother's support person should be seated by the mother's head. Adolescent mothers especially need to be encouraged to remain calm and to work with the clinician to deliver the baby as smoothly as possible. The mother is often frightened by the process of labor and benefits from a calm, soothing voice. A primiparous adolescent is especially likely to have little understanding of what is happening and to be extremely anxious. The presence of a support person for the adolescent mother during labor and delivery is important because it helps calm the mother and improves the outcome for both mother and infant (5).

All personnel should follow universal precautions by wearing a gown, gloves, mask, cap, and goggles before proceeding with the delivery (see Chapter 8).

Initial Assessment

A brief history should be obtained to determine (a) the onset and frequency of contractions, (b) the gestational age of the fetus, (c) whether bleeding is present, (d) the possible rupture of membranes, (e) the prenatal care, (f) intercurrent illnesses, and (g) fetal activity (2). A brief physical examination should be performed and fetal heart tones should be recorded.

Vaginal Examination

If no vaginal bleeding is present, a manual vaginal examination should be performed to determine the position of the fetus and whether delivery is imminent. This evaluation should assess cervical effacement, dilatation, and fetal station (1). A vaginal examination should never be performed by anyone other than an obstetrician for a third-trimester gestation with vaginal bleeding. Inadvertent manipulation of a placenta previa may cause profuse and uncontrollable vaginal bleeding.

The mother should be positioned on a bedpan with her legs widely separated (1). The perineum should be cleansed with an antiseptic solution before the examination is begun. Scrubbing should be anterior to posterior, away from the vaginal introitus. The clinician should use the thumb and index finger of a sterile gloved hand to separate the labia. The index and third finger of the second hand (also sterile gloved) should be used to perform the vaginal examination. If complete dilatation and effacement of the cervix are evident and the infant's head is at the perineum, preparation for delivery should begin immediately.

Delivery of the Infant

The mother should be positioned supine on the stretcher, with legs bent at the knees and flexed and abducted at the hips (2). The clinician should stand or sit between the mother's legs. The mother's perineum should again be cleansed with povidone-iodine solution, wiped anterior to posterior, and the legs and abdomen should be covered with sterile drapes.

The adolescent mother should be encouraged to remain calm so that the delivery will proceed smoothly.

Spontaneous vaginal delivery of the infant presenting by vertex is divided into three phases: delivery of the head, delivery of the shoulders, and delivery of the body (1). Delivery is about to occur when the presenting part distends the vulva (crowning). Speed of delivery should be controlled to avoid forceful expulsion of the infant.

Delivery of an infant presenting breech (feet first) is more difficult, and the infant and the mother are at greater risk of injury. An obstetrician should be called immediately to manage breech deliveries.

Delivery of the Head

A gentle, gradual delivery is best for the mother and the infant. As the head advances, the clinician places one hand over the occiput to control delivery. The second hand, draped with a sterile towel to avoid fecal contamination, may apply gentle pressure on the perineum from the coccygeal region upward (modified Ritgen maneuver) (Fig. 100.2). This maneuver will help extend the head at the proper time, thus protecting the maternal perineal musculature.

In vertex presentations, the forehead is followed by the face, chin, and neck. After the head has been delivered, a finger should palpate the infant's neck to check for a loop of umbilical cord encircling the neck (nuchal cord). The umbilical cord encircles the neck in 20% to 25% of deliveries. If

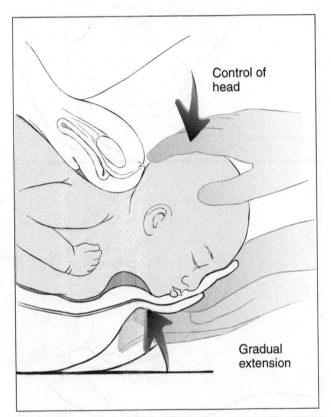

Figure 100.2 Gentle, upward pressure on the perineum protects the perineal musculature from injury.

a nuchal cord is present, it should be palpated to check for pulsation and then gently slipped over the infant's head. If the cord is tight, it should be clamped in two places and cut between the clamps; the remainder of the delivery should then proceed.

Once the head has been delivered, the infant's face should be wiped and the mouth and nose suctioned with a bulb syringe. Special maneuvers are necessary if thick meconium is present (Chapter 37).

Delivery of the Shoulders

Delivery of the shoulders also should proceed gradually. Gentle downward traction on the head will help deliver the anterior shoulder, followed by gentle upward traction, which delivers the posterior shoulder (Fig. 100.3). Forceful traction, especially with rotation, can cause injury to the infant's brachial plexus and great vessels.

Shoulder dystocia (shoulders unable to pass through the birth canal after delivery of the head) complicates 0.15% to 0.6% of all deliveries (2). This is an obstetrical emergency because the umbilical cord may become occluded, leading to fetal hypoxia. An obstetrician should be notified of shoulder dystocia immediately at the first suspicion that the shoulders may not pass. Exaggerated flexion and abduction of the maternal hips often resolves the problem in mild dystocia. Downward traction at the pubic symphysis also may dislodge the impacted anterior shoulder. Other maneuvers are occasionally necessary for more severe dystocia but are beyond the scope of this chapter.

Delivery of the Body and Extremities

The body and extremities should deliver easily after the head and shoulders have been delivered. The clinician must be prepared to control the remainder of the delivery and catch the newborn should it be expelled forcefully. Gentle traction may be necessary.

After the infant is delivered, the head should be held lower than the body at a 15-degree angle to allow drainage of secretions from the airway and to allow a small transfusion of blood from the placenta to the infant. The umbilical cord should be clamped within 1 minute of delivery to avoid excess transfusion of blood. Two Kelly clamps are placed 4 to 5 cm from the infant's abdomen, and the cord is cut between the clamps.

The infant should then be dried and placed under a radiant warmer to prevent cold stress. The nose and mouth may be suctioned again if necessary and the infant should be assessed by the second clinician at the delivery (6). This person should evaluate the infant's respiratory effort and heart rate and provide additional resuscitative measures as needed (see Chapter 36).

Delivery of the Placenta

After delivery of the infant, the uterus will continue to contract to allow the placenta to deliver. Placental separation from the

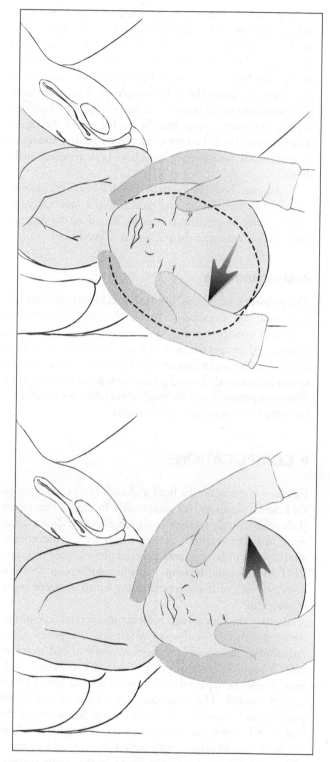

Figure 100.3 Delivery of the anterior and posterior shoulders.

uterine wall usually occurs within 5 minutes after delivery of the infant. Signs of placental separation include these: (a) the uterus becomes globular, (b) a small gush of blood occurs, (c) the umbilical cord protrudes further from the vagina, and (d) the uterus rises in the abdomen (1,7).

The mother should then be asked to bear down to expel the placenta. The placenta should not be delivered by pulling on the cord, because this may lead to uterine injury or tearing of the placenta, causing retained parts. Delivery of the placenta may be assisted by applying pressure to the abdomen just above the pubic symphysis. This will elevate the uterus into the abdomen and push the placenta into the vagina. The placenta may then be guided out of the vagina. The placenta should be kept in a basin for further inspection to ensure that no missing pieces have been retained in the uterus.

The uterus should be palpated after delivery of the placenta to stimulate contraction and reduce blood loss. Oxytocin (10 IU) may be given intravenously to aid in the contraction of the uterus after the placenta is delivered (4).

Postpartum Care

The perineum, vagina, and cervix should be inspected for lacerations. If any lacerations are noted, they should be repaired in a sterile manner by a clinician familiar with the techniques. This procedure can take place after transfer. After determining that the mother and infant are in stable condition, a maternity service is contacted, detailed information about the emergency delivery is provided, and the mother and infant are transferred for complete evaluation and admission.

▶ COMPLICATIONS

Excessive traction on the head and neck can cause injury to the brachial plexus and/or great vessels. Brachial plexus injury (Erb palsy) usually resolves over time. Shoulder dystocia can result in fractures of the clavicle, which are not uncommon after delivery of large infants. Brachial plexus injury and clavicle fracture should be suspected when a newborn does not move one arm or if asymmetry of the Moro or startle reflex is observed.

Postpartum hemorrhage is the most common type of obstetric hemorrhage and is an obstetrical emergency (2,8). An obstetrician should be notified while initial management is begun by the emergency physician. Intravascular volume should be replaced with crystalloid and blood products as needed. The most common causes of immediate postpartum hemorrhage are uterine atony, lacerations of the vagina and cervix, and retained placental fragments. Uterine atony may be treated with uterine massage and oxytocin (20 to 40 IU in 1 L of crystalloid). If the uterus remains boggy, an ergot preparation may be given to stimulate uterine contraction. Ergots may cause hypertension and should be avoided in women with pre-eclampsia or pre-existing hypertension. Any lacerations should be repaired, and the uterus should be inspected manually for fragments of placental tissue.

Infant distress is another complication that providers must be prepared to address (6). Clinicians must be prepared to treat an asphyxiated newborn, even if delivery is progressing without apparent complications (Chapter 36). An infant resuscitation tray should be available for all deliveries, and a provider should be assigned to the evaluation and treatment of the infant.

SUMMARY

1 Perform a brief assessment of the mother, including vital signs and fetal heart tones.

2 If the mother is in early labor, transfer her to a delivery suite.

3 If contractions are 2 to 3 minutes apart and the infant's head is distending the perineum, prepare for an emergency delivery.

4 Notify the obstetrician that assistance is needed immediately.

5 Assign one person for the mother and one for the infant; set up the equipment for delivery and newborn resuscitation.

6 Position the mother on her back with hips flexed and abducted and knees flexed; the mother's support person should be at the head of the bed.

7 Clean the perineum with povidone-iodine solution, and drape the abdomen and legs.

8 As head emerges, apply one hand to the head to control the speed of delivery; the other hand exerts upward pressure on the perineum (Fig. 100.2).

9 Check the neck for a loop of the umbilical cord—if present, slip over the infant's head; if the cord is tight, clamp in two places and cut between the clamps.

10 After the head is delivered, wipe the face and suction the nose and mouth.

11 Deliver the shoulders (Fig. 100.3) and the rest of body.

12 Clamp the umbilical cord in two places and cut between the clamps within 1 minute.

13 Assess the infant and provide resuscitation as needed.

14 Wait for the placenta to separate. Assist the mother in delivering the placenta with downward pressure on the abdomen—do not pull on the umbilical cord. Save the placenta for inspection.

15 Massage the uterus to stimulate contractions and prevent further bleeding; oxytocin (10 IU) can be given intravenously.

16 Check the cervix and perineum for lacerations.

CLINICAL TIPS

▶ The clinician should remain calm, even though this procedure is not commonly performed. Most deliveries proceed spontaneously without difficulty.

▶ Universal precautions should be observed.

▶ Neonatal resuscitation equipment should be ready to use.

▶ An isolette should be turned on before delivering the baby.

▶ A support person who can help the mother focus on the delivery should be included.

▶ SUMMARY

Delivery of a newborn is a procedure best done by the patient's obstetrical care provider. Whenever possible, the expectant mother should be transferred to a delivery suite or an obstetrician should be called to the scene of emergency delivery. Occasionally in emergency situations other clinicians may be called on to manage a delivery. The majority of vaginal vertex deliveries occur spontaneously, and the primary role of the clinician is to control the speed of delivery to avoid injury to the mother and the infant. Two clinicians should be available to attend the delivery—one for the mother and one for the infant. Equipment for resuscitation of the infant should be available, and universal precautions should be observed during the delivery.

▶ REFERENCES

1. Cunningham FG, Gant NF, Leveno KJ, et al., eds. *Williams Obstetrics.* 21st ed. New York: McGraw-Hill; 2001.
2. Doan-Wiggins LA. Emergency childbirth. In: Roberts JR, Hedges JR, eds. *Clinical Procedures in Emergency Medicine.* 4th ed. Philadelphia: WB Saunders; 2004:1117–1143.
3. Martin JA, Kochanek KD, Strobino DM, et al. Annual summary of vital statistics—2003. *Pediatrics.* 2005;115:619–634.
4. DeCherney AH, Nathan L, eds. *Current Obstetric and Gynecologic Diagnosis and Treatment.* 9th ed. New York: Lange Medical Books/McGraw-Hill; 2003.
5. Kennell J, Klaus M, McGrath S, et al. Continuous emotional support during labor in a U. S. hospital. *JAMA.* 1991;265:2197–2201.
6. Gausche-Hill M, Fuchs S, Yamamoto L, eds. *APLS: The Pediatric Emergency Medicine Resource.* 4th ed. Sudbury, MA: Jones and Bartlett Publishers; 2004:476–483.
7. Scherger JE. Management of normal labor and birth. *Prim Care.* 1993;20:713–719.
8. Stallard TC, Burns B. Emergency delivery and perimortem c-section. *Emerg Med Clin North Am.* 2003;21:679–693.

SECTION 14 ▶ ORTHOPAEDIC PROCEDURES
SECTION EDITOR: BRENT R. KING

101

JEAN E. KLIG

Splinting Procedures

▶ INTRODUCTION

Orthopaedic immobilization techniques utilize a wide range of devices to support musculoskeletal injuries. Splints are an essential part of this spectrum and are vital to the initial management of many injuries in children (1). The goal of splinting is to provide support at key points around an injury to allow for (a) decreased pain; (b) mechanical stabilization of bones, soft tissues, and neurovascular structures; (c) decreased risk of further injury to the affected area; and (d) decreased risk of additional swelling-related injuries such as a compartment syndrome. Splints are extremely versatile and can be used either for initial injury care or as definitive treatment in certain cases. They are commonly used for the early treatment of nondisplaced closed fractures in children. In the 24 to 48 hours after an injury, a splint provides support and immobilization as well as allowing the injured extremity to swell without significant risk of external compression. In contrast, a cast often allows little room for swelling and must be promptly opened when this occurs.

A splint can be used for up to 2 weeks following a nondisplaced closed fracture, after which a cast usually is applied. Use of a splint also offers a valuable temporizing measure with equivocal injuries initially diagnosed as joint sprains. In children, an acute "sprain" of any joint where an epiphysis is known to be unfused can in fact represent a nondisplaced Salter-Harris type I fracture, even when radiographs are unremarkable. It is therefore common practice to initially treat sprains in children as nondisplaced fractures, utilizing a splint until follow-up examination and/or radiographs are obtained. For older adolescents with closed epiphyses, splints may be used as definitive treatment for more severe joint sprains. The overall rule of "when in doubt, splint" is key to the treatment of many pediatric musculoskeletal injuries (2).

The splinting methods detailed in this chapter can be used for children of all ages and are appropriate for prehospital, emergency and ambulatory settings. Splint techniques can be performed by many types of skilled medical personnel.

▶ ANATOMY AND PHYSIOLOGY

Pediatric fractures differ greatly from those seen in adults, because the bones of a child are in a continual process of growth. A growing long bone has four anatomical parts: physis, epiphysis, metaphysis, and diaphysis (Fig. 101.1). Growth occurs in two regions. Increases in bone length occur at the growth plate (physis) via endochondral ossification, while increases in bone width occur at the periosteum by membranous ossification. The strongest parts of a child's bone are the periosteum and adjacent joint capsule and ligaments. By contrast, the growth plate is the weakest area of a child's bone and is therefore most vulnerable to injury (3). As a result, children are less likely than adults to have dislocations, sprains, and strain injuries but are more likely than adults to have fractures, which commonly involve the growth plate.

Certain fractures are unique to children. The greater strength of the periosteum as compared with the underlying

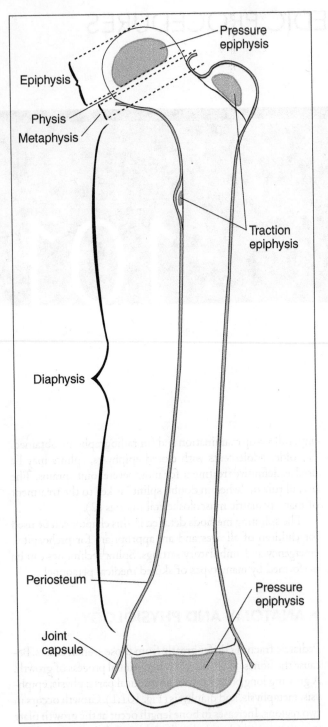

Epiphysis

Physis

Metaphysis

Pressure epiphysis

Traction epiphysis

Diaphysis

Periosteum

Pressure epiphysis

Joint capsule

Figure 101.1 Pediatric long bone. Children's bones are characterized by areas of growth, decreased rigidity (ossification), and a periosteum that is often stronger than the underlying bone trabecula. Fractures of the shaft often manifest as buckling (torus), bending (plastic), and/or fraying (greenstick). Multiple types of growth plate fractures occur.

bone trabecula results in buckling (torus) fractures, bending (plastic) fractures, and fractures that extend through the bone but only disrupt one side of the periosteum (greenstick). Fractures of the growth plate, which only occur in growing children, are delineated by the Salter-Harris classification

(Fig. 101.2). Five different forms of injury to the physis or growth plate region are defined by this classification. A type I fracture involves the zone of provisional calcification (physis) only, without fracture of the surrounding bone. A type II injury involves a slip at the epiphyseal plate with a fracture proximally through the metaphysis, while a type III involves a slip at the epiphyseal plate with a fracture distally to the articular surface of the bone. In a type IV injury, the fracture extends through the metaphysis and epiphyseal plate to the adjacent articular surface. Type V fractures are less common and involve compression of the growth plate.

Two key physiologic considerations relate to use of splints for pediatric patients. First, children tend not to suffer from significant muscle stiffness or spasm due to immobilization. Use of a splint for an "equivocal" fracture in a child until the presence (or absence) of a fracture can be verified therefore poses minimal risk of complications such as musculoskeletal rigidity. Second, the dynamics of bone growth allow for significant remodeling of angulated fractures. As a result, fractures with up to 20 degrees of angulation in the plane of joint motion can often be splinted without reduction. It is generally advisable to consult an orthopaedist for fractures with over 20 degrees of angulation even though a splint may be safely used (4).

▶ INDICATIONS

Splinting is an extremely versatile tool in the management of many pediatric extremity injuries and/or known fractures. The early diagnosis and treatment of a fractured extremity is vital to an optimal outcome in a child, given the swift rate at which pediatric bones grow and remodel. Clinical findings of a fractured extremity may include inability or reluctance to use the affected limb; pain with limb movement; reproducible bone tenderness to palpation (point tenderness); swelling, discoloration, or deformity at the fracture site; and crepitus (5).

Radiographs of the injured extremity should always be obtained when a child has positive or abnormal clinical signs. If the findings on a radiograph are unclear, then a similar view of the opposite uninjured extremity may be helpful. As mentioned previously, "negative" radiographs do not exclude the possibility of a fracture if the findings on physical examination suggest otherwise. Reproducible bone tenderness near a joint with an open epiphysis is suggestive of a Salter-Harris type I fracture and is a sufficient indication for splinting even without radiographic evidence of a fracture. Moreover, "sprains" are relatively rare in children and are commonly treated as Salter-Harris type I fractures until a follow-up assessment in 5 to 10 days (6,7).

Immediate evaluation by an orthopaedist is mandatory for any extremity fracture where signs of neurovascular compromise are present (see Chapter 106). These include extreme pain at rest, pain with passive movement, pallor, paralysis, and paresthesias. Orthopaedic consultation is also recommended for (a) open fractures, (b) elbow or femur fractures,

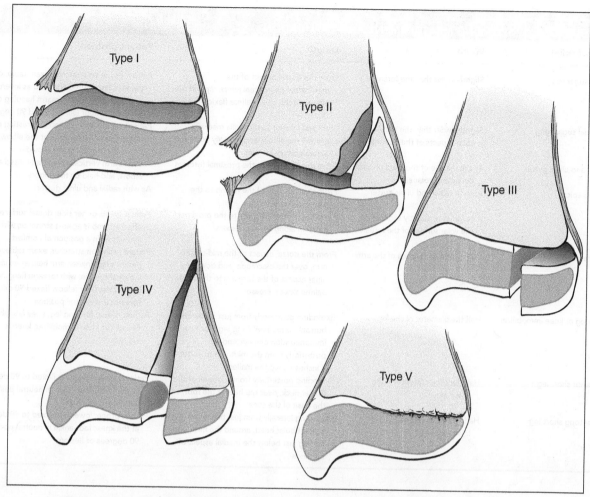

Figure 101.2 Salter-Harris classification for fractures in the growth plate region.

(c) fractures angulated greater than 20 degrees, (d) more severe Salter-Harris fractures (types III–V), and (e) unstable fractures. It is advisable to consult an orthopaedist when follow-up fracture care cannot be ensured within 2 weeks after the placement of a splint. Additionally, early placement of a temporary splint is indicated for injuries suspected to be unstable unless orthopaedic evaluation can be ensured within a brief time. In such cases, a splint can be loosely placed on the injured extremity to provide both temporary support and some pain relief, particularly during positioning for radiographs.

Finally, splints are sometimes used in children to immobilize areas where wound healing may be impaired by motion. This includes areas with multiple complex sutures, sutures over joint areas, burns, and dirty and/or infected wounds.

▶ EQUIPMENT

Although a wide range of prefabricated splints are available, many are not properly sized for children. Essential materials for splinting are listed below. Splints can be made with plaster, fiberglass, or prefabricated splint roll, which contains padding and fiberglass or plaster in one unit. Fiberglass is strong, durable, lightweight, and in many cases easier to apply than plaster.

Gauze roll or elastic (Ace) bandage
Cotton stocking material (stockinette)
Soft cotton roll (Webril)
Plaster roll or sheets or fiberglass roll
Commercial splint roll (optional)
Prefabricated splint (optional)

▶ PROCEDURES

General Principles

Guidelines for splint measurement and application are listed in Table 101.1. Most splints have four layers. A stockinette (layer 1) is placed against the skin for protection. This is optional but is often used for comfort. Webril (layer 2) is then placed around the stockinette to provide padding, especially at bony prominences (it can be omitted if commercial splint roll is used). Plaster, fiberglass, or commercial splint roll (layer 3) is

TABLE 101.1 | SPLINTING MEASUREMENT AND APPLICATION

Type of splint	Width	Length	Patient position
Distal sugar tong	Slightly wider than the forearm	From the dorsal aspect of the metacarpal-phalangeal joints, around the elbow, to the volar palmar flexion crease	Patient prone on stretcher, exam table, or parent's lap; injured arm held as inverted L over the edge, with forearm hanging down toward the floor (elbow flexed 90 degrees)
Proximal sugar tong	Slightly wider than the dorsal and volar aspects of the upper arm	From just inferior to the axilla medially, around the elbow, and laterally up to the acromioclavicular joint	Patient supine, with injured arm resting on the chest, flexed 90 degrees at the elbow, and internally rotated at the shoulder
Radial and ulnar gutter	To the midline of the hand on the dorsal and volar sides	From the nail base to the proximal forearm	Patient's arm vertically erect, stabilized at the elbow, and held by the fingers
Thumb spica	As with radial and ulnar gutter	From the nail base of the thumb to the proximal forearm	As with radial and ulnar gutter
Colles	As wide as or slightly wider than the volar surface of the forearm	From the proximal fingers to the proximal forearm along its volar aspect	Patient on his or her side; dorsal surface of affected limb is against stretcher, with fingers and elbow in a position of comfort
Long arm	Half the circumference of the arm	From the dorsal aspect of the mid-upper arm, over the olecranon, and down the ulnar aspect of the forearm to the distal palmar flexion crease	Patient prone on stretcher, exam table, or parent's lap; injured arm held as an inverted L over the edge, with forearm hanging down toward the floor (elbow flexed 90 degrees); forearm in a neutral position
Long leg or knee immobilizer	Half the diameter of the leg	Extending posteriorly from just below the buttock to the heel (long leg); for knee immobilization only, extending posteriorly from the midthigh to about 3 inches above the malleoli	Patient prone; for long leg, knee is slightly flexed; for knee immobilizer, knee is extended
Posterior short leg	Half the circumference of the lower leg	Extending posteriorly from the level of the fibular neck, over the heel of the foot, to the base of the toes	Patient prone; lower leg flexed to 90 degrees at the knee; foot-ankle in neutral position at 90 degrees of flexion
Sugar tong short leg	Half the circumference of the lower leg	Extending laterally from just below the level of the fibular head, around the heel, and ending just below the medial aspect of the knee	Patient prone; lower leg flexed to 90 degrees at the knee; foot-ankle in neutral position at 90 degrees of flexion

then placed to maintain the position of immobilization. An outer layer of elastic bandage (Ace wrap) or gauze wrap (layer 4) is rolled around the plaster, fiberglass or commercial splint roll to secure the splint to the limb and protect the firm layer.

Basic splinting procedures are shown in Figure 101.3, which demonstrates application of a distal sugar tong splint. After the necessary materials are obtained, the area is measured, and the splint material (stockinette and dry plaster, fiberglass, or commercial splint roll) is cut to an appropriate length (Fig. 101.3A). For convenience, the elastic bandage or gauze wrap can be used as a measuring tape to gauge the length of splint needed. Discomfort can be reduced by measuring the opposite, unaffected extremity. Areas where the splint will bend around joints can have notches cut at the edges to minimize folding of the plaster or fiberglass. As described above, the stockinette layer is optional, but if it is used, it is placed first by sliding it onto the extremity. The Webril layer is then placed by rolling it around the extremity (Fig. 101.3B). (Note: this step can be omitted if padded commercial splint roll is used.)

Next, the child's extremity is positioned for optimal plaster, fiberglass, or commercial splint roll application (Fig. 101.3C). Most splint material requires the application of water to initiate the curing process. Therefore, the operator should wet the

plaster, fiberglass, or commercial splint roll material and apply it carefully. Because the splint material releases heat as it cures, warm water should not be used to wet the splint material.

After the splint is applied, it is initially shaped at large joints. The clinician wraps the elastic bandage (Ace) or gauze wrap around the plaster or fiberglass (Fig. 101.3D). As mentioned, a layer of Webril can be applied to the outside of the plaster or fiberglass to prevent the elastic bandage or gauze wrap from sticking. The splint contours are then molded into their final form. The splint must be kept in position until the plaster, fiberglass, or commercial splint roll has completely hardened. If the splint has been applied to a young child, gentle restraint may be necessary.

Splinting in children requires preparation and patience. Four elements contributing to the successful application of a pediatric splint are pain control, positioning, molding, and adequate hardening. Before placing a splint, the clinician must be sure that the child has adequate pain control and/or distraction to create the best possible experience for all involved. The clinician should always ensure that the child is properly positioned for placement of the splint and has sufficient support or restraint to maintain that position while the splint is gently molded to the extremity. Once the splint is molded for proper joint positioning, an assistant or parent can support

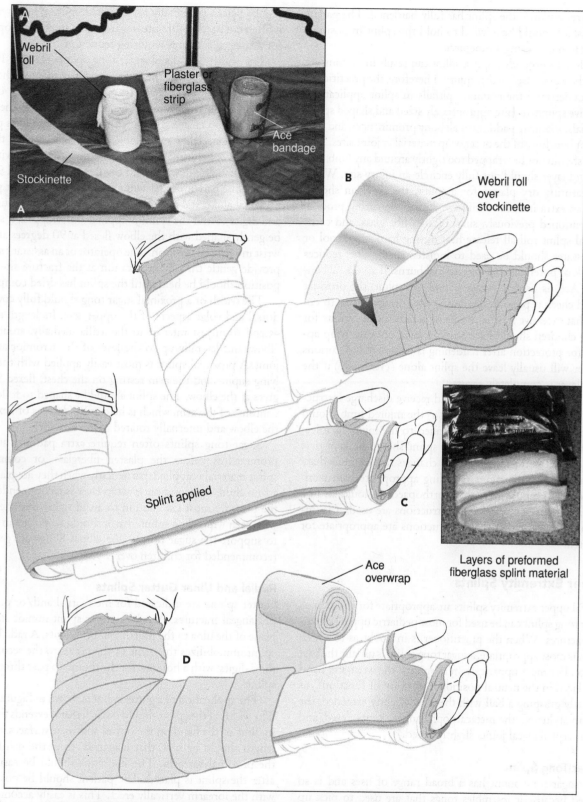

Figure 101.3 Basic splinting procedures (distal sugar tong splint).

A. Materials should be measured and prepared. The child should be appropriately positioned based on the type of splint applied.

B. Stockinette can be applied and the area wrapped with Webril for padding.

C. The plaster, fiberglass, or splint roll is moistened with cool or tepid water and applied for general splint shape.

D. Elastic bandage (Ace) or gauze roll is applied, and the splint is gently molded to its final shape. The patient (or parent) must hold the splint in position for approximately 20 minutes until it hardens.

the extremity until the splint has fully hardened. The parent or assistant should be advised to hold the splint in position for 20 minutes, using a timepiece.

Failure to properly apply a splint can result in discomfort or, in the worst case, further injury. Therefore, the practitioner must understand the common pitfalls in splint application. Effective splints require appropriately sized and shaped splint materials, adequate padding of all bony prominences, and care to limit bunching of the outer wrap material at joint sites. The splint should not be wrapped too tightly around any limb, and the rigid layer should not fully encircle an injury site. When premeasuring dry plaster for a splint, the clinician should allow an extra inch for shrinkage during the curing process. As mentioned previously, since plaster, fiberglass, and commercial splint roll all release heat during hardening, cool or tepid water should be used to moisten them. This reduces the risk of potentially serious dermal burns. If an elastic bandage (Ace) is used to wrap around the splint, the provider should check it periodically during the curing process to ensure that excessive heat is not being retained (8). Splints for young children should have an extra layer of outer wrap applied for protection after hardening is completed. A curious toddler will usually leave the splint alone (eventually) if the outer layer is completely secure.

All patients with splints should receive discharge instructions that include the following: (a) the injured limb should be elevated and ice should be applied to the injury as tolerated for up to 48 hours; (b) the splint should be kept dry; and (c) increased pain or sensory changes require immediate re-evaluation. Instructions regarding appropriate pain management and follow-up with an orthopaedist should also be given. If preprinted discharge instructions are used, it is important to ensure that these instructions are appropriate for children.

Upper Extremity Splints

Several upper extremity splints are appropriate for children. A sugar tong splint can be used for most pediatric upper extremity fractures. When the practitioner is in doubt as to which splint is most appropriate, a sugar tong splint is usually the best choice. For most upper extremity splints, the wrist and hand are placed in the neutral position ("position of function") as if gently grasping a ball with the wrist slightly extended, the thumb abducted, the metacarpophalangeal joints flexed, and the interphalangeal joints slightly flexed.

Sugar Tong Splint

The sugar tong splint has a broad range of uses and is so named because it resembles tongs that are used to pick up sugar cubes. The sugar tong splint provides the most effective immobilization of stable forearm and wrist fractures and is commonly used for these injuries. A double sugar tong—both a proximal and distal sugar tong splint combination applied at a 90-degree angle at the elbow—can be used to fully immobilize elbow injuries. The sugar tong splint can

also be placed proximally for humerus injuries; however, this is often not needed. Of note, sugar tong splints are not optimal for displaced fractures requiring reduction.

The width of a distal sugar tong splint (see Fig. 101.3) should slightly overlap the radial and ulnar edges of the arm. The length should extend from the dorsal aspect of the metacarpal-phalangeal joints, around the elbow, to the volar palmar flexion crease. To apply the splint, the child is placed prone on a stretcher, exam table, or parent's lap, and the injured arm is held like an inverted L over the edge, with the forearm hanging down toward the floor (elbow flexed 90 degrees). The parent or assistant should hold the arm at points proximal and distal to the splint area (e.g., proximal humerus and digits). After the splint is applied and wrapped, it should be gently shaped with the elbow flexed at 90 degrees and the wrist in a neutral position. The operator or an assistant should provide gentle three-point fixation at the fracture site. This position should be held until the splint has dried completely.

The width of a proximal sugar tong should fully cover the dorsal and volar aspects of the upper arm. Its length should extend from just inferior to the axilla medially, around the elbow, and laterally up to the level of the acromioclavicular joint. A proximal splint is most easily applied with the child lying supine and the arm resting on the chest, flexed 90 degrees at the elbow. The splint should be shaped to follow the contours of the arm, which is held at 90 degrees of flexion at the elbow and internally rotated at the shoulder.

Sugar tong splints often require extra padding at bony prominences before the plaster, fiberglass, or commercial splint material is applied, particularly when they are placed on a thin child. A second outer wrap layer is recommended, but the provider must use caution to avoid tightening the splint with each wrap. The splinted arm should be placed in a sling to support the sugar tong at the elbow. Slings are generally recommended for children over 4 years old.

Radial and Ulnar Gutter Splints

Gutter splints are indicated for metacarpal and/or proximal phalangeal fractures. An ulnar gutter splint immobilizes the plane of the ulna to the fourth and fifth digits. A radial gutter splint immobilizes the plane of the radius to the second and third digits, with a hole cut for the thumb to pass through the splint.

The application of a gutter splint is shown in Figure 101.4. The width of the splint should be such that it extends from the midline of the hand on the dorsal and volar surfaces, and the length should be such that it extends from the nail base to the proximal forearm. The fingertips should be easily seen after the splint is placed. The patient should be positioned with the forearm vertically erect. This is easily accomplished by seating a child in a parent's lap and having the parent hold the extremity at the elbow and by the uninjured fingers. Once the splint is wrapped, it should be shaped as follows: the wrist should be in a neutral position, the metacarpophalangeal joints should be in 70 degrees flexion, and the proximal interphalangeal joints in 20 to 30 degrees flexion. The parent should hold the splint in this position until it has dried completely.

A thin layer of padding can be placed between the fingers to minimize irritation from the gutter splint. An extra layer of outer wrap is recommended for children under 4 years old (or active children) to keep the splint dry and protected. Although optional, a sling can help to keep the injury elevated in children over 4 years old.

Thumb Spica Splint

A thumb spica splint is essentially a gutter splint adapted for the thumb. It is indicated for nondisplaced fractures of the first metacarpal bone, proximal phalanx of the thumb, or the scaphoid bone. The thumb spica splint is shown in Figure 101.5. Dimensions of the splint are the same as for the gutter splints, as is the position in which the child is held. After the outer wrap layer is applied, the operator should gently shape the splint as follows: the wrist should be placed in a neutral position, and the thumb should be abducted and in slight flexion at the metacarpophalangeal and interphalangeal joints ("wine glass" position of the thumb). The parent should be instructed to hold this position until the splint has dried completely. As with the gutter splints, use of a sling can help to keep the injury elevated and should be considered in children over 4 years old.

Colles Splint

A Colles splint provides volar support of the forearm and offers an alternative to the distal sugar tong splint for distal forearm and wrist fractures in older children. For young children, the sugar tong is recommended, because it provides both dorsal and volar stability. As shown in Figure 101.6, the width of a Colles splint should be such that it fully covers the volar aspect of the forearm, and the length should be such that it extends from the proximal fingers to the proximal forearm along the volar aspect. The child is positioned lying on his or her side with the dorsal aspect of the affected forearm against the stretcher. After the outer wrap layer is applied, the splint should be shaped with the wrist in a neutral position, and the digits should be slightly flexed at all joints. This position should be held until the splint has dried completely. A sling may be used, as previously described.

Long Arm Splint

A long arm splint is primarily used for stable injuries at or near the elbow. A double sugar tong splint is also an option for stable elbow injuries (see above). It is imperative that an orthopaedic consultation be obtained for patients with supracondylar fractures and other injuries that might compromise the function of the joint or neurovascular structures.

The long arm splint is shown in Figure 101.7. The width of a long arm splint should be such that it covers half of the arm circumference, and the length should be such that it extends from the dorsal aspect of the mid-upper arm over the olecranon and down the ulnar aspect of the forearm to the distal palmar flexion crease. The patient should be placed

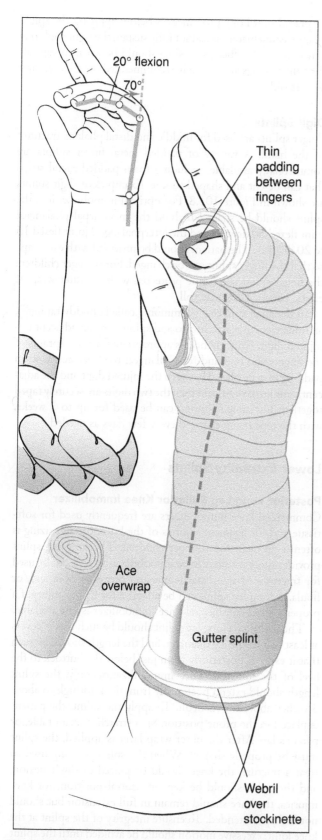

Figure 101.4 Ulnar gutter splint. A radial gutter splint is applied to the opposite (radial) side with a hole cut for the thumb to pass through.

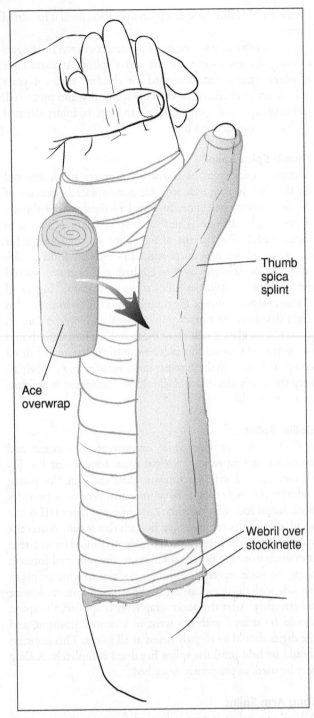

Thumb
spica
splint

Ace
overwrap

Webril over
stockinette

Figure 101.5 Thumb spica splint.

be placed over bony prominences before applying the splint. Many casting materials cannot fully sustain the right angle that is needed at the elbow, so a sling should be worn to support the splint. Slings are generally recommended for children over 4 years old.

Digit Splints

Finger splints are used for middle and distal phalanx fractures of the hand. A variety of padded metal finger splints are commercially available, including foam padded metal strips that can be cut and shaped to size. Examples of digit splints are shown in Figure 101.8. For optimal immobilization, the splint should be shaped to hold the metacarpal-phalangeal joint flexed 50 degrees and the interphalangeal joint flexed 15 to 20 degrees. The patient should be provided with extra tape so that the finger splint can be changed. For younger children, the finger splint should be protected with an outer wrap of elastic bandage or gauze roll.

In dynamic splinting (commonly called "buddy taping"), an injured digit is attached to and splinted by an adjacent un-injured digit. This method is appropriate for joint sprains of the fingers and toes and for phalangeal toe fractures. Cotton padding may be placed between the injured digit and the adjacent, uninjured digit, and then the two digits are securely taped together. Dynamic splinting can be used for up to 3 weeks, with the tape being changed every few days as needed.

Lower Extremity Splints

Posterior Long Leg Splint or Knee Immobilizer

Commercial knee immobilizers are frequently used for soft-tissue and/or ligament injuries of the knee, though sizing is often a problem for younger children. The long leg splint provides more effective knee immobilization and can be used for fractures of the distal femur and proximal tibia and/or fibula. A long leg splint can be adapted for a knee injury if a properly sized commercial knee immobilizer is not available.

The width of a long leg splint should be such that it covers at least half of the leg diameter, and the length should be such that it extends posteriorly from just below the buttock to the heel of the foot. For knee immobilization only, the splint length should extend posteriorly from the midthigh to about 3 inches above the malleoli. To apply the splint, the patient is placed in the prone position on a stretcher, exam table, or parent's lap. After the outer wrap layer is applied, the splint must be properly shaped. When the splint is being used to treat a fracture, the knee should be placed in slight flexion, and the ankle should be kept in neutral position; for knee injuries, the knee should remain in full extension but should not be hyperextended. To ensure integrity of the splint at the knee joint, excessive motion should be avoided until the splint has dried completely.

For comfort, extra padding can be placed over bony prominences before applying the splint material. Crutch support on one or both sides is recommended for ease of ambulation. In

in the prone position on a stretcher, exam table, or parent's lap, and the injured arm is held like an inverted L over the edge, with the forearm hanging down toward the floor (elbow flexed 90 degrees). After the outer wrap layer is applied, the splint should be shaped with the elbow flexed 90 degrees and the forearm in a neutral position (see Fig. 101.5). The parent or assistant should hold this position until the splint has dried completely. To ensure comfort, extra padding can

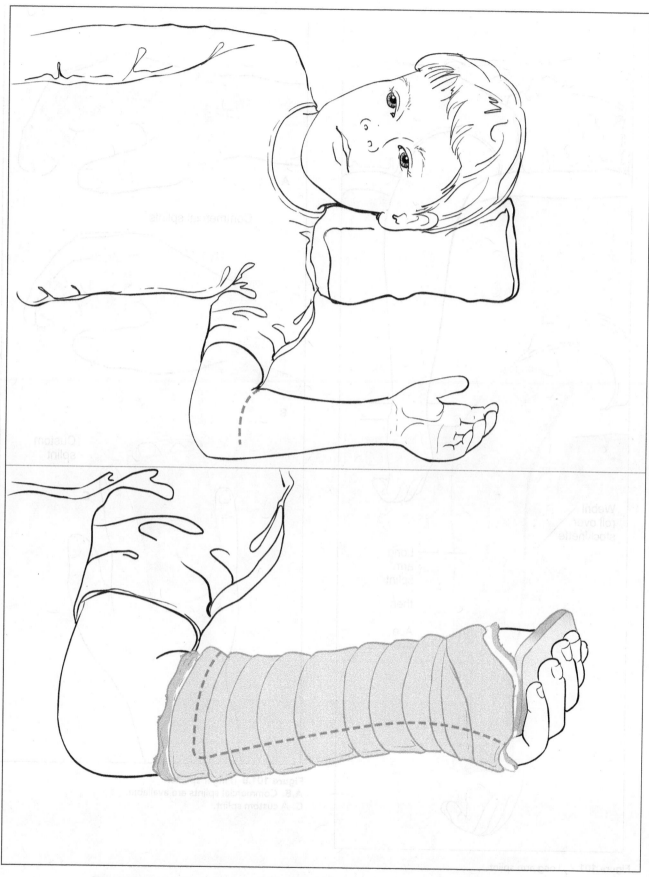

Figure 101.6 A Colles splint is used for older children. For younger children, a sugar tong splint is preferred precause it provides both dorsal and volar stability.

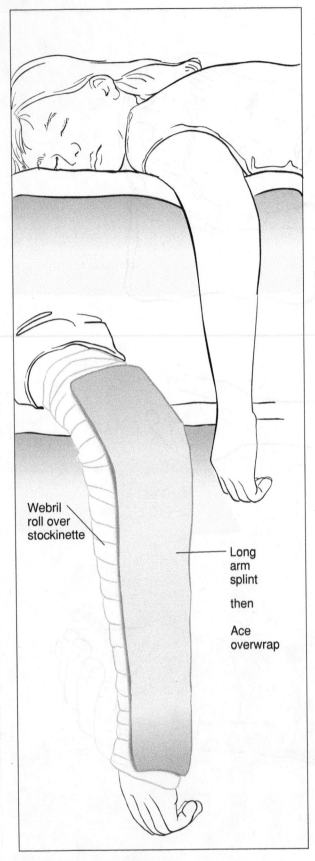

Webril
roll over
stockinette

Long
arm
splint

then

Ace
overwrap

Figure 101.7 Long arm splint.

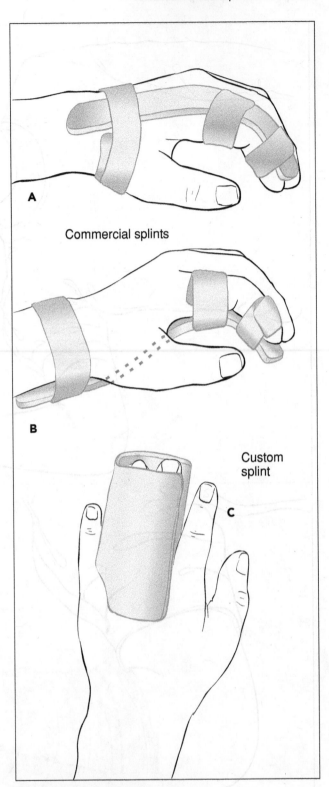

A

Commercial splints

B

Custom
splint

C

Figure 101.8 Finger splints.
A,B. Commercial splints are available.
C. A custom splint.

general, crutches should not be given to children under 6 years old, as they are unlikely to successfully coordinate crutch walking and are thereby at risk for further injury. Careful patient and parent education is advised when crutches are provided to young children over 6 years old. Without proper guidance, they are often misused and are therefore unsafe. The options are limited for children under 6 years old, as they must be transported by wheelchair or carried by an adult if they cannot ambulate with the long leg splint or knee immobilizer in place.

Posterior Short Leg Splint

A posterior leg splint is universally used to support injuries of the distal tibia and fibula, the ankle, and the foot. The stirrup splint (see below) is often combined with a posterior splint to stabilize ankle injuries.

Application of a posterior splint is shown in Figure 101.9A. The width of the splint should be such that it covers at least half of the leg circumference, and the length should be such that it extends posteriorly from the level of the fibular neck over the heel of the foot to the base of the toes. The splint should extend beyond the toes in younger children to avoid inadvertent injury (i.e., stubbed toes). The splint is applied with the child prone on a stretcher, exam table, or parent's lap, with the lower leg flexed to 90 degrees at the knee. After the outer wrap layer is applied, the splint is shaped with the foot-ankle in neutral position at 90 degrees of flexion. This position can be held by an assistant, or the child can be repositioned in a chair with the foot flat on the floor until the splint has dried completely.

For comfort, extra padding should be placed over bony prominences before the splint is applied. The clinician should avoid placing pressure near the fibular neck to reduce the risk of compression of the peroneal nerve. A second outer wrap layer is recommended to further protect the splint in young children. It is important, however, not to further tighten the splint when applying the second outer wrap layer. Crutches are recommended for ease of ambulation but, as discussed previously, should not be given to children under 6 years old.

Despite the best splint technique, the posterior leg splint often weakens at the ankle over time. The splint bends 90 degrees in this area (by design) and can be damaged by dorsiflexion or plantar flexion motions of the foot-ankle unit. Parents and older children should be warned to avoid all weight bearing on the splinted leg, and older children should be encouraged to use crutches. To reinforce the splint for younger children, fiberglass splint material should be used and a stirrup or sugar tong should be added to the outside of the splint, as described below.

Stirrup Splint (Sugar Tong, Ankle Brace)

Stirrup splints add lateral support for ankle soft tissue injuries. Commercial stirrup splints are valuable tools for dynamic splinting of the ankle and are widely available. Of note, a stirrup splint alone cannot be used to manage an ankle frac-

ture. However, a stirrup splint can be added around a posterior splint to fully stabilize this type of injury.

A stirrup splint is shown in Fig. 101.9B. The width of a stirrup splint should be such that it covers at least half of the leg circumference, and the length should be such that it extends laterally from just below the level of the fibular head and around the heel, ending just below the medial aspect of the knee. The splint is applied with the patient positioned as described above for a posterior splint.

Stirrup splints alone can fit in a loose shoe and can therefore allow for weight bearing to be initiated. If a commercial splint is not available, fiberglass material is recommended so that the splint can endure some weight bearing. Crutches should be provided if full weight bearing is contraindicated in children over 6 years old. Stirrup splints are not recommended for children under 6 years old except in combination with a posterior splint.

▶ COMPLICATIONS

Splints that are properly used rarely have significant complications. Two well-described problems can, however, be avoided through proper splinting technique. First, swelling commonly occurs around fracture areas and, if severe, can compromise neurovascular structures. Such complications can be avoided if the clinician is careful to (a) never fully encircle an injury with rigid splint material, (b) keep the outer wrap layer

---

 SUMMARY

1 Cut dry plaster or fiberglass and stockinette to fit the area to be splinted; use the opposite, unaffected extremity to measure the materials when possible.

2 Slide stockinette on extremity.

3 Roll Webril around the stockinette.

4 Position the child's extremity for optimal plaster or fiberglass application.

5 Wet the plaster or fiberglass material and apply; avoid using overly warm water because the splint will release additional heat as it hardens.

6 Perform initial splint shaping at large joints.

7 Overwrap the plaster or fiberglass with an elastic bandage (Ace) or gauze wrap; consider applying a layer of Webril to the outside of the plaster or fiberglass to prevent sticking to the elastic bandage or gauze wrap.

8 Shape the splint contours to the final form.

9 Maintain the splint position (or have parents hold) until the plaster or fiberglass has completely hardened.

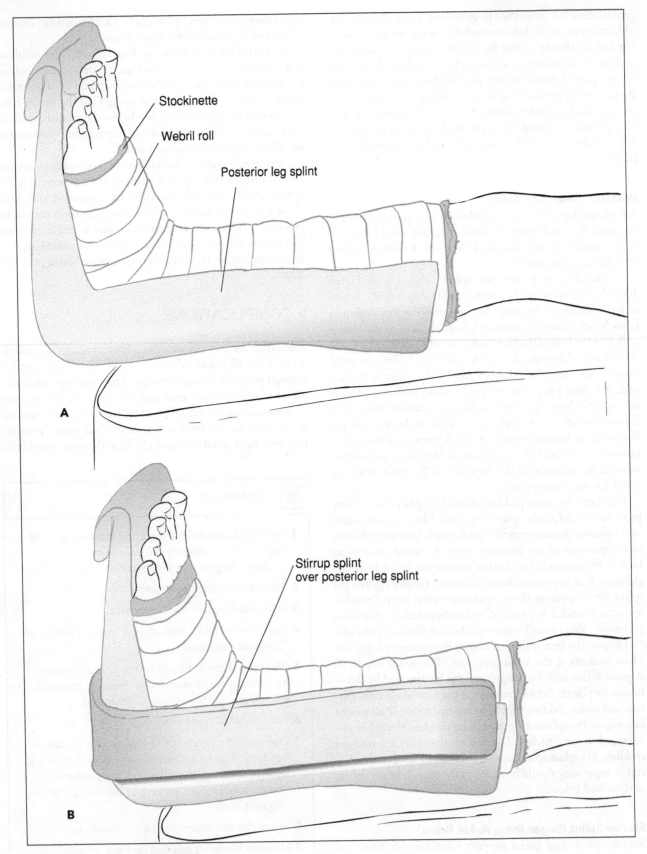

Stockinette

Webril roll

Posterior leg splint

A

Stirrup splint
over posterior leg splint

B

Figure 101.9
A. Posterior leg splint.
B. A stirrup applied for added lateral stability. The plastic or fiberglass is wrapped
with one or two layers of elastic (Ace) wrap.

CLINICAL TIPS

▶ If there is doubt about whether a child has a fracture, a splint should be applied, and a follow-up examination with possible repeat radiographs should be arranged.

▶ Adequate pain control should be provided before a splint is applied, especially in a young child.

▶ The appropriate length of a splint should be measured using the opposite, noninjured limb.

▶ Cool or tepid water should be used when making a splint to avoid thermal burns.

▶ Factors that contribute to making a functional and durable splint include properly positioning the patient, molding the plaster or fiberglass carefully, and allowing adequate drying time before the patient is discharged.

▶ Areas where the splint will bend around joints can have notches cut laterally to minimize folding of the plaster or fiberglass.

▶ For upper extremity splints that are heavy or involve the elbow, slings are often beneficial, although they are not generally tolerated by children under 4 years of age.

▶ The patient and/or parents should always be provided with discharge instructions regarding pain control, warning signs, and follow-up care.

snug but not tight, and (c) use verbal and written instructions to explain the importance of limb elevation in the first 48 hours after an injury. Signs of compartment syndrome should be reviewed in all cases but are especially important for those with fractures at or near a joint. Second, although much less common than with adults, prolonged immobiliza-

tion can eventually cause limb stiffness in children. Plans for follow-up orthopaedic care should be clearly outlined on discharge so that the splint can be removed or replaced in a proper time frame.

▶ SUMMARY

Splints are an essential tool for the management of acute fractures that do not require immediate surgical intervention. Splints also provide definitive treatment for many soft-tissue injuries and sprains and for some minor fractures. Because of the possibility of growth plate fractures that may be invisible on x-ray, the adage "when in doubt, splint" is a prudent guideline for most extremity injuries in children. Knowledge of splinting techniques is therefore a basic skill for all practitioners who care for injured children. Children's bones generally heal at a very rapid pace. Reasonable precision in the diagnosis, initial management, and follow-up treatment of a pediatric extremity injury will ensure that the best possible outcome is achieved. The importance of thorough discharge instructions and follow-up information cannot be overemphasized.

▶ REFERENCES

1. Bachman D, Santora S. Orthopedic trauma. In: *Textbook of Pediatric Emergency Medicine.* 4th ed. Baltimore: Lippincott Williams & Wilkins; 2000:1435–1478.
2. Shaw D. Principles and techniques of splint musculocutaneous injuries. *Emerg Med Clin North Am.* 1984;2:391–407.
3. Simon R. *Emergency Orthopaedics.* 3rd ed. Norwalk CT: Appleton & Lange; 2000.
4. Do TT, Strub WM, Foad SL, et al. Reduction versus remodeling in pediatric distal forearm fractures: a preliminary cost analysis. *J Pediatr Orthop.* 2003;12:109–120.
5. Beaty JH, Kasser JR. *Rockwood and Wilkins' Fractures in Children.* Baltimore: Lippincott Williams & Wilkins; 2001.
6. Lorell WW, Winter RB, Morrissey RT, et al. *Lorell and Winter's Pediatric Orthopaedics.* 5th ed. Philadelphia: Lippincott Williams & Wilkins; 2001.
7. Howes D. Plaster splints: techniques and indications. *Am Family Practice.* 1984;30:215–221.
8. Kaplan S. Burns following application of plaster splint dressings. *J Bone Joint Surg.* 1981;63A:670–672.

102

DAVID T. BACHMAN

Short Arm and Short Leg Casts

▸ INTRODUCTION

The use of emergency casting as a treatment for orthopedic injuries can be traced to Antonius Mathysen, a Dutch military surgeon, who in 1851 used dressings impregnated with dehydrated gypsum in the management of fractures (1). Today, casting, whether with plaster or synthetic materials, remains the most common method of immobilizing and stabilizing fractures so that healing can occur. In most instances, casting is the definitive treatment. It must be remembered, however, that even a properly applied cast is not a substitute for fracture reduction when needed.

Applying a short arm or short leg cast is within the scope of practice of family physicians, pediatricians, and emergency physicians who have a strong understanding of acute orthopedic injuries in the pediatric age group as delineated in standard reference texts (1,2). With proper training and supervision, personnel working in the ambulatory setting—including physician assistants, nurse practitioners, registered nurses, and technicians—can apply simple casts. It should be noted that a properly applied splint can provide immobilization comparable to that afforded by a cast (see Chapter 101). Consequently, when orthopedic referral is readily available, splinting is generally the initial treatment of choice for those whose experience with casting is limited. The growing popularity among youths of such activities as skateboarding, roller skating, and scooter riding will likely ensure a steady stream of pediatric fractures, affording ample opportunity for clinicians in the acute care setting to gain splinting and casting experience (3).

▸ ANATOMY AND PHYSIOLOGY

Distinct differences exist between children and adults in both the nature and management of skeletal injuries. Most differences reflect the fact that unlike the bones of an adult (i.e., anyone who has reached skeletal maturity), those of a child are growing (see also Fig. 101.1). The periosteum of the bones of a child is physiologically quite active. As a result, the potential for healing and, in many instances, for significant remodeling is high. With distal forearm fractures, the remodeling capability is such that injuries with as much as 15 degrees of angulation and 1 cm of shortening will completely remodel without functional sequelae using immobilization alone (4). Nonunion essentially never occurs. Conversely, fractures in children frequently involve the growth plate, posing a risk to ongoing bone growth without proper management (see also Fig. 101.2) (5). Many growth plate injuries result from mechanisms that in adults would cause a ligamentous injury. For example, a severe valgus injury to the knee will often result in a fracture through the distal femoral physis in a child; an adult will usually have only a strain of the medical collateral ligament. With any extremity injury in a child, therefore, the clinician must be highly suspicious of the possibility of a fracture.

Clearly, the most common indication for applying a cast is treatment of a fracture. In all instances, it must first be determined that the position of the fracture is satisfactory. Despite the potential for fracture remodeling in children, it is not correct to assume that remodeling can correct all deformities. Bowing and rotational deformities in particular have limited potential for remodeling.

Instances also occur in which clinical findings suggest a fracture but radiographic studies are negative. When this occurs, it is recommended that the involved extremity be immobilized until a definitive diagnosis can be established. A subtle fracture may be missed, or a nondisplaced Salter-Harris type I fracture at a growth plate may be radiographically invisible. Splinting is generally adequate in this setting. However, in some cases, such as a suspected toddler's fracture in a young child, a cast may be preferred. Similarly, it may be preferable to cast rather than splint certain soft-tissue injuries, such as a severe ankle sprain.

▶ INDICATIONS

Specific injuries for which a nonorthopedist can consider applying a short arm or short leg cast are listed below. As mentioned, proper splinting will generally provide equally satisfactory treatment on a temporary basis. The decision to cast rather than splint should be made only after the nature of any accompanying soft-tissue injuries (e.g., abrasions that require dressing changes) and the potential for ongoing swelling are evaluated. Whenever there is a likelihood of significant swelling, application of a readily removable or adjustable splint rather than a cast is recommended to minimize the potential for neurovascular compromise. Additionally, certain fractures merit urgent orthopedic consultation, including complete fractures of the radius, ulna, and tibia as well as fractures with significant displacement or growth plate involvement. All open fractures warrant emergent orthopedic consultation and evaluation. Even when the nonorthopedist does choose to provide the initial treatment and apply a cast, he or she should always ensure prompt referral to an orthopedic specialist for follow-up care.

The following are indications for a short arm cast (Fig. 102.1): (a) torus fractures of the radius and ulna; (b) nondisplaced Salter-Harris type I fractures of the distal radius (may be a clinical rather than a radiographic diagnosis); (c) clinically suspected scaphoid (navicular) fractures (thumb spica cast) (Fig. 102.2), although an overt fracture on x-ray warrants consultation with a hand specialist first if possible; and (d) nondisplaced, stable metacarpal fractures. The following are indications for a short leg cast (Fig. 102.3): (a) minor fibula fractures (including suspected Salter-Harris type I fractures of the distal fibula), (b) toddler's fractures, (c) severe ankle sprains, (d) stable fractures of metatarsals, and (e) fractures of the mid- and hindfoot.

▶ EQUIPMENT

Stockinette, 2-, 3-, and 4-inch widths
Cast padding (Webril), 2-, 3-, and 4-inch widths
Plaster or fiberglass rolls, 2-, 3-, 4-, and 6-inch widths
Plaster strips (splints), 3″ × 15″, 4″ × 15″, and 5″ × 30″ sizes
Felt padding
Bucket
Gloves, gowns, shoe covers, drapes (towels)
Cast knife
Cast bender
Cast saw
Cast spreader
Cast shoes (canvas overboots)

In general, successful application of a cast depends more on proper technique than on the specific brand of materials used. Certain types of cast padding are easier to work with than others, but all are satisfactory. The primary decision for the clinician is whether to use plaster or synthetic (fiberglass) casting material. Of the two, plaster is less expensive, has a longer shelf life, and is easier to apply. Fiberglass is lighter, provides superior strength, dries and cures more rapidly, resists water much better, and is unlikely to cause thermal burns. The material chosen usually reflects availability and clinician experience and preference.

▶ PROCEDURE

Certain steps must first be taken in applying all casts (6–8). Before applying any cast, it is important to assemble all the necessary materials. Running out of casting material midway through the procedure can adversely affect the quality of the cast provided. The amount and width of stockinette, cast padding, and casting material needed depends on the size of the patient and the type of cast applied. The patient and parents should be prepared for the procedure. Proper positioning is crucial. The help of an assistant is often necessary, especially with younger children. With adequate explanation and reassurance—and if a parent is allowed to remain—most children will cooperate fully. Draping is also important, both to protect patient clothing and modesty. The clinician, too, should take steps to protect his or her clothing. Gowns and shoe covers are recommended. Gloves are essential when working with fiberglass, as fibers on the skin can cause prolonged and extremely uncomfortable itching.

Before the cast is applied, the skin of the involved extremity should be washed with soap and water and thoroughly dried. All superficial wounds should be carefully cleansed and then covered with a thin, sterile dressing. If the wounds are more than minor, the clinician must consider initial splinting rather than casting until satisfactory wound healing has begun. Once cleaned, the extremity should be placed in the position in which it will be casted. Proper positioning must be maintained for the duration of the procedure if ridging of the casting materials and pressure points are to be avoided.

Next, stockinette can be applied (Fig. 102.1A). Its use, although favored by many, is not an essential step, but it does allow for smoother trimming at the ends of the cast. When used, it can be applied as one continuous piece overlying the whole portion of the extremity to be casted or as two segments at the upper and lower ends of the cast only. When it is applied in two segments, stretching and tension over bony prominences must be avoided. If it is applied as a single piece, care should be taken to cut off any folds or wrinkles that result.

The cast padding is the next layer to be applied. The padding should be rolled onto the extremity distally to proximally, each turn overlapping the previous one by half (Fig. 102.1B,C). Overpadding is to be avoided, as it will result in a

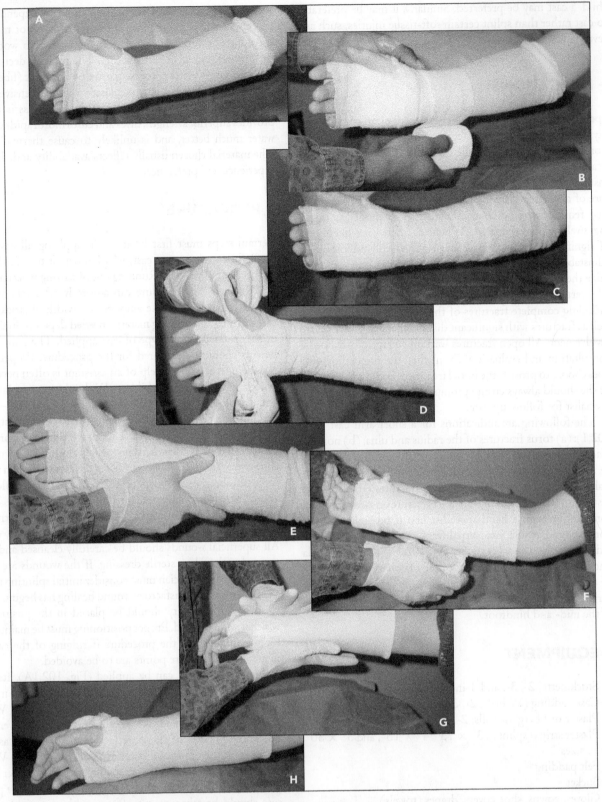

Figure 102.1 Applying a short arm cast.

    A. The casting position is maintained and the stockinette (optional) is applied.

B,C. Cast padding (Webril) is wrapped distal to proximal, overlapping by half each turn.

    D. Plaster rolls are similarly wrapped distal to proximal.

    E. The plaster is smoothed using the palms and thenar eminences (not the fingers).

F,G. The ends of the stockinette are folded over to provide smooth ends for the cast.

    H. Positioning of the extremity is maintained until the cast is hardened.

If hot water is used, the drying time is too fast to permit successful application, and the exothermic reaction of the plaster hardening can cause thermal burns. The end of the roll is easier to find if it is folded back before immersion. When there are no more air bubbles, the rolls should be removed and then squeezed (but not wrung out completely) to remove water. The more water removed, the faster the drying time. Pinching the ends of the roll together prevents "telescoping" during application.

Beginning distally, the plaster rolls should be applied in the same direction as the padding, again overlapping by half (Fig. 102.1D). The rolls must be held close to the extremity, using the thenar eminence to push the roll around the limb while wrapping under moderate tension. The free hand should be used to make pleats or tucks as needed to guide the roll and to accommodate the changing diameter of the limb. When one roll is finished, the next should begin at the same point. Two turns should not be taken at the same point other than at the upper and lower ends of the cast.

After one to two rolls of plaster have been applied, and when the plaster is the consistency of wet cardboard, smoothing and shaping should be done using the flat of the hand and the thenar eminence (Fig. 102.1E) (I). Additional rolls can then be applied until a cast of uniform thickness (0.25 inches) has been achieved. No more than six to seven layers of plaster are generally needed. The cast should not be any thicker at the fracture site than elsewhere. Rubbing and smoothing should continue to ensure that all layers of the cast fuse together into one strong unit. Of note, too much rubbing too late in the drying phase will cause the plaster to crumble. At all times during the process of smoothing, extreme care must be taken to avoid any focal indentations or pressure points. Before applying the final roll of plaster, the ends of the stockinette should be folded over and then covered with cast material so as to provide smooth ends for the cast (Fig. 102.1F,G). Alternatively, the ends of the stockinette can be folded over and held in place using shorter strips of cast material.

When using fiberglass casting materials, the same basic considerations apply, with some notable exceptions. First, cold water must always be used to wet the rolls. Second, as it is not possible to make tucks as readily as with plaster, it is recommended that rolls of narrower width be used. Two-inch rolls are generally adequate given the superior strength of fiberglass.

Once the cast is complete, positioning of the extremity must be maintained until adequate hardening occurs (Fig. 102.1H). Any movement during this time—when the interlocking of the plaster crystals is occurring—causes considerable loss of strength. (It takes 48 hours for a plaster cast to cure completely.) Once the cast hardens, the patient should be reexamined and questioned about pain relief, pressure points, and possible circulatory compromise. Written instructions regarding cast care and signs of complications should be provided and reviewed. A return for a formal cast check at 12 to 24 hours is suggested. Prescriptions for appropriate analgesics should be written and follow-up appointments planned.

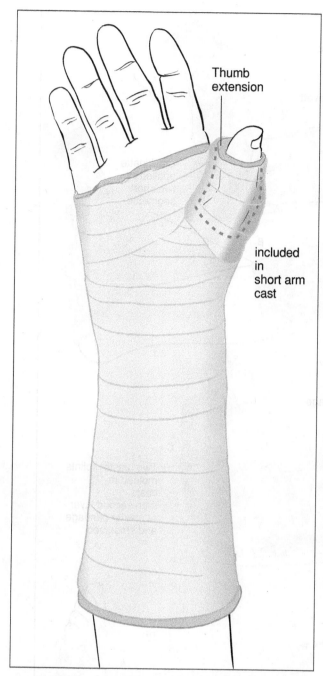

Figure 102.2 Thumb spica cast. The same approach is used as for a short arm cast, except that the (extended) thumb is included in an extension of the cast. To wrap the thumb itself, 2-inch cast padding can be cut to a 1-inch size.

loose cast. Extra padding should be applied over bony prominences such as the ulnar styloid, the malleoli, and the heel. Small pieces of felt can be used for this purpose if needed. Smooth application of the cast padding is essential; wrinkles should be cut or torn away.

If plaster is used, all the rolls needed to cast the injured extremity should be set on end in water deep enough to cover them completely. Using tepid or cool water is recommended.

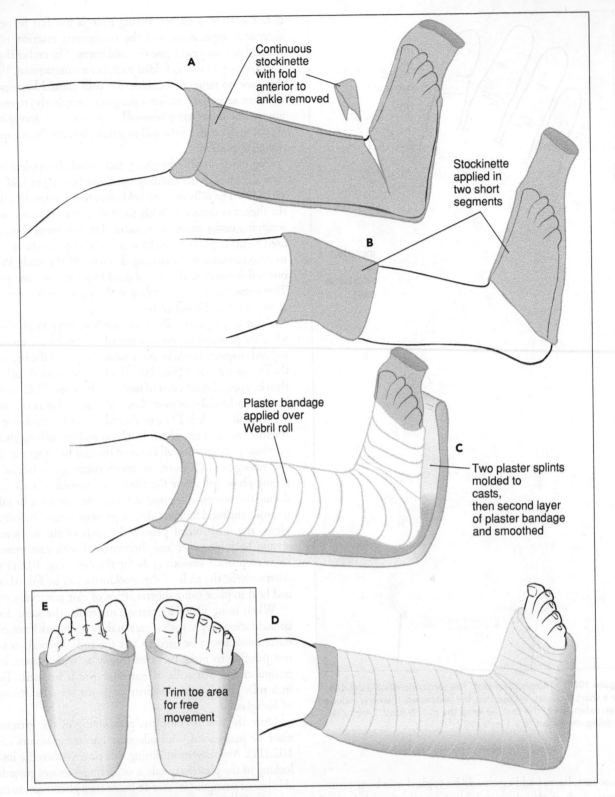

Figure 102.3   Applying a short leg cast.
   A,B. Stockinette (optional) is applied in either one continuous piece or two short segments at the
            proximal and distal ends of the cast. Cast padding (Webril) is then rolled distal to proximal
            over the extremity, overlapping by half each turn.
   C. The cast material is similarly wrapped distal to proximal. For a large child or if weight bearing is
          anticipated, plaster splints can be molded to the cast posteriorly and then overwrapped with
          another layer of plaster.
   D. The plaster is smoothed and shaped appropriately.
   E. The cast should be trimmed if necessary to allow for flexion and fanning of all the toes.

SUMMARY: SHORT ARM CAST

1 Assemble the materials. Two rolls of plaster are usually adequate; use 2- to 3-inch size for a child, 4-inch for an adult. With fiberglass, use narrower rolls.

2 Position the patient supine, with the extremity abducted 90 degrees and the elbow flexed 90 degrees.

3 Apply stockinette (optional) with thumbhole; avoid wrinkles.

4 Apply cast padding. Wrap from the proximal palmar crease to about 1 inch below the flexion crease of the elbow. Make a transverse tear in the padding before wrapping around the thumb webspace. Apply additional padding over the ulnar styloid.

5 Apply the cast material rolls by rolling from distal to proximal (do not begin too distally). A total of four to six layers of plaster or three layers of fiberglass are usually sufficient. Twist 180 degrees when wrapping through the thumb webspace. Before applying the second roll, fold over the ends of the stockinette. Allow for 90 degrees flexion at the metacarpal-phalangeal joints for fanning of fingers and for opposition of the thumb to the index and little fingers.

6 Smooth and shape (begin rubbing when the plaster is the consistency of wet cardboard). Mold to the shape of the forearm using palms and thenar eminences, not fingers. The shape should be cylindrical, not round.

7 Maintain immobilization during the drying. Reassess for pressure points, pain relief, and neurovascular compromise. Trim the ends of the cast as needed to allow for adequate finger and thumb motion.

8 For a thumb spica splint, use the same approach, except include the thumb (extended) in the cast. Cut 2-inch cast padding to a 1-inch size for use around the thumb itself.

 SUMMARY: SHORT LEG CAST

1 Assemble the materials. Three rolls of plaster are usually adequate. Use 3- to 4-inch size for a child, 6-inch for an adult. With fiberglass, use narrower rolls.

2 Position the patient and extremity as follows:

  a Patient sitting, knee flexed to 90 degrees,
     -OR-

  b Patient supine, hip and knee flexed to 90 degrees, assistant supporting leg,
     -OR-

  c Patient prone, knee flexed to 90 degrees.

3 Apply stockinette (optional). If single piece, cut away the transverse fold in front of the ankle (it is usually better to apply two short segments at the proximal and distal ends of the cast).

4 Apply cast padding, wrapping from the level of the distal metatarsals to one fingerbreadth below the tibial tubercle. Apply additional padding over the malleoli and heel.

5 Apply cast material, rolling from distal to proximal (do not begin too distally). A total of five to seven layers of plaster or three layers of fiberglass are usually sufficient. For a larger child or if weight bearing is intended, add reinforcing splints when using plaster:

  a Incorporate two plaster splints posteriorly, folding back last 1 to 2 inches at the level of the distal metatarsals.
     -OR-

  b Fold 4-inch plaster splints in half longitudinally, placing one posteriorly and one as a stirrup (U-shape from medial to lateral).

6 Smooth and shape (begin rubbing when the plaster is the consistency of wet cardboard). Mold to the shape of the lower leg using palms and thenar eminences, not fingers. Allow for flexion and fanning of all the toes.

7 Maintain immobilization during drying. Reassess for pressure points, pain relief, and neurovascular compromise. Fit the patient for a cast boot or crutches as needed. Prescribe no weight bearing for a minimum of 24 hours.

CLINICAL TIPS

▶ Cool or tepid water should be used when making a cast to avoid the possibility of thermal burns resulting from the exothermic reaction that occurs as plaster hardens.

▶ Using the widest roll of cast material practical for the size of the extremity will speed the application and allow for a more even cast.

▶ A splint should be used instead of a cast whenever significant delayed tissue swelling is a concern.

▶ Patients and parents should be carefully instructed to return immediately for evaluation of signs or symptoms of neurovascular compromise (e.g., increasing pain, paresthesias, numbness).

▶ COMPLICATIONS

Virtually all complications that can occur after the application of a cast can be prevented by careful adherence to technique. Fracture displacement occurs when a cast is applied too loosely or improperly molded or when the wrong type of cast altogether is chosen. For example, a complete midshaft fracture of the radius and ulna is likely to displace in a short arm cast because a well-applied long arm cast is needed for this type of fracture. Pressure sores and skin necrosis can be prevented if adequate padding is provided and care is taken to avoid creating pressure points during the molding and smoothing steps. A cast that is too loose can also prove problematic by allowing excessive movement between the cast and the underlying skin (5). It should be remembered that patients often first complain of burning pain or discomfort as a pressure sore develops. In such cases, a window should be cut in the cast or the cast should be removed and replaced. Thermal burns can be avoided if cool or cold water is used when making a plaster cast and if overly thick casts (more than eight layers) are not applied. Care should be taken not to cover the cast with a pillow or other insulating material during the drying phase.

Neurovascular compromise, leading eventually to frank compartment syndrome, is the most serious potential complication of casting (see also Chapter 106). As mentioned previously, a splint better allows for tissue swelling and is generally preferable to a cast when significant delayed swelling is a concern. If neurovascular compromise is suspected after cast placement, the cast should be "bivalved" (cut into two halves) *and* the underlying padding should be cut. Leaving the padding intact may not alleviate compression. It should be emphasized that the presence of distal pulses is no guarantee against the presence of compartment syndrome. Progressively increasing pain, especially pain with passive stretching of muscle, is the earliest sign of compartment syndrome and must not be ignored. Immediate orthopedic consultation should be sought when this complication is suspected.

▶ SUMMARY

With an understanding of the principles of both pediatric orthopedics and cast application, the family physician, pediatrician, or emergency physician can perform initial casting for a number of simple fractures. Complications can occur but are avoidable if proper technique is followed and families are given appropriate instructions regarding signs and symptoms that require immediate re-evaluation.

▶ REFERENCES

1. Wenger DR, Pring ME, Rang M. *Rang's Children's Fractures*. 3rd ed. Philadelphia: Lippincott Williams & Wilkins; 2005.
2. Bachman DT, Santora SD. Orthopaedic trauma. In: Fleisher GR, Ludwig S, Henretig F, eds. *Textbook of Pediatric Emergency Medicine*. 5th ed. Philadelphia: Lippincott Williams & Wilkins; 2006.
3. Zalavras C, Nikolopoulou G, Essin D, et al. Pediatric fractures during skateboarding, roller skating, and scooter riding. *Am J Sports Med*. 2005;33:568–573.
4. Do TT, Strub WM, Foad SL, et al. Reduction versus remodeling in pediatric distal forearm fractures: a preliminary cost analysis. *J Pediatr Orthop B*. 2003;12:109–115.
5. Perron AD, Miller MD, Brady WJ. Orthopedic pitfalls in the ED: pediatric growth plate injuries. *Am J Emerg Med*. 2002;20:50–54.
6. Iversen LD, Clawson DK. *Manual of Acute Orthopaedic Therapeutics*. 4th ed. Boston: Little, Brown & Co.; 1995.
7. Lewis RC. *Handbook of Traction, Casting, and Splinting Techniques*. Philadelphia: JB Lippincott Co.; 1977.
8. Wu KK. *Techniques in Surgical Casting and Splinting*. Philadelphia: Lea & Febiger; 1987.

PETER M. ANTEVY AND RICHARD A. SALADINO

103

Management of Finger Injuries

▶ INTRODUCTION

Finger injuries occur frequently in children and may have significant functional or cosmetic morbidity associated with them. These injuries are often treated in an outpatient setting but are usually painful and almost always frightening to the child. For all such injuries, age-appropriate restraint may be necessary and should be considered for young or uncooperative patients. This chapter discusses the outpatient management of common finger injuries, including subungual hematomas, subungual foreign bodies, nail bed lacerations and avulsions, and the mallet finger deformity.

▶ ANATOMY

An understanding of the anatomy of the nail bed allows the clinician to appropriately plan treatment and/or repair injuries to the fingertip. The nail bed is a thin layer of epithelial tissue overlying the cortex of the distal phalanx (Fig. 103.1). The germinal matrix is the proximal element of the nail bed responsible for most of the nail formation (1). The distal end of the germinal matrix is marked by the lunula, the light semicircular area extending just distal to the eponychium. The eponychium is the fold of skin that covers the proximal nail. The sterile matrix is the distal tissue of the nail bed and is responsible for a small amount of nail growth. The nail is tightly adherent to the sterile matrix but loosely held to the germinal matrix. The lateral margins of the nail are held in place by the lateral skin folds of the fingertip.

Managing the injuries discussed in this chapter also requires knowledge of the motor and neurovascular anatomy of the finger. Extension of the finger is provided by the extensor tendon that inserts onto the epiphysis of the distal phalanx. Flexion of the fingertip occurs via the insertion of the flexor

digitorum profundus tendon distal to the epiphyseal plate of the volar aspect of the distal phalanx. The flexor digitorum superficialis tendon divides and inserts on the bodies of the middle phalanges of the second through the fifth digits. A rich blood supply is afforded the fingertip by numerous branches of the ulnar and radial elements of the digital arteries. The pad of the fingertip is composed of fatty and soft tissues with dense sensory innervation.

▶ EXAMINATION OF THE DIGITS

It is important to perform (and document) a thorough examination of the injured finger in order to plan appropriate treatment (Fig. 103.2). In most cases, once the sensory examination and the parts of the functional examination that require intact sensation have been performed, appropriate local anesthesia (see Chapter 35) and, if necessary, sedation (see Chapter 33) can be administered. Judicious use of sedation and local anesthesia will result in a more comfortable examination and will increase the likelihood that a child will cooperate with the remainder of the examination. The examination is focused on evaluation of motor function and neurovascular integrity. In particular, it is important to examine the fingers and hand both in the anatomic position and in the position of injury. Injured structures underlying a laceration, such as a tendon or joint capsule, may not be visible in the anatomic position but may move into the site of the laceration when the finger is placed in the position of injury.

Motor function of the fingers is assessed by testing both muscle strength and tendon function. With a cooperative child, the child is asked to place his or her hand on the examination table with the palm facing upward. The clinician then places two fingers on the involved finger just proximal to the distal interphalangeal joint, holding the finger firmly

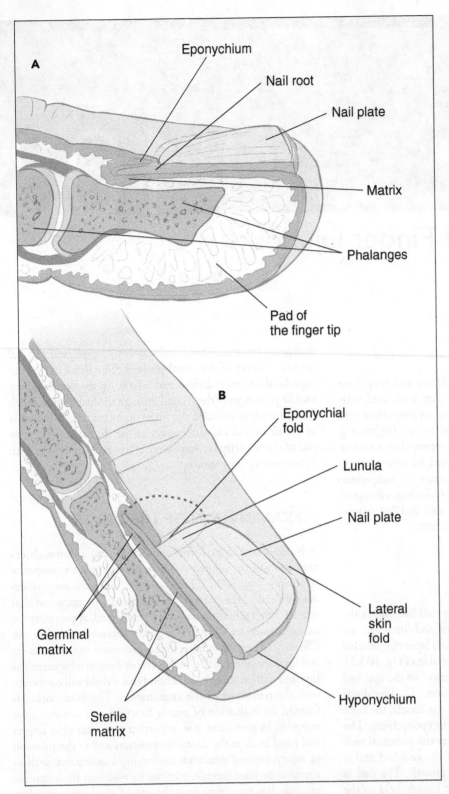

Figure 103.1 Anatomy of the finger and nail bed.

against the table (Fig. 103.2A). The patient is then asked to flex the tip of the finger. If function is normal, the maneuver is repeated against resistance. In this way, both distal muscle strength and integrity of the flexor digitorum profundus tendon are assessed. Proximal muscle strength and integrity of the flexor digitorum superficialis tendon are then tested by

holding the child's noninjured fingers against the examination table and again asking the child to flex the injured finger, first passively, then against resistance (Fig. 103.2B). Pain associated with these maneuvers in the presence of a laceration on the palmar or lateral portion of the finger may indicate a tendon injury. In younger children who are less likely to cooperate,

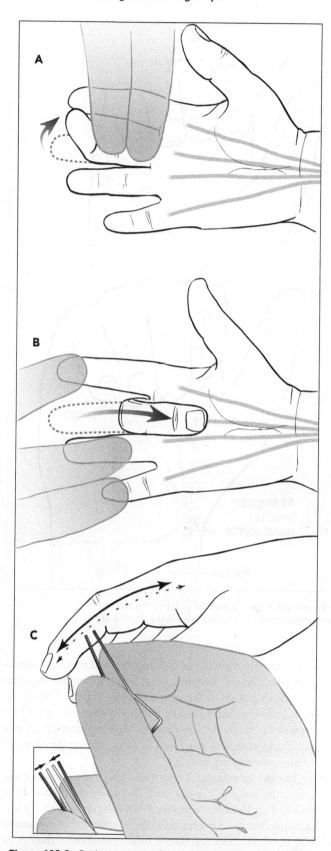

Figure 103.2 Basic sensory and motor examination of the digits.
A. Assessing flexion at the distal interphalangeal joint.
B. Assessing function at the proximal interphalangeal joint.
C. Testing two-point discrimination.

merely holding the child's hand against the examination table may cause the child to flex the appropriate fingers. It may, however, be impossible to know whether associated pain is present. Consequently, lacerations of the palmar or lateral aspects of the fingers of young or uncooperative children must be thoroughly explored. Extensor tendon injuries do not require immediate repair in many cases, but a careful exam should be performed nonetheless to detect these injuries. Cooperative children are asked to close and open their hand or to curl and uncurl the affected finger. Pain or weakness with this maneuver raises the suspicion of extensor tendon injury.

Injuries to the fingers commonly result in phalangeal fractures. Midshaft phalangeal fractures should be evaluated thoroughly for rotational deformity, angulation, or displacement and these findings clearly documented. To assess for rotational deformity, the patient is asked to slowly make a fist with the palm facing upward. As the fingertips approach the palm, they should all point toward the radial styloid. If the tip of the fractured finger points elsewhere, then a rotational abnormality is present (Fig. 103.3). Midshaft phalangeal fractures without rotation or displacement can be splinted using a dorsal foam splint that immobilizes joints on either side of the fracture. Those patients with rotational abnormalities or displacement should be referred to a hand surgeon to prevent permanent disability.

Evaluation of the sensory function of the fingers is also vitally important. In a finger with normal motor function but impaired sensation, the impairment may significantly limit the overall function of the individual digit and may affect the function of the hand itself. This part of the examination must obviously be performed prior to the administration of local anesthetic. In older children, two-point discrimination is tested using a paper clip opened and bent into a caliper with the points at 10 mm (see Fig. 103.2C). The child is asked to close his or her eyes, and the paper clip points are placed against the skin along the long axis of the finger. The touch should be relatively light so as to minimize the stimulation of pressure receptors. The patient is asked, "Do you feel one or two points?" The points of the paper clip are gradually brought closer together, and the test is repeated until the child reports feeling only one point. Two-point discrimination of 6 to 10 mm is normal for most children. It is important to assess sensation on both the radial and ulnar aspects of the finger as well as the dorsal and palmar sides. In cooperative younger children, it may only be possible to test light touch by asking the child whether he or she feels the touch of a finger or cotton-tipped swab on all aspects of the finger. With very young or uncooperative children, the clinician may not be able to discern the presence or absence of nerve injury. Indirect evidence of intact sensory innervation may be obtained by placing the finger in a bowl of warm water for 5 minutes. Intact innervation is indicated by wrinkling of the skin of the finger, whereas nerve injury results in persistence of smooth skin.

Vascular supply to the fingers is tested by assessing the capillary refilling time for the nail bed or fingertip pad. The tissue is compressed until it blanches and is then released. The

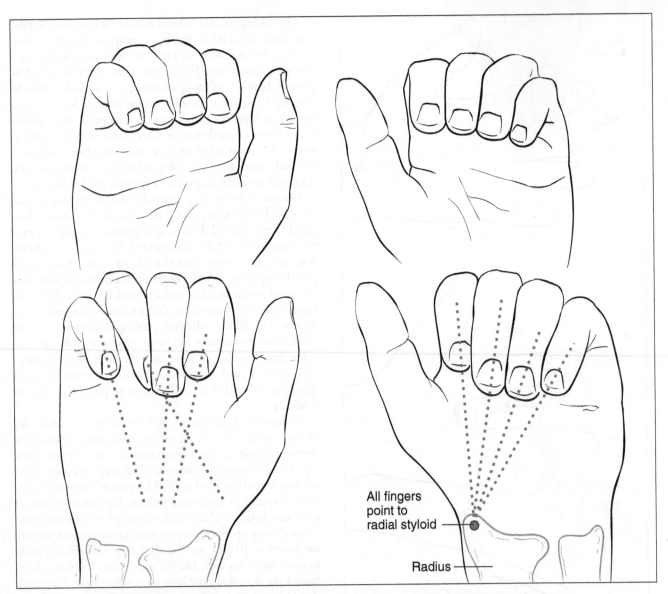

Figure 103.3 Finger rotational deformity. When flexed, the fingers should all point to the radial styloid. Upper row shows normal fingers. Lower row shows rotational deformities in the fingers of the right hand.

All fingers point to radial styloid

Radius

amount of time that it takes for the pink color to return is noted. Normal capillary refilling time is less than 2 seconds. In addition, if a sensory defect is noted in the context of a laceration, a vascular injury can be assumed.

▶ SUBUNGUAL HEMATOMA

A subungual hematoma is an acute, painful collection of blood between the fingernail and the nail bed, typically the result of blunt trauma to the fingertip. A subungual hematoma collects when the highly vascular nail bed is transiently crushed and extravasation of blood occurs, creating a blue-black discoloration beneath the nail. The nail and its margins usually remain intact. Often, as the hematoma enlarges, pressure beneath the nail increases, which compresses highly sensitive

nerve fibers in the nail bed and fingertip and results in significant pain. Typical mechanisms include trapping the fingertip in a closing door or window and blunt trauma from hammers and other heavy objects. Subungual hematomas are best treated by timely decompression. Nail trephination affords rapid and complete relief and is easily accomplished in an office or emergency setting.

In cases of subungual hematomas with disruption of the nail or its margins, the nail itself should be removed and the nail bed explored for lacerations requiring repair (2). An underlying distal phalanx fracture may be present, but hematoma size bears no direct correlation to the presence or absence of an underlying fracture (3). Any injury suspicious for fracture should be evaluated by plain radiography, as these injuries require immobilization (typically splinting). A displaced fracture of the distal phalanx can significantly disrupt the nail bed. Historically, subungual hematomas larger than 50% of the nail plate were thought to require nail removal to assess and repair any underlying nail bed lacerations (4–6). However, a more recent study demonstrated that otherwise uncomplicated subungual hematomas of virtually any size can be adequately treated with trephination alone (3). No subsequent cosmetic deformities or complications were noted in this study, even in the presence of underlying nondisplaced fractures. Another study reported nail bed injuries in 11 of 94 patients with subungual hematoma, yet these injuries did not correlate with hematoma size or the presence of a fracture (7).

A subungual hematoma usually remains liquefied for 24 to 36 hours (8). Therefore, drainage will still afford pain relief even if presentation is delayed. Relief of pain occurs rapidly once the hematoma is drained, and this should be performed as expeditiously as possible. However, trephination is unlikely to be successful beyond 48 hours after injury.

Equipment

Syringe with 27-gauge needle
Bupivacaine (0.25%) without epinephrine
Lidocaine (0.5% or 1%) without epinephrine
Antiseptic prep solution
Restraints (as needed)
Electrocautery device or, alternatively, a paper clip, butane lighter, and hemostats
Protective dressing

Procedure

Nail trephination involves creating a hole in the nail over the hematoma to allow drainage of the underlying blood (Fig. 103.4). If the hole is too small, blood can clot within it, preventing complete drainage and adequate pain relief. A hole of 3 or 4 mm in diameter is usually adequate, and one large hole is better than several small ones, each of which may clot (2). Anesthetic blockade of the finger (see Chapter 35) should be considered for a highly anxious child or for a child with underlying fractures in whom pain will persist. Most children easily tolerate drainage, however, especially when performed quickly with an electrocautery wire device (9,10).

The overlying nail should be gently cleaned with antiseptic solution. If alcohol is used, it must be allowed to dry, as it can ignite when heated. The electrocautery wire is held perpendicular to the nail over the subungual hematoma (Fig. 103.4A). When the wire has heated sufficiently, gentle downward pressure is used to trephinate the nail. Blood will rapidly exit through the hole, and the remainder may be extruded by gentle pressure on the nail bed. A high-speed nail drill can also be used in a similar fashion. As an alternative, the clinician can apply an 18-gauge needle perpendicular to the nail plate and spin it back and forth between the fingers with gentle downward pressure until the nail is penetrated. While slower and more likely to cause pain to an unanesthetized finger, this method is effective. Finally, a paper clip held by hemostats

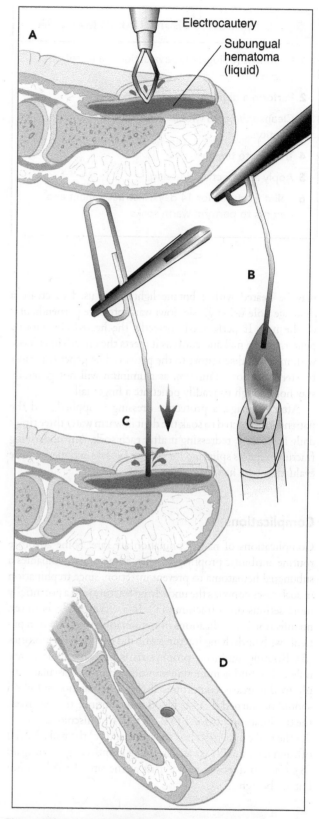

Figure 103.4 Nail trephination.
  A. A battery-powered heating element can be used to trephinate the nail and evacuate a subungual hematoma.
B,C. A paper clip is heated and used for nail trephination.
  D. One large hole is less likely to become occluded by clotted blood than multiple small holes.

SUMMARY: SUBUNGUAL HEMATOMA

1 Perform a radiographic evaluation if a fracture is suspected.

2 Perform a digital nerve block if necessary.

3 Cleanse the area with an antiseptic preparation solution.

4 Trephinate the nail.

5 Apply a protective dressing.

6 Splint fractures for 14 days; instruct patient and parents to perform warm soaks.

may be heated with a butane lighter and used to create a drainage hole using gentle downward pressure perpendicular to the nail. If performed correctly, the heated clip rapidly penetrates the nail and cools as it meets the underlying blood, with minimal discomfort to the patient. The paper clip must be steel and not aluminum, as aluminum will not generally stay hot enough to readily penetrate a fingernail.

After drainage, a protective dressing is applied, and the patient is instructed to soak the digit in warm water three times daily for 2 days, redressing it after each soak. Any underlying fracture requires splinting for at least 14 days and may require evaluation by a hand specialist.

Complications

Complications of nail trephination are rare. Some advocate routine antibiotic prophylaxis when a fracture accompanies a subungual hematoma to prevent infection, since trephination in such cases converts the underlying fracture into a potentially more serious open fracture (11). In a recent study, however, no infectious complications of trephination were noted in patients with underlying fractures who did not receive antibiotics (3). Routine antibiotic prophylaxis is probably unnecessary unless the child is immunocompromised or the vascular supply to the area is compromised (8). The parents and child should be warned that (a) blood may continue to ooze from the trephination site for 1 to 2 days; (b) the discoloration under the nail can persist days to weeks; and (c) the nail may fall off, and if so, it will take at least 3 to 4 months to grow in again (8). Carbon deposits may persist at the site of trephination but are benign (2).

▶ SUBUNGUAL FOREIGN BODY

Foreign bodies lodged under the nail of either a finger or toe are painful and are a nidus for infection. Removal of the foreign

body offers relief from pain, reduces the risk of infection, and can be performed in most outpatient settings.

Subungual foreign bodies are typically wedged between the nail and the nail bed, although penetration of either can occur. Mixed bacteria accompany the foreign body beneath the nail and can cause infection. This is especially true of wooden foreign bodies. When a wooden foreign body is allowed to remain beneath the nail, subsequent infection is common.

The nail bed is highly innervated. Therefore, while removal of a subungual foreign body brings significant pain relief, inflammation of the nail bed typically results in some persistent discomfort. Importantly, timely removal limits the risk of infection. Radiographs are obtained to document the presence of a radiopaque foreign body or when a fracture is suspected. Consultation with a hand surgeon is advised for foreign bodies that are clearly infected, for foreign bodies that cannot be removed, or if concern exists regarding bony injury and possible subsequent osteomyelitis due to deep nail bed penetration.

Equipment

Syringe with 27-gauge needle
Bupivacaine (0.25%) without epinephrine
Lidocaine (0.5% or 1%) without epinephrine
Restraints as needed
Hemostats or fine forceps
Fine-tipped scissors
No. 11 scalpel blade
Sterile protective dressing

Procedure

The finger with the foreign body is immobilized by taping the involved digit and adjacent finger(s) to a small pediatric arm board. The technique for removing the foreign body depends on the position of the foreign body beneath the nail (Fig. 103.5).

SUMMARY: SUBUNGUAL FOREIGN BODY

1 Perform a radiographic evaluation as needed to confirm the presence of a foreign body.

2 Perform a digital nerve block if necessary.

3 Remove the foreign body using appropriate technique based on nature of the object.

4 Clean and irrigate thoroughly.

5 Apply a protective dressing.

6 Prescribe antibiotic if there are signs of infection; instruct patient and parents to perform warm soaks.

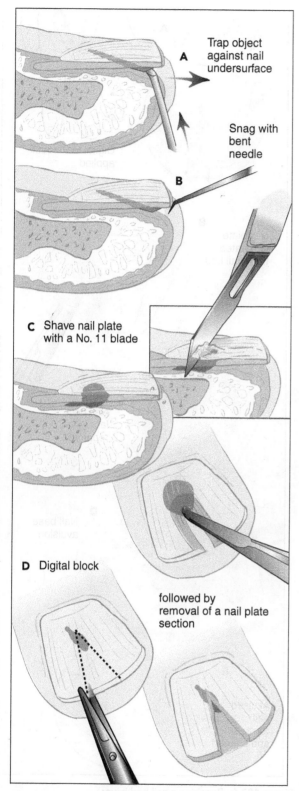

A Trap object against nail undersurface

Snag with bent needle

B

C Shave nail plate with a No. 11 blade

D Digital block

followed by removal of a nail plate section

Figure 103.5 Removing subungual foreign bodies.
A. The foreign body can be trapped against the nail using a needle and slowly withdrawn.
B. For a more deeply embedded foreign body, a needle with the tip bent can be used to "snag" the object and remove it.
C. The nail can be shaved down with a scalpel blade to allow removal of a foreign body.
D. A digital block and wedge resection of the nail can be performed.

A subungual foreign body that protrudes beyond the end of the nail is grasped with a hemostat or a pair of fine forceps and gently removed. If the protruding stump of the foreign body is not easily grasped at its distal aspect, it is pinned against the nail using the tip of fine-tipped scissors, a needle, or a No. 11 scalpel blade point. The foreign body is then gently drawn forward until it is out from beneath the nail (Fig. 103.5A).

Several methods can be used to remove a distal foreign body that cannot be grasped. A 25- or 27-gauge needle is bent at its tip to a 90-degree angle using a hemostat. The needle is inserted under the nail, rotated slightly to snag the object, and then gently withdrawn (Fig. 103.5B) (12). Alternatively, a No. 11 blade is held horizontally perpendicular to the nail and scraped proximally to distally across the nail overlying the foreign body (Fig. 103.5C). This procedure shaves down the nail until the foreign body is exposed and can be grasped and removed (10). Most children tolerate these methods without anesthesia.

Deeper or firmly embedded foreign bodies and any procedures resulting in significant nail bed manipulation will require a digital block (see Chapter 35). After adequate anesthesia, the nail may be lifted on either side of the foreign body using the sharp point of a pair of fine-tipped scissors to separate the nail from the nail bed. The scissors tip is oriented such that the point is angled slightly dorsally; the point is run along the undersurface of the nail to avoid damaging the nail bed. Two to three tracts of blunt dissection parallel to the long axis of the finger should release enough of the nail from the nail bed to allow the foreign body to be grasped with forceps and removed (10). For objects that cannot be removed by release of the fingernail as previously described, a V-shaped wedge is cut from the elevated nail overlying the foreign body to allow access for removal (Fig. 103.5D) (8).

Heavily contaminated or large wooden foreign bodies that have fragmented are most easily removed by first removing the entire nail (see "Nail Bed Injury"). This procedure requires a digital block, allowing full access to the site for débridement and irrigation. Débridement of the nail bed tissue itself should be minimized. Thorough cleaning and irrigation with several hundred milliliters of sterile saline via a large syringe and an 18-gauge plastic catheter minimizes residual bacteria and foreign body particles. The entire nail can be removed with fine-tipped scissors using the blunt dissection technique described above, but in this case the scissor tracts are extended to the proximal and lateral limits of the nail. The dorsal eponychial fold is similarly released from the proximal nail, and the lateral skin folds freed from the nail. The scissor tracts are kept parallel to the long axis of the finger. Foreign debris is removed, and the nail bed is irrigated and very gently scrubbed. A hole should be made in the center of the nail with either an electrocautery device, 18-gauge needle, or scissor tip. The proximal aspect of the nail is then placed beneath the eponychial fold. Two methods of securing the nail in situ have been described. Two 5.0 nylon sutures are placed through the nail at its midlateral positions and through the lateral skin.

The sutures are removed in 3 weeks. Alternatively, after the proximal aspect of the nail is placed beneath the eponychial fold, the nail is secured in anatomic position with a very small volume of tissue adhesive placed along the junction of the nail and the lateral folds.

A sterile, nonadherent dressing with antibiotic ointment beneath serves to protect the underlying tissue, promote healing, and prevent infection. The dressing should be removed in 12 to 24 hours, and the finger soaked in warm water two to three times daily, with redressing after each soak. Antibiotics are not indicated unless the wound is already infected, the foreign body was heavily contaminated, or deep penetration of the nail bed with possible bony inoculation has occurred. In such cases, a 5- to 7-day course of an antibiotic effective against staphylococcal and streptococcal species (e.g., cephalexin) should be prescribed.

Complications

Complications are rare and are mainly infectious. Retained wooden foreign bodies are more likely to cause infection, but the chance of infection is minimized by ensuring that the entire foreign body and small particulates are removed.

A foreign body that deeply penetrates the nail bed can inoculate the distal phalanx and result in osteomyelitis (8). The patient and parents should be warned to return immediately for increasing pain, tenderness, redness, swelling, or fever.

▶ NAIL BED INJURY

Significant trauma to the fingertip often results in avulsion of the fingernail and laceration of the underlying nail bed. Appropriate repair at the time of injury yields the best results (Fig. 103.6). Normal nail growth following a nail bed laceration requires a smooth nail bed. Irregular nail beds heal with scar formation, as do nail beds with avulsed tissue that are allowed to heal by secondary intention. Scar tissue will not produce new nail tissue or bind to the new nail, resulting in an abnormally formed or split fingernail or a nail that fails to adhere to the underlying nail bed (1,13,14). Likewise, the eponychial and lateral skin folds must remain open to prevent scarring between the skin folds and the underlying nail bed.

It is important to remember that many injuries to the fingertip do not require extensive exploration or repair. For example, uncomplicated subungual hematomas are usually associated with small nail bed lacerations, and these are best treated with nail trephination alone, as discussed previously. However, in cases of nail disruption, partial nail avulsion, or skin margin laceration, the nail must be removed completely for adequate examination and repair (6,13).

A few basic principles govern strategies for repair of nail bed injuries. Final outcome often depends on the initial care of the wound. Meticulous repair of the nail bed will minimize undesirable outcomes such as a split or nonadherent fingernail. Minimal débridement (or none) of the nail bed should be

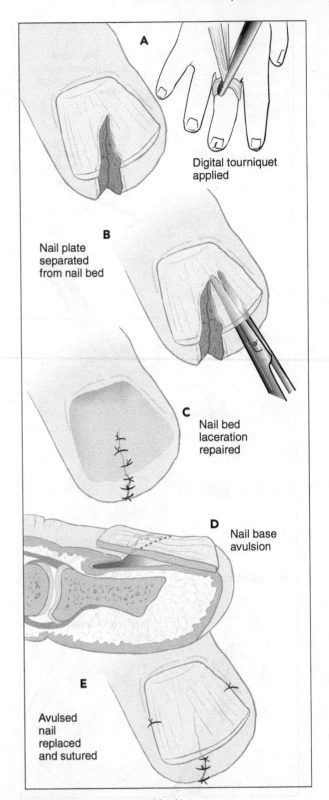

Figure 103.6 Repairing a nail bed injury.
A. A digital tourniquet is applied to provide a bloodless field.
B. Fine-tipped scissors are used to separate the nail from the nail bed by careful blunt dissection.
C. The skin and nailbed are sutured.
D. Nail base avulsion necessitates removal of the nail.
E. The nail is replaced into the eponychial fold and sutured in place or secured with tissue adhesive.

attempted, as nail bed tissue heals well when sutured back into place. As few sutures as necessary are used to close a nail bed laceration. Reattachment of avulsed nail bed tissue is vital to optimal outcome.

Significant fingertip injuries should be evaluated radiographically for evidence of underlying fractures. Any displacement must be corrected, and if the fracture is unstable, a hand surgeon should be consulted. Stability of all underlying fractures must be ensured to prevent recurrent damage to the nail bed caused by movement of unstable bone fragments. This may require Kirschner wiring (4,6). Finally, a thorough examination of the tendon function must be performed, as tendon injuries can be overlooked.

Equipment

Syringe with 27-gauge needle
Bupivacaine (0.25%) without epinephrine
Lidocaine (0.5% or 1%) without epinephrine
Restraints as needed
Antiseptic preparation solution
Tourniquet
Suture kit
Absorbable suture (5.0 or 6.0 chromic gut)
Magnifying eyewear
No. 15 scalpel blade
Dressing and splint
Electrocautery device

Procedure

A digital nerve block is effective anesthesia for repair of the fingertip (see Chapter 35). If the child is unable to tolerate the procedure with local anesthesia alone, procedural sedation should be considered (see Chapter 33).

A bloodless field is desirable for optimal repair and can be achieved using a digital tourniquet. After aseptic preparation of the entire finger, a sterile Penrose drain may be wrapped snugly around the base of the finger, stretched slightly, and clamped with a hemostat (Fig. 103.6A). Alternatively, the finger of a sterile glove can be cut and used as a substitute for a Penrose drain (13). A pneumatic tourniquet also can be used. The upper arm is first wrapped with several layers of padding such as cotton or gauze wrap, and the tourniquet is applied and inflated above the systolic pressure. A blood pressure cuff may similarly be used, but these devices are not designed for prolonged inflation and therefore tend to loose pressure during use. Regardless of the method chosen, tourniquet time and pressure should be minimized. If the pneumatic cuff is used, the patient should be warned that the involved arm will become numb once the cuff is inflated and will become uncomfortable (paresthesias) when the tourniquet is released but that these sensations will resolve. The arm will become painful after the cuff has been inflated for approximately 20 minutes, limiting the time available for repair. Finally, repair of a nail bed laceration is facilitated by using magnifying eyewear.

The fingernail is removed to fully expose the nail bed. The nail is gently separated from the underlying adherent nail bed with the end of a fine-tipped scissors (Fig. 103.6B). The tip is held parallel to the finger, angled slightly dorsally, then inserted between the nail and nail bed and advanced slowly. The tip is maintained against the underside of the nail to avoid injuring the nail bed. The scissor tip is moved proximally in several tracts until the nail is freed by blunt dissection from the underlying nail bed. Similarly, the eponychial and lateral folds are freed from the nail by inserting the scissor tip between the skin folds and the fingernail. The fingernail may have avulsed nail bed tissue attached to it; this should be saved for reimplantation onto the nail bed. Once the nail is removed, the nail bed is gently irrigated with several hundred milliliters of sterile saline using a large syringe and an 18-gauge plastic catheter.

Nail bed lacerations may be linear or stellate, but results are generally good if approximation and suturing of the nail bed tissues are precise (Fig. 103.6C). All lacerations should be repaired with fine absorbable suture on side-cutting needles (6.0 chromic gut suture is commonly used) (4,6). Any adjacent skin lacerations should be repaired with absorbable suture (e.g., 5.0 chromic gut) or nonabsorbable suture (e.g., 5.0 nylon). The nail itself can be trimmed but a tear or laceration of the nail does not need to be sutured. The nail is replaced to provide a physiologic dressing and to splint open the eponychium so that a new nail will grow in place.

More proximal lacerations may extend beneath the eponychium. If this is suspected, the germinal matrix must be exposed. The eponychium is cut back several millimeters perpendicular to its edges at the point that it curves distally. Retraction of this eponychial skin fold then allows adequate access to the proximal germinal matrix for inspection and repair (4,6,14). Once the germinal matrix is repaired, the eponychial incision sites are closed with 5.0 or 6.0 suture.

Nail bed avulsions often occur proximally when the fingertip is crushed, pulling the less adherent proximal nail out from beneath the eponychium so that it rests above the skin (Fig. 103.6D). In this case, the nail is removed and the nail bed examined for lacerations or tissue avulsions (13). Complete or distal nail avulsions also must be fully examined.

Nail bed tissue may adhere to the avulsed nail. Small fragments are best left attached to the nail and replaced as a unit with the nail. The nail with the attached nail bed fragments is replaced, supported with adhesive wound closure tape, and sutured into place to provide adequate immobilization (15). Larger fragments are gently trimmed off the nail with a No. 15 scalpel blade and sutured back into place with fine absorbable suture (14). Large injuries with absent, destroyed, or heavily contaminated tissues will require nail bed grafting, and therefore a hand surgeon should be consulted (4,6,14). Occasionally a nail avulsion will tear the germinal matrix proximally and pull it out from beneath the eponychium while it remains attached distally. These wounds also are best managed by a hand surgeon (6). Lacerations to the lateral or eponychial skin folds should be repaired with 5.0 or 6.0 chromic gut using standard skin closure techniques, with care taken to maintain the eponychial fold and approximate the skin edges precisely.

The repaired nail bed should be splinted, ideally with the original nail. Splinting protects the sensitive nail bed while keeping open the eponychium so that a new nail will grow in place. The nail is gently cleaned and trephinated at its center to allow for drainage. The nail is replaced into position beneath the eponychium and sutured in place through the lateral skin folds with two 5.0 sutures (Fig. 103.6E)(4,6,13,14). Another method is to use a nail stitch. This is similar to the two-stitch method, but one strand of each of the stitches is left long; the two long strands are then tied together across the nail to provide greater stability and self-tamponading pressure.

Recent data support the use of tissue adhesive to secure the nail plate into position beneath the eponychial fold. Two studies found that the application of tissue adhesive to the perionychium (eponychium and lateral folds) held the nail plate in place until it was pushed out by the newly formed nail (16,17). In a prospective randomized trial, Weil found that the time of nail bed repair was significantly shorter using tissue adhesive and resulted in comparable cosmesis when compared to traditional suture repair (17).

If the original nail cannot be used or was lost, a nonadherent splint of Silastic, mesh gauze, or the sterile foil from a suture packet may be secured beneath the eponychial fold and left in place for 3 weeks (13,14). A protective dressing and finger splint is then applied and left in place until a follow-up visit in 24 hours.

Complications

Failure to provide a smooth, well-approximated nail bed may result in a split or nonadherent nail (1,4,6,8,13,14). Scar tissue formation may also result in a hyperaesthetic nail bed and fingertip (14). Allowing the eponychial fold to scar may also result in a split nail or pain as the nail grows through the adhesion (13). Lateral fold scarring may result in ingrown nails (13). Fractures must be anatomically reduced to prevent recurrent nail bed injury due to bony motion or permanent abnormal anatomic alignment (4,6). Infection is rare and usually occurs only in wounds heavily contaminated with organic matter. Five days of an antibiotic effective against staphylococcal and streptococcal species (e.g., cephalexin) are warranted in such cases (6,13).

▶ FINGERTIP AVULSION OR AMPUTATION

Fingertip avulsions and amputations in children are often managed in an outpatient setting by emergency physicians and other clinicians. Partial or full fingertip amputations typically occur when a finger is caught in a closing door, although knives, slicers, power tools, and lawn mowers also cause these injuries. Unlike in the case of adults, distal amputations and partial avulsions often heal extremely well in children, especially before adolescence. In particular, the literature indicates that children younger than 2 years of age are very likely to demonstrate complete distal tip regeneration after amputation when managed conservatively (18).

In general, avulsions of only distal soft tissue or with a small amount of exposed bone are managed conservatively, whereas amputations at or proximal to the distal interphalangeal joint should be microsurgically reimplanted (4). In children, more distal amputations of the fingertip can generally be repaired by a nonsurgeon who is proficient in suturing skills (see below). Exposed bone need not be shortened unless extensive soft-tissue loss has occurred or the patient is over 12 years of age (4,10). Teenagers should have these wounds cared for similar to adults, with bone shortening and the creation of a skin flap to cover the bone. All injuries should be evaluated radiographically. Any finger that is contaminated or requires a flap or shortening procedure requires consultation by a hand surgeon.

Equipment

Syringe with 27-gauge needle
Bupivacaine (0.25%) without epinephrine
Lidocaine (0.5% or 1%) without epinephrine
Suture set
Rongeur to shorten bone (if necessary)
Absorbable suture (5.0 or 6.0 chromic gut)
Irrigation supplies
Dressings and splints

 SUMMARY: NAIL BED INJURY

1 Perform a radiographic evaluation if a fracture is suspected.

2 Perform a digital nerve block.

3 Remove the nail.

4 Clean and irrigate thoroughly.

5 Apply a digital tourniquet.

6 Repair the nail bed.

7 Repair any adjacent skin laceration.

8 Insert and suture the nail (or a small piece of Silastic, mesh gauze, or foil from the suture package).

9 Apply a sterile dressing with antibiotic ointment.

10 Splint the finger 10 to 14 days; ensure hand surgeon follow-up; prescribe antibiotics if indicated.

Digital tourniquet
Restraints as needed
Antibiotics

Procedure

For all distal amputations or partial avulsions, a digital block should be performed (see Chapter 35). A bloodless field is obtained with a digital tourniquet (see "Nail Bed Injury"). Regardless of the age of the patient, wounds involving avulsion limited to the distal skin and pulp are best managed conservatively with thorough irrigation, débridement of devitalized tissues, and a nonadherent sterile dressing that is changed each day (4,8,10). Wounds involving no or minimal exposed distal bone are likewise managed conservatively (4). Injuries with significant bone exposure require consultation with a hand surgeon. The bone is trimmed with a rongeur, and a skin flap is created to cover the bone. The skin is closed with 5.0 or 6.0 absorbable (chromic gut) suture, creating a shortened but closed digit (8).

Partial or complete fingertip avulsions frequently survive as a composite graft in children younger than 2 years of age (Fig. 103.7.A,B) (8,14). These injuries are first cleaned, irrigated, and débrided. The nail bed and skin are then approximated with 5.0 or 6.0 absorbable suture (Fig. 103.7C–E). In older children and adolescents, such wounds are managed conservatively (débrided, irrigated, dressed), as the likelihood that a skin flap will survive falls rapidly with age. A delayed free graft may be applied several days later if necessary (4,11). Contam-

inated wounds in adolescents should not be closed primarily; rather, a delayed closure or grafting should be performed (11).

Antibiotics are recommended for all exposed fractures of the distal phalanx. A first parenteral dose should be given at the time of initial care, followed by a 5- to 7-day oral course (8). Cleanliness and serial dressing changes must be stressed to the parents and appropriate follow-up with a hand surgeon ensured.

Complications

Complications are primarily due to infections. These are limited by thorough débridement, irrigation, and delayed closure or grafting if the wound is heavily contaminated. Frequent changes of sterile occlusive dressings and prophylactic antibiotics also increase the likelihood of a good outcome.

▶ MALLET FINGER DEFORMITY

The mallet finger deformity typically occurs when an extended finger is struck by an object (e.g., a baseball) with an axial force. Lacerations to the dorsal aspect of the finger at the level of the distal interphalangeal joint can also produce a similar deformity. The mallet deformity occurs when the extensor tendon separates from the distal phalanx so that the fingertip can no longer be straightened. In young children, the epiphyseal plate separates while the proximal epiphysis remains attached to the extensor tendon. In adolescents, whose epiphyseal plate has fused, the tendon pulls off the distal phalanx with or without a portion of the dorsal lip of the distal phalanx. Consultation with a hand surgeon is recommended if (a) the extensor tendon is lacerated or (b) a dorsal lip or epiphysis has avulsed off the proximal aspect of the distal phalanx, as such injuries occasionally require open repair (8,10).

Equipment

Radiographs
Splinting materials
0.25% bupivacaine without epinephrine
Lidocaine (0.5% or 1%) without epinephrine
Syringe with 27-gauge needle
Alcohol prep swab

Procedure

A closed mallet finger injury without fracture heals well with splinting (Fig. 103.8). A dorsal foam finger splint is applied with the distal interphalangeal joint in full extension to bring the extensor tendon and distal phalanx into juxtaposition. Full flexion should be allowed at the proximal interphalangeal joint. The splint is maintained for 6 to 8 weeks. If the distal interphalangeal joint falls into flexion at any time, the tenuous healing of tendon to bone may be

---

SUMMARY: FINGERTIP AVULSION OR AMPUTATION

1 Perform a radiographic evaluation if a fracture is suspected.

2 Perform a digital nerve block.

3 Débride soft tissue conservatively.

4 Clean and irrigate thoroughly.

5 For younger children, perform reimplantation of the fingertip.

  a Suture the skin, aligning landmarks.

  b Repair the nail bed injury.

  c Insert and suture the nail (or a small piece of Silastic, mesh gauze, or foil from the suture package).

6 Trim back bone in a teenager or if significant bony exposure in younger children.

7 Splint the finger 10 to 14 days; ensure hand surgeon follow-up; prescribe antibiotics if indicated.

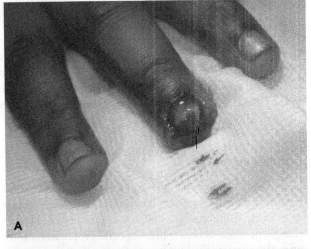

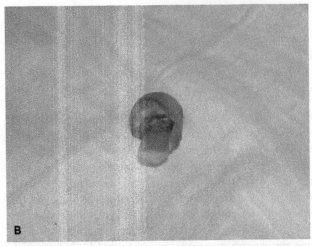

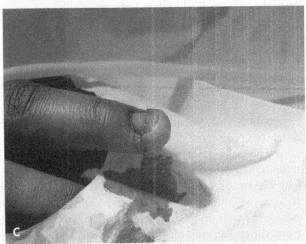

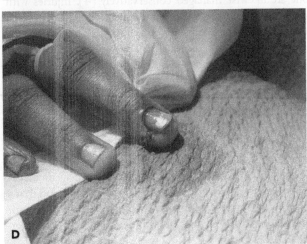

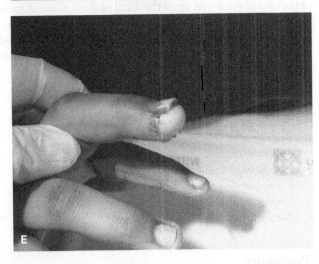

Figure 103.7 Repair of a distal fingertip amputation.
A,B. With a fingertip amputation, the avulsed nail often remains attached to the amputated distal fingertip.
C. The amputated distal fingertip is reattached. Both the skin and the nail bed should be sutured.
D. The nail is reinserted and secured with stitches or tissue adhesive.
E. In the worst-case scenario, the flap serves as a temporary "physiologic" dressing. With young children, the flap often remains viable and results in a good functional and cosmetic outcome.

lost. In this case, the splint is reapplied and the time course for splinting reinitiated. The splint may be carefully removed when wet or dirty, but the parents and child must be warned to ensure constant extension at the distal interphalangeal joint until the new splint is applied (8). Newer, commercially avail-

able thermoplastic splints maintain a low profile and minimize moisture between the splint and the skin.

Mallet finger deformities associated with fractures or epiphyseal separations may need operative repair. A splint is applied, as previously described, until the patient is evaluated by

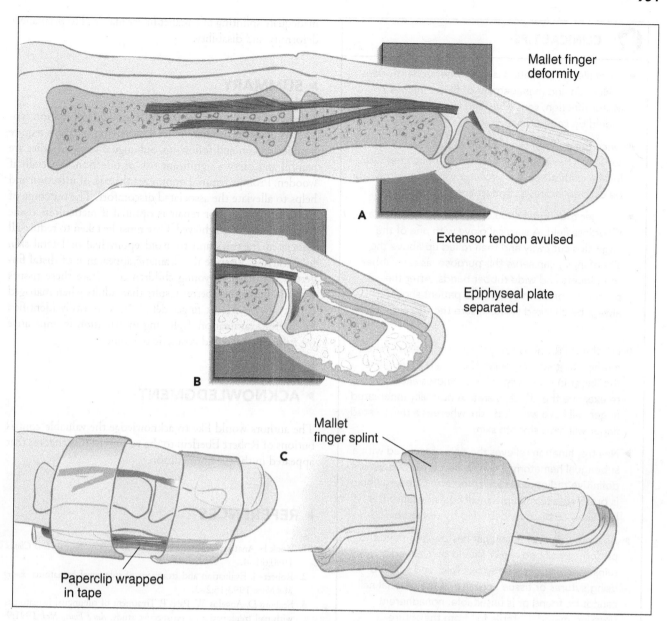

Mallet finger deformity

Extensor tendon avulsed

Epiphyseal plate separated

Mallet finger splint

Paperclip wrapped in tape

Figure 103.8 Splinting a closed mallet finger injury.

a hand surgeon (10). Mallet finger deformities due to tendon laceration need suture fixation of the tendon, which should be performed by an experienced nonsurgeon clinician or a hand surgeon (8). If repair of the tendon cannot be performed immediately, the wound should be thoroughly cleansed and irrigated, the skin loosely closed with 5.0 suture, and a splint applied. The patient is then referred to a hand surgeon for subsequent tendon repair. A 5-day course of oral antibiotics is generally recommended despite limited data showing clinical efficacy.

After splinting, all patients with a mallet finger deformity are instructed to elevate the injury for 48 hours. Appropriate analgesia should be prescribed. Follow-up within 7 days to assess appropriate extension of the joint in the splint must be ensured. Patients and parents should be warned that

SUMMARY: MALLET FINGER DEFORMITY

1 If open, repair extensor tendon laceration (if experienced with this procedure) and close wound,
  -OR-
  Close wound and refer tendon repair to hand surgeon.

2 Splint distal interphalangeal joint in extension; allow full movement of proximal interphalangeal joint.

3 Keep finger in full extension (even when the splint is changed) 10 to 14 days; ensure hand surgeon follow-up; prescribe antibiotics if indicated.

CLINICAL TIPS

▶ A detailed examination is the cornerstone of the evaluation and management of finger injuries. Motor function, sensation, and vascular integrity should be carefully assessed.

▶ Once the parts of the evaluation that require intact sensation have been performed and documented, local anesthetic and, if necessary, light sedation can be used to improve comfort and cooperation.

▶ A finger tourniquet should be used to establish a bloodless field. A surgical glove with one of the fingertips cut away and then rolled up above the site of injury can serve this purpose, as can rubber tourniquets and wide rubber bands. After the procedure or examination, the patient should always be checked to make sure the tourniquet has been removed.

▶ For the child who is too young to cooperate, one method of assessing nerve function is to immerse the finger in warm water for 5 minutes and then re-examine the affected area. A normally innervated finger will have wrinkled skin, whereas a denervated finger will have smooth skin.

▶ Nail trephination relieves the pain associated with a subungual hematoma and can be performed before definitive radiographs are complete. One large hole is preferable to multiple small holes because it is less likely to become occluded by clotted blood.

▶ An avulsed nail or a nail that has been removed to perform a nail bed repair should be cleaned, reinserted into the eponychial fold, and secured using sutures or tissue adhesive. If the original nail cannot be found or is unsuitable, nonadherent dressing material, sterile foil from the suture package, or a small piece of Silastic can be used instead.

▶ With young children, amputations of the fingertip (distal to the distal interphalangeal joint) can be treated by suturing the amputated piece back into place. The flap may remain viable, but even if it becomes nonviable, it serves as a "physiologic" dressing during healing.

▶ Patients with midshaft metacarpal fractures should always be checked for rotational abnormalities.

inadequate splinting of a mallet finger may lead to permanent deformity and disability.

▶ SUMMARY

Subungual hematomas are painful, but nail trephination typically provides immediate relief. Underlying fractures require immobilization and follow-up. Subungual foreign bodies are painful and carry a significant risk of infection, especially if wooden. Prompt removal minimizes the risk of infection and helps to alleviate the associated discomfort. The outcome of nail bed injuries after repair is optimal if meticulous tissue reapproximation is achieved. Care must be taken to reduce all associated fractures and to avoid eponychial or lateral skin fold scarring. Despite the dramatic appearance of distal fingertip amputations, young children regenerate these tissues well and have much better results than adults when managed conservatively. Mallet finger deformities are easily identified by careful examination. Splinting in extension is imperative for full functional and cosmetic outcome.

▶ ACKNOWLEDGMENT

The authors would like to acknowledge the valuable contributions of Robert Eberlein to the version of this chapter that appeared in the previous edition.

▶ REFERENCES

1. Zook E. Anatomy and physiology of the perionychium. *Hand Clinics.* 1990;6:1–4.
2. Roberts J. Evaluation and treatment of subungual hematoma. *Emerg Med News.* 1993;15:2–3.
3. Seaburg D, Angelos W, Paris P. Treatment of subungual hematomas with nail trephination: a prospective study. *Am J Emerg Med.* 1991;9: 209–213.
4. Tintinalli J, Krome R, Ruiz E. *Emergency Medicine: A Comprehensive Study Guide.* 6th ed. New York: McGraw-Hill; 2004.
5. Simon R, Wolgin M. Subungual hematoma: association with occult laceration requiring repair. *Am J Emerg Med.* 1987;5:302–305.
6. Van Beek A, Kassen M, Adson M, et al. Management of acute fingernail injuries. *Hand Clinics.* 1990;6:23–28.
7. Meek S, White M. Subungual haematomas: is simple trephining enough? *J Accid Emerg Med.* 1998;15:269–270.
8. Roberts J, Hedges J. *Clinical Procedures in Emergency Medicine.* 4th ed. Philadelphia: WB Saunders; 2004.
9. Milstein D, Milstein S. Letter to the editor. *Emerg Med News.* 1993;15:5.
10. Fleisher G, Ludwig S. *Textbook of Pediatric Emergency Medicine.* 4th ed. Baltimore: Williams & Wilkins; 2000.
11. Carter P. Common hand injuries and infections. Philadelphia: WB Saunders; 1983.
12. Davis L. Letter to the editor. *J Fam Pract.* 1980;11:5.
13. Roberts J. Fingernail avulsion and injury to the nail bed. *Emerg Med News.* 1993;15:3–4.

14. Shepard G. Management of acute nail bed avulsions. *Hand Clinics.* 1990;6:39–46.

15. Zook E. Discussion of "Management of acute nail bed avulsions." *Hand Clinics.* 1990;6:57–58.

16. Richards A, Crick A, Cole R. A novel method of securing the nail following nail bed repair. *Plast Reconstr Surg.* 1999;103:7–9.

17. Weil W. Prospective, Randomized, controlled trial of Dermabond versus suture repair in nail bed injuries [abstract]. Annual Meeting of the American Academy of Orthopaedic Surgeons; February 23–27, 2005; Washington, DC.

18. Rosenthal L, Reiner M, Bleicher M. Nonoperative management of distal fingertip amputations in children. *Pediatrics.* 1979;64:1–4.

104

DANIEL A. GREEN AND CHARLES G. MACIAS

Arthrocentesis

▶ INTRODUCTION

All pediatric patients who present with complaints of joint pain or swelling should be thoroughly examined to confirm or exclude the presence of an acute arthritis. The presence of warmth, swelling, tenderness, effusion, or erythema on physical examination indicates joint disease. Although there are many common causes of arthritis in childhood, the emergency physician must be vigilant to assess for the possibility of septic arthritis, especially in patients with monoarticular involvement. Elements of the history, persistence of fever, physical exam findings, and laboratory analysis may aid in making the diagnosis. Inadequately treated septic arthritis carries a high rate of long-term morbidity (1,2). Arthrocentesis (the aspiration of synovial fluid from a joint cavity using a needle and syringe) is the only way to establish a definitive diagnosis of an acute arthritis. Arthrocentesis can be performed by emergency physicians safely, inexpensively, and painlessly with the judicious use of topical and local anesthetics and procedural sedation (1,3–5).

▶ INDICATIONS

Any child with an acutely warm, tender, swollen, or erythematous joint requires immediate evaluation. Detecting an effusion is an important part of the physical examination. The knee is perhaps the simplest joint to evaluate for effusion, and knowledge of the technique for examination of this joint will aid the clinician in identifying other joint effusions. To properly examine the knee, the patient is placed in the supine position. Under normal circumstances, there is a concavity on the medial surface of the knee posterior to the medial patellar margin. If this concavity is absent, an effusion is present. The extremity should be externally rotated 30 to 40 degrees. Joint

fluid should then be milked from the medial aspect to the dependent lateral aspect of the joint space using the fingers of both hands. Using both thumbs, the operator then presses the fluid back toward the medial side. A positive "bulge sign," indicating the presence of a knee effusion, occurs when a delayed medial bulge is observed (3,6). Obese patients and patients with tense joints may have large effusions that are difficult to detect using this method. Balloting the patella (i.e., firmly pressing the center of the bone posteriorly) may cause a "click" as the patella contacts the underlying femur. In these patients, ballottement may be a superior method for detecting an effusion (3).

Several laboratory tests may assist the clinician in defining the risk for septic arthritis and thus the need for arthrocentesis. An elevated white blood cell count (WBC), an elevated erythrocyte sedimentation rate (ESR), or an elevated C-reactive protein (CRP) may be useful (7–11). A plain radiograph of the joint in question showing a wide joint space (or a widened joint space compared to the contralateral side) or ultrasound-proven effusion is also consistent with septic arthritis (12). However, normal or mild to moderate increases in lab values should not deter the clinician from performing joint aspiration if the clinical presentation raises the suspicion of infection. Therefore, arthrocentesis should be performed in virtually every patient with monarthritis at risk for septic arthritis in order to rule out infection.

There are no absolute contraindications to arthrocentesis, only relative contraindications. The presence of known or suspected cellulitis or skin lesions, which may harbor pathogenic organisms, should not keep the clinician from aspirating the joint. Although some authors recognize that this may introduce infection into a joint space, the benefits to the patient must be weighed against the risks of the potential morbidity of undiagnosed septic arthritis (5,13). More importantly, however, there are other points of entry into the joint that may bypass the lesion overlying the area of the commonest approach. Some authors recommend that if the needle must penetrate the joint through a potential source of infection, the patient should be admitted to the hospital to receive intravenous antibiotics (5). As septic arthritis is thought to be caused primarily by hematogenous spread, arthrocentesis may theoretically seed a sterile joint in patients with bacteremia (5,14,15). Nevertheless, if septic arthritis is suspected in such patients, joint aspiration should be performed (16).

Landmarks and scar tissue in patients with artificial joints may make the procedure difficult, although aspiration may be clinically warranted because of an increased risk of septic arthritis (5). Given the rarity of pediatric patients with artificial joints, orthopedic consultation should be sought for these patients prior to arthrocentesis.

Arthrocentesis may be indicated in patients with hemophilia and other coagulopathies for painful, tense traumatic hemarthroses and is indicated if septic arthritis is suspected (4,13,17). However, the coagulation defect should be corrected prior to performing the procedure. Additionally, the physician should consider consultation with the hematologist and/or orthopedist who cares for the child prior to performing arthrocentesis for hemarthrosis.

▶ EQUIPMENT

Saline solution or other cleansing agents
Marking pen
Alcohol sponges or wipes
Povidone-iodine solution
Sterile gauze dressings (2″ × 2″ and 4″ × 4″)
Sterile syringes
Needles
    18- to 20-gauge (shoulder, elbow, knee, and ankle joints)
    22- to 23-gauge (wrist and small joints)
Specimen collection tubes
Local anesthetics (vapocoolant, 1% lidocaine)
Sterile drapes and gloves
Adhesive bandage
Procedural sedation equipment (see Chapter 33)

▶ PROCEDURE

Several general considerations relevant to arthrocentesis at any joint will first be reviewed, followed by information needed to perform the procedure for specific joints (4–6,13,14,18–21). Prior to beginning, the operator should prepare the equipment for the procedure. Next, he or she should attempt to select the best site. The site should be as far as possible from other body structures (tendons, large nerves, blood vessels) and in a location that maximizes the chances of successful entry into the joint space. Before prepping and draping, the bony landmarks should be identified. This may be done with the

joint in the best position for insertion or in a position better suited to the identification of the landmarks, with subsequent repositioning for insertion. As repositioning and draping can cause these landmarks to be obscured (to vision and touch), the insertion site can be marked prior to prepping. Marking can be done with indelible ink or by indenting the skin with a needle cap or a similar object. The joint should be positioned to maximize the size of the joint cavity (e.g., by distraction) and to stretch the capsule and ligaments so that the needle tip does not penetrate any significant structures.

An important standard of pediatric practice is providing safe and effective analgesia and/or sedation for any painful procedure (see Chapter 33). If sedation is contraindicated and local anesthetics (see Chapter 35) are used alone, immobilization should be considered to avoid excessive patient movement during the procedure, because such movement may damage the articular cartilage (4). A papoose or tightly wrapped sheet may assist with this in the younger child whose developmental level precludes cooperation.

There are several available local anesthetics recommended for providing control of pain. Topical anesthetics such as ice, vapocoolants (ethyl chloride), and lidocaine-prilocaine paste (EMLA) may provide a variable degree of anesthesia and may be considered on a case-by-case basis. If subcutaneous injection of a local anesthetic such as 1% lidocaine is used, the clinician must be careful to avoid having the anesthetic enter the joint cavity, as it may alter the synovial fluid analysis (18). The use of bicarbonate buffer to minimize the burning sensation of the injection has not been studied in arthrocentesis.

Sterile technique should be observed at all times to avoid introducing infection into the joint. All debris, skin oils, and dirt should be removed from the skin over the joint and the immediate surrounding area using any combination of plain soap and water, alcohol wipes, chlorhexidine scrub, and povidone-iodine scrub. Antiseptics such as povidone-iodine solution are frequently used in successive passes using scrub brushes, impregnated swabs, or solution. Adequate drying after the final pass of povidone-iodine facilitates the full bactericidal effect of the solution. The antiseptic should be wiped from the immediate area overlying the aspiration site to prevent its introduction into the joint cavity. Drapes and gloves are used to avoid contamination and to practice universal precautions.

The needle should be inserted from a direction of penetration that minimizes damage to the articular cartilages and avoids damage to ligaments. The largest needle that can aspirate a joint without trauma should be used to overcome the difficulty with aspiration of viscous joint fluid. Finally, the joint should be aspirated. This is accomplished by drawing back on the plunger of the syringe while advancing the needle toward the space. If synovial fluid stops flowing into the syringe but joint fluid still remains, aspiration can be continued by repositioning the needle or reinjecting some of the joint fluid and aspirating again. Additionally, some operators apply pressure to the contralateral side of the joint in hopes of moving fluid toward the needle.

▶ SPECIFIC JOINTS

Knee via Superolateral Approach (Preferred Approach) (Fig. 104.1)

Position of patient: The patient's knee should be extended as much as tolerated.

Approach and insertion: The needle is inserted slightly lateral to the superolateral border of the patella (along the lateral and proximal borders).

Direction: The needle should be directed slightly inferiorly and slightly posteriorly to pass underneath the patella toward the middle of the medial side of the joint.

Knee via Medial Approach (Fig. 104.2)

Position of patient: The patient's knee should be extended as much as tolerated or flexed to no greater than 45 degrees.

Approach and insertion: The needle is inserted at the midpoint of the patella just below (posterior to) its medial border.

Direction: The needle should be guided underneath the patella toward the opposite patellar midpoint.

Ankle at Tibiotalar Joint (Fig. 104.3)

Position of patient: The patient should be in the supine position with his or her ankle in plantar flexion.

Approach and insertion: The needle is inserted anterior to the medial malleolus, in the hollow just medial to the anterior tibialis tendon.

Direction: The needle should be directed posterolaterally.

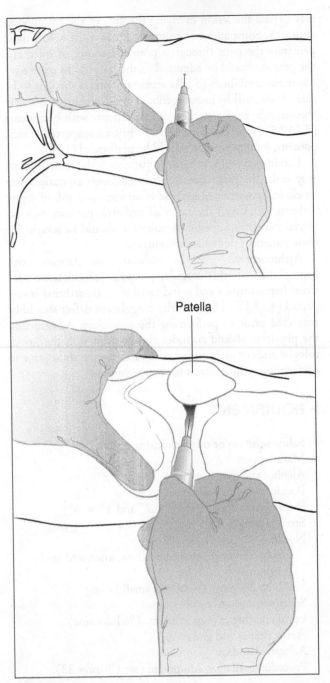

Patella

Figure 104.2 Arthrocentesis of knee via superolateral medial approach.

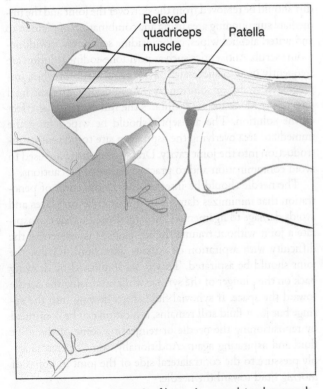

Relaxed quadriceps muscle

Patella

Figure 104.1 Arthrocentesis of knee via superolateral approach.

Ankle at Subtalar Joint (Fig. 104.4)

Position of patient: The patient's ankle is placed in the neutral position with slight inversion.

Approach and insertion: The needle should be inserted distal to the tip of the lateral malleolus (anterior to the tip of the fibula and proximal to the sinus tarsi).

Direction: The needle is directed horizontal to the subtalar joint toward the medial malleolus.

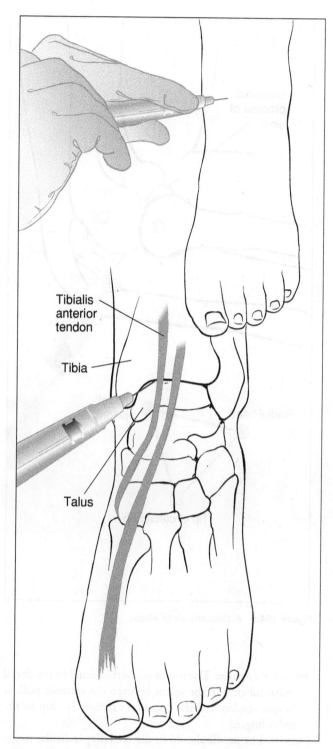

Tibialis
anterior
tendon

Tibia

Talus

Figure 104.3 Arthrocentesis of ankle at tibiotalar joint.

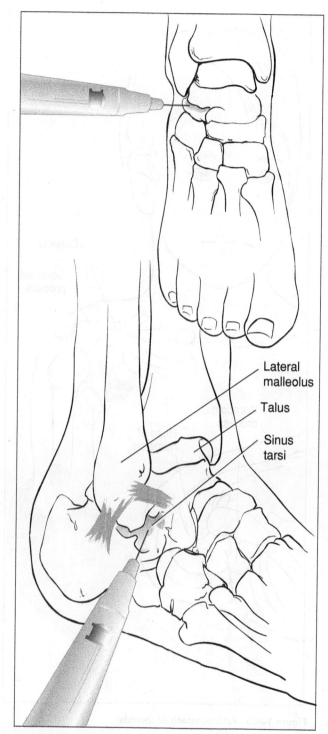

Lateral
malleolus

Talus

Sinus
tarsi

Figure 104.4 Arthrocentesis of ankle at subtalar joint.

Shoulder (Fig. 104.5)

Position of patient: The patient should be seated in an upright
position with the arm in slight external rotation and with
the hand in the lap, palm facing upward.

Approach and insertion: The needle is inserted inferior and lateral
to the coracoid process.

Direction: The needle should be directed posteriorly or posteriorly and slightly superiorly and laterally.

Elbow (Fig. 104.6)

Position of patient: The patient's elbow should be flexed to 70 to
90 degrees. It is preferable to rest the arm on a table.

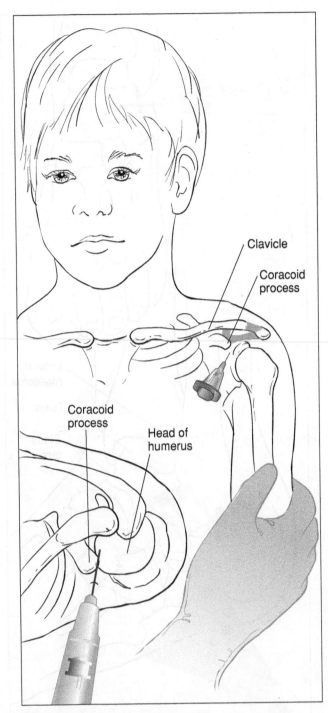

Figure 104.5 Arthrocentesis of shoulder.

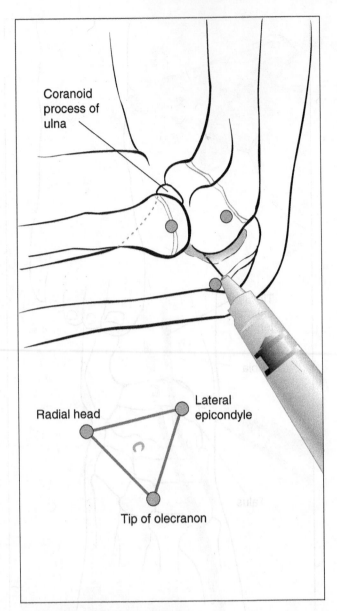

Figure 104.6 Arthrocentesis of elbow.

Approach and insertion: The needle should be inserted in the center of the anconeus triangle (between the lateral epicondyle of the humerus, the radial head, and the olecranon).

Direction: The needle is directed medially and slightly anteriorly toward the coronoid process of the ulna.

Wrist (Fig. 104.7)

Position of patient: The patient's wrist should be placed in 30 degrees of flexion and maximal ulnar deviation.

Approach and insertion: The needle is inserted distal to the dorsal radial tubercle in the sulcus between the extensor pollicis longus tendon and the common extensor tendon to the index finger.

Direction: The needle should be directed perpendicular to the skin.

Metacarpophalangeal and Interphalangeal Joints (Fig 104.8)

Position of patient: The patient's finger should be placed in 15 to 20 degrees of flexion.

Approach and insertion: The needle is inserted dorsally, just medial or lateral to the extensor tendon.

Direction: The needle is directed perpendicular to the finger.

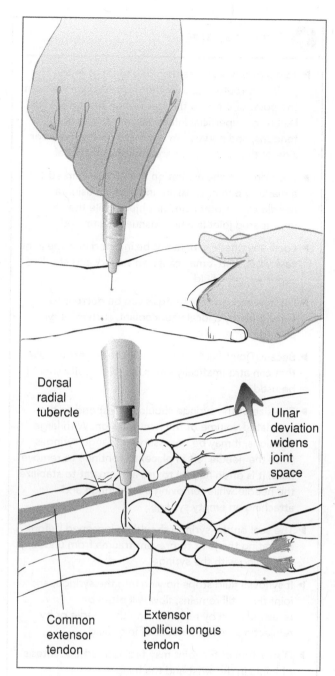

Figure 104.7 Arthrocentesis of wrist.

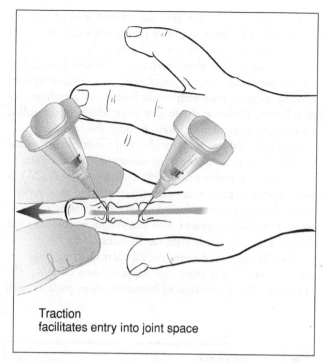

Figure 104.8 Arthrocentesis of metacarpophalangeal and interphalangeal joints.

▶ COMPLICATIONS

With adherence to the tenets previously listed and a cautious approach, there are few potential complications to performing arthrocentesis. The most significant potential complications are those associated with procedural sedation (Chapter 33). However, one must recognize the need to minimize movement

Thumb at First Carpometacarpal Joint (Fig 104.9)

Position of patient: The thumb can be placed in the palm, inside of a closed fist, or opposed with the little finger.

Approach and insertion: The needle is inserted proximal to the prominence, which is palpable at the base of the first metacarpal on the palmar side of the abductor pollicis longus tendon.

Direction: The needle is directed toward the base of the fourth metacarpal.

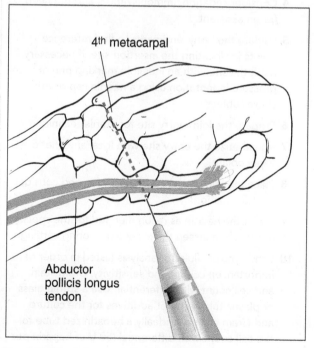

Figure 104.9 Arthrocentesis of thumb at carpometacarpal joint.

of the patient while providing the greatest level of comfort possible. It is for this reason that procedural sedation is commonly used for arthrocentesis in children (22).

Introduction of an inoculum into a sterile joint is unlikely if careful aseptic technique is practiced. Controversies exist concerning arthrocentesis with needle insertion through an area of cellulitis. However, the lack of comprehensive controlled trials investigating arthrocentesis through infected skin, especially in light of the growing incidence of community-acquired methicillin-resistant *Staphylococcus aureus* as a causative agent in septic arthritis, makes risk-benefit decisions difficult (23). If joint aspiration must occur through an infected area, conservative management would dictate that the patient be admitted to the hospital and treated with intravenous antibiotics until the certainty of a sterile joint can be assured (5).

A small amount of traumatic capsular bleeding often occurs, but bleeding is rarely significant unless a coagulopathy is present. The prevention of hemarthrosis in patients with

---

 CLINICAL TIPS

▶ Joints may have more than one route of entry. The preferred route is usually the shortest distance from the point of entry to the joint space and avoids skin lesions or superficial infections, major vessels, tendons, and nerves. An approach on the extensor side of the joint usually accomplishes this goal.

▶ The skin over the aspiration site can be marked with a marking pen or pressure indentation using a needle cap or other similar object while the unprepared joint is being manually examined.

▶ Local anesthetic should not be injected into the joint cavity because it may cause an artifact and sterilize septic synovial fluid.

▶ Discomfort of arthrocentesis can be decreased sufficiently by a local vapocoolant, such as ethyl chloride.

▶ Because joint fluid is so viscous, the largest needle that can atraumatically enter the joint cavity should be used.

▶ The size of the syringe should correspond to the estimated volume of the joint effusion. With large effusions, it may be necessary to change syringes (with the needle left in place) to continue to remove fluid. It is often helpful to use a hemostat to stabilize the needle while removing a full syringe and attaching an empty syringe.

▶ The seal on the syringe should be loosened before aspirating the joint to prevent trauma from undue struggling with the syringe.

▶ If synovial fluid stops flowing into the syringe, and joint fluid still remains, flow will often be re-established by repositioning the needle or by reinjecting a small amount of joint fluid.

▶ Distraction of the joint may facilitate arthrocentesis of joints in the wrist and the hand.

▶ Synovial fluid, like any other body fluid, should be considered infectious.

 SUMMARY

1 Discuss the procedure with the parents and child and obtain informed consent.

2 Review the technique for arthrocentesis of the specific joint by studying the appropriate text and figure. Remember to note the joint positioning, the insertion sites based on the bony landmarks, and the direction the needle should be inserted.

3 Gather the necessary equipment.

4 Consider sedation, immobilization, and the need for an assistant.

5 Palpate the bony landmarks to find reference points for locating the insertion site. If necessary, mark the site with an indelible marking pen or with pressure indentation using a needle cap or other similar object.

6 Prepare the joint entry site for sterile technique.

7 Anesthetize the entry site with local anesthetic or vapocoolant.

8 Place the joint in the correct position and consider joint distraction.

9 Direct the needle as recommended for the specific approach to lessen the chance of scoring cartilage.

10 Send synovial fluid for analysis (listed in order of importance): culture and sensitivity, Gram stain, and cell count with differential. Use a sterile glass or plastic tube without additives for the culture and Gram stain and ideally a heparinized tube for the cell count with differential (50 U of heparin per milliliter of synovial fluid).

---

bleeding disorders can be avoided by administering clotting factor prior to the procedure. Hypersensitivity and untoward reactions to antiseptics, local anesthetics or sedation, and analgesic agents can be minimized by the taking of a careful history prior to beginning the procedure.

▶ LABORATORY ANALYSIS

Along with historical and physical examination elements, the clinical suspicion of septic arthritis is further increased by abnormal laboratory and radiographic analyses. In determining the cause of arthritis, however, analysis of synovial fluid plays perhaps the most important role. Analysis of synovial fluid should include a Gram stain, as it may yield a presumptive diagnosis (24). The white blood cell count may reflect the degree of inflammation and joint destruction as well as suggest the likelihood of infection. Leukocyte counts greater than 80,000 to 100,000 and with greater than 70% to 75% polymorphonuclear neutrophils are consistent with septic arthritis, although it should be noted that septic arthritis has been demonstrated in patients with leukocyte counts of 50,000 per milliliter or less (24). Low glucose levels (one third serum glucose) have also been described with septic arthritis; however, some studies have found no reductions in glucose levels in the majority of patients with septic arthritis (24). Synovial fluid cultures are positive in approximately 65% of patients (25,26). Many children have negative cultures but clinical and synovial similarities to children with positive cultures, and therefore treatment should proceed similarly even in the absence of a causative agent (26).

The utility of protein, enzymes, immune complexes, rheumatoid factor, Lyme titers, and antinuclear antibody in children is controversial. However, should consultation with a rheumatologist be required later to evaluate possible noninfectious causes of arthritis, this may be facilitated if additional fluid is obtained during arthrocentesis for further testing.

▶ SUMMARY

When a child presents with signs and symptoms suggestive of arthritis, the emergency physician must rapidly determine whether it is septic arthritis. Arthrocentesis is the test of choice in such circumstances. Arthrocentesis in children may be safely performed in the emergency department with adequate attention to patient comfort and cooperation, preparation of the necessary materials, and careful adherence to proper technique. Procedural sedation may be performed to facilitate the procedure. The physician must understand and take steps to minimize the already rare complications of the procedure. The evaluation of joint fluid independently or in consultation with appropriate subspecialists will aid in making an accurate diagnosis.

▶ ACKNOWLEDGMENTS

The authors wish to acknowledge the valuable contributions of Mark C. Clark and Steven G. Rothrock for their contributions to the original version of this chapter in the first edition of this textbook.

▶ REFERENCES

1. Baker DG, Schumacher HR Jr. Acute monarthritis. *N Engl J Med.* 1993;329:1013–1020.
2. Morrey BF, Bianco AJ, Rhodes KH. Septic arthritis in children. *Orthop Clin North Am.* 1975;6:923–934.
3. Gatter RA, Schmacher HR Jr. Joint aspiration: indications and technique. In: Gatter RA, Schumacher HR Jr, eds. *A Practical Handbook of Synovial Fluid Analysis.* Philadelphia: Lea & Febiger; 1991:14–23.
4. Ezell SL, Kobernick ME, Benjamin GC. Arthrocentesis. In: Roberts JR, Hedges JR, eds. *Clinical Procedures in Emergency Medicine.* 2nd ed. Philadelphia: WB Saunders; 1991:847–859.
5. Reichman EF, Waddell R. Arthrocentesis. In: Reichman EF, Simon RR, eds. *Emergency Medicine Procedures.* New York: McGraw-Hill; 2004:559–584.
6. Siva C, Velazquez C, Mody A, et al. Diagnosing acute monoarthritis in adults: a practical approach for the family physician. *Am Fam Phys.* 2003;68:83–90.
7. Nelson JD, Koontz WC. Septic arthritis in infants and children: a review of 117 cases. *Pediatrics.* 1966;38:966–971.
8. Del Beccaro MA, Champoux AN, Bockers T, et al. Septic arthritis versus transient synovitis of the hip: the value of screening laboratory tests. *Ann Emerg Med.* 1992;21(12):14–18.
9. Kocher MS, Zurakowski D, Kasser JR. Differentiating between septic arthritis and transient synovitis of the hip in children: an evidence-based clinical prediction algorithm. *J Bone Joint Surg Am.* 1999;81:1662–1670.
10. Levine MJ, McGuire KJ, McGowan KL, et al. Assessment of the test characteristics of C-reactive protein for septic arthritis in children. *J Pediatr Orthop.* 2003;23:373–377.
11. Kallio MJT, Unkila-Kallio L, Aalto K, et al. Serum C-reactive protein, erythrocyte sedimentation rate and white blood cell count in septic arthritis of children. *Pediatr Infect Dis J.* 1997;16:411–413.
12. Bureau NJ, Chhem RK, Cardinal E. Musculoskeletal infections: US manifestations. *Radiographics.* 1999;19:1585–1592.
13. Samuelson CO, Cannon GW, Ward JR. Arthrocentesis. *J Fam Pract.* 1985;20:169–184.
14. Gatter RA. Arthrocentesis technique and intrasynovial therapy. In: McCarty DG, Koopman WJ, eds. *Arthritis and Allied Conditions.* 12th ed. Philadelphia: Lea & Febiger; 1993:711–720.
15. Goldenberg DL, Reed JI. Bacterial arthritis. *N Engl J Med.* 1985;312:764–771.
16. Dooley DP. Aspiration of the possibly septic joint through potential cellulitis: just do it! [letter]. *J Emerg Med.* 2002;23:210.
17. Hampers LC, Manco-Johnson M. Emergency department management of musculoskeletal injuries in children with inherited bleeding disorders. *Clin Pediatr Emerg Med.* 2002;3:138–144.
18. Hasselbacher P. Arthrocentesis and synovial fluid analysis. In: Schumacher HR Jr, ed. *Primer on the Rheumatic Diseases.* 9th ed. Atlanta: Arthritis Foundation; 1988:55–60.
19. Leversee JH. Aspiration of joints and soft tissue injections. *Primary Care.* 1986;13:579–599.
20. Miller JA. Joint paracentesis from an anatomic point of view, II: hip, knee, ankle, and foot. *Surgery.* 1957;41:999–1011.
21. Cardone DA, Tallia AF. Diagnostic and therapeutic injection of the hip and knee. *Am Fam Phys.* 2003;67:2147–2152.
22. Flood RG. Procedural sedation and analgesia for children in the emergency department. *Emerg Med Clin North Am.* 2003;21:121–139.
23. Gonzalez BE, Martinez-Aguilar G, Julten KG, et al. Severe staphylococcal sepsis in adolescents in the era of community-acquired methicillin-resistant *Staphylococcus aureus. Pediatrics.* 2005;115:642–648.
24. Fink CW, Nelson JD. Septic arthritis and osteomyelitis in children. *Clin Rheum Dis.* 1986;12:423–435.
25. Welkon CJ, Long SS, Fisher MC, et al. Pyogenic arthritis in infants and children: a review of 95 cases. *Pediatr Infect Dis.* 1986;5:669–676.
26. Bonhoeffer J, Haeberle B, Schaad UB, et al. Diagnosis of acute haematogenous osteomyelitis and septic arthritis: 20 years experience at the University Children's Hospital Basel. *Swiss Med Wkly.* 2001;131:575–581.

105

FREDERICK C. JOHNSON AND PAMELA J. OKADA

Reduction of Common Joint Dislocations and Subluxations

▶ INTRODUCTION

Extremity injuries are a common reason for children to visit the emergency department (ED). When a joint is involved, a range of injuries are possible. The patient may sustain a simple subluxation or dislocation or may have an open fracture through the joint space. The focus of this chapter is the management of subluxations and dislocations. In most cases, these injures can be definitively managed by the emergency physician, while in other cases the emergency physician must perform a limb-saving reduction before transferring the patient to a specialist for further management. The methods of reduction likewise range from the simplest of maneuvers to rather complex techniques requiring multiple operators and muscle relaxants. Before proceeding with a description of the injuries and reduction techniques, two important definitions should be understood. The subluxation of a joint refers to an incomplete disruption where there is partial communication of the articular surfaces. The dislocation of a joint refers to a complete dissociation of its articular surfaces.

▶ RADIAL HEAD SUBLUXATION

Radial head subluxation is one of the most common upper extremity injuries in children (1). The classic history involves a child who has traction applied to an arm and then refuses to use that arm. This can occur after a caretaker pulls the arm to prevent a fall, pulls the child up after a fall, pulls the arm of a stubborn toddler, or swings the child by both arms. This has led to the common term "nursemaid's elbow." However, it should be noted that the classic history of traction is often not elicited; in many cases, the mechanism of injury appears to be a simple fall. Radial head subluxation is commonly seen in toddlers, although it has been reported in infants younger than 6 months as a result of rolling over in bed (2). An increased incidence in females has also been reported (3,4). The left arm is more commonly injured than the right, perhaps reflecting the fact that a right-handed caretaker is most likely to grasp a child's left arm. The recurrence rate is up to 33% (3). It most commonly recurs in children 24 months of age or younger. Sex, family history, and the elbow involved in the initial episode are not risk factors for recurrence (5).

Anatomy and Physiology

Radial head subluxation typically occurs in children 1 to 4 years of age as a result of a sudden forceful longitudinal traction on the hand or wrist while the forearm is extended and pronated. The pulling episode is immediately followed by acute onset of pain and resistance to using the arm. The abrupt force affects the humeroradial articulation between the capitellum of the humerus and the head of the radius. Normally, the capitellum fits into the cupped surface of the radial head. A fan-shaped ligament known as the "radial collateral ligament" attaches proximally to the lateral epicondyle of the humerus and distally blends into the annular ligament of the radial head. The abrupt axial tension on the forearm pulls the radial head distally, tearing the distal attachment of the annular ligament and causing the radial head to pull out of the torn annular ligament. The distal aspect of the annular ligament, which slips free from the periosteum of the radial neck, becomes entrapped between the head of the radius and the capitellum. The child holds the forearm in pronation because supination is painful. Forced supination brings the annular ligament into its appropriate position over the radial head by using the radius as a lever (6).

Indications

The physical examination typically reveals a nondistressed child with a flexed elbow and slightly pronated wrist held to the side in the absence of significant point tenderness, ecchymosis, or focal edema. The child will appear content and normal, with the exception of a refusal to use the injured arm. Clinical diagnosis of radial head subluxation can be made when a typical history and physical examination is obtained, and these are usually sufficient grounds to perform the reduction maneuver without first obtaining radiographs. Even in those cases in which a child presents with a nonclassic history, there is little risk of fracture as long as the child has the typical physical examination findings of mild flexion of the elbow and pronated wrist position (7).

Equipment

No equipment is required for reduction of a radial head subluxation.

Procedure

Three reduction techniques are commonly employed. Supination at the wrist followed by flexion at the elbow is the classically taught and most commonly used method. The supination technique is performed by first gripping the patient's elbow using the nondominant hand, with the clinician's thumb on the patient's radial head. Using the dominant hand, the clinician grasps the patient's wrist, applies mild traction, and then in one swift movement supinates the wrist and flexes the forearm up toward the shoulder (Fig. 105.1A–D).

The effectiveness of the second technique, hyperpronation with flexion at the elbow, has been reported in multiple series (3,8,9). This maneuver involves gripping the patient's elbow using the nondominant hand, forcefully hyperpronating the child's wrist, and then flexing the forearm toward the shoulder (Fig. 105.2). This technique has shown superior success rates compared with supination-flexion (3,9). Furthermore, when used for the first reduction attempt, the pronation technique appears to be significantly less painful than the supination-flexion method (9). In fact, reduction often occurs with pronation alone.

A third option involves moving the elbow to a 90-degree position, supinating the wrist, and then extending the forearm (10). Regardless of the technique used, an audible or palpable "pop" usually indicates a successful reduction (4). Typically, the child will begin to use the arm within 5 to 10 minutes, although in many cases the child must be enticed to do so with a toy or other desired object (9).

Complications

The main pitfall involves overlooking a radial or humeral fracture. The patient must be carefully examined before attempting reduction. Radiographs should be obtained if external signs of trauma, such as swelling, abrasions, or ecchymosis are present. Additionally, failed attempts at reduction warrant radiographs of the elbow to look for signs of a fracture. On radiographs, elevation of the posterior fat pad or misalignment of the intersection of the anterior humeral line and the central radial line away from the middle third of the capitellum should raise suspicion of a fracture (Fig. 105.3) (11). Fractures in children who present with classic history and examination findings are rare; however, if a fracture is present, the reduction techniques will neither return function of the arm nor relieve the pain.

▶ DIGIT DISLOCATIONS

Digit dislocations are common among physically active adolescents and school-age children. The direction of the displacement of the middle or distal phalanx determines the type of dislocation for the proximal interphalangeal (PIP) or distal interphalangeal (DIP) joint, respectively. They are categorized as dorsal, volar, or lateral dislocations.

Dislocation of the DIP joint is less common than dislocation of the PIP joint. This is related to the additional stability provided to the DIP by the insertion of the flexor and extensor tendons to the proximal aspect of the distal phalanx. Closed reduction of the DIP and PIP joints is done in a similar fashion using a combination of traction and either extension or flexion.

Prior to any attempt at reduction of a suspected subluxed or dislocated joint, a thorough joint examination should be performed. Stability of the joint can be determined by testing the range of motion of the interphalangeal and metacarpophalangeal joints of the hand. As with all aspects of the physical examination, range of motion is influenced by pain, so accurate assessment typically requires a digital or wrist block (Chapter 35).

Active range of motion is tested by having the patient move the digit. Completing full range of motion without displacement of the phalanges demonstrates adequate joint stability. Passive joint stability is assessed by applying gentle radial and ulnar stress to each collateral ligament. Passive hyperextension is used to assess volar plate integrity. Stress testing should be done in both extended and moderately flexed positions to eliminate the stabilizing effect of the volar plate. The inability to actively extend the flexed PIP joint against resistance suggests a rupture of the central band of the extensor tendon, which can progress to a boutonniere deformity. Comparison with the same joint of the uninvolved hand may assist in the diagnosis. Thorough examination should occur after any successful joint reduction to ensure stability (12).

Regardless of the type of dislocation, pre- and postreduction radiographs are required to ascertain the presence of a fracture. Radiographic examination should include an anteroposterior (AP) and lateral image. Failure to obtain a true lateral radiograph may result in missing a fracture or a loose body in the joint.

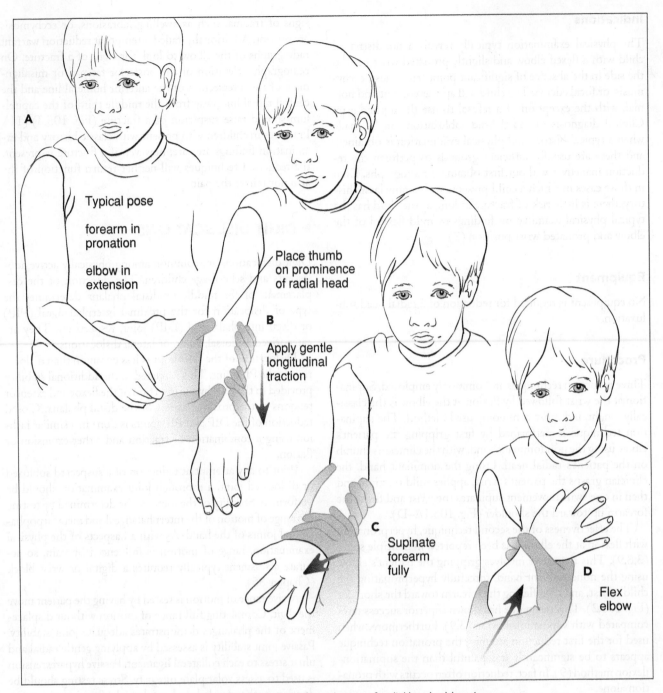

Figure 105.1 Procedure for reduction of radial head subluxation.

Anatomy and Physiology

The metacarpophalangeal joints are condyloid joints that allow flexion, extension, abduction, adduction, and circumduction. The joints are enclosed by a fibrous capsule. They are strengthened on each side by a triangular collateral ligament that extends from the sides of the head of the proximal bone to the sides of the base of the distal bone. The collateral ligaments are attached to the palmar ligaments, which are strong, thick plates that are firmly attached to the phalanx and loosely attached to the metacarpal. This volar plate is a dense fibrous

connective tissue that simultaneously provides support and allows for flexion at the joint (6). The interphalangeal joints are uniaxial hinge joints that only permit flexion and extension. The articulations join the head of one phalanx with the base of the more distal one. Like the metacarpophalangeal joints, they have collateral and palmar ligaments; however, they are reinforced dorsally by the extensor expansions of the digits (Fig. 105.4) (6).

Dorsal dislocations are the most common, resulting from some combination of hyperextension, longitudinal compression, and dorsal translation. Hyperextension of the PIP joint

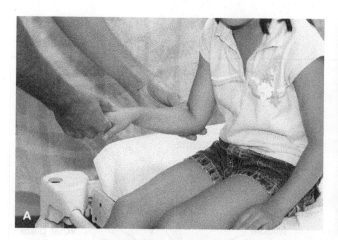

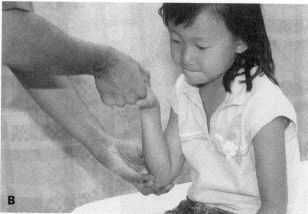

Figure 105.2 Pronation with flexion technique for reduction of radial head subluxation. Reduction of the radial head involves hyperpronation of the forearm (**A**) followed by flexion of the elbow (**B**).

can cause an avulsion of the volar plate from the middle phalanx (13,14). Volar dislocations of the PIP joint are rare. The most common mechanism is a rotational longitudinal compression force on a semiflexed middle phalanx that results in unilateral disruption of a collateral ligament and partial avulsion of the volar plate (15,16). This force can cause the distal aspect of the proximal phalanx to interpose itself between the central and lateral bands of the extensor tendon. Additionally, it can disrupt the central band as it inserts onto the proximal aspect of the middle phalanx. Because volar dislocations of the PIP joint can be very difficult to reduce, some specialists advocate an orthopaedic consultation for further evaluation and possible open reduction.

Indications

An interphalangeal joint subluxation is usually associated with forced hyperextension or hyperflexion of the digit during participation in physical activities. The patient presents with acute pain, deformity, and swelling. Radiographs are used to confirm the joint dislocation, identify fractures, and document successful reduction.

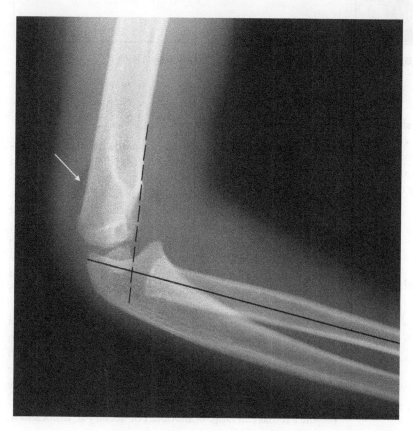

Figure 105.3 Lateral view radiograph of elbow reveals posterior fat pad sign (*arrow*) and slight posterior displacement of capitellum relative to anterior humeral line (*dashed line*), indicative of supracondylar fracture. The radiocapitellar line (*solid line*) in this patient is normal.

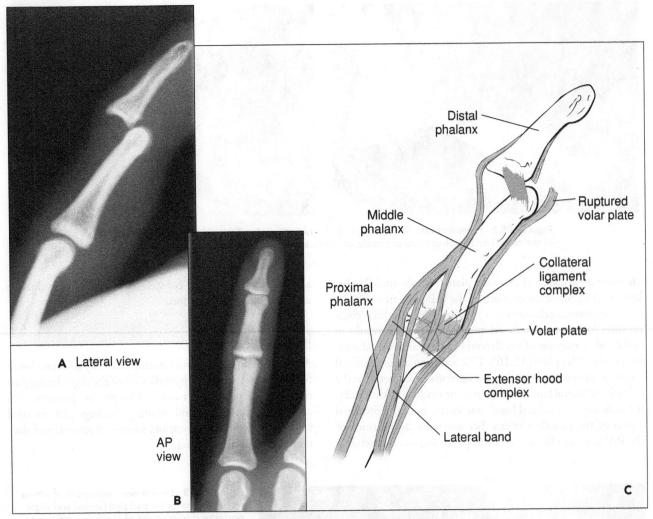

Figure 105.4 Radiographic (**A, B**) and schematic (**C**) representation of an interphalangeal joint dislocation.

Consultation with an orthopaedic surgeon should occur when findings consistent with neurovascular compromise, joint instability, or fracture are present. Additionally, an orthopaedist should be consulted when a lateral or volar PIP joint dislocation occurs. These subluxations may require open reduction and internal fixation (17).

Equipment

For digital block anesthesia:
Antiseptic solution (povidone-iodine or alcohol swabs)
Lidocaine 1% without epinephrine
Sodium bicarbonate 8.4%
27- or 30-gauge, 0.63-inch needle

For reduction:
Gauze pad

For immobilization:
Foam-padded malleable splint, appropriately sized
Tape

Procedure

Prior to reduction, digital block anesthesia should be provided. If rings are present on the affected digit, these should be removed. The reduction technique for a dorsal dislocation consists of three maneuvers. First, the affected joint is hyperextended. Then longitudinal traction is applied to the distal phalanx while hyperextension is maintained. Finally, the dislocated phalanx is gently pushed into its proper position (Fig. 105.5A–D). In some cases, the distal phalanx may be more easily grasped by first wrapping a 4″ × 4″ gauze pad around the finger. Postreduction radiographs are needed to re-evaluate for fracture.

After reduction, stabilization can be accomplished by a variety of means. Many operators choose to apply a splint such as a foam-padded, malleable digit splint. Should this option be chosen, the type of splint applied should be tailored to the injury. Splints for DIP dislocations are applied so that only the DIP is immobile. The DIP is splinted in extension, and the PIP has full range of motion. For dorsal PIP dislocations,

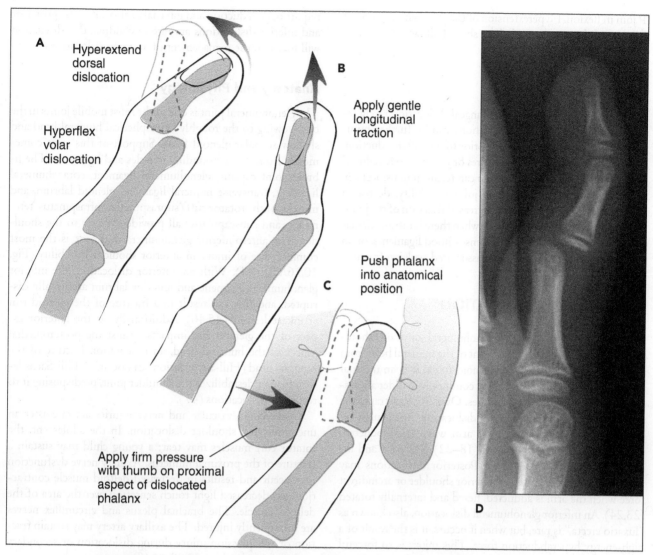

A Hyperextend dorsal dislocation

Hyperflex volar dislocation

B Apply gentle longitudinal traction

C Push phalanx into anatomical position

Apply firm pressure with thumb on proximal aspect of dislocated phalanx

D

Figure 105.5 Procedure for reduction of dorsal DIP joint dislocation (**A–C**). Radiograph of PIP joint dislocation (**D**).

the splint is applied dorsally, with the joint in 20 to 30 degrees of flexion. Splints applied for PIP dislocation should remain in place for 14 to 21 days, whereas those for DIP dislocations should remain in place for 10 to 14 days. Buddy taping to an adjacent finger is an acceptable alternative for younger children (13,14). If the dislocation is irreducible or unstable after reduction, referral to an orthopaedic or hand subspecialist is advised.

The reduction of a volar dislocation is more complex than a dorsal reduction. The typical maneuver of longitudinal traction can create a noose around the interposed proximal phalanx and hinder reduction. Some specialists advocate flexing the metacarpophalangeal and PIP joints, followed by gentle traction of the middle phalanx. Because the phalanx can be trapped between the extensor tendons, other specialists view this dislocation as irreducible and requiring open reduction (13,15).

Lateral dislocation of the PIP joint occurs when a radial- or ulnar-directed force leads to disruption of the collateral lig-

aments and a portion of the volar plate. Reduction is achieved with longitudinal traction and gentle maneuvering of the dislocated segment back into its normal position. The PIP joint is usually stable after reduction and can be treated with buddy taping or splinting. Patients should be referred to a hand specialist for follow-up (13,15).

Dislocation of the interphalangeal (IP) joint of the thumb is similar to dislocation of the DIP joints of the other phalanges. Dorsal dislocation of the thumb is more common than volar dislocation. The mechanism of injury is commonly hyperextension of the joint that results in a rupture of the proximal portion of the volar plate and at least a portion of the collateral ligaments. Reduction involves hyperextension and gentle traction on the distal phalanx (13,15).

Dislocation of the metacarpophalangeal joint of the thumb results from a hyperextension force that ruptures the volar plate, joint capsule, and a portion of the collateral ligament. Reduction is achieved by relaxing the hand with the wrist in flexion, the first metacarpal in flexion and adduction, and the

IP join in flexion. Hyperextension of the joint with continued traction of the proximal phalanx should allow reduction of the joint (13,15).

Complications

Timely reduction of an interphalangeal dislocation rarely results in complications. Complications can be further minimized by obtaining radiographs prior to and after reduction. Radiographs should detect fractures or incompletely reduced joints. Inadequate immobilization can result in redislocation. Delayed reduction can result in joint instability, decreased range of motion of the joint, or decreased function of the joint. Unsuccessful reduction can occur when there is intra-articular entrapment of the volar plate, extensor hood ligaments, or an osteochondral fragment from an associated avulsion fracture.

▶ SHOULDER DISLOCATION

Traumatic dislocation of the glenohumeral joint, or "shoulder dislocation," is the displacement of the humeral head from its normal articulation in the glenoid fossa. It is an unusual injury in children and occurs most commonly in older adolescents involved in sporting activities. Over 90% of traumatic shoulder dislocations are anterior dislocations and usually result from a force applied to the arm when it is abducted, extended, and externally rotated (18–22). Posterior and inferior dislocations occur rarely. Posterior dislocations may result from direct force to the anterior shoulder or an indirect force when the arm is adducted, flexed and internally rotated (23,24). An inferior glenohumeral dislocation, also known as "luxatio erecta," is rare, but when it occurs, it is the result of a high-energy hyperabduction force. This injury is so forceful that the humeral head may be driven through the soft tissues of the axilla, producing an open injury (25–28).

Although many methods have been described for reduction of a shoulder dislocation, few are appropriate for the child or adolescent. Maneuvers using leverage (Kocher) (29,30), overhead traction (Milch, Cooper) (31–34), external rotation (35,36), or lateral traction (Eskimo) (37,38) are not recommended in children. Reduction by these techniques is associated with complications that include further neuromuscular, vascular, and soft-tissue injury; fractures of the humeral neck and glenoid rim; and spiral fractures of the humeral shaft.

For the pediatric patient, reduction by forward flexion with gravity (Stimson) (39,40), scapular manipulation (Anderson) (41–43), or traction-countertraction (modified Hippocrates) are recommended. These reduction techniques are 70% to 90% effective on the first attempt and are commonly performed by emergency physicians in the ED (38).

In general, immediate orthopaedic consultation is required for posterior and inferior dislocations and for dislocations involving neurovascular compromise, humeral neck fractures, or intra-articular bony fragments. Intra-articular fractures often require open reduction and internal fixation. Because posterior and inferior dislocations are rare in children, this discussion will focus on the management of anterior dislocations.

Anatomy and Physiology

The glenohumeral joint is one of the most mobile joints in the body, owing to the roughly hemispherical humeral head and shallow scapular glenoid fossa. Support of this joint comes mostly from the surrounding muscles and ligaments. The fibrous joint capsule, glenohumeral ligament, coracohumeral ligament, transverse humeral ligament, glenoid labrum, and muscles of the rotator cuff (supraspinatus, infraspinatus, teres minor, and subscapularis) all provide stability to the shoulder. The anteroinferior glenohumeral ligament is the most common site of injury in anterior shoulder instability (Fig. 105.6A,B) (44). With an anterior dislocation, the inferior glenohumeral ligament and anterior labrum are usually disrupted, and this can result in a fracture of the glenoid rim (Bankart lesion) (45,46). Additionally, as the anterior aspect of the glenoid rim impacts against the posteromedial aspect of the humeral head, an indentation fracture of the humeral head (Hill-Sachs lesion) can occur. A Hill-Sachs lesion further destabilizes the shoulder joint, predisposing it to recurrent dislocations (47).

In the child, vascular and nerve injuries are rare after an uncomplicated shoulder dislocation. In the adolescent, the rotator cuff muscles may tear; a young child may sustain a fracture of the proximal humerus. Axillary nerve dysfunction may occur and results in decreased deltoid muscle contraction and decreased light touch sensation over the area of the deltoid muscle. The brachial plexus and circumflex nerves are infrequently injured. The axillary artery may sustain traction or compression injury during dislocation or secondary to forceful reduction (22,38,44,48).

The forward flexion and abduction maneuvers for reducing an anterior shoulder dislocation use the traction-countertraction principle to lever the humeral head into the glenoid fossa. Both maneuvers fatigue the shoulder girdle muscles, relax the biceps muscle, protect neurovascular structures, and help prevent humeral head impaction on the glenoid. The forward flexion technique allows spontaneous reduction using gravity, time, and muscle relaxation. The abduction technique applies active opposing forces.

Scapular manipulation causes the glenoid to release the humeral head impaction and allow reduction. When the humeral head dislocates from forced abduction and external rotation, the glenoid fossa is forced medially, and the inferior tip of the scapula is abducted. Although scapular manipulation has not been studied in patients younger than 17 years, this technique is atraumatic, uses minimal force, and has no reported complications in adults (41–43).

Traumatic shoulder dislocations are acutely painful. With anterior dislocations, the arm is held in slight abduction and external rotation. Movement of the arm is extremely painful

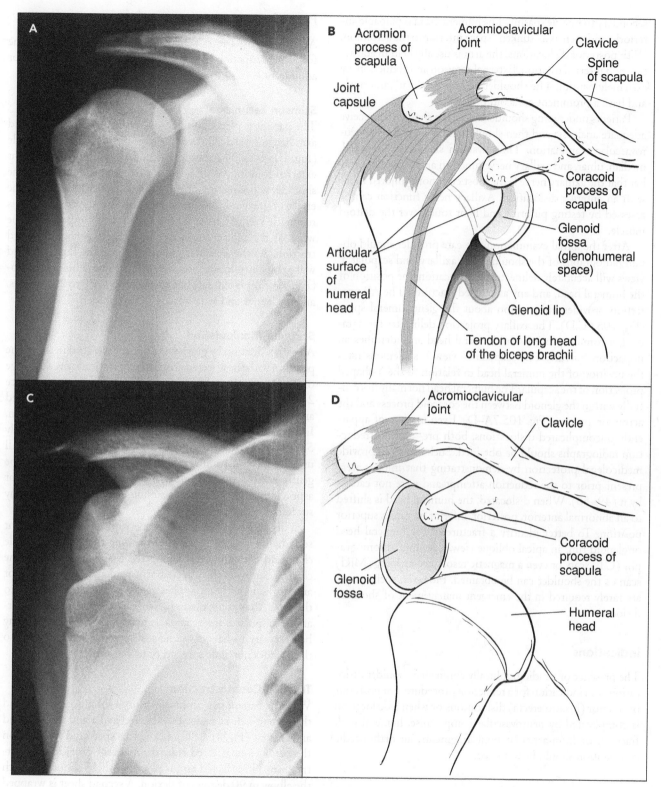

Figure 105.6
A, B. Normal shoulder joint.
C, D. Anterior dislocation of the shoulder.

secondary to muscle spasms. The humeral head is palpable anteriorly, and there is a "sunken" space inferior to the acromion. With posterior dislocations, the arm is usually held in adduction and internal rotation. External rotation and abduction are extremely painful. The shoulder will appear "flat" anteriorly and have a prominent coracoid process.

Patients undergoing shoulder reduction should first receive adequate analgesia and then should undergo a complete neurovascular examination. The physician should assess radial, median, ulnar, and axillary nerve function and should remember that the axillary nerve is the most commonly injured nerve with an anterior dislocation. Axillary nerve function can be assessed by testing pinprick and light touch over the deltoid muscle.

After the initial examination, the care provider should obtain radiographs of the shoulder. AP, axillary, and scapular Y views will accurately delineate the dislocation, the position of the humeral head, and any associated fractures. The AP projection provides information about the glenohumeral space (Fig. 105.6C,D). The axillary projection delineates the coracoid, acromion process, and humeral head and identifies an impaction fracture. The scapular Y view best demonstrates the position of the humeral head in relation to the Y-shaped projection of the scapula. The humeral head normally lies centrally within the glenoid between the coracoid process and the acromion process (Fig. 105.7A–D). Even in cases of apparently uncomplicated dislocations, both pre- and postreduction radiographs should be obtained. Such films can provide medicolegal protection by demonstrating that injuries were present prior to the reduction attempt and were not caused by it (49–53). When dislocated, the humeral head is shifted to an abnormal anterior, posterior, inferior or, rarely, superior position. To better identify a fracture of the humeral head or glenoid rim, an apical oblique view, a computed tomography (CT) scan, or even a magnetic resonance imaging (MRI) scan of the shoulder can be obtained. However, such images are rarely required in the emergent management of shoulder dislocations.

Indications

The presence of a radiographically confirmed shoulder dislocation is an indication for a reduction procedure. For posterior or inferior (luxatio erecta) dislocations or when a dislocation is complicated by neurovascular compromise, humeral neck fracture, or intra-articular bony fragments, an orthopaedic consultation should be obtained.

Equipment

Medications for procedural sedation
Monitoring equipment
Weights, 2 to 5 kg
Two sheets
Sling and swathe
Shoulder immobilizer

Procedure

After interposed intra-articular fragments are excluded, the following reduction maneuvers are appropriate for a child or adolescent.

Stimson Technique

The patient is placed in the prone position with the affected arm hanging vertically over the edge of the examination table (Fig. 105.8A). The shoulder is in forward flexion and slight external rotation. With adequate sedation and analgesia, the shoulder will sometimes reduce spontaneously due only to the effect of gravity. However, in most cases additional weight is required. Weights from 2 to 5 kg can be strapped onto the wrist of the affected arm to provide additional downward traction. As the shoulder muscles fatigue, the humeral head will gradually relocate into the glenoid fossa. This gentle procedure is simple and safe but may take up to 20 to 25 minutes, and analgesics and sedatives are often required.

Scapular Manipulation

As with reduction by gravity, the patient is placed in the prone position with the affected arm hanging vertically over the edge of the examination table (Fig. 105.8B). The operator can place 2- to 5-kg weights hanging from the wrist of the affected arm or have an assistant provide gentle downward traction. In either case, traction should be applied for approximately 5 minutes. When the patient's muscles relax, the scapula will usually become readily visible beneath the skin. It can be gently rotated by pushing its tip medially and its superior aspect laterally. A palpable or audible "clunk" may accompany successful reduction.

This procedure may also be performed with the patient seated. The patient is positioned facing the back of a stable chair and with the chest supported against the back of the chair. Then with the affected arm held parallel to the floor anteriorly, an assistant applies gentle longitudinal traction to the arm. After approximately 5 minutes of traction, the operator manipulates the scapula as previously described. It may be necessary to have a second assistant stabilize the chair so that it does not slide forward or to the side.

Traction-Countertraction

With the patient in a supine position, a sheet is placed around the patient's chest under the affected axilla and then around an assistant (Fig. 105.8C). Using this sheet and standing on the patient's unaffected side, the assistant provides countertraction. The affected arm is placed in slight abduction, with the elbow in 90 degrees of flexion. A second sheet is wrapped around the patient's flexed forearm just distal to the elbow and then is wrapped around the operator's body. The operator is positioned on the affected side approximately even with the patient's waist. Once adequate sedation is achieved, longitudinal traction is applied by pulling the sheet attached to the affected arm laterally and caudally while keeping the patient's arm abducted and elbow flexed. Both the operator

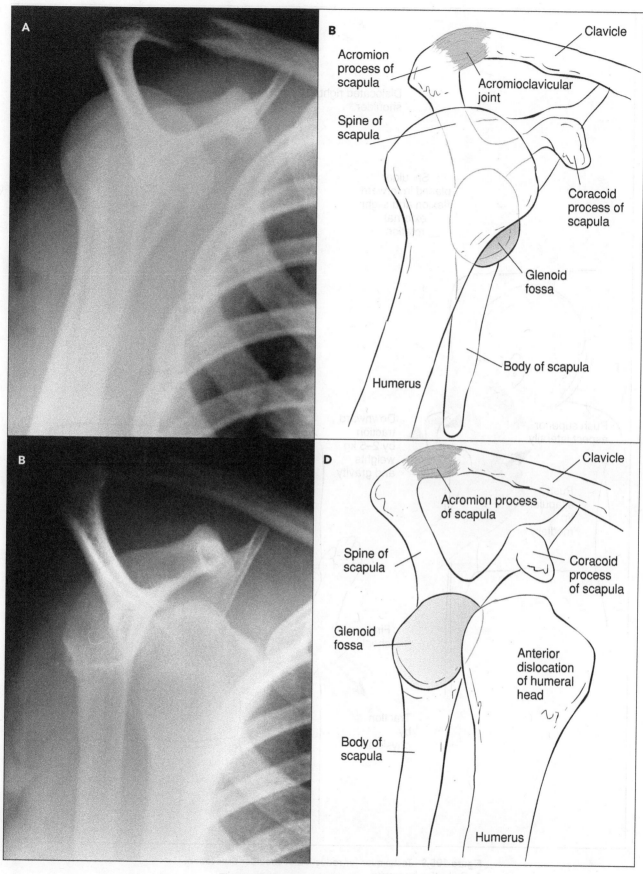

Figure 105.7 Scapular Y view of shoulder.
A, B. Normal.
C, D. Anterior dislocation.

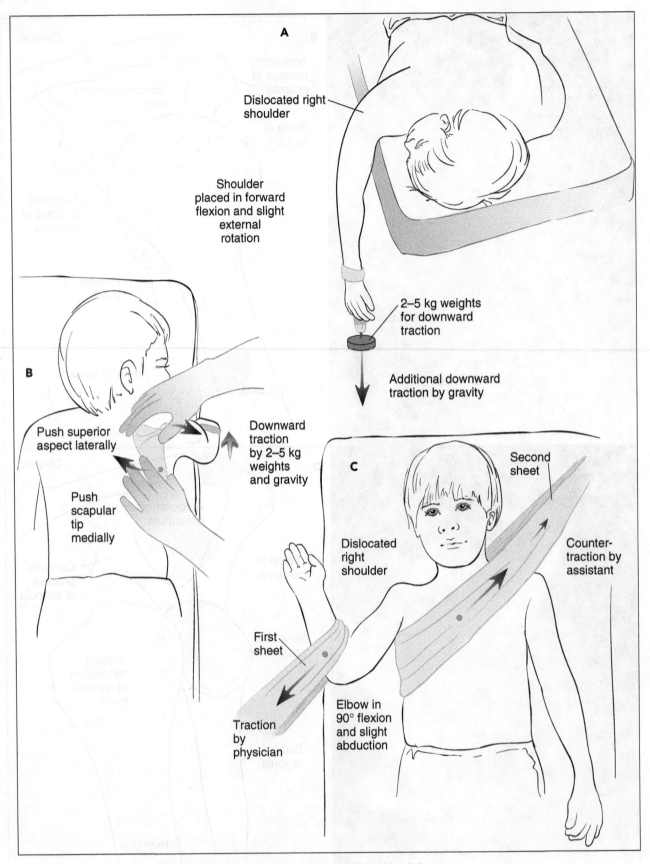

A

Dislocated right shoulder

Shoulder placed in forward flexion and slight external rotation

2–5 kg weights for downward traction

Additional downward traction by gravity

B

Push superior aspect laterally

Push scapular tip medially

Downward traction by 2–5 kg weights and gravity

C

Second sheet

Counter-traction by assistant

Dislocated right shoulder

First sheet

Traction by physician

Elbow in 90° flexion and slight abduction

Figure 105.8 Techniques for reduction of shoulder dislocation.
A. Reduction by gravity.
B. Reduction by scapular manipulation.
C. Reduction by traction-countertraction.

and the assistant can gain mechanical advantage by leaning back against the sheet. As traction causes the muscles to fatigue, gentle internal and external rotation will often help to disengage the humeral head. Reduction of the humeral head into the glenoid fossa is usually obvious and may be associated with an audible "clunk." This procedure is effective for both anterior and posterior dislocations.

Internal Rotation Technique

The patient is placed in a reclined or seated position. This procedure may require an assistant to aid in the reduction. The operator faces the patient and applies constant anteroposterior pressure using one hand placed over the patient's distal clavicle at the level of the humeral head. The affected arm is held flexed at the elbow and in slight abduction and internal rotation at the shoulder and is supported in this position by the operator or an assistant. After adequate sedation and analgesia, continuous longitudinal traction is applied to the affected arm, and it is gradually abducted to 90 degrees. The affected arm is brought toward the midline and then to the opposite side so that the hand is gently forced to touch the opposite shoulder. This maneuver is performed with a smooth arclike motion of the arm, and reduction usually occurs as the hand nears the opposite shoulder. This approach is useful in anterior dislocations.

Following any successful reduction, active motion and a normal contour of the shoulder are usually evident immediately. Distal neuromuscular status should be assessed after reduction to identify brachial plexus or vascular injury. AP and scapular Y radiographs should also be obtained to confirm successful reduction and evaluate for subtle fractures of the humeral head, glenoid tip, or humeral tip. A sling and swathe or shoulder immobilizer should be applied for 1 to 3 weeks (it can be removed for bathing). Immobilization allows healing of the anterior capsule and glenoid ligaments. The patient should be referred for orthopaedic evaluation and physical rehabilitation within 1 to 2 weeks of the reduction and should not participate in sports or other vigorous activities for 3 to 6 weeks.

Complications

The most common complication of traumatic shoulder dislocation is recurrent shoulder instability. This is due to a stretched subscapular tendon and to capsular laxity. Young age appears to be the highest predictor of recurrence. If a child has a shoulder dislocation before 10 years of age, the recurrence rate is 100%; if the first dislocation occurs between the ages of 10 and 20 years, the recurrence rate is 80% to 90%; and if the first dislocation occurs after age 20 but before age 30, the recurrence rate is 64% to 70% (18). Glenoid rim fractures and humeral head impaction fractures (Hill-Sachs) also increase the rate of recurrence (18,39,54–60). In some cases, soft tissues (e.g., the long head of the biceps tendon) or boney fragments within the joint prevent closed reduction. These patients usually require operative intervention.

Other rare but reported complications include fractures, neuromuscular injuries, and, rarely, osteonecrosis of the humeral head. Nerve injury involving the brachial plexus occurs in 10% to 25% of cases, most commonly involving the axillary nerve. In younger children, avascular necrosis of the humeral head, axillary artery injury, or degenerative arthritis can occur. Complications of the reduction technique, although infrequent, result from excessively forceful traction and compression on neurovascular structures in the axilla. Humeral neck and spiral humeral shaft fractures occur rarely from an overly forceful reduction and can be avoided with adequate sedation, analgesia, and muscle relaxation (36,38,46,48,54,61).

▶ PATELLA DISLOCATION

Patellofemoral instability is a common cause of ED visits in the adolescent population. Contrary to the stereotype of an overweight, sedentary child with patellar dislocation after little or no trauma, most patellar dislocations occur in athletically active children. Injuries can occur from either indirect or direct trauma to the knee, although a noncontact mechanism is more common (62–64). The average annual incidence of first-time patellar dislocation is 5.8 per 100,000. Females aged 10 to 17 years are at the greatest risk for first-time dislocation, with an annual incidence of 33 per 100,000 (62). Patients with a first-time dislocation were found to have a recurrence rate of 17%, whereas patients with a history of multiple dislocations had a recurrence rate of 49% (62).

Anatomy and Physiology

The patellofemoral articulation is a complex joint that relies on both bones and soft tissues for stability. The medial patellofemoral ligament (MPFL) and the vastus medialis muscle provide the greatest amount of resistance to lateral patellar movement. The MPFL runs from the medial femoral epicondyle to the superomedial aspect of the patella. This is the structure that is almost universally injured in lateral patellar dislocations. The patella commonly dislocates in a lateral direction and is frequently associated with injury to the MPFL and the cartilaginous surfaces of both the patella and femur (Fig 105.9A–D) (65).

Most patients describe a history of an acute, traumatic event and present with a painful and swollen knee (65). Patellar dislocation commonly occurs when the foot is planted and lower extremity internal rotation occurs while the knee is in valgus position. This action produces a significant lateral force on the patella that can exceed the strength of the MPFL, resulting in a lateral dislocation of the patella (66). Medial dislocations occur almost exclusively in patients with a history of surgery for instability (65).

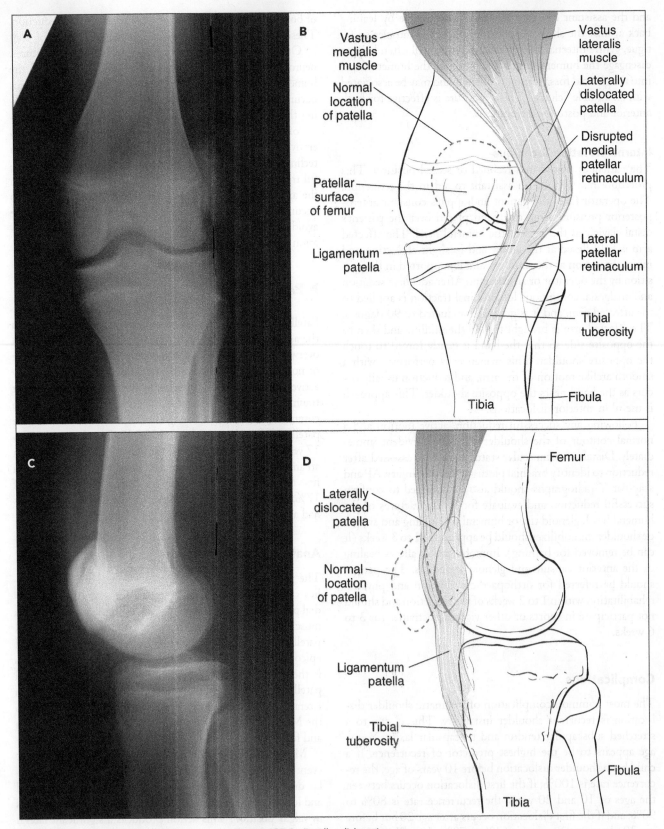

Figure 105.9 Patellar dislocation.

Imaging of the knee allows detection of intra-articular abnormalities and associated injuries that occur as a direct result of the dislocation. Additionally, it also allows for the identification of factors that might have predisposed the child to injury, such as patella alta or trochlear dysplasia (65). MRI is the preferred modality to image the injured joint because soft-tissue and osteochondral damage can be detected; however, to accurately explore articular injury, arthroscopic or macroscopic examination should be performed. Articular cartilage injury has been seen in as many as 77% of patients studied (67). However, neither of these techniques is practical in the acute care setting, and the emergency physician will in most cases have to rely on plain radiographs. The dislocated patella is easily seen on standard AP and lateral films. Additional information regarding the integrity of the patella itself can be gained from an infrapatellar ("sunrise") view. It should be remembered that the patella is not fully ossified until five years of age, and therefore the infrapatellar projection is most useful in the evaluation of older children. When diagnosis of patellar dislocation is made by physical examination, radiographs can be deferred until after reduction. However, as described for shoulder dislocation, prereduction films can provide both information regarding pre-existing injuries and medicolegal protection. Failure of the reduction attempt is also an indication for radiographs.

Indications

As mentioned, most patellar dislocations occur in athletically active children. Patients describe a history of an acute, traumatic event with a painful and swollen knee. The majority of dislocations spontaneously reduce with full knee extension. Persistence of a fixed dislocation is rare and seen in fewer than 10% of dislocations (66). These patients usually present with an acutely painful knee held in flexion and with extreme apprehension regarding movement of the involved patella. The femoral condyles are palpable medially, and the patella is visualized laterally as a mass (65). Injury to the MPFL can be determined by tenderness at its origin at the adductor tubercle of the femur or by a palpable deformity at its patellar attachment (66). In the acute setting, arthrocentesis, which reveals hemarthrosis and fatty globules, is diagnostic and can be therapeutic because the presence of a hemarthrosis may prevent reduction (see Chapter 104) (66). Once the hemarthrosis has been drained, reduction can proceed as described below. In the nonacute setting, patients will have tenderness over the origin of the MPFL. Osteochondral fractures have been associated with as many as 72% of lateral patellar dislocations (67). These injuries occur on the medial patellar facet or the lateral femoral epicondyle and can be detected by direct palpation (65).

Equipment

For reduction:
None (consider medications for sedation and analgesia)

For immobilization:
Standard knee immobilizer (appropriately sized) or a plaster splint
Crutches

Procedure

Nonoperative management involves reduction of the patella to avoid secondary injury to the articular surface. Because most patellar dislocations reduce spontaneously, reduction in the ED is rarely necessary. If the patella has not reduced, closed reduction is indicated. Sedation may be needed to allow patient relaxation and enhance cooperation with the reduction maneuver. The first step involves flexing the hip to relax the quadriceps femoris muscle. The reduction is achieved by slowly extending the knee with gentle medially directed pressure applied to the patella (Fig. 105.10) (68,69). On rare occasions, the patella may become tilted and locked against the lateral femoral epicondyle. In these instances, initial downward pressure on the lateral patella followed by medial translation allows reduction (65,70).

Radiographs should be taken to identify loose bodies within the joint, as these are an indication for arthroscopy (65). Aspiration of the joint may be considered to relieve pain and allow for a more thorough examination (see Chapter 104) (65). If osteochondral injury is not identified, the patient should be placed in an extended knee brace and provided with crutches (65). Orthopaedic follow-up should be scheduled within a week following the injury.

Complications

As described above, many patients who sustain a patellar dislocation will experience recurrence. Other potential complications include injuries to the anterior cruciate ligament, medial cruciate ligament, and meniscus that can occur by a similar deceleration and rotation movement. These should be evaluated with appropriate physical examination such as AP drawer testing or Lachman's test. Injuries to the medial retinaculum and fractures of the lateral femoral condyle and patella can also complicate patellar dislocation. Rarely, the patella will not be reducible because it is rotated, has become entrapped by the femoral condyle, or is locked in the joint space. In such cases, the patient is likely to require operative management, and therefore orthopaedic consultation is indicated.

▶ HIP DISLOCATION

Traumatic dislocation of the hip is an orthopaedic emergency that mandates immediate intervention. Fortunately, children account for less than 10% of all traumatic hip dislocations, so this injury is uncommon in the pediatric population (71–73). Traumatic hip dislocations are classified according to the position of the displaced femoral head in relation to the acetabulum: posterior, anterior, central, and inferior. Traumatic

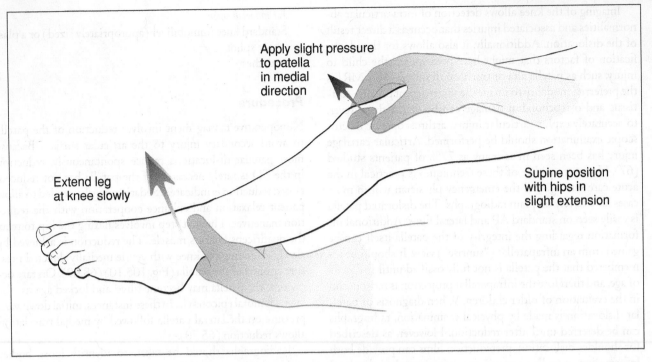

Apply slight pressure
to patella
in medial
direction

Extend leg
at knee slowly

Supine position
with hips in
slight extension

Figure 105.10 Technique for reduction of patellar dislocation.

hip dislocations in children are serious injuries requiring emergency treatment to minimize long-term complications. Early reduction decreases the risk of complications such as coxa magna, osteoarthritis, and avascular necrosis of the femoral head.

Two main mechanisms of injury result in hip dislocations. In the younger child (usually less than 5 years of age), a hip dislocation can result from a trivial fall either while running or from a low height. It is postulated that this occurs because of the generalized laxity of the ligaments surrounding the hip joint and the soft cartilaginous acetabulum. In the older child and adolescent, hip dislocations are often the result of high-energy trauma such as a motor vehicle crash or a sports-related injury (72,74,75).

Posterior hip dislocations are more commonly seen than anterior dislocations (85% to 90% vs. 10% to 15%). Rarely, inferior dislocations (luxatio erecta femoris) (76,77) or central dislocations through the ruptured triradiate cartilage of the acetabulum occur (78,79). In young children, associated acetabular fractures are rare (4% to 18%) compared with their frequency in adults, again partly because of ligamentous laxity and a cartilaginous acetabulum. In the adolescent, acetabular fractures or ipsilateral long bone fractures are more common (75,80–83).

Anatomy and Physiology

The hip joint is a ball and socket joint; the spherical head of the femur articulates with the cuplike acetabulum of the bony pelvis (Fig. 105.11). The strength and stability of this joint is dependent on the depth of the acetabulum and the strength of the surrounding ligaments and muscles. Important ligaments include the iliofemoral ligament, the pubofemoral ligament, the ligament of the head of the femur, and the ischiofemoral ligament. The iliofemoral ligament is a very strong, thick band that covers the anterior aspect of the hip joint and is shaped like an inverted Y. The apex is attached proximally to the anterior inferior iliac spine and the acetabular rim. The base is attached to the intertrochanteric line of the femur. Its main function is to prevent overextension of the hip during standing. Because of its strength, the iliofemoral ligament is rarely torn when the hip is dislocated. The ischiofemoral ligament surrounds the fibrous capsule posteriorly. It originates from the ischial portion of the acetabular rim and turns as it attaches to the superolateral aspect of the neck of the femur. The other ligaments around the hip joint, such as the pubofemoral ligament and the ligament of the head of the femur, are relatively weak and are therefore subject to failure during dislocation (72).

The acetabulum is a cup-shaped cavity that is formed by the ilium, ischium, and pubis. Before the age of 15 to 18 years, the three bones are not fused but are joined by a Y-shaped hyaline cartilage called the "triradiate cartilage." Growth of the acetabulum progresses in a centrifugal direction, and the acetabulum is completely developed by 15 to 18 years of age. Trauma to the triradiate cartilage or the occurrence of a central dislocation during childhood could result in acetabular dysplasia in adulthood (78,79).

Dislocation of the hip joint results from an acute force that thrusts the femoral head into the acetabulum. As previously stated, dislocations are described and classified based on the direction in which the femoral head is dislocated relative to

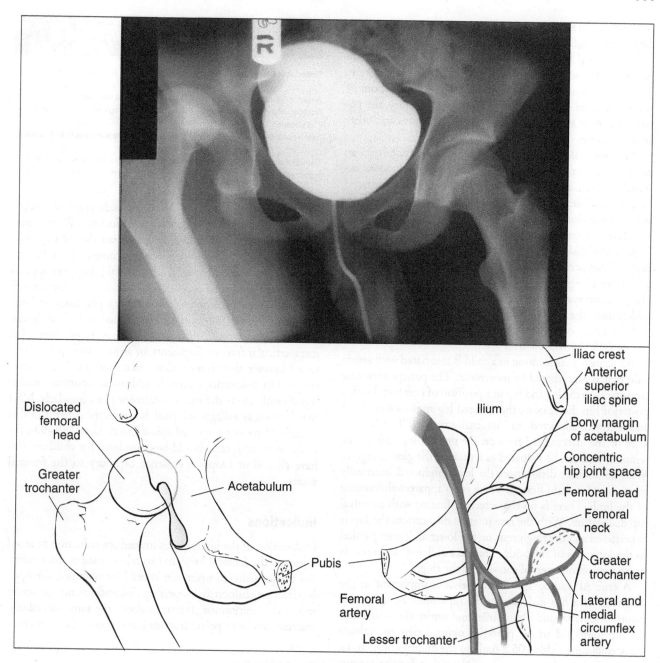

Figure 105.11 Normal (*left*) and dislocated (*right*) hip.

the acetabulum. Seventy-five percent to 90% of hip dislocations are posterior. A posterior hip dislocation can either be
an iliac posterior dislocation (the femoral head is posterior
and superior along the lateral aspect of the ilium) or an ischial posterior dislocation (the femoral head is posterior and
adjacent to the sciatic notch) (75,80,84).

With a posterior hip dislocation, the ligamentum teres is
avulsed, the posterior hip capsule is torn, the posterior acetabular rim is fractured, and the labrum may be avulsed. The
lateral hip rotator muscles (obturator internus, piriformis,
obturator externus, and quadratus muscles) may be partially
or completely torn as well. Because of the close proximity of
the sciatic nerve (L4, L5, S1, S2, and S3) to the hip joint,

it may also be injured (85). Before exiting the pelvis, the sciatic nerve divides into a tibial branch and peroneal branch.
The tibial branch is more commonly affected in traumatic hip
dislocations.

Anterior hip dislocations result in tearing of the ligamentum teres and the anterior joint capsule. The anterior muscles
of the hip joint may be torn or stretched. Because of proximity
of the femoral nerve and artery, injury to these structures may
also occur.

Posterior dislocation of the femoral head results from axial
load applied to the distal femur when the hip is in flexion,
adduction, and internal rotation. As mentioned previously, a
trivial fall onto both knees may cause a hip dislocation in a

young child. In an older child or adolescent, a posterior dislocation is typically the result of a high-energy mechanism. An example would be a child whose knee strikes the dashboard or back of the seat during a front impact motor vehicle crash. The impact would force the femoral head posteriorly, out of the acetabulum. Because this is a high-energy injury, the patient may have associated lower extremity fractures and other serious injuries (86).

Anterior dislocations of the femoral head result from an anteriorly directed force applied to the hip in abduction, external rotation, and extension. The femoral head is displaced forward and usually lies external to the obturator foramen between the ilium and pubis. Compression of the femoral vessels or inguinal structures may occur as a result of this injury. Central dislocations with an acetabular fracture, although unusual, can occur. The most common mechanisms would be a fall from a height or a motor vehicle crash (72,73,76). While classification systems for hip dislocations in children are not widely used, the Stewart-Milford classification of hip fracture dislocations is occasionally utilized in the adolescent patient (Table 105.1) (87).

An acute hip dislocation in a child is associated with severe pain that is exacerbated by movement. The patient therefore tends to keep the leg and hip in a position of comfort. With a posterior hip dislocation, the affected leg appears shortened and is flexed, adducted, and internally rotated. The foot or knee of the affected leg rests on the normal leg. Often, the femoral head can be palpated as a mass in the gluteal region. With an anterior dislocation, the leg is abducted, externally rotated, and in mild flexion. There is no apparent shortening of the limb. There is no characteristic finding with a central hip dislocation. With the rare inferior dislocation, the hip is hyperflexed and the thigh rests on the lower abdomen parallel to the long axis of the body. The knee is flexed, and there is no abduction or external rotation of the thigh.

A true AP radiograph of the pelvis is important in the diagnosis of a hip dislocation; the hips must be in neutral position. One should obtain inlet and outlet views to assess the hip joint and an AP posterior oblique view to evaluate the acetabulum. Table 105.2 outlines the findings likely to be seen on a true AP radiograph of the pelvis for the various types of hip dislocations.

TABLE 105.1	CLASSIFICATION OF TRAUMATIC HIP DISLOCATION
Grade I	A dislocation with or without an insignificant chip fracture from the acetabular rim
Grade II	A dislocation with one or more large fragments from the acetabular rim but with a sufficient socket remaining to ensure stability after reduction
Grade III	A dislocation with a blast fracture and disintegration of the acetabular rim that produces gross instability
Grade IV	A dislocation combined with a fracture of the neck or head of the femur

TABLE 105.2	FINDINGS ON A TRUE AP PELVIS RADIOGRAPH
Posterior dislocation	Femoral head lies superior and lateral to the acetabulum
Anterior dislocation	Femoral head lies medial to the acetabulum
Anterior inferior dislocation	Femoral head rests in the region of the obturator foramen
Inferior dislocation	Femoral head lies below the acetabulum and lateral to the ischial tuberosity
Central dislocation	Femoral head protrudes through the acetabulum

Following reduction, an AP pelvic radiograph should be obtained to document a concentric reduction. When interpreting postreduction films, the physician should pay close attention to the medial joint space and compare it to the normal contralateral joint space. If the medial joint space appears wider than the normal contralateral side, a postreduction CT study should be obtained to assess for trapped tissue or bony fragments within the joint. A postreduction CT study can also be used to assess for a fracture of the acetabulum or knee, intra-articular fracture fragments, or an associated pelvic fracture. However, there is no evidence that routine CT scans after simple hip dislocations provide additional information that significantly alters the initial treatment plan. Similarly, MRI may be used as a diagnostic tool; however, the benefits of this modality have not been well studied in children (88–93). Finally, an arteriogram should be considered for children who have clinical or Doppler evidence of injury to the femoral artery.

Indications

Dislocation of the hip requires immediate reduction to avoid injury to the femoral head and to relieve patient discomfort. An orthopaedic consultation should be obtained for open hip fracture-dislocations, open hip dislocations, neurovascular injury or compromise, fractures about the joint (acetabular fracture, femur or pelvic fracture), and central dislocations.

Equipment

Medications for procedural sedation (consider general anesthesia)
Monitoring equipment
Minimum of two assistants
Leg traction device or materials for spica cast

Procedure

Reduction of a hip dislocation follows initial trauma resuscitation in the patient with multiple injuries. A successful reduction requires adequate analgesia and muscle relaxation. In a hemodynamically unstable trauma patient, administration of sedation may further compromise the patient, and reduction under general anesthesia in the operating suite should

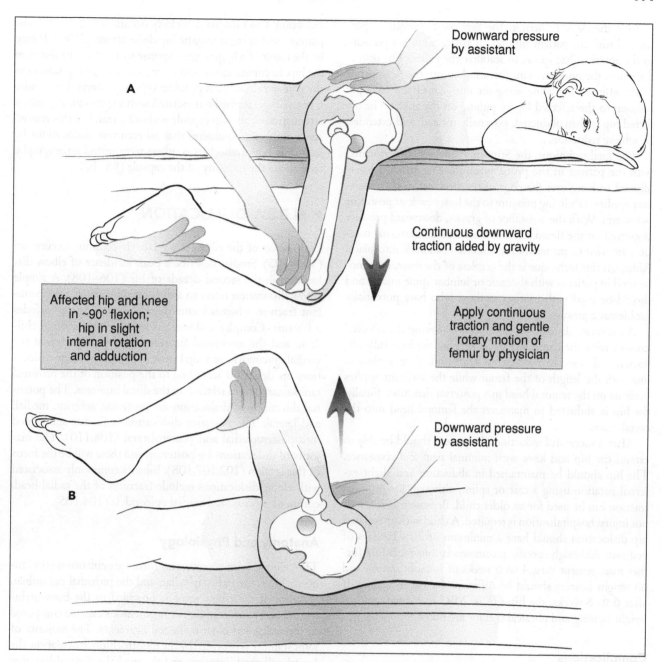

Downward pressure by assistant

A

Affected hip and knee in ~90° flexion; hip in slight internal rotation and adduction

Continuous downward traction aided by gravity

Apply continuous traction and gentle rotary motion of femur by physician

Downward pressure by assistant

B

Figure 105.12 Techniques for reduction of hip joint dislocation.

be considered for these children. Likewise, reduction under general anesthesia should be considered for younger children.

Once the patient is stabilized and is able to tolerate reduction of the hip, the physician must decide on a reduction technique (Fig. 105.12). Closed reduction of a posterior dislocation can be accomplished using the Allis (94), Stimson (95), or Bigelow (96) technique. All of these techniques work by maneuvering the femoral head laterally and then anteriorly back into the acetabulum. Of the three, the Allis maneuver is the most commonly used.

For the Allis maneuver, the patient is placed in the supine position. An assistant stabilizes the pelvis by applying direct pressure over both of the anterior superior iliac crests. The

affected hip and knee are flexed to 90 degrees while the hip is adducted and internally rotated. Next, the operator places a forearm behind the flexed knee and applies continuous traction to the distal femur. Continuous traction fatigues the muscle and overcomes muscle spasm. If continued resistance is met, the femur is gently rotated medially and the hip adducted to relax the hip joint capsule. The assistant can also apply anteriorly directed pressure on the femoral head to aid in the reduction. This rotary motion is used to guide the femoral head over the posterior acetabular rim and into the acetabulum. In some cases, it might be necessary for the physician to mount the stretcher in order to achieve the mechanical advantage necessary to reduce the dislocation.

Like the Allis maneuver, the Bigelow technique is performed with the patient supine. An assistant applies pressure to the anterior iliac spines to stabilize the pelvis. The operator places the nondominant forearm beneath the flexed knee of the affected leg while using the dominant hand to apply traction to the affected leg by pulling on the ankle. The affected hip is then abducted, externally rotated, and extended to achieve reduction.

The final technique, the Stimson maneuver, is performed with the patient in the prone position. The affected leg is allowed to hang over the edge of the stretcher, and an assistant applies stabilizing pressure to the lower back or posterior pelvic rim. With the assistance of gravity, downward pressure is exerted on the flexed knee, and internal and external rotation are used to maneuver the femoral head back into place. Although this technique is the gentlest of the three, it cannot be used in patients with thoracic or lumbar spine injures and should be used with caution in those who have potentially problematic airways.

An anterior dislocation is reduced by flexing the affected knee to relax the hamstring while keeping the hips fully abducted and flexed to 90 degrees. Traction is then applied in line with the length of the femur while the assistant applies pressure on the femoral head in a posterior direction. Finally, the hip is abducted to maneuver the femoral head into the acetabulum.

After a successful reduction, the patient should be able to extend the hip and knee with minimal pain and resistance. The hip should be maintained in abduction and slight external rotation using a cast or splint, although longitudinal traction can be used for an older child. Because this is a serious injury, hospitalization is required. A child with an isolated hip dislocation should have a minimum of 7 to 10 days of bed rest. Although specific recommendations regarding further management vary, 4 to 6 weeks of immobilization and no weight bearing should be sufficient for tissue healing. If after 6 to 8 weeks, the hip CT or MRI is normal, gradual weight bearing and physical therapy are initiated.

Complications

Complications following traumatic dislocation of the hip include avascular necrosis of the femoral head, sciatic nerve palsy, degenerative arthritis, coxa magna deformity, and recurrent posttraumatic dislocation of the hip (94–97). Avascular necrosis of the femoral head is the most common serious complication, with a reported incidence of 5% to 58%. This wide variation in incidence depends on the severity of injury and the timing between injury and successful reduction. A recent study demonstrated that reductions delayed more than 6 hours were associated with a 20 times higher risk of avascular necrosis (101). The incidence of degenerative arthritis in children is unknown, because long-term follow-up studies are lacking. Degenerative changes typically occur 5 to 20 years after the initial injury. Like avascular necrosis, degenerative arthritis appears to be associated with a delay in

reduction. Coxa magna deformity occurs in 13% to 47% of patients sustaining traumatic hip dislocations (71,98). It may be the result of a hyperemic response to a soft-tissue injury in the hip. Recurrent dislocations are a common complication in the younger child. This problem typically affects those under 6 years of age. It may be associated with a tear in the capsule or attenuation of the hip capsule without a tear. For this reason, some authors recommend that all recurrent dislocations be surgically explored, whereas others recommend arthrography to evaluate the integrity of the capsule (98–101).

▶ ELBOW DISLOCATION

Dislocation of the elbow is a relatively common occurrence (102–105). Studies describe a peak incidence of elbow dislocation in the second decade of life (106–108). A simple elbow dislocation refers to a dislocation without a concomitant fracture, whereas a complex elbow dislocation includes a fracture. Complex dislocations are more common in children, and the associated fractures are typically seen at the medial epicondyle or radial neck (103,109). Elbow dislocations are described according to the position of the proximal radioulnar joint in relation to the distal humerus. The potential directions of dislocation are posterior, anterior, medial, and lateral. The posterior dislocation is further subdivided into posteromedial and posterolateral (104,110). The majority of dislocations are posterior, and these will be the focus of this section (102,107,108). Injuries commonly associated with elbow dislocations include fractures of the radial head, coronoid process, and medial epicondyle (104,105).

Anatomy and Physiology

The elbow joint comprises three articulations: the ulnotrochlear, the radiocapitellar, and the proximal radioulnar. Stability of the elbow joint is provided to the bony architecture and reinforced by the ligamentous capsule composed of the radial and ulnar collateral ligaments. The majority of joint stability is provided by the ulnotrochlear articulation, the lateral collateral ligament, and the medial collateral ligament (110). In flexion, posterior dislocation is prevented by the support of the radial head against the capitellum and of the coronoid process against the trochlea. In extension, stability is provided by the interaction of the coronoid process with the trochlea and the locking of the olecranon process into the olecranon fossa.

Dislocation of the elbow can occur after a fall onto an outstretched hand. Typically, the forearm is supinated and extended, with a resulting valgus deformity. Hyperextension occurs, and the force of the fall is transmitted along the forearm to the coronoid process, which is displaced posterolaterally. This mechanism results in a spectrum of ligamentous injuries ranging from disruption of the lateral (or ulnar) collateral ligament with posterolateral subluxation and spontaneous reduction to complete disruption of the lateral and medial (or radial) collateral ligaments and consequent complete posterior dislocation and significant joint instability after reduction (103,110,113,114).

Indications

The history often involves a classic story of falling on an outstretched arm during some physical activity. The elbow typically has considerable swelling, and the affected forearm is held in a semiflexed position, usually supported by the opposite hand. The forearm appears shorter than the unaffected forearm. There is significant deformity of the elbow, with prominence of the ulna both medially and posteriorly (115). AP and lateral radiographs of the injured elbow aid in the diagnosis. Because of their relationship to the elbow, the brachial artery, median nerve, and ulnar nerve are at risk for injury from elbow dislocation.

Equipment

For reduction:
Medications for sedation and analgesia (consider general anesthesia)

For immobilization:
Casting material for a posterior splint
Sling

Procedure

Prompt reduction of a posterior elbow dislocation is paramount when vascular compromise threatens ischemic injury. A careful neurovascular assessment must be completed and documented before and after any reduction maneuvers. Several effective closed reduction techniques have been described, and closed reduction of simple elbow dislocations appears to be just as effective as operative reduction (112,115). However, regardless of the technique chosen, it is important to realize that multiple reduction attempts may result in further injury to the joint, and therefore involvement of an orthopaedist may be required if a reasonable number of initial efforts are unsuccessful. Finally, as with all major joint dislocations, reduction is facilitated by the appropriate use of procedural sedation and analgesia (see Chapter 33).

The initial maneuver involves manipulation of the upper extremity along the axes of the humerus and forearm. With the patient sitting upright, the affected elbow is held in 90 degrees of flexion with hypersupination of the forearm in order to release the radial head. While an assistant applies a posteriorly directed stabilizing force on the patient's affected forearm, the physician first applies traction to the proximal forearm along the long axis of the humerus by placing downward pressure on the volar surface of the proximal forearm. This movement is done to overcome the contraction of the biceps, brachialis, and triceps muscles. This is followed by traction along the axis of the forearm to bring the coronoid process distal to the

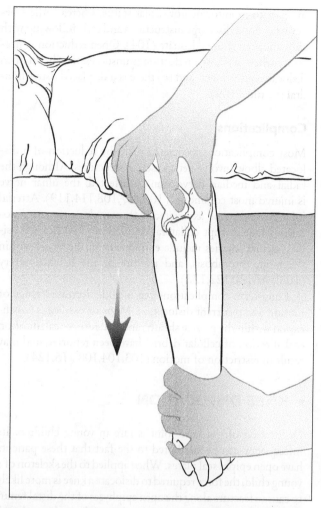

Figure 105.13 Technique for reduction of elbow joint dislocation.

humerus. The reduction is completed with flexion at the elbow while longitudinal traction and pressure on the volar aspect of the forearm are maintained (104,114,116). A variation of the technique places the patient in either the supine or prone position (117).

A second technique involves placing the patient prone, with the affected forearm dangling over the edge of the stretcher or examination table (Fig. 105.13). The wrist is then grasped, and slow traction is applied along the long axis of the forearm. This is done in order to induce muscular relaxation, which usually occurs within 10 minutes. Once the muscles around the elbow are relaxed, the olecranon is then grasped with the thumb and forefinger or pushed by the thumb and guided to a position just distal to the humerus (118).

After successful reduction, it is important to assess the range of motion and stability of the joint and to obtain radiographic images to ensure adequate reduction. Once this is done, the arm is placed in a posterior splint with the elbow flexed to 90 degrees and the forearm in midpronation. The arm should be supported in a sling. Some practitioners prefer to admit all patients who have sustained an elbow dislocation in order to monitor neurovascular status, whereas others believe that good discharge instructions and early follow-up with an orthopaedist are adequate (104). Open reduction is necessary when (a) closed reduction is unsuccessful, (b) an open dislocation is present, and (c) there is a displaced osteochondral fracture (109).

Complications

Most complications associated with the reduction of a dislocated elbow involve neurovascular structures. Although the radial and median nerves can be affected, the ulnar nerve is injured most commonly (102,107,108,114,119). Arterial injuries tend to be associated with complex or open dislocations that disrupt collateral circulation (120,121). Possible vascular injuries include entrapment of the vessel within the joint, thrombosis, and rupture of the brachial artery (103,107,120,122,123).

Long-term complications can include decreased range of motion and recurrent dislocation. Myositis ossificans (ossification within the muscle sheath) and heterotopic calcification (calcification of cellular debris) have been reported and may result in restriction of motion (103,104,108,115,124).

▶ KNEE DISLOCATION

Dislocation of the knee joint is rare in young children. Its infrequency can be attributed to the fact that these patients have open epiphyseal plates. When applied to the skeleton of a young child, the force required to dislocate a knee is more likely to cause a fracture along the open epiphyses of the distal femur or proximal tibia. However, once the epiphyses have closed, these same forces are more likely to cause a dislocation. In practical terms, this means that most pediatric patients who sustain knee dislocations will be adolescents (125–127). Knee dislocations are generally associated with high-energy trauma, such as motor vehicle crashes, and these patients often have injuries involving multiple organ systems (128).

Anatomy and Physiology

The knee joint is a simple hinge joint composed primarily of the articulation between the tibia and the femur. The joint is stabilized by the cruciate and collateral ligaments (129). Dislocation of the knee traditionally has been defined as a disruption of the tibiofemoral articulation (126,130). More recent studies have expanded this definition to include any knee subjected to a significant force that results in anterior and posterior cruciate ligament injury (128,129,131).

The clinical deformity associated with an unreduced dislocated knee makes diagnosis simple; however, when a dislocated knee is reduced in the prehospital setting (as many dislocated knees are), the diagnosis is much more challenging. Patients in this latter group typically present with a painful and swollen knee and have significant joint instability. The typical injury pattern includes damage to the anterior and posterior cruciate ligaments as well as the medial collateral ligament. Whenever a patient presents with findings suggestive of a serious knee injury, these ligaments must be assessed for damage (128,129,132,133). Should injuries to these structures be identified in the absence of a knee dislocation, the clinician must consider the possibility that the knee might have been dislocated and then relocated. If the possibility that the knee might have been dislocated is not considered, associated injuries, with potentially serious consequences, may not be discovered.

Most of the concern regarding knee dislocations centers upon injury to the neurovascular bundle (comprising the popliteal artery and vein and the peroneal nerve) that runs behind the knee. These structures lie in a relatively fixed position within the popliteal fossa and are therefore easily injured when the knee is dislocated. Perhaps the most devastating injury associated with dislocation of the knee is damage to the popliteal artery (128,129). This injury complicates 20% to 40% of knee dislocations (130,134). If the popliteal artery is damaged, there is not sufficient collateral blood flow to compensate, and lower extremity circulation is profoundly compromised. If repair is delayed for more than 6 hours, there is an increased risk of compartment syndrome and amputation (130,135,136). Given the high incidence of neurovascular injury, emergent orthopaedic consultation should be obtained when the results of examination suggest the possibility of knee dislocation. After reduction, management may include observation, angiography, and/or surgical exploration (128,130,131,136).

Like the artery, the vein and the nerve can be seriously injured when the knee is dislocated. In fact, the peroneal nerve is injured in approximately 50% of knee dislocations (126,136,137). Rapid assessment of the peroneal nerve includes evaluating dorsiflexion of the ankle and sensation along the dorsum of the foot.

Indications

Reduction of a dislocated knee should occur when physical findings are consistent with the diagnosis. Typically, the patient will present with a grossly deformed knee, most commonly with the tibia in an anterior position relative to the femur. Radiographs should be obtained and a careful neurovascular examination performed before and after the reduction. All patients with knee dislocation and vascular compromise require immediate reduction to improve circulation to the leg (136,137). When a patient presents with a history of significant trauma along with knee swelling and significant joint laxity, a reduced dislocation should be suspected, and a careful neurovascular examination should be performed.

Equipment

Medications for sedation and analgesia
Long leg immobilizer

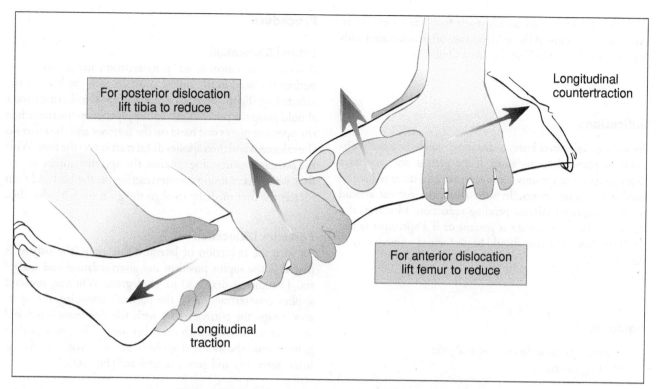

For posterior dislocation lift tibia to reduce

Longitudinal countertraction

For anterior dislocation lift femur to reduce

Longitudinal traction

Figure 105.14 Technique for reduction of knee joint dislocation.

Procedure

Adequate analgesia and sedation should be provided for the patient. The reduction technique is based on traction-countertraction. The patient is placed in the supine position. An assistant provides axial traction along the patient's thigh while the primary operator pulls along the tibiofemoral axis (Fig. 105.14). This maneuver is typically all that is required; however, if necessary, the tibia can be manipulated into its anatomic position to complete the reduction. After the reduction, radiographs should be obtained, and the neurovascular examination should be repeated. The knee should be immobilized with a posterior splint in 15 degrees of flexion to avoid tension on the popliteal artery (132,136,138).

Complications

Indications for reduction in the operating room include inability to reduce the knee, open dislocation, and continued signs of ischemia (127,136,137). Complications found with reduction include development of deep venous and arterial thromboses, compartment syndrome, and pseudoaneurysms (136). Additionally, care must be taken to avoid further hyperextension or pressure on the popliteal space, as this could exacerbate popliteal artery and peroneal nerve injury.

▶ ANKLE DISLOCATION

Ankle injuries, particularly sprains, are common. Like most other traumatic injuries, they are more common among active young males. However, dislocations of the ankle are unusual and are most often the result of a high-force injury. Like all high-force injuries, ankle dislocations are often associated with fractures and injuries to other areas of the body. Once diagnosed, they can be reduced in the ED by the emergency physician or an orthopaedic surgeon.

Anatomy and Physiology

Although it has a fairly extensive range of motion, the ankle is an inherently stable joint. The major articulations of the ankle occur between the talus, tibia, and fibula. The bones are held in position by a series of ligaments. Laterally, these include the anterior and posterior tibiofibular ligaments and the calcaneofibular ligament. The medial ligaments are the anterior and posterior tibiotalar ligaments, the tibiocalcaneal ligament, and the tibionavicular ligament. Ankle dislocations are generally the result of complete disruption of all or most of these ligaments, which allows the tibia and fibula to move from their normal relationship with the talus. Because several boney projections are in close association with these ligaments, it is not unusual for ankle dislocations to be complicated by factures, primarily factures of the malleoli and/or of the margins of the bones.

Several types of ankle dislocation can occur. Posterior dislocation is common and is the result of forced plantar flexion. Forced dorsiflexion often causes an anterior dislocation, but this injury can also be caused by a direct, forceful blow to the heel when the foot is in dorsiflexion. Although medial and lateral dislocations can also occur, medial dislocations are more common. These injuries usually result from forced inversion, eversion, or rotation of the ankle and are often associated with fractures of the malleoli or the distal fibula.

Indications

As with a dislocated knee, a dislocated ankle is usually obvious on physical examination. If the patient does not have neurovascular compromise, it is acceptable to defer reduction until a specialist arrives. In such cases, the patient should receive adequate analgesia pending reduction. However, if a neurovascular compromise is present or if a specialist is not available, then reduction should be performed immediately in the ED.

Equipment

Medications for sedation and analgesia
Splinting materials

Procedure

Lateral Dislocation

After administration of adequate sedation and analgesia, the patient is placed in the supine position with the knee of the affected leg slightly flexed by a pillow or towel roll. An assistant should grasp the patient's calf and apply countertraction while the operator places one hand on the forefoot and the other on the calcaneus and then applies distal traction on the foot. With the assistant maintaining traction, the operator dorsiflexes the foot while maintaining countertraction on the heel and then rotates the foot medially to align the great toe with the tibia.

Posterior Dislocation

As with the reduction of lateral dislocations, the patient is placed in the supine position and given sedation and analgesia. The knee is flexed 30 to 45 degrees. While an assistant applies countertraction to the patient's lower leg, the operator grasps the patient's heel with the dominant hand and the patient's forefoot with the other hand. The operator then plantar flexes the foot and applies traction. Finally, the foot is lifted anteriorly and gently dorsiflexed (Fig. 105.15).

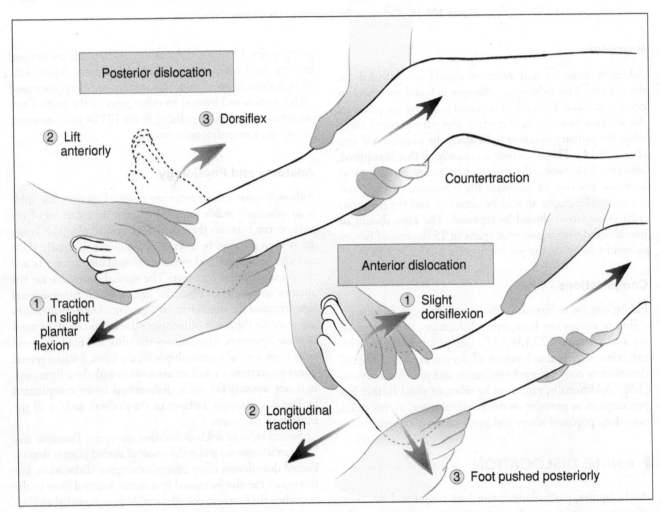

Figure 105.15 Technique for reduction of ankle joint dislocation.

SUMMARY

Radial Head Subluxation

1 Have the child sit comfortably in the caretaker's lap.

2 Support the child's arm in the nondominant hand, applying moderate pressure on the radial head with the thumb or fingers.

3 Hold the child's wrist in the dominant hand, placing the fingers on the volar aspect of the wrist and thumb on the dorsal aspect.

4 Apply gentle longitudinal traction to the arm.

5A (*Traditional*) *supination and flexion technique:* While maintaining traction, in one motion supinate the arm, then fully flex it.

5B *Pronation technique:* While maintaining traction, gently hyperpronate the arm. In many cases, reduction occurs with pronation alone, but some authorities recommend that the arm be maintained in pronation and flexed to complete the procedure.

6 A reduction click may be heard or felt.

7 If the procedure is successful, the child should be using the arm within 20 to 30 minutes.

8 If several appropriate attempts fail, radiographs should be obtained.

9 If the radiographs are normal, the arm should be placed in a sling, and the child referred to an orthopaedist. Spontaneous reduction may occur in a day or two.

Digit Dislocation

1 Remove all rings from the affected finger, and achieve anesthesia with a digital block.

2 Securely brace the affected hand or foot.

3 Apply gentle traction to the affected digit.

4 For dorsal dislocation, the joint is gently hyper-extended; for volar dislocation, it is hyperflexed.

5 Push the dislocated phalanx into its proper position.

6 Obtain radiographs after the reduction and splint the digit.

Shoulder Dislocation

A Reduction by Gravity

1 Use appropriate analgesia and sedation and monitor the patient.

2 Have the patient lie on a stretcher in the prone position with the affected arm dangling over the side.

3 Attach 2 to 5 kg of weight to the arm.

4 Allow the arm to hang for 20 to 40 minutes.

5 After the reduction, the arm will swing freely and painlessly in the forward position.

B1 Reduction by Scapular Manipulation—Prone Position

1 Use appropriate analgesia and sedation and monitor the patient.

2 Have the patient lie on a stretcher in the prone position with the affected arm hanging over the side.

3 Attach 2 to 5 kg of weight to the arm or have an assistant apply downward traction to the arm.

4 Gently rotate the scapula by simultaneously pushing its tip medially and its superior aspect laterally.

5 An audible or palpable "clunk" may occur with successful reduction.

B2 Reduction by Scapular Manipulation—Seated Position

1 Use appropriate analgesia and sedation, if needed.

2 Have the patient sit in a chair facing the back of the chair.

3 While an assistant applies forward traction to the affected arm, the scapula is rotated as described in B1.

C Reduction by Traction-Countertraction

1 Use appropriate analgesia and sedation and monitor the patient.

2 The patient is placed in the supine position with the elbow of the affected side in slight abduction and 90 degrees of flexion.

3 A sheet is looped around the flexed forearm distal to the elbow, then around the clinician (the clinician should be standing next to the hip on the affected side).

4 Have an assistant loop a second sheet about him- or herself and then around the patient's chest under the axilla on the affected side.

5 Exert continuous longitudinal traction on the affected arm, gradually increasing the force until reduction is achieved. It may be necessary to lean back against the sheets to gain mechanical advantage.

SUMMARY (*Continued*)

Patella Dislocation

1 Use appropriate analgesia and sedation and monitor the patient.

2 Place the patient in the supine position with the hips in flexion.

3 Bring the knee joint to full extension while gradually applying medial pressure on the patella to achieve reduction.

4 Appropriately immobilize the knee after an examination.

Hip Dislocation

A Supine Position (Allis)

1 Use appropriate analgesia and sedation and monitor the patient.

2 Place the patient in the supine position with both the hip and the knee in 90 degrees flexion and the hip in slightly internal rotation and adduction.

3 Have an assistant stabilize the pelvis with downward pressure applied to both iliac crests.

4 Apply continuous traction to the distal femur in line with the deformity.

5 Use a gentle rotary motion of the femur to gradually bring the femoral head over the posterior acetabular rim and into the acetabulum.

6 Postreduction radiographs should be obtained. Casting may be needed for appropriate immobilization.

B Prone Position (Stimson)

1 Use appropriate analgesia and sedation and monitor the patient.

2 Place the patient in the prone position with the thigh hanging vertically from the stretcher.

3 Apply downward vertical traction on the distal femur until reduction is achieved.

4 Postreduction radiographs should be obtained. Casting may be needed for appropriate immobilization.

Posterior Elbow Dislocation

1 Use appropriate analgesia and sedation and monitor the patient.

2 Apply traction to the proximal forearm with the elbow slightly flexed.

3 Apply forward and downward pressure to the olecranon while flexing the elbow.

4 Apply appropriate immobilization.

Knee Dislocation

1 Use appropriate analgesia and sedation as needed and monitor the patient.

2 Place the patient in the prone position.

3A *Anterior dislocation:* Lift the femur anteriorly or push the proximal tibia posteriorly.

3B *Posterior dislocation:* Apply longitudinal traction, then extend the knee while lifting the proximal tibia into reduced position.

4 Perform angiography after reduction.

5 If no vascular injury is present, immobilize appropriately.

Ankle Dislocation

1 Use appropriate analgesia and sedation as needed and monitor the patient.

2 Place the patient in the supine position.

3 Apply traction to the foot while an assistant applies countertraction to the lower leg; the dominant hand should hold the heel, and the nondominant hand should hold the forefoot.

4A *Lateral dislocation:*

    i Apply traction with the foot in dorsiflexion.

    ii Rotate the foot medially to align the great toe with the tibia.

4B *Posterior dislocation:*

    i Apply traction with the foot in a slight plantar flexion.

    ii Lift the foot anteriorly while gently dorsiflexing it.

4C *Anterior dislocation:*

    i Apply traction with the foot in slight dorsiflexion.

    ii Further dorsiflex foot and then push it posteriorly while plantar flexing it gently.

5 Immobilize the ankle appropriately.

CLINICAL TIPS

▶ Procedural sedation and analgesia should be used when appropriate.

▶ Restraint may sometimes be required.

▶ Patients should be appropriately monitored.

▶ The possibility of neurovascular compromise should always be investigated for elbow, knee, and ankle dislocations.

▶ Orthopaedic consultation should be obtained for dislocations with significant potential morbidity. However, if a consultant cannot provide assistance in a timely fashion, reduction should be attempted by the available personnel.

▶ After a successful reduction, the joint should be appropriately immobilized.

Anterior Dislocation

The patient is medicated and positioned as described above for posterior dislocation. With an assistant providing counter-traction, the operator grasps the patient's heel with the dominant hand and the patient's forefoot with the nondominant hand. The patient's foot is dorsiflexed as traction is applied. The ankle is then pushed back into its correct position and the foot is gently plantar flexed (Fig. 105.15).

Successful reduction should be confirmed by radiographs, and the ankle should be immobilized with a splint. The patient should be referred to an orthopaedic surgeon for follow-up evaluation and management.

Complications

Injuries to the anterior and posterior tibial vessels are common complications of ankle dislocation. Many victims have subsequent avascular necrosis of the talus. Likewise, many develop posttraumatic arthritis, recurrent subluxation of the peroneal tendons, or instability of the ankle (139–142).

▶ ACKNOWLEDGMENT

The authors would like to acknowledge the valuable contributions of Grace M. Young to the version of this chapter that appeared in the previous edition.

▶ REFERENCES

1. Schutzman SA, Teach S. Upper-extremity impairment in young children. *Ann Emerg Med.* 1995;26:474–479.
2. Newman J. "Nursemaid's elbow" in infants 6 months and under. *J Emerg Med.* 1985;2:403–404.
3. Macias CG, Bothner J, Wiebe R. A comparison of supination/flexion to hyperpronation in the reduction of radial head subluxation. *Pediatrics.* 1998;102:e10–14.
4. Quan L, Marcuse EK. The epidemiology and treatment of radial head subluxation. *Am J Dis Child.* 1985;139:1194–1197.
5. Teach SJ, Schutzman SA. Prospective study of recurrent radial head subluxation. *Arch Pediatr Adolesc Med.* 1996;150:164–166.
6. The upper limb. In: Moore KL, ed. *Clinically Oriented Anatomy.* 3rd ed. Baltimore: Williams & Wilkins; 1992:501–635.
7. Macias CG, Wiebe R, Bothner J. History and radiographic findings associated with clinically suspected radial head subluxations. *Pediatr Emerg Care.* 2000;16:22–25.
8. Jones J, Cote B. Irreducible nursemaid's elbow. *Am J Emerg Med.* 1995;13:491.
9. McDonald J, Whitelaw C, Goldsmith LJ. Radial head subluxation: comparing two methods of reduction. *Acad Emerg Med.* 1999;6:715–718.
10. Schunk JE. Radial head subluxation: epidemiology and treatment of 87 episodes. *Ann Emerg Med.* 1990;19:1019–1023.
11. Fick DS, Lyons TA. Interpreting elbow radiographs in children. *Am Fam Phys.* 1997;55:1278–1282.
12. Ufberg J, McNamara R. Management of common dislocations. In: Roberts JR, Hedges JR, eds. *Clinical Procedures in Emergency Medicine.* 4th ed. Philadelphia: Elsevier; 2004:946–988.
13. Lee SJ, Montgomery K. Athletic hand injuries. *Orthop Clin North Am.* 2002;33:547–554.
14. Young CC, Raasch WG. Dislocations: diagnosis and treatment. *Clin Fam Pract.* 2000;2:613–635.
15. Antosia RE, Lyn E. Hand. In: Marx JA, ed. *Rosen's Emergency Medicine: Concepts and Clinical Practice,* 5th ed. St. Louis: Mosby; 2002:493–534.
16. Palmer RE. Joint injuries of the hand in athletes. *Clin Sports Med.* 1998;17:513–531.
17. Jobe MT. Fracture and dislocations of the hand. In: Gustilo RB, Kyle RF, Templeman DC, eds. *Fractures and Dislocations.* St. Louis: Mosby; 1993:611–644.
18. Rowe CR. Prognosis in dislocation of the shoulder. *J Bone Joint Surg Am.* 1956;38:957–977.
19. Rowe CR. Anterior dislocations of the shoulder: prognosis and treatment. *Surg Clin North Am.* 1963;43:1609–1614.
20. Asher MA. Dislocations of the upper extremities in children. *Orthop Clin North Am.* 1976;7:583–591.
21. Heck CC. Anterior dislocation of the glenohumeral joint in a child. *J Trauma.* 1981;21:174–175.
22. Yu J. Anterior shoulder dislocations. *J Fam Pract.* 1992;35:567–571, 575–576.
23. Samilson RL, Miller E. Posterior dislocations of the shoulder. *Clin Orthop.* 1964;32:69–86.
24. Boyd HB, Sisk TD. Recurrent posterior dislocation of the shoulder. *J Bone Joint Surg Am.* 1972;54:779–786.
25. Davids JR, Talbott RD. Luxatio erecta humeri: a case report. *Clin Orthop.* 1990;252:144–149.
26. Davison BL, Orwin JF. Open inferior glenohumeral dislocation. *J Orthop Trauma.* 1996;10:504–506.
27. Freundlich BD. Luxatio erecta. *J Trauma.* 1983;23:434–436.
28. Mallon WJ, Bassett FH III, Goldner RD. Luxatio erecta: the inferior glenohumeral dislocation. *J Orthop Trauma.* 1990;4:19–24.
29. Hussein MK. Kocher's method is 3000 years old. *J Bone Joint Surg Br.* 1968;50:669–671.
30. Nash J. The status of Kocher's method of reducing recent anterior dislocation of the shoulder. *J Bone Joint Surg.* 1934;16:535–544.
31. Milch H. Treatment of dislocation of the shoulder. *Surgery.* 1938;3:732–740.
32. Milch H. The treatment of recent dislocations and fracture dislocations of the shoulder. *J Bone Joint Surg Am.* 1949:31:173–180.

33. Janecki CJ, Shahcheragh GH. The forward elevation maneuver for reduction of anterior dislocations of the shoulder. *Clin Orthop.* 1982;164:177–180.

34. Beattie TF, Steedman DJ, McGowan A, et al. A comparison of the Milch and Kocher techniques for acute anterior dislocation of the shoulder. *Injury.* 1986;17:349–352.

35. Eachempati KK, Dua A, Malhotra R, et al. The external rotation method for reduction of acute anterior dislocations and fracture dislocations of the shoulder. *J Bone Joint Surg Am.* 2004;86:2431–2434.

36. Plummer D, Clinton J. The external rotation method for reduction of acute anterior shoulder dislocation *Emerg Med Clin.* 1989;7165–175.

37. Poulson SR. Reduction of acute shoulder dislocation using the Eskimo technique: a study of 23 consecutive cases. *J Trauma.* 1988;28:1382–1383.

38. Riebel GD, McCabe JB. Anterior shoulder dislocation: a review of reduction techniques. *Am J Emerg Med.* 1991;9:180–188.

39. Stimson LA. *A Practical Treatise on Fractures and Dislocations.* Malvern, PA: Lea & Febiger; 1912.

40. Stimson LA. An easy method of reducing dislocations of the shoulder and hip. *Med Rec.* 1900;57:356–357.

41. Kothari RU, Dronen SC. Prospective evaluation of the scapular manipulation technique in reducing anterior shoulder dislocations. *Ann Emerg Med.* 1992;21:1349–1352.

42. Anderson D, Zvirbulis R, Cicollo J. Scapular manipulation for reduction of anterior shoulder dislocations. *Clin Orthop.* 1982;164:181–183.

43. McNamara RM. Reduction of anterior shoulder dislocation by scapular manipulation. *Ann Emerg Med.* 1993;22:1140–1144.

44. Tachdjian MO. Glenohumeral dislocations. In: *Pediatric Orthopaedics.* 3rd ed. Vol. 3. Philadelphia: WB Saunders; 2002:2128–2132.

45. Bankart ASB. Recurrent or habitual dislocation of the shoulder joint. *BMJ.* 1923;2:1132–1133.

46. Bankart ASB. The pathology and treatment of recurrent dislocation of the shoulder joint. *Br J Surg.* 1938;26:23–29.

47. Hill HA, Sachs MD. The grooved defect of the humeral head: a frequently unrecognized complication of dislocations of the shoulder. *Radiology.* 1940;35:690–700.

48. Travlos J, Goldberg I, Boome RS. Brachial plexus lesions associated with dislocated shoulders. *J Bone Joint Surg Br.* 1990;72:68–71.

49. Harvey RA, Trabulsy ME, Roe L. Are post reduction anteroposterior and scapular Y views useful in anterior shoulder dislocations? *Am J Emerg Med.* 1992;10:149–151.

50. Kornquth PJ, Salazar AM. The apical oblique view of the shoulder: its usefulness in acute trauma. *AJR Am J Roentgenol.* 1987;149:113–116.

51. Silfverskiold JP, Staehley DJ, Jones WW. Roentgenographic evaluation of suspected shoulder dislocation: a prospective study comparing the axillary view and the scapular Y view. *Orthopaedics.* 1990;13:63–69.

52. Garth WP, Slappey CE, Ochs CW. Roentgenographic demonstration of instability of the shoulder: the apical oblique projection: a technical note. *J Bone Joint Surg Am.* 1984;66:1450–1453.

53. Ceroni D, Sadri H, Leuenberger A. Radiographic evaluation of anterior dislocation of the shoulder. *Acta Radiol.* 2000;41:658–661.

54. Hoelen MA, Burgers AMJ, Rozing PM. Prognosis of primary anterior shoulder dislocation in young adults. *Arch Orthop Trauma Surg.* 1990;110:51–54.

55. Marans HJ, Angel KR, Schemitsch EH, et al. The fate of traumatic anterior dislocation of the shoulder in children. *J Bone Joint Surg Am.* 1992;74:1242–124.

56. Lawton RL, Choudhury S, Mansat P, et al. Pediatric shoulder instability: presentation, findings, treatment, and outcomes. *J Pediatr Orthop.* 2002;22:52–61.

57. Deitch J, Mehlman CT, Foad SL, et al. Traumatic anterior shoulder dislocation in adolescents. *Am J Sports Med.* 2003;31:758–763.

58. Davy AR, Drew SJ. Management shoulder dislocation: are we doing enough to reduce the risk of recurrence? *Injury.* 2002;33:775–779.

59. Walton JW, Paxinos A, Tzannes A, et al. The unstable shoulder in the adolescent athlete. *Am J Sports Med.* 2002;30:758–767.

60. Rowe CR. Complicated dislocations of the shoulder: guidelines in treatment. *Am J Surg.* 1969;117:549–553.

61. Winmoon C, Sathira-Angura V, Kunakornsawat S, et al. Fracture-dislocation of the glenohumeral joint in a 2 year old child: case report. *J Trauma.* 2003;54:372–375.

62. Fithian DC, Paxton EW, Stone ML, et al. Epidemiology and natural history of acute patellar dislocation. *Am J Sports Med.* 2004;32:1114–1121.

63. Nietosvaara Y, Aalto K, Kallio PE. Acute patellar dislocation in children: incidence and associated osteochondral fractures. *J Pediatr Orthop.* 1994;14:513–515.

64. Atkin DM, Fithian DC, Marangi KS, et al. Characteristics of patients with primary acute lateral patellar dislocation and their recovery within the first 6 months of injury. *Am J Sports Med.* 2000;28:472–479.

65. Beasley LS, Vidal AF. Traumatic patellar dislocation in children and adolescents: treatment update and literature review. *Curr Opin Pediatr.* 2004;16:29–36.

66. Hinton RY, Sharma KM. Acute and recurrent patellar instability in the young athlete. *Orthop Clin North Am.* 2003;34:385–396.

67. Nomura E, Inoue M, Kurimura M. Chondral and osteochondral injuries associated with acute patellar dislocation. *Arthroscopy.* 2003;19:717–721.

68. Zionts LE. Fractures and dislocations about the knee. In: Green NE, Swiontkowski MF, eds. *Skeletal Trauma in Children,* 3rd ed. Philadelphia: Elsevier; 2003:439–471.

69. Ufberg J, McNamara R. Management of common dislocations. In: Roberts JR, Hedges JR, eds. *Clinical Procedures in Emergency Medicine.* 4th ed. Philadelphia: Elsevier; 2004:946–986.

70. Beynnon BD, Johnson RJ, Coughlin KM. Knee. In: DeLee JC, Drez D, eds. *DeLee and Drez's Orthopaedic Sports Medicine: Principles and Practice.* 2nd ed. Philadelphia: Elsevier; 2003:1577–2154.

71. Hougaard K, Thomsen PB. Traumatic hip dislocation in children: follow-up of 13 cases. *Orthopedics.* 1989;12:375–378.

72. Tachdjian MO. Hip dislocations. In: *Pediatric Orthopaedics.* 3rd ed. Vol. 3. Philadelphia: WB Saunders; 2002:2273–2283.

73. Barquet A. Traumatic hip dislocation in childhood. *Acta Orthop Scand.* 1979;50:549–553.

74. Vialle R, Odent T, Pannier S, et al. Traumatic hip dislocation in childhood. *J Pediatr Orthop.* 2005;25:138–144.

75. Thompson VP, Epstein HC. Traumatic dislocation of the hip: a survey of two hundred and four cases covering twenty-one years. *J Bone Joint Surg Am.* 1951;33:746–778.

76. Beauchesne R, Kruse R, Stanton RP. Inferior dislocation (luxatio erecta) of the hip. *Orthopedics.* 1994;17:72–75.

77. Brogdon BG, Woolridge DA. Luxatio erecta of the hip: a critical retrospective. *Skeletal Radiol.* 1997;26:548–552.

78. Brooks E, Rosman M. Central fracture-dislocation of the hip in a child. *J Trauma.* 1988;28:1590–1592.

79. Bucholz RW, Ezaki M, Ogden JA. Injury to the acetabular triradiate physeal cartilage. *J Bone Joint Surg Am.* 1982;64:600–609.

80. Hughes MJ, D'Agostino J. Posterior hip dislocation in a five-year old boy: a case report, review of the literature, and current recommendations. *J Emerg Med.* 1996;14:585–590.

81. Craig CL. Hip injuries in children and adolescents. *Orthop Clin North Am.* 1980;11:743–754.

82. Rieger H, Penning D, Kein W, et al. Traumatic dislocation of the hip in young children. *Arch Orthop Trauma Surg.* 1991;110:114–117.

83. Pearson DE, Mann RJ. Traumatic hip dislocation in children. *Clin Orthop Relat Res.* 1973;92:189–194.

84. Kutty S, Thornes B, Curtin WA, et al. Traumatic posterior dislocation of hip in children. *Pediatr Emerg Care.* 2001;17:32–35.

85. Cornwall R, Radomisli TE. Nerve injury in traumatic dislocation of the hip. *Clin Orthop.* 2000;377:84–91.

86. Offierski CM. Traumatic dislocation of the hip in children. *J Bone Joint Surg Br.* 1981;63:194–197.

87. Stewart MJ, Milford LW. Fracture dislocation of the hip: an end result study. *J Bone Joint Surg Am.* 1954;36:342.

88. Frick SL, Sims SH. Is computed tomography useful after simple posterior hip dislocation? *J Orthop Trauma.* 1995;9:388–391.

89. Godley DR, Williamams RA. Traumatic dislocation of the hip in a child: usefulness of MRI. *Orthopedics.* 1993;16:1145–1147.

90. Hougaard K, Lindequist S, Nielsen LB. Computerised tomography after posterior dislocation of the hip. *J Bone Joint Surg Br.* 1987;69:556–557.

91. Rubel IF, Kloen P, Potter HG, et al. MRI assessment of the posterior acetabular wall fracture in traumatic dislocation of the hip in children. *Pediatr Radiol.* 2002;32:435–439.

92. Elder G, Harvey EJ. Imaging in musculoskeletal trauma: the value of magnetic resonance imaging for traumatic pediatric hip dislocations. *J Can Chir.* 2004;47:290–291.

93. Vialle R, Pannier S, Odent T, et al. Imaging of traumatic dislocation of the hip in childhood. *Pediatr Radiol.* 2004;34:970–979.

94. Allis O. An inquiry into the difficulties encountered in the reduction of dislocation of the hip. Philadelphia; 1896.

95. Stimson L. *Treatise on Dislocation.* Philadelphia: Lea Brothers & Co.; 1888.

96. Bigelow H. *The Mechanics of Dislocation and Fracture of the Hip with the Reduction of the Dislocations by the Flexion Method.* Philadelphia: Henry C. Lea & Co.; 1869.

97. Mehlman CT, Hubbard GW, Crawford AH, et al. Traumatic hip dislocation in children: long-term follow-up of 42 patients. *Clin Orthop.* 2000;376:68–79.

98. Salisbury RD, Eastwood DM. Traumatic dislocation of the hip in children. *Clin Orthop.* 2000;377:106–111.

99. Pennsylvania Orthopaedic Society, Scientific Research Committee. Traumatic dislocation of the hip joint in children. *J Bone Joint Surg Am.* 1968;50:79–88.

100. Funk FJ. Traumatic dislocation of the hip in children: factors influencing prognosis and treatment. *J Bone Joint Surg Am.* 1962;44:1135–1145.

101. Barquet A. Natural history of avascular necrosis following traumatic hip dislocation in childhood. *Acta Orthop Scand.* 1982;53:815–820.

102. Royle SG. Posterior dislocation of the elbow. *Clin Orthop.* 1991;269:201–204.

103. Ogden JA. Elbow. In: Ogden JA, ed. *Skeletal Injury in the Child.* 3rd ed. New York: Springer; 2000:542–566.

104. Thompson GH. Dislocations of the elbow. In: Beaty JH, Kasser JR, eds. *Rockwood and Wilkens' Fractures in Children.* 5th ed. Philadelphia: Lippincott Williams & Wilkins; 2001:705–739.

105. Rettig AC. Traumatic elbow injuries in the athlete. *Orthop Clin North Am.* 2002;33:509–522.

106. Josefsson PO, Nilsson BE. Incidence of elbow dislocation. *Acta Orthop Scand.* 1986;57:537–538.

107. Carlioz H, Abols Y. Posterior dislocation of the elbow in children. *J Pediatr Orthop.* 1984;4:8–12.

108. Neviaser JS, Wickstrom JK. Dislocation of the elbow: a retrospective study of 115 patients. *South Med J.* 1977;70:172–173.

109. Canale ST. Fractures and dislocations in children. In: Canale ST, ed. *Campbell's Operative Orthopaedics.* 10th ed. St. Louis: Mosby; 2003:1391–1565.

110. O'Driscoll SW, Jupiter JB, King GJ, et al. The unstable elbow. *J Bone Joint Surg Am.* 2000;82:724–738.

111. Linscheild RL, Wheeler DK. Elbow dislocations. *JAMA.* 1965;194:113–118.

112. Josefsson PO, Gentz CF, Johnell O, et al. Surgical versus non-surgical treatment of ligamentous injuries following dislocation of the elbow joint. *J Bone Joint Surg Am.* 1987;69:605–608.

113. O'Driscoll SW, Morrey BF, Korinek S, et al. Elbow subluxation and dislocation: a spectrum of instability. *Clin Orthop.* 1992;280:186–197.

114. Gomez JE. Upper extremity injuries in youth sports. *Pediatr Clin North Am.* 2002;49:593–626.

115. Josefsson PO, Johnell O, Gentz CF. Long-term sequelae of simple dislocation of the elbow. *J Bone Joint Surg Am.* 1984;66:927–930.

116. Osborne G, Cotterill P. Recurrent dislocation of the elbow. *J Bone Joint Surg Br.* 1966;48:340–346.

117. Parvin RW. Closed reduction of common shoulder and elbow dislocations without anesthesia. *Arch Surg.* 1957;75:972–975.

118. Meyn MA, Quigley TB. Reduction of posterior dislocation of the elbow by traction on the dangling arm. *Clin Orthop.* 1974;103:106–108.

119. Galbraith KA, McCullough CJ. Acute nerve injury as a complication of closed fractures or dislocations of the elbow. *Injury.* 1979;11:159–164.

120. Louis DS, Ricciardi JE, Sprengler DM. Arterial injury: a complication of posterior elbow dislocation: a clinical and anatomical study. *J Bone Joint Surg Am.* 1974;56:1631–1636.

121. Rubens MK, Auliciano PL. Open elbow dislocation with brachial artery disruption: case report and review of the literature. *Orthopaedics.* 1986;9:539–542.

122. Wilmshurst AD, Millner PA, Batchelor AG. Brachial artery entrapment in closed elbow dislocation. *Injury.* 1989;20:240–241.

123. Hoffammann KE, Moneim MS, Omer GE, et al. Brachial artery disruption following closed posterior elbow dislocation in a child: a case report with review of the literature. *Clin Orthop.* 1984;184:145–149.

124. Borris LC, Lassen MR, Christensen CS. Elbow dislocation in children and adults: a long-term follow-up of conservatively treated patients. *Acta Orthop Scand.* 1987;58:649–651.

125. Sponseller PD, Stanitski CL. Fractures and dislocations about the knee. In: Beaty JH, Kasser JR, eds. *Rockwood and Wilkens' Fractures in Children.* 5th ed. Philadelphia: Lippincott Williams & Wilkins; 2001:981–1076.

126. Gartland JJ, Benner JH. Traumatic dislocations in the lower extremity in children. *Orthop Clin North Am.* 1976;7:687–700.

127. Zionts LE. Fractures and dislocations about the knee. In: Green NE, Swiontkowski MF, eds. *Skeletal Trauma in Children.* 3rd ed. Philadelphia: Elsevier; 2003:439–471.

128. Wascher DC, Dvirnak PC, DeCoster TA. Knee dislocation: initial assessment and implications for treatment. *J Orthop Trauma.* 1997;11:525–529.

129. Fanelli GC, Feldmann DD, Edson CJ, et al. The knee: the multiple ligament-injured knee. In: DeLee JC, Drez D, eds. *DeLee and Drez's Orthopaedic Sports Medicine: Principles and Practice.* 2nd ed. Philadelphia: Elsevier; 2003:1577–2154.

130. Green N, Allen B. Vasculature injuries associated with dislocation of the knee. *J Bone Joint Surg Am.* 1977;59:236–239.

131. Merrill KD. Knee dislocations with vascular injuries. *Orthop Clin North Am.* 1994;25:707–713.

132. Ufberg J, McNamara R. Management of common dislocations. In: Roberts JR, Hedges JR, eds. *Clinical Procedures in Emergency Medicine.* 4th ed. Philadelphia: Elsevier; 2004:946–988.

133. Musgrave DS, Mendelson SA. Pediatric orthopedic trauma: principles in management. *Crit Care Med.* 2002;30:s431–443.

134. Varnell RM, Coldwell DM, Sangeorzan BJ, et al. Arterial injury complicating knee disruption. *Am Surg.* 1989;55:699–704.

135. Dart CH, Braitman HE. Popliteal artery injury following fracture or dislocation at the knee. *Arch Surg.* 1977;112:969–973.

136. Antosia RE, Lyn E. Knee and lower leg. In: Marx JA, ed. *Rosen's Emergency Medicine: Concepts and Clinical Practice*, 5th ed. St. Louis: Mosby; 2002:675–706.

137. Perryman JR, Hershman EB. The acute management of soft tissue injuries of the knee. *Orthop Clin North Am.* 2002;33:575–585.

138. Roberts DM. Emergency department evaluation and treatment of knee and leg injuries. *Emerg Med Clin North Am.* 2000;181:67–84.

139. Moehring HD, Tan RT, Marder RA, et al. Ankle dislocation. *J Orthop Trauma.* 1994;8:67–172.

140. Daffner RH, Ankle trauma. *Semin Roentgenol.* 1994;29:134–151.

141. Vander Griend RA, Savoie FH, Hughes JL. Fractures of the ankle: dislocations of the ankle. In: Rockwood CA, Green DP, Bucholz RW, eds. *Rockwood and Green's Fractures in Adults.* 3rd ed. Vol. 2. Philadelphia: JB Lippincott; 1991:2030.

142. Wroble RR, Nepola JV, Malvitz TA. Ankle dislocation without fracture. *Foot Ankle.* 1988;9:64–74.

106

Approach to Fractures with Neurovascular Compromise

▶ INTRODUCTION

Neurovascular compromise should be considered whenever a child presents with an injured extremity. Although children with cool, pale, or cyanotic injured extremities are of obvious concern, serious injuries also can be subtle (1,2). It is essential that individuals who care for children in either the prehospital setting or the emergency department (ED) be adept in the evaluation and initial management of the injured extremity. Depending on the circumstances, such as a lengthy prehospital extrication or transport, it may be several hours before the child receives definitive orthopaedic care. Emergency personnel therefore may be expected to perform limb-saving procedures, including fracture reduction or limb manipulation in a neurovascularly impaired extremity. When the clinician is confronting the rare but serious entity of compartment syndrome, expedient diagnosis and management are essential. The emergency physician must be able to measure intracompartmental pressures if an orthopaedic surgeon is not available to do so.

This chapter highlights specific orthopaedic injuries in children that may be limb threatening (3–7). All pediatric age groups may be affected, but due to the nature of certain injury patterns, school-age children and adolescents are the usual victims. Specific information about splinting (Chapter 101), casting (Chapter 102), and exsanguinating hemorrhage (Chapter 28) is provided elsewhere in this text and will not be discussed in detail in this chapter.

▶ ANATOMY AND PHYSIOLOGY

A comprehensive review of the musculoskeletal anatomy of each neurovascular structure of interest is beyond the scope of

this chapter. The reader is referred to a basic clinical anatomy textbook or atlas should more detail be desired (8,9).

Upper Extremity

The forearm is divided into an anterior (volar) and posterior (dorsal) compartment by a fascial sheath, interosseus membrane, and intermuscular septum. Each compartment contains its own muscle groups, innervation, and blood supply. An injury to the forearm that causes an elevation in compartmental pressures can result in the development of compartment syndrome. A detailed discussion of compartment syndrome (8,9) is provided later in this chapter. Table 106.1 lists the anatomic structures and their functions in the forearm and leg compartments.

The elbow joint is a complex synovial hinge joint between the distal humerus and the proximal radius and ulna. The spool-shaped trochlea and the rounded capitulum of the humerus articulate with the trochlear notch of the ulna and the cupped radial head, respectively. In evaluating children, one must be knowledgeable of the age at which the ossification centers first appear and fuse so as not to confuse an ossification center with a fracture. This is particularly challenging when interpreting radiographs of the elbow. "CRITOE" is a commonly used mnemonic that can help the clinician remember the ossification centers of the elbow and the ages at which they appear and fuse (Table 106.2). In girls, the centers of ossification fuse at age 14 to 15 years, whereas in boys fusion occurs at around 18 to 21 years of age.

An additional important feature of the bones of the elbow has to do with the actual structure of the supracondylar region of the humerus. In children, the distal metaphysis of the humerus is flared and flat. Posteriorly it is indented due

TABLE 106.1	COMPARTMENT STRUCTURES OF THE FOREARM AND LEG

FOREARM

Anterior (Volar) Compartment

Muscles: pronator teres, flexor carpi radialis, palmaris longus, flexor carpi ulnaris, flexor digitorum superficialis, flexor pollicis longus, flexor digitorum profundus, pronator quadratus

Blood supply: ulnar and radial arteries

Nerve supply: all muscles supplied by median nerve and its branches, except flexor carpi ulnaris and medial part of flexor digitorum profundus supplied by ulnar nerve. Principal action: flexion and pronation, intrinsic finger function (abduction, adduction), cutaneous sensation to palmar surface of hand.

Posterior (Dorsal) Compartment

Muscles: extensor carpi radialis brevis, extensor digitorum, extensor digiti minimi, extensor carpi ulnaris, anconeus, supinator, abductor pollicis longus, extensor pollicis brevis and longus, extensor indicis

Blood supply: posterior and anterior interosseous arteries

Nerve supply: deep branch radial nerve. Principal function: wrist and finger extension; essentially no sensory function.

LEG

Anterior Compartment

Muscles: tibialis anterior, extensor digitorum longus, peroneus tertius, extensor hallucis longus

Blood supply: anterior tibial artery

Nerve supply (principal): deep peroneal nerve. Principal function: cutaneous distribution of the anterior web space between the first and second toe, dorsiflexes foot and toes, inverts foot at ankle.

Lateral Compartment

Muscles: peroneus longus and peroneus brevis

Blood supply: branches of the peroneal artery

Nerve supply: superficial peroneal nerve. Principal function: cutaneous distribution of the front of the leg and dorsum of the foot, foot and ankle eversion.

Deep Posterior Compartment

Muscles: popliteus, tibialis posterior, flexor digitorum and hallucis longus

Blood supply: posterior tibial and peroneal arteries

Nerve supply: posterior tibial and peroneal nerves. Principal action: toe plantar flexion and assist in foot inversion, sensation to plantar aspect foot.

Superficial Posterior Compartment

Muscles: gastrocnemis, soleus, plantaris longus.

Nerve supply: sural nerve. Principal function: sensation to dorsal lateral portion of foot and ankle. Gastroc-soleus complex is chief ankle and foot plantar flexor though supplied by tibial nerve (deep posterior compartment structure).

to the olecranon fossa, and anteriorly it is thinned due to the coronoid fossa. The supracondylar region is a relatively weak section of bone that is somewhat susceptible to fracturing, especially when the ossification centers are not fused. The brachial artery and its branches, the radial and ulnar

TABLE 106.2	OSSIFICATION CENTERS OF THE ELBOW

Ossification Center	Age of Appearance
Capitulum	1–2 y
Radial head	5–7 y
Internal (medial) humeral epicondyle	5–9 y
Trochlea	9–10 y
Olecranon	9–11 y
External (lateral) humeral epicondyle	11–14 y

arteries, and the median and radial nerves are the principal neurovascular structures that could be damaged in a complex supracondylar elbow fracture.

Lower Extremity

The lower limb consists of four parts: the pelvis, consisting of the hip bones (fusion of the ilium, ischium, and pubis) and their connections between the vertebral column and the femur; the thigh, containing the femur connecting the knee and hip; the lower leg, containing the tibia and fibula connecting the ankle and the knee; and the foot and the connection to the ankle. Because the greatest risk for neurovascular injuries in the lower extremity involves the knee and the compartments of the leg, much of the discussion will focus on these areas.

Knee

As with the elbow, the knee is a synovial hinge joint. Articulation at the knee is between the large rounded condyles of the distal femur, the flattened condyles of the proximal tibia, and the facets of the patella. Principal movement of the knee is flexion and extension, but some lateral and medial rotation is also possible.

Important neurovascular structures that traverse from the thigh to the calf lie deep within the popliteal fossa and are generally well protected from damage by a strong, thick fascial covering. However, with knee dislocations, displaced fractures through the physes of the proximal tibia or distal femur, or penetrating injuries to the fossa, there is a relatively high risk of concomitant neurovascular injuries to the leg and foot. The popliteal artery and vein, the small saphenous vein, the tibial and common peroneal nerves, and the end branch of the posterior femoral cutaneous nerve all are contained in the fossa.

If the popliteal artery is damaged (severed or partially lacerated or undergoing vasospasm), circulation to the leg could be compromised, with resultant ischemic damage. The primary structures that innervate the leg and foot pass through the popliteal fossa. The tibial nerve supplies articular branches to the knee and motor branches to the muscles of the posterior leg and the plantar flexors of the foot. It joins a branch of the common peroneal nerve to form the sural nerve, which innervates the lateral aspect of the ankle and sole of the foot. The common peroneal nerve supplies articular branches to the knee and proximal tibiofibular joints, motor branches to the dorsiflexor and evertor muscles of the foot, and cutaneous sensory branches that innervate the skin of the calf.

Lower Leg

A deep sheath of fascia encapsulates the leg by surrounding its contents and attaching to the medial and lateral borders of the tibia. Two intermuscular septa together with an interosseous membrane between the tibia and fibula divide the leg into three compartments: anterior, posterior, and lateral (Fig. 106.1B). The posterior compartment is further subdivided into a superficial and deep compartment by a transverse intermuscular

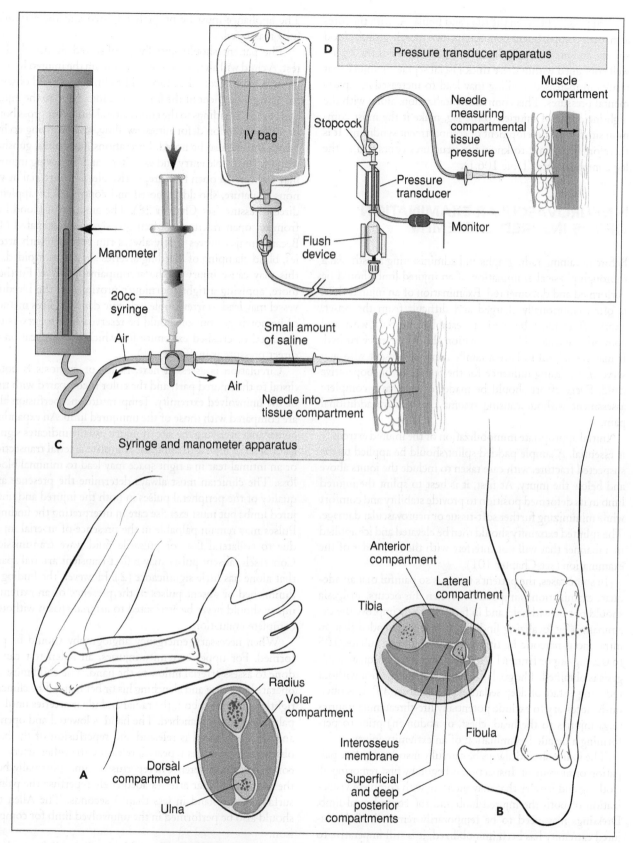

Figure 106.1
A. Forearm compartments.
B. Lower leg compartments.
C. Syringe and manometer setup for compartment pressure measurement.
D. Pressure transducer setup for compartment pressure measurement.

septum passing between the tibia and fibula. As with the fore-arm, each compartment contains its own muscle group, blood supply, and nerve supply. Because the structures of the leg are well contained within these thick fascial septae, an injury that results in increased swelling may lead to increased compartmental pressures. This compartmentalization, along with the high incidence of injuries to the leg, make it the most common site for the development of compartment syndrome. It is therefore important to know the structures contained in the leg compartments (Table 106.1).

▶ NEUROVASCULAR EXAMINATION OF THE INJURED EXTREMITY

Before obtaining radiographs and administering anesthesia, a thorough physical examination of an injured limb should be performed and documented. Examination of an injured child is often emotionally charged and difficult from the onset. Every effort must be made to establish rapport with and comfort the child. The examination should never be rushed. It may be helpful to have a family member present who will serve as a calming influence for the fearful or uncooperative child. Every effort should be made to perform a complete assessment without causing trauma or excessive additional pain.

Initial appropriate immobilization of the injured extremity is essential. A simple padded splint should be applied to the suspected fracture, with care taken to include the joints above and below the injury. At first, it is best to splint the injured limb in its deformed position to provide stability and comfort while minimizing further soft-tissue or neurovascular damage. The splinted extremity should then be elevated and ice applied in a manner that will not interfere with the remainder of the examination (see Chapter 101).

In some cases, the patient's injury is so painful that an adequate examination is impossible. When this occurs, analgesia should not be withheld and in fact will likely improve the examination by localizing findings. It is recommended that an intravenous narcotic be titrated (e.g., morphine sulfate 0.05 to 0.2 mg/kg or fentanyl 1 to 3 μg/kg) until adequate analgesia is obtained. The goal is to decrease pain and fear without inducing a state of deep sedation (see Chapter 33). It is obviously necessary to exclude potentially life-threatening injuries (e.g., injuries to the head, chest, or abdomen) prior to performing a detailed examination of an extremity injury.

The injury should always be carefully inspected before palpation or movement. Inspection is begun by first removing all clothing and jewelry that may interfere with complete visualization of both the injured limb and the contralateral limb. Dressings may need to be temporarily removed. If the injured extremity has been immobilized, it is still imperative to perform a complete neurovascular examination. The splint or traction device may have been inadequately applied, and a long bone fracture may be improperly aligned, shortened, or excessively stretched, with resulting neurovascular compromise.

The appliance must be properly adjusted and the extremity fully reassessed.

The patient should initially be observed undisturbed at rest. A child will always attempt to maintain the injured limb in a position of maximal comfort. The clinician should observe for active movement of the fingers and toes distal to the injury and compare findings to the contralateral limb. Any gross bony or musculotendon deformities, swelling, and overlying ecchymoses should also be noted. Lacerations, punctures, gunshot wounds (probable entry and exit sites), and degloving injuries may indicate an open fracture. Active bleeding, arterial or venous in nature, should be noted and controlled by applying direct pressure (see Chapter 28). The amount of blood loss from an open fracture is often grossly underestimated (1). Because major nerves nearly always run together with arteries, blind clamping of bleeding arteries should be avoided, as this may cause injury to the accompanying nerve. Furthermore, applying a tight tourniquet proximal to the bleeding vessel may lead to irreversible ischemic damage. This method of hemorrhage control should be reserved for an irreversibly damaged or crushed extremity for which the application of direct pressure is ineffective (1).

Circulation is assessed next. Pallor or cyanosis is noted distal to the injured part, and the color is compared with that of the uninvolved extremity. Temperature and perfusion also are compared with those of the uninjured limb. An expanding hematoma overlying the site of injury usually indicates significant arterial injury. In contrast, complete arterial transection or an intimal tear in a tight space may lead to minimal blood loss. The clinician must always determine the presence and quality of the peripheral pulses in both the injured and uninjured limbs but must exercise care in interpreting the findings. Pulses may remain palpable in the presence of arterial injury due to collateral flow or pulsatile fluid wave transmission. Conversely, absent pulses may reflect transient arterial spasm that alone has little significance (2). However, the finding of diminished or absent pulses in the presence of an extremity injury should never be attributed to arterial spasm without a complete evaluation.

When necessary, emergency angiography should be performed. For upper extremity injuries, an Allen test can be done to assess arterial inflow to the hand. The child must cooperate by raising and clenching his or her hand. The clinician tightly compresses both the radial and ulnar arteries until the palmar surface is blanched. The hand is lowered and opened, and then one vessel is released and reperfusion of the hand observed. The test is repeated, releasing the other artery and comparing the difference in reperfusion time. Normally, both the radial and ulnar arteries adequately reperfuse the palmar surface of the hand in less than 3 seconds. The Allen test should also be performed in the uninvolved limb for comparison.

Sensation should be assessed by localizing light touch using a cotton wisp. Two-point discrimination is done using the blunt ends of a paper clip, one centimeter apart. It may not be possible to reliably assess sensation by either of these methods in a nonverbal or uncooperative child. Still, the clinician should almost never use painful discrimination for the examination of the young child, as it is itself painful and rarely provides useful information (10,11). It is still possible to assess sensation in the hand of the infant or fearful child. Because autonomic nerve fibers travel in nerve bundles, the wrinkle test can be done to assess sensation to the hand. The hand is first submerged in warm water for 5 to 10 minutes. The hand and fingers are then inspected for wrinkling. Those areas with impaired sensation will not wrinkle (10).

Motor function is next evaluated in both the injured and uninjured extremities. Function and strength are carefully assessed and compared. In the evaluation for compartment syndrome, it is imperative to passively stretch and have the child actively flex the limb and the muscle group of concern. For example, the anterior compartment of the leg is the most common site for development of compartment syndrome. The primary nerve supply is via the deep peroneal nerve that serves in foot dorsiflexion by innervating the tibialis anterior and extensor digitorum longus muscles. In the event of compartment syndrome, these muscles are weakened and active foot dorsiflexion and toe extension are impaired. Furthermore, passive flexion of the toes results in severe pain due to ischemia resulting from increased intracompartmental pressure. Once the examination is complete, anesthesia (local, regional, or general) should be provided as necessary before radiographs are obtained or the wound is explored.

In the special case of the obtunded and/or comatose child, the physician must have a higher index of suspicion for neurovascular impairment and consequently a lower threshold for intervention (e.g., measuring intracompartmental pressures) (12). Any orthopaedic injury that leads to neurovascular compromise represents a potentially limb-threatening emergency. Insufficient arterial blood flow to a distal extremity can result from either vessel transection or laceration caused by a bony fragment or projectile missile (e.g., gunshot wound). Arterial spasm or compression caused by extrinsic pressure from the fractured bone or edematous tissue also may lead to ischemic damage. Venous obstruction is usually the result of tissue swelling from the injury or from tightly applied circumferential casts or dressings. If unrecognized or untreated, this can also lead to the development of compartment syndrome (12).

Nerve injury may be temporary due to stretching, and nerve dysfunction generally resolves within 6 months. However, permanent dysfunction can result from ischemic necrosis in late compartment syndrome. Nerves, like vessels, also can be transected. It is therefore essential to perform a rapid, accurate assessment and appropriate intervention to prevent permanent functional impairment or loss of the involved limb.

The proximity of the brachial artery to the elbow, the proximity of the popliteal artery to the knee, and the proximity of the pudendal artery to the pelvis make these three areas (elbow, knee, pelvis) particularly vulnerable to vascular compromise following a significant injury. The radial, median, and ulnar nerves around the elbow and the tibial and common peroneal nerves at the knee are at relatively high risk for nerve impairment. Therefore, much attention will be focused on recognizing and treating supracondylar humeral fractures and severe knee injuries. It must be stressed, however, that any complicated fracture or dislocation may be unstable and lead to associated vascular ischemia or nerve damage. A brief overview of unstable pelvic, femoral shaft, and complex tibia-fibula and ankle fractures is included. Features that aid in the prompt recognition, diagnosis, and management of compartment syndrome are highlighted first.

▶ COMPARTMENT SYNDROME

Pathophysiology

Generally speaking, insufficient blood flow to an extremity may lead to ischemic damage as early as 4 hours after an injury (3,13,14). Irreversible damage can occur 6 to 12 hours after onset of compromised vascular perfusion (4,11,15,16).

Compartment syndrome can be caused by any condition that leads to elevated tissue pressure within muscle groups enveloped by fascial sheaths. The actual incidence of compartment syndrome in children is unknown, but it is safe to say that it is a rare entity (12). Still, due to the potentially grave consequences if unrecognized and untreated, it is prudent to consider the diagnosis of compartment syndrome when faced with an extremity at risk.

The pathophysiology of compartment syndrome has been well studied (3,4,12–22). The increased pressure within the confined space leads to restriction of blood flow distally, with subsequent ischemic insult to the extremity. It was previously believed that the ischemia leading to compartment syndrome was secondary solely to impaired arterial blood flow. Acute compartment syndrome, however, is known to occur in the presence of palpable distal arterial pulses. Current theory holds that it is narrowing of the arterial-venous pressure gradient, either by increased venous pressure or decreased arterial pressure, that causes hypoperfusion and ischemic injury. Subsequent reperfusion within the compartment leads directly to elevated pressure from increased flow in the restricted space and indirectly to increased pressure from local tissue edema. Further ischemia develops, leading to necrosis and limb dysfunction.

A myriad of conditions may lead to compartment syndrome (3,12). Again, the basic principle is either (a) the contents within the confined sheath unduly swell or (b) the envelope surrounding the muscle group is overly constricting. Bleeding directly into the compartmental space secondary to blunt trauma (fractures, contusions), penetrating trauma (gunshot wounds) with arterial injury, primary limb surgery, joint dislocations, or fracture reduction may lead to the development of compartment syndrome. Excessively tight MAST suits, casts, air splints, and dressings may lead to compartment syndrome by excessive external constricting pressure. Intraosseous infusions, snakebites, burns, and cardiac catheterizations may result in an increased compartmental volume from intravenous fluid infiltration or capillary leak and are known causes of compartment syndrome in children.

A chronic or recurrent form of compartment syndrome may develop from prolonged, excessive muscle use. Its pathogenesis is not well understood, and the physician must have a high clinical suspicion for the diagnosis. If this entity is being considered, acute management involves cessation of exercise and referral to an orthopaedic specialist (3,4). Supracondylar fractures of the humerus, combined radius and ulnar fractures, femur fractures with skin traction, and tibial fractures are the most common mechanisms of injury leading to compartment syndrome in children (12).

The clinician should always consider the diagnosis of compartment syndrome when a child presents with complaints of pain seemingly out of proportion to that expected from the nature of injury (12). A nonverbal or especially fretful, uncooperative child makes diagnosis more difficult and often requires more careful scrutiny. Discretion and care must be given to the administration of heavily sedating analgesia that may interfere with serial examinations. As mentioned, severe pain elicited by actively flexing or passively stretching the suspected muscle groups is an especially sensitive sign and should heighten the clinician's concern. Paresthesias may be caused by ischemia to nerves traversing and innervating the suspected compartmental region. Decreased sensation to light touch or to two-point discrimination are reliable in defining distal sensory impairment. Swelling and palpable tenderness over the muscle group rather than the fracture site have been described by some as the earliest physical findings in compartment syndrome (14). As previously noted, palpable distal pulses and intact capillary perfusion *do not* rule out the diagnosis of compartment syndrome. Absent pulses and delayed perfusion are generally late findings and heighten the likelihood that myonecrosis has already occurred.

Early recognition and diagnosis via tissue pressure measurement allows for timely therapeutic intervention (i.e., emergency fasciotomy and prevention of permanent limb dysfunction). A multiply injured child who is obtunded or comatose is especially difficult to evaluate because of the inability to perform a complete neurologic examination. An infant or highly uncooperative child may similarly be difficult to evaluate thoroughly. As noted, the only reliable signs on examination may be a tensely swollen, exquisitely tender extremity.

Because many patients will present in a cast, splint, or bandage, all appliances should be removed if the clinician suspects compartment syndrome. The involved limb is then iced and elevated. If improvement is not observed within 1 hour, an orthopaedic surgeon must be emergently consulted. If one is not readily available (within 4 hours of the onset of symptoms), the ED physician must consider measuring compartmental pressures.

Measurement of Intracompartmental Pressures

Normal intramuscular resting pressure approximates zero (3,16). As pressure within a compartment increases, perfusion

decreases. No one standard recommendation represents the lowest accepted pressure above which performing a fasciotomy is always warranted. Rather, abnormally high pressures range from 30 to 45 mm Hg. Some authorities recommend surgical decompression when the intracompartmental pressure approaches 10 to 30 mm Hg of the diastolic blood pressure (4). A general rule to follow would be to consult an orthopaedic surgeon when the diagnosis is suspected on clinical grounds. If tissue pressures measure greater than 30 mm Hg, surgical decompression should likely be performed (3,4,12,13).

In animal investigations, 6 hours of warm ischemia resulted in irreversible damage in 50% of the muscles studied. Eight to 12 hours of severe ischemia led to near complete and irreversible damage (16). It is thus imperative to act quickly in the face of a potentially devitalized compartment. When the orthopedist is not available to measure compartment pressures, the emergency physician must be prepared to measure pressures to either assist a local orthopaedist in making the diagnosis or expedite transfer to an available accepting facility.

Any method used to measure intracompartmental pressures involves insertion of relatively large bore needles into, at times, multiple sites in the injured part. It is imperative that the patient be provided moderate procedural sedation to alleviate the pain and anxiety associated with needle insertion and to improve the chances for patient cooperation and successful measurement (see Chapter 33). Whitesides et al. (3,4,16,17,21,23) have described a relatively straightforward technique for tissue pressure monitoring that can be done entirely with equipment and material found in the ED or office setting.

Equipment

Plastic extension tubes (2)
18-gauge needles (2)
20-mL syringe
Three-way stopcock
Vial of bacteriostatic normal saline
Mercury manometer
Local anesthesia

The skin over the involved compartment is first prepared by cleansing with a povidone-iodine solution. The site of needle insertion is anesthetized with local anesthetic. It is important to avoid injection into the suspected compartment, as this may further raise the pressure.

The manometer measurement device is assembled as shown in Figure 106.1C. First, intravenous extension tubing is connected to the front and rear ports of a three-way stopcock, and a 20-mL syringe with the plunger at the 15-mL mark is connected to the upper port. A sterile 18-gauge needle is used to release the vacuum of a bottle of bacteriostatic normal saline. Once the vacuum has been released, this needle is connected to the front port of the stopcock. The front port of the stopcock is opened, and the plunger of the syringe slowly withdrawn until saline fills approximately half of the length of

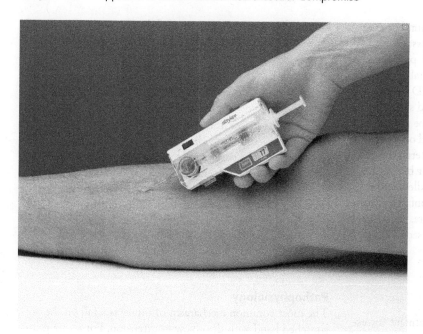

Figure 106.2 STIC intracompartmental pressure monitor system (Stryker Instruments, Kalamazoo, MI).

the tubing attached to the front port. It is important to withdraw the saline from the bottle slowly and smoothly so as to minimize bubble formation within the extension tubing and ensure that the saline only fills half of the extension tubing; the syringe should contain only air. The stopcock is then used to close the front port, and the needle is removed from the saline bottle. This needle is carefully removed and replaced with a new sterile needle. Keeping the front port stopcock closed during needle transfer will prevent loss of saline from the extension tubing.

Next, the extension tubing attached to the rear port is connected to the manometer. The needle is inserted into the desired muscle compartmental space, and the stopcock is opened to both extension tubes and to the syringe. This produces a closed system whereby air is free to flow into both extension tubes as the pressure increases. Next, the plunger is depressed slowly, forcing a rise in pressure within the system. As this is done, the mercury column within the manometer will slowly rise until the pressure within the system is equivalent to that within the tissue compartment. Then, as the pressure within the system surpasses the tissue pressure, the saline contained within the extension tubing will be forced toward the needle, which will cause visible movement of the saline within the extension tubing. The reading on the mercury manometer at the time the saline begins to move represents the compartmental pressure. If more than one compartment pressure is to be measured, the system is reclosed, and a new 18-gauge sterile needle is used each time.

Other techniques for measuring compartmental pressure include the wick catheter and the slit catheter methods (3,4,15–19). Both offer the advantage of continuous pressure monitoring but are cumbersome and not practical in either the ED or office setting. Another option is the STIC intracompartmental pressure monitor system (Stryker Instru-

ments, Kalamazoo, MI) (Fig. 106.2), a handheld, battery-operated, lightweight device that is relatively simple to use, requiring only the attachment of a needle and syringe apparatus and zeroing of the monitor before insertion in the injured limb. After injection of no more than 0.3 mL of saline into the compartment, the pressure can be read directly from the monitor. Finally, certain types of electronic equipment commonly found in EDs can be used to measure intracompartmental pressure. The two most often used are intravenous pumps and monitors with arterial line capabilities.

To use an intravenous pump, the pump must have an internal electronic manometer that reports the pressure within the system. A bag of normal saline is first placed onto the pump apparatus using the same technique as would be used for intravenous infusion. Next, a needle appropriate for measuring intracompartmental pressure (see above) is attached to the distal end of the infusion tubing, occupying the location normally occupied by the intravenous catheter. If the intravenous pump can be moved up and down, it should be placed level with the involved extremity. Then the pump should be set to infuse a small volume of fluid (e.g., 2 to 5 mL/hr). The baseline pressure within the system is recorded by pressing and holding the pressure button on the infusion pump. (Ideally, the baseline pressure should be zero, but often it is not.) Notably, many pumps have a limit to the amount of negative pressure that they are able to report, and pressures below the limit are inaccurately reported. If the baseline pressure reported is negative, this should be taken into consideration. After the baseline pressure is recorded, the needle is inserted into the compartment as previously described. The pressure button on the infusion pump is pressed and held, and the pressure reading shown on the pump display is noted. Positive baseline pressures and those negative baseline pressures that are within the limits of the machine's reporting ability are added to or subtracted from the reported number as appropriate to obtain the intracompartmental pressure.

To use a monitor for recording compartment pressure, the monitor and infusion system is set up for arterial line monitoring but with two exceptions (see Fig. 106.1D). First, the fluid to be infused need not be heparinized, and second, it is not necessary for a bag of intravenous fluid to be placed into the pressure bag. As described, a needle is placed on the distal end of the infusion setup instead of an intra-arterial catheter. The system is then zeroed, just as would occur before measuring an intra-arterial pressure. When the needle is inserted into the compartment, the pressure reading obtained from the monitor is the intracompartmental pressure. This pressure reading is displayed in the area normally used to display the blood pressure from an arterial line.

Fasciotomy

Operative fasciotomies represent definitive treatment for established compartment syndrome. The basic principle involves incising through the overlying skin and enveloping fascial sheaths of each involved compartment to release the constricted tissues and muscles. Needless to say, the variety of fasciotomies requires extensive knowledge of local anatomic structures. Details of the operative techniques and fine anatomy are beyond the scope of this book but are described in other texts (3,4,12,13,20).

Complications

Complications of neurovascular ischemia may be acute or delayed (13). When compartment syndrome develops and goes unrecognized or untreated, the consequences can be devastating. Volkmann's ischemia is defined as the neurologic sequelae of compartment syndrome, i.e., the pain from passively stretching the involved muscle groups and the sensory and motor deficits that result from the neurovascular compromise. Volkmann's ischemic contracture is the functionless limb that results from untreated ischemia. It may occur following fractures of the elbow, forearm, wrist, tibia, and femur.

The claw hand deformity is Volkmann's contracture resulting from untreated forearm ischemia. In its most severe form, ischemic necrosis causes flexor contractures in the elbow, forearm, wrist, hand, and fingers, and nerve damage causes intrinsic paralysis in the hand and wrist. This results in elbow flexion and forearm pronation. Characteristic findings in the hand and wrist are wrist flexion, hyperextension of the metacarpophalangeal joints, flexion of the interphalangeal joints, and thumb contracture—thus the claw hand appearance (14).

When myonecrosis progresses, several consequences may occur (2,13,14). The necrotic limb is at risk for bacterial gangrene infection and the associated serious complications of overwhelming sepsis. One of the more common occurrences of muscle breakdown is myoglobinuria. If the patient's hydration status is not optimal and myoglobin production exceeds

kidney filtration capacity, renal failure may develop. Death can result from either of these serious complications.

▶ FRACTURES AND DISLOCATIONS

As discussed below, the emergency physician is expected to recognize fractures and dislocations for which an emergent reduction must be performed to salvage a limb from neurovascular compromise and serious complications. Clearly, any time a reduction is performed by the emergency physician, the patient should be seen by an orthopaedic surgeon on a timely basis for re-evaluation and additional care.

Supracondylar Humeral Fractures

Pathophysiology

The most common mechanism of injury is a fall on the outstretched hand with the elbow in extension. Forces are transmitted proximally up the elbow, fracturing the supracondylar region. If enough force is generated, the proximal fragment is driven posteriorly and the distal fragment displaced anteriorly. This type of extension injury represents 95% to 99% of all supracondylar humeral fractures. Due to the nature of this injury, it is always important to adequately evaluate the wrist and shoulder for an associated injury (5,24–33).

A direct blow to the flexed elbow and a resultant fracture will cause anterior displacement of the proximal fragment of the humerus and posterior displacement of the distal fragment. This injury is far less common than the extension type.

The elbow joint is traversed by the brachial artery and the median, radial, and ulnar nerves. It is therefore not uncommon for neurovascular compromise to develop in the forearm or hand as a complication of this injury. With the extension injury, if the distal fragment is displaced medially, the radial nerve may be stretched and tented over the laterally displaced proximal fragment. If the distal fragment is displaced laterally, as when the lateral periosteum remains intact, the median nerve is pulled tautly over the medially placed proximal fragment. The medial displacement pattern occurs more frequently, and thus radial nerve injuries are more common. With the flexion-type injury, the ulnar nerve is more commonly stretched and injured because it is tightly bound to the medial intermuscular septum proximal to the fracture fragment and the cubital tunnel distal to the fracture. In a review of 4,520 fractures, 7% had concomitant nerve injuries, of which 45% were radial nerve injuries, 32% median nerve injuries, and 23% ulnar nerve injuries (25). In another report, there was a 12% incidence of peripheral neuropathies that developed after supracondylar humeral fractures (26). The anterior interosseus nerve was the most commonly injured branch of the median nerve that resulted in loss of flexion of the distal phalanges of the thumb and index finger. Because nearly all nerve injury is from traction, full recovery can generally be expected within 6 months after injury.

Although the brachial artery may be completely transected, arterial spasm is far more common. In fact, neurovascular compromise commonly occurs after a fracture even when no displacement of the distal fragment has occurred. Swelling and hemarthrosis in the cubital fossa may lead to arterial spasm and/or occlusion. Compartment syndrome can develop if ischemia is prolonged (5,20,23–30).

Equipment

Appropriate sedative and/or hypnotic agents
Monitors and resuscitation equipment
Splinting material
Doppler transducer

Procedure

Because it has a significant risk of neurovascular injury, reduction of the extension-type fracture with posterior displacement of the distal humeral fracture fragment will be detailed here. When a supracondylar humeral fracture of the elbow leads to neurovascular compromise in the forearm or hand, an orthopaedic surgeon must be emergently consulted. The arm should be immobilized, elevated, and iced. If the specialist is unavailable and the condition does not improve, it is the responsibility of the emergency physician to reduce the fracture to restore flow and function to the distal arm.

Procedural sedation should be administered to the child (see Chapter 33). The goal is to provide sufficient relief of pain and muscle relaxation so the child does not struggle and the muscles do not spasm during fracture reduction and immobilization. Once ready, an assistant immobilizes the arm proximal to the fracture site. The physician exerts longitudinal traction at the wrist until the arm length is approximately normal. The elbow is slightly hyperextended to release any locked fracture fragments. This is done while pressure is applied in the anterior direction against the distal humeral fragment. At this point, medial and lateral angulation should be corrected. The assistant applies gentle posterior traction on the proximal humerus while this is being done. The elbow is then flexed to maintain proper alignment, and posterior pressure is applied to the distal fragment. Distal pulses are assessed. If diminished or absent, the brachial artery may have spasmed due to tenting of the artery over the anteriorly displaced proximal bony fragment. If the fingers remain nonedematous, warm, pink, well perfused, and fully functional, these findings are far more significant than the presence or absence of a radial pulse. Slightly flexing the extremity to approximately 5 to 15 degrees should restore circulation and the distal pulse. If pulse and perfusion remain abnormal, arteriography and/or surgical exploration are required (26,27). Continuous pulse oximetry of an ipsilateral finger during the procedure is a quick way to ascertain whether perfusion is intact distally (28–30).

A long arm posterior splint is then applied (see Chapter 101). If the distal fragment was displaced medially, the elbow should be slightly pronated for splinting. Conversely, if the distal fragment was laterally displaced, the forearm should be immobilized in supination. A sling is then applied, and the patient is hospitalized for careful neurovascular checks.

If reduction of the fracture fails once, it should not be repeated due to the risk of more substantial brachial artery damage with excessive manipulation. In this case, an overhead olecranon reduction apparatus must be applied by an experienced orthopaedist. In fact, any nerve or vascular injury warrants overhead traction (27).

Postreduction radiographs should be obtained to document elbow position. Peripheral pulses, color, temperature, perfusion, and movement in the fingers and hand are repeatedly assessed and recorded. Emergent angiography is obtained should vascular injury be suspected. Inability to maintain a closed reduction or limb-threatening neurovascular damage may be an indication for an open, surgical reduction (27,29).

Complications

Malunion is a complication that can result after any healed displaced fracture. With a supracondylar humeral fracture in children, cubitus varus ("gunstock" deformity) and valgus deformities are seen. The most frequent cause is malposition of the distal humeral fragment. Elbow stiffness and impaired function are complications from prolonged immobilization more often seen in adults. As noted previously, a clawhand deformity is a complication resulting from untreated compartment syndrome in the forearm (14,24–31).

Distal Upper Extremity Injuries

Although potentially less serious than supracondylar fractures, injuries to the distal forearm are far more common. The mechanism of injury is similar to that previously described (i.e., a fall onto an outstretched arm). The resulting injuries usually involve the distal radius and ulna (e.g., Colles fracture). In most cases, this type of injury does not result in neurovascular compromise, but in cases of extreme angulation of the bones or significant local edema, the arterial supply and/or nerve supply to the hand may be compromised. Therefore, all patients presenting to the ED with these types of injuries should have a careful examination of the hand, as described previously.

If the examination demonstrates that either the blood supply or innervation to the hand is compromised, emergency reduction is appropriate. After adequate analgesia has been administered, an assistant grasps the upper arm above the elbow to stabilize it. The physician then exerts gentle longitudinal traction on the arm distal to the fracture (Fig. 106.3A,B). The procedure is successful if circulation to the hand is restored. Definitive reduction need not be accomplished until later.

Injuries Around the Knee

In children, physis (growth plate) fractures (Salter type) occur with greater frequency than ligamentous injuries due to the relative weakness of the growth plate compared with the

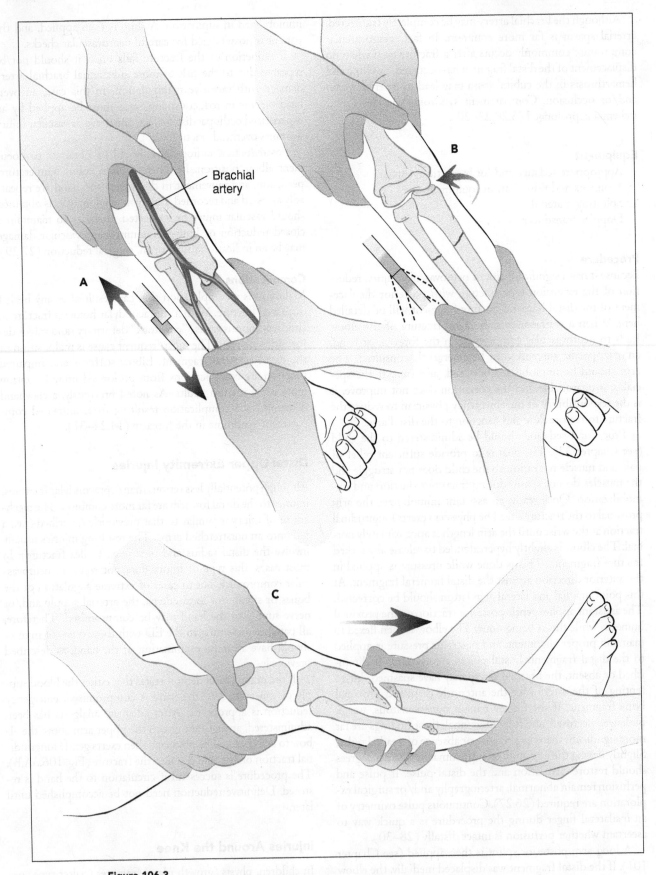

Figure 106.3
A, B. Technique for emergency reduction of forearm fracture with neurovascular compromise.
C. Technique for reduction of lower leg fracture with neurovascular compromise.

supporting ligaments. A frontal blow to a fixed thigh with the knee hyperextended may drive the lower leg forward. The result may be a fracture through the growth plate of the distal femur and anterior displacement of the distal epiphysis.

Occurring less frequently is a fracture-separation at the proximal tibial growth plate. The physis of the proximal tibia is well protected laterally by the fibula and anteriorly by the overhanging epiphyseal tubercle. Additionally, the insertion of the surrounding knee ligaments and musculotendons offers further protective support to the growth plate. However, a violent, direct blow to the proximal tibial epiphysis (e.g., motor vehicle running over the lower leg) may cause a fracture through the physis and posterior displacement of the proximal metaphysis into the popliteal fossa. More common, though still rare, is an indirect mechanism involving a blow to the hyperextended lower leg with the knee fixed. This injury may occur in an adolescent after a sports injury or in a preadolescent after a fall or motor vehicle accident, and it may result in fracture-separation through the tibial growth plate and similar posterior displacement of the proximal tibial metaphysis. A knee dislocation without fracture is a rare event in children. All three types of injuries, however, are discussed due to their relatively high associated risk of vascular compromise (2,20).

The popliteal artery is tightly secured at the popliteal fossa because it is anchored proximally at the adductor hiatus and distally at the soleus muscle. It provides primary circulation to the lower leg. Its tributaries provide poor collateral circulation at the popliteal fossa. Because the artery is firmly fixed in place, a fracture-separation around the hyperextended knee may posteriorly displace a fracture fragment and cause it to impinge on the popliteal artery. The nerve supply, principally composed of the tibial and common peroneal nerves, is more loosely attached than the artery, and therefore nerve injury is much less likely than vascular damage (7,34).

A meticulous examination of the leg and foot is mandatory whenever any of these injuries is suspected. Evaluation should include assessment for associated femur and pelvic fractures, which may not be immediately apparent. Both dorsalis pedis and posterior tibial pulses should be palpated or Doppler measured and should be compared with those on the uninjured side. The foot may be cold or pale. The lower leg may be cyanotic and exhibit delayed capillary refill if venous return is impaired. Muscle function and sensation in the lower leg, foot, and toes must be carefully assessed. If marked pain, muscle belly tenderness, and swelling are noted, a diagnosis of compartment syndrome should be considered. Elevated compartment pressures in the lower leg confirm the diagnosis.

Penetrating injuries around the knee also warrant special attention. Because late complications include development of arteriovenous fistulas and pseudoaneurysms, noninvasive duplex studies of the lower extremity are required even in the face of apparent vascular competence. An emergency angiogram should be obtained in all cases of severe knee injuries that risk involving the popliteal artery. This is especially important because distal pulses may appear normal immediately after the injury (3,7,34).

Chapter 105 details the procedure for reduction of a knee dislocation (see also Fig. 105.14). The principles are generally the same when dealing with a neurovascularly compromised leg from a fracture-separation through the physis of the distal femur or proximal tibia.

Unstable Pelvic Fractures

An unstable pelvic fracture is most commonly the result of a high-impact force (e.g., motor vehicle accident or fall) directly crushing the pelvis. Similarly by a fall from a great height, an indirect blow may be transmitted up through the femurs, driving the femoral heads back into and fracturing the pelvic ring.

Any pelvic fracture has the potential for significant bleeding, leading to hemodynamic compromise and shock. Serial hematocrit measurements should be obtained to assess blood loss. Evaluation for associated bladder and abdominal visceral injuries is always performed (1,12,35,36). Definitive treatment for these injuries generally involves either external fixation or angiographic embolization of bleeding vessels. These techniques require resources beyond those usually available in the ED, which may create a considerable delay in treatment. If a trauma victim is hemodynamically compromised due to blood loss from an unstable pelvic fracture, an immediately available, acceptable intervention must be employed pending further management. One formerly suggested method is to apply the pelvic portion of a pneumatic antishock garment, but this is now rarely performed for pediatric patients, and many emergency medical services (EMS) units and EDs no longer have these devices available. There are, however, three alternative approaches.

The first and simplest is the "sheet wrap" technique. In this technique, a standard bedsheet is folded lengthwise so that it is approximately the same width as the patient's pelvis. The sheet is passed underneath the patient at the level of his or her pelvis so that it crosses the lateral portions of the iliac crest and approximately equal lengths of sheet extend from either side of the patient. Standing on opposite sides of the patient, the operator and an assistant pass one another the ends of the sheet so that the sheet crosses in front of the patient at about the level of the symphysis pubis. The operator and assistant then apply traction on their respective sheet ends so that medially directed forces are applied from either side, pressing the pelvis back into a more normal position. When the desired tension has been achieved, the sheet can be tied or (preferably) secured with towel clips.

The second technique involves the use of a commercial pelvic binder. This device is applied around the pelvis in much the same way as the sheet, but the commercial binder has clips, straps, and/or buckles that secure it in place and straps or laces that allow it to be tightened. The commercial binders offer the advantage of causing less tissue necrosis when used for protracted periods (e.g., during interfacility transport) and do not require the use of metal towel clips, which can affect radiographs.

Finally, there is a commercially available vacuum device that uses a bean bag–type splint to stabilize the pelvis. The device is placed around the patient, and then vacuum is applied to realign the pelvis.

Femoral Shaft Fractures

Fractures of the femoral shaft that impair circulation distally may be manifested by a cool, pale, pulseless foot. Alternatively, even with a grossly displaced fracture, no neurovascular injury may be observed. However, gentle longitudinal traction in line with the long axis should be attempted when circulation is impaired. As traction is being applied, the leg is turned gradually from the deformed position. Once circulation is restored in the foot, the leg is immobilized in a traction splint. Splinting is always performed for displaced femur fractures to minimize hemorrhage into the thigh and prevent further neurovascular or soft-tissue injury.

Doppler arterial pressures should be obtained in both the affected and uninjured leg using a blood pressure cuff. A decrease in systolic arterial pressure of greater than or equal to 20 mm Hg in the injured leg as compared with the uninjured leg may indicate significant arterial compromise. Many authorities recommend an intraoperative arteriogram at this point. In the case of obvious circulatory compromise, an emergency arteriogram must be obtained. Serial hematocrits also need to be obtained, as significant and insidious hemorrhage may develop after a displaced femur fracture (1,12).

Tibia and Fibula Shaft Fractures

The great majority of tibia and fibula shaft fractures are nondisplaced or incompletely displaced. A rare but significant event is fracture through both the tibia and fibula, with complete displacement. Should limb-threatening vascular compromise occur, emergency reduction by gentle longitudinal traction is required (see Fig. 106.3C). As with a femoral shaft fracture, the leg may need to be turned from the plane of deformity while applying traction. When aligning a tibial fracture, the second toe should align with the tibial tubercle. This may need to be done even before radiographs are obtained (e.g., in

---

 SUMMARY

1 Stabilize the patient; follow the ABCs under the ATLS protocol.

2 Remove all clothing (including footwear) and jewelry covering and distal to the injured extremity.

3 Stop active bleeding with a direct pressure dressing.

4 Observe the child and inspect the injury. Note the preferred position of the extremity and note gross deformities, findings consistent with an open fracture, and the color. Always examine the contralateral limb in the same manner.

5 Unless obvious neurovascular compromise is present, gently apply a temporary, simple, padded splint to the injured part, initially leaving it in its deformed position. Include joints above and below the suspected fracture to provide adequate stability. Elevate and ice the injured limb (if neurovascular compromise is present, see 12 and 14 below).

6 Observe movements distal to the injury. Have the child move fingers and toes. Assess radial nerve function via finger and wrist extension. Test the median nerve with thumb to fingers apposition. The ulnar nerve can be assessed by spreading and adducting the fingers. For lower extremity injuries, have the child dorsiflex and plantarflex the toes.

7 Palpate the extremity distal to the injury and assess the temperature, capillary perfusion, and quality of the distal pulses.

8 Carefully palpate the injured part, noting the deformity pattern, hematoma, or crepitus. Listen for bruits. For upper extremity injuries, pay careful attention to the cubital fossa. For lower extremity injuries, closely examine the popliteal fossa. Evaluate for tenderness and swelling over associated compartments.

9 Assess sensation distal to the injury. In the upper extremity, test on the dorsum of the hand (radial nerve), thumb or index finger (median nerve), and fifth finger (ulnar nerve). In the leg, always assess sensation in the web space between the first and second toes (deep peroneal nerve).

10 Passively stretch the injured part to evaluate further for compartment syndrome.

11 Administer anesthesia if not already done and if the child is in pain.

12 Adequately splint the injured part. If neurovascular impairment exists before splinting, an attempt should be made to reduce the fracture. Reassess neurovascular status after a traction splint or appliance is in place to ensure that no new deficits are present.

13 Obtain appropriate radiographs with comparison views as needed.

14 Consult an orthopaedic surgeon if compartment syndrome is a concern.

CLINICAL TIPS

▶ It is important not to focus on the injured extremity at the expense of the ABCs.

▶ Dressings and splints applied elsewhere should be removed to ensure a good examination.

▶ The clinician should not be hesitant to attempt reduction of a fracture that is causing vascular compromise, particularly when an orthopaedic surgeon will not be available in a timely fashion.

▶ When reducing a fracture that is causing vascular compromise, the goal is restoration of blood flow, not definitive reduction.

▶ When unsure how to reduce such a fracture, gentle longitudinal traction is usually the most effective technique.

▶ The presence of distal pulses does not exclude the possibility of compartment syndrome.

a prehospital setting), as in the case of an obviously deformed lower leg with a pale, cool, pulseless foot.

Once a dorsalis pedis or posterior tibial pulse is obtained and perfusion restored to the foot, a posterior splint is applied (see Chapter 101) and orthopaedic consultation obtained. These patients may require arteriography and need close observation for signs of developing compartment syndrome (1,10).

Ankle Fractures

Another rare but significant injury in the pediatric population (most common in adolescents) is a severely displaced ankle fracture with associated dislocation. Such an injury may result in neurovascular impairment around or distal to the ankle joint. If prompt orthopedic care is unavailable and neurovascular impairment exists, as evidenced by a cool, pale, or pulseless foot, fracture-dislocation reduction should be performed. An assistant should apply steady, gentle proximal countertraction, and the injured ankle should be carefully rotated for proper alignment. As described for tibia and fibula shaft fractures, the second toe should be aligned with the tibial tubercle. A splint is applied, with care taken to avoid pressure over the bony prominences, and neurovascular status is reassessed (1,10).

▶ SUMMARY

Recognition and diagnosis of major arterial injury is relatively straightforward when pain, pulselessness, pallor, paralysis, and poikilothermia are present. In such cases, immediate surgical

intervention is mandatory in an attempt to restore vascular flow for limb salvage (2). In fact, by the time an injured extremity is cool and functionless, irreversible damage has likely already occurred (16).

Often the presentation is more subtle and complex. Signs of arterial injury include significant bleeding, an expanding hematoma, diminished or absent pulses, a bruit, distal ischemia, unremitting pain, and impaired distal sensation. The findings for arterial intimal tears may initially include a normal pulse. Perfusion also may be normal distally unless small vessel collapse occurs. For these reasons, frequent neurovascular reassessments are required. An understanding of regional anatomy, a knowledge of the mechanism of injury, and a high index of suspicion are needed when evaluating for vascular injury. As detailed in this chapter, significant injuries around the elbow or knee should be carefully and serially evaluated for signs of neurovascular impairment. Unstable pelvic fractures and displaced femur fractures may lead to significant blood loss and require immediate orthopaedic evaluation. Evaluation of penetrating extremity trauma may include Doppler flow noninvasive studies and/or angiography.

All children who sustain a fracture or dislocation require a thorough neurovascular examination. A complete examination includes assessment of color, temperature, capillary refill, pulses, movement, and sensation. Neurovascular compromise in the face of an orthopaedic injury is defined as impairment in blood flow or motor function or sensation in a distal extremity. Lack of cooperation and equivocal findings due to the child's developmental stage, fear, and pain warrant serial examinations and more careful observation. A neurovascularly compromised limb warrants emergent orthopaedic consultation.

▶ REFERENCES

1. Extremity trauma. In: American College of Surgeons, eds. *Advanced Trauma Life Support Course.* Chicago: American College of Surgeons; 1989:181–200.

2. Chervu A, Quiñonez-Baldrich WJ. Vascular complications in orthopaedic surgery. *Clin Orthop Relat Res.* 1988;235:275–288.

3. Mubarak SJ, Hargens AR. *Compartment Syndromes and Volkmann's Contracture.* Philadelphia: WB Saunders; 1981.

4. Van Ryn DE. Compartmental syndrome. In: Roberts JR, Hedges JR, eds. *Clinical Procedures in Emergency Medicine.* Philadelphia: WB Saunders; 1991:859–866.

5. Niemann KMW, Gould JS, Simmons B, et al. Injuries to and developmental deformities of the elbow in children. In: Bora FW, ed. *The Pediatric Upper Extremity: Diagnosis and Management.* Philadelphia: WB Saunders; 1986:213–246.

6. Moore KL. *Clinically Oriented Anatomy.* 2nd ed. Baltimore: Williams & Wilkins; 1985:626–793.

7. Beaty JH, Roberts JM. Fractures and dislocations of the knee. In: Rockwood C, Wilkens K, King R, eds. *Fractures in Children.* 3rd ed. Philadelphia: JB Lippincott; 1991:1171–1205.

8. Snell R, Smith M. *Clinical Anatomy for Emergency Medicine.* St. Louis: Mosby; 1993:575–739.

9. Netter FH. *Musculoskeletal System.* Summit, New Jersey: Ciba-Geigy Corporation; 1987:30–108. *The Ciba Collection of Medical Illustrations;* Vol. 8.

10. Bucknam CA. Vascular complications of fractures and dislocations. In: Gossling HR, Pillsbury SL, eds. *Complications of Fracture Management.* Philadelphia: JB Lippincott; 1984:123–140.

11. Dieckmann RA, Markison RE. Hand trauma. In: Grossman M, Dieckmann RA, eds. *Pediatric Emergency Medicine.* Philadelphia: JB Lippincott; 1991:300–304.

12. Simon R, Koenigsknecht S. *Emergency Orthopaedics: The Extremities.* 2nd ed. East Norwalk, CT: Appleton & Lange; 1987.

13. Willis RB, Rorabeck CH. Treatment of compartment syndrome in children. *Orthop Clin North Am.* 1990;21:401–412.

14. Moore RE, Friedman RJ. Current concepts in pathophysiology and diagnosis of compartment syndromes. *J Emerg Med.* 1985;7:657–662.

15. Lapuk S, Woodbury D. Volkmann ischemic contracture: a case report. *Orthop Rev.* 1988;17:618–624.

16. Allen MJ, Stirling AJ, Crawshaw CV, et al. Intracompartmental pressure monitoring of leg injuries. *J Bone Joint Surg Br.* 1985;67:53–57.

17. Whitesides TE, Haney TC, Morimoto K, et al. Tissue pressure measurements as a determinant for the need of fasciotomy. *Clin Orthop Relat Res.* 1975;113:43–51.

18. Garrett WV, Thompson JE, Talkington CM, et al. The role of fasciotomy in the acutely ischemic lower extremity. In: Kempczinksi RF, ed. *The Ischemic Leg.* Chicago: Year Book Medical Publishers; 1985:483–493.

19. Matsen FA, Mayo KA, Sheridan GW, et al. Monitoring of intramuscular pressure. *Surgery.* 1976;79:702–709.

20. Mubarak SJ, Hargens AR, Owen CA, et al. The wick catheter technique for measurement of intramuscular pressure. *J Bone Joint Surg Am.* 1976;58:1016–1020.

21. Nogi J. Common pediatric musculoskeletal emergencies. *Emerg Med Clin North Am.* 1984;2:409–422.

22. Rang M. Fractures with vascular damage. In: Rang M, ed. *Children's Fractures.* Philadelphia: JB Lippincott; 1983:44–48.

23. Whitesides TE Jr, Haney TC, Hiranda H, et al. A simple method for tissue pressure determination. *Arch Surg.* 1975;110:1311–1313.

24. Sherk H, Black JD. Orthopaedic emergencies. In: Fleisher GR, Ludwig S, eds. *Pediatric Emergency Medicine.* Baltimore: Williams & Wilkins; 1993:1397–1398.

25. Harris IE. Supracondylar fractures of the humerus. *Orthopaedics.* 1992;15:811–817.

26. McGraw JJ, Akbarnia BA, Hanel DP, et al. Neurologic complications resulting from supracondylar fractures of the humerus in children. *J Pediatr Orthop.* 1986;6:647–650.

27. Furrer M, Mark G, Ruedi T. Management of displaced supracondylar fractures of the humerus in children. *Injury.* 1991;22:259–262.

28. Vasli LR. Diagnosis of vascular injury in children with supracondylar fractures of the humerus. *Injury.* 1988;19:11–13.

29. Clement DA. Assessment of a treatment plan for managing acute vascular complications associated with supracondylar fractures of the humerus in children. *J Pediatr Orthop.* 1990;10:97–100.

30. Ray SA, Ivory JP, Beavis JP. Use of pulse oximetry during manipulation of supracondylar fractures of the humerus. *Injury.* 1991;22:103–104.

31. Klassen RA. Supracondylar fractures of the elbow in children. In: Morrey BF, ed. *The Elbow and Its Disorders.* Philadelphia: WB Saunders; 1985:182–221.

32. Worlock PH, Colton C. Severely displaced fractures of the humerus in children: a simple method of treatment. *J Pediatr Orthop.* 1987;7:49–53.

33. Alburger PD, Weidner PL, Betz RR. Supracondylar fractures of the humerus in children. *J Pediatr Orthop.* 1992;12:16–19.

34. Montgomery J. Dislocation of the knee. *Orthop Clin North Am.* 1987;18:149–156.

35. Smith WR, Oakley M, Morgan SJ. Current issues: pediatric pelvic fractures. *J Pediatr Orthop.* 2004;24:130–135.

36. Heetveld MJ, Harris I, Schlaphoff G, et al. Guidelines for the management of haemodynamically unstable pelvic fracture patients. *ANZ J Surg.* 2004;74:520–529.

JAMES M. CALLAHAN AND M. DOUGLAS BAKER

107

General Wound Management

▶ INTRODUCTION

Traumatic injuries are commonly encountered in pediatric patients. Ten million patients present to emergency departments (EDs) in the United States each year for treatment of traumatic wounds (1). A significant percentage of these patients are children. The goals of therapy in dealing with cutaneous wounds include restoration of function and structural integrity, prevention of infection, and production of cosmetically acceptable healing. These goals are interrelated, and adherence to sound principles of general wound management will lead to achieving them.

Effective wound management can be initiated by either emergency medical services (EMS) personnel or parents at the scene of an injury and is continued by nursing and medical personnel in the ED. The aim of therapy is to prevent secondary tissue damage or the development of infection so that the wound can heal primarily. Adequate preparation of equipment and a well-established treatment plan are among the keys to success.

General surgical principles, including adherence to standard aseptic techniques (Chapter 7), apply to all traumatic wounds. Appropriate restraint (Chapter 3) and anesthesia, sedation, and pain control (Chapters 33 to 35) will lead to improved outcomes. Preparation of the wound is an important prelude to actual wound closure, which is discussed in Chapters 108 and 109.

▶ ANATOMY AND PHYSIOLOGY

A working knowledge of both skin biomechanics and the mechanisms of soft-tissue trauma is necessary to manage wounds effectively. In addition, many factors can modify the overall effect and outcome of a particular injury in a given patient. Knowledge of these factors also is important.

The skin is remarkably resistant to traumatic forces (2) and is highly elastic due to its high content of elastin fibers. It also has a large number of collagen fibers, which give it added strength (2). A significant amount of force is required to cause tissue disruption.

The skin is constantly under static and dynamic tension. Static tension is caused by the force exerted on the skin by the underlying tissues at rest and the natural tension of the skin itself (3). Dynamic tension is caused by joint movement, muscle contraction, and gravity (3). Wounds under a large amount of tension tend to heal with wide, unattractive scars (3). Wound edges that retract more than 5 mm are thought to be under strong static tension (4). Wounds under low tension (edge retraction less than 5 mm) tend to heal with minimal scars. Wounds that cross joints or are perpendicular to wrinkle lines often lead to unattractive scars regardless of the repairer's skill (4). Patients and their families should be warned about these issues before repairs are made.

The skin is inhabited by micro-organisms, which can be a source of endogenous infection when trauma causes tissue disruption. Most of the bacteria in the skin reside in the horny layer of dead skin cells, which are in the process of being sloughed off. The stratum corneum below this layer is composed of tightly packed, viable cells that act as a barrier to bacteria (1). Exogenous sources of bacteria also can lead to wound infections.

The amount of bacteria present on the skin varies by anatomic location. Three distinct zones are characterized by the density of residing microorganisms (1). Moist areas (i.e., axillae, perineum, web spaces, and intertriginous areas) have extremely high bacterial concentrations and therefore are prone to infection when disrupted traumatically. Dry areas (i.e., back, chest, abdomen, arms, and legs) have low bacterial concentrations. Exposed areas (i.e., face, head, hands, and feet) have high bacterial concentrations, with the exception of the palms and dorsal surfaces of the hand where concentrations are low (1). Lacerations caused by contact with the oral cavity, especially the teeth (i.e., bite wounds), are highly contaminated and particularly prone to infection. Wounds that contact vaginal secretions or feces also will usually become infected.

It is important to consider the mechanism of injury in the management of soft-tissue trauma. Wounds are caused by mechanical or thermal forces (Chapter 113). Mechanical forces are of three types: shearing, tension, and compression (2).

Shearing occurs when forces of equal magnitude are applied to the skin in opposite directions along parallel planes (Fig. 107.1A) (2). A cut caused by an object with a sharp edge (e.g., a knife or glass) is an example of a shearing force. Little energy is transmitted to surrounding tissues, and therefore little devitalization of adjacent areas is seen. These wounds have a low potential for infection. Low-velocity missiles (e.g., .22-caliber rimfire bullets and bullets from handguns other than the .44 magnum pistol) usually cause a shear and compression injury that is confined to the actual missile tract (1). Direct injuries to internal organs or major vessels account for the morbidity and mortality associated with these wounds.

High-velocity missiles (including rifled slugs from a shotgun at a range of less than 45 meters) cause not only a shearing injury along the wound tract but also devitalization of adjacent tissues secondary to compression and the entrainment of large amounts of skin bacteria and debris. These wounds are highly prone to infection. They should be managed by extensive and repeated débridement of the wound in the operating room to remove devitalized tissue (1).

Tension injuries occur when the skin is struck with a blunt or semiblunt object at an angle of less than 90 degrees (Fig. 107.1B). Avulsion injuries and flap lacerations are common (2). Usually these injuries are associated with a larger force applied to the skin than is seen with shearing injuries. Devitalized tissue is more often seen adjacent to the wound. In addition, the vascular supply to a flap may be compromised, leading to necrosis. Tension wounds are more difficult to repair and more prone to infection.

Compression injuries, usually caused by blunt trauma directed at an angle of 90 degrees against skin that often overlies bones, cause the most tissue disruption (Fig. 107.1C) (2).

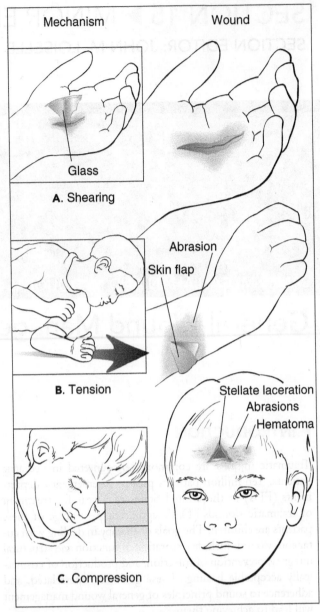

Figure 107.1 Common mechanisms of injury and resulting wounds.
A. Shearing injury.
B. Tension injury.
C. Compression injury.

Stellate lacerations with adjacent hematomas and abrasions are commonly seen. Large areas of devitalized tissue can result, and infection rates 100 times higher than those seen with shearing injuries have been reported (1).

Tissue damage caused by an object is directly related to the amount of kinetic energy the object transmits to the tissues involved. The kinetic energy of an object is described by the equation

$$KE = \tfrac{1}{2} mv^2$$

where m equals the mass of the object and v equals the object's velocity. Increasing the velocity, therefore, has a greater impact on the amount of tissue damage caused than increasing the mass of the object. Whether the material reacts with the biologic tissue or is relatively inert will determine if it will potentiate the development of infection. The configuration or shape of the object also will determine the nature of the wound it causes (2).

The environment in which the wounding event occurs will greatly modify the nature of the wound. Swamps, marshes, and other wet environments tend to have high bacterial loads. Wounds occurring on farms may be contaminated by animal feces. Further, soil and dirt have been shown to inhibit the infection-fighting capabilities of both the cellular and humoral immune systems (1). Organic components and inorganic clay components of soil inhibit white blood cell phagocytic and killing mechanisms and the bactericidal nature of human serum (1,5–7). These same elements also inactivate many antibiotics (8). Soil from swamps and similar areas have a high proportion of organic materials. Sand, a large-grained, inert component of soil, and the black dirt found on the surface of highways do not seem to have the same inhibitory effects (1).

Finally, characteristics of the patient will influence both the type of wound caused by a particular insult and the healing process. Patient age, general health, and intercurrent illnesses or medication can affect skin integrity and the processes involved in wound healing. Malnutrition, shock states, severe anemia, and uremia lead to delayed healing and increased infection rates (2). Chronic use of steroids can cause thinning of the skin analogous to the aging process, leading to large, shallow avulsions or flap injuries (2). These drugs can also impair healing mechanisms and increase infection rates.

The mechanism of injury, the characteristics of the wounding object, the environment in which the wound was sustained, and the health status of the patient are important to consider in the approach to general wound management. Developing an appropriate treatment plan based on the characteristics of the wound and the patient will improve the outcome. Characteristics that lead to increased areas of devitalization, delayed healing, or increased infection rates require specialized approaches to wound management.

▶ INDICATIONS

All wounds will benefit from some management. The clinician must determine the level of care necessary for the particular injury. Local cleansing and irrigation is important in almost all wounds, whereas additional interventions must be considered frequently but are only indicated in specific situations. Absolute contraindications to wound closure are few in number and include the presence of signs and symptoms of secondary bacterial infection, evidence of primary healing, and lack of cosmetic or functional need for closure.

Certain situations indicate the need for the removal of a foreign body within a wound (Chapter 111). In general, objects that are easily seen and grasped, objects likely to cause

intense inflammation, objects in close proximity to vital structures, and objects detected due to the development of a soft-tissue infection should be removed (9). Relatively inert foreign bodies that cause little tissue reaction and are not threatening because of their position or potential for migration may be left in place, especially if exploration would lead to further tissue damage (2,10). Other foreign bodies, especially those that are organic in nature, cause an intense tissue reaction and inflammation, which impairs the wound's ability to resist infection. These types of foreign bodies (e.g., wood, thorns, cactus spines, fabrics, devitalized skin, rooster spurs) must be diligently sought and removed or devastating infections may result (9,11,12). Metals vary in the amount of tissue reaction and inflammation they cause, which depends on their ability to be oxidized. Sometimes elusive foreign bodies may be more easily located and removed once they are encapsulated by scar tissue.

In grossly contaminated wounds and wounds with a large amount of devitalized tissue, débridement can decrease wound infections and complications by removing bacteria, debris, and devitalized tissue (see also discussion in Chapter 108). Devitalized tissue has been shown to impair the wound's ability to resist infection by acting as a culture medium that promotes bacterial growth, by inhibiting phagocytosis by leukocytes, and by limiting other leukocyte functions through the development of an anaerobic environment (13). Devitalized skin, fat, and muscle have been shown to cause comparable amounts of infection.

It is important to use débridement only when it is necessary, so as to not "make the wound *your* wound." Jagged-edged, uneven wounds have a much longer wound edge than straight lacerations. Jagged-edged wounds, if closed carefully, have a decreased amount of tension per unit length of wound edge and lead to better wound edge approximation (1). Converting such wounds to straight-edged wounds by débridement of skin and underlying tissue increases the amount of tension required to keep the wound edges approximated and therefore the width of the scar (1). Débridement of facial fat should be avoided, as unsightly depressions may result at the site of repair.

Fluid in a wound cavity, whether blood, pus, or serous fluid, will damage the defense mechanisms of the wound and lead to an increased risk of infection. Drains can be used to evacuate these fluids and improve healing. Drains should not be used prophylactically, however, as they actually may increase infection rates by damaging wound resistance to infection and permitting retrograde contamination of the wound by surface bacteria (14).

Wounds particularly prone to infection should be considered for delayed closure, as detailed in Chapter 108. These include markedly contaminated wounds, wounds with purulent material already present, wounds more than 12 to 19 hours old, missile wounds, wounds secondary to severe crush injury, wounds caused by human or animal bites, and wounds that have come into contact with feces, saliva (bites), or vaginal fluids. Such wounds, if cleaned appropriately and managed in an open fashion for 4 to 5 days, will develop a marked resistance

TABLE 107.1	TETANUS-PRONE WOUNDS

Wounds contaminated with soil, feces, saliva
Bite wounds
Crush wounds
Puncture wounds
Avulsion wounds
Missile wounds
Burns and frostbite

to infection and can undergo delayed closure at that time (15,16). It is important to keep in mind that clinical signs and symptoms of secondary bacterial infection are not clinically evident until at least 12 hours following contamination with pathogens (17).

All wounds carry the risk of tetanus as a potential complication. Contaminated wounds (especially involving soil or feces), wounds with devitalized tissue, and deep puncture wounds are particularly prone to contamination with *Clostridium tetani* (18). Patients who have not received at least three previous doses of tetanus toxoid or whose primary immunization status is unknown should receive 250 IU of tetanus immune globulin (TIG) intramuscularly if the wound is tetanus prone (Table 107.1). Recommendations for using TIG and tetanus toxoid based on the number of previous doses of toxoid, the type of wound, and the length of time since the last toxoid are provided in Table 107.2.

Increasing numbers of rabies cases have been reported among wild animals in recent years (19,20). Skunks, foxes, raccoons, and bats have a significant prevalence of rabies depending on their geographic location. Transmission of infection to stray and domestic dogs and cats, cattle, and even people has been reported. Bites by known, healthy, provoked domestic pets (dogs and cats) are unlikely to transmit rabies. Bites by unknown or unavailable animals or by skunks, foxes, raccoons, and bats should be treated as if the animal was rabid. Animals that can be observed and remain healthy for 10 days after biting a person could not have transmitted the virus. The virus has been transmitted in an aerosolized fashion in

TABLE 107.3	INDICATIONS FOR RABIES PROPHYLAXIS

1. Bites of wild carnivores (especially bats, foxes, raccoons, skunks, and woodchucks)
2. Bites of unknown or unavailable dogs and cats in rabies endemic areas
3. Bites of ill-appearing dogs and cats pending testing (may be discontinued if testing negative) or of animals who become ill during a 10-day observation period. Animals who are healthy and can be observed for 10 days do not need to be sacrificed and initial prophylaxis can wait until the animal develops symptoms.
4. Individual cases of bites by cattle, rodents, and lagomorphs (rabbits and hares, although they almost never transmit rabies)

Immunoprophylaxis is indicated if the animal is acting strangely (very aggressive behavior or nocturnal animals out during daylight hours).

caves inhabited by bats (19,20) and in enclosed rooms within dwellings in which bats have been found. Wounds for which rabies prophylaxis is indicated are listed in Table 107.3.

Wound repair that will require the open reduction of fractures, reanastomosis of vascular structures, or nerve or tendon repair should be taken to the operating room, where more controlled conditions allow for better wound healing (1). Extremely large wounds or wounds requiring extensive repairs in sensitive areas (e.g., wounds in the perineum, wounds in the medial canthus of the eye, extensive intraoral wounds) also should be considered for management in the operating room.

▶ EQUIPMENT

Sterile gloves and mask
Manual sphygmomanometer to aid hemostasis
Hair clippers or scissors for scalp wounds
Iodophor- or chlorhexidine-based solution for skin cleansing
Sterile saline solution for irrigation
Syringe, 35 mL for irrigation
Splashshield device for irrigation (may use 19-gauge needle or Angiocath)
High-porosity sponge
Sterile drapes
Gauze sponges
Antibiotic ointment, water-based
Microporous polypropylene dressings
Microporous tape
Cotton-tipped applicators
Needle driver
Scissors and/or scalpel
Forceps and/or skin hooks (may be made from 25-gauge needle and applicators)
Wound closure and anesthetic materials as needed (Chapters 35 and 108)

It is important, especially with pediatric patients, to have all of the equipment ready at the outset. Delays caused by the need to get equipment will only heighten the anxiety of the

TABLE 107.2	TETANUS PROPHYLAXIS				
No of doses of tetanus toxoid	Time since last dose	Clean wound		Tetanus-prone wound	
		TIG	dT*	TIG	dT*
<3 or unknown	<5 y	No	Yes	Yes	Yes
	5–10 y	No	Yes	Yes	Yes
	≥10 y	No	Yes	Yes	Yes
≥3	<5 y	No	No	No	No
	5–10 y	No	No	No	Yes
	≥10 y	No	Yes	No	Yes

*In children under 7 years of age, DTP or pediatric DT (if pertussis vaccine is contraindicated) should be given.

child as he or she waits for the procedure to begin. Instruments that may look threatening should be prepared out of the child's sight. The equipment should be appropriate for the degree of involvement and complexity of the procedure.

Protective equipment for health care personnel is extremely important (Chapter 8). Universal precautions should be followed by all personnel in dealing with wounds. Wound irrigation, hemostasis, and wound closure present opportunities for potentially contaminated blood to come into contact with the skin or mucous membranes of personnel involved in the procedure. A study in an adult ED population showed that 4% of patients who had blood drawn had unrecognized human immunodeficiency virus (HIV) infection. Patients with penetrating trauma had an increased seroprevalence rate independent of other known risk factors (21). Although the seroprevalence rate in children would be expected to be lower, it could approach 4%, depending on the age of the child (adolescents have increased rates) and the local incidence.

Splash guard devices can facilitate high-pressure irrigation while providing protection for physicians, nurses, and ancillary personnel. They are disposable and easy to use. They also are less threatening in appearance to a toddler or young school-age child than a needle or intravenous catheter. The Zerowet Splashshield (Zerowet, Los Angeles, CA) attaches to both Luer-Lok and slip-tip syringes and has a 19-gauge aperture that produces an adequate flow of irrigating solution.

For approximating skin edges, skin hooks, which can be fashioned from 25-gauge needles bent with a needle driver or hemostat and attached to the end of a cotton-tipped applicator, cause much less tissue trauma than forceps. Forceps (rather than fingers) should be used to catch suture needles that have been driven through a wound. Disposable instrument trays can be custom ordered to include the equipment most often required at a particular institution. Disposable trays are usually less expensive than recleaning, resterilizing, and packing reusable instruments. Good quality, standard instruments are available in disposable packages. Particularly fine instruments or instruments that are for specialized procedures and will only be used occasionally are more readily available and usually of better quality when purchased as reusable, surgical quality instruments.

▶ PROCEDURES

Hemostasis

As with any traumatic injury, the patient's overall status first should be assessed. Critical, life-threatening injuries should receive the highest priority. The airway and breathing should be assessed and stabilized. Vascular access should be obtained if the patient is hemodynamically unstable. Bleeding needs to be controlled. Even with minor wounds, a thorough secondary survey must be completed to ensure that concurrent injuries are not missed because the clinician's attention is drawn to the potentially disfiguring but not life-threatening laceration.

Control of bleeding, if it is significant, is an important part of the primary survey. Smaller wounds can wait until primary issues are addressed. Direct pressure followed by the application of a pressure dressing will lead to effective hemostasis in the vast majority of traumatic wounds (3,4) (see Fig. 28.1). EMS or ED personnel should ensure that all kinked or twisted flaps of tissue are returned to their original anatomic position to decrease the chance of vascular compromise.

Applying saline-soaked gauze pads will decrease heat loss from the wound while preventing desiccation of the wound edges, which in turn decreases the amount of devitalized tissue, lowers the chance of infection, and improves wound healing. If hemostasis cannot be achieved with direct pressure and the wound is on an extremity, the extremity should first be elevated for 1 minute. A sphygmomanometer placed proximal to the wound can then be inflated to a pressure just above the patient's systolic blood pressure (see Fig. 28.2). Tissue damage will not occur for approximately 2 hours following inflation (4).

Emergency Department Evaluation

The ED evaluation begins with the taking of an adequate history and the performance of a thorough physical examination using aseptic techniques (1) (Chapter 7). The mechanism and time of injury, characteristics of the wounding material, and location of the patient when the injury occurred should be noted. The possibility of a foreign body in the wound should be ascertained from the history. The patient's general health status, medication use, and immunization status, especially with regard to tetanus, should be determined.

A good physical examination of the injury requires hemostasis so that blood does not obscure the clinician's view. A sphygmomanometer can be used, as previously noted. Distal function is tested first. Neurovascular integrity and the function of all tendons possibly involved in the injury must be examined cautiously before anesthesia is used. Bones underlying or near the wound should be carefully palpated to elicit crepitus, instability, or tenderness, which could indicate the presence of a fracture. Radiographs should be obtained as indicated.

After the initial physical examination, the wound should be anesthetized (Chapter 35). When adequate anesthesia is obtained, *every* wound should be explored, even those that will not be sutured. The clinician should place the patient in a position that makes the wound easily accessible and should use adequate lighting. Appropriate anesthesia and hemostasis should provide a nearly bloodless and painless environment in which the clinician can work.

Exploration of extremity injuries should be performed through a full range of motion of the affected area. The examination also should be done in the position in which the injury occurred. Vascular structures, nerves, and tendons must be examined for incomplete injuries even if the distal examination seemed normal. The wound examination also should include a search for foreign bodies and devitalized tissues.

Foreign Bodies

The clinician must judge the likelihood that a foreign body is contained in the wound based on the history of the injury and the physical examination. Foreign bodies are rarely discovered unless they are anticipated by the person caring for the patient (9). Thorough exploration may reveal a foreign body in the wound but does not guarantee that one does not exist. Foreign bodies may be larger than the wound defect, especially if the wound extends into fatty tissue. Seeing the bottom of the wound decreases but does not eliminate the chance that a foreign body is present (22). Physical examination alone cannot exclude the presence of a foreign body in fatty tissues.

Wounds suspicious for the presence of foreign bodies should be radiographed. Multiple projections, surface markers, proper film exposure techniques (use of soft-tissue penetration settings), and the use of fluoroscopy can increase the sensitivity of radiographs in detecting foreign bodies (9). Most radiopaque objects, even if small, are easily demonstrated. All types of glass should be detectable on appropriately exposed radiographs regardless of their lead or heavy metal content (23). Glass fragments as small as 0.5 mm can be visualized on radiographs (24). Multiple projections will cast the shadow away from overlying bones and can result in alignment of the long axis of the foreign body with the long axis of the radiograph beam, increasing the chance of detection. Using xeroradiographs, computed tomography scans, and ultrasound (Chapter 135) may increase the probability of detecting less radiopaque foreign bodies (9). Nonradiopaque foreign bodies may present as filling defects, or air may be evident surrounding them on films (9).

Once a foreign body is detected, a decision must be made as to whether it will be removed based on its location and degree of reactivity. Removal of foreign bodies is discussed in Chapter 111.

Wound Cleansing and Irrigation

Using antiseptic solutions for wound cleansing is somewhat controversial. Certainly the intact skin surrounding a wound should be cleansed with an antiseptic solution (usually an iodophor-, hexachlorophene-, or chlorhexidine-containing solution). Obvious dirt or other foreign materials should be removed from the wound by irrigation or gentle scrubbing (Fig. 107.2A). Experimental evidence in laboratory animals suggests that using antiseptic solutions within the wound may damage tissue defenses and actually potentiate the development of infection (25,26). In these studies, the detergent component of scrub solutions seemed to be especially damaging to wound defenses. Povidone-iodine in the absence of detergents did not seem to increase infections but offered no therapeutic benefit over saline alone (26).

In contrast, a clinical trial showed that gently scrubbing wounds with a 1% povidone-iodine solution for 60 seconds reduced the incidence of wound infections when compared with saline irrigation alone (27). Most authorities recommend

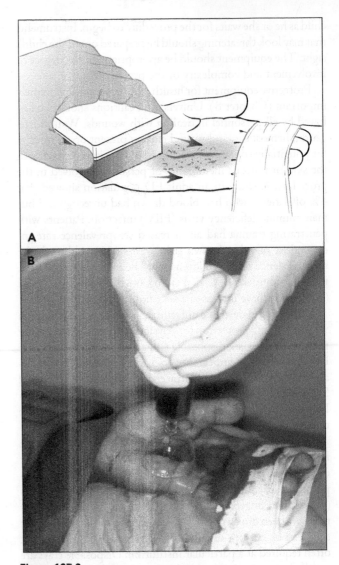

Figure 107.2
A. Gentle mechanical scrubbing of contaminated wound.
B. High-pressure irrigation using a Zerowet Splashshield.

using only saline or nontoxic surfactants within wounds to effect cleansing (25,26,28–30). "The only solution that should be placed in a wound is one that can be safely poured in the physician's eye" is a good axiom to follow (31), although testing various solutions in this way is not recommended.

Saline irrigation of wounds has become a standard practice in treating contaminated or dirty wounds. However, studies have not shown any benefit from the use of sterile saline over the use of plain tap water in terms of rates of infection (32,33). High-pressure irrigation of at least 8 lb/in^2 is required to remove most foreign material (Fig. 107.2B) (28,34). High-pressure irrigation of this magnitude can be accomplished using a 35-mL syringe and a 19-gauge plastic vascular catheter. Using 50 to 100 mL of fluid per centimeter of length of the laceration has been recommended (35). It has been shown that irrigation fluid disseminates laterally through the sides of the wound but does not penetrate beneath the wound bed (34).

Bacteria contaminating the wounds did not seem to be carried with the irrigating fluid in this model. Irrigation damaged tissue defenses in experimentally infected wounds. Therefore, this technique should only be used in contaminated wounds where the benefits of cleansing outweigh the consequences of tissue damage (34).

Irrigation also can be hazardous for medical personnel irrigating the wound. A splash of blood and possibly infective agents into the eyes or mucous membranes of the irrigator may transmit HIV, hepatitis B, and other bloodborne infections. As mentioned previously, studies have shown surprisingly high seroprevalence rates for these infections in urban, adult ED populations (2,36). Using splash shields has been shown to effectively decrease splatter onto the face and chest of the irrigator, and correctly using the Zerowet Splashshield eliminated all facial splash (37).

Irrigation can effectively eliminate large particles, soil, and loose pieces of devitalized tissue but not bacteria and small particles. Mechanical scrubbing of wounds with sponges is an effective way to remove bacteria but can lead to tissue damage and decreased resistance to infection. Sponges with a low porosity are more damaging, and soaking the sponge in saline does not decrease the damage caused (38). Various surfactant compounds in the polyol family have been developed for use with sponges, including Pluronic F-68 (Shur Medical Corp., Beaverton, OR) and Poloxamer 188 (Calgon Corp., St. Louis, MO) (28–30,38). These compounds have been shown to be effective and safe and do not potentiate tissue damage. Scrubbing should be used in particularly contaminated wounds and when irrigation may distort the wound edges and compromise the cosmetic result (e.g., in the periorbital area, where the loose areolar tissue is easily distended by lateral dissemination of irrigation fluids) (28,30). Facial and scalp wounds tend to have low infection rates. Irrigation of these wounds has not been shown to significantly alter infection rates or cosmetic outcomes when compared with simply washing the wound with normal saline and gauze (39).

Hair Removal

Hair has long been regarded as a potential source of wound contamination, and data in the surgical literature support this view (1,40). Hair also can make both the placement and removal of sutures difficult and, in the case of removal, more painful. Razor removal of hair has resulted in increased rates of postoperative infections in surgical patients (41,42). Removal of hair with electric clippers has led to decreased infection rates (41). The blade assemblies of electric clippers need to be adequately sterilized after each use (41), which can be difficult in a busy ED, especially if multiple scalp lacerations are being treated at the same time. Alternatively, petroleum jelly can be used to keep unruly hairs out of the wound while suturing takes place, or a small area adjacent to the wound edges may be trimmed close to the scalp with scissors. Eyebrows should never be shaved or clipped, as they serve as important landmarks for wound alignment during

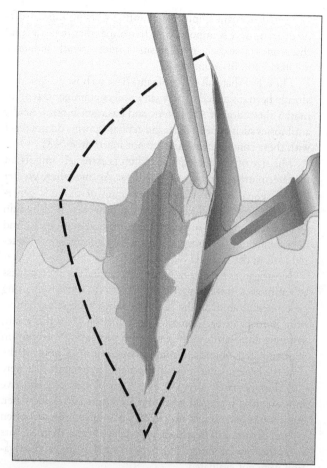

Figure 107.3 Wound débridement is performed to remove heavily contaminated or non-viable tissue.

repair; also, once shaved (or clipped), they may not grow back.

Débridement

Débridement can be an important step in wound management. It should be used to remove heavily contaminated tissue and also to remove devitalized tissue that will foster bacterial growth (Fig. 107.3) (13). However, débridement can also cause problems with wound healing. Excessive removal of tissue results in increased tension at the wound margins and, subsequently, increased scarring. If complete débridement of the wound is contraindicated because of the presence of vital structures or the probability of a poor cosmetic result, high-pressure irrigation should be used. This should be followed by meticulous débridement of all clearly nonviable tissue (13).

Antibiotics

One major goal of wound care is to prevent infection, which will lead to a decreased rate of complications and a more aesthetically pleasing scar. The rate of infection in properly cleansed nonbite wounds is generally quite low (less than 1%). Nevertheless, using prophylactic antibiotics has been advocated in many clinical situations involving minor soft-tissue trauma. It is important to remember that many wound characteristics and the mechanism of injury greatly influence the likelihood of an infection.

The effect that soil contaminants have on host defenses has already been discussed. These same soil contaminants tend to inhibit the action of amphoteric and basic antibiotics. Acidic antibiotics such as penicillins and cephalosporins do not react with these contaminants and are not inactivated (43).

The size of the bacterial inoculum is extremely important in determining if infection develops. An inoculum greater than or equal to 10^5 bacteria per gram of tissue is generally necessary to produce infection in otherwise healthy skin (44). Cleansing the wound (irrigation and scrubbing) and débridement, if necessary, are intended to decrease the bacterial load in the wound.

Investigators have attempted to determine the effectiveness of antibiotics in reducing wound infections. One study using experimental animals showed that, to be successful, antibiotics must be given soon after the injury (45). In this study, systemic antibiotics were effective in preventing infection in contaminated wounds if administered within 1 hour of the time the experimental wound was made. In wounds that were closed immediately after the injury, antibiotics were effective in preventing infection when initiated up to 24 hours later. Antibiotics had almost no effect (75% infection rate) when wound closure and treatment were delayed more than 3 hours from the time of injury. The benefits of cleansing and irrigation were not evaluated.

This research also showed that wounds left open exhibit an increase in their vascular permeability, which leads to a buildup of a protein exudate in the wound. Fibrin is deposited and envelops the bacteria in the wound, shielding it from the effects of antibiotics. Proteases delivered into the wound (trypsin or Travase) will break down these fibrinous deposits and may potentiate the beneficial effects of antibiotics (43,45).

By 3 to 6 hours, the bacterial concentration within wounds reaches 10^6 per gram of tissue, and infection rates increase greatly. Some clinical studies have shown that time to repair has a marked impact on infection rates, suggesting that the institution of antibiotic therapy has little effect on infection rates in wounds not closed before 3 to 6 hours (46,47). These studies support the work performed with animals. However, other clinical studies have found no difference in infection rates for pediatric wounds closed more than 6 hours after injury and those closed earlier (48).

Increased rates of infection have been found in wounds involving the hands and feet (47,49). The higher rates seem related more to the types of injury seen in these regions and to the level of bacterial contamination than to a decreased biologic resistance to infection inherent in these sites (15). Despite this finding, randomized clinical trials have failed to show any benefit of prophylactic antibiotics in wounds involving the hand (50,51). No studies have addressed the efficacy of prophylactic antibiotics in lower extremity wounds. Despite the lack of convincing data that prophylactic antibiotics are

TABLE 107.4	INDICATIONS FOR PROPHYLACTIC ANTIBIOTICS

1. Patient prone to development of infective endocarditis
2. Immunosuppressed patients (relative indication)
3. Soft-tissue lacerations occurring in previously lymphedematous tissue
4. Wounds judged to be contaminated or dirty by the clinician (especially in dependent areas)
5. Stellate lacerations with adjacent abrasions resulting from high impact
6. Delayed wound cleansing and repair (between 6 and 18 hours after injury, bacterial colony counts reach potentially infective concentrations, and therefore open management and delayed closure should be considered)
7. Wounds contaminated by saliva, feces, vaginal fluids (open management and delayed closure should be considered)
8. Missile wounds

efficacious in treating minor soft-tissue injuries, most experts suggest certain indications for using antibiotics in soft-tissue injury (Table 107.4) (15).

If the decision is made to give an antibiotic, one that has a broad spectrum and is effective against staphylococci and streptococci as well as facultative organisms should be chosen. Cephalexin is an inexpensive, well-tolerated, and effective choice. Oxacillin, dicloxacillin, and amoxicillin-clavulanic acid also are effective. Penicillin-sensitive patients can be cautiously treated with cephalosporins. If the patient also had a history of cephalosporin sensitivity, erythromycin, erythromycin-sulfisoxazole, and clindamycin are acceptable alternatives. Antibiotics are not a substitute for meticulous wound care and aseptic techniques.

Drains

Drains should be placed to evacuate any fluid-filled wound cavities. Vented, closed suction drainage is the most efficacious system (52). If a complex wound needs draining, a surgical consultation regarding the details of optimal drain choice and placement may be warranted.

Animal and Human Bites

Bite wounds are especially prone to infection due to the high inoculum of bacteria usually accompanying them and to the fact that many are puncture wounds or crush-type injuries. Puncture wounds require specific wound management techniques, which are described in Chapter 110. Bite wounds are common injuries. Over one million people are bitten by dogs each year in the United States, most of them children, and dog bites account for about 1% of ED visits (19,53,54). The incidence of cat, human, and other mammalian bites is lower but still significant.

Dog bites become infected somewhat more frequently than lacerations in general (54). However, with meticulous wound preparation, including high-pressure irrigation and débridement of devitalized tissues, most can be safely sutured to effect primary closure. *Staphylococcus*, *Streptococcus*, and

Bacteroides species, anaerobic cocci, and *Pasteurella canis* are the most common infecting organisms (54–56). Obviously infected wounds should be cultured and antibiotic therapy directed by sensitivities. Prophylactic antibiotics are probably indicated for dog bites of the hand, bites more than 12 hours old, and bites that inflict a deep puncture wound.

Amoxicillin-clavulanic acid is an excellent choice for use in animal bite wounds. When appropriate per-kilogram doses are used and given at least 6 hours apart (with food), gastrointestinal side effects can be minimized. Erythromycin has been used in patients who are penicillin sensitive (57). Some practitioners prefer dicloxacillin or cephalexin because these cost less and produce fewer side effects. They argue that although the in vitro activity of dicloxacillin and cephalexin against *P. canis* is inadequate, the clinical outcome with these agents in dog and cat bites is good (58). Clindamycin is another alternative agent for use in patients with allergies to penicillin.

Cat bites have a higher incidence of infection (56,59) and should not be closed if at all possible (14). These are usually small-caliber puncture wounds that result in the inoculation of bacteria relatively deep below the skin surface. The microbiology of the infecting organisms is similar to that seen in dog bites, although *P. multocida* (rather than *P. canis*) is implicated in up to 50% of infected cat bites (54,56,58). All cat bite wounds should receive meticulous irrigation and débridement as well as prophylactic antibiotics. Irrigation and débridement may be difficult to achieve due to the small size of the break in the skin.

Animal bites also raise the issue of rabies prophylaxis. Soap and water cleansing of wounds will decrease the transmission of rabies. Wounds at risk for rabies infection should not be sutured (20,60). Bites that carry a risk of rabies (see Table 107.3) require passive and active immunization. Human rabies immune globulin (RIG) is administered in a dose of 20 IU/kg. It is currently recommended that the entire dose of RIG be infiltrated around the margins of the wound. When impractical, most clinicians will infiltrate half the dose around the wound and administer the remainder intramuscularly at a site distant from the site of active immunization. Injection in the gluteal area is recommended. In instances when local infiltration is either impractical or particularly painful, the entire dose may be given intramuscularly.

Human diploid cell vaccine (HDCV) or another brand of active vaccine should be given in a dose of 1 mL intramuscularly on the initial day of treatment and repeated on days 3, 7, 14, and 28 (20,60). The deltoid area is the preferred injection site. RabAvert is an alternative to HDCV. It is considered equivalent in terms of safety and efficacy and is given in the same dose and according to the same schedule as HDCV.

Human bites have traditionally been thought of as having a high infection rate (57,61). Yet it has been argued that this is related more to the site and mechanism of injury and to delays in seeking treatment than any unique characteristics of human bites or their microbiology (56). Human bites often involve a high-impact mechanism of injury (e.g., fist fights, sports injuries), which results in tissue crushing and devitalization. This might partially explain why injuries to the dorsum of the hand (closed-fist injuries) have a much higher infection rate than other bite wounds. Wounds to the dorsal metacarpophalangeal joints should be considered bite wounds until proven otherwise, as the patient is often reluctant to admit involvement in an altercation. It is especially important to examine these wounds through a full range of motion, including full flexion, for penetration of the joint capsule or extensor tendons. A tendon injury that occurred when the fist was clenched may not be visible in the wound field when the fingers are extended.

Staphylococci, streptococci (including group A streptococci), *Bacteroides* species, anaerobic cocci, and *Eikenella corrodens* are organisms implicated in infections caused by human bites (54,58,59). Human bite wounds should not be closed unless on the face or in a well-vascularized area and then only if they are thoroughly irrigated and débrided (57). All persons with puncture wounds or lacerations resulting from human bites should be treated with prophylactic antibiotics. Most human bites in children result only in abrasions or contusions that require only surface cleansing. For human bite wounds requiring antibiotic treatment, amoxicillin-clavulanic acid is again an excellent choice (56). If dicloxacillin or cephalexin is used, penicillin must be added to cover *E. corrodens*. Giving a patient two medicines instead of one is likely to decrease patient compliance.

Tetanus Prophylaxis

All wounds should be assessed for the risk of tetanus as a potential complication, and the immunization status of all patients should be determined. When indicated, 250 IU of TIG should be administered intramuscularly for tetanus-prone wounds (see Table 107.1). Also when indicated, a single dose of tetanus toxoid should be administered intramuscularly as soon as possible after the injury (see Table 107.2).

Postrepair Wound Care

Dressings are an important part of wound care. An effective dressing will prevent contamination of the wound by exogenous bacteria and promote epithelial migration and healing (1). As long as the outer surface of the dressing remains dry, it is an effective barrier to bacteria. By day 3 after primary closure, wounds are remarkably resistant to infection from external contamination.

Drying of the wound impairs healing. A dressing that prevents evaporation of water will keep the eschar and dermis at the wound site moist and promote rapid re-epithelialization (Fig. 107.4A) (1). Nonwoven, microporous polypropylene dressings are recommended and should be attached to the skin by side strips of microporous tape (1). Water-based antibiotic ointments under the dressings keep wound edges moist, which facilitates both healing and suture removal.

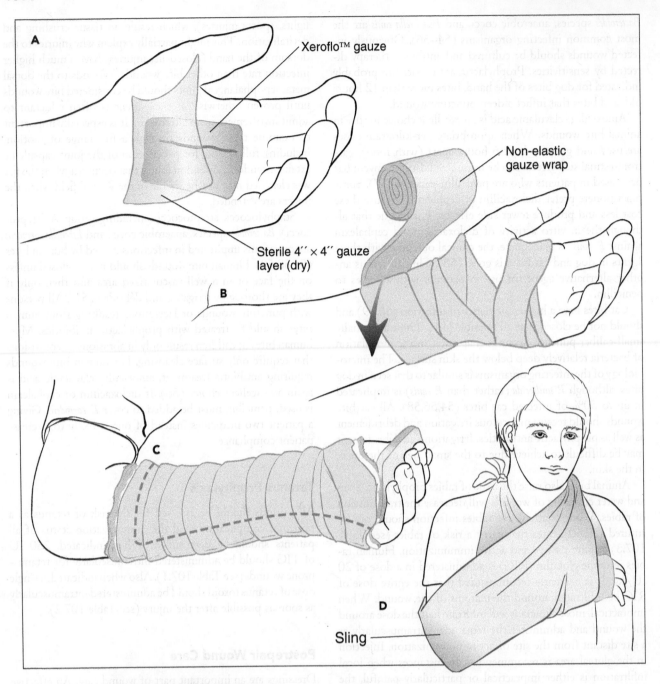

Figure 107.4 Wound dressing.
A. Application of a moist nonadherent dressing followed by a dry covering.
B. Application of a nonelastic gauze wrap.
C. Application of a splint.
D. Wound elevation.

Facial wounds do not need to be dressed. To remove blood clots along the wound edge, which will potentiate scar development, these wounds should be swabbed with half-strength hydrogen peroxide three to four times per day until suture removal (I). Abraded skin should be coated with water-soluble ointments. Wounds in cosmetically sensitive areas, especially abrasions, should be covered with sunblock with a protection factor of at least 15 for 6 months after injury to prevent the development of hyperpigmented scars.

Pressure dressings with nonelastic gauze wrap can prevent fluid accumulation in wounds, thereby inhibiting the development of infection (Fig. 107.4B). The amount of pressure applied proximal to extremity wounds is decreased to prevent edema development. Immobilization improves the ability of a wound to resist infection (I). Extremity wounds should be elevated and immobilized by slings and splints as needed (Fig. 107.4C,D). Wounds that are closed primarily can be washed and gently patted dry after 48 hours. Vigorous rubbing should

SUMMARY

1 Obtain hemostasis with direct pressure to the wound, or elevate the extremity for 1 minute and then apply a sphygmomanometer (see Chapter 28 and Figs. 28.1 and 28.2).

2 Obtain adequate history, including:
- ▶ Mechanism of injury
- ▶ Wounding object—mass, velocity, characteristics
- ▶ Environment in which the injury occurred
- ▶ Time of injury
- ▶ General health of the patient
- ▶ Medications
- ▶ Allergies
- ▶ Immunization status

3 Perform thorough physical examination, including:
- ▶ Assessment of distal neurovascular function
- ▶ Assessment of tendon integrity
- ▶ Palpation of adjacent bony structures

4 Anesthetize the wound.

5 Explore the wound through the full range of motion and in the position of injury.

6 Prepare all necessary equipment in advance.

7 Evaluate for the presence of foreign bodies.

8 Remove all reactive foreign bodies (vegetable materials, wood, organic materials, clothing) and foreign bodies near vital structures or with the potential to migrate.

9 Cleanse the wound using high pressure irrigation.

10 Use mechanical scrubbing for particularly contaminated wounds.

11 Débride obviously contaminated wounds and all devitalized tissue.

12 Consider using antibiotics for:
- ▶ Contaminated wounds
- ▶ Bite wounds
- ▶ Crush wounds
- ▶ Foot wounds
- ▶ Other indications (Table 107.4)

13 Place drains if fluid is present.

14 Administer appropriate tetanus and rabies prophylaxis.

15 Apply a dressing.

16 Immobilize the wound.

17 Elevate the wounded area when possible.

 CLINICAL TIPS

- ▶ Threatening instruments should be kept out of the child's sight.
- ▶ Overzealous débridement must always be avoided.
- ▶ Wounds to the metacarpophalangeal joints should be considered bite wounds until proven otherwise.
- ▶ Foreign bodies are not always visible in the wound.
- ▶ The probability of wound infection is influenced by the location of the wound, the mechanism of injury, the characteristics of the patient, and the environment in which the wound occurred.
- ▶ When used in wound care, prophylactic antibiotics should be initiated as early as possible.
- ▶ Antibiotics are not a substitute for meticulous irrigation and débridement.
- ▶ Moist dressings that face the wound improve healing. Dry dressings that face the environment prevent infection.
- ▶ Healing wounds are more sensitive to and need protection from sun exposure.

be avoided, as this can damage healing edges of the wound and lead to dehiscence and/or increased scarring.

▶ COMPLICATIONS

Complications from the general wound management techniques covered in this chapter should be minimal. Poor results, including wound infections and less than optimal scars, are more likely to occur if these principles are not followed. Meticulous and thorough wound preparation, including a complete and detailed history and physical examination, is as important as the actual wound closure. As mentioned previously, antibiotics are never a substitute for thorough wound cleansing, débridement, and proper aseptic techniques. Overzealous débridement, especially in cosmetically important areas and areas under high amounts of static skin tension, will lead to scars that are wider than necessary and unsightly. Using antiseptic scrub solutions and other foreign substances in wounds may actually potentiate wound infections.

▶ SUMMARY

General wound management techniques are often as important as actual wound closure in determining the eventual outcome in cases of soft-tissue trauma. A working knowledge of skin biomechanics and wounding mechanisms will provide the basic information necessary for developing a rational treatment plan for each individual patient and injury. Adequate preparation and attention to detail throughout the process will minimize the risk of wound infection and maximize the chances of an optimal wound repair.

▶ REFERENCES

1. Edlich RF, Rodeheaver GT, Morgan RF, et al. Principles of emergency wound management. *Ann Emerg Med.* 1988;17:1284–1302.
2. Trott A. Mechanisms of soft tissue trauma. *Ann Emerg Med.* 1988;17:1279–1283.
3. Thacker JG, Stolnecker MC, Allaire PE, et al. Practical applications of skin biomechanics. *Clin Plast Surg.* 1977;4:167–171.
4. Edlich RF, Rodeheaver GT, Thacker JG. The evaluation of wounds in the emergency department. In: Tintinalli JE, Krome RL, Ruiz E, eds. *Emergency Medicine: A Comprehensive Study Guide.* 3rd ed. New York: McGraw-Hill; 1992:1027-1030.
5. Haury BB, Rodeheaver GT, Pettry D, et al. Inhibition of nonspecific defenses by soil infection potentiating factors. *Surg Gynecol Obstet.* 1977;144:19–24.
6. Dougherty SH, Fiegel VO, Nelson RD, et al. Effects of soil potentiating factors on neutrophils in vitro. *Am J Surg.* 1985;150:306–311.
7. Rodeheaver GT, Pettry D, Turnbull V, et al. Identification of wound potentiating factors in soil. *Am J Surg.* 1974;128:8–14.
8. Roberts AH, Rye DG, Edgerton MT, et al. Activity of antibiotics in contaminated wounds containing clay soil. *Am J Surg.* 1979;137:381–383.
9. Lammers RL. Soft tissue foreign bodies. *Ann Emerg Med.* 1988;17:1336–1347.
10. Anderson MA, Newmeyer WL III, Kilgore ES Jr. Diagnosis and treatment of retained foreign bodies in the hand. *Am J Surg.* 1982;144:63–67.
11. Cooler JO, Kleiman MB, West K, et al. Retained spur following a rooster attack. *Pediatrics.* 1992;90:106–108.
12. Cracchiolo A III. Wooden foreign bodies in the foot. *Am J Surg.* 1980;140:585–587.
13. Haury B, Rodeheaver G, Veusko J, et al. Débridement: an essential component of traumatic wound care. *Am J Surg.* 1978;135:238–242.
14. Magee C, Rodeheaver GT, Golden GT, et al. Potentiation of wound infection by surgical drains. *Am J Surg.* 1976;131:547–549.
15. Edlich RF, Kenney JG, Morgan RF, et al. Antimicrobial treatment of minor soft tissue lacerations: a critical review. *Emerg Med Clin North Am.* 1986;4:561–580.
16. Edlich RF, Rogers W, Kasper G, et al. Studies in the management of the contaminated wound, I: optimal time for closure of contaminated open wounds; II: comparison of resistance to infection of open and closed wounds during healing. *Am J Surg.* 1969;117:323–329.
17. Talan DA, Citron DM, Abrahamian FM, et al. Bacteriologic analysis of infected dog and cat bites. Emergency Medicine Animal Bite Infection Study Group. *N Engl J Med.* 1999;340:85–92.
18. American Academy of Pediatrics. Tetanus. In: Pickering LK, ed. *Red Book: 2003 Report of the Committee on Infectious Diseases.* 26th ed. Elk Grove Village, IL: American Academy of Pediatrics; 2003:611.
19. Schmidt MJ, Olson JG, Krebs JW. Rabies goes wild. *Contemp Pediatr.* 1993;10(8):36–46.
20. Fishbein DB, Robinson LE. Rabies. *N Engl J Med.* 1993;329:1632–1638.
21. Kelen GD, Fritz S, Qaqish B, et al. Unrecognized human immunodeficiency virus infection in emergency department patients. *N Engl J Med.* 1988;318:1645–1650.
22. Avner JR, Baker MD. Lacerations involving glass: the role of routine roentgenograms. *Am J Dis Child.* 1992;146:600–602.
23. Felman AH, Fisher MS. The radiographic detection of glass in soft tissue. *Radiology.* 1969;92:1529–1531.
24. Tandberg D. Glass in the hand and foot: will an x-ray film show it? *JAMA.* 1982;248:1872–1874.
25. Custer J, Edlich RF, Prusak M, et al. Studies in the management of the contaminated wound, V: an assessment of the effectiveness of PHisoHex and Betadine surgical scrub solutions. *Am J Surg.* 1971;121:572–575.
26. Rodeheaver GT, Bellamy W, Kody M, et al. Bactericidal activity and toxicity of iodine-containing solutions in wounds. *Arch Surg.* 1982;117:181–186.
27. Gravett A, Sterner S, Clinton JE, et al. A trial of povidone-iodine in the prevention of infection in sutured lacerations. *Ann Emerg Med.* 1987;16:167–171.
28. Edlich RF, Rodeheaver GT, Thacker JG. Wound preparation. In: Tintinalli JE, Krome RL, Ruiz E, eds. *Emergency Medicine: A Comprehensive Study Guide.* 3rd ed. New York: McGraw-Hill; 1992:1037–1039.
29. Rodeheaver GT, Kurtz L, Kircher BJ, et al. Pluronic F-68: a promising new skin wound cleanser. *Ann Emerg Med.* 1980;9:572–576.
30. Bryant CA, Rodeheaver GT, Reeum EM, et al. Search for a nontoxic surgical scrub solution for periorbital lacerations. *Ann Emerg Med.* 1984;13:317–321.
31. Branemark PI, Albrektsson B, Lindstrom J, et al. Local tissue effects of wound disinfectants. *Acta Chir Scand.* 1966;357(suppl):166–176.
32. Moscati R, Mayrose J, Fincher L, et al. Comparison of normal saline with tap water for wound irrigation. *Am J Emerg Med.* 1998;16:379–381.
33. Valente JH. Wound irrigation in children: saline solution or tap water? *Ann Emerg Med.* 2003;41:609–616.
34. Wheeler CB, Rodeheaver GT, Thacker JG, et al. Side effects of high pressure irrigation. *Surg Gynecol Obstet.* 1976;143:775–778.
35. Knapp JF. Updates in wound management for the pediatrician. *Pediatr Clin North Am.* 1999;46:1201–1213.
36. Kelan GD, Green GB, Prucell RH, et al. Hepatitis B and hepatitis C in emergency department patients. *N Engl J Med.* 1992;326:1399–1404.
37. Pigman EC, Karch DB, Scott JL. Splatter during jet irrigation cleansing of a wound model: a comparison of three inexpensive devices. *Ann Emerg Med.* 1993;22:1563–1567.
38. Rodeheaver GT, Smith SL, Thacker JG, et al. Mechanical cleansing of contaminated wounds with a surfactant. *Am J Surg.* 1975;129:241–245.
39. Hollander JE, Richman PB, Werblud M, et al. Irrigation in facial and scalp wounds: does it alter outcome? *Ann Emerg Med.* 1998;31:73–77.
40. Dineen P, Druisin L. Epidemics of postoperative wound infections associated with hair carriers. *Lancet.* 1973;2:1157–1159.
41. Alexander JW, Fischer JE, Boyajian M, et al. The influence of hair removal methods on wound infections. *Arch Surg.* 1983;118:347–352.
42. Masterson TM, Rodeheaver GT, Morgan RF, et al. Bacteriologic evaluation of electric clippers for surgical hair removal. *Am J Surg.* 1984;144:301–302.
43. Edlich RF, Rodeheaver GT, Thacker JG. Antibiotics and drains in wound management. In: Tintinalli JE, Krome RL, Ruiz E, eds. *Emergency Medicine: A Comprehensive Study Guide.* 3rd ed. New York: McGraw-Hill; 1992:1040–1042.
44. Magee C, Hauvy B, Rodeheaver GT, et al. A rapid slide technique for quantitating wound bacterial count. *Am J Surg.* 1977;133:760–762.

45. Edlich RF, Smith QT, Edgerton MT. Resistance of the surgical wound to antimicrobial prophylaxis and its mechanism of development. *Am J Surg.* 1973;126:583–591.

46. Morgan WJ, Hutchinson D, Johnson HM. The delayed treatment of wounds of the hand and forearm under antibiotic cover. *Br J Surg.* 1980;67:140–141.

47. Thirlby RC, Blair J III, Thal ER. The value of prophylactic antibiotics for simple lacerations. *Surg Gynecol Obstet.* 1983;156:212–216.

48. Baker MD, Lanuti M. The management and outcome of lacerations in urban children. *Ann Emerg Med.* 1990;19:1001–1005.

49. Rutherford WH, Spence RAJ. Infection in wounds sutured in the accident and emergency department. *Ann Emerg Med.* 1980;9:350–352.

50. Grossman JAI, Adams JP, Kunec J. Prophylactic antibiotics in simple hand lacerations. *JAMA.* 1981;245:1055–1056.

51. Haughey RE, Lammers RL, Wagner DK. Use of antibiotics in the initial management of soft tissue hand wounds. *Ann Emerg Med.* 1981;10:187–192.

52. Golden GT, Roberts TL, Rodeheaver GT, et al. A new filtered sump tube for wound drainage. *Am J Surg.* 1975;129:716–717.

53. Rest JG, Goldstein EJC. Management of human and animal bite wounds. *Emerg Med Clin North Am.* 1985;3:117–126.

54. Brook I. Microbiology of human and animal bite wounds in children. *Pediatr Infect Dis J.* 1987;6:29–32.

55. Callaham M. Dog bite wounds. *JAMA.* 1980;244:2327–2328.

56. Aghababian RV, Conte JE Jr. Mammalian bite wounds. *Ann Emerg Med.* 1980;9;2:79–83.

57. Trott A. Care of mammalian bites. *Pediatr Infect Dis J.* 1987;6:8.

58. Callaham M. Controversies in antibiotic choices for bite wounds. *Ann Emerg Med.* 1988;17:1321–1329.

59. Edlich RF, Spengler MD, Rodeheaver GT, et al. Emergency department management of mammalian bites. *Emerg Med Clin North Am.* 1986;4:595–604.

60. American Academy of Pediatrics. Rabies. In: Pickering LK, ed. *Red Book: 2003 Report of the Committee on Infectious Diseases.* 26th ed. Elk Grove Village, IL: American Academy of Pediatrics; 2003:514–521.

61. Baker MD, Moore SE. Human bites in children. *Am J Dis Child.* 1987;141:1285–1290.

108

ROBERT McNAMARA AND MICHAEL DeANGELIS

Laceration Repair with Sutures, Staples, and Wound Closure Tapes

▶ INTRODUCTION

A laceration is a traumatic tear or opening in the skin surface. The goal of laceration repair is to reduce the risk of wound infection by restoring the skin's protective barrier and ultimately to achieve a functional and cosmetically pleasing scar.

Over one third of injuries in children involve a laceration, making it the most common specific injury for which care is sought in a pediatric emergency department (1,2). In addition, a significant number of these patients seek treatment in primary care clinics (3). Laceration repair accounts for half of all procedures performed on injured children (4).

The incidence of lacerations in children is strongly correlated with the developmental level of the child. The initial rise in incidence occurs with the ability to ambulate. Lacerations peak at 2 years of age, when the child has attained greatest mobility but lacks equivalent motor coordination. Half of childhood lacerations occur in children under 5 years of age, and these lacerations frequently involve falls on broken glass bottles, wooden furniture, asphalt, or concrete (2,4). Lacerations resulting from assaults or altercations are more common in adolescents.

Animal bites also are a frequent source of lacerations in children. This is especially true in the preschool and early school years, when inadvertent provocation can result in an attack by the animal.

Common sites of lacerations in children are the head (60%), the upper extremities (23%), and the lower extremities (15%) (5). Lacerations of the head or face are proportionately greater in children under 2 years of age, as older children are more likely to break a fall by extending an arm or leg.

The majority of childhood lacerations can be treated without subspecialty assistance (4). The need for consultation depends on a number of factors, including the level of skill and experience of the clinician, the complexity of the laceration and involvement of underlying structures, the location of the laceration, and the ability of the child to cooperate.

Considering the frequency of lacerations during childhood, the importance of early repair, and the straightforward methods required for the majority of these injuries, every clinician treating acute injuries in children should be capable of repairing lacerations

▶ ANATOMY AND PHYSIOLOGY

Knowledge of the anatomy and regenerative properties of the skin is crucial to performing an optimal laceration repair. The layers of the skin are depicted in Figure 108.1. The epidermis is the outermost layer and is composed of epithelial cells, whose function is to protect deeper tissues from infection and desiccation. Immediately beneath the epidermis is the dermis, which contains blood vessels, nerve endings, collagen, and fibroblasts. Below the dermis is the subcutaneous layer, which is composed primarily of fat cells. Hair follicles, nerve fibers, and blood vessels are also located in this layer. The subcutaneous layer is bounded below by a sheet of connective tissue called the fascia, which protects the underlying muscle and helps prevent superficial infection from spreading to deeper tissues.

The depth of the wound and the particular layers that have been disrupted are important factors in determining the best type of closure. Early contraction at the deeper levels

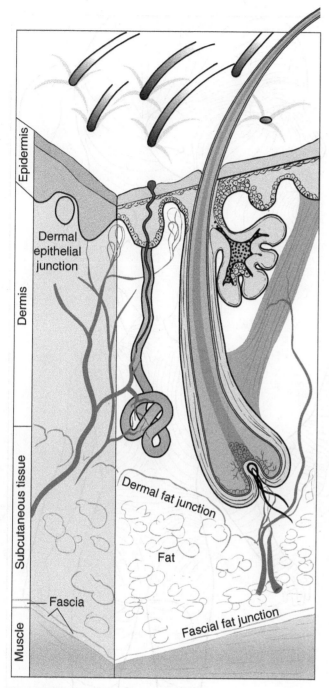

Figure 108.1 Anatomy of the skin layers.

Intact skin is under constant tension. This tension has both a static component and a dynamic component. The skin in a particular location of the body possesses an intrinsic amount of tension that is determined partly by the underlying muscles and joints. Relaxed skin tension lines (RSTLs) lie perpendicular to the underlying muscle and are accentuated by contraction of the muscle (Figure 108.2) (6–8). They are best identified by gently pinching the skin and observing the furrows and ridges that are formed. Tension adjacent to these lines determines the initial extent of separation that occurs along a laceration and the ultimate width of the scar. Sutures provide temporary support until the skin can regenerate tissue capable of overcoming this tension and maintaining closure of the wound (2). Lacerations running perpendicular to these lines tend to gape more and require stronger sutures over a longer period to provide adequate support. Consequently, these lacerations are at increased risk for scarring. Lacerations that run parallel to these lines can be expected to heal more rapidly and with better cosmetic results.

The normal healing process of skin occurs over a prolonged period and involves multiple, sometimes overlapping, stages. The healing process is typically divided into coagulation, inflammation, epithelialization, angiogenesis, collagen formation, and wound contraction (9,10).

Coagulation occurs within the first hours following injury and involves vasospasm, platelet aggregation, and fibrous clot formation. Platelets also release factors that help trigger the response of inflammatory cells.

The inflammatory phase, which peaks at 24 hours after the injury, is marked by increased capillary permeability, which allows leukocytes to migrate into the wound. Neutrophils and macrophages act as scavengers to rid the wound of debris and bacteria. Macrophages also release chemotactic substances that stimulate fibroblast replication.

Epithelialization occurs as new epithelial cells grow and migrate across the wound edges. In a sutured laceration, complete bridging of the wound occurs within 48 hours (10). The placement of sutures creates a new wound through the epithelium, and the new epithelial cells will migrate along the track of the suture. These cells frequently disappear once the suture is removed; however, when sutures are left in place for prolonged periods of time or are placed under excessive tension, these epithelial cells are more likely to remain and form punctate scars along the edge of the wound.

Angiogenesis is the process of new blood vessel formation. The various stages of wound healing depend on the delivery of substrates, including nutrients, oxygen, and inflammatory cells, to the site of injury. Angiogenesis is crucial for providing the means of delivery for these substrates.

Collagen, the principal structural protein of most tissues in the body, is essential for restoring the tensile strength of the skin. Fibroblast deposition of collagen components begins within 48 hours after the injury (2). Various enzymatic processes result in the formation of fibrils. Subsequent crosslinking of these fibrils gives the collagen its maximal strength. Although the process of collagen synthesis reaches a peak in

following injury frequently results in an inaccurate estimate of wound depth. The wound must be explored thoroughly for this reason. Certain layers retain sutures best: the fascial-fat junction, the dermal-fat junction, and the level just below the dermal-epidermal junction (Fig. 108.1). Adequate support of the affected tissue is a prerequisite for optimal closure and requires approximation of each involved layer. Improper alignment of the skin layers results in an uneven surface, which may cause shadowing and more obvious scarring.

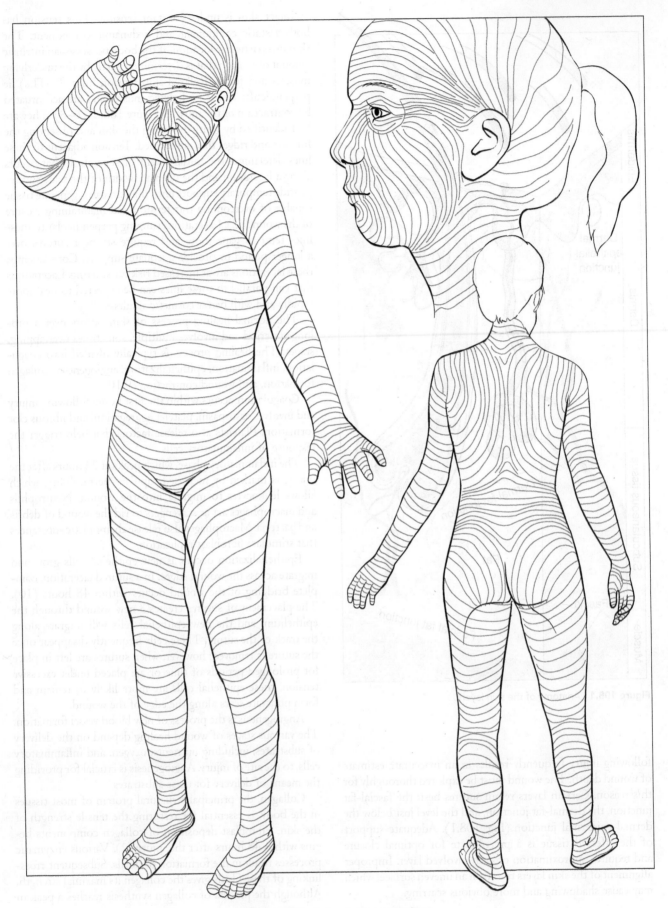

Figure 108.2 Relaxed skin tension lines.

the first week, remodeling continues for up to 12 months. A new scar will reach only one quarter of its ultimate strength by 3 weeks and less than two thirds by 4 months (10).

Wound contraction is a poorly understood process in which the full wound thickness moves toward the center of the wound. This occurs 3 to 4 days following the injury and appears to be independent of epithelialization and collagen formation. This process is considered an important part of wound healing and should not be confused with the contracture that results from scar shortening.

Various factors, both internal and external, will inhibit the normal process of healing. Underlying immune deficiencies or prolonged steroid use can affect the inflammatory stage. The presence of crushed tissue or debris surrounding the laceration, as frequently occurs with blunt trauma, will significantly impede epithelial cell growth. Epithelialization is, therefore, optimized by meticulous attention to wound cleansing, débridement, and foreign body removal (Chapters 107 and 111). Collagen synthesis is a complex process that depends on the presence of a number of trace minerals, vitamins, and plasma proteins as well as an adequate supply of oxygen. Poor nutrition, underlying illness, or vascular disease will adversely affect this process.

As the microscopic process of healing proceeds, the appearance of the wound also undergoes predictable stages of evolution and remodeling. What may initially appear to be a cosmetically appealing result following suture removal often will go through a stage in which it becomes increasingly thickened, reddened, and elevated. This occurs during the active period of fibrous tissue production and remodeling, which lasts approximately 3 months. Over the next 3 months, the scar can be expected to fade and recede as capillaries collapse and the cellular content is replaced by connective tissue. The look of the scar 6 months following the initial laceration is essentially its final appearance (2).

Hypertrophic scarring and keloid formation are the result of abnormal healing, which can occur despite proper wound management and closure (11). Hypertrophic scars are composed of red, raised, pruritic tissue, which is the result of excessive collagen deposition occurring within the original boundaries of the wound. Keloids are nodular masses of scar tissue that also contain increased amounts of immature collagen and migrate beyond the original extent of the wound. Keloids occur with greater incidence in dark-skinned individuals and have a higher propensity for certain areas of the body, such as the sternum, deltoid, and mandible.

Children appear to have advantages in healing ability over adults. Studies suggest that in adults the stages of healing begin later, occur at a slower rate, and do not reach the same level as in children. With increasing age, collagen biosynthesis and cross-linking are decreased (12), the rate of epithelialization is reduced (13), and the proliferative capacity and contractility of fibroblasts are diminished (14). The underlying reason for these changes is difficult to determine due to the presence of multiple confounding factors. It is unclear whether these changes in wound healing are the result of prolonged environmental exposure or underlying disease or are simply part of the natural process of aging.

▶ INDICATIONS

The basic goals of wound repair are to restore the integrity of injured tissue and to achieve a functional and aesthetically pleasing scar. These goals are best achieved by reducing tissue contamination, débriding devitalized tissue, restoring perfusion, and establishing a well-approximated skin closure (15).

Minor soft-tissue wounds are a common, unavoidable part of pediatric emergency care. Anxiety of the patient and family surrounding the repair of these injuries can be a source of much stress for the clinician. For these reasons, the ability to approach this situation in a clearly planned and confident manner is essential to the clinician's long-term survival in pediatric emergency care. Skilled minor wound care can be a source of great patient and personal satisfaction and should receive major consideration in the education of emergency care providers.

Reasons to Seek Consultation

Not every wound should be repaired by the emergency physician. Consultation should be considered for the following kinds of wounds (16):

Wounds involving an open fracture or joint space disruption

Wounds involving tendons, nerves, or blood vessels

Wounds involving specialized structures (e.g., parotid duct, lacrimal duct, tarsal plate)

Wounds that would be better treated under general anesthesia due to their extent or location

Wounds that the emergency physician considers beyond his or her own level of expertise

The consulting service will vary with the injury and can range from general surgery for a wound complicated only by its extent to plastic surgery, otolaryngology, oral surgery, or orthopaedics for more specialized circumstances. If the initial receiving hospital does not have the appropriate specialist available, transfer may be necessary.

A difficult situation arises when the family insists on a plastic surgeon for a relatively minor wound that is well within the capacity of the emergency physician. To readily consult plastic surgery in all such cases is a poor strategy. Often a simple closure yields a wholly acceptable result, and the expense of a plastic surgeon and the time delay caused by such consultation is inappropriate for the situation (17). The clinician should reason with and inform the family that he or she is capable of handling the wound. The clinician also should inform the family that revision is unlikely to be needed but, if required, can be performed without difficulty at a later date under more favorable conditions.

With complicated wounds, immediate repair even by an experienced plastic surgeon may not always be the best strategy (18). A complicated repair in the acute phase is considered less desirable by some authorities for the following reasons: (a) a higher risk of infection may necessitate suture removal and undermine the initial effort; (b) it is more difficult to make the proper cuts for Z-plasty, etc., in damaged tissue as opposed to the firm scar base that will be present at a later date; (c) less time is available to study the natural tendencies of the wound; and (d) the patient has no basis of comparison with which to judge the outcome of plastic surgery (18).

Some emergency physicians will feel comfortable with extensor tendon repair; however, the requirement for close follow-up and patient compliance, coupled with the potential for significant disability, make referral a strong consideration in these cases. The emergency physician also must be aware that delayed repair of certain injuries, including nerve and tendon transection and complicated facial lacerations, is an acceptable response on the part of a contacted consultant (17).

Infectious Considerations

The risk of infection in a wound depends on the interaction of patient factors, the wound environment, and the care provided by the physician (6,9,19–22). When wound evaluation indicates that primary closure would be associated with a high risk of infection, it is recommended to leave the wound open for delayed primary closure or to allow healing by secondary intention (6,9,21). Loosely closing a wound should never be considered. The infectious risk with this method is generally the same as with primary closure (9).

Because the rate of wound infection in children is quite low, delayed primary closure is rarely used in the management of pediatric wounds. Studies examining all types of pediatric lacerations repaired with primary closure report infection rates as low as 1% to 2%. Bites, complex or long lacerations (greater than 3 cm), and wounds of the lower extremities seem to be at higher risk for infection (23–25). It is important to realize that if primary repair fails due to wound infection, the subsequent management is similar to delayed primary closure (22).

Patient Factors

Patient factors associated with an increased rate of infection include the presence of diabetes, renal failure, liver failure, immunosuppression, connective tissue disorders, obesity, and malnutrition (16,26). Wound infection rates for pediatric patients with these conditions are generally unknown, as wound studies typically exclude such patients. The presence of an underlying illness should not be the sole reason for avoiding wound closure, and the majority of wounds in these patients are amenable to primary repair. It is important, however, to pay close attention to wounds in such patients and to ensure adequate follow-up.

Local Factors

Local factors associated with the wound itself are the main source of wound problems in the ED (9,19). The clinician should always consider the following factors before wound closure.

Time Delay

Time is a variable factor in the closure of wounds, as some, such as a highly contaminated puncture wound, should never be closed, and others may be safely closed at almost any time after the injury (22). The "golden period" of wound repair is frequently mentioned, but this period is dependent on the characteristics of each individual wound. Although there is a strong relationship between the timing of wound closure and the risk of subsequent infection, the length of the "golden period" is highly variable (16,25,27).

Several studies have demonstrated that if a wound contains greater than 10^5 bacteria per gram of tissue, the probability of infection will be high (28–30). The mean time to achieve this level of contamination in one study was 5.17 hours, leading some authorities to consider the "golden period" to be quite short (29). Actual clinical studies, however, have produced results that support individual evaluation of wounds to determine if the time delay for closure is acceptable. No difference was found in infection rates for pediatric wounds sutured more than 6 hours after injury as compared with those repaired earlier (25). A study of wounds in a Third World setting found that it was safe to close general wounds for a period up to 19 hours, whereas scalp and facial wounds could be closed at any time (27). In one study evaluating hand wounds, time was not a factor in infection for a period up to 18 hours (30).

The primary determinant of a patient's ability to resist wound infection is most likely the local circulation to the wound site (31). For that reason, injuries to well-vascularized areas such as the scalp, face, and tongue may be comfortably repaired many hours after presentation (19,31). In the previously mentioned Third World study, 97% of scalp wounds that were closed after 19 hours healed without complications (27).

Wound Contamination and Crush Injury

The degree of contamination is an important determinant of wound infection (6,28–30). Any foreign matter in the wound decreases resistance to infection. Soil components damage host defenses and raise the infective potential of bacteria. Saliva and feces are composed of concentrations of bacteria that greatly exceed the numbers needed to produce infection (6,9). The presence of devitalized tissue alone in a wound is considered a major risk factor for wound infection (6,31,32). Experimentally, inserting devitalized fat, muscle, or skin into a wound increases the infection rate (32). This occurs through inhibition of leukocyte function, creation of an anaerobic environment, and the support of bacterial growth by the "culture medium" nature of the devitalized tissue (32).

Crush injuries are generally considered to be at higher risk for infection due to the presence of devitalized tissue and, more importantly, disturbances of local blood flow (33). Although this makes intuitive sense, clinical series supporting this hypothesis are limited. Separate studies on hand injuries demonstrated conflicting results when comparing infection rates in crush versus laceration-type injuries (29,34). In areas where the vascular supply is good, such as the scalp, the overall infection rate will be low regardless of the mechanism of injury (27,35).

The ability to sharply débride devitalized or heavily contaminated tissue will have a major impact on the decision to close a wound primarily (15,19,21). Débridement can convert a crushed, dirty wound into a clean, sharply incised laceration suitable for primary repair. Similarly, adequate wound irrigation can be expected to reduce the bacterial contamination of a wound and decrease the rate of subsequent infection (Chapter 107).

Wound Location

Although the wound location itself will usually not preclude primary repair, some general issues are pertinent to remember in evaluating wounds. Most studies demonstrate an increased rate of wound infection in injuries to the lower extremities (24,25,35). This is thought to be due to the relatively poor blood supply to the lower extremities (24,31). The foot may be at a particularly high risk (6). Upper extremity wounds also are considered to be at higher risk for infection, particularly hand wounds, for reasons similar to those that apply to the lower extremities (31,35).

Areas with significant exposure to endogenous bacteria such as the mouth, vagina, and perianal area are theoretically at high risk for infection (6). These same areas, however, also have an excellent vascular supply, counterbalancing the increased bacterial exposure (31). Closure of wounds in the mouth is generally considered acceptable if no major time delay has occurred (36,37). The low rate of infection of episiotomy incisions indicates some margin of safety for primary wound repair in the perineum. If in doubt about closure in one of these areas, consultation should be considered.

Location of a wound also may influence where the repair is best undertaken. Lacerations of the perineum may require closure in the operating room for the best result in terms of patient fear and anxiety. Wounds in inaccessible areas of the oral cavity also may require such management.

Bite Wounds

Mammalian bites account for approximately 5% of all traumatic wounds evaluated in the ED and up to 1% of all ED visits (38–40). Considerable controversy exists surrounding the proper management of both human and animal bite wounds. The clinician's decision regarding closure in the case of a bite wound must weigh the various factors related to wound in-

fection together with the supposition that the wound is contaminated with bacteria (19). The important considerations then become the vascular supply to the area and the ability of the clinician to adequately clean the wound and decrease the bacterial contamination present (16,23,41).

In all types of bite wounds, the hand is at an especially high risk for infection (42–48). The hand contains many poorly vascularized structures that do not resist infection well. Also, because the fascial spaces and tendon sheaths closely communicate, infection can spread quickly through the entire hand (41). In contrast, wounds of the head and neck have a much lower risk of infection. The location of the wound should also be assessed for cosmetic and functional significance. Although the hand is important functionally, wounds should generally be managed without primary closure. For cosmetic reasons, facial wounds are typically repaired immediately (16,23).

Dog Bites

Dog bites account for approximately 0.4% of all ED visits and 60% to 90% of all bite injuries treated in the ED (49). Children and young adults are the most frequent victims of dog bites, and most of their injuries occur on the head, neck, and upper extremities (40,49). Because the larger teeth of dogs facilitate the tearing of tissue, dog bites are more likely to result in lacerations than puncture wounds (50). Consequently, most of the bite wounds considered for suturing in the ED are caused by dogs. These wounds are assumed to be contaminated, although it has been stated that meal-eating (as opposed to meat-eating) dogs do not have sufficient oral bacteria to create an inoculum at the level of 10^5 bacteria per gram of tissue (19). As with human bites, dog bites to the hand are at higher risk for infection regardless of the use of antibiotics (45,46).

Although dog bite wounds are generally considered contaminated, recent investigations support primary closure of selected injuries (38,50–53). In one randomized clinical trial, the infection rate in 169 dog bite lacerations was the same for those sutured as for those left to heal by secondary intention (7.7%) (51). This was true even for dog bites of the hand. Other observational studies have also demonstrated equivalent infection rates for sutured and nonsutured dog bite lacerations (38,52). In one series of 91 patients with primary closure of dog bites lacerations, investigators reported an infection rate of only 4.4% (52). Another study reported an infection rate of 5.7% in 88 dog bite lacerations repaired primarily. The infection rates in this study did not differ between patients discharged with and without prophylactic antibiotics (38).

In general, dog bite lacerations of the face should be repaired primarily. If coupled with excellent wound care and meticulous closing technique, suturing of facial dog bite wounds can safely be accomplished with minimal risk of infection. In 145 pediatric facial dog bite wounds repaired after pressure irrigation and wound edge excision, an infection rate of only 1.4% was reported even though no antibiotics were administered (53).

Cat Bites

Cat bites account for approximately 5% to 18% of all animal bites treated in the ED (48,54). Because of a cat's thin, sharp teeth, most bites result in puncture wounds (57% to 86%). Lacerations are much less common (5% to 17%) (48,54). The majority of these bites occur on the hand (48). Cat bites have a much greater risk of infection than dog bites. Their teeth are more likely to penetrate tendons, joints, and bone, resulting in deeper inoculation of bacteria. Also, the wound is difficult to explore and irrigate. The reported incidence of infection is as high as 30% to 50% (41,48,54).

Data are limited regarding the treatment of cat bite wounds with primary closure. Lacerations on the face may be considered for suturing, but in general sutures should be avoided in other locations. In one small study of cat bite lacerations on the face repaired with primary closure, there were no reported infections (48). Another study that included cat bite wounds located primarily on the head, neck, and upper extremities found an infection rate of only 4.4% after primary closure (38).

Human Bites

Human bites are the third most common mammalian bite in the United States, with the hand being involved in 60% to 75% of the cases (16). The notorious reputation of human bites is primarily based on one specific injury to the hand, the closed fist injury, or "fight bite." This injury occurs when the closed fist strikes the teeth of another person, most commonly during a fight (16). The forces involved to create the skin break are generally sufficient to inoculate the tendon and its coverings, which lie just under the skin in this area. Frequently, deeper injury occurs to the bone, cartilage, and joint space. When the hand is subsequently extended, the bacteria are carried into areas not accessible to routine cleansing in the ED (42). In the pediatric age group, these wounds are usually infected by the time of presentation (44,45). Admission to the hospital and intravenous antibiotic therapy are generally indicated for an infected closed fist injury (16,41,42,45).

All patients presenting with a wound over the metacarpal head should be considered to have a human bite wound until proven otherwise. It is prudent to treat each wound in this location as a bite wound regardless of the history provided by the patient. If the wound is not infected at presentation, it should be thoroughly evaluated by wound exploration and radiographic study to detect any underlying injury that would prompt hospitalization. Patients scheduled for outpatient treatment must have their wounds thoroughly cleansed, left open, and elevated. These patients are routinely treated with antibiotics and must be capable of early follow-up (42).

In children, human bites usually occur with fighting (62%) or playing (26%). Most of these bites result in superficial abrasions (75%), which do not generally get infected (41,44). The literature on suturing human bite lacerations in children is limited. One small series suggested that the placement of deep sutures was associated with an increased rate of infection (44). However, primary closure of wounds in well-vascularized areas

that can be adequately cleansed should not present a problem (23,38,55). The typical small forehead laceration that is caused by a playmate's tooth is one example of a bite wound that should not be closed unless the wound is surgically extended for proper cleansing (44).

Other Animal Bites

Rodent bites account for up to 7% of all animal bites treated in the ED (54,56). Most of these bites result in small puncture wounds with a very low risk of wound infection. Lacerations caused by monkeys have a notorious reputation based on anecdotal reports, whereas those caused by large herbivores such as horses will be associated with significant crush injury (57). Recommendations on primary closure of these wounds are lacking given their relative infrequency.

Foreign Bodies and Wound Closure

The presence of a nonirritant foreign body such as a small piece of metal or glass is not a contraindication to primary wound closure (58). Such wounds can be closed and managed expectantly if the foreign body is difficult to remove, is not in a critical area (e.g., a joint space or near a vital structure), and is not positioned so that it would be a likely source of ongoing irritation for the patient. Certainly, the patient and family should be informed of the presence of a foreign body and the rationale for the planned course of action.

Irritant foreign bodies such as wooden splinters or thorns should be removed at the time of presentation to avoid infectious complications (Chapter 111) (58). The presence of even minute amounts of soil in a wound invites infection, and thus wounds with suspected remaining soil should not be closed primarily (6,9).

Gunshot and Stab Wounds

Low-velocity gunshot wounds that do not damage underlying structures can be managed on an outpatient basis. The traditional care of these wounds includes open treatment (no sutures) and basic wound care without using antibiotics (59,60). These wounds generally heal well without antibiotic therapy despite retained metallic fragments in the wound (59,60).

Stab wounds must be evaluated for depth and involvement or penetration of underlying structures before closure. This frequently necessitates surgical consultation. These wounds may be categorized as puncture wounds or simple, sharply incised lacerations. In the latter slashing-type injuries, the wounds may be closed like any other. Deeper puncture-type injuries are traditionally managed in an open fashion (Chapters 107,110).

Dead Space

Eliminating any pocket or "dead space" in the depths of a wound that could collect blood or serum and thereby potentiate infection is often accepted as an essential step in wound management. This must be distinguished from the technique of a layered closure to decrease tension on the wound edge, which has cosmetic advantages (6,61). Although theoretically useful, the suture closure of dead space to decrease infection has not been clearly shown to be beneficial and may actually be detrimental (62–66). Animal studies suggest that deep sutures increase the risk of infection in contaminated wounds (63,65,66). In clean, noncontaminated wounds, however, this was not shown to be the case (65,66). Sutures through the adipose layer should be avoided. These sutures do not help to relieve tension, and they increase the rate of infection (61,62,64).

▶ EQUIPMENT

Basic surgical tool requirements useful for wound repair are listed below.

Needle holder. The size of the needle holder should match the size of the needle selected for suturing. An excessively large needle holder will flatten a small needle after only a few uses (67).

Tissue forceps. Tissue should be manipulated gently with forceps to avoid any crushing effects. An alternative to forceps is a single- or double-pronged skin hook (67).

Tissue scissors. A sharp, tightly cutting pair is essential for débridement (68).

Hemostats. These may be useful in situations when bleeding vessels will require ligation (68).

Scalpel. A No. 10 or 15 blade may be necessary for sharp débridement (68).

Sterile drapes. An adequate amount of drapes should be used to keep the wound area sterile. In the repair of facial wounds, the hole in the drape should not be so small as to obscure useful landmarks (36,67). Drapes over the face can be forgone if they cause excess anxiety in a child.

Sterile gauze. A ready and sufficient supply of gauze pads is frequently overlooked in setting up for laceration repair.

Sterile gloves. Although the use of sterile gloves (as opposed to clean, nonsterile gloves) has never been proven to reduce the rate of wound infection, this practice is still generally recommended. Of note, a recent multicenter, randomized clinical trial reported no difference in wound infection rates when clean, nonsterile gloves were used instead of sterile gloves for wound closure (69).

Mask. A mask is important for reducing contamination of the wound and protecting the clinician from mucous membrane exposure (6,68). One study, however, did not find any significant difference in wound infection rates when comparing lacerations repaired by clinicians with and without masks (70).

Light. An adequate light source is essential and should preferably be directed into the wound unobstructed from above.

Bed. The patient and bed should be positioned in such a way as to maximize the comfort of both the patient and the clinician during the procedure. Using arm extensions and pillows should be considered, and the height of the bed should be raised to a workable level.

Suture material (6,15,67,71–76). Sutures are divided into two general classes, absorbable and nonabsorbable, based on their rate of degradation. Sutures that undergo rapid degradation, losing their tensile strength within 60 days, are considered "absorbable." Sutures that maintain their tensile strength for greater than 60 days are considered "nonabsorbable."

Several types of nonabsorbable sutures are available for percutaneous suturing; however, the general choice for emergency physicians will be a synthetic monofilament type such as nylon (Dermalon, Ethilon) or polypropylene (Prolene). The monofilament sutures are preferred over braided or multifilament sutures, which are thought to increase the risk of wound infection by providing interstices for bacteria to be shielded from leukocytes. Most synthetic sutures possess a low coefficient of friction that allows the them to pass smoothly through tissue. This same property, however, lessens the stability of the knot, and therefore the clinician should use at least four throws when tying knots with synthetic material. Silk is more reactive than synthetic suture material, which limits its usefulness for general wound repair. The relatively soft feel of silk and its workability make it a consideration for repairs of the eyelid or mouth. In these areas, silk sutures are usually removed in a few days, thus lessening the reactivity problem.

Absorbable sutures are typically used to approximate the dermal area in deeper lacerations. Synthetic absorbable sutures are generally less reactive and have greater tensile strength than sutures from natural sources, such as catgut. Two commonly used synthetic absorbable sutures are polyglycolic acid (Dexon) and polyglactin (Vicryl). The use of absorbable sutures for skin closure has traditionally been discouraged because of the material's greater tissue reactivity and potential for increased scar formation. Recent studies, however, suggest that cosmesis is equivalent for wounds closed with absorbable and nonabsorbable sutures (74–76). One study, comparing the use of plain gut and nylon sutures in the repair of 95 uncomplicated pediatric lacerations, found no difference in cosmesis at 4 months (75). Another study comparing the use of rapid ("fast") absorbing gut versus nylon sutures in 84 patients with facial lacerations found no significant difference in cosmesis at 9 months (76). The primary advantage offered by the use of absorbable sutures for skin closure is that a return visit for suture removal is not required.

The size (diameter) of the suture material is a measure of its tensile strength. The appropriate suture size chosen for a repair depends on the tensile strength of the tissue being approximated. The clinician should select the smallest size suture that will adequately hold the tissues in place and thus minimize the amount of foreign material in the wound. In decreasing order of size and tensile strength, the sutures commonly used in the ED run from 3-0 to 6-0. In general, 3-0 and 4-0 absorbable and nonabsorbable sutures are used for fascial closure, 4-0 and 5-0 absorbable sutures for dermal closure, and 4-0 to 6-0 nonabsorbable sutures for skin closure. 6-0 sutures are used for the repair of facial wounds, whereas the use of 3-0 sutures is usually limited to the repair of wounds of the scalp or other areas of significant tension (e.g. wounds overlying joint surfaces).

Needles. The reverse cutting needle is the best choice for general wound repair in the ED. This needle has its cutting edge situated on the outside of the curve of the needle so that the cut is made away from the wound edge, which prevents the suture material from further cutting into the tissue along the path of the needle cut.

▶ PROCEDURE

Wound Preparation

General wound preparation and cleansing is critical for optimal wound repair, and this topic is detailed in Chapter 107. The repair of lacerations is perhaps the most common indication for using procedural sedation in the young child, and this technique is detailed in Chapter 33.

Anesthesia

Adequate anesthesia is essential for proper wound evaluation and closure (16,31). The application of local and regional anesthesia is detailed in Chapter 35. A few additional comments are herein emphasized. Complete anesthesia of the affected area must be accomplished before wound manipulation. It is the fault of the clinician and not the patient if the anesthesia is not satisfactory. If the anesthesia is inadequate, the clinician must retreat and start over to ensure a wound repair that is least distressing for both the patient and family.

The most common form of anesthesia used for laceration repair remains local infiltration. Although this method is the most reliable, local infiltration is painful and subjects the clinician to the risk of an inadvertent needle stick. Many strategies have been suggested to reduce the pain associated with infiltration. These include using small-gauge needles, buffered solutions, warmed solutions, a slow rate of injection, injection through the wound edges, subcutaneous rather than intradermal injection, and pretreatment with topical anesthetics (16,23,77–85).

An alternative method for the administration of local anesthesia is topical application of local anesthetics. Several such anesthetics have been used, including a combination of lidocaine, epinephrine, and tetracaine (LET). The major advantage of these agents is painless application and reduced patient anxiety (86–91). Although the onset of anesthesia is more delayed than with local infiltration, the application of topical anesthetics has been shown to significantly reduce the total treatment time in children with simple lacerations (92).

Hemostasis

Maintaining hemostasis is essential at every stage of laceration repair. Persistent bleeding often obscures the view of the clinician and thus hinders wound exploration and closure. Hematoma formation in a closed wound impairs healing and increases the risk of dehiscence and infection (68). Hemostasis usually can be achieved with direct pressure. If bleeding persists despite direct pressure, a blood pressure cuff can be placed proximal to the injury and inflated just above the patient's systolic pressure to help control bleeding (6,16). Vasoconstrictors, such as epinephrine, may also be used in combination with local anesthetics to reduce bleeding within the wound. The use of vasoconstrictors is discouraged in areas with end organ blood supply (e.g., fingers, nose, penis, toes) (16).

Exploration

Exploring the full extent of every wound is necessary to identify hidden foreign bodies and particulate matter embedded in the wound as well as injuries to underlying structures that may need repair. The clinician should avoid the temptation to initially probe a wound with a finger in search of foreign bodies. Exploration with a metal probe and the liberal use of radiographs constitute a much safer approach (68). It is essential to explore wounds of the extremities through their full range of motion and to be meticulous in examining them in the position of injury. For example, the typical knee wound is often approached with the patient's leg in full extension even though most injuries occur in some degree of flexion. Exploration of injuries to the plantar surface of the foot may be facilitated by laying the patient prone on the stretcher and elevating the foot into view.

The clinician should have little hesitation about extending a wound using a scalpel if needed for adequate visualization and wound exploration. The resultant added length to the wound should heal in an acceptable fashion given the sharply incised nature of the wound extension. If a foreign body is identified within a wound, this should be a signal to the clinician that more lies in wait for discovery. If the clinician is contemplating primary repair, he or she must continue to explore the wound until assured that no soil or irritant foreign bodies remain (6,58,68).

Débridement

Removing devitalized or heavily contaminated tissue from a wound is a fundamental principle of wound care (6,31,32,68). Sharp débridement of a contaminated wound may allow closure of a wound that would otherwise be treated with delayed primary closure (21). Débridement may be accomplished by excising the entire wound, sometimes referred to as "wound ellipsing," or in a more selective fashion. Wounds that are amenable to excision are those in areas lacking vital underlying structures and where there is sufficient excess tissue available to allow closing the wound without undue tension (6,68).

Although it decreases the likelihood of infection, excision can worsen the eventual cosmetic result. Excision should generally follow the relaxed skin tension lines (RSTLs), as described previously (see Fig. 108.2) (93–95). In fact, it is wise only to undertake an excision that can be easily done and where the wound closely parallels the RSTLs (6,93). An excision performed on a jagged wound that is not parallel to the RSTLs may produce a straight edge but will have a wide scar due to the tension on the wound. The same jagged laceration with multiple components running in different directions will essentially be a natural Z-plasty (93). Such a wound will have some segments following the RSTLs and will likely heal in a more acceptable manner than the "clean" excision (6,93).

Débridement of facial wounds should be conservative (36,93). Given the excellent blood supply of the face, it is difficult to be sure tissue is truly devitalized. It is wiser to refrain from débridement rather than to sacrifice tissue that may live (93). Loss of tissue is the most significant limiting factor to the success of later plastic scar revision (94). An important cosmetic structure such as the philtrum should never be débrided (36).

If a wound is excised, the effect of the natural contraction of the wound on surrounding structures must be anticipated. For example, a wide horizontal excision on the forehead may heal with a thin scar but displace the eyebrow upward on that side (30).

Certain areas are less amenable to excision and débridement. These areas include the nose, lip, hand, forearm, anterior lower leg, and foot (21,32,60). When excising in a hair-bearing region such as the eyebrow, all cuts must be angled parallel to the direction of the hair shafts to avoid excess follicle loss and a wide hairless scar (36,94).

The technique of wound excision involves making a smooth, elliptical cut around the wound area to be excised (Fig. 108.3). This usually will encompass the entire wound.

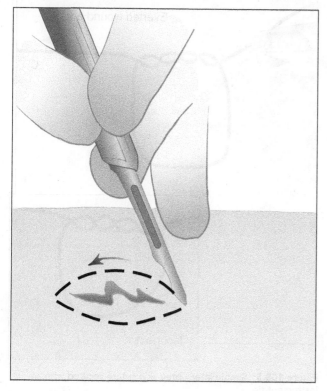

Figure 108.3 Elliptical incision of a jagged laceration.

It is recommended that the eventual length of the excision exceed the width by a factor of three (60). It is wise to mark the desired path of the skin cut. Two general methods are recommended for completing the excision. The skin can be scored with a scalpel and the cut completed with a pair of sharp tissue scissors (60) or the entire depth of the cut may be made with one stroke of the scalpel (95). With either technique, it is important to obtain a perpendicular cut completely through the dermis.

Minimizing Scar Formation

Although at times even the best of efforts will result in an unsightly hypertrophic scar (96), several important techniques are used to minimize excess scar formation. The width of a scar is primarily determined by the tension on the wound at the time of closure (6,73,95,97). The orientation of the laceration related to the RSTLs is the major determinant of the tension on the wound, and this is most simply ascertained by observing it at rest to see how far apart the wound edges gape (61).

If a laceration is significantly angled or perpendicular in relation to the RSTLs, it will likely heal with a wide scar (6,36,95). As previously mentioned, this is a primary consideration when contemplating wound excision. It is important to remember that the RSTLs in the individual patient do not always follow the book (61,94). The wrinkle lines that are so useful in adults to determine the orientation of the RSTLs are not as evident in children. The orientation of skin tension can be determined by simply pinching the skin and observing which direction has the longest furrows and hence the least tension (96).

When a wound is under tension, certain methods are used to counteract this influence and reduce the eventual width of the scar. The primary method to counteract tension is to place subcutaneous sutures before percutaneous sutures (60). Techniques such as Z-plasty and W-plasty to reduce the tension on less favorably placed wounds are used by plastic surgeons, and their performance is beyond the scope of this chapter (36,93,94). A relatively simple technique for reducing tension is to undermine the adjacent soft tissue to decrease the natural static tensions of the surrounding skin. A paucity of clinical studies of this technique exists; however, a wound study in a porcine model found that undermining generally decreased the forces required to close a wound (98).

Undermining is generally carried out in the plane of the subcutaneous fat for a distance of several millimeters or up to twice the width of the wound (Fig. 108.4; see also Fig. 111.2) (60,95). A pair of scissors or a scalpel is used to loosen the subdermal fatty tissue. The goal is to allow the skin edges to be brought together with very little tension. A note of caution has been raised about using undermining in contaminated wounds (6). The disruption in blood supply potentially caused by this largely unproven technique may lead to an increased risk of infection and offset any cosmetic improvement (6).

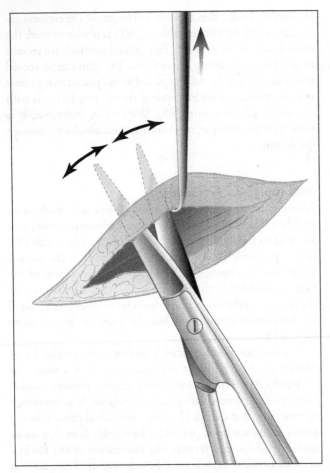

Figure 108.4 Undermining a wound reduces the degree of tension present after repair.

Scars that are most visible are characterized by abnormal color or an uneven surface that casts a shadow (60). Good technique can help minimize the latter problem by producing a flatter scar through eversion of skin edges, matching skin heights, proper suture placement, and care in handling tissue.

Wound edges must be everted at the time of closure (60,73,95). Eversion is accomplished by placing the percutaneous suture so that its depth is greater than its width (Fig. 108.5) (60,73). Alternatively, a mattress-type suture can be used to produce eversion of the wound edge (60,95). The difficulty with mattress sutures, however, is their tendency to cause ischemia of the wound edge (19). As discussed later in this chapter, using the lateral mattress suture for eversion may be preferable in this situation (95).

Absolute matching of the skin heights must be accomplished when a laceration is sutured (60). Going in and out of each wound edge separately, using two passes with the suture needle, is the best strategy in wounds that are uneven (6). For precise approximation of the wound edges in jagged or stellate lacerations, meticulous placement of individual sutures is recommended (6,73).

Most scar formation is a natural reaction to tissue injury, and therefore the tissue to be repaired should be handled

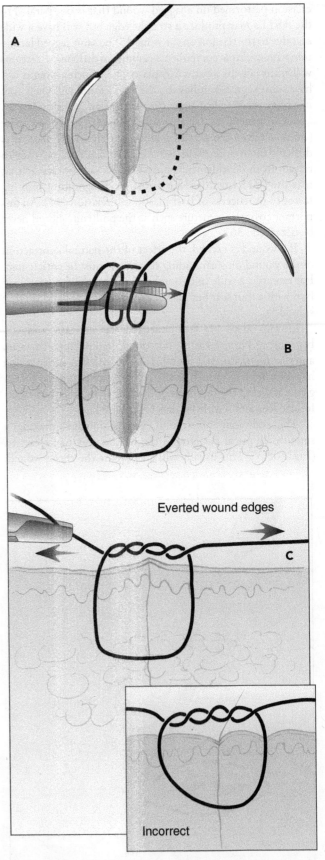

Everted wound edges

Incorrect

Figure 108.5 Simple interrupted skin suture secured with an instrument tie.

as gently as possible (21,95). This can be ensured by using noncrushing forceps and by using only fingers or skin hooks to handle the skin edges (21,67,94).

It is important for the clinician to be aware of circumstances when unsightly scarring is likely. For example, curved or U-shaped flap lacerations, often termed "trapdoor" lacerations, tend to yield poor results by virtue of the natural contraction of the wound to a central point in the flap (67,97). When these are encountered in cosmetic areas, such as the forehead, it is wise to consider referral or to warn the parents of the likely need for revision.

Suturing Techniques

General Principles

Key principles to remember regarding the use of sutures include the following:

1 Every suture is a foreign body. Therefore, the least amount of suture material should be used for the shortest period of time that is sufficient for wound healing. Corollaries to this include using deep sutures only when necessary, limiting the number of knots in a buried suture to three, and using the smallest size and number of sutures necessary for percutaneous closure (61,71,72).

2 Tight sutures increase the risk of infection by causing ischemia of the wound edge (6). If the suture is tight enough to necrose tissue, the hold of the suture will be weakened (99). It is important to anticipate swelling in the wound area and to approximate the tissue rather than tightly close it.

3 In general, the number of sutures placed for a given wound is the number required to ensure that no gaps appear between the wound edges. The distance of each suture from the wound edge (bite) is usually equal to the distance between sutures. Wounds under greater tension should have more skin sutures placed (so that each suture is under less tension), and thus the sutures should be closer to the wound edge (60,67).

4 Two general approaches to suturing a laceration are recommended. Some authorities advocate dividing the laceration into segments, starting with a central stitch and then bisecting each subsequent segment (67,95). Others insist on approaching the laceration from one end and using special techniques to remove any excess tissue that results in a "dog ear" at the far end of the wound (60,67).

Basic Use of Tools

The needle chosen should be appropriately sized to allow the desired depth of penetration into the wound edge. For the novice practitioner, use of a needle holder should be carefully studied because the majority of time wasted in wound repair relates to its use (100). The needle is best held perpendicular to the needle holder, and the position where the needle is grasped can be varied according to the clinician's needs. For soft-tissue repair, it is generally best to grab the needle relatively close to the thread end (swage). This hold will allow for more of the needle to be passed through the tissue and will make it easier to retrieve the needle using the needle holder or forceps (100). This position, however, allows for greater risk of needle breakage and makes it more difficult to apply force. If the tissue to be penetrated is tough, the needle must be grasped closer to the point (100). When using the needle holder, the clinician should make every effort to position the needle only once at each step to increase efficiency.

Wound edges should be manipulated in a gentle manner using only the fingers, a skin hook, or nontraumatic tissue forceps (21,60,68). To avoid damage to the epidermal layer, the forceps should be used to grasp the dermal-fat junction when suturing (60). The needle should be retrieved only with the needle holder or a pair of forceps to avoid injury to the clinician. For similar reasons, the clinician should not use the fingers to help push the tissue over the needle.

Types of Stitches

Simple Interrupted Skin Sutures

Because the simple interrupted skin suture is most commonly used, this technique should be mastered first. As mentioned previously, it is essential to obtain eversion of the wound edges to minimize scar formation. Eversion means that the wound edges are rolled slightly outward with the two edges of the wound lined up exactly. To achieve wound edge eversion, the path of the needle must be directly down or angled slightly away from the wound edge (see Fig. 108.5A) (60,73). Additionally, the depth of the suture path must be greater than the width. The entire depth of the wound edge can be pulled perpendicular to the skin by grasping the fat-dermal junction with forceps and driving the needle straight down (60). The needle must trace an equal path through both sides of the laceration to ensure accurate apposition of the wound. This is often accomplished with a single pass in small wounds with relatively apposed wound edges (Fig. 108.5) but is most easily achieved in more gaping wounds by driving the needle through one side and out through the center of the wound before re-entering on the opposite side of the wound.

Another technique for obtaining wound edge eversion is to pucker the wound edges in an everted manner with finger and thumb pressure before passing the needle completely through both sides of the wound (67). This technique does, however, put the clinician at risk for a needle stick. Eversion can be more safely achieved by applying slight pressure to the wound edges with tissue forceps.

Knot tying can be a source of frustration but is easily mastered with practice. The technique most useful for knot tying in the ED is the instrument tie (Fig. 108.5). This is best accomplished by pulling most of the suture through the wound, leaving a short (free) end at the insertion site. The remaining longer (needle) end of the thread is then grasped in the nondominant hand. The needle holder, still held in the dominant hand, is placed across the longer length of thread, and the thread is then looped twice over the tip (Fig. 108.5B). The needle holder then grasps the free end of the thread and pulls it through the double loop. The free end should be pulled away from the side of the wound where it initially entered, which will encourage the knot to lie flat across the wound (Fig. 108.5C). The knot is tightened so that the skin edges just come together. Further tightening beyond this point risks wound edge ischemia. The process is now reversed, with the needle holder again placed across the longer length of suture, which is then looped once under the tip. The needle holder then grasps the free end of the suture and returns it to the initial needle entry side of the wound, while the longer length of suture is carried back to the initial needle exit side of the wound. This alternating "over and under" method of tying produces a surgeon's knot. For monofilament sutures, this should be repeated first in the over and then in the under manner for a total of four throws to secure the knot.

Most skin repair will be performed with monofilament sutures that, due to their low coefficient of friction, allow for further loosening or tightening of previously tied knots (72). This takes some pressure off the need for perfect wound edge approximation at placement of the first throw in tying. This same property, however, can cause knots to loosen excessively during the attempt to secure them. To combat slippage of the first knot, a locking technique may be used. In this technique, after the first double knot is laid flat, the pull of the hands is immediately reversed to lock the knot (100). To retain the lock, the next throw must be placed without tension on the segments.

Excess knots will actually weaken the suture and should be avoided (73). The ends of the suture should be cut long enough to allow easy handling for removal.

Subcutaneous Sutures

Subcutaneous sutures are used to reapproximate the deeper layers of the skin and do not penetrate the epidermis. Although typically placed within the dermal layer, these sutures are traditionally referred to as "subcutaneous" sutures. The primary reason to place subcutaneous sutures is to counteract tension on the wound and thus decrease the width of the subsequent scar. If a deep, gaping laceration is closed without approximation of the underlying tissue, a depression may develop at the site of the wound. Using synthetic absorbable sutures to close the deeper tissues will decrease the tension on the wound (6,60,61,95). Placing such sutures in the dermal layer is especially important; however, the fascial layer overlying the muscle is also important to close (6,61,60,67). It is essential in repairing injured muscle that the fascia is incorporated in the suture, as the muscle itself will not hold a stitch (36,61).

When dermal sutures are placed, it is generally recommended that the knot be inverted or buried (i.e., located at the base of the wound) to keep as much foreign material as possible away from the healing wound edge (60,73,95). This is especially true in areas where the skin is thin or cosmesis is

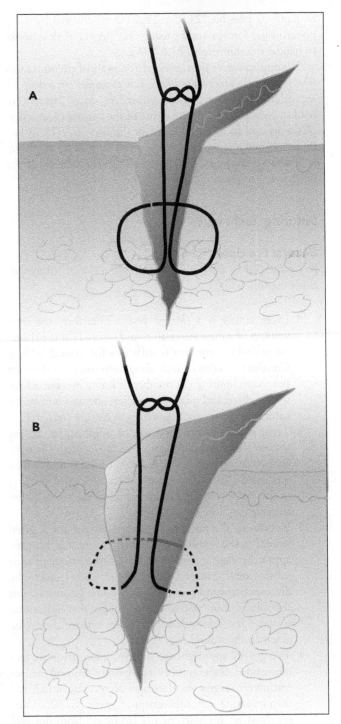

Figure 108.6
A. Buried subcutaneous suture.
B. Horizontal dermal stitch.

important. The initial insertion point of these sutures will be in the depths of the wound, typically at the dermal-fat junction (Fig. 108.6A). Exposure of the correct entry point can be facilitated by using tissue forceps or a skin hook. The needle is then rotated up through the tissue to exit in the dermis close to the dermal-epidermal junction. At this point, it is essential to pause and make sure that the second insertion point in the opposing dermis is at the same vertical and horizontal level as the exit point of the first pass. Once this is established, the downward pass of the suture becomes a mirror image of the first pass, exiting at the same level as the original insertion. The edges of the wound can then be closely apposed by pulling the two ends of suture in the same direction along the axis of the wound (67). Finally, the knot is tied, generally with only three throws to minimize the amount of suture material within the wound (72). The ends of the suture should be cut short to minimize the amount of suture material left in the wound.

A simple but useful variation of the traditional subcutaneous suture is the horizontal dermal stitch (Fig. 108.6B) (67). In this technique, the dermis is aligned by placing a simple suture in a horizontal plane. The loop and knot are at the same level in the dermal tissue. This suture provides a nice approximation of the wound edges before skin closure but carries the disadvantage of an inability to bury the knot. This suture is most practical when nearing the end of a subcutaneous closure and room is limited to maneuver for an additional inverted suture.

Interrupted Mattress Sutures

The three basic types of mattress sutures are the vertical, the horizontal, and the half-buried horizontal (Fig. 108.7). These suturing techniques, especially the vertical mattress suture, are useful in providing eversion of the wound edges. The traditional vertical mattress suture involves taking a large deep bite with the first pass of the needle and then reversing direction and taking a more superficial bite closer to the wound edge (Fig. 108.7A). If the superficial stitch is placed first, the wound edges can be pulled upward while the deeper stitch is placed, ensuring wound eversion in less time than with the traditional technique (101). Of note, the vertical mattress suture is more likely to cause ischemia of the wound edges than either simple interrupted or continuous sutures. Therefore, it is important to avoid the tendency to apply excess tension when tying these knots (19). The horizontal mattress suture closes a greater length of the wound than the vertical mattress suture but usually results in less accurate approximation of the wound edges (Fig. 108.7B). This suture may be helpful in areas where eversion is desirable but there is little subcutaneous tissue (67). The half-buried horizontal mattress suture combines an interrupted skin stitch with a buried dermal stitch (Fig 108.7C). This technique can be used to effectively join the edges of a skin flap to the edges of a recipient site (67). The dermal stitch is typically placed through the skin flap. The advantage of the half-buried horizontal mattress suture is that it halves the number of skin punctures and decreases the amount of tension on the free edge of the wound opposite the knot (43).

Corner Stitch and V-Y Advancement Flap

The corner stitch is simply a variation of the half-buried horizontal mattress suture. In executing the corner stitch, the dermal component of the half-buried suture is passed through

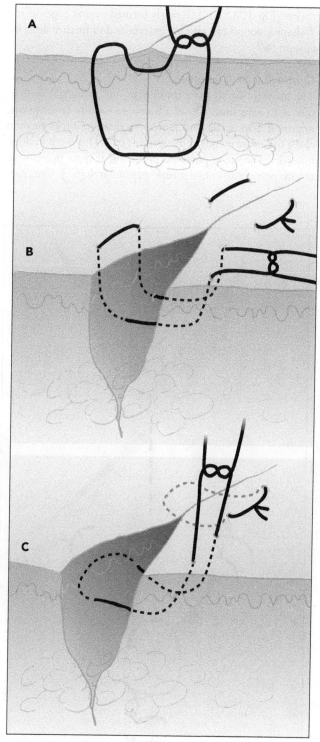

Figure 108.7 Mattress sutures.
A. Vertical mattress suture.
B. Horizontal mattress suture.
C. Half-buried horizontal mattress suture.

the very tip of the flap. The suture is tied with just enough tension to pull the flap snugly into the corner without blanching the flap (67). When applying this type of suture, it is often wise to extend the apex of a V-shaped laceration to form a Y configuration, which will release some of the tension on the corner (Fig. 108.8B). The newly formed wound edges of the Y-shaped wound can also be undermined to further decrease tension (67).

Continuous Skin Sutures

The main reason to use a continuous, or "running," skin suture is to save time. Other advantages include fewer knots, improved hemostasis, and more even distribution of tension along the entire length of the wound (67). This method does, however, pose some potential problems. If there is breakage at any point, the entire suture may unravel (67). Continu-

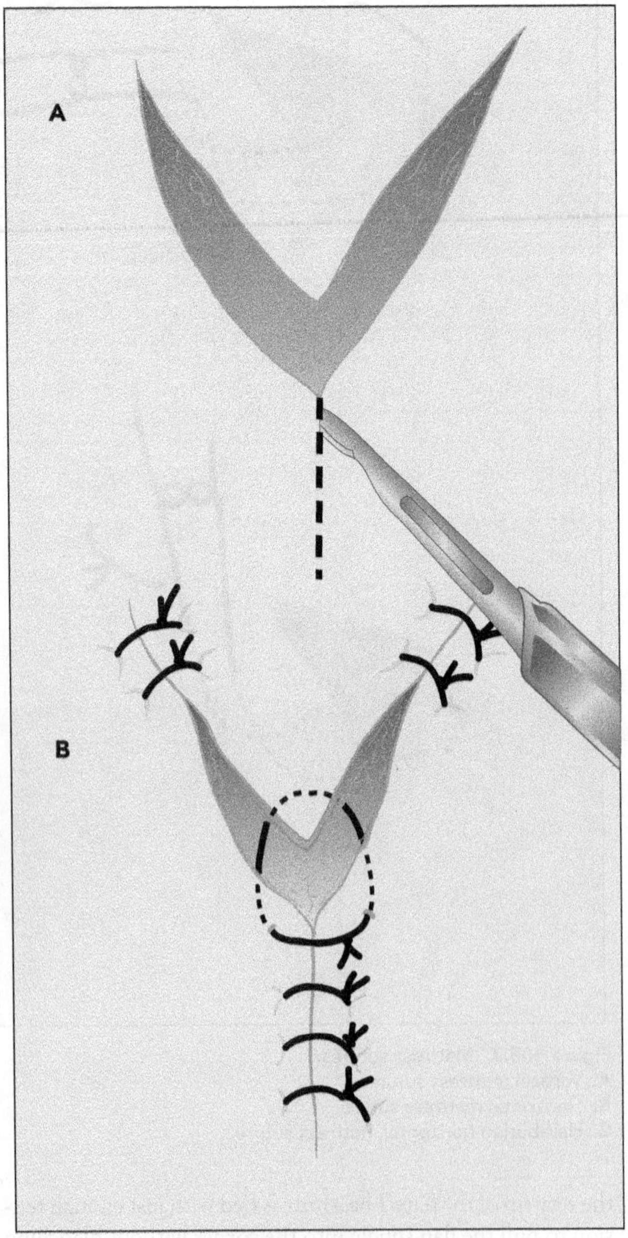

Figure 108.8 Corner stitch and V-Y advancement flap.
A. Extension of the wound at the apex of the V.
B. Half-buried horizontal mattress suture and simple interrupted stitches in the repair of a Y-shaped laceration.

ous sutures also may increase the risk of wound ischemia or early formation of stitch marks if pulled too tight (67,102). Ischemia is more likely to be a problem if an interlocking method is used. Many feel that continuous sutures are especially problematic in the setting of a focal wound infection; however, the suture can be cut and unwound from the infected area and secured with skin tape (102). In general, continuous sutures are recommended for straight, relatively clean wounds under little or no tension (67). Although most prefer interrupted sutures for cosmetic areas, careful placement of the individual stitches in a continuous suture can yield an excellent result (60).

The most useful continuous skin suture is the simple running stitch (Fig. 108.9A) (67). A simple interrupted stitch is first placed at one end of the wound, and only the free tail of the suture is cut. The clinician then performs sequential passes perpendicularly across the wound the same distance apart as normally placed interrupted sutures. After each pass, the thread is pulled to close the wound, and the placement is evaluated before proceeding to the next pass. If the placement is unacceptable, the needle can be backed out through the stitch site and the pass reattempted. Slight tension should be maintained on the thread with the clinician's nondominant hand so that the entire wound does not have to be reapproximated after each pass. Once the wound is closed, the running stitch is most simply ended by reversing the direction of the needle pass using an entry site close to the previous exit site. This forms a narrow loop on one side that can be tied with a final pass to the opposite side (Fig. 108.9A).

The continuous interlocking stitch is conducted in virtually the same manner as the simple running stitch except that the needle is also passed through a loop created by pulling a length of thread down in the direction the clinician is suturing (Fig. 108.9B). The interlocking loops that result prevent slippage as the suturing proceeds down the length of the wound (67). Another variation of the continuous suture is the running lateral mattress stitch or continuous half-buried horizontal stitch (Fig. 108.9C). This technique takes advantage of the more effective skin eversion provided by a mattress suture. It is generally recommended that a loop be intermittently run over the top of the wound to facilitate removal of the suture (95).

Continuous Subcuticular Sutures

The advantage of continuous subcuticular sutures is that there are no stitch marks, and therefore the sutures may be left in place for several weeks (94). Running subcuticular sutures are useful in wounds requiring an extended period of support, in wounds covered by casts, in patients prone to keloid formation, and in young children who may be frightened by suture removal (67). Unlike the other continuous suturing techniques, the running subcuticular technique does not offer much of a time-saving advantage, as it requires precise placement from side to side. These sutures are generally not recommended in wounds at increased risk for infection and should be avoided in wounds under significant tension (6,67,103).

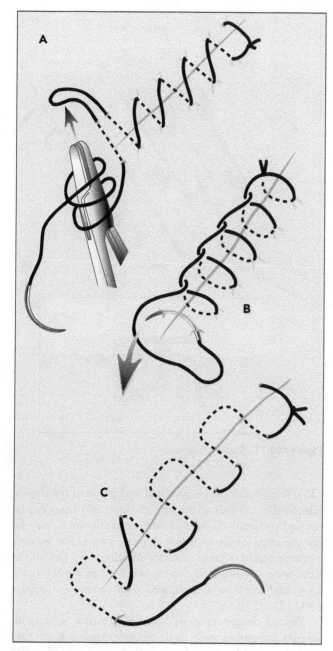

Figure 108.9 Continuous skin sutures.
A. Simple running skin stitch.
B. Continuous interlocking skin stitch.
C. Running lateral mattress stitch or continuous half-buried horizontal mattress stitch.

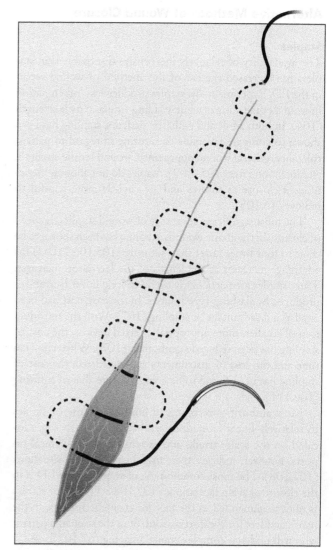

Figure 108.10 Running subcuticular stitch.

Because there are no stitch marks, running subcuticular sutures are often used for cosmetic closures. Exact alignment of the wound heights, however, can be difficult. Furthermore, in cosmetic areas, sutures are generally removed in 3 to 4 days, well before the risk period for stitch marks (31,73,96).

The running subcuticular stitch is usually started by passing the suture through the skin at one end of the wound and exiting within the dermis (Fig. 108.10). The wound is then closed by making small passes, less than 1 cm in width, on alternating sides of the wound in the dermal layer just below the skin surface. To ensure adequate alignment, each pass is usually begun slightly behind the exit point of the previous pass (67). Placement of each pass must be at the same level throughout the wound to ensure a good result. If the clinician must suture a long distance, it is advisable to bring the suture up to the surface on occasion to allow for easier removal (Fig. 108.10). The clinician can complete the suture by bringing it out through the skin surface. The two ends of exposed suture are then secured to the skin surface with wound tape. If the clinician is worried about the security of the repair, he or she can initiate the process with an interrupted suture and end with the looping back placement, as described with the simple running stitch (Fig. 108.9A). Skin tapes can be used to correct surface unevenness and to provide more accurate apposition of the epidermis (67).

Alternative Methods of Wound Closure

Staples

The availability of relatively inexpensive disposable skin sta-
plers has increased the use of this method of wound repair
in the ED. Experimentally, staples produce less inflammation
in wounds than sutures while yielding similar tensile strength
(104). In both adult and pediatric patients, stapling has been
shown to compare favorably to suturing in regard to patient
tolerance, general wound appearance, wound tensile strength,
and infection rates (105–109). Staples do not allow as meticulous a closure as sutures and are slightly more painful to
remove (16,105).

The most significant advantage of wound stapling is speed
of closure. In traumatic wounds, stapling has been shown to be
three to four times faster than suturing (105,106,110). This
advantage increases as the length of the laceration increases.
Thus, staples are particularly useful in long linear lacerations
produced by slashing-type injuries. In the past, cost had been
cited as a disadvantage of stapling (107). With the introduction of smaller, more appropriately sized devices, the cost of
stapling has been reduced significantly (107). When clinician
time and the cost of instruments are considered, the cost of
stapling has been found to be comparable to that of suturing
(106,111).

Most authorities recommend limiting the use of staples
to relatively linear lacerations with straight, sharp edges located on the scalp, trunk, and extremities (67). Clinical reports, however, indicate their usefulness in other situations
(107,108). The most common use of staples in the ED is in
the closure of scalp lacerations (107,108). The use of staples
is not recommended in the face for cosmetic reasons, in the
hands and feet for comfort reasons, or in the scalp of a patient
who will undergo complex cranial imaging (67,107).

The wound is prepared for staple placement in the same
manner as for traditional suture placement. This includes using subcutaneous sutures when needed to reduce tension. The
placement of staples is best achieved when an assistant everts
the wound edges with tissue forceps or finger pressure (67).
Once the edges are held in eversion, the stapling device is
centered over the wound, and with squeezing of the device's
handle, a staple is advanced in the wound and bent to the
proper configuration (Fig. 108.11A). If placed properly,
the crossbar of the staple is elevated a few millimeters above
the wound (Fig. 108.11B) (67).

A staple remover is a simple device that is often needed to
correct inaccurate placement of a staple at the time of repair.
This device can be given to the patient to bring to the follow-
up visit for staple removal. Staples are generally left in place
for a period of time similar to that for sutures in the same
area (16,67).

Wound Closure Tapes

The use of wound closure tapes, or "skin tapes," in pediatric
emergency care is common. One study reported that 20% of
lacerations in children were closed with wound closure tapes

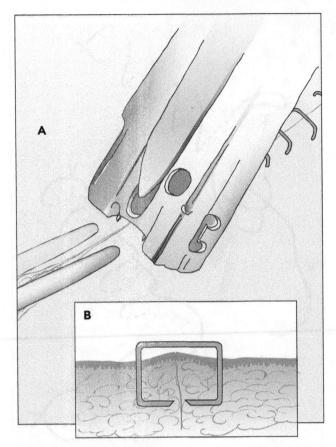

Figure 108.11   Staple placement.

(25). If a wound can be evaluated and prepared for closure
adequately with only a topical anesthetic, skin tapes can be
applied painlessly. Wound closure tapes, therefore, may be
the preferred choice in young children with minor wounds
not expected to require significant suturing (67). One of the
other main advantages of skin tapes is their greater resistance
to wound infection as compared with sutures and staples
(20,112).

Wound closure tapes are best used to close superficial,
straight lacerations under little tension. Areas that are particularly suited for tape closure include the forehead, malar
eminence, chin, chest, and nonjoint areas of the extremities
(67). Wound closure tapes are also useful in reinforcing other
repairs, such as a running subcuticular closure (6). To avoid
stitch marks in cosmetic areas, sutures can be removed in 2 to
3 days and replaced with skin tapes (67,95). If sutures appear
to be under significant tension at any time, their removal and
replacement with skin tapes is recommended (61,95). Wound
closure tapes should not be used in moist or hair-bearing areas
such as the scalp, axilla, palms, and soles (6,67).

After wound preparation, the technique of tape application
is fairly simple. This requires cleansing, drying, and applying
an adhesive adjunct (e.g., tincture of benzoin) to the surrounding skin before tape placement. The adhesive should not be
allowed to spill into the wound, as it may increase the risk
of infection (113). The skin heights must be approximated

carefully to ensure a good result. The skin tapes are placed perpendicularly across the wound, leaving some space for the wound to drain. Additional tapes can be placed across the ends of the previously placed strips to help prevent skin blisters caused by unsupported tape ends (67). There are various wound closure tapes available, with differing degrees of adhesion, porosity, breaking strength, and elasticity (114). One study, which compared several different types of wound closure tapes, noted that Steri-Strip, Curi-Strip, and Nichi-Strip tapes had the best overall performance (115). When the skin was treated with tincture of benzoin, Steri-Strip tapes outperformed all of the other wound closure tapes (115).

Tissue Adhesives

In 1998, the U.S. Food and Drug Administration (FDA) approved 2-octylcyanoacrylate (OCA; Dermabond, Ethicon) as the first tissue adhesive for use in the United States. The use of tissue adhesives is detailed in Chapter 109. A few comments are emphasized here. Several studies that compared OCA and conventional methods of wound closure suggested that with OCA the time needed for skin closure was shorter, its infection and dehiscence rates were comparable to those of conventional methods, and its cosmetic outcomes were equally good (116). Further, the use of adhesives is rapid and relatively painless, eliminates the risk of needle sticks, decreases the need for instruments and supplies, and does not require a return visit for suture removal (16,23). In addition, the adhesive itself has antimicrobial effects and can serve as its own wound dressing. There are, however, certain limitations. Tissue adhesives should not be used near the eyes, over joints, on mucosal surfaces, in dense hair-bearing areas, or on wounds under significant static or dynamic tension (67,74). Due to its liquid nature, runoff is a common problem (74). This can result in the inadvertent bonding of uninvolved tissues or other objects. Ointments or acetone can be used to remove tissue adhesive from areas of unintentional runoff (67,74).

Hair Ties

The closure of scalp wounds with the hair-tying method may be used as an alternative means of closure in small, superficial scalp wounds (117,118). The advantage of this technique is that it is relatively painless, surgical instruments are not required, and no foreign material is placed in the wound (67). In one study, when compared with standard suturing of scalp wounds, hair tying was found to be as effective, less painful, and less distressing to the patient. There was, however, mild wound separation noted in 8% of the patients (118).

The hair-tying method begins by separating the hair on each side of the laceration and then twisting it to form "ropes" of hair. The ropes of hair are then tied across the wound to tightly appose the skin edges. As the wound heals, the knot will grow away from the wound edge and can be cut free in 2 to 4 weeks.

Another method that has been described is the hair apposition technique (HAT), which involves securing the twisted hairs along the wound with tissue adhesive as opposed to using an actual knot (119). This method is noted to have the same advantages of traditional hair tying without the need for knot cutting several weeks later (119). However, the HAT method was not found to be as effective at achieving hemostasis and wound eversion (119).

Delayed Primary Closure

Delayed primary closure has been shown to be a safe alternative to immediate primary closure (120,121). If proper technique is used, overall healing time is not affected and the risk of infection is reduced. The technique of delayed primary closure is based on experimental studies of contaminated wounds. In one study, the infection rate for experimentally contaminated wounds was high if they were closed on the first day but low if closure was delayed until after 4 days (122). In general, this technique is not used as often in pediatric wound care because heavily contaminated wounds and crush injuries are infrequent in this population (24).

When a wound is being prepared for delayed primary closure, it should be irrigated and débrided in the same manner as for immediate primary closure. The wound cavity is then packed with sterile fine mesh gauze and covered with a bulky dressing. The wound is then left completely undisturbed for 4 to 5 days unless pain, fever, or other signs of wound infection develop (21,61,121). If the wound remains uninfected at the end of the waiting period, it is then approximated with sutures or wound closure tapes. These wounds will heal with excellent tensile strength, as the injury will just be entering the active phase of regeneration (121).

To avoid the need for repeat anesthesia of the wound, sutures can be placed in healthy tissue away from the wound edge during the first visit and then tied during the follow-up visit (21,61). Alternatively, on day 4 or 5, rather than just apposing the wound edges, the clinician may opt to sharply incise both edges to create a freshly cut surface for approximation (21). This delayed wound excision is primarily used to improve the cosmetic result, as a direct closure should heal without problems.

Approach to Specific Areas

Scalp

Lacerations of the scalp are common and generally heal without problems due to the scalp's extensive blood supply. The scalp is composed of five layers: skin, superficial fascia, galea aponeurotica, subgaleal (subaponeurotic) loose connective tissue, and periosteum. The superficial fascia contains a rich network of blood vessels that promote wound healing but also may lead to profuse bleeding even in the simplest of scalp lacerations (67). The subgaleal layer of loose connective tissue contains emissary veins that drain into the venous sinuses of the cranial hemispheres. Bacteria may be carried by these vessels to the meninges and intracranial sinuses. Careful approximation of the galeal layer protects against the spread of infection (67).

Emergency physicians must not be cavalier in their approach to scalp wounds, as significant underlying injury may be present. It is wise to explore all scalp wounds both visually and digitally to exclude the presence of a fracture or foreign body. Care should be taken to look under any flap of tissue (36). Débridement is generally not as high a priority, as the excellent blood supply of the scalp will ensure the survival of even heavily contused tissue (36). Bleeding vessels are best managed with direct pressure and expeditious wound closure. It is usually not necessary to tie off individual bleeders (36).

Scalp wounds are generally prepared in the same manner as other wounds, with the obvious obstacle of the hair. These wounds can usually be closed without hair removal. However, this may cause technical difficulties in suture placement and removal (123). Although the clinician is warned that unnecessary hair removal may increase the risk of infection, this recommendation is based on studies of preoperative patients (31). Clipping the hair rather than shaving it is a reasonable approach to scalp wounds (31). Vaseline-based ointments can also be used to mat down the hair adjacent to the wound (67).

Closure of the galea is generally recommended to prevent the development of a subgaleal hematoma and to minimize the risk of infection. Two general methods have been proposed for this. Some authorities feel that the galea should be closed together with the adjacent structures by taking one large bite through the involved layers (67). Others advocate separate closure of the galea with absorbable sutures (67,107,108,123). Although separate closure may provide a more secure approximation of the galea, the introduction of additional suture material into the wound may adversely affect wound healing.

In general, most scalp wounds can be repaired with percutaneous sutures or wound staples. Simple interrupted or vertical mattress sutures using 4-0 or 3-0 nonabsorbable nylon or polypropylene suture material are effective. The blue coloring of Prolene offers the advantage of easier identification at the time of removal. Wound stapling is a fast and cosmetically acceptable alternative to suturing for simple scalp lacerations (105–110). As previously mentioned, hair tying may be a reasonable alternative in suitable scalp wounds (117–119).

Forehead

Forehead lacerations are common in children. Most of these lacerations are simple, and few require plastic surgery consultation. The forehead is one of the easiest areas to predict wound tension because the RSTLs run transversely across the forehead. Lacerations that are horizontally oriented tend to heal well, while lacerations that are vertically oriented tend to heal with wider scars (36). In general, any laceration angled greater than 35 degrees from the RSTLs is more likely to heal with a poor result (93). For anatomical reasons, vertical lacerations situated in the midline are less likely to be problematic (36). Curved flap lacerations on the forehead may heal poorly secondary to the trapdoor effect caused by central contraction of the scar (67,94).

The effect of skin tension must be appreciated in all forehead lacerations. Efforts to counteract skin tension, includ-

ing undermining and deep suture placement, should always be considered. Deeper lacerations involving the deep fascia, frontalis muscle, and periosteum should be closed in layers. Wound closure tapes may be used to provide additional support while sutures are in place and after they are removed. Even small vertical forehead lacerations will be under tension and therefore should not be closed simply with wound closure tapes or tissue adhesives. Many people have small but unsightly forehead scars acquired as a result of an ED repair during youth. Extra care in the initial management and follow-up of these wounds will decrease the likelihood of such a result.

Windshield injuries are common and typically present with multiple lacerations, abrasions, and areas of tissue loss. Each individual laceration must be explored for the presence of glass (36). Multiple small wounds can be handled by a combination of loose single stitches, taping, or minor wound excision (36,94). Subsequent dermabrasion or dermaplaning may be necessary for such injuries (94).

Eyebrows

The eyebrow is a major cosmetic landmark, and therefore reapproximation must be exact (94). Shaving the eyebrow should generally be avoided because correct alignment of the eyebrow after it is shaved is difficult if not impossible. Furthermore, regrowth of eyebrow hair after it is shaved is slow and unpredictable (2,36,67). Débridement of the eyebrow, as with other facial structures, should be conservative (36,93). If débridement is necessary, excisional cuts must be angled parallel to the direction of hair follicle growth. Perpendicularly placed excisional cuts will damage an excessive number of hair follicles, leaving a wide hairless area (2,36,67). In closing the wound, the eyebrow margins should be sutured first to avoid a visible step-off.

Eyelids

Most eyelid lacerations are simple transverse wounds of the upper eyelid easily managed by the emergency physician. More complicated lacerations, however, must be recognized. The following lacerations are considered complex and require immediate ophthalmologic consultation (2,36,67):

Lacerations through the orbital septum. The presence of fat within the wound confirms this diagnosis.

Lacerations of the free margins. Meticulous repair is required to prevent deformity and disability.

Lacerations involving the levator palpebrae muscle or tendon. Ptosis is noted on exam.

Lacerations involving the medial canthal ligament.

Lacerations involving the lacrimal duct (these typically involve the medial third of the upper or lower lid). The duct must be probed through the punctum with fine suture material, and the wound examined for visualization of the suture to confirm duct injury. Failure to recognize and repair the lacrimal duct can lead to chronic tearing.

Nose

Although blunt nasal trauma is common, lacerations of the nose are relatively infrequent. Lacerations of the superior aspect of the nose are handled like other facial wounds. Lacerations of the inferior aspect of the nose are more difficult to repair. Because the skin overlying the inferior aspect of the nose is tight and stiff, it is often difficult to approximate gaping wounds in this location (2,36). In addition, suture material will often slice through the skin and pull out.

Full-thickness lacerations should be closed in layers. Absorbable sutures are used to repair the mucosal surface (36). The nasal cartilage, when involved, rarely requires sutures. The skin is usually closed with simple interrupted 6-0 nonabsorbable sutures. The skin of the distal nose does not hold stitches well and is prone to forming stitch marks and abscesses. For this reason, some authorities recommend subcuticular sutures for this area (67). Alternatively, simple interrupted sutures can placed initially with early removal and subsequent application of wound closure tapes. Skin taping, however, is difficult with adolescents, as the skin of the nose is quite oily (67). The free rim of the nares is an important cosmetic landmark and must be closed carefully (2).

Fractures commonly accompany nasal lacerations. Although the patient will ultimately be referred to an otolaryngologist, primary repair of the laceration can usually be completed by the emergency physician.

Ears

The primary goal in treating ear lacerations is to protect the underlying cartilaginous structures (Chapter 55). Repair of simple lacerations not involving the cartilage proceeds as with other wounds. If the cartilage has been violated, it must be covered to prevent subsequent infection (2,36,37,67). If skin loss is significant and a large amount of cartilage is exposed, early consultation should be sought for possible removal and preservation of the cartilage in a subcutaneous pocket for later use.

If at all possible, the wound should be closed without suturing the cartilage to decrease the risk of infection (37). The cartilage can be left unrepaired if the injury to the cartilage is small and the edges are well apposed before suturing. If repair of the underlying cartilage is necessary, sutures must be placed through the adjacent perichondrium, as the cartilage will not hold a stitch. In through-and-through ear lacerations, the skin on the posterior aspect of the ear may be closed with absorbable sutures to avoid excessive bending of the ear upon suture removal.

After an ear laceration is repaired, a conforming dressing should be applied (Chapter 55) (67). Moistened cotton balls are used to fill in the ear concavities as well as the space behind the ear. A large compression wrap is then applied around the head, and the dressing is left in place for 2 days. Upon removal of the dressing, the wound should be evaluated for a subperichondrial hematoma. If a hematoma is present, consultation with an otolaryngologist or plastic surgeon is recommended for drainage.

Lips

The principles of lip closure are few and include conservative débridement, excluding débridement of the philtrum, layered closure, and exact approximation of the vermillion border (Chapter 67) (2,36,37,67,94).

Tongue and Intraoral Lacerations

Most lacerations of the tongue and intraoral mucosa in children will heal well without sutures (Chapter 67). Lacerations of the tongue that are deep or involve a division of the free edge should be closed to avoid entrapment of food, prolongation of healing, or subsequent disability (2,67). Repair of intraoral mucosal lacerations is necessary only for deep lacerations to accelerate healing and to avoid complications. These lacerations must be evaluated closely to ensure that there are no injuries to the salivary ducts or facial nerves.

Other Facial Areas

Evaluation for injuries to underlying structures, particularly the parotid duct and facial nerve, is essential for lacerations involving the lateral aspects of the face.

Due to the underlying bony prominence, the cheek area is prone to a particular type of injury. A small laceration secondary to blunt trauma may actually be associated with significant muscle violation beneath the surface. If this is not recognized and repaired, an unsightly depressed scar may result (94). Palpation of a soft-tissue defect under the small laceration may be a clue to this injury. Extension of the skin wound may be necessary to allow adequate visualization and determine if a complex repair is needed.

The chin is a common area for lacerations in children, and the mechanism is virtually always blunt trauma from a fall. These wounds are tempting to débride, but débridement is usually not necessary (36). If the wound is not under significant tension, as appreciated by visualizing the wound at rest, wound closure tapes can be used.

Extremity Lacerations

In general, it is best to avoid deep sutures whenever possible in extremity lacerations because the overall incidence of wound infection is higher (36). The higher rate of infection in lower extremity wounds calls for careful evaluation of the need for any sutures at all in these wounds (24,25,35). This may be particularly pertinent with lacerations of the foot (6).

Lacerations over joints, especially the knee, will require prolonged immobilization of the joint if sutures are placed. Sutures may be forgone in some minor wounds in these areas to allow the patient to avoid the inconvenience and expense of joint immobilization.

Lacerations through the tip of the finger are common in young children and often caused by a closing door (Chapter 103). These injuries can appear dramatic but usually heal well. Significant bony involvement should prompt consultation with an orthopaedic or hand surgeon, but most of these injuries can be handled by the emergency physician.

Continued Wound Care

Dressings

Dressings play an important part in continued wound care (Chapter 107). An effective dressing will absorb wound secretions, protect the wound from further trauma, and prevent contamination from external sources (2,68,124). Wounds are susceptible to infection from surface contamination in the first 2 days after wound repair (68). Dressings, therefore, should remain in place for 24 to 48 hours, after which epithelialization is usually sufficient to protect the wound from gross contamination (2,16). Although dressings are universally recommended, clinical studies have not demonstrated an increased rate of infection in wounds that are not dressed (124). For most simple wounds, it is adequate to cover the wound with dry sterile gauze (2). A nonadherent material (Xeroform, Adaptic) may also be used to cover the wound surface to keep the wound from sticking to the dry gauze (68). Dressings should be changed if they become soiled, wet, or saturated with drainage because the wet dressing may itself become a source of infection (2).

Some studies indicate that the application of topical antibiotic ointments may reduce infection (125). These agents also help keep the wound moist and prevent scab formation. Maintenance of a moist environment encourages more rapid wound healing by increasing the rate of epithelialization. Preventing scab formation is also important because if a scab is allowed to become interposed in the wound edges, it will be replaced by scar tissue (6). Patients whose lacerations are closed with tissue adhesives should not have topical ointments applied to the wound. These agents may loosen the tissue adhesive and result in wound dehiscence (16).

Pressure dressings may be used to prevent fluid accumulation in certain wounds, thereby inhibiting the development of infection. The amount of pressure applied proximally to an extremity wound should be minimized to prevent wound edema (6). It may be necessary to splint a wound, especially if it overlies a joint. The injured extremity should also be elevated to provide comfort and reduce edema (2). A common oversight is failure to elevate hand injuries with the use of a simple sling. Likewise, prescribing crutches for lower extremity injuries often encourages the patient to remain in a more erect position. Local heat application increases blood flow to wounds and therefore may have a role in wound healing and the prevention of wound infections (126).

Antibiotics

Prophylactic antibiotics should not be prescribed routinely following laceration repair (Chapter 107). Several clinical studies have found that there is no benefit to prophylactic antibiotics in the management of simple lacerations (127). In fact, some evidence indicates the opposite effect (128). Some authorities suggest the use of antibiotics for wounds only when the predicted infection rate is greater than 10% (4). This strategy, however, has never been proven in a clinical

trial, and the rate of infection in routine pediatric lacerations is well below this threshold (24,25).

Intraoral and perioral lacerations are considered to be contaminated wounds due to the high bacterial counts of saliva (6). Studies, however, have shown that prophylactic antibiotics have little or no effect on the rate of infection in most of these wounds (129). Antibiotics are generally recommended in full-thickness intraoral wounds and those considered to be heavily contaminated. If a clinician chooses to use an antibiotic, penicillin is an adequate choice (129). Other high-risk wounds include those on the hands, feet, or perineum and those involving exposed cartilage on the nose or ear. Regarding hand lacerations, several studies indicate no significant benefit from using antibiotics (34,130,131).

The use of prophylactic antibiotics does not appear to reduce the rate of infection in dog or cat bite wounds (132). However, it does appear to reduce the risk of infection in human bites and all mammalian bites of the hand (132). Human bite wounds of the hand are at even greater risk for infection, particularly those from a closed fist injury (57). It is recommended that all such hand wounds receive antibiotics (57). Penicillin is a reasonable choice in noninfected wounds, as it covers oral flora adequately. If a wound becomes infected, staphylococcal coverage must be added, with the continuation of penicillin to cover *Eikenella corrodens*, a common organism in human bite wound infections (57). Bites in areas other than the hands generally heal well if they can be adequately cleansed and do not routinely require antibiotics. Although many physicians feel the need to prescribe antibiotics for such wounds, little scientific basis for this practice exists. (133).

Suture Removal

The general schedule for suture removal is 3 to 5 days for the face, 7 days for the scalp and anterior trunk, and 7 to 10 days for the extremities and back (2,16,36,37,67). Sutures subject to high tension, such as those over joints, should be left in place for 10 to 14 days. Increased pull on sutures may lead to early formation of stitch marks. If wound edema causes significant tension on any sutures, they should be removed and replaced with skin tapes (25). When a laceration is repaired primarily with wound closure tapes, follow-up is not necessary for removal. The tape strips will fall off spontaneously in 7 to 10 days. Tissue adhesive sloughs off in a similar time period.

▶ COMPLICATIONS

Any disruption of the skin involving the dermis will heal by the formation of scar tissue. A primary goal in suturing lacerations should be to minimize the size and visibility of the scar. Formation of keloids and hypertrophic scars are the unavoidable result of an abnormal healing process; however, a poorly or incorrectly performed step in wound closure will increase the likelihood of producing an unsightly scar.

An uneven skin surface resulting from an elevation or depression of scar tissue will cast a shadow across the skin,

SUMMARY

Wound Preparation

1 Use conscious sedation as needed.

2 Anesthetize the wound.

3 Control bleeding.

4 Explore the wound for foreign bodies or injuries to underlying structures.

5 Remove contaminated or devitalized tissue through débridement and excision.

6 Cleanse the wound thoroughly.

7 Undermine the wound edges when necessary to reduce tension.

Using a Needle Holder

1 Grasp the needle away from the swage and closer to the tip for tougher tissue.

2 Hold the needle perpendicular to the needle holder.

3 Enter the skin perpendicular to the surface.

4 Stabilize or manipulate the skin edges with a skin hook or nontraumatic forceps.

5 Retrieve the needle after each pass with the needle holder or forceps.

Instrument Tie

1 Pull the suture through the wound, leaving a small tail at the insertion site.

2 Grasp the longer (needle) end of the suture in the nondominant hand.

3 Loop the suture twice *over* the tip of the needle holder.

4 Grasp the shorter (free) end of the suture with the needle holder.

5 Pull the free end through the loops and away from the side of the wound initially entered.

6 Tighten the knot so that the skin edges just come together.

7 Loop the needle end of the suture once *under* the tip of the needle holder.

8 Grasp the free end of the suture with the needle holder.

9 Pull the free end through the loop and back to the initial needle entry side of the wound.

10 Repeat the single loop tie first in the over and then in the under manner for a total of four throws.

11 Cut both ends of the suture, allowing adequate length to retrieve the suture at the time of removal.

Simple Interrupted Skin Sutures

1 Enter the skin with the needle directed downward or angled slightly away from the wound edge.

2 Drive the needle to a depth greater than the width of the stitch.

3 Trace a symmetric path through both sides of the wound.

4 Secure the suture with an instrument tie.

Subcutaneous Sutures

1 Insert the needle from within the wound at the fat-dermal junction.

2 Rotate the needle up through the tissue and exit in the dermis.

3 Insert the needle in the opposing dermis at an equal vertical and horizontal level.

4 Rotate the needle down through the tissue and exit at the fat-dermal junction.

5 Bring both ends of the suture to the same side of the loop.

6 Secure the suture with a knot consisting of three throws only.

7 Cut the suture ends short.

Interrupted Mattress Sutures

Vertical Mattress

1 Place a wide, deep stitch across the wound—use two steps (retrieving the needle from within the wound) when necessary.

2 Reverse directions from the previous stitch, entering the same side as the recent exit but at a point closer to the wound edge and in line with the previous pass.

3 Complete a smaller and shallower pass on the same side as the initial entry site and the same distance from the wound edge as the second entry site.

4 Tie a knot on the side of the wound that was initially entered.

(continued)

SUMMARY (CONTINUED)

Horizontal Mattress

1 Place an initial stitch of the same dimensions as a simple interrupted suture pass.

2 Re-enter the skin lateral to the exit point and equidistant from the wound edge.

3 Perform a second pass, reversing directions from the previous stitch and exiting at a point lateral to the initial entry site and equidistant from the wound edge.

4 Tie a knot on the side of the wound that was initially entered.

Half-Buried Mattress or Corner Stitch

1 Enter the skin below and just lateral to the point of the V.

2 Exit within the wound.

3 Evert the tip of the flap with skin hooks or forceps.

4 Pass the needle through the dermis of the flap tip, parallel to the skin surface.

5 Enter the wound on the opposite side of the point of the V.

6 Exit through the skin at a point below and lateral to the point of the V, symmetrically across from the initial insertion site.

7 Secure the suture with an instrument tie.

Continuous Skin Sutures

Simple Running Stitch

1 Place a simple interrupted suture at one end of the laceration without cutting the needle end of the suture.

2 Travel the length of the laceration performing sequential passes perpendicular to the laceration and equidistant from each other.

3 Maintain tension on the needle end of the suture following each pass.

4 Reverse the direction of the needle pass once the end of the laceration is reached.

5 Enter the skin close to the previous exit site, and leave a narrow loop on that side by only partially pulling the suture through.

6 Secure the end of the suture with an instrument tie using a narrow loop at the free end of the suture.

Running Subcuticular Stitch

1 Pass the suture through the skin at one end of the wound and exit in the dermis.

2 Travel the length of the wound making small passes (less than 1 cm in width) within the dermis and parallel to the skin surface.

3 Alternate sides of the wound, with each entry site slightly behind the previous exit point and at the same vertical level of the dermis.

4 Complete the suture by bringing the needle out through the skin surface at the end of the wound.

5 Cut the needle from the suture.

6 Tape the free ends of suture to the skin surface using skin tape.

Staples

1 Evert the wound edges with a forceps or finger pressure.

2 Center the stapling device over the wound and apply gentle pressure to the wound surface.

3 Slowly squeeze the device trigger to eject the staple into the tissue.

4 Pull back the wrist to disengage the staple from the device.

Wound Closure Tapes

1 Clean and dry the skin surrounding the laceration.

2 Apply skin adhesive to the surrounding area.

3 Place skin tapes perpendicularly across the wound, leaving some space for oozing.

4 Place extra skin tapes across the ends of previous strips and parallel to the wound.

Delayed Primary Closure

1 Anesthetize the wound.

2 Explore the wound.

3 Débride and excise the wound as needed.

4 Thoroughly cleanse the wound.

5 Fill the wound cavity with sterile, fine mesh gauze.

6 Cover the wound with a bulky dressing.

7 Remove the dressing in 4 to 5 days and approximate the wound edges with sutures or skin tapes if no infection or devitalized tissue is evident.

CLINICAL TIPS

▶ Adequate immobilization and anesthesia are key to successful laceration repair in children.

▶ Natural landmarks should always be used. Shaving the eyebrow or using epinephrine in anesthetizing the vermilion border obscures two important landmarks.

▶ Shaving the hair is generally unnecessary in the repair of scalp wounds.

▶ The intrinsic forces across a laceration must be considered when planning wound closure.

▶ The use of delayed closure should be based on the location and the degree of contamination of the wound.

▶ Only skin hooks, nontraumatic forceps, or fingers should be used in handling wound edges.

▶ The fewest number of sutures should be used for the shortest period of time sufficient for wound healing.

▶ Three layers support sutures best: the fascial-fat junction, the dermal-fat junction, and the level just below the dermal-epidermal junction. Fat and muscle will not hold a stitch.

▶ Wounds under greater tension should have more skin sutures placed, and these should be closer to the wound edge.

▶ Wound edges should be approximated to accommodate edema that occurs after closure. Strangulation of tissue must be avoided.

▶ Wound edges should always be everted, not inverted.

▶ A pass that is wider at the base than at the surface ensures eversion of the edges.

▶ The use of colored sutures in hair improves visibility for eventual removal.

▶ Suture ends should be cut long enough to allow easy handling for removal.

▶ Parents should be told that the healing process and scar appearance will not be complete until 6 months after the repair.

▶ Leaving sutures in place for prolonged periods of time or under excessive tension results in stitch marks.

▶ Skin tapes can provide useful reinforcement to sutures or continued support following suture removal.

▶ The general schedule for suture removal is 3 to 5 days for the face, 7 days for the scalp and anterior trunk lacerations, and 10 to 14 days for the extremities and back.

▶ U-shaped or "trap door" lacerations are prone to scarring.

▶ Using fingers to push tissue over the needle risks injury to the clinician.

▶ Running subcuticular sutures are useful in wounds requiring an extended period of support, in wounds covered by casts, in patients prone to keloid formation, and in young children who may be frightened by suture removal.

▶ Vaseline-based ointments can be used to mat down hair and improve the exposure of scalp wounds.

making the defect more obvious. This may result from a failure to adequately align the skin layers or from inverting rather than everting the epidermal layer during closure. Formation of a hematoma in the subcutaneous layers can result in a depression of the skin surface once the hematoma has been absorbed. This may be avoided through closure of all skin layers.

Failure to accurately align natural landmarks such as the eyebrow or the vermillion border of the lip will be noticeable no matter how invisible the actual scar.

So-called "dog ears" result from excess tissue on one edge of the wound that is gathered at the end of the laceration. This may be a consequence of inaccurate alignment of wound edges by the clinician or the inevitable result of a laceration with avulsed tissue that leaves unequal lengths of opposing wound edges. The clinician can avoid malalignment by sewing

inward from both ends or by throwing an initial suture in the center of a long laceration dividing it into two smaller, more manageable lacerations. Additional corrective methods are possible in instances when the formation of a dog ear is unavoidable.

Optimal healing depends on the transport of oxygen and nutrients to the site of injury. Excessive undermining or rough handling of tissue can disrupt this process, resulting in the death of tissue and increased scar formation.

Sutures also can produce scars. Excessive tension placed on the sutures will result in strangulation and ischemia of the tissue. Sutures may actually tear through the wound margin. Healing will occur by formation of more scar tissue rather than the natural regeneration of the epithelium. Sutures that are left in place for excessive periods also will leave permanent stitch marks. Knots of subcutaneous sutures will increase tissue reaction at the skin surface and may even break through the surface if not buried.

Functional impairment can result from undue tension imposed by sutures placed across a laceration that occurs in a location requiring a significant degree of mobility, such as a joint. Contractures occur when inadequate tissue is available to allow full mobility following healing. They also can occur as a result of the abnormal continuation of the normal process of wound contraction. Contractures occasionally can be averted through using splints that allow the laceration to heal in the position of greatest extension. In certain instances, it may be preferable to allow the wound to heal by secondary intention.

▶ SUMMARY

Because lacerations occur commonly in children, laceration repair is an essential skill for the clinician treating acute injuries in the pediatric population. Additional expertise is sometimes necessary, but the majority of wound closures do not require a subspecialist. Careful attention to the mechanism of injury, the location of the wound, and the overall risk of infection will help the clinician determine the best method of closure. The clinician should possess a thorough understanding of skin anatomy and the orientation of relaxed skin tension lines. Exploration of the wound, proper cleansing and preparation, and appropriate follow-up wound care are also essential for optimizing function and minimizing scar formation. The best results are obtained when adequate immobilization, sedation, and analgesia are achieved.

▶ ACKNOWLEDGMENT

The authors would like to acknowledge the valuable contributions of John M. Loiselle to the version of this chapter that appeared in the previous edition.

▶ REFERENCES

1. McCraig LF, Ly N. *National Hospital Ambulatory Medical Survey: 2000 Emergency Department Summary.* Hyattsville, MD: National Center for Health Statistics; 2002. Advance Data from Vital and Health Statistics No. 326.
2. Selbst SM, Attia MW. Minor trauma: lacerations. In: Ludwig S, Fleisher GR, Henretig FM, eds. *Textbook of Pediatric Emergency Medicine.* 5th ed. Philadelphia: Lippincott Williams & Wilkins; 2006: 1571–1588.
3. Hambidge SJ, Davidson AJ, Gonzalez R, et al. Epidemiology of pediatric injury-related primary care office visits in the United States. *Pediatrics.* 2002;109:559–565.
4. Krauss BS, Herakal T, Fleisher GR. General trauma in a pediatric emergency department: spectrum and consultation patterns. *Pediatr Emerg Care.* 1993;9:134–138.
5. Baker MD, Selbst SM, Lanuti M. Lacerations in urban children: a prospective 12-January study. *Am J Dis Child.* 1990;144:87–92.
6. Edlich RF, Rodeheaver GT, Morgan RF, et al. Principles of emergency wound management. *Ann Emerg Med.* 1988;17:1284–1302.

7. Borges AF. Relaxed skin tension lines. *Dermatol Clin.* 1989;7:169–177.
8. Burns JL, Blackwell SJ. Plastic surgery. In: Townsend CM, Beauchamp RD, Evers BM, eds. *Sabiston Textbook of Surgery,* 17th ed. Philadelphia: Elsevier Saunders; 2004:2181–2203.
9. Simon B, Hern HG. Soft tissue injuries. In: Marx JA, Hockberger RS, Walls RM, eds. *Rosen's Emergency Medicine: Concepts and Clinical Practice.* 5th ed. St. Louis: Mosby; 2002:738–751.
10. Hunt TK. The physiology of wound healing. *Ann Emerg Med.* 1988;17:1265–1273.
11. Tredget EE, Nedelec B, Scott PG, et al. Hypertrophic scars, keloids, and contractures: the cellular and molecular basis for therapy. *Surg Clin North Am.* 1997;77:701–730.
12. Uitto J. Connective tissue biochemistry of the aging dermis: age-related alterations in collagen and elastin. *Dermatol Clin.* 1986;4: 433–446.
13. Holt DR, Kirk SJ, Regan MC, et al. Effect of age on wound healing in healthy human beings. *Surgery.* 1992;112:293–297.
14. Kono T, Tanii T, Furukawa M, et al. Correlation between aging and collagen gel contractility of human fibroblasts. *Acta Derm Venerol.* 1990;70:241–244.
15. Hollander JE, Singer AJ. State of the art: laceration management. *Ann Emerg Med.* 1999;34:354–367.
16. Capellan O, Hollander JE. Management of lacerations in the emergency department. *Emerg Med Clin North Am.* 2003;21:205–231.
17. McDowell AJ. Extravagant treatment of garden variety lacerations. *Plast Reconstr Surg.* 1979;63:111–112.
18. Borges AF. Timing of scar revision techniques. *Clin Plast Surg.* 1990;17:71–76.
19. Robson MC. Disturbances of wound healing. *Ann Emerg Med.* 1988;17:1274–1278.
20. Hunt TK. Disorders of repair and their management. In: Hunt TK, Dunphy JE, eds. *Fundamentals of Wound Management.* New York: Appleton-Century-Crofts; 1979:68–168.
21. Burke JF. Infection. In: Hunt TK, Dunphy JE, eds. *Fundamentals of Wound Management.* New York: Appleton-Century-Crofts; 1979: 170–240.
22. Berk WA, Welch RD, Bock BF. Controversial issues in clinical management of the simple wound. *Ann Emerg Med.* 1992;21:72–80.
23. Knapp JF. Emergency medicine: updates in wound management for the pediatrician. *Pediatr Clin North Am.* 1999;46:1201–1213.
24. Rosenberg NM, DeBaker K. Incidence of infection in pediatric patients with laceration. *Pediatr Emerg Care.* 1987;3:239–241.
25. Baker DM, Lanuti M. The management and outcome of lacerations in urban children. *Ann Emerg Med.* 1990;19:1001–1005.
26. Heinzelmann M, Scott M, Lan T. Factors predisposing to bacterial invasion and infection. *Am J Surg.* 2002;183:179–190.
27. Berk WA, Osbourne DD, Taylor DD. Evaluation of the "golden period" for wound repair: 204 cases from a Third World emergency department. *Ann Emerg Med.* 1988;17:496–500.
28. Robson MC, Duke WF, Krizek TJ. Rapid bacterial screening in the treatment of civilian wounds. *J Surg Res.* 1973;14:426–430.
29. Marshall KA, Edgerton MT, Rodeheaver GT, et al. Quantitative microbiology: its application to hand injuries. *Am J Surg.* 1976;131:730–733.
30. Nylen S, Carlsson B. Time factor, infection frequency and quantitative microbiology in hand injuries. *Scand J Plast Reconstr Surg.* 1980;14:185–189.
31. Edlich RF, Rodeheaver G, Thacker JG, et al. Technical factors in wound management. In: Hunt TK, Dunphy JE, eds. *Fundamentals of Wound Management.* New York: Appleton-Century-Crofts; 1979: 364–454.
32. Haury B, Rodeheaver G, Vensko J, et al. Debridement: an essential component of traumatic wound care. *Am J Surg.* 1978;135:238–242.

33. Cardany CR, Rodeheaver G, Thacker J, et al. The crush injury: a high risk wound. *JACEP.* 1976;5:965–970.

34. Haughey RE, Lammers RL, Wagner DK. Use of antibiotics in the initial management of soft tissue hand wounds. *Ann Emerg Med.* 1981;10:187–192.

35. Rutherford WH, Spence RAJ. Infection in wounds sutured in the accident and emergency department. *Ann Emerg Med.* 1980;9:350–352.

36. Dushoff IM. About face. *Emerg Med.* November 1974:24–77.

37. Crow RW. Sports-related lacerations: promoting healing and limiting scarring. *Phys Sports Med.* 1993;21:143–147.

38. Chen E, Hornig S, Shepherd SM, et al. Primary closure of mammalian bites. *Acad Emerg Med.* 2000;7:157–161.

39. Hollander JE, Singer JS, Valentine S, et al. Wound registry: development and validation. *Ann Emerg Med.* 1995;25:675–685.

40. Wiley JF. Mammalian bites: review of evaluation and management. *Clin Pediatr.* 1990;29:283–287.

41. Weber EJ, Callaham ML. Mammalian bites. In: Marx JA, Hockberger RS, Walls RM, eds. *Rosen's Emergency Medicine: Concepts and Clinical Practice.* 5th ed. St. Louis: Mosby; 2002:774–785.

42. Callaham ML. Human and animal bites. *Top Emerg Med.* April 1982:1–13.

43. Lindsey D, Christopher M, Hollenbach J, et al. Natural course of the human bite wound: incidence of infection and complications in 434 bites and 803 lacerations in the same group of patients. *J Trauma.* 1987;27:45–48.

44. Baker DM, Moore SE. Human bites in children: a 6-year experience. *Am J Dis Child.* 1987;141:1285–1290.

45. Schweich P, Fleisher G. Human bites in children. *Pediatr Emerg Care.* 1985;1:51–53.

46. Boenning DA, Fleisher GR, Campus JM. Dog bites in children: epidemiology, microbiology, and penicillin prophylactic therapy. *Am J Emerg Med.* 1983;1:17–21.

47. Cummings P. Antibiotics to prevent infections in patients with dog bite wounds: a meta-analysis of randomized trials. *Ann Emerg Med.* 1994;23:535–540.

48. Dire DJ. Cat bite wounds: risk factors for infection. *Ann Emerg Med.* 1991;20:973.

49. Weiss HB, Friedman DI, Coben JH. Incidence of dog bite injuries treated in emergency departments. *JAMA.* 1998;279:51–53.

50. Dire DJ. Emergency management of dog and cat bite wounds. *Emerg Clin North Am.* 1992;10:719–736.

51. Maimaris C, Quinton DN. Dog bite lacerations: a controlled trial of primary wound closure. *Arch Emerg Med.* 1988;5:156–161.

52. Dire DJ, Hogan DE, Riggs MW. A prospective evaluation of risk factors for infections from dog bite wounds. *Acad Emerg Med.* 1994;1:258–266.

53. Guy RJ, Zook EJ. Successful treatment of acute head and neck dog bite wounds without antibiotics. *Ann Plast Surg.* 1986;17:45–48.

54. Aghababian RV, Conte JE. Mammalian bite wounds. *Ann Emerg Med.* 1980;9:79–83.

55. Donkor P, Bankas DO. A study of primary closure of human bite injuries to the face. *J Oral Maxillofac Surg.* 1997;55:479–481.

56. Kizer K. Epidemiologic and clinical aspects of animal bite injuries. *JACEP.* 1979;8:134–141.

57. Callaham M. Controversies in antibiotic choices for bite wounds. *Ann Emerg Med.* 1988;17:1321–1330.

58. Davies D, Smith R. Plastic and reconstructive surgery. The hand II. *Br Med J.* 1985;290:1729–1734.

59. Brunner RG, Fallon WF. A prospective, randomized clinical trial of wound débridement versus conservative wound care in soft tissue injury from civilian gunshot wounds. *Am Surg.* 1990;56:104–107.

60. Ordog GI, Wasserberger J, Balasubramanium S, et al. Civilian gunshot wounds: outpatient management. *J Trauma.* 1994;36:106.

61. Dushoff IM. A stitch in time. *Emerg Med.* January 1973:1–16.

62. Edlich RF. Technical considerations in closure of skin wounds. In: Sparkman RS, ed. *The Healing of Surgical Wounds.* Pearl River, NY: Davis & Geck; 1985:2–19.

63. DeHoll D, Rodeheaver G, Edgerton MT, et al. Potentiation of infection by suture closure of dead space. *Am J Surg.* 1974;127:716–720.

64. Milewski PJ, Thomson H. Is a fat stitch necessary? *Br J Surg.* 1980;67:393–394.

65. Austin PE, Dunn KA, Eily-Cofield K, et al. Subcuticular sutures and the rate of inflammation in noncontaminated wounds. *Ann Emerg Med.* 1995;25:328–330.

66. Mehta PH, Dunn KA, Bradfield JF, et al. Contaminated wounds: infection rates with subcutaneous sutures. *Ann Emerg Med.* 1996;27:43–48.

67. Lammers RL, Trott AT. Methods of wound closure. In: Roberts JR, Hedges JR, eds. *Clinical Procedures in Emergency Medicine.* 4th ed. Philadelphia: WB Saunders; 2004:655–693.

68. Lammers RL. Principles of wound management. In: Roberts JR, Hedges JR, eds. *Clinical Procedures in Emergency Medicine.* Philadelphia: WB Saunders; 2004:623–654.

69. Perelman VS, Francis GJ, Rutledge T, et al. Sterile versus nonsterile gloves for repair of uncomplicated lacerations in the emergency department: a randomized controlled trial. *Ann Emerg Med.* 2004;43:363–370.

70. Ruthman JC, Hendrickson D, Miller RF, et al. Effect of cap and mask on infection rates. *Ill Med J.* 1984;165:397–399.

71. Swanson NA, Tromovitch TA. Suture materials, 1980s: properties, uses, and abuses. *Int J Dermatol.* 1982;21:374–378.

72. Capperauld I. Sutures in wound repair. In: Westaby S, ed. *Wound Care.* St. Louis: Mosby; 1986:47–57.

73. Macht SD, Krizek TJ. Sutures and suturing: current concepts. *J Oral Surg.* 1978;36:710–712.

74. Schremmer RD. New concepts in wound management. *Clin Ped Emerg Med.* 2004;5:239–245.

75. Karounis H, Gouin S, Eisman H, et al. A randomized, controlled trial comparing long-term cosmetic outcomes of traumatic pediatric lacerations repaired with absorbable plain gut versus nonabsorbable nylon sutures. *Acad Emerg Med.* 2004;11:730–735.

76. Holger JS, Wandersee SC, Hale DB. Cosmetic outcomes of facial lacerations repaired with tissue adhesives, absorbable, and nonabsorbable sutures. *Am J Emerg Med.* 2004;22:254–257.

77. Bartfield JM, Gennis P, Barbera J, et al. Buffered versus plain lidocaine as a local anesthetic for simple laceration repair. *Ann Emerg Med.* 1990;19:1387–1389.

78. Scarfone RJ, Jasani M, Gracely EJ. Pain of local anesthetics: rate of administration and buffering. *Ann Emerg Med.* 1998;31:36–40.

79. Brogan GX, Giarrusso E, Hollander JE, et al. Comparison of plain, warmed, and buffered lidocaine for anesthesia of traumatic wounds. *Ann Emerg Med.* 1995;26:121–125.

80. Mader TJ, Playe SJ, Garb JL. Reducing the pain of local anesthetic infiltration: warming and buffering have a synergistic effect. *Ann Emerg Med.* 1994;23:550–554.

81. Krause RS, Moscatti R, Filice M, et al. The effect of injection speed on the pain of lidocaine infiltration. *Acad Emerg Med.* 1997;4:1032–1035.

82. Kelly AM, Cohen M, Richards D. Minimizing the pain of local infiltration anesthesia for wounds by injection into wound edges. *J Emerg Med.* 1994;12:593–595.

83. Bartfield JM, Sokaris SJ, Raccio-Robak N. Local anesthesia for lacerations: pain of infiltration inside versus outside the wound. *Acad Emerg Med.* 1998;100–104.

84. Morris R, McKay W, Mushlin P. Comparison of pain associated with intradermal and subcutaneous infiltration with various local anesthetic solutions. *Anesth Analg.* 1987;66:1180–1182.

85. Bartfield JM, Lee FS, Raccio-Roback N, et al. Topical tetracaine attenuates the pain of infiltration of buffered lidocaine. *Acad Emerg Med.* 1995;2:104–108.

86. Pryor GJ, Kilpatrick WR, Opp DR. Local anesthesia in minor lacerations: topical TAC versus lidocaine infiltration. *Ann Emerg Med.* 1980;9:568–571.

87. Daya MR, Burton BT, Schleiss MR, et al. Recurrent seizures following mucosal application of TAC. *Ann Emerg Med.* 1988;17:646–648.

88. Dailey RH. Fatality secondary to misuse of TAC solution. *Ann Emerg Med.* 1988;17:159–160.

89. Schilling CG, Bank DE, Borchart BA, et al. Tetracaine, epinephrine (adrenaline), and cocaine (TAC) versus lidocaine, epinephrine, and tetracaine (LET) for anesthesia of lacerations in children. *Ann Emerg Med.* 1995;25:203–208.

90. Zempsky WT, Karasic RB. EMLA versus TAC for topical anesthesia of extremity wounds in children. *Ann Emerg Med.* 1997;30:163–166.

91. Krief W, Sadock V, Tunik M, et al. EMLA versus LET for topical anesthesia in wound repair [abstract]. *Acad Emerg Med.* 2002;9:398.

92. Priestley S. Application of topical local anesthetic at triage reduces treatment time for children with lacerations: a randomized controlled trial. *Ann Emerg Med.* 2003;42:34–40.

93. Borges AF. Timing of scar revision techniques. *Clin Plast Surg.* 1990;17:71–76.

94. Borges AF. Scar analysis and objectives of revision procedures. *Clin Plast Surg.* 1977;4:223–237.

95. Robinson DW. Simple revision of scars. *Clin Plast Surg.* 1977;4:217–222.

96. Davies DM. Scars, hypertrophic scars, and keloids. *Br Med J.* 1985;190:1056–1058.

97. Wray RC. Force required for wound closure and scar appearance. *Plast Reconstr Surg.* 1973;72:380–382.

98. McGuire MF. Studies of the excisional wound, I: biomechanical effects of undermining and wound orientation on closing tension and work. *Plast Reconstr Surg.* 1980;66:419–427.

99. Westaby S. Wound closure and drainage. In: Westaby S, ed. *Wound Care.* St. Louis: Mosby; 1986:32–46.

100. Anderson RM, Romfh RF. *Technique in the Use of Surgical Tools.* New York: Appleton-Century-Crofts; 1980.

101. Jones JS, Gartner M, Drew G, et al. The shorthand vertical mattress stitch: evaluation of a new suture technique. *Am J Emerg Med.* 1993;11:483.

102. McLean NR, Fyfe AHB, Flint EF, et al. Comparison of skin closure using continuous and interrupted nylon sutures. *Br J Surg.* 1980;67:633–635.

103. Irvin TT. Simple skin closure. *Br J Hosp Med.* 1985;33:325–333.

104. Roth JH, Windle BH. Staple versus suture closure of skin incisions in a pig model. *Can J Surg.* 1988;31:19–20.

105. George TK, Simpson DC. Skin wound closure with staples in the accident and emergency department. *J R Coll Surg Edinb.* 1985;30:54–56.

106. Shuster M. Comparing skin staples to sutures in an emergency department. *Can Fam Physician.* 1989;35:505.

107. Brickman KR, Lambert RW. Evaluation of skin stapling for wound closure in the emergency department. *Ann Emerg Med.* 1989;18:1122–1125.

108. Ritchie AJ, Rocke LG. Staples versus sutures in the closure of scalp wounds: a prospective, double-blind, randomized trial. *Injury.* 1989;20:217–218.

109. Khan AN, Dayan PS, Miller S, et al. Cosmetic outcomes of scalp wound closure with staples in the pediatric emergency department: a prospective, randomized trial. *Pediatr Emerg Care.* 2002;18:171–173.

110. Kanegaye JT, Vance CW, Chan L, et al. Comparison of skin stapling devices and standard sutures for pediatric scalp lacerations: a randomized study of cost and time benefits. *J Pediatr.* 1997;130:808.

111. Orlinsky M, Goldberg RM, Chan L, et al. Cost analysis of stapling versus suturing for skin closure. *Am J Emerg Med.* 1995;13:77–81.

112. Connolly WB, Hunt TK, Zederfelt B, et al. Clinical comparison of surgical wounds closed by suture and adhesive tapes. *Am J Surg.* 1969;117:318–322.

113. Panek PH, Presak MP, Bolt D, et al. Potentiation of wound infection by adhesive adjuncts. *Am Surg.* 1972;38:343–345.

114. Rodeheaver GT, Halverson JM, Edlich RF. Mechanical performance of wound closure tapes. *Ann Emerg Med.* 1983;12:203–206.

115. Rodeheaver GT, Spengler MD, Edlich RF. Performance of new wound closure tapes. *J Emerg Med.* 1987;5:451.

116. Singer AJ, Thode HC. A review of the literature on octylcyanoacrylate tissue adhesive. *Am J Surg.* 2004;187:238–248.

117. Officer C. Scalp lacerations in children. *Aust Fam Physician.* 1981;10:970.

118. Davies MJ. Scalp wounds: an alternative to suture. *Injury.* 1988;19:375–376.

119. Hock MO, Ooi SB, Saw SM, et al. A randomized controlled trial comparing the hair apposition technique with tissue glue to standard suturing in scalp lacerations (HAT study). *Ann Emerg Med.* 2002;40:19–26.

120. Tobin GR. An improved method of delayed primary closure: an aggressive management approach to unfavorable wounds. *Surg Clin North Am.* 1984;64:659–666.

121. Dimick AR. Delayed wound closure: indications and techniques. *Ann Emerg Med.* 1988;17:1303–1304.

122. Edlich RF, Rogers W, Kasper G, et al. Studies in the management of the contaminated wound, I: optimal time for closure of contaminated open wounds; II: comparison of resistance to infection of open and closed wounds during healing. *Am J Surg.* 1969;117:323–329.

123. Howell JM, Morgan DO. Scalp laceration repair without prior hair removal. *Am J Emerg Med.* 1988;6:7–10.

124. Chrintz H, Vibits H, Cordtz TO, et al. Need for surgical wound dressing. *Br J Surg.* 1989;76:204–205.

125. Dire DJ, Coppola M, Dwyer DA, et al. Prospective evaluation of topical antibiotics for preventing infections in uncomplicated soft-tissue wounds repaired in the ED. *Acad Emerg Med.* 1995;2:4–10.

126. Rabkin JM, Hunt TK. Local heat increases blood flow and oxygen tension in wounds. *Arch Surg.* 1987;122:221–225.

127. Cummings P, Del Beccaro MA. Antibiotics to prevent infection of simple wounds: a meta-analysis of randomized studies. *Am J Emerg Med.* 1995;13:396–400.

128. Day TK. Controlled trial of prophylactic antibiotics in minor wounds requiring suture. *Lancet.* 1975;2:1174–1176.

129. Armstrong BD. Lacerations of the mouth. *Emerg Med Clin North Am.* 2000;18:471–480.

130. Roberts SHN, Teddy PJ. A prospective trial of prophylactic antibiotics in hand lacerations. *Br J Surg.* 1977;64:394–396.

131. Grossman JAI, Adams JP, Kunec J. Prophylactic antibiotics in simple hand lacerations. *JAMA.* 1981;245:1055–1056.

132. Turner WS. Evidence-based emergency medicine/systematic review abstract. Do mammalian bites require antibiotic prophylaxis? *Ann Emerg Med.* 2004;44:274–276.

133. American Academy of Pediatrics. *Red Book: Report of the Committee on Infectious Diseases.* 26th ed. Elk Grove Village, IL: American Academy of Pediatrics; 2003:182.

109

JUDD E. HOLLANDER

Use of Tissue Adhesives in Laceration Repair

▶ INTRODUCTION

Cyanoacrylate tissue adhesives are liquid monomers that polymerize into a stable bond when they come into contact with wounds. They are applied topically to the apposed wound edges and should not be introduced into the wound. The tissue adhesives offer many advantages over standard wound closure devices: They may be applied rapidly and painlessly to any easily approximated laceration. Because they slough off spontaneously within 5 to 10 days, they do not require a follow-up visit for suture removal. This is particularly important in the young child, for whom removal of sutures may be as anxiety provoking as the initial placement. The tissue adhesives are roughly equivalent in strength to 5-0 sutures but should not be used alone for wounds otherwise requiring stronger wound closure devices (such as high-tension wounds). They can be used in conjunction with deep sutures. The cyanoacrylates form an occlusive dressing that serves as a barrier to microbial penetration (1) and have been shown to have inherent antibacterial properties and reduce infection rates in experimental animal models (2). Clinical trials comparing wounds closed with octylcyanoacrylate to those closed by sutures have consistently demonstrated similar scar appearance (3–5).

The disadvantages of tissue adhesives are that (a) they have less tensile strength than 5-0 sutures and staples and thus cannot be used for wounds under high tension and (b) they are less resistant to moisture than sutures and staples and thus must be used with caution in patients who will be swimming or exposed to water.

Application of tissue adhesives is a manual skill that is easily acquired (6). In contrast, 1 to 2 years of experience are required before a practitioner becomes proficient at suturing traumatic

lacerations (7). Tissue adhesives can be stored and are easily applied in the office, urgent care, or emergency department setting.

▶ INDICATIONS

Cyanoacrylate tissue adhesives are indicated for the closure of noncontaminated wounds that are under minimal tension. They should be used only when the wound edges can be easily approximated. Most wounds occur in the head and neck, and this area has low wound infection rates and low tension, making cyanoacrylates the ideal wound closure device. Octylcyanoacrylates may also be safely used on the torso and in areas of the extremities that are not subject to significant tension. In areas that are subject to moderate tension, placement of deep sutures may allow easy approximation of skin edges and subsequent skin closure with tissue adhesives. Even when deep sutures are placed, tissue adhesives offer advantages because they will still reduce time requirements and eliminate the need for follow-up and suture removal. Tissue adhesives are also useful for closing various skin flaps, where the addition of sutures may further compromise vascular supply. Finally, tissue adhesives may be used to close lacerations over fragile skin that is easily torn by sutures, such as the skin over the lower leg, especially in elderly patients.

▶ CONTRAINDICATIONS

Cyanoacrylates are contraindicated for patients with allergies to cyanoacrylate or formaldehyde, a breakdown product. Tissue adhesives are also contraindicated when there is an increased risk of infection or poor wound healing, such as in areas of poor vascularity. They are contraindicated in wounds that cannot be easily apposed, with or without deep sutures. Relative contraindications to application of tissue adhesives include wounds involving mucocutaneous borders, areas with dense hair, and areas routinely exposed to bodily fluids.

▶ EQUIPMENT

Tissue adhesive
Gloves
Petrolatum gel
Sterile gauze

▶ PROCEDURE

Proper wound selection, evaluation, and preparation prior to closure are critical (8,9). The wound should be cleaned, irrigated, and débrided as necessary (Chapter 107). A topical anesthetic will minimize discomfort if applied prior to wound cleaning. The clinician should make sure that the wound edges are apposed so that the adhesive does not enter the wound. When adhesive is placed between the wound edges, it prevents epithelialization and may result in inflammatory reactions (10). Tissue adhesives should be applied to relatively dry skin. Hemostasis can be obtained by applying pressure with sterile gauze or by dripping a topical epinephrine solution (alone or in combination with lidocaine) into the wound. When hemostasis cannot be obtained, the wound should be closed with sutures or staples instead.

Patient positioning at the time of tissue adhesive application is important to prevent run of tissue adhesive away from the wound. Restraint may also be necessary in the young child who is unable to hold still for the procedure (Chapter 3). The patient should be positioned so that the wound surface is parallel to the floor. This will greatly reduce runoff. Important structures (e.g., the eye) adjacent to the wound should be covered with dry gauze to prevent tissue adhesive migration into the area. The wound may also be surrounded by a rim of petrolatum gel or topical antibiotic ointment to block adhesive runoff. Another "trick" is to gently squeeze and release pressure on the vial to control the amount of adhesive that is expressed. Avoiding excessive expression of the adhesive also minimizes the chances that the practitioner's fingers will get stuck to the wound. If the practitioner's gloved hand has come in contact with the adhesive and might be getting stuck to the patient's skin, the other hand should be used to reinforce wound apposition while the original hand is gently pulled away from the wound.

Long lacerations or incisions or lacerations with multiple limbs may be divided into discrete segments and closed in stages. Use of surgical adhesive tapes to secure the wound at various intervals may also facilitate closure of a long lacera-

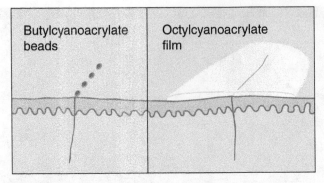

Figure 109.1 With the butylcyanoacrylates, the adhesive is applied as discrete bead (*left*). With the octylcyanoacrylates, the adhesive is applied as one continuous film across the entire wound (*right*).

tion. Areas of the laceration can then be closed sequentially, mimicking closure of multiple smaller lacerations.

There are differences in application technique depending on the type of tissue adhesive being used. Butylcyanoacrylates polymerize rapidly on contact with the skin, usually within 10 to 15 seconds. As a result, they are applied in a pattern of discrete drops along the wound surface, like spot welding (Fig. 109.1). To apply histoacryl blue, the tip of the vial is cut off and the adhesive is expressed either directly from the tip of the vial or through a 25-gauge needle that is attached to the hub of the vial. The needle allows more precise application. With Indermil, another type of butylcyanoacrylate, the adhesive is expressed directly from the tip of the applicator. Butylcyanoacrylates are indicated only for small linear lacerations (less than 4 cm) on the face.

Octylcyanoacrylate (Dermabond, Ethicon, Somerville, NJ) is supplied in a glass vial within a plastic container. The vial should be gently crushed between the thumb and forefinger and the adhesive expressed through the tip of the applicator by gently squeezing the container. This kind of adhesive forms a thin, flexible bond that typically sets in 30 to 60 seconds. This adhesive should be applied over the entire wound extending out 5 to 10 mm on either side of the wound (Fig. 109.2). After allowing the first layer to partially polymerize for 30 to 60 seconds, the practitioner should apply another two or three layers of adhesive, allowing 10 to 15 seconds between each application. High-viscosity Dermabond does not require three layers and will polymerize more rapidly. It also has less runoff.

Octylcyanoacrylates and butylcyanoacrylates are not interchangeable. The increased flexibility and tensile strength of the octylcyanoacrylates offer an advantage for most wounds (Table 109.1) because butylcyanoacrylates are more likely to crack.

▶ POSTOPERATIVE WOUND CARE

Wounds should be kept clean and dry to avoid premature sloughing of the adhesive (Table 109.2). The wound can get

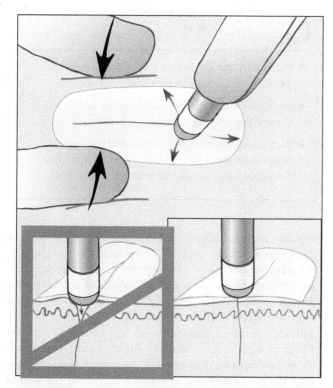

Figure 109.2 The wound edges are held in apposition with the fingers of the nondominant hand, and adhesive is applied evenly across the entire wound, including a margin of at least 5 to 10 mm on either side of the wound. The left-lower panel depicts incorrect placement of adhesive into the wound, which should be avoided.

wet briefly during showering or bathing, but patients should avoid scrubbing or soaking the wound. Swimming should be avoided because it can result in premature sloughing of the adhesive.

TABLE 109.1	COMPARISON OF TYPES OF CYANOACRYLATE ADHESIVES	
	Octylcyanoacrylate	Butylcyanoacrylate
Number of carbons in side chain	8	4
Breaking strength	Moderate	Low
Flexibility	Great	Poor
Color	Transparent	Opaque
Indications	Most facial lacerations, any type of wound surface (flat or irregular contour), wounds subject to minimal or moderate tension	Short facial lacerations, flat surfaces, wounds subject to minimal tension
Length restrictions	None	Limited to short lacerations (<4 cm)

Adapted from Singer AJ, Quinn JV. Tissue adhesives. In: Singer AJ, Hollander JE, eds. *Lacerations and Acute Wounds: An Evidenced-Based Guide.* Philadelphia: FA Davis; 2002:83–97.

TABLE 109.2	SAMPLE INSTRUCTIONS FOR WOUND CARE FOLLOWING CLOSURE WITH TISSUE ADHESIVES

▶ Check your wound daily. Contact your doctor or return to the ED if there is significant swelling, redness, warmth, or pus.
▶ Return if your wound opens up. As long as it is not infected, it may be repaired again with either adhesive or sutures (stitches).
▶ You may cover your wound with a dry bandage.
▶ Do not scratch, rub, or pick at the adhesive.
▶ You may shower or bathe, but do not scrub or soak your wound.
▶ Do not place any tape directly on your wound.
▶ Do not apply any ointment on the adhesive.
▶ The adhesive will fall off on its own within 5 to 10 days.

Adapted from Singer AJ, Quinn JV. Tissue adhesives. In: Singer AJ, Hollander JE, eds. *Lacerations and Acute Wounds: An Evidenced-Based Guide.* Philadelphia: FA Davis; 2002:83–97.

Tissue adhesives form their own dressing; however, some patients may prefer an additional clean, dry dressing. These dressings should not be applied until the tissue adhesive has completely dried. Ointments, such as topical antibiotics, should not be applied; they may loosen the adhesive.

▶ COMPLICATIONS

Most failures of tissue adhesives are caused by practitioner error in management. They include improper wound preparation, failure to anticipate runoff, and poor patient selection (Table 109.3).

The major potential pitfall of using tissue adhesives is that the practitioner can be tempted to spend inadequate time evaluating, selecting, and preparing the wound. The fact

TABLE 109.3	POTENTIAL PROBLEMS WITH TISSUE ADHESIVES
Problem	Ways to avoid the problem
Runoff	Position patient with wound parallel to floor.
	Circumscribe wound with ointment.
Spillage into eyes	Cover patient's eyes with gauze barrier.
	Position patient so that wound is not above eye.
	Apply petrolatum gel barrier before applying adhesive.
Wound dehiscence	Avoid adhesive use for high-tension wounds.
	Use deep sutures or immobilization for high-tension wounds.
Wound infection	Use adhesives only for properly selected wounds.
	Use proper wound preparation, including irrigation, exploration, and (when necessary) débridement.
Getting stuck to the wound	Express small amounts of adhesive and control runoff.
	Switch hands used to appose wound edges prior to polymerization of the adhesive.

Adapted from Singer AJ, Quinn JV. Tissue adhesives. In: Singer AJ, Hollander JE, eds. *Lacerations and Acute Wounds: An Evidenced-Based Guide.* Philadelphia: FA Davis; 2002:83–97.

that tissue adhesives are easy to use should not result in the practitioner skipping basic steps in wound management. The wound will still need to be cleansed prior to closure. Although anesthesia may not be required for wound closure with tissue adhesives, it may still be needed for wound exploration and cleansing. Obviously, proper cleansing is paramount for preventing infection. It may be tempting to close wounds with tissue adhesives without exploring, débriding, or irrigating them, but this should not be done.

Failure to close the wound while the wound is in a horizontal position will result in tissue adhesive runoff. If adhesive runs into the eye, the patient must open the eyelids widely to avoid matting of the eyelashes. If the eyelids become matted

CLINICAL TIPS

▶ Protecting the eye with a petrolatum barrier or gauze reduces the risk of eyelid adhesion.

▶ Gently squeeze and release pressure on the vial to control the amount of adhesive expressed.

▶ Surgical adhesive tape can be used to provide temporary apposition of long wound edges while the adhesive is applied in sequential segments.

together, an ophthalmic ointment, such as erythromycin or bacitracin, should be applied to help accelerate sloughing of the adhesive, and the eye can be patched. The cyanoacrylates are not toxic to the globe and will not cause any long-term damage to the eye. Matted eyelids do not need to be surgical separated or cut. With the application of a topical ophthalmic antibiotic ointment, matted eyelids will be able to separate within a couple of days (at most). Anticipation of runoff will allow the practitioner to properly position the patient, consider the use of adjuvant materials to surround the wound site, and have gauze available to wipe off migrating adhesive at the earliest possible time.

Wound dehiscence is usually the result of improper wound selection, improper adhesive application, or both. Wounds that cannot be easily approximated should not be closed with tissue adhesives alone, regardless of patient request. Premature sloughing of the tissue adhesive with dehiscence may also occur with recurrent friction and exposure to moisture. If the patient will not be able to keep the wound relatively dry for at least 5 to 7 days, tissue adhesives should not be used.

In the event that the practitioner's glove gets stuck to the patient, gentle traction, if applied early may be all that is necessary. If gentle traction is not sufficient, the tip of gloved finger that is adherent to the patient can be cut off and a topical antibiotic ointment applied. This will expedite the separation of the skin from the adherent glove.

▶ SUMMARY

Because lacerations occur commonly and laceration repair is a frightening experience for children, minimizing the pain and duration of the repair is important. Tissue adhesives are a well-studied, efficacious method of wound closure that results in an excellent cosmetic outcome in a painless and time-efficient manner. Careful attention to general wound preparation techniques (cleansing, exploration, and anesthesia) is important to ensure an optimal outcome. The infrequent complications of tissue adhesive use are generally avoidable with proper techniques. As a result, use of tissue adhesives is the ideal method of wound closure for simple, easily approximated lacerations regardless of length.

SUMMARY

1 Determine that the wound is appropriate for the use of tissue adhesives.

2 Anesthetize the wound as needed for irrigation.

3 Clean, irrigate, and débride the wound as indicated.

4 Obtain hemostasis with sterile gauze or the application of a topical epinephrine solution.

5 Position and restrain the patient to minimize adhesive runoff.

6 Protect important structures such as the eyes.

7 Manually approximate the wound edges.

8 Apply the adhesive.

  a Butylcyanoacrylates:

    i Apply drops along wound surface.

  b Histoacryl blue:

    i Cut the vial tip.

    ii Express the adhesive through the tip or a 25-gauge needle.

    iii Apply the adhesive linearly along the wound margins.

  c Octylcyanoacrylate:

    i Gently crush the glass vial within the plastic container.

    ii Express the adhesive until the applicator tip is saturated.

    iii Apply the adhesive over the entire wound extending out to the sides.

    iv Repeat the application for an additional 2 to 3 layers unless using a high-viscosity adhesive.

9 Wipe away any migrating adhesive with gauze as quickly as possible.

▶ REFERENCES

1. Singer AJ, Nable M, Cameau P, et al. Evaluation of a liquid occlusive dressing for excisional wounds (abstract). *Acad Emerg Med.* 2002;8:449.
2. Quinn JV, Maw JL, Ramotar K, et al. Octylcyanoacrylate tissue adhesive wound repair versus suture wound repair in a contaminated wound model. *Surgery.* 1997;122;69–72.
3. Quinn JV, Wells GA, Sutcliffe T, et al. A randomized trial comparing octylcyanoacrylate tissue adhesive and sutures in the management of lacerations. *JAMA.* 1997;277:1527–1530.
4. Singer AJ, Hollander JE, Valentine SM, et al. Prospective randomized controlled trial of a new tissue adhesive (2-octylcyanoacrylate) versus standard wound closure techniques for laceration repair. *Acad Emerg Med.* 1998;5:94–98.
5. Singer AJ, Quinn JV, Hollander JE, et al. Closure of lacerations and incisions with octylcyanoacrylate: a multi-center randomized clinical trial. *Surgery.* 2002;131:270–276.
6. Hollander JE, Singer AJ. Application of tissue adhesive: rapid attainment of proficiency. *Acad Emerg Med.* 1998;5:1012–1017.
7. Singer AJ, Hollander JE, Valentine SM, et al. Association of training level and short-term appearance of repaired lacerations. *Acad Emerg Med.* 1996;3:378–383.
8. Quinn JV. *Tissue Adhesives in Wound Care.* Hamilton, Canada: BC Decker; 1998.
9. Singer AJ, Quinn JV. Tissue adhesives. In: Singer AJ, Hollander JE, eds. *Lacerations and Acute Wounds: An Evidenced-Based Guide.* Philadelphia: FA Davis; 2002:83–97.
10. Singer AJ, Berruti L, McClain SA. Comparative trial of octylcyanoacrylate and silver sulfadiazine for the treatment of full-thickness skin biopsies. *Wound Repair Regen.* 1999;7:356–361.

110

HAZEL GUINTO-OCAMPO

Management of Plantar Puncture Wounds

▸ INTRODUCTION

The feet are the most common site for puncture wounds (1). The vast majority of plantar puncture wounds are caused by nails and generally occur during the summer (2,3). These injuries are common among children and account for 0.8% of emergency department (ED) visits (2). With the exception of hand puncture wounds, plantar puncture wounds have a higher complication rate than puncture wounds elsewhere in the body (1). These complications include soft-tissue infections, mostly caused by *Staphylococcus* and *Streptococcus* species, and osteomyelitis, of which 90% are caused by *Pseudomonas* species (2,4–17). The development of infectious complications has been associated with retained foreign bodies (4,18). Puncture wounds through sneakers have been implicated in pseudomonal infections (13,19).

When evaluating plantar puncture wounds, the following information should be obtained and documented: history of immunocompromise; tetanus immunization status; size, nature, and condition of the object that caused the puncture; potential for contamination or presence of a foreign body; prehospital care; site of injury; footwear and clothing penetrated; and elapsed time since the injury.

Coring or enlargement of the puncture site may be beneficial in contaminated wounds or those with a possible foreign body by allowing improved visualization, irrigation, and drainage. Physicians or other health care providers in the office or ED setting can easily perform this procedure.

▸ ANATOMY AND PHYSIOLOGY

The foot can be divided into three zones (20) (Fig. 110.1). Because of the close proximity of the tarsal bones to the skin surface and the greater force exerted on this weight-bearing area, puncture wounds in Zone 1 penetrate deeper and have the highest risk of infectious complications (21,22), followed by Zone 2 and, lastly, Zone 3. Complications include cellulitis, soft-tissue abscess, foreign body granuloma, pyarthrosis, and osteomyelitis. Infections occurring in the first few days following the puncture are most commonly due to *Staphylococcus aureus* or group A streptococci (5). Pyarthrosis and osteomyelitis secondary to puncture wounds are overwhelmingly due to *Pseudomonas aeruginosa* (9–19). The incidence of infections is reportedly as high as 15% (2), with the incidence of osteomyelitis estimated to be 0.4% to 0.6% (23). It should be noted that such estimates are likely high, as a large percentage of patients do not seek medical attention for superficial puncture wounds (24). Patients presenting late (7 days or more) are at increased risk for infectious complications (2). In addition, children appear to be at greatest risk for permanent sequelae as a result of these infections (3). Most puncture wounds are considered to be tetanus prone and thus require tetanus prophylaxis (see Table 107.2).

▸ INDICATIONS

The management of plantar puncture wounds is controversial (1,23,25). Exploration of plantar puncture wounds for foreign bodies is technically difficult. Plantar skin is thick, relatively rigid, and sensitive. Because of the narrowness of puncture wounds, they are difficult to effectively irrigate, and locating foreign bodies that penetrate the plantar fascia is almost impossible (1). Management strategies include expectant therapy, surface cleansing without exploration (26), simple probing and grasping, trimming jagged epidermal skin edges (27), and wound exploration through coring or

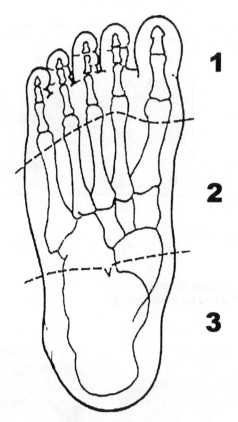

Figure 110.1 Puncture zones of the foot.

intense and excessive inflammation and should be removed as soon as possible (1).

Imaging studies should be obtained if the history suggests a retained foreign body or if exploration is inconclusive. Plain radiographs will reveal retained metal, pencil graphite, most glass, certain plastics, gravel, sand, some wood, and some aluminum (32–38). Ultrasound (Chapter 135) (4,34,36,39–42), computed tomography (4,43–46), or magnetic resonance imaging (4) may be required for visualization of nonradiopaque retained foreign objects.

Surgical consultation should be obtained for wounds with deep or unrecoverable foreign bodies or wounds complicated by an abscess, pyarthrosis, or osteomyelitis (11,23,25).

▶ EQUIPMENT

Lidocaine, 1% to 2% without epinephrine
Syringes, 10 and 30 mL
Needle, 25 or 27 gauge, 1.5 inch
Scalpel blade (No. 11) or 4-mm disposable punch biopsy corer
Forceps
Normal saline
Povidone-iodine solution, 10%
Angiocath or splash shield, 18 gauge
Iodoform gauze, 0.25 inch
Gauze dressing
Adhesive strips
Sterile gloves

▶ PROCEDURE

The area around the puncture wound should be cleansed with povidone-iodine (Fig. 110.2A). Soaking the foot in an antiseptic solution has not been proven to be useful (47). If coring is undertaken, local anesthesia should be used and consideration given to administering a peroneal nerve block (see Chapter 35). Procedural sedation and use of age-appropriate restraints are recommended for young children and older children who are unable to cooperate (Chapters 3 and 33). The procedure is best performed with the child in the prone position and with the plantar surface facing up. Blind probing and grasping should be avoided since foreign bodies may be forced deeper into the wound and underlying nerves and vessels damaged. With a No.11 scalpel blade (or 4-mm punch biopsy corer or cuticle scissors), a 2-mm circular rim of full-thickness skin is removed (Fig. 110.2B). Irrigation of the wound tract with normal saline may be performed (Fig. 110.2C) using a 30-mL syringe and an 18-gauge Angiocath or splash shield. Any debris or foreign objects should be cautiously removed using a pair of forceps. Packing the tract with iodoform gauze (Fig. 110.2D) before applying a bulky dressing is optional.

Patients should be instructed to avoid weight bearing over the next 5 days and to keep the foot elevated when possible.

enlargement of the puncture wound by removal of a block of tissue (11,28,29). The percentage of foreign bodies that are discovered and successfully removed and the percentage of infections averted following wound exploration are unknown. High-pressure wound irrigation, deep probing, and extensive tissue débridement have not been shown to improve outcome (2,23,28,30). The potential for delayed wound healing and the discomfort associated with wound exploration and débridement must be weighed against the benefit of preventing infectious complications.

Clean, superficial wounds with no suspicion for a retained foreign body may be managed expectantly after surface cleansing. Jagged epidermal skin edges should be trimmed. Grossly contaminated puncture wounds and those suspicious for foreign body should be explored. Coring is the preferred method, since simple probing and blind grasping have unknown false-positive rates (23) and may force foreign bodies deeper into the wound (31).

When a foreign body is discovered, the risk of leaving it should be weighed against the potential harm of attempted removal. Foreign bodies should be removed if they are visible and readily accessible, cause pain, or threaten vital structures (25). Small, inert, deeply embedded objects that cause no symptoms may be left in place. The removal of glass, metal, and plastic, which are relatively inert, may be postponed if necessary. Vegetative or contaminated foreign bodies cause

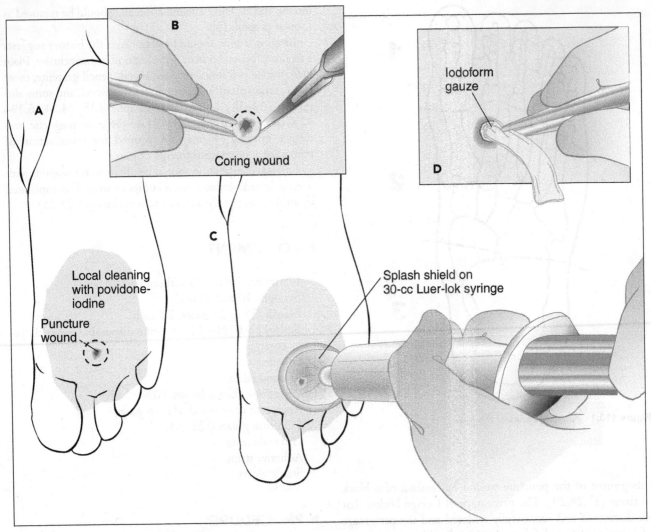

B

Coring wound

Iodoform gauze

D

A

Local cleaning with povidone-iodine

Puncture wound

C

Splash shield on 30-cc Luer-lok syringe

Figure 110.2 Coring a plantar puncture wound (see text for description).

 SUMMARY

1 Obtain radiographs to identify potential foreign bodies or fractures or to evaluate for osteomyelitis if late presentation.

2 Consider procedural sedation and the use of age-appropriate restraints for young children and older children who are unable to cooperate.

3 Place the patient in the prone position.

4 Prepare the wound in an antiseptic fashion.

5 Administer a local or peroneal block.

6 Through the use of coring, remove a 2-mm rim of full-thickness skin from around the puncture site.

7 Remove any debris or foreign bodies.

8 Irrigate the wound with saline under high pressure.

9 Pack the wound with iodoform gauze (optional).

10 Apply a bulky dressing.

11 Administer tetanus toxoid and tetanus immune globulin when indicated.

12 Encourage non-weight-bearing for 5 days and elevation of the extremity.

13 Administer antistaphylococcal antibiotics if there is evidence of cellulitis.

14 Refer the patient for surgical management for wounds with a retained foreign body or if a deep abscess, pyarthrosis, or osteomyelitis is present.

15 Arrange for patient follow-up in 24 to 48 hours.

CLINICAL TIPS

▶ Coring is not indicated for clean or superficial wounds.

▶ Wounds in Zone 1 and those that present late are more likely to become infected.

▶ There should be a high index of suspicion for osteomyelitis in wounds that present late, especially if there is a retained foreign body. When osteomyelitis is suspected, antimicrobials active against *Pseudomonas* species should be initiated.

Close follow-up within 48 hours is essential (26) because even wounds that are properly managed may become infected. In addition, patients and/or parents should be warned to watch out for symptoms or signs of osteomyelitis, which may take from days to weeks to manifest. They should be advised to seek prompt re-evaluation if pain or tenderness around the puncture site or pain with weight bearing develops (11), even if coring has been performed. Tetanus toxoid and tetanus immune globulin should be administered before discharge when indicated (Chapter 107).

The use of prophylactic antimicrobial therapy for plantar puncture wounds is controversial (1,48). Many authors believe that it does not compensate for inadequate initial wound care, is ineffective in wounds with retained foreign bodies, and may contribute to the development of a Gram-negative infection. However, prophylactic antimicrobial therapy should be considered in high-risk patients and in patients with wounds in Zone I (20,29,49). For wounds that are obviously infected at presentation, antimicrobial therapy should be initiated (23,45,50–52). Most infections respond well to first-generation cephalosporins or amoxicillin-clavulanate (3,23,53). Pseudomonal infections in older children can be treated with fluoroquinolones (54).

▶ COMPLICATIONS

Painful scarring may result from coring. Damage to underlying vessels, nerves, and fascia can occur with excessive débridement or coring. Limiting the amount of probing and the depth of the tract will minimize the incidence of this complication. Wound re-examination within 24 to 48 hours aids in early recognition of potential problems.

▶ SUMMARY

Plantar puncture wounds are a common problem during childhood. Wounds that are grossly contaminated and those suspected of harboring a foreign body may benefit from coring or enlargement of the wound site for improved irrigation and foreign body removal. Close follow-up is mandatory to recognize the potential complications of cellulitis, abscess, pyarthrosis, and osteomyelitis.

▶ ACKNOWLEDGMENT

The authors would like to acknowledge the valuable contributions of E. Howard Dixon III to the version of this chapter that appeared in the previous edition.

▶ REFERENCES

1. Capellan O, Hollander JE. Management of lacerations in the emergency department. *Emerg Med Clin North Am.* 2003;21:205–231.
2. Fitzgerald RH, Cowan DE. Puncture wounds of the foot. *Orthop Clin North Am.* 1975;6:965–972.
3. Jarvis JG, Skipper MD. Pseudomonas osteochondritis complicating puncture wounds in children. *J Pediatr Orthop.* 1994;14:755–759.
4. Imoisili MA. Toothpick puncture injuries of the foot in children. *Pediatr Infect Dis J.* 2004;23:80–82.
5. Eidelman M. Plantar puncture wounds in children: analysis of 80 hospitalized patients and late sequelae. *Isr Med Assoc J.* 2003;5:268–271.
6. Laughlin RT. Calcaneal osteomyelitis caused by nail puncture wounds. *Foot Ankle Int.* 1997;18:575–577.
7. Mader J, Ortiz M, Calhoun J. Update on the diagnosis and management of osteomyelitis. *Clin Podiatr Med Surg.* 1996;13:701–724.
8. Joseph W, Kosinski M. Prophylaxis in lower extremity infectious diseases. *Clin Podiatr Med Surg.* 1996;13:647–660.
9. Toohey JS. Pseudomonas osteomyelitis following puncture wounds of the foot. *Kans Med.* 1993;94:325–326.
10. Miron D. Infections following nail puncture wound of the foot: case reports and review of the literature. *Isr J Med Sci.* 1993;29:194–197.
11. Inaba AS, Zukin DD, Perro M. An update on the evaluation and management of plantar puncture wounds and *Pseudomonas* osteomyelitis. *Pediatr Emerg Care.* 1992;8:38–44.
12. Jacobs R, McCarthy R, Elster J. *Pseudomonas* osteochondritis complicating puncture wounds in children. *J Pediatr Orthop.* 1989;14:755.
13. Riley D. *Pseudomonas* osteomyelitis can occur in the foot after puncture wounds. *Practitioner.* 1988;232:296, 298.
14. Riley D. Pseudomonas osteomelitis can occur in the foot after puncture wounds. *Practitioner.* 1988;232:296–298.
15. Graham B, Gregory D. *Pseudomonas aeruginosa* causing osteomyelitis after puncture wounds of the foot. *South Med J.* 1984;77:1228–1230.
16. Das DE S. *Pseudomonas* osteomyelitis following puncture wounds of the foot in children. *Injury.* 1981;12:334–339.
17. Chusid M, Jacobs W, Sty J. *Pseudomonas* arthritis following puncture wounds of the foot. *J Pediatr.* 1979;94:429–431.
18. Starosta D, Sacchetti A, Sharkey P. Calcaneal fracture with compartment syndrome of the foot. *Ann Emerg Med.* 1988;17:856–858.
19. Fisher M, Goldsmith J, Gilligan P. Sneakers as a source of *Pseudomonas aeruginosa* in children with osteomyelitis following puncture wounds. *J Pediatr.* 1985;106:607–609.
20. Patzakis MJ, Wilkins J, Brien WW, et al. Wound site as a predictor of complications following deep nail punctures to the foot. *West J Med.* 1989;150:545–547.
21. Ho K, Abu Laban R, Rosen P, et al. *Emergency Medicine Concepts and Clinical Practice, Ankle, and Foot.* 4th ed. St. Louis: Mosby-Year Book; 1998:821.

22. Markiewitz A, Karns D, Brooks P. Late infections due to incomplete removal of foreign bodies: a report of two cases. *Foot Ankle.* 1994;15:52.

23. Chisholm CD, Schlesser JF. Plantar puncture wounds: controversies and treatment recommendations. *Ann Emerg Med.* 1989;18:1352–1357.

24. Weber EJ. Plantar puncture wounds: a survey to determine the incidence of infection. *J Accid Emerg Med.* 1996;13:274–277.

25. Wedmore IS, Charett J. Orthopedic emergencies. *Emerg Med Clin North Am.* 2000;18:85–113.

26. Schwab RA, Powers RD. Conservative therapy of plantar puncture wounds. *J Emerg Med.* 1995;13:291–295.

27. Mahan KT, Kalish SR. Complications following puncture wounds of the foot. *J Am Podiatr Assoc.* 1982;72:497–504.

28. Riegler HF, Routson GW. Complications of deep puncture wounds of the foot. *J Trauma.* 1979;19:18–22.

29. Edlich RF, Rodeheaver GT, Horowitz JH, et al. Emergency department management of puncture wounds and needlestick exposure. *Emerg Med Clin North Am.* 1986;4:581–582.

30. Chudnofsky C, Sebastian S. Special wounds: nail bed, plantar puncture, and cartilage. *Emerg Med Clin North Am.* 1992;10:801–822.

31. Reinherz RP, Hong DT, Tisa LM. Management of puncture wounds in the foot. *J Foot Surg.* 1985;24:288–292.

32. Chisholm CD, Wood CO, Chua G, et al. Radiographic detection of gravel in soft tissue. *Ann Emerg Med.* 1997;29:725–730.

33. Ellis G. Are aluminum foreign bodies detectable radiographically? *Am J Emerg Med.* 1993;11:12–13.

34. Jacobson JA, Powell A, Craig JG, et al. Wooden foreign bodies in soft tissue: detection at ultrasound. *Radiology.* 1998;206:45–48.

35. Lammers RL. Soft tissue foreign bodies. *Ann Emerg Med.* 1988;17:47–45.

36. Schlager D, Sanders AB, Wiggins D, et al. Ultrasound for the detection of foreign bodies. *Ann Emerg Med.* 1991;20:189–191.

37. Courter BJ. Radiographic screening for glass foreign bodies: what does a "negative" foreign body series really mean? *Ann Emerg Med.* 1990;19:997–1000.

38. Felman AH, Fisher MS. The radiographic detection of glass in soft tissue. *Radiology.* 1969;92:1529–1531.

39. Hill R, Conron R, Greissinger P, et al. Ultrasound for the detection of foreign bodies in human tissue. *Ann Emerg Med.* 1997;29:353–356.

40. Manthey DE, Storrow AB, Milbourn JM, et al. Ultrasound versus radiography in the detection of soft-tissue foreign bodies. *Ann Emerg Med.* 1996;28:7–9.

41. DeFlaviis L, Scaglione P, Del Bo P, et al. Detection of foreign bodies in soft tissues: experimental comparison of ultrasonography and xeroradiography. *J Trauma.* 1988;28:400–404.

42. Gilbert FJ, Campbell RSD, Bayliss AP. The role of ultrasound in the detection of non-radiopaque foreign bodies. *Clin Radiol.* 1990;41:109–112.

43. Bauer AR, Yutani D. Computed tomographic localization of wooden foreign bodies in children's extremities. *Arch Surg.* 1983;118:1084–1086.

44. Kuhns LR, Borlaza GS, Seigel RS, et al. An in vitro comparison of computed tomography, xerography, and radiography in the detection of soft-tissue foreign bodies. *Radiology.* 1979;132:218–219.

45. Roobottom CA, Weston MJ. The detection of foreign bodies in soft tissue: comparison of conventional and digital radiography. *Clin Radiol.* 1994;49:330–332.

46. Rhoades CE, Soye I, Levine E, et al. Detection of a wooden foreign body in the hand using computed tomography. *J Hand Surg.* 1982;7:306–307.

47. Verdile VP, Freed HA, Gerard J. Puncture wounds to the foot. *J Emerg Med.* 1989;7:193–199.

48. Pennycook A, Makower R, O'Donnell AM. Puncture wounds of the foot: can infective complications be avoided? *J R Soc Med.* 1994;87:581–583.

49. Joseph W, Lefrock J. The use of oral antibiotics in lower extremity infections. *Clin Podiatr Med Surg.* 1996;13:647–660.

50. Rahn KA, Jacobson FS. *Pseudomonas* osteomyelitis of the metatarsal sesamoid bones. *Am J Orthop.* 1997;26:365–367.

51. Joseph WS, LeFrock JL. Infections complicating puncture wounds of the foot. *J Foot Surg.* 1987;26:S30–33.

52. Miller EH, Semian DW. Gram-negative osteomyelitis following puncture wounds of the foot. *J Bone Joint Surg Am.* 1975;57:535–537.

53. Simon R, Koenigsknecht S. *Emergency Orthopedics: The Extremities.* 3rd ed. Norwalk, CT: Appleton & Lange; 1995:491.

54. Raz R. Oral ciprofloxacin for treatment of infection following nail puncture wounds of the foot. *Clin Infect Dis.* 1995;21:194–195.

JOHN A. BRENNAN AND HOWARD FRIEDLAND

Subcutaneous Foreign Bodies

111

▶ INTRODUCTION

Lacerations and puncture wounds are common presentations to the emergency department (ED). Most of these wounds are minor, but a significant number can be complicated with foreign bodies. It is important to have a high index of suspicion and thoroughly evaluate all wounds for foreign bodies. A wound that does not heal appropriately or develops an abscess should be evaluated for a retained foreign body (1–7).

Retained foreign bodies place children at a higher risk for infection and scarring. Foreign bodies can migrate, thereby causing neurological problems or other injuries.

Retained foreign bodies account for a significant number of malpractice claims. The management of foreign bodies is both high risk and very common, highlighting the importance of proper management of these patients.

The types and locations of foreign bodies change with age. Infants crawl on all fours, so their hands and knees are at risk for foreign bodies. As children begin to walk, they are at risk for puncture wounds to their feet. These injuries occur during adolescence, but teenagers may also be involved in violence and thus are at risk for foreign bodies from trauma, including bullets, knives, and other sharp objects.

As with all wound management, a thorough history and physical examination is necessary to determine the risk of foreign bodies as well as what type of foreign bodies might be encountered. The history and physical will be dependent on the patient's age and ability to cooperate.

Once the presence of a foreign body has been confirmed, a determination must be made as to the most appropriate procedure, optimal setting, and best clinician to perform the foreign body removal. There are a number of factors involved in making such decisions. The patient's ability to cooperate with the procedure is paramount. An attempt to remove a foreign body from an uncooperative patient is likely to fail

and can be dangerous. The location of the foreign body will also dictate where the removal should be accomplished as well as by whom. If there is a superficial foreign body that is visualized and in a safe anatomical location, it can be removed by the physician in the ED. If the foreign body is located next to vital or easily injured structures, it should be removed by the appropriate surgical subspecialist under controlled conditions with the use of procedural sedation and analgesia or in the operating room. If the emergency physician decides to proceed with the removal of the foreign body, a time limit should be set, usually 30 minutes, and strictly followed. The entire plan should be discussed with the parents, as well as the alternative course if the initial procedure is unsuccessful.

▶ ANATOMY AND PHYSIOLOGY

Foreign bodies vary in their ability to cause inflammation in the body. The majority of the subcutaneous foreign bodies are glass, wood, or metal. Glass and metal are usually benign and do not cause significant acute inflammation. They can cause injury due to migration as well as lacerate tendons, nerves, or muscles as they enter the body. They may cause chronic inflammatory changes over time, which may appear as osteolytic lesions or pseudotumors on x-rays (8,9). Even benign foreign bodies can cause infection if they are contaminated with bacteria or bring bacteria from the skin as they enter the body.

The body's reaction to a subcutaneous foreign substance depends on the degree of inflammatory response that is stimulated. Polymorphonuclear neutrophils represent the body's initial reaction. These cells release hydrolytic enzymes that cause destruction of the foreign body and pustule formation. This reaction can result in the extrusion of the foreign body or lead to infection and abscess formation. Less inflammatory foreign bodies will cause granuloma formation as macrophages wall off the foreign body with fibrin and collagen. Granulomas may still become infected due to chronic inflammation.

Wooden foreign bodies cause inflammatory reactions in most patients (9,10). If not immediate, there will eventually be inflammatory changes. Other plant material, including thorns and spines from cacti, is also likely to trigger significant inflammation (10). These foreign bodies are at high risk for infection and may also carry fungi, leading to phycomycoses.

Graphite foreign bodies, usually from a pencil, can lead to tattooing of the tissue. Embedded silica can cause granulomas months and even years after implantation (11). A commonly encountered foreign body is rubber from the sole of a shoe, usually a sneaker. Rubber is an excellent growth medium for bacteria, especially *Pseudomonas* organisms (12). Puncture wounds through a sneaker are at high risk for infection, including cellulitis, perichondritis, and ultimately osteomyelitis.

The location of the foreign body affects the difficulty of finding and removing it as well as influences potential complications. The hand is one of the most common areas where foreign bodies are found. There are multiple structures and tissue planes in the hand. This makes locating foreign bodies by exam or imaging difficult. The mobility of the hand can cause a foreign body to enter in one location but quickly relocate a distance away from the entrance wound. The number of relatively superficial tendons, ligaments, nerves, and vessel also make attempts at foreign body removal more difficult and potentially more dangerous. The foot, especially the sole, is also a common location for foreign bodies. Often the foreign body will be contaminated with additional material. A puncture wound from a nail can leave a foreign body in the soft tissue, such as the nail, a portion of the shoe, sock material, or dirt. These wounds are at high risk for infection. Most skin infections are due to *Staphylococcus aureus* or group A streptococci. Puncture wounds of the feet, especially through sneakers, are also at risk for infections with *Pseudomonas aeruginosa*. Other organisms that cause foreign body–associated infections include non–group A streptococci, clostridia, and various fungal species. The thickness of the sole of the foot makes the examination harder and the removal of any foreign bodies difficult.

► INDICATIONS

Locating a foreign body is often a difficult process. It begins with entertaining the suspicion of a foreign body. The first step is to obtain an adequate history. A physical examination will identify some foreign bodies and give clues to the possible presence of others. A foreign body is often not obvious on the first inspection of the wound. For example, glass is very difficult to visualize in a wound. Still, wounds less than 5 mm in depth are unlikely to retain a glass foreign body (13). Physical examination findings suspicious for a foreign body include

pain out of proportion to the wound, pain on deep palpation over the wound, pain with passive movement of the area, pain over a palpable mass, and skin discoloration. Wounds most likely to have a glass foreign body include puncture wounds, wounds to the head or feet, and wounds from a motor vehicle collision (14).

An important adjunct in determining the presence of or helping to localize a foreign body is imaging. The best modality depends on the type of foreign body suspected as well as its location. The most commonly utilized modality is plain radiography.

Plain radiographs are able to identify most glass or metallic foreign bodies. Aluminum is difficult to detect on radiographs when ingested, but aluminum subcutaneous foreign bodies are usually visible. Glass is usually visible down to 1 to 2 mm in size. Overlying bone reduces the ability to visualize glass foreign bodies (15–19). Gravel 1 to 2 mm in diameter can be visualized in 97% of cases, but gravel less than 0.5 mm in diameter can seen in fewer than 75% of cases (20). Wood, vegetable material, and plastic are only rarely visible on plain radiographs (15%). Wood is virtually impossible to visualize after 48 hours because the air trapped in the wound is absorbed and the density of the wood then matches the surrounding tissue. Subcutaneous air on a radiograph may be indicative of the location of a foreign body that is itself not visible (21). It is important to obtain multiple views at opposite angles to allow localization in multiple planes. Underpenetrated images are often helpful in visualizing foreign bodies. Digital radiography systems can adjust the brightness and contrast to improve visualization. Radiopaque surface markers at the entrance site can also be helpful in localizing the foreign body. Useful markers include ECG electrodes, paper clips, and needles.

Fluoroscopy is a less frequently used form of plain radiography. Because fluoroscopy provides continuous images, localizer needles can be placed and moved to the foreign body under direct imaging. Once the foreign body is localized, it can be removed by following the localizing needles down to where it is. The disadvantages of fluoroscopy include the lack of availability, the high radiation dose, and the prolonged time required for the procedure.

Computed tomography (CT) also uses x-rays, but it is better able to detect small differences in density. Foreign bodies that are not visible in plain radiographs may be visible on a CT scan. Because of the three-dimensional ability of CT, it is able to visualize foreign bodies behind bone and more accurately locate foreign bodies near vital structures. CT is the modality of choice for foreign bodies of the head (22).

Magnetic resonance imaging (MRI) also allows three-dimensional imaging. Since it does not use x-rays, it is useful for locating foreign bodies that have a density similar to that of the surrounding tissue. Wood, vegetable matter, and plastic are much better visualized on an MRI scan. Surrounding inflammation or edema are also better visualized. MRI is a poor choice for metallic foreign bodies, since they may cause significant artifact. Of more concern is the potential of MRI scanning to cause the migration of metallic foreign bodies. MRI should be used with caution in locating foreign bodies in the head, eye, or neck (22,23).

A disadvantage of both CT and MRI is that they require a still and cooperative patient. In some cases, the patient may require sedation, which can make these imaging techniques complicated and prolonged. CT scanning and sometimes MRI scanning require separation of the child from the parents as well, which can make a cooperative child uncooperative. CT and MRI should be reserved for high-risk patients or in cases where plain radiography is inconclusive.

Ultrasound is emerging as one of the most important techniques for locating foreign bodies. It is excellent at visualizing radiolucent subcutaneous foreign bodies. The sensitivity and specificity of ultrasound in locating foreign bodies exceed 90% in many studies. Because ultrasound can be performed in real time, it allows direct visualization of instruments moving toward the foreign body. Another advantage is that neither the patient nor the operator are exposed to radiation. The disadvantages include a high degree of operator dependence and difficulty visualizing objects close to bone or in wounds that contain gas in the tissue (Chapter 135) (24–28).

Once a foreign body has been located by exam and imaging, the next step is to determine the risks and benefits of removal. This is a multifactorial process. Not all foreign bodies require removal. The benefits of removal include reduced risk of infection, often decreased pain, and decreased risk of late sequelae. These benefits are fairly consistent, so the primary question is, What is the risk of this specific foreign body to the patient? The answer will depend on the type of foreign body and its location. After determining whether the patient would benefit from the removal, the next question is, What risks are involved in removing the object? The risks of removal will depend on the location of the foreign body and its proximity to vital structures. The decision to remove it will be based on the type of foreign body and its location (Table 111.1).

Foreign bodies with a high risk for injury or infection should be removed. These include objects that are highly inflammatory, potentially toxic, or infectious. Foreign bodies that involve important structures, including tendons, ligaments, nerves, and blood vessels, or that might migrate to those structures should be removed. Foreign bodies involving a joint space or an open fracture also should be removed. Foreign bodies that may cause an allergic reaction, continued pain, or cosmetic deformity should be removed as well. Small, inert foreign bodies in a benign location can usually be left in place.

The parents and child should be apprised of the risks and benefits of removal and must be involved in the decision to leave a foreign body alone. The younger the patient is, the longer the opportunity for even benign foreign bodies to develop negative long-term sequelae. Clinicians should therefore have a lower threshold for the removal of foreign

TABLE 111.1	INDICATIONS FOR REMOVING FOREIGN BODIES

Reactive materials likely to cause inflammation or infection (e.g., thorns, spines, wood, other vegetable material, and clothing)
Heavy bacterial contamination
Toxicity (e.g., spines with venom, heavy metals)
Impingement on or damage to tendons, vessels, or nerves
Impairment of mechanical function
Intra-articular location
Proximity to fractured bone
Potential for migration toward important anatomic structures
Intravascular location
Persistent pain
Established inflammation or infection
Allergic reaction
Cosmesis or psychological distress

Reproduced with permission from Iammers RL, Magill T. Detection and management of foreign bodies in soft tissue. *Emerg Med Clin North Am.* Reproduced 1992;10:767–781.

bodies in children (1,4). Any child discharged with a retained foreign body should be provided with instructions for local wound care and follow-up with the appropriate surgical specialist (depending on the location of the foreign body).

Once a decision to remove the foreign body is reached, the next question is whether the procedure can be safely performed in an ED or office setting. Removal of foreign bodies in the neck, chest, or abdomen should not be performed in this setting. The risk of vital structures being involved is too high. These cases are best managed in the operating room. The surgeon will be able to adequately dissect the tissue, visualize the adjacent structures, and control any bleeding. Additionally, general anesthesia will ensure a cooperative patient, and the sterile environment of the operating room will minimize further contamination of deep structures.

If the patient is able to cooperate or appropriate is for sedation and the foreign body is in an amenable location, the process of removal can begin. Prior to removing the foreign body, a time limit, usually 30 minutes, should be set. The parents should be advised that if the foreign body cannot be removed in that time frame, all attempts would stop. The patient will then require referral to the appropriate surgical specialist. This may need to occur immediately or could be arranged as close outpatient follow-up, depending on the specifics of the foreign body. It is easy to get caught up in the desire to complete the procedure. Prolonged attempts are not more likely to be successful, and they put the patient at increased risk for injuries to surrounding tissue. Not all foreign bodies can or will be removed in the ED of office setting. If the patient is unable to cooperate during the procedure, the attempt should be stopped, for the safety of both the patient and the clinician. If the patient can be reassured or appropriately sedated, an additional attempt can be made. If the patient is still unable to cooperate, further attempts should be not be initiated, and a surgical referral should be made, as described above.

▶ EQUIPMENT

Tourniquet or blood pressure cuff

Gauze pads

Needle (25-gauge needle or smaller)

Syringe

Anesthesia: lidocaine 1% or 2% or bupivacaine 0.5% or 1% with or without epinephrine, depending on wound location

Irrigation and preparation solution

Drapes for sterile field

Sterile needles or paper clips for localization during radiography

Scalpel, No. 15 blade for enlarging wound or en bloc removal of foreign body

Forceps, with and without teeth, for grasping object and skin

Hemostat, curved and straight, for grasping object

Large syringe with 18-gauge needle, Angiocatheter, or splash shield

Sterile normal saline for irrigation

40% salicylic acid for superficial splinters

Elmer's glue for small cactus spines

Dressings, bandages, and ointments

▶ PROCEDURE

The first step in removing a foreign body is to identify and localize the object, as detailed above. To reiterate briefly, several radiologic techniques can assist in localizing foreign bodies that cannot be directly visualized. Metallic markers should be placed at 90-degree angles to each other over the surface of a wound before obtaining a plain radiograph. Multiple views can be taken to localize a foreign body in two or more planes. If the foreign body is radiopaque but not able to be localized using this technique, fluoroscopy or CT may help identify the object and aid in its removal (23). If the foreign body is not radiopaque, ultrasonography (Chapter 135) or CT guidance can be used for localization and removal (29,30). Finally, metal detectors have been used successfully to assist with metallic foreign body removal from extremities (31).

Before beginning any procedure, all equipment should be assembled and prepared. Before and after manipulation or application of anesthesia to a wound, the clinician should assess tendon function, nerve function, and the vascular status of the involved extremity. The wound is examined while the underlying tendons and muscles are extended and flexed through their entire range of motion in order to reproduce all relationships of the wound to the underlying structures. To ensure appropriate visualization of the wound, anesthesia, complete immobilization, and proper lighting are critical. It is generally recommended that local anesthetic agents that contain epinephrine be avoided on digits and end organs. This medical axiom is, however, being challenged. A tourniquet applied

proximally to the wound or a blood pressure cuff inflated to 20 mm Hg above the systolic blood pressure will provide adequate hemostasis. Neither a tourniquet nor an inflated cuff should be used for more than 30 minutes at a time. Alternately, if a wound only involves a finger, a sterile glove (sized for the patient's hand) may be applied to the involved hand. The fingertip of the glove covering the involved digit is cut and rolled to the base of the finger, which limits blood flow to the finger during examination of the wound and maintains a sterile field (32). Cleansing the area surrounding the wound with povidone-iodine and placing sterile drapes around the wound will minimize contamination from skin flora.

If the foreign body is not readily visible, extending or enlarging the wound with a No. 15 scalpel blade should be considered. If only superficial dermis and epidermis are incised, the risk of damaging underlying structures will be minimized when enlarging the wound. If possible, the clinician should attempt to incise along the natural skin folds and not perpendicular to skin creases (see Fig. 108.2). The wound can be carefully explored by spreading the soft tissue with a hemostat. Blind probing with any instrument should be avoided,

SUMMARY: PREPARATION FOR FOREIGN OBJECT REMOVAL

1 Use appropriate imaging technique and surface markers to identify possible foreign bodies.

2 Examine the extremity proximal and distal to the wound to ensure that tendon function, neurologic function, and vascular status are intact.

3 Examine the tendons through their entire range of motion to ensure that potential overlapping tissue planes present during the injury are reproduced

4 Provide adequate local analgesia, consider procedural sedation, and immobilize the patient and extremity.

5 Control for hemostasis by applying a proximal tourniquet or blood pressure cuff expanded to 20 mm Hg above systolic blood pressure for no more than 30 minutes at a time.

6 Cleanse the area around the wound with povidone-iodine and place sterile drapes around the wound.

7 Set a time limit of 30 minutes for exploration of the wound.

8 Explore the wound so that the entire foreign body location is determined, including any anatomic relationships with important structures.

9 Remove the entire foreign body, including devitalized or infected tissue.

especially in areas where vital structures are located, such as the hand, foot, or face. Blind probing with a finger should never be done because of the risk of injury to the examiner. In children, vital structures are closer to the skin and to each other and have a higher risk of injury during manipulation of a wound.

Once the foreign body is located, examination of its entire length and identification of its exact anatomic location will ensure that important structures are not involved. If the foreign body is metal or glass, it can be grasped with forceps or a hemostat and removed as one piece. Following removal, re-exploration of the wound will ensure that no important structures were damaged during removal and that no pieces of the foreign body were left behind. If the wound is clean, does not contain particulate matter or devitalized tissue, and is less than 12 to 24 hours old, it should be thoroughly irrigated with sterile saline and sutured. For older or contaminated wounds, débridement of devitalized tissue, placement of a Penrose drain, or delayed primary closure is indicated.

Difficult-to-find, relatively clean embedded objects that are parallel to the skin, such as a long, thin needle or a piece of glass, are best approached by incising the skin perpendicular to the midpoint of the object's long axis (4). Gentle spreading of tissues with a hemostat will aid in locating the object. The object can then be grasped with the hemostat and removed via its original entrance site or through the newly created incision (Fig. 111.1). The incision is then closed.

If the foreign body enters perpendicular to the skin and is difficult to find, attempted localization through a linear incision is not recommended. This will displace the foreign body to one side of the wound. Instead, a small elliptical incision (large enough to ensure that the foreign body can be removed) should be made, with the entrance site of the foreign body in its center (Fig. 111.2). Then, with a No. 15 scalpel blade, the skin is undermined below the dermis 0.5 cm in all directions. The foreign body can be displaced into the middle of the wound by compressing the surrounding skin surface (Fig. 111.2). The object can then be grasped and removed with a hemostat. If no contamination is evident, thorough irrigation followed by wound closure should be performed.

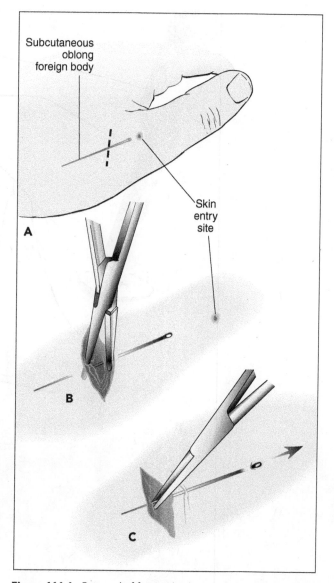

Figure 111.1 Removal of foreign body oriented parallel to skin surface.

 SUMMARY: REMOVAL OF FOREIGN BODY ORIENTED PARALLEL TO SKIN SURFACE

1 Incise the skin perpendicular to midpoint of the object's long axis with a No. 15 scalpel blade.

2 Spread tissues with a hemostat to locate the object.

3 Grasp the object with the hemostat and remove through the original entrance site or a new incision.

 SUMMARY: REMOVAL OF FOREIGN BODY ORIENTED PERPENDICULAR TO SKIN SURFACE

1 Using a No. 15 scalpel blade, make an elliptical incision, with the entrance site of the foreign body in the center.

2 Undermine the surrounding skin 0.5 cm in all directions.

3 Compress the adjacent skin surface to displace the foreign body into the center of the wound.

4 Grasp and remove the foreign body with a hemostat.

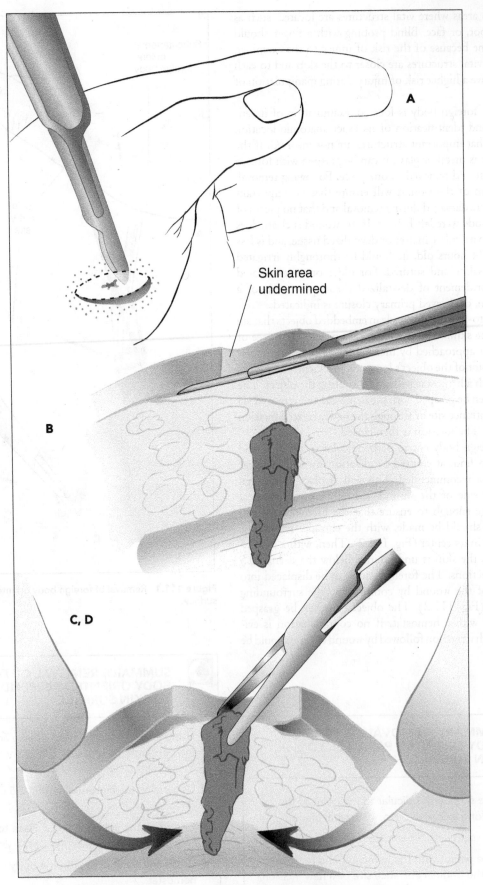

Skin area
undermined

Figure 111.2   Removal of foreign body oriented perpendicular to skin surface.

Removing vegetable matter and wooden splinters requires special care. If the end of a splinter or piece of wood is grasped, it often fragments, leaving multiple pieces in the wound. If the piece is already fragmented or cannot be removed without fragmentation, either an incision down the entire long axis of the foreign body should be made or en bloc removal of the material and surrounding tissue should be performed. To cut down to the foreign body, an incision is made over its entire long axis, and removal via the new skin incision rather than through the entrance wound is indicated. Thorough irrigation of the entire tract and removal of all foreign debris should follow.

Before performing en bloc removal of a foreign body and surrounding tissue, the clinician must first ensure that no tendons, nerves, or vessels are present in the surgical field. An elliptical incision is then made around the wound to a depth below the foreign body. The surrounding skin is undermined 0.5 cm. in all directions with a No. 15 scalpel blade. The entire block of tissue then can be removed by grasping the piece of tissue with a toothed forceps or hemostat and applying upward traction (Fig. 111.3). If this technique is performed properly, no fragments will be left behind, and contaminated tissue will be excised. En bloc removal also should be considered for superficial objects that are difficult to visualize or have the potential to stain, infiltrate, damage, or irritate surrounding tissue.

Superficial splinters also can be removed using keratolytic agents. Salicylic acid hydrates the stratum corneum, loosens the cell margins of the dermis, and detaches the splinter fragment (33). Applying 40% salicylic acid and then covering the area with an occluding adhesive strip is successful in removing subcutaneous splinters parallel to the skin surface in 3 out of 4 cases by 72 hours and in 100% of cases by 7 days (33).

Cactus spines make up a unique class of foreign bodies that present problems with removal. Large and medium spines that do not have barbs on their tip can be removed with the same technique as embedded long needles (34). Traction can be applied to the long axis of the spine because cactus needles do not fracture easily. Small cactus spines are more difficult to remove. Patients with punctures due to small cactus spines can have over 1,000 embedded spines. Several techniques can be used for removal. Toothless forceps can be used alone or in combination with the application of a thin layer of glue (Elmer's) covered with a single layer of gauze. Once the glue is dry, the gauze is lifted, removing most of the spines (34). Less successful techniques include applying a facial peel, adhesive tape, cellophane sealing tape, or ostomy cement, waiting for it to dry, and then pulling most of the spines off at once (34,35).

Although few prospective studies have addressed the utility of antibiotics in preventing infections in patients undergoing foreign body removal, it is generally recommended that patients with wounds that are devitalized (dusky appearing with a tenuous or poor blood supply), older than 12 to 24 hours, or contaminated (with dirt or vegetable or particulate matter) or patients who are immunocompromised receive prophylactic antibiotics. A penicillinase-resistant penicillin derivative, erythromycin, or a first-generation cephalosporin is commonly used for this purpose (2,7). Because of the serious nature of hand infections, an antibiotic for most hand wounds that previously contained a foreign body is recommended. Until further studies are performed, physicians should consider these factors and tailor treatment to each particular case.

A 1- or 2-day follow-up of all patients already infected or at risk for developing an infection will aid in detecting potential complications before any serious sequelae occur.

▶ COMPLICATIONS

Complications of wound exploration and foreign body removal parallel those of retained foreign bodies. Prolonged manipulation of and resulting damage to tissue can lead to superficial and deep wound infections, including cellulitis, abscesses, lymphangitis, septic arthritis, and osteomyelitis. Conversely, infections can occur if foreign material is left behind (especially foreign material such as wood, vegetable matter, or graphite). Physicians must weigh the risk of introducing an infection through extended exploration against the risk of a retained foreign material causing an infection.

Repeated wound handling can directly damage nearby structures, including nerves, arteries, tendons, muscle, and bone. This is especially true in younger patients, whose smaller size makes these consequences more likely. Scarring may occur if dermal or subcutaneous tissue is crushed or devitalized during exploration. To minimize this damage, a time limit for exploration should be set and tissue handled as little as possible during the procedure.

 SUMMARY: EN BLOC REMOVAL OF FOREIGN BODY AND SURROUNDING CONTAMINATED TISSUE

1 Make sure no tendons, nerves, or vessels are within surgical field.

2 Make an elliptical incision around the wound with a No. 15 scalpel blade.

3 Undermine the surrounding skin 0.5 cm in all directions.

4 Extend the initial incision to a depth greater than that of the foreign body.

5 Remove the block of tissue with a hemostat or toothed forceps by applying gentle traction.

6 Re-explore the wound to ensure that there is no damage to important structures or any remaining fragments of the foreign body.

7 Irrigate and consider closing the wound if it is not old or dirty.

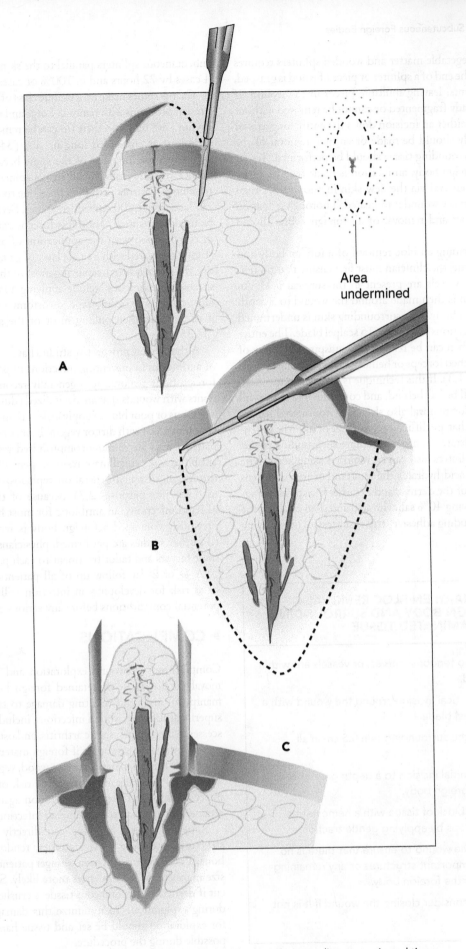

Area
undermined

Figure 111.3 En bloc removal of foreign body and surrounding contaminated tissue.

CLINICAL TIPS

▶ The possibility of a retained foreign body should be considered in every laceration and puncture wound.

▶ A persistent infection, draining sinus, and culture-negative abscess should be assumed to be caused by a foreign body until definitively proven otherwise.

▶ A normal plain radiograph does not rule out the presence of a nonradiopaque foreign body.

▶ Use appropriate radiographic techniques and surface markers to identify and localize a possible foreign body.

▶ Examination of tendon, neurologic, and vascular function should be performed before the administration of any anesthetic or sedating agent as well as before and after wound exploration.

▶ Examine tendons through their entire range of motion to ensure that potential overlapping tissue planes present during injury are reproduced.

▶ Provision of adequate analgesia and immobilization allows the wound to be thoroughly evaluated without patient movement or discomfort.

▶ Set a time limit of 30 minutes for exploration of a wound.

▶ Control for hemostasis by applying a proximal tourniquet or blood pressure cuff expanded to 20 mm Hg above systolic blood pressure for no more than 30 minutes at a time.

▶ Explore the wound so that the entire foreign body location is known, including any anatomic relationships with important structures.

▶ Remove the entire foreign body, including devitalized or infected tissue.

▶ Consultants should be involved if the exploration involves complex structures or will take a prolonged amount of time.

Techniques to limit bleeding can compromise arterial flow to the involved area. Vasoconstricting agents are contraindicated near end organs such as fingers, toes, nose, ears, and penis and for tissue that has a compromised arterial supply (e.g., partially devitalized skin). Application of a tourniquet or blood pressure cuff should not exceed 20 to 30 minutes at a time. The tourniquet or cuff should be released for 1 to 2 minutes at regular intervals to limit pain and tissue hypoperfusion. Neuropraxia, intimal vascular damage, vascular thrombosis, and gangrene have been reported with use of tourniquets, primarily if left on for more than 2 continuous

hours (36,37). The technique of rolling the fingertip of a glove to the base of the involved finger can lead to pressures as high as 1,000 mm Hg if the glove is too small. An appropriate size glove for the patient's hand provides adequate hemostasis with lower pressures and less risk of damage (32).

▶ SUMMARY

The ability to remove subcutaneous foreign bodies is an important skill physicians must possess when dealing with injured pediatric patients. Although this procedure has many potential complications, knowledge of a variety of alternative techniques will increase the clinician's ability to successfully remove foreign bodies. Properly preparing the pediatric patient and the wound for exploration will save time and effort and decrease potential complications from this procedure. Immobilization, anesthesia, and analgesia are important factors that physicians must address in young and often apprehensive children before any attempt at foreign body removal. Finally, setting a time limit and handling tissue as little as possible will reduce the risk of injuring tissue and important adjacent structures.

▶ ACKNOWLEDGMENT

We would like to thank Dr. S. Rothrock for his contribution to the version of this chapter in the first edition of this text.

▶ REFERENCES

1. Baker MD, Lanuti M. The management and outcome of lacerations in urban children. *Ann Emerg Med.* 1990;19:1001–1006.
2. Chisholm CD, Schlesser JF. Plantar puncture wounds: controversies and treatment recommendations. *Ann Emerg Med.* 1989;18:1352–1357.
3. Fitzgerald RH, Cowan JD. Puncture wounds of the foot. *Orthop Clin North Am.* 1975;6:965–972.
4. Lammers RL, Magill T. Detection and management of foreign bodies in soft tissue. *Emerg Med Clin North Am.* 1992;10:767–781.
5. Anderson MA, Newmeyer WL 3rd, Kilgore ES Jr. Diagnosis and treatment of retained foreign bodies of the hand. *Am J Surg.* 1982;144:63–67.
6. Morgan WJ, Leopold T, Evans R. Foreign bodies in the hand. *J Hand Surg.* 1984;9:194–196.
7. Langsam A. Solid foreign bodies in the soft tissue: diagnosis and management. *Del Med J.* 1985;57:701–702.
8. Swischuk LE, Jorgenson F, Jorgenson A. Wooden splinter induced "pseudo-tumor" and "osteomyelitis-like lesions" of bone and soft tissue. *Am J Roentgenol Radium Ther Nucl Med.* 1974;122:176–179.
9. Epstein WL, Fukuyama K. Mechanisms of granulomatous inflammation. *Immunol Ser.* 1989;46:687–721.
10. Chow D, Cooke TD, Feltis T. Thorn-induced synovitis. *Can Med Assoc J.* 1987;136:1057–1058.
11. Mowry RG, Sams WM Jr, Caulfield JB. Cutaneous silica granuloma: a rare entity or rarely diagnosed? Report of two cases with review of the literature. *Arch Dermatol.* 1991;127:692–694.

12. Fisher M, Goldsmith J, Gilligan P. Sneakers as a source of *Pseudomonas aeruginosa* in children with osteomyelitis following puncture wounds. *J Pediatr.* 1985;106:607–609.

13. Avner JR, Baker D. Lacerations involving glass. *Am J Dis Child.* 1992;146:600–602.

14. Montano JB, Steele MT, Watson WA. Foreign body retention in glass-caused wounds. *Ann Emerg Med.* 1992;21:1360–1363.

15. Flom LL, Ellis GL. Radiologic evaluation of foreign bodies. *Emerg Med Clin North Am.* 1992;10:163–177.

16. Courter BJ. Radiographic screening for glass foreign bodies: what does a "negative" foreign body series really mean? *Ann Emerg Med.* 1990;19:997–1000.

17. de Lacey G, Evans R, Sandin B. Penetrating injuries: how easy is it to see glass (and plastic) on radiographs? *Br J Radiol.* 1985;58(685):27–30.

18. Tandberg D. Glass in the hand and foot: will an x-ray film show it? *JAMA.* 1982;248:1872–1874.

19. Pond GD, Lindsey D. Localization of cactus, glass, and other foreign bodies in soft tissues. *Ariz Med.* 1977;34:700–702.

20. Chisholm CD, Wood CO, Chua G, et al. Radiographic detection of gravel in soft tissue. *Ann Emerg Med.* 1997;29:725–730.

21. Brewer TE Jr, Leonard RB. Detection of retained wood following trauma. *N C Med J.* 1986;47:575–577.

22. Bodne D, Quinn SF, Cochran CF. Imaging foreign glass and wooden bodies of the extremities with CT and MR. *J Comput Assist Tomogr.* 1988;12:608–611.

23. Lewis TT, Case A, Troughton A, et al. Metallic foreign body localization with magnetic resonance imaging. *Radiol Today.* 1991;57:16–17.

24. Banerjee B, Das RK. Sonographic detection of foreign bodies of the extremities. *Br J Radiol.* 1991;64:107–112.

25. Blyme PJH, Lind T, Schantz K, et al. Ultrasonographic detection of foreign bodies in soft tissue: a human cadaver study. *Arch Orthop Trauma Surg.* 1990;220:24–25.

26. Crawford R, Matheson AB. Clinical value of ultrasonography in the detection and removal of radiolucent foreign bodies. *Injury.* 1989;20:341–343.

27. Gilbert FJ, Campbell RS, Bayliss AP. The role of ultrasound in the detection of nonradiopaque foreign bodies. *Clin Radiol.* 1990;41:109–112.

28. Manthey DE, Storrow AB, Milbourn JM, et al. Ultrasound versus radiography in the detection of soft-tissue foreign bodies. *Ann Emer Med.* 1996;28:7–9.

29. Bissonnette RT, Connell DG, Fitzpatrick DG. Preoperative localization of low-density foreign bodies under CT guidance. *Can Assoc Radiol J.* 1988;39:286–287.

30. Bradley M, Kadzombe E, Simms P, et al. Percutaneous ultrasound guided extraction of nonpalpable soft tissue foreign bodies. *Arch Emerg Med.* 1992;9:181–184.

31. West A, Glucksman E. The use of a metal locator in an accident and emergency department. *Arch Emerg Med.* 1987;4:57–61.

32. Barnett A, Pearl RM. Readily available, inexpensive finger tourniquet. *Plast Reconstr Surg.* 1983;71:134–135.

33. Copelan R. Chemical removal of splinters without epidermal toxic effects. *J Am Acad Dermatol.* 1989;20:697–698.

34. Lindsey D, Lindsey WE. Cactus spine injuries. *Am J Emerg Med.* 1988;6:362–369.

35. Martinez TT, Jerome M, Barry BC, et al. Removal of cactus spines from the skin: a comparative evaluation of several methods. *Am J Dis Child.* 1987;141:1291–1292.

36. Dove AF, Clifford RP. Ischemia after use of a finger tourniquet. *Br Med J (Clin Res Ed).* 1982;284:1162–1163.

37. Pedowitz RA. Limb tourniquets during surgery. *Acta Orthop Scand.* 1991;62[Suppl 245]:17–33.

JOHN M. LOISELLE AND KATHLEEN M. CRONAN

112

Hair Tourniquet Removal

▶ INTRODUCTION

"Hair-thread tourniquet syndrome" refers to conditions in which an appendage (e.g., finger, toe, or penis) is circumferentially constricted by a hair or thread, leading to impairment of lymphatic and eventually venous return (1,2). Cases involving entrapment of other body parts, such as the female genitalia (clitoris and labia), though unusual, have also been reported (3). Hair tourniquets most frequently occur in the first few months of life, although they occasionally occur in toddlers. Normal perfusion is restored by unraveling the hair or cutting the constricting band and thereby eliminating the vascular compression. Principles that should be adhered to when releasing the constricting band include protecting entrapped soft tissue from harm and avoiding injury to the neurovascular and tendon structures of the appendage. The removal procedure in most cases can be performed in the ambulatory office or the emergency department. This procedure is usually performed by an emergency physician, general pediatric practitioner, or family physician, but if significant edema has occurred, with ensuing distortion of tissues, surgical consultation may be necessary.

▶ ANATOMY AND PHYSIOLOGY

Anatomic structures involved in a digital hair tourniquet include the layers of the skin as well as the nerves, blood vessels, and lymphatics (Fig. 112.1). The neurovascular bundles of the fingers and toes are located on the dorsal and palmar or plantar aspects of both the radial and ulnar margins. The major neurovascular structures of the penis and clitoris are located on the dorsal surface at the 12 o'clock position. Deeper structures of the penis that may become involved include the dorsally located corpora cavernosum and also the corpus spongiosum, which is located on the ventral surface and surrounds the urethra (4).

Hair tourniquets have been associated with postpartum hair loss (telogen effluvium), mothers with long hair (particularly blonde hair in the case of a Caucasian child), use of mittens or booties in infants, and hair shed in the bathtub (2,5–7). Child abuse must be considered, especially in cases involving the penis, as several reports have been made of tourniquets being placed intentionally (2,8). It is postulated that often the offending hair is wet when it first becomes wrapped around the appendage. The hair contracts as it dries, leading to the initial constriction (1,5,9,10).

Constriction of venous and lymphatic vessels, with inhibition of venous return, by a hair tourniquet leads to edema and progressive swelling. This compounds the compression of the vessels and compromises distal perfusion in a vicious cycle. If the constricting agent remains in place long enough, it can cut through the skin layers. Epithelialization may then occur, obscuring the hair beneath an overlying skin bridge. Injury may be caused by ischemia and by direct damage to structures through the cutting action of the tourniquet. Necrosis and gangrene of digits (5,6,8) and erosion through the urethra, with resulting fistula formation, have been reported (11–13).

▶ INDICATIONS

The child with a constricting band of hair or thread may present in several ways. Most frequently, the child has an erythematous, swollen, painful appendage. When inspected carefully, the appendage exhibits a sharp, circumferential demarcation beyond which it is affected. At the point of demarcation, an extra crease or indentation is noted. Because of the difficulty in localizing a source of pain in the infant, it is

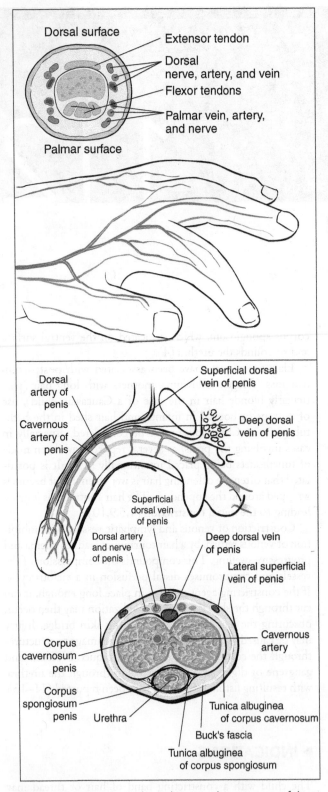

Figure 112.1 Neurovascular and structural components of the fingers and penis.

important not to overlook this as a possible diagnosis when evaluating the presentation of irritability and crying (3).

A number of other processes may present in a similar fashion. Hair tourniquets involving the penis may initially be confused with a paraphimosis in the uncircumcised male (6) or with balanitis, a localized infection of the glans penis. Similarly, a hair tourniquet on the digit may mimic infectious processes such as a cellulitis, felon, and paronychia. Rarely encountered entities resulting in bandlike constrictions around the digits include congenital amniotic bands and ainhum, a rare condition of spontaneous bandlike constriction and ischemia occurring in the toes of dark-skinned people (1,2).

Frequently, the hair or thread is visible and may simply be cut or unwrapped. There are case reports of the use of depilatory agents for successfully removing entrapped hairs (14). When the strand is not visible or has eroded through the dermis and involves underlying structures, or if uncertainty exists regarding completeness of removal, a surgical or urologic consult may be necessary.

▶ EQUIPMENT

Local or regional anesthesia materials (Chapter 35)
Scalpel blade, No. 15
Povidone-iodine solution
Fine-tipped forceps
Ear curette
Ophthalmic spud or spoon curette
Fine-tipped hemostat
Blunt probe
Fine-tipped scissors

▶ PROCEDURE

The technique used for removing a hair tourniquet and the need for involving specialists depend on the perceived risk to the appendage, the involvement of underlying structures, the depth of the hair, and the appendage involved. If a loose end of the constricting hair can be located, it may simply be necessary to grasp it firmly with gloved fingers, fine forceps, or a hemostat and gently unwind it. It should be noted that a single strand may have broken into several and that this process may need to be repeated.

In cases when the constricting band does not seem too deeply imbedded in the soft tissue, a blunt probe or metal ear wax curette may be gently inserted beneath the constriction (Fig. 112.2). Insertion is facilitated when performed in a proximal to distal direction while applying traction to the skin. The hair generally penetrates less deeply and may be more accessible on the dorsal aspect of the fingers or toes. Once the strand is isolated with a metal object, it can be cut with fine-tipped scissors. Alternatively, a scalpel blade may be used to cut through the hair onto the probe or curette, which serves to protect the underlying skin.

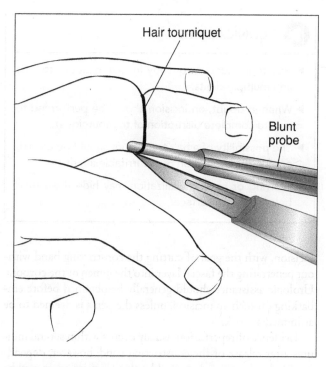

Figure 112.2 Removal of a hair tourniquet with a blunt probe.

In situations in which the degree of edema or depth of penetration of the hair makes this technique impossible, direct incision of the band to ensure release is necessary. Surgical consultation should be considered at this point.

Incisional Approach

Digits

A digital nerve block is performed (Chapter 35), and the digit and surrounding area are prepped and draped in a sterile fashion. The major consideration when determining the best site for an incision in the removal of a hair tourniquet is the location of underlying structures. Because the neurovascular bundles lie at the dorsal and palmar aspects of the radial and ulnar portions of the digits, one recommended approach is to make the incision between the bundles using a No. 15 scalpel blade at either the 3 o'clock or 9 o'clock position (Fig. 112.3A). A short incision should be made longitudinally along the digit with the blade perpendicular to the strand and the skin surface. The incision is made in a proximal to distal direction and should be extended to the bone to ensure incision of the fiber.

An incision on the dorsal surface provides an acceptable alternative approach (Fig. 112.3A) (2,15). Although this may result in an incision into the extensor tendon, a longitudinal incision parallel to the direction of the tendon fibers should heal well with splinting and general wound care. This incision has the advantage of avoiding the neurovascular bundles entirely.

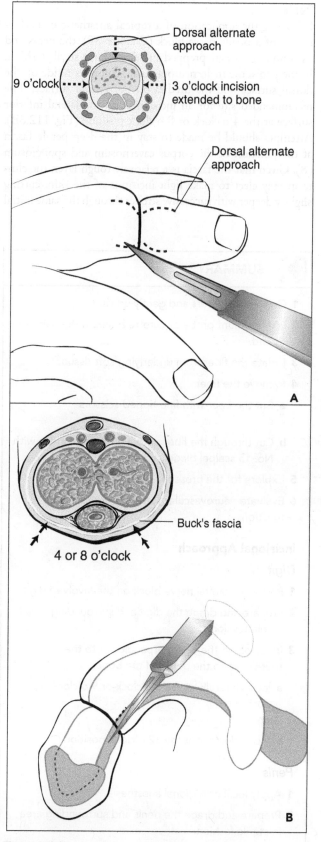

Figure 112.3
A. Incisional removal of a hair tourniquet from a digit.
B. Incisional removal of a hair tourniquet from a penis.

Penis

Following the application of a topical anesthetic or performance of a penile nerve block (Chapter 35), the penis and surrounding area are prepped and draped in a sterile fashion. In the penis, the main neurovascular structures reside on the dorsal surface and the urethra on the ventral surface. The recommended site for an incision is on the lateral inferior surface at the 4 o'clock or 8 o'clock position (Fig. 112.3B). Attempts should be made to stay in the deep penile fascia at the junction of the corpus cavernosum and spongiosum (8). Given that the fascia is a relatively tough layer, the clinician may elect to make light incisions of the skin, cutting slightly deeper with successive strokes through the same initial

SUMMARY

1 Grasp loose fibers and gently unwind.

2 Insert a blunt probe or curette beneath the hair or thread.

3 Isolate the fiber from underlying soft tissue.

4 Remove the fiber:

   a Cut the fiber with fine-tipped scissors
      or

   b Cut through the fiber onto a probe or curette with No. 15 scalpel blade.

5 Explore for the presence of additional strands.

6 Evaluate neurovascular status and tendon function.

Incisional Approach

Digit

1 Perform a digital nerve block on the involved digit.

2 Prepare and drape the digit and surrounding area in sterile fashion.

3 Incise along the digit perpendicular to the tourniquet to the depth of the bone:

   a Incise laterally at the 3 o'clock or 9 o'clock position
      or

   b Incise dorsally at the 12 o'clock position.

Penis

1 Apply local or regional anesthesia.

2 Prepare and drape the penis and surrounding area in sterile fashion.

3 Incise the lateral inferior surface at either the 4 o'clock or 8 o'clock position.

CLINICAL TIPS

▶ Hair tourniquets frequently involve multiple strands and multiple digits.

▶ When in doubt, an incision should be performed to ensure complete disruption of the tourniquet.

▶ The possibility of a hair tourniquet should be considered in the evaluation of the irritable infant.

▶ Scarring or re-epithelialization may hide the strand below the skin surface.

incision, with the goal of cutting the constricting band without penetrating the fascial layer into the lumen of the corpora. Urologic assistance should generally be obtained before embarking on such an incision, unless the penis is deemed to be at immediate risk.

Evidence of reperfusion usually occurs within several minutes after release of the constricting band; however, depending on the tissue insult caused by the constriction, it may be days before normal perfusion has returned completely. When any question remains as to whether the circumferential constriction has been completely removed, surgical consultation should be obtained.

Neurovascular status and tendon function should be documented following the procedure. The need for tetanus prophylaxis should be addressed. An extremity should be placed in an elevated position to allow for passive drainage. Re-evaluation in 24 hours will help to ensure that all constricting bands have been removed and that the soft tissue has adequate perfusion and is free from infection.

▶ COMPLICATIONS

Damage to neurovascular structures may be the result of prolonged ischemia, the cutting action of the tourniquet, or the incision. Similarly, injuries to the corpus cavernosum, corpus spongiosum, or urethra are possible with incisional removal of hair tourniquets involving the penis. Dorsal incisions in the fingers and toes generally do not cause functional damage to tendons, but tenosynovitis may result from injury to the tendon sheath. Once penetration of the superficial layers of the skin has occurred, whether by the hair or the incision, infection is a risk.

▶ SUMMARY

Diagnosis of a hair or thread wrapped around an appendage such as a finger, a toe, or the penis may be obvious or may test the diagnostic skills of an astute clinician. In the uncomplicated case, removal is a simple matter of unwinding the offending hair. If the hair has been present for a prolonged period, progressive edema and penetration into deeper layers of skin may necessitate an incisional approach to ensure complete removal. A consultant is frequently necessary at this point. Although serious consequences have been reported with delay in recognizing and removing such objects, successful removal generally results in reperfusion with few, if any, complications.

▶ ACKNOWLEDGMENT

The authors would like to acknowledge the valuable contributions of Richard T. Cooke, Jr. to the version of this chapter that appeared in the previous edition.

▶ REFERENCES

1. Alpert JJ, Filler R, Glaser HH. Strangulation of an appendage by hair wrapping. *N Engl J Med.* 1965;273:866–867.
2. Barton DJ, Sloan GM, Nichter LS, et al. Hair-thread tourniquet syndrome. *Pediatrics.* 1988;82:926–929.
3. Pawel BB, Henretig FM. Crying and colic. In: Fleisher G, Ludwig S, Henretig FM, eds. *Textbook of Pediatric Emergency Medicine.* 5th ed. Philadelphia: Lippincott Williams & Wilkins; 2006:229–232.
4. Gross CM, ed. *Gray's Anatomy.* 28th ed. Philadelphia: Lea & Ferbiger; 1966.
5. Mariani PJ, Wagner DK. Topical cocaine prior to treatment of penile tourniquet syndrome. *J Emerg Med.* 1986;4:205–208.
6. Wang M, Schott J, Tunnessen WW Jr. Head-thread tourniquet syndrome [picture of the month]. *Arch Pediatr Adolesc Med.* 2001;155:515–516.
7. Strahlman RS. Toe tourniquet syndrome in association with maternal hair loss. *Pediatrics.* 2003;111:685–687.
8. Kerry RL, Chapman DD. Strangulation of appendages by hair and thread. *J Pediatr Surg.* 1973;8:23–27.
9. Haddad FS. Penile strangulation by human hair: report of three cases and review of the literature. *Urol Int.* 1982;37:375–388.
10. Summers JL, Guira AC. Hair strangulation of the external genitalia. *Ohio State Med J.* 1973;69:672–673.
11. Toguri AG, Light RA, Warren MW. Penile tourniquet syndrome caused by hair. *South Med J.* 1979;72:627–628.
12. Harrow BR. Strangulation of penis by a hidden thread [letter]. *JAMA.* 1967;199:171.
13. Press S, Schnachner I, Paul P. Clitoris tourniquet syndrome. *Pediatrics.* 1980;66:781–782.
14. Douglas DD. Dissolving hair wrapped around an infant's digit [letter]. *J Pediatr.* 1977;91:162.
15. Serour F, Gorenstein A. Treatment of the toe tourniquet syndrome in infants. *Pediatr Surg Int.* 2003;19:598–600.

113

KATHY N. SHAW AND MARC H. GORELICK

Burn Management

▶ INTRODUCTION

In 2002, there were more than 163,000 emergency department (ED) visits for burn injuries (1). Most of these burns occurred in the home, and the majority were preventable. Young children less than 4 years of age have the highest incidence of injury from burns. They are most at risk for scald burns requiring hospitalization and for death in house fires. Overall, burn injuries are the third leading cause of accidental death in children (2–3). Burns also are a significant mechanism of child abuse (4).

Four different types of burns may occur, depending on the source of injury. Thermal burns are the most common type of burn injury seen in children (2). They occur as a result of scalds, contact burns, or flame injuries. Chemical burns in children usually involve ingestion or contamination with acids or alkalis found in household products. Electrical burns are usually low-voltage injuries that occur in toddlers mouthing electrical cords or playing with sockets. Although rare, high-voltage injuries may be seen, typically in older children or adolescents. Radiation burns in children are usually due to sunburn (5).

Most burns are minor and can be treated in an outpatient setting. In order to make decisions regarding management, the physician must be able to determine the depth or degree of the burn, the percentage of body surface area involved, whether the pattern of injury is typical of abuse, and whether deformity or loss of function may occur. Once a burn is determined to be minor, trained nursing or emergency medical services (EMS) personnel can often provide local care. The care the minor burn patient receives is crucial to the ultimate outcome. Many of the same principles apply to burns as those discussed under basic wound care (Chapter 107). The goals are to relieve pain, prevent infection and additional trauma, and minimize scarring and contracture.

Treatment of the major burn victim should be performed by physicians trained in burn management. The initial care of the major burn victim is critical to both immediate survival and the ultimate outcome (6,7). Expert pediatric respiratory management is often needed for major burn victims with smoke inhalation. Mortality for these children is much higher than for those children with comparable burns but no smoke inhalation (8).

▶ ANATOMY AND PHYSIOLOGY

The skin is the largest organ in the body and has many important functions. It acts as a barrier to infection and loss of body water, as a thermal regulator, as a sensory organ, and as an excretory organ. Of the skin's three layers (Fig. 113.1), the dermis contains the blood vessels, nerves, and epithelial appendages (e.g., hair) as well as sebaceous and sweat glands that are necessary for most of the skin's primary functions and for self-repair. The depth of the burn injury therefore determines the extent of the damage to this organ and its ability to heal (Table 113.1). Superficial or first-degree burns affect only the epidermis or tough protective barrier. A mild sunburn is a typical example. Partial-thickness or second-degree burns extend into the dermis. Deep second-degree burns may mimic third-degree burns, as most of the skin elements are destroyed. Healing is prolonged, and hypertrophic scarring may occur. Full-thickness or third-degree burns involve the entire dermis, including neurovascular structures. Fourth-degree burns extend into the muscle, fascia, or bone.

Both the depth and degree of the burn and the extent of skin involvement determine the severity of the injury and affect the skin's ability to maintain its physiologic functions. First-degree burns are not included in calculations of the extent of involvement unless the area exceeds 25% to 30% of the

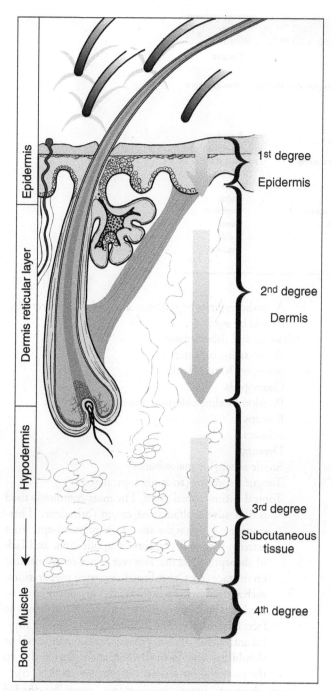

Figure 113.1 Skin layers and corresponding classification of burn depths.

body surface area. Estimates of body surface area (BSA) involvement in babies and young children cannot be done using the "rule of 9s" because they have a proportionately larger head and smaller lower extremities (Fig. 113.2). Emergency departments should have access to tables listing BSA by body part and age of the child, such as the Lund and Browder charts (9). For smaller burns, the area can be estimated by comparing the child's palm size, which is 1% of BSA, with the burned area.

▶ INDICATIONS

Treatment of burns depends on the severity of injury, location, characteristics of the child, and mechanism of injury (Table 113.2). A first-degree burn is identified by pain, erythema, and subsequent peeling, but healing occurs without scarring. A typical second-degree burn is painful, red, blanches with pressure, has weeping blisters, and usually heals with minimal or no scarring. Deep second-degree burns may appear white and be anesthetic but often will blanch with pressure. Third-degree burns are dry, leathery, white or charred in appearance, painless, and require grafting because the dermis has been destroyed. The depth of the burn sometimes can be difficult to determine in the first few hours and may require repeated examinations.

Minor burns are usually treated in the ED or office by trained personnel, including nurses and emergency medical technicians (EMTs) under the supervision of a physician. A minor burn is defined as a second-degree burn that covers less than 10% of BSA in children under 6 years of age and less than 15% in older children and adults or a third-degree burn that covers less than 2% of the BSA. Exceptions include burns that may cause loss of function or severe deformity or are associated with a higher risk of infection, such as burns of the hands, face, eyes, ears, feet, perineum, or genitalia. In addition, burns should not be classified as minor if the child has an underlying disease that may affect the healing process, if the burn is suspected to have occurred from child abuse or neglect, if the caretaker is unable to care for the burn, or if the burn is circumferential and may require escharotomy or crosses a flexion crease indicating a more severe injury.

Major burns include second-degree burns greater than 20% of BSA and third-degree burns greater than 10% of the BSA in children. In addition, burns associated with smoke inhalation or major trauma or high-voltage electrical burns should be considered major burns. When concern arises about the healing process, the clinician also should consider it a major burn. These should be treated by a physician knowledgeable in burn care. General or plastic surgeons should be consulted as needed and when available, especially for procedures such as escharotomy and treatment of burns that may cause disability or disfigurement. Most major burns require the special facilities and personnel of a burn center. Transfer to a center with pediatric intensive care should be considered for children with inhalational or high-voltage electrical injuries regardless of the extent of the burns. Most burns of moderate extent also require hospitalization or close follow-up by a physician knowledgeable in burn management.

▶ EQUIPMENT

Standard resuscitation equipment, including airway equipment, supplemental oxygen, intravenous access, and isotonic intravenous fluids, such as lactated Ringer's.

TABLE 113.1	CHARACTERISTICS OF BURNS BY DEGREE		
Degree	**Symptoms/physical examination**	**Healing**	**Causes**
First (superficial)	Pain 48–72 hr Erythema Mild edema Blanches	Epithelium may peel in 5–10 days No scarring	Ultraviolet light
Second (partial thickness)	*Superficial* Painful Bright red Weeping Blisters *Deep* White/yellow or mottled +/– anesthetic	*Superficial* 10–14 days Minimal or no scarring *Deep* 25–35 days Hypertrophic scarring Requires grafting	*Superficial* Short flash Brief scald *Deep* Scalds Short flash
Third (Full thickness)	Dry, leathery Anesthetic Pearly white ⟶ charred Thrombosed veins visible		Flame Scald Electrical

A cardiorespiratory monitor and pulse oximeter also should be available.

Cleaning and débridement
  Sterile saline or water
  Syringes, 30 to 60 mL
  Gauze pads
  Povidone-iodine solution, one-quarter strength
  Forceps
  Scissors
  Dressing
  Sterile sheet (for major burns)
  Tongue depressor (to apply topical agents)
  Topical antimicrobial agent. The most commonly used is 1% silver sulfadiazine cream (Silvadene, Thermazene). This has the advantages of broad-spectrum activity, ease and comfort of application, and lack of absorption. Its use, however, is not recommended on the face (6). Other broad-spectrum preparations, such as bacitracin/polymyxin B (Polysporin), may be used for small burns, particularly those involving the face. Mafenide acetate (Sulfamylon) is another topical antimicrobial cream that is occasionally used but should be avoided in the outpatient setting due to the potential for serious systemic side effects (6).

Inner dressing. Inner dressings are generally divided into conventional and synthetic (10,11). Conventional dressings are those made from cotton gauze. The gauze may be plain or impregnated with a greasy material such as petrolatum to render it nonadherent; examples include Aquaphor, Vaseline, and Adaptic. Xeroform gauze also incorporates 3% bismuth tribromophenate as an antibacterial agent.

A wide variety of synthetic materials also are available. These have been designed to render frequent dressing changes unnecessary. Some dressings commonly available in the United States include semipermeable polyurethane films, such as OpSite and Tegaderm (adhesive) and Epi-Lock (nonadhesive); hydrocolloid

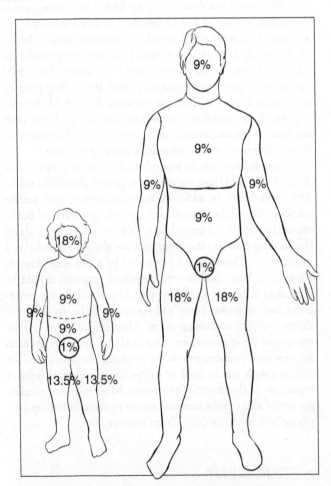

Figure 113.2 Differences in the percentage of body surface area distribution between a child and an adult. Note that the percentages for the torso refer to the front only or the back only; the percentages for the head and extremities refer to the entire region.

TABLE 113.2	CLASSIFICATION OF BURNS IN CHILDREN		
Classification	**Burn**		**Associated factors**	**Disposition**

Classification	Burn		Associated factors	Disposition
Major	2°: >20% BSA		Potential loss of function	Burn center
	3°: >10% BSA	or	Increased risk of infection	
	Circumferential		Severe deformity	
	Crosses flexion crease		e.g., burns of hands, face, ears, nose, feet, perineum, genitalia	
			e.g., immunosuppressed child	
			High-voltage injury	Pediatric intensive care
		or	Smoke inhalation	
Moderate	2°: 10% to 20%	+	None of above	Hospitalization or close follow-up by specialist
	3°: 2% to 20%	or	Parental inability to care for burn	
		or	Child abuse suspected	
Minor	2°: <10% BSA	+	None of above	Outpatient treatment
	3°: <2% BSA			

dressings, such as DuoDerm; and composites, including Biobrane and Epigard.

A number of investigators have failed to demonstrate the clear superiority of any of the various types of dressings—all provide satisfactory results when properly used (12–19). Conventional dressings continue to be the most widely used and have the advantages of being readily available and simple to apply. Moreover, most health care providers are familiar with their use. Synthetic dressings, by obviating the need for frequent dressing changes, may make home care easier and may minimize patient discomfort. Several studies comparing different dressings have found total costs to be similar (12,16). Thus, the choice of dressing method is largely a matter of patient and physician preference.

Outer dressing
    Cotton gauze rolls
    Stockinette or burn netting
    Tape
Miscellaneous
    Scalpel, No. 10 or 15 for escharotomy
    Splinting materials (Chapter 101)

▶ PROCEDURE

Major Burns

Initial Resuscitation Measures

Treatment of major burns begins with appropriate prehospital care. The clinician should focus primary attention on management of the airway, breathing, and circulation. The cervical spine should be immobilized if concomitant trauma is suspected. The burn wound may initially be immersed in cool water to provide rapid return to normal temperature. Ice, however, should be avoided, as excessive cold leads to potentiation of ischemic damage (20). Chemical burns should be vigorously irrigated with water. Appropriate dressings include a dry, sterile sheet or saline-soaked gauze; both provide immediate pain relief and some degree of protection of the wound. Home remedies such as butter or other ointments are not indicated.

In the ED, sterile technique must be meticulously practiced from the outset in the care of patients with major burns, including masks and gowns for medical personnel (Chapters 7 and 8). Resuscitation continues, with particular attention to fluid management. Large-bore intravenous access is mandatory, preferably through unburned skin. Isotonic crystalloid, such as normal saline or lactated Ringer's, is administered in boluses of 20 mL/kg as needed to restore circulatory stability. A number of formulas for estimating fluid needs of burned children over the first 24 hours have been developed, the details of which are beyond the scope of this book (21–27). Children with electrical burns must be monitored for cardiac dysrhythmias. Importantly, such patients frequently have internal injuries more extensive than those suggested by the external appearance of the burn.

Emergent Escharotomy

A problem unique to the burn victim is compromised ventilation or regional circulation due to restrictive eschar in circumferential full-thickness burns of the chest or extremities, respectively. In such cases, incisional decompression or escharotomy is performed emergently as a palliative measure (7,28,29). With a No. 10 or 15 scalpel, a single incision is made that extends the full length of the burn and is carried down through the eschar to the layer of the subcutaneous fat; occasionally, extension down to the deep fascia is necessary. Anesthesia or analgesia is not required, as the nerve fibers have been destroyed, and bleeding is typically minimal. The preferred site of the escharotomy incision is along the lateral or medial aspect of the limb or bilaterally in the anterior axillary line on the chest (Fig. 113.3). Extension along the costal margins also may be necessary. Following decompression, rapid improvement in chest excursion or limb perfusion should be observed. If not, the incision should be checked for adequacy of length and depth.

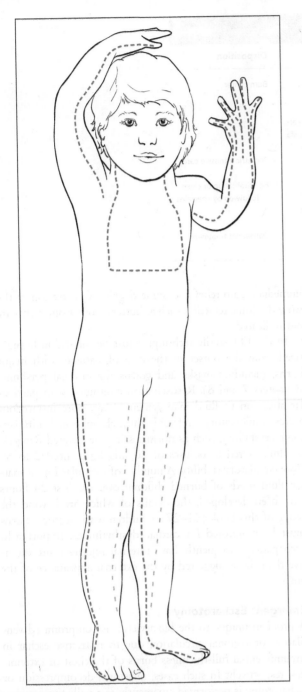

Figure 113.3 Escharotomy incision sites in a child.

Burn Preparation

Care of the burn itself in the ED is similar to that described for the prehospital setting. Because the burned child is typically in a great deal of pain, analgesia must be provided as early as possible (30). All clothing is removed from burned areas. Adherent molten material such as tar should be cooled with water but left in place. The burns are then irrigated and protected with dry, sterile sheets or saline-soaked gauze. It should be noted that prolonged use of saline-soaked gauze can cause discomfort for the patient from cooling. In addition, small infants may need to be placed under an overhead

warmer to prevent hypothermia due to evaporative heat loss. Further wound care, such as débridement or application of any topical agents, should be left to the discretion of the surgeon who will assume further care of the child with major burns (31). Supportive measures in the ED include any necessary ongoing resuscitative interventions, maintenance of analgesia, and tetanus immunoprophylaxis as needed.

Minor Burns

The treatment of minor partial-thickness burns is directed toward providing an optimal environment for wound healing to occur (32). A number of approaches that meet this goal are possible. While considerable debate exists in the literature on various points of burn care, most burns can be managed successfully using one of several methods. The choice of approach in a specific case depends on a number of factors, including characteristics of the burn and of the patient and physician preference.

Burn Preparation and Débridement

In all cases, the wound must be prepared. Clothing should be removed from the burned area. Chemical burns are irrigated with large amounts of water or saline; a small child may be placed in a sink for this purpose. As with major burns, if adherent tar is present, it should be left in place. Applying a solvent ointment such as petrolatum or Aquaphor allows easy removal of the tar after 24 to 48 hours (7).

The process of preparing and dressing a partial-thickness burn can be quite painful. Adequate pain control, which usually requires narcotics, must be provided before proceeding. For larger burns, procedural sedation may be necessary (Chapter 33).

First-degree burns require no débridement, and the eschar of a full-thickness burn also should be left undisturbed at the initial ED encounter. Any loose, necrotic, or clearly nonviable tissue should be débrided from partial-thickness burns using a forceps and scissors (Fig. 113.4A). Topical application of an anesthetic (e.g., viscous lidocaine) over small burns may help limit pain. The toxic dose of anesthetic must not be exceeded. Overzealous débridement at the initial visit should be avoided. Great controversy exists over the management of intact blisters, but firm evidence in support of the various approaches is scarce (7,31,33–35). Generally, blisters should be left intact in fresh burns (less than 24 hours old). Large bullae (greater than 5 cm), especially those crossing joints, are best opened and débrided at the time of the first dressing change, whereas small blisters are left intact. Ruptured blisters are generally unroofed, particularly if the wound appears dirty, to prevent bacterial infection beneath the open epithelium, although some evidence exists that débridement is unnecessary (35). Aspiration of blisters is to be avoided.

After the burn is débrided, it is gently but thoroughly cleansed with a bland soap or dilute (quarter-strength) solution of povidone-iodine using 4″ × 4″ cm gauze pads. Gentle

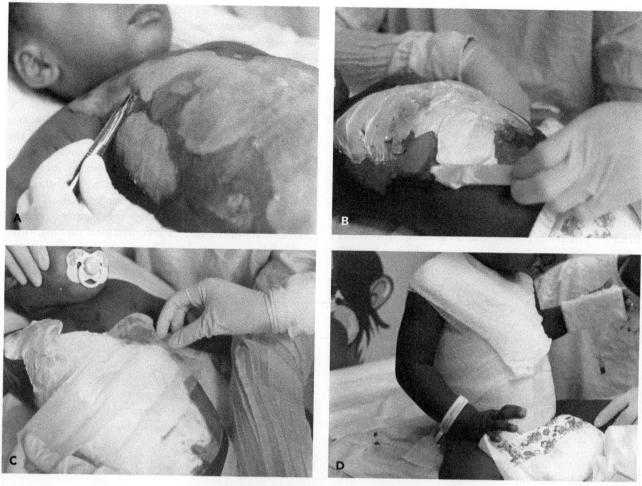

Figure 113.4 Conventional burn dressing.
A. Débridement.
B. Application of topical antimicrobial agent.
C. Nonadherent inner dressing.
D. Absorbent outer dressing.

saline irrigation is followed by pat drying with sterile sponges before application of a dressing. Sterile technique must be adhered to during all stages of burn care.

Burn Dressings

The simplest method of burn treatment is the open or exposure method, in which the exposed wound itself provides a natural dressing—blister, crust, or eschar. Because of the difficulty in keeping open wounds clean in children, the open method is usually reserved for burns less than 1 cm or burns of the face or neck, where dressing application is problematic (31). Following preparation of the burn as previously described, a topical antibacterial ointment such as bacitracin/polymyxin B is applied. This ointment is more cosmetically acceptable for an undressed burn than silver sulfadiazine. The patient or parent is then instructed to clean the burn and reapply ointment one or two times a day until healed.

Most burns in children are treated with some type of closed dressing (36). Two basic approaches are described here. In the

first approach, the clinician uses a conventional gauze-type dressing. Antibacterial cream such as silver sulfadiazine is applied to the cleansed and débrided wound to a thickness of approximately 2 to 3 mm (0.063 inch) using a sterile tongue blade so that it covers the entire surface (Fig. 113.4B). The burn is then covered with a layer of gauze sponges. Alternatively, the antibiotic cream may be applied first to the gauze or a nonadherent type of gauze dressing may be used, with or without an antibacterial agent (Fig. 113.4C). This first layer is then wrapped in several layers of roller gauze to create a bulky, absorbent outer dressing (Fig. 113.4D). In burns of the hand, wads of gauze can be placed between the fingers and in the palm to create a protective bulky dressing. Finally, the entire dressing is covered with stockinette, elastic bandage, or burn netting to keep the child from unwrapping it. A glove or shirt can be fashioned from these materials for burns of the extremities or trunk.

Conventional dressings are usually changed once daily (12). Some authorities prefer to have most patients return in 24 hours for the first dressing change. Home care consists of removing the dressing, removing all antibacterial cream, cleansing with a mild soap and water, and reapplying the dressing as previously outlined. Outpatient analgesics such as acetaminophen with codeine should be supplied for the first few dressing changes. Follow-up visits with a primary care provider at 3 and 7 days are recommended, with more frequent visits for supervised dressing changes if compliance is a problem. The parent is instructed to return if signs of infection develop.

As an alternative to conventional dressing materials, a variety of synthetic dressings intended to serve as temporary skin substitutes are available (13–19,37). The burn is prepared in the manner described. The dressing material is cut to fit the burn, overlapping the adjacent healthy skin by 1 to 2 cm. The dressing is placed over the wound under moderate tension, any wrinkles are smoothed out, and any air or fluid underneath the dressing is pressed out. Dressings without adhesive (e.g.,

Biobrane, Epi-Lock) are secured with paper tape or adhesive strips along the margins. The inner dressing is then covered with roller gauze and stockinette, as with the conventional dressings.

Synthetic dressings should be re-examined in 24 hours. If the dressing is not adhering to the skin, it must be removed. If the wound has remained clean, it may be redressed in the same manner. Failure to adhere after 48 to 72 hours (two or three attempts) requires a change in management. If the synthetic dressing is adhering properly, only the outer dressing is changed. The inner dressing is kept in place until healing is complete (approximately 14 days for a partial-thickness burn). The outer dressing can be changed daily at home, with less frequent changes needed as the quantity of exudate decreases. As in the case of a conventional dressing, twice weekly follow-up visits should be made with the primary care provider.

 SUMMARY

Major Burns

1 Initiate necessary resuscitation measures.

2 Provide adequate analgesia.

3 Remove clothing from burned areas.

4 Perform an emergent escharotomy if indicated.

   a Incise the full length of each burn down to subcutaneous fat.

   b Incise along the lateral or medial aspect of the limb or bilaterally in an anterior axillary line for the chest.

5 Irrigate the burns with saline.

6 Cover the burns with sterile dry sheets or saline-soaked gauze.

7 Maintain body temperature with overhead warmers as needed.

8 Administer tetanus immunoprophylaxis when indicated.

9 Contact a burn center as necessary.

Minor Burns

1 Provide adequate analgesia.

2 Prepare the wound.

   a Irrigate the burns with saline.

   b Débride necrotic or clearly nonviable tissue using a forceps and scissors.

   c Gently clean the burns with mild soap or quarter-strength povidone-iodine.

   d Pat dry with sterile sponges.

3 Apply a wound dressing.

   a Open:

      i Apply antibiotic ointment (e.g., bacitracin-polymyxin B) to face, neck, or small (less than 1 cm) extremity burns.

   b Closed:

      i Apply inner dressing.

         (1) Conventional:

            (a) Coat the burn with a layer of silver sulfadiazine.

            (b) Cover the area with sterile gauze.

         (2) Synthetic:

            (a) Cut material to fit the burn with a slight overlap of adjoining healthy skin.

            (b) Apply the material without wrinkles or trapped air.

            (c) Secure the material with tape.

      ii Apply outer dressing.

         (1) Wrap the inner dressing in several layers of roller gauze.

         (2) Cover the dressing with a stockinette or elastic bandage.

4 Splint extremities with partial- or full-thickness burns that extend across joints.

5 Administer tetanus immunoprophylaxis when indicated.

Splinting

Joints crossed by extensive partial- or full-thickness burns should be splinted in the position of function using standard splinting techniques (Chapter 101). This is particularly important when synthetic dressings are used, as minimizing motion will increase the chance of successful adherence. Patients with such burns should be referred to a surgeon for follow-up.

▶ COMPLICATIONS

With the loss of the epidermal barrier, burn wounds are commonly colonized with micro-organisms, which may lead to local or even systemic infection. The rate of burn wound infection is greatest in children and the elderly. Certain burns are more prone to infection: deep partial-thickness and full-thickness burns, burns of the lower extremities and perineum, and burns involving greater than 30% of BSA (37). When infection occurs, healing is delayed and extension of the depth of injury is possible. Preventing infection is therefore paramount and is best accomplished by careful attention to appropriate technique. Prophylactic systemic antibiotics are not indicated (38).

The risk of hypothermia in children with extensive burns may be increased with the application of saline-soaked gauze if efforts to maintain body heat are not followed. This is especially critical in young infants, who have a larger ratio of BSA to volume.

Extensive fluid and blood loss and resulting cardiovascular instability may be triggered by overaggressive early débridement of extensive burns. Débridement of major burns should be performed under controlled conditions and in consultation with specialists in burn management.

CLINICAL TIPS

- ▶ Appropriate burn management depends on the depth and extent of the burns.

- ▶ Burns in children may be a manifestation of abuse.

- ▶ Most major burns in children require the expertise of a burn center.

- ▶ Initial resuscitation measures should be addressed before definitive burn care.

- ▶ Analgesia should be provided as early as possible.

- ▶ Aspiration of blisters should be avoided.

- ▶ A final covering of stockinette or burn netting limits the ability of the young child to remove the dressing.

- ▶ The young burn victim is at significant risk for heat loss due to the relatively high ratio of BSA to volume.

▶ SUMMARY

The vast majority of burns can be effectively managed in the outpatient setting; however, the physician must be capable of categorizing and classifying burns to provide optimal burn care for children. Recognition of child abuse, risk factors for poor burn healing, and associated injuries are important when deciding care and disposition. The focus for minor burns is on relief of pain, prevention of infection and additional trauma, and minimization of scarring and contracture. ED care for the major burn patient may affect survival and ultimate prognosis. Knowledge of when to seek consultation and transfer to tertiary care facilities is crucial. Finally, the ED personnel should consider burn prevention counseling as an important aspect of burn care of young children.

▶ REFERENCES

1. McCaig LF, Burt CW. *National Hospital Ambulatory Medical Care Survey: 2002 Emergency Department Summary.* Hyattsville, MD: National Center for Health Statistics; 2004. Advance Data from Vital and Health Statistics no. 340.
2. Centers for Disease Control. Childhood injuries in the United States. *Am J Dis Child.* 1990;144:627–646.
3. Malek M, Chang B. The cost of medical care for injuries to children. *Ann Emerg Med.* 1991;20:997–1005.
4. Hyden PW, Gallagher TA. Child abuse intervention in the emergency room. *Pediatr Clin North Am.* 1992;39:1053–1081.
5. Schonfeld N. Outpatient management of burns in children. *Pediatr Emerg Care.* 1990;6:249–253.
6. Hettiaratchy S, Papini R. Initial management of a major burn, I: overview. *BMJ.* 2004;328:1555–1557.
7. Baxter CR, Waeckerle J. Emergency treatment of burn injury. *Ann Emerg Med.* 1988;17:1305–1315.
8. Thompson PB, Herndon DN, Traber DL, et al. Effect on mortality of inhalation injury. *J Trauma.* 1986;26:163–165.
9. Lund CC, Browder NC. The estimation of areas of burns. *Surg Gynecol Obstet.* 1944;79:352–358.
10. Quinn KJ, Courtney JM, Evans JH, et al. Principles of burn dressings. *Biomaterials.* 1985;6:369–377.
11. Queen D, Evans JH, Gaylor JDS, et al. Burn wound dressings: a review. *Burns.* 1987;13:218–228.
12. Warden GD. Outpatient care of thermal injuries. *Surg Clin North Am.* 1987;67:147–157.
13. Stair TO, D'Orta J, Altieri MF, et al. Polyurethane and silver sulfadiazine dressings in treatment of partial thickness burns and abrasions. *Am J Emerg Med.* 1986;4:214–217.
14. Afilalo M, Dankoff J, Guttman A, et al. Duoderm hydroactive dressing versus silver sulfadiazine/Bactigras in the emergency treatment of partial skin thickness burns. *Burns.* 1992;18:313–316.
15. Cockington RA. Ambulatory management of burns in children. *Burns.* 1989;15:271–273.
16. Gerding RL, Emerman CL, Effron D, et al. Outpatient management of partial thickness burns: Biobrane versus 1% silver sulfadiazine. *Ann Emerg Med.* 1990;19:121–124.
17. Gerding RL, Imbembo AL, Fratianne RB. Biosynthetic skin substitute versus 1% sulfadiazine for treatment of inpatient partial thickness thermal burns. *J Trauma.* 1988;28:1265–1269.
18. Waffle C, Simon RR, Joslin C. Moisture-vapour-permeable film as an outpatient burn dressing. *Burns.* 1988;14:66–70.

19. Wyatt D, McGowan DN, Najarian MP. Comparison of a hydrocolloid dressing and silver sulfadiazine cream in the outpatient management of second degree burns. *J Trauma*. 1990;30:857–865.

20. Purdue GF, Layton TR, Copeland CE. Cold injury complicating burn therapy. *J Trauma*. 1985;25:167–168.

21. Finkelstein JL, Schwartz SB, Madden MR, et al. Pediatric burns: an overview. *Pediatr Clin North Am*. 1992;39:1145–1163.

22. Carvajal HF. A physiologic approach to fluid therapy in severely burned children. *Surg Gynecol Obstet*. 1980;150:379–384.

23. Graves TA, Cioffi WG, McManus WF, et al. Fluid resuscitation of infants and children with massive thermal injury. *J Trauma*. 1988;28:1656–1659.

24. Hettiaratchy S, Papini R. Initial management of a major burn, II: assessment and resuscitation. *BMJ*. 2004;329:101–103.

25. O'Neill JA. Fluid resuscitation in the burned child: a reappraisal. *J Pediatr Surg*. 1982;17:604–607.

26. Demling RH. Fluid replacement in burned patients. *Surg Clin North Am*. 1987;67:15–30.

27. Merrell SW, Saffle JR, Sullivan JJ, et al. Fluid resuscitation in thermally injured children. *Am J Surg*. 1986;152:664–669.

28. Bennett JE, Lewis E. Operative decompression of constricting burns. *Surgery*. 1958;43:949–955.

29. Pruitt BA, Dowling JA, Moncrief JA. Escharotomy in early burn care. *Arch Surg*. 1968;96:502–507.

30. Osgood PF, Szyfelbein SK. Management of burn pain in children. *Pediatr Clin North Am*. 1989;36:1001–1013.

31. Griglak MJ. Thermal injury. *Emerg Med Clin North Am*. 1992;10: 369–383.

32. Zawacki BE. Reversal of capillary stasis and prevention of necrosis in burns. *Ann Surg*. 1974;180:98–102.

33. Forage AV. The effects of removing the epidermis from burnt skin. *Lancet*. 1962;690–693.

34. Rockwell WB, Ehrlich HP. Should burn blister fluid be evacuated? *J Burn Care Rehabil*. 1990;11:93–95.

35. Andrejak M, Davion T, Gineston JL, et al. Management of blisters in minor burns. *Br Med J*. 1987;295:181.

36. Hudspith J, Rayatt S. First aid and treatment of minor burns. *BMJ*. 2004;328:1487–1489.

37. Dodd D, Stutman HR. Current issues in burn wound infections. *Adv Pediatr Infect Dis*. 1991;6:137–162.

38. Boss WK, Brand DA, Acampora D, et al. Effectiveness of prophylactic antibiotics in the outpatient treatment of burns. *J Trauma*. 1985;25:224–227.

LAUREN DALY AND YAMINI DURANI

114

Incision and Drainage of a Cutaneous Abscess

▶ INTRODUCTION

A cutaneous abscess is a localized cavity of purulent material in the superficial skin and soft tissue. It causes a fluctuant swelling or mass, with inflammatory changes in the surrounding soft tissue. The abscess may progress to a spontaneous discharge of its contents through its external or internal surface (1–3).

The preferred treatment for the cutaneous abscess is surgical incision and drainage (1–5). Percutaneous needle aspiration alone inadequately drains an abscess cavity and often results in persistent or recurrent abscess formation. Incision and drainage of an abscess likely mitigates potential bacteremic dissemination or extension into important adjacent tissues (e.g., vascular structures). The procedure is simple, may be done quickly, and is usually curative for all age groups. It is commonly performed by physician and physician extenders in the emergency or outpatient setting.

Evaluation and treatment of superficial abscesses accounts for 1% to 2% of all emergency and outpatient visits (1–5). Although cutaneous abscesses are among the most common soft-tissue infections, only a few controlled studies of their treatment in adults and children have been carried out.

▶ ANATOMY AND PHYSIOLOGY

A cutaneous abscess occurs after disruption of the normal barriers of the skin that prevent natural bacterial colonization from becoming an infection. Localized cellulitis first develops when bacteria proliferate within the skin and subcutaneous tissues. As bacterial enzymatic activity produces necrosis, liquefaction, and a leukocytic response, pus forms and an abscess results. Cellulitis generally resolves with antibiotic therapy, whereas an abscess usually does not respond to antibiotics alone without open drainage of the pus.

Common causes for the disruption of the normal skin barriers to infection include direct trauma to or a foreign body in the skin or soft tissues; injection or accumulation of bacterial inoculum (e.g., injury from cat bite or rusty nail); decreased or inadequate blood or lymphatic circulation (e.g., necrosis, hemorrhage); and poor host systemic immunity (e.g., debilitating disease, immunocompromised host). Proliferation of bacteria subsequently occurs and may progress to an abscess. Often a keratin plug will sufficiently obstruct the normal outflow of a secretory gland to prevent the normal clearance of bacterial colonization. Areas prone to such obstruction are the axilla, groin, perineum, and breast (4). In the infant or younger child, common sites also include the perianal area from mucocutaneous infection or enterocutaneous fistula (3) and the digits from finger sucking or biting (6).

Overall, *Staphylococcus aureus* is the predominant organism isolated from most abscesses, especially as a single isolate. In many communities, methicillin-resistant *S. aureus* (MRSA) is an established organism that accounts for as many as half of the *S. Aureus* isolates in soft-tissue infections (7). The causative organism usually reflects the indigenous flora of the specific site. Oral flora are found in abscesses that result from prolonged or repeated contact with the mouth, as in the fingers or toes of infants (see Chapters 115 and 116). Mixed aerobic and anaerobic flora predominates in the abscesses of the head and fingers in children because they are typically associated with oral or perianal flora. The organisms commonly isolated include *Escherichia coli* and anaerobic organisms, such as *Peptostreptococcus*, *Bacteroides*, *Fusobacterium*, and *Clostridium* species (4–7). Fecal flora is usually isolated from abscesses of the anogenital, vulvovaginal, inguinal, and perirectal areas. These bacteria are most commonly mixed aerobic and anaerobic organisms: *E. coli*, group D streptococci, *Neisseria gonorrhoeae*, or *Peptostreptococcus*, *Enterobacter*, or *Bacteroides* species. Abscesses of the axilla are commonly caused by Gram-negative aerobic organisms, *E. coli* or *Enterobacter* species. Aerobic organisms indigenous to the skin and secretory gland typically cause abscesses distant from the oral or anogenital areas in the general population; they include *S. aureus*, coagulase-negative staphylococci, and α- and β-hemolytic streptococci (4–7).

▶ INDICATIONS

Clinically, both cellulitis and an abscess may appear as a localized area of pain (dolor), erythema (rubor), warmth (calor), edema (tumor), or induration; the patient usually complains of localized pain and swelling without fever. Fluctuance on physical examination with or without spontaneous drainage usually indicates the presence of an abscess (2,5). A definitive diagnosis of an abscess can be made based on successful percutaneous needle (18-gauge) aspiration of pus from the site (2).

The treatment for a cutaneous abscess is surgical incision and drainage (1–4). Optimal management of cutaneous abscesses in the emergency or outpatient setting requires the following appropriate conditions: (a) the inflammatory mass is an acute, superficial, and localized cutaneous abscess without extension to deeper structures; (b) the child will be adequately cooperative when the procedure is performed under local or regional anesthesia; and (c) the child has no other apparent medical condition that precludes outpatient management, such as airway or anatomical anomalies. If these conditions are not met, or if the depth, extent, or cosmetic implications of the abscess are questionable, a pediatric surgical consultation and treatment under general anesthesia may be more appropriate.

There are contraindications to performing incision and drainage of an abscess in an emergency setting. Cellulitis without abscess should not be surgically managed. Tinea capitis infrequently produces an inflammatory response called a "kerion," which presents as a tender, boggy, erythematous scalp mass. Congenital neck masses that often become infected include branchial cleft cyst, thyroglossal duct cyst, and cystic hygroma. Tuberculous cervical adenitis (scrofula) and mycotic aneurysm occur rarely in children. Other causes include viral inflammation (herpetic whitlow or zoster), chemical inflammation (insect or arachnid toxins), and idiopathic inflammation (autoimmune disorders). These masses do not benefit from incision and drainage and should not be incised in the outpatient setting without further diagnostic evaluation.

Certain abscesses may require surgical consultation secondary to a high rate of potential complications and need for intraoperative management. Abscesses within the central triangle of the face (bridge of nose to corners of mouth), which may drain into the cavernous sinus, have high potential for morbidity, including development of septic phlebitis and in-

tracranial extension. Certain abscesses of the hand, especially those involving distal digits and deep perianal abscesses, may also require subspecialty evaluation.

▶ EQUIPMENT

For sterile preparation and dressing of abscess cavity:
> Antiseptic solution (povidone-iodine)
> Gauze (4″ × 4″)
> Sterile drapes
> Gauze packing strips (plain, iodoform) and/or Penrose drain
> Cloth tape

For local or regional anesthesia:
> Lidocaine 1% to 2% without epinephrine
> Needle, 27 or 25 gauge, 1 inch
> Syringe, 3 or 5 mL

For incision of abscess cavity, probing the cavity, clearing loculations, grasping skin edges, and manipulating gauze packing strip and dressing:
> Culture swabs
> Scalpel blades, No. 11 for small stab incision and No. 15 for larger cutaneous incision
> Hemostat clamps, small
> Forceps, toothed
> Scissors

For irrigation of abscess cavity:
> Syringe, 20 mL with 18-gauge intravenous catheter
> Irrigation solution (normal saline or sterile water)
> Monitoring equipment if parenteral sedation is used

▶ PROCEDURE

To increase the success of adequate drainage, direct visualization and access to the abscess site must be optimized by careful positioning and selective immobilization. An assistant or papoose may be helpful in restraining the patient. The site is cleansed with antiseptic solution and draped using sterile technique (Chapter 7). The surrounding noninfected skin and subcutaneous tissue are first anesthetized using 1% to 2% lidocaine without epinephrine by local infiltration (Fig. 114.1) or regional block (Chapter 35). The roof of the abscess is then anesthetized by intradermal injection along the linear course of the proposed incision (Fig. 114.2). A regional block is preferred over local infiltration because local anesthetics are less effective in the acidic milieu of an abscess. For a larger abscess or one in a more difficult location, the child may benefit from parenteral sedation and analgesia. Unfortunately, pain often is unavoidable despite appropriate anesthesia, especially during the spreading and breaking of loculations. For most children, pain diminishes with the drainage of pus and relief of pressure from the abscess. Topical ethyl chloride alone is usually ineffective for this procedure (2).

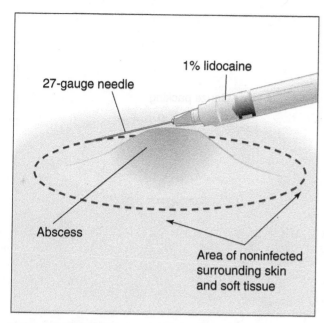

Figure 114.1 Administration of local anesthesia to a subcutaneous abscess.

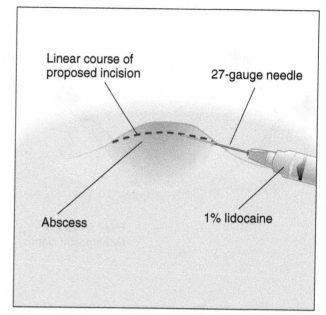

Figure 114.2 Anesthetic administration along proposed incision site.

Organisms for culture and identification should be obtained by percutaneous needle aspiration from the abscess after sterile preparation (2). Pus obtained from an open incision may preclude the isolation of anaerobic bacteria. Gram stain of the pus may be helpful in the choice of antibiotics if prescribed. In the past, routine Gram stain and culture were generally not indicated in the uncomplicated abscess, however, with the surge in MRSA, routine Gram stain and culture are now recommended for all abscesses (8).

The abscess cavity is incised with the scalpel blade; a linear incision parallel to the skin folds (Fig. 114.2) minimizes sub-

sequent scarring. The incision should extend the entire length of the cavity to permit optimal drainage. For a smaller abscess (less than 1 cm), the No. 11 scalpel blade is used to make a stab opening at the point of maximal fluctuance, followed by one swift upward motion of the blade to complete the incision (Fig. 114.3). For a very large abscess, the No. 15 scalpel blade may be used to make an elliptical excision (Fig. 114.4) of thin, nonviable, or necrotic overlying skin to facilitate drainage. An opening sufficiently wide to allow complete drainage of pus is crucial to the successful treatment of the abscess cavity.

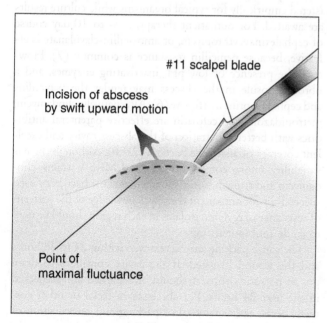

Figure 114.3 Linear incision of a cutaneous abscess.

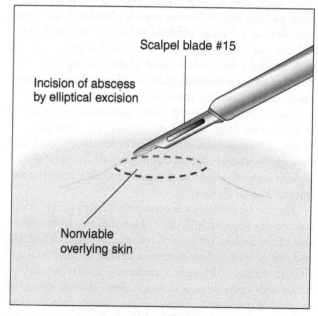

Figure 114.4 Elliptical incision of a cutaneous abscess.

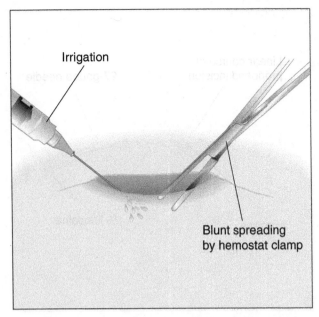

Figure 114.5 Removal of loculations and irrigation of an abscess.

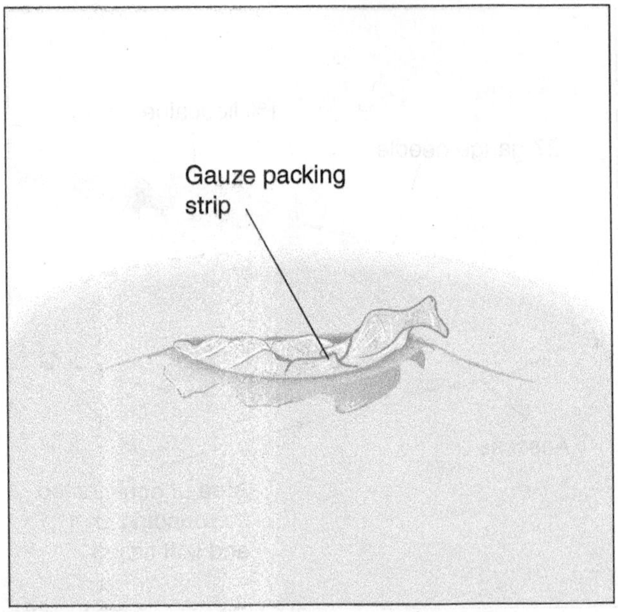

Figure 114.6 Placing a gauze packing strip in the abscess cavity.

Elliptical excisions are, however, not advised routinely or in cosmetically sensitive areas.

After the abscess is incised, the cavity is probed with the goal of breaking down loculations, identifying foreign bodies, and ensuring proper drainage of pus. Loculations of pus and necrotic debris are cleared by blunt spreading with a hemostat clamp (Fig. 114.5). Copious irrigation of the abscess with normal saline or sterile water follows to remove all the pus and necrotic tissue. Retained blood, plasma, and cellular debris sustain continued infection and should be continuously drained after this initial procedure. Many superficial abscesses empty completely after incision and irrigation and have no remaining cavity. These require warm soaks to keep the incision open until healing commences. If a cavity remains, a gauze packing strip or Penrose drain is placed within it to ensure continued drainage of blood and coagulum (Fig. 114.6). A 1-cm end is left external to the wound edges to act as a wick and aid subsequent removal of the packing strip. The choice of drainage material, plain or iodine-laden (iodoform) gauze, is not based on scientific evidence but rather on the mechanical process of a wick. Some authorities prefer that a small Penrose drain, split along one side to ensure patency, be placed instead, usually held there by an absorbable suture through the wound edge, as this may afford less painful subsequent removal. Layers of dry gauze and tape complete the external wound dressing.

The use of antibiotics is controversial, even in this era of community-acquired MRSA (9). Host defense, depth and extent of the abscess, patterns of community-acquired MRSA, and risk of endocarditis determine the use of adjunctive antibiotic therapy. Although a cutaneous abscess usually resolves with open surgical drainage alone, there is debate as to whether transient bacteremia does accompany the incision and drainage procedure (6,7,10,11). Oral antibiotics may be effective for abscesses with surrounding areas of mild cellulitis or lymphangitis. Parenteral antibiotic therapy is warranted for an abscess that is associated with systemic symptoms and signs of toxicity, that involves deeper tissue structures (e.g., tenosynovitis, fascitis, pyomyositis), or that occurs in a person predisposed to infection (e.g., immunocompromise, insulin-dependent diabetes, autoimmune disease, immunosuppression from high-dose steroid therapy or chemotherapy) (1,4–5). American Heart Association guidelines are recommended for endocarditis prophylaxis (11).

The choice of antibiotics varies with the site of the abscess, identification of the bacterial organism, and patterns of susceptibility. Broad-spectrum antibiotics may be administered empirically for typical organisms while culture results are awaited. For outpatient therapy, a 5- to 10-day course of cephalexin, erythromycin, or amoxicillin-clavulanate is effective, because penicillin resistance is common (7). However, the presence of low pH, inactivating enzymes, and a fibrotic capsule in the abscess may render the penicillins and cephalosporins ineffective (6). Alternatively, clindamycin, metronidazole, and cefoxitin are effective parenteral antibiotics with better penetration of the abscess cavity and excellent coverage of anaerobic bacteria (2,4,6). Although there is variability among community-acquired MRSA strains, clindamycin and trimethoprim-sulfamethoxazole have been used successfully for outpatient therapy. Knowledge of the patterns of resistance of *S. Aureus* isolates in each region should be used to guide antibiotic therapy.

The gauze packing strip is removed within 24 to 48 hours and the wound irrigated. If the cavity continues to drain pus or necrotic debris, it should be repacked and rechecked in the next 24 hours. For abscesses in facial or other cosmetic areas, earlier removal of packing and re-evaluation of the wound is best. After the packing is removed, warm soaks

SUMMARY

1 Optimize the approach to and visualization of the abscess site.

2 Anesthetize around the abscess site and along the proposed incision course by intradermal infiltration with 1% to 2% lidocaine without epinephrine.

3 Perform percutaneous needle aspiration for Gram stain and culture.

4 Incise the entire length of the abscess cavity.

5 Spread open the abscess cavity with a hemostat clamp or fingers. Clear all loculations of purulent material. Irrigate copiously and evacuate the cavity completely.

6 Place a gauze packing strip (or Penrose drain slit on one side and held in place with an absorbable suture) and cover with a dry gauze dressing.

7 Consider the need for antibiotics.

8 Provide tetanus toxoid immunization when indicated.

9 Change the gauze packing strip and check the wound within 24 to 48 hours.

10 Encourage warm soaks 15 to 20 minutes several times daily after the gauze packing strip is removed.

11 Re-evaluate frequently.

 CLINICAL TIPS

▶ Evaluation of the inflammatory mass is necessary to ensure that it is an acute, superficial, and localized cutaneous abscess without extension to deeper structures. Incision and drainage of an inflamed mass that is not an abscess should be avoided.

▶ General anesthesia and an intraoperative procedure should be considered for the child who is uncooperative or has other conditions that may preclude outpatient management.

▶ A sufficiently wide incision with adequate blunt spreading and copious irrigation are necessary to ensure complete drainage of the abscess cavity. The risk of progression or recurrence of an abscess increases with suboptimal incision and drainage.

▶ Oral or parenteral antibiotics may be indicated.

▶ Close follow-up should be emphasized.

applied for 15 to 20 minutes several times daily for the next 4 to 5 days should be sufficient to maintain open wound edges and allow for continued drainage. Healing usually occurs in 7 to 10 days (2). Inadequate tetanus immune status requires appropriate immunization (see Table 107.2). Finally, close follow-up care ensures optimal management and decreases complications after incision and drainage of an abscess.

▶ COMPLICATIONS

Few complications arise from this procedure, and those that do occur are most commonly from inadequate or overly aggressive drainage. Inadequate drainage may lead to local extension, causing secondary problems such as osteomyelitis, septic thrombosis, and fistula formation. Abscesses in the cervical, axillary, and inguinal areas may be adjacent to neurovascular structures. These lesions may worsen after inappropriately proceeding with an incision and drainage in the outpatient setting without further diagnostic evaluation. Injury may occur to these adjacent structures with overly aggressive incision.

Other complications may arise from failure to recognize the child who may be predisposed to endocarditis or bacteremia (e.g., valvular heart disease, immunocompromise, immunosuppression). As with any wound healing process, scar and keloid formation may follow (Chapter 108).

Patients should be instructed to notify a health care provider if secondary signs of infection occur, such as fever, chills, pain, redness, red streaks, increased swelling, and reaccumulation of pus.

▶ SUMMARY

Surgical incision and drainage of the uncomplicated cutaneous abscess generally prevents progression or bacteremic dissemination of the infection. After optimal anesthesia and analgesia, the abscess cavity is incised with a scalpel over its entire length, probed with a hemostat clamp to clear all loculations, and irrigated to ensure adequate drainage. Gauze packing strips and antibiotics are used if indicated. Optimal management includes close follow-up care.

▶ ACKNOWLEDGMENT

The authors would like to acknowledge the valuable contributions of Grace M. Young to the version of this chapter that appeared in the previous edition.

▶ REFERENCES

1. Llera JL, Levy RC. Treatment of cutaneous abscess: a double-blind clinical study. *Ann Emerg Med.* 1985;14:15–19.

2. Halvorson GD, Halvorson JE, Iserson KV. Abscess incision and drainage in the emergency department. Pt I. *J Emerg Med.* 1985;3: 227–232.

3. Meislin HW. Pathogen identification of abscesses and cellulitis. *Ann Emerg Med.* 1986;15:329–332.

4. Meislin HW, Lerner SA, Graves MH, et al. Cutaneous abscesses: anaerobic and aerobic bacteriology and outpatient management. *Ann Intern Med.* 1977;87:145–149.

5. Llera JL, Levy RC, Staneck JL. Cutaneous abscesses: natural history and management in an outpatient facility. *J Emerg Med.* 1984;1: 489–493.

6. Brook I, Frazier EH. Aerobic and anaerobic bacteriology of wounds and cutaneous abscesses. *Arch Surg.* 1990;125:1445–1451.

7. Brook I, Finegold SM. Aerobic and anaerobic bacteriology of cutaneous abscesses in children. *Pediatrics.* 1981;67:891–895.

8. Sattler CA, Mason EO, Kaplan SL. Prospective comparison of risk factors and demographic and clinical characteristics of community-acquired, methicillin-resistant versus methicillin-susceptible *Staphylococcus aureus* infection in children. *Pediatr Infect Dis J.* 2002;21:910–916.

9. Lee MC, Rio AM, Aten MF, et al. Management and outcome of children with skin and soft tissue abscesses caused by community-acquired methicillin-resistant *Staphylococcus aureus*. *Pediatr Infect Dis J.* 2004;23:123–127.

10. Brobrow BJ, Pollack CV, Gamble S, et al. Incision and drainage of cutaneous abscesses is not associated with bacteremia in afebrile adults. *Ann Emerg Med.* 1997;29:404–408.

11. Dajani AS, Taubert KA, Wilson W, et al. Prevention of bacterial endocarditis: recommendations by the American Heart Association. *JAMA.* 1997;277:1794–1801.

ESTHER M. SAMPAYO AND FRED M. HENRETIG

115

Incision and Drainage of a Paronychia

▶ INTRODUCTION

A paronychia is a superficial infection of the soft-tissue epithelium bordering the base of the nail fold. It is one of the most frequently encountered hand infections in all age groups and is sometimes, though less commonly, located on the toes. When a paronychia evolves to a closed pocket of pus (abscess), proper treatment involves adequate drainage. Several techniques are commonly recommended for treating the varying stages of this process. Recent overviews of paronychia have appeared (1–6), although no controlled studies comparing various treatment approaches are found. Successful management of common acute paronychia in children of any age relies on accurate and early diagnosis. Commencement of treatment is well within the repertoire of emergency physicians and pediatricians and is typically performed in the ambulatory setting.

▶ ANATOMY AND PHYSIOLOGY

The structure of the nail complex is illustrated in Figure 115.1A. When the seal between the proximal nail fold and the nail plate is disrupted, invading bacteria gain entry and infection ensues (Fig. 115.1B). The bacterial etiology of both pediatric and adult paronychias has been studied and reflects both skin (staphylococcal and streptococcal species) and typical oral flora. Most infections are mixed, and more than 70% include oral anaerobes (7,8). In infants, typical insults include the grasp reflex, which can cause recurrent finger paronychias and ingrown nails; tight-fitting sleeper outfits, which can cause toe paronychias; and overzealous nail trimming, which can lead to the involvement of both fingers and toes (9). Digital sucking and nail biting account for most paronychias in toddlers, preschool, and school-age children. Nail biting, hangnails, minor trauma related to work, antiretroviral therapy and artificial nails have been implicated in acute paronychias in adolescents and adults (10–12).

A paronychia develops over a few hours and begins laterally when a nail fold becomes painful, red, and swollen. As infection evolves, pus may accumulate under the eponychium (cuticle) and under the nail fold along the sides of the nail plate (Fig. 115.2). With further extension, pus may dissect under the nail plate, potentially compromising the ventral floor of the germinal matrix, which is primarily responsible for nail growth. Ultimately, the infection may spread to contiguous structures, causing a felon, osteomyelitis, septic tenosynovitis, or pyarthrosis (4). Adequate drainage of enclosed purulence will relieve pain, hasten resolution, and usually obviate such complications.

▶ INDICATIONS

A paronychia may begin as cellulitis with redness, swelling, and tenderness along the edge of the nail but without frank pus accumulation. At this stage, treatment may be nonsurgical, including warm soaks, elevation, splinting, and appropriate antibiotics. Any appearance of frank pus or fluctuance warrants a drainage procedure, and little is lost by erring on the side of early drainage in uncertain cases. For small pockets of pus at the base of the nail (the most common pediatric situation), simple lifting of the eponychium off the base of the nail is sufficient. When pus accumulates below the base or side of the nail plate, additional drainage is afforded by the removal of proximal and lateral strips of nail, respectively. It is not necessary or desirable to incise periungual skin as part of the initial approach to acute paronychias. By contrast, failure of a paronychia to resolve appropriately after treatment or chronic-recurrent paronychia usually necessitates referral to a hand specialist for consideration of more

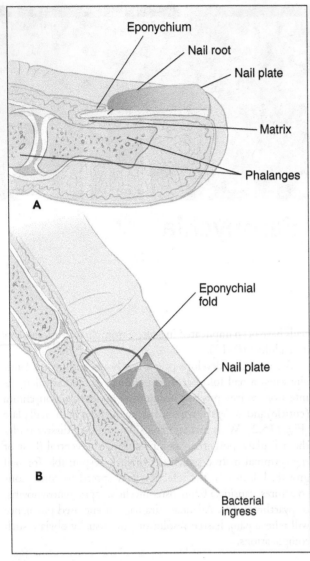

Figure 115.1
A. Structure of the nail.
B. Course of bacterial infection.

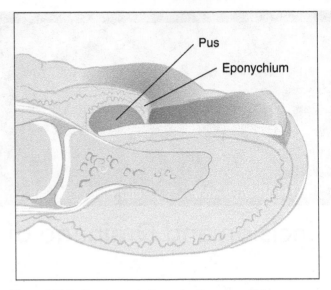

Figure 115.2   Pus accumulation under the eponychium.

aggressive surgery (e.g., eponychial marsupialization and nail plate removal) (13).

▶ EQUIPMENT

Ethyl chloride spray
Lidocaine 1% to 2% without epinephrine
Syringe and needle, 25 to 27 gauge
Antiseptic prep solution (e.g., Betadine)
Scalpel blade, No. 11
Small hemostat or clamp
Gauze strip packing
Scissors, small
Gauze pads

▶ PROCEDURE

For most patients who require only the lifting of a small area of eponychium, anesthesia beyond patient distraction and possibly ethyl chloride spray is usually unnecessary. Children who require extensive drainage and/or nail plate incision will need digital block anesthesia (Chapter 35). Brief soaking of the digit may soften the eponychium and facilitate the procedure. After superficial disinfectant is applied and anesthesia (if indicated) is undertaken, the child should be restrained momentarily as appropriate for age (Chapter 3). A No. 11 scalpel blade or the tip of a small hemostat is introduced under the eponychial fold parallel to the surface of the nail plate and is extended proximally into the depth of the enclosed pocket of pus (Fig. 115.3A). Since the overlying tissue involved is usually thin and devitalized, this can often be done with one quick pass of the scalpel blade or hemostat, causing a minimal amount of pain. For more extensive paronychias involving most of the nail base, the blade or hemostat tips may be fanned through the range of the pocket (Fig. 115.3B). When pus is encountered below the lateral edge of the nail, the nail fold skin should be gently lifted, and a thin longitudinal strip of nail is incised and removed (Fig. 115.4). If the pus has dissected below the proximal base of the nail (a subungual abscess), the proximal one third of the nail is removed in a strip perpendicular to the long axis of the nail. A small superficial incision in the eponychium in the longitudinal plane at the corner of the nail may facilitate lifting the nail plate (Fig. 115.5).

When the nail plate is so incised, or if a deep pocket remains after simple lifting of a large proximal paronychia, a small strip of gauze packing should be left in place to ensure continued drainage. The wound should then be dressed with sterile, dry gauze. Warm soaks also will promote drainage and should be initiated the same day if no packing is used

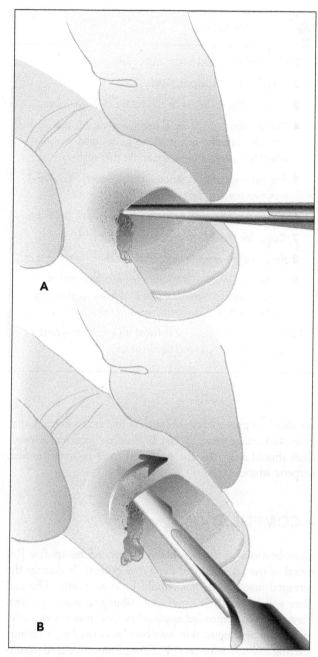

Figure 115.3 Drainage of the paronychia.

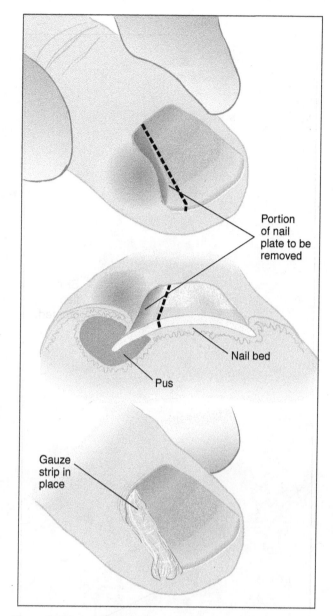

Figure 115.4 Involvement below the lateral nail edge and removal of the lateral nail.

or after the packing has been removed. Packing removal is typically performed at 24 hours after simple eponychial elevation or at 48 hours when both eponychial lifting and partial nail plate removal have been used. Some authorities prefer to begin warm soaks the same day regardless of whether packing is used. Local antibiotic ointments are unproven in efficacy, but may facilitate compliance with soaks. Systemic antibiotics are likewise of uncertain additional benefit but often are prescribed. Amoxicillin-clavulanate for 5 to 7 days would be a logical choice given the typical mixed flora (8). Suspicion for community-acquired methicillin-resistant *Staphylococcus au-*

reus (MRSA) infections can be treated with clindamycin or trimethoprim-sulfamethoxazole (cotrimoxazole) (14).

Follow-up evaluation generally is warranted at 24 to 48 hours for any paronychia treatment with an extended drainage procedure and/or packing. Most patients will have resolution in 5 to 7 days; persistence beyond 10 days or continued recurrence should prompt consideration of evaluation for osteomyelitis and subspecialty referral. In cases of chronic paronychia (duration longer than 6 weeks), it is important that the patient avoid possible irritants or inciting trauma. Most cases of chronic paronychia are fungal in etiology, and treatment options include the use of topical antifungal agents and steroids and surgical intervention (6). Patients with chronic paronychias that are unresponsive to therapy should be

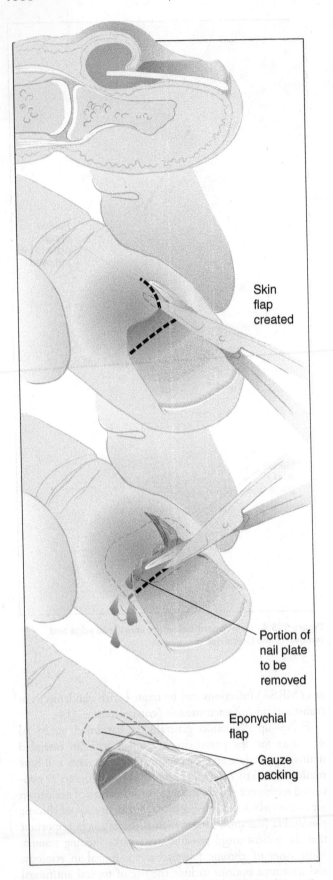

Skin flap created

Portion of nail plate to be removed

Eponychial flap

Gauze packing

Figure 115.5 Involvement below the proximal base of the nail and removal of the proximal nail.

SUMMARY

1 Restrain the child when necessary.

2 Prepare an antiseptic field.

3 Apply ethyl chloride or digital block anesthesia.

4 For proximal, superficial involvement, lift the eponychium and use packing as needed. Minimal anesthesia may be necessary in this setting.

5 For subungual purulence, lift the eponychium and remove part of the nail plate.

6 Cover the site with an outer bulky gauze dressing.

7 Consider local and/or oral antibiotics.

8 Encourage warm soaks (when packing is removed).

9 Follow up in 24 to 48 hours for more complex procedures to evaluate site and remove packing and/or in 5 to 7 days for resolution.

10 Refer to a subspecialist for persistence beyond 10 days or continued recurrence.

evaluated for potential causes, such as immunodeficiency, diabetes, and malignancy (15,16). In children, recurrent paronychias should also raise the suspicion for a common mimic, herpetic whitlow.

▶ COMPLICATIONS

Complications of the recommended procedures are few. Removal of the proximal nail plate may potentially damage the germinal matrix and thus should be done gently. The nail plate will lift easily if significant subungual pus is present. Previously recommended approaches that involved extensive incision of periungual skin have been associated with chronic scarring and nail deformity (1). Complications related to contiguous spread of infection generally are related to delayed or

CLINICAL TIPS

▶ Early drainage of pus is the basic intervention—err on side of early procedure.

▶ For the majority of small, localized paronychia, simple lifting of the edge of the cuticle can be accomplished without anesthesia.

▶ Follow-up is critical, as complications may occur even when the treatment is optimal.

inadequate drainage but may in rare instances develop despite appropriate treatment; hence the need for good follow-up.

▶ SUMMARY

Paronychia is the most common hand infection in children. Management usually can be accomplished entirely within the ambulatory setting by emergency physicians or pediatricians familiar with the procedure. The mainstay of treatment is the timely provision of adequate drainage and close attention to follow-up.

▶ REFERENCES

1. Canales FL, Newmeyer WL 3d, Kilgore ES Jr. The treatment of felons and paronychias. *Hand Clin.* 1989;5:515.
2. Silverman RA. Diseases of the nail in infants and children. *Adv Dermatol.* 1990;5:153–170.
3. Hausman L. Hand infections. *Orthop Clin North Am.* 1992;23:171.
4. Mack GR. Common problems of the hand. *Adv Dermatol.* 1992;7:315–351.
5. Rockwell PG. Acute and chronic paronychia. *Am Fam Physician.* 2001;63:1113–1116.
6. Jebson PJ. Infections of the fingertip: paronychias and felons. *Hand Clin.* 1998;14:547–555.
7. Brook I. Bacteriologic study of paronychia in children. *Am J Surg.* 1981;141:703–705.
8. Brook I. Aerobic and anaerobic microbiology of paronychia. *Ann Emerg Med.* 1990;19:994–996.
9. Matsui T, Kidou M, Ono T. Infantile multiple ingrowing nails of the fingers induced by the grasp reflex: a new entity. *Dermatology.* 2002;205:25–27.
10. Mowad CM, Ferringer T. Allergic contact dermatitis from acrylates in artificial nails. *Dermatitis.* 2004;15:51–53.
11. Roberge RJ, Weinstein D, Thimons MM. Perionychial infections associated with sculptured nails. *Am J Emerg Med.* 1999;17:581–582.
12. Sibel S, Macher A, Goosby E. Paronychia in patients receiving antiretroviral therapy for human immunodeficiency virus infection. *J Am Podiatr Med Assoc.* 2000;90:98–100.
13. Bednar MS, Lane LB. Eponychial marsupialization and nail removal for surgical treatment of chronic paronychia. *J Hand Surg [Am].* 1991;16:314–317.
14. Ladhani S, Garbash M. Staphylococcal skin infections in children: rational drug therapy recommendations. *Paediatr Drugs.* 2005;7:77–102.
15. Kapellen TM, Galler A, Kiess W. Higher frequency of paronychia (nail bed infections) in pediatric and adolescent patients with type I diabetes mellitus than in non-diabetic peers. *J Pediatr Endocrinol Metab.* 2003;16:751–758.
16. Yip KM, Lam SL, Shee BW, et al. Subungual squamous cell carcinoma: report of 2 cases. *J Formos Med Assoc.* 2000;99:646–649.

116

HAZEL GUINTO-OCAMPO

Incision and Drainage of a Felon

▶ INTRODUCTION

A felon is an abscess of the distal pulp or pad of the fingertip (1–7). The most commonly affected digits are the thumb and index finger (8). Unlike a paronychia, a felon is a deep soft-tissue infection that involves the distal pulp of a finger or thumb and may not communicate with skin until late in the course. Incision and drainage are often required to prevent the spread of infection to bone and to relieve pain. Several techniques have been advocated, all of which involve surgical drainage with as little interruption to the vascular, neurologic, and structural components as possible. No technique has been definitively shown to be best.

A felon may occur in any age group. The emergency or primary care physician with experience in minor surgical procedures may perform the procedure on the cooperative patient with regional anesthesia alone. For uncooperative patients, procedural sedation may be necessary (see Chapter 33).

▶ ANATOMY AND PHYSIOLOGY

The distal finger consists of a relatively closed compartment bounded by the nail and skin on the dorsal and distal aspects, by skin on the palmar surface, and by the flexion crease of the distal interphalangeal joint proximally (Fig. 116.1). The pulp of the fingertip is divided into small compartments by 15 to 20 fibrous septae that run from the periosteum to the skin. These septae are most dense at the flexor crease, at the fingertip, and on each side at the dorsal-palmar junction. The septae are least dense at the center of the touch pad. The flexor digitorum profundus tendon inserts at the proximal one third to middle of the distal phalanx. Blood is supplied by digital arteries, which lie parallel and lateral to

the phalanx. The digital nerves lie palmar and superficial to the arteries. Both arteries and nerves begin to arborize just beyond the distal phalangeal epiphysis.

A felon is caused by inoculation of bacteria into the fingertip from a minor puncture wound, splinter, or fissure and can go unnoticed by the patient until the severe throbbing pain and localized swelling begin. A felon may arise when an untreated paronychia spreads into the pad of the fingertip (4). Cases have also been reported of iatrogenic felon formation as the result of repeated finger sticks (4,9). Young children and diabetic patients, who commonly undergo finger sticks to obtain blood, are therefore at increased risk for developing a felon.

Infection in the pulp of the fingertip may progress in several ways. Inflammation and edema cause increased pressure in the relatively noncompliant compartments. As pressure rises, the arteries collapse, and tissue necrosis, including necrosis of the periosteum and cancellous bone (osteitis), may ensue (10). The epiphysis is spared, as its blood supply is outside the closed space, which allows regeneration of eroded bone in children. The extent of regeneration depends on the virulence of the organism and the patient's age (10). The fibrous septae, being least dense in the central area of the finger pad, may allow abscess extension to overlying skin. In this case, a draining sinus may result (1). Rarely, the abscess located deep in the pulp may dissect around the side of the phalanx and cause an associated paronychia.

Although the bacteriology in children has not been extensively studied, the primary pathogens consist of skin flora, especially *Staphylococcus aureus*. Oral flora are also common in children who suck their fingers or thumb. Recently, methicillin-resistant *S. aureus* has been reported in felons (11,12). Complications of an untreated felon include tenosynovitis, flexion contracture, septic arthritis, and osteomyelitis (13–17).

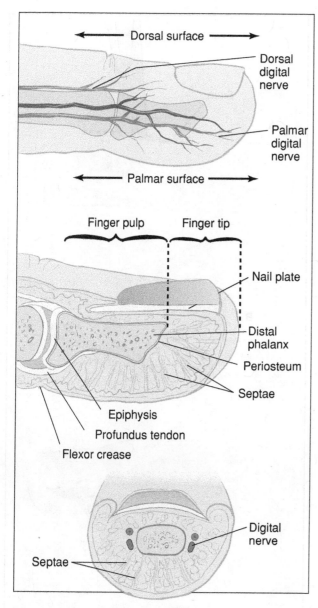

Figure 116.1 Anatomy of the fingertip.

▶ INDICATIONS

Felons are characterized by intense throbbing pain made worse by dependent position and localized distal pulp swelling and redness. Compared to a paronychia, the pain caused by a felon is usually more intense. The swelling does not extend proximal to the distal interphalangeal joint (1). Differential diagnoses include herpetic whitlow (18) (distinguished by the presence of vesicles and a history of recurrence), osseous metastasis (19), and superficial abscess extension from a paronychia.

Early in the infection, before frank pus formation, the need for incision and drainage may be obviated with immobilization, elevation, oral antibiotics, and warm water or saline soaks (4,8,17,20,21). A tense fingertip should be surgically decompressed even when no frank pus drainage

or fluctuance is present, as ischemic necrosis of deep tissues may precede skin necrosis and pus drainage (21,22). Once abscess formation has occurred, treatment of this deep space infection involves timely incision and drainage, appropriate antibiotic therapy, elevation and immobilization, and close follow-up. "Fish mouth," through-and-through, "hockey stick" or "J," and transverse palmar incision techniques are not recommended, as they are more likely to result in painful sensitive scars and damage to neurovascular structures (4,20,23,24).

Radiographs should be obtained if osteomyelitis or a foreign body is suspected. Tetanus prophylaxis should be administered when necessary.

Significant lymphangitis or tenosynovitis or suspicion of osteomyelitis should prompt hand surgery referral for admission, intravenous antibiotic therapy, and operative incision and drainage.

▶ EQUIPMENT

Sterile gloves
Tongue depressor
Tape
Digital tourniquet, sterile Penrose drain with hemostat
Scalpel blade, No. 11
Fine hemostat
Syringe, 20 mL with sterile saline for irrigation
Catheter, 18-gauge, intravenous or splash shield
Iodophor gauze or sterile umbilical tape, 0.25 inch
Zinc oxide (optional)
Bandage material, adaptic gauze fluffs, Kerlix
Digital splint, plaster or preformed
Sling

▶ PROCEDURE

A comfortable, well-lit area, an assistant, and fine sterile instruments are required for the procedure. Older children may cooperate with metacarpal or digital nerve block placement (Chapter 35) using lidocaine or bupivacaine. Procedural sedation and age-appropriate restraints are recommended for younger children (Chapters 3 and 33). The digit may be secured to a tongue depressor at the level of the middle phalanx and again more proximally on the hand to minimize movement of the tip (Fig. 116.2). After the nerve block, the involved digit is sterilely prepared and draped. A bloodless field is achieved with a digital tourniquet such as a Penrose drain clamped at the base of the finger or using simple manual pressure along the radial and ulnar digital arteries. The tourniquet should be released briefly every 20 to 30 minutes to avoid prolonged ischemia of the finger.

The volar longitudinal incision or the high lateral incision is the preferred technique (1–4,7,8,20,23), depending on the

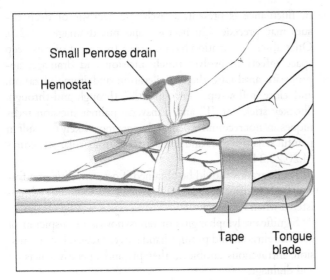

Figure 116.2 Immobilization and hemostasis of the finger.

area of greatest fluctuance, which may be identified with a blunt probe. A felon with maximal tenderness at the center of the terminal pulp is drained using a volar longitudinal incision using a No. 11 scalpel blade (Fig. 116.3A). The incision starts no closer than 3 to 5 mm from the distal interphalangeal (DIP) joint flexor crease and extends to the end of the distal phalanx. The incision should be made as deep as the dermis. Using a fine hemostat, the subcutaneous tissues are gently dissected and explored, necrotic tissue is excised, and loculations are gently disrupted. A small amount of pus may be expressed. Dissecting proximally may extend the process to the tendon sheath of the flexor digitorum profundus and should be avoided. The wound is irrigated with saline through an 18-gauge intravenous catheter or a splash shield. A sterile gauze wick (plain or antibiotic-impregnated umbilical tape or 0.25-inch iodophor gauze) is loosely placed in the depth of the wound. Zinc oxide ointment may be applied to help keep the wound open and draining (7). The digital tourniquet is removed, and a sterile bulky dressing, finger splint, and sling are applied.

A felon with maximal fluctuance located on the lateral aspect of the distal pulp is incised using a high lateral incision with a No. 11 scalpel blade with the bevel facing distally (Fig. 116.3B). The incision starts 5 mm distal to the flexor DIP crease and is extended parallel to the lateral border of the nail plate, with approximately 5 mm maintained between the incision and the nail plate border to avoid the more volar neurovascular structures. The incision ends just distal to the attached portion of the nail plate. The wound is dissected and explored using a fine hemostat (Fig. 116.3C), and the abscess is decompressed and irrigated as above. The wound is packed with a gauze wick (Fig. 116.3D), the tourniquet is removed, and a sterile bulky dressing, finger splint, and sling are applied.

A sample of the drained pus is collected and sent for Gram stain and culture to identify infection from emerging organisms such as methicillin-resistant *S. aureus.*

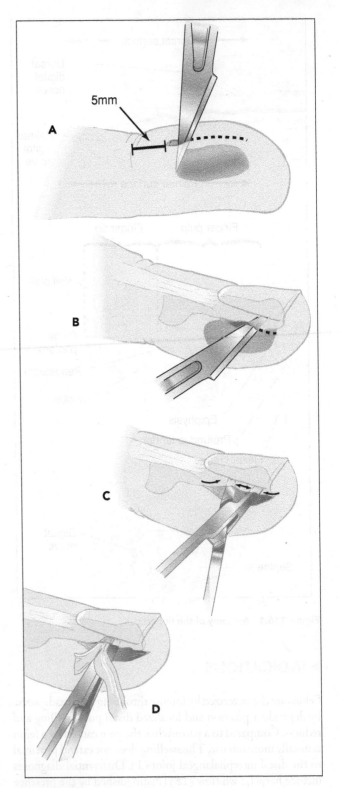

Figure 116.3
A. Volar longitudinal incision.
B. High lateral incision.
C. Disruption of loculations in a felon.
D. Wick placement.

Follow-up evaluation in 24 to 48 hours for wick removal and wound inspection is mandatory. The wound is allowed to close by secondary intention. Postoperative care includes splinting, strict elevation for at least 24 hours, twice daily warm soaks beginning the next day, dry dressing changes, and range-of-motion activities to facilitate healing and reduce discomfort (4). Antistaphylococcal antibiotics are recommended (1–7,14–17,21), and the duration of therapy varies from 5 to 14 days, depending on the severity of the infection and the clinical response (4,23). The choice of antibiotics can be tailored once the organism is identified from the pus culture. Prolonged healing or persistent drainage and/or pain necessitate hand surgery consultation.

 SUMMARY

1 Administer procedural sedation as needed.

2 Immobilize the involved digit.

3 Perform digital or metacarpal nerve block of the affected digit.

4 Sterilely prepare and drape the digit.

5 Apply a tourniquet to provide hemostasis.

6 Incise the area of maximal tenderness with a No. 11 scalpel blade.

  a Use a volar longitudinal incision if fluctuance is located at the center of the terminal pulp.

  b Use a high lateral incision on a plane parallel to the fingernail when fluctuance is lateral to the distal pulp.

7 Gently dissect the subcutaneous tissues with a fine hemostat.

8 Disrupt abscess loculations gently with a fine hemostat.

9 Collect sample of pus and send for Gram stain and culture.

10 Irrigate the wound with sterile saline using an 18-gauge intravenous catheter or splash shield.

11 Place a gauze wick in the wound.

12 Remove the tourniquet.

13 Apply a bulky dressing, splint, and sling.

14 Prescribe an antistaphylococcal antibiotic.

15 Arrange follow-up at 24 to 48 hours to remove gauze wick and inspect the wound.

16 Allow the wound to heal by secondary intention.

 CLINICAL TIPS

▶ A tense, swollen, red, very tender fingertip or a fingertip with a fluctuant abscess requires incision and drainage and antibiotic therapy.

▶ The following incision techniques are not recommended since they are more likely to result in damage to neurovascular structures and painful, sensitive fingertip pads: "fish mouth," "hockey stick" (or "J"), and transverse palmar.

▶ A volar longitudinal or high lateral incision is preferred, and the point of maximum fluctuance determines the incision type.

▶ The incision should be at least 3 to 5 mm distal to the DIP joint flexor crease to avoid the flexor digitorum profundus insertion and flexor sheath.

▶ Sending drained purulent material for culture and sensitivity will identify infections caused by emerging organisms that cause soft-tissue infections, such as methicillin-resistant *Staphylococcus aureus.*

▶ COMPLICATIONS

Flexor tenosynovitis may arise as a direct result of felon formation, but more commonly it arises from iatrogenic injury to the tendon or sheath. An unstable touch pad may result from disruption of the septae. A painful scar may occur when the digital nerve is injured. This may be prevented by making the incision just beneath the nail and dissecting carefully along the periosteum of the tuft. An anesthetic fingertip or a neuroma may occur from damage to both digital nerves as a result of through-and-through incisions. Knowledge of the relevant anatomy, use of proper technique, sterile procedure, and appropriate antibiotic coverage, with the provision of close follow-up and prompt referral when complications are identified, minimize the risk of iatrogenic complications.

▶ SUMMARY

Felons usually require incision and drainage and antistaphylococcal antibiotic coverage. The incision should be located at the point of maximal fluctuance and should allow for adequate drainage while avoiding injury to the fingertip septae and neurovascular bundle. Close follow-up is essential. Hand surgery referral should be sought for any complications from the felon or from the incision and drainage procedure.

▶ ACKNOWLEDGMENT

The authors would like to acknowledge the valuable contributions of Courtney A. Bethel to the version of this chapter that appeared in the previous edition.

▶ REFERENCES

1. Clark DC. Common acute hand infections. *Am Fam Physician.* 2003;68:2167–2176.
2. Harrison BP, Hilliard MW. Orthopedic emergencies: emergency department evaluation and treatment of hand injuries. *Emerg Med Clin North Am.* 1999;17:793–822.
3. Ablove RH, Moy OJ, Peimer CA. Pediatric surgery for the primary care pediatrician, II: pediatric hand disease: diagnosis and treatment. *Pediatr Clin North Am.* 1998;45:1507–1524.
4. Jebson PJ. Infections of the fingertip: paronychias and felons. *Hand Clin.* 1998;14:547–555.
5. Nathan R, Taras JS. Common infections in the hand. In: Hunter JM, Mackin E, Callahan AD, eds. *Rehabilitation of the Hand: Surgery and Therapy.* 4th ed. St. Louis: Mosby; 1995:251–260.
6. Hausman MR, Lisser SP. Hand infections. *Orthop Clin North Am.* 1992;23:171–185.
7. American Society for Surgery of the Hand. *The Hand: Primary Care of Common Problems,* 2nd ed. Philadelphia: Churchill Livingstone; 1990:77–79.
8. Stern PJ. Selected acute infections. *Instr Course Lect.* 1990;39:539–546.
9. Perry A, Gottlieb L, Zachary L. Fingerstick felons. *Ann Plast Surg.* 1988;20:249–251.
10. Flatt AE. *Infections: The Care of Minor Hand Injuries.* 3rd ed. St. Louis: Mosby; 1972:247–250.
11. Connolly B, Johnstone F, Gerlinger T, et al. Methicillin-resistant *Staphylococcus aureus* in a finger felon. *J Hand Surg [Am].* 2000;25:173–175.
12. Karanas YL, Bogdan MA, Chang J. Community acquired methicillin-resistant *Staphylococcus aureus* hand infections: case reports and clinical implications. *J Hand Surg [Am].* 2000;25:760–763.
13. Watson PA, Jebson PJ. The natural history of the neglected felon. *Iowa Orthop J.* 1996;16:164–166.
14. Leddy JP. Infections of the upper extremity. In: Bora FW, ed. *Pediatric Upper Extremity Diagnosis and Management.* Philadelphia: WB Saunders; 1986:362–363.
15. Canales FL, Newmeyer WL, Kilgore ES. The treatment of felons and paronychias. *Hand Clin.* 1989;5:515–523.
16. Mann RJ. *Infections of the Hand.* Philadelphia: Lea & Febiger; 1988;1–84.
17. Kilgore ES, Brown LG, Newmeyer WL, et al. Treatment of felons. *Am J Surg.* 1975;130:194–198.
18. Szinnai G. Multiple herpetic whitlow lesions in a 4-year old girl: case report and review of the literature. *Eur J Pediatr.* 2001;160:528–533.
19. Gilhuis R. Three patients with a malignant felon. *Neth J Surg.* 1984; 36:144–146.
20. Brown DM, Young VL. Hand infections. *South Med J.* 1993;85:56–66.
21. Bolton H, Fowler P, Jepson R. Natural history of pulp space infection and osteomyelitis of the distal phalanx. *J Bone Joint Surg Br.* 1949;31:499–504.
22. Carter PR. *Common Hand Injuries and Infections: A Practical Approach to Early Treatment.* Philadelphia: WB Saunders; 1983;216–219.
23. Moran GJ, Talan DA. Hand infections. *Emerg Med Clin North Am.* 1993;11:601–619.
24. Lewis RC. Infections of the hand. *Emerg Med Clin North Am.* 1985;3:263–275.

JULIETTE QUINTERO-SOLIVAN AND SHARI L. PLATT

117

Ingrown Toenail Repair

▶ INTRODUCTION

Onychocryptosis, or ingrown toenail, is a common condition frequently managed in the emergency department or primary care setting. Although more common in adults, this condition is seen in adolescents and, rarely, in children (1–3). It principally affects the great toes, and patients often seek attention early due to the intensity of pain and its effect on ambulation (1).

An ingrown toenail occurs when the lateral edge of the nail plate impinges on the lateral skin fold and traumatizes the skin. The result is varying degrees of pain, inflammation, granulation tissue formation, and infection. Therefore, management is aimed at relieving pain, minimizing further injury, preventing recurrence, and identifying and treating infection and complications. Predisposing factors include tight-fitting shoes, trauma, trimming nails in a curved fashion, picking and tearing nail edges, and nail or digit deformities (4,5).

Management is best tailored to the individual patient (4). In most situations, conservative management involving basic foot care and relief of pain is sufficient (4,6). In others, with higher degrees of injury or chronic or recurrent symptoms, surgical repairs are indicated (6).

▶ ANATOMY AND PHYSIOLOGY

The "nail" itself, or nail plate, is a thickened convex structure made of consecutive layers of keratinized cells. The nail plate is supported by the nail unit, which is divided into four components: the nail bed, the proximal nail fold, the hyponychium, and the nail matrix (4,7). The deep nail plate layer is firmly attached to the nail bed. At the distal end of the digit, the nail bed and plate separate, and the skin thickens to become the fingertip. The junction between the free edge of

the nail plate and the skin of the fingertip is the hyponychium, which forms a seal between these two layers (4). Proximally, the nail plate inserts into the proximal nail fold and is sealed dorsally by the eponychium, or cuticle. Within the proximal nail fold is found the nail germinal matrix (Fig. 117.1; see also 115.2A). The matrix extends from the distal edge of the lunula (the white crescent shape at the base of the nail) and lateral edges of the nail plate to the most proximal extent of the nail root, the nail apex (4). The nail predominantly grows distally from the germinal matrix at a rate of approximately 2 mm per month (7).

The main pathophysiology of this condition occurs when a hard nail spicule, acting like a foreign body, imbeds into the lateral skin fold and causes reactive inflammation and ultimately secondary infection. Three stages of disease have been proposed by Heifitz: stage I, mild edema and erythema along the lateral nail fold; stage II, increased pain, edema, and erythema, with evidence of drainage; stage III, chronic inflammation with marked granulation tissue formation and lateral fold hypertrophy (8).

▶ INDICATIONS

Management of ingrown toenails ranges from nonsurgical (conservative) treatment to multiple surgical options, depending on the stage of disease, the chronicity of symptoms, the etiology, and existing comorbid conditions (7). Stage I and mild stage II lesions are best managed by conservative means (4). However, for higher grade lesions, treatment failures, and recurrences, more aggressive minor surgical procedures are employed, such as angular nail plate resection (wedge resection), partial nail resection, complete nail plate resection, wedge excision of the nail fold, plastic nail wall reduction, partial onychectomy, complete onychectomy, and Syme amputation

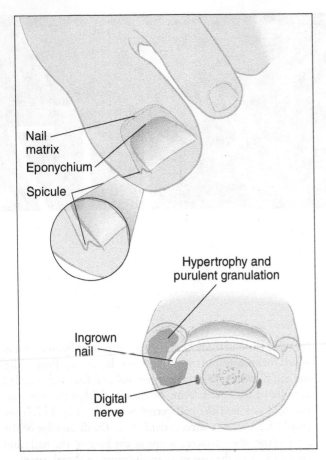

Nail
matrix

Eponychium

Spicule

Hypertrophy and
purulent granulation

Ingrown
nail

Digital
nerve

Figure 117.1　Anatomy of an ingrown toenail.

of the toe (4,9). Simpler surgical interventions are easily performed in the emergency department or outpatient setting, depending on practitioner comfort level and experience; however, management of more complicated lesions may require more specialized care.

In mild cases, these interventions may be curative, but in more severe cases, these procedures are palliative and should be performed in conjunction with more permanent solutions, such as chemical or surgical matricectomy (3,4,7). The ultimate goal of all treatment is to alleviate the nail spicule impaction and prevent recurrences, which will subject the patient to multiple painful surgical procedures. Despite extensive experience and literature on management approaches, much disagreement and therefore variability exists among practitioners (6). Regardless of the management employed, all patients should be instructed on proper foot hygiene, horizontal nail trimming, and avoidance of tight-fitting shoes (10).

▶ EQUIPMENT

Digital block anesthesia
1% or 2% lidocaine without epinephrine

Syringe with 25- or 27-gauge needle
Digital tourniquet, quarter-inch Penrose drain
Povidone-iodine or antiseptic cleanser
Sterile gauze 4″ × 4″
Sterile cotton or petrolatum gauze
Isopropyl alcohol or collodion
Scalpel blade, No. 11
Nail cutter or splitter
Hemostat, small
Antibacterial ointment
Nail file, small
Suture material for wedge resection
Silver nitrate sticks
Mini-curette

▶ PROCEDURES

Nonsurgical Treatment

Mild to moderate lesions (minimal to moderate pain, erythema, no discharge) can be managed conservatively (4,7,9,11). This is the most frequently used management approach to stage I lesions (4). Manipulation of an exquisitely tender ingrown toenail often requires a digital nerve block (Chapter 35). Use of topical local anesthetic cream such as EMLA prior to digital nerve block for ingrown toenail surgery was not shown to provide clinical benefit in one study (12). However, many practitioners continue to use it prior to the digital nerve block until more definite data exist. Bleeding may be minimized by applying a digital tourniquet before any procedure. A mini-curette can then be used to remove any visible debris or nail spurs. If the nail is curved to form a central peak, the central portion of the nail surface may be filed down until the nail bed matrix is visible through the thinned nail, which allows for release of the curvature pressure. The affected nail edge is then grasped with a hemostat and lifted out of the nail groove by rotating away from the nail fold (Fig. 117.2). The nail plate must be handled with care to avoid fracturing it. Debris is again removed by curettage, and granulation tissue may be ablated via application of a silver nitrate stick for no longer than 1 minute. A small piece of cotton soaked in alcohol or petrolatum gauze is then firmly packed under the nail edge. The patient may replace the alcohol-soaked swab daily. Another similar approach is to pack a wisp of cotton under the nail edge and soak it with collodion. This may remain in place for 3 to 6 weeks and then should be replaced until the nail grows beyond the distal aspect of the nail fold. The patient must be instructed to follow strict foot hygiene habits consisting of warm water soaks of the affected toe, trimming of the nail transversely as it grows, and wearing of loose-fitting footwear. This procedure, with good patient compliance, is associated with a success rate as high as 96% in patients with stage I and mild stage II disease (3,13–18).

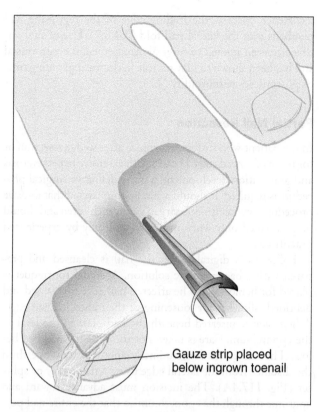

Figure 117.2 Conservative management of an ingrown toenail.

Angular Nail Resection with Débridement

In more severely affected stage II patients or in mildly affected stage II patients who fail to perform the rigorous postprocedural foot care required with conservative management, a more aggressive mode of therapy may be required.

The least invasive surgical procedure is a wedge resection of the distal portion of the affected nail, which includes removal of the nail spicule. A digital block is required for anesthesia before this procedure. A quarter-inch Penrose drain or the equivalent applied proximally on the digit may be used as a digital tourniquet to minimize bleeding. The toe is prepped with povidone-iodine and covered with a sterile drape. The nail edge is raised by carefully inserting a hemostat or an equivalent instrument beneath the nail plate and advancing it with a gradual side-to-side motion. Care is taken to not injure the delicate nail bed below. The nail is again cleansed and a triangular wedge or oblique segment of nail is excised with sharp pointed scissors to a point one third to one half the distance to the proximal nail fold, as shown in Figure 117.3 (3). The nail wedge and the nail spicule must be completely removed. The remaining nail edge should be filed down so that it may grow smoothly along the nail groove. The exposed nail matrix should be débrided and cleansed. Trauma to the nail groove must be avoided, as this can lead to scarring and obliteration. All keratotic material must be removed with a sharp blade. The nail bed should be dressed with antibacterial ointment and nonadherent gauze with dressing. Close follow-up for 48 hours should be arranged to check the wound (3). The patient should be instructed on basic foot hygiene and foot care techniques. This procedure is usually palliative and is curative in many mild stage II cases. A significant risk of

---

⊙ SUMMARY: NONSURGICAL TREATMENT

1 Administer digital nerve block anesthesia.

2 Clean the nail groove with an alcohol pad.

3 File the central nail peak as needed.

4 Elevate the nail edge from the groove with a hemostat.

5 Remove debris from the nail groove with curettage and débridement.

6 Apply silver nitrate to granulation tissue as needed.

7 Pack cotton or gauze beneath the nail edge.

8 Apply a bulky dressing.

9 Emphasize follow-up home care.

   a Change the packing as needed until the nail extends beyond the distal aspect of the nail fold.

   b Initiate warm water soaks after 24 hours.

   c Trim the nail transversely.

   d Wear loose-fitting shoes.

10 Follow-up with a physician for wound evaluations at 24 to 48 hours and again after 1 to 2 weeks.

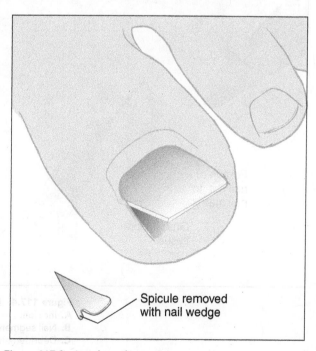

Figure 117.3 Angular nail resection.

SUMMARY: ANGULAR NAIL RESECTION

1 Administer digital nerve block anesthesia.

2 Clean the nail groove with an alcohol pad.

3 Apply a digital tourniquet as needed.

4 Prepare and drape the toe in sterile fashion.

5 Lift the nail edge with a hemostat.

6 Cut a triangular wedge from the distal nail with sharp pointed scissors.

7 Remove the nail wedge and spicule.

8 File the remaining nail edge.

9 Remove debris from the nail groove with curettage and débridement.

10 Apply an antibacterial ointment.

11 Apply a bulky dressing.

12 Emphasize follow-up home care as for the nonsurgical method.

13 Follow-up with physician for wound evaluations at 24 to 48 hours and again after 1 to 2 weeks.

recurrence exists as the leading edge of the regrowing nail reimbeds into the lateral nail fold (3,4,6,7). Use of oral antibiotics as an adjunct to surgical management is controversial and has been shown to play no role in decreasing healing time or postprocedure morbidity (12).

Partial Nail Resection

In the patient who suffers recurrence after wedge resection or for more advanced stage II cases with extensive hyperkeratosis and granulation development, a more definitive surgical procedure is required. It should again be emphasized that invasive procedures are rarely necessary in younger children and should be performed only when indicated and only by experienced practitioners.

Following a digital block, the nail is cleansed and prepared with a bacteriostatic solution. A digital tourniquet is placed for hemostasis. The affected nail edge is cleansed and débrided, allowing for loosening of the imbedded nail edge. A hemostat is inserted beneath the nail plate to the level of the eponychium. Care is taken not to injure the nail bed below. The nail is cut longitudinally approximately one third the distance from the lateral edge using a nail cutter or splitter (Fig. 117.4A). The incision must advance toward and continue through the eponychium so that the entire nail portion inclusive of the nail root may be resected, as shown. The resected nail strip is then removed using a hemostat via

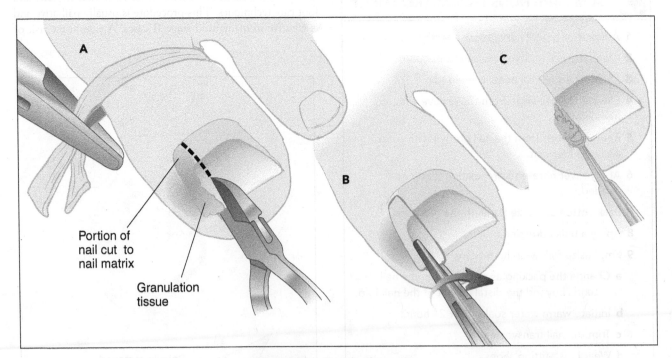

Figure 117.4 Partial nail resection.
A. Incision.
B. Nail segment removal.
C. Débridement.

a slow, steady rotating motion toward the intact nail edge to minimize damage to the nail bed (Fig. 117.4B). The exposed nail bed is then gently débrided and cleansed to remove all the keratotic material and granulation tissue (Fig. 117.4C). Additional pressure may be applied during this procedure to ensure hemostasis (3,16). Some recommend placing a cotton wisp beneath the growing nail plate edge to elevate the edge and prevent a recurrence (4). This is to be done by the patient until the nail edge grows beyond the nail groove (4).

To prevent recurrences, definitive management often involves ablation of the matrix (matricectomy) to prevent growth of the lateral nail edge (7). This is accomplished by surgical or chemical means (phenol, sodium hydroxide, nitric acid, or carbon dioxide laser vaporization) (19). Indications for ablation are less common in children and should be performed by a surgical or podiatric specialist. Patients should be instructed to keep the toe dry for the initial 24 hours and then initiate daily or twice daily washings or soakings followed by antibacterial ointment application and dry dressing changes (3). Wound healing is often associated with serous drainage (3). Use of oral antibiotics as an adjunct to surgical management is controversial and has been shown to play no role in decreasing healing time or postprocedure morbidity in most patients (20). Oral antibiotics should be considered for patients who present with additional signs of infection, such as a purulent exudate or cellulitis; immunocompromised patients; and patients at risk for poor wound healing. Wound follow-up is essential at 48 hours (3–5).

Partial nail resection is often successful if it is followed by rigorous nail hygiene and appropriate trimming. The ultimate long-term success of partial nail resection *without* an ablative procedure involves healing of the lateral hypertrophied fold and resolution of edema before the leading edge of the regrowing nail is close to being re-embedded. In most cases not involving ablative procedures, the nail will regrow in a normal manner, leaving little or no deformity.

Complete Nail Resection

Removal of the entire nail plate is rarely indicated but may be necessary for extensive lesions involving both the medial and lateral nail fold edges. This procedure is often best reserved for surgeons or podiatric surgeons. Complete nail resection will give definite relief of symptoms; however, it is associated with a high risk of recurrence. The procedure involves a technique similar to that for partial nail resection except that the entire nail plate is separated from the nail bed and proximal nail fold and removed. The toe is dressed as usual, with similar care instructions given. Elevation of the regrowing nail plate edge by cotton wisp packing is recommended as a means to prevent a recurrence (4). The nail bed will re-epithelialize within weeks (4).

Alternative Surgical Procedures

Wedge excision of the subcutaneous skin of the lateral nail fold is performed by surgeons or podiatric surgeons to reduce the convexity of the lateral fold skin. The procedure involves a soft-tissue wedge resection of a triangular segment just lateral to the affected nail groove (Fig. 117.5). This technique, in conjunction with removal of the nail plate, has been shown to have a high cure rate, less postoperative pain, and a low risk of infection (19).

Occasionally more invasive procedures, such as onychectomies, may be carried out by surgeons or podiatric surgeons. In these procedures the matrix and nail fold are removed to ensure permanent removal of the toenail. These procedures are rare and best carried out after infection and inflammation have subsided (4). A Syme amputation of the distal phalanx has been described but is reserved for older patients with chronic disease (4). In these procedures, poor aesthetic outcome is the main concern.

As previously mentioned, a child requiring any of these more aggressive surgical interventions normally should be referred for podiatric consultation and follow-up, as these procedures require a significant level of experience and skill.

 SUMMARY: PARTIAL NAIL RESECTION

1 Administer digital nerve block anesthesia.

2 Clean the nail groove with an alcohol pad.

3 Prepare and drape the toe in sterile fashion.

4 Place a digital tourniquet for hemostasis.

5 Insert a hemostat beneath the nail plate to the level of the eponychium.

6 Cut the nail longitudinally through the eponychium with a nail cutter or splitter.

7 Remove the resected nail edge with a hemostat ensuring total nail root removal.

8 Remove debris from the nail groove with curettage and débridement.

9 Consider ablation of the matrix to prevent recurrence.

10 Apply antibacterial ointment.

11 Apply a bulky dressing.

12 Consider oral antibiotics.

13 Emphasize follow-up home care, as previously discussed.

14 Follow-up with a physician for wound evaluations at 24 to 48 hours and again after 1 to 2 weeks.

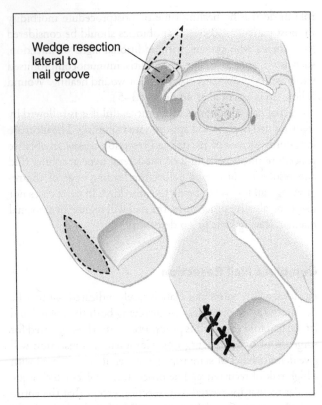

Wedge resection
lateral to
nail groove

Figure 117.5 Wedge excision of nail fold.

SUMMARY: WEDGE EXCISION OF NAIL FOLD

1 Administer digital nerve block anesthesia.

2 Clean the toe with povidone-iodine and place a sterile drape.

3 Apply a digital tourniquet for hemostasis.

4 Make an elliptical incision through the granulation tissue lateral to the affected nail groove.

5 Extend the incision in a wedge-shaped fashion.

6 Remove the resulting triangular-shaped segment of tissue.

7 Bring together the opposing sides of the wound with sutures.

8 Apply antibacterial ointment.

9 Apply a bulky dressing.

10 Emphasize follow-up home care, as previously discussed.

11 Follow-up with a physician for wound evaluations at 24 to 48 hours and again after 1 to 2 weeks.

CLINICAL TIPS

▶ Surgical approaches in children should be avoided when possible.

▶ Digital block anesthesia should be considered even with the most conservative treatment.

▶ Nail edge elevation with gauze packing is effective for most patients.

▶ Wedge or lateral nail plate resections should be reserved for the more severe cases.

▶ Patients who have ingrown toenail recurrences and require nail resection with surgery of the lateral nail fold or germinal matrix ablation should be referred to podiatric consultants for treatment and/or follow-up.

▶ COMPLICATIONS

Bleeding is frequently associated with procedures involving full or partial removal of the nail. Placement of a digital tourniquet will generally provide adequate hemostasis during a procedure. Additional applied pressure may be required once the tourniquet is removed. Prolonged application of the tourniquet may result in distal toe ischemia, which may result in ulceration, necrosis, and poor healing (I). Infection may be a complication of the disease process itself or may be a post-surgical complication. As mentioned previously, recurrence of ingrowth is often unavoidable, especially in the more severe cases. Any surgical intervention or overaggressive débridement may result in abnormal or absent nail regrowth due to damage to the nail groove or matrix. In addition, care must be taken not to damage underlying fascia and periosteum below the nail bed (I).

▶ SUMMARY

Ingrown toenails are commonly seen in the ambulatory setting. The physician should be familiar with the various treatment options outlined in this chapter. Treatment must be individualized for each patient based on the patient's age and the severity and chronicity of the condition. As in all procedures, the patient and/or legal guardian should be made well aware of potential complications and possible aesthetic outcomes as well as the risk of recurrence. In children, a conservative approach is encouraged, and good foot hygiene and footwear usage must always be stressed.

▶ ACKNOWLEDGMENT

The authors would like to acknowledge the valuable contributions of George L. Foltin to the version of this chapter that appeared in the previous edition.

▶ REFERENCES

1. Zuber TJ. Ingrown toenail removal. *Am Fam Physician*. 2002;65:2547–2558.

2. Katz AM. Congenital ingrown toenails. *J Am Acad Dermatol*. 1996;34:519–520.

3. McGee D. Ingrown toenail. In: Roberts JR Hedges JR, eds. *Clinical Procedures in Emergency Medicine*. 4th ed. Philadelphia: WB Saunders; 2004:1015–1018.

4. Coughlin MJ. Conditions of the forefoot: abnormalities of the toenail. In: DeLee JC, Drez D, eds. *DeLee and Drez's Orthopedic Sports Medicine*. 2nd ed. Philadelphia: WB Saunders; 2003:2521–2531.

5. Goldstein BG, Goldstein AO. Paronychia, herpetic whitlow, and ingrown toenail. 2005. www.uptodateonline.com. Accessed July 3, 2007.

6. Rounding C, Hulm S. Surgical treatments for ingrown toenails. *The Foot*. 2001;11:166–182.

7. Ikard RW. Onychocryptosis. *J Am Coll Surg*. 1998;187:96–102.

8. Heifitz CJ. Ingrown toenail: a clinical study. *Am J Surg*. 1937;38:298–315.

9. Connolly B, Fitzgerald RJ. Pledgets in ingrowing toenails. *Arch Dis Child*. 1988;63:71–72.

10. Murtagh J. Ingrowing toenails. *Aust Fam Physician*. 1993;22:206.

11. Senapati A. Conservative outpatient management of ingrowing toenails 1986. *J R Soc Med*. 79:339–340.

12. Serour F, Ben-Yehuda Y, Boaz M. EMLA cream prior to digital nerve block for ingrown nail surgery does not reduce pain at injection of anesthetic solution. *Acta Anesth Scand*. 2002;46:203–206.

13. Jackson JL, Linakis JG. Ankle and foot injuries. In: Barkin RM, ed. *Pediatric Emergency Medicine Concepts and Clinical Practice*. St. Louis: Mosby; 1992:374.

14. Seibert JS, Mann RA. Dermatology and disorders of the toenails. In: Mann RA ed. *DuVries' Surgery of the Foot*. St. Louis: Mosby; 1978:498–504.

15. Coughlin MJ. Toenail abnormalities. In: Mann RA, Coughlin MJ, eds. *Surgery of the Foot and Ankle*. St. Louis: Mosby; 1993:1049–1071.

16. Reijnen JA, Goris RJ. Conservative treatment of ingrowing toenails. *Br J Surg*. 1989;76:955–957.

17. Murray WR. Management of ingrowing toenail. *Br J Surg*. 1989;76:883–884.

18. Ilfeld FW. Ingrown toenail treated with cotton collodion insert. *Foot Ankle*. 1991;11:312–313.

19. Persichetti P, Pierfranco S, Li Vecchi G, et al. Wedge excision of the nail fold in the treatment of ingrown toenail. *Ann Plast Surg*. 2004;52:617–620.

20. Reyzelman AM, Trombello KA, Vayser DJ, et al. Are antibiotics necessary in the treatment of locally infected ingrown toenails? *Arch Fam Med*. 2000;9:930–932.

118

DOUGLAS S. DIEKEMA

Fishhook Removal

▶ INTRODUCTION

Removal of a fishhook can pose a challenge to those working in the emergency department (ED). Most frequently the hook will find its way into a finger or foot. The barb on the end of the hook prevents easy removal, but several time-honored techniques provide effective means of extraction. No clinical trial has compared the most common methods, although all have been the subject of colorful discussion in letters to the editor of various medical journals (1–7). Fishermen have used the string technique of fishhook removal in the field for years, a testimony to its reliability and straightforward nature. But other methods, as described in this chapter, have their ardent supporters as well.

▶ ANATOMY AND PHYSIOLOGY

Because most fishhooks embed in skin and subcutaneous tissue, understanding the anatomy of the skin and of the hook facilitates successful removal. Important anatomic and physiologic characteristics of the skin are described in detail in Chapters 107, 108, and 113. Most fishhooks consist of an eyelet at the end of a straight shank and a curved belly that ends in a barb (Fig. 118.1). The barb is usually located on the inner curve of the hook, pointed away from the hook's tip. When the sharp point of the hook enters tissue, the barb engages and prevents the hook from being pulled back through the entrance site. Atraumatic removal of the hook requires that the barb be disengaged from the surrounding tissue.

▶ INDICATIONS

The location of the fishhook may determine which of the three methods described in this chapter will best accomplish

removal. The push-through method is most effective when the point of the hook is near the surface of the skin, allowing it to be pushed through easily. This method is less useful when the tip is buried deep, as pushing it through would cause additional significant tissue damage. The rapidity, painlessness, and lack of dependence on special tools make the string technique ideal for use in the field or when local anesthesia is not available or desirable. It may also be the best technique for deeply embedded hooks. For it to be performed successfully, however, the body part containing the hook must be immobilized during the removal procedure. Therefore, the string technique should not be used on body parts that cannot be fully immobilized, such as ears or eyelids. This technique also may be contraindicated for fishhooks located near the eye, as the airborne hook might injure the patient's eye. Finally, the needle technique can be used in the ED for those hooks embedded superficially. The more deeply embedded the hook, however, the more difficult it may be to find the barb with the needle tip.

Although the vast majority of fishhooks can be easily removed in the field, office, or ED, fishhooks that have penetrated the globe require immediate consultation with an ophthalmologist. Involvement of the eyelid should alert the clinician of the possibility of corneal or globe involvement, and no manipulation of the hook should be attempted before involvement of the eye has been ruled out. Likewise, consultation with a surgeon may be judicious for those hooks that have embedded near vital structures. This may apply to fishhooks in the neck, near the radial artery, and in the genitals.

▶ EQUIPMENT

Gloves
Wire cutter
Antiseptic prep solution (e.g., povidone-iodine)

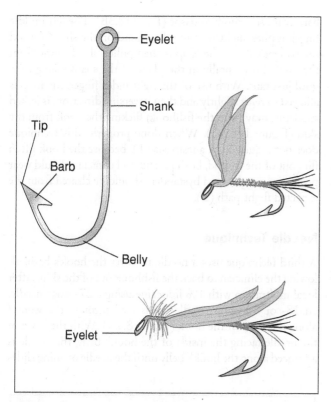

Figure 118.1 Structure of a fishhook.

Lidocaine 1% to 2% without epinephrine (for push-through and needle techniques)
Syringe and needle for local anesthesia (27 gauge)
Safety goggles (for string technique)
String, fishing line, or 1.0 silk (for string technique)
Needle, 18 gauge (for needle technique)

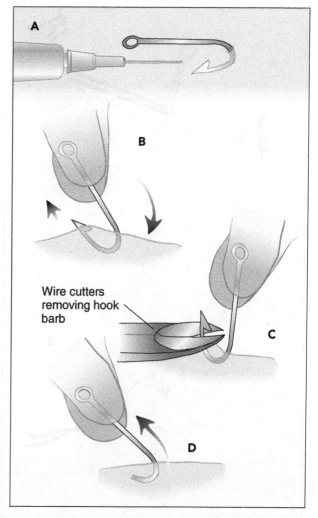

Wire cutters removing hook barb

Figure 118.2 Push-through method of fishhook removal.

▶ PROCEDURE

Before removing the embedded barb, the clinician should remove multiple hooks or attached lures if present. Often, lures and additional hooks can be unscrewed while grasping the embedded hook with a hemostat. A wire cutter can be used to isolate the embedded hook from other hooks attached to the same shaft. Once the embedded hook has been disconnected from any attachments, the skin and fishhook should be prepared with povidone-iodine, and the barbed hook can be removed from the skin using one of the following techniques.

Push-Through Method

The push-through method of removal requires a digital block or local infiltration of the skin overlying the point of the hook with 1% lidocaine (Fig. 118.2A). The point of the hook is then advanced and pushed through the skin (Fig. 118.2B), the barb clipped off with a wire cutter (Fig. 118.2C), and the remainder of the shank and belly backed out of the entry wound (Fig. 118.2D). On occasion, particularly with

a multiple-barbed hook, it might be easier to cut the eye of the hook and then advance the belly and shank forward through the exit wound (5,6). The exit site is usually small and therefore suturing is not indicated.

String Technique

The string technique begins by securing the body part containing the fishhook firmly against a table or flat surface to prevent movement during the procedure. A piece of string (e.g., silk suture) about 3 feet long should be looped around the belly of the fishhook (Fig. 118.3A). Using two loops around the belly of the fishhook increases the likelihood of the fishhook remaining attached to the string after the procedure. If the shank has been cut, the remaining portion of the shank can be grasped with a strong hemostat, which then will act as a substitute shank. The ends of the string should be wrapped securely around the clinician's right index finger (or left finger if the clinician is left-handed). The eye and shank of the fishhook should be firmly grasped between the clinician's left index finger and thumb and then depressed, disengaging the

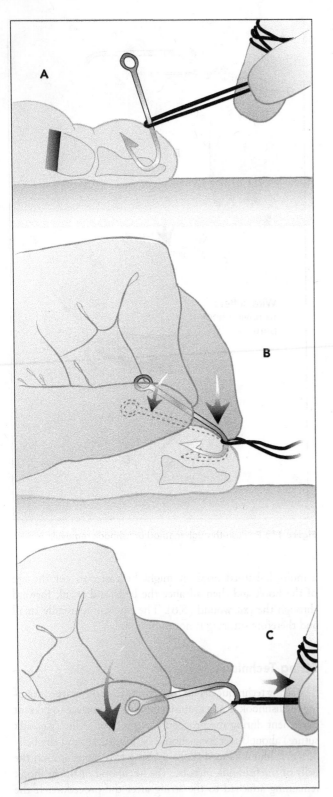

Figure 118.3 String technique of fishhook removal.

barb from surrounding tissue (Fig. 118.3B). The left middle finger applies slight pressure downward on the shank toward the patient's skin. The loop is then pulled slowly away from the hook, horizontally in the plane of the shank's long axis, until just taut. With use of the right index finger, the loop is allowed to relax slightly and then, reversing direction, is jerked suddenly away from the fishhook, flicking the hook from the skin (Figure 118.3C). When done properly, this technique does not require local anesthesia (1). Because the hook often flies out of the wound, both patient and clinician should wear protective goggles, and bystanders should be cleared from the expected flight path (2).

Needle Technique

A third technique uses a needle to cover the hook's barb, allowing the clinician to back the fishhook out of the skin. After local infiltration with 1% lidocaine using a 27-gauge needle, an 18- or 20-gauge needle is inserted through the wound along the shaft of the hook (Fig. 118.4A). With the bevel of the needle facing the inside of the hook's belly, the needle is advanced along the hook's belly until the needle opening slides

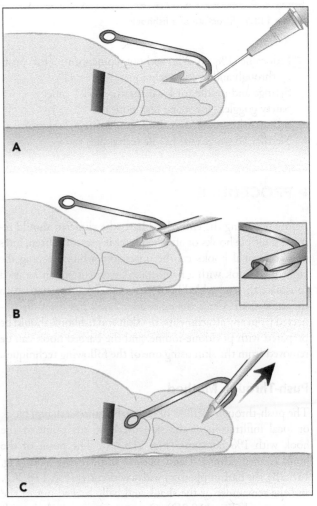

Figure 118.4 Needle technique of fishhook removal.

SUMMARY

1 Remove attached lures and additional hooks from the embedded hook.

2 Prepare the field in antiseptic fashion.

3 Inject local anesthesia or perform a digital block if needed.

4 Push-through method:

  a Push the tip of the hook through the anesthetized skin.

  b Clip the barb.

  c Back the shank and belly of the fishhook out of the entry wound.

  d If the hook has multiple barbs, cut the eye of the hook and then pull the belly and shaft out through the exit wound.

5 String technique:

  a Secure the body part involved.

  b Loop string around the belly of the fishhook.

  c Wrap the ends of the string securely around the index finger.

  d Depress the shank of the hook with the opposite index finger and thumb.

  e Forcefully jerk the string to remove the hook.

6 Needle technique:

  a Insert an 18-gauge needle along the inside of the fishhook belly.

  b Engage the barb with the needle opening.

  c Back the needle and hook out of the skin together.

7 Irrigate, cleanse, and dress the wound.

8 Administer a tetanus booster if indicated.

 CLINICAL TIPS

▶ The push-through method works best when the point of the hook is near the skin surface, minimizing additional tissue damage as the barb is advanced through the skin.

▶ The needle technique works best when the hook is superficially embedded.

▶ The string technique is simple enough to be done in the field, and when performed correctly, it requires no anesthesia.

▶ The provider staff should take care to be out of the line of flight and thus avoid eye injury when employing the string technique.

---

over (engages) the barb of the hook (Fig. 118.4B). Once the barb has been covered, the needle and hook are held firmly together while backing the hook and needle out of the wound as a unit (Fig. 118.4C).

Following removal of the fishhook, routine wound care should be performed. The wound should be cleansed and a tetanus booster given if necessary. Antibiotics are not generally indicated (1,3).

▶ COMPLICATIONS

Complications are rare when these procedures are performed properly. As with any wound, infection is a rare complica-

tion (4,5). The wound should be thoroughly irrigated and cleansed, and the patient instructed to return if any signs of infection arise. The push-through technique may cause additional tissue damage as the needle is advanced through intact skin: the deeper the needle, the higher the risk of causing significant damage. The string technique is effective and safe when done properly. If the body part containing the fishhook is not properly secured, however, movement when the hook is jerked can result in tissue damage and pain. Most failures of this technique are thought to be due to the lack of a quick and confident yank on the string. As mentioned, the patient and clinician should both wear protective goggles to prevent eye injury. It is also wise for the clinician and any bystanders to position themselves away from the expected flight path of the fishhook so that it does not become embedded in someone else after it is free of the patient. Finally, the needle technique is more difficult to perform without causing excessive local trauma when the fishhook is deeply embedded.

▶ SUMMARY

Personnel familiar with the procedures outlined in this chapter can easily accomplish removal of an embedded fishhook in the field, in the office, or in the ED. After removal of the hook, cleansing the wound, updating tetanus coverage, and follow-up care should suffice.

▶ ACKNOWLEDGMENT

The author would like to acknowledge the valuable contributions of Linda Quan to the version of this chapter that appeared in the previous edition.

▶ REFERENCES

1. Friedenberg S. How to remove an imbedded fishhook in five seconds without really trying. *N Engl J Med.* 1971;284:733–734.
2. David SS. Fish hook removal. *Lancet.* 1991;338:1463–1464.
3. Cooke T. How to remove fish hooks with a bit of string. *Med J Aust.* 1961;48:815–816.
4. Barnett RC. Removal of fish hooks. *J Hosp Med.* 1980;70:56–57.
5. Doser C, Cooper WL, Ediger WM, et al. Fishhook injuries: a prospective evaluation. *Am J Emerg Med.* 1991;9:413–415.
6. Eldad S, Amiram S. Embedded fishhook removal. *Am J Emerg Med.* 2000;18:736–737.
7. Gammons M, Jackson E. Fishhook removal. *Am Fam Physician.* 2001;63:2231–2236.

SUSAN M. FUCHS

119

Ring Removal

▶ INTRODUCTION

Occasionally children try on a parent's ring or toy jewelry, only to realize that the ring cannot be removed. By the time the child arrives in the emergency department or office, several attempts to remove the ring have often been made, resulting in increased swelling of the affected finger. Another scenario is an adolescent who injures a finger distal to a ring. In these cases, the injury (possibly a fracture) results in swelling that does not allow removal of the ring. With continued swelling, ring removal is often necessary to avoid vascular compromise to a digit. Although this chapter focuses on rings, other round objects (washers, metal nuts) can be treated in a similar manner.

▶ ANATOMY AND PHYSIOLOGY

The degree of vascular compromise of the finger depends on the magnitude and duration of swelling. Initial swelling is usually due to injury or attempts at ring removal and does not compromise circulation. Further swelling of the finger can result in obstruction of venous and lymphatic drainage, which in turn exacerbates the swelling. The risk of complete obstruction of circulation and gangrene can occur in 10 to 12 hours (1).

Acute swelling of a finger also can result from an allergic reaction, insect bite, or burn to the finger, in which case edema is the primary problem. When a finger is injured due to a fracture or dislocation, the deformity can itself prevent ring removal with or without significant swelling. Compared to those of an adult, the fingers of a young child tend to be chubby, which may further exaggerate the effects of swelling. The time to presentation also will affect the amount of swelling but does not necessarily correlate directly.

▶ INDICATIONS

A child often will present with a complaint about a painful finger, whereas an adolescent may be more stoic. Conversely, finger injury may be the initial presentation, only to have ring removal discovered as a secondary problem.

Several methods can be attempted to save the ring; however, if the digit is already ischemic or if a displaced fracture or a dislocation occurs distal to the ring, the ring should be cut off immediately.

Perfusion of the finger is in doubt when it is pale and mottled and has diminished or absent capillary refill. If perfusion is questioned, a pulse oximeter lead can be attached to the fingertip (Chapter 75). If a reading is obtained (a pulse wave form), perfusion is still present (2).

Assuming there is no circulatory compromise to the finger, one factor in determining the best removal method is the type of ring (e.g., plastic versus metal, narrow band versus wide band, inexpensive versus expensive or irreplaceable). It may be easier to cut a plastic ring with a ring cutter than attempt another technique, whereas if the ring is a broad, strong metal band, the string method may be a better starting point, assuming no vascular compromise has occurred.

▶ EQUIPMENT

Water-soluble lubricant (e.g., KY jelly or lidocaine jelly if available)
2.0 or 3.0 silk suture, string, or umbilical tape, 20 inches long
Ribbon gauze, 1.25 cm wide, 20 inches long
Rubber band
Hemostats or mosquito clamps
Surgical glove to fit patient
Ring cutter (manual or battery powered)

Elastic tape, 1 inch wide (intravenous tourniquet or Penrose drain)

Blood pressure cuff

Monitoring equipment if conscious sedation has been administered

It is beneficial to have all equipment available for the various methods rather than to begin searching for the ring cutter after other methods fail.

▶ PROCEDURE

Because some of these methods may be upsetting and painful for an infant or child, consideration should be given to (a) letting the parent hold the child during the procedure (Chapter 2), (b) administering a digital block to provide pain relief (Chapter 35), and/or (c) possibly using conscious sedation (Chapter 33).

Before beginning any of the methods described in this chapter, the procedure should be explained to the child and parents, and the equipment demonstrated. Any needles should be shielded from the child's view. The parent can assist the child in elevating the affected hand. While preparing the equipment, the parent or child should apply ice to the finger for 5 minutes to limit further swelling. The hand and finger are then cleansed with sterile water, with the hand kept elevated as much as possible during the procedure.

Depending on the methods attempted at home or en route to the hospital, the degree of swelling, the duration of swelling, and the desire to preserve the ring, one or more of the following techniques can be performed (see "Indications").

Glove Method

The finger portion of a surgical glove is placed on the patient's finger. A portion of the glove is passed underneath the ring using forceps or a hemostat. This portion should be circumferential and long enough to turn inside out and over the ring. This portion of the glove is pulled toward the fingertip. A twisting motion may be necessary. The glove should not be pulled so hard that it rips or the remainder of the glove slips under the ring (Fig. 119.1) (3).

String Pull or Rubber Band Method

With the string pull, one end of the suture (string) or a rubber band is slipped beneath the ring and pulled through until both ends are of equal length. A hemostat may be used to grasp the suture or rubber band under the ring. The ring and distal finger are then lubricated. Both ends of the suture or rubber band are grasped with the clinician's fingers or a hemostat and pulled in a circular motion. The suture or rubber band should be rotated around to different sections of the ring and pulled along the axis of the finger to gradually advance the ring off (Fig. 119.2) (4,5).

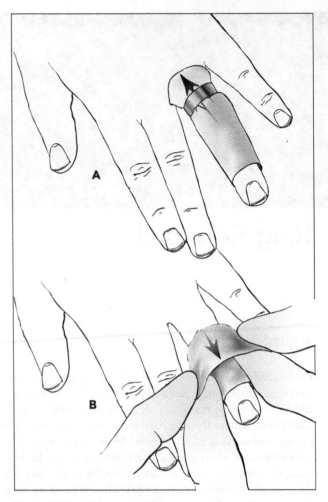

Figure 119.1 Glove method of ring removal.

If this method is not successful, a digital block should be administered before the next maneuver. If the block is performed with medication deposited into the web space or via a volar metacarpal approach, no significant additional swelling of the finger should occur.

String Wrap Method (Performed with Suture, Umbilical Tape, or Ribbon Gauze)

With the string wrap, one end of thick silk suture (or umbilical tape or ribbon gauze) is passed under the ring so that 5 inches remains on the proximal side of the finger. A hemostat may be used to slide the suture under the ring. The remaining suture (tape, gauze) is wrapped tightly around the swollen finger beginning just distal to the ring. Each loop of the suture (or umbilical tape) should touch so that no tissue bulges between loops (each loop of gauze should overlap a half width). The wrap should be continued just beyond the proximal interphalangeal joint (PIP) (Figs. 119.3 and 119.4) (1,2,4,6–8). When the wrap is complete, the proximal piece of string (under the ring) is pulled toward the fingertip with the clinician's fingers or a hemostat. As the string (tape, gauze) gradually unwinds, it should ease the ring over the PIP joint and off the

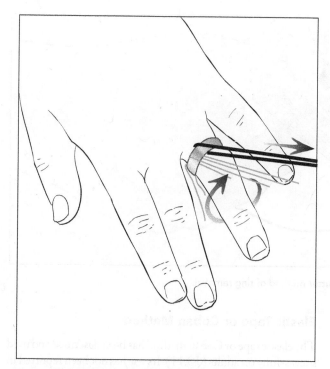

Figure 119.2 String pull method of ring removal.

finger. If the string (tape, gauze) was not long enough or the wrapping not tight or close enough, this procedure may have to be repeated (4,7,8).

Ring Cutters

Manual

The ring cutter has a guard over the wheel to prevent cutting the skin, and this characteristic should be explained to the child and parent. The ring cutter should be examined to ensure that the sawtooth wheel of the ring cutter is sharp,

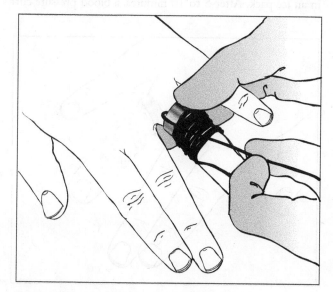

Figure 119.3 String wrap method of ring removal.

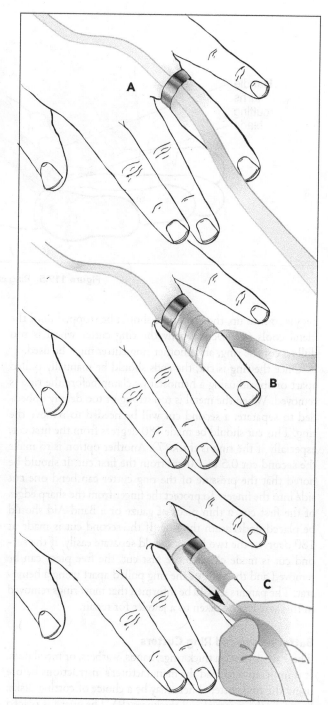

Figure 119.4 Ribbon gauze method of ring removal.

approximates the cutter guard, and turns easily. It should then be cleaned with alcohol and dried with gauze. Next the cutter guard is placed under the ring. Due to swelling of the tissue, this frequently causes pain. The easiest place to cut is the thinnest portion of the ring, but the best position to perform this procedure is usually on the palmar surface. If possible, the ring should be turned until the thinnest section is on the palmar surface. The wheel is placed on the ring, the handle of the ring cutter is grasped, and pressure is applied while the wheel is turned (Fig. 119.5) (4,7,9). If the ring

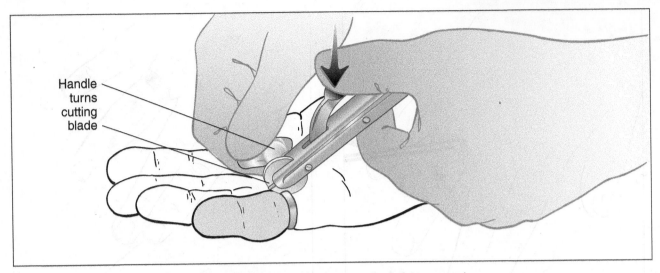

Figure 119.5 Ring cutter method of ring removal.

begins to heat up, the procedure should be stopped until the metal cools (4). Occasionally the ring cutter wheel is too dull to cut the ring, and another ring cutter must be used.

Once the ring is cut, the ends should be manually pulled apart or spread using a hemostat or clamp before the ring is removed. When the metal is too strong or too deeply imbedded to separate, a second cut will be needed to remove the ring. This cut should be made 180 degrees from the first cut, especially if the ring is thick (7). Another option is to make the second cut 0.5 to 1.0 cm from the first cut. It should be noted that the pressure of the ring cutter can bend one cut side into the finger. To protect the finger from the sharp edges of the first cut, a thin piece of gauze or a Band-Aid should be placed underneath the ring. If the second cut is made at 180 degrees, the two halves should separate easily. If the second cut is made close to the first cut, the free piece can be removed and the ends of the ring pulled apart using a hemostat. The parents should be informed that most rings removed in this way can be taken to a jeweler for repair.

Battery-Powered Ring Cutters

These work best on thick rings, bands, washers, or metal nuts. It is imperative to read the manufacturer's instructions before using the ring cutter. There may be a choice of cutting disks, based on the material and thickness (9). The guard is placed under the patient's ring, and the finger and ring are lubricated with a water-soluble lubricant. Goggles or eye shields should be worn when using the ring cutter. The cutter is turned on and swept gently across the ring surface. Each pass removes a layer of metal. It may take several passes to completely cut the ring. There is no need to press down hard. When the ring is cut, the ends should be manually pulled apart or spread using a hemostat or clamp before the ring is removed. Occasionally a second cut will be needed to remove the ring. A cut made 180 degrees from the first cut allows the ring to fall off, but a cut made 0.5 to 1.0 cm from the first cut may make jewelry repair easier (7,9).

Elastic Tape or Coban Method

The elastic tape or Coban method has been described and used successfully on adults (10,11). Its use has not been reported in children or adolescents but may prove beneficial when severe swelling occurs and the ring cannot be cut. It should not be used if there is a finger fracture or dislocation and one needs to remove the ring prior to reduction. The procedure actually exsanguinates the finger as a way of reducing the edema. It is similar to the string wrap method but uses elastic tape or Coban and a blood pressure cuff. Before this method is attempted, sedation will probably be necessary.

Either 1-inch wide elastic tape, Coban, an intravenous tourniquet, or a 1-inch Penrose drain is wrapped tightly around the finger from the tip of the finger to the ring (i.e., in a distal to proximal direction). Note that this is opposite the direction used for the string wrap method (Fig. 119.6). The hand is then elevated above the head, and the finger wrapped in an ice pack. After 5 to 10 minutes, a blood pressure cuff

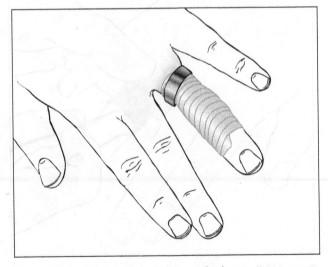

Figure 119.6 Elastic tape or Coban method.

SUMMARY

1 Explain the procedure to the child and parents.

2 Elevate the hand.

3 Apply ice to the finger for 5 minutes to see if the swelling diminishes.

4 Cleanse the area with sterile water and keep the hand elevated as much as possible during the procedure.

Glove Method

5 Place the finger portion of a glove on the patient's finger.

6 Pass the proximal portion of the glove underneath the ring using a forceps or hemostat.

7 Grasp the glove with the fingers or hemostat.

8 Pull the glove edges towards the tip of the finger.

String Pull Method

5 Slip one end of a suture or string beneath ring and pull through until both ends are of equal length. A hemostat may be used to grasp the suture under the ring.

6 Lubricate the ring and the distal finger.

7 Grasp both ends of the suture with fingers or a hemostat.

8 Pull in a circular motion. Slip the suture around to different sections of the ring and pull as the ring gradually moves off of the finger.

9 Clean the finger and reassess perfusion (color, capillary refill).

String (Suture, Umbilical Tape, Gauze Ribbon) Wrap Method

5 Administer a digital block.

6 Pass the end of a suture or string under the ring so that 5 inches remains on the proximal side of the finger. A hemostat may be used to slide the suture under the ring.

7 Wrap the remaining suture in a tight spiral around the swollen finger beginning just distal to the ring.

8 Continue the wrap beyond the proximal interphalangeal (PIP) joint.

9 Pull the proximal end of the string toward the fingertip with fingers or a hemostat. As the string gradually unwinds, it should ease the ring over the PIP joint and off of the finger.

10 Remove the suture from the finger.

11 Repeat the procedure as needed.

12 Clean the finger and assess perfusion (color, capillary refill).

Ring Cutter Method (Manual)

5 Administer a digital block.

6 Examine the ring cutter to ensure that the sawtooth wheel is sharp, approximates the cutter guard, and turns easily.

7 Clean the ring cutter with alcohol and then dry with gauze.

8 Turn the ring, if possible, until the thinnest section is on the palmar surface of the finger.

9 Place the cutter guard under the ring.

10 Place the wheel on the ring, grasp the handle of the ring cutter, and apply pressure while turning wheel. If the ring begins to heat up, stop until the metal cools.

11 When the ring is cut, manually pull apart the ring or spread the ends using a hemostat or clamp, and remove the ring.

12 When it is necessary (as is common with thick rings), make a second cut 180 degrees from the first cut (a cut 0.5 to 1.0 cm from the first cut may be made instead). Protect the finger from the sharp edges of the first cut with a thin piece of gauze or a Band-Aid slipped underneath the ring. Once the second cut is complete, the ring will come off if the cut was made 180 degrees from the first cut; if the second cut was made close to the first cut, remove the free piece and pull the ends of the ring apart using a hemostat.

13 Examine the finger for cuts, clean the finger, and check perfusion.

14 Take the ring to a jeweler for repair.

Elastic Tape or Coban Method

5 Wrap 1-inch wide elastic tape, Coban, an intravenous tourniquet, or a Penrose drain tightly around the finger from the tip of the finger to the ring.

6 Elevate the hand above the head and wrap in an ice pack.

7 After 5 to 10 minutes, apply a blood pressure cuff to the forearm and inflate to systolic pressure plus 100 mm Hg.

8 Remove the tape.

9 Attempt removal with one of the previous methods.

10 If the finger is still too swollen, repeat steps 5 to 8.

CLINICAL TIPS

▶ The ring cutter should be tested before beginning the procedure. The test should include either a visual inspection of the ring cutter or a test cut on a piece of plastic.

▶ The patient and/or parents should be informed before the procedure that one of the options includes cutting the ring. Some will prefer that this be tried first.

▶ The decision to use a digital block should be based on the patient's degree of discomfort and level of cooperation and the likelihood of ring removal by the first method chosen. With young children, the use of string or ring cutters can outweigh the threat of a needle.

is applied to the patient's forearm and inflated to systolic pressure plus 100 mm Hg. The tape is then removed. If the edema is reduced sufficiently to remove the ring, one of the previously discussed methods can be used. If the finger is still too swollen, this procedure can be repeated until the swelling is reduced enough to permit ring removal (10,11).

Following ring removal using any of these techniques, the patient should be reminded not to place a ring on the affected finger until all swelling has resolved. The digit should be cleaned and perfusion reassessed (color, capillary refill). If flow does not appear to be restored after ring removal, it should be checked using a pulse oximeter. If no flow is evident after 5 to 10 minutes or all efforts at removal have failed, a hand or vascular surgeon should be consulted.

▶ COMPLICATIONS

Trauma to the digit in the form of a cut or bruise can occur during ring removal. Cleansing and a dressing (Band-Aid) are all that is needed. If a digital block was used, the patient may experience a throbbing pain as the anesthetic wears off.

▶ SUMMARY

Although the order in which ring removal has been outlined takes into account the desire to save the ring, if this is not a priority, using a ring cutter is the most reliable method. Obviously the decision regarding which method to use depends on the patient, the degree of swelling, the presence or absence of vascular compromise, the presence of an injury distal to the ring, and the type of ring.

▶ REFERENCES

1. Young JR. Unring a finger. *Emerg Med.* 1982;15:107–108.
2. Jastremski MS. Ring removal. In: Jastremski MS, Dumas MS, eds. *Emergency Procedures.* Philadelphia: WB Saunders; 1992:141–143.
3. Inoue S, Akazawa S, Fukuda H, et al. Another simple method for ring removal. *Anesthesiology.* 1995;83:1133–1134.
4. Carlson DW, DiGiulio GA, Gewitz MH, et al. Illustrated techniques of pediatric emergency procedures. In: Fleisher GR, Ludwig S, Henretig FM, eds. *Textbook of Pediatric Emergency Medicine.* 5th ed. Philadelphia: Lippincott Williams & Wilkins; 2006:1928.
5. McElfresh EC, Peterson-Elijah RC. Removal of a tight ring by the rubber band technique. *J Hand Surg [Br].* 1991;16:225–226.
6. Mizrahi S, Lunski I. A simplified method for ring removal from an edematous finger. *Am J Surg.* 1986;151:412–413.
7. Stone DB, Koutouzis TK. Foreign body removal. In: Roberts JR, Hedges JR, eds. *Clinical Procedures in Emergency Medicine.* 4th ed. Philadelphia: WB Saunders; 2004:711–713.
8. Thilagarajah M. An improved method of ring removal. *J Hand Surg [Br].* 1999;24B:118–119.
9. Ramponi DR. Don't get uptight about ring removal. *Nursing.* 2002;32:56–57.
10. Cresap CR. Removal of a hardened steel ring from an extremely swollen finger. *Am J Emerg Med.* 1995;13:318–320.
11. Mullett STH. Ring removal from the oedematous finger. *J Hand Surg [Br].* 1995;20:496.

A. FELIPE BLANCO AND JAMES F. WILEY, II

120

Intramuscular and Subcutaneous Injections

▶ INTRODUCTION

Since its introduction in the second half of the 19th century, intramuscular injection has been a main route of drug delivery for the prophylaxis and treatment of disease (1). This mode of drug administration is most useful when the patient's disease and/or the pharmacokinetic properties of the drug preclude oral dosing and an intravenous route is unavailable or unnecessary. The technique is straightforward and may be used for patients of all ages. New drugs and new applications for current drugs have increased the variety and frequency of agents delivered by this route.

Subcutaneous injection predates intramuscular injection in medical history. One of its first uses was for the prophylactic injection of cowpox to provide immunity against smallpox in the mid-18th century (1). Subcutaneous injection serves a more limited but still important role in drug delivery for pediatric care.

▶ ANATOMY AND PHYSIOLOGY

Site selection for intramuscular injection involves several considerations. The site should avoid major nerves and blood vessels. The muscle mass should be large enough to allow retention and absorption of the injected drug, and anatomic landmarks used for injection should remain consistent from patient to patient. In children, the four sites for intramuscular injection are the anterolateral thigh (vastus lateralis muscle), the ventrogluteal area (gluteus medius muscle), the upper arm (deltoid muscle), and the buttock (gluteus maximus muscle) (Fig. 120.1). Site preference depends on age and nutrition status of the child, as shown in Table 120.1 (2). Malnour-

ished children may have decreased muscle mass at one or more injection sites and therefore require special consideration.

Intramuscular injection creates a depot for drug absorption from the muscle into the systemic circulation. However, this route does not always ensure rapid or complete bioavailability. Absorption depends on the lipophilic properties and concentration of the drug, on the total surface area available, and on blood flow at the injection site. Absorption varies by injection site: it is most rapid from the deltoid muscle, slowest from the gluteal muscles, and intermediate from the vastus lateralis muscle (3). Injected drug absorption increases with exercise and decreases or stops with circulatory disturbances such as shock, hypotension, congestive heart failure, and myxedema.

Intramuscular injection presents the delivered drug as a potential antigen to macrophages and T cells within the muscle. Furthermore, intramuscular injection causes tissue injury, which leads to a migration of many inflammatory cells of different types to the area. As a result, an amnestic response may occur within T lymphocytes, leading to a type IV immunologic response after re-exposure to the drug. Thus, intramuscular injection may predispose an individual to hypersensitivity and allergic reactions to the drugs received.

Intramuscular injection causes direct tissue injury and pain. Muscle enzymes (aspartate transaminase, creatine phosphokinase) are elevated by injection. This is especially true when large volumes are used, when the drug is intrinsically irritating, and when the pH of the injectant is far from physiologic range (3). Inadvertent injection into an artery or vein compounds the potential for tissue injury. Arterial injection may cause subsequent vasospasm and potential drug toxicity in the distal tissues. Arterial or venous injection also carries the risk of untoward systemic effects with certain agents, such as

1113

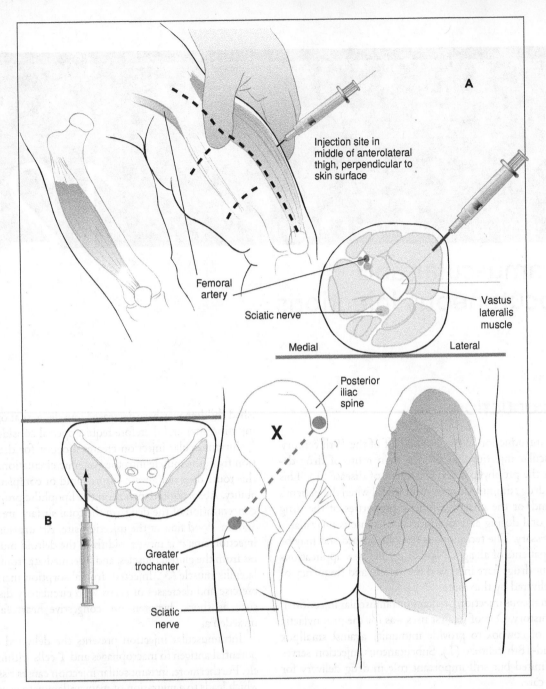

Figure 120.1 Intramuscular injection sites.

A. Anterolateral thigh (vastus lateralis muscle). Technique: Pinch the muscle belly (not the skin) with free hand if necessary to stabilize and expose more muscular mass. Insert the needle 90 degrees to the skin in the anterolateral aspect of the thigh, at the junction of the middle and distal thirds, at an angle of 45 degrees to the long axis of the thigh.

B. Dorsogluteal (maximus, medius, minimus gluteal muscles). Technique: With the patient prone, locate the head of the greater trochanter of the femur and the posterior iliac spine. The line between these two points divides the gluteal area into upper outer and lower inner portions. Insert the needle superior and lateral to this line, at approximately halfway between the two anatomical points mentioned. The needle must go in perpendicular to the stretcher, not to the patient's skin.

C. Upper lateral arm (deltoid muscle). Technique: Expose the arm from the shoulder to the elbow. Pinch the deltoid muscle belly (not the skin) with free hand if necessary to stabilize and expose more muscular mass. Insert the needle perpendicular to the skin at a point halfway from the acromion process of the scapula to the deltoid tuberosity of the humerus.

D. Ventrogluteal (gluteus medius, tensor fasciae latae muscles) (von Hochstetter's site). Technique: Locate the anterior iliac spine with left index finger on the right side of the patient, or vice versa. Extend the middle finger of the same hand to the most superior point of the iliac crest forming a triangle between these two fingers and the iliac crest. Insert the needle in the center of the triangle perpendicular to the skin.

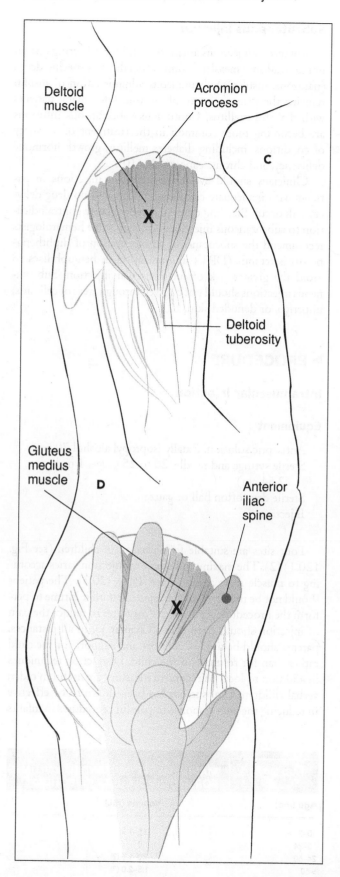

| TABLE 120.1 | PREFERRED INJECTION SITES |

Age (y) or clinical status	Sites (muscle)*
<2	Anterior lateral thigh (vastus lateralis)
	Ventral gluteal (gluteus medius)
2–10	Anterior lateral thigh
	Ventral gluteal
	Upper arm (deltoid)
>10	Upper arm
	Anterior lateral thigh
	Ventral gluteal
	Dorsal gluteal (gluteus maximus)
Malnourished	Anterior lateral thigh
	Ventral gluteal

* Sites listed in descending order of preference.

lidocaine. Table 120.2 lists drugs commonly injected via the intramuscular route and their potential for tissue injury.

The goal of subcutaneous injection is to deliver the drug into the adipose tissue, which lies below the dermis layer of the skin and above the muscle layer. The optimal sites for this

Route/agent	Pain	Tissue injury
Intramuscular administration		
Vaccines		
Acellular DPT	++	+
Hepatitis B	+	+
Haemophilus influenzae type B conjugate vaccine	+	+
Pneumococcal conjugate vaccine	+	+
Antibiotics		
Penicillin g procaine	+++	++
Penicillin g benzathine	+++	++
Ceftriaxone	++++	++
Ampicillin sodium	++	+
Analgesics		
Morphine sulfate	+	+
Hydromorphone hydrochloride	+	+
Anticonvulsants		
Phenobarbital sodium	+	+
Midazolam	+	+
Sedation medications		
Ketamine	+	+
Diphenhydramine hydrochloride	+	+
Haloperidol	+	+
Antidote/other emergency		
Epinephrine	+++	+
Naloxone hydrochloride	+	+
Atropine sulfate	+	++
Pralidoxime	+	++
Subcutaneous administration		
Insulin	+	+
Morphine sulfate	+	+
MMR	++	++

task are the upper lateral shoulder, the anterior thighs, and the abdomen, because they have a relative abundance of fat and few surface veins. The adipose layer has a smaller blood supply relative to the muscle layer; therefore, drug absorption after subcutaneous injection is less consistent and slower than after intramuscular injection. Drugs given subcutaneously, such as growth hormone and insulin, are best absorbed from the abdomen, followed by the arms, thighs, and buttocks (4,5). The potential for allergic reactions and tissue injury discussed above for intramuscular injections also exists, although to a lesser extent, in the case of subcutaneous injections. Table 120.2 also lists the agents commonly delivered by subcutaneous injection.

▶ INDICATIONS

Intramuscular Injection

Common reasons for using intramuscular injections in the ambulatory setting include immunization, infectious prophylaxis, treatment of existing infection, pain management, and sedation (Table 120.2). The need for intramuscular epinephrine to treat anaphylaxis and the need for intramuscular anticonvulsants for prolonged seizures in patients in whom intravenous access cannot be obtained are two emergency indications for intramuscular injection (6,7). This route of drug delivery ensures compliance and avoids first-pass metabolism. With some infectious diseases (e.g., streptococcal pharyngitis and certain gonococcal infections), a single intramuscular shot of antibiotic has proven as efficacious as a multiple-day, orally administered drug regimen (8,9). Potential advantages of intramuscular drug administration, however, should be weighed against the pain of the procedure and potential risks of local injury and allergic reaction when used in the outpatient setting. Intramuscular injections should be avoided in patients with bleeding dyscrasias and circulatory instability. Hematoma formation and hemorrhage can cause extensive local tissue damage in patients with hemophilia, thrombocytopenia, von Willebrand disease, disseminated intravascular coagulation, and other clotting disorders. In addition, patients in shock do not absorb drugs well from intramuscular injections and may suffer complications from erratic drug delivery.

Intramuscular injections should not be given near cutaneous vascular malformations because these sites increase the risk of inadvertent intravascular injection. Injection through denuded skin or near a skin infection (impetigo, cellulitis) risks internal spread of a local infection. Drugs that have a high likelihood of precipitation at the site and incomplete bioavailability should not be administered. Phenytoin and digoxin, for example, are not recommended for injection for this reason. Other drugs that precipitate to varying degrees at the injection site include ampicillin, diazepam, and quinidine (3).

Subcutaneous Injection

Subcutaneous injections are most useful for delivering certain immunizations (measles, mumps, rubella) and specific drugs (naloxone, insulin). Subcutaneous administration of insulin remains the primary route of treatment for many patients with diabetes mellitus. Continuous subcutaneous infusions are becoming more common in the treatment of a variety of conditions, including diabetes mellitus, growth hormone deficiency, and chronic cancer pain (10).

Clinicians should avoid subcutaneous injections in patients with inadequate circulation, as little to no drug delivery will occur. Bleeding dyscrasias are a relative contraindication to subcutaneous injection, although some hematologists recommend the subcutaneous administration of diphtheria-pertussis-tetanus (DPT) immunization in hemophiliacs to avoid the greater risk of intramuscular injection. Subcutaneous injections should not be given through areas of cellulitis, impetigo, or denuded skin.

▶ PROCEDURE

Intramuscular Injection

Equipment

> Antiseptic solution, usually isopropyl alcohol 70%
> Sterile syringe and needle, 20 to 25 gauge, 1 inch (2.54 cm)
> Sterile dry cotton ball or gauze
> Injectant

Four sites are suitable for injection in children (see Fig. 120.1) (2). The maximum volume of injection varies according to muscle mass and age (see Table 120.3). The patient should not be informed of the injection until it is time to perform the procedure. Appropriate measures to reduce the pain of injection should commence (Chapter 1). In all instances, parents should be used as comfort and support for the child rather than for restraint of the child. Distraction techniques in addition to local pain control measures are useful in older, verbal children. Oral sucrose has been shown to be effective in reducing the pain response to painful procedures in infants

TABLE 120.3	MAXIMUM RECOMMENDED VOLUMES FOR INTRAMUSCULAR INJECTION
Age (mo)	**Volume (mL)**
0–3	0.5–1.0
3–24	1.0
24–60	1.0–1.5 (?)
>60	1.5–2.0 (?)

Note: Reduced volumes are indicated for patients with decreased muscle mass.

SUMMARY: INTRAMUSCULAR INJECTION

1 Provide pain reduction and distraction techniques.

2 Draw up the injectant using a large-gauge (18 to 21) needle out of view of the patient.

3 Remove the large needle and attach the injecting needle; ensure that the needle is tightly connected to syringe hub.

4 Remove remaining air from the syringe.

5 Restrain the patient as appropriate.

6 Cleanse the skin with an antiseptic solution and allow it to dry.

7 Quickly insert the needle down to the muscle (hub of the syringe at the skin surface) and aspirate to ensure that the needle is not in a blood vessel. In smaller children, first bunch the deltoid or anterolateral thigh muscle mass by pinching the muscle belly (not the skin), as necessary.

8 Inject the solution and remove the needle.

9 Apply a cotton ball or gauze over the site with moderate pressure.

CLINICAL TIPS: INTRAMUSCULAR INJECTION

▶ The drug should be appropriate for the intramuscular route.

▶ The patient should be assessed for contraindications to the procedure (bleeding dyscrasia, cellulitis).

▶ Techniques should be used to reduce psychological stress and pain.

▶ A safe age-appropriate site should be chosen (Table 120.1).

▶ Needles should be switched after drawing up the injectant.

▶ The smallest diameter needle that will permit free flow of the injectant should be used (not less than 25 gauge to ensure aspiration of blood if a vein or artery is inadvertently entered).

▶ An appropriate needle length should be used (usually 7/8 of an inch to 1 inch, although longer for obese or adolescent patients).

▶ The antiseptic should be dry before the skin is penetrated.

▶ The injection solution should be warmed to room temperature.

▶ In smaller children with little deltoid or anterolateral thigh muscle mass, first pinching the muscle belly may assist intramuscular positioning of the needle tip.

▶ The needle should be inserted quickly through the skin to minimize pain.

▶ The plunger of the syringe should not be depressed during needle insertion.

▶ Aspiration for blood before injection ensures the needle is not in a blood vessel.

▶ Slow and steady injection reduces pain.

▶ Irritating injectants (e.g., ceftriaxone) may be mixed with 1 mL of 1% lidocaine before injection.

▶ Alternating sites for subsequent injections reduces the risk of muscle contractures.

▶ Premature infants, young infants, and malnourished infants or children deserve extra caution.

(II). The injectant is drawn up, out of view of the patient, using a large needle (18 to 21 gauge). The large needle is removed, and an injecting needle (23 to 25 gauge) is attached to the syringe. The injecting needle is tightly connected to the syringe hub to avoid leakage of the drug during injection. Air should be expelled from the syringe with the needle pointing upward. The need for the injection should be explained in an age-appropriate fashion. The patient is restrained as appropriate for age (Chapter 3), and the skin cleansed with an antiseptic solution, which is allowed to dry.

A site is selected that has no visible superficial veins, no cutaneous vascular malformations, no signs of trauma, and no signs of infection or inflammation. For deltoid and anterolateral thigh injections in younger children, the muscle belly may be bunched up by pinching with the nondominant hand to stabilize and expose more muscle mass, but care should be taken to avoid pinching skin and subcutaneous tissue inadvertently, and thus converting an intended intramuscular injection into an unintended subcutaneous one. The needle is quickly inserted down to the muscle (the hub of the syringe should be at the skin surface) and aspirated to ensure that the needle is not in a blood vessel. The direction and angle of the needle depends on the intramuscular site chosen (see Fig. 120.1A–D). The solution is injected slowly and the needle removed. A cotton ball or gauze is then applied over the site with moderate pressure.

Subcutaneous Injection

Equipment

Antiseptic solution, usually isopropyl alcohol 70%
Sterile tuberculin or insulin syringe with 27-gauge, 0.5-inch needle
Sterile dry cotton ball or gauze
Injectant

The injection should not be discussed with the child until just before it is administered. The needle should be tightly connected to the syringe. The injectant is drawn up in the syringe out of view of the patient. Measures to reduce pain should be applied (Chapter 35). In all instances, parents should be used as comfort and support for the child rather than for restraint of the child. Distraction techniques in addition to local pain control measures are useful in older, verbal children. Oral sucrose has been shown to be effective in reducing the pain response to painful procedures in infants (11). Next the need for the injection is explained in an age-appropriate fashion. A site is selected (upper outer arm, lateral thigh, or abdomen) that has no visible superficial veins, no cutaneous vascular malformations, no signs of trauma, and no signs of infection or inflammation (Fig. 120.2). The skin is cleansed with an antiseptic solution, which is allowed to dry. In thinner children, the skin and subcutaneous tissue may be bunched up by pinching with the nondominant hand

---

CLINICAL TIPS: SUBCUTANEOUS INJECTION

▶ Psychological stress may be avoided with a variety of distraction techniques.

▶ Topical pain relievers may reduce or eliminate the discomfort of the procedure.

▶ Overlying blood vessels must be avoided.

▶ Quick needle insertion reduces pain.

▶ In thinner children, first bunching the skin and subcutaneous tissue by pinching the site may help avoid inadvertent intramuscular injection.

▶ Rotating injection sites prevents lipodystrophy, lipoatrophy, and subcutaneous nodules or scarring.

---

to minimize the risk of unintended intramuscular injection. The needle is quickly inserted into the subcutaneous layer at a 45-degree angle to the skin. After aspiration to ensure there is no blood return, the drug is injected and the needle withdrawn. A gauze or cotton ball is applied to the site until bleeding stops.

▶ COMPLICATIONS

Complications following intramuscular injection arise from the needle wound, incorrect technique, and the substance delivered to the tissue. In one multihospital study of 12,123 patients who received intramuscular injections, the local complication rate was 0.4%, with abscess formation being most frequent complication (12). Most information derives from case reports that highlight the serious potential for injury but provide no incidence data for each complication. Main complications arising from the needle wound are infection and inadvertent puncture of vital structures. Reports exist of cellulitis with abscess formation (staphylococcal, clostridial, and sterile), clostridial myositis, and frank gangrene associated with intramuscular injections (13–15). Using sterile disposable needles, giving attention to site cleansing before the procedure, and avoiding sites with adjacent infection usually will prevent such complications.

Repetitive injections can cause muscle contracture, permanent muscle fibrosis, and intramuscular hemorrhage with hematoma formation despite correct technique. Rotating injection sites in children who receive multiple injections and avoiding obviously traumatized areas prevent these complications (16,17).

Permanent nerve injury and intra-arterial injection with vascular damage necessitating skin grafting or limb amputation have occurred from incorrect needle positioning before

---

SUMMARY: SUBCUTANEOUS INJECTION

1 Provide pain reduction and distraction techniques.

2 Draw up the injectant using a 27-gauge, 0.5-inch needle out of view of the patient; ensure that a tight connection exists between the needle and syringe.

3 Remove remaining air from the syringe.

4 Restrain the patient as appropriate.

5 Choose an injection site with no overlying superficial veins or vascular malformations.

6 Cleanse the skin with an antiseptic solution and allow it to dry.

7 Quickly insert the needle at a 45-degree angle through the skin down to the hub of the syringe. Aspirate to ensure no blood return. In thinner children, first bunch the skin and subcutaneous tissue by pinching the site, as necessary.

8 Inject the solution and remove the needle.

9 Apply a cotton ball or gauze over the site with moderate pressure.

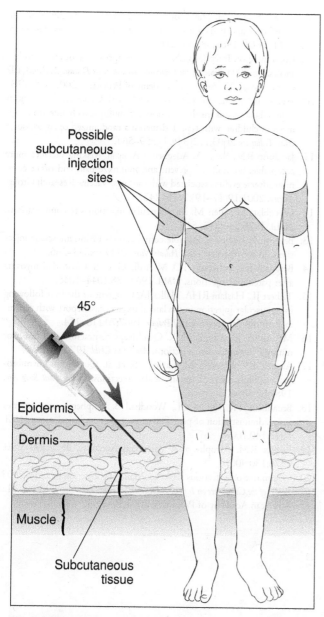

Possible subcutaneous injection sites

45°

Epidermis

Dermis

Muscle

Subcutaneous tissue

Figure 120.2 Subcutaneous injection.

injection. Premature or small infants and malnourished children are at particular risk for these dreaded complications. Needle aspiration before injection and adherence to suggested injection sites, needle length, and injectant volumes will prevent these rare but potentially disastrous outcomes.

Of the four intramuscular sites, the dorsal gluteal area most often is associated with significant nerve or vascular injury. The most frequent complication at this site is sciatic nerve injury, but superior gluteal nerve damage, posterior femoral cutaneous nerve damage, and pudendal nerve damage have been reported from injections at this site (16). In the upper arm, radial nerve injuries result from injections to the lower portion of the proximal third of the arm, and axillary nerve damage has followed deltoid injection with excessively long

needles (18). The lateral thigh and ventral gluteal regions appear to be safer for injection than the upper arm and dorsal gluteal area. However, femoral artery thrombosis in an infant has been reported after an intramuscular injection in the anterolateral thigh with a longer needle than recommended (15). No neuromuscular complications have yet been reported from the ventral gluteal area.

Inadvertent subcutaneous injection can cause a large red site of inflammation as the injected drug spreads through the subcutaneous layer. Differentiation between subcutaneous injection and cellulitis may be difficult. Subsequent lipodystrophy and skin pigmentation can occur, depending on the irritative characteristics of the injectant (19). This complication often follows injection with a short needle, drug delivery during the initial skin puncture, and early withdrawal of the needle while drug is still being injected.

Intramuscular drug injection can also create a significant immunologic response that predisposes patients to severe allergic reactions and anaphylaxis. Allergic reactions to drugs are unpredictable. For this reason, *all* children receiving intramuscular injections on an outpatient basis should be observed for a minimum of 30 minutes following injection to ensure no signs of an acute allergic response appear before discharge.

Pain is an unavoidable adverse effect of an intramuscular injection. Immediate pain, however, can be minimized by preparing the child psychologically, administering local anesthesia at the site, using distraction techniques in the older child, and performing rapid skin puncture. With current recommendations, some children are receiving up to 5 intramuscular immunizations at a single well child visit. Every attempt to reduce the pain of injection is warranted in these patients. Additionally, measures to reduce pain and anxiety include simultaneous injection of multiple vaccines, positioning of the limb to induce muscle relaxation, and Z-tracking of the immunization (see Fig. 86.3) (20). Delayed pain can be due to (a) aseptic irritation and necrosis, which varies in degree with the different substances given; (b) an immune response to the injectant; (c) infection; or (d) muscle spasm. Of these, only avoidance of infection is within control of the care provider. Pretreatment with acetaminophen or a nonsteroidal anti-inflammatory drug 30 minutes before injection may blunt the delayed pain due to tissue reaction.

Compared with intramuscular injection, complications of subcutaneous injection are less severe. Local infection, allergic reaction, and abscess may occur, but muscle contracture, intra-arterial injection, and nerve injury are highly unlikely due to the shorter needle used and the recommended sites of injection. Untoward systemic effects may follow inadvertent intravenous injection. Care should be taken to avoid superficial veins when performing a subcutaneous injection. Finally, subcutaneous nodules and scarring may form after repetitive subcutaneous injections to a particular site. These nodules may alter the absorption of the drug. This problem is most frequent in diabetics who do not carefully rotate sites. In these patients, insulin injection into subcutaneous nodules hampers insulin delivery to the circulation, resulting in poor glucose homeostasis. Rotating injection sites and avoiding pre-existing scars prevent this complication.

▶ SUMMARY

Intramuscular and subcutaneous injection of substances is commonly performed in a variety of clinical settings. With knowledge of technique, the procedures are straightforward and cause minimal complications. Small infants and malnourished children are more prone to adverse effects and require special care when receiving injections.

▶ REFERENCES

1. Howard-Jones N. The origin of hypodermic medication. *Sci Am.* 1971;224:96–102.
2. Bergson P, Standford S, Kaplan A. Intramuscular injections in children. *Pediatrics.* 1982;70:944–948.
3. Greenblatt DJ, Koch-Weser J. Drug therapy: intramuscular injection of drug. *N Engl J Med.* 1976;295:542–546.
4. Beshyah SA, Anyaoku V, Niththyananthan R, et al. The effect of subcutaneous injection site on absorption of human growth hormone: abdomen versus thigh. *Clin Endocrinol.* 1991;35:409–412.
5. Bantle JP, Weber MS, Rao S, et al. Rotation of the anatomic regions used for insulin injections and day-to-day variability of plasma glucose in type I diabetic subjects. *JAMA.* 1990;263:1802–1806.
6. Lieberman P. Use of epinephrine in the treatment of anaphylaxis. *Curr Opin Allergy Clin Immunol.* 2003;3:313–318.
7. Rey E, Treluyer JM, Pons G. Pharmacokinetic optimization of benzodiazepine therapy for acute seizures: focus on delivery routes. *Clin Pharmacokinet.* 1999;36:409–424.
8. Rajan VS, Sng EH, Thirumorthy T, et al. Ceftriaxone in the treatment of ordinary and penicillinase-producing strains of *Neisseria gonorrhoeae.* *Br J Vener Dis.* 1982;58:314–316.
9. Committee on Infectious Diseases. Appropriate use of antimicrobial agents. In: *2003 Report of the Committee on Infectious Disease.* 26th ed. Elk Grove Village, IL; American Academy of Pediatrics; 2003:695–718.
10. Weintrob N, Benzaquen H, Galatzer A, et al. Comparison of continuous subcutaneous insulin infusion and multiple daily injection regimens in children with type I diabetes: a randomized open crossover trial. *Pediatrics.* 2003;112[3 Pt I]:559–564.
11. Jacobson RM, Swan A, Adegbenro A, et al. Making vaccines more acceptable: methods to prevent and minimize pain and other common adverse events associated with vaccines. Vaccine Research Group. *Vaccine.* 2001;19(17–19):2418–2427.
12. Greenblatt D, Allen M. Intramuscular injection site complications. *JAMA.* 1978;240:542–544.
13. Beecroft P, Redick S. Possible complications of intramuscular injections on the pediatric unit. *Pediatr Nurs.* 1989;15:333–336.
14. Berggren RB, Batterton TD, McArdle G, et al. Clostridial myositis after parenteral injections. *JAMA.* 1964;188:1044–1048.
15. Talbert JL, Haslam RHA, Haller JA. Gangrene of the foot following intramuscular injection in the lateral thigh: a case report with recommendations for prevention. *J Pediatr.* 1967;70:110–114.
16. McCloskey JR, Chung SMK. Quadriceps contracture as a result of multiple intramuscular injections. *Am J Dis Child.* 1970;131:416.
17. Alvarez EV, Munters M, Lavine LS, et al. Quadriceps myofibrosis: a complication of intramuscular injections. *J Bone Joint Surg Am.* 1980;62:58–60.
18. Broadbent TR, Odom GL, Woodhall B. Peripheral nerve injuries from administration of penicillin: report of four clinical cases. *JAMA.* 1948;140:1008.
19. Buchta RM. Atrophy after parenteral injection. *Am J Dis Child.* 1976;130:900.
20. Committee on Infectious Diseases. Managing injection pain. In: *2003 Report of the Committee on Infectious Disease.* 26th ed. Elk Grove Village, IL: American Academy of Pediatrics; 2003:20–21.

MICHELE McKEE AND FRED M. HENRETIG

121

Use of Atropine and Pralidoxime Autoinjectors

▶ INTRODUCTION

Military chemical weapons of the nerve agent type are currently considered a significant terrorist threat to civilian populations worldwide in the aftermath of the Tokyo sarin attack in 1995 by a religious extremist cult and, of course, the incidents of September 11, 2001, and the subsequent intentional mail-borne anthrax outbreak in the United States in October 2001. The Iraqi chemical weapons attacks on the Kurdish population of northern Iraq in the late 1980s are believed to have involved numerous pediatric victims. Children may be victims of terrorism as well, as was witnessed in the 1995 Oklahoma City bombing. The potential use of such potent poisons as terrorist weapons has resulted in the search for management strategies that would allow for the rapid treatment of mass casualties resulting from exposure to these agents (1,2).

▶ PATHOPHYSIOLOGY

Nerve agents are organophosphorus compounds that act as potent inhibitors of acetylcholinesterase, similarly to organophosphate pesticides (3–5). After exposure, the inhibition of these agents becomes irreversible after a variable period of time, a process termed "aging." Four compounds are currently recognized as military nerve agents: tabun, sarin, soman, and VX ("Venom X"). With soman, aging occurs within minutes, while with the others, it takes several hours. This is relevant because, in a mass casualty scenario, rapidly treating large numbers of critical patients in the field or soon after arrival at a hospital may result in many lives saved and considerably less long-term morbidity if treatment can be provided prior to the onset of the aging phenomenon.

Nerve agent–induced anticholinesterase inhibition results in the accumulation of acetylcholine at neural junctions, resulting initially in stimulation of cholinergic transmission. However, the impact on the neuromuscular junction of somatic nerves is relatively unique, with initial stimulation followed shortly by paralysis. In addition to the neuromuscular junction, cholinergic synapses are found in the central nervous system (CNS); several autonomic sites, including both sympathetic and parasympathetic nerve endings; and sympathetic and parasympathetic ganglia. The resulting cholinergic syndrome is classically divided into central, nicotinic (neuromuscular junction and sympathetic ganglia), and muscarinic (smooth muscle and exocrine gland) effects.

The clinical presentation for a given patient will depend on the dose and route of exposure (3,4). Children may be more susceptible due to heavier exposure (living "closer to the ground"; all nerve agents are heavier than air), higher minute ventilation, and possibly greater susceptibility to CNS manifestations (1,6–8).

With low-dose vapor exposures, toxic manifestations include eye findings, particularly dimmed vision and miosis, as well as rhinorrhea, mild dyspnea, and wheezing. As the dose increases, more severe respiratory effects, nausea, vomiting, and muscle weakness are expected. Exposure to very high vapor concentrations results in rapid onset of paralysis and seizures; death due to respiratory arrest may occur within minutes.

▶ INDICATIONS

Diagnosis of nerve agent toxicity is primarily achieved by clinical recognition and response to antidotal therapy. The overall

1121

treatment approach for these agents should focus on airway and ventilatory support, aggressive use of antidotes, prompt control of seizures with a benzodiazepine (or even empiric benzodiazepine therapy in severe cases before seizures have occurred), and decontamination as necessary (see also Chapter 128). Atropine, in relatively large doses, is used for its antimuscarinic effects, and pralidoxime chloride (2-PAM) serves to reactivate of acetylcholinesterase if aging has not yet occurred. Atropine counteracts bronchospasm and excess bronchial secretions, bradycardia, the gastrointestinal effects of nausea, vomiting, diarrhea, and cramps and may lessen seizure activity. However, atropine does not improve skeletal muscle paralysis. 2-PAM dissociates organophosphate from the cholinesterase, and its effects are observed predominantly at the neuromuscular junction, with improved muscle strength. The recommended initial dose of atropine is 0.05 mg/kg (minimum dose 0.1 mg, maximum 5 mg) administered intravenously or intramuscularly for moderate to severe toxicity, which can be repeated every 2 to 5 minutes as needed until bronchospasm and excess respiratory secretions are relieved. 2-PAM in doses of 25 mg/kg administered intravenously or intramuscularly (maximum dose 1 g intravenously, 2 g intramuscularly) is recommended promptly in all serious cases, along with concomitant atropine treatment. This can be repeated in 30 to 60 minutes for severe cases and then again every hour for 1 to 2 additional doses in cases with persistent weakness or high atropine requirement.

In individual cases of severe organophosphate poisoning, atropine and 2-PAM are optimally administered intravenously. However, animal data suggest that intravenous atropine may provoke arrhythmias in hypoxic animals, and so hypoxia should be corrected, if possible; otherwise intramuscular use is preferable initially (4). In all cases, the intramuscular route is acceptable if intravenous access is not readily available, which might be of considerable relevance in a pediatric mass casualty incident.

▶ EQUIPMENT

Autoinjectors of atropine and pralidoxime, 10-cc sterile saline vial, emptied
Filter needle
3-cc syringe
23- or 25-gauge needle for injection

Most U.S. emergency medical services teams now stock intramuscular autoinjectors of atropine and 2-PAM. These are spring-loaded injector devices that can be easily used by both medical and nonmedical personnel. Many clinicians are familiar with this technology, which is used in an epinephrine autoinjector, or "EpiPen." Such autoinjectors inject medications more forcefully than traditional syringe and needle intramuscular injections, with an enhanced rate of absorption (2-PAM) and onset of clinical effects (atropine) observed

| TABLE 121.1 | USE OF ATROPINE AND PRALIDOXIME AUTOINJECTORS: SUGGESTED INITIAL DOSES FOR NERVE AGENT VICTIMS |

Atropine dosing (1 injector of each appropriate size)*

Age	Weight	Autoinjector size
<6 mo	<15 lb (<7 kg)	0.25 mg
6 mo–4 y	15–40 lb (7–18 kg)	0.5 mg
5–10 y	41–90 lb (18–41 kg)	1 mg
>10 y	>90 lbs (>41 kg)	2 mg

Pralidoxime dosing (using 600-mg adult-intended injectors)†

Age	Weight	No. of autoinjectors	Pralidoxime (dose range in mg/kg)
3–7 y	13–25 kg	1	24–46
8–14 y	26–50 kg	2	24–46
>14 y	>51 kg	3	35 or less

* FDA guidelines list the doses by weight in pounds.
†Pediatric autoinjectors of pralidoxime are not FDA approved or available at this time. While not approved for pediatric use, the 600-mg adult-sized pralidoxime autoinjector might be considered as initial treatment in dire (especially prehospital) circumstances for children with severe, life-threatening nerve agent toxicity who lack intravenous access and for whom more precise milligrams-per-kilogram intramuscular dosing would be logistically impossible. Suggested dosing guidelines are offered; note potential excess of the initial pralidoxime dose for age or weight, although within general guidelines for the recommended total over the first 60 to 90 minutes of therapy for severe exposures. Adapted from Henretig FM, Cieslak TJ, Madsen JM, et al. Emergency department awareness and response to incidents of biological and chemical terrorism. In: Fleisher GF, Ludwig S, Henretig FM, eds. *Textbook of Pediatric Emergency Medicine.* 5th ed. Philadelphia: Lippincott Williams & Wilkins; 2006:135–162.

(9–12). Currently, there is little clinical experience to draw from regarding the efficacy of autoinjector therapy for mass casualty exposures to a nerve agent, let alone specific pediatric experience. However, in dire circumstances, these autoinjectors would seem to offer an optimal route of rapid antidote administration in children. An atropine autoinjector (AtroPen) has recently been approved by the U.S. Food and Drug Administration (FDA) for pediatric use in just this context and is manufactured in 0.25-, 0.5-, and 1-mg doses in addition to the adult-sized dose of 2 mg (Table 121.1). The AtroPen delivers one dose only in a total volume of up to 0.7 mL and is nonrefillable. It employs a 22-gauge needle that delivers the atropine in a circular field of distribution with a 0.2- to 0.78-inch depth of insertion. The adult-intended 2-PAM autoinjector contains 600 mg in a 2-mL volume.

▶ PROCEDURE

In mass casualty situations, prior skin preparation is not necessary. The autoinjector can even be used through outer clothing. It is deployed by removing the safety cap and then applying it with firm pressure at a 90-degree angle to the anterolateral aspect (vastus lateralis muscle) of the midthigh (Fig. 121.1). The needle will automatically extend and begin the injection. Steady pressure should be held for 10 seconds to allow for

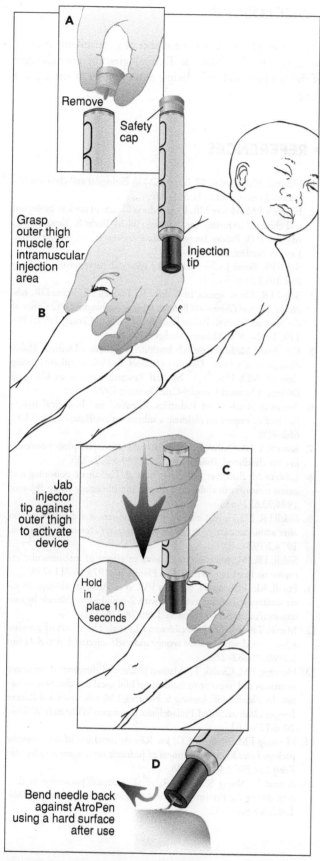

Figure 121.1 AtroPen 0.25-mg autoinjector.

complete emptying of the canister. In small or thin infants, the muscle mass itself may be grasped and bunched up to provide a thicker area of injection, although pinching of skin and subcutaneous tissue, resulting in conversion of the intended intramuscular injection to a subcutaneous one, must be avoided. The needle remains visible after the drug is dispensed and should be disposed of carefully. Military doctrine recommends that the needle be bent back and then used to pin the empty canister through a soldier's uniform as a means of recording administered dose, but in civilian mass casualty scenarios this practice might result in subsequent health care provider needle stick injury and thus should be approached cautiously.

Pediatric-sized 2-PAM autoinjectors are not currently available, but these are expected to win FDA approval in the foreseeable future. Even the adult-intended 2-PAM injectors (600 mg) might be useful in children over 2 to 3 years of age or 13 kg in weight (see Table 121.1) (13). If 2-PAM injectors are used, they should probably be administered away from the site of atropine injection, as there may be slowed atropine absorption with concomitant 2-PAM injection at the same site (10,11). For infants, one might consider using the adult pralidoxime autoinjector as a convenient source of concentrated (300 mg/mL) pralidoxime solution suitable for syringe or needle intramuscular injection. This can be effected by discharging the contents of one or more autoinjectors into an emptied 10-cc sterile saline vial and then withdrawing the solution through a filter needle into syringes suitable for small-volume intramuscular injections (Chapter 120) (14). Repeat doses of both atropine and 2-PAM can be administered as needed, within established guidelines (see Table 121.1).

SUMMARY

1. In critical nerve agent–poisoned children, consider emergent therapy with autoinjected atropine and 2-PAM as well as a benzodiazepine.

2. In mass casualty scenarios, the autoinjectors may be deployed without skin preparation and even through outer clothing.

3. Remove the autoinjector safety cap.

4. Place the autoinjector perpendicular to the anterolateral midthigh surface and press firmly for 10 seconds.

5. Carefully dispose of the empty canister and exposed needle.

6. Give repeat doses as needed (Table 121.1).

7. Inject atropine and 2-PAM in separate sites if possible.

CLINICAL TIPS

▶ In small, thin infants, muscle mass (not just skin and subcutaneous tissue!) may be grasped and bunched up to allow a thicker injection site.

▶ Used autoinjectors may be pinned to a patient's clothing after the needle is bent back as a field expedient way of containing the device and accounting for dose administration, but caution is necessary to avoid inadvertent needle stick injuries.

▶ Adult-intended autoinjectors can used in children in dire circumstances, particularly those over 2 to 3 years of age and 13 kg in weight (Table 121.1).

▶ Adult-intended 2-PAM autoinjectors can serve as a convenient source of concentrated 2-PAM for use in syringe and needle injection into young infants.

▶ COMPLICATIONS

Israel has for some years provided autoinjectors of atropine and an oxime similar to 2-PAM to all its citizens, intended for self-use in a wartime or terrorist context. During the 1990–1991 Gulf War, 240 Israeli children were evaluated for accidental autoinjection of atropine, none of whom were exposed to a nerve agent (15). The doses encountered were as high as 17 times the dose recommended for age. Systemic anticholinergic effects occurred in nearly half of victims, but seizures, severe dysrhythmias, and deaths did not occur. Thus, autoinjected atropine, even in excess dosage and in the absence of nerve agent toxicity, was fairly well tolerated in this pediatric cohort.

▶ SUMMARY

Autoinjectors provide a convenient and likely safe and effective route of critical nerve agent antidote administration. Although never tested in a pediatric mass casualty scenario, most authorities would recommend their use for such an incident were it ever to occur, and atropine autoinjectors are now available and FDA-approved for just such an indication in pediatric sizes. The potential use of adult-intended 2-PAM autoinjectors is also discussed and recommended for severely affected children over 2 to 3 years of age or 13 kg in weight. It is possible that 2-PAM autoinjectors will also become available in pediatric sizes.

▶ DISCLOSURE

Dr. Henretig has served as a member of a consultant advisory board to Meridian Medical Technologies, the manufacturer of the atropine and pralidoxime autoinjectors in the United States.

▶ REFERENCES

1. Henretig FM, Cieslak TJ, Eitzen EM Jr. Biological and chemical terrorism. *J Pediatr.* 2002;141:311–326.
2. Henretig FM, McKee MR. Preparedness for acts of nuclear, biological and chemical terrorism. In: Gausche-Hill M, Fuchs S, Yamamoto L, eds. *APLS: The Pediatric Emergency Medicine Resource.* 4th ed. Sudbury, MA: Jones & Bartlett; 2004:568–591.
3. Sidell FR, Borak J. Chemical warfare agents, II: nerve agents. *Ann Emerg Med.* 1992;21:865–871.
4. Sidell FR. Nerve agents. In: Sidell FR, Takafuji ET, Franz DR, eds. *Medical Aspects of Chemical and Biological Warfare.* Washington, DC: Office of the Surgeon General, Walter Reed Army Medical Center; 1997:129–179. Textbook of Military Medicine No. 8.
5. U.S. Army Medical Research Institute of Chemical Defense. *Medical Management of Chemical Casualties Handbook.* 3rd ed. Aberdeen Proving Ground, MD: U.S. Army Medical Research Institute of Chemical Defense, Chemical Casualty Care Division; 1999.
6. American Academy of Pediatrics. Chemical and biological terrorism and its impact on children: a subject review. *Pediatrics.* 2000;105: 662–670.
7. Sofer S, Tal A, Shahak E. Carbamate and organophosphate poisoning in early childhood. *Pediatr Emerg Care.* 1989;5:222–225.
8. Lifshitz M, Rotenberg M, Sofer S, et al. Carbamate poisoning and oxime treatment in children: a clinical and laboratory study. *Pediatrics.* 1994;93:652–655.
9. Sidell FR, Markis JE, Groff W, et al. Enhancement of drug absorption after administration by an automatic injector. *J Pharmacokinet Biopharm.* 1974;2:197–210.
10. Sidell, FR. Modification by diluents of effects of intramuscular atropine on heart rate in man. *Clin Pharm Ther.* 1974;16:711–715.
11. Friedl, KE, Hannan CJ, Schadler PW, et al. Atropine absorption after intramuscular administration with 2-pralidoxime chloride by two autoinjector devices. *J Pharm Sci.* 1989;78:728–731.
12. Martin TR, Kastor JA, Kershbaum KL, et al. The effects of atropine administered with standard syringe and a self-injector device. *Am Heart J.* 1980;99:282–288.
13. Henretig FM, Cieslak TJ, Madsen JM, et al. Emergency department awareness and response to incidents of biological and chemical terrorism. In: Fleisher GF, Ludwig S, Henretig FM, eds. *Textbook of Pediatric Emergency Medicine.* 5th ed. Philadelphia: Lippincott Williams & Wilkins; 2006:135–162.
14. Henretig FM, Mechem CC, Jew RK. Potential use of auto-injector packaged antidotes for treatment of pediatric nerve agent toxicity. *Ann Emerg Med.* 2002;40:405–408.
15. Amitai Y, Almog S, Singer R, et al. Atropine poisoning in children during the Persian Gulf crisis: a national survey in Israel. *JAMA.* 1992;268:630–632.

122

LOUIS M. BELL AND NICHOLAS TSAROUHAS

Obtaining Biologic Specimens

▶ INTRODUCTION

Biologic specimens can be an important adjunct to the history and physical examination. Poorly obtained specimens not only may lead to erroneous diagnoses but also may cause undue morbidity. This chapter discusses the indications, materials, procedures, and complications involved in the collection of biologic specimens. The interpretation of these results is also addressed.

▶ BLOOD CULTURES

Blood cultures are the cornerstone to the diagnosis of bacteremia and sepsis. The Gram stain is of controversial benefit (1) and may have no value unless bacteremia is overwhelming (2). Consequently, most institutions do not routinely Gram stain blood specimens. For this reason, it is important to optimize the procedure for obtaining a proper blood culture. Isolation of the offending micro-organism is crucial to diagnosis and management of patients with bloodborne bacterial disease.

Anatomy and Physiology

Peripheral veins are the most common vessels from which blood cultures are drawn. The veins used most often in pediatric blood draws are those in the antecubital fossa. However, because of the occasional difficulty in obtaining blood specimens from young children and infants, other sites also are

frequently used (Chapter 73). Using the femoral vein, located medial to the femoral arterial pulsation and below the inguinal ligament, is sometimes discouraged because of the possible difficulty in appropriately cleaning the site. This difficulty is more of a problem in the adult patient, and therefore this site need not be excluded in the child.

Arteries are equally acceptable sites for blood cultures. The radial artery is most commonly used, but the ulnar, dorsalis pedis, and posterior tibial arteries and even the temporal artery are occasionally used (Chapter 72). In the newborn, the umbilical artery or vein is often used as a site from which to draw blood cultures. These cultures are most helpful if drawn at placement of the line (Chapter 38). Capillary collections are not acceptable as blood culture specimens.

Indications

The obvious indication for drawing a blood culture is a toxic-appearing child. Such patients should always have a blood culture drawn to rule out sepsis. Many additional scenarios, however, deserve special note.

Children with immunodeficiencies obviously are more susceptible to the development of serious bacterial infections. Examples include children with oncologic disease, acquired immunodeficiency syndrome, chronic renal failure, and sickle cell anemia. Patients on immunosuppressive medication also are at higher risk for sepsis. Neonates are immunocompromised by virtue of the immaturity of their immune systems. All febrile infants less than 2 months of age warrant a full sepsis evaluation. Additionally, other signs of illness, such as irritability, lethargy, poor feeding, and apnea, may indicate sepsis. Although fever often is the presenting symptom, it should be noted that some of these children may not have the ability to mount a febrile response. All of these scenarios require increased vigilance with respect to possible sepsis.

Much has been written in the pediatric literature regarding occult bacteremia. It is commonly described as the presence of bacteremia in a well-appearing child (usually less than 2 years of age) with a high fever (usually greater than 39.0°C to 39.4°C). Since routine immunization has been instituted against *Haemophilus influenzae* type b and, more recently, *Streptococcus pneumoniae*, the incidence of occult bacteremia has declined considerably. It is currently estimated to be 1.5% to 2%.

The optimal time to obtain a blood culture is when the micro-organisms are most likely to be recovered from the bloodstream. Although this may occur just before the onset of symptoms (fever, chills), it is obviously impossible to obtain a blood culture before the patient becomes symptomatic. Ideally, the blood culture should be obtained as close to the onset of symptoms as possible (3).

How many cultures are necessary? Li et al. found no significant difference in the yield of blood culture results in studies performed with two sets drawn simultaneously versus those done with an interval of time between them (4). In older infants and children, a single blood culture suffices for the majority of clinical scenarios. In neonates, however, two blood cultures may be beneficial, especially to distinguish between true coagulase-negative staphylococcus sepsis and simple contamination (5).

Endocarditis merits special consideration. In most cases, the bacteremia is continuous and the timing not so important. However, serial cultures may increase the yield and make the diagnosis easier (3). The micro-organisms usually implicated include *Streptococcus viridans*, *Staphylococcus aureus*, *Staphylococcus epidermidis*, and enterococci. Children with congenital heart disease, prosthetic valves, or a history of rheumatic fever are at highest risk. A high degree of suspicion should be maintained in any child with prolonged fever, especially in the presence of a new heart murmur.

Children who have long-term venous access catheters (Broviac or Hickman) and develop fever are commonly admitted to the hospital to rule out "line" infection. Most clinicians prefer peripheral and central venous catheter cultures to help in the management of line infections as well as to distinguish contaminants from true pathogens. Additionally, in immuno-compromised patients, such as those with oncologic diseases, many recommend that cultures be drawn from all lumens of multilumen catheters. It is believed that this increases the sensitivity of the blood culture (6).

Because of the potential seriousness of a line infection, these children are started on presumptive antibiotic therapy until culture results are known. The most common micro-organisms implicated in these infections are the Gram-positives *S. aureus* and *S. epidermidis*, although Gram-negative infections also occur. Any febrile child who has a central line and presents with chills, change in mental status, or hypotension should be presumed to have line sepsis. Oncology patients receiving long-term chemotherapy and children with gastrointestinal or nutritional disorders make up a large part of this population.

Immunocompetent children rarely develop pure anaerobic infections. When anaerobes are involved, the infection often is polymicrobial. Examples include dental infections, human bites, and abscesses. Some authorities believe that if an anaerobic infection is strongly suspected, a separate anaerobic blood culture should be obtained. However, there is no routine need for anaerobic cultures (3).

Fungi often are difficult to grow in routine blood cultures. In addition to sometimes taking several weeks to grow, special media and techniques often are required. For instance, *Malassezia furfur*, a lipid-dependent yeast, grows poorly in standard culture but well in media overlaid with olive oil (7). This species is known to cause systemic infection in babies with central venous catheters in neonatal intensive care units. The laboratory should be consulted when fungi are suspected.

Equipment

Peripheral Blood Culture

Iodine swabs
Alcohol swabs
Chlorhexidine
Blood culture tube or bottle
Tourniquet
Butterfly needle
Syringe, 3 to 5 mL
Gauze
Band-Aids
Sterile gloves

If Vacutainer system is used:
  Vacutainer needle and holder or
  Vacutainer butterfly and holder

If newly placed intravenous catheter is used:
  Peripheral intravenous catheter
  T-connector

Central Line Blood Culture

Steel clamp
Iodine swabs
Blood culture tube or bottle
Syringes, 5 mL
Sterile transfer needle
Heparin or saline flush
Sterile gloves
Sterile drape

Needleless Central Line Blood Culture

Steel clamp
Iodine swabs
Vacutainer tube (for discarded blood)
Vacutainer needle and holder
Needleless cannula
Vacutainer tube (for blood culture)
Heparin or saline flush
Sterile gloves
Sterile drape

Totally Implanted Venous Access System Blood Culture

Huber needle with a 90-degree bend
Extension tubing with side clamp
Gauze to stabilize needle
Equipment listed for central line blood culture

Poor skin preparation is the most common cause of blood culture contamination (3). The most frequently used disinfectants contain some combination of iodine, alcohol, and chlorhexidine. Many institutions use disposable swabs of povidone-iodine (Betadine). This preparation yields 1% available iodine. One large, randomized, crossover, investigator-blinded, prospective study compared four antiseptic solutions: 10% povidone-iodine, 70% isopropyl alcohol, tincture of iodine (2% iodine and 2.4% sodium iodide, diluted in ethanol), and povidone-iodine combined with 70% ethyl alcohol (a product called "Persist") (8). Of the 12,692 blood cultures drawn, 333 (2.6%) were contaminated. These investigators detected no significant differences in the contamination rate among the four disinfectants, although there was some suggestion that those antiseptics that contained alcohol might be slightly more efficacious. Another randomized, controlled study found alcoholic chlorhexidine to be more efficacious in reducing blood culture contamination rates than skin preparation with aqueous povidone-iodine (9). Similarly, another adult study compared 1% iodine pads with iodine tincture pads (2% iodine–47% ethanol) and found less contamination with the latter alcohol-containing pad (10).

Tubes and bottles are the two main types of receptacles used for blood cultures (Fig. 122.1). Tubes are used with media systems, whereas bottles are used with broth systems. A common media system uses the Isolator 1.5 microbial tubes. This system basically involves extracting the collected blood from the tube and then directly plating the collected blood onto media. With this technique, independent colonies can be counted and identified, which is one advantage of media systems over broth systems.

With broth systems (BACTEC or Pedi-BacT), the blood is inoculated into the bottle, and this culture is not disturbed unless bacterial growth is sensed by automated systems. The broths are enriched with mixtures to enhance bacterial growth (soybean-casein digest, brain heart infusion, etc.). Additionally, antibiotic-binding resins often are added.

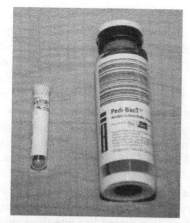

Figure 122.1 Blood culture tube and bottle.

Sodium polyanethol sulfonate (SPS) usually is added for its anticoagulant properties and its ability to counteract antibacterial factors in the blood (1).

Many authorities believe that the broth system is superior for a variety of reasons. Most important is that there are fewer contaminated specimens. The media system involves several processing steps that expose the culture, whereas the broth system is closed until a micro-organism is detected. Additionally, the broth system is more sensitive and quicker in the detection of a potential pathogen. Finally, the broth system, because it is automated, involves far less labor and therefore less cost.

Procedure

Peripheral Blood Culture

As with all pediatric procedures, the first step involves establishing a relationship with the child and parent. When possible (and when age appropriate), the procedure is explained to both child and parent, and the proper restraint technique is chosen (Chapter 3). The desired site is selected, and the tourniquet is applied. It is important to observe "universal precautions" regarding potential "exposure to bloodborne pathogens" as outlined by the Occupational Safety and Health Administration (OSHA) "to prevent contact with blood or other potentially infectious materials" (11). While it is optimal to use sterile gloves, this is often not practical, so care must be exercised not to recontaminate a sterilized area with palpation by a nonsterile glove (12).

The site should be sterilized by scrubbing with an alcohol wipe for at least 60 seconds. Next, a Betadine swab is used to wipe in concentric circles outward from the anticipated point of venipuncture. This is repeated with two more Betadine swabs. The clinician must now allow the Betadine to dry for 1 to 2 minutes. The most common breach of technique is not to wait at least 60 seconds for this important step (13). Alternatively, some clinicians reverse the order of the Betadine and the alcohol preparation. Again, it is important not to contaminate the area by repalpating the vein once the site has been sterilized.

With the site now prepared, the vein is punctured and the blood withdrawn (Chapter 73). The appropriate volume for blood culture depends on the institution's culture system. Many broth systems recommend up to 5 mL of blood. Of course, this is neither practical, nor prudent, in the majority of pediatric patients. In pediatric patients, the magnitude of the bacteremia may be greater than in adults; therefore, a lesser volume is sufficient (14). While it is possible to recover organisms from volumes less than 0.5 mL (15), most experts agree that 0.5 mL of blood is the minimum necessary for a good result.

Only one blood culture tube or bottle is sufficient for the vast majority of pediatric situations. Notable exceptions may include endocarditis, central line infections, and strong suspicion of anaerobic infections. The adult literature supports obtaining more than one blood culture in the majority of clinical circumstances (16).

The unclotted blood should be inoculated into the tube or bottle as quickly as possible after the draw. Studies done in children (13) and adults (17–19) have shown no benefit from changing needles between the one used for the blood draw and the one used to inoculate the tube or bottle. The former practice of changing needles is now agreed to be a "no-benefit, high-risk procedure" (20). Similarly, needles should not be recapped; they should be discarded immediately into a sharps container. It is estimated that one third of all needlestick injuries occur during recapping (21).

A common practice in many institutions involves drawing blood specimens through a newly placed peripheral intravenous catheter. While there is literature support for this practice (19,22), a larger, more recent study found blood contamination rates were lower when specimens were drawn from a separate site than when they were drawn through a newly inserted intravenous catheter (23). Nevertheless, if a blood culture is to be drawn through the catheter, the same technique to sterilize the site with three Betadine pads and one alcohol pad should be performed before the intravenous catheter is inserted. An assistant attaches a T-connector with syringe and then withdraws the blood. The T-connector is removed and a sterile needle is attached to the blood-filled syringe. It is important to dispense the first inoculum of blood into the blood culture receptacle.

Central Line Blood Culture

The technique for drawing blood is described in Chapter 74. The most important step is sterilizing the site. Betadine swabs are used to disinfect the connection between the extension tubing or cap and the hub. The tubing or cap is then disconnected, and the hub itself again is disinfected. A sterile syringe is attached, and 0.5 mL (infant) to 1 mL (child) is withdrawn for discard. Interestingly, while the "discard" step is generally recommended, a recent study found no benefit to this common practice (24). Another syringe is attached, and the blood culture specimen (0.5 to 1 mL) is collected. A sterile needle is attached to the syringe, and the blood is inoculated into the receptacle. Of note, the catheter should be flushed with heparin or saline when the blood draw is completed.

Needleless Central Line Blood Culture

The technique for drawing blood is described in Chapter 74. Here again, the most important step is sterilizing the site. The rubber cap of the central line is swabbed well with Betadine, as are the tops of the Vacutainer tubes. The needleless cannula, which is attached to the Vacutainer needle, is then pushed into the rubber cap of the central line. The Vacutainer tube for discard is now attached, and approximately 1 mL is withdrawn and discarded. The Vacutainer blood culture tube is now attached, and 1 to 2 mL of blood is collected. When the needleless cannula is removed, the rubber cap is swabbed with Betadine, and then the line is flushed with heparin or saline.

Totally Implanted Venous Access System Blood Culture

Blood cultures are just as easily performed with implanted systems as with standard central lines. The technique for drawing blood is described in Chapter 74. Once the subcutaneous cylinder is palpated, the overlying skin is disinfected with three Betadine swabs followed by an alcohol swab. After connecting the Huber needle to tubing and a syringe, it is inserted through the diaphragm to the back of the reservoir. Again, the first 1 to 2 mL of blood is discarded, and then the blood culture specimen is collected in a separate syringe. After the blood has been collected, the system is flushed with heparin or saline.

Interpretation of Results

A great deal has been written on the interpretation of blood culture results. Certain clues are useful to distinguish between infection and contamination. The most important factor is the clinical status of the patient. Recovery of a virulent micro-organism in a well child supports contamination. Growth factors that support contamination include an organism that takes several days to grow out, one that grows in only one of several collections, one that grows in the enrichment broth only, and a culture with multiple species present. Finally, certain micro-organisms (diphtheroids, coagulase-negative staphylococci, micrococci, and bacilli) are common contaminants in immunocompetent hosts with no "hardware" (i.e., indwelling prosthetic devices).

Another area of difficulty lies with determining central line infections. It often is problematic to determine if the cultured micro-organism (usually a staphylococcus or Gram-negative rod) is a primary line pathogen. This key distinction has great import for the therapeutic regimen. If the line is the source of infection and not merely of colonization, the clinician should consider line removal.

Many authorities believe that quantitative blood cultures are important in interpreting blood culture results. Yagupsky and Nolte (25), in an extensive review of quantitative studies, note a clear trend toward low colony counts in contaminated blood cultures compared with true positive cultures. Diagnosis of coagulase-negative staphylococcal sepsis in young infants may be aided through these techniques (26). Quantitative studies also may prove useful in monitoring antibiotic efficacy and predicting the severity of clinical disease (25,27). Several authorities believe that quantitative methods are important in diagnosing central line infections (28–30). Others note that this information has not been shown to be necessary for management or to correlate with outcome (31).

Quantitative blood cultures hold promise for resolving many of these issues of contamination, colonization, and infection. However, the most important information is gained from the history and physical examination of the patient. The clinical picture is always the crucial variable that dictates the therapeutic plan.

Complications

Complications related to the procurement of blood cultures are divided into two groups: those that can adversely affect the patient and those that can adversely affect the results. The latter mainly involve contaminated specimens. The blood culture may become contaminated from the patient's own normal skin flora, the blood drawer's hands, or the laboratory

---

 SUMMARY: BLOOD CULTURE

Peripheral Blood Culture

1 Establish rapport with the patient and family.

2 Consider topical analgesia and child life support to decrease the pain and anxiety associated with the procedure.

3 Restrain the child as for phlebotomy.

4 Apply a tourniquet and select a site.

5 Sterilize the site by scrubbing with alcohol for 60 seconds, followed by Betadine, swabbing three times concentrically starting at the center of the site.

6 Wait for the Betadine to dry 1 to 2 minutes and then obtain the culture while maintaining universal precautions and without repalpating the site.

7 Obtain at least 0.5 mL of blood and transfer to a blood culture tube or bottle without changing needles.

Central Line Blood Culture

1 Sterilize the cap, hub, or site depending on whether the central line is capped, needleless, or totally implanted, as per step 5 above.

2 Discard 0.5 mL (infant) to 1 mL (child) of blood drawn from the central line (Hickman) or discard 1 to 2 mL of blood from a needleless central line or a totally implanted device.

3 Obtain blood culture.

4 Flush the line, catheter, or system with heparin or saline.

 CLINICAL TIPS: BLOOD CULTURE

▶ The skin should be prepared properly so that blood culture contamination is avoided.

▶ Most children only need to undergo one blood culture, with the exception of patients with endocarditis, central line infection, or likely anaerobic infection.

▶ Obtaining blood cultures from an intravenous site should be avoided because the contamination rate may be increased.

▶ A broth system for detection of blood infection is preferred to media systems because of higher sensitivity, more rapid micro-organism detection, and decreased specimen contamination.

---

technician's respiratory droplets. The American Society of Microbiologists set 3% as the maximum acceptable blood culture contamination rate (32). Complications related to phlebotomy or accessing an indwelling line are discussed in Chapters 73 and 74.

▶ RESPIRATORY SPECIMENS

Respiratory infections are one of the most common reasons pediatric patients are brought to medical attention. Despite the advances in critical care pediatrics, these infections still cause a significant number of pediatric deaths each year. It is therefore of utmost importance to know which study is indicated, how to properly collect the specimen, and how to interpret the results. An accurate diagnosis is the cornerstone of a sound therapeutic plan.

Anatomy and Physiology

It is important to understand the anatomy of the respiratory system to know where to search for a pathogen, what normal flora and cells can be expected to be found, and what structures can be damaged by the procedure. A good nasopharyngeal sample yields a specimen with ciliated, columnar epithelial cells. The majority of respiratory viruses, *Chlamydia trachomatis*, and *Bordetella pertussis* are best recovered from here. The oropharynx is the area where group A β-hemolytic streptococci (GABHS) are detected. Although the palatine tonsils regress by puberty, any inflamed areas of the posterior pharyngeal wall may harbor these causative pathogens of tonsillitis.

The trachea, because of its position inferior to the pharynx, is not an ideal location to recover potential bacterial pathogens. Procedures to recover tracheal micro-organisms are invariably contaminated by pharyngeal flora. Furthermore, it usually is unclear if the recovered tracheal micro-organisms accurately reflect the etiology of the suspected pneumonia. The bronchoalveolar lavage (BAL) and protected respiratory brush (PRB) procedures attempt to sample as close as possible to the area of pulmonary pathology. Both techniques ideally sample secondary or tertiary bronchi. The PRB technique has the added advantage of eliminating much of the upper airway contamination.

Indications

The most common indication for the throat swab is the need to detect GABHS. "Strep throat" is a common cause of pharyngitis in the school-age child. Although usually seen in children 2 years of age and older, it can occur at any age. It commonly presents as sore throat with fever. Headache and abdominal pain are also common. Physical examination usually reveals pharyngeal erythema, often accompanied by tonsillar enlargement and exudate.

An important reason to culture even children with classic disease is for management of acute and postinfectious sequelae. Untreated patients may develop suppurative complications (otitis media, cervical adenitis, peritonsillar abscess) and nonsuppurative complications (rheumatic fever, glomerulonephritis). Scarlet fever, which can be recognized by its characteristic sandpaper-like erythematous rash, commonly occurs with pharyngitis and is caused by a group A streptococcal exotoxin.

Another reason for culturing patients is to appropriately manage contacts of the index patient who subsequently develop illness. Symptomatic family members should probably be cultured. Post-treatment cultures are indicated only in patients who are at high risk for rheumatic fever or who are persistently symptomatic.

Throat swabs also are commonly used to detect gonococcal pharyngitis. Gram stain and culture of an exudative pharyngitis are indicated in the appropriate clinical setting. Patients at risk include those who are sexually active and children who are suspected victims of abuse.

Another use of the swab culture is to screen the anterior nares (and other body sites) for *S. aureus* and its associated toxins. For example, some strains of *S. aureus* elaborate a toxic shock syndrome toxin (TSST-I). Demonstration of *S. aureus* carriage also is important for infection control purposes in newborn nurseries, hospital outbreaks, and interhospital transfers.

Many investigators have compared nasopharyngeal swab (NPS) with nasopharyngeal aspirate (NPA) for isolation of respiratory viruses. Heikkinen et al. found that the rate of detection of respiratory syncytial virus (RSV) was significantly higher with NPA than with NPS (33). This has been corroborated by several other studies. Interestingly, this same study found no difference between the two sampling methods with respect to any of the other viruses, although the numbers were small.

In the diagnosis of severe acute respiratory syndrome (SARS), Chan et al. found that pooled throat and NPS specimens provided a higher diagnostic yield than did NPA specimens (34). This is important in that the NPS procedure has a greater risk of generating infectious aerosols during its performance. Nevertheless, most experts now recommend the

use of NPA over NPS as the collection method of choice for most respiratory pathogens.

Interestingly, one small study done on 32 young military recruits with pneumonia in Finland found that a sputum sample was superior to both NPS and NPA for reliable detection of *Mycoplasma pneumoniae* by polymerase chain reaction (PCR) assay (35). Another study compared NPS and sputum from 50 adult patients with pneumonia for the detection of another common respiratory pathogen, *Chlamydia pneumoniae*, and found no difference between the two samples (36).

Tracheal aspiration is probably more useful as a therapeutic rather than a diagnostic procedure. It usually is done through an endotracheal tube to remove airway secretions and debris in order to optimize gas exchange and prevent atelectasis and infection. Diagnostically, the aspirate occasionally may be helpful in the investigation of infectious respiratory disease. Bacterial tracheitis is one such example.

A useful technique in diagnosing severe or unusual lower respiratory disease is BAL. One disease in which it has proven especially useful is *Pneumocystis carinii* pneumonia (PCP). This disease of immunocompromised patients is readily diagnosed by staining BAL washings. This early diagnosis avoids empiric therapy and leads to early treatment and improved outcome. Other common diseases of the immunocompromised also may be diagnosed with BAL; these include infections caused by cytomegalovirus, *Aspergillus fumigatus*, *Candida albicans*, and *Legionella pneumophila*. Additionally, other bacterial, mycobacterial, and viral diseases can be diagnosed by BAL.

The PRB technique has become popular in many intensive care settings. This procedure is a sensitive and specific approach to ventilated patients to determine the cause of pneumonia and differentiate between infection and colonization (37). It also may have a role in routine surveillance culturing of stable, mechanically ventilated patients (38).

Equipment

Throat Swab

Sterile Dacron- or rayon-tipped swabs, with or without self-contained medium for transport
Sheep blood agar for direct inoculation

 SUMMARY: THROAT SWAB

1 With a cooperative child, ask the patient to open his or her mouth, stick out the tongue, and say "ah."

2 With an uncooperative child, restrain with arms over head and use a tongue blade to get exposure of the posterior pharynx.

3 Swab the tonsils and posterior pharynx, especially areas of exudate or erythema.

4 Place a swab in the transport medium or holder and transport to the lab within 4 hours or gently swab agar growth plates at the bedside.

CLINICAL TIPS: THROAT SWAB

▶ The tongue or anterior part of the mouth should not be touched by the throat swab.

▶ With an uncooperative child, the nostrils may be occluded to induce the child to open his or her mouth.

▶ All patients who have a negative rapid antigen detection assay should have a throat culture sent.

SUMMARY: NASOPHARYNGEAL SWAB

1 Insert a swab a few centimeters into the nasopharynx.

2 Rotate the swab gently for several seconds.

3 Either place in an appropriate transport medium or streak onto a plate at the bedside.

Nasopharyngeal Swab

Calcium alginate or Dacron swab (aluminum shaft for *C. trachomatis*)

Regan-Lowe or Bordet-Gengou medium for *B. pertussis*

Tryptose phosphate broth with 5% bovine albumin, Hanks balanced salt solution with 5% gelatin, or 10% albumin or buffered sucrose phosphate for *C. trachomatis* (39)

Nasopharyngeal Aspirate

Lukens or mucus trap (Fig. 122.2)
Sterile suction catheter (Table 122.1)
Sterile, nonbacteriostatic saline
Suction source

SUMMARY: NASOPHARYNGEAL ASPIRATE

1 Attach a mucus trap to wall suction and then to a sterile suction catheter.

2 Remove the suction catheter wrapper and gently insert the catheter into the nasopharynx the length corresponding to the distance between the nasal tip and the tragus of the ear.

3 Apply suction and withdraw the catheter with a slow, twirling motion.

4 Seal the trap and transport expeditiously to the lab.

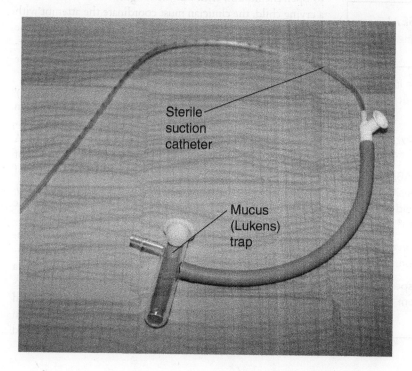

Figure 122.2 Mucus (Lukens) trap with sterile suction catheter attached.

TABLE 122.1	SUCTION CATHETERS AND PRESSURES	
Age	Catheter size*	Suction pressure†
Premature infant	6	80–100
Infant	8	80–100
Preschool age	10	100–120
School age	12	100–120
Adolescent	14	120–150

*Catheter sizes given use French system.
†Pressures are in millimeters of mercury.

Tracheal Aspirate

Same as for nasopharyngeal aspirate, with oxygen source and catheter with side holes in addition to end holes.

Bronchoalveolar Lavage

Same as for nasopharyngeal aspirate and tracheal aspirate; procedure may be aided by the use of a bronchoscope.

Protected Respiratory Brush

Telescoping, double-lumen brush catheter (Fig. 122.3)
Sterile scissors
Sterile specimen collection container
Betadine

CLINICAL TIPS: NASOPHARYNGEAL SWAB AND NASOPHARYNGEAL ASPIRATE

▶ The nasal catheter or nasal swab should be inserted toward the occiput when obtaining nasal secretions for analysis.

▶ *Bordetella pertussis* should be evaluated by nasopharyngeal aspirate instead of a nasal swab.

▶ The rapid fluorescent antibody method (FAB) of detection for *B. pertussis* may be more sensitive than culture, so both FAB and culture should be performed to maximize detection.

▶ ELISA detection is preferred to FAB when evaluating for respiratory syncytial virus (RSV) infection.

▶ If processing is delayed, nasopharyngeal specimens should be stored at 4°C and protected from ultraviolet radiation.

SUMMARY: TRACHEAL ASPIRATE AND BRONCHOALVEOLAR LAVAGE

1 Preoxygenate the endotracheally intubated patient with 100% FIO_2 for at least 1 minute using bag-valve ventilation.

2 Attach a sterile catheter to a mucus trap and suction source.

3 Remove the ventilation device and advance a sterile catheter until mild resistance is encountered and withdraw 1 to 2 cm (tracheal aspirate) or advance beyond carina until firm resistance is encountered (bronchoalveolar lavage).

4 Apply suction and collect the specimen using a slow, twirling motion.

5 Remove the catheter from the endotracheal tube.

6 Reoxygenate the patient using 100% oxygen and bag-valve breaths delivered by hand.

7 If secretions are thick, instill 2 to 5 mL of sterile, nonbacteriostatic saline into the endotracheal tube and provide several hand-ventilated breaths before obtaining the specimen.

8 Place the patient on previous ventilator settings.

Procedure

Throat Swab

With a cooperative child, the clinician first asks the patient to open the mouth, stick out the tongue, and say "ah." With a crying child, the clinician must coordinate the attempt with the patient's screaming. Either way, the goal is to swab the posterior pharynx, tonsils, and any areas of exudate or erythema. Care should be taken to avoid contact with the tongue or anterior oral cavity.

If a self-contained liquid transport medium is used, usually the base must be broken to saturate the swab that has been reinserted into its container. The container must be transported to the laboratory for processing within 4 hours. A recent study by Bourbeau and Heiter found that the use of swabs without transport medium increased the sensitivity of the test while lowering the cost of the transport device (40). If plates are used, the specimen is gently swabbed onto the appropriate medium at bedside.

The same swabs may be used to culture and then inoculate Thayer-Martin chocolate agar in the detection of *Neisseria gonorrhoeae*. This agar inhibits growth of normal flora and nonpathogenic *Neisseria* species found on mucosal surfaces. Additionally, a carbon dioxide pellet or vial is included with these plates to enhance growth. After the plate has been swabbed with the specimen, the carbon dioxide is dispensed

SUMMARY: PROTECTED RESPIRATORY BRUSH

1 Obtain a current anteroposterior chest radiograph for measurement if the procedure is being done blindly.

2 Measure the distance between tip of the endotracheal tube and the midpoint of the right mainstem bronchus.

3 Add additional length based on the child's weight as follows: 1 cm if less than 10 kg, 2 cm if 10 to 20 kg, and 3 cm if more than 20 kg.

4 Preoxygenate the endotracheally intubated patient at least 1 minute with 100% FIO_2 using a hand-ventilated bag-valve device.

5 Advance a protected respiratory brush device via the endotracheal tube to the premeasured distance or guide placement using a fiberoptic bronchoscope.

6 Advance the inner catheter out of the outer catheter by squeezing the inner and outer handles together.

7 Brush the bronchus several times using a back-and-forth motion of the thumb ring.

8 Retract the brush back into the catheter and withdraw the entire unit from the endotracheal tube rapidly.

9 Reoxygenate patient and resume mechanical ventilation using the previous settings.

10 Sterilize the inner and outer catheter using Betadine.

11 Expose the brush and collect into a sterile container by cutting the brush with sterile scissors.

by either adding the pellet or shattering the vial. The system should be sealed to prevent the release of the carbon dioxide.

Nasopharyngeal Swab

The NPS specimen is obtained by inserting the swab a few centimeters into the nasopharynx (Fig. 122.4) and then rotating it gently to maximize the number of ciliated columnar epithelial cells. The specimen is then placed in the appropriate transport medium or streaked onto a plate at the bedside.

Nasopharyngeal Aspirate

The NPA is set up by attaching the mucus trap to the suction source and then to the sterile suction catheter. The wrapper is removed from the catheter, which is now gently inserted into

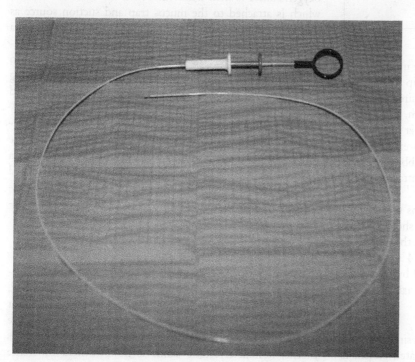

Figure 122.3 Protected respiratory brush.

CLINICAL TIPS: TRACHEAL ASPIRATE, BRONCHOALVEOLAR LAVAGE, AND PROTECTED RESPIRATORY BRUSH

▶ The patient should have cardiac and pulse oximetry monitoring throughout these procedures, and the procedures should be halted if significant bradycardia or hypoxemia occur.

▶ Intravenous or topical lidocaine administration should be considered prior to obtaining specimens in patients for whom increased intracranial pressure caused by gagging could be detrimental.

▶ These procedures should be performed expeditiously and with the proper catheter or brush size to avoid atelectasis.

▶ Bronchoconstriction may be caused by these procedures. .

▶ Catheter placement for bronchoalveolar lavage is greatly enhanced when the procedure is performed using a fiberoptic bronchoscope.

▶ The patient's clinical findings must be carefully correlated with tracheal aspirate results.

▶ Fiberoptic bronchoscopic-assisted bronchoalveolar lavage is considered the procedure of choice for identifying *Pneumocystis carinii* pneumonia.

▶ The most easily interpreted clinical information regarding bronchial tree infection is provided by protected respiratory brush specimens.

▶ Pneumothorax may be caused by the protected respiratory brush procedure.

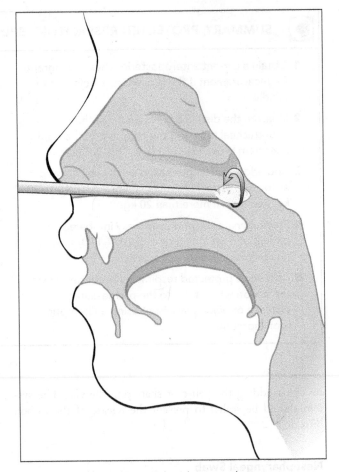

Figure 122.4 Nasopharyngeal swab in nasopharynx.

the nasopharynx (Fig. 122.5). An approximate measurement of the appropriate distance is that from the tip of the nose to the tragus. Once the catheter is in the desired location, suction is applied. Using a slow twirling motion, the catheter is withdrawn. Retained secretions in the catheter may be collected into the trap by suctioning a few milliliters of sterile, nonbacteriostatic saline. Finally, the original rubber tubing of the trap is disconnected from the catheter and attached to the trap to seal and close the system.

It is important to transport these specimens to the laboratory as quickly as possible. Viral specimens should not be frozen. If laboratory processing is to be delayed, the specimens should be stored (no longer than a few days) at 4°C. It should also be noted that that viruses are inactivated by ultraviolet light, so specimens should be shielded appropriately.

Tracheal Aspirate

The tracheal aspirate procedure (Fig. 122.6) is similar to that used for the NPA. The endotracheally intubated patient is

first preoxygenated with 100% oxygen for 1 minute. The oxygen source is then removed. The sterile suction catheter, which is attached to the mucus trap and suction source as described, is quickly guided into the endotracheal tube with a sterile gloved hand. The catheter is advanced until mild resistance is encountered (the carina) and is then withdrawn 1 to 2 cm. Suction is applied, and the specimen is collected using a slow twirling motion. The catheter is then withdrawn and removed.

The patient is immediately reoxygenated with 100% oxygen and placed on the previous ventilator settings. If the aspirate is difficult to collect because of thick secretions, a few milliliters of sterile, nonbacteriostatic saline are instilled into the endotracheal tube, the patient is given a few hand-ventilated breaths, and the above described procedure is repeated.

Bronchoalveolar Lavage

The BAL procedure is similar to the tracheal aspirate procedure. The patient is preoxygenated as previously described, and the suction catheter is advanced. The key difference is that the catheter is passed beyond the carina until firm resistance is met (ideally into a second- or third-generation bronchus). Sterile, nonbacteriostatic saline is now instilled by sterile

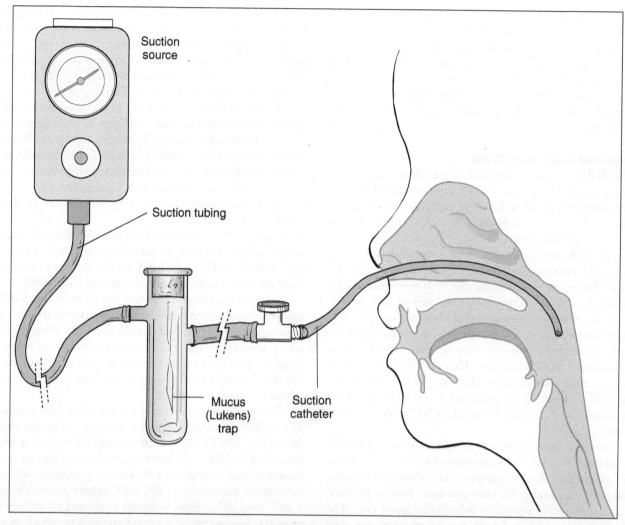

Figure 122.5 Nasopharyngeal aspirate in nasopharynx.

Figure 122.6 Tracheal aspirate performed by nurse.

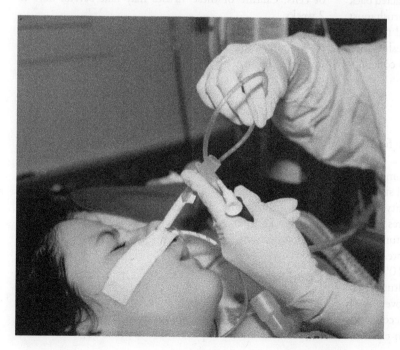

syringe through the catheter. The volume instilled is 1 to 2 mL/kg, with a maximum of 20 mL. The saline is allowed to dwell for several seconds and then is suctioned into a mucus trap, as described. Ideally, 80% of the volume instilled should be withdrawn. This lavage may be repeated, providing the patient tolerates the procedure. Catheter placement is greatly enhanced if this procedure is aided by a fiberoptic bronchoscope.

Protected Respiratory Brush

The PRB specimens are obtained using a telescoping, double-lumen brush catheter (Fig. 122.7). This apparatus has a distal polyethylene glycol occlusion to minimize contamination. Also needed are sterile scissors, a sterile specimen collection container, and Betadine.

The PRB procedure also can be done either with bronchoscopic assistance or blindly. If the procedure is to be done blindly, the distance that the PRB apparatus will be advanced must be premeasured. One method uses the patient's most recent anteroposterior chest radiograph (38). From this radiograph, the distance from the end of the endotracheal tube to the midpoint of the right mainstem bronchus is recorded. The PRB is advanced based on this measurement and the child's weight: if the child weighs less than 10 kg, the PRB is advanced an additional 1 cm; if 10 to 20 kg, an additional 2 cm; and if more than 20 kg, an additional 3 cm.

After measurement, the patient is preoxygenated. The PRB apparatus is then advanced into the endotracheal tube. At the desired distance, the inner catheter is advanced out of the outer catheter by squeezing the inner and outer handles together, which jettisons the protective polyethylene glycol plug. The clinician, using back and forth motion of the thumb ring, now brushes this bronchus several times with the previously protected brush. When completed, the brush is retracted back into the catheters, and the unit is withdrawn. The brush must now be sterilely recovered. The outer catheter and then the inner catheter are sterilized with Betadine. The brush is then exposed and cut with sterile scissors into a sterile container for transport to the laboratory (Fig. 122.7).

Interpretation of Results

Many institutions routinely perform a throat swab for rapid GABHS antigen detection along with the culture. This is usually a latex agglutination or an enzyme-linked immunosorbent assay (ELISA). The sensitivity of these rapid studies is reported at 70% to 90% (39), and the specificity is better than 98% (2). It is recommended that cultures be performed on rapid tests that are negative. The culture is the gold standard and takes 24 to 48 hours to incubate. Proper technique is the key to an accurate result. The 10% false-negative rate reported on properly performed cultures (41) is most likely due to antibiotic pretreatment and overgrowth of other micro-organisms. Carriers of GABHS account for most of the false positives. Considerable variation exists on

how physicians manage presumed streptococcal pharyngitis. For patients with negative rapid studies, some initiate treatment pending the culture results, whereas others opt to wait until the culture results are known. Some physicians do only cultures, whereas others do no studies and treat all patients fitting the clinical picture of GABHS infection.

Interpreting the throat swab for *N. gonorrhoeae* is less confusing. Although a Gram stain with Gram-negative diplococci associated with leukocytes may be helpful, most generally follow the results of the culture. The *S. aureus* screen of the anterior nares, however, must be interpreted with caution. Ten percent to 30% are colonized with *S. aureus*, and 10% of the normal *S. aureus* strains that colonize the nares can produce TSST-I (32).

Chlamydia and measles virus both may be detected by rapid antigen studies done on the nasopharyngeal swab. Fluorescent antibody (FAB) and ELISA are the two most common techniques used. Culturing either organism is difficult.

As mentioned, possible *B. pertussis* should be evaluated with nasopharyngeal aspirate rather than nasopharyngeal swab. Interestingly, the rapid method (usually the FAB), although relatively insensitive, still may be more sensitive than culture. *B. pertussis* is a fastidious bacterium that is difficult to recover. For this reason, many laboratories perform both FAB and culture to enhance detection.

The rapid detection of RSV is reported to have sensitivities of 80% to 90% (32) and a specificity of greater than 96% (42). The ELISA (which is easily automated) is preferred over the FAB, as the latter requires high-quality antisera, fluoresceinated conjugants, a fluorescent microscope, and an experienced microscopist (39). RSV culture generally takes 5 to 7 days. Adenovirus, influenza virus, and parainfluenza virus may be detected by the rapid methods previously mentioned. The key is for the NPA to collect a sufficient number of cells. Culture of these viruses may take several days to 2 weeks.

The difficulty with interpreting tracheal aspirates is due to contamination and colonization. A pure growth of one micro-organism with many neutrophils is highly suggestive but unfortunately rare. The patient's clinical status must be carefully considered when interpreting these results.

The excellent sensitivity and specificity of BAL has made it the diagnostic procedure of choice in diagnosing PCP. Most research, however, has centered on the bronchoscope-assisted BAL. It remains to be seen if the procedure, when performed blindly, is equally effective.

The PRB may offer the clinician the most easily interpreted information. When done properly, little contamination should occur. Again, more research needs to be done on blind collections.

Complications

Throat swab, nasopharyngeal swab, and nasopharyngeal aspirate have similar minor complications. Gagging is probably the most common complication. Occasionally, emesis occurs.

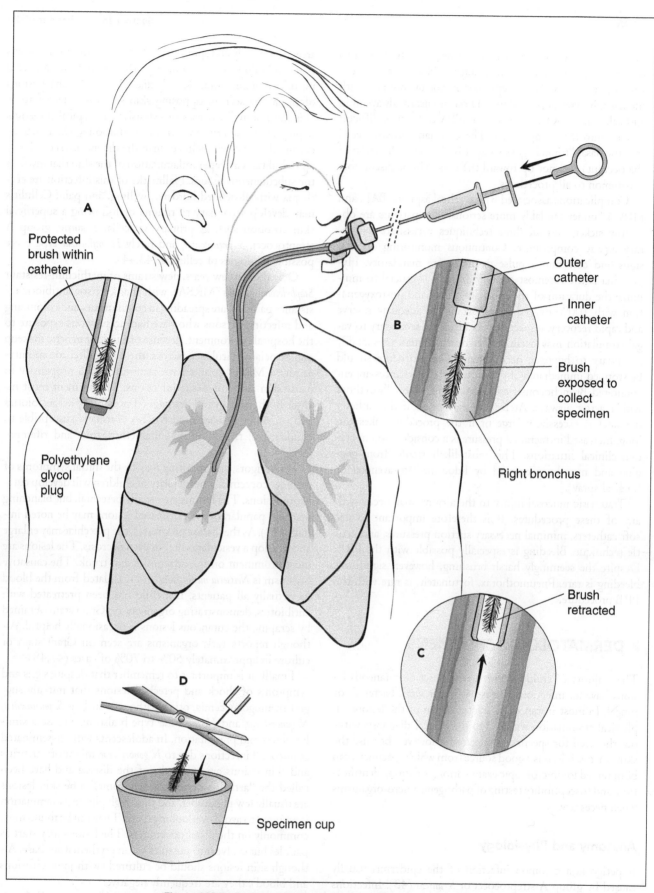

Figure 122.7 Protected respiratory brush procedure.
A. Catheter inserted into bronchus.
B. Brush advanced out of catheter to collect specimen.
C. Brush withdrawn back into catheter for removal.
D. Brush tip sterilely cut with scissors into specimen cup for transport.

Protected brush within catheter

Polyethylene glycol plug

Outer catheter

Inner catheter

Brush exposed to collect specimen

Right bronchus

Brush retracted

Specimen cup

Supine infants who vomit should immediately be turned to one side to prevent aspiration. Traumatic bleeding may occur with the throat swab, and epistaxis is not uncommon with the nasopharyngeal procedures. These are nearly always mild and self-limited. Occasionally, the NPA catheter is difficult to pass into the nasopharynx. The clinician needs to recall that the nasal "tunnel" goes straight back (in the direction of the occiput) and not up toward the eyes. Minor discomfort is common to all procedures.

Complications associated with tracheal aspirate, BAL, and PRB are understandably more serious. The patients are obviously sicker, and all three techniques necessitate temporary airway compromise. Continuous monitoring of vital signs and continuous pulse oximetry are mandatory. Hypoxemia is the foremost complication. It is crucial to minimize the duration of the procedure. Pre- and postoxygenation with 100% oxygen is important for adequate reserve and rapid recovery, respectively. Bradycardia secondary to vagal stimulation may occur. Other dysrhythmias, presumably secondary to hypoxia, occur rarely. The procedure should be stopped immediately if these rhythm disturbances are encountered. Bronchoconstriction may occur, especially in those with reactive airways. Atelectasis may result if the catheter diameter is excessively large or if the procedure takes too long. Increased intracranial pressure is a consideration in certain clinical situations. This most likely results from gagging and may be prevented by lidocaine (intravenous or tracheal spray).

Traumatic mucosal injury to the airways may occur with any of these procedures. It is therefore important to use soft catheters, minimal necessary suction pressures, and gentle technique. Bleeding is especially possible with the PRB. Despite the seemingly harsh brushing, however, significant bleeding is rare. Pneumothorax, fortunately, is rare with the PRB procedure.

▶ DERMATOLOGIC SPECIMENS

The majority of children with a new onset of cutaneous lesions have an infectious disease, whether viral, bacterial, or fungal. In most instances, characterization of the lesions on physical examination will lead to the correct diagnosis without the need for specimen collection. However, because the skin is accessible, it is a good source from which specimens can be obtained for microscopic examination, isolation, identification, and susceptibility testing of pathogenic micro-organisms when necessary.

Anatomy and Physiology

Impetigo is a common infection of the epidermis usually caused by group A streptococci or S. aureus (43). Infections start with thin-walled vesicles or pustules that easily rupture and release a cloudy yellow exudate. When dried, the fluid forms honey-colored crusts. The exudate may inoculate other areas of the body and spread the infection. In addition, S. aureus causes a bullous form of impetigo that begins with a flaccid pustule sometimes quite large in diameter (3 to 4 cm). Lesions often can be seen in opposing skin surfaces, referred to as "kissing lesions." In cases of extensive or atypical impetigo, wiping away the crusted exudate or unroofing the bullae to culture the fluid will help confirm the diagnosis (see below).

Cellulitis is a deeper inflammation of the skin that involves the subcutaneous tissues. Hallmarks of this infection are erythema with ill-defined borders, swelling, and pain. Cellulitis may develop secondary to trauma or following a superficial skin eruption such as primary varicella. S. aureus, group A streptococci, S. pneumoniae, and rarely H. influenzae type b are possible etiologies of cellulitis (43,44).

Over the last few years, new strains of methicillin-resistant Staphylococcus aureus (MRSA), with characteristic antibiotic resistance patterns, are spreading in communities and colonizing and infecting persons who have had no previous exposure to the hospital environment. Because of a unique genetic makeup and associated virulence factors, these so-called community-acquired MRSA strains have demonstrated a propensity to cause skin and soft-tissue infections. Management must include both incision and drainage (if possible) plus antibiotics (45). Community-acquired MRSA is usually susceptible to clindamycin, trimethoprim-sulfamethoxazole, and rifampin (46).

Fever, rigors, and vomiting may be the initial symptoms of meningococcemia. The majority of children will develop cutaneous lesions. The lesions are usually petechial, but blanching macular, papular, or even urticarial lesions may be noted initially (43). As the disease progresses, the petechiae may enlarge and develop a vesicular center or even necrosis. The lesions are most prominent on the extremities and trunk. The causative organism is Neisseria meningitidis and is isolated from the blood in virtually all patients. If a child has been pretreated with antibiotics, demonstrating organisms on Gram stain obtained by scraping the cutaneous lesions is occasionally helpful. Although reports vary, organisms are seen on Gram stain or culture in approximately 50% to 70% of cases (47,48).

Finally, it is important to remember that despite signs and symptoms of shock and petechial lesions that initially suggest meningococcemia, other pathogens such as S. pneumoniae, N. gonorrhoeae, and H. influenzae type b also may cause a similar illness and presentation. In adolescents with disseminated gonococcal infections due to N. gonorrhoeae, migratory arthritis and skin lesions are hallmarks of the disease and have been called the "arthritis-dermatitis syndrome." The skin lesions are usually few in number, and thorough physical examination is required to avoid overlooking them. They can be found most commonly on the distal extremities. The lesions may start as papules but evolve into pustules on an erythematous base. Although skin lesions should be cultured (with joint effusions and blood), they are frequently negative.

Only S. aureus, which belongs to phage group II (types 3A, 3B, 3C, 55, 71), can cause staphylococcal scalded-skin syndrome (SSSS) (43,44). An exfoliative exotoxin, often

SUMMARY: DERMATOLOGIC SPECIMENS

All Lesions

Check the specimen collection and processing requirements of the specific diagnostic laboratory that will be performing the test.

Pustules and Crusted Lesions

1 Choose an intact pustule or crusted lesion.

2 Lightly apply isopropyl alcohol to the lesion and allow it to dry prior to sampling.

3 Unroof the pustule with a 23-gauge needle or remove crust.

4 Rotate a sterile swab vigorously in the pustule or vigorously swab the base of the exposed crusted lesion with a sterile swab premoistened with sterile, nonbacteriostatic saline.

5 Send the specimen to the lab for Gram stain and culture or inoculate Thayer-Martin agar if *N. gonorrhoeae* is suspected.

6 Dress the site with topical antibiotic ointment and a sterile dressing (gauze or Band-Aid).

Petechiae, Purpura, or Ecthyma Gangrenosa

1 Select a suitable site (preferably a vesicle, bulla, or pustule or a new petechial or purpuric lesion).

2 Lightly apply isopropyl alcohol to the lesion and allow it to dry prior to sampling.

3 Obtain material from the margin of the lesion by scraping the lesion with a scalpel.

4 Place material on a sterile swab for Gram stain and culture and then on a glass slide for Gram stain.

5 Dress the site with a topical antibiotic ointment and sterile dressing (gauze or Band-Aid).

Unroofing Vesicles and Conjunctival Sampling

1 Select a new vesicle for sampling.

2 Lightly apply isopropyl alcohol to the lesion and allow it to dry prior to sampling.

3 Unroof the vesicle with a 23-gauge needle.

4 Roll a mini-tipped rayon or Dacron swab in the base of the lesion.

5 Roll the swab onto two locations of a glass microscope slide.

6 Allow the slide to air dry.

7 Send the slide for fluorescent monoclonal antibody testing and send the swab for viral culture.

8 For conjunctival sampling, gently stroke the lower conjunctival eye space five or six times with a mini-tipped rayon or Dacron swab; process the specimen as in steps 5 through 7 above.

Fungal Skin and Nail Scraping

1 Collect a scraping from the edge of a dry skin lesion using two glass slides or a toothbrush
-OR-
Swab wet or weeping lesions with a Dacron swab
-OR-
Gently pull loose hairs using a forceps
-OR-
Scrape underside of the protruding part of the nail using a scalpel.

2 Place specimen directly onto mycobiotic agar (Remel) or other fungal culturing and detection system.

Scraping for Scabies

1 Select a fresh papule or burrow for sampling.

2 Apply isopropyl alcohol lightly to skin and allow it to dry.

3 Apply a single drop of mineral oil to the site.

4 Abrade the superficial epidermis with a scalpel blade.

5 Transfer material to a slide and examine under 10× power.

---

originating at a distant site not on the skin, causes generalized bulla formation and exfoliation. Initially, the child may present with fever and erythroderma, which progresses shortly to large flaccid bullae filled with clear fluid. The upper layer of the epidermis appears wrinkled and may be removed with only light pressure (Nikolsky sign). The organism usually is not recovered from the areas of exfoliation. Instead, a primary

cellulitis, the nares, conjunctiva, stool, or blood should be cultured.

Occurring most frequently with *Pseudomonas* or fungal septicemia, ecthyma gangrenosa is characterized by a rounded, indurated, painless mass with a central necrotic black center. Notably, the border, which can be irregular, is usually red and nonblanching or purpuric. Gram-stained smear of the exudate

CLINICAL TIPS: DERMATOLOGIC SPECIMENS

▶ The success of sampling is highly dependent on the selection of the appropriate site that maximizes the yield of the suspected organism.

▶ Calcium alginate–tipped or wooden shaft cotton swabs should not be used for specimen collection because they inhibit the growth of some viruses, *Chlamydia*, and bacteria.

or scraping of the lesions will show either the Gram-negative rods of *Pseudomonas* or the large Gram-positive cocci of a fungal infection.

Herpes simplex virus (HSV) is one of the most common viral infections of humans. HSV infection is unique to humans, who serve as the only natural host for the virus. Herpesvirus hominis has two major groups, type 1 and type 2 (43). Children often exhibit the results of primary infection, including herpes gingivostomatitis, herpes keratoconjunctivitis, herpes vulvovaginitis and progenitalis (in sexually active adolescents), neonatal herpes, Kaposi varicelliform eruption (eczema herpeticum), and herpetic whitlow (primary cutaneous inoculation). Except for herpetic whitlow, the cutaneous and mucous membrane involvement is characterized by grouped or clustered vesicular lesions on an erythematous base. In the mouth, the lesions may coalesce into yellowish, painful plaques. In general, fever and pain accompany the primary infection. Herpetic whitlow is more commonly pustular in appearance and forms deep bullous swellings on the fingers. It often appears as deep, painful bubbles under the skin surrounded by erythema (43). Mucous membrane vesicle or conjunctival cultures can be collected to confirm the diagnosis (see below).

Another member of the herpes virus family, varicella-zoster virus (VZV), causes a common childhood disease, chicken pox. This primary infection is widespread, with attack rates of 85% among susceptible siblings and somewhat less among day-care attendees. Although common and easily recognized, it can be lethal in the immunocompromised host and can spread quite easily among susceptible hospitalized children. The incubation period following exposure is 10 to 21 days, with most children developing symptoms at 14 to 16 days. The infection begins with a prodrome of low-grade fever, headache, and malaise. The onset of rash begins as papules, which progress to vesicles, pustules, and finally crusted lesions. Two hallmarks of the disease are the characteristic appearance of the delicate vesicle described as a "dewdrop on a rose petal" and the fact that lesions are present in various stages (papules, vesicles, umbilicated pustules) simultaneously. Umbilicated vesicles and pustules also are common. The lesions involve

the scalp, face, trunk, and extremities and come in "crops," usually over the first 3 days after onset. The child is no longer infectious when all the lesions have crusted.

Herpes zoster, or shingles, occurs as VZV reactivates following the primary chicken pox illness and appears as characteristic grouped vesicles on an erythematous base in a dermatomal distribution. Factors that lead to reactivation of the latent VZV are currently being intensely researched. Although zoster is thought of as occurring only in adults, children also may present with shingles. These children usually have a history of chicken pox in the first year of life. The rash resolves in 7 to 14 days in 90% of children (43). In an otherwise healthy child with shingles, an immunologic evaluation is not indicated. Occasionally, depending on the circumstances, diagnosis may be confirmed with a culture and/or fluorescent monoclonal antibody test.

Superficial fungal skin infections are common in children. Their young age and normally close play predispose them to three common types of fungal infections: the dermatophytoses (tinea or ringworm), tinea versicolor, and candidiasis (thrush and diaper dermatitis). Tinea infections usually are caused by strains of *Microsporum* and *Trichophyton* (43,49). Tinea capitis is the most common dermatophytosis of childhood (43). Characteristically, hair loss occurs, with the hair shafts broken off close to the scalp in a circular pattern. Slight redness and scaling also may be noted. Diagnosis by Wood's lamp is less likely than in times past. *Microsporum audouinii* infection, once the most common cause of tinea capitis, causes the hair to fluoresce a brilliant green color. Currently, however, *Trichophyton tonsurans* causes the majority of cases and does not fluoresce under a Wood's lamp (43). Tinea corporis, because of its round or oval appearance and a raised scaling border, is often referred to as ringworm. However, lesions may present in many forms, including eczematous, vesicular, and pustular. Scrapings of the lesions for culture will confirm diagnosis. Onychomycosis (tinea unguium) is a common chronic fungal infection of the fingernails and toenails. It occurs primarily in adolescents and adults and is difficult to cure. Yet it should be noted that mucocutaneous candidiasis, associated with congenital immunodeficiency and endocrinopathy (e.g., hypoparathyroidism), can present in childhood with recurrent superficial *Candida* infections, especially onychomycosis.

Scabies is a contagious pruritic disease caused by the arachnid mite *Sarcoptes scabiei*, which is less than 0.5 mm in length. The mite burrows underneath the skin in the stratum corneum and deposits eggs. History reveals intense pruritus, especially at night, usually with multiple family members affected. The rash is characterized by pruritic papules, vesicles, pustules, and occasionally linear burrows associated with scaling (only 10% of cases) (50). Importantly, the distribution of the rash in infants and young children differs from its distribution in older children, adolescents, and adults. In infants and toddlers, the rash is often diffuse, with the axilla, lumbosacrum, groin, trunk, head, neck, palms, and soles commonly affected. In older children and adults, the head is almost never involved, and the rash is limited more to the extremities, interdigital webs, and flexures of the wrists and arms, although the breasts, areolae, genitalia, and waist can sometimes be involved. Diagnosis occasionally can be confirmed by a skin scraping, which might reveal the eggs or a mite. The yield of the skin scraping is frustratingly low in children, and often diagnosis is based purely on the history and physical examination (50).

Indications

As previously stated, obtaining specimens from the skin is not necessary in many cases, as the diagnosis is established during the history and physical examination. As listed in Table 122.2, obtaining dermatologic specimens in children includes four general indications. First is the immunocompetent child in whom the presentation is atypical and where a culture or rapid diagnostic test would be helpful in confirming the suspected diagnosis. Second is the immunocompromised child, who, in most cases, should have the diagnosis confirmed with specimen collection. These children are at risk for more extensive and/or atypical infections with opportunistic microorganisms. Special treatments may be needed in these cases. Third, any child who is severely ill (sepsis or shock) should have cutaneous specimens sent to the microbiology and/or

virology laboratories for Gram stain or rapid diagnostic tests. Obviously, resuscitation and antimicrobial therapy should be instituted before specimen collection. Fourth is any infection whose spread among hospitalized children is possible. For example, the use of a negative-pressure isolation room (such rooms are often few in number) usually justifies confirming the diagnosis of chicken pox. Virtually no contraindications exist for these procedures.

Equipment

Unroofing Pustules and Crusts

Isopropyl alcohol
Needle, 18 to 23 gauge
Tuberculin syringe
Sterile swab with self-contained transport medium

Petechiae, Purpura, Ecthyma Gangrenosa

Isopropyl alcohol
Scalpel, No. 11 blade
Glass slide
Sterile swab with self-contained transport medium

TABLE 122.2	INDICATIONS FOR DERMATOLOGIC PROCEDURES				
Infection	**Lesion type**	**Procedure**	**Procedure indicated**	**Comments***	**Tests**
Bacterial					
Impertgo	Pustules Crusted lesions	Unroofing	Rarely	2, 4	Gram stain and culture
Meningococcemia	Petechiae† Purpura†	Scraping	Always	3	Gram stain and culture
Staphylococcal scalded-skin syndrome	Bullae Pustules Exfoliation	Unroofing	Always	3; search for the primary site of infection	Gram stain and culture
Pseudomonal (or fungal) sepsis	Ecthyma Gangrenosa	Scraping	Always	3	Gram stain and culture
Viral					
Herpes simplex virus	Vesicles Pustules	Unroofing	Occasionally	1, 2; in neonates always obtain specimen	Rapid diagnostic slide; culture
Varicella	Vesicles Pustules	Unroofing	Rarely	1, 2	Rapid diagnostic slide; culture
Zoster	Vesicles Pustules	Unroofing	Rarely	1, 2	Rapid diagnostic slide; culture
Fungal					
Tinea corpous	Scaling papules	Scraping	Occasionally	2, 4	Agar plate
Tinea capitus	Alopecia	Scraping	Occasionally	2, 4	Agar plate
Onychomycosis	Vesicle, pustules	Scraping	Occasionally	2, 4	Agar plate
Scabies	Papules Pustules Vesicles	Scraping	Occasionally	1, 2, 4	Microscopic evaluation

*Comments
1. Obtain a specimen if child is admitted to the hospital for infection control purposes; the child should be placed in isolation pending results.
2. If diagnosis is unclear or if the child is immunocompromised, then obtain specimen.
3. Always obtain a specimen; the results of the culture may be important in treatment.
4. With extensive infection requiring hospitalization, culture may be helpful in determining appropriate treatment.
†Other cause of petechiae and purpura include *H. influenzae* type b, *N. gonorrhoeae*, *S. pneumoniae*, Rocky Mountain spotted fever, and purpura fulminans.

Unroofing Vesicles and Conjunctival Sampling

Isopropyl alcohol
Needle, 23 gauge sterile
Sterile mini-tip Dacron or rayon-tipped swab on a metal
    or plastic shaft
Glass slide
Viral transport medium
Chlamydia collection kit
Viral/*Chlamydia* collection medium

It is important to note that calcium alginate–tipped or wooden shaft swabs should not be used for collecting these specimens, because they inhibit growth of some viruses, *Chlamydia*, and bacteria (51,52). These specimens should be transported in viral transport medium. The medium includes gentamicin to inhibit bacterial overgrowth and nutrients (sucrose, L-glutamic acid, bovine albumin, etc.) to support viral and chlamydial growth (53).

Fungal Skin and Nail Scraping

Adhesive tape
Scalpel, No. 11 blade (for nails)
Toothbrush (for skin and scalp)
Sterile swab (for weeping lesions)
Wood's lamp

Scraping for Scabies

Isopropyl alcohol
Scalpel, No. 11 blade
Mineral oil
Glass slide

Procedure

Unroofing Pustules and Crusted Lesions

An intact pustule should be chosen. Alcohol should be lightly applied and allowed to dry completely. The pustule is unroofed with a 23-gauge needle (Fig. 122.8). The fluid and the basal cells are collected by rotating the swab vigorously in the pustule. If *N. gonorrhoeae* is suspected, Thayer-Martin agar is used for inoculation. The agar, with a carbon dioxide pellet or vial in an airtight pouch, will enhance the growth (54).

If the pustule is large, an 18-gauge needle on a tuberculin syringe can be used to puncture the pustule. The pustule fluid can be sent for Gram stain and culture. Crusted lesions will require crust removal. The moist base of the lesion should be vigorously swabbed with a premoistened sterile swab and sent to the microbiology laboratory for Gram stain and culture.

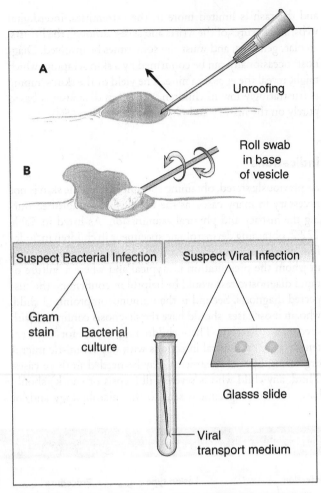

Figure 122.8 Procedure for unroofing a vesicle or pustule.

Petechiae, Purpura, Ecthyma Gangrenosa

Lesions should be carefully examined. Vesicles, pustules, or bullae are preferable. If none are present, a new petechial or purpuric lesion is selected. Enough specimen for Gram stain and culture will be obtained only by scraping vigorously into the skin to cause an abrasion and weeping. The material should be collected from the margin of a larger lesion. The material can then be transferred to a glass slide for Gram stain, and the swab is sent for Gram stain and culture (Fig. 122.9). Gram-stained smears from petechial skin lesions have been reported to show Gram-negative, bean-shaped diplococci consistent with meningococci in 50% to 70% of cases. Organisms can be demonstrated in endothelial cells and neutrophils. Although cultures from these scrapings are frequently negative, blood and/or CSF cultures are also frequently positive.

Unroofing Vesicles and Conjunctival Sampling

A new skin vesicle should be chosen and alcohol applied lightly. Vigorous wiping is avoided so as to not disrupt the vesicle integrity. The alcohol is allowed to dry completely. With a sterile 23-gauge needle, the vesicle is carefully unroofed, with care taken not to cause bleeding (see Fig. 122.8).

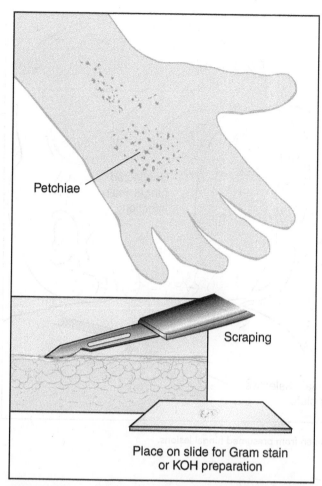

Petchiae

Scraping

Place on slide for Gram stain
or KOH preparation

Figure 122.9 Procedure for scraping petechiae and superficial fungal infections (tinea corporis, tinea capitis, onychomycosis).

After unroofing, the mini-tipped rayon or Dacron swab is rolled vigorously in the base of the lesion. The cells from the vesicle base are then transferred to the glass slide by rolling the swab onto the glass and spreading the cells over a small circular area (the diameter of a pencil eraser) in each of two locations on the slide (one for a control). The slide is allowed to air dry and then is submitted to the clinical virology laboratory. To test for both HSV and VZV, a separate slide should be prepared for each virus. The slides are air dried and labeled appropriately with the patient's name and collection date. The used swab should be placed in viral transport medium and sent for routine viral culture.

A fluorescent monoclonal antibody test can be performed on the slides. When adequate cells are present on the slides, the sensitivity and specificity are approximately 95% (50,52). These tests can be performed in 1 to 2 hours. It is important to remember that HSV grows in tissue culture as quickly as bacteria, usually within 72 hours. VZV takes much longer to be isolated in tissue culture (7 to 14 days).

Conjunctival swabs should be taken by stroking the lower conjunctival space of the eye five or six times with a cotton swab to obtain epithelial cells. To diagnose HSV or adenovirus, the swab is used to spread the cells over a small circular area (the diameter of a pencil eraser) in each of two separate areas of a glass microscope slide. The slides are air dried. A fluorescent monoclonal antibody test should be performed. The swab should be sent in viral transport medium for viral isolation (53).

If *Chlamydia* is suspected, the swab is dropped into viral/chlamydial transport medium. Specimens are inoculated onto tissue culture cells and stained with *Chlamydia*-specific monoclonal antibodies after 48 hours of incubation. Using a rapid antigen detection kit (e.g., Syva Microtrak) also is an option. Specimen collection is critical, and the kit instructions for collection and slide preparation should be strictly followed. Gross contamination of pus or discharge or a lack of epithelial cells will render the slide uninterpretable. Chlamydial culture remains the more sensitive procedure, and a specimen should be sent for routine culture when submitting a slide for rapid antigen detection (53).

Fungal Skin and Nail Scraping

A scraping is collected from the edge of a dry lesion using two glass slides or a toothbrush and is either directly transported to the diagnostic laboratory or placed directly onto mycobiotic agar (Remel) or other suitable fungal culturing or detection system (Fig. 122.10) (47). Wet or weeping skin lesions should be swabbed with a Dacron swab. The swab is inoculated by rolling over the agar surface. Forceps also can be used to collect hairs. Those that resist the pull should be left in place; those that are loose should be selected. The medium is inoculated by pressing the hairs gently against the agar surface. For onychomycosis, a scalpel should be inserted under the protruding nail and scraped. Currently at our institution, the lesions are vigorously brushed with a toothbrush, and the entire toothbrush is sent to the microbiology laboratory.

Scraping for Scabies

The most likely lesions to yield evidence of mite infestation (e.g., mite, ova, larval, or fecal material) are fresh papules or burrows. A bright light is helpful. Areas of excoriation are not suitable. Once the lesion is identified, alcohol is applied lightly to the skin and allowed to dry completely. A single drop of mineral oil is applied to the papule. The epidermis is superficially abraded with a scalpel blade, and the material is transferred to a slide and examined under a microscope with 10× power to identify signs of *Sarcoptes scabiei* (55).

Interpretation of Results

Proper specimen collection and handling are vital components of any good diagnostic laboratory. Each laboratory has slightly different requirements for handling specimens. The time and expense of performing these procedures for the diagnosis of bacterial, viral, and fungal infections necessitate an understanding of those requirements. Most diagnostic

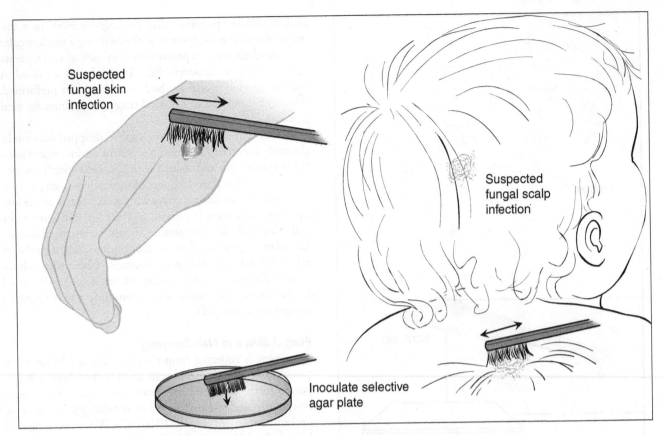

Figure 122.10 Collection of specimen from presumed fungal lesions.

laboratories have specimen collection and transport guidelines, which should be reviewed by the clinicians collecting the specimens.

Complications

Minimal complications are associated with these procedures. They are, therefore, rarely contraindicated. Possible complications include bleeding, pain, and subsequent infection at the site of the procedure. For the vast majority of patients, however, the complications are well tolerated.

▶ SUMMARY

The obtaining of biological specimens from patients with infections of the blood, respiratory tract, and skin should be performed with assiduous attention to proper technique. Blood culture contamination is avoided by careful cleansing with Betadine and obtaining the specimen without repalpating the blood vessel. Results from tracheal aspirates and BAL specimens should be interpreted carefully based on the patient's clinical condition, and the PRB technique may be employed if these simpler methods of determining the cause of

lower respiratory tract infection are equivocal. The quality of dermatological specimens is highly dependent on judicious selection of the best lesion for sampling. Proper methods employed in obtaining these specimens will ensure the best outcome and least morbidity for the patient.

▶ REFERENCES

1. Ackerman VP, Pritchard RC. Blood culture techniques: a survey in Australasian laboratories. *Pathology.* 1987;19:265–273.
2. Jui J, Brancato FP. Blood cultures and anaerobic culture techniques. In: Roberts JR, Hedges JR, eds. *Clinical Procedures in Emergency Medicine.* 2nd ed. Philadelphia: WB Saunders; 1991:1093–1099.
3. Mylotte JM, Tayara A. Blood cultures: clinical aspects and controversies [review]. *Eur J Clin Microbiol Infect Dis.* 2000;19(3):157–163.
4. Li J, Plorde JJ, Carlson LG. Effects of volume and periodicity on blood cultures. *J Clin Microbiol.* 1994;32:2829–2831.
5. Struthers S, Underhill H, Albersheim S, et al. A comparison of two versus one blood culture in the diagnosis and treatment of coagulase-negative staphylococcus in the neonatal intensive care unit [see comment]. *J Perinatol.* 2002;22:547–549.
6. Robinson JL. Sensitivity of a blood culture drawn through a single lumen of a multilumen, long-term, indwelling, central venous

catheter in pediatric oncology patients. *J Pediatr Hematol Oncol.* 2002;24:72–74.

7. Aschner JL, Punsalang A, Maniscalco WM, et al. Percutaneous central venous catheter colonization with *Malassezia furfur*: incidence and clinical significance. *Pediatrics.* 1987;80:535–539.

8. Calfee DP, Farr BM. Comparison of four antiseptic preparations for skin in the prevention of contamination of percutaneously drawn blood cultures: a randomized trial. *J Clin Microbiol.* 2002;40:1660–1665.

9. Mimoz O, Karim A, Mercat A, et al. Chlorhexidine compared with povidone-iodine as skin preparation before blood culture: a randomized, controlled trial. *Ann Intern Med.* 1999;131:834–837.

10. Strand CL, Wajsbort RR, Sturmann K. Effect of iodophor vs iodine tincture skin preparation on blood culture contamination rate. *JAMA.* 1993;269:1004–1006.

11. Occupational Safety and Health Administration. Occupational exposure to bloodborne pathogens: final rule (29 CFR Part 1910.1030). 58 *Federal Register* 64175–64182 (1991).

12. Washington JA. Collection, transport, and processing of blood cultures [review]. *Clin Lab Med.* 1994;14:59–68.

13. Isaacman DJ, Karasic RB. Lack of effect of changing needles on contamination of blood cultures. *Pediatr Infect Dis J.* 1990;9:274–278.

14. Weinstein MP. Current blood culture methods and systems: clinical concepts, technology, and interpretation of results. *Clin Infect Dis.* 1996;23:40–46.

15. Jawaheer G, Neal TJ, Shaw NJ. Blood culture volume and detection of coagulase negative staphylococcal septicaemia in neonates [see comment]. *Arch Dis Child Fetal Neonatal Ed.* 1997;76:F57–58.

16. Aronson MD, Bor DH. Blood cultures. *Ann Intern Med.* 1987;106:246–253.

17. Krumholz HM, Cummings S, York M. Blood culture phlebotomy: switching needles does not prevent contamination. *Ann Intern Med.* 1990;113:290–292.

18. Thamlikitkul V, Chokloikaew S, Tangtrakul T, et al. Blood culture: comparison of outcomes between switch-needle and no-switch techniques. *Am J Infect Control.* 1992;20:122–125.

19. Smart D, Baggoley C, Head J, et al. Effect of needle changing and intravenous cannula collection on blood culture contamination rates. *Ann Emerg Med.* 1993;22:1164–1168.

20. Leisure MK, Moore DM, Schwartzman JD, et al. Changing the needle when inoculating blood cultures: a no-benefit and high-risk procedure. *JAMA.* 1990;264:2111–2112.

21. Jagger J, Hunt EH, Brand-Elnaggar J, et al. Rates of needle-stick injury caused by various devices in a university hospital. *N Engl J Med.* 1988;319:284–288.

22. Isaacman DJ, Karasic RB. Utility of collecting blood cultures through newly inserted intravenous catheters. *Pediatr Infect Dis J.* 1990;9:815–818.

23. Norberg A, Christopher NC, Ramundo ML, et al. Contamination rates of blood cultures obtained by dedicated phlebotomy vs intravenous catheter. *JAMA.* 2003;289:726–729.

24. Everts R, Harding H. Catheter-drawn blood cultures: is withdrawing the heparin lock beneficial? *Pathology.* 2004;36:170–173.

25. Yagupsky P, Nolte FS. Quantitative aspects of septicemia. *Clin Microbiol Rev.* 1990;3:269–279.

26. St. Geme JW, Bell LM, Baumgart S, et al. Distinguishing sepsis from blood culture contamination in young infants with blood cultures growing coagulase-negative staphylococci. *Pediatrics.* 1990;86:157–162.

27. Marshall GS, Bell LM. Correlates of high grade and low grade *Haemophilus influenzae* bacteremia. *Pediatr Infect Dis J.* 1988;7:86–90.

28. Flynn PM, Shenep JL, Stokes DC, et al. In-situ management of confirmed central venous catheter-related bacteremia. *Pediatr Infect Dis J.* 1987;6:729–734.

29. Raucher HS, Hyatt AC, Barzilai A, et al. Quantitative blood cultures in the evaluation of septicemia in children with Broviac catheters. *J Pediatr.* 1984;104:29–33.

30. Wing WJ, Norden CW, Shadduck RK, et al. Use of quantitative bacteriologic techniques to diagnose catheter-related sepsis. *Arch Intern Med.* 1979;139:482–483.

31. Decker ND, Edwards KM. Central venous catheter infections. *Pediatr Clin North Am.* 1988;35:579–612.

32. Weinbaum FI, Lavie S, Danek M, et al. Doing it right the first time: quality improvement and the contaminant blood culture. *J Clin Microbiol.* 1997;35(3):563–565.

33. Heikkinen T, Marttila J, Salmi AA, et al. Nasal swab versus nasopharyngeal aspirate for isolation of respiratory viruses. *J Clin Microbiol.* 2002;40:4337–4339.

34. Chan PK, To WK, Ng KC, et al. Laboratory diagnosis of SARS. *Emerg Infect Dis.* 2004;825–831.

35. Raty R, Ronkko E, Kleemola M. Sample type is crucial to the diagnosis of *Mycoplasma pneumoniae* pneumonia by PCR. *J Med Microbiol.* 2005;54[Pt 3]:287–291.

36. Garnett P, Brogan O, Lafong C, et al. Comparison of throat swabs with sputum specimens for the detection of *Chlamydia pneumoniae* antigen by direct immunofluorescence. *J Clin Pathol.* 1998;51:309–311.

37. Chastre J, Viau F, Brun P, et al. Prospective evaluation of the protected specimen brush for the diagnosis of pulmonary infections in ventilated patients. *Am Rev Resp Dis.* 1984;130:924–929.

38. Clarke WR, Bell LM, Conte VH, et al. Blind endobronchial cultures: an alternative respiratory culturing method in children with chronic respiratory failure. *J Crit Care.* 1992;7:230–235.

39. Feigen RD, Cherry JD, eds. *Textbook of Pediatric Infectious Diseases.* 3rd ed. Philadelphia: WB Saunders; 1992.

40. Bourbeau PP, Heiter BJ. Use of swabs without transport media for the Gen-Probe Group: a strep direct test. *J Clin Microbiol.* 2004;42:3207–3211.

41. Bisno AL. The rise and fall of rheumatic fever. *JAMA.* 1985;254:538–541.

42. Ahluwalia GS, Hammond GW. Comparison of cell cultures and three enzyme-linked immunosorbent assays for the rapid diagnosis of respiratory syncytial virus from nasopharyngeal aspirate and tracheal secretion specimens. *Diagn Microbiol Infect Dis.* 1988;9:187–192.

43. Hurwitz S. Bacterial and protozoal infection of the skin (pp. 275–310); Viral diseases of the skin (pp. 318–341); Skin disorders due to fungi (pp. 372–400). In: *Clinical Pediatric Dermatology.* 2nd ed. Philadelphia: WB Saunders; 1993.

44. Weinberg AN, Swartz MN, Tsao H, et al. Soft tissue infections: erysipelas, cellulitis, gangrenous cellulitis, and myonecrosis. In: Freedberg IM, Eisen AZ, Wolff K, et al., eds. *Fitzpatrick's Dermatology in General Medicine.* 6th ed. New York: McGraw-Hill; 2003:1883.

45. Diep BA, Sensabaugh GF, Somboona NS, et al. Widespread skin and soft tissue infection due to methicillin-resistant *Staphylococcus aureus* strains harboring the genes for Panton-Valentine leucocidin. *J Clin Microbiol.* 2004;42:2080–2084.

46. Buescher SE. Community-acquired methicillin-resistant *Staphylococcus aureus.* *Pediatrics.* 2005;17:67–70.

47. Rogers MA. Bacterial infections. In: Schachner LA, Hansen RC, eds. *Pediatric Dermatology.* 3rd ed. New York: Mosby; 2003:1045.

48. Demis DJ. Bacterial infections. In: *Clinical Dermatology.* Vol. 3. Philadelphia: JB Lippincott; 1990:2–12.

49. Nelson MM, Martin AG, Heffernan MP. Superficial fungal infections: dermatophytosis, onychomycosis, tinea nigra, piedra. In: Freedberg IM, Eisen AZ, Wolff K, et al. *Fitzpatrick's Dermatology in General Medicine.* 6th ed. New York: McGraw-Hill; 2003:1883–1896.

50. McIntosh K, Pierik L. Immunofluorescence in viral diagnostics. In: Coonrod JD, Kunv LJ, Ferroro MJ, eds. *The Direct Detection of Microorganisms in Clinical Samples.* Orlando, FL: Academic Press; 1983:26–31.

51. Chernesky MA, Ray CG, Smith TF. Laboratory diagnosis of viral infections. *Cumitech.* 1982;15:1–17.

52. Greenberg SB, Krilov LR. Laboratory diagnosis of viral respiratory disease. *Cumitech.* 1986;21:1–16.

53. Lennette DA, Schmidt NJ. *Diagnostic Procedures for Viral, Rickettsial, and Chlamydial Infections.* 5th ed. New York: American Public Health Association; 1979.

54. Isenberg HD, Schoenkrecht FD, Graevenitz A. Collection and processing of bacteriological specimens. *Cumitech.* 1979;9:1–22.

55. Hurwitz S. Insect bites and parasitic infestations. In: *Clinical Pediatric Dermatology.* 2nd ed. Philadelphia: WB Saunders; 1993:405–413.

META CARROLL AND JAMES F. WILEY, II

123

Clinical Laboratory Procedures

▶ INTRODUCTION

This chapter deals with laboratory tests that may be commonly performed by a physician or other health care provider during the emergent care of a child. The focus is on the scientific background of each test, the equipment required, the procedure, and the interpretation of results. Since January 1995, with a recent update in 2003, significant federal oversight has governed the performance of all clinical laboratory tests. This chapter specifically deals with physician-performed microscopy that is not waived under federal regulation.

Regulations under the Clinical Laboratory Improvement Act (CLIA) of 1988 require that all sites of laboratory testing register with the Health Care Financing Administration (HCFA) and obtain a provider number. According to CLIA, tests are classified as waived, physician-performed microscopy, moderate complexity, and high complexity. Waived tests require certification only, without any further requirement except to agree to random inspection intended to ensure that only waived tests are being performed. Urine beta human choriogonadotropin, rapid urine dipstick, fecal occult blood, spun hematocrit, and HemoCue tests are some of the more common waived tests utilized in the emergency department (ED) (1). Laboratories performing physician-performed microscopy are subject to quality control and assurance regulations but are exempt from routine laboratory inspections. All other tests are classified as moderate complexity or high complexity and require external proficiency testing, establishment of written quality control and quality assurance procedures, special personnel requirements, and laboratory inspections every 2 years (2,3). In some instances, the hospital clinical laboratory can administer the satellite laboratory activities in the ED. This arrangement allows for resources to comply with CLIA regulations.

▶ INFECTIOUS DISEASE

Gram Stain

The Gram stain, named for Hans Christian Gram, differentiates two large groups of bacterial species: Gram-positive and Gram-negative organisms. The procedure requires applying crystal violet, a dye taken up by the bacterial cell wall, then Gram's iodine, which aids in bonding dye to the cell wall. Next, decolorization with an acetone-alcohol agent and counterstaining with safranin solution are performed. The Gram-positive organisms retain the crystal violet dye and resist decolorization, thus appearing purple in color. Gram-negative organisms take up the dye but are then susceptible to decolorization and on microscopic examination appear pink. The ability to resist decolorization is due to the cell wall composition of each organism. The Gram-positive cell wall contains a thick peptidoglycan layer with numerous teichoic acid cross-links. These cross-links contribute to cell wall resistance to alcohol decolorization. In contrast, the cell wall of the Gram-negative organism has a thin layer of peptidoglycan and a thick external coat of lipopolysaccharides and protein islands (4,5).

Other cells in a Gram-stained specimen include erythrocytes and leukocytes, which initially stain with the application of crystal violet; the stain then washes out with an application of decolorizer. Subsequent safranin counterstain results in a pink or red cell appearance. Yeast cells, resisting decolorization and staining purple, are Gram-positive in their Gram reaction, but fungal mycelia are Gram variable (4). This procedure is designated as moderately complex by the U.S. Food and Drug Administration (FDA) and thus requires proficiency testing, designated personnel, written quality control and assurance measures, and laboratory inspection every 2 years.

Equipment

Glass slide and coverslip

Crystal violet solution

Ethyl alcohol 95% (optional: acetone-ethyl alcohol mixture)

Gram's iodine

Safranin solution

Heat source (optional: 95% methanol)

Procedure

Gram staining requires specimen collection, preparation of the smear, staining, decolorization, counterstain application, drying, and finally microscopic examination. The primary goal of specimen collection is to obtain the body fluid or exudate material with minimal contamination. For example, careful cleaning of the surrounding skin before obtaining a wound exudate specimen helps to eliminate skin bacterial contaminants. Material collected in a syringe or plastic container is preferable to using cotton swabs, which can absorb components of the specimen. The specimen is thinly applied on a clean glass slide and air dried. Most specimens will adhere to the slide and do not require heat fixing. To heat-fix, the slide is passed over a gentle flame several times. The slide should feel warm to the touch and should not be overheated to avoid damaging the specimen. Alternatively, fixation can be performed with 95% methanol. The methanol is applied to the slide, allowed to run off for 1 minute, then air dried before staining. The following steps are then performed (5,6).

The slide is flooded with crystal violet solution for 30 to 60 seconds and rinsed with tap water. Then the slide is flooded with Gram's iodine solution for 30 to 60 seconds and rinsed with tap water. Next, the decolorizer agent (95% ethyl alcohol or acetone-ethyl alcohol mixture) is used to rinse the slide for 5 to 30 seconds, until the drops running off the slide are no longer blue. For decolorizing agents that have higher acetone content, the decolorization is much more rapid (5 to 10 seconds). The agent used will dictate the rinsing time required for adequate decolorization. Thicker smears also may require more time for decolorization. Finally, the slide is flooded with

safranin solution for 30 to 60 seconds, rinsed with tap water and air dried. If a paper towel or filter paper is used to facilitate drying the slide, it is important to ensure that the slide is blotted, as wiping may damage the specimen. The specimen is examined under first a low-power and then a high-power objective. Using an oil immersion lens allows better visualization of leukocytes, erythrocytes, and bacteria.

A more rapid method of Gram staining can be used. First, crystal violet is applied for a few seconds, followed by Gram's iodine solution for a few seconds. The slide is rinsed with decolorizing agent, and safranin solution (counterstain) is applied for a few seconds. The slide is then rinsed with tap water and dried.

Interpretation

Using the Gram stain technique serves two primary purposes: (a) classification of bacteria on the basis of the Gram reaction (i.e., Gram-positive vs. Gram-negative) and (b) identification of numbers and morphology of bacteria (e.g., cocci, bacilli, etc.). These two factors are valuable clues to the cause of disease and may help guide early treatment. Of note, appropriate antibiotic therapy should not be dictated by the Gram stain alone but should be chosen based on all available clinical information. Gram staining, as it provides an opportunity for direct examination of the specimen, also determines the adequacy of the specimen for culture. For example, a sputum sample with more than 10 epithelial cells per low-power field indicates contamination of the sample with oropharyngeal flora and is thus inadequate for culture.

The Gram stain is useful in many clinical settings, including infections of the lower respiratory tract, genitourinary tract, skin and soft tissues, and joint spaces. Bacterial morphology and Gram reaction may help guide therapy in cases of septic arthritis, cystitis, and skin infections. Gram stain findings for respiratory and gynecological pathogens are summarized in Table 123.1 (7,8). Gram stains of cerebrospinal fluid and the buffy coat of peripheral blood (in the setting of meningitis and septicemia, respectively) are generally performed in the hospital laboratory rather than the ED.

TABLE 123.1	GRAM STAIN FINDINGS	
Specimen source	**Organism**	**Gram stain**
Lower respiratory tract	• Contaminated specimen	• >10 epithelial cells/LPF, <25 neutrophils/LPF
	• Good quality specimen	• <10 epithelial cells/LPF, >25 neutrophils/LPF
	• *Streptococcus pneumoniae*	• GP cocci in pairs and chains; inflammatory cells
	• *Staphylococcus aureus*	• GP cocci singly, in pairs, chains, clusters; inflammatory cells
	• *Haemophilus influenzae*	• GN coccobacilli; inflammatory cells
	• Viral pathogen	• No predominant bacterial organism
	• *Mycoplasma*	• No predominant bacterial organism; mononuclear cells
Genital tract	• Normal flora (lactobacillus, gardnerella)	• Large GP rods with smaller Gram-variable rods
	• *Neisseria gonorrhoeae*	• GN intracellular diplococci, leukocytes
	• *Chlamydia trachomatis*	• Many leukocytes
	• *Candida albicans*	• Branched hyphae, budding yeast
	• *Gardnerella vaginalis*	• Mixed flora, Gram-variable rods, large GP rods in small numbers (0–5/HPF), clue cells, leukocytes

GN, Gram-negative; GP, Gram-positive.

The decolorizing step, as previously described, distinguishes Gram-positive from Gram-negative organisms. Failure to perform this step correctly yields erroneous results. Underdecolorization occurs when rinsing with the decolorizing agent is not performed an adequate length of time. Thus cellular elements retain the crystal violet dye even in the absence of the thick peptidoglycan layer of Gram-positive organisms. Overdecolorization also may occur. The specimen that is decolorized for too long a period (especially when using the rapid-acting, high–acetone content decolorizer) may remove crystal violet dye and lead to the erroneous interpretation of Gram-negative staining. Of note, any loss in cell wall integrity of Gram-positive organisms may allow the crystal violet to rinse away with the decolorizing step. The teichoic acid cross-links may be affected by such factors as antibiotic treatment, the action of autolytic enzymes, or the age of the organism itself (4,6). In light of the potential for misinterpretation and the frequent difficulty in obtaining an adequate, contaminant-free specimen, the Gram stain is always recommended as a diagnostic adjunct, not the sole determinant, in guiding appropriate presumptive antibiotic therapy.

Potassium Hydroxide Preparation

The potassium hydroxide (KOH) preparation provides direct microscopic examination of clinical specimens in suspected fungal infections. Fungi have a polysaccharide-containing cell wall. The KOH solution is an alkali that digests proteinaceous material, such as host cellular material, while leaving the fungal cell wall intact (4). Thus using the KOH preparation can help confirm the diagnosis in clinically suspected fungal infections. The KOH preparation is designated as a physician-performed microscopy procedure and requires proficiency testing, test management, and quality control and assurance policies.

Equipment

Glass slide and coverslip
Scalpel, No. 15 blade
KOH solution (10%)
Heat source (optional)

Procedure

The specimen is obtained and placed on a glass slide. For cutaneous infections, the site is cleaned with an alcohol swab and the active edge of the lesion is scraped with the edge of a microscope slide or scalpel blade (see also Chapter 122). If the infection involves scalp and hair, one may select a short broken hair and remove it using a hemostat or gently scrape the scalp using the slide or a scalpel. For vaginal infection, the specimen is collected using a cotton swab. Care must be used in viewing such specimens, as the cotton strands may resemble fungal hyphae on microscopic examination (9).

The specimen is covered with one to two drops of KOH solution and topped with the coverslip. Alternatively, the coverslip may be placed on the specimen and one drop of KOH solution placed at the edge of the preparation, allowing the solution to flow under the coverslip (9). One should wait at least 5 minutes before proceeding with the microscopic examination. If proteinaceous debris remains, potentially obscuring fungal elements, 5 to 10 minutes longer is allowed before re-examining the specimen microscopically. Alternatively, the clinician can pass the specimen quickly over a flame, which may speed the alkali digestion. It is important not to overheat or boil the material, as this will damage the specimen. The specimen is examined using a low-power objective (10× magnification), then high-power objective to identify fungal elements.

Interpretation

Fungi are divided into yeasts and molds, which differ in the macroscopic appearance of colonies formed on culture media, microscopic morphologic features, the mode of sporulation, and the characteristics of the spores produced. Most of the clinically significant fungi reproduce by asexual sporulation. Three types of spores—arthroconidia, chlamydospore, and blastoconidia—may be identified by microscopic examination (Table 123.2 and Fig. 123.1) (4,9).

As previously mentioned, care must be taken in preparing the specimen and interpreting microscopic findings. Overheating may damage the specimen and obliterate fungal elements. Foreign material such as the cotton fibers from a swab

TABLE 123.2	MICROSCOPIC EXAMINATION OF FUNGI	
Fungi	**Site**	**Microscopic appearance**
Dermatophytoses	Skin	Colorless, branched, septate hyphae (3–5 μm in diameter)
Microsporum spp.	Hair/scalp	Arthroconidia appear as square, rectangular, or barrel-shaped thick-walled cells:
Trichophyton spp.	Nails	– within the hair shaft
Epidermophyton spp.		– on the hair shaft periphery
		– in chains in skin and nails
Tinea versicolor	Skin	Round yeast cells (3–8 μm in diameter), dark, short, curved hyphae elements (2.5–4 μm in diameter)
Malassezia furfur		
Candidiasis	Skin	Branched, septate hyphae
Candida albicans	Nails	Blastoconidia
Candida spp.	Mucous membranes	• Individual round or oval budding yeast cells (3–4 μm in diameter)
	Blood	• Pseudohyphae, i.e., budding structures that are elongated and remain attached to mother cells
	Urine	(5–10 μm in diameter)

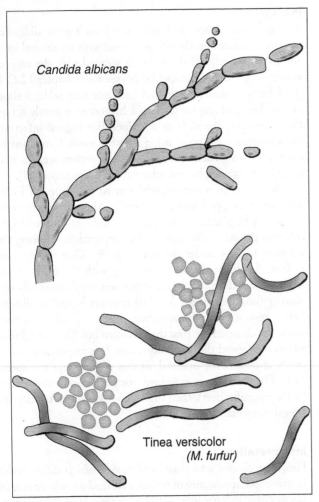

Figure 123.1 Identification of fungal elements (40× magnification).

may masquerade as hyphae. Inadequate time allowed for the KOH preparation may impair fungi visualization, as cellular debris obscures fungal elements. Such debris also may resemble fungal elements, further impeding accurate identification.

Cellophane Tape Preparation

The adult pinworm, *Enterobius vermicularis*, lives in the cecum, colon, appendix, and rectum. The female adult migrates to the perianal area and deposits her eggs on the skin at night. Thus, perianal pruritus that interferes with sleep characterizes *Enterobius* infection. Cellophane (or cellulose) tape applied to the perianal skin in the morning, before the patient washes or defecates, will pick up the deposited eggs, thus demonstrating infection. The pinworm examination is designated as a physician-performed microscopy procedure and requires proficiency testing, test management, and quality control and assurance policies.

Equipment

Cellulose tape
Glass slide
Small paper label (approximately 1 cm × 2 cm)

Wooden tongue depressor
Glass test tube (optional)
Toluene (for use with frosted tape)

Procedure

A small paper label is placed at one end of a 1 cm × 8 cm length of tape (Fig. 123.2). Then the tape strip is placed,

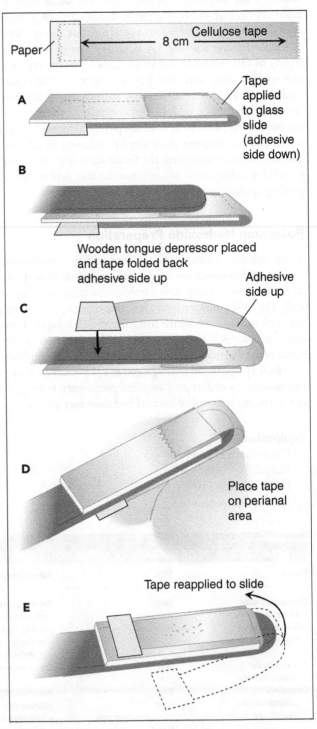

Figure 123.2 Collection of *Enterobius vermicularis* using tongue blade and cellophane tape.

adhesive side down, on a microscope slide with the free end of the tape wrapped over the opposite edge of the slide. Next, the slide and tape are placed on a wooden tongue depressor. The tape is peeled back holding the paper label end and wrapped (adhesive side out) over the end of the tongue depressor. While the slide is held against the tongue depressor, the tape is placed on the perianal area and the tongue depressor is pressed down firmly.

The tongue depressor is removed, then the tape is brought back over the slide edge (adhesive side down again) and placed back on the slide using firm pressure. The slide is examined under the low-power objective. When frosted tape is used, the tape is lifted, one drop of toluene is applied, and the tape is pressed onto the slide and examined microscopically to view eggs (10).

Alternatively, each end of a 1 cm × 8 cm strip of tape is folded over (with the adhesive side folded on itself) about 1 cm from the end. The tape is stretched, adhesive side out, over the butt end of a test tube, and each end is firmly held with the thumb and forefinger (Fig. 123.3). The tape is applied to the perianal area, rocking the tube back and forth to cover more skin area. The tape is removed, applied to the slide (adhesive side down), and viewed under the microscope (10). Toluene may again be required to delineate eggs. Occasionally, adult worms also can be demonstrated by tape preparation.

Interpretation

When the adult female lays eggs, the eggs are partially embryonated. Within a few hours (by the time the cellophane tape preparation is performed), the eggs may be fully embryonated and are infective. Characteristic eggs are 50 to 60 μm in length and 20 to 30 μm in breadth. They are flattened on one side and have a translucent, thick shell (8). Direct smears of fecal material may be prepared; tape preparations, however, better demonstrate the embryonated eggs. After treatment, follow-up tape preparations are obtained to demonstrate that the patient is free of infection. Tape preparations may be required for 3 to 4 consecutive days to confirm cure (11).

▶ GYNECOLOGY

Wet Mount/Wet Preparation

The wet preparation, useful in evaluating the patient with presumed vaginitis, cervicitis, or pelvic inflammatory disease, involves suspending a specimen in saline solution and then examining the preparation microscopically to identify inflammatory cells and organisms. The wet preparation of vaginal or cervical specimens is designated as a physician-performed microscopy procedure and requires proficiency testing, test management, and quality control and assurance policies.

Equipment

Glass test tube with 1 mL of sterile saline solution
Cotton-tipped swab
Glass slide and coverslip

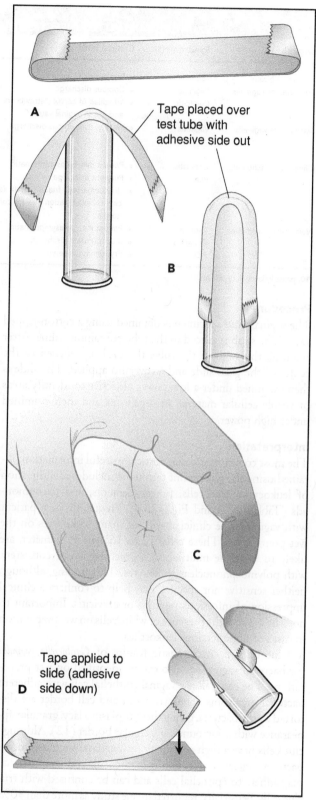

A

Tape placed over test tube with adhesive side out

B

C

D Tape applied to slide (adhesive side down)

Figure 123.3 Collection of *Enterobius vermicularis* using test tube and cellophane tape.

TABLE 123.3	SEXUALLY TRANSMITTED INFECTIONS IN THE PEDIATRIC PATIENT		
Organisms	**Syndrome(s)**	**Clinical findings**	**Laboratory findings**
Candida albicans	Vaginitis	• Erythema of vagina	• Branched and budding hyphae on KOH and wet preparation
Trichomonas vaginalis	Vaginitis	• Copious discharge	• Trichomonads and leukocytes on wet preparation
	Cervicitis	• Petechiae of cervix ("strawberry cervix") and upper vaginal vault	
Gardnerella vaginalis	Vaginitis	• Watery, malodorous discharge	• "Fishy" odor of specimen with addition of KOH due to release of amines
			• Clue cells on wet preparation
			• Vaginal pH >4.5
			• Wet preparation with many leukocytes
Chlamydia trachomatis	Cervicitis	• Patient may be asymptomatic	
	PID	• Purulent discharge	
		• Erythematous, friable cervix (although cervical examination may be completely normal)	
Neisseria gonorrhoeae	Vaginitis	• Patient may be asymptomatic	• Wet preparation with many leukocytes
	Cervicitis	• Mucopurulent discharge	• Gram stain with Gram-negative intracellular diplococci and leukocytes
	PID	• Erythematous cervix	

PID, pelvic inflammatory disease.

Procedure

The vaginal fluid specimen is obtained using a cotton-tipped swab. The swab is placed in the tube containing saline. After agitating the swab in the tube, the swab is touched to the center of the glass slide and a coverslip applied. The slide is then examined under a low-power objective to identify areas of visible cellular material or organisms and then examined under high power.

Interpretation

The most common and diagnostically useful information obtained using the wet mount technique includes identification of leukocytes, clue cells, fungal elements, and trichomonads (Table 123.3 and Fig. 123.4). Frequently in a patient with vaginitis, the clinician will see many leukocytes on the wet preparation. These cells, 12 to 15 μm in diameter, are likely to have the multilobed, segmented nuclei consistent with polymorphonuclear leukocytes. This finding, although neither sensitive nor specific, may help to confirm a clinical impression of infectious vaginitis or cervicitis. Important to note, however, is the presence of white cells on wet preparation in cases of noninfectious leukorrhea.

Clue cells, a characteristic feature of *Gardnerella vaginalis* (or bacterial vaginosis), also can be identified on wet preparations. The clue cell is a vaginal epithelial cell with adherent bacterial organisms. The cytoplasm and cell border are distorted by the bacteria, giving the cytoplasm a lacy, granular appearance with a surrounding irregular border (12). Although clue cells have a high specificity for bacterial vaginosis, other bacterial organisms (including lactobacilli and streptococci) may adhere to epithelial cells and can be confused with true clue cells. Sensitivity, reported in one study as more than 90%, has been shown in other studies to be lower and clearly dependent on clinician expertise in identifying the cells (13–15).

Trichomonads are the protozoa identified on wet preparation as small (5 to 15 μm in length) flagellated organisms that have jerky, nondirectional motility (10). Identification of the organism is specific and therefore diagnostic for trichomoni-

asis. In one study, however, protozoa were identified on wet preparations in only 60% of patients with culture-positive trichomoniasis (16). The low sensitivity may be related to several factors, most important of which include the rapid

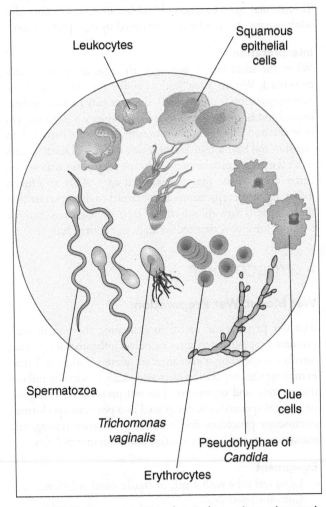

Figure 123.4 Wet preparation of vaginal secretions: microscopic findings (100× magnification).

loss of protozoan motility (within 30 to 60 minutes of specimen preparation) and other specimen material (epithelial cells, leukocytes, fungal elements) obscuring the organisms. Thus, culture, Pap test, or monoclonal antibody techniques may be necessary for definitive diagnosis (the latter two of which are not routinely performed in the ED setting).

Motile Sperm Microscopy

Microscopic examination of vaginal secretions to identify motile sperm is an important and rapidly performed laboratory procedure in the ED. This procedure often is used in cases of alleged sexual assault and abuse. Sperm may remain motile in the vagina for 6 to 12 hours and for an even longer period in the cervix. In controlled studies, 50% of sperm lost motility by 2 to 3 hours, providing the ED physician with a relatively narrow window of opportunity for visualizing motile sperm (17). In contrast, nonmotile sperm can be seen on microscopic examination of a specimen days after intercourse, a confounding factor in evaluating a sexual assault victim who may have had recent voluntary intercourse. Thus, this important microscopic finding is only identified by the initial examining physician; the forensic pathologist involved in a sexual assault case will likely first evaluate specimens many hours after collection, precluding identification of motile sperm (17,18). Motile sperm microscopy is designated as a physician-performed microscopy procedure and requires proficiency testing, test management, and quality control and assurance policies.

Equipment

- Sterile container (e.g., glass test tube)
- Small syringe or dropper
- Sterile, nonbacteriostatic saline solution
- Cotton-tipped swab
- Glass slide and coverslip
- Supravital stain (optional)
- Glacial acetic acid (optional)

Procedure

The clinician may obtain the specimen in the older pediatric patient by aspirating secretions pooled in the posterior fornix using a small syringe or dropper. Optionally, the clinician may wash the vagina with 5 to 10 mL of saline, aspirate the fluid, and place it in a sterile container. A third option, especially in the small child, is to place a cotton-tipped swab in the vaginal orifice and then in 2 to 3 mL of saline in a glass test tube.

Using a dropper or small syringe, a few drops of the specimen are placed on a clean glass slide and the coverslip applied. The specimen is then examined under low- and high-power objective to identify motile sperm. Often sperm may be obscured by cellular material, especially red blood cells. Using glacial acetic acid provides lysis of red blood cells. Of note, however, is that the acid will leave sperm immotile. Another option is to use supravital stain, which lyses red blood cells and

stains sperm blue for easier visualization. Supravital staining results in little loss of sperm motility (17,18).

Interpretation

The mature human spermatozoon is about 60 μm long and has two major components, the head (composed of acrosome and nucleus) and the tail (composed of neck, middle piece, principal piece, and end piece). The head is approximately 4.5 μm by 3.0 μm (in contrast to a polymorphonuclear neutrophil, which is approximately 12 to 15 μm in diameter). The principal piece is so named because it comprises the main portion of the flagellum or tail structure that propels the sperm (Fig. 123.5) (19).

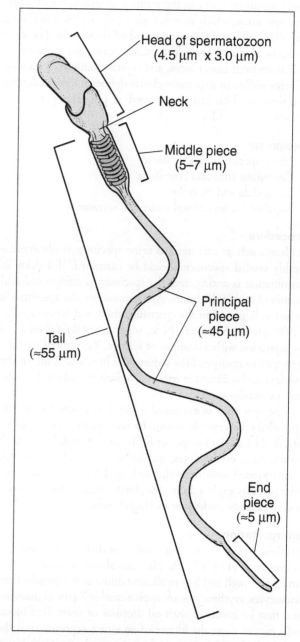

Figure 123.5 Spermatozoon anatomy (100× magnification).

False-negative interpretation of specimen occurs when inadequate sampling, specimen preparation, and/or interpretation occurs. For example, cellular material such as red blood cells may obscure sperm. Using glacial acetic acid, as previously described, results in immotile sperm. As described above, *Trichomonas vaginalis* is a motile protozoan found in vaginal secretions that may be confused with spermatozoa, yielding a false-positive result. However, this flagellated parasite can generally be distinguished based on size, as it is significantly smaller (5 to 15 μm in length) than the spermatozoon.

▶ MICROSCOPIC EXAMINATION OF URINE SEDIMENT

Urine sediment refers to the multiple constituents of a urinary specimen, which may include erythrocytes, leukocytes, epithelial cells, and casts composed of these cells. The constituents also may include bacteria, yeast, and parasites as well as spermatozoa, mucus, and crystals. Supravital staining of urine sediment may more clearly delineate these sediment constituents. This test is classified as physician-performed microscopy by CLIA.

Equipment

Urine specimen, freshly voided
Centrifuge tube and centrifuge
Glass slide and coverslip
Supravital stain (crystal violet and safranin)

Procedure

A clean catch or catheterized urine specimen is obtained; a freshly voided specimen should be examined. If a delay in examination is anticipated, the specimen is refrigerated and examined within 48 hours. At examination, the specimen is mixed well, placed in the centrifuge tube, and centrifuged at 1,500 rpm for 5 minutes. Next, supernatant fluid is removed by aspiration with a dropper or syringe. The centrifuge tube is tapped to resuspend the sediment. Then, 1 to 2 mL of the resuspended sediment is removed, a drop placed on the slide, and a coverslip applied.

The specimen is examined under low power to identify epithelial cells, crystals, mucus, bacteria, yeast, sperm, and artifacts. At least 10 low-power fields are reviewed. Under high power, casts, erythrocytes, and leukocytes can be identified. As mentioned, another option to help delineate cellular components is to apply a drop of supravital stain to the specimen and re-examine under low and high power.

Interpretation

Erythrocytes in the urine are colorless disks on microscopic examination (Fig. 123.6). The cells shrink in concentrated urine, and swell and lyse in alkaline dilute urine. Smaller than leukocytes, erythrocytes are approximately 7 μm in diameter and may be confused with oil droplets or yeast. Red blood cells cannot enter the filtrate of an intact nephron; thus the presence of erythrocytes in the urine is abnormal and may be associated with injury to the glomerular membrane or result from renal calculi, urinary tract infection, malignancies, damaged renal capillaries, vascular injury, and toxic- or allergy-mediated reactions. The appearance of erythrocytes in urine can also be caused by contamination due to vaginal bleeding or menstruation.

No visible erythrocytes on microscopic examination of sediment may indicate absence of bleeding, infection, or glomerular damage but may represent a false-negative result. Red blood cells can be disrupted or lysed, and only the hemoglobin is detectable by urine dipstick (chemical analysis) or by macroscopic appearance (red urine) in the presence of a negative microscopic examination. More than three red blood cells per high-power field is considered abnormal (20).

Pyuria, or white blood cells in the urine, occurs in the presence of infection, inflammation, or malignancy within the genitourinary system. Fewer than five white blood cells per high-power field can be found in a normal urine specimen. Leukocytes are easier to identify than erythrocytes due to their larger size (diameter approximately 12 μm) and cellular components (visible cytoplasm and nuclei). Nuclear details, especially the multilobed nucleus of the polymorphonuclear leukocyte, can be enhanced with supravital staining. Renal tubular epithelial cells may be confused with leukocytes, again necessitating staining techniques.

Casts are formed within the renal tubular lumen or collecting ducts and are generally cylindrical, with parallel sides and rounded ends. Cast formation may occur with urinary stasis, stress or exercise, pyelonephritis, glomerulonephritis, urinary tract infection, nephrotic syndrome, renal tubular damage, or chronic renal disease. A summary of the conditions associated with urinary casts is provided in Table 123.4.

Epithelial cells, sloughed from the cellular lining of the genitourinary system, are often found in normal urine specimens. Epithelial cells originate from the vagina and lower urethra (squamous epithelial cells); the renal pelvis, bladder, and upper urethra (transitional epithelial cells); and the renal tubules (renal tubular epithelial cells). Squamous cells are irregularly shaped, large cells that are easily identified under low power with a central nucleus (about the size of an erythrocyte) and abundant cytoplasm. They are frequently seen in a specimen that is obtained without adequate preparation, such as without use of the clean catch technique. Transitional epithelial cells are smaller than squamous cells, are round, and contain a central nucleus. In the absence of unusual morphology, these cells seldom indicate pathology. When large numbers of unusually shaped transitional epithelial cells are seen on microscopic examination of urine, renal carcinoma (and therefore cytologic examination) should be considered. Renal tubular cells are round and larger than leukocytes with a single round nucleus. When present in large numbers, these cells indicate tubular injury, as can be seen in infectious, inflammatory, toxin-mediated, and allergic processes. Tubular damage also occurs in renal transplant rejection. Staining techniques help distinguish leukocytes from renal tubular cells, particularly with respect to nuclear detail and morphology.

Bacteria in the urine are identified in cases of pyelonephritis, urinary tract infection, and contaminated urine specimens.

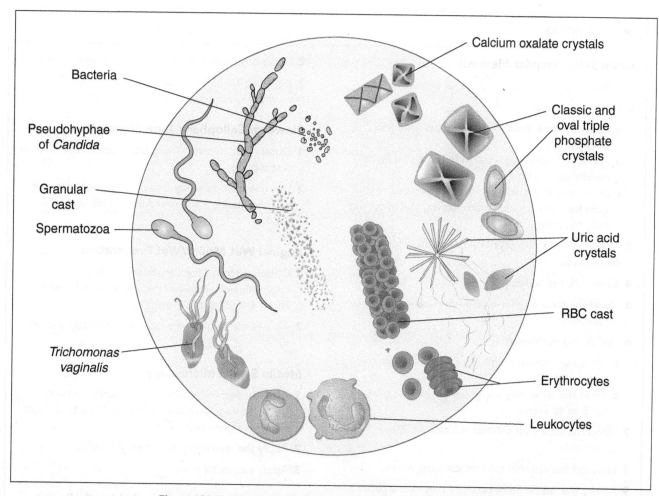

Figure 123.6 Urine sediment: microscopic findings (100× magnification).

The Gram-negative organisms are the most common pathogens and are most easily seen under high power using Gram-staining techniques. Specimens that remain at room temperature must be examined shortly after collection. With delay in microscopic examination, bacteria may represent multiplication of contaminant organisms rather than an acute infectious process.

Yeast cells (most commonly *Candida albicans*) seen in patients with vaginal candidiasis and/or diabetes may be confused with erythrocytes on microscopic examination of urine sediment. Another organism, *Trichomonas vaginalis*, the most commonly encountered parasite identified in urine, may resemble a leukocyte. Because of its flagellated structure and movement in urine, however, it is usually easily distinguishable. Finally, spermatozoa can be seen in urine, as mentioned previously.

Mucous threads seen on the examination of urine sediment are composed of protein material produced by cells of the genitourinary system. The threads are irregular in shape and better visualized under low light. Clumps of mucus can be similar to hyaline casts in appearance.

Crystals commonly seen in urine are present in healthy patients and patients with pathologic conditions. In acidic urine, urate crystals are reddish brown or yellow. These variously shaped crystals (rhomboid, wedge, needle, or rosette) can appear in urine specimens in the absence of disease, in patients with leukemia, and in some cases of arthritis. Calcium oxalate crystals, colorless prism shapes, and octahedral shapes that resemble envelopes may suggest ethylene glycol poisoning but also appear in normal acidic urine specimens. In alkaline urine, the triple phosphate crystal is a colorless prism resembling a coffin lid. Calcium phosphate crystals, also colorless, can appear as plates, needles, or thin prisms. Abnormal crystals in urine include cystine, cholesterol, leucine, tyrosine,

TABLE 123.4	EXAMINATION OF URINARY SEDIMENT: CASTS AND ASSOCIATED CONDITIONS
Cast	**Associated conditions**
Hyaline	Glomerulonephris, pyelonephritis, stress, exercise, chronic renal disease, congestive heart failure
Red blood cell	Glomerulonephritis, exercise
White blood cell	Pyelonephritis
Epithelial cell	Renal tubular damage
Granular	Urinary stasis, urinary tract infection, stress, exercise
Fatty	Nephrotic syndrome

SUMMARY

Gram Stain (Regular Method)

1 Collect the specimen with minimal contamination.

2 Fixation methods:

  a Apply the specimen to a clean glass slide and air-dry.

  b For heat fixation, pass the slide through a flame rapidly several times.

  c For chemical fixation, apply 95% methanol to the slide for 1 minute, dump the excess, and allow the slide to air-dry.

3 Flood the slide with crystal violet solution for 30 to 60 seconds.

4 Rinse with tap water.

5 Flood the slide with Gram's iodine solution for 30 to 60 seconds.

6 Decolorize as follows:

  a Rinse the slide with 95% ethyl alcohol for up to 30 seconds OR

  b Rinse the slide with acetone-ethyl alcohol mixture for 5 to 10 seconds.

7 Flood the slide with safranin solution for 30 to 60 seconds.

8 Rinse off the safranin solution with tap water.

9 Air-dry the specimen or carefully blot with a paper towel or filter paper.

Gram Stain (Rapid Method)

1 Collect the specimen and fix as for the normal method.

2 Apply crystal violet for a few seconds and drain.

3 Apply Gram's iodine for a few seconds.

4 Rinse with a decolorizing agent.

5 Apply safranin for a few seconds.

6 Rinse the slide with tap water.

7 Air-dry the specimen or carefully blot with a paper towel or filter paper.

KOH (Potassium Hydroxide) Preparation

1 Obtain the specimen by scraping onto a glass slide or applying from a cotton swab in the case of vaginal secretions.

2 Apply one to two drops of KOH 10% to the slide.

3 Either wait 5 to 10 minutes to view the specimen or pass the specimen quickly over a flame.

Pinworm Cellophane Tape Preparation

1 Obtain the specimen using tape applied to a slide or test tube.

2 Use one drop of toluene applied between the tape and slide to view the specimen if frosted tape is used.

Vaginal Wet Mount/Wet Preparation

1 Obtain a vaginal fluid specimen using a cotton-tipped swab and placing it in a tube with about 1 to 2 mL of saline.

2 Agitate the swab in the tube and then apply to the slide.

Motile Sperm Microscopy

1 Aspirate secretions from the posterior fornix or swab the vaginal orifice and place it in 2 to 3 mL of saline in a glass test tube.

2 Apply the specimen to a clean glass slide.

3 Apply supravital stain.

Microscopic Examination of Urine Sediment

1 Obtain the urine specimen.

2 Refrigerate if a delay in urine examination is anticipated.

3 Mix the specimen well.

4 Place the specimen in a centrifuge tube and centrifuge at 1,500 rpm for 5 minutes.

5 Remove supernatant by syringe or dropper aspiration.

6 Tap the centrifuge tube to resuspend the sediment.

7 Remove 1 to 2 mL of the resuspended sediment and place one drop on a slide.

CLINICAL TIPS

Gram Stain

▶ It is important not to overdecolorize or underdecolorize, because this reduces the ability to distinguish Gram-positive from Gram-negative bacteria.

▶ The Gram stain alone should not be used to dictate antibiotic therapy.

▶ Several factors diminish the staining of Gram-positive bacteria, including antibiotic therapy, aging of the specimen, and the presence of autolytic enzymes.

KOH (Potassium Hydroxide) Preparation

▶ Cotton fibers from a swab may masquerade as hyphae.

▶ Adequate time must be allowed for the KOH to break down nonfungal cellular elements.

▶ The slide should not be overheated to the point that the KOH boils.

Pinworm Cellophane Tape Preparation

▶ The tongue blade or test tube should be pressed firmly to obtain the specimen.

▶ The specimen should be handled with gloved hands, since the eggs are very likely to be infective.

Vaginal Wet Mount/Wet Preparation

▶ The wet mount is an important adjunct to clinical judgment and more definitive testing in establishing the etiology of a vaginal discharge.

▶ When properly identified, the wet mount has high specificity for the diagnosis of trichomoniasis and bacterial vaginosis.

▶ The absence of recognized clue cells or trichomonads on microscopic examination of the wet mount does not exclude these diagnoses.

Motile Sperm Microscopy

▶ Demonstration of motile sperm requires rapid specimen evaluation because sperm only remain motile in the vagina for 6 to 12 hours.

▶ Nonmotile sperm remain in the vagina for days after sexual intercourse.

▶ Supravital staining lyses red blood cells, stains sperm blue, and causes little loss of sperm motility.

Microscopic Examination of Urine Sediment

▶ Supravital staining may enhance the recognition of cellular components.

▶ Delay in specimen examination markedly reduces the ability to detect casts in urine sediment.

▶ Delay in specimen examination with the specimen at room temperature may cause bacterial overgrowth in contaminated specimens.

▶ Spermatozoa and trichomonads may be observed in urine sediment.

▶ Common artifacts include oil droplets, hair, fibers, and talcum powder. Proper specimen collection and the use of clean materials (droppers, slides, syringes, and coverslips) reduces their presence.

---

sulfonomides, radiographic dyes, bilirubin, and ampicillin (see Fig. 123.6).

Finally, artifactual material often is found in urine specimens, including oil droplets, hair, fibers, and talcum powder, reinforcing the need for proper specimen collection and the use of clean containers, droppers, syringes, slides, and coverslips (20,21).

▶ EMERGENCY DEPARTMENT LABORATORIES

Point-of-care testing in the ED holds promise for improving test turnaround time and shortening patient length of stay. Useful tests for ED care include KOH preparation, wet preparation of vaginal and cervical secretions, motile sperm mi-

croscopy, urine sediment microscopy, and Gram stain. However, these tests require a dedicated microscope, appropriate training, and, in the case of Gram stain, a high degree of laboratory oversight. The ED with a high patient volume may be best served by a "stat" laboratory within the department that has a dedicated laboratory technician who can perform a variety of tests in addition to those discussed in this chapter. An onsite stat laboratory has the advantages of test performance by a highly trained technician, rapid test turnaround, and the ability of the clinician to review test results easily with the technician. The principal drawbacks to an onsite stat laboratory concern cost and space. Waived tests, such as urine pregnancy, urine dipstick, and fecal occult blood, and rapid determination of hematocrit or hemoglobin are essential for any ED in order to provide the most timely care. The procedures for these tests vary by manufacturer. The practitioner should consult package inserts for the specific test. In hospital settings such as the ED, a test with a built-in quality control should be utilized.

▶ REFERENCES

1. Pub 100-04 Medicare Claims Processing Transmittal 102. Department of Health and Human Services. Centers for Medicare and Medicaid Services, February 20, 2004. Available at: http://www.cms.hhs.gov/manuals/pm_trans/R102CP.pdf. Accessed April 9, 2005.

2. Schuman AJ. Office labs: still worth it under CLIA? *Contemp Pediatr.* 1993;10:50–74.

3. Laessig RH, Ehrmeyer SS. CLIA 2003's new concept: equivalent quality control. *Med Lab Obs.* 2005;37:32–34.

4. Baron EJ, Finegold SM, eds. *Bailey and Scott's Diagnostic Microbiology.* 8th ed. St. Louis: Mosby; 1990.

5. Murray PR. Microscopy. In: Wentworth BB, ed. *Diagnostic Procedures for Bacterial Infections.* Washington, DC: American Public Health Association; 1987:681–683.

6. Quintiliani R, Bartlett RC. *Examination of the Gram-stained Smear.* Nutley, NJ: Hoffman-La Roche; 1985.

7. Farmer MY, Hook EW, Heald FP. Laboratory evaluation of sexually transmitted disease. *Pediatr Ann.* 1986;15:715–724.

8. Walsh RD, Cunha BA. Diagnostic significance of the sputum Gram stain in pneumonia. *Hosp Physician.* October 1992:37–44.

9. Larone DH. *Medically Important Fungi: A Guide to Identification.* 2nd ed. New York: Elsevier; 1987:173–177.

10. Markell EK, Voge M, John DT, eds. *Medical Parasitology.* 7th ed. Philadelphia: WB Saunders; 1992:72–74, 268–269, 421–422.

11. Garcia LS, Bruckner DA, Brewer TC, et al. Techniques for the recovery and identification of cryptosporidium oocysts from stool specimens. *J Clin Microbiol.* 1993;18:185–190.

12. Farmer MY, Hook EW, Heald FP. Laboratory evaluation of sexually transmitted diseases. *Pediatr Ann.* 1986;15:716–724.

13. Spiegel CA, Amsel R, Holmes KK. Diagnosis of bacterial vaginosis by direct Gram stain of vaginal fluid. *J Clin Microbiol.* 1983;18:170–177.

14. Spiegel CA. Vaginitis. In: Wentworth BB, Judson FN, eds. *Laboratory Methods for the Diagnosis of Sexually Transmitted Diseases.* Washington, DC: American Public Health Association; 1984:151–168.

15. Johnson J, Shew ML. Screening and diagnostic tests for sexually transmitted diseases in adolescents. *Semin Pediatr Infect Dis.* 1993;4:142–150.

16. Krieger JN, Tam MR, Stevens CE, et al. Diagnosis of trichomoniasis. *JAMA.* 1988;259:1223–1227.

17. Hoelzer M. Sexual assault. In: Tintinalli JE, ed. *Emergency Medicine: A Comprehensive Study Guide.* New York: McGraw-Hill; 1992:398–402.

18. Braen GR. Sexual assault. In: Rosen P, Barkin RM, eds. *Emergency Medicine Concepts and Clinical Practice.* St. Louis: Mosby; 1992:2003–2012.

19. Dym M. The male reproductive system. In: Weiss L, ed. *Histology Cell and Tissue Biology.* New York: Elsevier Biomedical; 1983:1014–1017.

20. Free HM, ed. *Modern Urine Chemistry.* Elkhart, IN: Miles Laboratories; 1986:44.

21. Strasinger SK. *Urinalysis and Body Fluids: A Self-Instructional Text.* 2nd ed. Philadelphia: FA Davis; 1989:46–50, 54–86.

124

ZACH KASSUTTO

Skin Testing

▶ INTRODUCTION

Intradermal injections can be used for the diagnosis of tuberculosis, for allergy testing, and for local anesthesia. The rationale for injecting into the dermis, as opposed to the subcutaneous layer of the skin or the muscle, is that it can elicit localized effects while limiting the systemic dispersion of the injected substances. Injecting into the dermis can also elicit specific immune responses that are easily detected by inspection and palpation. The procedure is quickly learned and is performed by a physician, nurse, or physician's assistant. Intradermal injections can be used with children in any age group.

The classic and most common application of this procedure is the intradermal injection of mycobacterium derivatives to diagnose previous mycobacterium infection. This procedure, first described by Mantoux in 1908 (1), is currently the most widely used and cost-effective tool for diagnosing tuberculosis. Because of the recent resurgence of tuberculosis in the United States, this diagnostic procedure is commonly used in the emergency department (ED) setting.

▶ ANATOMY AND PHYSIOLOGY

The skin is composed of three basic layers (see Fig. 128.1)—the epidermis, the dermis, and the subcutaneous tissue. The epidermis is a thin, superficial layer composed of an outer layer of dead, keratinized epithelial cells and an inner cellular layer. The dermis lies just beneath the epidermis and contains blood vessels, connective tissue, hair follicles, and sebaceous glands. The deeper subcutaneous layer contains mostly fat. This layer supports the blood vessels, nerves, and lymphatics that supply the more superficial layers. Sweat glands and roots of hair follicles also are found in the subcutaneous layer.

The tuberculin tests (tine and Mantoux) are the prototypes of a cell-mediated immune response (type IV hypersensitivity

reaction). In the nonimmunocompromised patient, exposure to an antigen (e.g., *Mycobacterium tuberculosis*) results in the development of sensitized lymphocytes. Re-exposure to the antigen (as in intradermal injection) causes these cells to release mediators at the site of re-exposure, which results in induration and erythema (a positive test). If no reaction occurs, the patient was not exposed to a significant load of the antigen previously or the patient is anergic. This type of reaction, called a "delayed hypersensitivity skin test," usually manifests within 48 to 72 hours. Table 124.1 lists other potential antigens available for intradermal skin testing.

Other antigens such as antibiotics result in an immediate hypersensitivity reaction mediated by IgE on presensitized mast cells in the dermis (type I hypersensitivity reaction). This type of reaction can detect sensitivity to a host of other antigens, including other drugs, microorganisms, pollens, animal dander, and helminths. A positive response is manifested by the triple response of Lewis et al. (2). Initially the skin becomes pale, followed by an erythematous flare and then a slight swelling or induration described as a "wheal." This dermal reaction to histamine usually begins within 5 minutes of allergen exposure and peaks at approximately 30 minutes. Occasionally, a late phase reaction occurs 3 to 24 hours later and manifests as ill-defined edema.

▶ INDICATIONS

The tuberculin skin test is based on the observation by Robert Koch that infection with *M. tuberculosis* caused cutaneous reactivity to tuberculin, the heat-killed, purified protein derivative (PPD) from cultures of *M. tuberculosis*. When tuberculin is introduced into the dermis with a syringe, the test is called a "tuberculin skin test" (TST) or "Mantoux test." This test is currently the only recommended skin test for detecting

TABLE 124.1	EXAMPLES OF SUBSTANCES INJECTED INTRADERMALLY

Tests for *Mycobacterium* infection
 Old tuberculin (OT)
 Purified protein derivative (PPD)
Antigens for anergy testing
 Tetanus toxoid antigen
 Diphtheria toxoid antigen
 Streptococcus antigen
 Candida antigen
 Trichophyton antigen
 Proteus antigen
Negative controls for hypersensitivity testing
 Normal saline solution
 Glycerine
Tests for evidence of infection
 Leprosy
 Lymphogranuloma venereum
 Mumps
 Cat scratch disease
 Chancroid
 Brucellosis
 Tularemia
 Glanders
 Toxoplasmosis
 Blastomycosis
 Histoplasmosis
 Coccidioidomycosis
 Trichonosis
 Filariasis
Allergy testing
 Horse serum based antivenin
 Drugs (including antibiotics)
 Pollens
 Animal dander
 Bee venoms
Local anesthesia
 Lidocaine or other local anesthetic

TABLE 124.3	RISK-ASSESSMENT QUESTIONNAIRE FOR TUBERCULOSIS

1. Was your child born outside the United States?
 If yes, this question would be followed by:
 Where was your child born?
 If the child was born in Africa, Asia, Latin America, or Eastern Europe, a tuberculin skin test (TST) should be placed.
2. Has your child traveled outside the United States?
 If yes, this question would be followed by:
 Where did the child travel, with whom did the child stay, and how long did the child travel?
 If the child stayed with friends or family members in Africa, Asia, Latin America, or Eastern Europe for ≥1 week cumulatively, a TST should be placed.
3. Has your child been exposed to anyone with TB disease?
 If yes, this question should be followed by questions to determine if the person had TB disease or LTBI, when the exposure occurred, and what the nature of the contact was. If confirmed that the child has been exposed to someone with suspected or known TB disease, a TST should be placed. If it is determined that a child had contact with a person with TB disease, notify the local health department per local reporting guidelines.
4. Does your child have close contact with a person who has a positive TB skin test?
 If yes, see Question 3 above for follow-up questions.

Risk-assessment questionnaires can include the following questions based on local epidemiology and priorities:

1. Does your child spend time with anyone who has been in jail (or prison) or a shelter, uses illegal drugs, or has HIV?
2. Has your child drank raw milk or eaten unpasteurized cheese?
3. Does your child have a household member who was born outside the United States?
4. Does your child have a household member who has traveled outside the United States?

Note: Adolescents can be asked these questions directly.
Reproduced from Pediatric Tuberculosis Collaborative Group, American Academy of Pediatrics. Targeted tuberculin skin testing and treatment of latent tuberculosis infection in children and adolescents. *Pediatrics.* 2004;114:1175–1201.

tuberculosis. It is indicated acutely in suspected mycobacterial infection or in patients with a significant tuberculosis exposure (Table 124.2). This diagnosis should be considered in children with chronic cough, pneumonia (especially of the upper lobes), adenopathy (particularly of the hilum) or adenitis (especially of the head or neck), or meningitis.

TABLE 124.2	PATIENTS AT RISK FOR TUBERCULOSIS INFECTION

1. Contacts of adults with infectious tuberculosis
2. Patient or parents from country with high prevalence of tuberculosis
3. Frequent exposure to high-risk adults (HIV-infected patients, homeless persons, drug abusers, poor and medically indigent city dwellers, nursing home residents, migrant farm workers)
4. Chest radiograph abnormalities suggestive of tuberculosis
5. Clinical evidence of tuberculosis
6. HIV seropositivity
7. Immunosuppressive disorders
8. Corticosteroids at immunosuppressive doses
9. Other medical risk factors (Hodgkin disease, lymphoma, diabetes, chronic renal failure, malnutrition)
10. Incarcerated adolescents

Adapted from Lewis T, Grant RT. Vascular reactions of the skin to injury. Pt. II. *Heart.* 1924;11:209.

Tuberculosis can involve virtually any body system, including the lungs, central nervous system, gastrointestinal system, cardiovascular system, bones, joints, skin, and eyes. In the primary care setting, a risk assessment questionnaire (Table 124.3) is used to identify patients with risk factors for TB who should be tested (3). TST is not indicated routinely for low-risk populations. The screening multiple puncture tests (including the commercial brands Monovacc, Aplitest, and Tine) are no longer recommended for the diagnosis of tuberculosis due to a high rate of false-positive responses (approximately 20%) and false-negative responses (up to 10%) (4). The only absolute contraindication for intradermal tuberculin placement is a severe skin reaction with prior testing. The patient will give a history of a bullous or necrotic-type reaction. Upon examination of the patient, it is also likely that residual scarring from such a reaction will be evident.

The Mantoux test is also useful for the diagnosis of diseases due to nontuberculous mycobacterium species (cervical adenitis is the most common example in children). These organisms share a number of common antigens with *M. tuberculosis* and account for many false-positive reactions when *M. tuberculosis* is being ruled out.

Skin testing also is used to test for allergic and anergic reactions. Tests other than intradermal injection are used by allergists to test for immediate hypersensitivity. These include the scratch test and the prick-puncture test. With the scratch test, a superficial scratch is made through the outer cornified layer of the skin. The allergen is then applied to the area. Nonspecific reactions can occur at the site in response to the local trauma alone, resulting in a false positive. This test is not recommended for routine use. In the prick-puncture test, allergen is applied to the skin surface, and then a needle is passed through the substance into the epidermis. The needle tip is then elevated to lift a small portion of the epidermis. The intradermal test is more sensitive and is therefore the test of choice in the ED. Skin tests for hypersensitivity to drugs or other substances are rarely, if ever, carried out in the emergency setting. In the rare event that a potential antigen needs to be given to a patient, an allergist can be consulted. In most cases, such as suspected antibiotic allergy, an alternative drug can be selected. If no alternative is available and the situation is life-threatening or the allergy history is vague, the drug is given with appropriate precautions in the event of anaphylaxis.

Intradermal injection also can be used for local anesthesia (Chapter 35) and for antitoxin allergy testing in cases of envenomations (Chapter 129).

▶ EQUIPMENT

Alcohol swab
Sterile, disposable tuberculin syringe
Intradermal needle, small gauge (26 or 27), short (0.25 to 0.50 inches), and beveled
Purified protein derivative (PPD)

PPD is introduced into the skin with a so-called "tuberculin syringe." The same size and type of equipment is used regardless of the patient's age. If multiple antigens are to be injected for anergy testing, an anergy panel is available (Multitest CMI). This device consists of a plastic applicator with multiple sterile test heads preloaded with skin antigens and a negative control. As with the injection of any chemical or biologic product, monitoring and resuscitative equipment should be available in the event of an adverse reaction such as anaphylaxis.

▶ PROCEDURE

This procedure is considered routine, and written consent is not required. The substance to be injected should not be outdated. The active fraction of tuberculin is easily absorbed by plastic or glass, and it should therefore be kept in a cool, dark place and not be transferred from one container to another. To avoid reduced potency, tuberculin should be injected as soon as possible after it is drawn into the syringe.

A site for injection free of hair, obvious superficial blood vessels, pigmented lesions, and infected or other skin lesions is selected. Because it may be scarred by the procedure, the location should have minimal cosmetic ramifications. The volar aspect of the forearm several inches distal to the elbow

is the most frequently used area. Infrequently, the patient's back is used. The diaphragm of the vial stopper is wiped with 70% alcohol, and then the substance to be injected is drawn into a tuberculin syringe. For an initial PPD, 0.1 mL or 5 TU (tuberculin units) is used. Air bubbles are removed from both the syringe and the lumen of the needle. Using circular motions, a 3-cm region of skin is cleansed with an alcohol swab. After the alcohol dries completely, the skin is stretched by placing thumb and forefingers at either side of the injection site. Alternatively, the forearm may be grasped from the posterior aspect, which secures the arm and stretches the skin at the same time.

The syringe is held nearly parallel to the skin, with the bevel of the needle directed up. The angle of the needle to the skin should be less than 15 degrees relative to the skin surface. The clinician then inserts the needle into the skin just past the opening in the bevel of the needle. The clinician pulls the plunger back to ensure that a blood vessel has not been entered. If blood is aspirated, the clinician should withdraw the needle and reattempt the procedure with a new syringe at a different location. The substance is injected while the skin is observed for the appearance of a wheal or a pale bleb (Fig. 124.1). Waiting several seconds after injecting the substance before removing the needle will minimize the amount of liquid that may seep through the injection site upon withdrawal of the needle. The needle is then removed slowly. The presence of a wheal confirms injection into the dermal layer. Absence of a wheal or more than a small amount of bleeding at the injection site indicates probable injection into the subcutaneous tissue (5).

The exact time and site of the injection is documented. The intradermal PPD test is standardized regarding both the dose of tuberculin injected and the definition of the diameter of a positive response. PPD that seeps out of the skin may falsely decrease the amount of a dermal response in a patient who is sensitized.

After the injection, the perimeter of the injection site may be marked with a waterproof pen or skin marker so that the site of injection is easily located when the patient returns for follow-up. For the injection of allergens, the patient should be observed for 30 minutes for possible allergic reaction.

Some authorities advocate using a control injection with sterile normal saline on the opposite forearm. Isopropyl alcohol, for example, can cause a reaction that may be misinterpreted as a response to antigen. This technique is often used when testing for immediate hypersensitivity, but it is not common for tuberculin testing.

For the Mantoux test, appropriate follow-up must occur at 48 to 72 hours. All results should be interpreted by qualified medical personnel and not by the patient or a family member. Induration of greater than or equal to 15 mm is a positive test. A reaction that is less than 5 mm is negative. Reactions between 5 and 15 mm are interpreted based on the patient's age and risk factors (Table 124.4). Repeat testing may be indicated 8 to 10 weeks after the first test. Of note, a negative TST does not exclude tuberculosis. About 10% of immunocompetent patients with culture-positive disease have a negative TST (6).

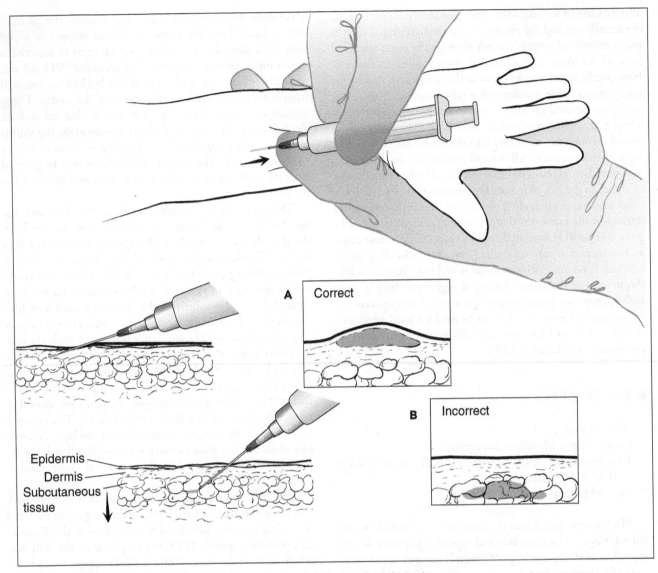

Figure 124.1   Proper positioning of syringe and hands for intradermal injection.
A. Using the appropriate angle and depth of needle insertion, the injectant is deposited in the intradermal layer.
B. With an incorrect angle and/or depth of needle insertion, the injectant may be deposited in subcutaneous tissue.

Many patients with tuberculosis demonstrate anergy early in the course of illness. Patients also may be anergic due to coinfections (especially with HIV), young age, and immunosuppression. Conversely, some patients may have an increased response to skin testing. These include patients who have received BCG (bacillus Calmette-Guerin) vaccination and patients exposed to mycobacterium species (including nontuberculous mycobacterium species) who have had repetitive skin testing. This so-called "booster phenomenon" cannot be differentiated from the response to natural infection.

The family should receive instructions to call or return at once if skin breakdown occurs or if the patient develops evidence of a systemic allergic reaction (e.g., hives or respiratory distress). Other family members also may require testing for tuberculosis if exposure was significant.

▶ COMPLICATIONS

Some hypersensitive patients may develop a severe reaction at the injection site, which can range from vesiculation to ulceration and necrosis. Such strongly positive tests can result in scarring. For this reason, areas of lesser cosmetic importance are chosen for this test. All patients receiving PPD need to be questioned regarding such a reaction, as it is a contraindication to standard PPD testing. Other less significant reactions include transient bleeding or immediate erythema at the puncture site. Some patients develop pain or pruritus at the test site, which may be relieved by cold packs or topical steroid preparations.

Anaphylaxis is rare with PPD but can occur with the intradermal injection of allergens. This type of reaction is more likely with injections to the skin layers deeper than the

TABLE 124.4	**DEFINITIONS OF POSITIVE TUBERCULIN SKIN TEST RESULTS IN CHILDREN AND ADOLESCENTS**

Induration ≥5 mm

1. Children or adolescents in close contact with a known or suspected infectious case of TB
2. Children or adolescents with suspected TB disease:
   a. Finding on chest radiograph consistent with active or previously active TB
   b. Clinical evidence of TB disease
   c. Children or adolescents who are immunosuppressed (e.g., receiving immunosuppressive therapy or with immunosuppressive conditions such as HIV infection)

Induration ≥10 mm

1. Children or adolescents at increased risk of disseminated disease:
   a. Patients <4 years old
   b. Patients with concomitant medical conditions (e.g., Hodgkin disease, lymphoma, diabetes mellitus, chronic renal failure, or malnutrition)
2. Children or adolescents with increased risk of exposure to cases of TB disease:
   a. Patients born in a country with a high prevalence of TB cases
   b. Patients who travel to a country with a high prevalence of TB cases or patients with parents born in a country with a high prevalence of TB cases
   c. Patients frequently exposed to adults with risk factors for TB disease (e.g., adults who are HIV-infected or homeless, users of illicit drugs, those who are incarcerated, or migrant farm workers)

Induration ≥15 mm

Children ≥4 years old with no known risk factors

Adapted from American Academy of Pediatrics. *Red Book: 2003 Report of the Committee on Infectious Diseases.* 25th ed. Elk Grove Village, IL: American Academy of Pediatrics; 2003:642–660.

 CLINICAL TIPS

▶ The substance to be injected should not be outdated.

▶ Proper storage of the injected substance must be ensured.

▶ The active component of PPD is easily absorbed onto plastic, so it should be promptly injected after being drawn out of the vial.

▶ The site of the injection can be marked with a waterproof marker to ease in later identification of the site.

▶ After injecting the substance, waiting several seconds before removing the needle will minimize the amount of liquid that may seep through the injection site upon withdrawal of the needle. This decreases the likelihood of a false-negative test.

dermis. A patient should be observed for approximately 30 minutes after receiving intradermal allergen. Complications can be minimized by taking a careful history and by using proper technique.

 SUMMARY

1 Select a site for injection, usually the volar aspect of the forearm.

2 Draw up the substance to be injected using sterile technique.

3 Cleanse the skin with a 70% alcohol swab and allow to dry.

4 Secure the arm and stretch the skin at the injection site.

5 Hold the syringe with the bevel up and nearly parallel to the skin; insert the needle into superficial layers of skin just past the tip of the needle.

6 Aspirate to ensure that a blood vessel has not been entered, then slowly inject the substance.

7 Slowly withdraw the needle and confirm intradermal placement by the presence of a wheal.

8 Document the site of injection and consider drawing a circle around the site with a waterproof marker.

9 Ensure follow-up with a physician or other health professional in 48 to 72 hours for interpretation.

▶ SUMMARY

A recent resurgence of tuberculosis has occurred in this country. The Mantoux test is easy to perform, relatively inexpensive, and effective in diagnosing tuberculosis. The procedure is learned quickly and has an important role in the ED setting.

▶ REFERENCES

1. Mantoux C. Intradermoreation de la tuberculose. *C R Acad Sci.* 1908;147:355.
2. Lewis T, Grant RT. Vascular reactions of the skin to injury, II: the liberation of a histaminelike substance in the injured skin, the underlying cause of factitious urticaria and of wheals produced by burning: and observations upon the nervous control of certain skin reactions. *Heart.* 1924;11:209.
3. Pediatric Tuberculosis Collaborative Group, American Academy of Pediatrics. Targeted tuberculin skin testing and treatment of latent tuberculosis infection in children and adolescents. *Pediatrics.* 2004;114:1175–1201.
4. Committee on Infectious Diseases, American Academy of Pediatrics. Screening for tuberculosis in infants and children. *Pediatrics.* 1994;93:131–134.
5. McConnell EA. Giving intradermal injections. *Nursing.* 1990;20(3):70.
6. Pickering LK, ed. *Red Book: 2003 Report of the Committee of Infectious Diseases.* 26th ed. Elk Grove Village, IL: American Academy of Pediatrics; 2003.

125

MARY A. HEGENBARTH AND GARY S. WASSERMAN

Gastric Lavage

▶ INTRODUCTION

Gastric lavage has been performed for almost two centuries, and it yet remains a controversial procedure. In 1812, Physick used a hollow tube to lavage twin infants with laudanum (tincture of opium) overdose (1). Determining the best approach for decontamination of the poisoned patient is a difficult task because there are many confounding variables (e.g., characteristics of the substance ingested, amount of ingestant, time since ingestion, unreliability of history, time for patient to seek medical care, and differences in techniques) (2–12). Despite the extensive use of gastric lavage, few reports have demonstrated improvement in patient outcomes (13–15). In recent years, the advisability of any gastric emptying procedure for most patients has been questioned, with many experts recommending activated charcoal as the primary treatment (4,5,10,12,16,17). Official position statements for gut decontamination of the poisoned patient were first published in 1997; gastric lavage guidelines were re-evaluated in 2004 and are essentially unchanged (18,19).

Since acute ingestions rarely cause fatality, especially in nonintentional childhood ingestions, practitioners must rapidly decide if gastric lavage has an acceptable risk-benefit ratio for a particular patient. Other methods of gut decontamination include activated charcoal and/or whole bowel irrigation (syrup of ipecac is no longer recommended). Consultation with a clinical toxicologist or poison center is highly recommended if the clinician is unsure about the best method of gastrointestinal decontamination for a particular patient; treatment should be individualized.

There has been a 85% decline in the utilization of gastric lavage from 1993 to 2005 (3.45% of all exposures to 0.51%) (20,21). Most pediatric patients requiring treatment for toxic ingestions are either young children less than 6 years of age with accidental poisoning or adolescents with intentional ingestions due to suicide attempts or illicit drug use. The procedure is similar to gastric intubation (Chapter 84) and is done in the hospital setting (primarily the emergency department) by physicians and/or nurses. Gastric lavage is moderately difficult to perform and requires attention to detail for optimal effectiveness and avoidance of complications. Gastric lavage should not be performed routinely in the management of the poisoned patient (19).

▶ ANATOMY AND PHYSIOLOGY

Small children obviously have smaller nasal and oral passageways, a shorter esophagus, and a smaller stomach than adults. Other factors that may make lavage relatively difficult in young children include a large tongue, loose primary teeth, and an uncooperative attitude regarding the procedure. Lavage tubes are easily inserted too far into children, which may cause serious malposition despite clinical signs of adequate placement

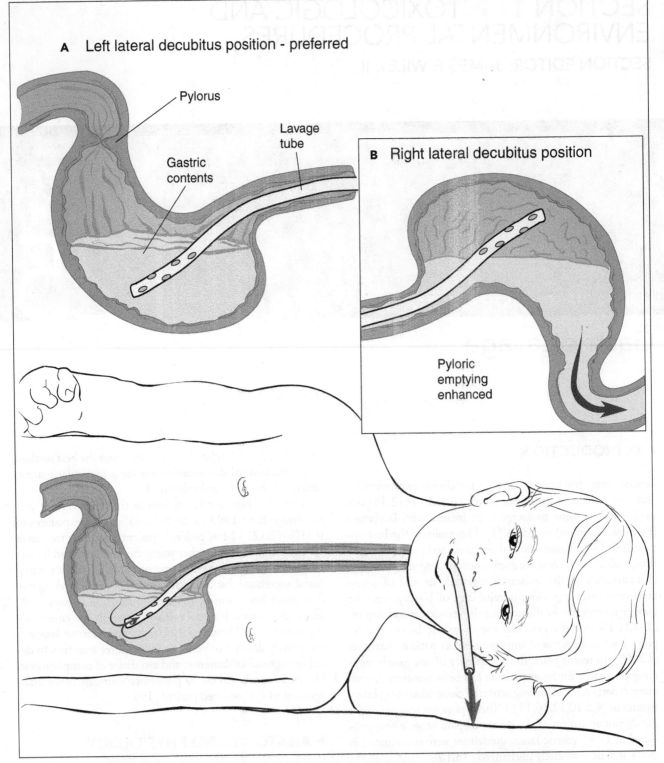

Figure 125.1 Effect of patient position on pyloric emptying and availability of gastric contents to lavage. (Adapted from Burke M. Gastric lavage and emesis in the treatment of ingested poisons: a review and a clinical study of lavage in 10 adults. *Resuscitation*. 1972;1:91–105.)
A. Left lateral decubitus (preferred). Access to gastric contents enhanced, pyloric emptying discouraged.
B. Right lateral decubitus. Pyloric emptying enhanced (undesirable).

(22). Proper insertion length has been found to correlate with patient height (22,23).

Gastric lavage aims to remove toxin from the stomach before absorption occurs; its effectiveness diminishes with increasing time since ingestion. Effectiveness also depends on the physical characteristics of the substance(s) ingested. Liquids are rapidly absorbed and are unlikely to be significantly recovered given the typical delay preceding lavage. Solid preparations are absorbed more slowly; absorption is further delayed with enteric-coated forms, substances that retard gastrointestinal motility (e.g., anticholinergic agents), and substances that tend to form concretions. Dogma suggests that gastric lavage may have the undesired effect of accelerating absorption by enhancing pyloric emptying into the duodenum (24). However, more recent studies contradict these earlier results and have discovered no evidence showing any increase in the amount of marker present in the small bowel after lavage compared with no intervention (25,26). Enhanced gastric emptying into the pylorus is more likely if the patient is lying on the right side or if large aliquots of cold fluids are used (27–29). Therefore, the left lateral decubitus position is preferred to maximize access of the tube to stomach contents and minimize pyloric emptying (Fig. 125.1). Young children are more susceptible to electrolyte changes than adults; normal saline or 0.45 normal saline is recommended rather than water. Using warmed or at least room temperature fluid will prevent iatrogenic hypothermia and may aid in slowing pyloric transit time (27). Gastric emptying from lavage is incomplete, as continued drug absorption occurs and drug concretions may form (14,30,31).

▶ INDICATIONS

Gastric lavage is indicated for life-threatening toxic ingestions in which the potential benefit of the procedure is felt to outweigh the substantial risks. Obtunded patients in one study who underwent gastric lavage within 1 hour of ingestion had improved outcome compared with those who received only activated charcoal (8). Lavage is most effective when performed within the first 30 to 60 minutes after ingestion, although drugs whose absorption is prolonged (e.g., aspirin, anticholinergics) may sometimes be recovered in significant amounts even after many hours. Specific indications for gastric lavage include the unconscious poisoned patient or ingestion of a highly toxic substance, especially one with rapid onset of central nervous system depression or seizures (e.g., cyclic antidepressants, clonidine, cyanide, camphor). Table 125.1 summarizes the contraindications to gastric lavage.

Consultation is recommended if the physician is unsure about the best method(s) of gastrointestinal decontamination. For the majority of children with mild to moderate potential toxicity, activated charcoal alone may be the safest, most effective treatment; observation is often adequate for asymptomatic patients (9).

TABLE 125.1	CONTRAINDICATIONS TO GASTRIC LAVAGE

▶ Airway compromise without prior endotracheal intubation (e.g., loss of gag reflex)
▶ Previous esophageal or gastric injury, surgery, or anomaly (e.g., stricture, tracheoesophageal fistula, gastric stapling, etc.); however, children with gastric fundoplication can be safely lavaged
▶ Time since ingestion exceeds 1 to 2 hours
▶ Ingestions likely to cause only mild toxicity (risks outweigh benefits)
▶ Patient at risk for hemorrhage (e.g., coagulopathy, medical condition)
▶ Most hydrocarbon ingestions unless unusually large volume or containing a highly toxic component (e.g., insecticide)
▶ Acid or alkaline caustic ingestion
▶ Plant or mushroom ingestions if fragments too large to pass

▶ EQUIPMENT

Orogastric lavage tube with side holes or closed system (Fig. 125.2)
Tape measure
Lubricant for tube
Oral airway or bite block
Rigid suction device with large openings to handle emesis
Funnel and/or wide-tipped syringe for instilling and withdrawing fluid
Lavage fluid, warmed or room temperature normal saline, at least 1 to 2 L
Basin for collecting drainage
Sterile specimen container for toxicologic analysis
Activated charcoal, if indicated
Restraint devices (e.g., papoose board, extremity restraints) for young or uncooperative patients
Protective clothing, eyewear, gloves for personnel
Resuscitative equipment, including oxygen, bag-valve-mask device, and airway equipment
Monitoring of vital signs, cardiac rhythm, and oxygen saturation if patient is unstable, intubated, or depressed level of consciousness

Large lavage tubes (24 to 50 French) are most effective for recovering solid fragments. The tube should be fairly rigid to prevent collapse and should have side holes. Tubes especially designed for gastric lavage are preferred rather than soft rubber or nasogastric tubes. A 24 French tube is commonly used for young children; 34 to 40 French tubes are recommended for adolescents and adults. The syringe used for infusing and draining fluid should have a large-bore opening or it will impede drainage. Commercially available kits for gastric lavage include appropriate tubes packaged with special wide-tipped syringes. More elaborate closed system sets also are available. Their contents vary and may include special bags for fluid infusion and/or drainage collection and adapters for direct charcoal administration (Easi-Lav, Kimberly-Clark, Irving, Texas; Tum-E-Vac, Ethox, Buffalo, NY). The Easi-Lav disposable closed system has unique one-way valves and simultaneous or separately operated dual plungers that simplify gastric lavage.

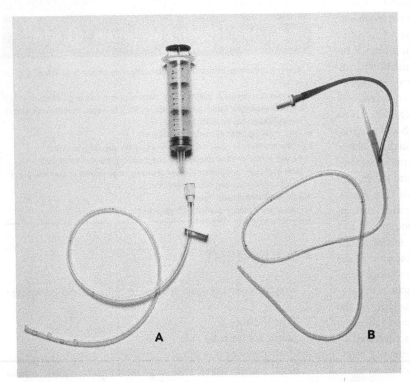

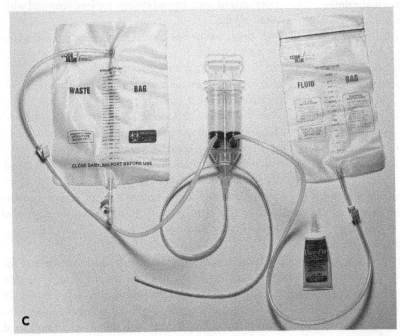

Figure 125.2
A. Orogastric tube with syringe.
B. Salem sump tube (not recommended).
C. Closed system for gastric lavage using dual syringes.

The closed system kits are more expensive than simple kits but are convenient for performing large-volume lavages (Fig. 125.2C).

▶ PROCEDURES

The oral approach is preferred in almost all instances, as it allows passage of a larger tube without trauma to the nasal mucosa and turbinates. The main disadvantages of the oral route are that gagging is increased and that the patient may bite on the tube. A bite block may be helpful but often causes gingival and oral trauma. Formal consent is not generally obtained before gastric lavage, but the indications, technique, and potential complications should be discussed with the parents and the procedure explained to the child (as appropriate for age).

Next, the patient's ability to protect the airway is assessed by checking the gag reflex and the level of consciousness. If the patient is unconscious and lacks a gag reflex, the airway should be protected by endotracheal intubation (Chapter 16).

However, intubation is rarely necessary, according to some authorities. Many children who appear somewhat sleepy are promptly awakened upon tube insertion and are able to fully protect their airway. If any question arises about the adequacy of airway protection, however, the patient should be intubated before attempting lavage.

Adequate restraint is essential—at least two persons are usually necessary to perform lavage in an uncooperative child. Suctioning equipment should be working and at hand. The distance for tube insertion is measured by placing the tube on the child and measuring from the teeth to the epigastrium, allowing for curvature of the tube along the tongue and oropharynx. Proper tube insertion length also can be determined using the patient's height (Fig. 125.3). Marking the distance for tube insertion with tape or ink is suggested. The patient is positioned in the left lateral decubitus position to minimize pyloric emptying; mild Trendelenburg positioning (head lower than feet at 20-degree tilt on the table) decreases the risk of aspiration. The distal tube is generously lubricated and inserted into the oropharynx. If cooperative, the patient is asked to swallow as the tube is gently advanced to the premarked length; tube insertion may be performed with the patient in the upright sitting position. Some authorities do not advise using topical anesthetic sprays or gels to ease passage, as they may interfere with the protective gag reflex. Do not apply force while passing the tube, especially if the patient is struggling. Flexing the neck may help pass the tube into the esophagus. In intubated patients, brief deflation of

the endotracheal tube cuff is advisable. The lavage tube should be removed if the patient develops respiratory distress, continual coughing, or inability to phonate or if the tube meets resistance or coils back through the mouth. Once the tube appears to have passed successfully, its position is determined by insufflating 5 to 20 cc of air with a syringe while listening for a rush of air over the stomach. If equivocal, air insufflation is repeated while listening in the axillary lung fields. Practitioners should be aware that air sounds are easily transmitted in young children, and care is needed to confirm gastric tube position. Gastric contents usually drain if the tube is properly positioned. If gastric contents do not return, an attempt can be made to advance the tube a few centimeters, as it may be in the distal esophagus. Although rarely needed, additional maneuvers to exclude inadvertent tracheal positioning of the tube may be performed if difficulty arises in confirming proper tube placement. One such test is to instill a few milliliters of saline into the tube, with coughing indicative of tracheal misplacement. Another method is to place the free end of the tube under water during expiration; if air bubbles are seen, the tube is in the trachea. Although seldom needed, radiographs may be helpful to ensure proper placement if tube position is still uncertain.

The stomach should be drained of its contents before beginning lavage, and the initial gastric aspirate saved for toxicologic analysis in a sterile specimen container. Aliquots of 10 mL/kg (about 100 mL in children, up to 200 mL in adolescents) of warm saline are used for lavage; water may

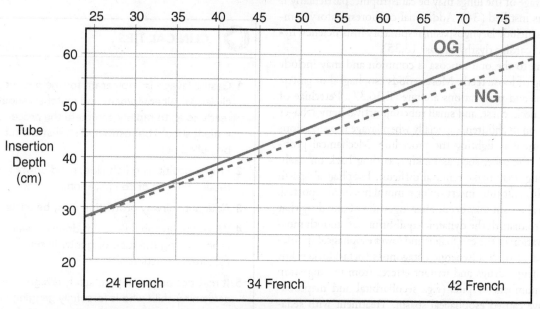

Figure 125.3 Estimation of gastric tube insertion depth based on patient height. OG, orogastric tube length; NG, nasogastric tube length. (Adapted from Scalzo AJ, Tominack RL, Thompson MW. Malposition of pediatric gastric lavage tubes demonstrated radiographically. *J Emerg Med.* 1992; 10:586. Used with permission of A. J. Scalzo.)

be substituted for adolescents and adults. The fluid may be infused by gravity or with a syringe, but rapid, forceful fluid injection should be avoided, as this may force stomach contents out the pylorus. Next, the lavage fluid is drained by gravity (by holding the end of the tube below the level of the stomach) or removed by syringe aspiration; the amount returned should approximate the amount infused. The procedure is continued until the return fluid is clear (minimum 1 L). In some patients, significant amounts of toxin can be recovered by further lavage after visual clearing (6). If concretions are suspected (e.g., aspirin), it may be helpful to flex the child's hips and gently massage the stomach (32). When using the dual-plunger system, the simultaneous inflow of lavage fluid and outflow of stomach contents tend to better agitate stomach contents, yielding more efficient lavage. However, one must be aware that solid materials (e.g., tablets, food) may obstruct the valves and require some plunger manipulation to correct. When lavage has been completed, regardless of the system, the tube may be used for installing activated charcoal before withdrawal. Retching or vomiting commonly occurs when the tube is removed. After lavage, the patient should be observed for any respiratory symptoms that might indicate pulmonary aspiration.

▶ COMPLICATIONS

Although rare, gastric lavage is associated with potentially serious complications. The most common serious complication is pulmonary aspiration, which may occur despite the presence of a gag reflex or a cuffed endotracheal tube (9,12,33). Inadvertent lavage of the lungs may be catastrophic, particularly if charcoal is instilled (34). Additional cardiorespiratory complications include laryngospasm, respiratory insufficiency, hypoxia, and cardiac dysrhythmias (13,35).

Trauma to the oral mucosa is common and may include dislodging of loose teeth. More serious esophageal or gastric lacerations and perforations are rare (8,36,37). Petechiae of the head, neck, chest, and small subconjunctival hemorrhages are common in children, especially when lavage is overzealous or the patient is fighting the procedure. Mechanical problems with the tube, such as kinking, curling back on itself, or knotting, may make removal difficult. Esophageal spasm causing difficult tube insertion or removal has been reported. Esophageal spasm may occur after ingestion of any drug that interacts to disturb the dynamic equilibrium of smooth muscle innervation of the esophagus and lower esophageal sphincter. Overdose of β-adrenergic antagonists (beta-blockers) or anticholinergic drugs and irritant effects from the ingestion of large numbers of pills (e.g., secobarbital and meprobamate) have caused esophageal spasm. Treatment with sedatives, glucagon, or nitroglycerin has been anecdotally effective (38,39). Electrolyte imbalance and hypothermia are potential problems in young children lavaged with cold or inappropriate lavage solutions.

SUMMARY

1 Ensure airway protection. Restrain and position the patient in the left lateral decubitus, head-down position. Have suction on at the bedside.

2 Measure the tube insertion distance and mark the tube (Fig. 125.3).

3 Lubricate the tube and insert gently through the mouth to the predetermined distance.

4 Confirm tube placement by auscultation of insufflated air over the stomach and by eventual return of gastric contents.

5 Lavage the patient using 10 mL/kg aliquots of saline (up to 200 mL) until the return is clear.

6 Instill activated charcoal before withdrawing the tube.

Respiratory complications can be minimized by giving careful attention to the airway and respiratory status, patient position, and accurate tube placement. Gentle technique with careful positioning of bite blocks and good lubrication minimizes trauma. Hypothermia and hyponatremia are prevented by using warmed saline for lavage. Food or drug concretions commonly block the lavage tube holes or obstruct at the narrow syringe connection to the lavage tube; manipulation of fluid flow may be required to keep the system patent.

CLINICAL TIPS

1 Gastric lavage is unpleasant for the patient and clinicians. All equipment and materials should be ready so as to rapidly complete the procedure. The patient should be restrained so that the tube cannot be pulled out.

2 Proper positioning (left side, head down) is vital to reduce the risk of complications.

3 Adequate airway protection must be ensured.

4 When the lavage fluid is not draining well, repositioning the tube or gently flushing it may restore its function.

5 It may not be possible to safely lavage an awake, screaming child who is forcefully gagging or vomiting around the tube. The procedure should be discontinued because the risks of aspiration and trauma are unacceptable.

▶ SUMMARY

In rare cases, gastric lavage may be useful in the child with a recent life-threatening ingestion. Airway protection must be ensured, and the child should be adequately restrained in the proper position, with working suction at hand. A large-bore orogastric tube should be used; tube insertion length should be premeasured and position confirmed after placement. Pulmonary aspiration is the most common among several serious complications. For this reason, careful consideration of the risk versus benefit of gastric lavage should occur before its performance.

▶ REFERENCES

1. Major RH. History of the stomach tube. *Ann Med Hist.* 1934;6:500–509.
2. Auerbach PS, Osterloh J, Braun O, et al. Efficacy of gastric emptying: gastric lavage versus emesis induced with ipecac. *Ann Emerg Med.* 1986;15:692–698.
3. Tandberg D, Diven BG, McLeod JW. Ipecac-induced emesis versus gastric lavage: a controlled study in normal adults. *Am J Emerg Med.* 1986;4:205–209.
4. Tenenbein M, Cohen S, Sitar DS. Efficacy of ipecac-induced emesis, orogastric lavage, and activated charcoal for acute drug overdose. *Ann Emerg Med.* 1987;16:838–841.
5. Underhill TJ, Greene MK, Dove AF. A comparison of the efficacy of gastric lavage, ipecacuanha and activated charcoal in the emergency management of paracetamol overdose. *Arch Emerg Med.* 1990;7:148–154.
6. Young WF, Bivens HG. Evaluation of gastric emptying using radionuclides: gastric lavage versus ipecac-induced emesis. *Ann Emerg Med.* 1993;22:1423–1427.
7. Tenenbein M. Inefficacy of gastric emptying procedures. *J Emerg Med.* 1985;3:133–136.
8. Kulig K, Bar-Or D, Cantrill SV, et al. Management of acutely poisoned patients without gastric emptying. *Ann Emerg Med.* 1985;14:562–567.
9. Merigian KS, Woodard M, Hedges JR, et al. Prospective evaluation of gastric emptying in the self-poisoned patient. *Am J Emerg Med.* 1990;8:479–483.
10. Kulig K. Initial management of ingestions of toxic substances. *N Engl J Med.* 1992;326:1677–1681.
11. Phillips S, Gomez H, Brent J. Pediatric gastrointestinal decontamination in acute toxin ingestion. *J Clin Pharmacol.* 1993;33:497–507.
12. Pond SM, Lewis-Driver DJ, Williams GM, et al. Gastric emptying in acute overdose: a prospective randomised controlled trial. *Med J Aust.* 1995;163:345–349.
13. Allan BC. The role of gastric lavage in the treatment of patients suffering from barbiturate overdose. *Med J Aust.* 1961;2:513–514.
14. Comstock EG, Faulkner TP, Boisaubin EV, et al. Studies on the efficacy of gastric lavage as practiced in a large metropolitan hospital. *Clin Toxicol.* 1981;18:581–597.
15. Ardagh M, Tait C. Limiting the use of gastrointestinal decontamination does not worsen the outcome from deliberate self-poisoning. *N Z Med J.* 2001;114:423–425.
16. Greensher J, Mofenson HC, Caraccio TR. Ascendancy of the black bottle (activated charcoal). *Pediatrics.* 1987;80:949–951.
17. Albertson TE, Derlet RW, Foulke GE, et al. Superiority of activated charcoal alone compared with ipecac and activated charcoal in the treatment of acute toxic ingestions. *Ann Emerg Med.* 1989;18:56–59.
18. American Academy of Clinical Toxicology and European Association of Poison Centres and Clinical Toxicologists. Gut decontamination [position statement]. *Clin Toxicol.* 1997;35:695–762.
19. American Academy of Clinical Toxicology and European Association of Poison Centres and Clinical Toxicologists. Gastric lavage [position statement]. *Clin Toxicol.* 2004;42:933–943.
20. Litovitz TL, Clark LR, Soloway RA. 1993 Annual Report of the American Association of Poison Control Centers Toxic Exposure Surveillance System. *Am J Emerg Med.* 1994;12:546–555.
21. Lai MW, Klein-Schwartz W, Rodgers GC, et al. 2005 Annual Report of the American Association of Poison Control Centers National Poisoning and Exposure Data Base. *Clin Toxicol.* 2006;44:803–932.
22. Scalzo AJ, Tominack RL, Thompson MW. Malposition of pediatric gastric lavage tubes demonstrated radiographically. *J Emerg Med.* 1992;10:581–586.
23. Strobel CT, Byrne WJ, Ament ME, et al. Correlation of esophageal lengths in children with height: application to the Tuttle test without prior esophageal manometry. *J Pediatr.* 1979;94:81–84.
24. Saetta JP, March S, Gaunt ME, et al. Gastric emptying procedures in the self-poisoned patient: are we forcing gastric content beyond the pylorus? *J R Soc Med.* 1991;84:274–276.
25. Shrestha M, George J, Chiu MJ, et al. A comparison of three gastric lavage methods using the radionuclide gastric emptying study. *J Emerg Med.* 1996;14:413–418.
26. Eddleston M, Juszczak E, Buckley N. Does gastric lavage really push poisons beyond the pylorus? A systematic review of the evidence. *Ann Emerg Med.* 2003;42:359–364.
27. Ritschel WA, Erni W. The influence of temperature of ingested fluid on stomach emptying time. *Int J Clin Pharmacol.* 1977;15:172–175.
28. Burke M. Gastric lavage and emesis in the treatment of ingested poisons: a review and a clinical study of lavage in 10 adults. *Resuscitation.* 1972;1:91–105.
29. Vance MV, Selden BS, Clark RF. Optimal patient position for transport and initial management of toxic ingestions. *Ann Emerg Med.* 1992;21:243–246.
30. Saetta JP, Quinton DN. Residual gastric content after gastric lavage and ipecacuanha-induced emesis in self-poisoned patients: an endoscopic study. *J R Soc Med.* 1991;84:35–38.
31. Sharman JR, Cretney MJ, Scott RD, et al. Drug overdoses: is one stomach washing enough? *N Z Med J.* 1975;81:195–197.
32. Bartecchi CE. A modification of gastric lavage technique. *JACEP.* 1974;3:304–305.
33. Matthew H, Mackintosh TF, Tompsett SL, et al. Gastric aspiration and lavage in acute poisoning. *BMJ.* 1966;1:1333–1337.
34. Harris CR, Filandrinos D. Accidental administration of activated charcoal into the lung: aspiration by proxy. *Ann Emerg Med.* 1993;22:1470–1473.
35. Thompson AM, Robins JB, Prescott LF. Changes in cardiorespiratory function during gastric lavage for drug overdose. *Hum Toxicol.* 1987;6:215–218.
36. Caravati EM, Knight HH, Linscott MS Jr, et al. Esophageal laceration and charcoal mediastinum complicating gastric lavage. *J Emerg Med.* 2001;20:273–276.
37. Wald P, Stern J, Weiner B, et al. Esophageal tear following forceful removal of an impacted oral-gastric lavage tube. *Ann Emerg Med.* 1986;15:80–82.
38. Rinder HM, Murphy JW, Higgins GL. Impact of unusual gastrointestinal problems on the treatment of tricyclic antidepressant overdose. *Ann Emerg Med.* 1988;17:1079–1081.
39. Panos RJ, Tso E, Barish RA, et al. Esophageal spasm following propranolol overdose relieved by glucagon. *Am J Emerg Med.* 1986;4:227–228.

126

MICHAEL SHANNON

Activated Charcoal Administration

▶ INTRODUCTION

The efficacy of activated charcoal in the treatment of poisoning was first described in the 1700s, although it was Tovery's survival after ingesting a strychnine and charcoal slurry before the French Academy of Medicine in 1831 that dramatized its life-saving effects (1,2).

Activated charcoal is created from the exposure of carbon-containing materials (usually low-ash wood) to steam and acids, producing a finely granular substance with a surface area of approximately 1,000 m²/g.

▶ ANATOMY AND PHYSIOLOGY

The microscopic pores of activated charcoal permit adsorption of drugs and other large-molecular-weight substances. Activated charcoal, in fact, effectively adsorbs almost all toxins, with notable exceptions including alcohol, metals and minerals, hydrocarbons, and cyanide. Maximal adsorption of toxins by charcoal occurs when the charcoal-drug ratio is 10:1.

Because of its effectiveness both in preventing systemic absorption of an ingested toxin (i.e., enhancement of pre-absorptive elimination) and in accelerating the elimination of already absorbed toxins (i.e., postabsorptive elimination enhancement), charcoal has become the most important intervention in the treatment of toxic exposures. Because gastric emptying and cathartic administration provide only modest benefit after toxic ingestion, increasing data support the administration of activated charcoal alone (3,4).

▶ INDICATIONS

Activated charcoal is indicated in two distinct circumstances. First, it should be considered after the ingestion of any toxin known to be adsorbed by activated charcoal. Second, it may be valuable in enhancing the elimination of drugs that can be removed by gastrointestinal dialysis (e.g., theophylline, phenobarbital, salicylates) or drugs that are known to have substantial elimination of parent compound and/or pharmacologically active metabolite through the bile (e.g., carbamazepine). In the case of theophylline and phenobarbital, oral charcoal will enhance the elimination of drug that has been administered intravenously (5,6).

The window of opportunity for clinical effectiveness depends on the absorption characteristics of the toxin. With toxins in which gut absorption is complete within 2 to 4 hours, activated charcoal has a clear role only if it is administered in that time frame. In contrast, for drugs with delayed gut absorption (e.g., drugs with anticholinergic activity), activated charcoal is potentially effective in preventing drug absorption for up to 12 hours postingestion. Current recommendations suggest that activated charcoal's benefit is maximal if given within 1 hour of ingestion.

Contraindications to activated charcoal are loss of airway control, ingestion of a caustic agent (because such victims should be NPO and because endoscopic evaluation cannot be easily performed after charcoal administration), and gastrointestinal obstruction or perforation.

▶ EQUIPMENT

Activated charcoal
Flavoring (cola or cherry syrup)
Cup with a lid
Straw
If patient is uncooperative:
Nasogastric tube (Chapter 84)

Activated charcoal is available in many forms. The simplest preparation is desiccated charcoal, which is reconstituted as needed for administration. However, the most common form of activated charcoal currently available consists of either charcoal suspended in water (with an added sweetener) or a cathartic, most commonly sorbitol. These preparations avoid the mess produced by the preparation of a charcoal slurry from powder. Activated charcoal–sorbitol mixtures should be avoided because (1) they are more emetogenic than charcoal alone, (2) sorbitol can produce dangerous fluid losses when administered to young children, and (3) cathartics have no proven efficacy in the management of the poisoned patient. Less commonly used but also available are charcoal capsules or tablets. These forms are difficult with children because many tablets must be ingested to achieve the minimally effective charcoal dose.

Activated charcoal is administered in a dose of 1 g/kg. Although many authorities advocate strict attention to the

10:1 activated charcoal–toxin ratio, with no ceiling dose, the maximal dose is typically 50 to 60 g. In circumstances where repetitive oral charcoal is administered, the typical dose is 1 g per kilogram of body weight (maximum 50 to 60 g) every 4 hours or 0.5 g/kg every 2 hours.

▶ **PROCEDURE**

Administration of activated charcoal to a child or adult is usually accomplished easily by having the patient slowly drink a charcoal slurry prepared in a vehicle of water or cathartic (Fig. 126.1). Flavoring agents have little effect on adsorptive characteristics and may be added. Placing the slurry in a covered cup and using a straw often makes the mixture more palatable. In the case of an infant or toddler, activated charcoal is rarely

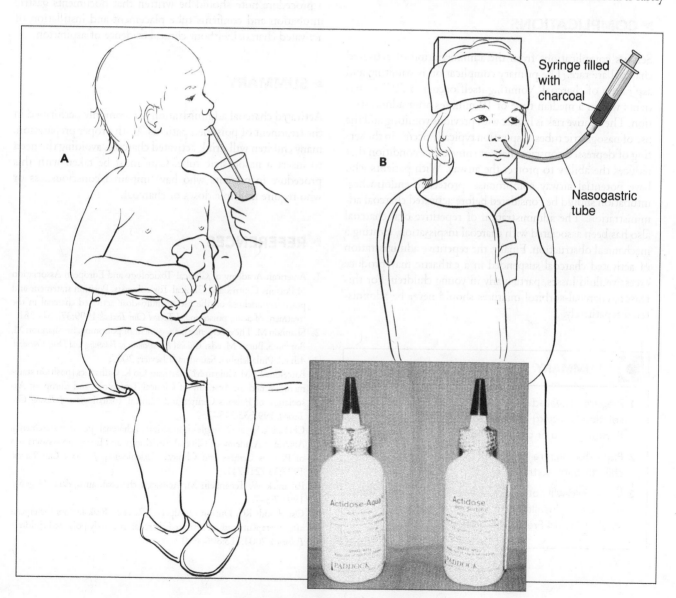

Figure 126.1 Activated charcoal administration.
A. Child voluntarily drinking an activated charcoal slurry.
B. Nasogastric administration.

taken voluntarily (although this may be initially attempted), requiring that it be administered via an orogastric tube (if gastric lavage is being first performed) or by a small nasogastric tube (if it is simple charcoal instillation).

Activated charcoal administration to the small child requires a 12 to 14 French nasogastric tube, sterile lubricant, catheter tip syringe, and restraining papoose. After the child is restrained and with the help of an assistant, the clinician inserts the nasogastric tube (Chapter 84). Tube placement should be confirmed ideally by return of gastric contents or by air insufflation which is heard after placing a stethoscope over the stomach. With the patient's head restrained, the activated charcoal is infused slowly. After infusion is complete, the nasogastric tube is removed and the child released from restraints.

▶ COMPLICATIONS

Serious complications from the administration of activated charcoal are rare. The primary complication is vomiting and aspiration of charcoal. Vomiting itself occurs in 20% of patients within a median time of 10 minutes after administration. The relative risk is higher with previous vomiting and the use of nasogastric tubes. Aspiration typically occurs in the setting of depressed consciousness or some other condition that reduces the ability to protect the airway. With patients who have potential airway compromise, protective endotracheal intubation should be considered before activated charcoal administration. The administration of repetitive oral charcoal also has been associated with charcoal inspissation, creating a mechanical obstruction. Finally, the repetitive administration of activated charcoal suspended in a cathartic may produce excessive fluid losses, particularly in young children. For this reason, charcoal-sorbitol mixtures should never be administered repetitively.

SUMMARY

1 Prepare activated charcoal by mixing an aqueous solution (1 mg/kg up to 50 to 60 g) and add flavoring (cola or cherry syrup) if desired.

2 Place the mixture in cup with a lid and offer to the child through a straw.

3 If the child will not drink the activated charcoal, then it should be instilled through an orogastric tube or a small (12 to 14 French) nasogastric tube.

CLINICAL TIPS

▶ Most children will drink the charcoal if it is prepared properly.

▶ Activated charcoal should not be administered to a child with an altered level of consciousness until the airway is protected.

▶ Multiple doses of activated charcoal require special attention to cathartic administration; cathartic should never be administered serially.

As with any procedure that has potential complications, a procedure note should be written that documents gastric intubation and confirms tube placement and instillation of activated charcoal without clinical evidence of aspiration.

▶ SUMMARY

Activated charcoal administration is commonly performed in the treatment of poisoned patients. With proper preparation, many children will drink activated charcoal, avoiding the need to insert a nasogastric tube. Care must be taken with this procedure in patients who have impaired consciousness or who require multiple doses of charcoal.

▶ REFERENCES

1. American Academy of Clinical Toxicology and European Association of Poisons Centres and Clinical Toxicologists. Position statement and practice guidelines on the use of multi-dose activated charcoal in the treatment of acute poisoning. *J Toxicol Clin Toxicol.* 1999;37:731–751.
2. Shannon M. The emergency management of poisoning. In: Shannon M, Borron S, Burns M, eds. *Clinical Management of Poisoning and Drug Overdose.* 4th ed. Philadelphia: Saunders/Elsevier; 2007.
3. Barceloux D, McGuigan M, Hartigan-Go K. Cathartics [position statement]. American Academy of Clinical Toxicology and European Association of Poisons Centres and Clinical Toxicologists. *J Toxicol Clin Toxicol.* 1997;35:743–752.
4. Chyka PA, Seger D. Single-dose activated charcoal [position statement]. American Academy of Clinical Toxicology and European Association of Poisons Centres and Clinical Toxicologists. *J Toxicol Clin Toxicol.* 1997;35:721–741.
5. Palatnick W, Tenenbein M. Activated charcoal: an update. *Drug Saf.* 1992;7:3–7.
6. Osterhoudt KC, Durbin D, Alpern ER, et al. Risk factors for emesis after therapeutic use of activated charcoal in acutely poisoned children. *Pediatrics.* 2004;113:806–810.

127

Whole-Bowel Irrigation

▶ INTRODUCTION

Whole-bowel irrigation (WBI) is a procedure intended to prevent the absorption of poisons by removing them from the gastrointestinal tract. It consists of the rapid enteral administration of large amounts of the special irrigation fluid polyethylene glycol electrolyte lavage solution (PEGELS) over several hours (1). It is routinely used in patients of all ages as a colonoscopy preparative procedure. It differs from the other gastrointestinal decontamination procedures, syrup of ipecac–induced emesis, gastric lavage, and single-dose activated charcoal administration in that it has the potential to decontaminate the intestines as well as the stomach. Although WBI has been shown to decrease the bioavailability of selected ingestants to a greater extent than these other procedures, it should be restricted to specific indications because it is both labor intensive and time consuming.

Prevention of absorption is a cardinal tenet of treating the acute overdose patient. The traditional approach was to use either ipecac-induced emesis or gastric lavage as the primary intervention, followed by activated charcoal as an adjunctive procedure. However, opinion has shifted to charcoal monotherapy (2–5), and current practice reflects this change.

Situations arise, however, when charcoal would be expected to be of limited benefit. These include ingestion of substances not adsorbed by charcoal (iron being the most important) and presentation of a patient several hours after the ingestion of delayed release pharmaceuticals. These drugs can persist for prolonged periods within the intestines and thus beyond the reach of ipecac, gastric lavage, and charcoal.

▶ ANATOMY AND PHYSIOLOGY

Drug absorption depends on such factors as dissolution of the pharmaceutical, ionization state (the ionized form of a drug is less well absorbed), location of the substance within the gastrointestinal tract (more surface area and blood flow to the proximal small intestine), and transit time for the toxin through the gastrointestinal tract. Most toxins are absorbed in the proximal small intestine. The rationale for using WBI is to hasten the transit of poison past the area of absorption and thus decrease its bioavailability (1).

Human bioavailability studies in volunteers receiving WBI have consistently shown decreases in drug absorption of 67% to 73% (6–8). This exceeds the performance of syrup of ipecac, gastric lavage, or a single dose of activated charcoal when performed at comparable times after ingestion. Only 3,500 molecular weight polyethylene glycol electrolyte solution should be used for WBI, because it was specifically designed to prevent fluid or electrolyte flux across the gastrointestinal epithelium (9).

▶ INDICATIONS

The indications for using WBI are the ingestion of substances not adsorbed by charcoal and the ingestion of delayed release pharmaceuticals (Table 127.1) (10). These types of pharmaceuticals can persist within the gut for many hours beyond the reach of the other decontaminating procedures. Of the toxins not adsorbed by activated charcoal, iron is most commonly ingested, and it has been shown to be removed by WBI (11). WBI should also be considered for the treatment of lithium (8), lead (12), and zinc (13) overdoses. Ingestion of very large amounts of toxic substances and delayed presentation after ingestion are potential indications (1); however, these specific situations are difficult to identify in the clinical setting. WBI is also of potential benefit for illicit drug body stuffers and packers (14). While this is an unlikely presentation in the pediatric age group, such cases have been reported (15).

1175

TABLE 127.1	INDICATIONS FOR WHOLE-BOWEL IRRIGATION

I. Strongly recommended . . .
    Iron
    Lithium
    Modified (sustained) release pharmaceuticals
II. Consider for . . .
    Heavy metals
        Lead salts
        Zinc salts
    Packets of illicit drugs

Contraindications for WBI are ileus, gastrointestinal hemorrhage, obstruction, and perforation. Compromised circulation also is a contraindication because of the need to elevate the head of the bed. An absent gag reflex is a relative contraindication because of the risk of pulmonary aspiration.

▶ EQUIPMENT

Polyethylene glycol electrolyte lavage solution
Nasogastric tube (10 to 12 French)
Intravenous pole
Reservoir bag used for tube feedings
Commode
Irrigation solution, which is available as a powder requiring reconstitution with tap water or as a ready-to-use product

▶ PROCEDURE

The nasogastric tube is passed into the stomach, and the gastric location is assessed by auscultation during air injection (Chapter 84). It is preferable to confirm that the tip of the tube is in the midportion of the stomach with an x-ray. The tube is then attached to a reservoir bag of irrigation solution, which is hung from an intravenous pole (Fig. 127.1). Mechanical infusion pumps are not recommended because most cannot achieve the high flow rates required for adequate WBI. The patient should be seated or the head of the bed elevated to at least 45 degrees. The desired rates of flow are 500 mL/hr for children less than 6 years, 1,000 mL/hr for children 6 to 12 years, and 1,500 to 2,000 mL/hr for children above 12 years. The endpoint is a clear rectal effluent, which takes many hours to achieve. A commode or similar receptacle is useful to collect the effluent.

A nasogastric tube is required because patients will not consume the irrigation fluid at the required rate. Only a small-bore tube is needed for this procedure, although such a tube would not be suitable for gastric lavage or even gastric aspiration. Pretreatment with syrup of ipecac is undesirable because this tends to cause vomiting of the irrigating solution. Placing the patient in an upright position promotes the settling of the

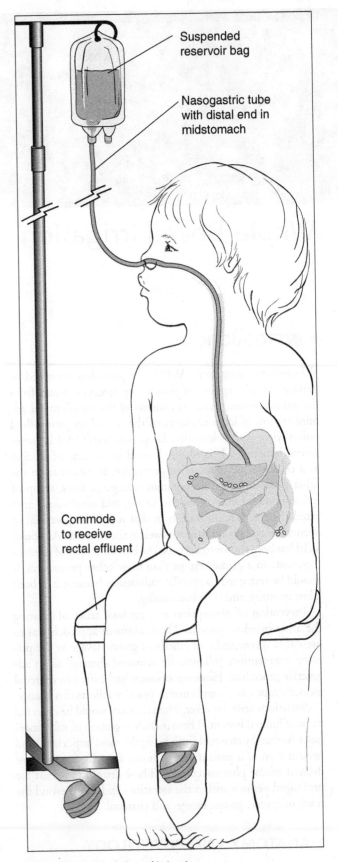

Suspended reservoir bag

Nasogastric tube with distal end in midstomach

Commode to receive rectal effluent

Figure 127.1 Whole-bowel irrigation.

ingestant into the distal portion of the stomach, decreases the likelihood of vomiting, and establishes a dependent relationship of the intestines to the stomach. These measures favor a more efficient irrigation.

Although not frequent, emesis may complicate this procedure. When it occurs, it is usually a consequence of the ingestant itself (e.g., theophylline or salicylate). Ingestant-induced emesis is best managed by the administration of an antiemetic, which must be given parenterally, as WBI interferes with the absorption of orally administered medications. Metoclopramide (initial dose 0.1 mg/kg every 6 hours, intravenously) is favored for both its antiemetic and its gastric-emptying properties. Keeping the upper half of the patient's body upright also decreases the likelihood of emesis. If emesis occurs despite these measures, the infusion rate may be decreased by 50% for 30 to 60 minutes with the intent of returning to the previous rate. These interventions control emesis in most situations.

A single dose of activated charcoal can be given before initiating WBI, but multiple doses of charcoal should not be given during the procedure. Charcoal adsorption of the ingestant may be blocked by the polyethylene glycol of the irrigating solution, which can occupy the binding sites on the charcoal. This has been shown to occur with the lower charcoal doses

CLINICAL TIPS

▶ Nasogastric administration of irrigation solution is required because even the most cooperative patient will not consume a sufficient amount at the required rate.

▶ Emesis is usually controlled by decreasing the rate of infusion for brief periods of time.

▶ Positioning the patient upright promotes a more efficient whole-bowel irrigation.

▶ A commode or similar receptacle is strongly recommended for collecting the effluent.

used in multiple-dose charcoal therapy to promote drug excretion but not with the larger initial dose that is used to prevent drug absorption (16).

Monitoring of WBI requires the usual nursing supervision for intravenous therapy; however, monitoring the patient's fluid or electrolyte status during the procedure is not necessary. The endpoint is a clear rectal effluent, which takes many hours to achieve. If WBI is being used to remove foreign bodies from the gastrointestinal tract, then the appearance of a clear rectal effluent may not be a valid endpoint. In such instances, the endpoint to consider is the absence of radiopaque foreign bodies on abdominal radiographs or the passage of the expected number of foreign bodies in the rectal effluent (17). After completion of WBI, two to three liquid bowel movements are expected.

SUMMARY

1 Pass a 12 French nasogastric tube into the stomach (Chapter 84).

2 Ensure gastric location by auscultation after air injection.

3 Radiologically confirm that the tip of the tube is in the midportion of the stomach.

4 Attach the proximal end of the tube to the nasogastric tube feeding bag.

5 Hang the bag on an intravenous pole.

6 Seat the patient or elevate the head of the bed to at least 45 degrees.

7 Place polyethylene glycol electrolyte lavage solution into the feeding bag and allow it to flow into the patient by gravity.

8 Desired rates of flow:

Less than 6 years old—500 mL/hr

From 6 to 12 years old—1,000 mL/hr

More than 12 years old—1,500 to 2,000 mL/hr

9 The endpoint is clear rectal effluent, which can take many hours to achieve.

10 Use a commode or other receptacle to collect the rectal effluent.

▶ COMPLICATIONS

To date, no major complications from properly performed WBI have been reported. Theoretical concerns exist for pulmonary aspiration after emesis or perforation of a viscus if WBI is given in the presence of ileus or gastrointestinal hemorrhage. However, relative to the other forms of gastrointestinal decontamination, WBI should be regarded as having a low risk-benefit ratio.

▶ SUMMARY

Whole-bowel irrigation is an effective but labor-intensive gastrointestinal decontamination procedure for poisoned patients. It is not a panacea for all overdose patients and should be reserved for its specific indications.

▶ REFERENCES

1. Tenenbein M. Whole-bowel irrigation as a gastrointestinal decontamination procedure after acute poisoning. *Med Toxicol.* 1988;3:77–84.

2. Kulig K, Bar-Or D, Cantrill SV, et al. Management of acutely poisoned patients without gastric emptying. *Ann Emerg Med.* 1985;14:562–567.

3. Albertson TE, Derlet RW, Foulke GE, et al. Superiority of activated charcoal alone compared with ipecac and activated charcoal in the treatment of acute toxic ingestions. *Ann Emerg Med.* 1989;18:56–59.

4. Merigian KS, Woodard M, Hedges JR, et al. Prospective evaluation of gastric emptying in the self-poisoned patient. *Am J Emerg Med.* 1990;8:479–483.

5. Kulig K. Initial management of ingestions of toxic substances. *N Engl J Med.* 1992;326:1677–1681.

6. Tenenbein M, Cohen S, Sitar DS. Whole-bowel irrigation as a decontamination procedure after acute drug overdose. *Arch Int Med.* 1987;147:905–907.

7. Kirshenbaum LA, Mathews SC, Sitar DS, et al. Whole-bowel irrigation versus activated charcoal in sorbitol for the ingestion of modified release pharmaceuticals. *Clin Pharmacol Ther.* 1989;46:264–271.

8. Smith SW, Ling LJ, Halstenson CE. Whole-bowel irrigation as a treatment for acute lithium overdose. *Ann Emerg Med.* 1991;20:536–539.

9. Davis GR, Santa Ana CA, Morawski SG, et al. Development of a lavage solution associated with minimal water and electrolyte absorption or secretion. *Gastroenterology.* 1980;78:991–995.

10. American Academy of Clinical Toxicology and European Association of Poisons Centres and Clinical Toxicologists. Whole bowel irrigation [position paper]. *J Toxicol Clin Toxicol.* 2004;42:843–854.

11. Tenenbein M. Whole-bowel irrigation in iron poisoning. *J Pediatr.* 1987;111:142–145.

12. Roberge RJ, Martin TG. Whole-bowel irrigation in an acute oral lead intoxication. *Am J Emerg Med.* 1992;10:577–583.

13. Burkhart KK, Kulig KK, Rumack B. Whole-bowel irrigation as treatment for zinc sulfate overdose. *Ann Emerg Med.* 1990;19:1167–1170.

14. Hoffman RS, Smilkstein MJ, Goldfrank LR. Whole-bowel irrigation and the cocaine body packer: a new approach to a common problem. *Am J Emerg Med.* 1990;8:523–527.

15. Beno S, Calello D, Baluffi A, et al. Pediatric body packing: drug smuggling reaches a new low. *Pediatr Emerg Care.* 2005;21:744–746.

16. Kirshenbaum LA, Sitar DS, Tenenbein M. Interaction between whole-bowel irrigation solution and activated charcoal: implications for the treatment of toxic ingestions. *Ann Emerg Med.* 1990;19:1129–1132.

17. Scharman EJ, Lembersky R, Krenzelok EP. Efficacy of whole-bowel irrigation with and without metoclopramide pretreatment. *Am J Emerg Med.* 1994;12:302–305.

DAVID C. LEE AND TADEUSZ KORZUN

128

Skin Decontamination

▶ INTRODUCTION

Similar to the patient who presents with multiple trauma, a child with a life-threatening dermal exposure can pose a dramatic challenge. Health care providers must not solely concentrate on the exposure and neglect the fundamentals of resuscitation. Furthermore, unlike in the case of the trauma patient, health care providers must follow hazardous materials (HAZMAT) procedures and policies for their own protection (Chapter 8) (1). The primary objective in decontamination is to rapidly remove the offending toxin, because, typically, the longer the contact, the greater the absorption. Fortunately, with nearly all dermal exposures, the aphorism "the solution to the pollution is dilution" is valid.

▶ ANATOMY AND PHYSIOLOGY

The skin is an extremely effective barrier to potentially toxic compounds. The ability of the skin to act as a barrier depends on the relative maturity and thickness of the epidermis, dermis, subcutaneous fat, and appendices (Fig. 128.1A) (2–4).

The epidermis is composed of four layers, which form a tough, water-insoluble covering. The rate-limiting step in the penetration of the skin for most substances is diffusion through the outermost layer (stratum corneum) (5). Because the dermis is more permeable than the epidermis, any disruption of the epidermis may lead to greater tissue injury and absorption. The thickness of the stratum corneum varies with age and location on the body (Fig. 128.1B). The preterm infant does not have a fully formed stratum corneum and is more susceptible to dermal absorption (2,3,5). Plantin et al. noted that dermal permeability is increased in premature infants but falls steadily until approximately the age of 10 days (6). The newborn infant has an average dermal thickness of

1.2 mm, compared with an average thickness of 2.1 mm in an adult (2). Epidermal and dermal thickness also differs in various areas of the body. Rates of absorption correlate proportionately with these variations (7). Vanrooij et al. showed that absorption of polyaromatic hydrocarbons was 69% greater in the groin compared to the palm. (Fig. 128.2) (8).

The dermis and subcutaneous fat, the two deeper layers of the skin, mainly act as a fibrous envelope and as an insulator. These layers and the deeper layers of the epidermis are rich in enzymes and can modify chemicals that penetrate the stratum corneum. The skin is capable of phase I oxidative, phase II conjugation, reduction, and hydrolytic reactions (8–10). Sweat gland ducts and hair follicle orifices may enable toxins to penetrate the skin. Their concentration also varies with age and anatomical site. The adult forehead has approximately 900 follicles per square centimeter, compared with none on the palms and soles.

The pediatric patient is more susceptible than the adult patient to suffering injury from dermal exposures, not only because of the differences in the structure of the skin but also because of the higher proportion of body surface area to body weight (11). Wester et al. showed that the neonate exhibits roughly three times greater absorption rates than the adult for an equal amount of exposure (12). Because infants have much less keratin in their skin, they are more susceptible to vesicants and caustics than are adults (13,14). Table 128.1 summarizes important factors that may enhance toxin absorption.

▶ INDICATIONS

The goals of decontamination are to prevent both absorption and systemic toxicity. No absolute contraindications exist for dermal decontamination. Life-saving procedures, however, should not be delayed by the need for skin decontamination.

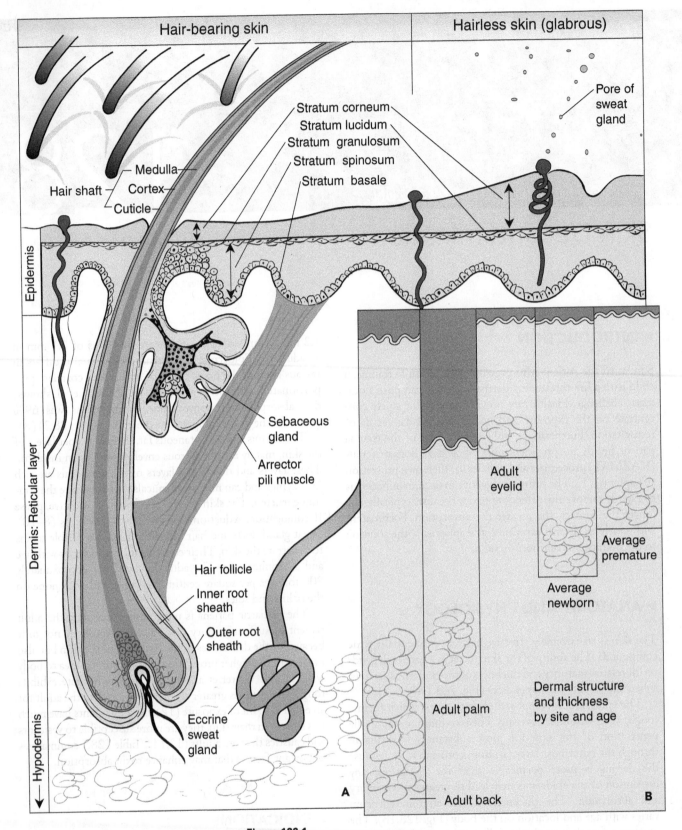

Figure 128.1
A. Anatomy of the skin.
B. Variation in dermal structure and thickness (7).

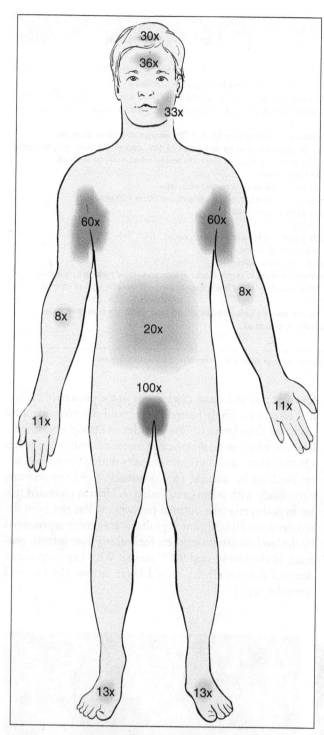

Figure 128.2 Absorption rates of parathion in male adults (7).

TABLE 128.1	FACTORS ENHANCING ABSORPTION

Host Properties
  Maturity of the dermis
  Integrity of the dermis
  Anatomical site
  Skin hydrations
Chemical Properties
  High lipid solubility
  Low molecular weight
  High chemical concentration
Physical Factors
  Occlusion or wrapping of the area
  Prolonged exposure
  Amount of surface area exposed
  Vehicle that toxin is dissolved in

Personal protective equipment (PPE) (in the hospital, not in the chemical release zone; see Chapter 8):
  Powered air-purifying respirator (PAPR) that provides a protection factor of 1,000 (respirator must be approved by the National Institute for Occupational Safety and Health [NIOSH])
  Combination 99.97% high-efficiency particulate air (HEPA)/organic vapor/acid gas respirator cartridges (also NIOSH-approved)
  Double-layer protective gloves
  Chemical-resistant suit
  Head covering and eye/face protection (if not part of the respirator)
  Chemical-protective boots
  Suit openings sealed with tape

▶ PROCEDURE

Before skin decontamination, health care personnel must ensure their safety by donning appropriate personal protective equipment (Chapter 8). The Occupational Safety and Health Administration (OSHA) has recently provided guidance for first receivers of potentially contaminated patients. This guidance identifies level C PPE as most appropriate for hospitals when they are operating outside of the area of incident (15,16). Resuscitative efforts aimed at addressing respiratory or circulatory compromise should not be delayed by skin decontamination. The patient should be placed in an area specifically designed for decontamination and should be dealt with using special procedures established to prevent contamination of other areas of the hospital with the exposure. The designated area should have a self-contained water drainage system (gurney with collection bottle or floor drain with a containment tank) and air ventilation that is filtered and goes to the outside. For mass casualty situations, the optimal site for decontamination may be outside of the hospital, with appropriate designation and maintenance of hot, warm, and cold zones (Fig. 128.3). However, in temperate zones with cold winters, specially constructed facilities

▶ EQUIPMENT

Established area for decontamination in the emergency department, as per HAZMAT protocols
Green soap or other mild soap
Lukewarm normal saline irrigant (Table 128.2 lists alternative irrigants for rare exposures)

TABLE 128.2	CHEMICALS REQUIRING SPECIFIC DECONTAMINATION	
Toxin	**Classification**	**Treatment**
Bitumen	Caustic	Copious irrigation with cold water until bitumen cools and hardens.
		Betumen that is adherent to blistered skin should be removed with blister epithelium. Bitumen adherent to unblistered skin should be covered liberally with a hydrocarbon solvent (e.g., mineral oil).
Chromic acid	Caustic with systemic toxicity	Standard decontamination with consideration of 10% ascorbic acid added to irrigant.
Hydrofluoric acid	Caustic with systemic toxicity	Standard decontamination followed by application of 10% calcium gluconate gel. Parenteral calcium administration by injection or venous or arterial infusion may be required.
		Patient at risk for hypocalcemia.
Lime (calcium oxide)	Caustic	Brush off as much as possible prior to contact with water.
Methyl mercury	Caustic with systemic toxicity	Standard decontamination with blister débridement and blister fluid removal.
Phenol	Caustic with systemic toxicity	Irrigate with polyethylene glycol (PEG) 400.
Phosphorus (elemental yellow phosphorus)	Caustic	Avoid exposure to air.
		Copious water irrigation, and keep covered with water.
Radiation	Acute radiation syndrome	Obtain radiation monitoring device.
		Protect personnel if patient is radioactive.
		Decontaminate from periphery to center of area of exposure. Avoid creating new breaks in the skin. Allow wounds to bleed freely. Collect urine and faces for signs of internal decontamination.
Reactive metals (e.g. elemental sodium, potassium, lithium)	Caustic	Apply mineral oil and remove visible particles with forceps, gauze or towels, then store removed particles in mineral oil.

Note: The treatment protocols given here are theoretically optimal, but decontamination efforts should not be delayed for a significant time to institute them.

adjacent to the main ED but structurally distinct and with separate ventilation systems may be useful (Fig. 128.4). Once stabilization procedures have been initiated, skin decontamination begins with the removal of all clothes and jewelry. The removal of clothing alone is estimated to accomplish as much as 90% of the decontamination in fully clothed individuals. These items should be handled carefully and placed in double plastic bags. Any solid or particulate matter is brushed off before washing. This prevents dissolution of solid matter and increased toxin absorption. Similarly, viscous liquid contaminants should be blotted off. Tepid water should be used at high volumes and low pressures to rinse the patient. Forceful irrigation could theoretically cause the dissolution of

fine particles and cause disruptions in the protective epidermal layer. Excessively heated water could theoretically cause increased dissolution of fine particles and peripheral vasodilatation, which in turn may cause increased toxin absorption. On the other hand, in colder climates during the winter, water needs to be warmed to a reasonably tepid temperature, particularly with infants and young children at increased risk for hypothermia (the optimal temperature has not been determined scientifically but is probably reasonably represented by the level chosen by mothers for bathing their infants, generally in the low to mid 90°F range). With large exposures, decontamination efforts should begin around the face and move distally.

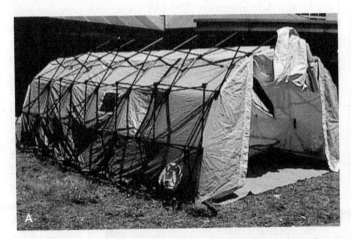
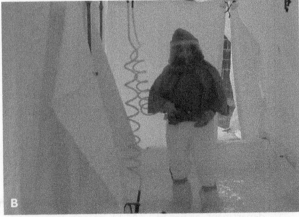

Figure 128.3 An easily deployable outdoor decontamination facility. (Reproduced with permission from Henretig FM, Cieslak TJ, Madsen JM, et al. Emergency department awareness and response to incidents of biological and chemical terrorism. In: Fleisher GR, Ludwig S, Henretig FM, eds. *Textbook of Pediatric Emergency Medicine.* 5th ed. Philadelphia: Lippincott Williams & Wilkins; 2006:150.)

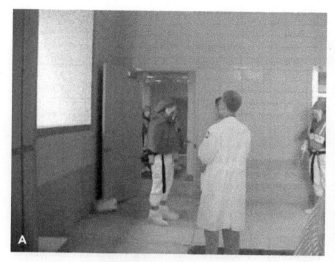
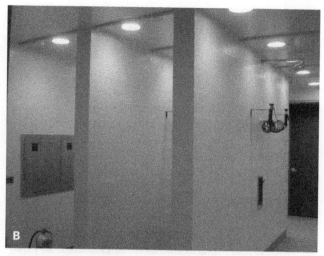

Figure 128.4
A. An indoor decontamination facility contiguous with but structurally separate from the main ED.
B. Parallel lanes allow capacity for both ambulatory and nonambulatory victims.
(Reproduced with permission from Henretig FM, Cieslak TJ, Madsen JM, et al. Emergency department awareness and response to incidents of biological and chemical terrorism. In: Fleisher GR, Ludwig S, Henretig FM, eds. *Textbook of Pediatric Emergency Medicine*. 5th ed. Philadelphia: Lippincott Williams & Wilkins, 2006:150.)

After rinsing the patient, tincture of green soap or other mild soap is used to wash off further residue. Exposed skin should be handled gently to avoid accidentally abrading the skin and thereby further increasing toxin exposure. Special attention should be paid to areas where contaminants may collect—hair, nails, orifices, intertriginous areas, and areas of high dermal absorption such as the face and genitalia.

On rare occasions, certain exposures require special irrigants and procedures (see Table 128.2). Toxins that are insoluble in water or those that create exothermic reactions when combined with water require decontamination with other solutions or by dry removal. For example, irrigating dry lime,

which contains calcium oxide, will create a caustic alkali solution of calcium hydroxide. Dry lime should be carefully brushed off the skin prior to contact with water. Another example is phenol, which may be better decontaminated with polyethylene glycol 400 than with water.

Antidotes and neutralizing agents can lead to exothermic reactions and may themselves increase toxicity. Furthermore, obtaining these antidotes often cause a delay in the decontamination. Some exceptions to this rule exist, as is evident in the treatment of hydrofluoric acid (HF), phenol, and phosphorus exposures.

⬤ SUMMARY

1 Place the patient in the proper area for decontamination; ensure adequate protection of health care personnel based on the toxic exposure.

2 Perform appropriate stabilization procedures and remove all clothing and jewelry.

3 Brush off solid matter and blot any viscous liquid on the skin.

4 Starting at the face and moving distally, rinse the skin with tepid water irrigant at high volume and low pressure (Table 128.2 lists exceptions).

5 Gently wash the patient with mild soap (tincture of green soap), with special attention to the hair, nails, intertriginous areas, and face.

6 Maintain temperature homeostasis throughout the procedure to avoid hypothermia.

▶ COMPLICATIONS

Hypothermia is the major potential complication of skin irrigation, requiring that tepid water be used, temperature be monitored closely, and warming be instituted as needed following decontamination (Chapter 131). Other problems associated with skin decontamination are failure to stabilize

◗ CLINICAL TIPS

▶ Hazardous materials protocols should be developed for any hospital area likely to receive contaminated patients.

▶ Airway, breathing, and circulation must be addressed before attempts at skin decontamination.

▶ Early facial decontamination avoids further exposure by ingestion or inhalation.

the patient before instituting irrigation and failure to protect health care personnel properly during decontamination.

▶ SUMMARY

As compared with the adult patient, the pediatric patient is more susceptible to injury from a toxic dermal exposure. Fortunately, the basics of decontamination are technically simple to perform and easy to remember.

▶ REFERENCES

1. Horton DK, Berkowitz Z, Kaye WE. Secondary contamination of ED personnel from hazardous materials events, 1995–2001. *Am J Emerg Med.* 2003;21:199–204.

2. Eady R, Goldsmith L, Dahl M. Structure and function. In: Schachner L, Hansen R, eds. *Pediatric Dermatology.* 3rd ed. New York: Mosby; 2003:3–42.

3. Rutter N. Physiology of the newborn skin. In: Harper J, Oranje A, Prose N, eds. *Textbook of Pediatric Dermatology.* London, UK: Blackwell Sciences; 2000:43–52.

4. Began D. Dermatologic principles. In: Flomenbaum N, Goldfrank L, Hoffman R, et al., eds. *Goldfrank's Toxicologic Emergencies,* 8th ed. New York: McGraw Hill Co; 2006:456–464.

5. McAuliffe DJ, Blank IH. Effects of UVA (320–400 nm) on the barrier characteristics of the skin. *J Invest Dermatol.* 1991;96: 758–762.

6. Plantin P, Jouan N, Karangwa A, et al. [Variations of the skin permeability in premature newborn infants: value of the skin vasocon-striction test with Neosynephrine]. *Arch Fr Pediatr.* 1992;49:623–625.

7. Maibach HI, Feldman RJ, Milby TH, et al. Regional variation in percutaneous penetration in man. Pesticides. *Arch Environ Health.* 1971;23:208–211.

8. VanRooij JG, De Roos JH, Bodelier-Bade MM, et al. Absorption of polycyclic aromatic hydrocarbons through human skin: differences between anatomical sites and individuals. *J Toxicol Environ Health.* 1993;38:355–368.

9. Guy R, Hadgraft J. Principles of skin permeability relevant to chemical exposure. In: Hobson D, ed. *Dermal and Ocular Toxicity: Fundamentals and Methods.* Boston: CRC Press; 1991:221–246.

10. Began D. Dermatologic principles. In: Goldfrank L, ed. *Goldfrank's Toxicologic Emergencies.* 7th ed. New York: McGraw-Hill; 2002:432–440.

11. Lynch EL, Thomas TL. Pediatric considerations in chemical exposures: are we prepared? *Pediatr Emerg Care.* 2004;20:198–208.

12. Wester RC, Noonan PK, Cole MP, et al. Percutaneous absorption of testosterone in the newborn rhesus monkey: comparison to the adult. *Pediatr Res.* 1977;11:737–739.

13. Rotenberg JS, Burklow TR, Selanikio JS. Weapons of mass destruction: the decontamination of children. *Pediatr Ann.* 2003;32:260–267.

14. Yu CE, Burklow TR, Madsen JM. Vesicant agents and children. *Pediatr Ann.* 2003;32:254–257.

15. OSHA best practices for hospital-based first receivers of victims from mass casualty incidents involving the release of hazardous substances. Occupational Safety and Health Administration, 2005. Available at: www.osha.gov/dts/osta/bestpractices/html/hospital_firstreceivers.html. Accessed May 13, 2005.

16. Scarfone R, Sullivan F, Henretig FM. Decontamination of the chemically contaminated patient in the pediatric emergency department. *Pediatr Emerg Care.* In press.

DIANE P. CALELLO, KEVIN C. OSTERHOUDT,
AND G. RANDALL BOND

129

Envenomation Management
and Tick Removal

▶ INTRODUCTION

Envenomation management procedures vary greatly by offending organism but generally involve some part of three
components: inactivation of venom, removal of envenomation apparatus or body parts, and local wound management.
This chapter deals with the procedures for managing North
American snakebites, North American scorpion stings, black
widow spider bites, jellyfish envenomation, and marine vertebrate envenomation as well as the procedures for tick removal.
Envenomation from exotic reptiles and arthropods occurs in
the United States, and guidance may be obtained from regional poison control centers.

▶ NORTH AMERICAN SNAKE BITES

Anatomy and Physiology

Venomous snakes are indigenous throughout the United
States, with the exception of Maine, Alaska, and Hawaii.
The most prominent native venomous snakes are members
of the Viperidae family (Crotalinae subfamily) and include
rattlesnakes, moccasins, and copperheads. These "pit vipers"
have hollow, hinged front fangs connected to venom glands,
which allow subcutaneous injection of venom much like a
syringe and needle. Rattlesnakes are the largest North American snakes and have the longest fangs, reaching a length of
3 to 4 cm. Although the potency and exact composition of
venom varies significantly among species, all have the ability
to cause local swelling, direct cellular injury, and shock (1).
Some species, such as the eastern diamondback rattlesnake,
primarily have hemorrhagic toxins, which cause the aggregation of platelets or degradation of fibrinogen and can result

in disseminated intravascular coagulation. Others, such as the
Mojave rattlesnake, have neurotoxins, which cause paresthesia,
weakness, and muscle fasciculation.

Coral snakes, which represent the other family (Elapidae)
of venomous snakes indigenous to the United States, are found
in the southeastern United States and the Sonoran desert of
Arizona. These brightly colored snakes can be identified by
the sequence of their rings: the coral snake has red rings adjacent to yellow rings, in contrast to the nonvenomous scarlet
king snake, also found in the area (thus the mnemonic "red
on yellow, kill a fellow; red on black, venom lack"). These
snakes are relatively shy, and no human bites have been reported in Arizona in several years. Coral snake venom, while
not causing the degree of tissue destruction seen with most
crotaline snakebites, contains potent neurotoxins, which can
cause severe manifestations such as cranial nerve dysfunction
and respiratory muscle paralysis (2).

Because a snake will deliver the same amount of venom
whether biting an adult or a child, the degree of envenomation by weight is greater for children, and therefore pediatric
patients are likely to present with more severe symptoms (3).
In addition, a deeper bite into the muscle is theoretically more
likely in children, although, as in adults, bites through the fascia leading to elevated compartment pressures are rare. Two
fang marks are typically seen after envenomation, although
single or multiple marks are possible.

Indications

The severity of envenomation and the need for intervention
vary dramatically depending on the species and quantity of
venom injected (1,3–21). Although toxicity may be delayed,
most victims present with symptoms or show signs within
the first 4 to 8 hours. All symptomatic patients should have

frequent vital signs, fluid support, and adequate analgesia. Affected extremities should be immobilized, and in the case of the hand, wrist, and forearm, a volar splint should be placed for comfort (Chapter 101). Elevation of the extremity is not advised before the administration of antivenom, as this will hasten systemic distribution of venom; the affected extremity, once immobilized, should be kept at or slightly below the level of the heart. A complete blood count with platelet count, prothrombin time (PT), partial thromboplastin time (PTT), fibrinogen, and urinalysis should be obtained in all patients.

The extent of tissue edema and the rapidity of its proximal spread following Crotalinae envenomation may be dramatic. At time of presentation to the emergency department (ED), the leading edge of edema and ecchymosis on the affected extremity should be marked; thereafter, repeated measurements of linear progression, as well as circumference, should be taken. If edema increases at a rate greater than 0.5 cm/h, antivenom administration should be strongly considered (see below). Because of the extent of swelling and tenderness with palpation or passive movement, the question of compartment syndrome involving the calf or forearm frequently arises. Fortunately, owing to the subcutaneous location of venom, a true compartment syndrome following rattlesnake envenomation is uncommon, particularly when antivenom is used (4,5,11). Because of the infrequent occurrence of a true compartment syndrome, any time this complication is suspected, direct measurements of compartment pressures should be obtained before performing fasciotomy (Chapter 106).

Supportive Management

Close monitoring of distal extremity perfusion is critical and can also guide antivenom therapy (see below) (6). The two most useful parameters, color and capillary refill, should be assessed at least hourly. Based on studies done with digital subtraction angiography, if color and capillary refill are questionable but the digit remains warm, perfusion is likely adequate (7). Alternatively, a pulse oximeter placed on the distal portion of the extremity (finger or toe) may be helpful: the presence of a waveform indicates pulsatile flow and perfusion. A nonperfused distal extremity warrants surgical consultation (7,10). When tissue perfusion to the distal extremity is good and perfusion is only questioned in the area immediately surrounding a more proximal bite, surgical intervention is not required. Significant tissue loss is uncommon, particularly with antivenom therapy (5,8,9).

The tetanus immunization status of all snakebite victims should be ascertained and tetanus toxoid administered as recommended (see Table 107.2) (22). The value of prophylactic antibiotic administration after snakebite is controversial. No benefit was found to support prophylactic antibiotics in a relevant study of crotaline bites (19), nor in a study of nonvenomous snakebites (23). However, the warmth, redness, swelling, and tenderness seen after Crotaline snake envenomation can be difficult to differentiate from secondary cellulitis or abscess. Skin blebs and soft-tissue necrosis should

be treated using standard principles of wound management. As noted above, caregivers should be mindful of tissue perfusion, but concerns regarding compartment syndrome should prompt aggressive antivenom therapy and the measurement of intracompartmental pressure before the decision to perform surgical fasciotomy is reached (24). The local tissue destructive effects of snake venom may be functionally disabling and merit physical rehabilitation therapy.

Antivenom

For crotaline envenomation, there are two antivenom products currently available. Antivenin Crotalidae Polyvalent (ACP, Wyeth Laboratories, Marietta, PA) is a horse serum–derived product that contains whole antibody fragments and carries a high risk of immune-mediated reactions (discussed below). Crotalidae Polyvalent Immune Fab (CroFab, Protherics Laboratories, Nashville, TN) is a sheep serum–derived antivenom that contains only the Fab antibody fragment and has a lower risk of side effects. Use of Antivenom Crotalidae Polyvalent has fallen dramatically since the introduction of Crotalidae Polyvalent Immune Fab and its availability is very limited. There is one antivenom available for North American elapid snakes.

The initial decision to give antivenom and how much to give has traditionally been based on the severity of envenomation. Mild crotaline envenomation is characterized by swelling and tissue changes limited to the local bite site. Moderate envenomation includes significant local swelling and rapid proximal spread. Severe envenomation is present when the entire extremity is affected or when systemic signs of envenomation, coagulopathy, weakness, muscle fasciculation, or hypotension are present.

Early administration of antivenom has the potential to reduce ultimate tissue injury. Delayed administration may reverse coagulopathy or neurotoxicity but has less effect on local tissue injury. Unfortunately, antivenom administration is associated with a 9% to 25% rate of acute hypersensitivity reaction and, in the case of Antivenom Crotalidae Polyvalent (equine origin), an almost universal experience of delayed reaction (serum sickness) (5,12,14–17,25–27). The decision to administer antivenom represents a risk versus benefit choice, and controversy exists regarding the management of moderate to severe swelling alone, particularly following a copperhead bite (4,5,8,9,12,13,28,29). Systemic reactions and local tissue necrosis are uncommon even in untreated patients with significant swelling following copperhead envenomation (8), which has led to less frequent use of antivenom in such cases.

In coral snake envenomation, no early findings predict which victims will have severe neurologic symptoms. In fact, very minimal local injury may be present with significant envenomation (2). Any patient confirmed to have been bitten by a coral snake should receive antivenom, if available, as soon as possible following the bite. Antivenom is available for the eastern and Texas coral snakes. This product may also be helpful in bites by Sonoran coral snakes.

Depending on the antivenom to be used, relative contraindications to administering antivenom include previous history of prolonged close contact with sheep or horses, previous exposure to horse serum–based products, wool, papaya or papain allergy, or a positive skin test (if performed). With full consideration of risks, antivenom may still be given (5,12,18). Concurrent use of beta-blockers should raise concern, as these drugs reduce the efficacy of intervention should anaphylaxis occur. The administration of snake antivenom is a complex procedure, and early involvement of physicians skilled in snakebite treatment is recommended.

Crotalidae Polyvalent Immune Fab (Ovine)

Equipment

Crotalidae Polyvalent Immune Fab antivenom
10 mL of Sterile Water for Injection USP or vial of antivenom
250 mL of 0.9% Sodium Chloride for Injection USP
Patent intravenous catheter
Intravenous infusion pump
Cardiorespiratory monitoring equipment
Additional drugs for potential resuscitation in case of anaphylaxis

CroFab is a purified preparation of Fab (monovalent) immunoglobulin fragments derived from the serum of sheep that have been hyperimmunized with the venom from four species of pit viper: *Crotalus adamanteus* (eastern diamondback rattlesnake), *Crotalus atrox* (western diamondback rattlesnake), *Crotalus scutulatus* (Mojave rattlesnake), and *Agkistrodon piscivorus* (cottonmouth, water moccasin). It is believed that cross-reactivity with the venom components of other crotaline snakes renders this antivenom effective in the management of envenomation by all North American Crotalinae species.

Procedure

Antivenom administration is a relatively dangerous procedure that merits continuous cardiorespiratory monitoring, frequent patient assessment, and the capability for immediate intervention and treatment for anaphylaxis. At least two patent intravenous lines are recommended. The ED and intensive care unit (ICU) are the most appropriate settings for performing this procedure. Tourniquets are not recommended in the first-aid treatment of North American pit viper envenomation. However, when a venous constricting band or compressive wrap has been applied in the prehospital setting, it may be beneficial to begin antivenom therapy prior to its removal.

Each vial of Crotalidae Polyvalent Immune Fab is reconstituted in 10 mL of sterile water. The antivenom will slowly solubilize with gentle swirling, but vials should not be shaken, as this can lead to foamy denaturing of protein. The manufacturer recommends that reconstituted vials of antivenom be utilized within 4 hours of preparation.

It is advantageous to administer crotaline antivenom as soon after envenomation as is clinically warranted (30). Anecdotally, correction of snake venom–derived coagulopathy has been described as late as 52 hours after envenomation (31). An initial dose of four to six vials of reconstituted antivenom is prepared by further dilution with 0.9% saline to a total volume of 250 mL. The intravenous tubing leading to the patient is primed with the antivenom preparation. This initial dose is then infused intravenously at a rate of 25 to 50 mL/h for 10 minutes, with rapid, methodical advancement over 15 minutes to a rate of 250 mL/h in the absence of symptoms or signs of allergic reaction. One hour after completion of the initial antivenom dose, the patient should be closely evaluated for the progression of local swelling and ecchymoses as well as the state of coagulopathy. Antivenom dosing may be supplemented in 2 to 4 vial increments, as necessary, to achieve control of the envenomation injury. As snake venom will continue to be released from tissue compartments over time, additional two-vial doses of antivenom are recommended at 6, 12, and 18 hours following the time that initial control was achieved. Additional two-vial doses may be administered, as needed, at the discretion of a treating physician with experience in the care of snake envenomation.

One of the most difficult aspects of envenomation treated with Crotalidae Polyvalent Immune Fab is the "recurrence phenomena" (25,30,32). Thrombocytopenia or hypofibrinogenemia may recur 2 or more days after initial treatment. Recurrent swelling has also been described. Patients otherwise recovered can be managed expectantly as outpatients with close follow-up (25,32). These recurrent manifestations may be less responsive to more antivenom. In the absence of clinical bleeding, isolated, mild to moderate thrombocytopenia or hypofibrinogenemia—but not both together— can be followed clinically without further antivenom. Patients must be informed of the associated risks and the potentially traumatic hobbies and elective surgery to be avoided. High-risk patients may require treatment with more antivenom and/or in-hospital observation (25,32).

If anaphylactic or anaphylactoid symptoms or signs (itching, urticaria, hypotension, respiratory distress or edema, etc.) occur during antivenom therapy, the infusion should be stopped immediately. Epinephrine (1:1000) at a dose of 0.01 mL/kg intramuscularly or subcutaneously (maximum dose 0.3 mL) is the most effective drug for halting anaphylaxis (33). Consideration may be given to concomitant treatment with histamine H_1 and H_2 blockers and/or corticosteroids. The resumption of antivenom therapy should be considered in relation to the increased risk involved; consultation with a medical toxicologist is advised. The prophylactic administration of histamine H_1 and H_2 blockers, corticosteroids, and/or epinephrine prior to antivenom therapy has not been subjected to cost-benefit analysis.

If the clinician determines that the patient should continue to receive antivenom after an allergic reaction occurs, many patients will tolerate the slow resumption and titration of antivenom infusion after histamine blockade and/or epinephrine injection without further adversity. More severe reactions may warrant an epinephrine infusion titrated from 0.05 µg/kg/min.

Antivenin (Crotalidae) Polyvalent (Equine Origin) and Antivenin (*Micrurus fulvius*) (Equine Origin) North American Coral Snake

Equipment

Antivenom skin testing (optional):
   Horse serum (1:10) from antivenom kit
   0.02 mL of 0.9% Sodium Chloride for Injection USP
   Tuberculin syringes with subcutaneous needles
   Isopropyl alcohol skin disinfectant
   Patent intravenous catheter

Antivenom preparation and administration:
   Polyvalent Crotalidae antivenom or coral snake–
      specific antivenom
   10 mL of Bacteriostatic Water for Injection USP
      (diluent provided in antivenom kit)
   250 mL of 0.9% Sodium Chloride for Injection USP
   Patent intravenous catheter
   Intravenous infusion pump
   Cardiorespiratory monitoring equipment
   Additional drugs for potential resuscitation in case of
      anaphylaxis

Wyeth Antivenin (Crotalidae) Polyvalent (equine origin) is a partially purified protein precipitate from the serum of horses that have been hyperimmunized with the venom from four species of pit viper: *Crotalus adamanteus* (eastern diamondback rattlesnake), *Crotalus atrox* (western diamondback rattlesnake), *Crotalus durissus terrificus* (tropical rattlesnake), and *Bothrops atrox* (fer-de-lance). Cross-reactivity with the venom components of other crotaline snakes allows this antivenom to be used in the management of envenomation by all North American and South American Crotalinae species.

Procedure

Skin Testing. Skin testing may be performed to assess the relative risk that an individual has prior hypersensitization to horse serum and may experience an IgE-mediated reaction during antivenom administration. Treatment with polyvalent antivenom carries a 0% to 33% risk of an acute hypersensitivity reaction (itch, hives, wheezing, anaphylaxis) (14–17). When the skin test is positive, reaction to the antivenom occurs 50% to 100% of the time. When skin testing is negative, reaction still occurs 10% to 28% of the time, because many of the reactions are not IgE mediated but are anaphylactoid (e.g., the result of direct activation of complement by polymerized immunoglobulin) (5,14,15).

Only those patients who will receive antivenom should have skin testing, because the test can sensitize patients for future antivenom administration. Some clinicians believe that skin testing is superfluous and just adds risk once a decision to proceed with antivenom therapy has been made. Careful car-

diorespiratory monitoring and preparation for treatment of anaphylaxis should be done, as described above for the administration of Crotalidae Polyvalent Immune Fab. A 0.02-mL volume of diluted horse serum (provided by manufacturer at 1:10) is injected intradermally on the volar aspect of the forearm, with avoidance of any veins or vascular malformations (see Fig. 124.1). The 1:10 horse serum may be further diluted to 1:100 before skin testing of individuals thought to be high risk for horse antigen sensitization (equestrians or farmworkers or those with previous treatment with equine-derived antivenoms). A control of 0.02 mL of sterile normal saline may be placed in a similar manner adjacent to the horse serum site to aid in interpretation. The clinician then observes the skin site, vital signs, respiration, and general patient condition for 15 to 20 minutes. A positive reaction consists of a wheal, erythema, urticaria, or systemic reaction.

Antivenom Preparation and Administration. As mentioned for crotaline Fab antivenom, antivenom administration should be performed in a setting, such as the ED or the ICU, in which continuous monitoring, frequent assessments, and prompt intervention are possible. Acute reaction rates with this product are higher than with the crotaline Fab antivenom.

Each vial of Crotalidae antivenom is reconstituted with the 10 mL of diluent provided. Care should be taken to direct the diluent directly at the lyophilized pellet rather than allow it to trickle down the side of the vial. Adequate dissolution of the lyophilized antivenom should be ensured by rolling each vial vigorously between the palms until no particles or powder are observed when the vial is held up to a light (small globules of lipid may be seen, but no powder should be undissolved). An initial dose of 5 to 10 reconstituted vials, depending on clinical severity of envenomation, is prepared by further dilution with 0.9% saline to a total volume of 250 mL, and the intravenous tubing leading to the patient is primed with the antivenom preparation. One approach to the infusion of equine-derived antivenom is to begin at a rate of 2 mL/h. The rate may then be doubled every 2 minutes to a maximum of 250 mL/h (achieved by 15 minutes after initiation of infusion). Before each increase, the patient should be assessed for any signs of an acute allergic reaction.

If an acute allergic reaction occurs, antivenom administration should be stopped immediately and treatment provided, as described for Crotalidae Polyvalent Immune Fab. If antivenom therapy is to proceed in the face of an acute hypersensitivity reaction, the antivenom should be further diluted to half the original concentration before infusion is resumed. Dilution, reduction of infusion rate, and treatment with antihistamines and low-dose epinephrine usually allow the infusion of antivenom without further complications (5,18).

If coagulopathy is present, the patient's PT, PTT, fibrinogen, and platelet count should be checked 30 to 90 minutes following the completion of antivenom administration. If the abnormalities have significantly corrected and the rate of swelling has slowed, no further antivenom is warranted. Coagulation parameters should then be rechecked in another 1 to 2 hours. If correction is not adequate or was only temporary, more antivenom may be administered. It is not unusual for significant envenomations to require 15 to 30 vials to correct the abnormalities. These should be given in 5 to 10 vial aliquots in the same manner that the patient has previously tolerated. Attention to tetanus prophylaxis and wound care are as previously described for Crotalidae Polyvalent Immune Fab.

Antivenin (*Micrurus fulvius*) (equine origin) North American Coral Snake is not an effective treatment for all species of North American coral snakes, and its administration is rare. As it is an equine-derived product, the principles of its administration are similar to those described for Antivenin (Crotalidae) Polyvalent (equine origin). The indications for antivenom therapy and the appropriate dose should be considered in consultation with an expert in coral snake envenomation treatment. Precise instructions for its use may be found on the package insert.

Complications

As discussed in the sections on antivenom administration procedures, acute anaphylactic and anaphylactoid allergic responses are the most concerning complications of antivenom therapy. For North American crotaline envenomations, Crotalidae Polyvalent Immune Fab (ovine) is now largely preferred to Antivenin (Crotalidae) Polyvalent (equine origin), despite its higher purchase price, because the incidence of these acute reactions is 0% to 14% with the Fab product compared with 23% to 56% with the equine whole-antibody product (24,25). Depending on the antivenom to be used, patients with a history of prolonged close contact with sheep or horses; previous antivenom administration; wool, papaya, or papain allergy; or a positive skin test should be considered to be at increased risk of allergic reaction to antivenom. Most patients who receive at least 5 to 10 vials of equine-derived whole-antibody antivenom will experience a delayed serum sickness reaction. Serum sickness usually occurs 3 to 23 days following envenomation therapy (18). When it occurs, serum sickness can be treated with antihistamines and corticosteroids. The incidence of serum sickness following therapy with ovine-derived Fab antivenom is approximately 7% (24,25,30).

Antivenin (Crotalidae) Polyvalent (equine origin) contains thimerosal, 0.005%, as a preservative, and Crotalidae Polyvalent Immune FAB (ovine) contains up to 0.11 mg of mercury in the form of thimerosal per vial.

Complications associated with coral snake horse serum–derived antivenom are similar to those outlined for Crotalidae antivenom. Coral snake antivenom may not reverse existing neurologic symptoms, particularly if administration is delayed. The clinician should be prepared to provide respiratory support to patients with existing weakness at the time of antivenom administration.

▶ SCORPION STINGS

Anatomy and Physiology

Although several species of scorpions are known to exist in the southwestern United States, only one has significant medical importance, the bark scorpion, *Centruroides exilicauda* (formerly *Centruroides sculpturatus*) (34). This scorpion makes its home primarily in the desert Southwest, almost exclusively in Arizona. Rare reports of envenomation have occurred in other parts of the United States when the scorpion has traveled from Arizona as a "hitchhiker" in luggage or in the trunk of a car (34). Young children usually manifest the most severe symptoms and therefore receive the most interventions, for reasons discussed below.

When a scorpion sting occurs, the most frequent symptom manifested, particularly in an older child or adult victim, is local pain. Local effects such as erythema, swelling, or blanching are absent. Often, a "tap test"—tapping over the often near-invisible bite to try to elicit pain—is positive. More severely affected individuals will experience pain and paresthesia of the affected extremity. When relatively more venom per kilogram of body weight is injected, as occurs in the case of small children, peripheral motor neuron and cranial nerve manifestations may occur. These include uncontrolled jerking movements of the extremities, peripheral muscle fasciculation, opsoclonus, tongue fasciculation, and facial twitching. Severe reactions may include agitation, extreme tachycardia, salivation, and respiratory distress (34–38), which may be misperceived as seizure activity. Respiratory distress is most likely due to a combination of excess salivation, loss of pharyngeal tone, and uncoordinated contraction of the diaphragm and intercostal muscles. Rarely, respiratory compromise of infants and toddlers will progress to a point that endotracheal intubation and mechanical ventilation are required. Without antivenom therapy, symptom duration may be up to 46 hours (39).

Management

Most victims of scorpion envenomation can be managed solely with supportive care (analgesia, sedation, and adequate airway support). One retrospective review of 33 patients demonstrated relief of agitation and abnormal motor activity with the use of high-dose midazolam infusion (mean initial dose 0.3 mg/kg, mean infusion rate 0.3 mg/kg/h) (40). Where supportive care alone is not sufficient, severe envenomation has been shown to respond well to therapy with a goat serum–derived *Centruroides* antivenom (34,35,39,41). Unfortunately, production of this antivenom has been discontinued by Arizona State University. A new antivenom is currently being tested.

▶ *LATRODECTUS* ENVENOMATION

Anatomy and Physiology

The black widow spider, of the genus *Latrodectus*, is found throughout most of the United States and in most locales worldwide. In North America, the most common species is *Latrodectus mactans*, which can be identified by the hourglass-shaped red mark on the ventral surface of the black abdomen of the female spider. The male spiders cannot envenomate humans. Black widow spider antivenom contains latrotoxins, whose neurotoxic activity arises from calcium-mediated synaptic release of acetylcholine, norepinephrine, and other neurotransmitters (42).

After a black widow spider bite, patients usually develop pain at the bite site, although some patients may be initially asymptomatic. Symptom onset usually begins within 30 minutes but may be delayed for 2 to 3 hours. A local wheal-and-flare "target lesion" may be visible over the bite, and a tap test may be positive (43). The most common signs after widow envenomation are pain at the bite site; abdominal pain; pain in the back, chest, shoulder, leg, or groin; diaphoresis; and muscle rigidity (43,44). Additional signs and symptoms include tachycardia, vomiting, and "regional" diaphoresis (involving just one extremity or the area overlying the bite). Severe hypertension may result. Other rare manifestations include priapism, compartment syndrome, and myocarditis (45–47). Untreated, symptoms may last several days, and rare fatalities do occur (43–45,48).

Management

A number of treatment options have been suggested for the management of widow spider envenomation. Calcium gluconate, theorized to mitigate calcium-mediated synaptic derangements, has repeatedly proved ineffective in reducing signs and symptoms of envenomation (43,45,48,49). Opioids and benzodiazepines are helpful in the management of pain and muscle fasciculations as well as anxiety. In one review, 55% of patients receiving opioids alone and 70% receiving combination opioid-benzodiazepine therapy experienced relief without further therapy (43).

Antivenom should be considered in patients with severe symptoms not managed by supportive care. In addition, any patients with potentially life-threatening manifestations of envenomation, such as a hypertensive crisis, are good candidates for antivenom therapy. Antivenom therapy has been reported to reverse most consequences of envenomation (46,48). Of note, antivenom therapy has provided relief of envenomation as late as 90 hours after a bite (48,49).

A horse-derived IgG antivenom to *Latrodectus mactans* is available for severe envenomations not responsive to supportive therapy (see above). Similar to crotaline antivenom, this heterologous serum product poses a risk of both acute and delayed reactions. While antivenom appears to provide rapid relief of symptoms and clinical improvement (43,46–49) and dramatically shortens the duration of envenomation (43), its use should be reserved for those with severe symptoms or potentially life-threatening complications. There are significant data to support the use of *L. mactans* antivenom in patients envenomated by other *Latrodectus* species, especially *L. hesperus*, indigenous to the southwestern United States (43,50).

Procedure

Instructions for reconstitution, skin testing, dilution, and administration of *Latrodectus* antivenom are as for crotaline antivenom administration. One vial is usually adequate for the relief of symptoms (43,46,48,49). Allergic reaction is an absolute indication for stopping antivenom administration and a contraindication to continued *Latrodectus* antivenom administration. Further care should be directed at the treatment of the allergic reaction and supportive care.

Complications

Although frequently used in the past, antivenom use has declined with improvements in supportive care and reports of severe reactions, including death. Although these reactions do not seem to occur as frequently as those associated with crotaline antivenom, in a review of 163 patients, acute reactions occurred in 5 of 58 receiving antivenom, one of which resulted in death (43). Serum sickness reactions may occur. Only patients with life-threatening reactions uncontrolled with supportive care and in whom there are no allergic contraindications should be considered candidates for antivenom.

▶ JELLYFISH STINGS

Anatomy and Physiology

Jellyfish tentacles contain thousands of stinging cells, or nematocysts, which are triggered by contact. When stimulated, nematocysts forcefully extrude a thin, threadlike appendage that can penetrate human skin and inject a toxic venom. Several species are found in North American and Hawaiian waters, including the cabbage head jellyfish (*Stomolophus meleagris*), the Chesapeake Bay sea nettle (*Chrysaora quinquecirrha*), and the Atlantic and Pacific Portuguese man-of-war (*Physalia physalis* and *Physalia utriculus*). The most dangerous species, the box jellyfish (*Chironex fleckeri*), is found only in Indian and South Pacific waters (51).

When jellyfish envenomation occurs, symptoms are almost immediate. Mild symptoms include itching, burning, urticaria, and local paresthesia. With more severe envenomation, significant pain radiates centrally. The contact point may demonstrate a whiplike tentacle print with subepithelial ecchymosis. Hemorrhagic vesicles may develop. Although most envenomations produce only a painful sting, systemic symptoms may occur, ranging from headache, vomiting, and malaise to syncope, delirium, coma, paralysis, renal failure, pulmonary edema, and cardiovascular collapse (51–54). Anaphylaxis has been reported (55). Deaths from North American jellyfish stings are exceedingly rare and completely confined to the *Physalia* (man-of-war) species (54). Severity of symptomatology depends on species, season, extent of contact, prior sensitization, and underlying health of the victim (51–54). Determining the species responsible for a given sting requires knowledge of jellyfish indigenous to the area.

Management

Suspected jellyfish stings may be treated as described in the "Procedure" without significant concern about complications.

Equipment

Gloves, two pairs
5% acetic acid (vinegar) or bicarbonate of soda paste (for Chesapeake Bay sea nettle stings)
Forceps
Shaving cream
Razor

Procedure

For jellyfish stings, supportive cardiorespiratory care should be provided and significant allergic reaction treated before focusing on wound treatment. In addition to supportive care and analgesia, intervention is directed at (a) deactivation of the nematocysts, (b) removal of retained tentacle fragments, and (c) skin care. The clinician should don two pairs of surgical gloves before handling the wound to avoid accidental envenomation from residual nematocysts. The sting site should not be washed with freshwater, rubbed, or wiped, as these maneuvers may cause further nematocyst discharge. When providing first aid at the scene, rinsing with seawater may help remove some nematocysts. Lesions from North American species, except the Chesapeake Bay sea nettle, should be soaked in a 5% acetic acid solution (vinegar) for 30 minutes to deactivate nematocysts (Fig. 129.1A) (56). Stings from the Chesapeake Bay sea nettle, which is found only in bays on the Atlantic coast, should be treated with a paste of sodium bicarbonate (baking soda) (52,53). Alternative first-aid measures, such as use of isopropyl alcohol or meat tenderizer, are not as effective as acetic acid or sodium bicarbonate and may cause further nematocyst discharge (51,52). Tentacle fragments should be removed with forceps (Fig. 129.1B). Additionally, shaving cream may be applied and the wound shaved to remove residual nematocysts (Fig. 129.1C). Local wound care includes daily application of Burrow's solution.

Although the above procedures will reduce further envenomation and pain, further measures for analgesia may be necessary. Aside from analgesic medications, the use of either cold packs or hot freshwater immersion has been suggested. Two studies comparing these methods have concluded that hot water immersion is superior for pain relief; further study is needed in this area (57,58).

The role of allergic reaction in the slow resolution of skin lesions is unclear (51,59). Many undischarged nematocysts have been found on a patient even after correct treatment as previously outlined (52). Therapy with topical corticosteroids is frequently recommended (51,52). Prophylactic antibiotics are not indicated.

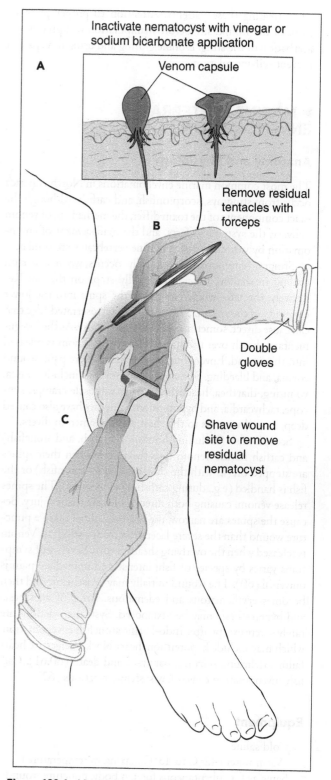

Figure 129.1 Management of jellyfish stings.

Complications

The main concerns in managing patients with jellyfish stings are to prevent inadvertent discharge of nematocysts, which causes further symptoms, and to avoid self-envenomation when treating these patients. Attention to proper pretreatment of the wound site before manipulation will prevent exacerbation of the sting. Double gloving and using forceps will prevent self-inoculation.

▶ MARINE VERTEBRATE ENVENOMATION

Anatomy and Physiology

The most common marine envenomations in North America occur from stingrays, scorpionfish, and catfish. Although the exact components of the toxin differ, the mechanism of venom delivery, the systemic effects, and the management of envenomation by various types of marine vertebrates are similar.

Stingray envenomation typically occurs when a person wading in shallow water accidentally steps on the ray. Reflexively, the tail "whips" to thrust the spine into the lower extremity of the victim. The spine has a retroserrated edge that can cause direct, sometimes severe, tissue injury. As the integumentary sheath over the spine is ruptured, venom is released into the wound. Envenomation results in severe pain, wound edema, and bleeding. Systemic manifestations include nausea, vomiting, diarrhea, headache, dizziness, muscle cramps, syncope, tachycardia, and hypotension. Stingrays have also caused deep, mortal wounds to the chest and abdomen in divers.

Scorpionfish (including lionfish, zebrafish, and stonefish) and catfish release venom into the victim when their spines are stepped on (as with the slow-moving scorpionfish) or the fish is handled (e.g., during catfishing excursions). The spines release venom, causing both direct and toxic tissue injury. Because the spines are narrow, the wound is more often a puncture wound than the severe laceration from a stingray. Venom is released when the overlying sheath is torn. Severity of symptoms varies by species of fish; intense and immediate pain is universal (60). The wound initially may be ischemic and then becomes erythematous and edematous. Areas of anesthesia and hyperesthesia may be juxtaposed. Systemic reactions are rarely severe except after Indo-Pacific stonefish envenomation, which may include hypotension, heart block, congestive heart failure, delirium, seizures, paralysis, and death (60,61). Catfish envenomation causes few systemic reactions (62).

Equipment

    Cold saline
    Warm water (42°C to 43°C maximum temperature)
    Same as for subcutaneous foreign body, puncture wounds, and laceration repair (Chapters 108, 110, and 111)

Procedure

The major components of marine envenomation management are (a) irrigation of the wound, (b) hot water immersion to neutralize the heat-labile venom proteins, (c) systemic and regional analgesia, and (d) adequate débridement and foreign body removal. Although antivenom exists for some particularly dangerous Indo-Pacific stonefish species, it is generally not available or indicated for other envenomations.

The wound should be irrigated as soon as possible with cold saline to remove residual venom and to inhibit venom absorption by vasoconstriction. Subsequently, the wound should be immersed in hot water, 40°C to 43°C for 30 to 90 minutes, to neutralize heat-labile venom proteins (60,63). Adequate analgesia should be provided; a local anesthetic or regional nerve block may be helpful (Chapter 35) (64). Great care should be taken in immersing an anesthetized extremity in hot water to prevent burns. Any obvious spine or sheath should be removed from the wound. After treating with warm water and achieving adequate pain control, the wound should be definitively explored and débrided. Radiographs are necessary following marine vertebrate envenomation to detect retained spines in wounds that may be difficult to adequately explore. Large wounds may require loose primary or delayed secondary closure (Chapters 107 and 108).

Complications

For patients with marine vertebrate injuries, the clinician must use caution during warm water immersion to avoid contact burns. Secondary infection (with or without retained foreign body) occurs frequently. Careful attention to wound management and early identification of a retained foreign body help reduce the likelihood of infection (Chapters 107 and 111). Close patient follow-up in 1 to 2 days will identify patients in need of antibiotic treatment. Prophylactic antibiotics at the first visit may be considered, but no evidence indicates that prophylactic antibiotics prevent subsequent wound infection after marine vertebrate envenomation. Wounds with a high risk of infection include large lacerations, deep puncture wounds (especially intra-articular), and wounds with retained foreign material (51).

▶ TICK REMOVAL

Anatomy and Physiology

Ticks are a common summertime finding on the skin of persons who live in or have recently visited rural areas. Ticks are most often found in moist or covered areas such as the scalp, axillae, groin, and genitalia. They usually fall off spontaneously after finishing their meal, but meals can last up to 14 days.

Indications

Because the likelihood of the transmission of tick-borne diseases such as Lyme disease, Rocky Mountain spotted fever, and tick paralysis is related to the duration of tick exposure, all ticks should be removed when discovered.

SUMMARY

Antivenom Skin Testing

1 Perform skin testing only after deciding to administer antivenom.

2 Perform skin testing only in a monitored environment.

3 Be prepared to treat an immediate hypersensitivity reaction.

4 Dilute provided horse serum 1:10 with normal saline or sterile water (crotaline antivenom) or reconstitute *Latrodectus* antivenom, one vial in 2.5 mL of sterile water.

5 Inject 0.02 mL of the antivenom serum intradermally in the volar aspect of the forearm.

6 Consider injecting 0.02 mL of a normal saline control adjacent to the antivenom site for comparison.

7 Observe the skin test site(s) for 15 to 20 minutes.

8 A positive reaction is any wheal, erythema, urticaria, or systemic reaction.

Antivenom Preparation and Administration

1 Only administer antivenom in a monitored environment (ED, ICU) and with immediate availability of physician intervention.

2 Reconstitute each vial of antivenom with 10 mL of sterile water or the diluent provided; for *Latrodectus* antivenom, reconstitute one vial in 2.5 mL of diluent, then add reconstituted solution to remainder of diluent (normal saline or D5W) for a total volume of 100 mL and skip to step 6.

3 Once diluent is added, roll each vial vigorously between palms for several minutes until no particles of powder can be observed when the vial is held up to the light. Small globules of lipid may be apparent but no powder should be undissolved.

4 For each vial to be given, remove 10 mL from a 250-mL bag of normal saline or D5W.

5 Add the vials of antivenom to the bag, making a reconstituted volume of 250 mL.

6 Use an infusion pump for antivenom delivery, ensuring that the antivenom is administered as close to the intravenous site as possible.

7 Start the infusion of the antivenom at 2 mL/h; double the rate of infusion every 2 minutes for the next 15 minutes (maximum rate: 250 mL/h).

8 Monitor the patient closely for signs of allergic reaction; if such occur, stop the infusion immediately and administer epinephrine, antihistamines, and corticosteroids as needed.

Continuation of Antivenom Administration in a Patient with an Allergic Reaction

1 Consultation with a medical toxicologist is advised.

2 Start a second intravenous line.

3 Administer diphenhydramine 1 mg/kg intravenously and ranitidine 2 mg/kg intravenously.

4 Give methylprednisolone 2 mg/kg intravenously to minimize delayed hypersensitivity reaction.

5 Start epinephrine infusion at 0.05 μg/kg/min; adjust the infusion as necessary to control allergic signs and symptoms during further antivenom administration.

6 Further dilute the antivenom to one half its original concentration.

7 Resume antivenom infusion at 2 mL/h and double every 3 to 5 minutes as tolerated.

Nematocyst Deactivation and Removal after Jellyfish Stings

1 Wear double gloves before handling the wound to avoid accidental envenomation.

2 Do not wipe or rub the wound.

3 Soak lesions from all species except Chesapeake Bay sea nettle in 5% acetic acid solution (vinegar) for 30 minutes to deactivate nematocysts.

4 Treat Chesapeake Bay sea nettle wounds with paste of bicarbonate of soda.

5 Remove tentacle fragments with a forceps.

6 Apply shaving cream and shave the wound to remove residual nematocysts.

Treating Marine Vertebrate Envenomation

1 Irrigate the wound as soon as possible with cold saline.

2 Provide analgesia. Often local anesthetic or regional nerve block is necessary.

3 Explore and débride the wound to remove residual elements of any sheath or spine.

4 Place the affected extremity in water as warm as can be tolerated by the victim (42°C to 43°C [110°F], maximum temperature) for 30 to 90 minutes.

(continued)

SUMMARY (CONTINUED)

5 Definitively explore and débride the wound after adequate pain control and detoxification.

6 Radiographs are necessary to detect retained spines.

7 Loose primary closure may be performed on large wounds.

Tick Removal

1 Grasp the tick as close to the skin as possible using a blunt, curved forceps held in a gloved hand.

2 Pull steadily and firmly directly away from the skin.

3 Examine the skin to be sure all tick parts have been removed.

4 Remove residual material with a forceps or excise it with large-gauge needle.

5 Thoroughly clean the skin with soap and water.

Equipment

Gloves
Forceps
Large needle (18 gauge)

Procedure

Several techniques for tick removal have been described, many of which come from American folklore (65). These "passive" techniques, which try to encourage the tick to self-detach,

 CLINICAL TIPS

Antivenom Administration

▶ Antivenom administration is most strongly indicated for persons who have suffered envenomation by rattlesnakes or neurotoxic snakes.

▶ Close assessment of the patient's physical findings and response to supportive measures helps to determine the need for antivenom except after a neurotoxic snakebite.

▶ Patients on β-adrenergic blockers should not receive antivenom unless their envenomation is life-threatening.

▶ Patients with positive skin reaction to *Latrodectus* antivenom should not undergo antivenom administration. *Crotalidae* antivenom administration after a positive skin test must be decided based on the severity of symptoms.

▶ Many patients will develop serum sickness 2 to 3 weeks after antivenom administration.

Jellyfish Stings

▶ Fresh water or isopropyl alcohol increases nematocyst discharge and should not be used.

▶ Meat tenderizer is commonly used but also may promote nematocyst discharge.

▶ Life-threatening anaphylactic reactions rarely occur from jellyfish stings in the United States.

▶ Delayed pruritus and hives localized to the sting site are common.

Marine Vertebrate Envenomations

▶ Adequate analgesia should be a high priority in the management of marine envenomations.

▶ Care should be taken to avoid contact burns during warm water immersion.

▶ Careful wound management is essential to a good outcome.

▶ Secondary infection occurs frequently, necessitating close patient follow-up.

Tick Removal

▶ Crushing the tick increases the potential exposure to the patient and clinician.

▶ All material must be carefully removed from the skin.

▶ Universal precautions should be observed to avoid contamination by human or tick secretions.

It is important to avoid crushing the tick to prevent exposing the host to more tick fluids. Because both human blood and tick secretions are potentially infectious, universal precautions should be observed, both during the procedure and afterward when handling the tick.

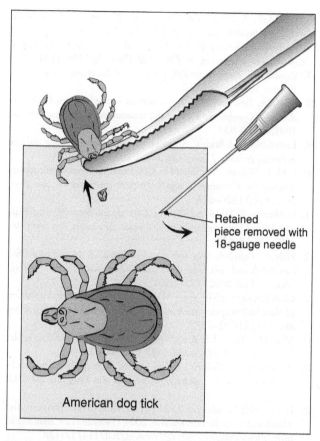

Figure 129.2 Tick removal.

▶ SUMMARY

Snake envenomations are infrequent but potentially life-threatening in children. Assessment of the wound, administration of antivenom as indicated, and treatment of systemic effects provide the best approach to these injuries. With spider bites and scorpion stings, symptomatic treatment is usually the best approach. Jellyfish stings can be alleviated by simple measures that can be administered on the beach, although victims should be watched carefully for signs of anaphylaxis. Marine vertebrate stings require appropriate wound management and warm water immersion. Tick attachment is a common pediatric problem requiring rapid removal that avoids further infectious exposure.

▶ REFERENCES

1. Russell FE, Carlson RW, Wainschel J, et al. Snake venom poisoning in the United States. *JAMA*. 1975;233:341–344.
2. Craig S, Kitchens MD, Van Mierop LHS. Envenomation by the eastern coral snake. *JAMA*. 1987;258:1615–1618.
3. White RR, Weber RA. Poisonous snakebite in central Texas. *Ann Surg*. 1991;213:466–472.
4. Hurlbut KM, Dart RC, Spaite D, et al. Reliability of clinical presentation for predicting significant pit viper envenomation [abstract]. *Ann Emerg Med*. 1988;17:438.
5. Swindle GM, Seaman KG, Arthur DC, et al. The six-hour observation rule for grade I crotalid envenomation: is it sufficient? Case report of delayed envenomation. *J Wilderness Med*. 1992;3:168–172.
6. Wingert WA, Chan L. Rattlesnake bites in southern California and rationale for recommended treatment. *West J Med*. 1988;148:37–44.
7. Curry SC, Kraner JC, Kunkel DB, et al. Noninvasive vascular studies in management of rattlesnake envenomation to extremities. *Ann Emerg Med*. 1985;14:1081–1084.
8. Burch JM, Agarwal R, Mattox KL, et al. The treatment of crotalid envenomation without antivenom. *J Trauma*. 1988;28:35–43.
9. Downey DJ, Omer GE, Moneim MS. New Mexico rattlesnake bites: demographic review and guidelines for treatment. *J Trauma*. 1991;31:1380–1386.
10. Roberts RS, Csencsitz TA, Heard CW Jr. Upper extremity compartment syndromes following pit viper envenomation. *Clin Orthop Relat Res*. 1985;193:184–188.
11. Garfin SR, Mubarak SJ, Akeson WH. Role of surgical decompression in treatment of rattlesnake bites. *Surg Forum*. 1979;30:502–504.
12. Wingert WA, Sullivan JB, Sinkinson CA. Snakebite management: which approach to use. *Emerg Med Rep*. 1984;5:37–44.
13. Kunkel DB, Curry SC, Vance MV, et al. Reptile envenomation. *J Toxicol Clin Toxicol*. 1984;21:503–526.

include covering the tick with petroleum jelly, coating with fingernail polish, applying rubbing alcohol, and touching a hot object (e.g., a just-extinguished match) to the hind part. When objectively examined, none of these techniques resulted in successful removal, even after several hours (65). In addition, if the tick self-detaches, the cement secreted by the mouthparts will remain in the skin, with ongoing infection risk. Mechanical removal is the only recommended technique (65,66).

To accomplish this, the tick should be grasped by the mouthparts as close to the skin as possible using blunt, curved forceps held in a gloved hand (Fig. 129.2). The tick is then pulled out of the skin using a firm, steady motion directed perpendicular to the body. The skin should be closely examined to ensure that all tick parts have been removed. Any remaining material should be removed with forceps, or the site should be excised with an 18-gauge needle using a method similar to removing a splinter (Chapter 111). Finally, the site should be thoroughly cleansed with soap and water.

Complications

Care must be taken in the removal of the tick to ensure that no tick body parts are left in the skin.

14. Spaite DW, Dart RC, Hurlbut K, et al. Skin testing: implications in the management of pit viper envenomation [abstract]. *Ann Emerg Med.* 1988;17:389.

15. Jurkovich GJ, Luterman A, McCullar K, et al. Complications of *Crotalidae* antivenin therapy. *J Trauma.* 1988;28:1032–1037.

16. Jamieson R, Pearn J. An epidemiologic and clinical study of snakebites in childhood. *Med J Aust.* 1989;150:698–701.

17. Curro V, Stabile A, Michetti V. Antivenom treatment in snake bites [letter]. *Acta Pediatr Scand.* 1988;77:597–597.

18. Burgess JL, Dart RC. Snake venom coagulopathy: use and abuse of blood products in the treatment of pit viper envenomation. *Ann Emerg Med.* 1991;20:795–801.

19. Clark RF, Selden BS, Furbee B. The incidence of wound infection following crotalid envenomation. *J Emerg Med.* 1993;11:583–586.

20. Karlson-Stiber C, Persson H, Heath A, et al. Clinical experiences with specific sheep Fab fragments in the treatment of *Vipera berus* bites: a preliminary report [abstract]. *Vet Hum Toxicol.* 1993;35:333.

21. Smilkstein MJ. Therapy for toxicologic emergencies. *Acad Emerg Med.* 1994;1:126–129.

22. Pickering LK, ed. Tetanus. In: *Red Book: 2003 Report of the Committee on Infectious Disease.* 26th ed. Elk Grove Village, IL: American Academy of Pediatrics; 2003:611–616.

23. Weed HG. Nonvenomous snakebite in Massachusetts: prophylactic antibiotics are unnecessary. *Ann Emerg Med.* 1993;22:220–224.

24. Gold BS, Dart RC, Barish RA. Bites of venomous snakes. *New Engl J Med.* 2002;347:347–356.

25. Ruha AM, Curry SC, Beuhler M, et al. Initial postmarketing experience with Crotalidae Polyvalent Immune Fab for treatment of rattlesnake envenomation. *Ann Emerg Med.* 2002;39:609–615.

26. Clark RF, McKinney PE, Chase PB, et al. Immediate and delayed allergic reactions to Crotalidae Polyvalent Immune Fab (ovine). *Ann Emerg Med.* 2002;39:671–676.

27. Holstege CP, Wu J, Baer AB. Immediate hypersensitivity reaction associated with the rapid infusion of Crotalidae Polyvalent Immune Fab (ovine). *Ann Emerg Med.* 2002;39:677–679.

28. Lavonas EJ, Gerardo CJ, O'Malley G, et al. Initial experience with Crotalidae Polyvalent Immune Fab (ovine) antivenom in the treatment of copperhead snakebite. *Ann Emerg Med.* 2004;43:200–206.

29. Caravati EM. Copperhead bites and Crotalidae Polyvalent Immune Fab (ovine): routine use requires evidence of improved outcomes. *Ann Emerg Med.* 2004;43:207–208.

30. Dart RC, Seifert SA, Boyer LV, et al. A randomized multicenter trial of Crotalinae Polyvalent Immune Fab (ovine) antivenom for the treatment for the crotaline snakebite in the United States. *Arch Int Med.* 2001;161:2030–2036.

31. Bebarta V, Dart RC. Effectiveness of delayed use of Crotalidae Polyvalent Immune Fab (ovine) antivenom. *J Toxicol Clin Toxicol.* 2004;42:321–324.

32. Boyer LV, Seifert SA, Cain JS. Recurrence phenomena after immunoglobulin therapy for snake envenomations, II: guidelines for clinical management with crotaline Fab antivenom. *Ann Emerg Med.* 2001;37:196–201.

33. Joint Task Force on Practice Parameters; American Academy of Allergy, Asthma and Immunology; American College of Allergy, Asthma and Immunology; Joint Council of Allergy, Asthma and Immunology. The diagnosis and management of anaphylaxis: an updated practice parameter. *J Allergy Clin Immunol.* 2005;115:S483–523.

34. Curry SC, Vance MV, Ryan PJ, et al. Envenomation by the scorpion *Centruroides sculpturatus. J Toxicol Clin Toxicol.* 1984;21:417–449.

35. Bond GR. Antivenin administration for *Centruroides* scorpion sting: risks and benefits. *Ann Emerg Med.* 1992;21:788–791.

36. Rachesky IJ, Banner W, Dansky J, et al. Treatment for *Centruroides elixicauda* envenomation. *Am J Dis Child.* 1984;138:1136–1139.

37. Rimsza ME, Zimmerman DR, Bergeson PS. Scorpion envenomation. *Pediatrics.* 1980;66:298–302.

38. Berg RA, Tarantino MD. Envenomation by the scorpion *Centruroides elixicauda* (*C sculpturatus*): severe and unusual manifestations. *Pediatrics.* 1991;87:930–933.

39. LoVecchio F, McBride C. Scorpion envenomations in young children in central Arizona. *J Toxicol Clin Toxicol.* 2003;41:937–940.

40. Gibly R, Williams M, Walter FG. Continuous intravenous midazolam infusion for *Centruroides exilicauda* scorpion envenomation. *Ann Emerg Med.* 1999;34:620–625.

41. LoVecchio F, Welch S, Klemens J, et al. Incidence of immediate and delayed hypersensitivity to *Centruroides* antivenom. *Ann Emerg Med.* 1999;34:615–619.

42. Hahn I, Lewin NA. Arthropods. In: Goldfrank LR, Flomenbaum NE, Lewin NA, et al., eds. *Goldfrank's Toxicologic Emergencies.* 7th ed. New York: McGraw-Hill; 2002:1573–1588.

43. Clark RF, Kestner SW, Vance MV. Clinical presentation and treatment of black widow spider envenomation: a review of 163 cases. *Ann Emerg Med.* 1992;21:782–787.

44. Moss HS, Binder LS. A retrospective review of black widow spider envenomation. *Ann Emerg Med.* 1987;16:188–192.

45. Pneumatikos IA, Galiatsou E, Goe D, et al. Acute fatal toxic myocarditis after black widow spider envenomation. *Ann Emerg Med.* 2003;41:158.

46. Hoover NG, Fortenberry JD. Use of antivenin to treat priapism after a black widow spider bite. *Pediatrics.* 2004;114:e128–129. Available at: http://www.pediatrics.org/cgi/content/full/114/1/e128.

47. Cohen J, Bush S. Case report: compartment syndrome after a suspected black widow spider bite. *Ann Emerg Med.* 2005;45:414–416.

48. O'Malley GF. Successful treatment of latrodectism with antivenin after 90 hours. *New Engl J Med.* 1999;340:657.

49. Sunthorntham S, Roberts JR, Nilsen GJ. Dramatic clinical response to the delayed administration of black widow spider antivenin. *Ann Emerg Med.* 1994;24:1198–1199.

50. Isbister GK, Graudins A, White J, et al. Antivenom treatment in arachnidism. *J Toxicol Clin Toxicol.* 2003;41:291–300.

51. Auerbach PS. Marine envenomation. *N Engl J Med.* 1991;325:486–493.

52. Roson CL, Tolle SW. Management of marine stings and scrapes. *West J Med.* 1989;150:97–100.

53. Burnett JW, Calton GJ. Jellyfish envenomation syndromes updated. *Ann Emerg Med.* 1987;16:1000–1005.

54. Stein MR, Marraccini JV, Rothschild NE, et al. Fatal Portuguese man-of-war (*Physalia physalis*) envenomation. *Ann Emerg Med.* 1989;18:312–315.

55. Togias AG, Burnett JW, Kagey-Sobotka A, et al. Anaphylaxis after contact with a jellyfish. *J Allergy Clin Immunol.* 1985;75:672–675.

56. Turner B, Sullivan P, Pennefather J. Disarming the bluebottle, treatment of *Physalia* envenomation. *Med J Aust.* 1980;2:394–395.

57. Lopez EA, Weisman RS, Bernstein J. A prospective study of the acute therapy of jellyfish envenomations [abstract]. *J Toxicol Clin Toxicol.* 2000;38:512.

58. Nomura JT, Sato RL, Ahern RM, et al. A randomized paired comparison trial of cutaneous treatments for acute jellyfish (*Carybdea alata*) stings. *Am J Emerg Med.* 2002;20:624–626.

59. Fisher AA. Toxic versus allergic reactions to jellyfish. *Cutis.* 1984;34: 450–454.

60. Kizer KW, McKinney HE, Auerbach PS. *Scorpaenidae* envenomation: a five-year poison center experience. *JAMA.* 1985;253:807–810.

61. Lehmann DF, Hardy JC. Stonefish envenomation. *N Engl J Med.* 1993;329:510–511.

62. Zeman MG. Catfish stings: a report of three cases. *Ann Emerg Med.* 1989;18:211–213.

63. Isbister GK. Venomous fish stings in tropical northern Australia. *Am J Emerg Med.* 2001;19:561–565.

64. Garyfallou GT, Madden JF. Lionfish envenomation [letter]. *Ann Emerg Med.* 1996;28:456–457.

65. Needham GR. Evaluation of five popular methods for tick removal. *Pediatrics.* 1985;75:997–1002.

66. Bowles DE, McHugh CP, Spradling SL. Evaluation of devices for removing attached *Rhipicephalus sanguineus* (Acari: Ixodidae). *J Med Entomol.* 1992;29:901–902.

130

RHETT LIEBERMAN AND VALERIE McDOUGALL KESTNER

Cooling Procedures

▶ INTRODUCTION

The spectrum of heat-related illness includes those that are rel-atively benign and self-limited and those that are potentially more serious and life-threatening. Benign and self-limiting heat-related illnesses include heat cramps, heat edema, and heat syncope. However, these can be an indication of a more serous condition. Heat edema is a mild form of heat-related illness, while heat cramps are painful spasms of skeletal mus-cles of the extremities and abdomen and may be a sign of impending heat exhaustion (1). The more serious conditions in the spectrum of heat-related illness include heat exhaustion and heatstroke. Heat exhaustion typically occurs at core body temperatures of 38.0°C to 40.5°C and has symptoms such as progressive lethargy, headache, nausea, vomiting, lighthead-edness, and myalgias. Heatstroke is classically differentiated from heat exhaustion by the presence of both a core tempera-ture greater than 40.5°C and an acute neurological or mental status change (2). The neurological manifestations of heat-stroke include ataxia, psychosis or irrational behavior, seizures, opisthotonos, posturing, and coma (3).

Rapid cooling is an intervention that can reduce morbidity and mortality in the pediatric patient with heatstroke. The appropriate cooling procedures are for the most part simple to perform and can be done by any health care worker. Some can be accomplished in the prehospital phase of care of the child, such as moving the patient to a cool, shaded environment, removal of clothing, rest, and oral fluid replacement. This chapter focuses on management strategies for cooling in an emergency care setting.

▶ ANATOMY AND PHYSIOLOGY

All humans produce heat as a byproduct of metabolism and muscle activity. Recognition of hyperthermia requires a rectal measurement of temperature in order to adequately assess core body temperature, as oral, axillary, and otic temperatures tend to underestimate core body temperature (4).

There are four mechanisms of heat transfer in the body: evaporation, radiation, convection, and conduction (Fig. 130.1). Normally, body heat is transferred from the core to the skin via cutaneous blood flow, where heat can be lost through the four heat transfer mechanisms. Radiation, the transfer of heat into the environment by means of photons of light, accounts for 55% to 65% of heat loss. This method of heat transfer is dependent on a gradient of heat between two sources; in heat-related illness, this is a gradient between core and ambient temperatures as well as the amount of exposed body surface area. Since heat-related illness often occurs when ambient temperature is above body temperature, heat loss oc-curs more by evaporation of water from perspiration from the skin and the evaporative cooling from exhaled moisture than from radiation. Evaporation is an important mechanism of heat loss to the environment while preserving skin blood flow and thus is the major means of heat reduction in the hyperthermic patient.

Convection and conduction account for 15% of the body's heat transfer. Convection can be defined, in the context of cooling a hyperthermic patient, as the transfer of heat by particles of air or water having contact with the patient, and it is often used in conjunction with evaporation. Conduction can be defined as the direct transfer of heat from one object to another, and it is the mechanism at work when a patient is immersed in ice water. Since evaporation of water allows for more loss of heat than conduction, it is understandable that some human studies have shown evaporation techniques to be more effective in lowering core body surface temperature than ice water immersion (5).

Often, heat-related illness occurs when the ambient tem-perature exceeds the core body temperature. Although children

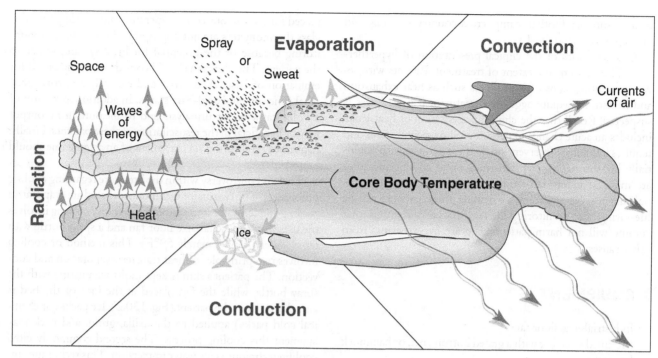

Figure 130.1 Methods of heat transfer.

have a greater ratio of body surface area to mass than adults, they often lack the understanding or ability to remove themselves from an overheated environment. Evaporation becomes the primary mechanism of heat transfer in these environments. However, in humid conditions, evaporative heat loss is rendered ineffective and results in a rising core temperature.

Children who are risk for heat-related illnesses include patients with cystic fibrosis, heart disease, eating disorders/malnutrition/obesity, diabetes (increased water loss), congenital absence of sweat glands, familial dysautonomia (temperature instability), and cerebral palsy (6–9). Dehydration in conjunction with electrolyte abnormalities and situations involving strenuous exercise, lack of fluid intake, and poor feeding contribute to hyperthermia. In addition, neonates and infants have a limited ability to perspire and therefore are significantly hampered in their ability to lose heat in hot, humid weather.

The pathophysiology of thermoregulation occurs centrally in the hypothalamus. Heat-sensitive areas in the hypothalamus respond to a rising core temperature through sympathetic tone and autonomic mechanisms that utilize cholinergic pathways to the sweat glands. As the temperature rises, cholinergic stimulation causes sweat to be released from the glands. It is important to recall that young children possess a limited number of sweat glands and thus are limited in their response to a rising core temperature in this way. Sympathetic tone changes in arterioles and subcutaneous arteriovenous anastomoses increases blood flow to the skin surface in response to overheating. Flow through the skin can comprise up to 30% of cardiac output and effectively transfer heat from the body core to the skin surface. Vasodilatation dissipates heat by convection, and sweat dissipates it by evaporation (10).

Core body temperature increases occur secondary to any combination of excess metabolic heat production, excessive environmental heat, and altered heat dissipation. In hyperthermia, the central hypothalamic set point is *normal* but overwhelmed, as peripheral mechanisms are unable to maintain the body's temperature at that set point. Fever is differentiated from hyperthermia, despite their clinical similarities, in that during fever cytokines and other biochemical reactants cause the central hypothalamic set point to be elevated. Therefore, it is necessary to emphasize that drugs with antipyretic effects are not beneficial in treating hyperthermia, as their mechanism of action is to lower the central set point that has been elevated (10).

▶ INDICATIONS

Patients presenting with heat-related illness require cooling management. Risk factors for hyperthermia based on a patient's medical history, age, and the preceding environment will help in determining appropriate management. Infants, because of factors such as limited sweat glands and the inability to remove themselves from a potentially harmful situation, are at high risk in hot environments, as when they are left inside a closed automobile. Children and adolescents who are subjected to strenuous activity in a hot and humid environment increase their risk of heat illness. A preadolescent's or poorly trained athlete's ability to transport muscle-generated heat and to produce sweat is less than the ability of an older child or better trained athlete. Examples of common settings for heat-related illnesses in the pediatric population include summer football camp, cross-country running, and marching in a band (8–13).

Characteristics of the clinical presentation of hyperthermia will determine the extent of treatment. Patients with severe presenting signs of heat illness such as heat exhaustion and heatstroke require aggressive treatment if heat illness is suspected. Recall that the clinical presentation of heatstroke includes an acute change in neurological or mental status and requires immediate intervention. In these patients with potentially life-threatening hyperthermia, rapid cooling measures are initiated before lab studies are obtained or a differential diagnosis is entertained. Treating these patients can be life-saving, and monitoring the temperature will ensure that cooling will not harm patients who are hyperthermic from other causes.

▶ EQUIPMENT

Industrial-size floor fan
Modified stretcher with a grated bottom, net, or hammock
Ice packs
Spray bottle with tepid water (15°C, 59°F) (5)
Water-resistant monitor leads

▶ PROCEDURE

When a heatstroke victim presents to the emergency department, the clinician should begin treatment with attention to both immediate temperature reduction and the resuscitation basics of airway, breathing, and circulation. The patient should be attached to a cardiac a monitor with water-resistant leads and should be placed on a bed with a grated bottom or netting to allow for maximal heat transfer. A hyperthermic patient should receive supplemental oxygen and have two large-bore intravenous catheters placed. Hydration, electrolyte balance, and coagulation status must be determined expeditiously. Typical laboratory tests in severe cases might include complete blood count, prothrombin and partial thromboplastin times, serum electrolytes, blood urea nitrogen, creatinine, creatine phosphokinase, calcium, phosphorus, urinalysis with urine myoglobin, and arterial blood gas analysis. For patients requiring intravascular volume support, up to 20 mL/kg of lactated Ringer solution or normal saline is infused rapidly. Further cardiovascular support may be provided as needed, with inotropes such as low-dose dopamine and/or dobutamine, which enhance myocardial contractility while maintaining peripheral vasodilation. Subsequent fluid therapy (or initial treatment for more stable patients) is begun with 5% dextrose in 0.2% saline at an appropriate maintenance rate. Patients with hyperthermia are not often severely dehydrated and thus may not require large volumes of intravenous fluid. However, the clinician should monitor and support the cardiovascular system to maintain perfusion. The patient's clothing should be removed, and a rectal temperature probe should be

placed for continuous core temperature monitoring. Of note, glass thermometers are not appropriate for continuous monitoring because of the potential for breakage and injury to the patient. The clinician should consider drawing blood for evaluation of basic chemistries and electrolyte disturbances, renal function, and acid-base status. In addition, insertion of a Foley catheter for urinalysis and to measure urine output may be beneficial in the resuscitation of these patients. Finally, continued monitoring via placement of an arterial line should be considered.

There is controversy within the literature regarding cooling procedures. The two major techniques debated are evaporative cooling and ice water immersion. Evaporative cooling involves the use of an industrial-size floor fan and a spray bottle with tepid water (approximately 59°F). This method of cooling involves two principles of heat transfer: evaporation and convection. The patient's skin is kept moist via misting with the spray bottle, while the fan placed at the foot of the bed is aimed directly at the patient (Fig. 130.2). Ice packs (or chemical cold packs) applied to the axilla, groin, and neck may augment this cooling process. The second commonly cited cooling technique is ice water immersion. This technique employs conduction as its heat transfer mechanism and is accomplished by placing the patient in ice water at approximately 1°C to 3°C.

Most clinical studies suggest that evaporative cooling is superior to ice water immersion (5,14–19). The evaporative cooling technique has achieved cooling rates between 0.07°C and 0.3°C per minute in adults. It is believed to be superior to ice water immersion for several reasons. One is that ice water immersion has the undesired effect of peripheral vasoconstriction, which minimizes heat transfer and increases shivering. In addition, ice water immersion is more difficult to use in the uncooperative, agitated, psychotic, or comatose patient. Finally, monitoring and managing the airway is technically more difficult in a patient immersed in ice water.

Evaporative cooling techniques such as those using a spray bottle and fan provide heat exchange comparable to ice water immersion but with fewer undesired effects. Furthermore, evaporation and convection are more efficient heat exchange mechanisms than conduction. In evaporative cooling, skin blood flow is preserved, and overall it is more comfortable for the patient. It has the benefits of increased ease of application, monitoring, stabilization, and treatment by staff. Evaporative methods carry no contraindications and can be quickly and easily performed in an emergency department with a written protocol and availability of appropriate equipment.

Other cooling techniques have been suggested in the literature. Sponge baths with alcohol should be avoided due to risk of alcohol toxicity and rebound hyperthermia (2,15). Cold humidified oxygen has not proven to be efficacious and risks bronchospasm. The cooling rates for iced peritoneal lavage and for evaporative cooling have been found to be equivalent in canine models (15,20). The cooling rates for iced gastric lavage have been shown to be inferior to those for evaporative cooling in canine models (15,21). Use of an intravascular

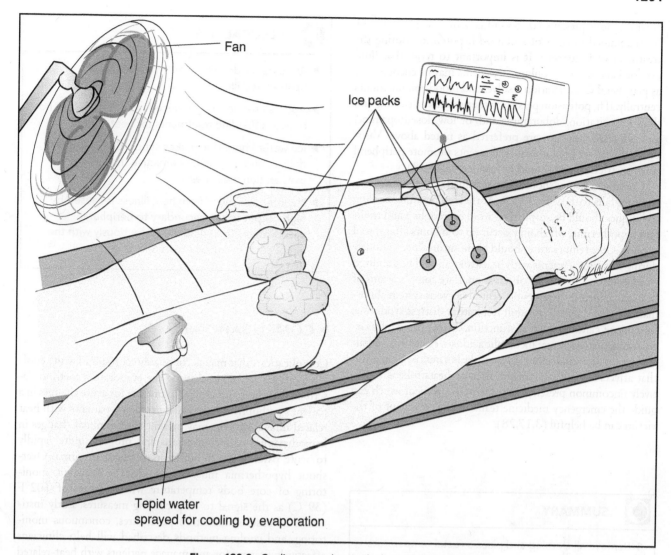

Figure 130.2 Cooling procedure in the hyperthermic patient.

cooling catheter has demonstrated improvement in patients with central nervous system disease; however, it has not yet been studied in heatstroke (15,22–24).

Currently there are no recommendations for routine administration of cold peripheral intravenous fluids in the emergency management of heat-related illnesses. The use of pharmacological agents such as dantrolene for cooling has also been investigated, although most of the literature concerns hyperthermia due to anesthetic agents. In randomized, controlled trials in humans, one study showed short-term improvement in cooling rate with the use of dantrolene, while others suggest that its administration did not change survival rates and was found to be ineffective; consequently, dantrolene use at present is controversial (15,25–28).

Complications that may occur as a direct result of acute cooling methods are minimal using the evaporation method described. However, there are potential complications encountered in the overall presentation and treatment of heat-related illness. Shivering, shaking, fasciculations, or con-

vulsions may occur during cooling. Benzodiazepines are the treatment of choice for these symptoms (e.g., diazepam at 0.1 to 0.3 mg/kg/dose) and are additionally recommended as treatment for those patients who have agitation or psychosis as a manifestation of their heat-related illness (13). Antipsychotics are not appropriate for the treatment of agitation in the setting of heat-induced illness because they may lower the seizure threshold and cause dystonia. Also, haloperidol has been suggested as a complicating factor in some cases of death from heatstroke and therefore should be avoided (17).

Hypotension is a common clinical manifestation of heatstroke. It is the consequence of shunting of blood through dilated skin vessels, which results in high-output cardiac failure and is not typically a reflection of hypovolemia or dehydration. This hypotension typically responds to cooling procedures and often does not require fluid boluses. However, ongoing circulatory management with measurement of vital signs, urine output, intra-arterial blood pressure, and central venous pressure (or Swan-Ganz measurements) must be maintained in cases of sustained hypotension during the treatment of heatstroke. It is important to recall that fluid overload and resultant pulmonary edema may be encountered as peripheral vasodilatation resolves and blood volume shunts centrally. If hypotension persists in the presence of cooling and fluid resuscitation, dobutamine and/or low dose dopamine, as vasopressor therapy, are preferred as noted above. Vasopressors that are predominantly α-agents promote peripheral vasoconstriction and should be avoided (3,15,18).

Cooling measures should be maintained until the core temperature falls to 102°F (39°C). At this temperature, cooling techniques should be stopped to avoid overcooling and resultant hypothermia, which may occur up to 6 hours after initial cooling. Core temperature should be monitored continuously during this time. Patients with heatstroke should be admitted to a monitored setting for observation. Late complications of heatstroke include: irreversible central nervous system abnormalities, rhabdomyolysis, adult respiratory distress syndrome, liver injury, cardiovascular dysfunction, disseminated intravascular coagulation, severe metabolic acidosis, electrolyte imbalance, and acute renal failure. Heatstroke is a multisystem insult that affects almost every organ. Because heatstroke is a relatively uncommon presentation, a written protocol which can guide the emergency medicine teams' acute treatment of the victim can be helpful (3,17,28).

SUMMARY

1 Remove all clothing and place a rectal temperature probe for continuous core temperature monitoring.

2 Place the patient on a modified stretcher with a grated bottom, net, or hammock to maximize heat dissipation.

3 Liberally spray the patient with tepid water (15°C, 59°F).

4 Place the patient in the air stream of an industrial-size floor fan.

5 Consider the application of ice packs to the axilla, groin, and neck to augment temperature reduction.

6 Control shivering, seizures, and agitation with appropriate doses of benzodiazepines.

7 Carefully administer fluids to avoid pulmonary edema as the core body temperature falls; consider monitoring central venous pressure.

8 Stop cooling measures when the core body temperature falls to 39°C (102°F).

CLINICAL TIPS

▶ Antipyretics do not lower hyperthermia of heat-related illness.

▶ Agents used for drug-induced hyperthermia are not effective first-line treatments for heatstroke.

▶ Ice water immersion makes supportive care more difficult and may be less effective than using evaporation measures.

▶ Hypotensive shock from heat illness is caused by high-output failure secondary to peripheral vasodilation. Treat fluid losses cautiously with the aid of central venous pressure monitoring.

▶ **COMPLICATIONS**

Complications that may occur as a direct result of acute cooling methods are minimal using the evaporation method described. However, it is crucial to prepare for acute changes in a patient's pathophysiology when managing patients with heat related illness. Patients may present with minimal changes in hemodynamics or mental status and progress quite rapidly to acute psychosis with agitation, seizures, or coma. Overshoot hypothermia must be avoided by constant monitoring of core body temperature with a target of 102°F (39°C) as the signal to stop cooling measures. Early institution of basic stabilization procedures, continuous monitoring, and cooling methods described will help clinicians effectively prepare for and manage patients with heat-related illness.

Patients who experience heatstroke have altered hypothalamic responsiveness to heat stress for up to 1 year. During this time, they must avoid hot climates and excessive exertion.

▶ **SUMMARY**

Heat exhaustion and heatstroke requires immediate, aggressive treatment if suspected. While cooling measures are in progress, the clinician must keep a broad differential diagnosis for the etiology of the hyperthermia and perform a thorough clinical evaluation to find the true cause of the patient's malady. Rapid cooling by the evaporation method is a simple, safe, comfortable, and noninvasive technique for treating hyperthermia. Further, it is easier to monitor and treat the victim of heat illness while using evaporative cooling. Benzodiazepines are recommended for controlling common complications encountered such as seizures, shivering, and agitation.

▶ ACKNOWLEDGMENT

The authors would like to acknowledge the valuable contributions of John J. Kelly to the version of this chapter that appeared in the previous edition.

▶ REFERENCES

1. Sandor RP. Heat illness. *Phys Sportsmed.* 1997;25:35–40.
2. Khosla R, Guntupalli KK. Heat-related illnesses. *Crit Care Clin.* 1999;15:251–263.
3. Tek D, Olshaker JS. Heat illness. *Emerg Med Clin North Am.* 1992;10:299–310.
4. Banitalebi H, Bangstad HJ. Measurement of fever in children: is infrared tympanic thermometry reliable? *Tidsskr Nor Laegeforen.* 2002;122:2700–2701.
5. Weiner J, Khogali M. A physiologic body cooling unit for treatment of heatstroke. *Lancet.* 1980;2:276–278.
6. Avery ME. Heat-induced illness. In: Avery ME, First LR, eds. *Pediatric Medicine.* Baltimore: Williams & Wilkins; 1989.
7. Wexler RK. Evaluation and treatment of heat-related illnesses. *Am Fam Physician.* 2002;65:1439–1440.
8. Smith NJ. The prevention of heat disorders in sports. *Am J Dis Child.* 1984;138:786–790.
9. Ewald MB, Baum CR. Environmental emergencies. In: Fleisher GR, Ludwig S, Henretig FM, eds. *Textbook of Pediatric Emergency Medicine.* Philadelphia: Lippincott Williams & Wilkins; 2006:1017–1021.
10. Simon HB. Hyperthermia. *N Engl J Med.* 1993;329:483–487.
11. Dankes DM, Webb DW, Allen J. Heat illness in infants and young children: a study of 47 cases. *Br Med J.* 1962;2:287.
12. Bar-Or O. Thermoregulation and fluid electrolyte needs. In: Smith NJ, ed. *Sports Medicine: Health Care for Young Athletes.* Evanston, IL: American Academy of Pediatrics; 1983.
13. Bytomski JR, Squire DL. Heat illness in children. *Curr Sports Med Rep.* 2003;2:320–324.
14. Wyndham CH, Strydom NB, Cooke HM. Methods of cooling subjects with hyperpyrexia. *J Appl Physiol.* 1959;14:771–776.
15. Hedad E, Rav-Acha M, Heled Y, et al. Heatstroke: a review of cooling methods. *Sports Med.* 2004;34:501–511.
16. Kielblock AJ, Van Rensburg JP, Franz RM. Body cooling as a method for reducing hyperthermia: an evaluation of techniques. *S Afr Med J.* 1986;69:378–380.
17. Knochel JP. Heat illness. In: Callahan ML, ed. *Current Practice of Emergency Medicine.* Philadelphia: BC Decker; 1991.
18. Callahan M. Heat illness. In: Rosen P, et al., eds. *Emergency Medicine.* St. Louis: Mosby; 1988.
19. Armstrong LE, Crago AE, Adams R, et al. Whole-body cooling of hyperthermic runners: comparison of two field therapies. *Am J Emerg Med.* 1996;14:355–358.
20. White JD, Kamath R, Nucci R, et al. Evaporation versus iced peritoneal lavage treatment of heatstroke: comparative efficacy in a canine model. *Am J Emerg Med.* 1993;11:1.
21. White JD, Riccobene E, Nucci R, et al. Evaporation versus iced gastric lavage treatment of heatstroke: comparative efficacy in a canine model. *Crit Care Med.* 1987;15:748–750.
22. Mack WJ, Huang J, Winfree C, et al. Ultrarapid, convection-enhanced intravascular hypothermia: a feasibility study in nonhuman primate stroke. *Stroke.* 2003;34:1994–1999.
23. Schmutzhard E, Engelhardt K, Beer R, et al. Safety and efficacy of a novel intravascular cooling device to control body temperature in neurologic intensive care patients: a prospective pilot study. *Crit Care Med.* 2002;30;2481–2488.
24. Inderbitzen B, Yon S, Lasheras J, et al. Safety and performance of a novel intravascular catheter for induction and reversal of hypothermia in a porcine model. *Neurosurgery.* 2002;50:364–370.
25. Channa AB, Seraj MA, Saddique AA, et al. Is dantrolene effective in heatstroke patients? *Crit Care Med.* 1990;18:290–292.
26. Bouchama A, Cafege A, Devol EB, et al. Ineffectiveness of dantrolene sodium in the treatment of heatstroke. *Crit Care Med.* 1991;19:176–180.
27. Hadad E, Cohen SY, Heled Y, et al. Clinical review: treatment of heatstroke: should dantrolene be considered? *Crit Care.* 2005;9:86–91.
28. Bouchama A, Knochel JP. Medical progress: heat stroke. *N Engl J Med.* 2002;346:1978–1988.

131

Warming Procedures

▶ INTRODUCTION

Hypothermia is defined as a core temperature below 35°C (95°F). The most common cause of hypothermia in the pediatric population is exposure to cold environments (cold water drowning, "found outside" in winter, etc.). Children, especially very young children, are relatively susceptible to hypothermia because of their large surface area to mass ratio, immature judgment, and lack of behavioral defense mechanisms. Less commonly, chronic disease, malnourishment, fatigue, and intoxication are important risk factors in children.

▶ ANATOMY AND PHYSIOLOGY

Hypothermia can be categorized as mild (core body temperature 32°C to 35°C [89.6°F to 95°F]), moderate (28°C to 31°C [82.4°F to 87.8°F]), or severe (less than 28°C [82.4°F]). Clinical deterioration roughly parallels these divisions. Patients with mild hypothermia have intact thermoregulatory responses (vasoconstriction, shivering) and mild alterations in muscle control, coordination, and mental status. Moderate hypothermia is accompanied by a decreased level of consciousness, ineffective or absent shivering, and dysrhythmias, often heralded by the appearance of a J wave on EKG (Fig. 131.1). Severe hypothermia is accompanied by loss of consciousness, absent shivering, and ventricular fibrillation or asystole.

Although hypothermia can cause death, it also has a powerful neuroprotective effect when it occurs rapidly. Thus, in contrast to normothermic arrest, hypothermic arrest can be successfully reversed even if the arrest is prolonged (1 to 2 hours). Children with profound accidental hypothermia and even apparent clinical death have been successfully resuscitated with good neurologic outcomes (1–3), and patients with rec-

tal temperatures as low as 16.0°C have survived with little or no demonstrable morbidity. Thus, the techniques described in this chapter are truly life-saving techniques that pediatricians and emergency medicine providers should be prepared to institute in appropriate conditions.

Warming techniques can be categorized as passive or active. Passive techniques encourage endogenous generation of heat and are the treatment of choice for patients who can shiver. Passive techniques include encouraging exercise and providing warm clothes, insulation (blankets), and food (Fig. 131.2) (4–6). Active techniques include exogenous application of heat to external organs (skin) or internal organs. Common procedures are listed in Table 131.1. One important complication of active external warming is "afterdrop." Afterdrop is a fall in core temperature caused, in part, by vasodilation and improved circulation to cold extremities, with return of cooled blood to the body's core. Thus, some experts recommend limiting active external warming to the trunk and avoiding it altogether in patients with intact shivering (external warming can suppress shivering and may be less efficient than shivering). However, forced air warmers can be very effective in children and are less likely to cause afterdrop than the other techniques. Forced air warmers use circulating warm air to heat the body by convection (heat transfer by a moving body of gas or liquid). Another major advantage of forced air warmers is that they are commonly used in operating rooms and can be easily transported to the emergency department (ED) for emergent use. Thus, forced air warmers are increasingly used for even unstable patients. Indeed, forced air warmers have been used successfully to warm children with severe hypothermia and cardiac arrest (Fig. 131.3) (3).

Active internal warming requires establishing access to an internal body cavity. Many of the necessary procedures are described elsewhere in this textbook. Closed thoracic lavage and peritoneal lavage require chest tube and peritoneal catheter

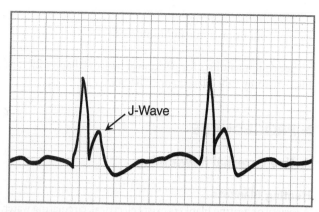

Figure 131.1 ECG change with hypothermia, including presence of J wave.

TABLE 131.1	COMMON WARMING PROCEDURES

Active External Warming
Electrical heating blankets
Forced air
Hot water bottles
Radiant warmers
Warm water bath

Active Internal Warming
Bladder lavage
Closed thoracic lavage
Extracorporeal warming
Gastric lavage
Mediastinal (open thoracic) lavage
Peritoneal lavage
Warm inhaled air
Warm i.v. fluids

placement and are attractive techniques for utilization in the ED because pediatric emergency care providers are relatively experienced in them (Chapters 27 and 29). Gastric lavage and bladder lavage have limited effectiveness because of the small surface area of these organs. Likewise, warmed intravenous fluid and warmed inhalation therapy have modest heat exchange and are best considered techniques to prevent additional heat loss rather than techniques to provide heat. The most effective therapy, and the preferred therapy for severely

hypothermic patients with nonperfusing cardiac rhythms, is extracorporeal support. One series from an experienced team reports long-term survival following extracorporeal bypass in 15 of 32 patients presenting with a mean core temperature of 21.8°C and a mean time between discovery and bypass of 141 minutes (7). The major disadvantage of extracorporeal support is the need for specialized equipment and trained personnel.

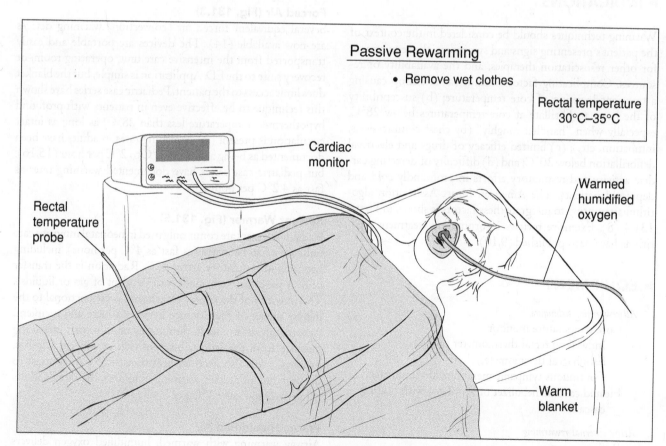

Figure 131.2 Passive rewarming.

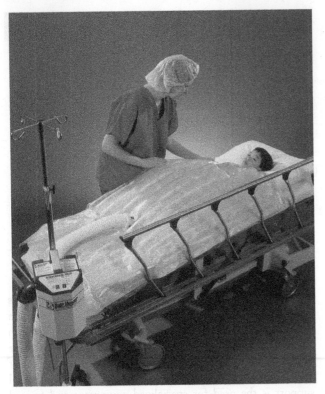

Figure 131.3 Child in a forced air warming device.

► INDICATIONS

Warming techniques should be considered in the context of the patient's presenting signs and symptoms, the requirement for other resuscitation therapies, and the availability of resources. Complicating factors include (a) afterdrop causing a transient lowering of core temperature; (b) susceptibility of the heart to fibrillate at core temperatures below 28°C, especially when "handled roughly" (by chest compressions, intubation, etc.); (c) limited efficacy of drugs and electrical defibrillation below 30°C; and (d) difficulty of detecting cardiac activity and respiratory efforts in profoundly cold and depressed patients. The American Heart Association algorithm attempting to integrate these factors is shown in Figure 131.4 (8). Extensive reviews incorporating treatment algorithms have been published (9,10).

► EQUIPMENT

All rewarming techniques
> Core temperature monitor
>> Indwelling rectal thermometer probe
>> Esophageal thermometer
>> Continuous tympanic membrane thermometer
> Heated cascade nebulizer or ventilator with heating cascade

Active external rewarming
> Radiant warmer
> Warmed blankets or forced air rewarmer

Active internal rewarming
> Rapid intravenous fluid infuser

See equipment lists for peritoneal lavage (Chapter 27) and thoracostomy tube placement (Chapter 29).

► PROCEDURES

Active External Rewarming

Heating Blankets

A variety of heating blankets exist (electrical, circulating water, resistive). Heating blankets work by direct, contact-to-contact heat transference (conduction). Blankets should be placed on top of the patient to maximize heat transfer. Placement of heating blankets under the patient is less effective because compression of the dependent vascular beds attenuates heat transfer (6), and 90% of ongoing losses are lost from nondependent areas of the body (5). Accordingly, when warming blankets are placed on top of the patient, there is little difference in efficacy between the various blankets (11,12), and warming rates may be comparable to convective warming devices (13). The need for ongoing patient resuscitation may limit the effectiveness of this technique due to the need to uncover the patient.

Forced Air (Fig. 131.3)

Several equivalent forced air (convection) warming devices are now available (14). The devices are portable and easily transported from the intensive care unit, operating room, or recovery suite to the ED. Application is simple, but the blanket does limit access to the patient. Pediatric case series have shown this technique to be effective even in patients with profound hypothermia (temperature less than 28°C) as long as intact circulation is present (3). Warming rates in adults have been documented as being as slow as 1°C to 2°C per hour (15,16), but pediatric case series have documented warming rates as fast as 4.2°C per hour (3).

Radiant Warmer (Fig. 131.5)

Radiant warmers are commonly used in neonatal intensive care units to warm neonates (as fast as 4°C per hour), including neonates in circulatory arrest (17). Radiation is the transfer of heat waves through space (independent of gas or liquids). The intensity of the energy transferred is proportional to the inverse square of the distance between source and recipient. Accordingly, heat energy diminishes rapidly with increasing distance from the lamps. Interposition of objects (clothes, bandages) will also decrease heat transfer (5). In contrast to the high rate of radiant warming in infants, the rate in adults is relatively low, at ~1°C per hour (18).

Warm, Humidified Air

Airway warming with warmed, humidified oxygen delivers oxygen to the potentially hypoxic patient as well as prevents

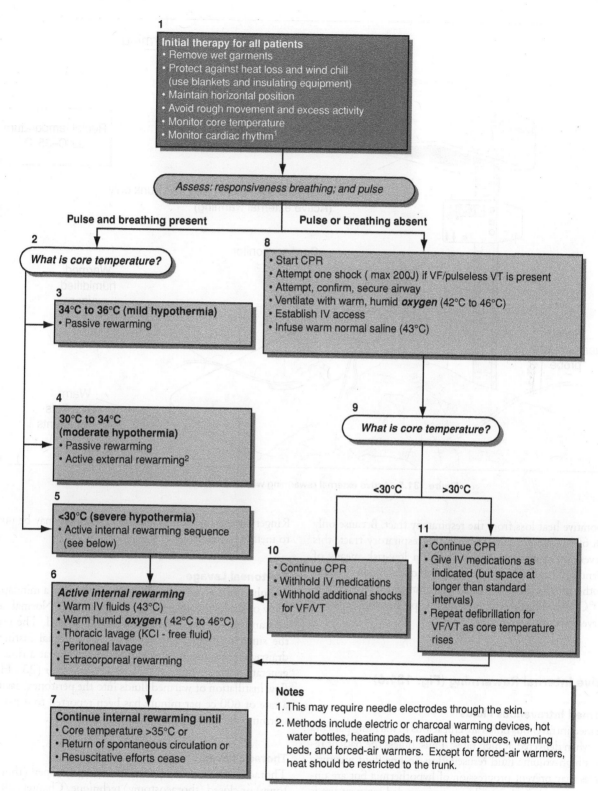

Figure 131.4 Algorithm for treatment of hypothermia. (Adapted from *Special resuscitation circumstances, I: hypothermia.* In: Cummins RO, Field JM, Hazinski MF, eds. *ACLS for Experienced Providers.* Dallas, TX: American Heart Association; 2003:83–93.)

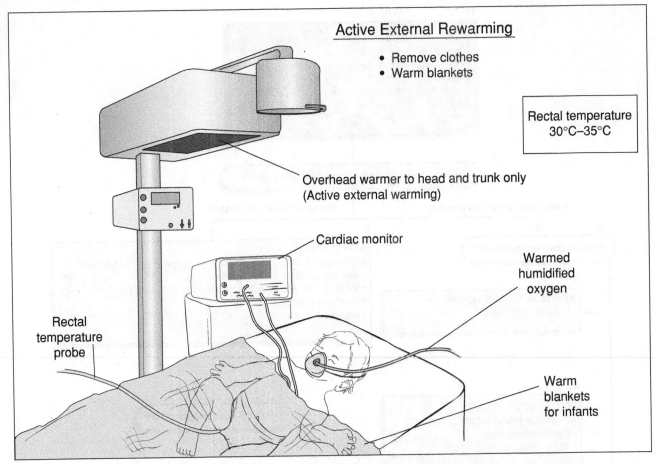

Figure 131.5 Active external rewarming with an overhead warmer.

evaporative heat loss from the respiratory tract. Because only 10% of heat loss occurs through the respiratory tract, this intervention may be better viewed as a low-risk means of preventing heat loss rather than a technique to actively warm hypothermic patients (6,19). The recommended temperature is 40°C. Warming rates of less than 1°C per hour are generally achieved with this technique (19).

Active Internal Rewarming (Fig. 131.6)

Warmed Intravenous Fluids
Warmed intravenous fluids are efficacious in warming patients only when delivered at high rates. Thus, unless the patient requires high-volume fluid resuscitation, in-line fluid warming devices may prevent progression of hypothermia but are unlikely to correct it (6,20). The recommended temperature is 40°C to 42°C. If an in-line warming device is not available, intravenous bags can be warmed in a microwave oven (average 2 minutes for a 1-L bag of crystalloid) (21,22). However, care should be taken to calibrate this to the microwave being used, and the fluids should be mixed thoroughly to distribute "hot spots" caused by imperfections in the oven. Red blood cells should not be microwaved. Normal saline is preferred to

Ringer lactate solution because the cold liver may be unable to metabolize lactate.

Peritoneal Lavage
A multihole dialysis catheter is placed through a minilaparotomy or percutaneous puncture (Chapter 27). Normal saline or standard dialysate solution at 40°C is used. The use of the single-catheter technique with conventional instill and drainage techniques to instill 10 to 15 cc/kg at a time will generate warming rates of 2°C to 4°C per hour (23). High-flow instillation of warmed fluids into the peritoneal cavity at a rate of 600 cc per minute has been reported to generate a warming rate of up to 8°C in 45 minutes (24).

Thoracic Lavage
Thoracic lavage can be performed using an open (thoracotomy) or closed (thoracostomy) technique (Chapters 29 and 31). Both techniques should be reserved for extreme cases involving cardiac arrest or instability. Thoracotomy and open thoracic irrigation allows "bathing" of mediastinal structures with warmed solutions as well as the potential for open cardiac massage if necessary (25). It is not necessary to open the pericardium. The physician bathes the heart for several minutes in 1 to 2 L of warmed (40°C) isotonic solution,

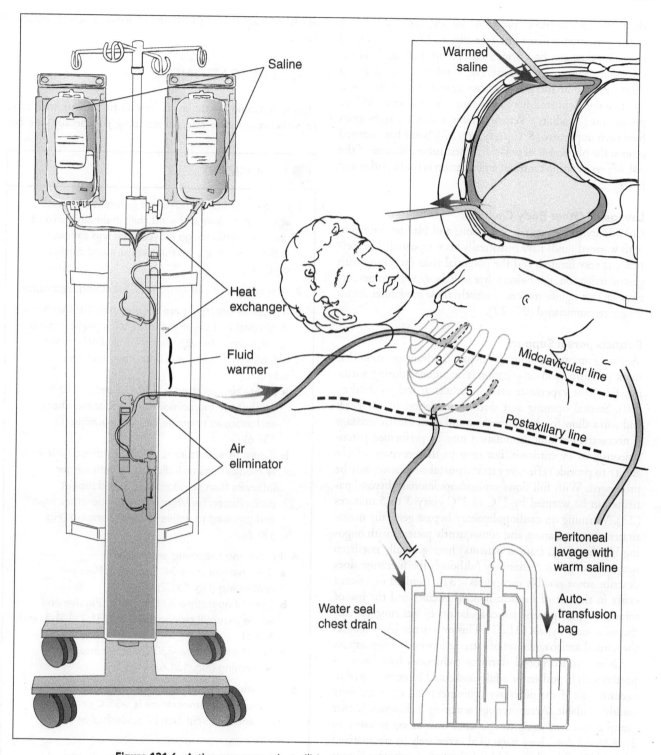

Figure 131.6 Active core rewarming utilizing peritoneal lavage and thoracic cavity lavage.

removes the solution with suction, and repeats as necessary. Open cardiac massage should be used as necessary, but blood flow will be limited in a cold, contracted heart. Internal defibrillation should be attempted on a fibrillating heart once the myocardial temperature reaches 26°C to 28°C. Physician comfort with thoracotomy and repair must exist for the use of this technique.

Closed thoracic irrigation can be accomplished through either single or multiple chest tubes (26). If a single chest tube is used, 200- to 300-cc aliquots (in an adult-size patient) of warmed isotonic fluid (40°C to 42°C) is instilled and then withdrawn (a Y-connector can facilitate the transfer). Alternatively, one chest tube (for infusion) can be placed in the third intercostal space at the midclavicular line and another chest tube (for drainage) placed in the fifth intercostal space at the posterior axillary line (see Fig. 131.6). The infused isotonic saline can be warmed and pumped through an in-line countercurrent fluid infuser (rapid infuser). The draining chest tube can be suction or gravity drained into a water seal chest drain. Reported flow rates range from 180 to 550 cc per minute (in adults). Warming rates with these techniques have been impressive (8°C per hour) (27). Some have warned against the placement of left-sided chest tubes (because of the risk of precipitating ventricular fibrillation in the hypothermic heart) (23).

Lavage of Other Body Cavities

Colonic irrigation, gastric irrigation, and bladder irrigation with warmed fluids have historically been reported. Their efficacy is very limited, and the potential risks (vomiting with gastric irrigation, fluid-electrolyte imbalance with colonic irrigation) are significant; consequently, these modalities are no longer recommended (27–29).

Extracorporeal Support

Warming on cardiopulmonary bypass is advantageous in that tissue perfusion and oxygenation is maintained during warming. Extensive experience exists in adults as well as children (30). Sternal opening and direct cannulation of the heart and aorta allow for direct warming and open cardiac massage if necessary. Femoral cannulation may be performed percutaneously or by cutdown, but time to the provision of (or ability to provide) effective extracorporeal circulation may be prolonged. With full flows on cardiopulmonary bypass, patients can be warmed by 1°C to 2°C every 3 to 5 minutes (23). Warming on cardiopulmonary bypass generally necessitates anticoagulation, and consequently patients with ongoing bleeding (e.g., trauma patients) have generally not been warmed using this technology (although the literature does describe some notable exceptions) (31). Limited experience exists in the use of heparin-bonded circuits and the use of minimal or no patient anticoagulation in warming on cardiopulmonary bypass (31,32). This experience likely reflects the natural anticoagulation of extreme low body temperature.

Other extracorporeal warming techniques have been reported with hypothermic adults and could be extrapolated to pediatric use if the necessary equipment and expertise were readily available. Arteriovenous warming techniques (either pump assisted or using the patient's own blood pressure to drive blood flow) have been used extensively in traumatized adults (33). The flow of blood through a warming device (40°C) is dependent on having large enough arterial and venous access catheters to achieve high blood flows (200 to 400 cc per minute) (33). Local (not systemic) anticoagulation is often sufficient to prevent circuit thrombosis (33). Warming rates of 3°C per hour can be achieved (33). Less but successful experience has been reported with venovenous warming devices in adults (warming rates of 2°C per hour when extracorporeal flows of 150 to 400 cc per minute across a 40°C heat exchanger were achieved) (32,34). Successful warming

via hemodialysis has also been reported in several children (35).

▶ COMPLICATIONS

Passive warming is safe but is limited to patients with mild hypothermia. Active external warming is generally safe but

---

 SUMMARY

1 For all patients: Remove wet garments; protect against heat loss and wind chill; maintain horizontal position; avoid rough movements and excess activity; monitor core temperature and cardiac rhythm.

2 Assess level of consciousness, breathing, and pulse.

3 If pulse or breathing are absent, start CPR with one defibrillation if VF or pulseless VT is present; secure airway; ventilate with warm, humidified oxygen; establish IV access; and infuse warmed normal saline.
  a If core temperature is <30°C, continue CPR, withhold IV medications and additional shocks, and proceed to active internal warming (Fig. 131.6)
  b If core temperature is >30°C, continue CPR, give IV medications as indicted but with longer intervals than standard ACLS, and repeat defibrillation for VF or VT as temperature rises and proceed to active internal warming (Fig. 131.6).

4 If pulse and breathing are present:
  a Core temperature 34°C to 36°C: Passive rewarming (Fig. 131.2)
  b Core temperature 30°C to 34°C: Passive and active external rewarming (Fig. 131.2, 131.3, and 131.5)
  c Core temperature <30°C: Active internal rewarming (Fig. 131.6)

5 For patients requiring active internal rewarming, continue until temperature is >35°C or return of spontaneous circulation or resuscitative efforts cease.

6 Passive rewarming includes: Warm clothes, blankets, exercise, and food.

7 Active external rewarming includes: Heating blankets, forced warm air devices, radiant warmers, and warm humidified air.

8 Active internal warming includes: Warmed IV fluids, peritoneal lavage, thoracic lavage, and extracorporeal support.

CLINICAL TIPS

▶ Hypothermic cardiac arrest can be reversed even if prolonged.

▶ External active rewarming may result in "afterdrop," although this complication is rarely encountered with the use of forced air warmers, which are especially useful in children.

▶ Active internal rewarming for severe hypothermia may be effected with commonly practiced procedures and available equipment, such as peritoneal and closed thoracic lavage.

▶ The most effective technique for treatment of severe hypothermia, especially complicated by nonperfusing cardiac rhythm, is cardiopulmonary bypass.

---

is not without risk. Risks of external warming include iatrogenic ventricular fibrillation, mismatch of metabolic demands and perfusion, and afterdrop. Ventricular fibrillation can be precipitated by excess stimulation of the severely hypothermic patient (4). Thus, patients should be transported gently, and a careful evaluation to exclude any signs of perfusing cardiac activity should be done prior to initiating chest compressions. The mismatch between metabolic activity and perfusion may be exacerbated in unstable patients treated with active external warming. In theory, the benefits of remaining in a "metabolic icebox" may be lost if body temperature increases enough to increase tissue metabolism in the absence of improved perfusion. Accordingly, some centers avoid external warming in severely hypothermic patients that are being transported to cardiopulmonary bypass centers (2). The phenomenon of afterdrop has been well documented. External warming–mediated skin vasodilatation can contribute to afterdrop when cold blood returns to the central circulation (23). Afterdrop has not been documented in association with external warming by forced-air devices, perhaps because the high heat transfer in these devices compensates for vasodilatory effects. All conduction and radiant warming devises carry a risk of causing burns. Ischemic skin (from hypothermic shunting) can be susceptible to burns, even in the absence of equipment malfunction (36). Internal warming techniques (peritoneal or thoracic irrigation) carry risks for organ injury or viscous perforation, hemorrhage, and infection. Extracorporeal support carries risks of anticoagulation, infection, and air-bubble thrombosis.

SUMMARY

Hypothermia is a common and often avoidable cause of morbidity and mortality in infants and children. When active treatment for hypothermia is necessary, it can usually be read-

ily performed in the ED with commonly available equipment (i.e., forced air rewarmers, radiant heaters, or warming blankets). The management of severe hypothermia with hemodynamic instability may benefit from the expertise and equipment available in the operating room or intensive care setting so that aggressive rewarming via cardiac bypass, peritoneal lavage, or thoracic cavity lavage can be performed. Good patient outcomes can be achieved with timely application of these procedures, even in patients who at first appear unsalvageable.

▶ ACKNOWLEDGMENT

The authors would like to acknowledge the valuable contribution of Julie Lange Varga to the version of this chapter that appeared in the previous edition.

▶ REFERENCES

1. Letsou GV, Kopf GS, Elefteriades JA, et al. Is cardiopulmonary bypass effective for treatment of hypothermic arrest due to drowning or exposure? *Arch Surg.* 1992;127:525–528.

2. Antretter H, Dapunt OE, Mueller LC. Survival after prolonged hypothermia. *N Engl J Med.* 1994;330:219.

3. de Caen A. Management of profound hypothermia in children without the use of extracorporeal life support therapy. *Lancet.* 2002; 360(9343):1394–1395.

4. Larach MG. Accidental hypothermia. *Lancet.* 1995;345(8948):493–498.

5. Sessler DI. Complications and treatment of mild hypothermia. *Anesthesiology.* 2001;95:531–543.

6. Lenhardt R. Monitoring and thermal management. *Best Pract Res Clin Anaesthesiol.* 2003;17:569–581.

7. Walpoth BH, Walpoth-Aslan BN, Mattle HP, et al. Outcome of survivors of accidental deep hypothermia and circulatory arrest treated with extracorporeal blood warming. *N Engl J Med.* 1997;337:1500–1505.

8. Cummins RO. Special resuscitation circumstances, I: hypothermia. In: Cummins RO, Field JM, Hazinski MF, eds. *ACLS for Experienced Providers.* Dallas: American Heart Association; 2003:83–93.

9. Giesbrecht GG. Cold stress, near drowning and accidental hypothermia: a review. *Aviat Space Environ Med.* 2000;71:733–752.

10. Danzl DF. Accidental hypothermia. In: Auerbach P, ed. *Wilderness Medicine.* St. Louis: Mosby; 2001:135–177.

11. Taguchi A, Ratnaraj J. Effects of a circulating-water garment and forced-air warming on body heat content and core temperature. *Anesthesiology.* 2004;100:1058–1064.

12. Sessler DI, Moayeri A. Skin-surface warming: heat flux and central temperature. *Anesthesiology.* 1990;73:218–224.

13. Matsuzaki Y, Matsukawa T, Ohki K, et al. Warming by resistive heating maintains perioperative normothermia as well as forced air heating. *Br J Anaesth.* 2003;90:689–691.

14. Perl T, Brauer A, Timmermann A, et al. Differences among forced-air warming systems with upper body blankets are small: a randomized trial for heat transfer in volunteers. *Acta Anaesthesiol Scand.* 2003;47:1159–1164.

15. Kornberger E, Schwarz B, Lindner KH, et al. Forced air surface rewarming in patients with severe accidental hypothermia. *Resuscitation.* 1999;41:105–111.

16. Koller R, Schnider TW, Neidhart P. Deep accidental hypothermia and cardiac arrest: rewarming with forced air. *Acta Anaesthesiol Scand.* 1997;41:1359–1364.

17. Currie AE. How cold can you get? A case of severe neonatal hypothermia. *J R Soc Med.* 1994;87:293–294.

18. Weyland W, Weyland A, Hellige G, et al. Efficiency of a new radiant heater for postoperative rewarming. *Acta Anaesthesiol Scand.* 1994;38:601–606.

19. Frank SM, Hesel TW, El Rahmany HK, et al. Warmed humidified inspired oxygen accelerates postoperative rewarming. *J Clin Anesth.* 2000;12:283–287.

20. Petrone P, Kuncir EJ, Asensio JA. Surgical management and strategies in the treatment of hypothermia and cold injury. *Emerg Med Clin North Am.* 2003;21:1165–1178.

21. Aldrete JA. Preventing hypothermia in trauma patients by microwave warming of i.v. fluids. *J Emerg Med.* 1985;3:435–442.

22. Leaman PL, Martyak GG. Microwave warming of resuscitation fluids. *Ann Emerg Med.* 1985;14:876–879.

23. Danzl DF, Pozos RS. Accidental hypothermia. *N Engl J Med.* 1994;331:1756–1760.

24. Papenhausen M, Burke L, Antony A, et al. Severe hypothermia with cardiac arrest: complete neurologic recovery in a 4-year-old child. *J Pediatr Surg.* 2001;36:1590–1592.

25. Kangas E, Niemela H, Kojo N. Treatment of hypothermic circulatory arrest with thoracotomy and pleural lavage. *Ann Chir Gynaecol.* 1994;83:258–260.

26. Iversen RJ, Atkin SH, Jaker MA, et al. Successful CPR in a severely hypothermic patient using continuous thoracostomy lavage. *Ann Emerg Med.* 1990;19:1335–1337.

27. Brunette DD, Biros M, Mlinek EJ, et al. Internal cardiac massage and mediastinal irrigation in hypothermic cardiac arrest. *Am J Emerg Med.* 1992;10:32–34.

28. Brunette DD, Sterner S, Robinson EP, et al. Comparison of gastric lavage and thoracic cavity lavage in the treatment of severe hypothermia in dogs. *Ann Emerg Med.* 1987;16:1222–1227.

29. Brunette DD, McVaney K. Hypothermic cardiac arrest: an 11 year review of ED management and outcome. *Am J Emerg Med.* 2000;18:418–422.

30. Farstad M, Anderson KS, Koller ME, et al. Rewarming from accidental hypothermia by extracorporeal circulation: a retrospective study. *Eur J Cardiothorac Surg.* 2001;20:58–64.

31. von Segesser LK, Garcia E, Turina M. Perfusion without systemic heparinization for rewarming in accidental hypothermia. *Ann Thorac Surg.* 1991;52:560–561.

32. Gregory JS, Bergstein JM, Aprahamian C, et al. Comparison of three methods of rewarming from hypothermia: advantages of extracorporeal blood warming. *J Trauma.* 1991;31:1247–1251.

33. Gentilello LM, Cobean RA, Offner PJ, et al. Continuous arteriovenous rewarming: rapid reversal of hypothermia in critically ill patients. *J Trauma.* 1992;32:316–325.

34. Brauer A, Wrigge H, Kersten J, et al. Severe accidental hypothermia: rewarming strategy using a veno-venous bypass system and a convective air warmer. *Intensive Care Med.* 1999;25:520–523.

35. Owda A, Osama S. Hemodialysis in management of hypothermia. *Am J Kidney Dis.* 2001;38(2):E8.

36. Dewar DJ, Fraser JF, Choo KL, et al. Thermal injuries in three children caused by an electrical warming mattress. *Br J Anaesth.* 2004;93:586–589.

132

JOHN M. LOISELLE

General Principles of Emergency Department Ultrasonography

▶ INTRODUCTION

The beginning of ultrasonography can be traced to the development of sonar in World War II. Applications in the field of medicine became apparent as early as the 1950s. Although ultrasonography was initially considered a tool of radiologists, its use has spread to different subspecialties, notably cardiology and obstetrics, where it is now a routine and required skill. More recently, its benefits have been demonstrated for specific applications within emergency medicine. The American College of Emergency Physicians (ACEP) has issued position papers endorsing the 24-hour availability of ultrasound technology within the emergency department (ED) and its use by appropriately trained, experienced, and credentialed emergency physicians (1). In addition, a report by the American Institute of Ultrasound in Medicine agreed that ultrasound examinations may be performed by appropriately trained emergency physicians in (a) certain immediate or life-threatening situations in which ultrasound examination is needed and other ultrasound physicians are not available, (b) certain urgent conditions in which ultrasound physicians cannot provide timely service on a 24-hour-a-day, 7-day-a-week basis, and (c) situations in which ultrasound guidance may enhance the performance of certain procedures (2).

Emergency medicine residency programs are required to provide formal training in the emergent use of ultrasound as part of the core curriculum (1,3,4). Fellowships specializing in the use of ultrasound by emergency physicians already exist. It is now clear that the use of ultrasonography in the ED for specific indications is rapidly becoming a necessary skill.

The role of ultrasonography in the ED differs significantly from its previously recognized roles in other areas of medicine. For diagnostic purposes, ultrasound is generally used in the ED to answer a specific question, such as whether products of conception are clearly identifiable in the uterus. Its uses are limited to specific areas, and it is not intended to replace the more complete ultrasound studies typically performed by other specialists. Diagnostic ultrasonography has distinct advantages in the ED, where rapid, immediately available studies are crucial. It is possible to obtain adequate examinations even during the performance of cardiopulmonary resuscitation (5).

Ultrasound not only functions as a diagnostic tool in the ED but also provides guidance in the performance of various invasive procedures. It improves success rates and decreases complications in procedures commonly performed blindly (6–12). Ultrasound facilitates these procedures by allowing the clinician to visualize a needle or probe as it approaches the target, mark the skin surface above the target, or measure the distance from the skin surface to the target.

Uses of ultrasound in the ED have been studied in a number of applications specific to pediatric patients. Benefits have been demonstrated in all pediatric age groups, including neonates (13). Investigators have evaluated its usefulness in cases involving pediatric trauma, removal of foreign bodies, adolescent pregnancies, pulseless electrical activity, and vascular line placement (10–18).

The chapters in this section are intended to serve not as a comprehensive instructional aid in the use of ultrasound technology but as an introduction to and review of the various techniques. As in the use and interpretation of any diagnostic procedure, routine standards must be applied. The clinician must develop understanding and competency in the areas of application, visualization, and interpretation of ultrasound images. Specific indications must be developed to avoid overuse of this technique. Definitive expertise in ultrasonography requires several years of subspecialty training. This is clearly not the goal for emergency physicians. However, training emergency physicians to perform and interpret ultrasound examinations for specific indications is possible in a reasonable period of time (18–21). ACEP has recommended minimum numbers of studies to be performed for proficiency in specific applications, and other authorities have suggested minimum hourly requirements in formal instruction, hands-on training, review of the literature, and formal review of studies with skilled sonographers (1,22,23). These suggested requirements are consistent with those currently recommended in other nonradiologic specialties utilizing ultrasound (23). Ongoing review and quality assurance are a necessary part of maintaining proficiency in ED ultrasonography.

▶ ANATOMY AND PHYSIOLOGY

Ultrasonography, like sonar, is based on the generation of sound waves and relies on the ability of tissues within their path to propagate and reflect these waves in order to produce a two-dimensional image of objects in its field. The ultrasound transducer converts electrical energy to sound energy, which propagates through body tissues (Fig. 132.1A). The denser the tissue, the better the sound waves are propagated. Sound waves propagate poorly through gas and do not reach structures separated from the transducer by a gas interface. This presents a problem for the unprepped patient with intestinal air who requires an abdominal scan. Wave propagation through bone is so rapid that ultrasound units are unable to accommodate it, and therefore objects behind bone cannot be detected.

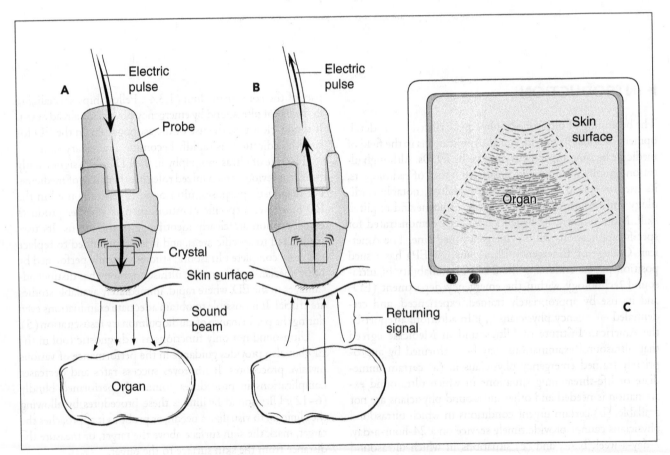

Figure 132.1
A. Generation of an ultrasound beam by transducer.
B. Detection of a reflected ultrasound beam by transducer.
C. Corresponding image production on ultrasound screen.

Waves are reflected by interfaces of tissues of differing densities, producing echoes (Fig. 132.1B). These echoes are detected by the transducer and converted back into electrical energy from which an image is constructed (Fig. 132.1C). Echogenic or hyperechoic objects reflect most ultrasound waves and appear white on the ultrasound screen. Anechoic objects mainly transmit ultrasound waves and appear black on the screen. Objects of intermediate densities both transmit and reflect ultrasound waves and appear as varying shades of gray.

An acoustic window is an anechoic structure through which ultrasound waves can be transmitted to underlying structures of interest. A fluid-filled bladder is a commonly used acoustic window. Acoustic shadowing occurs when the ultrasound beam strikes a highly reflective surface, such as a renal stone or other calcified object, resulting in a dark shadow beyond the object. This may be helpful in identifying foreign bodies or a hindrance if distal objects become hidden within the shadow. Artificial acoustic windows can be used when the area of interest is superficial and below the normal focal zone of the transducer. A standoff pad or intravenous fluid bag can be placed against the surface of the body to increase the distance to the object under study while avoiding an air interface.

The resolution of ultrasound images depends on multiple factors. The strength of the echo, and therefore the image resolution, is proportional to the difference in density or acoustic impedance of adjacent tissues. Larger differences in tissue densities produce greater signal reflections and therefore greater resolution. Sound waves that strike perpendicular to the structure's surface rather than at an angle produce less scatter and a stronger echo, thereby providing greater resolution. Sound waves lose energy as they penetrate through a greater amount of tissue, and this beam attenuation results in lower resolution for distant objects.

The focal zone of a transducer is the depth at which its image resolution is greatest and is determined by the frequency of the sound waves emitted. Higher frequencies produce greater resolution but penetrate less deeply below the body surface. Clinically relevant frequencies used in ultrasonography range from 2 to 9 megahertz (MHz). Transducers are available that produce specific frequencies within this range. A transducer that produces sound waves at a frequency of 2.25 MHz has optimal resolution capabilities at a depth of 8 to 12 cm. A 3.5-MHz transducer has a focal zone at 4 to 8 cm, and a 5- or 7.5-MHz transducer at 2 to 5 cm.

Ultrasonography is a noninvasive means of providing immediate bedside assessment of both anatomy and function. The image on the screen is rapidly and continuously updated, similar to the operation of a home television set, resulting in a real-time display that, to the clinician's eye, appears to move exactly as the body structures move.

As children and adults are susceptible to different disease processes, there are different indications and possibilities for the use of ED ultrasonography in different age groups. Using ultrasound in children offers both advantages and disadvantages. Children in general possess less adipose tissue, and the depth to structures from the skin surface is not as great, which allows improved resolution of most structures in the body. Certain disease processes that are well known to complicate ultrasound studies (e.g., COPD, ascites) rarely occur in children. However, the smaller body of a child can make using a standard "adult" transducer impossible. Narrow rib interspaces limit the possible windows and transducer sizes that can be used. Moreover, organs and structures are smaller and therefore harder to find and evaluate.

▶ INDICATIONS

Ultrasound studies by emergency physicians are not intended to replace the physical examination, alternate studies, or ultrasound studies by a more experienced practitioner when available. Within the realm of the ED and the requirements of the emergency physician, several uses have been established for ultrasound. Its use in the ED is optimal for (a) relatively common conditions in which proficiency can be maintained, (b) conditions in which emergent diagnosis is essential in dictating management, (c) situations in which no better diagnostic modality is available, (d) conditions in which ultrasound provides reasonable sensitivity and specificity in the hands of trained emergency physicians, and (e) conditions in which a rapid, focused study can deliver findings that are readily detected and interpreted.

Currently, a number of uses are established for pediatric ultrasonography by emergency physicians, several of which are discussed in detail in the remaining chapters of this section. In addition, certain ED ultrasound procedures that have been demonstrated as effective in adults are currently being evaluated for extrapolation to pediatric patients (3). A number of investigational uses also exist, although these are not discussed.

The quality of the study in pediatric patients may be limited by a number of factors, including agitation and lack of cooperation by the young child, tenderness with pressure from the transducer, inability to achieve proper positioning for the study, the small size of the child, and the size of the available equipment. It should be emphasized that ED ultrasonography must not interfere with procedures or evaluations of higher priority.

▶ EQUIPMENT

The proper ultrasound machine and other specific equipment options will depend on the anticipated applications within the ED.

Ultrasound machine—optimally a unit capable of being upgraded and compatible with the different transducers necessary for anticipated uses. Many machines are equipped with standard features and numerous options, most of which are unnecessary for intended uses in the ED. The unit must be portable for rapid bedside deployment. A screen size of at least 5 inches diagonally is recommended for adequate visualization. The screen should be capable of displaying the image with a minimum of 64 shades of gray (24). Standard controls on an ultrasound machine include these:

Overall gain—controls the power output or strength of the ultrasound signal and acts in a manner comparable to the brightness control on a television set.

Time gain compensation—accounts for beam attenuation by controlling beam strength at different levels to produce a consistent, uniform image. Near gain controls dampen the signals of superficial structures, whereas far gain controls allow for enhancement of distant echoes. These are controlled automatically on some units. Others have multiple controls for different depths in a graphic equalizer format.

Zoom—provides image magnification.

Freeze frame—provides a still image for evaluation. This may be important when scanning structures in motion such as the heart or when measurements or a hard copy are desired.

Electronic calipers—allow accurate measurements of objects being scanned.

Doppler—provides the capability to detect motion due to changes in wavelengths produced by an object moving toward or away from the transducer. Generally used to detect blood flow. Flow characteristics are depicted on-screen using color.

Transducers—ultrasound waves are produced by a vibrating quartz crystal within the transducer by means of a piezoelectric effect. The alignment of these piezoelectric elements determines the focal length of the transducer. As described previously, the higher the frequency of sound wave produced, the better the resolution but the more superficial the sound wave penetration. The common frequencies available are 3.5 MHz for use in abdominal scanning, 5 MHz for cardiac examinations, and 7.5 MHz for superficial scanning, such as subcutaneous foreign body detection. Varying sizes and shapes of transducers make them useful for particular types of scanning, such as endovaginal, abdominal, and transesophageal scans (Fig. 132.2). Some are the size of a fingertip for use in tight spaces. Transducers should be selected according to the likely uses of the machine in the ED.

Printer—essential for providing documentation of ultrasound findings both for the medical record and for future quality review. Most units have the capability of labeling the printout with identifying information.

Videotape recorder—useful in providing additional documentation and for subsequent review of the study. It is a necessary part of a quality assurance program.

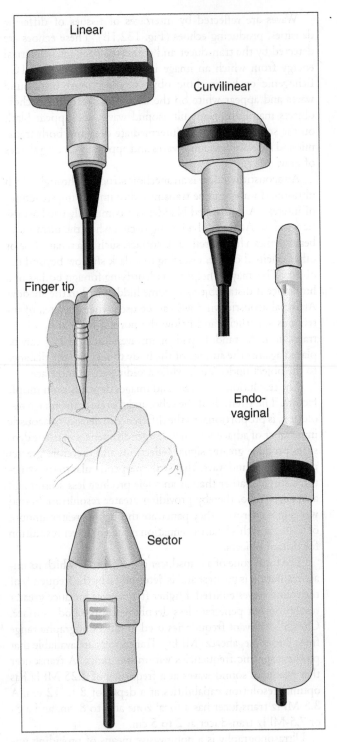

Figure 132.2 Transducer types.

Acoustic gel—provides an interface between the skin and the transducer by conducting sound waves.

Acoustic standoff pads—act as an artificial acoustic window intended to provide additional distance to superficial structures so that structures remain within the transducer's focal zone. An intravenous fluid bag often provides an acceptable alternative.

▶ PROCEDURE

The procedure should be explained to the child when maturational age and circumstances allow. Reassurance that the examination is noninvasive and painless should lower anxiety and in most cases will improve the child's compliance. This is especially important for procedures such as endovaginal scanning in the adolescent.

The position of the patient on the examining table will vary depending on the intended area to be scanned. Optimal positioning is discussed for each procedure in the relevant chapter. Correct positioning will provide the best and most accurate views of certain structures and will frequently determine the difference between an adequate and inadequate scan. Inability to position the patient properly due to lack of cooperation or contraindications to moving the patient may limit or preclude scanning in particular cases.

The position of the clinician also is an important aspect of the examination. For each application, the clinician should have a routine, comfortable position; should ensure the screen is easily visible and accessible; and should be close enough to the patient to enable the transducer to be readily manipulated to the desired position. The clinician must assume a position in which no interference occurs with the ongoing evaluation or management of the patient. In most cases, the clinician will have his or her dominant side toward the patient, with the area to be examined approximately at elbow level (Fig. 132.3A).

The unit itself may require time to warm up and should be turned on as soon as it becomes apparent that ultrasonography may be used. Initial standard control settings should be determined for specific scans before actual use, and the clinician should check that these settings are in place before proceeding. Fine-tuning can then be performed as necessary. Common errors include not allowing adequate time for the

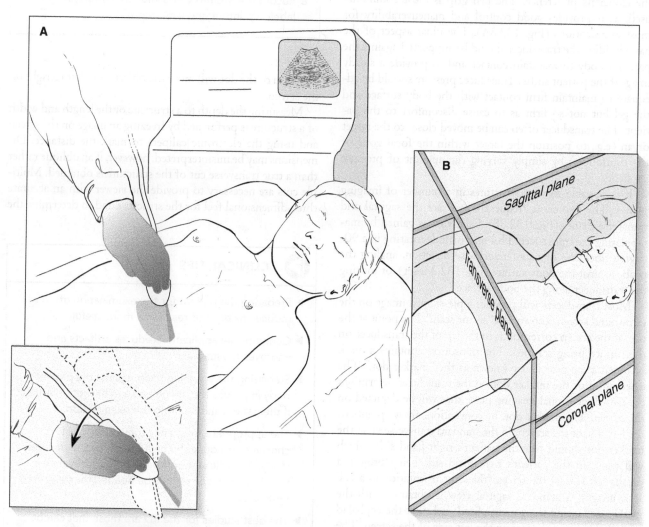

Figure 132.3
A. Recommended position of clinician in relation to supine patient and ultrasound unit.
B. Sagittal and transverse imaging planes. Alternating between the two planes is performed by rotating transducer 90 degrees. Angling the transducer changes the transverse imaging plane (*inset*).

unit to warm up and manipulating contrast and gain knobs excessively. Overuse of the gain to increase contrast will result in more artifacts and produce an inaccurate depiction of tissue densities (24). The gain should be adjusted using organs of known sonodensity for comparison.

The clinician should apply a generous amount of gel either to the body surface above the structure to be scanned or directly to the transducer. Inadequate amounts of gel result in poor transmission of sound waves, known as "contact artifact," as well as interference from bubbles within the gel.

Transducer frequency should be selected according to the desired use. The focal zone of the transducer should be equivalent to the estimated depth of the structure of interest. As mentioned previously, acoustic standoff pads may be used to provide additional distance between the transducer and superficial target structures (see Fig. 136.2). Several methods of gripping the transducer are possible, and which one is chosen depends on the type of examination being performed and the clinician's preference. The pen grip is most commonly used, as it provides good control and maneuverability for most examinations (Fig. 132.3A). The ulnar aspect of the hand holding the transducer should be supported against the patient's body to maintain contact and to provide a steady image if the patient shifts. Transducer pressure should be adequate to maintain firm contact with the body surface and the gel but not so firm as to cause discomfort to the patient. The transducer often can be moved closer to the target organ (e.g., to position the target within the focal zone of the transducer) by simply varying the amount of pressure applied.

It is possible to view structures in a number of imaging planes. The two most frequently used are the sagittal and transverse planes (Fig. 132.3B). Each view is gained by manipulating the transducer. This may include rotating in a 90-degree clockwise or counterclockwise direction, angling the probe against the body surface (Fig. 132.3 inset), or moving the transducer along the body surface.

Most transducers will produce a pie-shaped image on the ultrasound screen, known as a "sector scan." The point at the top of the screen corresponds to the tip of the transducer on the surface being scanned. The transducer contains a mark or indentation near its tip known as the "marker dot." The orientation of the marker dot on the transducer determines the two-dimensional imaging plane that will be depicted on the screen. The marker dot, by convention, always points to the left side of the screen. In the standard transverse view, the marker dot should face the patient's right-hand side, which will result in the patient's right-hand side being projected on the left side of the screen (the same orientation as a CT scan image). A standard sagittal view is obtained with the marker dot facing the patient's head such that the cephalad part of the image appears on the left side of the screen. The ability to position the structure of interest within the screen is rapidly gained through experience. Angling the probe so that the marker dot points upward or moving the probe in the

direction of the dot will move the object from left to right on the screen.

Measuring the depth to a structure or the length and width of a structure is performed by freezing an image on the screen and using the electronic calipers to mark the distance. Dimensions may be misinterpreted, however, if an oblique rather than a true transverse cut of the structure is obtained. Multiple cuts are necessary to provide the viewer with an accurate three-dimensional feel for the structure and to determine the

SUMMARY

1 Prepare the patient for the specific examination.

2 Warm up the ultrasound unit with proper initial settings.

3 Position the patient appropriately for the examination.

4 Apply gel to the body surface overlying the structure of interest.

5 Grip the transducer in a comfortable manner and orient the marker dot.

6 Image the structure in multiple planes using angling and sweeping movements as necessary.

7 Measure depth to structure and/or overall size as necessary.

8 Record the desired views with an appropriately labeled printout and videotape.

CLINICAL TIPS

▸ Preparing the patient for the examination often will reduce anxiety and result in a more useful scan.

▸ Generous gel application reduces artifacts and improves the image.

▸ Stabilizing the scanning hand against the patient's body improves the image and avoids motion artifact if the patient shifts during the examination.

▸ The appropriate frequency transducer must be chosen to produce the best image for the desired study. Acoustic standoff pads (or an intravenous fluid bag) may sometimes be needed for superficial structures.

▸ The best studies for the ED are those that can be performed rapidly, are easily interpreted, and are goal directed.

optimal view. All photographed or recorded images should be labeled with the patient's identifying information, the structure visualized, and the imaging plane used.

▶ COMPLICATIONS

No harmful effects of ultrasound have been documented on patients or clinicians at energy levels that are used clinically (25). Current recommendations call for using the lowest energy level necessary to provide adequate visualization of objects and minimizing the exposure to which individual patients are subjected. Excessive force or pressure, as in any physical examination, has the possibility of inflicting soft-tissue injury and the potential to precipitate injuries, such as the rupture of an intra-abdominal abscess or cyst.

▶ SUMMARY

ED bedside ultrasonography for pediatric patients is a modality still relatively early in its development, but it has already been demonstrated as a useful adjunct to the physician's ability to accurately diagnose and treat conditions in acutely ill and injured children. It can both avoid unnecessary invasive procedures and decrease the complications of others. It is not intended to replace a thorough history and physical examination or a more complete ultrasound study performed by other specialists. A number of studies have shown its accuracy for specific indications in the hands of properly trained emergency physicians. Structured training, credentialing, and quality assurance programs are important in acquiring and maintaining this skill.

▶ REFERENCES

1. American College of Emergency Physicians. Emergency ultrasound guidelines—2001. *Ann Emerg Med.* 2001;38:470–481.
2. Initial report of the American Institute of Ultrasound in Medicine, Ad Hoc Committee on Ultrasound in Emergency Medicine.
3. Hegenbarth M. Bedside ultrasound in the pediatric emergency department: basic skill or passing fancy? *Clin Pediatr Emerg Med.* 2004;5:201–216.
4. Cardenas E, Galli RL. Lower transabdominal endovaginal ultrasonography by emergency medicine residents. *Ann Emerg Med.* 1993;22:920.
5. Bocka JJ, Overton DT, Hauser A. Electromechanical dissociation in human beings: an echocardiographic study. *Ann Emerg Med.* 1988;17:450–452.
6. Callahan JA, Seward JB, Tajik AJ, et al. Pericardiocentesis assisted by two-dimensional echocardiography. *J Thorac Cardiovasc Surg.* 1983;85:877–879.
7. Kuhn G, Burton J, Zelenka J. Central venous access using portable ultrasound in the emergency department. *Ann Emerg Med.* 1993;22:922.
8. Bradley M, Kadzombe E, Simms P, et al. Percutaneous ultrasound guided extraction of nonpalpable soft tissue foreign bodies. *Arch Emerg Med.* 1992;9:181–184.
9. Alderson PJ, Burrows FA, Stemp LI, et al. The use of ultrasound to evaluate internal jugular vein anatomy and to facilitate central venous cannulation in pediatric patients. *Br J Anaesth.* 1993;70:145–148.
10. Chu RWP, Wong YC, Luk SH, et al. Comparing suprapubic urine aspiration under real-time ultrasound guidance with conventional blind aspiration. *Acta Pediatr.* 2002;91:512–516.
11. Donaldson JS, Morello FP, Junewick JJ, et al. Peripherally inserted central venous catheters: US-guided vascular access in pediatric patients. *Radiology.* 1995;197:542–544.
12. Schlager D, Sanders AB, Wiggins D, et al. Ultrasound for the detection of foreign bodies. *Ann Emerg Med.* 1991;20:189–191.
13. Gochman RF, Karasic RB, Heller MB. Use of portable ultrasound to assist urine collection by suprapubic aspiration. *Ann Emerg Med.* 1991;20:631–635.
14. Mutabagani KH, Coley BD, Zumberge N, et al. Preliminary experience with focused abdominal sonography for trauma (FAST) in children: is it useful? *J Pediatr Surg.* 1999;34:48–54.
15. Holmes JF, Brant WE, Bond WF, et al. Emergency department ultrasonography, I: the evaluation of hypotensive and normotensive children with blunt abdominal trauma. *J Pediatr Surg.* 2001;36:968–973.
16. Chen L, Hsiao AL, Moore CL, et al. Utility of bedside bladder ultrasound before urethral catheterization in young children. *Pediatrics.* 2005;115:108–111.
17. Pershad J, Chin T. Early detection of cardiac disease masquerading as acute bronchospasm: the role of limited echocardiography by the emergency physician. *Pediatr Emerg Care.* 2003;19:e1–3.
18. Denys BG, Uretsky BF, Reddy PS, et al. An ultrasound method for safe and rapid central venous access. *N Engl J Med.* 1991;324:566.
19. Ma OJ, Mateer JR, Ogata M, et al. Prospective analysis of a rapid trauma ultrasound examination performed by emergency physicians. *J Trauma.* 1995;38:879–885.
20. Schlager D, Lazzareschi G, Whitten D, et al. A prospective study of ultrasonography in the ED by emergency physicians. *Am J Emerg Med.* 1994;12:185–189.
21. Jehle D, Davis E, Evans T, et al. Emergency department sonography by emergency physicians. *Am J Emerg Med.* 1989;7:605–611.
22. Olson DW. Gynecological applications of ultrasonography. In: *Diagnostic Ultrasonography for Emergency Medicine ACEP.* St. Louis: Mosby; 1993.
23. Mateer J, Plummer D, Heller M, et al. Model curriculum for physician training in emergency ultrasonography. *Ann Emerg Med.* 1994;23:95–102.
24. Heller M, Jehle D. *Ultrasound in Emergency Medicine.* Philadelphia: WB Saunders; 1995.
25. American Institute of Ultrasound in Medicine. Official statement on clinical safety. March 1988.

133

JOHN M. LOISELLE

Ultrasound-Assisted Suprapubic Bladder Aspiration

▶ INTRODUCTION

Suprapubic bladder aspiration of urine is a means of obtaining urine in a sterile fashion by passing a needle through the abdominal wall directly into the urinary bladder. This technique is most commonly used to collect urine from incontinent children as part of a sepsis evaluation when isolating an organism from the urinary tract may be of paramount importance. A urine culture obtained by a suprapubic aspiration is considered the gold standard for detecting bacteruria (1). The suprapubic approach avoids potential contamination from organisms present on the perineum or in the distal urethra. Numerous studies have demonstrated the superiority of suprapubic bladder aspiration compared with other techniques of collecting urine for culture in infants and toddlers (2–8). Although the technique is inherently invasive, few serious complications have been reported with suprapubic bladder aspiration (9–11).

Reported rates of successfully obtaining urine by suprapubic bladder aspiration vary from 23% to 90% (1,2,5,7,8,12–15). Despite the straightforward nature of the technique, suprapubic bladder aspiration performed in an emergency department (ED) setting is often unsuccessful. Experience with the technique improves the success rate (13,15), but a primary factor for failure to obtain urine is the lack of urine in the bladder at the time of the attempt.

Ultrasound was first described as a useful adjunct to suprapubic aspirations in infants in the early 1970s (16). The advent of relatively low cost, portable ultrasound devices has expanded the availability of this noninvasive diagnostic technique to a variety of clinical settings. Ultrasound can be used to determine the presence of urine within the bladder before suprapubic bladder aspiration or to guide the needle during the procedure. Several studies demonstrate that ultrasound can accurately predict the volume of urine in the infant bladder (17,18) and improve the success rate in obtaining urine specimens when compared with blind aspiration (12,13,15,19,20). In addition to the ED setting, this technique may prove valuable in neonatal intensive care units and other areas where suprapubic bladder aspiration is performed regularly.

Suprapubic bladder aspiration is usually performed by a physician and can be done in most inpatient and outpatient settings. Physicians with no formal training in ultrasonography have been able to assess bladder volume accurately (12,18). The relative ease of learning and performing the ultrasound procedure allows trained physician assistants, nurse practitioners, and nurses to use it as well.

▶ ANATOMY AND PHYSIOLOGY

The urinary bladder is an intra-abdominal organ in infants and children under 2 years of age, making it easily accessible by suprapubic bladder aspiration. As a child grows, the bladder recedes into the pelvis and, in older children, enters the abdomen only when full. When suprapubic bladder aspiration is performed in the midline along the suprapubic crease, the needle passes through skin, rectus muscle, and the anterior wall of the bladder. When viewed by ultrasound, these tissues create a lighter background than the full bladder, which appears as a black ovoid structure (Fig. 133.1).

▶ INDICATIONS

Suprapubic bladder aspiration may be indicated in incontinent children less than 2 years of age when the collection

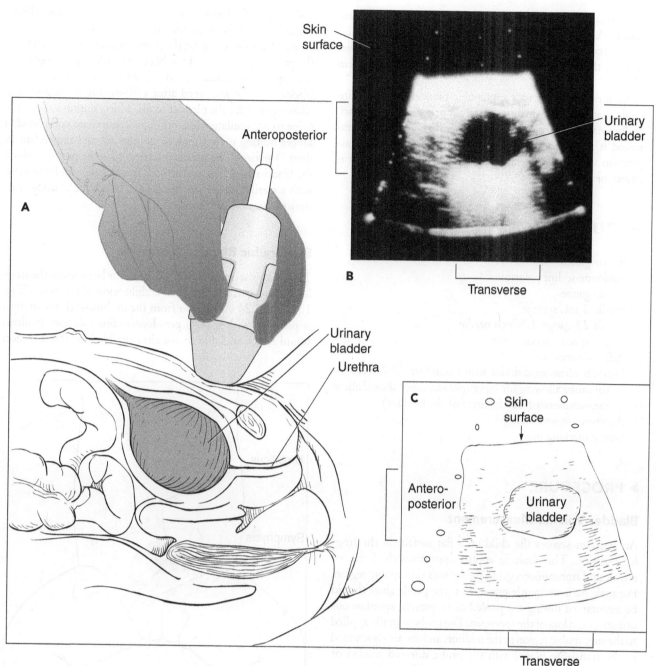

Figure 133.1
A. Position of the patient and ultrasound probe for scanning the bladder.
B. Ultrasound image of a full urinary bladder in an infant.
C. Schematic depiction of an ultrasound image.

of sterile urine is necessary and urethral contamination must be avoided. A common clinical situation that may necessitate suprapubic bladder aspiration is the sepsis evaluation in a febrile infant. A urinary tract infection is a common source of bacterial infection in these infants, and obtaining uncontaminated urine that allows identification of a true pathogen is imperative. Aspiration of the bladder may also be used when uncontaminated urine must be obtained from the incontinent child who has gastroenteritis and frequent diarrheal stools.

Urethral catheterization is widely used in lieu of suprapubic bladder aspiration, and it is the procedure of choice in most facilities. Urethral catheterization is more often successful in obtaining an adequate volume of urine for culture than suprapubic aspiration (21) and is less painful for the infant (22). However, the incidence of contamination is higher in cultures obtained by urethral catheterization than in those obtained by suprapubic aspiration (1). At times, anatomic considerations limit the opportunities for urethral catheterization. It is occasionally difficult to find the urethral orifice in the infant female. A suprapubic aspiration may be the preferred method of urine collection in the young female infant with labial adhesions or the male infant with a minimally retractable foreskin (1).

Contraindications to a suprapubic bladder aspiration include anatomic abnormalities of the gut or genitourinary tract, abdominal wall infection, and bleeding diatheses (21). Ultrasound is indicated as an adjunct to suprapubic bladder aspiration when the clinician is unsure whether the bladder is empty or full.

▶ EQUIPMENT

Sterile gloves
Povidone-iodine solution
Sterile gauze
Sterile 5-mL syringe
22- or 23-gauge, 1.5-inch needle
Sterile specimen container
Adhesive bandage
Portable ultrasound device with a standoff 7.5-MHz sector probe allowing for superficial scanning (should allow measurement of the diameter of the bladder)
Acoustic transmission gel
Sterile marking pen

▶ PROCEDURE

Bladder Volume Measurement

An assistant secures the child on a flat surface in the frog-leg position. The clinician applies approximately 5 mL of ultrasound transmission gel to the infant's suprapubic region. For male patients, gentle pressure on the penile shaft should be maintained during the procedure to prevent spontaneous urination and loss of the specimen. The probe is gently applied to the suprapubic region in the midline, and the area is scanned in the transverse plane, with the probe directed caudad or cephalad as needed to maximize the size of the bladder image (Fig. 133.1A). The bladder appears as an anechoic (black) structure below the brighter reflections of the rectus muscle and anterior bladder wall.

The image is frozen at the maximum bladder size, and the anteroposterior (AP) and transverse internal bladder diameters are measured to the nearest 0.5 cm. The bladder is considered to be full if both the maximum AP and transverse diameters are 2 cm or more and empty if either diameter is less than 2 cm. These parameters have resulted in successful obtainment of greater than 2 mL of urine in more than 75% of attempts (13). Other studies have utilized additional measurements to estimate urinary volumes (14,15,17,18). Some ultrasound scanners display bladder volume rather than an ac-

tual image (20). Greater success may be expected when larger bladder diameters are identified.

After ultrasonography, the probe and gel are removed from the patient's abdomen. If the bladder is full, suprapubic bladder aspiration should be attempted at once. If empty, the bladder may be rescanned after a 30-minute waiting period, allowing time for the bladder to fill. Thirty minutes allows for urine to accumulate while other procedures are completed; a longer waiting period may be impractical and imprudent in the ED setting. The needle insertion site (the point at which the bladder is closest to the abdominal wall) can be marked with a sterile pen, or the needle can be advanced using real-time ultrasound guidance.

Suprapubic Bladder Aspiration

The child is securely restrained on his or her back in the frog-leg position, which facilitates stabilization of the pelvis (Fig. 133.2) (23,24). The skin from the umbilicus to the urethra is prepared with a 10% povidone-iodine solution. If ultrasound is not available to visualize the bladder, the insertion

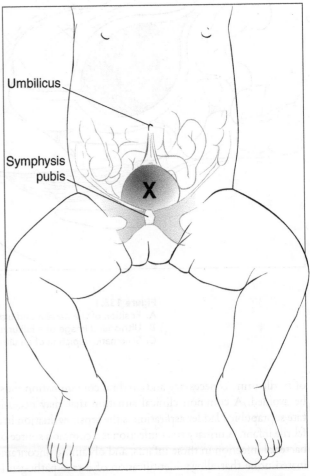

Figure 133.2 Frog-leg position and identification of insertion site.

site should be in the midline 1 to 2 cm above the pubic symphysis on the abdominal wall. The site can be draped with a sterile cloth, and if desired, local anesthetic such as 1% lidocaine may be infiltrated at the site. This is an optional part of the procedure, because needle insertion for the procedure is probably less painful than local infiltration anesthesia. Alternatively, a topical anesthetic such as eutectic mixture of local anesthetic cream (EMLA) can be applied (see Chapter 35), although the need for urgency may make this step impractical. Next, the urethral opening should be occluded. This is achieved by applying gentle pressure to the base of the penis against the pubic symphysis in the boy or by applying pressure directly to the urethral meatus in the girl.

The skin is punctured, and the needle is advanced in a cephalad direction angled approximately 20 degrees from the vertical while applying mild negative pressure to the syringe (Fig. 133.3). In this way, the needle will puncture the center of a full bladder. A distinct change in resistance may be felt as the needle passes through the bladder wall. When the needle enters the bladder cavity, urine will be aspirated. If the bladder is partially empty, however, this angle of entry may cause the needle to pass over the top of the bladder and thus result in unsuccessful aspiration. In such cases, the needle is withdrawn but not removed from the skin. The procedure is the repeated with the needle reoriented vertically so that a lower part of the abdominal cavity will be entered. If still unsuccessful, the clinician should delay at least 1 hour before a repeated attempt. During this time, the child is hydrated with fluids to fill the bladder.

Suprapubic Aspiration Using Ultrasound Guidance

Once the sterile field has been prepared, a sterile sheath is placed over the ultrasound probe and proximal cable.

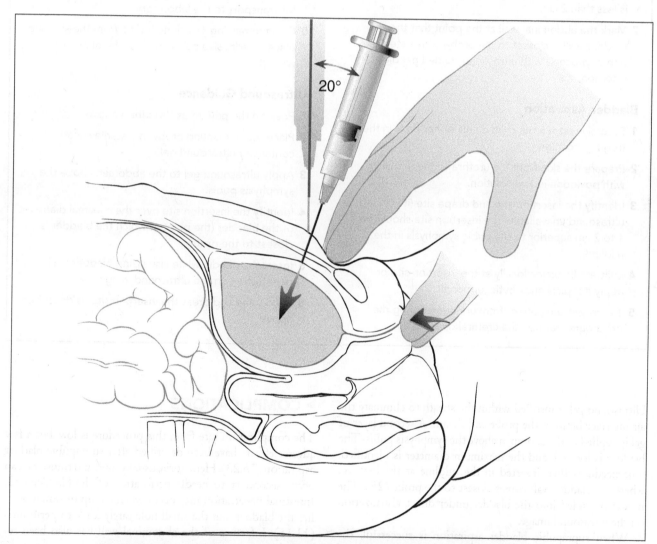

Figure 133.3 The skin is punctured and the needle advanced in a cephalad direction angled approximately 20 degrees from the vertical while mild negative pressure is applied to the syringe. Gentle pressure is applied to the urethral meatus.

SUMMARY

Ultrasound Bladder Measurement

1 Immobilize the child in a supine, frog-leg position.

2 Apply ultrasound transmission gel to the infant's suprapubic region.

3 Apply gentle pressure to the penile shaft in male patients or over the urethral meatus in female patients.

4 Scan in the transverse plane until the maximum size bladder image is obtained.

5 Remove the transmission gel and proceed with suprapubic aspiration if both maximum AP and transverse diameters are 2 cm or more.

6 Repeat the scan after 30 minutes if either diameter is less than 2 cm.

7 Mark the abdominal wall at the point that the bladder wall is closest to the probe with a sterile pen or proceed with ultrasound-guided needle insertion.

Bladder Aspiration

1 Securely restrain the child on his or her back in the frog-leg position.

2 Prepare the skin from the urethra to the umbilicus with povidone-iodine solution.

3 Identify the insertion site and drape site (if ultrasound unavailable, the insertion site should be 1 to 2 cm superior to the pubic symphysis in the midline).

4 Infiltrate lidocaine locally at the insertion site or apply a topical anesthetic (optional).

5 To prevent the patient from urinating during the procedure, occlude the urethral opening by applying pressure at the base of the penis in boys or to the urethral meatus in girls.

6 Insert the needle through the abdominal wall in a slightly cephalad direction approximately 20 degrees from vertical and apply negative pressure to the syringe as the needle is advanced.

7 If unsuccessful, withdraw the needle without removing it from the abdominal wall and reinsert it at the same site oriented perfectly upright (vertical).

8 If still unsuccessful, hydrate the child for at least 1 hour or until the bladder is full (ideally confirmed by ultrasound measurement) before reattempting the procedure.

9 When urine is obtained, place it in a sterile container for transport to the laboratory.

10 Clean remaining povidone-iodine from the site and place an adhesive bandage over the puncture wound.

Ultrasound Guidance

1 Position the patient as described above.

2 Place the ultrasound probe in a sterile sheath containing ultrasound gel.

3 Apply ultrasound gel to the abdomen above the symphysis pubis.

4 Identify the insertion site over the maximal diameter of the bladder (the point at which the bladder is closest to the probe).

5 Insert the needle while visualizing bladder wall penetration on the ultrasound image.

6 Send urine and dress the insertion site as described above.

Ultrasound gel is instilled within the sheath to eliminate the air interface between the probe and sheath. A second layer of gel is applied to the abdomen above the symphysis pubis. The bladder is located, and the maximum diameter is identified. The needle is then inserted in the midline at the location where the bladder wall comes closest to the probe (25). The needle is guided into the bladder under direct visualization on the ultrasound image.

When suprapubic bladder aspiration is successful, the urine is placed in a sterile container, which is transported promptly to the laboratory. Betadine around the insertion site is then cleaned from the skin, and a small adhesive bandage is placed over the puncture wound.

▶ COMPLICATIONS

The complication rate from this procedure is low, but a few adverse effects have been described after suprapubic bladder aspiration (15,23). Hematuria, usually mild and transient, can occur secondary to needle perforation of the bladder wall. Intestinal penetration may occur when a loop of bowel overlies the bladder, but the small hole rarely leads to peritonitis (11,15). Infection of the abdominal wall has also been reported.

These complications of suprapubic bladder aspiration are not common but are difficult to avoid. The best way to ensure the lowest complication rate is to carefully identify the

CLINICAL TIPS

▶ The incidence of successful bladder aspiration increases with ultrasound identification of larger bladder diameters.

▶ Gentle pressure to occlude the urethra should be maintained during ultrasound to inhibit spontaneous urination and resulting loss of specimen.

▶ Having an assistant hold the probe during ultrasound-guided aspiration allows the operator greater control over the procedure.

▶ A topical or infiltrative anesthetic may reduce patient pain and movement during the procedure.

▶ An empty bladder should be rescanned after 30 minutes to allow time for urine to accumulate.

landmarks for insertion and introduce the needle only 1 to 2 cm above the pubic symphysis on the abdominal wall. Infection is best prevented by strict adherence to aseptic technique (see Chapter 7). The insertion site should be carefully prepared with povidone-iodine before the procedure and then cleaned and dressed after the needle has been removed.

The application of pressure with the ultrasound probe against the lower abdomen in the setting of a full bladder may trigger urination and loss of the specimen (14,20). Applying minimal pressure with the probe while manually occluding the urethra can reduce this possibility. No additional risk of complication is associated with the use of ultrasound. On the contrary, visualizing the bladder as empty or full before suprapubic bladder aspiration should minimize the number of attempts and subsequent complications (12,13).

▶ SUMMARY

Although largely supplanted by urethral catheterization in recent years, suprapubic bladder aspiration remains a safe and effective procedure for obtaining sterile urine from an incontinent child. Complications from this procedure are rare. In addition, suprapubic bladder aspiration offers the advantage of being easily and quickly performed while avoiding contamination during insertion of a catheter, as often occurs when urethral catheterization is attempted with a struggling child. Suprapubic aspiration is a valuable but underutilized technique that is perhaps most useful for obtaining an uncontaminated urine specimen from the infant undergoing a sepsis evaluation.

Portable ultrasonography is an easily learned technique for identifying the urinary bladder. Unlike other applications of ultrasonography, identifying a full bladder requires little expertise. Because the empty bladder is a potential space that only becomes visible as it fills, it is, quite simply, either there or not there. Ultrasound-assisted suprapubic bladder aspiration is useful for confirming that the patient has a full bladder. Ultrasound can also be used for direct guidance of the needle when penetrating the bladder. The adjunctive use of ultrasound enhances the success rate of suprapubic bladder aspiration and limits the number of attempts.

▶ REFERENCES

1. American Academy of Pediatrics Committee on Quality Improvement Subcommittee on Urinary Tract Infection. Practice parameter. The diagnosis, treatment, and evaluation of the initial urinary tract infection in febrile infants and young children. *Pediatrics.* 1999;103:843–852.
2. Aronson AS, Gustafson B, Svenningsen NW. Combined suprapubic bladder aspiration and clean-voided urine examination in infants and children. *Acta Paediatr Scand.* 1973;62:396–400.
3. Bonadio WA. Urine culturing techniques in febrile infants. *Pediatr Emerg Care.* 1987;3:75–78.
4. Edelmann CM Jr, Ogwo JE, Fine BP, et al. The prevalence of bacteriuria in full-term and premature newborn infants. *J Pediatr.* 1973;82:126–132.
5. Nelson JD, Peters PC. Suprapubic aspiration of urine in premature and term infants. *Pediatrics.* 1965;36:132–134.
6. Pryles CV. Percutaneous bladder aspiration and other methods of urine collection for bacteriologic study. *Pediatrics.* 1965;36:128–131.
7. Pryles CV, Atkin MD, Morse TS, et al. Comparative bacteriologic study of urine obtained from children by percutaneous suprapubic bladder aspiration of the bladder and by catheter. *Pediatrics.* 1959;24:983–991.
8. Saccharow L, Pryles CV. Further experience with the use of percutaneous suprapubic bladder aspiration of the urinary bladder. *Pediatrics.* 1969;43:1018–1024.
9. Morrell RE, Duritz G, Oltorf C. Suprapubic aspiration associated with hematoma. *Pediatrics.* 1982;69:455–457.
10. Lanier B, Daeschner CW. Serious complication of suprapubic bladder aspiration of the urinary bladder. *J Pediatr.* 1971;79:711.
11. Polnay L, Fraser AM, Lewis JM. Complication of suprapubic bladder aspiration. *Arch Dis Child.* 1975;50:80–81.
12. O'Callaghan C, McDougall PN. Successful suprapubic bladder aspiration of urine. *Arch Dis Child.* 1987;62:1072–1073.
13. Gochman R, Karasic R, Heller M. Use of portable ultrasound to assist urine collection by suprapubic aspiration. *Ann Emerg Med.* 1991;20:631–635.
14. Chu RW, Wong YC, Luk SH, et al. Comparing suprapubic urine aspiration under real-time ultrasound guidance with conventional blind aspiration. *Acta Paediatr.* 2002;91:512–516.
15. Ozkan B, Kaya O, Akdag R, et al. Suprapubic bladder aspiration with or without ultrasound guidance. *Clin Pediatr.* 2000;39:625–626.
16. Goldberg BB, Meyer H. Ultrasonically guided suprapubic urinary bladder aspiration. *Pediatrics.* 1973;51:70–74.
17. Chen L, Hsiao AL, Moore CL, et al. Utility of bedside ultrasound before urethral catheterization in young children. *Pediatrics.* 2005;115:108–111.
18. Milling TJ, Amerongen RV, Melville L, et al. Use of ultrasonography to identify infants for whom urinary catheterization will be unsuccessful because of insufficient urine volume: validation of the urinary bladder index. *Ann Emerg Med.* 2005;45:510–513.

19. Kiernan SC, Pinckert TL, Keszler M. Ultrasound guidance of suprapubic bladder aspiration in neonates. *J Pediatr.* 1993;123:789–791.

20. Munir V, Barnett P, South M. Does the use of volumetric bladder ultrasound improve the success rate of suprapubic aspiration of urine? *Pediatr Emerg Care.* 2002;18:346–349.

21. Pollack CV, Pollack ES, Andrew ME. Suprapubic bladder aspiration versus urethral catheterization in ill infants: success, efficiency, and complication rates. *Ann Emerg Med.* 1994;23:225–230.

22. Kozer E Rosenbloom E, Goldman D, et al. Pain in infants who are younger than 2 months during suprapubic aspiration and transurethral bladder catheterization: a randomized, controlled study. *Pediatrics.* 2006;118(1):e51–56.

23. Ruddy R. Suprapubic bladder aspiration. In: Fleisher GR, Ludwig S, eds. *Textbook of Pediatric Emergency Medicine.* 5th ed. Baltimore: Williams & Wilkins; 2006:1920.

24. Abbott GD, Shannon FT. How to aspirate urine suprapubically in infants and children. *Clin Pediatr.* 1970;9:277–278.

25. Loiselle JM, McCans K. Urinary bladder ultrasound. In: Fleisher GR, Ludwig S, eds. *Textbook of Pediatric Emergency Medicine.* 5th ed. Baltimore: Williams & Wilkins; 2006:1952.

KATHLEEN A. LILLIS AND DIETRICH JEHLE

134

Emergent Cardiac Ultrasonography

▶ INTRODUCTION

Ultrasonography is a valuable recent addition to the diagnostic armamentarium of emergency physicians. Bedside sonography allows for more rapid diagnosis and treatment of patients with potentially life-threatening illnesses while using a noninvasive modality. Because of advances in the quality of the imaging and in the portability of ultrasonography, the use of echocardiography by emergency physicians is now standard practice in the management of various acute cardiovascular disease processes (1).

Limited emergency cardiac ultrasound performed at the bedside can provide valuable life-saving information in seconds. Studies have demonstrated that with little formal training emergency physicians are capable of using ultrasound to diagnose specific emergent conditions and that they display acceptable technical skill and interpretive acumen (2). The optimal amount of training required to accurately detect such conditions and the frequency of examinations necessary to maintain proficiency for emergency physicians have not yet been definitively determined. However, using recorded photographic images or hard copy and videotaped examinations provides a means of quality assurance (see Chapter 132). Emergent echocardiography is most useful in pediatric patients to confirm the diagnoses of cardiac tamponade, pulseless electrical activity, and cardiac trauma (3,4).

▶ ANATOMY AND PHYSIOLOGY

Cardiac tamponade results from the accumulation of fluid, pus, or blood within the pericardial sac. This restricts cardiac filling, limits stroke volume, and reduces blood pressure. If tamponade remains uncorrected, it can result in cardiovascular insufficiency, shock, and eventually death.

Infection is the most common cause of pericarditis and the accumulation of pericardial fluid in children. Bacterial etiologies are more likely to result in cardiac tamponade. Up to 15% of patients develop pericardial effusions 1 to 3 weeks following cardiac surgery in a condition known as postpericardiotomy syndrome (5). Trauma, both penetrating and blunt, is increasingly seen as a cause of tamponade in older children and adolescents. Other causes include collagen vascular and oncologic disease.

Pulseless electrical activity (PEA) or electromechanical dissociation (EMD) is said to exist in the patient who displays electrical cardiac activity on a monitor but has no detectable pulse. PEA in children has multiple causes, including severe hypovolemia (e.g., blood loss), cardiac tamponade, severe hypoxemia, tension pneumothorax, hypothermia, and ingestions. Detection of cardiac motility in the setting of PEA is crucial for determining the prognosis, underlying causes, and possible therapeutic interventions.

Impediments in adult echocardiography such as obesity, difficulty with positioning, and chronic obstructive pulmonary disease are less likely to pose limitations to ultrasound scanning in children. However, the smaller size of the child may present more of a problem in gaining access to the chest without interrupting ongoing management.

For purposes of ultrasound evaluation, the heart can be divided into three planes: the long-axis plane, the short-axis plane, and the four-chamber plane. The long-axis plane transects the heart parallel to the long axis of the left ventricle. The short-axis plane is obtained by transecting the heart perpendicular to the plane of the long axis. The four-chamber plane is a special coronal plane that transects the heart nearly parallel to the dorsal and ventral surfaces of the body (6).

The pericardium is a dense tissue that forms a sac completely surrounding the heart and a proximal part of the aorta and pulmonary artery. This tissue is highly echogenic and is visualized as the outer border of the heart on ultrasound. The pericardium is composed of two layers—the visceral pericardium and the parietal pericardium. Fluid between these layers is seen on ultrasound as an anechoic space between the two more reflective echoes. A small amount of fluid is normally present in this potential space and serves to lubricate the membranes. Generally, fluid is not visible anteriorly or in the nondependent areas of the supine patient. Any anterior displacement of the parietal pericardium represents an abnormal collection of fluid. Effusions tend to collect initially around the more dependent and mobile ventricles and later in the area of the less mobile atria. The minimal quantity of fluid detected with echocardiography varies with the size of the patient and the frequency of the probe; however, the amount of fluid required to produce hemodynamic changes is very easily visualized. Pericardial fat, pleural effusions, and subdiaphragmatic fluid may be confused with pericardial fluid. These anechoic stripes are not circumferential and do not demonstrate the normal variation in size between systole and diastole seen with pericardial fluid.

Hemopericardium is the most common feature of cardiac injury and is also seen as a circumferential echo-free space within the pericardium. An acute hemopericardium may present as a pericardial hematoma that has echogenic components. Any significant intrapericardial collection—either echo-free or echodense—in the setting of penetrating injury is presumed to represent penetrating cardiac injury.

Myocardial rupture is a rare complication of blunt chest trauma. Most patients die at the scene. In patients entering the emergency medical services (EMS) system alive, however, rapid diagnosis and treatment is essential for survival. Usually the pericardial sac contains the rupture, and these patients present with hemopericardium and some degree of cardiac tamponade.

▶ INDICATIONS

The role of pediatric cardiac ultrasound by the emergency physician is restricted to a few specific conditions in which it can provide immediate and unequivocal findings. It is in no way intended to supplant the role of a comprehensive echocardiographic examination. Currently, this procedure has three main applications: (i) detection of a pericardial effusion in the appropriate clinical setting, (ii) detection of a hemopericardium or cardiac rupture associated with chest trauma, and (iii) detection of the presence of any cardiac motion associated with PEA.

Suspicion of cardiac tamponade must be acted on within seconds. In an adolescent who has sustained a penetrating chest wound, an emergent echocardiographic examination can provide information regarding the extent of injury before a patient deteriorates. Emergent cardiac ultrasound gives the physician the ability to immediately look inside the chest to confirm or refute the diagnosis at the bedside.

Cardiac tamponade in a child may present with a number of physical findings. Hypotension, especially when associated with evidence of increased central venous pressures; the presence of a pulsus paradoxus; chest pain; poor peripheral perfusion; and distended neck veins may all be signs of tamponade. However, no clinical findings associated with tamponade are 100% sensitive or specific. The classic triad of distant heart sounds, hypotension, and elevated central venous pressure are rarely present in a child, making tamponade a difficult clinical diagnosis.

Standard available tests also are nonspecific in diagnosing cardiac tamponade. ECG changes or increased heart size on a chest radiograph may suggest pericardial fluid; however, normal results do not exclude its presence. The size of the cardiac silhouette on chest radiograph depends on the amount of fluid in the effusion and the distensibility of the pericardial sac. Effusions of acute onset generally do not result in a significant increase in the cardiac shadow. Echocardiography is therefore the procedure of choice in detecting the presence of a pericardial effusion (7). Limited ultrasound in the ED may provide important additional information, especially when there is limited time available before the need for intervention.

Ultrasound also may be useful in the setting of blunt or penetrating chest trauma in cases of suspected hemopericardium or cardiac rupture. Its role may be restricted to those patients with symptoms or extended to those with a significant mechanism of injury in an attempt to anticipate potential deterioration. The Focused Assessment with Sonography for Trauma (FAST) has been shown in one small study to be 100% sensitive and specific in determining cardiac injury in patients with pericardial effusions following penetrating chest trauma (see Chapter 138) (8).

Using ultrasound to diagnose cardiac trauma is not intended to replace other standard tests currently available. It should be used as a noninvasive, rapidly available modality to complement other clinical tools and to determine the presence of specific cardiac injury in a patient who has suffered chest trauma (9). Two-dimensional echocardiography performed in the ED for identifying penetrating cardiac injuries has decreased the time to diagnosis and has improved the survival rate and neurologic outcome of survivors (10).

In the setting of PEA, ultrasound may be used to determine whether cardiac function is truly absent or if the heart is pumping but unable to generate adequate stroke volume to register a blood pressure. In the former case the prognosis is essentially the same as for asystole, whereas in the latter instance a treatable cause may be determined and more aggressive interventions indicated (7).

Using cardiac ultrasonography for more advanced studies in the ED setting, such as diagnosis of a particular congenital heart disease in neonates, is not feasible. Although cardiac ultrasound by emergency physicians may demonstrate abnormal anatomy, determining a definitive diagnosis for the particular congenital lesion is unlikely. The level of education and expertise necessary to reliably make such a diagnosis is usually attained only by the pediatric cardiologist.

▶ EQUIPMENT

The scanner must have adequate image quality. It should be capable of displaying the image in at least 64 shades of gray. Fewer shades will significantly compromise identification and will impair the quality of a hard copy produced. The screen size must be at least 5 inches diagonally. Equipment with a small screen size is impractical for use in the ED and makes it difficult for more than one physician to view the screen at once. Any machine used in the ED must be portable and compact. Measurement capabilities with an on-screen caliper system are necessary to make quantitative distinctions between normal and abnormal anatomy. Ultrasound machines used in the ED must be able to produce hard copies for permanent records. A freestanding printer that prints the screen image on specially treated paper is the most practical. Videotaping capabilities allow subsequent viewers to visualize ventricular wall or valvular motion that is not appreciated on a paper image. Doppler ultrasound is an option that provides flow information simultaneously with the anatomic information displayed on the screen. Color Doppler maps different velocities and direction of flow with the use of color. This information is advantageous when scanning the heart, aorta, and other vascular structures. However, Doppler ultrasound is not required for identifying pericardial effusions or assessing myocardial contractility for pediatric patients in the ED. Transducers with frequencies of 3.5 and 5.0 MHz should be available. The 3.5-MHz transducer should have a narrow footplate to allow imaging between the ribs in young children. Ultrasound gel is used to provide an acoustic interface between the chest wall and the transducer.

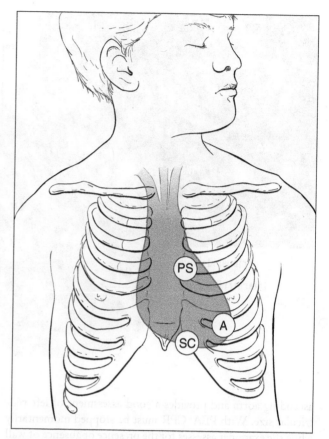

Figure 134.1 Transducer locations for standard windows. PS, parasternal; A, apical; SC, subcostal.

▶ PROCEDURE

To perform a limited examination of the heart using ultrasound, four standard views are normally visualized. Each view is a two-dimensional image of the heart, in either the long- or short-axis plane or the coronal plane, obtained through one of three windows (Fig 134.1). A window refers to a location on the body through which the transducer can image the heart. The four standard views for an ED study are the subcostal four-chamber view, the left parasternal short-axis view, the left parasternal long-axis view, and the apical four-chamber view.

The subcostal four-chamber view often provides the most important information for a single-view examination (11). To obtain this view, the patient should be in the supine position. Ultrasound gel is applied, and the transducer is placed at the left infracostal margin at the level of the xiphoid. The beam is aimed at the left shoulder and the marker dot pointed toward 9 o'clock. By rotating the transducer, the clinician can obtain the desired four-chamber view (Fig. 134.2). The structures closest to the transducer appear nearest the top of the display, and the marker points toward the left side of the screen. A small amount of hepatic parenchyma lies directly below the transducer. The right-sided chambers are posterior to the liver. The visceral and parietal pericardia are seen as single bright reflecting surfaces. Fluid between these two pericardial layers can be seen as a separation of the bright echoes. The subcostal four-chamber view can provide essential information in a short period and therefore should be used early in the ultrasound examination of the heart. The subcostal four-chamber view quickly screens for pericardial fluid while causing minimal interference with ongoing cardiopulmonary resuscitation (CPR). Cardiac wall motion can be assessed grossly in most cases. A limited, goal-directed examination may be performed within 1 minute (11,12).

The next two views are obtained by placing the transducer in the left parasternal window, which is immediately adjacent to the sternum between the second and fourth intercostal spaces (see Fig. 134.1). Both left parasternal views may occasionally require positioning the patient in the left lateral decubitus position. These views may be difficult to obtain in poorly compliant or critically ill patients. The left parasternal long-axis view is obtained by rotating the transducer so that the plane of the beam is parallel to a line drawn from the right shoulder to the left hip (Fig 134.3). The marker dot must therefore be pointed at approximately 4 o'clock. This view allows visualization of the aortic valve and proximal

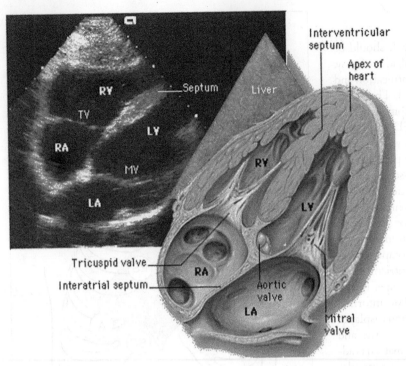

Figure 134.2 Subcostal view demonstrates the four chambers of the heart and both the mitral and tricuspid valves. LA, left atrium; LV, left ventricle; MV, mitral valve; RA, right atrium; RV, right ventricle; TV, tricuspid valve. (Copyright 2005, Yale Center for Advanced Instructional Media, Yale University.)

ascending aorta and provides a good assessment of left ventricular size. With PEA, CPR must be stopped momentarily while the examiner assesses for the presence or absence of wall and valve motion.

The left parasternal short-axis view is obtained by rotating the transducer so that the plane of the beam is perpendicular to the long axis of the heart (marker dot pointing at approx-

imately 8 o'clock). By angling the transducer from the left hip to the right shoulder, the clinician can visualize sections extending from the apex through the mitral valve to the aortic valve (Figs. 134.4 and 134.5).

The apical four-chamber view requires the patient to be in the supine or left lateral decubitus position. This view is obtained by placing the transducer directly over the point of

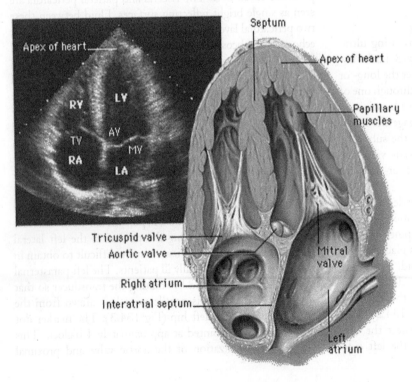

Figure 134.3 The left parasternal long-axis view provides an excellent image of the left ventricular wall and septum. AV, aortic valve; LA, left artium; LV, left ventricle; LVOT, left ventricular outflow tract; MV, mitral valve; RVOT, right ventricular outflow tract. (Copyright 2005, Yale Center for Advanced Instructional Media, Yale University.)

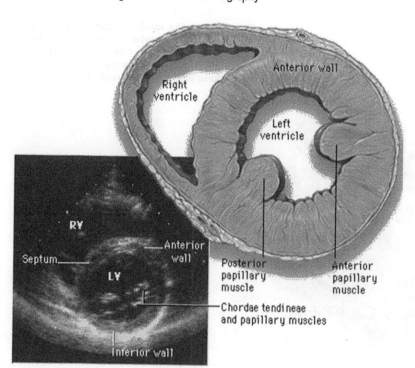

Figure 134.4 The left parasternal short-axis view is shown here at the level of the mitral valve. LV, left ventricle; RV, right ventricle. (Copyright 2005, Yale Center for Advanced Instructional Media, Yale University.)

maximum impulse and directing the beam toward the right shoulder. The marker dot should be pointing at approximately 8 o'clock. The transducer may need to be angled and/or rotated to obtain the desired view (Fig. 134.6).

Although these standard views can provide essential information, it may be necessary to visualize other, more useful planes by manipulating the transducer during the examination. The best view is the one that provides the desired information.

The subcostal four-chamber view is the best for visualizing a pericardial effusion, followed by the left parasternal long-axis view. Once evidence of a pericardial effusion is demonstrated by ultrasound, clinical correlation is generally necessary to make the diagnosis of cardiac tamponade. A hyperdynamic heart with diastolic collapse of the right atrium and ventricle indicates that intrapericardial pressures from the effusion have exceeded intracardiac pressures, confirming

Figure 134.5 The left parasternal short-axis view demonstrates the three leaflets of the aortic valve. RV, right ventricle (Copyright 2005, Yale Center for Advanced Instructional Media, Yale University.)

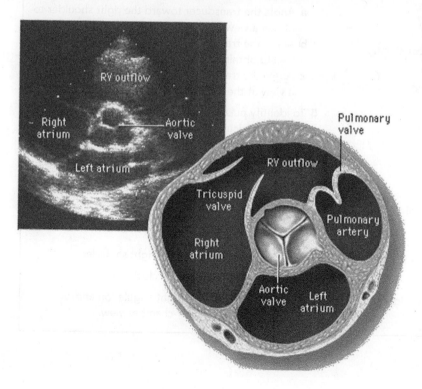

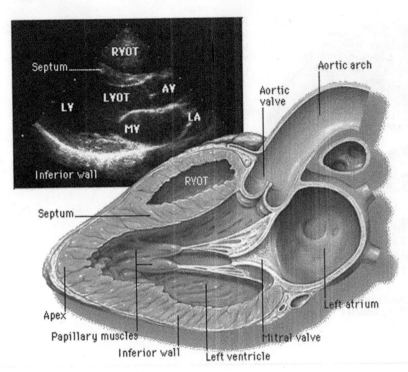

Figure 134.6 The apical four-chamber view. LA, left atrium; LV, left ventricle; MV, mitral valve; RA, right atrium; RV, right ventricle; TV, tricuspid valve. (Copyright 2005, Yale Center for Advanced Instructional Media, Yale University.)

 SUMMARY

Subcostal Window

1 Place the patient in the supine position.

2 Place ultrasound gel and the transducer at the left infracostal margin at the level of the xiphoid.

3 Aim the transducer at the left shoulder.

4 Point the marker dot at 9 o'clock.

5 Adjust the image by rotating the transducer slightly to obtain a four-chamber view.

6 Identify the echogenic visceral and parietal pericardial layers.

7 Scan for echo-free space, representing fluid separating pericardial layers.

Parasternal Window

1 Place the patient in the supine or left lateral decubitus position.

2 Place ultrasound gel and the transducer at the left parasternal area between the second and fourth intercostal spaces.

3 Aim the transducer down at the heart and slightly angled toward the right shoulder.

4 *Left parasternal long-axis view:* orient the transducer so that the marker dot is pointed to 4 o'clock; *left parasternal short-axis view:* orient the transducer so that the marker dot is pointed at 8 o'clock:

  a Angle the transducer toward the right shoulder to obtain a view at the aortic level.

  b Angle the transducer perpendicular to the chest wall to obtain a view at the mitral valve level.

  c Angle the transducer toward the left hip to obtain a view at the papillary muscle level.

5 To identify pulseless electrical activity, stop CPR and assess ventricular wall motion.

Apical Window

1 Place the patient in the supine or left lateral decubitus position.

2 Place ultrasound gel and the transducer at the point of maximal impulse.

3 Direct the transducer at the right shoulder.

4 Point the marker dot at 8 o'clock.

5 Adjust the image with slight angulation and/or rotation to obtain a four-chamber view.

the presence of cardiac tamponade. Respiratory variations of chamber diameters provide visual evidence of the mechanisms responsible for the paradoxical pulse. However, these observations require extensive ultrasound experience and are not easily demonstrated on ED studies.

The left parasternal long-axis view allows the physician visual access to the left ventricle and is the preferred view for determining PEA. The apical four-chamber view and the subcostal four-chamber view are good alternative views.

▶ COMPLICATIONS

No complications are associated with performing cardiac ultrasounds in children. However, limitations obviously exist. The accuracy of the procedure and subsequent decisions based on the results depend on the physician performing the examination. Pericardial fat, pleural effusions, and subdiaphragmatic fluid may be confused with pericardial fluid. Such a misinterpretation may lead to unnecessary pericardiocentesis. These anechoic stripes differ from effusions in that they are not circumferential. Previous experience has actually shown a decreased incidence of unnecessary pericardiocentesis and its associated risks (1). For limited studies such as these, the accuracy of trained emergency physicians has been excellent,

without significant misinterpretations (2). Additionally, to make the diagnosis of PEA, cardiac ultrasound will need to be performed on a child who is being resuscitated. However, it is unlikely that the brief cessation of CPR necessary to evaluate cardiac motion will have a significant detrimental effect on the patient.

▶ SUMMARY

Echocardiography provides invaluable information to emergency physicians. Limited bedside cardiac ultrasound performed on children and adolescents is a noninvasive, immediately available method of examining the heart. Ultrasonography is most useful in the ED setting for diagnosing cardiac tamponade and pulseless electrical activity. The technique can be learned quickly and provides a high degree of accuracy for these indications. Early diagnosis and treatment of these conditions in the pediatric patient may be life-saving.

▶ REFERENCES

1. Ciccone TJ, Grossman SA. Cardiac ultrasound. *Emerg Med Clin North Am.* 2004;22:621–640.
2. Mayron R, Gaudio FE, Plummer D, et al. Echocardiography performed by emergency physicians: impact on diagnosis and therapy. *Ann Emerg Med.* 1988;17:150–154.
3. Jehle D, Davis E, Evans T, et al. Emergency department sonography by emergency physicians. *Am J Emerg Med.* 1989;7:605–611.
4. Lanoix R, Leak LV, Gaeta T, et al. A preliminary evaluation of emergency ultrasound in the setting of an emergency medicine training program. *Am J Emerg Med.* 2000;18:41–45.
5. Gewitz MH, Woolf PK. Cardiac emergencies. In: Ludwig S, Fleisher GR, eds. *Textbook of Pediatric Emergency Medicine.* 5th ed. Philadelphia: Lippincott Williams & Wilkins; 2006:717–758.
6. Hagan AD, DeMaria AN, eds. *Clinical Applications of 2D Echocardiography and Cardiac Doppler.* Boston: Little, Brown; 1989:19–63.
7. Mazurek B, Jehle D, Martin M. Emergency department echocardiography in the diagnosis and therapy of cardiac tamponade. *J Emerg Med.* 1991;9:27–31.
8. Tayal VS, Beatty MA, Marx JA, et al. Fast (Focused Assessment with Sonography in Trauma) accurate for cardiac and intraperitoneal injury in penetrating anterior chest trauma. *J Ultrasound Med.* 2004;23:467–472.
9. Beggs CW, Helling TS, Hays LV. Early evaluation of cardiac injury by two-dimensional echocardiography in patients suffering blunt chest trauma. *Ann Emerg Med.* 1987;16:542–545.
10. Plummer D, Brunette D, Asinger R. Emergency department echocardiography improves outcome in penetrating cardiac injury. *Ann Emerg Med.* 1992;21:709–712.
11. Heller M, Jehle D. *Ultrasound in Emergency Medicine.* Philadelphia: WB Saunders; 1995:126–134, 184–194.
12. Rubin M. Cardiac ultrasonography. *Emerg Med Clin North Am.* 1997;15:745–762.

CLINICAL TIPS

▶ Echocardiography is the procedure of choice for detecting the presence of a pericardial effusion. Displacement of the parietal pericardium or presence of an anechoic fluid space suggests the presence of a pericardial effusion.

▶ The subcostal four-chamber view is best for detecting a pericardial effusion.

▶ The left parasternal long-axis view is best for detecting cardiac motion in the presence of pulseless electrical activity.

▶ The subcostal four-chamber view is the most convenient and least interruptive when CPR is in progress.

▶ The left lateral decubitus position brings the heart closer to the chest wall and out from under the sternum and may improve visibility.

▶ The transducer should have a narrow footplate to allow imaging between the ribs in young children.

135

VERENA T. VALLEY AND JAMES R. MATEER

Ultrasound Evaluation of Potential Ectopic Pregnancy

▸ INTRODUCTION

More than one million ectopic pregnancies were estimated to have occurred among women in the United States from 1970 to 1989, with teenagers having the highest mortality rate (1). This hospital-based estimate may be falsely low due to the impact of medical advancement in diagnosis and treatment and a concurrent shift from inpatient treatment to multiple outpatient visits (2). Black adolescents and other minorities had the highest mortality rate for ectopic pregnancy—almost five times that for white teenagers (3). Furthermore, adolescent females and young women have the highest rate of *Chlamydia trachomatis* infection, which is a risk factor for subsequent ectopic pregnancy (4).

By definition, an ectopic pregnancy occurs when a fertilized ovum implants at a site other than the endometrial lining of the uterus. A heterotopic pregnancy is the combination of an ectopic pregnancy and an intrauterine pregnancy (IUP). This is believed to occur in only 1 in 30,000 pregnancies (5) but may have a higher incidence in patients taking fertility drugs or patients with extensive tubal disease. Studies have shown that over 40% of ectopic pregnancies may be initially missed (6,7). Improved methods of early diagnosis for ectopic pregnancy are needed to reduce the morbidity and mortality associated with this condition.

Ultrasound is a rapid and effective diagnostic tool for evaluating ectopic pregnancy. The main value of ultrasound is to determine the presence and viability of an IUP. By proving the presence of an IUP, diagnosis of an ectopic pregnancy is essentially excluded. The lack of an IUP on ultrasound, however, suggests the possibility of an ectopic pregnancy, especially if associated with an adnexal mass or significant free pelvic fluid.

Ultrasonography using a portable unit can usually be performed without difficulty in standard emergency department (ED) pelvic examination rooms. The number of examinations required for clinical competence has not been extensively studied. Reports in the primary care literature, however, suggest that a physician can be trained to perform a limited obstetrical ultrasound examination with a program that includes 40 to 75 training scans (8,9).

▸ ANATOMY AND PHYSIOLOGY

Normal Pelvic Anatomy

Ultrasonographic characteristics of the postpubertal adolescent female are not significantly different from those of an adult female (10). For transabdominal scanning, the full bladder is used to displace bowel gas and serves as an acoustic window to the pelvis. The normal shape of the distended bladder is rectangular on transverse views and is teardrop-shaped on longitudinal views.

In the immediate premenarcheal period, the ovaries and the uterus enlarge rapidly and attain a mean volume by menarche that approaches adult size (11). The maximum uterine size for nulliparous adults is 7 cm in length and approximately 4 × 5 cm in anteroposterior and transverse dimensions. For multiparous patients, these dimensions are increased by 1 to 2 cm in all planes. With an empty bladder, the normal anteverted uterus lies at about 90 degrees to the plane of the vagina, whereas a fully distended bladder can position the uterus almost parallel to the vagina. The cervix is usually midline; however, the fundus is commonly tilted slightly to the right or left of midline. The endometrium is visualized within the uterus as a central bright echo, called the "endometrial stripe." The

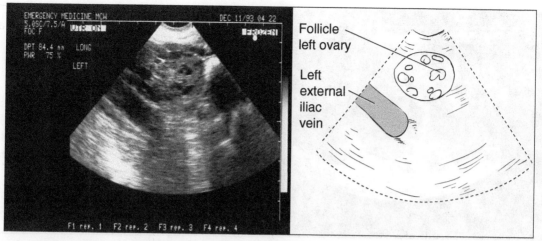

Figure 135.1 Longitudinal view of the left ovary demonstrating the characteristic follicular pattern. The ovary normally lies medial to the external iliac vein.

sonographic size and appearance of the endometrial stripe vary during the menstrual cycle, with a normal width of 2 to 4 mm in the proliferative phase and 5 to 6 mm in the secretory phase. In addition, the endometrial stripe becomes more echogenic during the secretory phase. When searching for an early IUP, the entire endometrial stripe must be visualized. Uterine anomalies, including bicornuate and septate uteruses, are occasionally seen. These often are first noted in early pregnancy when the gestational sac forms in one horn of the uterus.

The normal size of the ovary is 2 × 2 × 3 cm in young adults. Identification is facilitated when the characteristic multiple follicles (0.5 to 1.0 cm in diameter) are visualized around the periphery of the ovarian cortex (Fig. 135.1). When follicle size exceeds 2.5 cm, a physiologic cyst or other abnormality should be considered. The position of the ovaries is variable, but they are most commonly located near the posterior lateral pelvic wall, just anterior to the internal iliac vessels and medial to the external iliac vessels.

The vagina is a hypoechoic tubular structure caudad to the cervix and immediately posterior to the bladder on a transabdominal scan. This structure is recognized by a central echogenic stripe, which is formed by the opposing mucosal interface. The posterior fornix is closely related to the posterior cul-de-sac. The cul-de-sac is located posterior to the uterus and upper vagina. A small amount of fluid in the cul-de-sac is normal during midcycle.

Ultrasound Findings of Intrauterine Pregnancy

Recognizing an IUP is critical. The embryologic features of a normal IUP include (in chronological order of ultrasound appearance) the gestational sac, the yolk sac, the double decidual sac sign, the fetal pole, and fetal cardiac activity (Fig. 135.2 and Table 135.1).

In obstetrics, gestational age is traditionally defined based on the menstrual age—the time from the beginning of the last normal menses. Ultrasound imaging also follows this convention for references to gestational age. Gestational age can be determined by ultrasound as early as 5 weeks based on measurements of the internal diameter of the gestational sac. For more advanced early pregnancy (6 to 12 weeks' gestation), a crown-rump length can be determined by measuring the maximal length of the embryo excluding extremities and the yolk sac. The crown-rump length of the embryo during the first trimester is the most accurate measurement of gestational age that can be obtained by ultrasound during a pregnancy.

Gestational Sac

The gestational sac is the first developmental marker that can be imaged and has been reported to be 5 mm by the fifth gestational week (12). It can be seen at 4.5 to 5 weeks' gestation with endovaginal ultrasound and at 5.5 to 6 weeks' gestation using the transabdominal approach. The ultrasonic appearance is that of a round, anechoic (echo-free or dark) sac measuring greater than 5 mm internal diameter, surrounded by a thick concentric echogenic ring, and located within the endometrial echo.

Yolk Sac

The yolk sac has a characteristic appearance consisting of a bright, ring-like structure with an anechoic center. It is

TABLE 135.1	ULTRASONOGRAPHIC GESTATIONAL MARKERS FOR INTRAUTERINE PREGNANCY	
Structure	**Transabdominal**	**Endovaginal**
Gestational sac	5.5–6 wk	4.5–5 wk
Yolk sac (secondary)	6–6.5 wk	5–5.5 wk
Embryo (fetal pole)	7 wk	5.5–6 wk
Cardiac activity	7 wk	6 wk
Fetal parts	8+ wk	8 wk

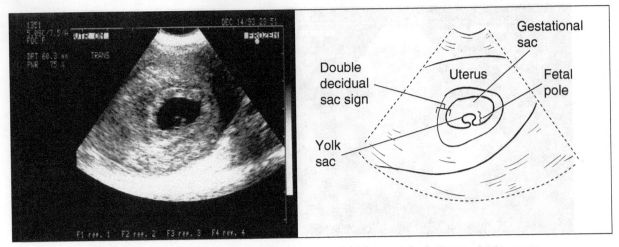

Figure 135.2 Transverse view of the uterus demonstrating features of an early intrauterine pregnancy.

attached to the fetal umbilicus by a narrow stalk. It is the first structure that can be accurately identified within the gestational sac. It also is the earliest reliable sign of an IUP. Endovaginal ultrasound is the preferred method for evaluating an early or atypical intrauterine sac. The presence of a yolk sac is associated with a 62% incidence of a normal pregnancy (liveborn infant) (13). It can be seen at 5 to 5.5 weeks' gestation on endovaginal ultrasound and at 6 to 6.5 weeks' gestation on transabdominal ultrasound. It usually is not seen after 12 weeks gestational age.

The presence of a yolk sac virtually eliminates the possibility that an intrauterine gestational sac represents a pseudogestational sac of ectopic pregnancy (14). A pseudogestational sac, or pseudosac of ectopic pregnancy, is a saclike structure inside the uterus of a patient with an ectopic pregnancy. It is related to endometrial hormonal stimulation with edema fluid or blood accumulation. It can be differentiated from an early IUP by its lack of embryonic contents, absence of a double decidual sac, and lack of a definite thick, brightly echogenic decidual reaction.

Double Decidual Sac Sign

The double decidual sac sign consists of two concentric echogenic rings surrounding the gestational sac. The inner ring represents the decidua capsularis, chorionic villi, and chorion surrounding an anechoic area. The outer ring represents the decidua vera or endometrium of the uterus. The ring between these layers is anechoic and is the remnant of the uterine cavity. The presence of a double decidual sac has been described as a sign of IUP; however, it is a less reliable sign for the diagnosis of a normally developing pregnancy (15). The presence of a double decidual sac sign is therefore suggestive of an IUP but is not by itself diagnostic.

Fetal Pole

The fetal or embryonic pole is recognized sonographically as a thickened area adjacent to the yolk sac and often can be seen

when the embryo is 2 mm. It can be seen at 5.5 to 6 weeks' gestation on endovaginal ultrasound and 7 weeks' gestation on transabdominal ultrasound.

Fetal Cardiac Activity

A fetal heart beat always should be present in a normally developing embryo at about 6.5 weeks' gestation and can generally be seen in a 2- or 3-mm fetus. Identification of cardiac activity is of particular importance, as 97% of embryos with cardiac activity have a normal outcome (liveborn infant) (15–18). Cardiac activity is reliably seen at 6 to 6.5 weeks' gestation on endovaginal ultrasound and at 7 weeks' gestation on transabdominal ultrasound but often can be identified as soon as an embryonic pole is visible.

Ultrasound Findings of Ectopic Pregnancy

Findings on an ultrasound examination that suggest an ectopic pregnancy include a definitive ectopic pregnancy or a positive HCG level and no definitive IUP.

Definitive Ectopic Pregnancy

A definitive ectopic pregnancy is defined as the presence of a sac larger than 5 mm (maximum internal diameter) with a thick, concentric echogenic ring visualized outside the endometrial echo and containing a definite yolk sac or an obvious fetal pole (with or without fetal pulsations).

No Definitive Intrauterine Pregnancy

Diagnosis of an ectopic pregnancy must be strongly considered in the face of a serum human chorionic gonadotropin (HCG) level above the discriminatory zone and no IUP noted on the ultrasound examination. Serum HCG levels correlate with the size and gestational age of the embryo. The discriminatory zone of HCG (i.e., the level above which a normal IUP is reliably visualized) was first described in 1981 (15). For transabdominal sonography, this level has been most recently set at an HCG concentration of 3,600 mIU/mL using the first international reference preparation (IRP) (equals 1,800 mIU/mL via the second international standard [IS]), which correlates to a gestational age of approximately 6 weeks. With the advent of endovaginal sonography, the discriminatory zone of HCG is currently as low as 1,025 mIU/mL IRP (approximately 500 mIU/mL second IS), consistent with 5 weeks' gestation. The absolute minimum value of HCG identifying the discriminatory zone depends on the equipment used and the sonographer's technique. This value should ideally be established separately for each institution. The lack of an IUP when the HCG is above the discriminatory zone, therefore, represents either an ectopic pregnancy or a recent abortion. This category accounts for the majority of ectopic cases diagnosed in an ED setting (19).

For patients with no IUP and an HCG below the discriminatory zone, an early IUP is likely, but an early ectopic or a recent abortion with falling HCG levels cannot be excluded. For patients who lack an IUP, have no significant incidental findings, and have an HCG level below the discriminatory zone, the current standard of care is outpatient follow-up in 2 to 3 days for a repeat HCG level and ultrasound. Many patients in this category have an early IUP. This is confirmed by a 66% or greater increase in HCG level within 48 hours and identification of an IUP once the HCG is above the discriminatory zone.

Incidental Findings Suspicious for Ectopic Pregnancy

Certain ultrasound findings, although not the primary focus of a limited study in the ED, raise the index of suspicion for the presence of an ectopic pregnancy. Significant incidental findings on ultrasound include fluid in the cul-de-sac, adnexal masses, tubal rings, a myomatous uterus, and an intrauterine device (IUD). Such findings require consultation with an obstetrician-gynecologist.

Fluid in the Cul-de-Sac
Moderate to large amounts of fluid that extend into the adnexa or the paracolic gutters suggest hemorrhage from a ruptured ectopic pregnancy or cyst.

Adnexal Masses
Masses greater than 2.5 to 3.0 cm in diameter that are not simple cysts and are tender to palpation with the probe are suggestive of an ectopic pregnancy. Fetal heartbeats within masses have been observed in as many as 23% of cases (1). Additionally, these masses may contain amorphous material that is thought to represent blood, blood clots, and gestational material. This amorphic appearance was noted in 40% of tubal pregnancies (20).

Tubal Rings
Tubal rings are echogenic rings found outside the uterus that may indicate an early ectopic pregnancy. A tubal ring usually

can be differentiated from a common corpus luteum cyst by its thick, round, brightly echogenic ring. A corpus luteum cyst is surrounded by less echogenic ovarian tissue, which may contain characteristic follicles.

Myomatous Uterus
Fibroids can interfere with ultrasound examination due to acoustic shadowing. Findings in the ED may therefore be impossible to interpret.

Intrauterine Device
An IUD will cast a characteristic shadow on sonography and may interfere with imaging of the uterus.

▶ INDICATIONS

Considerable overlap exists between the clinical presentation for a spontaneous or threatened abortion and that for an ectopic pregnancy. This is one reason why so many patients with ectopic pregnancy are initially misdiagnosed. It is therefore essential that the clinician first consider the possibility of ectopic pregnancy before a patient's condition is labeled as a spontaneous or threatened abortion. Bedside ultrasound can greatly facilitate differentiating these conditions in conjunction with other diagnostic tests and, as appropriate, close outpatient follow-up.

Indications for pelvic sonography include patients presenting with a positive urine pregnancy test and lower abdominal pain, an adnexal mass or tenderness, vaginal bleeding, orthostasis, and any other risk factor for ectopic pregnancy. A "rule-out ectopic" protocol integrating the use of bedside ultrasonography in the ED has been shown to significantly reduce the incidence of discharged patients with subsequent ectopic pregnancy rupture (Fig. 135.3) (21).

For the ED evaluation, the endovaginal approach is preferred over the transabdominal approach due to its higher image resolution in early pregnancy. In addition, the patient usually has an empty bladder, having recently submitted a urine sample for a pregnancy test. Advantages and disadvantages of each technique are listed in Table 135.2.

Endovaginal ultrasonography should not be performed if the diagnosis of vaginal bleeding due to a vaginal tear is suspected based on the history or physical examination. An obstetrician-gynecologist should be consulted in this scenario.

TABLE 135.2	ADVANTAGES AND DISADVANTAGES OF TRANSABDOMINAL AND ENDOVAGINAL ULTRASOUND
Transabdominal	**Endovaginal**
Better overview	Better resolution
Less invasive	More comfortable than pelvic examination
Easier image orientation	Image orientation may be confusing
Requires full bladder	Best done with empty bladder

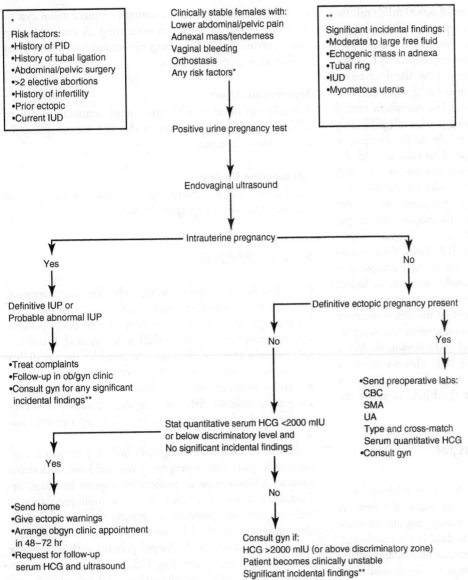

Figure 135.3 Summary of rule-out ectopic protocol.

Risk factors:
• History of PID
• History of tubal ligation
• Abdominal/pelvic surgery
• >2 elective abortions
• History of infertility
• Prior ectopic
• Current IUD

Clinically stable females with:
Lower abdominal/pelvic pain
Adnexal mass/tenderness
Vaginal bleeding
Orthostasis
Any risk factors*

Significant incidental findings:
• Moderate to large free fluid
• Echogenic mass in adnexa
• Tubal ring
• IUD
• Myomatous uterus

Positive urine pregnancy test

Endovaginal ultrasound

Intrauterine pregnancy

Yes → Definitive IUP or Probable abnormal IUP
• Treat complaints
• Follow-up in ob/gyn clinic
• Consult gyn for any significant incidental findings**

No → Definitive ectopic pregnancy present

No → Stat quantitative serum HCG <2000 mIU or below discriminatory level and No significant incidental findings

Yes →
• Send home
• Give ectopic warnings
• Arrange obgyn clinic appointment in 48–72 hr
• Request for follow-up serum HCG and ultrasound

No → Consult gyn if:
HCG >2000 mIU (or above discriminatory zone)
Patient becomes clinically unstable
Significant incidental findings**

Yes →
• Send preoperative labs:
CBC
SMA
UA
Type and cross-match
Serum quantitative HCG
• Consult gyn

▶ EQUIPMENT

Ultrasound machine—a two-dimensional, real-time, black-and-white machine with hard copy (printer capabilities) is suggested.

Probes—a 3.5- to 5.0-MHz mechanical sector, annular array, or curved array probe is necessary for transabdominal ultrasound. A 5.0- to 7.5-MHz mechanical sector, annular array, or curved array endovaginal probe is necessary for endovaginal ultrasound.

Ultrasound gel

Disposable probe covers—required to avoid transmitting infection. Condoms are frequently used, although latex gloves also can be used to cover the endovaginal probe.

Probe disinfectant—a number are available (22). Probe manufacturers provide information about safe and ef-

fective cleaning and disinfecting, as a particular disinfectant may be safe for some probes and destructive for others. Bleach wipes are acceptable for many probes.

Sterile gloves—necessary for the endovaginal examination.

Videotape recording capabilities—a highly recommended option for quality assurance and case review purposes.

▶ PROCEDURE

The clinician should position the ultrasound machine next to the pelvic examination table in such a way that the machine keyboard can be easily and comfortably accessed throughout the examination. Often the patient will want to see the screen; the machine can be easily adjusted so as to accommodate the patient's view. The clinician should avoid placing the patient in the Trendelenburg position, as any fluid present can help outline pelvic organs and tubes. Using a slightly reversed Trendelenburg position is recommended.

The ultrasound equipment should be ready to use before the actual scanning. For example, the patient's name (or medical record number) should be entered into the ultrasound machine, and the videotape recorder should be on and ready to record. In addition, it is often helpful to label the initial screen as the longitudinal (or long) view, as this is the first view in the scanning sequence. Placing the videotape recorder on both "Record" and "Pause" will allow the clinician to simply take the machine off of "Pause" to record the different anatomic views.

Transabdominal Imaging

A full bladder is necessary to displace bowel gas out of the pelvis and provide a homogenous sonographic window. It is possible for the bladder to be overfilled and thus displace the uterus and ovaries beyond the focal zone of the probe. When this occurs, the patient should be asked to partially empty the bladder. If it is necessary to rapidly fill the bladder, this can be accomplished via retrograde introduction of sterile saline through a Foley catheter. Introduction of air bubbles should be avoided, as this could interfere with imaging.

Imaging with transabdominal ultrasound is performed in the longitudinal (sagittal), transverse, and oblique planes. The image orientation in obstetrics and gynecology traditionally refers to the position of the probe with respect to the organ or structure of interest. Thus, a true longitudinal view of the ovary or of a tilted uterus may be oblique to the long axis of the patient.

The ultrasound gel is applied to the patient's lower abdomen. A 3.5- to 5.0-MHz probe is placed in the midline immediately above the pubic symphysis. The orientation marker, or marker dot, on the probe should be directed at the patient's head (Fig. 135.4A). This position should provide a longitudinal view of the uterus directly below the anechoic bladder. The endometrial stripe is visualized using a side-to-side sweeping motion performed by angling the "tail" of the probe. With an anteverted uterus, the cervix and cul-de-sac can be detected by angling the probe in a caudal direction. From the midline longitudinal view, a slow sweeping motion laterally can be used to obtain longitudinal views of the ovaries (Fig. 135.4B).

Beginning again from the midline longitudinal view, rotating the probe 90 degrees counterclockwise will produce a transverse view of the uterus. The entire anteverted uterus from the fundus to the cervix can be viewed by angling the probe first cephalad and then caudad. A transverse view of the adnexa can be obtained by beginning with the transverse view of the uterus at the level of the fundus. The probe is angled laterally to aim at the adnexa. A slow sweep cephalad and then caudad will provide a view of the adnexa from top to bottom. The uterus and adnexa are carefully scanned for the presence of a gestational sac. The scan should be videotaped for further review.

Endovaginal Imaging

The patient should be given a short explanation of the procedure. It is helpful to mention that the probe is smaller than most specula and is only inserted a short distance. Therefore, the endovaginal ultrasound examination may be more

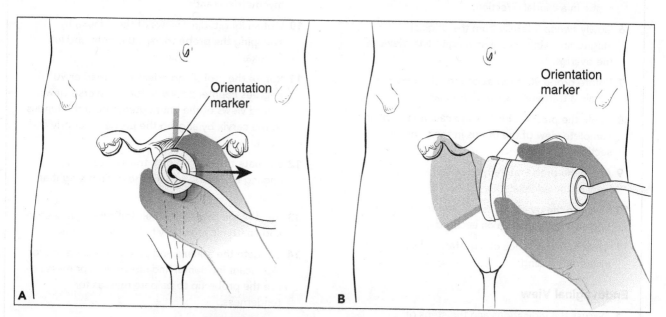

Figure 135.4
A. Initial positioning of the transabdominal probe.
B. Transabdominal sweep of the right adnexa.

comfortable than the speculum examination. The option of having the patient place the tip of the probe into the vagina may make the patient less anxious. Complete emptying of the urinary bladder is indicated to increase patient comfort with the procedure and to bring the uterus closer to the vaginal transducer.

The probe must be disinfected before each use with a commercially available preparation (Fig. 135.5A). Ultrasound gel is applied to the tip of the probe. All air bubbles are removed

as the probe is covered with a latex condom, probe cover, or a digit of a surgical latex glove (Fig. 135.5B). A small amount of gel applied to the outside of the probe cover facilitates insertion into the vagina. The examination is performed most easily with the patient on a pelvic examination table in a slightly reversed Trendelenburg position.

Standard imaging planes in an endovaginal scan are longitudinal and transverse to the uterus. The transverse plane is generally semicoronal to the body axis. Oblique planes are

---

◉ SUMMARY

1 Arrange the ultrasound machine next to the patient and examination table.

2 Enter patient identification, label the image for the initial view, and prepare the videotape recorder.

3 Place the patient supine and in a slightly reversed Trendelenburg position.

Transabdominal View

1 Begin the examination when the patient's bladder is full.

2 Apply ultrasound gel to the patient's lower abdomen.

3 Place the ultrasound probe above the pubic symphysis with the orientation marker pointed toward the patient's head.

4 Define the entire endometrial stripe using a side-to-side sweeping motion.

5 Visualize the cervix and cul-de-sac by angling the probe in a caudal direction.

6 Slowly sweep laterally from the original longitudinal view to obtain longitudinal views of the ovaries.

7 Rotate probe 90 degrees counterclockwise to obtain a transverse view of uterus.

8 Angle the probe cephalad and caudad to obtain a complete view of the uterus in the transverse section.

9 Angle the probe laterally to obtain a transverse view of the adnexa.

10 Visualize the ovaries by sweeping from top to bottom of the adnexa on each side.

11 Record the presence of a gestational sac or any incidental findings.

Endovaginal View

1 Discuss the indications and the steps of examination with the patient.

2 Instruct the patient to empty the bladder.

3 Prepare the probe with an approved disinfectant.

4 Place ultrasound gel into the condom or suitable probe cover.

5 Displace any bubbles from between the probe tip and condom and lubricate the outer probe tip with a small amount of gel.

6 Place the index finger on the probe orientation marker and align the marker upward.

7 Slowly insert the probe into the vaginal vault approximately 3 to 4 inches.

8 Identify and align the endometrial stripe and record the view using a printer or videotape recorder.

9 Assess the entire endometrium for the presence of a gestational sac and contents (yolk sac, fetal pole, or fetal heart activity); evaluate the position of the gestational sac within uterus, with attention to the myometrial mantle.

10 Obtain longitudinal views of the adnexa by sweeping the probe toward the right and left adnexa.

11 Rotate the probe and orientation marker 90 degrees counterclockwise for transverse views; record views of the entire uterus from the fundus to the cervix by angling the probe anteriorly and posteriorly.

12 Evaluate the adnexa on a transverse view by angling the probe toward the patient's right and left.

13 Identify the ovaries by their follicular appearance and anatomic proximity to the iliac vessels.

14 Evaluate the adnexa and posterior cul-de-sac for significant incidental findings of fluid or masses; use the probe tip to palpate masses for tenderness.

15 Remove the probe slowly from the vagina.

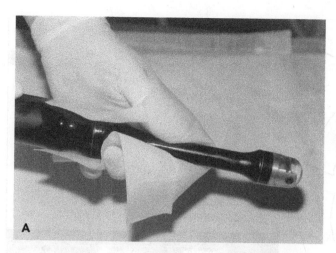

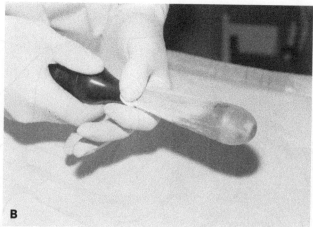

Figure 135.5
A. Disinfecting the endovaginal probe.
B. Application of the probe cover.

used as needed to visualize the adnexa. Pelvic structures can be guided toward the probe with the abdominal hand, and the probe tip can be used to localize areas of tenderness detected by the bimanual pelvic examination.

 CLINICAL TIPS

▶ The diagnosis of ectopic pregnancy should be entertained despite a normal physical examination.

▶ The adnexa should be adequately visualized even if an intrauterine pregnancy is present.

▶ All views should be obtained before commenting to the patient regarding any findings.

▶ The follicular appearance and anatomic landmarks (ileac vein) aid in identification of the ovaries.

▶ Loops of bowel may mimic a mass; however, observation of the mass for a short period usually reveals peristalsis if it is bowel.

▶ The tip of the probe can be used to palpate suspicious and/or tender masses.

▶ It is often difficult to describe findings to consultants if the images are not labeled.

▶ Videotaping the examination is the optimal way to document scans for quality assurance review and for educational purposes.

▶ Allowing the patient to insert the endovaginal probe may decrease the level of anxiety associated with the examination.

▶ The abdominal hand can be used to guide structures toward the endovaginal probe.

The probe is held with the index finger on the probe orientation marker. The probe is slowly inserted approximately 3 to 4 inches into the vaginal vault with the orientation marker pointing up (Fig. 135.6A). This orients the probe in the longitudinal position. The endometrial stripe is located on the ultrasound monitor and aligned by moving the probe either in the lateral or anteroposterior planes to visualize its full extent. In a normally positioned or anteverted uterus, the fundus should appear on the left side of the ultrasound monitor screen (Fig. 135.6B). Often the uterus does not lie perfectly in the longitudinal plane, and the probe must be rotated or angled until the endometrial stripe is seen. The endometrial stripe is then followed to the cervix. The entire endometrium is assessed for the presence of a gestational sac and contents (yolk sac, fetal pole, or fetal heart activity). The position of a gestational sac within the uterus is carefully noted, with attention given to the amount of myometrium surrounding it (myometrial mantle).

Longitudinal sweeps of the adnexa are done from the midline position to either side (Fig. 135.7), which is accomplished by slowly angling the whole probe toward the lateral side wall of the pelvis while maintaining the orientation marker in the upright position. The longitudinal views of the adnexa are labeled "left" or "right" and videotaped for documentation and review.

The orientation marker and probe are then rotated 90 degrees counterclockwise for the transverse views (Fig. 135.8). The endometrium again can be visualized from the fundus to the cervix. The probe is angled so that it is pointing toward the patient's anterior to view the fundus of the uterus, assuming an anteverted uterus. The probe is then gently angled posteriorly to visualize the body of the uterus and cervix. This maneuver ensures that the entire uterus is visualized. These views should be labeled "transverse" and videotaped for subsequent review.

The adnexa and posterior cul-de-sac are evaluated for the presence of significant incidental findings of fluid or masses.

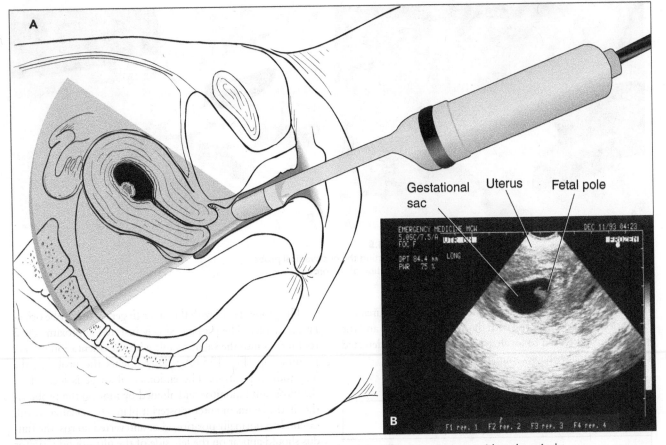

Figure 135.6 Longitudinal view of the uterus and early intrauterine pregnancy with endovaginal ultrasound.
A. Endovaginal probe orientation and scanning field.
B. Ultrasound image.

The adnexa are evaluated in the transverse plane by angling the probe toward the patient's right and left. As mentioned previously, the ovaries often are found adjacent to the external iliac vein (Fig. 135.1). After locating the iliac vein, the probe can be rotated or slightly angled anteriorly to image the ovary. The ovary has a very characteristic follicular appearance that aids in its sonographic identification. Any masses should be assessed for tenderness with the probe tip.

The fallopian tubes may or may not be visualized. Normal tubes are difficult to image because of their small size. They are usually located lateral to the uterus behind the ovaries or in the cul-de-sac. The pathologic tube is more easily identified due to the accumulation of fluid, pus, or blood in the lumen or in the adjacent area.

The cul-de-sac should also be evaluated for the presence of fluid or blood clots. Using a high-resolution probe may make a small amount of fluid in the cul-de-sac appear falsely large to the novice sonographer due to magnification. A small amount of free fluid is normally present, especially in midcycle (23). Should the clinician find a large amount of fluid in the cul-de-sac, a transabdominal view of the pelvis may provide a more accurate estimation of fluid accumulation. Other intraperitoneal gutters where fluid may accumulate are also best investigated using the transabdominal approach.

Magnification of the ultrasound images can help to identify structures and is a function found on the ultrasound keyboard. Zooming out (less image magnification) is often helpful when initially imaging the endometrial stripe and cervix or when determining the presence of fluid in the cul-de-sac. Zooming in (greater image magnification) provides better detail of intrauterine contents, especially fetal structures such as the fetal pole and yolk sac. The largest possible magnification that still enables orientation and recognition of the organs or pathology should be used.

Pitfalls

Many pitfalls are associated with ultrasound diagnosis of early pregnancy. For example, it is incorrect to assume that an HCG below the discriminatory zone excludes significant ultrasound findings. Many ectopics have been diagnosed with low HCG levels. The absolute level and rate of rise of HCG with an ectopic is variable and depends on the available vascular supply.

Fortunately, a combined IUP and ectopic pregnancy (heterotopic pregnancy) is quite rare (1/30,000). Of note, however, it is less rare in patients taking fertility drugs (up to 1/5,000) and patients with tubal abnormalities. For this reason, the ultrasound examination should not be considered

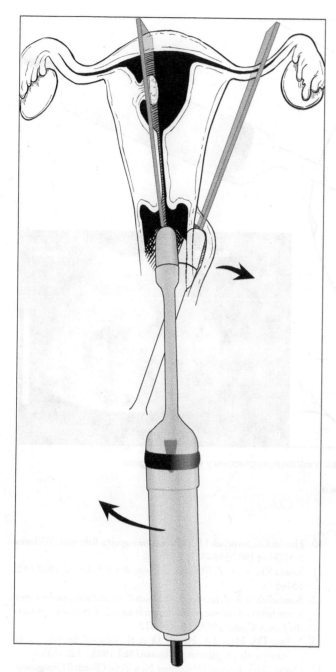

Figure 135.7 Longitudinal sweep of the left adnexa with an endovaginal probe.

centrally located in the uterus. Diagnosis is confirmed by the lack of a complete, symmetric myometrial mantle around the entire gestational sac. In other words, with a normal intrauterine gestation, a uniform rim of solid tissue should represent the myometrial mantle around the gestational sac. Interstitial pregnancies may appear intrauterine or extrauterine on the ultrasound study.

Advanced ectopics (8 or more weeks) have been misdiagnosed as an IUP when the gestational sac and contents appear normal. To avoid this pitfall, it is important to routinely determine if the gestational sac lies within the endometrial echo and has a complete myometrial mantle surrounding it.

Cervical ectopic pregnancy is rare and may be confused with the more common finding of an abortion in progress (with a low-lying gestational sac) or a large nabothian or cervical gland cyst. Endovaginal ultrasound and follow-up examinations are often needed to further evaluate this potential diagnosis.

Videotaping the ultrasound examination with careful image and orientation labeling may decrease the need for repeat ultrasound examinations. If the ultrasound is abnormal, the videotape can be reviewed with consultants, and the decision whether to perform a repeat ultrasound may be based on their recommendations.

▶ COMPLICATIONS

Currently no known risks to the patient or fetus are associated with the ultrasound energy used during the transabdominal or endovaginal ultrasound. Nevertheless, the power output of the machine should be maintained at the lowest possible level that produces a good image during ultrasound examination of the pregnant uterus.

▶ SUMMARY

With the high rate of adolescent pregnancies, the possibility of ectopic pregnancy is an ongoing concern. The presence of an ectopic pregnancy is a difficult diagnosis to make based on the physical examination alone. Using bedside ultrasonography can enhance the emergency physician's diagnostic accuracy (19). The recognition of an intrauterine pregnancy with careful examination of the adnexa can exclude the diagnosis of an ectopic pregnancy. The lack of an intrauterine pregnancy with an HCG above the discriminatory zone should be considered to indicate an ectopic pregnancy until proved otherwise. The possibility of an ectopic pregnancy must be entertained before diagnosing a spontaneous or threatened abortion, as much overlap exists between these clinical presentations. An understanding of the utility and limitations of ultrasonography in conjunction with careful patient follow-up may ultimately decrease the morbidity and mortality associated with ectopic pregnancy.

finished as soon as an IUP is identified. The clinician must routinely examine the adnexa and cul-de-sac for significant masses or fluid to exclude this possibility.

Interstitial pregnancies are a subset of ectopic pregnancies with implantation in the intrauterine portion of the fallopian tube or that portion of the tube that passes through the wall of the uterus. This subset is associated with a higher incidence of mortality because of the tendency to progress further before rupture and the increased likelihood of exsanguination at this highly vascular and muscular site (24). This type of ectopic pregnancy is suspected when the gestational sac is not

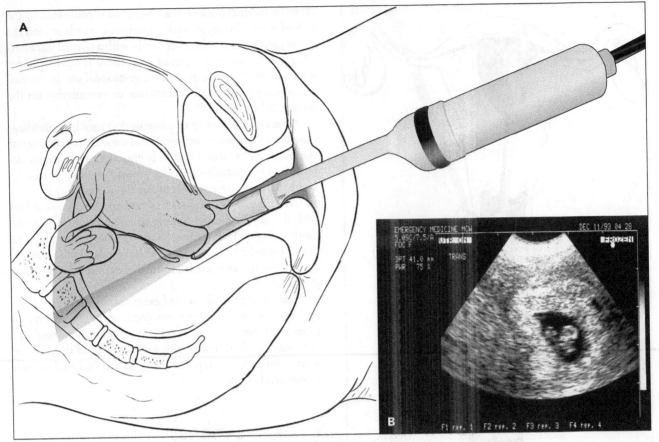

Figure 135.8 Transverse view of the uterus and early intrauterine pregnancy with endovaginal ultrasound.
A. Endovaginal probe orientation and scanning field.
B. Ultrasound image.

▶ REFERENCES

1. Goldner TE, Lawson HW. Surveillance for ectopic pregnancy–United States, 1970–1989. *MMWR CDC Surveill Summ.* 1993;42(6):73–85.
2. Zane SB, Kieke BA, Kendrick JS, et al. Surveillance in a time of changing health care practices: estimating ectopic pregnancy incidence in the United States. *Matern Child Health J.* 2002;6:227–236.
3. Centers for Disease Control. Ectopic pregnancy surveillance—United States, 1970–1987. *MMWR CDC Surveill Summ.* 1939(4):9–17.
4. Centers for Disease Control. Chlamydia screening among sexually active young female enrollees of health plans—United States, 1999–2001.
5. DeVoe RW, Pratt JH. Simultaneous intrauterine and extrauterine pregnancy. *Am J Obstet Gynecol.* 1948;56:1119–1123.
6. Stovall TG, Kellerman AL, Ling FW, et al. Emergency department diagnosis of ectopic pregnancy. *Ann Emerg Med.* 1990;19:1098–1103.
7. Abbott J, Emmans LS, Lowenstein SR. Ectopic pregnancy: ten common pitfalls in diagnosis. *Am J Emerg Med.* 1990;8:515–522.
8. Hahn R, Roi LD, Ornstein SM, et al. Obstetric ultrasound training for family physicians: results from a multisite study. *J Fam Pract.* 1988;26:553–558.
9. Smith CB, Sakornbut EL, Dickinson LC, et al. Quantification of training in obstetrical ultrasound: a study of family practice residents. *J Clin Ultrasound.* 1991;19:479–483.
10. Hayden CK, Swischuk LE. *Pediatric Ultrasonography.* Baltimore: Williams & Wilkins; 1987:359–371.
11. Krantz KE, Atkinson JP. Gross anatomy. *Ann N Y Acad Sci.* 1967;142:551–575.
12. Bernaschek G, Rudelstorfer R, Csaicsich P. Vaginal sonography versus serum human chorionic gonadotropin in early detection of pregnancy. *Am J Obstet Gynecol.* 1988;158:608–612.
13. Nyberg DA, Mack LA, Harvey D, et al. Value of the yolk sac in evaluating early pregnancies. *J Ultrasound Med.* 1988;7:129–135.
14. Dodson MG. *Transvaginal Ultrasound.* New York: Churchill Livingstone; 1991:173–175.
15. Kadar N, DeVore G, Romero R. Discriminatory hCG zone: its use in the sonographic evaluation for ectopic pregnancy. *Obstet Gynecol.* 1981;58:156–161.
16. Stabile I, Campbell S, Brudzinskas JG. Ultrasonic assessment of complications during the first trimester of pregnancy. *Lancet.* 1987;2:1237–1240.
17. Mantoni M. Ultrasound signs in threatened abortion and their prognostic significance. *Obstet Gynecol.* 1985;65:471–475.
18. Cashner KA, Christopher CR, Dysert GA. Spontaneous fetal loss after demonstration of a live fetus in the first trimester. *Obstet Gynecol.* 1987;70:827–830.
19. Mateer JR, Aiman EJ, Brown M, et al. Ultrasonographic examination by emergency physicians of patients at risk of ectopic pregnancy. *Acad Emerg Med.* 1995;2:867–873.

20. Rottem S, Thaler I, Levron J, et al. Criteria for transvaginal sonographic diagnosis of ectopic pregnancy. *J Clin Ultrasound.* 1990;18:274–279.

21. Mateer JR, Valley VT, Aiman EJ, et al. Outcome analysis of a protocol including bedside endovaginal sonography in patients at risk for ectopic pregnancy. *Ann Emerg Med.* 1996;27:283–289.

22. Odwin CS, Fleischer AC, Kepple DM, et al. Probe covers and dis-

infectants for transvaginal transducers. *J Diagn Med Sonography.* 1990;6:130–135.

23. Davis FA, Gaines BB. Fluid in the female pelvis: cystic patterns. *J Ultrasound Med.* 1986;5:75–80.

24. Telmus L, Pedowitz P. Intersitial pregnancy: a survey of 45 cases. *Am J Obstet Gynecol.* 1953;66:1271.

136

BARBARA M. G. PEÑA

Ultrasonographic Foreign Body Localization and Removal

▶ INTRODUCTION

Children commonly present to the emergency department (ED) with a subcutaneous foreign body (splinter, glass, etc.). Although rarely life-threatening, subcutaneous foreign bodies can be a source of frustration to patients, parents, and physicians, as well as being associated with potentially significant complications (1–4). Undetected foreign bodies often lead to repeat visits to the ED, additional expense, surgery, and, in extreme cases, substantial morbidity (5). In addition, missed foreign bodies comprise the second most frequent basis for malpractice claims filed against emergency physicians (6).

The detection and removal of subcutaneous foreign bodies is becoming easier and more efficient due to the increasing availability of portable, handheld ultrasonography in the ED. As more EDs become equipped with these devices, there is a need for emergency physicians to become well versed in their use. Ultrasonography has historically been used effectively for detecting ocular foreign bodies; evaluating extremities by delineating muscle groups, tendons, and vascular structures; and localizing foreign bodies preoperatively (7–14). It also has been used to localize and remove both radiopaque and nonradiopaque materials from extremities (1,10,14–19). More recently, studies have proved the utility of ultrasonography in evaluating foreign bodies in the mouth, head, and neck (20,21). Techniques for removing subcutaneous foreign bodies without the aid of ultrasound localization are discussed fully in Chapter 111.

Ultrasound offers the emergency physician an accurate, safe, and painless means of (a) determining if a foreign body is present, particularly if nonradiopaque; (b) performing precise preoperative three-dimensional localization; and (c) maintaining visualization during foreign body removal (7,9,13,16,22,23). It is particularly useful for confirming the presence of a foreign body in the pediatric population, as these patients are often unable or unwilling to provide a thorough history. In addition, once the foreign body is removed, ultrasonography can be used to determine whether it has been removed in its entirety (21), as wood, thorns, and some cactus spines tend to fragment both with the initial skin puncture and during removal (4,24).

Although it is not difficult to search for foreign bodies with ultrasonography, it does require patience, training, and the proper equipment. Definitive identification and removal of a foreign body with ultrasound requires practice. However, it has been demonstrated that physicians with no formal training in ultrasonography can be highly effective in detecting foreign bodies in clinical simulations (22).

▶ ANATOMY AND PHYSIOLOGY

The response of the body to a foreign object depends, in part, on the type of material present in the wound. If the body is unable to expel the foreign material, macrophages will attempt to digest it. If these mechanisms fail, fibroblasts will form a collagen capsule around it, resulting in a granuloma with associated hypervascularity and neovascularity (18). It is thought that subsequent capsular disruption secondary to trauma can result in delayed or recurrent inflammation (3,25).

Over time, retained subcutaneous foreign bodies can have variable effects on the surrounding tissues. Foreign body type and location affect potential complications. Glass, metal, and plastics are relatively inert and may produce minimal sequelae in the body. Conversely, organic materials, such as wood, tend to cause a pronounced inflammatory response. In addition, foreign bodies can migrate and result in neuropraxia, delayed rupture of nerves and tendons, and vascular injury (26–29).

They can also enter the circulation. Other complications are discussed in Chapter 111.

▶ BASIC PRINCIPLES OF ULTRASOUND

Whereas the visibility of objects on roentgenograms and CT scans depends on their density, ultrasonography detects differences in acoustic impedance between different tissues. The density of a medium multiplied by the velocity of sound through that medium determines its acoustic impedance. The greater the difference in acoustic impedance between two media, the more sound waves are reflected back toward the transducer to help produce an image. For example, the difference in acoustic impedance at the air-tissue interface at the surface of the skin is so great that virtually 100% of the sound is reflected and no image is produced. Thus, gel is used as a coupler to allow sound to enter into the tissues (3,30–32).

The ultrasound transducer not only produces sound waves but also serves as a receiver of the reflected waves. Objects in the path of the beam either reflect, absorb, or transmit sound. The stronger the reflected sound (echoes) returning from an object, the brighter the image produced. When the beam of ultrasound is perpendicular to the foreign material, more sound is reflected back to the transducer, and the dots comprising the image are brighter. Hence, a better image or a better artifact is usually seen when the beam is perpendicular to the object. Furthermore, when the reflection of sound is strong secondary to large differences in acoustic impedance, some returning sound is repeatedly reflected between the transducer and the object, much like the repeating echo heard when a person shouts in a canyon. This recurring reflection of sound between the transducer and the object is a reverberation that produces a "comet tail" artifact. Its appearance can be so striking that its presence can serve as a clear indication that a foreign body is present. This artifact, however, also can occur when air is present in the tissues, as the air-tissue interface represents a significant difference in acoustic impedance (3,9,15,30,31,33).

Small changes in beam orientation can have a great impact on the appearance of shadows, artifacts, or the imaging of the foreign object itself. For instance, tendons may appear echogenic if the beam is perpendicular or hypoechoic if the beam is oblique to the tendon. The size, shape, orientation of the object in relationship to the surface of the skin, and whether the object is in the focal zone of the transducer also will affect its ultrasonographic visibility (5,16,32,34,35). Although vessels are visible with gray-scale imaging, the addition of Doppler makes their identification much easier (9,11,16,36).

It cannot be overemphasized that the clinician needs to be familiar with the ultrasound equipment, the normal anatomy of the extremities, and the appearance of a variety of foreign bodies in longitudinal and transverse sections. The skin interface appears bright, with the soft tissues represented as more hypoechoic. Practice on normal hands and feet will increase comfort with the appearance of tendons, vessels, muscles, and

bones. Scanning should be performed both at rest and with active range of motion (9,11,13). Differences can be noted in the appearance of a tendon or object when the ultrasound beam is oblique versus perpendicular to the normal anatomy. Beef or chicken models may be used to observe the characteristic echo patterns produced by different materials. As mentioned previously, these patterns can alert the ultrasonographer that a foreign body is present and also may provide clues as to the composition of the object. For instance, metal and glass are often associated with reverberation artifacts, whereas wood, pebbles, and sand can cause distal shadows (Fig. 136.1) (5,15,16,22,34,35). Organic materials often cause an intense inflammatory response, which can highlight the echogenic object by creating a contrasting darker background around the object. These hypoechoic halos around objects also can represent fibrinous exudates, collagenous capsule formation, abscesses, and granulation tissue (1,2,4,16,18). Further discussion of clinically important concepts in ultrasonography can be found in Chapter 132.

▶ INDICATIONS

Foreign bodies are sometimes overlooked in the initial evaluation of soft tissue wounds in the ED (17). Physical examination usually identifies foreign bodies that are superficial and can be seen or palpated. Radiographs commonly identify those that are radiopaque. Radiopaque materials are commonly missed on initial examination because radiographs were never ordered (37). The history of an injury (e.g., an injury involving a thin or breakable object) or a physical examination consistent with retained foreign material, as well as the patient's subjective opinion that a foreign body is present, are the best means for determining if a diligent search, including imaging studies, is necessary. Clinical findings associated with retained objects include localized tenderness, sharp pain with palpation, pain associated with a mass, discoloration beneath the surface of the skin, a chronic draining sinus, a nonhealing wound, an abscess with sterile purulent cultures, and persistent sterile monoarticular arthritis (2–4,23,28,38).

A number of factors determine the need for foreign body removal. Foreign bodies that cause pain, affect function, or pose a risk of potential damage to underlying structures should be removed. In addition, those causing (or likely to cause) toxic, inflammatory, or hypersensitivity reactions should be removed. A more complete discussion of indications for removing foreign bodies is provided in Chapter 111.

Most large studies have reported wood to be the most common foreign material found in the extremities, followed by either glass or metal (5,16,34,37,39). Glass visualization on plain films depends on size and proximity to bone. Most glass fragments, regardless of lead content and pigmentation, and virtually all metal objects can be visualized with plain radiographs (37,40,41). Wood, however, is only visualized 5.5% to 15% of the time (2,37,36). Undetected wooden foreign bodies can cause significant morbidity,

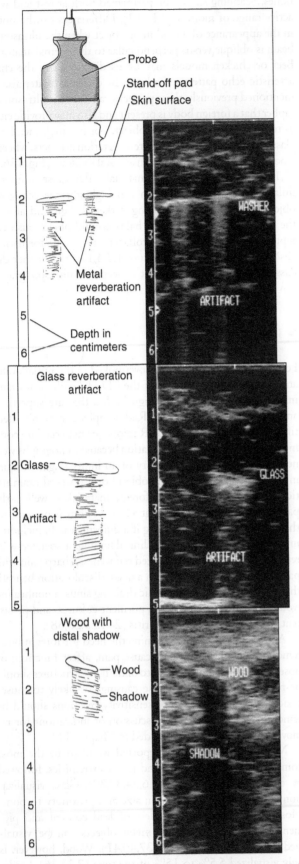

Figure 136.1 Ultrasound images of various embedded materials: metal washer (*top*), glass (*middle*), and wood (*bottom*).

including pain, abscess, and infection. Sometimes secondary changes caused by foreign bodies, such as a filling defect, bony changes, or the introduction of air into the soft tissues, can be appreciated even when the object itself cannot be seen with plain films (28,37,42). Ultrasonography, however, has been shown to detect numerous nonradiopaque materials, including vegetable matter, sea urchin spines, thorns (rose, cactus, palm, blackthorns), sutures, fish bones, gauze, and plastic (1,14,15,36,43–45). In addition, studies on the use of portable handheld ultrasonography have shown its effectiveness for the detection of nonopaque and semiopaque foreign bodies with a diameter greater than 4 mm (46).

The effectiveness of plain films in the localization of radiopaque foreign bodies is limited primarily by overlying bone and the size and density of the foreign bodies. In addition, although radiographs outline the shape of foreign bodies, they are not particularly useful for three-dimensional localization or visualization of nearby neurovascular structures and tendons (3,4,9,13). By underpenetrating the film or using a soft-tissue technique, the resulting contrast between a foreign body and its surroundings can be enhanced, allowing better visualization. Plain radiographs do poorly at demonstrating organic matter, especially if enough time has elapsed to permit saturation of the object by blood and tissue fluid (4,13,23,28,37,42). Use of bedside ultrasound and the patient's perception of a foreign body—that is, a "foreign body sensation" reported by the patient—may be as effective as plain radiography for initial screening (47).

Xeroradiography and fluoroscopy, although enhancing the likelihood of detection, are most effective for imaging radiopaque objects and expose the patient to higher doses of radiation. CT can often detect foreign bodies not seen with other modalities; however, because of its cost and radiation dose, it is not recommended as a routine screening tool for foreign bodies. As with plain films and xeroradiography, small foreign bodies and saturated wood can be missed. MRI cannot be used for metallic objects or if a metal implant is nearby. Gravel also produces significant artifacts secondary to ferromagnetic particles, and thus MRI is not recommended for wounds containing gravel. Both CT and MRI are expensive, require specialized personnel for their operation, and are generally impractical for foreign body detection in the ED. Furthermore, children may require sedation for these modalities. CT and MRI are therefore recommended only in appropriate circumstances and when other modalities fail (3,4,22, 36,48).

Ultrasonography offers several advantages over other imaging techniques. It often can visualize radiopaque and organic foreign bodies with the use of portable or handheld equipment in the ED. It does not expose the patient to radiation and offers information for three-dimensional localization of the object and on the object's relationship to surrounding structures. Ultimately, this decreases operating time and incision size and allows the emergency physician to choose an optimal site for the incision.

▶ EQUIPMENT

Ultrasound machine (handheld or conventional)

Ultrasound transducer or probe—image resolution in both the axial and lateral planes depends on the probe used. The higher the frequency of the probe (7.5 to 10 MHz), the better the axial and lateral resolution and the clearer the image produced. As frequency increases, however, the imaging depth decreases. This is not usually a problem, since the foreign bodies that emergency physicians are generally interested in removing are relatively superficial. Smaller transducer heads are better for areas that are difficult to image, such as web spaces. Probe heads vary in size from a fingertip version to ones measuring approximately 6 × 1.5 cm (see Fig. 132.2). The clinician must balance the advantages of a smaller probe, which can be used in tight spaces, against those of a larger probe, which can provide a more adequate field of view.

Standoff pad or gel pad—not all probes are capable of imaging the first few millimeters beneath the surface of the skin, in which case a standoff pad or bag of saline is useful. The standoff or gel pad (Fig. 136.2) permits sound transmission and can be cut with a scalpel to the size and thickness necessary to allow the near zone on the monitor to include these first few millimeters beneath the skin's surface. They also are useful when scanning irregular surfaces or near bony prominences (49).

Ultrasound transmission gel

Standard equipment for removing a subcutaneous foreign body (see Chapter 111)

Optional equipment:

Printer or videotape connection (useful for documenting findings)

Doppler capabilities (useful when working in highly vascular areas)

▶ PROCEDURE

Identification

Ultrasound scanning for a foreign body generally does not require initial administration of anesthesia. A small amount of ultrasound transmission gel is applied to the skin surface above the location most likely to contain the foreign material. When scanning over broken skin or near secretions, the clinician can place a small amount of gel into the fingertip of a sterile glove or condom and place the transducer inside to avoid contamination. The glove is smoothed against the transducer head to eliminate any air bubbles.

Slow and methodical scanning is recommended, especially when the object is believed to be small. The search should be performed in a number of planes, as it is easy to miss a small, thin object such as a needle or toothpick when viewed only in transverse section (Fig. 136.3). Studies have shown the use of power Doppler imaging to aid in the detection of foreign bodies by increasing the visibility of the hypoechoic halo and the foreign body itself (18). The hypervascularity immediately surrounding foreign bodies has been shown on power Doppler imaging to correlate with granulation tissue and neovascularity.

A reasonable time limit should be set for detecting the object. Plain films should be obtained if a possibility exists that the object might be radiopaque. Plain radiographs generally provide a larger field of view than can be easily scanned with ultrasound; they can therefore be used as a guide to focus the search. Plain films and ultrasound are obviously not mutually exclusive and should be used together to detect objects that might be missed when using either modality alone (16–24). Foreign materials may appear as distinct objects or as one of numerous artifacts or shadows, as previously stated.

Localization

The image should correspond to the image expected in both longitudinal and transverse views. As shown in Figure 136.3, a typical sewing needle would appear to be approximately 3 to 5 cm in length, with a comet tail artifact, when viewed in longitudinal section. In transverse section, it would appear as a pinpoint but have the same distal artifact. Such artifacts may not be well visualized if the orientation of the beam is oblique to the object. Foreign bodies also may be more elusive when not perpendicular to the surface of the skin (4,16).

Once the foreign object is located in at least two planes, the skin can be marked in a variety of ways. Using a marker, pen, or sterile tape, the skin is marked over the ends of an object,

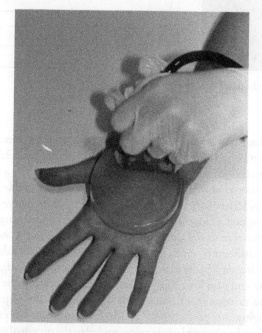

Figure 136.2 Use of a standoff or gel pad to scan for a shallow foreign body.

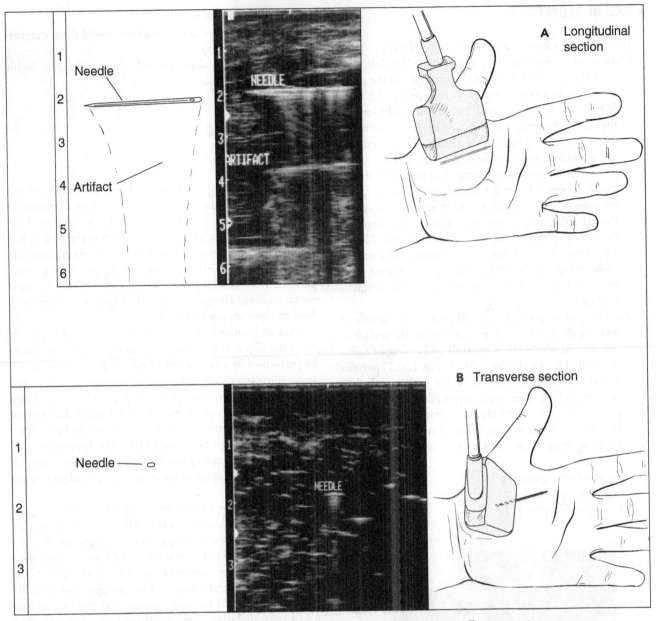

Figure 136.3 Probe orientation and appearance of an embedded needle in different scanning planes.

noting the depth listed on the ultrasound screen to the object at each point and the presence of any intervening structures. Alternatively, the skin over a foreign body is anesthetized and a localization needle is guided ultrasonographically to the object. When the needle contacts the foreign material, resistance or a grating sensation is frequently noted (7,16,23,50). The skin surface can be marked using radiographic markers called Beekley spots, which are small metallic beads on an adhesive disc that can be easily repositioned (Fig. 136.4) (16).

Removal

Once the precise depth and orientation of the object are known, this information can be used to plan the site for incision. For example, it may be advantageous to remove a foreign body from the lateral aspect of the heel, if feasible, as opposed to the weight-bearing plantar surface. Again, a time limit should be set for the procedure itself. An acceptable time limit is 15 to 30 minutes, considering that it is often necessary to maintain a bloodless field (16,23,24). Prolonged attempts at removal in the ED are impractical and usually unsuccessful.

Anesthesia is applied to the area requiring manipulation (see Chapter 35). By making a perpendicular incision adjacent to the end of a long, thin object, the transducer can be held in the nondominant hand, with the image of the object in a longitudinal projection (Fig. 136.5). Forceps or hemostats can then be observed while being guided to the proximal end of the foreign body through the incision. Traction applied along

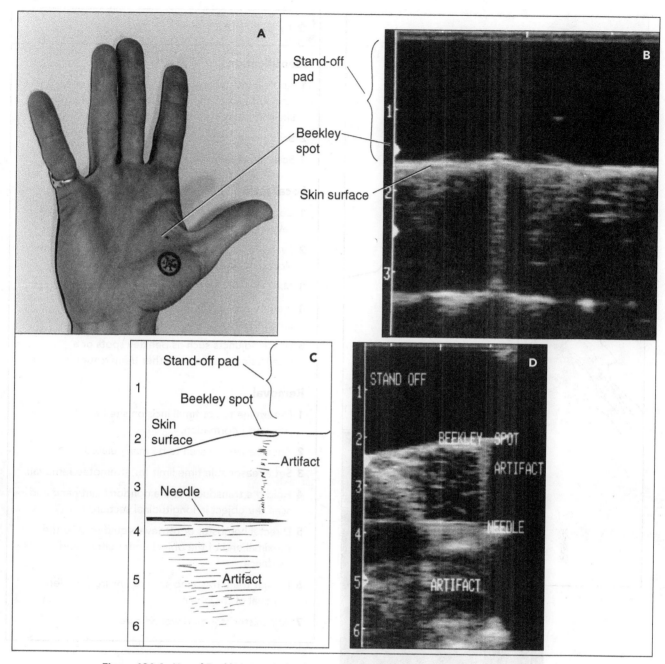

Figure 136.4 Use of Beekley spots in localizing subcutaneous foreign bodies.

the longitudinal axis of the object will decrease the incidence of fragmentation. It is best to visualize both the foreign body and the hemostat in the longitudinal plane (4,16). Structures such as tendons can be evaluated by putting the extremity through a range of motion while visualizing the structure on the monitor.

The decision to remove a foreign body and the approach chosen must be based on the specifics of each situation. If material is being removed that is likely to break upon its removal, the ultrasound and/or the plain films should be repeated to ensure that all of it has been removed. After removal, standard wound care is administered (see Chapter 107). If no remaining material is detected, patients should be advised to return

to the ED if pain persists or infection develops, because a foreign body may still be present in the wound (3,4,23,51).

▶ COMPLICATIONS

The most frequently encountered problems with this procedure are generally the same for the removal of any foreign body (Chapter 111). The addition of ultrasound to this common procedure poses no known additional biologic hazards at the intensities used for diagnostic purposes (30).

A few pitfalls, however, are associated with using ultrasound. Not all foreign bodies will be seen with ultrasound. It

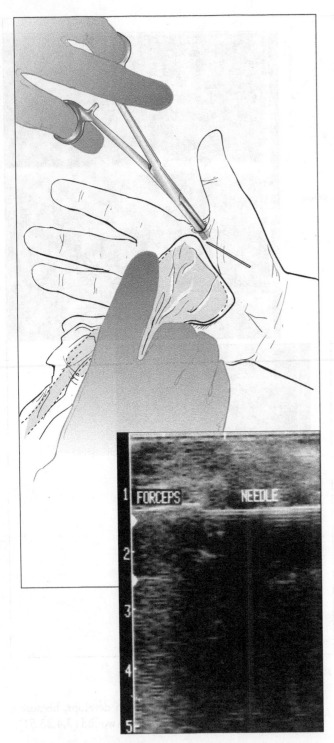

Figure 136.5 Ultrasound guidance in the removal of a subcutaneous foreign body.

Identification

1 Apply ultrasound gel, a transducer, and/or a standoff pad to the area overlying the site most likely to contain a foreign body.

2 Scan slowly and methodically.

3 Scan the area in a number of planes.

Localization

1 Confirm the object's size and shape by viewing it in several planes.

2 Evaluate the depth of the object at several points along its length.

3 Mark the skin surface at sites overlying the object.

4 Identify surrounding or overlying anatomic structures.

5 Utilize adjuncts such as Beekley spots or a localization needle to further demarcate the object.

Removal

1 Determine the optimal incision site based on previous information.

2 Anesthetize the area to be manipulated.

3 Set a reasonable time limit for attempted removal.

4 Hold the transducer in the nondominant hand and scan the object in longitudinal section.

5 Direct a hemostat or retrieval equipment to the proximal end of the object under ultrasound guidance.

6 Repeat the ultrasound scan to ensure complete removal of the object.

7 Administer standard wound care.

Another potential problem concerns misidentification of an image, which could result in time spent removing what appeared to be a foreign body but was not. This carries with it the possible surgical complications associated with removing any foreign object. False positives mentioned in the literature include fresh hematomas, calcifications, scars, cysts, keratin plugs, and atypical sesamoid or other small bones. Partially ossified cartilage in children can be mistaken for a foreign body, so care must be taken to avoid this type of misidentification (1,2,4,8,9,13,16,34,36). Such errors can be minimized by careful scanning in multiple planes. The entire length of an echogenic structure should be scanned to ensure that it does not represent the head of a metacarpal bone. Similar

is important to take the time to perform a slow and careful examination. If one foreign body is detected, the possibility that a second or third foreign body may be present must be considered. A foreign body with a large shadow or artifact may obscure a more distal, smaller object. Objects also may be obscured by tendon, bone, or granulation tissue (3,4,35).

CLINICAL TIPS

- ▶ Scanning should always be performed in several planes.

- ▶ Anatomic structures such as tendons can be detected with real-time scanning during motion of the extremity.

- ▶ Practice in detecting foreign bodies can be obtained by scanning pieces of meat with imbedded objects.

- ▶ Normal anatomic variants may be identified through comparative scanning of the uninvolved extremity.

- ▶ Radiographs often provide a useful adjunct when scanning radiopaque objects.

structures in the same area or findings on plain films may suggest that ossified cartilage is being imaged. By using needle localization, the tissue can be incised to the suspicious site to visualize hematoma, scar tissue, or calcifications in soft tissue. With localization using a finder needle, bone hardness is useful in correctly identifying sesamoid and metacarpal bones. If it is not clear that a particular image represents a foreign body, comparative scanning of the opposite extremity can be helpful (8,16). Additionally, an x-ray with the localization needle in place may complement the ultrasound.

An oblique beam can change the appearance of a structure. Tendons may be mistaken for foreign bodies when scanned at a perpendicular angle. The same tendon may appear relatively hypoechoic and be mistaken for an area of inflammation when the beam is oblique to the tendon. An abnormality or foreign body should always be confirmed in two planes. Air can be introduced into the tissue at the time of injury or surgical exploration. This can cause reverberation artifacts that may be incorrectly assumed to have been created by the presence of a foreign body; it can also make the ultrasound examination impossible. A wound recheck in 48 hours would allow time for air absorption, and a repeat ultrasound examination could be performed at that time (1–4,15,34).

Using ultrasound may in fact reduce the complication rate associated with subcutaneous foreign body removal. Because surrounding structures are visualized, complications associated with blind surgical exploration can be avoided. Furthermore, no ionizing radiation is used (2,7,9–13,16,36).

▶ SUMMARY

As the natural curiosity of children often prompts exploration of their environment, pediatric patients commonly present to the ED with a possible subcutaneous foreign body. Ultrasonography offers an advantage over plain films for the management of such cases, as it can visualize a number of nonradiopaque materials. In addition, because ultrasonography does not involve radiation, it often appeals to parents. Whereas the use of both plain radiographs and fluoroscopy often ends up necessitating blind surgical exploration, ultrasonography offers precise three-dimensional localization of the object and neighboring structures. This allows the physician to plan for an optimal incisional site and to remove the object under direct visualization. Considering that retained foreign materials may be associated with significant morbidity and liability, ultrasound can represent a valuable tool by providing the emergency physician with a simple, safe, noninvasive method of localizing and retrieving foreign objects.

▶ ACKNOWLEDGMENT

The author would like to acknowledge the valuable contributions of Barbara J. Abrams to the version of this chapter that appeared in the previous edition.

▶ REFERENCES

1. Banerjee B, Das RK. Sonographic detection of foreign bodies of the extremities. *Br J Rad.* 1991;64:107–112.
2. Kobs JK, Hansen AR, Keefe B. A retained foreign body in the foot detected by ultrasonography. *J Bone Joint Surg.* 1992;71:296–298.
3. Lammers RL. Soft tissue foreign bodies. *Ann Emerg Med.* 1988;17: 1336–1347.
4. Lammers RL, Magill T. Detection and management of foreign bodies in soft tissue. *Emerg Med Clin North Am.* Philadelphia: WB Saunders; 1992;10:767–781.
5. Graham DD. Ultrasound in the emergency department: detection of wooden foreign bodies in the soft tissues. *J Emerg Med.* 2002;22:75–79.
6. Dunn JD. Risk management in emergency medicine. *Emerg Med Clin North Am.* 1987;5:51–69.
7. Coombs CJ, Mutimer KL, Slattery PG, et al. Hide and seek preoperative ultrasonic localization of nonradiopaque foreign bodies. *Aust N Z J Surg.* 1990;60:989–991.
8. Fornage BD, Rifkin MD, Touche DH, et al. Sonography of the patellar tendon: preliminary observations. *AJR Am J Roentgenol.* 1984;143:179–182.
9. Fornage BD, Schernberg FL. Sonographic diagnosis of foreign bodies of the distal extremities. *AJR Am J Roentgenol.* 1986;147:567–569.
10. Fornage BD, Schernberg FL. Sonographic preoperative localization of a foreign body in the hand. *J Ultrasound Med.* 1987;6:217–219.
11. Fornage BD, Schernberg FL, Rifkin MD. Ultrasound examination of the hand. *Radiology.* 1985;155:785–788.
12. Fornage BD, Touche DH, Segal P, et al. Ultrasonography in the evaluation of muscular trauma. *J Ultrasound Med.* 1983;2:549–554.
13. Gooding GAW, Hardiman T, Sumers M, et al. Sonography of the hand and foot in foreign body detection. *J Ultrasound Med.* 1987;6:441–447.
14. Gordon D. Nonmetallic foreign bodies [letter]. *Br J Radiol.* 1985;58: 574.
15. DeFlaviis L, Scaglione P, Del Bo P, et al. Detection of foreign bodies in soft tissues: experimental comparison of ultrasonography and xeroradiography. *J Trauma.* 1988;28:400–404.

16. Shiels WE, Babcock DS, Wilson JL, et al. Localization and guided removal of soft tissue foreign bodies with sonography. *AJR Am J Roentgenol.* 1990;155:1277–1281.

17. Blankstein A, Cohen I, Heiman Z, et al. Ultrasonography as a diagnostic modality and therapeutic adjuvant in the management of soft tissue foreign bodies in the lower extremities. *Isr Med Assoc J.* 2001;3:411–413.

18. Davae KC, Sofka CM, Di Carlo E, et al. Value of power Doppler imaging and the hypoechoic halo in the sonographic detection of foreign bodies: correlation with histopathologic findings. *J Ultrasound Med.* 2003;22:1309–1313.

19. Porter MD, Schriver JP. Ultrasound-guided Kopans' needle location and removal of a retained foreign body. *Surg Endosc.* 2000;14:500.

20. Charron F, Callonnec F, Thiebot J, et al. Imaging of a foreign body in the submandibular space. *J Radiol.* 2002;83:1773–1774.

21. Ng SY, Songra AK, Bradley PF. A new approach using intraoperative ultrasound imaging for the localization and removal of multiple foreign bodies in the neck. *Int J Oral Maxillofac Surg.* 2003;32:433–436.

22. Schlager D, Sanders AB, Wiggins D, et al. Ultrasound for the detection of foreign bodies. *Ann Emerg Med.* 1991;20:189–191.

23. Barnett RC. Soft tissue foreign body removal. In: Roberts JR, Hedges JR, eds. *Clinical Procedures in Emergency Medicine.* Philadelphia: WB Saunders; 1991:581–591.

24. Lindsey D, Lindsey WE. Cactus spine injuries. *Am J Emerg Med.* 1988; 6:362–369.

25. Peacock EE. *Wound Repair.* 3rd ed. Philadelphia: WB Saunders; 1984: 1–14.

26. Rachman R. Soft tissue injury by mercury from a broken thermometer. *Am J Clin Pathol.* 1974;61:296–300.

27. Yu JC. Migration of broken sewing needle from left arm to heart. *Chest.* 1975;67:626–627.

28. Cracchiolo A. Wooden foreign bodies in the foot. *Am J Surg.* 1980;140: 585–587.

29. Kleinman MB, Elfenbein DS, Wolf EL, et al. Periosteal reaction due to foreign body-induced inflammation of soft tissue. *Pediatrics.* 1977;60: 638–641.

30. Kremkau FW. *Diagnostic Ultrasound: Principles, Instruments and Exercises.* 3rd ed. Philadelphia: WB Saunders; 1989:10–56, 226–230.

31. Pinkney N. *A Review of the Concepts of Ultrasound: Physics and Instrumentation.* 4th ed. Deer Park, NY: Sonicor; 1990:1–14.

32. Slasky BS, Lenkey JL, Skolnick ML, et al. Sonography of soft tissues of extremities and trunk. *Semin Ultrasound.* 1982;3:288–330.

33. Ziskin MC, Thickman DI, Goldenberg NJ, et al. The comet tail artifact. *J Ultrasound Med.* 1982;1:1–7.

34. Gilbert FJ, Campbell RSD, Bayliss AP. The role of ultrasound in the detection of nonradiopaque foreign bodies. *Clin Radiol.* 1990;41: 109–112.

35. Suramo I, Pamilo M. Ultrasound examination of foreign bodies. *Acta Radiol Diag.* 1986;27:463–466.

36. Crawford R, Matheson AB. Clinical value of ultrasonography in the detection and removal of radiolucent foreign bodies. *Injury.* 1989;20:341–343.

37. Anderson MA, Newmeyer WL, Kilgore ES. Diagnosis and treatment of retained foreign bodies in the hand. *Am J Surg.* 1982;144:63–65.

38. Swischuk LE, Jorgenson F, Jorgenson A, et al. Wooden splinter induced "pseudotumors" and "osteomyelitis-like lesions" of bone and soft tissue. *AJR Am J Roentgenol.* 1974;122:176–179.

39. Morgan WJ, Leopold T, Evans R. Foreign bodies in the hand. *J Hand Surg [Br].* 1984;9:194–196.

40. Courter BJ. Radiographic screening for glass foreign bodies: what does a "negative" foreign body series really mean? *Ann Emerg Med.* 1990;19:997–1000.

41. Tandberg D. Glass in the hand and foot: will an x-ray film show it? *JAMA.* 1982;248:1872–1874.

42. Mucci B, Stenhouse G. Soft tissue radiography for wooden foreign bodies: a worthwhile exercise? *Injury.* 1985;16:402–404.

43. Chau WK, Wu SSM, Wang JY. Ultrasonic detection of an intraabdominal foreign body. *J Clin Ultrasound.* 1985;13:130–131.

44. Ginsburg MJ, Ellis GL, Flom LL. Detection of soft-tissue foreign bodies by plain radiography, xeroradiography, computed tomography, and ultrasonography. *Ann Emerg Med.* 1990;19:701–703.

45. de Lacey G, Evans R, Sandin B. Penetrating injuries: how easy is it to see glass (and plastic) on radiographs? *Br J Radiol.* 1985;58:27–30.

46. Levy AD, Harcke HT. Handheld ultrasound device for detection of non-opaque and semi-opaque foreign bodies in soft tissues. *J Clin Ultrasound.* 2003;31:183–188.

47. Friedman DI, Forti RJ, Wall SP, et al. The utility of bedside ultrasound and patent perception in detecting soft tissue foreign bodies. *Pediatr Emerg Care.* 2005;21:487–492.

48. Russell RC, Williamson DA, Sullivan JW, et al. Detection of foreign bodies in the hand. *J Hand Surg [Am].* 1991;16:2–11.

49. Nault P. Applying ultrasound to irregular surfaces. *PT Mag.* 1993;1:94.

50. Bernardino ME, Jing BS, Thomas JL, et al. The extremity soft-tissue lesion: a comparative study of ultrasound, computed tomography, and xeroradiography. *Diagn Radiol.* 1981;139:53–59.

51. Smoot EC, Robson MC. Acute management of foreign body injuries to the hand. *Ann Emerg Med.* 1983;12:434–437.

SUSANNE I. KOST

137

Ultrasound-Assisted Venous Access

▶ INTRODUCTION

Intravenous catheter placement for pediatric patients is a critically important technical skill for health care professionals in the emergency department (ED). A combination of small veins, moving targets, "baby fat," and dehydration may preclude successful venous cannulation even by experienced professionals. The use of ultrasound technology has been shown to improve rates of successful intravenous cannulation in both the central (1,2) and peripheral (3,4) circulation. In fact, evidence-based recommendations from the Agency for Healthcare Research and Quality (AHRQ) suggest that ultrasound guidance for placement of central venous catheters should become standard procedure (5).

When indicated for the pediatric patient, access to the central circulation can be achieved via the internal and external jugular, subclavian, basilic, umbilical, and femoral veins. The internal jugular, subclavian, and femoral veins are traditionally located using landmark-based approaches (see Chapter 19). Anatomic variation, thrombus, accidental arterial cannulation, and risk of injury to surrounding structures pose significant barriers to success using the blind approach. Ultrasound guidance has been shown to increase the rate of successful central venous cannulation via the internal jugular vein in adults and infants and via the subclavian and femoral veins in adults (1,2). Despite limited evidence currently available regarding ultrasound-assisted central access using the subclavian or femoral veins in children, it is likely that the improved success rates seen in adults would extend to the pediatric population.

Literature supporting ultrasound-assisted peripheral access has generally focused on the placement of peripherally inserted central catheters ("PICC lines"), usually via basilic or cephalic veins in the antecubital fossa or upper arm, and success rates approaching 99% have been reported (3,6). In theory, the same principles should apply when cannulating any large (greater than 3 mm) peripheral vein, even with a standard intravenous catheter.

Ultrasound-assisted central line placement should be regarded as a minor surgical procedure to be performed by an experienced physician. It should be done in an appropriate hospital setting such as the ED, operating room, cardiac catheterization laboratory, or intensive care unit. The technique is quickly learned and has been shown to reduce both the time and number of needle insertions required to successfully cannulate central veins. To date, little evidence exists on the use of ultrasound-assisted peripheral access in pediatrics, but the increased success rates achieved with central venous access may prove to be applicable in accessing larger peripheral veins as well.

▶ ANATOMY AND PHYSIOLOGY

Veins may be distinguished ultrasonographically from arteries by the fact that they have thinner walls, are more easily compressed, and lack arterial pulsations. In addition, veins are distended by maneuvers that impede venous return, such as dependent placement, application of tourniquets, and the Valsalva maneuver, whereas arterial diameter will remain relatively constant in response to these maneuvers (Fig. 137.1). While a "standard" location can be described for most large veins (see Chapters 19 and 73), considerable anatomic variability exists among individuals. Visualization of the vein provided by ultrasound improves success by removing the "blind" component of the initial puncture. For example, ultrasound studies have demonstrated that in approximately 6% of patients the internal jugular vein is thrombosed, absent, or unexpectedly small on one side. The vein also may be located more laterally in the neck than expected, whereas in 10% of children it runs directly anterior to the carotid artery (7,8).

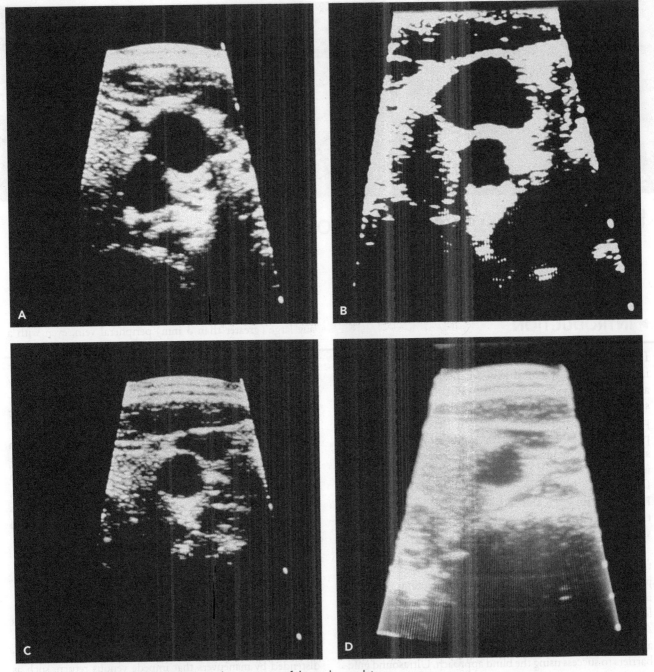

Figure 137.1   Ultrasound appearance of the neck vasculature.
  A. Normal anatomy.
  B. Increased internal jugular vein size with Valsalva maneuver.
  C, D. Decreased internal jugular vein size with skin compression by transducer (C, gentle compression; D, more compression). (Reproduced with permission from Site-Rite II, Dymax Corporation, Pittsburgh, PA.)

Another important ultrasonographic concept is that of Doppler flow, which can be appreciated both audibly and visually, depending on the ultrasonographic equipment. Venous flow produces a uniform pattern, likened audibly to a windstorm or radio static, whereas arterial flow has a definite pulsatile quality (Fig. 137.2). Two-dimensional ultrasound visualization of the vein has proven superior to Doppler flow alone in facilitating central venous access, but using Doppler flow as an adjunct to two-dimensional visualization provides confirmation that the target is a vein rather than an artery.

▸ INDICATIONS

Ultrasound-assisted venous access may be indicated in any situation where venous access is expected to be difficult and

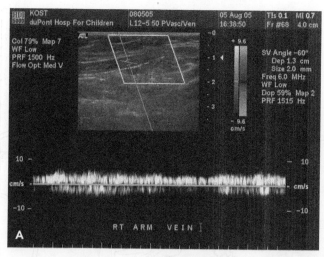
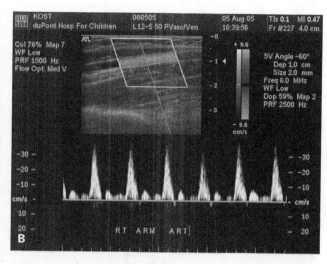

Figure 137.2
A. Doppler image across a vein with a continuous flow pattern.
B. Doppler image across an artery demonstrating pulsatile flow pattern.

a practitioner familiar with the use of two-dimensional ultrasound is available. As mentioned above, evidence-based recommendations from AHRQ suggest that ultrasound guidance for placement of central venous catheters should become standard practice (5). Landmark-based central venous catheter placement can be complicated by the inadvertent selection of an absent, small, or thrombosed vessel. Such problems are clearly revealed by ultrasound scanning and thereby may be avoided.

It should be noted, however, that even with the use of ultrasound guidance, obtaining central venous access in a younger

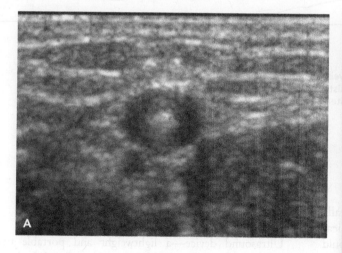
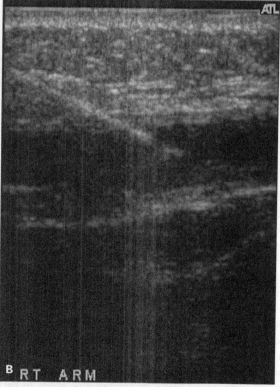

Figure 137.3
A. Transverse (short-axis) view of vein with penetrating needle.
B. Longitudinal (long-axis) view of vein with penetrating needle. Turning the transducer 90 degrees clockwise or counterclockwise will move from one view to the other.

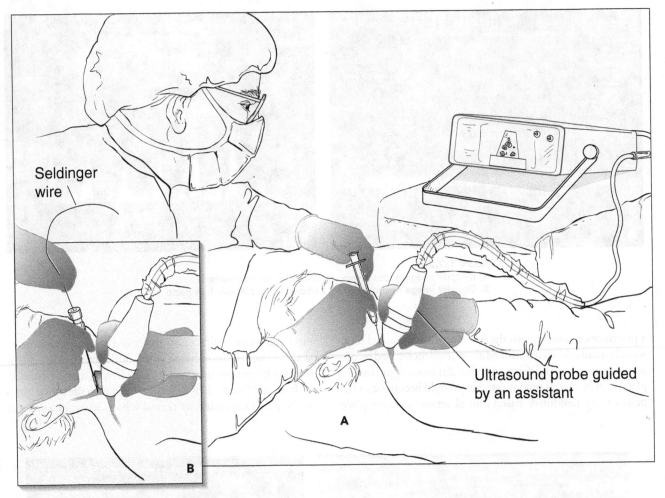

Figure 137.4
A. Ultrasound-monitored internal jugular vein catheterization. Note the sterile sheath on the ultrasound probe and the role of the assistant.
B. Use of a needle guide in ultrasound-assisted internal jugular vein catheterization. Note the use of the Seldinger wire.

child via the internal jugular or subclavian vein is technically difficult and is associated with significant potential complications (see Chapter 19). Consequently, these procedures should only be attempted by experienced clinicians. For those with less experience, it may be preferable to perform ultrasound-assisted central venous access via the proximal femoral vein (i.e., at the groin).

Ultrasound can be a valuable adjunct even for peripheral access with obese patients, intravenous drug abusers, chronically ill or often hospitalized patients, or any patient with a history of difficult intravenous access. Ultrasound-assisted access, when available, offers an alternative to central venous access, surgical cutdowns, or intraosseous access in patients who need simple venous access but have no visible or palpable peripheral veins (4).

▶ EQUIPMENT

Ultrasound device—a lightweight and portable two-dimensional ultrasound scanner is preferred. It should be noted that Doppler ultrasound alone can be used to locate patent arteries and veins. Although the detailed information provided by a two-dimensional ultrasound scan concerning the depth, size, and anatomical relationships of the relevant vein will not be available, the Doppler technique will allow the clinician to avoid absent or thrombosed vessels and to this extent provide guidance in central line placement.

Transducer probe—the higher the operating frequency, the better the lateral and axial resolution of the scan. Higher ultrasonic frequencies, however, are absorbed more strongly by human tissues, so deeper planes cannot be imaged without using extremely high power levels. In practice, a transducer with an operating frequency of 6 to 10 MHz appears satisfactory. A small linear transducer is preferred over the larger curvilinear transducer typically used in abdominal imaging. Although the curvilinear transducer may be used to visualize vascular structures, the curved edges tend to distort the lateral aspects of the screen, thus potentially compromising the accurate advancement of the needle into the vein. For portable systems limited to an endovaginal transducer or a curvilinear transducer, the former is probably superior for vascular imaging.

Ultrasound gel
Needle guide
Sterile sheaths for the transducer probe
Skin marking pen
Sterile povidone-iodine ointment
Standard equipment for central or peripheral venous access as indicated

▶ PROCEDURE

Standard intravenous access preparation, including patient and parent education as well as personnel and equipment requirements, also applies in the setting of an ultrasound-guided procedure. If central access is the goal, the pediatric patient will have to remain still, and inevitably some children will require procedural sedation (see Chapter 33). However, many children requiring emergent central line placement will be severely compromised and have a depressed sensorium, making sedation unnecessary. Positioning is of considerable importance, and sight lines from the operator to the ultrasound screen should be considered prior to positioning the patient and the machine. Although central venous access via the internal jugular vein is primarily described below, the principles discussed are equally applicable to the proximal femoral vein (see also Chapter 19). The three levels of increasing sophistication in using ultrasound are localization, monitoring, and needle guidance.

Localization

At the simplest level, the ultrasound scan is used to plan the procedure by visualizing the relevant vascular anatomy. Ultrasound gel is applied to likely venipuncture sites, and the vessels are examined with the transducer probe. Veins may be visualized in two dimensions—the short axis and the long axis (Fig. 137.3). Turning the transducer by 90 degrees allows the operator to move from one view to the other.

For central access via the internal jugular vein, initial placement of the probe should be above the clavicle and within the groove between the two heads of the sternocleidomastoid

muscle. The internal jugular vein is generally located anterolaterally to the carotid artery. Ultrasound localization of the subclavian vein is significantly complicated by the clavicle, as ultrasound waves will not pass through bone. Alternatives include moving the transducer medially to use a low internal jugular vein approach or moving it laterally to access the subclavian via the axillary vein. The latter approach has been used successfully with landmark-based localization in children (9).

A suitable skin puncture site can be marked (or the course of the selected vein mapped) on the overlying skin with a waterproof pen. The ultrasound gel and transducer probe are then removed, and the standard procedure for venous cannulation is performed.

Monitoring

At the next level of expertise, the ultrasound scan is used not only to plan the procedure but also to monitor the position of the venipuncture needle in real time. The ultrasound probe needs to be positioned close to the chosen puncture site so that the venipuncture needle passes within the scan plane. This means that the probe will impinge on the sterile field and must therefore be contained within a sterile sheath. Alternatively, sterile povidone-iodine ointment may be used as the ultrasound conductive medium, since it is easier to apply this to the skin than to maintain a pool of sterile ultrasound gel between the sheath and the transducer probe. A well-placed rubber band around the sheath and the head of the transducer may aid in maintaining the gel over the transducer tip. The probe is positioned in such a way that the vessel image is centered on the ultrasound screen. The puncture site is anesthetized with 1% lidocaine, and the needle is inserted and advanced with continuous aspiration using ultrasound guidance (Fig. 137.4A).

The advantage of this procedure is that the venipuncture needle is highly reflective of ultrasound and produces a white trace, which can be observed advancing toward and then penetrating the lumen of the selected vessel (see Fig. 137.3). At the point of contact with the vessel, the needle will be seen to indent the anterior surface of the vessel. Once access has been confirmed through the aspiration of blood into the syringe, the transducer is removed and the vessel is cannulated.

Needle Guidance

The final level of sophistication relies on the use of a suitable needle steering attachment or needle guide. Such a device is designed to restrict the movement of the venipuncture needle to a predetermined path in the image plane. The needle will therefore achieve venipuncture if inserted when the vein is visualized and transected by the electronically generated puncture line indicating the needle path. Either the probe and needle guide are both contained within the sterile sheath or the needle steering guide is sterilized in glutaraldehyde and clipped onto the ensheathed probe.

SUMMARY

1 Check equipment and ensure that the patient is appropriately monitored.

2 Utilize sedation as needed.

3 For central internal jugular or subclavian access, place the patient in the Trendelenburg position with a roll under the shoulders and the head turned away from the side to be cannulated.

4 Apply ultrasound gel and transducer.

5 Localize the vessel to be cannulated in the transverse and longitudinal planes.

6 Modify the position of the patient or the chosen route of access based on the findings.

Localization

1 Mark the position of the vein on the skin surface.

2 Remove the ultrasound gel and transducer.

3 Perform standard central venous catheterization using the markings as a guide.

Monitoring

1 Prepare and drape the patient before the ultrasound scan.

2 Place the probe and ultrasound gel in a sterile sheath or apply povidone-iodine ointment directly

to the skin as the ultrasound conductive medium.

3 Identify the vein and center the image on the ultrasound screen.

4 Anesthetize the puncture site with 1% lidocaine as needed.

5 Insert the needle on a syringe and advance with continuous aspiration.

6 Observe the needle penetrate the vein on the ultrasound monitor.

7 Remove the transducer and complete cannulation in standard fashion.

Needle Guidance

1 Prepare and drape the patient in sterile fashion.

2 Connect a needle guide to the transducer.

3 Center the image of the vein on ultrasound screen and within the electronically generated puncture line.

4 Hold the needle in the needle guide with the thumb.

5 Advance the needle while monitoring its progress on the ultrasound screen.

6 Remove the transducer once penetration of the vessel lumen has been visualized.

The initial approach is identical to the monitoring method described above. Once the vein has been identified and centered on the monitor, the needle is held within the needle guide with the thumb of the hand holding the transducer and slowly advanced through the anesthetized skin with the free hand. The progress of the needle is viewed on the ultrasound monitor while the vein image is maintained within the electronically generated puncture line. Once penetration of the vessel lumen by the needle is visualized and blood aspirated, the transducer and attached needle guide are removed, and the procedure is completed in the standard fashion.

If the venipuncture is observed in real time by means of ultrasound, it is possible to dispense with the usual syringe on the needle and instead use a Seldinger guidewire as a stylet (Fig. 137.4B). This prevents possible dislodgment of the needle from the vein when the syringe is disconnected to thread the Seldinger wire and also minimizes the risk of air embolism.

▶ COMPLICATIONS

As described in Chapter 19, the incidence of complications during central line placement can be high, and such complications may have serious consequences. The most likely reason for complications such as arterial puncture and pneumothorax during internal jugular line placement is that the venipuncture is performed blindly. It is therefore expected that using two-dimensional ultrasound will reduce the complication rate associated with the placement of such central lines. Certainly the rate of carotid puncture during internal jugular venous cannulation in adults has been shown to be significantly reduced (10), but large pediatric studies have yet to be performed. No complications unique to ultrasound use during central line placement have been reported. As discussed previously, central venous access in younger pediatric patients via the internal jugular and subclavian veins requires a high degree of technical expertise and should therefore only be performed by experienced personnel.

CLINICAL TIPS

▶ Familiarity with the ultrasound appearance of veins and arteries in children should be gained before attempting to place central lines with ultrasound assistance. Veins may be compressed by the ultrasound probe, whereas arteries show faint wall pulsations.

▶ A Valsalva maneuver or Trendelenburg positioning will increase the diameter of the internal jugular vein but will not affect the thick-walled carotid artery.

▶ The clinician should place the ultrasound device where the monitor is easily visible during the procedure.

▶ Bubbles must be eliminated from the ultrasound conductive medium, as air causes ultrasound artifacts.

▶ Marker pens should contain ink that will not be wiped off by the preparation solution used.

▶ Excess pressure on the transducer may collapse the vein so that it is not visible on the monitor.

▶ SUMMARY

Two-dimensional ultrasound clarifies the vascular anatomy and helps the clinician to both optimize the positioning of the patient and select a suitable puncture site. It is then possible to guide a peripheral catheter or, in the case of central access, a finder needle into the chosen vein and to visualize threading of a guidewire in real time. Using ultrasound reduces the time needed to achieve venous access and increases the likelihood of a complication-free procedure.

▶ ACKNOWLEGMENT

The author would like to acknowledge the valuable contributions of Peter J. Alderson, who authored the chapter on ultrasound-assisted central line placement in the first edition.

▶ REFERENCES

1. Abboud PC, Kendall JL. Ultrasound guidance for vascular access. *Emerg Clin North Am.* 2004;22:749–773.
2. Hind D, Calvert N, McWilliams R, et al. Ultrasonic locating devices for central venous cannulation: meta-analysis. *BMJ.* 2003;327: 361–364.
3. Donaldson JS, Morello FP, Junewick JJ, et al. Peripherally inserted central venous catheters: US-guided vascular access in pediatric patients. *Radiology.* 1995;197:542–544.
4. Brannam L, Blaivas M, Lyon M, et al. Emergency nurses' utilization of ultrasound guidance for placement of peripheral intravenous lines in difficult-access patients. *Acad Emerg Med.* 2004;11: 1361–1363.
5. Agency for Healthcare Research and Quality. Making health care safer: a critical analysis of patient safety practices. *Evid Rep Technol Assess (Summ).* 2001;43:i–x, 1–668.
6. Sofocleous CT, Schur I, Cooper SG, et al. Sonographically guided placement of peripherally inserted central venous catheters: review of 355 procedures. *AJR Am J Roentgenol.* 1998;170:1613–1616.
7. Alderson PJ, Burrows FA, Stemp LI, et al. The use of ultrasound to evaluate internal jugular vein anatomy and to facilitate central venous cannulation in pediatric patients. *Br J Anaesth.* 1993;70: 145–148.
8. Denys BG, Uretsky BF. Anatomical variations of internal jugular vein location: impact on central venous access. *Crit Care Med.* 1991;19: 1516–1519.
9. Metz RI, Lucking SE, Chaten FC, et al. Percutaneous catheterization of the axillary vein in infants and children. *Pediatrics.* 1990;85: 531–533.
10. Denys BG, Uretsky BF, Reddy PS, et al. An ultrasound method for safe and rapid central venous access. *N Engl J Med.* 1991;324: 566.

138

ANDREW DEPIERO

Focused Abdominal Sonography for Trauma

▶ INTRODUCTION

Focused abdominal sonography for trauma (FAST) is used as a rapid assessment tool for patients with severe blunt abdominal trauma. The use of bedside ultrasound in the diagnostic evaluation of trauma originated in Europe. By the early 1990s, FAST was being increasingly used in North America. Several reports concluded that FAST is a rapid and effective means of evaluating an adult after blunt abdominal trauma (1–4). FAST examinations are usually performed by surgeons or emergency physicians. In its policy statement, the American College of Emergency Physicians supports the use of emergency ultrasound (5). FAST is now considered an alternative to diagnostic peritoneal lavage or abdominal computed tomography (CT) in the Advanced Trauma Life Support course (6). The procedure offers several advantages: (a) it is rapid and non-invasive; (b) it can be performed at the bedside during the secondary survey and simultaneously with other diagnostic and therapeutic interventions; and (c) it is relatively easy to learn (particularly important for clinicians who are not imaging specialists), as the test does not focus upon the imaging of any particular organ. FAST may potentially identify organ pathology or injury, but the examination itself is limited only to the detection of fluid. The role of FAST in penetrating trauma is unclear.

Despite its advantages, the utility of FAST has been questioned in terms of its sensitivity and in regard to both the experience and training of the operator (7–11). Some argue that hemoperitoneum is an inadequate indicator of abdominal visceral injury. In a series of 575 adult patients with abdominal visceral injuries, 157 (34%) had no evidence of hemoperitoneum either on CT scan or at the time of surgery. The FAST examination was falsely negative in 26 cases (17%) (12). Additional controversy surrounds the use of FAST

for children. Some studies have reported excellent sensitivity (92.5% to 100%) in pediatric patients and have strongly advocated its use (13,14). Others have reported much less favorable results, with sensitivities ranging from 30% to 55% (15–18). These studies report a number of significant injuries not detected by the FAST examination, including bowel injuries (with and without intraperitoneal air), liver laceration, adrenal hematoma, renal laceration, splenic laceration, and perinephric hematoma. Such conflicting literature has resulted in considerable debate as to whether FAST should be utilized at all in pediatric trauma patients, but the issue remains to be settled. Certainly, there is evidence indicating that a FAST examination should be interpreted with caution with pediatric patients, and the interpretation of a negative examination should include careful correlation with other clinical information.

▶ ANATOMY AND PHYSIOLOGY

The goal of the FAST examination is to identify fluid (blood) in specific areas within the chest and abdomen. Blood collects in the dependent regions of the abdomen—the right upper quadrant, the left upper quadrant, and the pouch of Douglas. When the patient is erect, any fluid in the abdomen drains to the pelvis. For the supine trauma patient presenting to the hospital, free peritoneal blood will usually flow in the superior or inferior direction. If the bleeding is from above the bony pelvis, blood flows superiorly. The protective properties of the pelvis are such that most injuries, and therefore most bleeding, will be from above the pelvis. The internal anatomy of the abdomen is such that blood tends to collect in the right upper quadrant. Patients with severe thoracoabdominal trauma may also have blood in the pericardial space, potentially leading to cardiac tamponade.

The Subxiphoid View

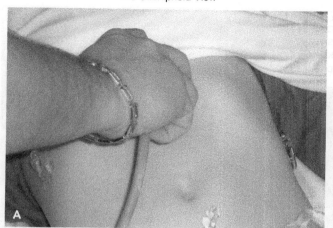

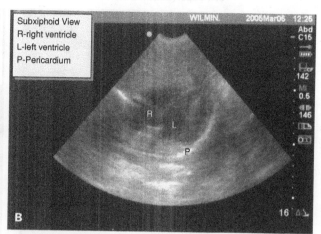

Subxiphoid View
R-right ventricle
L-left ventricle
P-Pericardium

Figure 138.1
A. Subxiphoid view.
B. Normal heart examination.

As described in Chapter 132, the ultrasound image is generated based on the pulse-echo principle. The ultrasound machine delivers short electrical pulses into the body. The image is created from the energy reflected back to the machine from the various body structures. When blood is not clotted, it allows transmission of ultrasound waves without echoes. As a result, these areas will appear black. Solid organs have different echogenicities and will appear as different shades of grey. These echogenicities may also reveal particular organ pathology or organ injury. This, however, is considered beyond the scope of the FAST examination.

▶ INDICATIONS

There is no absolute indication for a FAST examination in the pediatric trauma patient. A FAST examination may be considered appropriate for the detection of intraperitoneal fluid in the pediatric patient with blunt abdominal trauma. The FAST examination should never pre-empt a thorough primary survey, nor should it delay the initiation of any necessary interventions identified by this initial assessment. The FAST examination is unnecessary when indications already exist for abdominal operative intervention.

Right Upper Quadrant View

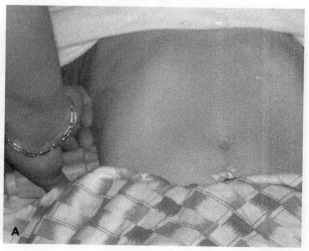

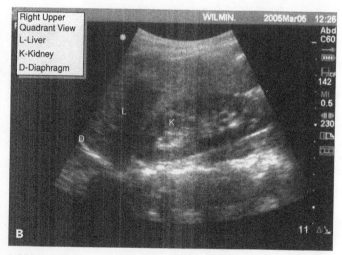

Right Upper
Quadrant View
L-Liver
K-Kidney
D-Diaphragm

Figure 138.2
A. Right upper quadrant view.
B. Normal right upper quadrant examination.

Left Upper Quadrant View

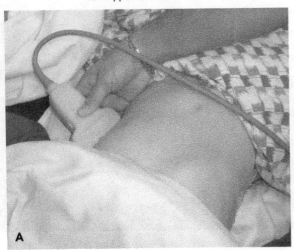

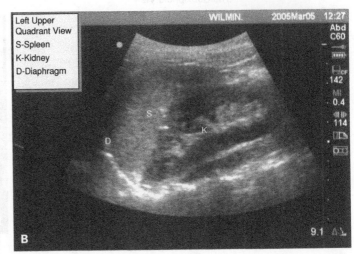

Figure 138.3
A. Left upper quadrant view.
B. Normal left upper quadrant examination.

▶ EQUIPMENT

Portable ultrasound unit—videotape and hard copy capabilities are preferred for permanent records and quality assurance.
Abdominal probe (2 to 5 MHz)
Ultrasound gel

▶ PROCEDURE

The patient is examined in the supine position, with the clinician standing on the patient's right side. Many ultrasound devices allow the entry of patient identifiers. Ultrasound gel is applied to the abdomen in four regions: the pericardial area,

the right upper quadrant, the left upper quadrant, and the suprapubic area. The order in which the regions are scanned is determined by the preference of the clinician.

The heart and pericardial region are examined from the subxiphoid view (Fig. 138.1). The probe should be positioned just under the xiphoid parallel to the skin surface and should be aimed toward the patient's left shoulder and oriented for sagittal sections. The goal of the examination is to evaluate the pericardial space for blood (see also Chapter 134). The right upper quadrant is examined with the transducer parallel to the ribs in the midclavicular line, typically between the 11th and 12th ribs (Fig. 138.2). This approach should allow evaluation of the liver, kidney, diaphragm, and Morrison's pouch for blood. The spleen and kidney are examined with the transducer positioned parallel to the ribs in the left posterior

Suprapubic View

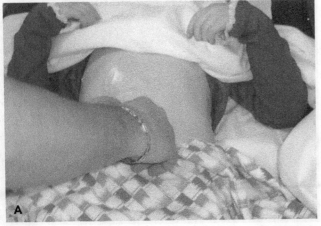

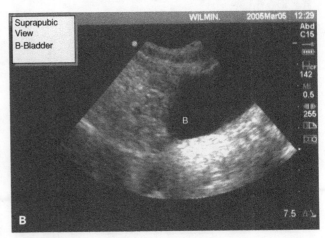

Figure 138.4
A. Suprapubic view.
B. Normal suprapubic examination.

SUMMARY

1 Examine the patient in the supine position.

2 Apply ultrasound gel to the subxiphoid area, right upper quadrant, left upper quadrant, and suprapubic area.

3 Place the probe under the xiphoid parallel to the skin surface and aimed at the left shoulder.

4 Identify the pericardial sac and four chambers of the heart.

5 Place the probe in the right midclavicular line parallel to the rib and between the eleventh and twelfth ribs.

6 Identify liver, right kidney, diaphragm, and Morrison's pouch.

7 Position the transducer in the left posterior axillary line parallel to the ribs.

8 Identify the diaphragm, spleen, and left kidney.

9 Place the transducer above the symphysis pubis.

10 Identify the bladder.

axillary line (Fig. 138.3). The diaphragm is also visualized in this view. Especially in this region of the abdomen, all structures may not be visualized in a single view, and multiple images may be necessary for a complete examination of the spaces between the diaphragm and spleen and between the spleen and kidney. The examination of the suprapubic area requires that the transducer be placed just above the symphysis pubis and be angled for transverse sections (Fig. 138.4). The probe should be directed so as to allow examination of the retrovesical space and provide a transverse view of the bladder.

CLINICAL TIPS

▶ Clinicians who plan to use the FAST examination should practice obtaining the correct views and identifying normal structures on colleagues.

▶ FAST should not interfere with or delay the trauma resuscitation.

▶ The interpretation of the FAST exam should be limited to the presence or absence of fluid.

▶ Clinical management must depend on ultrasound findings as well as the clinical evaluation.

▶ Catheterization and infusion of saline may improve bladder imaging.

Filling an empty bladder with a Foley catheter may enhance the quality of the study.

▶ COMPLICATIONS

The procedure itself is not associated with any adverse effects. Complications may arise as a result of the potential limitations of the technique or from any delay in definitive surgical care.

▶ SUMMARY

FAST is a rapid bedside technique for the detection of intra-abdominal or pericardial bleeding in the setting of blunt abdominal trauma. The FAST examination has been used by emergency physicians and general surgeons with success in adult trauma patients. Although it has become more commonly used in pediatric patients in trauma centers, its role in the management of pediatric trauma patients remains controversial and is still undergoing evaluation.

▶ ACKNOWLEDGMENT

The author thanks Dr. Paul Sierzenski for his assistance with the ultrasound images.

▶ REFERENCES

1. Kimura A, Otsuka T. Emergency center ultrasonography in the evaluation of hemoperitoneum: a prospective study. *J Trauma.* 1991;31: 20–23.

2. Ma OJ, Mateer JR, Ogata M, et al. Prospective analysis of a rapid trauma ultrasound examination performed by emergency physicians. *J Trauma.* 1995;38:879–885.

3. Rozycki GS, Ochsner MG, Schmidt JA, et al. A prospective study of surgeon-performed ultrasound as the primary adjuvant modality for injured patient assessment. *J Trauma.* 1995;39:492–498.

4. Boulanger BR, McLellan BA, Brenneman FD, et al. Emergent abdominal sonography as a screening test in a new diagnostic algorithm for blunt trauma. *J Trauma.* 1996;40:867–874.

5. *Emergency Ultrasound Guidelines.* Dallas, TX: American College of Emergency Physicians; 2001. ACEP policy statement.

6. *Abdominal Trauma in Advanced Trauma Life Support for Doctors.* Chicago: American College of Surgeons; 1997:157–175. Student course manual.

7. Ma OJ, Gaddis G, Steele MT, et al. Prospective analysis of the effect of physician experience with the FAST examination in reducing the use of CT scans. *Emerg Med Aust.* 2005;17:24–30.

8. Jang T, Sineff S, Naunheim R, et al. Residents should not independently perform focused abdominal sonography for trauma after 10 training examinations. *J Ultrasound Med.* 2004;23:793–797.

9. Kirkpatrick AW, Sirois M, Ball CG, et al. The hand-held ultrasound examination for penetrating abdominal trauma. *Am J Surg.* 2004; 187:660–665.

10. Miller MT, Pasquale MD, Bromberg WJ, et al. Not so FAST. *J Trauma.* 2003;54:52–59.

11. Gracias VH, Frankel HL, Gupta R, et al. Defining the learning curve for the focused abdominal sonogram for trauma (FAST) examination: implications for credentialing. *Am Surg.* 2001;67:364–368.

12. Shanmuganathan K, Mirvis SE, Sherbourne CD, et al. Hemoperitoneum as the sole indicator of abdominal visceral injuries: a potential limitation of screening abdominal US for trauma. *Radiology.* 1999;212:423–430.

13. Suthers SE, Albrecht R, Foley D, et al. Surgeon-directed ultrasound for trauma is a predictor of intra-abdominal injury in children. *Am Surg.* 2004;70:164–167.

14. Soudack M, Epelman M, Maor R, et al. Experience with focused abdominal sonography for trauma (FAST) in 313 pediatric patients. *J Clin Ultrasound.* 2004;32:53–61.

15. Emery KH, McAneney CM, Racadio JM, et al. Absent peritoneal fluid on screening trauma ultrasonography in children: a prospective comparison with computed tomography. *J Pediatr Surg.* 2001;36: 565–569.

16. Coley BD, Mutabagani KH, Martin LC, et al. Focused abdominal sonography for trauma (FAST) in children with blunt abdominal trauma. *J Trauma.* 2000;48:902–906.

17. Patel JC, Tepas JJ 3rd. The efficacy of focused abdominal sonography for trauma (FAST) as a screening tool in the assessment of injured children. *J Pediatr Surg.* 1999;34:44–47.

18. Mutabagani KH, Coley BD, Zumberge N, et al. Preliminary experience with focused abdominal sonography for trauma (FAST) in children: is it useful? *J Pediatr Surg.* 1999;34:48–52.

Page numbers followed by *b* indicate boxes; *f* indicate figures; page numbers followed by *t* indicate tables.